Rosen's Emergency Medicine

Concepts and Clinical Practice

Volume Two

Rosen's EMERGENCY MEDICINE

Concepts and Clinical Practice

Fifth Edition

Editor-in-Chief

JOHN A. MARX, M.D.
Chair,
Department of Emergency Medicine,
Carolinas Medical Center,
Charlotte, North Carolina;
Clinical Professor of Emergency Medicine,
University of North Carolina School of Medicine,
Chapel Hill, North Carolina

Senior Editors

ROBERT S. HOCKBERGER, M.D.
Chair,
Department of Emergency Medicine,
Harbor-UCLA Medical Center,
Torrance, California;
Professor of Medicine,
UCLA School of Medicine,
Westwood, California

RON M. WALLS, M.D.
Chairman,
Department of Emergency Medicine,
Brigham and Women's Hospital;
Associate Professor of Medicine (Emergency Medicine),
Harvard Medical School,
Boston, Massachusetts

Editors

JAMES ADAMS, M.D.
Chief, Division of Emergency Medicine,
Northwestern Memorial Hospital;
Professor of Medicine,
Division of Emergency Medicine,
Northwestern University Medical School,
Chicago, Illinois

ROGER M. BARKIN, M.D.
Professor of Surgery,
Division of Emergency Medicine,
University of Colorado Health Sciences Center;
Vice President for Pediatric and Newborn Programs,
HealthONE,
Denver, Colorado

WILLIAM G. BARSAN, M.D.
Professor and Chair,
Department of Emergency Medicine,
University of Michigan,
Ann Arbor, Michigan

DANIEL F. DANZL, M.D.
Professor and Chairman,
Department of Emergency Medicine,
University of Louisville School of Medicine,
Louisville, Kentucky

MARIANNE GAUSCHE-HILL, M.D., FACEP, FAAP
Associate Professor of Medicine,
UCLA School of Medicine;
Director, Emergency Medical Services,
Department of Emergency Medicine,
Harbor-UCLA Medical Center,
Torrance, California

GLENN C. HAMILTON, M.D., MSM
Professor and Chair,
Department of Emergency Medicine,
Wright State University School of Medicine,
Dayton, Ohio

LOUIS J. LING, M.D.
Professor of Emergency Medicine,
University of Minnesota;
Medical Director,
Hennepin Regional Poison Center;
Associate Medicine Director for Medical Education,
Emergency Medicine Staff Physician,
Hennepin County Medical Center,
Minneapolis, Minnesota

EDWARD NEWTON, M.D., FACEP
Associate Professor of Emergency Medicine,
Keck and USC School of Medicine,
Vice Chairman,
Department of Emergency Medicine,
Los Angeles County and University of Southern California Medical Center,
Los Angeles, California

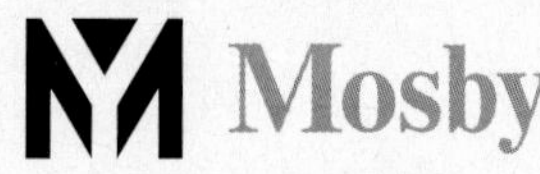

An Affiliate of Elsevier

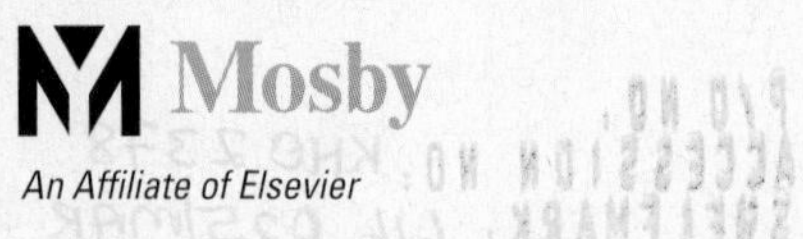

Senior Managing Editor: Kathy Falk
Project Manager: Pat Joiner
Senior Production Editor: David Stein
Designer: Mark Oberkrom

Fifth edition

NOTICE

Pharmacology is an ever-changing field. Standard safety precautions must be followed, but as new research and clinical experience broaden our knowledge, changes in treatment and drug therapy may become necessary or appropriate. Readers are advised to check the most current product information provided by the manufacturer of each drug to be administered to verify the recommended dose, the method and duration of administration, and contraindications. It is the responsibility of the licensed prescriber, relying on experience and knowledge of the patient, to determine dosages and the best treatment for each individual patient. Neither the publisher nor the editor assumes any liability for any injury and/or damage to persons or property arising from this publication.

Mosby, Inc.
An Affiliate of Elsevier
11830 Westline Industrial Drive
St. Louis, Missouri 63146

Printed in China

International Standard Book Number 0-323-01185-3

04 05 GW/RRD-W 9 8 7 6 5 4 3 2

Contributors

Cynthia K. Aaron, M.D., FACEP, FACMT
Associate Professor, Department of Emergency Medicine,
University of Massachusetts Medical School,
Director, Toxicology Services, Attending Physician,
Emergency Department,
UMass Memorial Medical Center,
Worcester, Massachusetts
157: Pesticides

Jean T. Abbott, M.D., FACEP
Associate Professor, Department of Surgery,
Division of Emergency Medicine,
University of Colorado School of Medicine;
Attending Physician, Emergency Department,
University Hospital,
Denver, Colorado
172: Acute Complications of Pregnancy

Norman S. Abramson, M.D.
Professor of Emergency Medicine,
University of Pittsburgh School of Medicine;
Attending Physician,
Mercy Hospital,
Pittsburgh, Pennsylvania
6: Brain Resuscitation

Riyad B. Abu-Laban, M.D., MHSc, FRCPC
Assistant Clinical Professor,
Division of Emergency Medicine, Department of Surgery,
University of British Columbia;
Attending Physician and Research Director,
Department of Emergency Medicine,
Vancouver General Hospital,
Vancouver, British Columbia, Canada
51: Ankle and Foot

Kumar Alagappan, M.D.
Associate Professor, Department of Emergency Medicine,
Albert Einstein College of Medicine,
Bronx, New York;
Associate Chairman, Department of Emergency Medicine,
North Shore-Long Island Jewish Health System,
New Hyde Park, New York
97: Headache

James T. Amsterdam, M.D., DMD, MMM
Professor of Emergency Medicine,
Department of Emergency Medicine,
University of Minnesota,
Minneapolis, Minnesota;
Head, Emergency Medical Department,
Health Partners Regions Hospital,
St. Paul, Minnesota
65: Oral Medicine

Deirdre Anglin, M.D., MPH
Associate Professor,
Department of Emergency Medicine,
University of Southern California,
Los Angeles, California
63: Elder Abuse and Neglect
64: Youth, Gangs, and Violence

Felix Ankel, M.D., FACEP
Assistant Professor of Emergency Medicine,
Department of Emergency Medicine,
University of Minnesota,
Minneapolis, Minnesota;
Director, Emergency Medicine Residency,
Regions Hospital/Healthpartners Institute for Medical Education,
St. Paul, Minnesota
80: Aortic Dissection

Robert E. Antosia, M.D., MPH
Instructor in Medicine,
Harvard Medical School;
Attending Physician,
Department of Emergency Medicine,
Brigham and Women's Hospital,
Boston, Massachusetts
43: Hand
50: Knee and Lower Leg

John David Armstrong, II, M.D., MA
Professor, Department of Pulmonary Sciences and Critical Care Medicine,
Associate Director,
The Center for Health Care Ethics, Humanities and Law,
University of Colorado Health Sciences Center,
Denver, Colorado
199: End of Life

Chandra D. Aubin, M.D.
Clinical Instructor,
Division of Emergency Medicine
Washington University School of Medicine,
St. Louis, Missouri
10: Clinical Decision Making

Tom P. Aufderheide, M.D., FACEP
Associate Professor, Department of Emergency Medicine,
Medical College of Wisconsin,
Milwaukee, Wisconsin
73: Acute Ischemic Coronary Syndromes
82: Peripheral Arteriovascular Disease

Paul E. Austin, M.D.
Attending Physician, Department of Emergency Medicine,
Durham Regional Hospital,
Durham, North Carolina
160: General Approach to the Pediatric Patient

Trimble L. Bailey, B.S.
Burn and Wound Healing Laboratory,
University of Virginia Health Sciences Center,
Charlottesville, Virginia
56: Thermal Burns
57: Chemical Injuries

Adam Z. Barkin
Vanderbilt University School of Medicine
Nashville, Tennessee
132: Sepsis Syndromes

Roger M. Barkin, M.D.
Professor of Surgery, Division of Emergency Medicine,
University of Colorado Health Sciences Center;
Vice President for Pediatric and Newborn Programs,
HealthONE,
Denver, Colorado
161: Fever
166: Infectious Diarrheal Disease and Dehydration
170: Sudden Infant Death Syndrome

Theodore M. Barnett, M.D.
Assistant Professor of Pediatrics,
University of Missouri–Kansas City School of Medicine;
Chief, Section of Emergency Medicine,
Childrens Mercy Hospital,
Kansas City, Missouri
60: Child Abuse

William G. Barsan, M.D.
Professor and Chair,
Department of Emergency Medicine,
University of Michigan,
Ann Arbor, Michigan
84: Esophagus, Stomach, and Duodenum
95: Stroke

Bruce M. Becker, M.D., MPH, FACEP
Associate Professor, Department of Community Health,
Brown University School of Medicine;
Attending Physician, Department of Emergency Medicine,
Rhode Island Hospital;
Attending Physician,
Department of Pediatric Emergency Medicine,
Hasbro Children's Hospital,
Providence, Rhode Island
127: Parasites

Edward Bernstein, M.D.
Professor and Vice Chair for Academic Affairs,
Department of Emergency Medicine,
Boston University School of Medicine,
Boston, Massachusetts
197: Multiculturalism and Care Delivery

Judith Bernstein, RNC, Ph.D.
Assistant Professor,
Department of Maternal and Child Health,
School of Public Health and Emergency Medicine,
School of Medicine,
Boston University,
Boston, Massachusetts
197: Multiculturalism and Care Delivery

Howard A. Bessen, M.D.
Professor of Medicine,
UCLA School of Medicine,
Los Angeles, California;
Director, Emergency Medicine Residency Program,
Harbor-UCLA Medical Center,
Torrance, California
81: Abdominal Aortic Aneurysm

Elisabeth F. Bilden, M.D.
Fellow in Medical Toxicology,
Department of Emergency Medicine,
University of Arizona Health Sciences Center;
Attending Physician,
University Hospital,
Tucson, Arizona
145: Antidepressants

Timothy J. Bill, M.D.
Resident in Plastic Surgery,
University of Virginia Health Sciences Center,
Charlottesville, Virginia
56: Thermal Burns
57: Chemical Injuries

Diane M. Birnbaumer, M.D.
Associate Professor of Medicine,
UCLA School of Medicine,
Los Angeles, California;
Associate Residency Director,
Department of Emergency Medicine,
Harbor-UCLA Medical Center,
Torrance, California
33: Geriatric Trauma
176: The Elder Patient

Michelle H. Biros, M.D., MS
Associate Professor,
Department of Emergency Medicine,
Hennepin County Medical Center and the University of Minnesota;
Research Director,
Department of Emergency Medicine,
Hennepin County Medical Center,
Minneapolis, Minnesota
34: Head

Robert A. Bitterman, M.D., JD, FACEP
Director of Risk Management and Managed Care,
Department of Emergency Medicine,
Carolinas Medical Center,
Charlotte, North Carolina
89: Acute Gastroenteritides
90: Large Intestine
200: Medicolegal and Risk Management

Kenneth E. Bizovi, M.D.
Assistant Professor, Department of Emergency Medicine,
Oregon Health Sciences University;
Assistant Professor, Oregon Poison Center,
Portland, Oregon
142: Acetaminophen

Thomas Blackwell, M.D.
Clinical Assistant Professor,
Department of Emergency Medicine,
University of North Carolina School of Medicine,
Chapel Hill, North Carolina;
Medical Director, The Center for Prehospital Medicine,
Department of Emergency Medicine,
Carolinas Medical Center;
Medical Director, Merklenburg EMS Agency,
Charlotte, North Carolina
186: Principles of Emergency Medical Services Systems

Andra L. Blomkalns, M.D.
Chief Resident, Department of Emergency Medicine,
University of Cincinnati,
Cincinnati, Ohio
55: Venomous Animal Injuries

Frederick C. Blum, M.D., FACEP, FAAP
Associate Professor of Emergency Medicine,
Department of Emergency Medicine,
West Virginia University,
Morgantown, West Virginia
11: Fever

Ira J. Blumen, M.D., FACEP
Associate Professor of Clinical Medicine,
Section of Emergency Medicine,
Department of Medicine,
Pritzker School of Medicine,
University of Chicago;
Program and Medical Director,
University of Chicago Hospitals Aeromedical Network,
University of Chicago Hospitals,
Chicago, Illinois
187: Air Medical Transport

J. Stephen Bohan, M.D., FACP, FACEP
Clinical Director, Department of Emergency Medicine,
Brigham and Women's Hospital,
Boston, Massachusetts
190: Guidelines and Clinical Pathways

Edward B. Bolgiano, M.D., FACEP, FACP
Chairman, Department of Emergency Medicine,
Bon Secours Hospital;
Assistant Professor,
Department of Medicine and Surgery,
University of Maryland School of Medicine,
Baltimore, Maryland
128: Tick-Borne Illnesses

Laura J. Bontempo, M.D.
Instructor of Medicine, Department of Internal Medicine,
Harvard University;
Emergency Physician,
Department of Emergency Medicine,
Brigham and Women's Hospital,
Boston, Massachusetts
121: Rhabdomyolysis

Marc Borenstein, M.D., FACEP, FACP
Clinical Associate Professor, Department of Medicine,
Columbia University College of Physicians and Surgeons,
New York, New York;
Chairman and Residency Program Director,
Department of Emergency Medicine,
Newark Beth Israel Medical Center,
Newark, New Jersey
117: Selected Oncologic Emergencies

Andrea Bracikowski, M.D., FAAP, FACEP
Director, Pediatric Emergency Medicine,
Departments of Emergency Medicine and Pediatrics,
Vanderbilt University School of Medicine,
Nashville, Tennessee
165: Gastrointestinal Disorders

John C. Bradford, D.O., FACEP
Associate Professor, Department of Emergency Medicine,
Northeastern Ohio University College of Medicine,
Rootstown, Ohio;
Director, Emergency Medicine Residency,
Department of Emergency Medicine,
Akron General Medical Center,
Akron, Ohio
28: Vaginal Bleeding

William J. Brady, M.D.
Assistant Professor, Department of Emergency Medicine,
University of Virginia;
University of Virginia Health System,
Department of Emergency Medicine,
University of Virginia;
Assistant Professor, Department of Internal Medicine,
University of Virginia,
Charlottesville, Virginia
14: Confusion
73: Acute Ischemic Coronary Syndromes

Sabina Braithwaite, M.D., FACEP
Assistant Professor of Clinical Emergency Medicine,
Department of Emergency Medicine,
University of Virginia Health System,
Charlottesville, Virginia
18: Dyspnea

David F.M. Brown, M.D.
Instructor, Division of Emergency Medicine,
Harvard Medical School;
Assistant Chief, Department of Emergency Medicine,
Massachusetts General Hospital,
Boston, Massachusetts
15: Coma and Depressed Level of Consciousness
53: Foreign Bodies

James E. Brown, M.D.
Assistant Professor, Department of Emergency Medicine,
Wright State University School of Medicine,
Dayton, Ohio
19: Chest Pain

Douglas D. Brunette, M.D.
Department of Emergency Medicine,
Hennepin County Medical Center,
Minneapolis, Minnesota
66: Ophthalmology

Keith K. Burkhart, M.D.
Associate Professor of Medicine and Pharmacology,
Department of Emergency Medicine,
Pennsylvania State University,
Milton S. Hershey Medical Center,
Hershey, Pennsylvania
154: Lithium

Michael J. Burns, M.D., FACEP, FACP
Clinical Professor of Medicine,
Division of Emergency Medicine,
University of California Irvine College of Medicine,
Irvine, California;
Attending Physician, Emergency Department,
University of California Medical Center,
Orange, California
177: The Immunocompromised Patient

John D. Cahill, M.D., DTM and H
Clinical Instructor in Medicine, Department of Medicine,
Brown University School of Medicine;
Chief Resident in Emergency Medicine,
Department of Emergency Medicine,
Rhode Island Hospital,
Providence, Rhode Island
127: Parasites

Michael L. Callaham, M.D.
Professor, Department of Medicine,
Chief, Division of Emergency Medicine,
University of California–San Francisco,
San Francisco, California
54: Mammalian Bites

Bruce Campana, M.D., FRCPC, FACEP
Emergency Consultant,
Department of Emergency Medicine,
King Faisal Specialist Hospital,
Riyadh, Saudi Arabia
47: Soft Tissue Spine Injuries and Back Pain

Richard M. Cantor, M.D., FAAP, FACEP
Vice Chair for Pediatric Emergency Medicine,
Associate Professor of Pediatrics and Emergency Medicine,
Department of Emergency Medicine,
Upstate Medical University,
Syracuse, New York
32: Pediatric Trauma

Stephen V. Cantrill, M.D., FACEP
Associate Director,
Department of Emergency Medicine,
Denver Health Medical Center;
Assistant Professor,
Division of Emergency Medicine,
Department of Surgery,
University of Colorado Health Sciences Center,
Denver, Colorado
35: Face

Stuart M. Caplen, M.D., FACEP
Chief, Department of Emergency Medicine,
Englewood Hospital and Medical Center,
Englewood, New Jersey
168: Neurologic Disorders

Grace L. Caputo, M.D., MPH
Pediatric Residency Program Director,
Department of Pediatrics,
Phoenix Children's Hospital/Maricopa Medical Center,
Phoenix, Arizona
163: Reactive Airways Disease and Pneumonia

Andrea Carlson, M.D.
Fellow in Medical Toxicology,
Toxikon Consortium,
Cook County Hospital and University of Illinois at Chicago,
Chicago, Illinois
159: Sedative Hypnotics

Dennis Chan, M.D.
Assistant Clinical Professor,
Department of Emergency Medicine,
University of California, San Diego;
Emergency Physician, Emergency Medicine,
Sharp Memorial Hospital,
San Diego, California
129: Tuberculosis

Dane M. Chapman, M.D., FACEP
Director of Emergency Medical Education and Training;
Associate Professor of Emergency Medicine,
Division of Emergency Medicine,
Washington University School of Medicine,
St. Louis, Missouri
10: Clinical Decision Making

Douglas M. Char, M.D., FACEP
Residency Program Director,
Assistant Professor of Emergency Medicine,
Division of Emergency Medicine,
Washington University School of Medicine;
Attending Physician,
Department of Emergency Medicine,
Barnes-Jewish Hospital;
Attending Physician,
Department of Emergency Medicine,
St. Louis Children's Hospital,
St. Louis, Missouri
10: Clinical Decision Making

Carl R. Chudnofsky, M.D.
Chair, Department of Emergency Medicine,
Albert Einstein Medical Center,
Philadelphia, Pennsylvania
183: Sedation and Analgesia for Procedures

Richard F. Clark, M.D., FACEP
Associate Professor of Medicine,
Director, Division of Medical Toxicology,
Department of Emergency Medicine;
Medical Director,
San Diego Division, California Poison Control System,
San Diego, California
150: Hallucinogens

Phillip A. Clement, M.D.
Department of Emergency Medicine,
East Carolina University School of Medicine,
Greenville, North Carolina
24: Diarrhea

Wendy C. Coates, M.D., FACEP
Associate Professor of Medicine,
UCLA School of Medicine,
Los Angeles, California;
Director, Medical Education,
Department of Emergency Medicine,
Harbor-UCLA Medical Center,
Torrance, California
91: Anorectum

Stephen A. Colucciello, M.D., FACEP
Assistant Clinical Professor,
Department of Emergency Medicine,
University of North Carolina at Chapel Hill
Chapel Hill, North Carolina;
Assistant Chairperson,
Department of Emergency Medicine;
Director of Clinical Services and Trauma Coordinator,
Carolinas Healthcare Systems,
Charlotte, North Carolina
109: Suicide
180: Substance Abuse

Edward E. Conway, Jr., M.D., MS, FCCP, FAAP, FCCM
Associate Professor,
Department of Pediatrics and Anesthesiology,
Albert Einstein College of Medicine,
Bronx, New York;
Chief, Division of Pediatric Critical Care,
Hyman-Newman Institute of Neurology and Neurosurgery,
Beth Israel Medical Center,
New York, New York
168: Neurologic Disorders

Mary Ann Cooper, M.D.
Associate Professor,
Department of Emergency Medicine, Neurology, and Bioengineering,
University of Illinois at Chicago,
Chicago, Illinois
136: Electrical and Lightning Injuries

William H. Cordell, M.D.
Director, Section of Research,
Department of Emergency Medicine,
Indiana University School of Medicine,
Indianapolis, Indiana
196: Information Technology in Emergency Medicine

Natalie Cullen, M.D.
Assistant Professor, Department of Emergency Medicine,
Wright State University,
Dayton, Ohio
25: Constipation

A. Adam Cwinn, M.D., FRCPC
Associate Professor, Division of Emergency Medicine,
University of Ottawa;
Director, General Campus,
Department of Emergency Medicine,
Ottawa Hospital,
Ottawa, Ontario, Canada
48: Pelvis

Rita K. Cydulka, M.D., FACEP
Associate Professor, Department of Surgery,
Case Western Reserve University;
Attending Physician, Emergency Department,
MetroHealth Medical Center;
Consultant, Department of Emergency Medicine,
Cleveland Clinic Foundation,
Cleveland, Ohio
114: Dermatologic Presentations
120: Diabetes Mellitus and Disorders of Glucose Homeostasis
181: Evaluation of the Developmentally and Physically Disabled Patient

Robert H. Dailey, M.D., FACEP
Staff Emergency Physician,
San Ramon Regional Medical Center,
San Ramon, California
69: Chronic Obstructive Pulmonary Disease

Daniel F. Danzl, M.D.
Professor and Chairman,
Department of Emergency Medicine,
University of Louisville School of Medicine,
Louisville, Kentucky
133: Frostbite
134: Accidental Hypothermia

Christine D. Darr, M.D.
Chairman, Department of Pediatric/Newborn Medicine,
Rose Medical Center;
Pediatric Emergency Physician,
Swedish Medical Center,
Denver, Colorado;
Medical Director, Pediatric Division,
Carepoint, PC,
Aurora, Colorado
163: Reactive Airways Disease and Pneumonia

Robert Dart, M.D.
Assistant Professor,
Department of Emergency Medicine,
Boston University School of Medicine;
Attending Physician,
Department of Emergency Medicine,
Boston Medical Center,
Boston, Massachusetts
27: Acute Pelvic Pain

Mohamud Daya, M.D., MS
Associate Professor, Department of Emergency Medicine,
Oregon Health Sciences University,
Portland, Oregon
46: Shoulder

Robert A. De Lorenzo, M.D., FACEP
Lieut. Colonel, Medical Corps, United States Army,
Department of Emergency Medicine,
Brooke Army Medical Center,
Ft. Sam Houston, Texas
20: Syncope

Kathleen A. Delaney, M.D.
Professor, Division of Emergency Medicine,
University of Texas Southwestern Medical School;
Emergency Department Medical Director,
Parkland Memorial Hospital,
Dallas, Texas
144: Anticholinergics
151: Heavy Metals

Theodore R. Delbridge, M.D., MPH
Assistant Professor of Emergency Medicine,
University of Pittsburgh;
Medical Director, STAT MedEvac;
Assistant Medical Director, Pittsburgh EMS,
Pittsburgh, Pennsylvania
74: Dysrhythmias

Jeff D. Disney, M.D.
Department of Emergency Medicine,
University of California–San Diego,
San Diego, California
118: Acid-Base Disorders

Susan M. Dunmire, M.D., FACEP
Associate Professor of Emergency Medicine,
University of Pittsburgh School of Medicine;
Attending Physician, Emergency Department,
UPMC Presbyterian University Hospital,
Pittsburgh, Pennsylvania
78: Infective Endocarditis and Valvular Heart Disease

Edward Rivers Eastman, M.D.
Chief Resident, Department of Emergency Medicine,
University of Florida Health Science Center Jacksonville,
Jacksonville, Florida
94: Selected Urologic Problems

Marc Eckstein, M.D., FACEP
Assistant Professor of Emergency Medicine,
Department of Emergency Medicine,
University of Southern California School of Medicine;
Director of Prehospital Care,
Department of Emergency Medicine,
Los Angeles County and University of Southern California Medical Center;
Medical Director, Los Angeles City Fire Department,
Los Angeles, California
38: Thorax
173: Chronic Medical Illness During Pregnancy

Richard F. Edlich, M.D., Ph.D.
Distinguished Professor of Plastic Surgery and Professor of Biomedical Engineering,
University of Virginia Health Sciences Center,
Charlottesville, Virginia
56: Thermal Burns
57: Chemical Injuries

Mary A. Eisenhauer, M.D., FRCPC
Associate Professor, Department of Medicine,
University of Western Ontario;
Medical Director of Research, Emergency Medicine,
London Health Sciences Center,
London, Ontario, Canada
44: Wrist and Forearm

Javier I. Escobar, II, M.D.
Pediatric Emergency Medicine Fellow,
Department of Emergency Medicine,
University of Florida HSCIJ,
Jacksonville, Florida
94: Selected Urologic Problems

Jay L. Falk, M.D., FACEP, FCCM
Clinical Professor,
Department of Medicine and Emergency Medicine,
University of Florida College of Medicine,
Gainesville, Florida;
Academic Chairman, Department of Emergency Medicine,
Orlando Regional Healthcare System,
Orlando, Florida
76: Heart Failure

Craig F. Feied, M.D., FACEP, FAAEM
Director,
National Center for Emergency Medicine Informatics;
Director of Informatics,
Washington Hospital Medical Center,
Department of Emergency Medicine;
Associate Clinical Professor,
Department of Emergency Medicine,
George Washington University Medical Center,
Washington, DC
83: Venous Thrombosis and Pulmonary Embolism

Kim M. Feldhaus, M.D.
Assistant Professor,
Department of Surgery,
University of Colorado Health Sciences Center;
Attending Physician,
Department of Emergency Medicine,
Denver Health Medical Center,
Denver, Colorado
139: Submersion

Madonna Fernández-Frackelton, M.D.
Assistant Professor of Medicine,
Department of Emergency Medicine,
UCLA School of Medicine;
Assistant Professor of Medicine,
Department of Emergency Medicine,
Harbor-UCLA Medical Center,
Torrance, California
123: Bacteria

John T. Finnell, M.D., FACEP
Assistant Professor of Clinical Emergency Medicine,
University of Minnesota School of Medicine,
Minneapolis, Minnesota;
Assistant Residency Director,
Department of Emergency Medicine,
Health Partners Regions Hospital,
St. Paul, Minnesota
179: Acute and Chronic Alcoholism

Marsha D. Ford, M.D., FACEP, FACMT
Clinical Professor,
Department of Emergency Medicine,
University of North Carolina,
Chapel Hill, North Carolina;
Director, Division of Medical Toxicology,
Assistant Chairman, Department of Emergency Medicine,
Carolinas Medical Center;
Director, Carolinas Poison Center,
Charlotte, North Carolina
155: Antipsychotics

E. John Gallagher, M.D.
University Chair, Department of Emergency Medicine,
Professor of Emergency Medicine, Medicine, Epidemiology and Social Medicine,
Albert Einstein College of Medicine;
Chair, Department of Emergency Medicine,
Montefiore Medical Center,
Bronx, New York
101: Peripheral Nerve Disorders

Marianne Gausche-Hill, M.D., FACEP, FAAP
Associate Professor of Medicine,
UCLA School of Medicine;
Director, Emergency Medical Services,
Department of Emergency Medicine,
Harbor-UCLA Medical Center,
Torrance, California
170: Sudden Infant Death Syndrome

Joel M. Geiderman, M.D.
Clinical Professor,
Department of Emergency Medicine,
UCLA School of Medicine;
Chair, Ruth and Harry Roman Emergency Department,
Department of Emergency Medicine,
Burns and Allen Research Institute,
Cedars-Sinai Medical Center,
Los Angeles, California;
Medical Director, Beverly Hills Fire Department,
Beverly Hills, California
42: General Principles of Orthopedic Injuries
45: Humerus and Elbow

Michael A. Gibbs, M.D.
Residency Program Director,
Department of Emergency Medicine,
Carolinas Medical Center;
Medical Director, MedCenter Air;
Assistant Clinical Professor of Emergency Medicine,
University of North Carolina at Chapel Hill,
Chapel Hill, North Carolina
49: Femur and Hip
119: Electrolyte Disturbances

W. Brian Gibler, M.D.
Richard C. Levy Professor of Emergency Medicine,
Chairman, Department of Emergency Medicine,
University of Cincinnati College of Medicine;
Director, Center for Emergency Care,
University of Cincinnati Hospital;
Medical Director, Emergency Services,
The Greater Cincinnati Health Alliance;
President, Vanguard Medical, Inc.;
President, EMCREG-International,
Cincinnati, Ohio
73: Acute Ischemic Coronary Syndromes
127: Parasites

Brian P. Gilligan, M.D.
Fellow, Pediatric Emergency Medicine,
Department of Emergency Medicine,
University of Florida;
Department of Emergency Medicine,
Shands Jacksonville,
Jacksonville, Florida
8: Pediatric Resuscitation

Susan L. Gin-Shaw, M.D., FACEP
Education Director, Department of Emergency Medicine,
Maricopa Medical Center;
Attending Physician, Division of Internal Medicine,
Arizona Heart Hospital,
Phoenix, Arizona
30: Multiple Trauma

Claudia R. Gold, M.D., FACEP
Clinical Instructor,
Department of Emergency Medicine,
Los Angeles County–USC Medical Center,
Los Angeles, California;
Chair, Department of Emergency Medicine,
Children's Hospital of Orange County,
Orange, California
61: Sexual Assault

Richard Goldberg, M.D.
Associate Clinical Professor,
Department of Emergency Medicine,
University of Southern California Medical Center,
Los Angeles, California;
Staff Physician, Department of Emergency Medicine,
Saint Joseph Medical Center,
Burbank, California
201: Wellness, Stress, and the Impaired Physician

James A. Gordon, M.D., MPA
Director, MEC Program in Medical Simulation and Instructor in Medicine,
Harvard Medical School;
Attending Physician,
Department of Emergency Medicine,
Massachusetts General Hospital,
Boston, Massachusetts
195: The Social Role of Emergency Medicine

John E. Gough, M.D.
Associate Professor,
Department of Emergency Medicine,
East Carolina University School of Medicine,
Greenville, North Carolina
24: Diarrhea

Louis Graff, M.D., FACP, FACEP
Associate Professor,
Traumatology and Emergency Medicine,
Associate Professor of Clinical Medicine,
University of Connecticut School of Medicine,
Farmington, Connecticut;
Assistant Clinical Professor,
Division of Emergency Medicine,
Department of Surgery,
Yale University School of Medicine,
New Haven, Connecticut;
Associate Chief, Emergency Medicine,
New Britain General Hospital,
New Britain, Connecticut
192: Observation Medicine/Clinical Decision Units

Timothy A.D. Graham M.D., CCFM (EM)
Clinical Lecturer
Division of Medicine and Dentistry
University of Alberta
Alberta, Canada
3: Monitoring the Emergency Patient

Richard O. Gray, M.D.
Assistant Professor,
Department of Emergency Medicine,
University of Minnesota School of Medicine;
Staff Physician and Director of Medical Student Education,
Department of Emergency Medicine,
Hennepin County Medical Center,
Minneapolis, Minnesota
79: Hypertension

John A. Guisto, M.D., FACEP
Associate Professor, Department of Emergency Medicine,
University of Arizona Health Sciences Center;
Clinical Director, Emergency Department,
University Medical Center,
Tucson, Arizona
131: Soft Tissue Infections

David D. Gummin, M.D.
Clinical Assistant Professor,
Medical College of Wisconsin;
Associate Medical Director,
Children's Hospital of Wisconsin,
Milwaukee, Wisconsin
156: Opioids

Daniel E. Gurr, M.D.
Director of International Medicine Fellowship,
Department of Emergency Medicine,
Harvard Medical School;
Director of Student Programs,
Brigham and Women's Hospital,
Boston, Massachusetts
49: Femur and Hip

David A. Guss, M.D.
Professor of Clinical Medicine and Surgery,
Chair, Department of Emergency Medicine,
University of California–San Diego Medical Center,
San Diego, California
85: Liver and Biliary Tract

Leon Gussow, M.D., ABMT
Senior Attending Physician,
Department of Emergency Medicine,
Cook County Hospital;
Consultant, Illinois Poison Center,
Chicago, Illinois
159: Sedative Hypnotics

Rania Habal, M.D., FACEP
Assistant Professor,
Department of Emergency Medicine,
New York Medical College,
Valhalla, New York;
Attending Physician,
Department of Emergency Medicine,
Metropolitan Hospital,
New York, New York
174: Drug Therapy and Substance Abuse

Tenagne Haile-Mariam, M.D.
Assistant Professor,
Department of Emergency Medicine,
George Washington University Medical Center,
Washington, DC
124: Viruses

Glenn C. Hamilton, M.D., MSM
Professor and Chair, Department of Emergency Medicine,
Wright State University School of Medicine,
Dayton, Ohio
19: Chest Pain
115: Anemia, Polycythemia, and White Blood Cell Disorders
116: Disorders of Hemostasis

Christina E. Hantsch, M.D.
Assistant Professor,
Department of Surgery,
Division of Emergency Medicine,
Loyola University Chicago;
Medical Director,
Illinois Poison Center,
Chicago, Illinois;
Attending Physician,
Emergency Medicine and Medical Toxicology,
Loyola University Medical Center,
Maywood, Illinois
156: Opioids

Stephen W. Hargarten, M.D., MPH
Professor and Chairman,
Department of Emergency Medicine,
Medical College of Wisconsin,
Milwaukee, Wisconsin
58: Injury Prevention and Control

David W. Harrison, M.D., CCFP (EM), FCRPC
Associate Clinical Professor,
Department of Emergency Medicine,
University of British Columbia;
Attending Physician,
Department of Emergency Medicine,
Vancouver General Hospital,
Vancouver, British Columbia, Canada
185: The Difficult Patient

Ann L. Harwood-Nuss, M.D.
Professor, Associate Dean,
Department of Emergency Medicine,
University of Florida,
Jacksonville, Florida
94: Selected Urologic Problems

William Heegaard, M.D., MPH
Assistant Professor,
Department of Emergency Medicine,
University of Minnesota School of Medicine;
Associate Staff Physician,
Department of Emergency Medicine,
Hennepin County Medical Center,
Minneapolis, Minnesota
34: Head

Timothy Heilenbach, M.D.
Clinical Instructor, Department of Emergency Medicine,
Chicago Medical School,
North Chicago, Illinois;
Associate Director of Education,
Department of Emergency Medicine,
Mount Sinai Hospital,
Chicago, Illinois
21: Nausea and Vomiting

Katherine L. Heilpern, M.D., FACEP
Assistant Professor and Assistant Dean, Medical Education,
Department of Emergency Medicine,
Emory University School of Medicine,
Atlanta, Georgia
26: Jaundice

Robin R. Hemphill, M.D.
Associate Program Director and Assistant Professor,
Department of Emergency Medicine,
Vanderbilt University Medical Center,
Nashville, Tennessee
86: Pancreas

Sean Henderson, M.D., FACEP, FAAEM
Assistant Professor of Emergency Medicine,
Department of Emergency Medicine,
Keck School of Medicine,
University of Southern California;
Los Angeles County and University of Southern California Medical Center,
Los Angeles, California
38: Thorax
175: Labor and Delivery

Philip L. Henneman, M.D.
Clinical Professor and Chair,
Department of Emergency Medicine,
Tufts University School of Medicine;
Chair, Department of Emergency Medicine,
Baystate Health System,
Springfield, Massachusetts
23: Gastrointestinal Bleeding
87: Small Intestine
88: Acute Appendicitis

Gregory L. Henry, M.D.
Clinical Professor, Department of Emergency Medicine,
The University of Michigan Medical School;
Staff Physician, Department of Emergency Medicine,
Saint Joseph Mercy Hospital;
CEO, Medical Practice Risk Assessment, Inc.,
Ann Arbor, Michigan
17: Headache

H. Gene Hern, Jr., M.D.
Faculty, Department of Emergency Medicine
Alameda County Medical Center,
Highland General Hospital,
Oakland, California
52: Wound Management Principles

Kendall Ho, M.D., FRCPC
Assistant Professor, Division of Emergency Medicine,
Department of Surgery;
Associate Dean,
Division of Continuing Medical Education,
University of British Columbia;
Attending Staff, Department of Emergency Medicine,
Vancouver General Hospital,
Vancouver, British Columbia, Canada
51: Ankle and Foot

Robert S. Hockberger, M.D.
Chair,
Department of Emergency Medicine,
Harbor-UCLA Medical Center,
Torrance, California;
Professor of Medicine
UCLA School Of Medicine,
Westwood, California
36: Spine
104: Thought Disorders

Gwendolyn L. Hoffman, M.D., FACEP
Associate Professor, Department of Emergency Medicine,
Michigan State University College of Human Medicine,
East Lansing, Michigan;
Residency Director, Department of Emergency Medicine,
Spectrum Health/MSU Program in Emergency Medicine,
Grand Rapids, Michigan
5: Blood and Blood Components

Robert S. Hoffman, M.D.
Assistant Professor of Clinical Surgery,
Department of Emergency Medicine,
New York University School of Medicine;
Director, New York Poison Control Center;
Attending Physician, Bellevue Hospital;
Attending Physician, NYU Medical Center,
New York, New York
148: Cocaine, Amphetamines, and Other Sympathomimetics
153: Inhaled Toxins

Benjamin Honigman, M.D., FACEP
Head, Division of Emergency Medicine,
Associate Professor, Department of Surgery,
University of Colorado Health Sciences Center;
Attending Physician, Department of Emergency Medicine,
University of Colorado Hospital;
Medical Director, Emergency Medical Services,
Division of EMS and Injury Prevention,
Colorado Department of Public Health and Environment,
Denver, Colorado
138: High-Altitude Medicine
199: End of Life

Mark A. Hostetler, M.D., MPH
Instructor, Department of Pediatrics,
Instructor, Department of Surgery,
Division of Emergency Medicine,
Washington University School of Medicine,
St. Louis Children's and Barnes-Jewish Hospitals,
St. Louis, Missouri
165: Gastrointestinal Disorders

Debra Houry, M.D., MPH
Residency in Emergency Medicine,
Denver Health Medical Center,
Denver, Colorado
172: Acute Complications of Pregnancy

J. Stephen Huff, M.D.
Associate Professor, Department of Emergency Medicine,
University of Virginia;
University of Virginia Health System,
Emergency Medicine, University of Virginia;
Associate Professor, Department of Neurology,
University of Virginia,
Charlottesville, Virginia
14: Confusion
100: Spinal Cord Disorders

H. Range Hutson, M.D.
Assistant Professor, Department of Emergency Medicine,
Brigham and Women's Hospital,
Harvard Medical School,
Boston, Massachusetts
63: Elder Abuse and Neglect
64: Youth, Gangs, and Violence

Kenneth V. Iserson, M.D., MPA, FACEP
Professor, Department of Emergency Medicine,
University of Arizona College of Medicine;
Emergency Physician and Bioethics Committee Chair,
University Medical Center;
Director, Arizona Bioethics Program,
University of Arizona College of Medicine,
Tucson, Arizona
198: Bioethics

Kenneth C. Jackimczyk, M.D.
Associate Chairman, Department of Emergency Medicine,
Maricopa Medical Center,
Phoenix, Arizona
184: The Combative Patient

Andrew Jagoda, M.D.
Associate Professor/Associate Residency Director,
Department of Emergency Medicine,
Mount Sinai School of Medicine;
Attending Physician, Department of Emergency Medicine,
Mount Sinai Hospital,
New York, New York
102: Neuromuscular Disorders

Thea James, M.D.
Clinical Instructor, Department of Emergency Medicine,
Boston University School of Medicine;
Clinical Instructor, Department of Emergency Medicine,
Boston Medical Center,
Boston, Massachusetts
197: Multiculturalism and Care Delivery

Timothy G. Janz, M.D.
Associate Professor, Department of Emergency Medicine,
Pulmonary/Critical Care Division,
Department of Internal Medicine,
Wright State University School of Medicine,
Dayton, Ohio
115: Anemia, Polycythemia, and White Blood Cell Disorders
116: Disorders of Hemostasis

James B. Jones, M.D., PharmD
Associate Director,
Emergency Medicine Research Program;
Clinical Assistant Professor,
Department of Emergency Medicine,
Indiana University School of Medicine,
Indianapolis, Indiana
29: Back Pain

Robert C. Jorden, M.D., FACEP
Department of Emergency Medicine,
Phoenix Baptist Medical Center,
Phoenix, Arizona
30: Multiple Trauma

Nicholas J. Jouriles, M.D.
Attending Physician, Department of Emergency Medicine,
MetroHealth Medical Center and Cleveland Clinic Foundation;
Associate Professor, Department of Emergency Medicine;
Residency Director,
Case Western Reserve University,
Cleveland, Ohio
77: Pericardial and Myocardial Disease

Louise W. Kao, M.D.
Methodist Hospital Emergency Medicine Residency,
Indiana University School of Medicine,
Indianapolis, Indiana
184: The Combative Patient

Gabor D. Kelen, M.D.
Professor and Chairman,
Department of Emergency Medicine,
The Johns Hopkins University,
Baltimore, Maryland
126: AIDS and HIV

Eugene E. Kercher, M.D.
Associate Clinical Professor of Medicine,
UCLA School of Medicine,
Los Angeles, California;
Chair, Department of Emergency Medicine,
Kern Medical Center,
Bakersfield, California
106: Anxiety Disorders

Kelly E. King, M.D.
Lieutenant Commander, Medical Corps,
United States Navy,
Assistant Professor, Department of Military and Emergency Medicine,
Uniformed Services University,
Bethesda, Maryland
22: Abdominal Pain

Susan Kirelik, M.D.
Medical Director, Pediatric Emergency Medicine,
Medical Center of Aurora;
Carepoint, PC,
Aurora, Colorado
163: Reactive Airways Disease and Pneumonia

Kevin J. Kirshenbaum, M.D.
Clinical Instructor, Department of Radiology,
Rush Medical College;
Director of Residency-Diagnostic Radiology,
Illinois Masonic Medical Center,
Chicago, Illinois
36: Spine

Eileen Klein, M.D., MPH
Assistant Professor, Department of Pediatrics,
University of Washington;
Attending Physician, Department of Emergency Medicine,
Children's Hospital and Regional Medical Center,
Seattle, Washington
9: Neonatal Resuscitation

Jeffrey A. Kline, M.D.
Clinical Assistant Professor of Emergency Medicine,
University of North Carolina School of Medicine,
Chapel Hill, North Carolina;
Assistant Director of Research,
Department of Emergency Medicine,
Carolinas Medical Center,
Charlotte, North Carolina
4: Shock

Kristi L. Koenig, M.D., FACEP
Clinical Professor of Emergency Medicine,
George Washington University Medical Center;
Director, Emergency Management Strategic Healthcare Group,
Department of Veterans Affairs,
Washington, DC
188: Disaster Preparedness
189: Weapons of Mass Destruction

Dina Halpern Kornblau, M.D.
Assistant Clinical Professor, Department of Pediatrics,
Weill Medical College of Cornell University,
New York, New York;
Attending Physician, Department of Pediatrics,
Saint Barnabas Hospital,
Bronx, New York
168: Neurologic Disorders

Joseph Kosnik, M.D., FACEP, FAAEM
Adjunct Assistant Professor,
Department of Emergency Medicine,
Wayne State University School of Medicine,
Detroit, Michigan;
Attending Physician,
Emergency Department,
MidMichigan Medical Center,
Midland, Michigan
149: Toxic Alcohols

Joshua M. Kosowsky, M.D.
Attending Physician, Department of Emergency Medicine,
Brigham and Women's Hospital,
Boston, Massachusetts
72: Pleural Disease

Rashmi Kothari, M.D.
Associate Professor, Department of Emergency Medicine,
Michigan State University/Kalamazoo Center for Medical Studies,
Borgess Research Institute,
Kalamazoo, Michigan
95: Stroke

Theodore K. Koutouzis, M.D.
Attending Physician,
Department of Emergency Medicine,
Northwestern Memorial Hospital,
Chicago, Illinois
111: Tendonitis and Bursitis

Ken Kulig, M.D., FAACT, FACMT
Associate Clinical Professor,
Division of Emergency Medicine and Trauma,
University of Colorado Health Sciences Center;
Director, Porter Regional Toxicology Center,
Denver, Colorado
141: General Approach to the Poisoned Patient

Thomas G. Kwiatkowski, M.D.
Associate Professor, Department of Emergency Medicine,
Albert Einstein College of Medicine,
Bronx, New York;
Chairman, Department of Emergency Medicine,
North Shore-Long Island Jewish Health System,
New Hyde Park, New York
97: Headache

Christ G. Kyriakedes, D.O., FACEP
Assistant Professor of Clinical Emergency Medicine,
Department of Emergency Medicine,
Northeastern Ohio University College of Medicine,
Rootstown, Ohio;
Assistant Program Director,
Department of Emergency Medicine,
Akron General Medical Center,
Akron, Ohio
28: Vaginal Bleeding

Mark I. Langdorf, M.D., MHPE, FACEP
Division Chief and Residency Director,
Associate Professor of Clinical Emergency Medicine,
Division of Emergency Medicine,
University of California–Irvine,
Irvine, California;
Medical Director, Emergency Department,
UCI Medical Center,
Orange, California
177: The Immunocompromised Patient

Frank W. Lavoie, M.D.
Chief, Department of Emergency Medicine,
Southern Maine Medical Center,
Biddeford, Maine
103: Central Nervous System Infections

Eric J. Lavonas, M.D., FACEP
Clinical Instructor of Emergency Medicine,
Department of Emergency Medicine,
University of North Carolina at Chapel Hill,
Chapel Hill, North Carolina;
Division of Medical Toxicology,
Department of Emergency Medicine,
Carolinas Medical Center,
Charlotte, North Carolina
155: Antipsychotics

James M. Leaming, M.D.
Assistant Professor and
Residency Program Director,
Department of Emergency Medicine,
University of Alabama at Birmingham,
Birmingham, Alabama
32: Pediatric Trauma

David C. Lee, M.D.
Director of Research, Department of Emergency Medicine,
North Shore University Hospital,
Manhasset, New York
152: Hydrocarbons

Roger J. Lewis, M.D., Ph.D.
Associate Professor, Department of Medicine,
University of California, Los Angeles,
Los Angeles, California;
Director of Research, Department of Emergency Medicine,
Harbor-UCLA Medical Center,
Torrance, California
191: Medical Literature and Evidence-Based Medicine

Mark Lowell, M.D.
Clinical Assistant Professor,
Department of Emergency Medicine,
University of Michigan Medical Center,
Ann Arbor, Michigan
84: Esophagus, Stomach, and Duodenum

Douglas W. Lowery, M.D.
Assistant Professor of Emergency Medicine,
Department of Emergency Medicine,
Emory University School of Medicine;
Medical Director, Emergency Department,
Emory University Hospital,
Atlanta, Georgia
110: Arthritis
178: The Organ Transplant Patient

Marie M. Lozon, M.D.
Clinical Assistant Professor,
Division Director, Pediatric Emergency Medicine,
Departments of Emergency Medicine and Pediatrics,
University of Michigan,
Ann Arbor, Michigan
183: Sedation and Analgesia for Procedures

Robert C. Luten, M.D.
Professor,
Department of Pediatrics and Emergency Medicine,
University of Florida;
Department of Emergency Medicine,
Shands Jacksonville,
Jacksonville, Florida
8: Pediatric Resuscitation

Everett Lyn, M.D., MS
Director of Education,
Attending Physician,
Department of Emergency Medicine,
Brigham and Women's Hospital;
Harvard Medical School,
Boston, Massachusetts
43: Hand
50: Knee and Lower Leg

Richard L. Maenza, M.D., FACEP
Associate Clinical Professor of Emergency Medicine,
Department of Emergency Medicine,
University of Pittsburgh,
Pittsburgh, Pennsylvania;
Attending Emergency Physician,
Department of Emergency Medicine,
The Medical Center of Beaver County,
Beaver, Pennsylvania
92: Renal Failure

Malcolm Mahadevan, M.D., MRCP, FRCSEd
Registrar, Department of Emergency Medicine,
National University Hospital,
Singapore;
Instructor, Traumatology and Emergency Medicine,
University of Connecticut School of Medicine,
Farmington, Connecticut
192: Observation Medicine/Clinical Decision Units

William K. Mallon, M.D., FACEP, FAAEM
Associate Professor of Clinical Emergency Medicine,
Keck School of Medicine,
University of Southern California;
Director of Residency Training,
Department of Emergency Medicine,
Los Angeles County and
University of Southern California Medical Center,
Los Angeles, California
175: Labor and Delivery

Diku P. Mandavia, M.D., FACEP, FRCPC
Clinical Assistant Professor,
Department of Emergency Medicine,
University of Southern California;
Attending Staff Physician,
Ruth and Harry Roman Emergency Department,
Cedars-Sinai Medical Center,
Los Angeles, California
69: Chronic Obstructive Pulmonary Disease

Mariann Manno, M.D., FAAP
Assistant Professor, Department of Pediatrics,
University of Massachusetts Medical School;
Director, Pediatric Emergency Medicine,
Childrens Medical Center,
University of Massachusetts Memorial Health Care,
Worcester, Massachusetts
162: Upper Airway Obstruction and Infection

Catherine A. Marco, M.D.
Assistant Professor, Department of Surgery,
Medical College of Ohio;
Attending Physician, Department of Emergency Medicine,
Saint Vincent Mercy Medical Center,
Toledo, Ohio
126: AIDS and HIV

Vincent Markovchick, M.D.
Professor, Division of Emergency Medicine,
Department of Surgery, University of Colorado;
Director of Emergency Medical Services,
Department of Emergency Medicine,
Denver Health,
Denver, Colorado
38: Thorax
140: Radiation Injuries

John A. Marx, M.D.
Chair,
Department of Emergency Medicine,
Carolinas Medical Center,
Charlotte, North Carolina;
Clinical Professor of Emergency Medicine,
University of North Carolina School of Medicine,
Chapel Hill, North Carolina
39: Abdominal Trauma

James Mathews, M.D.
Assistant Dean, Graduate and Continuing Medical Education;
Professor of Medicine,
Northwestern University Medical School,
Chicago, Illinois
79: Hypertension

Maureen McCollough, M.D., MPH, FACEP
Assistant Professor of Medicine,
UCLA School of Medicine,
Los Angeles, California;
Director of Pediatric Emergency Medicine,
Department of Emergency Medicine,
Olive View-UCLA Medical Center,
Sylmar, California
167: Renal and Genitourinary Tract Disorders

David B. McMicken, M.D., FACEP
Clinical Assistant Professor of Family and Preventive Medicine,
Emory University School of Medicine,
Atlanta, Georgia
179: Acute and Chronic Alcoholism

Kemedy K. McQuillen, M.D.
Attending Physician,
Department of Emergency Medicine,
Advocate Christ Hospital and Medical Center,
Oak Lawn, Illinois
169: Musculoskeletal Disorders

Harvey W. Meislin, M.D., FACEP
Professor and Chief, Division of Emergency Medicine,
Associate Chairman, Department of Surgery,
Director, Arizona Emergency Medicine Research Center,
University of Arizona Health Sciences Center,
Tucson, Arizona
131: Soft Tissue Infections

Frantz R. Melio, M.D., FACEP
Clinical Associate Professor,
Department of Emergency Medicine,
University of North Carolina at Chapel Hill,
Chapel Hill, North Carolina;
Chair/Medical Director,
Department of Emergency Medicine,
WakeMed,
Raleigh, North Carolina
70: Upper Respiratory Tract Infections

Gregory P. Moore, M.D., JD
Associate Clinical Professor,
Department of Emergency Medicine,
Indiana University School of Medicine;
Attending Physician,
Department of Emergency Medicine,
Methodist Hospital,
Indianapolis, Indiana
67: Otolaryngology
184: The Combative Patient

Gregory J. Moran, M.D., FACEP
Associate Professor of Medicine,
Department of Emergency Medicine and Division of Infectious Diseases,
UCLA School of Medicine,
Los Angeles, California;
Research Director, Department of Emergency Medicine,
Olive View-UCLA Medical Center
Sylmar, California
71: Pneumonia

Laurie J. Morrison, M.D., FRCPC, M.Sc.
Director, Division of Emergency Medicine,
Department of Medicine,
University of Toronto;
Research Director, Division of Prehospital Care,
Department of Emergency Services,
Sunnybrook and Women's College Health Sciences Center,
Toronto, Ontario, Canada
171: General Approach to the Pregnant Patient

Robert L. Muelleman, M.D., FACEP
Chief, Section of Emergency Medicine,
Nebraska Health Systems,
Omaha, Nebraska
113: Allergy, Hypersensitivity, and Anaphylaxis

Kathryn L. Mueller, M.D., MPH, FACEP, FACOEM
Associate Professor,
Department of Surgery, Division of Emergency Medicine,
University of Colorado Health Sciences Center;
Medical Director,
Colorado Division of Worker's Compensation,
Denver, Colorado
193: Occupational Health in the Emergency Department

Deborah A. Mulligan-Smith, M.D., FAAP, FACEP
Associate Clinical Professor,
Community Health and Family Medicine,
University of Florida;
Associate Clinical Professor,
Pediatric Department,
Nova Southeastern College of Medicine;
Medical Director of Pediatric Services and EMSC,
North Broward Hospital District,
Ft. Lauderdale, Florida
93: Genital Infections

Michael F. Murphy, M.D.
Associate Professor,
Departments of Emergency Medicine and Anesthesiology,
Dalhousie University,
Halifax, Nova Scotia, Canada
3: Monitoring the Emergency Patient

Lindsay Murray, M.D., MBBS, FACEM
Senior Lecturer in Emergency Medicine,
Department of Surgery,
University of Western Australia;
Medical Director,
Western Australian Poisons Information Center;
Consultant Emergency Physician,
Department of Emergency Medicine,
Sir Charles Gairdner Hospital,
Perth, Western Australia, Australia
143: Aspirin and Nonsteroidal Agents

Lewis S. Nelson, M.D.
Assistant Professor of Clinical Surgery,
Department of Emergency Medicine,
New York University School of Medicine;
Director, Fellowship in Medical Toxicology,
New York City Poison Control Center;
Associate Director, New York City Poison Control Center;
Attending Physician, Bellevue Hospital;
Attending Physician, NYU Medical Center,
New York, New York
153: Inhaled Toxins

John D.G. Neufeld, M.D.
Staff Emergency Physician,
Department of Emergency Medicine,
Rockyview General Hospital,
Calgary Regional Health Authority,
Calgary, Alberta, Canada
31: Trauma in Pregnancy

Robert W. Neumar, M.D., Ph.D.
Assistant Professor, Department of Emergency Medicine,
Hospital of the University of Pennsylvania,
Philadelphia, Pennsylvania
7: Adult Resuscitation

Edward Newton, M.D., FACEP
Associate Professor of Emergency Medicine,
Keck and USC School of Medicine;
Vice Chairman,
Department of Emergency Medicine,
Los Angeles County and University of Southern California Medical Center,
Los Angeles, California
41: Peripheral Vascular Injury
173: Chronic Medical Illness During Pregnancy

Kim Newton, M.D., FACEP
Director, Emergency-Ambulatory,
Assistant Professor of Clinical Emergency Medicine,
Keck School of Medicine,
University of Southern California,
Los Angeles, California
37: Neck

James T. Niemann, M.D., FACEP, FACP
Professor of Medicine,
UCLA School of Medicine,
Los Angeles, California;
Department of Emergency Medicine,
Harbor-UCLA Medical Center,
Torrance, California
75: Implantable Cardiac Devices

Eric K. Noji, M.D.
Senior Medical Officer,
World Health Organization,
Geneva, Switzerland
188: Disaster Preparedness

Richard Nowak, M.D., MBA, FACEP
Professor, Department of Medicine,
Case Western Reserve University Medical School,
Cleveland, Ohio;
Vice-Chairman, Department of Emergency Medicine,
Henry Ford Hospital,
Detroit, Michigan
68: Asthma

John F. O'Brien, M.D., FACEP
Associate Professor, Department of Emergency Medicine,
University of Florida College of Medicine,
Gainesville, Florida;
Assistant Residency Director,
Department of Emergency Medicine,
Orlando Regional Medical Center,
Orlando, Florida
76: Heart Failure

Jonathan S. Olshaker, M.D.
Professor of Surgery and Medicine,
University of Maryland School of Medicine;
Chief, Emergency Care Services,
Veterans Affairs Medical Center,
Baltimore, Maryland
13: Dizziness and Vertigo

Edward J. Otten, M.D., FACEP
Professor of Emergency Medicine and Pediatrics,
Director, Division of Toxicology,
University of Cincinnati,
Cincinnati, Ohio
55: Venomous Animal Injuries

Arthur M. Pancioli, M.D.
Assistant Professor, Department of Emergency Medicine,
University of Cincinnati College of Medicine;
Director, Division of Cerebrovascular Research,
University of Cincinnati College of Medicine,
Cincinnati, Ohio
99: Brain and Cranial Nerve Disorders

Paul M. Paris, M.D., FACEP, LLD(Hon.)
Professor and Chairman,
Department of Emergency Medicine,
University of Pittsburgh School of Medicine;
Chief Medical Officer,
Center for Emergency Medicine of Western Pennsylvania,
Pittsburgh, Pennsylvania
182: Pain Management

Stephen J. Parker, M.D.
Fellow Medical Toxicology/Clinical Instructor Emergency Medicine,
Department of Emergency Medicine,
Oregon Health Sciences University–Oregon Poison Center;
Fellow Medical Toxicology,
Department of Emergency Medicine,
Oregon Poison Center,
Portland, Oregon
142: Acetaminophen

Debra Perina, M.D.
Associate Professor, Emergency Medicine,
Director, Prehospital Care Division,
University of Virginia Health Sciences Center,
Charlottesville, Virginia
18: Dyspnea

Andrew D. Perron, M.D.
Assistant Professor of Emergency Medicine and Orthopaedic Surgery,
Department of Emergency Medicine,
University of Virginia Health System,
Charlottesville, Virginia
100: Spinal Cord Disorders

Michael A. Peterson, M.D.
Director, Emergency Ultrasound Program,
Department of Emergency Medicine,
Harbor-UCLA Medical Center,
Torrance, California
90: Large Intestine

James A. Pfaff, M.D., FACEP
Colonel, United States Army,
Chairman, Department of Emergency Medicine,
Brooke Army Medical Center,
San Antonio Uniformed Services Health Education Consortium,
Emergency Medicine,
San Antonio, Texas
67: Otolaryngology

Michael Alan Polis, M.D., MPH
Clinical Professor,
Department of Emergency Medicine,
George Washington University Medical Center,
Washington, DC;
Senior Investigator,
Laboratory of Immunoregulation,
National Institute of Allergy and Infectious Diseases,
Bethesda, Maryland
124: Viruses

Charles V. Pollack, Jr., M.D., MA, FACEP
Associate Professor,
Department of Emergency Medicine,
University of Pennsylvania School of Medicine;
Chairman, Department of Emergency Medicine,
Pennsylvania Hospital,
Philadelphia, Pennsylvania
2: Mechanical Ventilation and Noninvasive Ventilatory Support
16: Seizures
96: Seizures

Emily S. Pollack, M.D., FAAP, FACEP
Bryn Mawr, Pennsylvania
96: Seizures

Timothy G. Price, M.D., FACEP, FAAEM
Assistant Professor of Emergency Medicine,
Department of Emergency Medicine,
University of Louisville School of Medicine,
Louisville, Kentucky
136: Electrical and Lightning Injuries

Thomas B. Purcell, M.D.
Adjunct Assistant Professor,
Department of Medicine,
UCLA School of Medicine,
Los Angeles, California;
Residency Director,
Department of Emergency Medicine,
Kern Medical Center,
Bakersfield, California
107: Somatoform Disorders
108: Factitious Disorders and Malingering

Linda Quan, M.D.
Professor, Department of Pediatrics,
University of Washington;
Director, Department of Emergency,
Childrens Hospital and Regional Medical Center,
Seattle, Washington
9: Neonatal Resuscitation

Tammie E. Quest, M.D.
Assistant Professor, Department of Emergency Medicine,
Emory University School of Medicine,
Atlanta, Georgia
26: Jaundice

Rama B. Rao, M.D.
Assistant Clinical Professor, Emergency Medicine and Forensic Pathology,
Consultant, New York City Poison Control Center and Office of Chief Medical Examiner of the City of New York;
Residency Research Codirector,
Bellevue Hospital Center/NYU Medical Center,
New York, New York
148: Cocaine, Amphetamines, and Other Sympathomimetics

Robert C. Reiser, M.D., MS
Assistant Professor, Department of Emergency Medicine;
Medical Director, Emergency Medicine,
University of Virginia,
Charlottesville, Virginia
12: Weakness

Christopher F. Richards, M.D.
Instructor, Department of Emergency Medicine,
Harvard Medical School;
Attending Physician, Department of Emergency Medicine,
Brigham and Women's Hospital,
Boston, Massachusetts
111: Tendonitis and Bursitis

John Richards, M.D.
Assistant Professor, Department of Emergency Medicine,
University of California–Davis Medical School,
Sacramento, California
104: Thought Disorders

David J. Roberts, M.D., ABMT
Clinical Associate Professor,
University of Minnesota,
Minneapolis, Minnesota;
Consulting Toxicologist,
North Memorial Health Care,
Robbinsdale, Minnesota;
Associate Medical Director,
Hennepin Regional Poison Center,
Hennepin County Medical Center,
Minneapolis, Minnesota
146: Common Cardiovascular Drugs

Howard Rodenberg, M.D.
Medical Director, Volusia County EMS;
Adjunct Professor of Human Factors,
Embry-Riddle Aeronautical University,
Daytona Beach, Florida
187: Air Medical Transport

Kevin G. Rodgers, M.D.
Associate Clinical Professor of Emergency Medicine,
Co-Program Director,
Emergency Medicine Residency,
Department of Emergency Medicine,
Indiana University School of Medicine,
Indianapolis, Indiana
29: Back Pain

Richard E. Rothman, M.D., Ph.D.
Assistant Professor,
Department of Emergency Medicine,
The Johns Hopkins University,
Baltimore, Maryland
126: AIDS and HIV

David H. Rubin, M.D., FAAP
Associate Clinical Professor, Department of Pediatrics,
Weill Medical College of Cornell University;
Division Chief, Department of Pediatrics,
New York Presbyterian Hospital,
New York, New York;
Chairman, Department of Pediatrics,
Saint Barnabas Hospital,
Bronx, New York
168: Neurologic Disorders

Douglas A. Rund, M.D.
Professor and Chairman,
Department of Emergency Medicine,
The Ohio State University,
Columbus, Ohio
105: Mood Disorders

Jeffrey W. Runge, M.D., FACEP
Administrator,
National Highway Traffic Safety Administration,
Washington, DC;
Director, Carolinas Center for Injury Prevention and Control,
Assistant Chairman, Department of Emergency Medicine,
Carolinas Medical Center,
Charlotte, North Carolina
58: Injury Prevention and Control

Sudha Russell, M.D., FAAP
Associate in Pediatrics,
Janet Weis Children's and Women's Hospital,
Geisinger Health System,
Lewisville, Pennsylvania
163: Reactive Airways Disease and Pneumonia

Patricia R. Salber, M.D., MBA, FACEP, FACP
Medical Director, Managed Care,
General Motors Corp in Conjunction with the Permanente Company;
Co-President and Co-Founder,
Physicians for a Violence Free Society
Larkspur, California
62: Intimate Partner Violence and Abuse

Sally A. Santen, M.D.
Assistant Professor and Assistant Residency Director,
Department of Emergency Medicine,
Vanderbilt University Medical Center,
Nashville, Tennessee
86: Pancreas

John R. Saucier, M.D.
Associate Clinical Professor, Department of Surgery,
University of Vermont,
Burlington, Vermont;
Attending Faculty, Department of Emergency Medicine,
Maine Medical Center,
Portland, Maine
103: Central Nervous System Infections

Diane Sauter, M.D., FACEP
Chairman, Department of Emergency Medicine,
Greater Southeast Community Hospital,
Washington, DC
174: Drug Therapy and Substance Abuse

Neil Schamban, M.D.
Department of Emergency Medicine,
University of Connecticut Integrated Residency Emergency Medicine,
Farmington, Connecticut
117: Selected Oncologic Emergencies

Robert E. Schneider, M.D.
Clinical Assistant Professor,
Department of Emergency Medicine,
University of North Carolina School of Medicine,
Chapel Hill, North Carolina;
Academic Faculty,
Department of Emergency Medicine,
Carolinas Medical Center,
Charlotte, North Carolina
40: Genitourinary System

Sandra M. Schneider, M.D., FACEP
Professor, Department of Emergency Medicine;
Chair, Department of Emergency Medicine,
University of Rochester,
Rochester, New York
147: Caustics

Carl H. Schultz, M.D., FACEP
Professor, Department of Medicine,
Division of Emergency Medicine,
University of California–Irvine College of Medicine,
Irvine, California;
Attending Faculty,
Department of Emergency Medicine,
University of California–Irvine Medical Center,
Orange, California
188: Disaster Preparedness
189: Weapons of Mass Destruction

Sara A. Schutzman, MD
Assistant in Medicine (Emergency Medicine) and Assistant Professor,
Department of Emergency Medicine,
Harvard Medical School,
Boston, Massachusetts
163: Reactive Airways Disease and Pneumonia

Donna L. Seger, M.D., FACEP, FAACT
Assistant Professor,
Department of Medicine and Emergency Medicine,
Vanderbilt University Medical Center;
Chief and Fellowship Director, Medical Toxicology,
Department of Medicine, VUMC;
Medical Director,
Middle Tennessee Poison Center,
Nashville, Tennessee
143: Aspirin and Nonsteroidal Agents

Jennifer Seirafi, M.D.
Department of Emergency Medicine,
George Washington University Medical Center,
Washington, DC
98: Organic Brain Syndrome

Clare T. Sercombe, M.D., FACEP
Department of Emergency Medicine,
North Memorial Medical Center,
Robbinsdale, Minnesota
112: Systemic Lupus Erythematosus and the Vasculitides

Joseph Sexton, M.D., FACEP
Attending Physician,
Emergency Medicine Department,
Hunterdon Medical Center,
Flemington, New Jersey
128: Tick-Borne Illnesses

Nathan I. Shapiro, M.D.
Harvard Affiliated Emergency Medicine Residency,
Department of Emergency Medicine,
Brigham and Women's Hospital,
Massachusetts General Hospital,
Boston, Massachusetts
132: Sepsis Syndromes

Ghazala Sharieff, M.D., FACEP
Assistant Clinical Professor of Medicine and Pediatrics,
University of California San Diego;
Director of Pediatric Emergency Medicine,
Palomar-Pomerado Health System,
San Diego, California
167: Renal and Genitourinary Tract Disorders

Peter Shearer, M.D.
Clinical Assistant Professor/Assistant Residency Director,
Department of Emergency Medicine,
Mount Sinai School of Medicine;
Attending Physician, Department of Emergency Medicine,
Elmhurst Hospital Center;
Attending Physician, Department of Emergency Medicine,
Mount Sinai Hospital,
New York, New York
102: Neuromuscular Disorders

Robert Shesser, M.D., MPH
Professor and Chair,
Department of Emergency Medicine,
George Washington University Medical Center,
Washington, DC
76: Heart Failure

Richard D. Shih, M.D.
Residency Director, Department of Emergency Medicine,
Morristown Memorial Hospital,
Morristown, New Jersey
158: Plants, Mushrooms, and Herbal Medications

Lee W. Shockley, M.D.
Associate Professor, Department of Surgery,
Division of Emergency Medicine, University of Colorado Health Sciences Center;
Residency Program Director,
Department of Emergency Medicine,
Denver Health Medical Center,
Denver, Colorado
137: Scuba Diving and Dysbarism

Jonathan Siff, M.D., MBA
Senior Clinical Instructor,
Case Western Reserve Instructor;
Attending Physician, Department of Emergency Medicine,
Metrohealth Medical Center,
Cleveland, Ohio
120: Diabetes Mellitus and Disorders of Glucose Homeostasis

Robert Silbergleit, M.D.
Assistant Professor,
Department of Emergency Medicine,
University of Michigan,
Ann Arbor, Michigan
6: Brain Resuscitation

Barry Simon, M.D.
Chairman, Department of Emergency Medicine,
Alameda County Medical Center,
Highland General Hospital,
Oakland, California;
Assistant Clinical Professor,
Department of Internal Medicine,
University of California–San Francisco,
San Francisco, California
52: Wound Management Principles

Jonathan I. Singer, M.D., FAAP, FACEP
Professor of Emergency Medicine and Pediatrics,
Vice Chair, Department of Emergency Medicine,
Wright State University School of Medicine;
Staff Physician, Childrens Medical Center,
Dayton, Ohio
168: Neurologic Disorders

Martin J. Smilkstein, M.D.
Associate Professor, Department of Emergency Medicine,
Oregon Health Sciences University;
Associate Director, Medical Toxicology Fellowship Program,
Oregon Poison Center,
Oregon Health Sciences University,
Portland, Oregon
142: Acetaminophen

Jeffrey Smith, M.D., MPH
Associate Professor, Department of Emergency Medicine,
George Washington University Medical Center,
Washington, DC
98: Organic Brain Syndrome

William S. Smock, M.D., MS, FACEP
Assistant Professor,
Director of Clinical Forensic Medicine,
Department of Emergency Medicine,
University of Louisville School of Medicine,
Louisville, Kentucky
59: Forensic Emergency Medicine

Maria Stephan, M.D., FAAP
Assistant Professor, Department of Emergency Medicine,
Case Western Reserve University School of Medicine;
Staff Physician, Department of Emergency Medicine,
Meno Health Medical Center,
Cleveland, Ohio
181: Evaluation of the Developmentally and Physically Disabled Patient

Mary H. Stewart, M.D., FACEP
Director, Emergency Department,
Allen Memorial Hospital;
Attending Physician, MetroHealth Medical Center;
Assistant Professor, Case Western Reserve University,
Cleveland, Ohio
114: Dermatologic Presentations

David A. Talan, M.D., FACEP, FIDSA
Professor of Medicine, UCLA School of Medicine,
Los Angeles, California;
Chairman, Department of Emergency Medicine;
Faculty, Division of Infectious Diseases,
Olive View-UCLA Medical Center,
Sylmar, California
71: Pneumonia

Ellen Taliaferro, M.D.
Associate Professor,
Division of Emergency Medicine,
The University of Texas Southwestern Medical Center,
Dallas, Texas
62: Intimate Partner Violence and Abuse

Vivek S. Tayal, M.D.
Clinical Assistant Professor of Emergency Medicine,
Department of Emergency Medicine,
University of North Carolina at Chapel Hill,
Chapel Hill, North Carolina;
Director of Ultrasound,
Director of Quality Assurance,
Department of Emergency Medicine,
Carolinas Medical Center,
Charlotte, North Carolina
119: Electrolyte Disturbances

Jonathan M. Teich, M.D., Ph.D.
Assistant Professor,
Division of Emergency Medicine,
Department of Medicine,
Harvard Medical School;
Attending Physician,
Department of Emergency Medicine and Director,
Center for Applied Medical Information Systems,
Brigham and Women's Hospital,
Boston, Massachusetts
196: Information Technology in Emergency Medicine

Stephen H. Thomas, M.D., MPH
Instructor in Medicine,
Department of Medicine (Emergency Medicine),
Harvard Medical School;
Director, Undergraduate Education,
Department of Emergency Medicine,
Massachusetts General Hospital,
Boston, Massachusetts
53: Foreign Bodies

William C. Toepper, M.D., FAAP, FACEP
Attending Physician, Illinois Masonic Medical Center;
Clinical Assistant Professor,
Pediatric Education Director,
Department of Emergency Medicine,
University of Illinois at Chicago,
Chicago, Illinois
164: Cardiac Disorders

Glenn Tokarski, M.D.
Department of Emergency Medicine,
Henry Ford Hospital,
Detroit, Michigan
68: Asthma

Christian Tomaszewski, M.D.
Clinical Assistant Professor of Emergency Medicine,
University of North Carolina at Chapel Hill,
Chapel Hill, North Carolina;
Department of Emergency Medicine,
Carolinas Medical Center,
Charlotte, North Carolina
180: Substance Abuse

Susan P. Torrey, M.D.
Assistant Clinical Professor of Emergency Medicine,
Department of Emergency Medicine,
Tufts University School of Medicine,
Boston, Massachusetts;
Associate Residency Director,
Department of Emergency Medicine,
Baystate Medical Center,
Springfield, Massachusetts
87: Small Intestine

T. Paul Tran, M.D.
Section of Emergency Medicine,
Nebraska Health Systems,
Omaha, Nebraska
113: Allergy, Hypersensitivity, and Anaphylaxis

Thomas W. Turbiak, M.D., FACEP
Chairman and Senior Medical Director,
Department of Emergency Medicine and Ambulatory Care Service,
Manchester Memorial Hospital/Rockville General Hospital,
Manchester, Connecticut
123: Bacteria

Karen Van Hoesen, M.D.
Associate Clinical Professor,
Department of Emergency Medicine;
Director, Hyperbaric Medicine Fellowship;
Director, Diving Medicine Center,
UCSD Medical Center,
San Diego, California
194: Hyperbaric Medicine

Michael V. Vance, M.D., FACEP
Formerly, Department of Medical Toxicology,
Samaritan Regional Poison Center,
Phoenix, Arizona
157: Pesticides

Marshall G. Vary, M.D.
Assistant Professor of Clinical Psychiatry,
Department of Psychiatry,
The Ohio State University;
Vice President/Medical Director,
Behavioral Health Services,
Grant/Riverside Methodist Hospital;
Chair, Department of Psychiatry,
Riverside Methodist Hospitals,
Columbus, Ohio
105: Mood Disorders

Larissa I. Velez, M.D.
Assistant Clinical Instructor,
Emergency Medicine Division, Department of Surgery,
University of Texas Southwestern Medical Center;
Parkland Health and Hospital System,
Emergency Medicine Division, Department of Surgery;
Toxicology Fellow,
Dallas, Texas
151: Heavy Metals

Salvator Vicario, M.D., FACEP, FAAEM
Associate Professor,
Department of Emergency Medicine,
University of Louisville School of Medicine,
Louisville, Kentucky
135: Heat Illness

Robert J. Vissers, M.D., FRCPC, FACEP
Assistant Professor,
University of North Carolina;
Residency Director,
Department of Emergency Medicine,
University of North Carolina Hospitals,
Chapel Hill, North Carolina
185: The Difficult Patient

Ron M. Walls, M.D.
Chairman,
Department of Emergency Medicine,
Brigham and Women's Hospital;
Associate Professor of Medicine (Emergency Medicine),
Harvard Medical School,
Boston, Massachusetts
1: Airway

Frank G. Walter, M.D., FACEP, FACMT, FAACT
Associate Professor of Emergency Medicine,
Chief of Medical Toxicology,
University of Arizona College of Medicine;
Director of Clinical Toxicology,
Department of Emergency Medicine,
University Medical Center,
Tucson, Arizona
145: Antidepressants

David G. Ward, M.D., ABP
Staff Physician, Emergency Department,
Heartland Regional Medical Center,
St. Joseph, Missouri
166: Infectious Diarrheal Disease and Dehydration

Kevin R. Ward, M.D.
Assistant Professor,
Department of Emergency Medicine and Physiology;
Director of Research,
Department of Emergency Medicine;
Associate Director,
Virginia Commonwealth University Reanimation Engineering for Shock Center,
Richmond, Virginia
7: Adult Resuscitation

Paul M. Wax, M.D., FACMT, FACEP
Associate Professor, Department of Emergency Medicine,
University of Rochester;
Attending Physician, Emergency Department,
University of Rochester Medical Center;
Assistant Medical Director,
Finger Lakes Regional Poison Control Center,
Rochester, New York
147: Caustics

Ellen J. Weber, M.D., FACEP
Associate Clinical Professor, Division of Emergency Medicine, Department of Medicine,
University of California San Francisco;
Associate Director, Department of Emergency Medicine,
University of California San Francisco Medical Center,
San Francisco, California
54: Mammalian Bites
125: Rabies

Jim Edward Weber, DO
Assistant Professor,
Department of Emergency Medicine,
University of Michigan Medical Center,
Ann Arbor, Michigan;
Director of Emergency Medicine Research,
Hurley Medical Center,
Flint, Michigan
130: Bone and Joint Infections

Suzanne R. White, M.D.
Associate Professor,
Departments of Emergency Medicine and Pediatrics,
Wayne State University School of Medicine;
Medical Director,
CHM Regional Poison Control Center,
Detroit Medical Center,
Detroit, Michigan
149: Toxic Alcohols

John M. Wightman, EMT-T/P, M.D., MA
Lieutenant Colonel, United States Air Force,
Medical Corps,
Associate Professor, Department of Military and Emergency Medicine,
Uniformed Services University,
Bethesda, Maryland
22: Abdominal Pain

Saralyn R. Williams, M.D.
Assistant Professor of Medicine,
Division of Medical Toxicology,
Department of Emergency Medicine,
San Diego Division, California Poison Control System,
San Diego, California
150: Hallucinogens

John M. Wogan, M.D., FACEP
Chairman, Department of Emergency Medicine,
Greater Baltimore Medical Center,
Baltimore, Maryland
122: Selected Endocrine Disorders

Jeannette M. Wolfe, M.D., FACEP
Assistant Clinical Professor,
Department of Emergency Medicine,
Tufts School of Medicine,
Baystate Hospital,
Springfield, Massachusetts
88: Acute Appendicitis

Richard E. Wolfe, M.D.
Assistant Professor, Division of Emergency Medicine,
Harvard Medical School;
Chief, Department of Emergency Medicine,
Beth Israel Deaconess Medical Center,
Boston, Massachusetts
15: Coma and Depressed Level of Consciousness

Allan B. Wolfson, M.D., FACEP, FACP
Professor, Department of Emergency Medicine,
University of Pittsburgh Medical Center;
Program Director, University of Pittsburgh Affiliated Residency in Emergency Medicine,
Pittsburgh, Pennsylvania
92: Renal Failure
119: Electrolyte Disturbances

David W. Wright, M.D.
Assistant Professor,
Department of Emergency Medicine;
Assistant Director,
Emergency Medicine Research Center,
Emory University School of Medicine,
Atlanta, Georgia
178: The Organ Transplant Patient

Barry Yarbrough, M.D., FACEP
Physician,
Centennial Medical Center and St. Thomas Hospital,
Nashville, Tennessee
135: Heat Illness

Michael Yaron, M.D., FACEP
Associate Professor, Department of Surgery,
Division of Emergency Medicine,
University of Colorado Health Sciences Center;
Attending Physician, Emergency Department,
University Hospital,
Denver, Colorado
138: High-Altitude Medicine

Donald M. Yealy, M.D., FACEP
Professor and Vice Chair,
Department of Emergency Medicine,
University of Pittsburgh School of Medicine,
Pittsburgh, Pennsylvania
74: Dysrhythmias
182: Pain Management

Kelly D. Young, M.D.
Assistant Clinical Professor, Department of Pediatrics,
University of California, Los Angeles,
Los Angeles, California;
Assistant Clinical Professor,
Department of Pediatrics and Emergency Medicine,
Harbor-UCLA Medical Center,
Torrance, California
191: Medical Literature and Evidence-Based Medicine

Gary D. Zimmer, M.D.
Chief Resident,
Department of Emergency Medicine,
Harvard Affiliated Emergency Medicine Residency;
Brigham and Women's Hospital;
Massachusetts General Hospital,
Boston, Massachusetts
132: Sepsis Syndromes

Brian J. Zink, M.D.
Associate Professor,
Department of Emergency Medicine,
Assistant Dean for Medical Student Career Development,
University of Michigan Medical School,
Ann Arbor, Michigan
130: Bone and Joint Infections

D. Demetrios Zukin, M.D., FAAP
Clinical Assistant Professor, Department of Pediatrics,
University of California San Francisco,
San Francisco, California;
Attending Physician, Department of Emergency Medicine,
Children's Hospital Oakland,
Oakland, California
161: Fever

Preface to the Fifth Edition

We three have had the very remarkable privilege of serving as authors for the first two editions, editors for the next two, and now, senior editors of this fifth edition of *Rosen's Emergency Medicine: Concepts and Clinical Practice.* This makes for a span of more than two decades, extending from our residency training years to our current places in three corners of this country. It is fair to say that we and this textbook have grown up hand-in-hand. During this time, we have endeavored to help shape and mend the book under Peter's direction. It has been an ongoing commitment to meet the dynamic and substantive needs of emergency medicine's academicians and clinicians alike.

This fifth edition has evolved considerably from its predecessor. The book's chapters and sections have been organized according to the emergency physician's precept, beginning with *Critical Management Principles* and ending with *Philosophic Issues of Practice.* The three volumes have been divided and marked as pragmatically and clearly as possible. The chapters themselves have been formatted according to one of three templates. These templates, their newly worked pedagogy, and a second highlighting color have been applied thoroughly and consistently, a process intended to assist the author as well as the reader. The chapters have been prepared by emergency medicine authorities, often those who lead the investigative endeavors in the field about which they write. This latest iteration of the textbook contains 201 chapters, 27 more than the fourth edition, yet within roughly the same confines of space. This was accomplished in part by sharply paring back the references to contain mostly new vintage and strong evidence-based citations with a few classic investigations included. Two noteworthy sections have been added. Chapters within the *Special Populations* section address the differing clinical and disposition needs of unique groups. The *Cardinal Presentations* section provides brief, complaint-based chapters for those symptoms and signs we face most often. These are algorithm-driven, containing focused differentials and empiric management schemata. They are meant to parallel the thinking and action process of the emergency physician. Comprehensive coverage of pathophysiology, epidemiology, and the like is found in clinical chapters elsewhere in the book. The entire text will be available on CD-ROM, complete with full search capability as well as the self-assessment questions and answers prepared by Hal Thomas, M.D., and his colleagues. Finally, a website for the textbook is under development. This will provide chapter updates and communication exchanges between readers, authors, and editors, among other features.

What remains constant is the mission of the book. There is a "biology" of emergency medicine, to quote our editor emeritus. That biology continues to grow and shift, and it is a biology with which this text strives to keep pace. Among many changes, we have innovative airway management techniques, new and more aggressive pharmacologics for cardiovascular and neurologic disorders, the emergence of ultrasound, and the increasing governmental influence on our specialty to consider. Emergency physicians are applying increasingly comprehensive diagnostic and management strategies in the ED in concert with the emphasis on resource-efficient outpatient management, and emergency medicine continues to minister to all persons, irrespective of their medical calamity, their social condition, or their ability to pay. For what changes and for what remains the same, there is the same call for the evidence of sound practice and research, and for a textbook to reflect those data.

We are indebted to the many authors for scribing their wisdom, as well as to our band of resolute editors who oversaw the proceedings with such painstaking care. We are also thankful to a few who worked behind the scenes and without whose sustenance this book would not have passed the most formative stage. Kathy Falk has given colossal effort and has been our steadying influence, always coaxing and prodding, always mindful of the big picture. Laura DeYoung lent us vital direction and vision in the early going. Judy Fletcher has been responsive to each of our many calls for help and guidance all along the way. Finally, each of us has been fortunate to have the unyielding support and expertise of our administrative assistants, Phyllis Allen (JAM), Maria Figueroa (RSH), and Diane Pugh (RMW).

The inaugural edition of this book was dedicated to those physicians who had accepted the "responsibilities, challenges, and excitements" of emergency medicine, while the most recent was committed to those members of our specialty who were "on the front line of responsibility for the care of our society." We would like to dedicate this fifth edition to these same individuals, the pioneers of our specialty, as well as to those who have since joined the ranks. We are very proud to be numbered among them. Ultimately, we are humbled by and grateful for the chance to continue the lineage of this textbook.

JOHN A. MARX
ROBERT S. HOCKBERGER
RON M. WALLS

Preface to the First Edition

From the vision and foresight of a few physicians who perceived the need for a unique, disciplined, sensitive approach to the identification and stabilization of patients threatened with loss of life or limb, emergency medicine has rapidly developed into an exciting, academically recognized medical specialty. This textbook is dedicated to those who have accepted its responsibilities, challenges, and excitements.

We have attempted to define in depth the material on which our practice is based. There have been a number of efforts to write about emergencies, but we believe that this is the first to call solely on those people who themselves practice the specialty. In every chapter theory and knowledge pertinent to the practice of emergency medicine are presented.

This book is not an easy one; it was written based on published literature, not anecdote or prejudice. In many instances where the data are not available, both sides are presented with a suggested practice. The book is intended for all with a serious interest in or a need to know emergency medicine, including those who do not practice full-time emergency medicine, as well as the dedicated specialists who do.

The book is organized into two main sections—trauma and nontrauma. This division is artificial but does correspond to the first major decisions made in patient evaluations, because trauma usually affects individual anatomic structures whereas nontrauma is more likely to affect systems.

Despite this artificial separation, long and detailed discussion and instruction to authors concerning content and style ensued. We realize that we could not tap all available talent for contributions to the book, but we have made an effort to represent different schools of thought and regions of the country.

There are deliberate omissions; for example, we elected not to include any procedures. There was not enough room to create an atlas, but it was our desire to cover the chosen topics in detail. No effort has been made to address administration, management, disaster planning, or technical requirements of emergency medicine supplies or design. Prehospital care has been included only as it relates to individual topics, not as suggested protocol or from the vantage point of technician training programs.

It would be impossible to write a book this long and present nothing controversial. In fact we ourselves find sections we cannot totally accept, but in the process of working with multiple authors, we cannot with intellectual honesty put ideas into their material. We have, however, achieved our goal of presenting an in-depth vision of emergency medicine written by specialists in emergency medicine. We hope you will find the reading of this book as stimulating and enjoyable as we have found its creation.

PETER ROSEN
FRANK J. BAKER II
G. RICHARD BRAEN
ROBERT H. DAILEY
RICHARD C. LEVY

Acknowledgments

I am indebted to our authors for their considerable expertise and intellect; to Jim, Roger, Bill, Dan, Marianne, Glenn, Louis, and Ed for the constant dedication and incredible craftsmanship; to Bob and Ron for their uncompromising devotion, faithfulness, and friendship; to Conner and Shelby whose unconditional love and encouragement were requisite to the task; and, of course, to Peter for creating, inspiring, and now, entrusting.

JAM

To Peter for entrusting his work and his vision to us; to John and Ron for making our collaboration a truly enjoyable, as well as educational, undertaking; to Kathy and Laura, for their invaluable advice and support; and to Patty, the love of my life.

RSH

This book has been a true labor of love; born of a great need to define the biology of emergency medicine, nurtured by the incredible contributions of those who walked before us, and strengthened each time by the exquisite intellects of our authors. To Peter, thanks for all of it. You know what it is and what it means. To my fellow editors, thanks for helping to make this book something of such singular value. To my faculty, residents, and students in Boston, thanks for your intellectual curiosity, willingness to challenge conventional wisdom, creativity in developing new knowledge through innovative research, and ability to deliver such incomparable emergency care, which inspire me to try to be better. To Diane, thanks for your extraordinary skill and focus. And to Barbara, Andrew, Blake, Alexa, Murphy, and Pasley, thank you for your unconditional love and for making me feel so complete that I am inspired to share.

RMW

With thanks to my loved ones, who inspire and rejuvenate me.

JA

The perspective, insight, and focus of our readers and authors continue to make this text relevant to the practicing emergency physician. A host of professionals have been instrumental and I am particularly appreciative of the efforts of Kathi Thompson of HCA-HealthONE in Denver and Kathy Falk of Harcourt. Suzanne Barkin, M.D., and my sons, Adam and Michael, have been supportive throughout the production of this book, providing support, suggestions, encouragement, and humor. They remain the motivation to push the boundaries of knowledge.

RMB

I would like to thank my children—David, Blake, and Anna—for putting up with me over the years and for being a constant source of inspiration to me. I think I have learned as much from them as they have from me. Most of all, I thank my wife and best friend, Mary, for her constant support and attention to everyone in our family. She is the glue that sticks us together and makes it all worthwhile.

WB

To my colleagues at the University of Louisville, and our 28 residency classes. Joanna, Maggie, and Julia—thanks for making things fun. And to my parents, Frank and Mary Ellen Danzl, thanks for everything; Dad, you almost made it for one more edition.

DD

To my husband, David Hill, for his love and support and to my children, Jeremiah and Katie, for always being there for me.

MGH

To the faculty, residents, and support staff of the Department of Emergency Medicine at Wright State University School of Medicine, my professional home and source of academic support for 20 years. To Lynda, James, Kate, and Liz, my personal support system and the ones who balance encouragement and motivation with patience and sacrifice. To Peter Rosen, who introduced me to the excitement of academic emergency medicine.

GCH

To emergency medicine residents and faculty everywhere, in their continued quest for knowledge, but especially those at Hennepin County Medical Center for continuously teaching me. I am grateful to all of the authors who shared their time, energy, and wisdom. Special thanks to my wife, Beth, and to Eric, Ali, and Amanda for their love, patience, and understanding.

LJL

I would like to thank my teachers: my parents and my children, professors and patients, colleagues and students, who have patiently taught me about medicine and life; and my steadfast companion and wife, Lynda, who has made the pursuit of wisdom possible.

EN

Contents

VOLUME ONE
PART ONE
FUNDAMENTAL CLINICAL CONCEPTS

SECTION I CRITICAL MANAGEMENT PRINCIPLES

SECTION II CARDINAL PRESENTATIONS

PART TWO TRAUMA

SECTION I GENERAL CONCEPTS

SECTION II SYSTEM INJURIES

SECTION III ORTHOPEDIC INJURIES

SECTION IV SOFT TISSUE INJURIES

SECTION V VIOLENCE AND ABUSE

VOLUME TWO

PART THREE
MEDICINE AND SURGERY

SECTION I HEAD AND NECK DISORDERS

SECTION II PULMONARY SYSTEM

SECTION III CARDIAC SYSTEM

SECTION IV VASCULAR SYSTEM

SECTION V GASTROINTESTINAL SYSTEM

SECTION VI GENITOURINARY SYSTEM

SECTION VII NEUROLOGY

VOLUME III

PART FOUR
ENVIRONMENT AND TOXICOLOGY

SECTION I ENVIRONMENTAL

SECTION II TOXICOLOGY

PART FIVE
SPECIAL POPULATIONS

SECTION I THE PEDIATRIC PATIENT

PART THREE

Medicine and Surgery

65 Oral Medicine

James T. Amsterdam

PERSPECTIVE

Patients with dental emergencies commonly present to the ED because of pain, anxiety, and fear of cosmetic deformity. Prompt management of dental emergencies affords the patient great relief and satisfaction.[1]

PRINCIPLES OF DISEASE

Anatomy

The stomatognathic system consists of the musculoskeletal unit of the mandible, maxilla, and muscles of mastication; the dental unit (teeth); the attachment apparatus that anchors teeth; and other soft tissues of the oral cavity.[2]

Musculoskeletal Unit The mandible is formed by two rami that divide into a horizontal and an ascending portion. The horizontal portion forms the body of the mandible. The ascending ramus divides into the coronoid process anteriorly and the condylar process posteriorly. The temporomandibular articulation is unique because it consists of a bilateral joint or diarthroses between the mandibular fossa and articular eminence of the mandible's temporal bone and condyle (Figure 65-1). An intervening layer of fibrous connective tissue separates the articulating surfaces. A fibrous capsule also surrounds the temporomandibular joint (TMJ) and is reinforced by capsular ligaments that help limit mandibular range of motion. Functionally, when the mandible opens, the condyles move inferiorly and anteriorly down the eminence; during closure, the mandible moves posteriorly along the eminence and superiorly into the fossa.[2]

The muscles of mastication are divided into the mandibular elevators (the supramandibular group) and depressors (the inframandibular group). The elevators, or "masseteric sling," consist of the masseters, medial pterygoids, and temporalis. The posterior-superior movement of the condyle during mandibular closure is the result of bilateral, simultaneous movement of this group. The muscles involved in the opening or depression of the mandible include the lateral pterygoid, digastric, geniohyoid, and mylohyoid. Bilateral activity of these muscles results in opening; unilateral contraction causes the mandible to deviate to the opposite side. At rest, the mandible assumes a position in which the mandibular and maxillary teeth are separated by a few millimeters of space. During functional activity, mandibular closure occurs as the action of the elevators predominates.

Teeth The pulp is the tooth's center and serves as its neurovascular supply. The primary purpose of the pulp is to provide sensation and to produce dentin, a microtubular structure that hydrates and cushions the tooth during mastication. The part of the tooth normally visible in the oral cavity is the coronal portion covered with enamel, the hardest substance in the body. The part that is not normally visible and anchors the tooth is called the root. The root is covered with cementum, which is much softer than enamel and not designed for exposure in the oral cavity (Figure 65-2).[2]

The normal primary or deciduous dentition consists of 10 mandibular and 10 maxillary teeth. The primary dentition is important for mastication, cosmetics, growth, and development and functions as a "physiologic space maintainer." Starting at the midline and moving posteriorly in any quadrant, the normal dentition consists of a central incisor, lateral incisor, canine, and two primary molars. The lower central incisor is the first tooth to erupt, at approximately 6 months of age; all primary teeth should be present by 3 years of age. If not, further investigation for developmental or endocrine abnormalities is warranted. The permanent dentition begins to erupt at approximately 5 to 6 years of age with the appearance of the first molar. Normally, the permanent dentition consists of 32 teeth: the central incisor, lateral incisor, canine, two premolars, and three molars. The third molars are the last to erupt, appearing at approximately 16 to 18 years of age, and are commonly called "wisdom teeth." Note that the primary molars are replaced by the permanent premolars (Figure 65-3, *A* and *B*).[3]

There are many numbering systems for teeth, but none are universal. Perhaps the most common system for the permanent dentition, however, consists of numbering the teeth from 1 to 32, starting with the upper right third molar (1) to the upper left third molar (16) to the lower left third molar (17) to the lower right third molar (32). Because there may be congenital absence of teeth or additional, supernumerary teeth, it is perhaps best for practitioners to anatomically describe which tooth is involved (e.g., the upper left second premolar or the lower right second molar).[2,4]

Specific terminology is used to describe aspects of dentition. The labial or buccal surface faces outside the oral cavity; the oral, palatal, or lingual surface faces the tongue; the medial surface is toward the midline; and the distal surface is toward the ramus of the mandible. The interproximal surface refers to the contacting area of adjacent teeth, and

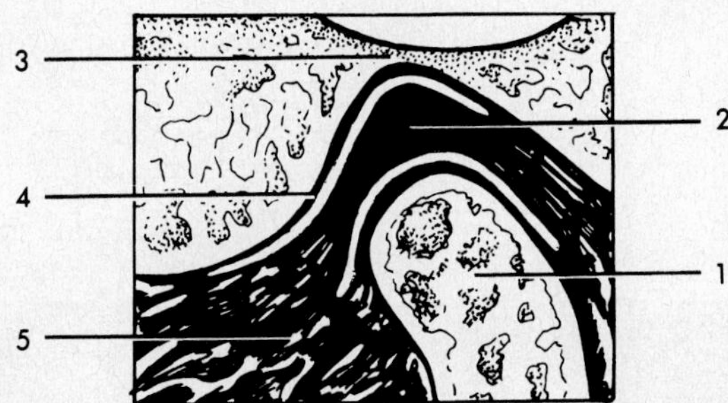

Figure 65-1. Temporomandibular joint structures in sagittal section: *1,* condyle; *2,* disk; *3,* mandibular (temporal-fossa); *4,* eminence; *5,* lateral pterygoid. *Modified from Weisgold AS et al: Dental medicine. In Kaye D, Rose LF, editors:* Fundamentals of internal medicine, *St Louis, Mosby.*

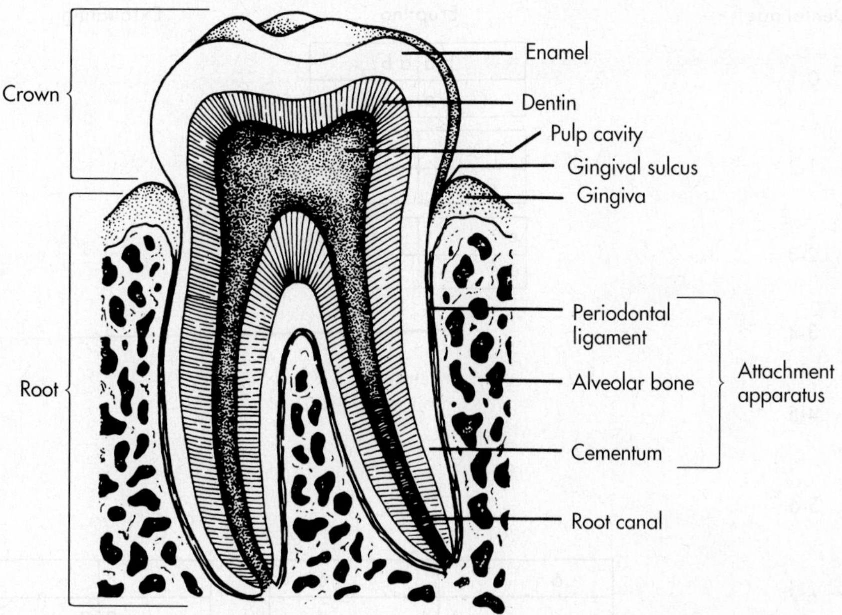

Figure 65-2. **The dental anatomic unit and attachment apparatus.**

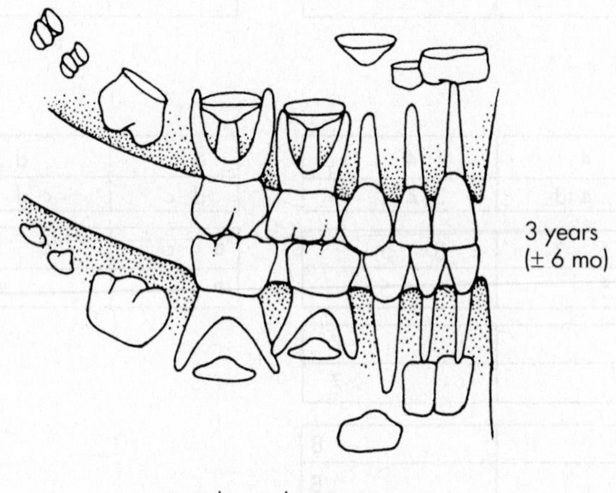

A

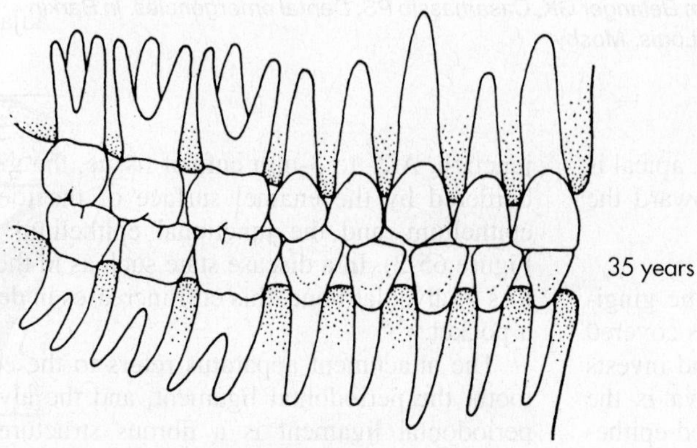

Figure 65-3. **A, Numbering and naming of deciduous and permanent dentition on the right side. Tooth numbering is in the more conventional upper right third molar (1) to lower right third molar (32).**

Continued

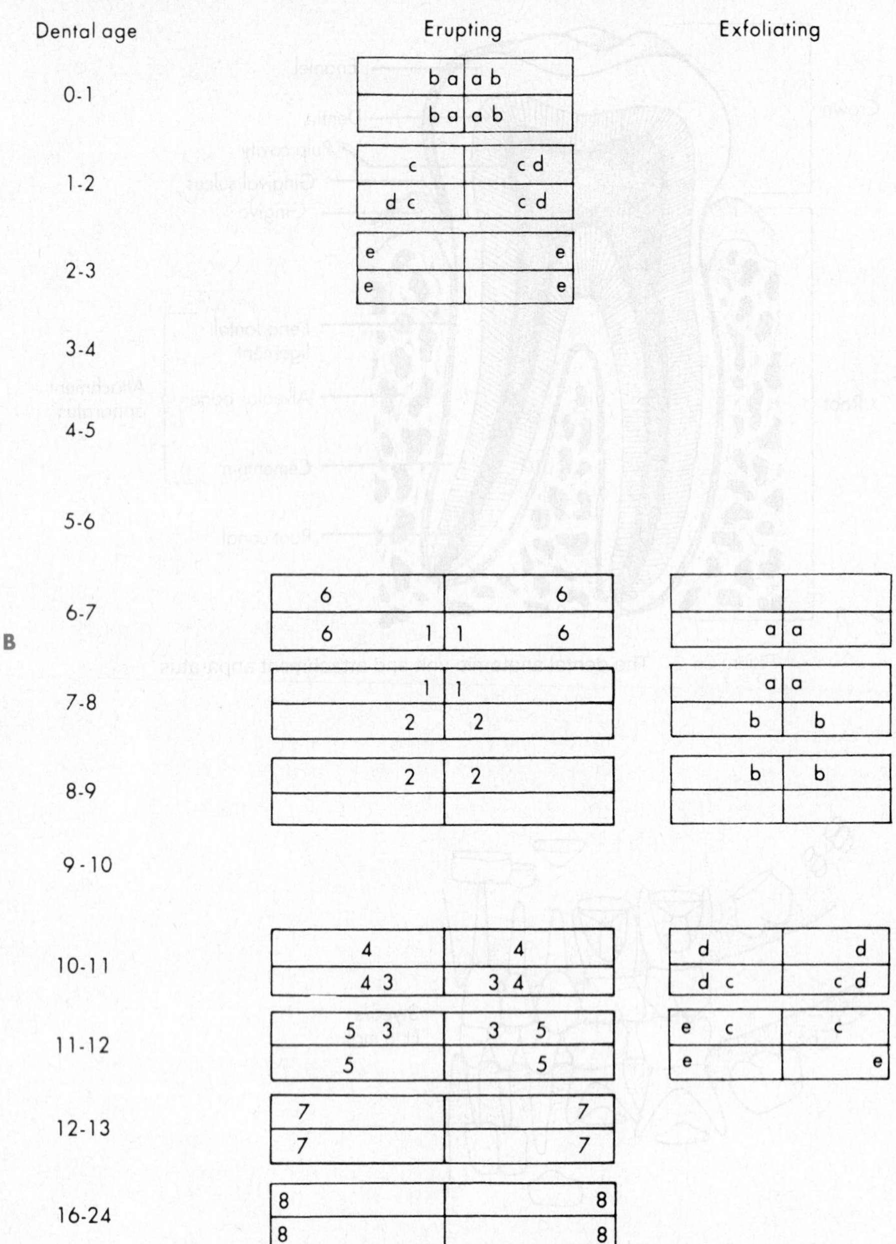

Figure 65-3, cont'd. **B,** **Most common pattern of dental development.** ***a-e,*** **Primary teeth;** ***1-8,*** **secondary (permanent) teeth.** ***B from Belanger GK, Casamassio PS: Dental emergencies. In Barkin R, editor:*** **Pediatric emergencies,** ***St Louis, Mosby.***

the occlusal surface refers to the biting area. Finally, apical is in the direction of the root, whereas coronal is toward the crown of the tooth.

Periodontium The periodontium consists of the gingival unit and the attachment apparatus. The gingiva is covered with keratinized, stratified, squamous epithelium and invests the tooth and alveolar bone. Apical to the gingiva is the alveolar mucosa, which is covered by nonkeratinized epithelium and is therefore more subject to trauma. In healthy individuals the gingiva is attached firmly to the tooth by connective tissue fibers inserting into the cementum, extending coronally from the alveolar bone to the cementoenamel junction. A 2- to 3-mm cuff of tissue, the gingival sulcus, is bordered by the enamel surface of the tooth, the gingival epithelium, and the junctional epithelium at its base (see Figure 65-2). In a disease state such as in the presence of the loss of alveolar bone, this cuff increases in depth and is called a pocket.[2,5,6]

The attachment apparatus refers to the cementum on the tooth, the periodontal ligament, and the alveolar bone. The periodontal ligament is a fibrous structure that surrounds the root of the tooth. It is the key structure that anchors the tooth because it serves as a double periosteum that lays down cementum on the tooth on one side and alveolar bone on its other side.

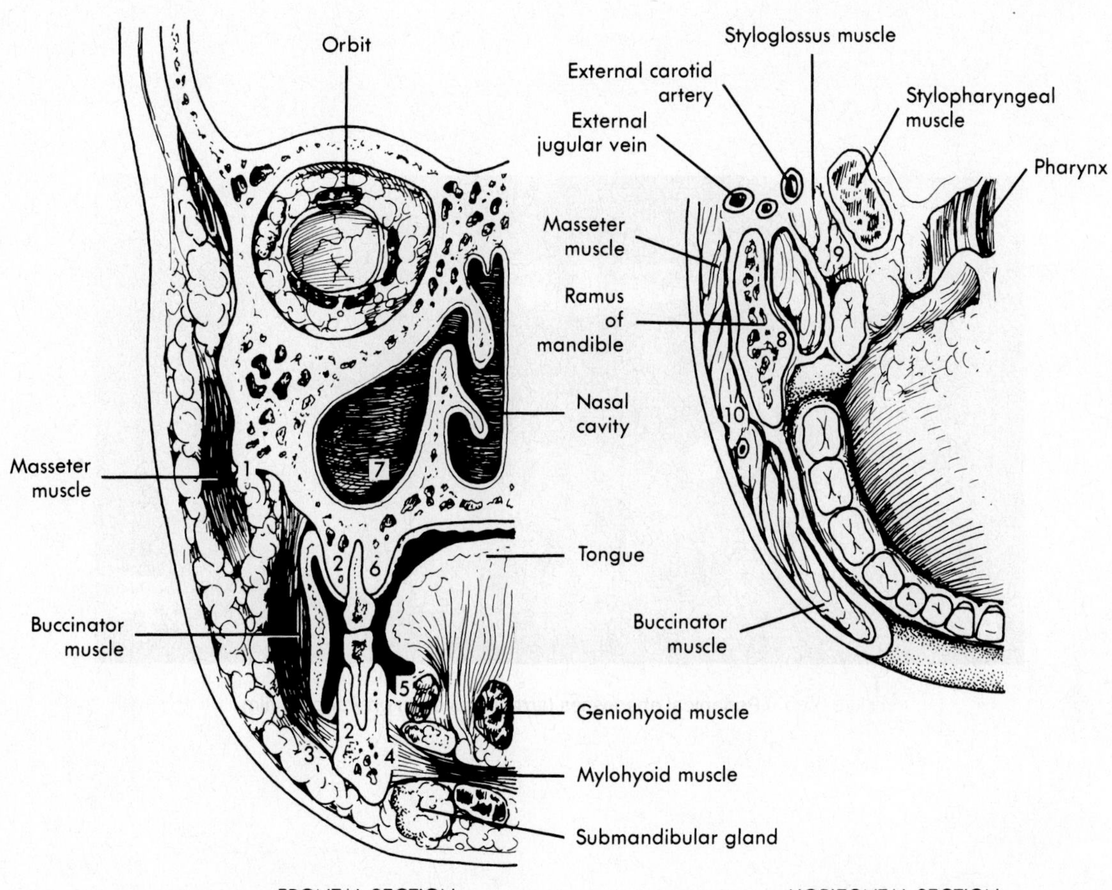

Figure 65-4. **Natural progression of dental infection. The pathways by which such infections may travel are: *1,* postzygomatic (from canine fossa in cuspid and bicuspid region; pterygomaxillary fossa communicates from rear); *2,* vestibular; *3,* facial; *4,* submandibular; *5,* sublingual; *6,* palatal; *7,* antral; *8,* pterygomandibular; 9, parapharyngeal; and *10,* masseteric. *Redrawn from Rose LF, Hendler BH, Amsterdam JT:* Consultant *22:*125, 1982.**

Fascial Planes of the Head and Neck The head and neck's fascial planes are defined as potential spaces filled with loose areolar tissue that separates the layers of fascia of the head and neck. The deep cervical fascia is most important in a discussion of the extension of oral infection to the head and neck (Figure 65-4). The deep cervical fascia consists of the superficial and investing layer, the pretracheal layer, the prevertebral layer, and the carotid sheath. The superficial and investing layer surrounds the entire neck; it splits as it attaches to the inferior border of the internal pterygoid muscles at the mandible's ascending ramus. This split forms the masticator space. This space communicates superiorly above the level of the zygomatic arch with the superficial and deep temporal pouches.[7-9]

Other spaces of importance in the neck to which dental infection may spread include the lateral pharyngeal or parapharyngeal space, which is lateral to the pharynx and medial to the masticator space; the retropharyngeal space, which is between the deep cervical and prevertebral fascia; and the prevertebral space, which is posterior to the retropharyngeal space. The pharyngomaxillary space extends from the base of the skull to the hyoid bone and is especially important because it communicates with all deep spaces.

The mandible itself may be divided further. The mylohyoid muscle divides the superior sublingual and inferior submaxillary spaces.

Pathophysiology

Nontraumatic Dental Emergencies Two pathophysiologic processes affect the dental health of the majority of the population: (1) dental caries and (2) periodontal disease. Variables related in both disease states include oral environment consisting of the teeth, attachment apparatus, presence of local factors such as bacterial plaque and oral microflora, and substrate and host states, including immunocompromised diseases and nutritional status.

Factors such as water fluoridation, fluoride supplements, and plaque control techniques (e.g., flossing, brushing, and dental surgical procedures) have significantly decreased the prevalence of both dental caries and periodontal disease.[10-12]

Dental Caries Dental caries is a multifactorial disease involving a susceptible host, cariogenic oral flora, and a substrate. As early as 1890, it was proposed that caries resulted from the decalcification of enamel by the production of acids from bacteria.[8,9] In the presence of saliva and

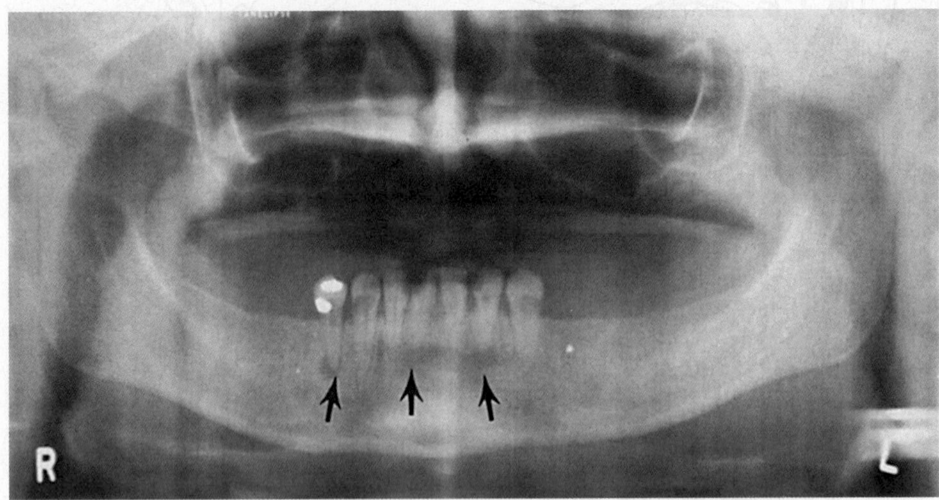

Figure 65-5. **Periapical abscesses (*arrows*) as seen on Panorex film.**

carbohydrate, cariogenic oral flora are able to develop a matrix called dental bacterial plaque. The bacteria metabolize the carbohydrate to form acids that decalcify the enamel.[10] After the carious process has invaded the enamel, the microporous dentin is able to transmit saliva, byproducts of the bacteria, and the bacteria themselves to the pulp. The pulp initially reacts with a hyperemic response, which continues to an inflammatory state, progressing to total degeneration and necrosis.

Pus then leaks from the apex of the root and forms an abscess; this is termed a periapical abscess. Periapical abscesses are confined within the alveolar bone (see Figure 65-5). The abscess may break through the cortical plate of either the mandible or maxilla and then spread subperiosteally. Subperiosteal extensions are generally well confined anatomically by muscle attachments; however, if the muscle attachments are violated either during a surgical procedure or by the natural extension of an infective process, the bacteria can gain access to the fascial planes of the head and neck.[13-17]

Infection extending to the submaxillary, sublingual, and submental spaces with elevation of the tongue is called Ludwig's angina. Ludwig's angina is one of the most serious of mandibular infections because of its potential for airway obstruction.

Space infections may also involve the face. The canine space is bounded by the orbicularis oris, the levator labii superioris, and the buccinator; abscessed anterior maxillary teeth commonly involve this space. Infection can extend to the periorbital area. The most serious complication of such space infections is cavernous sinus thrombosis as a result of contamination of the (valveless) facial venous system. The buccal space is superficial to the buccinator and limited by the anterior border of the masseter; maxillary molar infection commonly spreads to this space. The mental space is located at the anterior table of the mandible and is often infected by abscessed lower anterior teeth.[17]

CLINICAL FEATURES

Examination of the Oral Cavity

It is recommended that the examiner wear eye protection, a mask, and gloves for universal precautions when examining the oral cavity. Ideally, the patient should be placed in a dental/ENT chair or on a cart at a 45-degree angle. The pediatric patient should be placed in the parent's lap facing the parent. The examiner then sits in front of the parent. While the parent gently restrains the arms and legs, the emergency physician leans the child backward and locks the child's head between the physician's legs.

An overhead examination light, head light, or flashlight can be used for illumination. Other ancillary aids include a tongue depressor, 2×2 gauze, and possibly a dental mirror. To prevent the mirror from fogging it should be either warmed under hot water or a flame or moistened with the patient's saliva.

Examination of the oral cavity should be systematic, beginning with the soft tissues, including the tongue. The base of the tongue is examined for lesions, and Wharton's duct is milked. Stensen's duct, opposite the maxillary molars, should be examined on each side.

The teeth should then be examined. Percussing a tooth with a tongue blade or handle of a mirror is a good way to elicit tenderness.

Radiographic evaluation of teeth is best performed using dental (periapical) films; however, these are generally not available in the ED. A panoramic radiograph is a useful alternative (Figure 65-5).

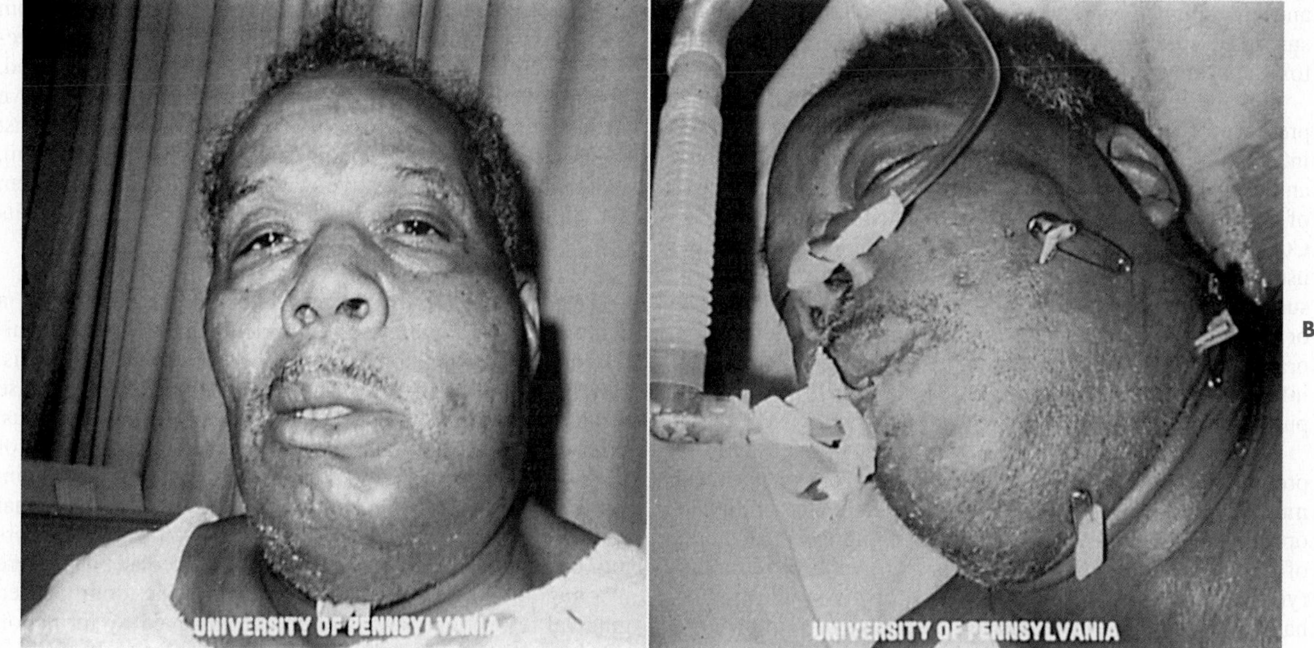

Figure 65-6. **Extensive spread of infection of odontogenic origin involving masseteric, sublingual, submental, and submandibular spaces with extension to mediastinum. A, Preoperative. B, Postoperative. Note drainage from mediastinum.** *From Guernsey LH: Practical problem solving in oral surgery. In Cohen DW, editor:* Continuing dental education, *vol 2, suppl 10, Philadelphia, 1979, University of Pennsylvania School of Dental Medicine.*

Signs and Symptoms

Dental Caries Dental caries is the most common cause for pain of odontogenic origin. The patient may give a variable history of a sudden or gradual onset of a sharp-to-dull throbbing pain. In most cases the patient can indicate the specific tooth involved, but at times the pain may be generalized. An early pulpitis is sensitive to changes in temperature and aggravated by lying down; a more advanced pulpitis is worsened by any stimulus, including air. Pain may be referred to the ear, temple, eye, neck, and rarely, the opposite jaw.

Physical examination may reveal a grossly decayed tooth; however, if the carious process is interproximal or did not result in destruction of the outer table of enamel, the offending tooth may not be obvious. Localization of the involved tooth may be made by percussing the teeth with a tongue blade or by having the patient bite on a piece of a tongue blade. Exquisite pain to percussion suggests an underlying periapical abscess, especially if the tooth is not sensitive to hot or cold. Palliative management is indicated for most odontalgia. Systemic analgesics such as nonsteroidal antiinflammatory drugs (NSAIDs) or synthetic opioid agents are indicated. Although NSAIDs should be sufficient for most pain resulting from carious teeth, a therapeutic dental block may also be helpful. Although synthetic opioids are useful, caution should be exercised because of their propensity for abuse.[18,19] A dental anesthetic nerve block is helpful.[20,21] A limited quantity of analgesics should be dispensed that will also encourage follow-up with a general dentist.

Patients with dental pain should be examined carefully for swelling caused by abscessed teeth. A periapical abscess, or a localized swelling of the gingiva adjacent to the apex of the tooth (called a parulis), may cause pain from distension of the tissues. More commonly, fluctuant abscesses are a result of periodontal abscesses and are best treated with an incision and drainage. The gingiva is anesthetized superficially with 2% lidocaine with 1:100,000 epinephrine. A conservative stab incision is made toward the alveolar bone and must extend through the periosteum; blunt dissection is carried out with a mosquito hemostat. Unlike other abscess drainage, it is unnecessary to open the abscess from end to end—such a large incision exposes too much alveolar bone. In the dental office, a simple curettage between the tooth and the gingiva would establish drainage. For physicians not trained in dental scaling and curettage, the simple stab incision is as sufficient. The cavity is irrigated, and assuming there is sufficient space, a Penrose or iodoform drain is placed and secured with a No. 4-0 silk suture.[2]

The patient is started on phenoxymethyl-penicillin or erythromycin and warm saline rinses and is referred to the oral maxillofacial surgeon or general dentist. Drains are removed in 24 to 48 hours, and antibiotics are continued for 7 to 10 days.[7]

The presence of cellulitis or swelling in the contiguous spaces of the head and neck indicates the spread of a localized infection. In the early stages of such an infection, the upper half of the face is generally involved, with extension of infection from maxillary teeth; cellulitis from mandibular teeth generally involves extension to the lower half of the face and the neck (Figure 65-6). More advanced infections may extend into any of the fascial planes of the head and neck down to the mediastinum. Fortunately, in the nondebilitated host, untreated dental infections tend to localize and spontaneously drain extraorally. In the presence of a compromised host or aggressive microorganisms, spread into the fascial planes is more common, with a potential for greater morbidity and mortality. General indications for admission include suspected spread of infection to fascial planes, high fever, toxic appearance, trismus, and an immunocompromised host.[7]

It is the role of the emergency physician to recognize the presence of such an infection and the potential for a given infection of odontogenic origin to spread to the fascial planes and deep spaces of the head and neck. The potential sequelae of sepsis and airway obstruction must be appreciated. Computed tomography scanning of the head and neck can be useful if the diagnosis is in doubt. However, any index of suspicion warrants an immediate consultation with the ENT or the oral maxillofacial surgeon. It is the role of the ENT or oral maxillofacial surgeon to compartmentalize the spread of infection and to determine the site of the initial focus so that pus can be evacuated.

Signs of infection peak in 3 to 5 days. Fever usually is present. Any irritation of the internal pterygoid or masseter muscles results in trismus. Trismus results in the ability to open the mouth only a few millimeters, limiting visualization of the pharynx and making diagnosis of lateral or retropharyngeal space involvement difficult. Difficulty swallowing or handling secretions increases the suspicion of retropharyngeal or parapharyngeal infection. Respiratory distress may be apparent or the airway may occlude rapidly.[7]

Ludwig's angina is a bilateral boardlike swelling involving the submandibular, submental, and sublingual spaces with elevation of the tongue. The most serious immediate sequela is airway obstruction. A characteristic brawny induration is present; there is no fluctuance for incision and drainage. Hemolytic streptococcus is most commonly responsible for the infection, although a mixed staphylococcal-streptococcal flora is not uncommon, and both may lead to an overgrowth of anaerobic gas-producing organisms, including *Bacteroides fragilis.* Treatment consists of admission to a unit capable of observing and managing the airway after airway maintenance. Cricothyrotomy may be necessary in these patients for emergent airway control.[9]

Administration of a high dosage of antibiotics, such as 15 to 20 million units of intravenous penicillin daily, is necessary to achieve good tissue penetration. *B. fragilis* infections may be highly resistant and a second- or third-generation cephalosporin, clindamycin, or metronidazole may be required to eradicate them.[8] If antibiotic therapy is not helpful, surgery is performed to eliminate etiologic factors and to explore for pockets of pus.

In general, the most important therapeutic treatment of orofacial infections is surgical drainage and removal of necrotic tissue. Involved teeth will require endodontic therapy if they are restorable or extraction if they are nonrestorable or have lost all alveolar support. Antibiotic therapy is useful for halting the spread of cellulitis and preventing hematogenous dissemination, but it is no substitute for the prompt evacuation of pus.[7]

Penicillin is the antibiotic of choice for treatment of orofacial infections. Minor infections respond to 250 to 500 mg penicillin VK qid. More serious infections such as Ludwig's angina require up to 12 million U penicillin G intravenously a day. Most oral bacteria are sensitive to penicillin, with the exception of some *Bacteroides* species. Second- or third-generation cephalosporins are useful in this case or in the patient allergic to penicillin, although care must be exercised for the potential of crossover sensitivity. Clindamycin is also effective when there is a predominance of anaerobes in the penicillin-allergic patient, or one in whom penicillin or third-generation cephalosporins seem ineffective. Potential side effects should be carefully monitored. Erythromycin is a potential alternative because it is active against most oral bacteria, but it is less active against anaerobic and microaerophilic streptococci, fusobacterium, and anaerobic gram-negative cocci. There is also a problem with long-term intravenous administration because of its irritant effects.[12]

Periodontal Disease Periodontal disease represents a continuum of pathology. Early periodontal disease is manifested by inflammation of the gingiva, termed gingivitis. Gingivitis is generally the result of an inflammatory response to an irritant such as dental bacterial plaque and calculus. With extension of inflammation, there is ultimately loss of alveolar bone, termed periodontitis. A physiologic space from the crest of the alveolar bone to the base of the junctional epithelium is maintained for the insertion of gingival fibers into cementum. In response to a loss of alveolar bone, there is a migration of gingiva down the root of the tooth, termed gingival resorption. This is often accompanied by formation of gingival pockets. Advanced periodontitis results from a continuation of this process and results in marked mobility of the teeth and eventual loss as the attachment apparatus is destroyed.[2,5,6]

Space infections of the head and neck occasionally result from periodontal disease. However, the combination of periodontal lesions and resultant pulpal pathology can create periapical abscesses with the same sequelae as those caused by dental caries alone.

Gingivitis and periodontitis in themselves rarely cause a patient to come to the ED unless there is sudden alarm at seeing blood on a toothbrush or the realization that certain teeth are loose. Occasionally, the patient complains about sensitive teeth. The patient can be advised to improve home care and see a dentist as soon as possible.

More commonly, a patient presents with pain from a periodontal abscess or swelling of the gingiva when food or pus becomes trapped in a "pocket." In the dental office, a periodontal abscess is treated with curettage to establish drainage. In the ED treatment consists of a small conservative stab incision at the most fluctuant point to establish drainage, saline rinses, and antibiotic coverage. Using tetracycline for patients more than 8 years of age is preferable because it provides better coverage for the gram-negative and anaerobic organisms found in the gingival pocket. The patient should be referred to the general dentist or periodontist for further treatment.[2,5,6]

Acute Necrotizing Ulcerative Gingivitis Unlike gingivitis, in which the gingiva becomes inflamed in response to an irritant such as bacterial plaque but is not invaded by bacteria, acute necrotizing ulcerative gingivitis (ANUG) is a periodontal lesion in which bacteria actually invade nonnecrotic tissue. ANUG lesions are commonly accompanied by systemic manifestations of fever, malaise, and regional lymphadenopathy.[2,5,6]

Whereas gingivitis is a painless condition, ANUG is characterized by painful edematous interdental papillae. The normally pointed interdental papillae are blunted and ulcerated. A gray pseudomembrane covers the tissue and leaves a bleeding surface when removed. The lesions can involve any

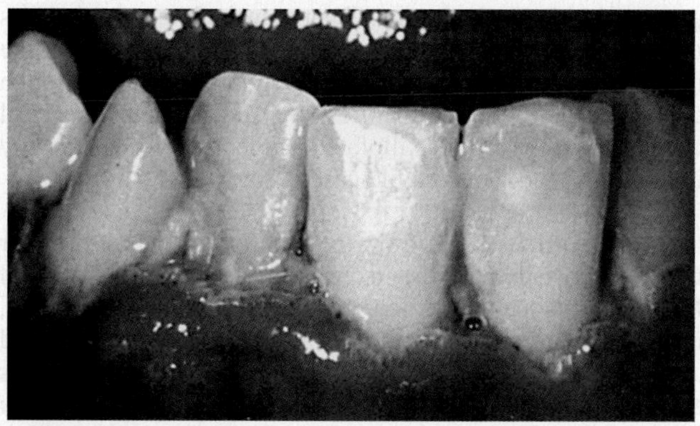

Figure 65-7. **Acute necrotizing ulcerative gingivitis (ANUG) involving lower anterior teeth.**

part of the gingiva but are more common in the anterior incisor and posterior molar regions. The patient complains of pain, a metallic taste, and foul breath (Figure 65-7).

Gingival crevices in ANUG show a predominance of fusobacteria and spirochetes. Electron microscopy reveals a layering pattern showing fusobacteria in superficial layers with spirochetes invading in deeper layers. Other necrotizing ulcerative oral diseases such as Vincent's angina (extension of ANUG to the fauces and tonsils), cancrum oris (extension of ANUG to the lips and buccal mucosa eroding through the teeth), and some pulmonary abscesses are also caused by fusospirochetes.[22]

Because ANUG results from an overgrowth of bacteria normally present in the gingival crevice, immunologic factors probably contribute to the disease. ANUG has been associated with immunocompromised hosts, fatigue, local trauma, emotional stress, and smoking. ANUG has the name "trench mouth" from its occurrence in large populations living in close quarters under significant stress, such as in the trenches in World War I, military barracks, and college dormitories.[23] Despite this, there is no evidence that ANUG is communicable.

ANUG treatment consists of prescribing warm saline rinses; systemic analgesics so that the patient can improve oral hygiene; and systemic antibiotics such as penicillin, erythromycin, or tetracycline.

Topical local anesthetics such as viscous lidocaine may provide some relief. Antibiotics provide dramatic relief within 24 hours, as do dilute (3%) hydrogen peroxide rinses. Although the patient will feel better, he or she should be advised to see a general dentist or periodontist for follow-up (this should be clearly documented on the chart). The soft tissue and alveolar bone destruction from ANUG predisposes the patient to further periodontal disease; corrective procedures are necessary to create an environment conducive to maintaining periodontal health.[5,6]

Oral Pain Although dental caries is the most common source of oral pain, the following disease entities may also cause oral or facial pain.

Root Canal Pain Endodontic or root canal therapy involves opening the pulp chamber of the tooth, removing pulp tissue from the chamber and the root portion of the tooth to the apex, irrigating and effectively sterilizing the canal, and sealing the pulp chamber to prevent ingress of saliva and contamination. After surgery, the patient may experience exquisite pain caused by irritation beyond the apex of the tooth from instrumentation or from the buildup of gas from the irrigation solutions. Swelling may cause the tooth to be elevated slightly out of the socket so that premature contact during chewing causes extreme pain. Such patients may have no relief with either systemic analgesics or anesthetic nerve blocks, presumably from the sensation of intense pressure. Treatment may consist of opening the canal to allow the gas or fluid to escape and of occlusal adjustment to take the tooth out of contact; therefore, the patient's general dentist or endodontist may have to be contacted.[24]

Cracked Tooth and Split Root Syndromes Patients with cracked teeth or a split root may report having a toothache. Pain occurs primarily with chewing or forced closure. The patient may have had an extensive dental restoration, previous endodontic therapy, or a history of having received an upward blow to the jaw. In the ED, the diagnosis is made from history and from having the patient bite on a piece of wood. In the dental office, the diagnosis will be made by removing a restoration and inspecting the cavity floor. Management is similar to that for carious teeth, including symptomatic pain medication and referral back to the dentist to consider possible causes.[2]

Maxillary Sinusitis Dental pain is often referred to the area of the sinuses; similarly, congested or inflamed sinuses in the proximity of the apices of the maxillary teeth may cause apparent odontogenic pain. The patient may complain of throbbing pain unrelated to changes in temperature and aggravated by lying down. On examination, there is no apparent dental cause. There may be tenderness over the maxillary sinuses or periorbital regions. Nasal discharge may be present. The Panorex film can screen for both dental and sinus pathology. See Chapter 67 for a detailed discussion.

Atypical Odontalgia Atypical odontalgia describes dental pain for which there is no dental cause. The patient may have a history of multiple dental procedures with no relief. The pain is chronic and occurs spontaneously. Percussion may elicit pain, and there may be thermal sensitivity as if a vital tooth were present. If paroxysmal pain of neuropathic origin is excluded, atypical odontalgia can be entertained. Similar to many chronic pain syndromes, treatment with tricyclic antidepressants may be efficacious. Such management is best left to the dentist or pain management consultant who will follow the patient on a long-term basis.

Postextraction Pain Pain after an extraction (i.e., immediate periosteitis) is common for approximately 24 hours. Systemic analgesics are usually adequate for pain control. Aspirin-containing compounds and NSAIDs are effective analgesics but can contribute to postoperative bleeding and oozing.

A much more painful condition, acute alveolar osteitis or dry socket, may occur approximately 3 to 4 days after an extraction. The patient has a pain-free interval followed by sudden onset of excruciating pain associated with a foul odor. The pathophysiology involves premature loss of the healing blood clot from the socket with a localized infection of the bone.[25]

Treatment of a dry socket consists of an anesthetic nerve block, gentle irrigation of the socket, and packing the socket with iodoform gauze saturated with a medicated dental paste such as "Seda-Dent," or barely dampened with eugenol (oil of cloves). The packing affords almost immediate relief. Patients with a dry socket require daily follow-up for pack changes until the condition resolves. Most dentists include oral antibiotic (e.g., penicillin or erythromycin) coverage, analgesics, and NSAIDs with this regimen until the condition resolves. It should be noted that although the condition is secondary to premature loss of the blood clot from the socket, no attempt should be made to stir up bleeding in the socket to form a new clot because this procedure is associated with a high incidence of osteomyelitis.[25]

Paroxysmal Pain of Neuropathic Origin Paroxysmal pain of neuropathic origin is most commonly caused by tic douloureux, trigeminal neuralgia. The diagnosis is made principally on the basis of history. The patient complains of paroxysmal episodes of an excruciating, lancinating pain, also described as recurrent bursts of an electric shock. The pain follows the anatomic distribution of the involved division of the fifth cranial nerve. On physical examination, the pain can sometimes be elicited by tapping specific areas of the face (the so-called trigger zones) in the region of the distribution of the nerve involved.[26]

Medical management for tic douloureux consists of carbamazepine, although some patients may be afforded no relief. Patients who fail medical management and are in significant distress may be candidates for neurosurgical procedures that ablate the nerve. The emergency physician should arrange close follow-up if treatment for tic douloureux is initiated in the ED. Patients taking carbamazepine require adjustment of the dosage to achieve therapeutic effect and also require monitoring for toxicity. Moreover, patients in whom the diagnosis is entertained need additional evaluation to exclude the presence of multiple sclerosis, cerebellopontine angle tumor, acoustic neuroma, or nasopharyngeal carcinoma. Patients with this condition commonly require a full dental, otolaryngologic, and neurologic evaluation to investigate correctable causes.

Other causes of orofacial pain of the paroxysmal type include headaches (see Chapter 17). Vascular headaches such as migraine and cluster headaches may have facial pain as their principal manifestation. Rheumatologic disorders such as giant cell arteritis and polymyalgia rheumatica in the elderly can result in facial pain. Dull pain in the lower jaw is not always of dental origin. Myocardial ischemia may cause isolated jaw pain.

Temporomandibular Myofascial Pain Dysfunction Syndrome The TMJ is a bilateral joint subject to almost continuous use. It is extremely sensitive to proprioceptive stimuli and can react to interferences in occlusion of only fractions of a millimeter. TMJ syndrome results from anatomic disharmony (see Figure 65-1) and occlusal disturbances. The condition is aggravated by trauma or clenching of the teeth or bruxism. Patients complain of pain in the region of the TMJ, usually unilateral. The pain is dull, worsens during the course of a day, and in extreme cases may result in trismus with palpable masseter and internal pterygoid spasm.[26-29]

TMJ radiographs are not helpful. Treatment consists of the external application of heat for 15 minutes 4 to 6 times per day, soft diet, analgesics including NSAIDs, and a muscle relaxant such as diazepam. Patients should be referred to a dentist specializing in TMJ disorders such as a periodontist or a periodontal prosthodontist. Treatment at this stage consists of continued physiotherapy, bite appliances that put the musculature at rest, and occlusal adjustment.[30] Although certain anatomic abnormalities are amenable to surgical correction, most oral maxillofacial surgeons consider surgery only for the most intractable cases.[28]

Pericoronitis Pain from the eruption of the third molar teeth (i.e., wisdom teeth) in the adult is common. Trapped food and plaque cause the gingiva surrounding crowded, malerupted, or impacted third molar teeth to become inflamed and swollen. This condition is called pericoronitis and is extremely painful because of repeated trauma from the opposing third molar biting on tender tissues and from distention of retromolar tissue on opening of the mandible. Pericoronitis is treated locally with warm saline irrigation, with or without hydrogen peroxide rinses. If the condition is severe or if there is a fever, an antibiotic is recommended. If fluctuant pus is present, an incision and drainage should be performed, exercising care not to track the infection posteriorly or to dissect deeply into distorted tissues, possibly encountering the internal carotid artery.[7]

Definitive treatment involves removal of the opposing third molar tooth for immediate relief and removal of the involved third molar tooth after the infection is resolved.[2] These patients should be referred to the oral maxillofacial surgeon.

Oral Manifestations of Systemic Disease Although the oral manifestations of many systemic diseases are nonspecific, several diseases have distinct oral presentations. In certain instances, recognition of the oral signs aids in the specific diagnosis. In other disease states, the oral condition is a contributing factor to the overall pathophysiology.[31]

Diabetes Mellitus Oral manifestations of diabetes mellitus are associated primarily with periodontal lesions. Diabetic patients appear to be more susceptible to periodontitis. Acute gingival abscess and sessile or pedunculated gingival proliferations have been described as being caused by or intimately associated with diabetes.[31]

Similar to other systemic manifestations of diabetes, the degree of control of the diabetes seems to correlate with its effects on the periodontium. Uncontrolled diabetes generally results in a greater periodontal disease. Control of diabetes helps decrease periodontal severity, although irreversible damage—such as bone loss—may result.

Although the severity of periodontal disease in diabetic patients is a function of the response to local factors such as plaque and calculus, there is also evidence to support the role of vascular changes and alterations in the role of polymorphonuclear leukocytes, monocytes, oral microflora, the patient's immune response, and genetic variables. Patients with diabetes who have advanced retinal changes have also been found to have more periodontal manifestations.

Maintenance of a healthy periodontium is important in the diabetic patient. Just as the degree of diabetic control affects the periodontium, so too does periodontal disease affect the degree of control. Patients with brittle diabetes or subject to repeated episodes of ketoacidosis might be thrown out of control from a simple periodontal abscess. The presence of advanced periodontal disease in a young patient, especially in the absence of local factors, should lead one to exclude the diagnosis of diabetes. A sudden change from a healthy

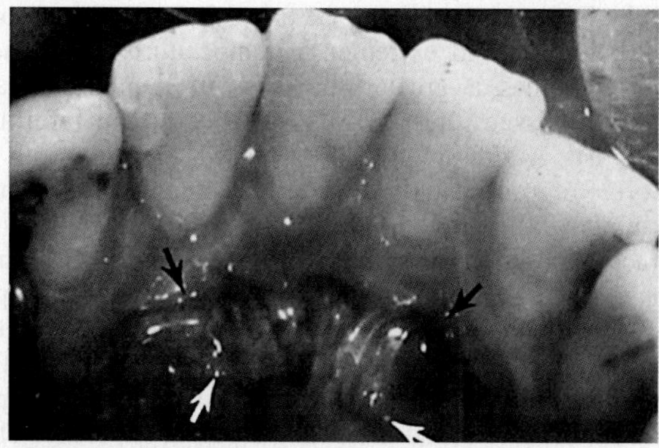

Figure 65-8. **Lesion *(arrows)* secondary to systemic lupus erythematosus involving the floor of mouth.**

periodontium to a diseased state would lead a physician to suspect a similar diagnosis in the adult. Human immunodeficiency virus (HIV) infection should also be ruled out.

Collagen Vascular Diseases Systemic lupus erythematosus is the most common collagen vascular disease to have oral manifestations. Patients commonly have large ulcerated intraoral lesions with necrotic borders. The lesions are usually secondarily infected and painful (Figure 65-8).

Scleroderma is usually recognized by the characteristic facies. The periodontal ligament may appear thickened on dental radiographs. Characteristic microscopic changes can be seen on gingival biopsy. Rare entities such as the midline lethal granuloma or Wegener's granulomatosis present with large intraoral ulcerative lesions, usually involving the hard palate.[31]

Granulomatous Diseases Oral manifestations of granulomatous diseases are fairly rare today, but are still seen. Tuberculosis may give rise to lesions of the tongue or tonsillar area. These lesions are most commonly confused with syphilitic ulcerations or infections caused by actinomycosis. A more common and benign entity is the pyogenic granuloma.[6] The pyogenic granuloma is a proliferation of highly vascular connective tissue in response to an irritant. The lesions range from sessile to pedunculated and have a warty texture. Pyogenic granulomas in the oral cavity are usually gingival in origin. They are especially common in pregnancy and are called pregnancy tumors. Pregnancy tumors generally resolve 2 to 3 months after delivery; those that do not resolve require surgical excision.

Blood Dyscrasias The gingiva may be massively infiltrated by leukemic cells in acute leukemic states, especially acute granulocytic. The gingiva is edematous, bluish-red, and may cover the teeth. These gingivae are compromised and may allow for the ingress of bacteria leading to sepsis. Chronic leukemic states have no specific gingival lesions, and leukemic states in remission are associated with normal gingiva. In addition to sepsis, gingival hemorrhage is a serious sequela. Gingival sequelae are more severe with underlying periodontal disease; therefore, during remissions it is imperative to maintain good periodontal health. Acute hemorrhage is controlled with the application of gauze pressure and hemostatic agents such as topical thrombin, absorbable gelatin powder, and oxidized regenerated cellulose.[2]

Thrombocytopenic purpura commonly presents with oral manifestations. Spontaneous gingival bleeding from trauma is characteristic. Acute hemorrhage is managed in a fashion similar to that discussed for acute leukemia. Less serious persistent oozing responds to treatment of the underlying state.

Drug-Induced Gingival Hyperplasias Dilantin hyperplasia was first described in 1939.[32] Of patients on dilantin, 40% showed some degree of gingival hyperplasia. Younger patients seem to be affected more often than older patients. The degree of gingival hyperplasia does not appear to be related to dosage. The disease ranges from slight enlargements of the interdental papillae to massive enlargement of the gingiva, which covers the crowns of the teeth and may actually move the teeth. The hyperplastic tissue is subject to infection. The presence of local irritants seems to make the hyperplasia worse.[5,6] Treatment of the condition includes removal of local irritants and surgical excision of the hyperplastic tissue. If the drug is not discontinued, hyperplasia is likely to recur, although less severely if good oral hygiene is maintained.

Drug-induced gingival hyperplasia is no longer unique to sodium diphenylhydantoin. Recently, a similar lesion has been recognized in patients receiving nifedipine therapy. Although only speculative, it may be the ability of both drugs to alter calcium metabolism that affects the gingival hypertrophy. The other widely used calcium antagonist, verapamil, has yet to be associated with gingival hypertrophy.[33-35]

Aphthous Stomatitis Patients may complain of recurrent small oral mucosal ulcers. The ulcers are approximately 2 to 3 mm in size with a white center. The lesions tend to be tender but rarely become infected.

Multiple ulcers that have coalesced can create an impressively large lesion. As much as one third of the population is thought to be affected by this condition, which is believed to be related to stress, nutrition, oral trauma, and hormonal etiologies. Treatment can be symptomatic (hydrogen peroxide rinse, topical dental preparations such as benzocaine and an emollient gel, 50:50 mixture of Benadryl and Kaopectate or Maalox) or prescription regimens such as steroid-antibiotic ointment (Kenalog in Orabase) or sucralfate, and oral antibiotics for secondary infection. A new topical agent, Debacterol, available only by prescription, can be applied to the ulcer; Debacterol seals the ulcer and promotes rapid healing. Ulcers that may appear similar to aphthous ulcers are those on the soft palate associated with hand-foot-and-mouth disease or lesions on the gingivae and tongue from herpetic stomatitis.[36,37]

TRAUMATIC DENTAL EMERGENCIES

Fractures of Teeth

The anterior teeth are commonly injured from falls or blows directly to the teeth. Forceful blows to the mandible directed superiorly may result in fractures of the premolars and molars caused by a wedgelike effect of the cusps of the mandibular teeth in the central fossae of the maxillary teeth. Many children have an anterior overbite, which makes this part of the dentition more prone to injury. Blunt trauma to the dentition may result in damage to the neurovascular supply to the tooth, bleeding within the tooth, fractures of the root or crown, loosening of the tooth, or actual expulsion of the tooth from its socket. Long-term sequelae of blunt trauma or reimplantation of teeth include resorption of the root.[2,38,39]

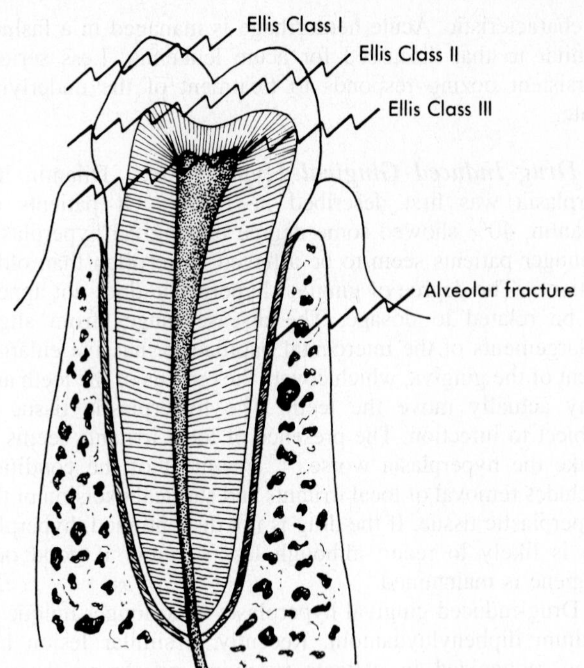

Figure 65-9. **Ellis classification for fractures of anterior teeth.** *From Tintinalli JE et al:* **Emergency medicine: a comprehensive study guide,** *ed 4, New York, 1996, McGraw-Hill.*

Fractures of the anterior teeth are managed on the basis of the type of fracture, its relation to the pulp of the tooth, and the patient's age. The Ellis classification system was used to describe fractures of anterior teeth; however, now it is the accepted practice to simply describe the anatomy involved.[40] Fractures involving enamel; enamel and dentin; and enamel, dentin, and pulp exposure have traditionally been referred to as Ellis I, II, and III, respectively (Figure 65-9).

The simplest and most common dental fracture involves only the enamel portion of the tooth leaving a chalky-white appearance. These injuries are usually minor unless a sharp portion of the tooth causes soft tissue trauma, in which case the sharp edge may be smoothed with an emery board. The patient or parents are usually concerned about the cosmetic deformity, but they can be reassured that the tooth can be restored to its natural appearance with the use of enamel-bonding plastic materials. Therefore referral to the dentist is necessary but not urgent.

Fractures involving the dentin have an ivory-yellow appearance. The pulp continually lays down dentin throughout the life of the tooth in response to normal and noxious stimuli. Therefore, in the child the pulp is relatively large in size and there is less dentin; the inverse is true in the adult. Because dentin is a microtubular tissue capable of allowing bacteria to percolate into the pulp chamber, fractures involving dentin are more serious in children and adolescents because there is little dentin to protect the pulp after it is exposed to the oral cavity.

In younger patients, the management of dentin fractures involves the immediate placement of a dressing of calcium hydroxide paste over the exposed dentin covered with dry foil, a metal band, or more commonly an enamel-bonded plastic. Early intervention may prevent contamination of the pulp and the need for subsequent root canal treatment. The pediatric or general dentist should be notified as soon as possible. Exposed dentin may be exquisitely sensitive, so the patient should avoid extremes in temperature. In the adult patient who has a greater thickness of dentin compared with pulpal tissue, there is less need for urgent referral to the dentist. A dressing can be placed on the tooth for comfort. Referral should be made to the dentist for the next working day.

Fractures of teeth resulting in pulp exposure are the most serious class of fractures of anterior teeth because the pulp chamber is immediately contaminated. Care should be taken to differentiate dentin exposure from the pulp. The tooth is wiped clean with a piece of gauze and examined for a pink blush or a drop of blood indicating a pulpal exposure. There may be excruciating pain from exposure of the nerve, or the shock of the trauma may have disrupted the neurovascular supply at the apex of the tooth, eliminating most sensitivity. This injury is often accompanied by serious fractures of the tooth, possibly involving the entire crown or root.[41]

Pulp exposures are true dental emergencies. In the primary dentition, exposure of the pulp can be treated by performing a pulpotomy, in which the pulp in the chamber is removed, the remaining tissue mummified with formocresol and covered with a layer of calcium hydroxide, and the tooth restored. In most cases, if there has been minimal contamination, the primary tooth lasts its natural lifetime. In the adult, the pulpotomy is not a successful procedure, and complete removal of all pulpal tissue from the crown and root must be performed. Although management of pulp exposures is more urgent in the child, endodontic therapy is less complicated and more successful in the adult if there is also a minimum of contamination; therefore, in the case of a pulpal exposure from a dental fracture, the general dentist, pedodontist, or endodontist should be notified immediately if possible, or follow-up instructed for the next working day. If no dentist is available, a piece of moist cotton can be placed over the exposed pulp and covered with a piece of dry foil or sealed with a temporary root canal sealant (e.g., Cavet).

Although some have advocated removal of the exposed pulpal tissue with a dental endodontic instrument called a barbed broach, this procedure is not recommended because these instruments break easily even in the hands of a skilled endodontist.[41] In cases of extreme pain, a dental anesthetic nerve block might be helpful.

Subluxated and Avulsed Teeth

Teeth that are loosened in their sockets as a result of a force are called subluxated. There may or may not be associated fractures. The diagnosis of subluxation can be made by gently tapping a tooth with two tongue blades. Any perceptible mobility is evidence for subluxation. There may be a ring of blood surrounding the gingival crevice. Minimally mobile teeth respond well to a soft diet for several days. Markedly mobile teeth require stabilization as soon as possible for 10 days to 2 weeks. Teeth can be stabilized (generally by a dentist) by means of Erich arch bars, wire ligation, enamel bonding plastics, or a combination of both.[3] Most of these techniques require an oral maxillofacial surgeon, hospital dentist, or pedodontist. They should be performed as soon as possible.[41]

As a temporizing measure, the patient can bite gently on a piece of gauze, or the teeth can be stabilized for up to 24 to 48 hours with the application of a periodontal pack such as "Coe-Pak."[42] A resin and catalyst paste are mixed together in

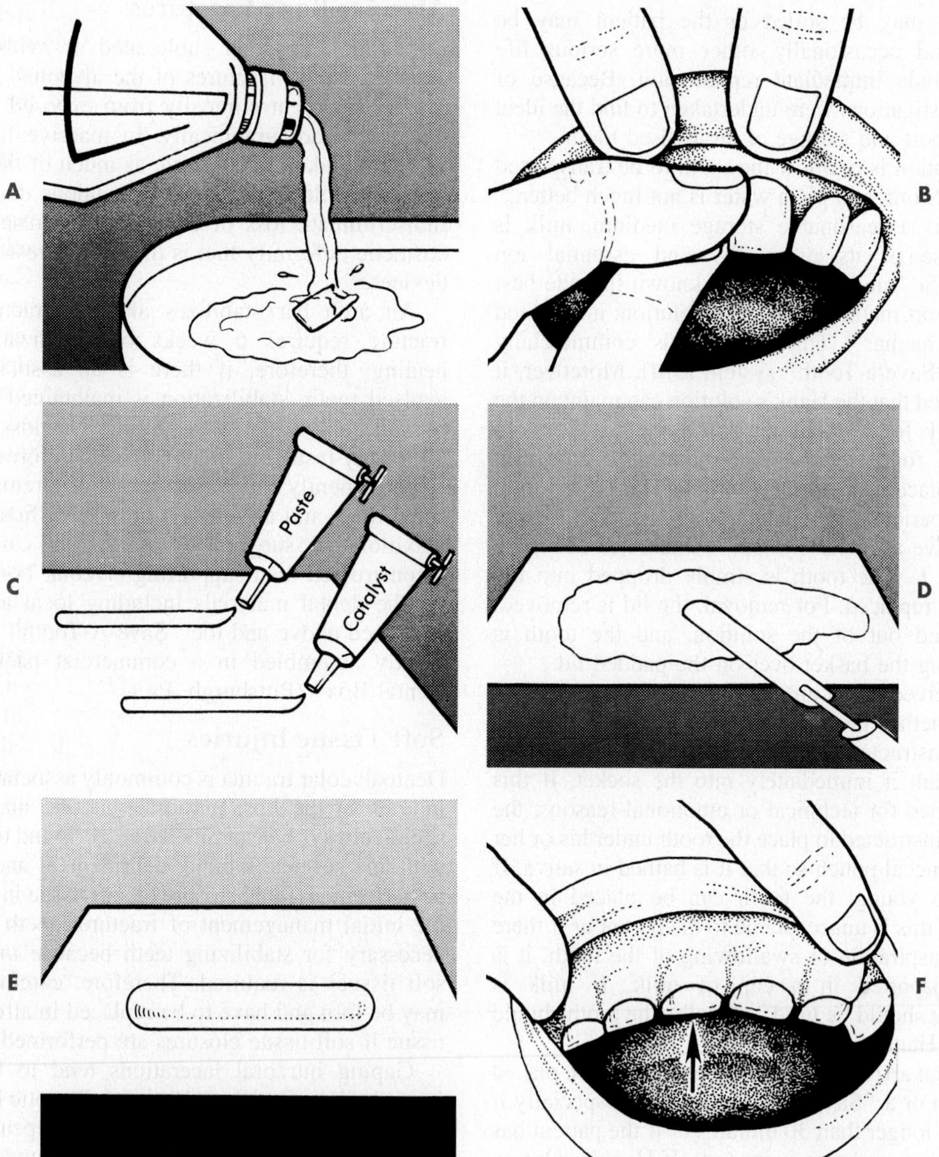

Figure 65-10. **Reimplantation and stabilization of an avulsed tooth. A, Tooth is rinsed. B, Tooth is placed back into socket. C and D, Periodontal pack is mixed. E, Splint material is ready for application. F, Packing is molded over reimplanted tooth and two adjacent teeth to either side.**

equal quantity to a firm consistency and molded over the anterior and posterior aspect of the involved tooth and two or three adjacent teeth on each side. The patient is asked to close the mouth while the mixture hardens (Figure 65-10). The patient is advised to avoid hot liquids that will soften the pack, eat a liquid-to-soft diet, and see the dentist as soon as possible.

Avulsed teeth are those completely torn from the socket and are a true dental emergency. The first question that should be asked is, "Where is the tooth?" If teeth are unaccounted for, the possibility of aspiration or entrapment in soft tissues should be considered.[46] Management of recovered avulsed teeth depends on the age of the patient and the length of time that the tooth has been absent from the oral cavity.[43] Avulsed primary teeth in the pediatric patient aged 6 months to 6 years are not replaced in the socket. Reimplanted primary teeth ankylose or fuse to the bone so that although the dentofacial complex grows downward and forward, the reimplantation site does not. There may also be interference with the eruption of the permanent tooth. Cosmetic deformity results in either case. Such patients should be referred to a pedodontist for consideration of a space maintainer or cosmetic appliance.

Avulsed permanent teeth require prompt intervention. When a tooth has been avulsed from its socket, the periodontal ligament fibers are torn; fragments remain attached both to the cementum on the root of the tooth and to the alveolar bone in the socket. Ideally, the best environment for an avulsed tooth is its socket, and it has been known since the mid-1960s that an avulsed tooth can be successfully replanted if it is returned to its socket within 30 minutes of the avulsion.[44-46] A 1% chance of successful replantation is lost for every minute that the tooth is outside of its socket; however, there is often difficulty with immediate replantation. On-site personnel (parents, teachers, trainers, paramedics) may be unfamiliar or uncomfortable with tooth replantation. The tooth may be soiled or the patient may be uncooperative. And occasionally, other more serious life threats may preclude immediate replantation. Because of these factors, investigations were undertaken to find the ideal medium for transport and storage of an avulsed tooth.

The worst situation is to allow the tooth to be transported in a dry medium. Storage in plain water is not much better.[47] Although saliva is a reasonable storage medium, milk is preferable because of its osmolarity and essential ion concentration of Ca^{++} and Mg^{++}.[47] It is known that the best storage and transport medium is Hank's solution: a balanced pH cell culture media.[48] This solution is commercially available as the "Save-a-Tooth" system (3M). Moreover, it has been determined that the Hank's solution can maintain the viability of the cells for 12 to 24 hours or more.[49] If the tooth has been avulsed for more than 30 minutes or has been allowed to dry, placement of the tooth in Hank's solution helps restore the periodontal ligament cells.[50,51]

Use of the "Save-a-Tooth" system is illustrated in Figure 65-11, *A* through *E*. The tooth is simply dropped into the basket and the lid replaced. For removal, the lid is removed, the basket is lifted out of the solution, and the tooth is retrieved by tipping the basket over on the padded lid.

If a call is received about an avulsed tooth, it should first be determined whether the tooth is permanent. If it is, the caller should be instructed to rinse the tooth off in saline or water and reimplant it immediately into the socket. If this cannot be performed for technical or emotional reasons, the patient should be instructed to place the tooth under his or her tongue or in the buccal pouch so that it is bathed in saliva. If the patient is too young, the tooth can be placed in the parent's mouth. If this is unacceptable to the parent or if there is concern about aspiration or swallowing of the tooth, it is then ideally transported in a cup of milk. If milk is unavailable, saline should be used.[51] Ideally, the tooth should be transported in Hank's solution.

When the patient arrives in the ED, the tooth can be placed in Hank's solution or a "Save-a-Tooth" system (especially if avulsion has been longer than 30 minutes or if the patient has other life threats that are being managed). If Hank's solution is not available, the tooth is rinsed with saline, the socket suctioned if necessary, and the tooth immediately implanted. Local anesthesia may be necessary. The tooth should be manipulated only by the crown, if possible, so that the remaining periodontal ligament fibers are not damaged. Stabilization must be performed immediately or the tooth will exfoliate. Stabilization is performed as described for markedly subluxated teeth (see Figure 65-10). The status of tetanus immunization should be checked, and the patient treated according to standard. The patient should be started on phenoxymethylpenicillin or erythromycin.[2,52]

The patient is placed on a liquid diet for several days and advanced to a soft diet for 1 week. Stabilization is maintained for approximately 2 weeks, and the tooth is gradually brought into function to prevent ankylosis. Teeth that have been avulsed for longer than 30 minutes will invariably require endodontic therapy.[43] Although there may be concern about the anatomic orientation of the tooth or more confusion about which socket to use when several teeth are avulsed, each tooth should be placed into a socket with the best fit so that the tooth remains in a good physiologic environment. The dentist can make any necessary readjustments before final stabilization.

Alveolar Bone Fractures

Dental fractures and subluxated or avulsed teeth may be associated with fractures of the alveolus. Alveolar fractures may be apparent clinically from exposed pieces of bone or diagnosed radiographically. In massive facial trauma, care should be taken to conserve as much of the alveolar bone as possible, unless there is a tremendous danger of aspiration. Indiscriminate loss of alveolar bone results in tremendous cosmetic deformity that is difficult to restore with prosthetic devices.[53]

An arch bar stabilizes alveolar fractures. An alveolar fracture requires 6 weeks of stabilization for adequate healing; therefore, if there is an associated subluxed or avulsed tooth, stabilization is maintained at the expense of possible ankylosis of the tooth. The loss of alveolar bone ultimately results in more cosmetic deformity for the patient. A permanently ankylosed tooth can remain functional for some time, and although it may be difficult for the oral and maxillofacial surgeon to remove, it can be more easily reconstructed than supporting alveolar bone.

The dental materials including local anesthesia supplies described above and the "Save-A-Tooth" system are conveniently assembled in a commercial package called "The Dental Box" (Pittsburgh, Pa.).

Soft Tissue Injuries

Dentoalveolar trauma is commonly associated with soft tissue injuries of the lips, intraoral mucosa, and tongue. Wounds should always be examined for debris and tooth fragments. As with any surgical wound, debridement and irrigation should be performed. Final closure of soft tissue injuries should await the initial management of fractured teeth or the procedures necessary for stabilizing teeth because manipulation of the soft tissues is required. Therefore, carefully placed sutures may be torn and have to be replaced in already compromised tissue if soft tissue closures are performed first.[54]

Gaping intraoral lacerations tend to become ulcerated, secondarily infected, and painful. Fibrotic healing results in a cumbersome scar that is subject to repeated trauma during chewing. A well-prepared mucosal wound is closed with No. 4-0 absorbable or black silk suture. Gingival and tongue lacerations are best closed with No. 4-0 black silk because this material is less irritating to the touch. Absorbable suture, such as 4-0 chromic, is excellent for children. Large tongue lacerations should be well approximated or a cleft will form during healing, necessitating a revision. Anesthesia can be achieved by either direct local injection or lingual block. Small (< 1 cm) lacerations are best left alone, especially in children. The management of through-and-through lacerations involving both skin and oral mucosa is controversial. With proper preparation, mucosa can be closed as described previously. Skin is closed with No. 6-0 or No. 7-0 synthetic nonabsorbable sutures that are removed in 3 to 4 days, depending on the amount of muscle tension on the wound. Intraoral silk closures are removed in approximately 7 days.[54]

Through-and-through lacerations and other significant intraoral wounds may benefit from prophylactic antibiotics (penicillin is the drug of choice).[52] The patient is advised to maintain oral hygiene, use saline rinses six times a day, place a triple antibiotic ointment over the skin closure, and watch carefully for infection. These patients should be seen in 48 to 72 hours to check for infection. Normal postoperative soft tissue swelling should not be mistaken for an infected wound.

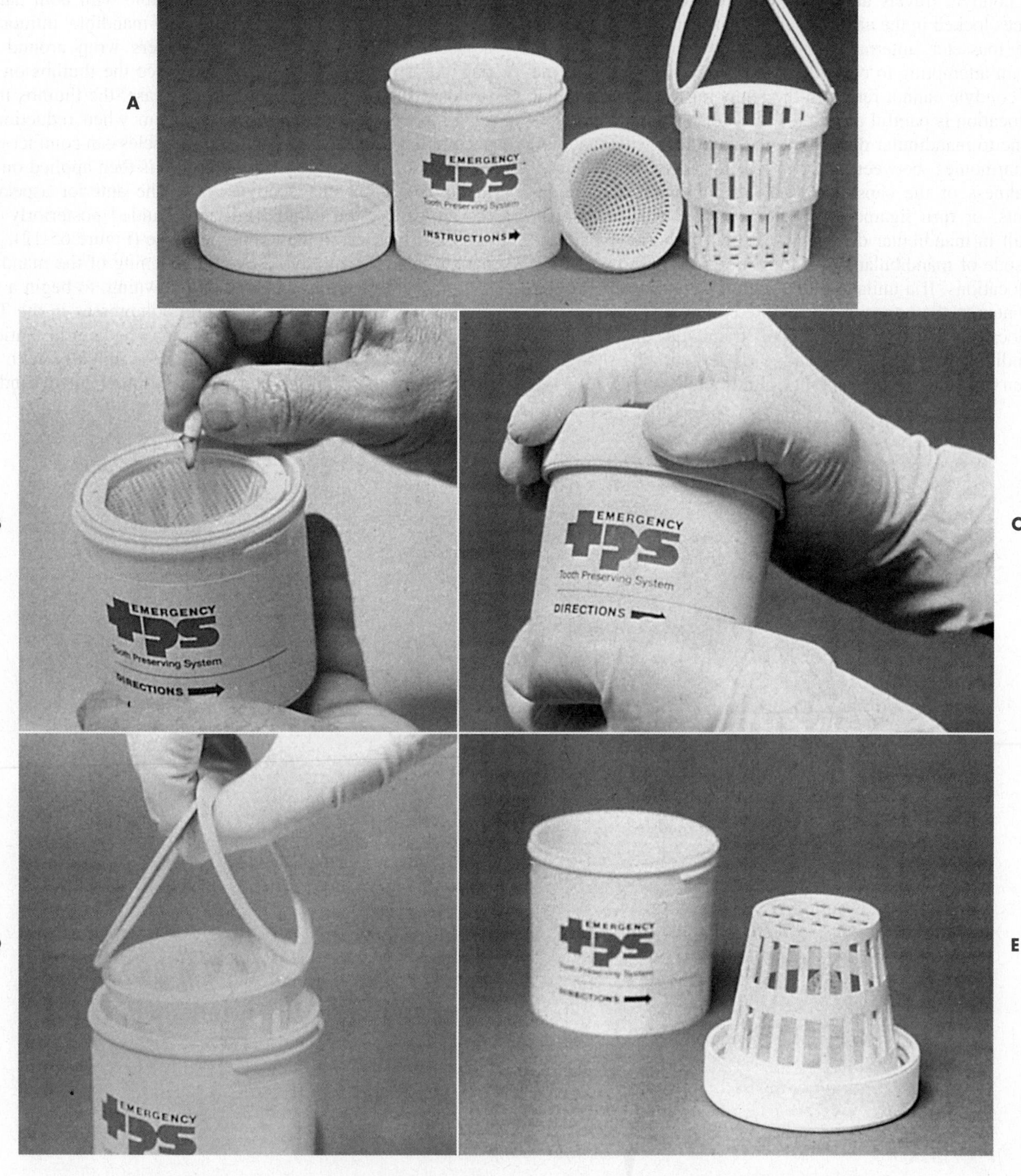

Figure 65-11. **A,** Tooth Preserving System—TPS. **B,** Each avulsed tooth is dropped into a separate TPS container of Hank's solution. **C,** Lid is tightly secured. Container can be gently swirled to clean tooth. **D,** Tooth is removed from container by lifting basket. **E,** Tooth is retrieved by turning basket over onto cushioned interior lining of lid. *Photos courtesy Paul Krasner, DDS, Biological Rescue Products, Inc., 566 High Street, Pottstown, PA.*

Temporomandibular Joint Dislocation

The mandibular condyles may dislocate from trauma, but more often follows extreme opening of the mandible such as occurs after a yawn or laughter. TMJ dislocation occurs when the condyle travels anteriorly along the eminence and becomes locked in the anterior superior aspect of the eminence. The masseter, internal pterygoid, and temporalis go into spasm attempting to close the mandible; trismus results, and the condyle cannot return to the temporal fossa. Mandibular dislocation is painful and frightening for the patient. Patients prone to mandibular dislocation include those with anatomic disharmonies between the fossa and articular eminence, weakness of the capsule and the temporomandibular ligaments, or torn ligaments. Dystonic reaction to drugs may result in mandibular dislocation. Patients who have had one episode of mandibular dislocation are predisposed to further dislocations. If a unilateral dislocation has occurred, the jaw deviates to the opposite side. More commonly, a symmetric dislocation occurs. In cases of traumatic dislocation, a mandibular series, Panorex, or TMJ radiographs should be taken to exclude the possibility of a fracture.[2,7,53-55]

Reduction of a dislocated mandible is fairly straightforward if one considers the anatomy of the TMJ. The patient usually requires midazolam for muscle relaxation and sedation. Either facing the patient or from behind, the emergency physician grasps the mandible with both hands; the thumbs rest on the ridge of the mandible intraorally adjacent to the molars, and the fingers wrap around the outside of the jaw. Some prefer to place the thumbs on the occlusal surfaces of the teeth; in this case, the thumbs must be wrapped with gauze to protect them when reduction is accomplished because the masseter muscles can contract with tremendous force. Downward pressure is then applied on the mandible to free the condyles from the anterior aspect of the eminence; the mandible is then guided posteriorly and superiorly back into the temporal fossae (Figure 65-12). The patient is advised to avoid extreme opening of the mandible such as occurs during laughing and yawning, to begin a soft diet for 1 week, and to apply warm compresses in the TMJ area. NSAIDs and muscle relaxants may be helpful. Patients with chronic dislocation may be helped initially with the application of a Barton bandage (elastic fabricated bandage

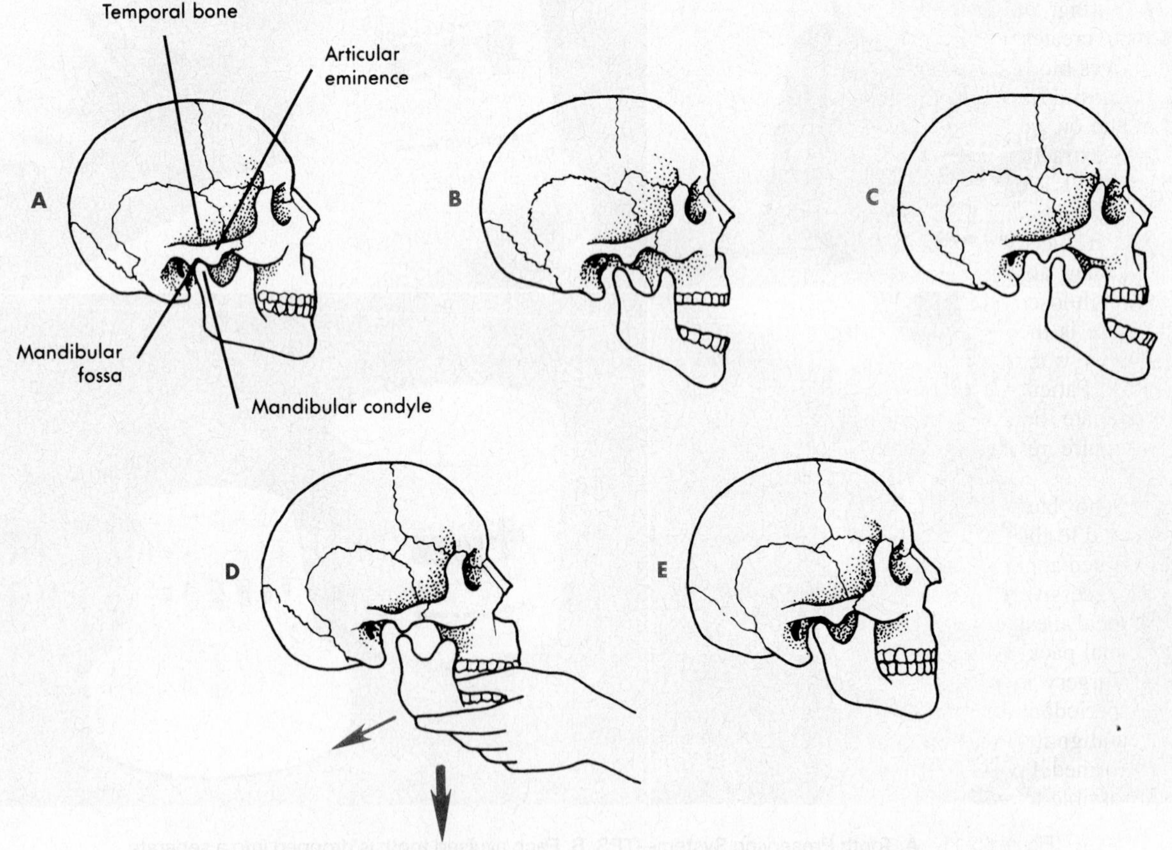

Figure 65-12. **Reduction of temporomandibular joint (TMJ) dislocation. This figure illustrates TMJ in normal and dislocated positions. A,** Closed position, with mandibular condyle resting in mandibular fossa behind articular eminence. **B,** In maximally open position, condyle is just under and slightly behind eminence. **C,** In dislocated position, condyle moves forward and upward slightly above eminence; muscle spasm then occurs. **D,** To reduce dislocation, thumbs are placed intraorally and lateral to lower molars, pressure is applied to lower molar ridge area near jaw angle in downward and backward direction. **E,** When condyle has cleared articular eminence, muscle contraction will return jaw to a normal closed position. *Redrawn from Rose LF, Hendler BH, Amsterdam JT:* Consultant *22:125, 1982.*

that wraps around the top of the head and mandible). Intermaxillary fixation with wire and elastics may be necessary. Those patients who have difficulty reducing themselves, or who are plagued by recurrences, may require surgical revision of the eminence for relief.[2,7]

Hemorrhage

Oral hemorrhage is a common complication of dental scalings, periodontal surgery, and dental extractions. Hemorrhage is controlled easily with local measures postoperatively. However, patients may have sustained or recurrent hemorrhage after these procedures and present to the ED. History should be obtained for recent dental procedures, drugs with antiplatelet activity such as aspirin, underlying coagulopathy, or a history of spontaneous bleeding. Spontaneous gingival hemorrhage without an inciting factor warrants a screen for coagulopathy and a complete blood count (CBC) and differential. Diseases that result in spontaneous gingival hemorrhage are discussed in the section on oral manifestations of systemic disease. Management of coagulopathies from factor deficiencies requires factor replacement and administration of aminocaproic acid if there has been a recent dental extraction or periodontal surgery.[2,7]

Bleeding after extraction is the most common cause for oral hemorrhage. Historic information of cigarette smoking, excessive spitting, or using straws is helpful information because each creates negative pressure in the oral cavity, which dislodges blood clots from the socket. Excessive clots should be removed from the oral cavity. The patient should be allowed to bite on gauze for 20 minutes. If bleeding has not stopped, the extraction site should be infiltrated with 2% lidocaine with 1:100,000 epinephrine so that the tissue blanches. Gauze pressure should then be repeated for another 20 minutes. If bleeding continues, the socket should be packed with an absorbable gelatin sponge or oxidized regenerated cellulose and secured with a No. 4-0 silk suture. Gauze pressure is then again applied. Failure to respond to these measures warrants an evaluation for an underlying coagulopathy. Patients who have had multiple extractions without adequate bone recontouring and soft tissue closure may require revision of the surgical site to achieve hemostasis.[2]

Patients who have bleeding after periodontal surgery usually respond to the local measures previously detailed, as well as continued application of gauze pressure. Patients who are bleeding excessively after a deep scaling may be helped by injection of local anesthetic with epinephrine or the placement of a periodontal pack. Patients who have recently undergone periodontal surgery involving gingival flaps may have dislodged the periodontal packs that were placed to ensure proper tissue alignment and wound healing. The periodontist should be informed if possible so that the pack can be replaced as soon as possible to ensure appropriate healing.

KEY CONCEPTS

- The most common nontraumatic dental emergencies are pain from dental caries, periodontal abscesses, and spread of infection of dental origin.
- The most important concern of dental infection is any compromise of the airway.
- Fractures of teeth are managed differently depending upon which structures are involved: enamel, dentin, or pulp exposure.
- Avulsed teeth must be implanted as quickly as possible and are best preserved in Hank's solution.
- Soft tissue injuries such as lip lacerations when involved with dental injuries should be managed after the teeth have been stabilized.

REFERENCES

1. Amsterdam JT, Wagner DW, Rose LF: Interdisciplinary training: hospital dental general practice/emergency medicine, *Ann Emerg Med* 9:310, 1980.
2. Amsterdam JT: Emergency dental procedures. In Roberts JR, Hedges J, editors: *Clinical procedures in emergency medicine,* ed 3, Philadelphia, 1998, WB Saunders.
3. Amsterdam JT: General dental emergencies. In Tintinalli JE, Krome RL, Ruiz E, editors: *Emergency medicine: a comprehensive study guide,* ed 4, New York, 1995, McGraw-Hill.
4. Meford HM: Acute care of avulsed teeth, *Ann Emerg Med* 11:559, 1982.
5. Genko, editor: *Contemporary periodontics,* St Louis, 2000, Mosby.
6. Linde J, editor: *Clinical periodontology and implant dentistry,* Copenhagen, 1997, Munksgaard.
7. Peacock WF: Face and jaw emergencies. In Tintinalli JE, Kelen GD, Stapczynski JS, editors: *Emergency medicine: a comprehensive study guide,* ed 5, New York, 2000, McGraw-Hill.
8. Mandell GL, Bennett JE, Dolin R, editors: *Principles and practice of infectious disease,* ed 3, Edinburgh, 2000.
9. Iwu CO: Ludwig's angina: a report of 7 cases and review of current concepts of management, *Br J Oral Maxillofac Surg* 28:189, 1990.
10. Amsterdam JT: Dental caries. In Honigman B, editor, *Emerg Index,* Denver, 1994, Emergency Information Center.
11. Orland FJ et al: Use of germ free animal techniques in the study of experimental dental caries. I. Basic observations on rats reared free of all microorganisms, *J Dent Res* 11:232, 1954.
12. Holloway PJ: The role of sugar in the etiology of dental caries, *J Dent* 11:189, 1983.
13. Rose LF, Hendler BH, Amsterdam JT: Temporomandibular disorders and odontic infections, *Consultant* 22:110, 1982.
14. Solinitsky U: The fascial compartments of the head and neck in relation to dental infections, *Bull Georgetown U Med Center* 7:86, 1954.
15. Barkin R, Todd JK, Amer J: Periorbital cellulitis in children, *Pediatrics* 62:390, 1978.
16. Dice WH, Pryor GJ, Kilpatrick WR: Facial cellulitis following dental injury in a child, *Ann Emerg Med* 11:541, 1985.
17. Karlin RJ, Robinson WA: Septic cavernous sinus thrombosis, *Ann Emerg Med* 13:449, 1984.
18. Ahmad N, Grad HA, Haas DA et al: The efficacy of non-opioid analgesics for postoperative dental pain: a meta-analysis, *Anesth Prog* 44:119, 1997.
19. Po AL, Zhang WY: Analgesic efficacy of ibuprofen alone and in combination with codeine or caffeine in post-surgical pain: a meta-analysis, *Eur J Clin Pharmacol* 53:303, 1998.
20. Amsterdam JT: Regional anesthesia of the head and neck. In Roberts JR, Hedges J, editors: *Clinical procedures in emergency medicine,* ed 3, Philadelphia, 1998, WB Saunders.
21. Bennett CR: *Monheim's local anesthesia and pain control in dental practice,* ed 6, St Louis, 1978, Mosby.
22. Laskin D: The role of the dentist in the emergency room, *Dent Clin North Am* 19:675, 1975.
23. Schluger S: Necrotizing ulcerative gingivitis in the army: incidence, communicability, and treatment, *J Am Dent Assoc* 38:174, 1949.
24. Ingle JI: *Endodontics,* Philadelphia, 1974, Lea & Febiger.
25. Colby RC: The general practitioner's perspective of the etiology, prevention, and treatment of dry socket, *Gen Dent* 45:461, 1997.
26. Brightman VJ: Chronic oral sensory disorders—pain and dysgeusia. In Lynch M, editor: *Burket's oral medicine, diagnosis and treatment,* Philadelphia, 1994, JB Lippincott.
27. Sicher H: Structural and functional basis for disorders of the temporomandibular articulation, *J Oral Surg* 13:275, 1955.
28. Alderman MM: Disorders of the temporomandibular joint and related structures. In Lynch M, editor: *Burket's oral medicine, diagnosis and treatment,* Philadelphia, 1994, JB Lippincott.

29. Alderman MM: Disorders of the temporomandibular joint and related structures: rationale for diagnosis, etiology, and management, *Alpha Omegan* 69:12, 1976.
30. Weisgold AS, Laudenbach KW: Occlusal etiology and management of disorders of the temporomandibular joint and related structures, *Alpha Omegan* 69:12, 1976.
31. Rose LF: General health affecting periodontal disease and therapeutic response. In Goldman HM, Cohen DW, editors: *Periodontal therapy,* ed 6, St Louis, 1980, Mosby.
32. Kimball OP: The treatment of epilepsy with sodium diphenylhydantoin, *JAMA* 112:1244, 1939.
33. Lederman D et al: Gingival hyperplasia associated with nifedipine therapy, *Oral Surg* 57:620, 1984.
34. Ramon Y et al: Gingival hyperplasia caused by nifedipine-a preliminary report, *Int J Cardiol* 5:195, 1984.
35. Cohen DW: Gingival hyperplasia—a new lesion for the cardiologist? *Int J Cardiol* 5:205, 1984.
36. Alpsoy E, Er H, Durusoy C et al: The use of sucralfate suspension in the treatment of oral and genital ulceration of Behcet disease: a randomized, placebo-controlled, double-blind study, *Arch Dermatol* 135:529, 1999.
37. Vincent SD, Lilly GE: Clinical, historical, therapeutic features of aphthous stomatitis: literature review and open clinical trials employing steroids, *Oral Surg Oral Med Oral Pathol* 74:79, 1992.
38. Andreason JO: *Traumatic injuries of the teeth,* Philadelphia, 1981, WB Saunders.
39. Coccia CT: A clinical investigation of root resorption rates in reimplanted young permanent incisors: a five year study, *J Endodontol* 6:413, 1980.
40. Johnson R: Descriptive classification of trauma: the injuries to the teeth and supporting structures, *J Ain Dent Assoc* 102:195, 1981.
41. Medford HM, Curbs JW: Acute care of severe tooth fractures, *Ann Emerg Med* 12:364, 1983.
42. Medford HM: Temporary stabilization of avulsed or luxated teeth, *Ann Emerg Med* 17:490, 1982.
43. Grossman LL Ship II: Survival rate of reimplanted teeth, *Oral Surg* 29:899, 1970.
44. Andreasen JO, Hjorting-Hansen E: Replantation of teeth. I. Radiographic and clinical study of 110 human teeth replanted after accidental loss, *Acta Odontol Scand* 24:263, 1966.
45. Andreasen JO, Hjorting-Hansen E: Replantation of teeth. II. Histological study of replanted anterior teeth in humans, *Acta Odontol Scand* 24:287, 1966.
46. Söder PO et al: Effect of drying on viability of periodontal membrane, *Scand J Dent Res* 85:164, 1977.
47. Blomlöf L: Milk and saliva as possible storage media for traumatically exarticulated teeth prior to replantation, *Swed Dent J* (Suppl) 8:1, 1981.
48. Lindskog S, Blömlof L: Influence of osmolality and composition of some storage media on human periodontal ligament cells, *Acta Odontol Scand* 40:435, 1982.
49. Kristerson L, Söder PO, Otteskog P: Transport and storage of human teeth in vitro for autotransplantation and replantation, *J Oral Surg* 34:13, 1976.
50. Matsson L et al: Ankylosis of experimentally reimplanted teeth related to extra-alveolar period and storage environment, *Pediatr Dent* 4:327, 1982.
51. Krasner P: Modern treatment of avulsed teeth by emergency physicians, *Am J Emerg Med* 12:241, 1994.
52. Steele MT et al: Prophylactic penicillin for intraoral wounds, *Ann Emerg Med* 18:847, 1989.
53. Irby WB, editor: *Facial trauma and concomitant problems,* St Louis, 1979, Mosby.
54. Hendler BH, Wagner D: Injury to the lip and oral mucosa: trauma rounds, *Emerg Med* 6:278, 1974.
55. Myall WT, Sandor GK, Gregory CE: Are you overlooking fractures of the mandibular condyle? *Pediatrics* 79:639, 1987.

66 Ophthalmology

Douglas D. Brunette

PERSPECTIVE

Background and Epidemiology

Two percent of ED patients have eye complaints, and the majority can be treated without ophthalmologic consultation.[1] Central retinal artery occlusion and caustic exposure require immediate therapy. Other ophthalmologic conditions can be evaluated with a history and examination before treatment.

Figures 66-1 and 66-2 are provided as brief reviews of normal ocular anatomy and funduscopic appearance.

OCULAR TRAUMA

Perspective

It is important to apply a systematic approach in the management of patients with ocular trauma. Many extraocular structures are found in close proximity, and concomitant, nonocular injury is common. Penetrating and blunt ocular trauma may involve several eye structures.

Nonpenetrating Trauma

Orbit and Lid

Clinical Features and Management

Contusion Blunt injury to the orbits and surrounding tissues results in ecchymosis, swelling, and an often-dramatic appearance. A thorough assessment should explore the possibility of other significant injury. Basilar skull fractures may present with bilateral ecchymosis (raccoon eyes). Underlying globe injury may be present, and complete examination impeded by swelling. The emergency physician should attempt to visualize and examine all structures underlying the eyelids and obtain an accurate visual acuity. This should be done soon after the patient presents, before further swelling occurs. Examining the structures underlying severely swollen eyelids is difficult. A Desmarres retractor may help avoid global pressure.

Treatment of isolated soft-tissue injury to the eyelids and surrounding area is symptomatic. Head elevation and cold

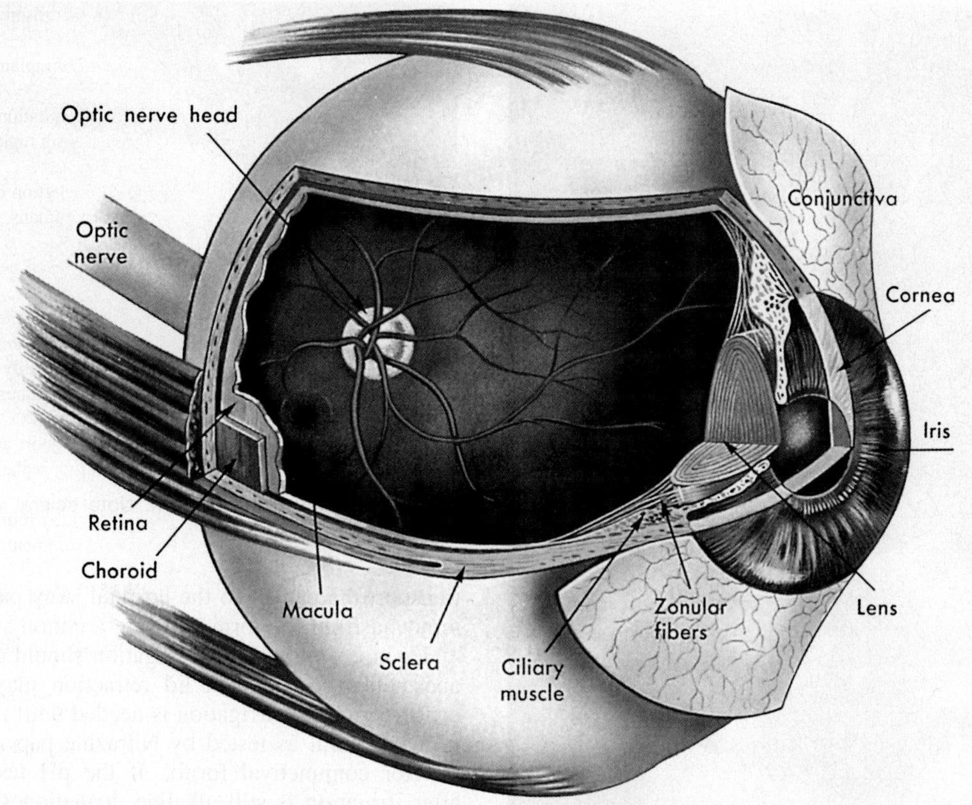

Figure 66-1. **Cutaway section of eye.** *From Stein-Slatt-Stein:* **Ophthalmic assistant,** *ed 5, St Louis, 1988, Mosby.*

compresses started in the ED should continue for 48 hours and will decrease the pain and swelling. Complete resolution takes 2 to 3 weeks. Patients should be instructed to seek follow-up care for any increase in signs or symptoms.

Orbital wall fractures When blunt force causes an acute rise in intraorbital pressure, prolapse of orbital soft tissues into the maxillary sinus may result because the orbital floor is generally the weakest point.[2] Entrapment of the inferior rectus and inferior oblique ocular muscles, orbital fat, and connective tissues results in enophthalmos, ptosis, diplopia, anesthesia of the ipsilateral cheek and upper lip, and limitation of upward gaze. Subcutaneous orbital emphysema may be palpable. Associated globe injuries occur in 10% to 25% of patients with orbital floor fractures.[3] Radiographic examination of the face can help but is imperfect. The teardrop sign, a bulge extending from the orbit into the maxillary sinus, and an air-fluid level in the maxillary sinus are indirect signs of orbital floor injury (Figure 66-3). If the fracture involves an infected sinus, treatment consists of nasal decongestants, broad-spectrum oral antibiotics, and ice packs to the orbit for 48 hours. Some ophthalmologists will use steroids to reduce swelling. Surgical repair is only for persistent diplopia or cosmetic concerns and is generally not performed until swelling subsides in 7 to 10 days.[4,5] Patients should be reevaluated by an ophthalmologist in 1 to 2 weeks.

Medial orbital wall fractures, through the lamina papyracea of the ethmoid bone, involve entry into the ethmoid sinus. Clinical features include orbital emphysema and epistaxis. Diplopia from medial rectus impingement can occur.[2] The finding of orbital emphysema should prompt the search for associated injury.[6] Rarely is orbital emphysema significant

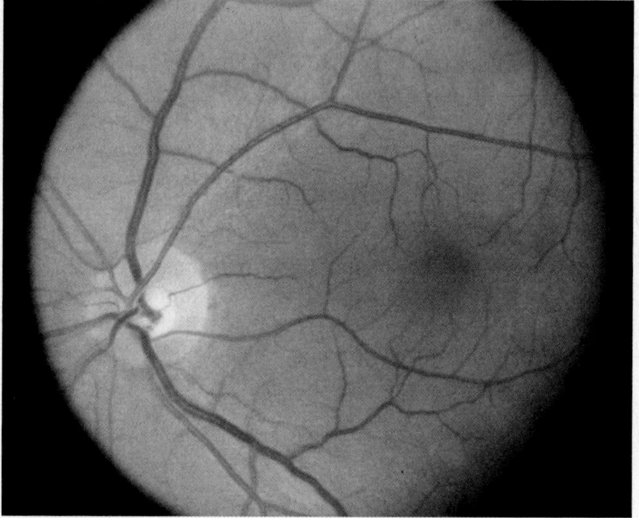

Figure 66-2. **Normal fundus.**

enough to compress the optic nerve and result in acute visual loss.[7] In most cases, orbital emphysema is a benign finding that resolves with time. Prophylactic antibiotics are not needed unless the fracture involves an infected sinus.[6,8]

Patients with orbital floor and medial orbital wall fractures should avoid blowing their noses and performing Valsalva maneuver to limit the extent of emphysema.

Orbital rim fractures are also common. They are a result of direct force.

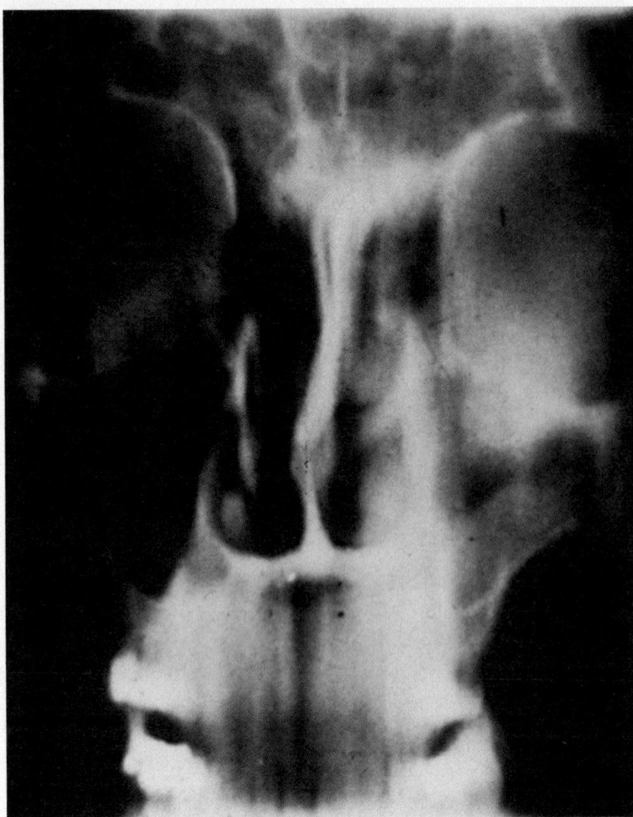

Figure 66-3. **Facial radiograph demonstrating teardrop sign in right maxillary sinus from orbital floor fracture.**

Retrobulbar Hemorrhage Orbital hemorrhage in the potential space surrounding the globe may occur after blunt trauma and injury to the orbital vessels. Significant hemorrhage results in an acute rise in intraorbital pressure that is transmitted to the globe and optic nerve. This may result in occlusion of the central retinal artery. Clinical findings include proptosis, limitation of ocular movement, visual loss, and increased intraocular pressure. An orbital computed tomography (CT) scan will demonstrate a hematoma.

When a retrobulbar hematoma compromises retinal circulation, immediate ophthalmologic consultation for decompression is warranted. Treatment of increased intraocular pressure includes carbonic anhydrase inhibitor, topical beta blocker, and intravenous (IV) mannitol. A lateral canthotomy can be done in the ED as a temporizing measure before definitive decompression.[2]

Cornea and Conjunctiva

Clinical Features and Management

Chemical burns Exposing the eye to chemicals is a true ocular emergency. Exposure to strong alkaline chemicals, found in drain cleaners, chemical detergents, industrial solvents, and as lime in plaster and concrete, produces a liquefactive necrosis that penetrates and dissolves tissues until the alkaline agent is removed. Acid burns tend to be less devastating than alkali burns because acidic exposure causes coagulation necrosis and the precipitation of tissue proteins limits the depth of the injury.

Treatment should begin at the scene with immediate irrigation using copious amounts of water. Irrigation should continue for at least 30 minutes before any attempt to

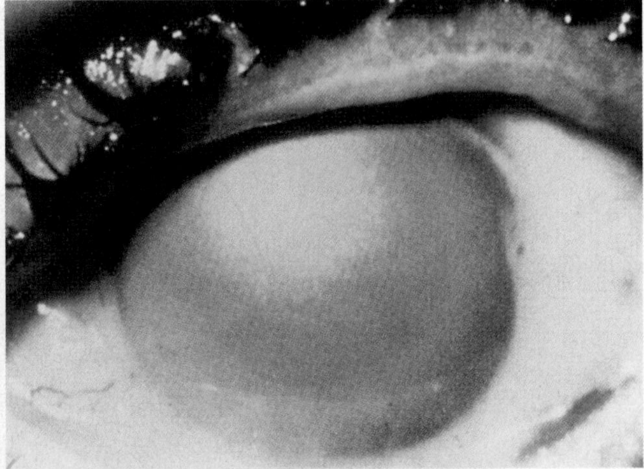

Figure 66-4. **Severe alkali burn. Note scleral whitening and the cloudy cornea.**

transport the patient to the hospital. Any particles should be removed from the fornices using a cotton swab.

Upon hospital arrival, irrigation should continue. Topical anesthetics and manual lid retraction may be needed for proper irrigation. Irrigation is needed until the pH of the tear film is neutral as tested by Nitrazine paper dipped into the inferior conjunctival fornix. If the pH tested immediately after irrigation is still alkaline, irrigation should be reinstituted. A normal pH should be checked again 10 minutes after the cessation of irrigation and periodically thereafter. Treatment after irrigation consists of a cycloplegic (avoid phenylephrine), topical antibiotics, treatment of increased intraocular pressure, and pain management.

Ophthalmologic consultation is indicated in all significant chemical exposures. Identification of the substance and its pH value is important. Although alkaline substances with a pH less than 12 and acidic substances with a pH greater than 2 are thought not to cause significant injury, concentration and contact time will alter this general rule.[9,10]

Severity can be judged by the degree of corneal cloudiness and scleral whitening (Figure 66-4).[11] Long-term complications include perforation, scarring, and neovascularization of the cornea; adhesions of the lids to the globe (symblepharon); glaucoma; cataracts; and retinal damage.

Miscellaneous irritants, solvents, detergents, and glues All exposures should initially be treated as though they were an alkali or acid exposure until the substance is identified. Detergents generally cause conjunctival irritation only. More irritating substances may denude the corneal epithelium and cause anterior chamber inflammation. After copious irrigation these injuries should be treated as corneal abrasions.

Aerosol exposures are common. Intraocular foreign bodies may result from the propellant. Exposure to the compounds found in personal defense devices (e.g., mace) should be treated in the same manner as other chemical injuries.

Super glue (cyanoacrylate adhesive) exposure is also common. These glues harden rapidly, and typically the eyelids are sealed shut. Misdirected lashes and the hardened super glue may act as a foreign body and cause corneal defects.[12] Gentle traction on the eyelids and separating glued eyelashes may open the eyelids. If the eyelids are sealed shut in a normal anatomic position and cannot be opened with gentle traction, the eye may be left alone, allowing time for

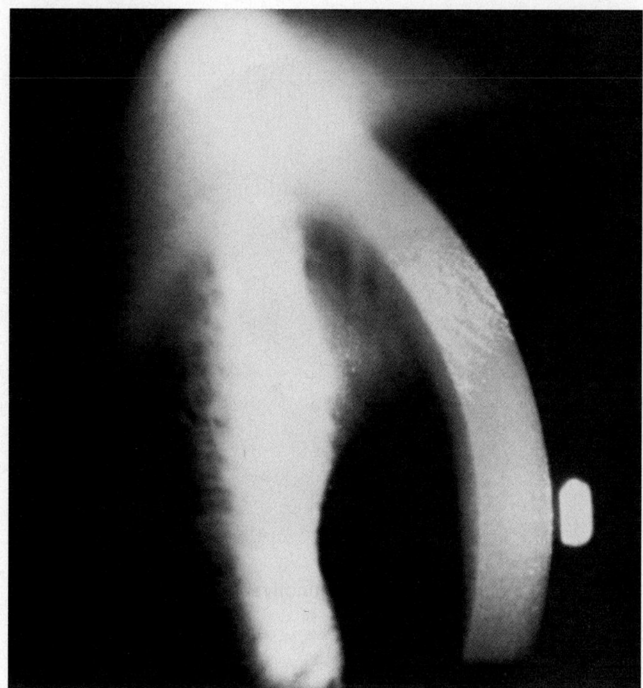

Figure 66-5. **Corneal abrasion demonstrated by slit-lamp examination.**

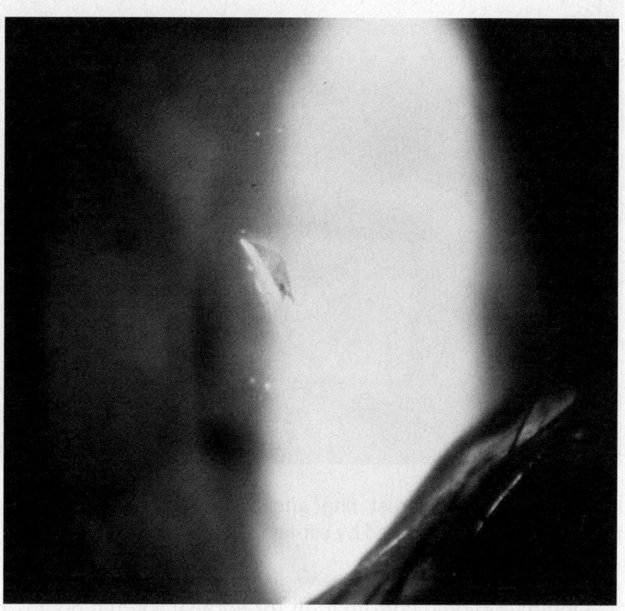

Figure 66-6. **Corneal foreign body (glass) seen by slit-lamp examination.**

the super glue to dissolve by physiologic mechanisms over several days.[13] If the eyelids are inverted and sealed shut, surgical intervention may be needed. Attempts to dissolve the super glue with other substances should be avoided. Ophthalmic consultation should be obtained for super glue exposures.

Thermal burns Thermal burns affect the eyelids more than the globe because of reflex blinking and Bell's phenomenon. Superficial eyelid burns can be treated by irrigation and topical antibiotic ophthalmic ointment. Second- or third-degree eyelid burns need ophthalmic consultation. Hot liquid splashes and cigarette ashes to the cornea usually result in a superficial corneal epithelial injury and are treated as corneal abrasions. Molten metals and other hot objects may result in globe perforation.

Radiation burns (ultraviolet keratitis) Ultraviolet light from sun lamps, tanning booths, high-altitude environments, or welder's arc results in direct corneal epithelial damage. After a latent period of 6 to 10 hours, patients develop a foreign body sensation, tearing, intense pain, photophobia, and blepharospasm.[14] Topical ophthalmic anesthetics facilitate physical examination. Examination reveals decreased visual acuity, injected conjunctiva, and diffuse punctate corneal lesions, often with a discrete lower border defining the cornea protected by the inferior lid. Treatment consists of a short-acting cycloplegic and a topical broad-spectrum antibiotic ointment. Eye patching may be used for patient comfort on the more affected eye. Oral narcotics are commonly needed. Patients should never be prescribed topical anesthetics because frequent use retards healing and can lead to corneal ulcer formation.[15] Patients should have ophthalmologic follow-up in 24 hours.

Mechanical corneal abrasions Patients complain of a foreign body sensation, pain, photophobia, and decrease in visual acuity. The degree of relief afforded by topical anesthesia can differentiate corneal injury from other causes of acute eye pain.[16] Physical examination reveals injected conjunctiva, decreased visual acuity if the defect is large or lies in the visual axis, and demonstration of the epithelial defect with slit-lamp examination using fluorescein (Figure 66-5). Foreign bodies of the lid conjunctiva must be identified. Treatment consists of cycloplegia, topical nonsteroidal antiinflammatory medications, and topical antibiotics. Contact lens patients should be treated with topical antibiotics with antipseudomonal coverage. Eye patching should be avoided, especially in injury involving vegetable matter or contact lens use. Data suggest that eye patching confers no benefit in healing small, uncomplicated corneal abrasions.[17,18] Patients with corneal abrasions should not wear their contact lenses. Oral pain medications may be needed. Patients should have ophthalmologic follow-up in 24 hours.

Corneal foreign bodies Patients with corneal foreign bodies experience pain, foreign body sensation, injected conjunctiva, tearing, and blepharospasm. Administration of a topical ophthalmic anesthetic facilitates physical examination. Diagnosis is made with slit-lamp examination (Figure 66-6). After a topical anesthetic is applied, the initial attempt at removing corneal foreign bodies should be with a stream of sterile saline solution. If this fails, the foreign body should be removed using a commercial eye spud or 25-gauge needle with a 1- to 3-ml syringe as a handle and magnification, generally the slit-lamp. The patient must be totally cooperative and the patient's head firmly stabilized within the slit-lamp.

Iron-containing corneal foreign bodies leave a residual rust ring (Figure 66-7). Removal of the rust ring should be left to the ophthalmologist at the 24-hour follow-up visit because the affected cornea gradually softens, and the rust migrates toward the corneal surface, making removal easier.

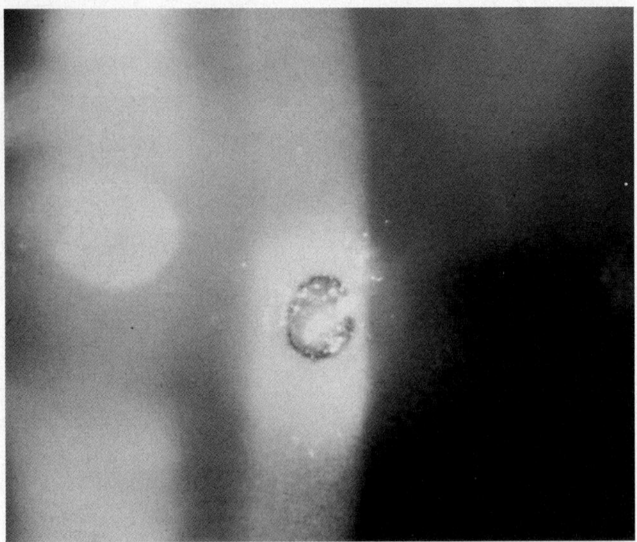

Figure 66-7. **Corneal rust ring after removal of iron-containing foreign body demonstrated by slit-lamp examination.**

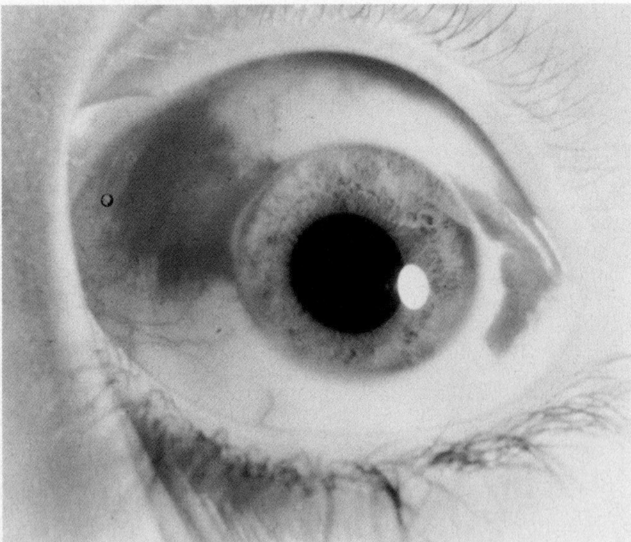

Figure 66-8. **Subconjunctival hemorrhage.**

Ophthalmologic consultation for corneal foreign bodies is recommended if a large area of the visual axis is involved, the object is deeply embedded within the cornea, the risk of perforation is increased for any reason, or there are multiple foreign bodies.

Treatment after foreign body removal is similar to that for corneal abrasion, with ophthalmologic follow-up within 24 hours.

Use of high-speed drills, saws, grinders, and pounding objects or involvement in explosions should alert the EP to the likelihood of an intraocular foreign body with perforation. Computed tomography (CT) can be used to rule out the diagnosis of an intraocular foreign body.

Conjunctival foreign body Conjunctival foreign bodies can be removed under topical anesthesia with a cotton-tipped applicator or fine forceps. Topical phenylephrine can be used to reduce the conjunctival bleeding.

Subconjunctival hemorrhage Rupture of small subconjunctival blood vessels is common and occurs as a result of trauma or Valsalva's maneuver, or without apparent cause. Patients complain of its appearance. Pain, diminished visual acuity, or photophobia suggests a more serious pathologic condition. Subconjunctival hemorrhage is flat, bright red, smooth, limited to the bulbar conjunctiva, and sharply demarcated at the limbus (Figure 66-8). Subconjunctival hemorrhage must be distinguished from bloody chemosis, which is indicative of more serious globe pathology. Bilateral or recurrent subconjunctival hemorrhage may require workup for bleeding diathesis. Treatment consists of local cold compresses for 24 hours, with resolution in 2 to 3 weeks.

Anterior Chamber and Iris

Clinical Features and Management

Traumatic hyphema Disruption of blood vessels in the iris or ciliary body results in hyphema. If the patient is sitting, the blood often layers and forms a meniscus with the aqueous humor. Hyphemas range from minimal blood seen only with the slit-lamp to the "eight ball," or total hyphema with blood that has clotted. Patients complain of pain, photophobia, and decreased visual acuity. The EP will see the blood directly or with the aid of the slit-lamp (Figure 66-9). There is generally no afferent pupillary defect present. Intraocular pressure may also rise.

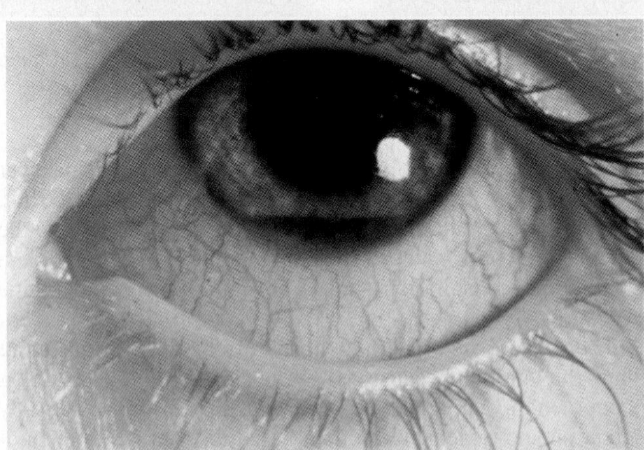

Figure 66-9. **Small hyphema layering out in the inferior portion of the anterior chamber.**

Management of hyphema must be individualized for a given patient. Selected low-grade hyphemas in reliable patients may be managed on an outpatient basis; all other patients should be admitted. General therapy includes elevating the bed 30 to 45 degrees, bed rest, and limiting eye movement such as reading.[11] Analgesics are appropriate, but have the patient avoid taking aspirin and other platelet inhibitors.[19] Antiemetics and sedatives should be used cautiously. Increased intraocular pressure occurs as a result of aqueous flow blockage from the blood present. In patients without sickle cell, initial treatment is a topical beta blocker; a topical alpha agonist or topical carbonic anhydrase inhibitor is added if needed. Oral acetazolamide or IV mannitol may also be used.

Specific treatment for hyphema with miotics, mydriatics, cycloplegics, steroids, and antifibrinolytics such as aminocaproic acid will vary depending on the specific clinical

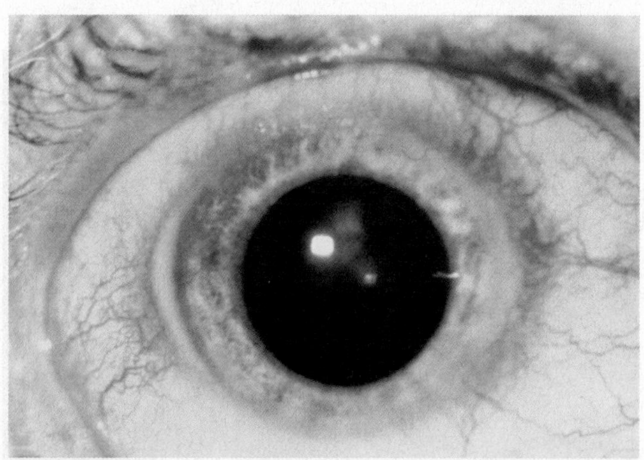

Figure 66-10. **Ciliary flush. Note that conjunctival injection is most prominent immediately around the limbus.**

situation, and is best left to the ophthalmologist.[11,20-22] Failure of medical therapy to control high intraocular pressure or for a large clot to resolve and corneal blood staining are indications for surgical intervention.[21] Case reports exist for the use of anterior chamber thrombolytics in those whose large clot fails to resolve.[19]

The major complication of hyphema is rebleeding, which occurs after 2 to 5 days when the initial clot retracts and loosens.[23] Rebleeding is more common in those with visual acuities of 20/200, initial hyphema covering more than one third of the anterior chamber, medical attention delayed more than 1 day after injury, and elevated intraocular pressure at the initial examination.[24] Other complications include corneal blood staining, acute or chronic glaucoma, and anterior or posterior synechia formation.

Patients with hemoglobinopathies (e.g., sickle cell disease, thalassemia) are at increased risk for hyphema complications. Red blood cells in the anterior chamber sickle in the relatively acidic and hypoxic environment,[25] which leads to decreased aqueous humor outflow and a rapid rise in intraocular pressure. Increased intraocular pressure in a sickle cell patient with a hyphema should be treated with topical beta blockers. All other antiglaucoma medications should be prescribed by an ophthalmologist only. If needed, methazolamide by mouth, and not acetazolamide, may be used.

Traumatic iridocyclitis Blunt injury of the globe may contuse and inflame the iris and ciliary body, resulting in ciliary spasm. Patients complain of photophobia and deep aching eye pain. Examination reveals perilimbal conjunctival injection (ciliary flush), cells and flare in the anterior chamber, and a small, poorly dilating pupil (Figure 66-10). These symptoms indicate white blood cells and protein as a result of the inflammation.

Treatment consists of paralyzing the iris and ciliary body with a long-acting cycloplegic agent, such as homatropine methylbromide 5%, given four times daily for 7 to 10 days.[26] Prednisolone acetate 1% may be given to help relieve the inflammation if there is no improvement after 5 to 7 days, but should be avoided in patients with a corneal epithelial defect. Resolution occurs within 1 week.

Traumatic mydriasis and miosis Blunt injury may result in either pupillary dilatation or constriction and may persist for days. For significant head trauma and altered mental status, a cranial nerve palsy must be ruled out before ascribing pupillary mydriasis to local contusion.

Permanent pupillary mydriasis may result from small radial tears in the pupillary sphincter muscle. The pupil margin may look irregular or scalloped. No specific ED treatment is warranted.

Iridodialysis Traumatic iridodialysis is a tearing of the iris root from the ciliary body, leading to the formation of a "secondary pupil." This injury often is the cause of a hyphema. If there is no associated hyphema present, no specific ED treatment is needed. Large tears can lead to monocular diplopia and may require surgical correction. Immediate ophthalmologic consultation is warranted when iridodialysis has caused a hyphema or a decrease in visual acuity.

Anterior chamber angle recession Blunt injury to the ciliary body may cause posterior displacement of the iris and surrounding tissues, deepening the anterior chamber, widening the anterior chamber angle, and causing potential damage to the trabecular meshwork that drains the aqueous humor. Severe damage can cause acute glaucoma.

Scleral and Lens Injuries

Clinical Features and Management

Cataract If the lens capsule is disrupted by either blunt or penetrating trauma, the relatively dehydrated stroma absorbs fluid, swells, and becomes cloudy. Acute glaucoma may develop from blockage of the aqueous humor flow through the pupil, necessitating surgical intervention. In less severe injury, cataract formation may occur over weeks to months.

Lens subluxation and dislocation Complete disruption of the lens zonule fibers from blunt trauma may result in anterior or posterior dislocation of the lens. Incomplete disruption of the lens zonule fibers results in subluxation of the lens. Lens dislocation may occur with minor trauma in patients with Marfan's syndrome, homocystinuria, tertiary syphilis, and other predisposing conditions. Patients complain of monocular diplopia or visual distortion with subluxation and marked visual blurring with dislocation. Examination reveals decreased visual acuity. The edge of a subluxated lens can be seen when the pupil is dilated. Iridodonesis is a trembling or shimmering of the iris after rapid eye movements and is a helpful sign of lens dislocation. Treatment ranges from observation to surgical removal and is dictated by the location of the dislocated lens and associated eye injury. Immediate ophthalmologic consultation is warranted.

Scleral rupture Blunt trauma causes scleral rupture by suddenly elevating intraocular pressure. Ruptures are most common at the insertions of the intraocular muscles or at the limbus, where the sclera is the thinnest.[27] The diagnosis of scleral rupture is obvious when intraocular contents are visualized; however, occult global rupture can be difficult to diagnose. Patients complain of eye pain and decreased vision. Examination may reveal a bloody chemosis or severe subconjunctival hemorrhage overlying the scleral rupture site. Uveal prolapse through the scleral wound, appearing as a brownish/black discoloration, can also be seen (Figure 66-11). Although a lower than normal intraocular pressure is

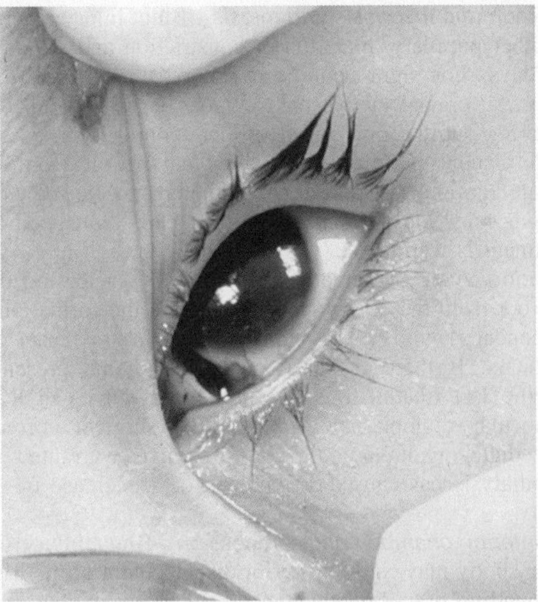

Figure 66-11. **Scleral laceration with penetrating globe injury. Note care being taken to not increase intraocular pressure with examiner's fingers.**

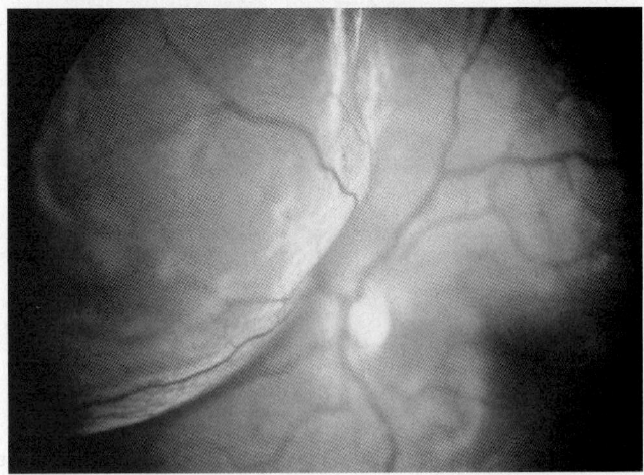

Figure 66-12. **Retinal detachment. Note large portion of retina billowing forward.**

a good indication of rupture, tonometry should never be performed in suspected globe rupture. Any maneuvers that increase intraocular pressure need to be avoided. A CT scan, ultrasonography, and indirect ophthalmoscopy all play a role in the diagnosis of occult globe rupture but may be left to the ophthalmologist.

Treatment in the ED for a known globe rupture includes avoidance of further examination or manipulation and the placement of a protective metal eye shield to prevent accidental pressure on the globe. The patient should be kept NPO, and a tetanus injection given as needed. Antiemetics should be given if the patient is nauseated. Broad-spectrum IV antibiotics should be instituted.[28]

Theoretical classic teaching states that the use of succinylcholine is contraindicated in the presence of a penetrating ocular injury due to the rise in intraocular pressure and potential for ocular extrusion. Increased intraocular pressure occurs 1 to 4 minutes after succinylcholine administration, and returns to baseline after 7 minutes.[29] The literature contains many conflicting studies on the efficacy of pretreatment with various agents including nondepolarizing muscle relaxants, gallamine, d-tubocurarine, diazepam, and others that reduce or attenuate the rise in intraocular pressure resulting from succinylcholine use.[29] However, one study reported on the use of succinylcholine after pretreatment with nondepolarizing agents in 100 patients with penetrating eye injury; no adverse events were found.[30] Given the need for rapid airway management in a patient with penetrating ocular injury, rapid sequence intubation with succinylcholine after pretreatment with nondepolarizing and sedative agents is appropriate.

Ophthalmologic consultation is required for all patients with suspected or proven globe rupture.

Posterior Segment Injuries

Clinical Features and Management

Vitreous hemorrhage Bleeding into the vitreous may occur from injuries to the retina and uveal tract and their associated vascular structures.

Patients complain of decreased visual acuity and "floaters." Floaters, described by the patient as dark dots or strands moving in their visual field in the direction of the preceding eye movement, are caused by vitreous blood.

There is a diminished red reflex and an inability to visualize the fundus clearly with the direct ophthalmoscope. With vitreous hemorrhage caused by blunt trauma, B scan ultrasonography is used to search for retinal injury and the need for operative repair.[31]

Treatment of vitreous hemorrhage includes elevating the head of the bed to allow for settling of the blood, avoiding platelet-inhibiting drugs and Valsalva's maneuver. Vitrectomy is performed for vitreous hemorrhage with an associated retinal detachment. Ophthalmologic consultation is warranted for acute traumatic vitreous hemorrhage.

Retinal injuries Blunt injury to the retina may result in hemorrhage, a tear or detachment, or commotio retinae.

Hemorrhage can occur in the preretinal (subhyaloid), superficial retinal, or deep (subretinal) spaces. Preretinal hemorrhage appears "boat shaped," superficial retinal hemorrhage "flame-shaped," and deep retinal as rounded and grape-purple in color.

Tears and detachments from blunt trauma are common. Symptoms include floaters from bleeding, "flashing lights" from stimulation of retinal neurons, and visual field cuts or decreased visual acuity. Retinal tears or detachments do not cause pain. Examination may reveal the hazy gray membrane of the retina billowing forward (Figure 66-12), but many tears are peripherally located and not seen with direct ophthalmoscopy. Visual acuity may be normal unless the macula is involved. Indirect ophthalmoscopy is warranted if historic clues to the presence of retinal tears are present.

Ophthalmologic consultation is warranted in all cases of suspected or proven retinal detachment. Treatment includes photocoagulation or operative repair; prognosis depends on the condition of the macula.

Commotio retinae occurs after recent ocular trauma. Patients may have decreased visual acuity or be asymptomatic. Examination reveals a cloudy whitening of the involved

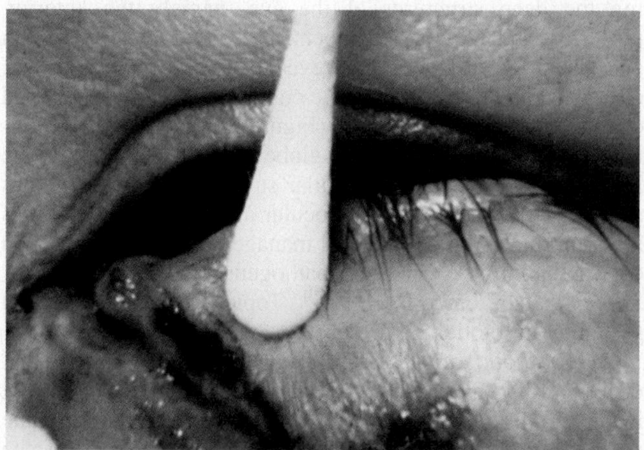

Figure 66-13. **Facial laceration near the medial canthus with involvement of the canaliculus.**

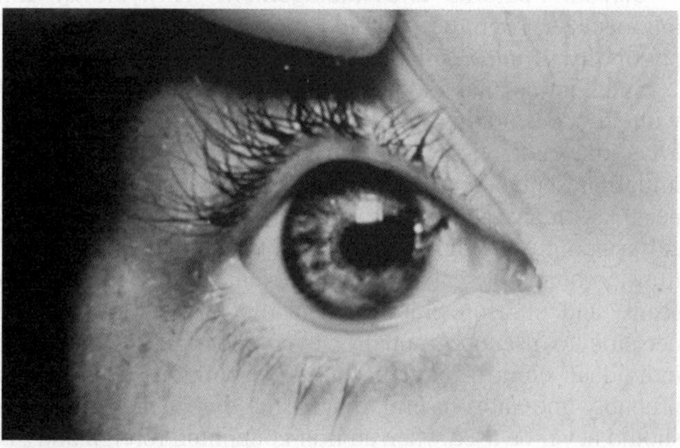

Figure 66-14. **Teardrop-shaped pupil demonstrating anterior chamber perforation through corneal laceration.**

area that will subside in a few weeks with no specific treatment. Serial follow-up is necessary to ensure that retinal tear or detachment has not occurred.

Optic nerve injury Significant blunt force to the orbital contents may avulse, transect, compress, or contuse the optic nerve. Fractures may extend into the orbital canal and cause optic nerve damage. Patients complain of visual field cuts or decreased visual acuity. Examination reveals an afferent pupillary defect, assorted visual field cuts, a decrease in visual acuity, or total blindness. The optic disc is normal initially, but pallor will eventually develop.[2] An orbital CT scan can help define the location and extent of injury. Management of traumatic optic neuropathy is controversial. High-dose methylprednisolone and surgical decompression have been used with varying degrees of success.[2] When edema or bleeding within the optic nerve is visualized, or with significant reduction in visual acuity, high-dose steroids can be used. Surgical decompression should be considered when decreasing visual acuity is occurring from a known orbital canal fracture.

Penetrating Trauma

Lacerations of the Eyelids

Clinical Features and Management Any laceration involving the eyelids should prompt a search for penetrating globe injury and, if indicated, a thorough search for a foreign body. Soft eye pads should be avoided to prevent increases in intraocular pressure.

Emergency physicians can manage simple horizontal or oblique partial-thickness lid lacerations. These can be closed primarily using 6-0 or 7-0 nylon interrupted sutures. Sutures should be removed in 3 to 5 days.

Several lid lacerations have a high likelihood of cosmetic or functional complications and should be managed by ophthalmologists or plastic surgeons skilled in this area. The following lid lacerations fall into the category of complex lid lacerations and need immediate referral.

1. Lacerations involving the lid margins
2. Lacerations involving the canalicular system. Injury to the canalicular system should be suspected in any laceration involving the medial lower eyelid area (Figure 66-13)
3. Lacerations involving the levator or canthal tendons
4. Laceration through the orbital septum. Orbital fat will protrude through septal lacerations into the wound. Because eyelids have no subcutaneous fat, the appearance of fat in a lid laceration confirms this diagnosis. These wounds are associated with a high incidence of globe penetration and intraorbital foreign bodies.
5. Lacerations with tissue loss

Conjunctival Lacerations

Clinical Features and Management Lacerations of the bulbar conjunctiva commonly have intraocular foreign bodies or underlying scleral perforation. Slit-lamp examination can distinguish superficial from deeper lacerations. Small, superficial lacerations require no suturing and heal quickly. Topical prophylactic ophthalmic antibiotics are advisable. Larger (> 1 cm) and deeper lacerations may require repair by an ophthalmologist.

Corneal and Scleral Lacerations

Clinical Features and Management

Corneal lacerations Signs of corneal perforation (full-thickness corneal lacerations) include loss of anterior chamber depth, teardrop-shaped pupil caused by iris prolapse through the corneal laceration, and blood in the anterior chamber (Figure 66-14). Small corneal lacerations can be difficult to diagnose. If aqueous humor is leaking from the corneal wound, it will appear as streaming fluorescent dye surrounded by an orange pool of solution on slit-lamp examination (Seidel test).[32] Full-thickness corneal lacerations are managed as described earlier for blunt traumatic globe rupture.

Superficial partial-thickness corneal lacerations without a widened wound can be treated with a cycloplegic, topical antibiotic and a pressure patch. Repairs of partial-thickness corneal lacerations requiring suture closure are performed in the operating room.

Scleral lacerations Penetrating scleral lacerations present with the signs and symptoms of blunt globe rupture. Globe perforation may be unrecognized in the absence of significant physical examination findings.

Orbital and Intraocular Foreign Bodies

Clinical Features and Management Any orbital and intraocular penetration should be approached with the possibility of intracranial injury.

Small intraocular and intraorbital foreign bodies can occur with any perforating injury and be difficult to diagnose. Physical examination of the eye may be completely normal at initial presentation. Occult foreign bodies should be suspected with any penetrating injury associated with mechanical grinding, sanding, drilling, and hammering. Plain orbital films, orbital CT scan, magnetic resonance imaging (MRI) scans, and ultrasonography aid in diagnosis. Although the decision to use one modality over another is dictated by individual clinical circumstances, an orbital CT scan is probably the most useful diagnostic tool. The MRI scan should never be used when an iron-containing foreign body is suspected.

Treatment of intraocular foreign bodies is dictated by clinical circumstances and is left to the ophthalmologist. Patients with acute intraocular foreign bodies should be hospitalized, made NPO, have a protective shield placed, and given antibiotics. Generally speaking, acute intraocular foreign bodies are surgically removed.[27] Plastic, glass, and many metals are relatively inert, and their nonacute removal is sometimes likely to cause more damage than their permanent presence. Organic foreign bodies are more important to remove because of their propensity for infection. Siderous oxidation of ocular tissues is a late complication of iron-containing intraocular foreign bodies that can lead to visual loss. Chalcosis, a sterile inflammatory reaction to copper-containing compounds, may occur, requiring removal of the offending object.

Complications of Ocular Trauma

Clinical Features and Management

Posttraumatic corneal ulcers Any defect in the corneal epithelium may become infected with bacteria or fungi. Ulcerations are surrounded by a cloudy white or gray appearing cornea (Figure 66-15). A reactive sterile hypopyon may be present in the anterior chamber. Emergent ophthalmologic consultation is needed. Treatment includes cycloplegia, topical antibiotics, and often admission to the hospital. Corneal perforation is a complication.

Endophthalmitis Endophthalmitis is an infection involving the deep structures of the eye, namely the anterior, posterior, and vitreous chambers. Patients complain of pain and visual loss. Examination reveals decreased visual acuity, chemosis, and hyperemia of the conjunctiva, and the infected chambers are hazy or opaque (Figure 66-16). Endophthalmitis is a complication of blunt globe rupture, penetrating eye injury, foreign bodies, and ocular surgery. Prompt diagnosis and early treatment with intraocular and systemic antibiotics are important in the successful management of posttraumatic endophthalmitis.[33] Common pathogens are *Staphylococcus, Streptococcus,* and *Bacillus.*[34] Topical, intravitreal, and systemic antibiotics all are used.

Sympathetic ophthalmia This is an inflammation that occurs in the uninjured eye weeks to months after the initial insult to the injured eye. It is thought to be an autoimmune response to the normally sequestered uveal tissues of the injured eye becoming exposed with injury. Patients have pain, photophobia, and decreased visual acuity. Treatment includes steroids and other immunosuppressive agents.[34] Enucleation of the blind injured eye can reduce symptoms even after the sympathetic ophthalmia has developed.

DISEASE OF THE CONJUNCTIVA

Clinical Features and Management

Conjunctivitis Conjunctivitis is an inflammation of the bulbar and palpebral conjunctiva caused by various viral, bacterial, mechanical, allergic, and toxic agents. When the cornea is also involved, it is known as keratoconjunctivitis. Multiple viral and bacterial pathogens are responsible for acute conjunctivitis. Adenovirus, Coxsackie, and enteroviruses have been isolated as causes of conjunctivitis. Common bacterial agents include *Streptococcus pneumoniae, Haemophilus influenzae, Staphylococcus* organisms, *Moraxella catarrhalis,* and *Neisseria gonorrhoeae.* Less common bacterial causes are *Klebsiella* and *Pseudomonas.*

Acute Bacterial Conjunctivitis Patients complain of pink eye, redness, a foreign body sensation, lid swelling, drainage, and eye crusting in the morning. Photophobia and visual loss are notably absent.

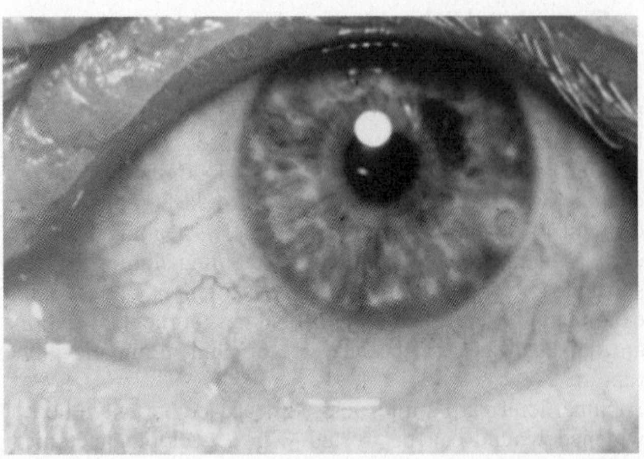

Figure 66-15. **Peripherally located corneal ulcer.**

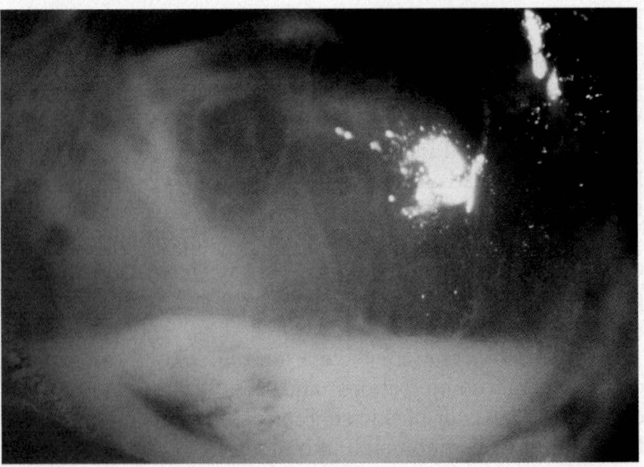

Figure 66-16. **Endophthalmitis resulting from globe rupture.**

Treatment of acute bacterial conjunctivitis includes warm compresses and topical ophthalmic antibiotics. In uncomplicated acute bacterial conjunctivitis, topical trimethoprim and polymyxin is a good initial selection.[35] Neomycin ophthalmic solutions should be avoided because of the high incidence of hypersensitivity reactions.[35] Medications should be continued for 7 days. Corticosteroids and eye patching should be avoided.

Cultures are indicated when symptoms are severe or when prior treatment has been inadequate or unsuccessful.[35] Complications of acute bacterial conjunctivitis include corneal ulcer formation, keratitis, and corneal perforation. Patients with complicated bacterial conjunctivitis should be referred to an ophthalmologist.

Acute bacterial infection caused by *N. gonorrhoeae* is uncommon but important because of its significant complications. Infection occurs from direct contact with individuals infected with urethritis or pelvic inflammatory disease. Signs and symptoms are markedly increased, including a copious purulent discharge. Gram's stain may reveal the diagnosis, although cultures are more sensitive.

Treatment is more aggressive than with other causes of bacterial conjunctivitis. Hospital admission for IV antibiotics, saline irrigation, and topical ophthalmic antibiotics is warranted in moderate and severe cases, and any patient with corneal involvement. Outpatient management may be done in selected mild cases with ceftriaxone 1 g intramuscularly (IM) as a single dose, topical erythromycin ointment, and saline solution irrigation of the conjunctiva.[35] A substantial proportion of patients will have concomitant *Chlamydia trachomatis* infection and should be treated with oral doxycycline, tetracycline, or erythromycin, or a single dose of 1 g azithromycin.[35]

Viral Conjunctivitis Viral infection is the most common cause of conjunctivitis. Viral conjunctivitis generally produces more redness, itching, eye irritation, and preauricular lymphadenopathy (Figure 66-17). It commonly occurs in the setting of other viral symptoms (e.g., fever, myalgias, malaise).

Viral conjunctivitis is very contagious for 10 to 12 days after onset and appropriate preventive measures should be taken. Treatment consists of artificial tears and cool compresses. A vasoconstrictor and antihistamine combination can be used if itching is severe.

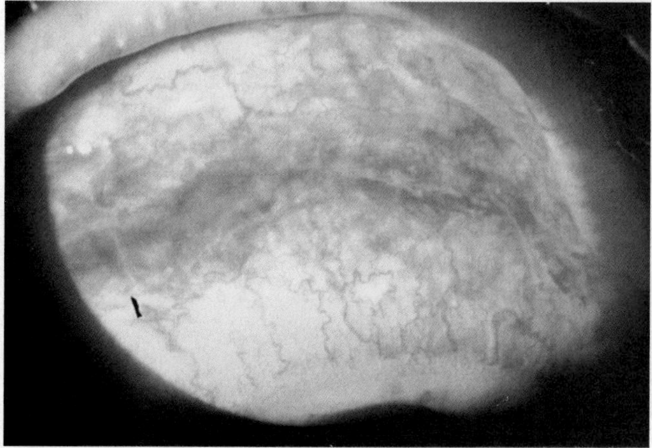

Figure 66-17. **Conjunctival injection from viral conjunctivitis.**

Ophthalmia Neonatorum Conjunctivitis that occurs within the first month of life is termed ophthalmia neonatorum and has several causes. A bacterial cause should be investigated with Gram's stain and cultures within the first 2 weeks of life. *N. gonorrhoeae* and *Chlamydia* are both transmitted from mother to infant via the birth canal.[35]

Infection with *N. gonorrhoeae* manifests within 2 to 4 days after birth. The infant should be carefully examined for evidence of systemic gonococcal infection. Hospitalization and blood and cerebrospinal fluid examination may be indicated. Nonsystemically infected neonates can be effectively treated with a single dose of ceftriaxone, 125 mg IM, topical polymyxin B/bacitracin ointment, and saline washes.[35] These patients should also be treated for ocular chlamydial infection. Close follow-up is needed.

Infants with chlamydial infection develop symptoms between 5 and 13 days after birth. Topical erythromycin ointment and oral erythromycin are the antibiotics used.[37] Treatment is for 14 days.

Chemical conjunctivitis from antibiotic ointment administration immediately after delivery occurs within 1 to 2 days of birth but should not be the diagnosis if the infant has significant symptoms, the time course is inappropriate, or other historic and physical examination parameters are not classic. In such cases, an assumption of a bacterial cause should be made.

In neonates with no information from stains or cultures and in whom an organism is not known or suspected, topical erythromycin ointment and oral erythromycin are utilized.

Miscellaneous Conjunctivitis Allergic conjunctivitis is common. Allergens include drugs, cosmetics, and environmental agents. Eye itching is generally more pronounced in patients with allergic conjunctivitis and tends to be bilateral. Artificial tears, cool compresses, combination topical ocular decongestants, topical vasoconstrictor/antihistamine combinations, and topical nonsteroidal agents may be used for treatment. Other causes of conjunctivitis include toxic conjunctivitis from topical ocular medications (aminoglycosides, antivirals, and preservatives), molluscum contagiosum, and chronic conjunctivitis.

DISEASE OF THE CORNEA

Differential Considerations

Clinical Features and Management

Pterygium/Pingueculum A pterygium is a wedge shaped area of conjunctival fibrovascular tissue that extends onto the cornea. A pinguecula is white or yellow, flat to slightly raised tissue on the conjunctiva, immediately next to but not on the cornea. Patients can be asymptomatic or present with irritation and redness. Treatment includes protection from wind, dust and sunlight, and artificial tears. An inflamed pinguecula can be treated with a short course of a topical nonsteroidal agent. Nonemergent referral to an ophthalmologist is recommended. Surgical removal is possible for selected individuals.

Superficial Punctate Keratitis These are superficial, multiple, pinpoint corneal epithelial defects. Patients present with pain, photophobia, redness, and a foreign body sensation. Superficial punctate keratitis is a nonspecific finding that is seen in many conditions. The most common precipitating conditions are ultraviolet burns (welders or sunlamps), conjunctivitis, topical eye drug toxicity (neomycin, gentamicin, drugs with preservatives including artificial tears), contact lens disorders, dry eye and exposure keratopathy, blepharitis, mild chemical injury, and minor trauma. Specific treatment is aimed at the underlying offending cause. Nonspecific treatment for a significant noncontact lens–associated superficial punctate keratitis includes nonpreserved artificial tears, topical antibiotics such as trimethoprim/polymyxin drops, and cycloplegia. Patients with a significant contact lens–associated superficial punctate keratitis should stop wearing their contact lenses, and be treated with a topical fluoroquinolone or tobramycin drops during the day, and ointment at night. Patients should receive ophthalmologic follow-up the next day.

Corneal Ulcers and Infiltrate from Infection Corneal infiltrates present as a focal white opacity without an epithelial defect. Corneal ulcers will have an overlying corneal epithelial defect that stains with fluorescein in addition to the corneal infiltrate. Patients present with pain, redness, photophobia, and decreased vision. The most common cause is bacterial, but fungal and herpes simplex infections are also possible. Patients should be immediately referred to an ophthalmologist for corneal culturing before treatment is initiated.

Herpes Simplex Infections Infection with herpes simplex may be either primary or reactivation of preexisting disease. Symptoms include foreign body sensation, tearing, photophobia, clear discharge, and decreased visual acuity. Physical examination reveals a red eye and may or may not include the classic herpetic vesicles located on the lids or conjunctiva. Corneal involvement is seen on slit-lamp examination, and may appear as a superficial punctate keratitis, ulcer, or the classic dendritic lesions (Figure 66-18). Treatment for epithelial keratitis consists of topical antiviral agents such as trifluridine 1% every 2 hours for 14 to 21 days.[38] Topical prophylactic antibiotics and cycloplegia are also employed. Topical steroids are contraindicated in corneal epithelial disease, but have proven to be beneficial in stromal disease.[38] Emergent ophthalmologic consultation is advised.

Herpes Zoster Infection Herpes zoster keratoconjunctivitis occurs as a result of activation of the virus along ophthalmic division of the trigeminal nerve. The rash follows dermatomal patterns, involves the forehead and upper eyelid, and produces significant pain. Involvement of the nasociliary nerve, manifested by zoster lesions on the tip of the nose (Hutchinson's sign), is associated with a 76% risk of ocular involvement versus 34% risk if the nerve is not involved.[39] Ophthalmic zoster mandates emergent ophthalmologic consultation. Treatment is complex, and depends upon the type, location, and degree of ocular involvement. Oral and topical antiviral and steroid agents as well as antibiotics are used.[36,40]

Contact Lens Complications The common complications of contact lens use involving the cornea include mechanical damage such as abrasions, corneal neovascularization, infections producing corneal ulcers, hypersensitivity or toxicity reactions to preservatives in solutions, and contact lens deposits. If no significant signs or symptoms exist that indicate corneal infection, the patient should discontinue contact lens use and follow up with his or her ophthalmologist. When corneal infection is present or suspected, immediate ophthalmologic consultation is indicated.

DISORDERS OF THE LIDS AND OCULAR SOFT TISSUES

Differential Considerations

Clinical Features and Management

Hordeolum/Chalazion Hordeolums and chalazions are localized, nodular, inflammatory processes of the eyelids. Symptoms and signs include pain, swelling, and redness (Figure 66-19). Spontaneous rupture may occur, and most resolve with warm compresses applied for 15 minutes 4 to 6 times each day. Topical antibiotics (erythromycin) may be used. Incision and drainage are indicated for chalazia unresponsive to conservative therapy.[41]

Dacryocystitis Dacryocystitis is an acute infection of the lacrimal sac from nasolacrimal duct obstruction. The most common organism is *S. aureus.* Symptoms and signs include pain, tenderness, swelling, and erythema over the lacrimal

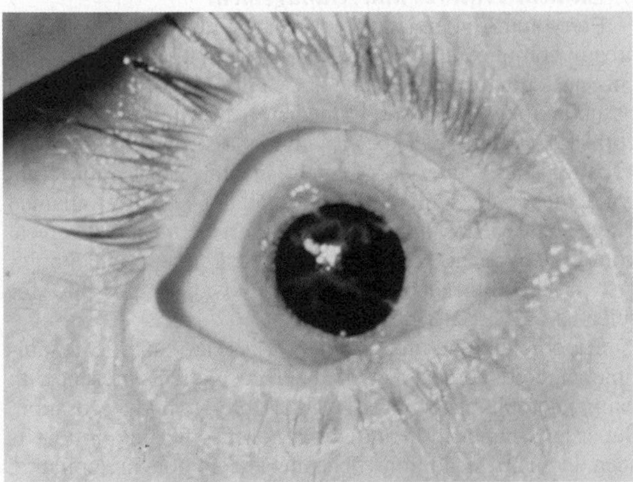

Figure 66-18. **Herpes simplex infection. Note typical dendritic pattern on cornea.**

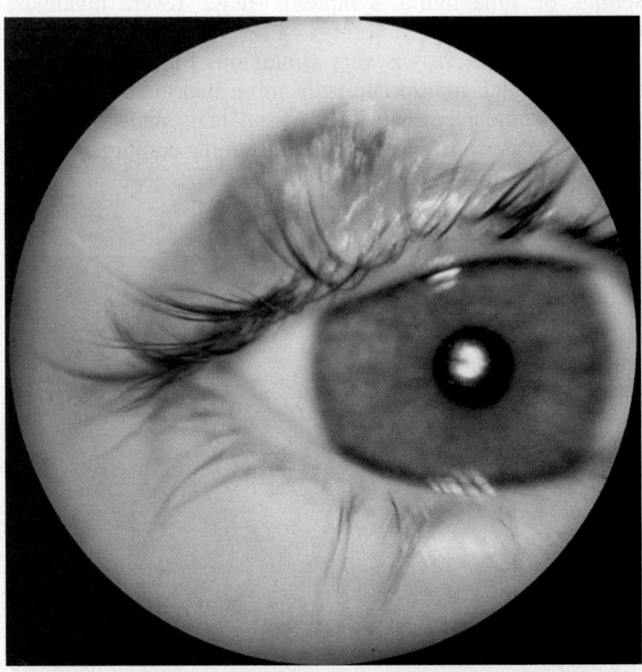

Figure 66-19. **Chalazion of the upper eyelid.**

sac (Figure 66-20). Pressure over the sac may express purulent material from the puncta. Treatment includes topical ocular and oral anti-*Staphylococcal* antibiotics and warm compresses. Gentle massage of the area during warm compress application may help decompress purulent material and relieve symptoms. Systemically ill patients should be hospitalized.

Blepharitis Patients present with thickened, mattered, red eyelid margins with pronounced blood vessels. Patients complain of burning, itching, tearing, foreign body sensation, and morning crusting of the eyelids. Treatment includes rubbing the eyelid margins with a mild shampoo using a cotton-tipped applicator or cloth twice per day, warm compresses, and artificial tears. Severe blepharitis can also be treated with topical antibiotic ointment applied at night.

Preseptal Cellulitis Patients present with lid erythema and warmth, tenderness, and swelling, and may have a low-grade fever. It is important to note the absence of findings associated with orbital (postseptal) cellulitis (i.e., proptosis, restriction of extraocular movements, pain with eye movement, and patient toxicity). If any of these findings are present, orbital cellulitis or abscess should be suspected and the patient managed more aggressively with imaging studies (CT scan of brain and orbits) and hospitalization. Preseptal cellulitis has a continuum of disease, and treatment is tailored for the degree of patient toxicity. Mild disease can be treated on an outpatient basis with oral antibiotics, but hospitalization with IV antibiotics may be needed for moderate to severe disease.

GLAUCOMA

Clinical Features and Management

Aqueous humor is produced by the ciliary processes. In addition to providing structural support to the eye, aqueous humor delivers oxygen and nutrients to the avascular lens and cornea, and removes their waste products. This fluid passes from the posterior chamber to the anterior chamber through the pupillary aperture. The aqueous humor is transported into the trabecular meshwork located at the anterior chamber angle formed by the junction of the root of the iris and the peripheral cornea. The trabecular meshwork serves as a one-way valve and filter for the aqueous humor into the canal of Schlemm, which in turn drains into episcleral veins.

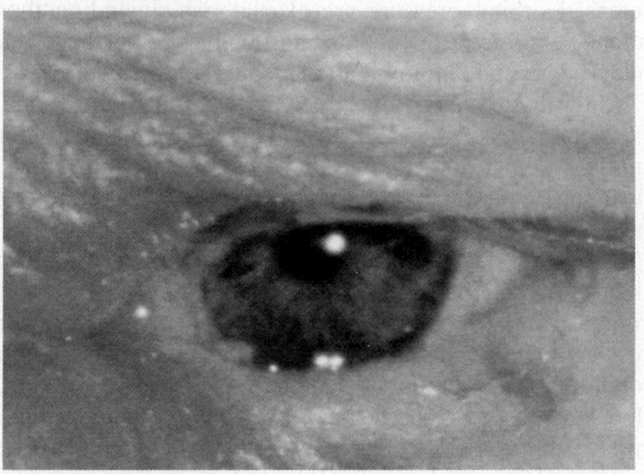

Figure 66-20. **Dacryocystitis.**

Intraocular pressure is determined by the rate of aqueous humor production relative to its outflow and removal. Normal intraocular pressure is between 10 and 20 mm Hg.[42]

Glaucoma is an optic neuropathy caused by increased intraocular pressure. Irreparable optic nerve damage can result. The simplest classification is to divide the glaucomas into primary or secondary, and open angle or closed angle. Secondary glaucoma is associated with another ocular or nonocular event, whereas primary glaucoma is not. Closed-angle glaucoma is caused when the anterior chamber angle is narrowed, reducing the outflow and removal of aqueous humor, whereas open-angle glaucoma occurs with a normal anterior chamber angle.

Patients vary in their susceptibility to a given level of intraocular pressure. Some may develop significant optic nerve findings despite a relatively low intraocular pressure (low-tension glaucoma), whereas others may have scant optic nerve changes despite relatively high intraocular pressure (ocular hypertension).[43]

Primary Open-Angle Glaucoma Primary open-angle glaucoma is the most common form of glaucoma and is a leading cause of blindness in the United States. There is increased resistance to aqueous humor outflow through the trabecular meshwork. Primary open-angle glaucoma is generally insidious, slowly progressive, chronic, bilateral, and painless. Advanced disease occurs before symptoms. Symptoms begin as visual field loss at the periphery that progresses centrally. Signs include an optic cup to optic nerve ratio of greater than 0.6.[44] Other findings include vertically oval, deep, and pale optic cups, with nasal displacement of blood vessels.

The three treatment options are medications, argon laser trabeculoplasty, and guarded filtration surgery. Initial treatment is generally with one or more topical agents. β Blockers, selective a2 receptor agonists, carbonic anhydrase inhibitors, prostaglandin agonists, miotics, and sympathomimetics are all used.

Topical ocular medications are absorbed and may produce significant systemic side effects.[45] Topical β blockers have produced asthma, heart block, congestive heart failure, hypoglycemia, and depression. Adrenergics have produced hypertension and cardiac dysrhythmias, whereas carbonic anhydrase inhibitors have produced renal calculi and hypokalemia. Complications may arise as a result of drug interaction. Prolonged apnea, for example, has resulted when succinylcholine has been given to a patient on topical ophthalmologic acetylcholinesterase inhibitors.[46]

Secondary Open-Angle Glaucoma Secondary open-angle glaucoma can have a number of causes, including lens induced, inflammatory, exfoliative, pigmentary, steroid induced, traumatic, angle recession, and ocular tumor.

Treatment is directed to the offending mechanism and includes the methods used for primary open-angle glaucoma.

Primary Angle Closure Glaucoma Primary angle closure glaucoma occurs in patients who have anatomically small and shallow anterior chambers. This anatomic variation results in the iris being nearly in contact with the lens, resulting in resistance to aqueous humor flow from the posterior to anterior chamber. This is called pupillary block.[47]

Attacks of primary angle closure glaucoma are precipitated by pupillary dilatation. Dimly lit rooms, emotional upset, and various anticholinergic and sympathomimetic medications are common precipitating events. The dilatation of the pupil increases the degree of pupillary block, leading to an accumulation of aqueous humor in the posterior chamber. The iris bulges forward, obliterating the angle between the cornea and iris, obstructing the trabecular meshwork, decreasing outflow, and leading to a rapid rise in intraocular pressure.[48]

A second, less common mechanism of acute angle closure glaucoma, produced without pupillary block, is caused by a flat or plateau iris. This leads to a narrow angle recess. Dilatation of the pupil causes the iris to fold and bunch over the angle, blocking aqueous humor outflow into the trabecular meshwork.

Symptoms are abrupt in onset, and include severe eye pain, blurred vision, headache, nausea, vomiting, and occasionally abdominal pain. Patients see a halo around lights. Signs include conjunctival injection and a cloudy (steamy) cornea with a mid to dilated pupil that is sluggish or fixed (Figure 66-21). Visual acuity may be significantly decreased, and intraocular pressures will be markedly elevated.

Treatment should begin promptly. If visual acuity is markedly reduced (hand movements or less), a combination of all topical glaucoma medications with intravenous osmotics and acetazolamide should be utilized.[36] Intraocular pressures < 50 mm Hg without significant visual acuity change can be managed without the intravenous medications.[36] Topically administered timolol 0.5% decreases intraocular pressure within 30 to 60 minutes.[49] Pilocarpine 1% to 2% is topically administered, one drop every 15 minutes for two doses, and one drop may be placed prophylactically in the unaffected eye. A topical A2-agonist (apraclonidine 1.0%) for one dose, and topical steroid (prednisolone acetate 1% every 15 minutes for four doses) should be given.[36] In the setting of a severe attack, acetazolamide, a carbonic anhydrase inhibitor, is given in an intravenous dose of 250 to 500 mg, and mannitol 1 to 2 mg/kg over 45 minutes.[50] Sedatives and antiemetics may be administered as needed. Ophthalmologic consultation is warranted.

The definitive therapy for primary angle closure glaucoma is surgical.

Secondary Angle Closure Glaucoma Pupillary block may develop from a swollen or dislocated lens, or posterior synechia (adhesions between the iris and lens). Secondary angle closure glaucoma, without pupillary block, can be caused by intraocular tumors, central retinal vein occlusion, or postoperatively. Treatment is directed at the offending cause.

ACUTE VISUAL LOSS

Differential Considerations

Acute visual loss, usually in only one eye, occurs over a period ranging from a few seconds to a day or two. The vision is generally reduced to 20/200 or worse. Patients need to be quickly evaluated to determine whether a treatable lesion exists. The differential diagnosis of acute visual loss not related to trauma includes vascular occlusion, retinal detachment, vitreous hemorrhage, macular disorders, neuroophthalmologic disease, and hysteria. Most of these patients

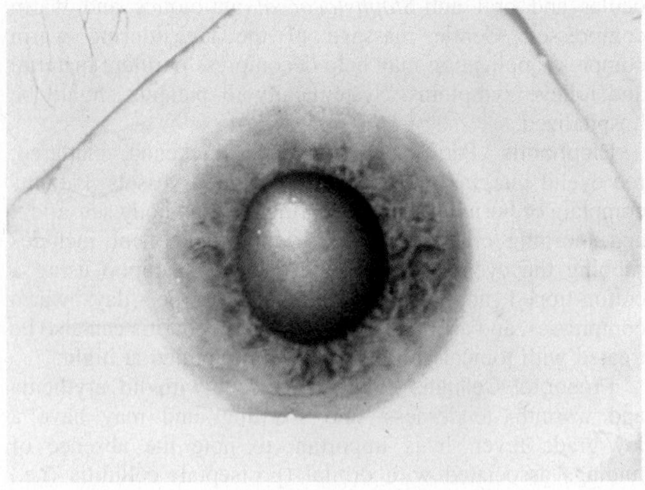

Figure 66-21. **Acute narrow-angle glaucoma. Note steamy appearance of cornea with a midpositioned and sluggish pupil.**

will need ophthalmic or neurologic referral for a complete workup.

Patients may complain of acute visual loss when they may have neither an acute process nor a visual loss caused by the eye itself. For example, a patient with a visual field cut secondary to a neuroophthalmologic lesion may have an acute visual loss when the patient discovers the field cut. A patient with a hemianopia usually will have normal visual acuity even though both eyes are affected. An accurate history about how the patient discovered the visual loss, as well as the timing of that loss, is vital.

Clinical Features and Management

Central Retinal Artery Occlusion Acute visual loss as a result of vascular occlusion of the central retinal artery is typically painless.

Central retinal artery occlusion causes an ischemic stroke of the retina. It occurs most commonly in those between 50 and 70 years of age, and 45% will have carotid artery disease.[51] Risk factors include hypertension, cardiac disease, diabetes, collagen vascular disease, vasculitis, cardiac valvular abnormality, and sickle cell disease. Patients with increased orbital pressure are also at risk, including those patients with acute glaucoma, retrobulbar hemorrhage, and endocrine exophthalmos. Patients complain of a severe loss of vision that develops over seconds. Examination reveals a markedly reduced visual acuity with a prominent afferent pupillary defect. On funduscopic examination, the retina is edematous with a pale gray-white appearance, and the fovea appears as a cherry-red spot (Figure 66-22).

Therapy should be instituted immediately and should be directed at dislodging the embolus, dilating the artery to promote forward blood flow, and reducing intraocular pressure to allow for an increase in perfusion gradient. Digital global massage should be begun immediately in the ED. Global massage is performed by applying direct digital pressure through closed eyelids. This pressure can be applied for 10 to 15 seconds, and followed by a sudden release.[52] Increases in P_{CO_2} lead to retinal artery vasodilation and

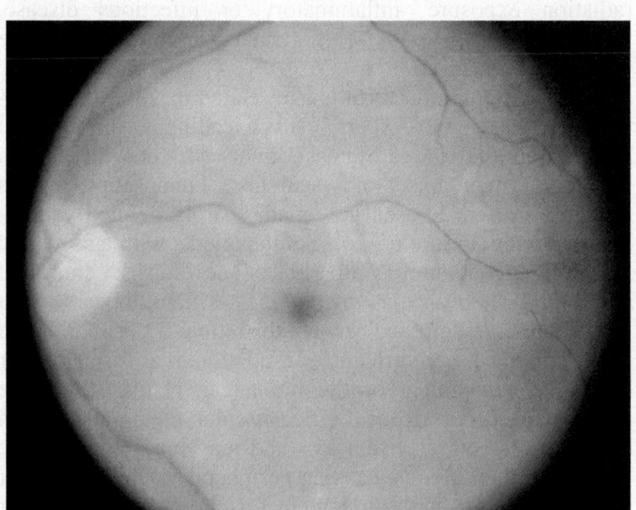

Figure 66-22. **Central retinal artery occlusion. Note cherry-red spot (fovea).**

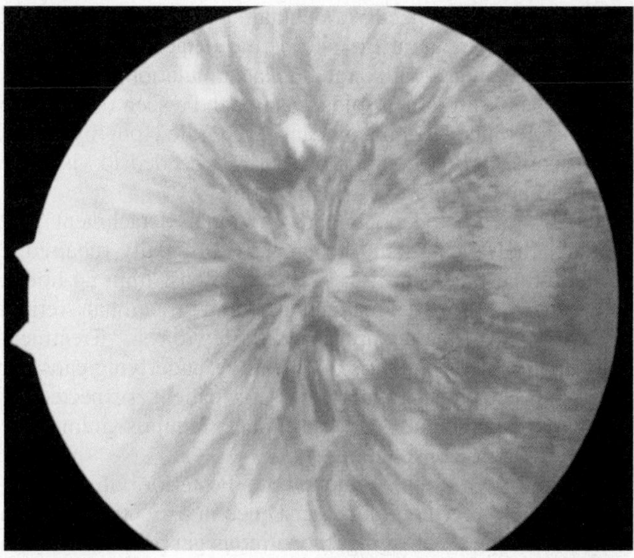

Figure 66-23. **Central retinal vein occlusion.**

increased retinal blood flow. Increases in P_{CO_2} are obtained by either rebreathing into a paper bag for 10 minutes each hour, or inhaling a 95% oxygen, 5% carbon dioxide mixture (carbogen). Intraocular pressure may be reduced by instilling timolol maleate 0.5% topically. Acetazolamide, 500 mg IV or by mouth will lower intraocular pressure as well as increase retinal blood flow.[53] Emergent ophthalmologic consultation should be obtained as anterior chamber paracentesis may be attempted. A recent study, however, failed to find any therapeutic benefit for patients who received anterior chamber paracentesis and inhaled carbogen.[54] Thrombolytic agents have been studied, but no clear guidelines for their use exist.[52] A complete medical evaluation is necessary since central retinal artery occlusion is usually an embolic event.

Central Retinal Vein Occlusion A painless loss of vision, central retinal vein occlusion leads to edema, hemorrhage, and vascular leakage. The wide spectrum of clinical appearances depends on the degree of venous obstruction present. Loss of vision can range from minimal to recognition of hand motion only. There are two types of central retinal vein occlusion, ischemic and nonischemic. The nonischemic type shows mild fundus changes and will not have an afferent pupillary defect. These patients tend to have less severe visual loss, with two thirds of the patients having 20/40 or better visual acuity without therapy.[55] Patients with ischemic central retinal vein occlusion have a marked decrease in visual acuity and often an afferent pupillary defect. Appearance can vary but classically includes dilated and tortuous veins, retinal hemorrhages, and disc edema (Figure 66-23). Branch retinal vein occlusions occur just distal to an arteriovenous crossing, and hemorrhages occur distal to the site of occlusion. The differential diagnosis of central retinal vein occlusion includes hypertension, diabetes mellitus, hyperviscosity syndromes, and papilledema. All of these are bilateral processes, whereas central retinal vein occlusion is generally unilateral. Neovascular glaucoma is the major complication of ischemic central retinal vein occlusion. Treatment is complex, and includes lowering of intraocular pressure, topical steroids, cyclocryotherapy, and photocoagulation.[55,56] Underlying medical disease should be managed as well. The prognosis depends on the degree of obstruction and resultant complications.

Retinal Breaks and Detachment The retina has two layers: the inner neuronal retina layer and the outer retinal pigment epithelial layer, which can be separated by fluid accumulation.

A retinal break is a tear in the retinal membranes and may or may not lead to retinal detachment. Retinal detachments occur by three mechanisms: rhegmatogenous, exudative, and tractional. Rhegmatogenous retinal detachment occurs as a result of a tear or hole in the neuronal layer, causing fluid from the vitreous cavity to leak between and separate the two retinal layers. Rhegmatogenous retinal detachment generally occurs in patients more than 45 years of age, is more common in men than women, and is associated with degenerative myopia.[57] Trauma may be associated with rhegmatogenous detachment by causing tears in the retina or by causing a disinsertion of the retina from its attachment at the ora serrata anteriorly. Traumatic retinal detachment can occur at any age. There is greater risk with severe myopia.

Exudative retinal detachment occurs as a result of fluid or blood leakage from vessels within the retina. Conditions leading to exudative retinal detachment include hypertension, toxemia of pregnancy, central retinal venous occlusion, glomerulonephritis, papilledema, vasculitis, and choroidal tumor.

Traction retinal detachment is a consequence of fibrous band formation in the vitreous and contraction of these bands. These fibrous bands result from the organization of inflammatory exudates or blood from prior vitreous hemorrhage.

Typically, patients complain of flashes of light related to the traction on the retina, floaters related to vitreal blood or pigmented debris, and visual loss. The visual loss is commonly described as a filmy, cloudy, or curtainlike appearance. Pain is absent. Visual acuity can be minimally changed to severely decreased. Visual field cuts relate to the location of the retinal detachment, and an afferent pupillary defect occurs if the detachment is large enough. When the detachment is visualized via ophthalmoscopy, the retina will appear out of focus at the site of the detachment. In large retinal detachments with large fluid accumulation, the bullous detachment, with retinal folds, easily can be seen (see Figure 66-12). Retinal detachment cannot be ruled out by direct funduscopy. Indirect ophthalmoscopy is needed to visualize the more anterior portions of the retina.

Acute rhegmatogenous and tractional detachment that threaten the fovea should be urgently surgically repaired.[36] Acute retinal breaks are surgically repaired within 24 hours. All other acute rhegmatogenous and tractional retinal detachments can be repaired within a few days.[36] Treatment of exudative detachment is aimed at the underlying cause or use of laser photocoagulation. Any patient suspected of having retinal break or detachment requires immediate ophthalmologic consultation.

Posterior Vitreous Detachment Posterior vitreous detachment is a very common occurrence in patients more than 60 years of age. With aging, the vitreous gel pulls away from the retina; this can lead to symptoms similar to retinal break, vitreous hemorrhage, and retinal detachment. No specific treatment is indicated for posterior vitreous detachment unless it is accompanied by a retinal break, vitreous hemorrhage, or retinal detachment.[36] Patients with a new posterior vitreous detachment should have prompt evaluation by an ophthalmologist to rule out these surgically amenable complications.

Vitreous Hemorrhage Vitreous hemorrhage results from bleeding into the preretinal space or into the vitreous cavity. The most common causes are diabetic retinopathy and retinal tears. Additional causes include neovascularization associated with branch vein occlusion, sickle cell disease, retinal detachment, posterior vitreous detachment, trauma, age-related macular degeneration, retinal artery microaneurysms, trauma, and intraocular tumor. Symptoms begin with floaters or "cobwebs" in the vision and may progress over a few hours to severe visual loss without pain. Direct ophthalmoscopy reveals a reddish haze in mild cases to a black reflex in severe cases. Details of the fundus are usually difficult to visualize. Vitreous hemorrhage by itself will not cause an afferent pupillary defect, which, if present, indicates a retinal detachment behind the vitreous hemorrhage. The hemorrhage may be evenly distributed throughout the vitreous or focal. Long-standing preretinal hemorrhage can become a white mass that may be misdiagnosed as a tumor, exudate, or infection. Initial therapy consists of bed rest with elevation of the head of the bed, and avoidance of anticoagulative medications. Definitive therapy is targeted at the underlying cause. Vascular retinopathy is treated with laser photocoagulation or cryotherapy, and retinal tears and detachments are repaired. If the cause of the hemorrhage is unknown, then prompt diagnostic work up is indicated to look for surgically correctable lesions. Ultrasonography can be used to determine whether a retinal detachment is present and may also determine the cause.[58] Vitrectomy is indicated in certain patients.

Macular Disorders Many disease processes cause acute changes in the macula leading to acute visual loss. The role of the EP is to recognize the maculopathy and refer the patient to an ophthalmologist. Keys to the diagnosis of macular dysfunction include loss of central vision with preservation of peripheral vision, complaints of central visual distortion, and anatomic changes in the retina.

Degenerative maculopathies occur as the result of trauma, radiation exposure, inflammatory or infectious disease, vascular disease, toxins, or hereditary disease, or may be idiopathic in nature.

The most common form is age related macular degeneration after the age of 65 years.[59] It is a leading reason for legal blindness in the United States. Patients present with either a gradual or rapid onset of visual loss. Funduscopy reveals scattered drusen. Drusen are small, sharply defined yellow-white masses (Figure 66-24). Some patients with age-related macular degeneration and drusen develop a choroidal (subretinal) neovascular membrane, which appears as a grayish-green membrane beneath the retina. If this membrane is left untreated, hemorrhage, transudation, scar formation, or exudative detachment of the retina can result. If a large hemorrhage occurs from the neovascular membrane, it can cause severe central visual loss and may break through the retina into the vitreous, causing peripheral visual loss. Laser photocoagulation is the treatment for choroidal neovascular membrane formation and should be performed as soon as possible.[59]

Inflammatory processes involving the retina may also cause visual loss, especially if the macula is involved. Bacterial, viral, and protozoal agents have been shown to cause maculopathy. The presenting symptoms and signs vary according to the disease process and severity. Inflammatory debris from exudative processes may fill the vitreous, leading to a cloudy appearance. Infections within the eye are often associated with severe pain, redness, and periocular edema. If the retina and choroid are obliterated, the lesions will appear white. Patients suspected of having an inflammatory maculopathy need emergent consultation and thorough medical evaluation.

Neuroophthalmologic Visual Loss Visual loss not readily explained by an obvious abnormality on physical examination is called neuroophthalmologic visual loss. Patients can be divided into those who complain of decreased vision and have a reduced visual acuity, and those patients who complain of visual loss, but have a normal visual acuity. It is imperative to conduct careful visual field testing in this latter group.

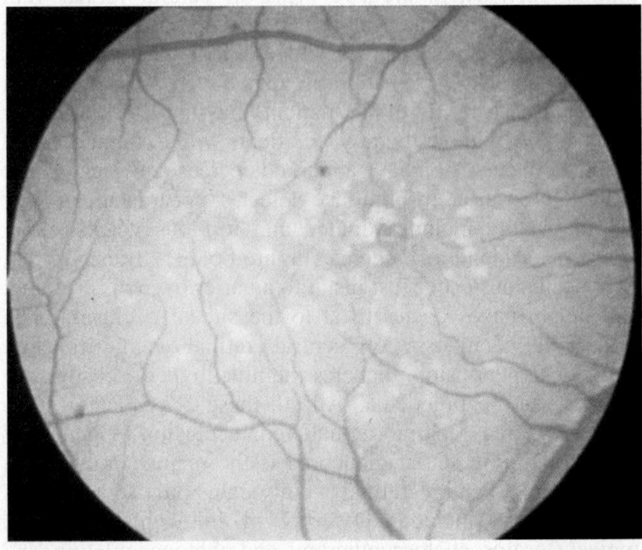

Figure 66-24. **Drusen occurring in macular degeneration.**

Neuroophthalmologic visual loss can be further divided into prechiasmal, chiasmal, or postchiasmal anatomic areas.

Prechiasmal visual loss Patients with prechiasmal disease have decreased visual acuity or visual field loss in the eye on the affected side. Prechiasmal disease may be a unilateral or bilateral process. The swinging flashlight test will reveal an afferent pupillary defect on the side involved, unless the process is bilateral. In such cases, the relative degree of afferent defect will determine the results. Visual field testing demonstrates a field defect that does not respect the vertical meridian and is often localized to the center of the visual field. Causes of prechiasmal visual loss include optic neuritis, ischemic optic neuritis, compressive optic neuritis, and toxic and metabolic optic neuritis.

Optic neuritis Optic neuritis is an acute monocular loss of vision caused by focal demyelination of the optic nerve. The patient's age ranges from 15 to 45 years. Symptoms include a progressive loss of vision over several hours or days and ocular pain with eye movement. Visual acuity can range from minimal loss to no light perception. An afferent pupillary defect is always present, and direct ophthalmoscopic examination reveals a normal or swollen disc.[60] The natural history of optic neuritis is for visual acuity to reach its poorest within 1 week, and then slowly improve over the next several weeks. Approximately 30% of patients presenting with acute optic neuritis will develop multiple sclerosis within 5 years.[61] In an initial study of patients with acute optic neuritis, treatment with a 3-day course of IV methylprednisolone reduced the rate of development of multiple sclerosis over a 2-year period.[62] However, 5-year follow-up of this same patient cohort revealed no significant differences among treatment groups in the development of multiple sclerosis.[61] Use of oral steroids for hastening optic neuritis is controversial. The Optic Neuritis Study Group had shown an increased risk of optic neuritis recurrences in those patients treated with oral prednisone.[61,62] However, a recent randomized and controlled study of high-dose oral methylprednisolone in acute optic neuritis showed improved recovery from optic neuritis at 1 and 3 weeks, but no effect at 8 weeks or on subsequent attack frequency.[63] Long-term visual outcome is no different than observation alone.

Ischemic optic neuropathy Ischemic optic neuropathy (ION) is the most common cause of optic neuropathy and one of the most common causes of visual loss past middle age. ION can be giant cell arteritis or idiopathic. Temporal arteritis (giant cell arteritis) is characterized by weight loss, malaise, jaw pain, headache, scalp tenderness, polymyalgia rheumatica, low-grade fever, and severe painless visual loss. It is extremely rare in people younger than 50 years of age, but the incidence rises with each subsequent decade. A significant proportion of patients will sustain visual loss, which can be sudden, severe, and bilateral.[64] Occasionally, visual loss will be preceded by episodes of amaurosis fugax. In one series of patients, visual loss was unilateral in 46%, sequential in 37%, and simultaneously bilateral in 17%.[65] There is a large afferent pupillary defect, visual loss, and a visual field defect that may respect the horizontal meridian. The optic disc has pallor and swelling. The diagnosis can be aided with an elevated erythrocyte sedimentation rate (ESR), but can be seen with normal sedimentation rates.[66] A guide to the upper limit of normal ESR is age/2 for men and (age+10)/2 for women.[36] The diagnosis is confirmed by temporal artery biopsy, although biopsy has been normal early in the disease. Treatment for temporal arteritis should be instituted when typical signs and symptoms, particularly visual loss, exist. The standard treatment is high-dosage corticosteroids, which should be started as soon as the diagnosis is suspected. Treatment should not wait for biopsy results. Biopsy should be performed within 1 week of diagnosis. Patients treated with oral prednisone are less likely to have visual improvement and more likely to develop fellow eye involvement when compared to high-dose IV methylprednisolone.[65] Patients with visual loss have a 34% chance of improvement with IV methylprednisolone.[65]

Nonarteritic ischemic optic neuropathy Nonarteritic ischemic optic neuropathy is much more common than temporal arteritis. These patients lack the classic symptoms of temporal arteritis and do not have an elevated ESR. Most of these patients will have systemic vascular disease, diabetes, or hypertension, and they tend to be younger. They have painless visual loss, afferent pupillary defects, disc swelling, and visual field defects that respect the horizontal meridian. The visual loss is less severe than with temporal arteritis, and improvement occurs in one third of patients. Steroids have been advocated, but the results are unclear. If there is any doubt about whether a particular patient has temporal arteritis or an idiopathic form of ischemic optic neuropathy, treatment with steroids should be started until a temporal artery biopsy is performed.

Compressive optic neuropathy Compressive optic neuropathy occurs at any age and can be caused by tumor, aneurysm, sphenoid sinusitis or mucocele, blunt trauma, and thyroid disorders. Although defined as a prechiasmal disorder, compression can occasionally occur far enough posteriorly to affect the optic chiasm. Patients with compressive optic neuropathy have visual loss that continues to progress beyond 7 days. Compressive optic neuropathies require neuroradiographic evaluation and rapid medical and surgical intervention. Optic neuritis can be difficult to distinguish from a compressive optic neuropathy, but compressive syndromes tend to involve other cranial nerves. If the signs and symptoms do not closely fit optic neuritis or ischemic optic neuropathy, a compressive lesion exists until proven otherwise.

Toxic and metabolic optic neuropathy A large number of toxic and metabolic neuropathies exists. Common toxic causes include barbiturates, chloramphenicol, emetine, ethambutol, ethylene glycol, isoniazid, heavy metals, and methanol. Causes of metabolic optic neuropathies include thiamine deficiency and pernicious anemia. These processes are bilateral, progressive, and symmetric. Visual loss can be severe, and visual field testing reveals central defects. Treatment is aimed at the underlying toxin or metabolite involved.

Chiasmal visual loss Chiasmal disease is the second category of neuroophthalmologic visual loss, most commonly caused by chiasmal compression from pituitary tumors, craniopharyngioma, or meningioma. Visual loss is gradual and progressive. Although formal visual field testing is necessary to stage the patient, the diagnosis usually can be made by confrontation visual field testing. The classic defect is a bitemporal hemianopsia; however, tumors often compress the optic chiasm and optic nerves asymmetrically, resulting in combined central and temporal defects. Any time a visual field defect respects the vertical meridian from a neuroophthalmologic visual loss, the lesion is out of the globe and must be either chiasmal or postchiasmal.

Postchiasmal visual loss Postchiasmal disease represents the third category of neuroophthalmologic visual loss. The most common causes are infarction, tumor, arteriovenous malformation, and migraine disorders. Patients complain of difficulty in performing a certain task, such as reading. Lesions can be located from the immediate postchiasmal optic tract to the occipital cortex. The classic visual field defect is homonymous hemianopsia. Patients with such lesions have a focal neurologic deficit and need neurologic consultation. Cortical blindness is a special cause of neuroophthalmologic visual loss that is most commonly caused by bilateral occipital infarction. Cortical blindness often is mistaken for functional blindness because patients will have both normal funduscopic examinations and intact pupillary reflexes. Anton's syndrome is characterized by bilateral blindness, normal pupillary reflexes, bilateral occipital lesions, and interestingly, denial of blindness. It is this denial of blindness that may be incorrectly assumed to be evidence for a functional process.

Functional visual loss Patients with functional visual loss fall into two categories: hysterical conversion reactions and malingering. Patients with hysterical conversion reactions have a nondeliberate, imagined visual loss. The patient will have a flatter affect than one would expect under the circumstances of acute visual loss. The patient might appear completely unaffected emotionally by the acute visual loss. The malingerer, on the other hand, is a patient who is well aware that no visual loss exists, yet deliberately feigns visual loss for secondary gain. This patient typically will be overemotional concerning the visual loss.

Examination of a patient with a suspected functional visual loss should be conducted in the exact manner as every other ophthalmologic examination, with particular attention paid to possible neuroophthalmologic deficits. Normal pupillary reflexes and the absence of an afferent pupillary defect, together with a normal funduscopic examination, point toward functional visual loss. Multiple tests can ascertain whether a visual loss is organic or functional. Patients with feigned visual loss will be hesitant to try to appose the index fingers of each hand and will often write their names in a disorderly fashion, whereas genuinely blind patients will be able to sign their name without difficulty. One effective test involves placing a large mirror directly in front of the patient's face, and asking the patient to look straight ahead. The mirror is then tilted slightly back and forth. Most patients will follow the reflection of their eyes in the mirror as it changes position, proving feigned visual loss. Some difficult cases require more sophisticated tests. If the diagnosis of feigned visual loss cannot be definitively made, consultation is required to rule out neuroophthalmologic visual loss.

ANISOCORIA

Clinical Features

Anisocoria in a patient with head trauma or decreased level of consciousness demands immediate and aggressive intervention. If a patient is awake and alert, has no signs of trauma, and has anisocoria of unknown cause, the first step is determining which pupil is abnormal. If one pupil constricts poorly to a light stimulus, it is likely to be the abnormal one. Anisocoria greater in dark suggests the abnormal pupil is the smaller pupil, whereas anisocoria greater in light suggests the abnormal pupil is the larger pupil. If anisocoria exists in a patient with a normal afferent visual system, either an innervational or structural defect in the iris sphincter exists. Most structural defects in the iris can be diagnosed by slit-lamp examination. If both pupils react well to light and no iris abnormalities are seen with slit-lamp examination, the next step is to determine whether the anisocoria increases in light or darkness. Adie tonic pupil, pharmacologic blockade, and third-nerve palsy will have anisocoria that increases in light, whereas benign anisocoria and Horner's syndrome will have anisocoria that increases in darkness.[36] Comparing pupillary size in a brightly and dimly lit room is the easiest method to evaluate the effect of lighting on anisocoria.

Adie Tonic Pupil With Adie tonic pupil, patients complain of blurred near vision but have normal distant vision. Adie syndrome is seen in young women 70% of the time and has associated symmetrically reduced deep tendon reflexes. Examination reveals poor accommodation with a very slow constriction to near testing. The pupil will redilate slowly when the vision is again made distant. Slit-lamp examination reveals sector palsies of the iris. The diagnosis is confirmed when a weak cholinergic agent (pilocarpine 0.1%) causes an intense pupillary constriction as a result of cholinergic supersensitivity in the affected pupil compared to the normal pupil. These patients need to be referred to an ophthalmologist on a nonemergent basis for cholinergic agent therapy.

Pharmacologic Mydriasis Pharmacologic mydriasis can be caused by the deliberate or inadvertent local administration of both sympathomimetic and parasympatholytic agents. Phenylephrine and cocaine are two sympathomimetic substances commonly used as a nasal premedicant for nasotracheal intubation; careless administration may lead to anisocoria. Parasympatholytic agents, such as atropine and scopolamine, have been implicated in the development of anisocoria. The transdermal scopolamine patches placed for the prevention of motion sickness can cause anisocoria. Pilocarpine 1.0% can be used in special circumstances to help differentiate a third-nerve palsy from pharmacologically mediated mydriasis. The administration of pilocarpine 1.0% will rapidly constrict the pupil that is dilated secondary to a third-nerve palsy, but will not produce miosis in a pupil dilated from anticholinergic agents.

Third-Nerve Palsy Patients with anisocoria that increases in light, without evidence of Adie tonic pupil or pharmacologic medication, should be suspected of having a third-nerve palsy. They almost always have other signs of third nerve involvement, including ptosis and extraocular muscle dysfunction. Patients will complain of diplopia, and the involved eye will be turned down and out. Patients may have ptosis and extraocular dysfunction with or without pupil dilatation. Any patient who has a new onset third-nerve lesion involving the pupil should be admitted to the hospital to rule out aneurysm.

Horner's Syndrome Horner's syndrome consists of ptosis, miosis, and facial anhydrosis resulting from an interruption of sympathetic innervation. The dilatation lag, a classic finding, results from the Horner's pupil requiring up to 15 seconds to fully dilate. The anisocoria will be greater at 3 to 5 seconds of darkness than at 15 seconds of darkness, although the anisocoria will still be more pronounced than in light. Topical ophthalmologic cocaine 10% can be used to aid the diagnosis. A Horner's pupil will dilate less than the normal pupil in reaction to topical cocaine. Central nervous system strokes and tumors, lung carcinomas, thyroid adenomas, Pancoast tumors, headache syndrome, carotid dissection, herpes zoster, otitis media, and congenital Horner's syndrome (trauma during delivery) are all causes of Horner's syndrome. Hydroxyamphetamine 1% administered 24 hours after the cocaine test can be used to determine the level of sympathetic interruption, and dictate the type of workup indicated. In general, patients with new onset Horner's syndrome should receive a thorough and immediate workup to determine the etiology.

Physiologic Anisocoria Twenty percent of the population may have anisocoria of greater than 0.4 mm at any given examination.[67] This anisocoria may be transient or prolonged and may alternate pupils. Although the anisocoria increases in darkness, there is no dilatation lag as seen with Horner's syndrome.

ABNORMAL OPTIC DISC

Clinical Features and Differential Considerations

An important acquired cause for an abnormal optic disc is papilledema. Papilledema refers to the changes in the optic disc from increased intracranial pressure. Causes include intracranial tumor, pseudotumor cerebri, intracranial hematomas from trauma, subarachnoid hemorrhage, brain abscess, and meningitis or encephalitis. There is swelling of the optic disc and blurring of the disc margins, hyperemia, and loss of physiologic cupping. Flame-shaped hemorrhages and yellow exudates appear near the disc margins as the edema progresses. Patients may have significant headaches or be completely asymptomatic. Visual acuity is not affected until the papilledema is longstanding. Brief obscurations of vision, enlargement of the physiologic blind spot, and inferior nasal visual field loss are common. Papilledema is a bilateral process, but may be asymmetric. Any patient with newly diagnosed papilledema should be admitted to the hospital for immediate neuroradiographic evaluation.

There are many conditions that may mimic papilledema, including central retinal vein occlusion, papillitis, hypertensive retinopathy, ischemic optic neuropathy, optic disc vasculitis, and diabetic papillitis with retinopathy.

NYSTAGMUS

Clinical Features and Differential Considerations

Clinically significant nystagmus is an oscillation of the eyes that occurs within 30 degrees of the midline. Pendular nystagmus is of equal velocity in both directions. With jerk nystagmus, the velocity is faster in one direction. The pathologic component is the slow movement, but the nystagmus is named according to the direction of the fast component. Nystagmus can also be divided into monocular or binocular, conjugate (both eyes moving in the same direction) or disconjugate (eyes moving in opposite directions), and primary gaze position or gaze position nystagmus. Important questions include the presence of tinnitus, nausea, vomiting, oscillopsia, and vertigo.

Congenital nystagmus is noted at birth or within the perinatal period and is usually horizontal, conjugate, bilateral, symmetric, and pendular. On lateral gaze, this nystagmus may become jerky in nature but remains horizontal despite upward or downward gaze. Congenital nystagmus is damped by convergence, increased with fixation, accentuated by covering one eye, and abolished with sleep. These patients do not have oscillopsia, nor do they have other neurologic complaints. Almost all of these patients will have recognized their nystagmus previously, and the diagnosis is generally straightforward.

There are many causes of acquired nystagmus. General categories of disease that result in nystagmus include toxic exposure, defective retinal impulses, diseases of the labyrinths or of the vestibular nuclei, and lesions of the brain stem or cerebellum controlling ocular posture. The workup includes drug and toxic screening, and neuroradiologic testing with a CT or MRI scan.

DISORDERS OF EXTRAOCULAR MOVEMENT

Clinical Features and Differential Considerations

Patients complain of diplopia produced or exacerbated by certain eye movements. The first step is to determine whether the diplopia is monocular or binocular. Binocular diplopia disappears with either eye covered. Monocular diplopia is less concerning, caused most commonly by refractive errors, dislocated lens, iridodialysis, and feigned disease.

Binocular diplopia from misalignment of the eyes has a multitude of causes. Local mechanical defects such as hematoma, orbital floor fractures, or abscess and cranial nerve palsy of CN III, IV, or VI can lead to motility problems. Thyroid disease, progressive ophthalmoplegia, extraocular muscle fibrosis syndrome, multiple sclerosis, and myasthenia gravis all can lead to newly acquired extraocular movement dysfunction.

The most common cause is cranial nerve palsy. Patients with brain stem disease will often have involvement of other cranial nerves, disturbances in level of consciousness, and sensorimotor loss. Isolated third-nerve lesions will produce a palsy in which the patient develops ptosis, an inability to turn the eye inward or upward, and pupillary mydriasis. The causes of third-nerve palsy are varied and require aggressive and immediate neurologic and radiologic examination.

Isolated fourth-nerve palsy is an easily missed disorder. Patients complain of double vision, which is made worse in downgaze, or gaze away from the paretic side. These patients typically have a head tilt to the opposite shoulder to compensate for the vertical extorsion, and will have weakness in downward gaze. Trauma and vascular disease account for most cases of isolated fourth-nerve palsy, but aneurysm, intracranial tumor, and myasthenia gravis have been implicated.

Sixth cranial nerve palsies are the most commonly reported ocular motor palsies. Patients with sixth cranial nerve palsies have an esotropia that is worsened by lateral gaze and will often turn their heads laterally toward the paretic side to compensate. Sixth-nerve palsy is caused by a variety of diseases. Aneurysm, vascular disease (diabetes, hypertension, atherosclerosis), trauma, neoplasm, multiple sclerosis, meningitis, thyroid eye disease, and increased intracranial pressure may all cause dysfunction. Workup consists of careful neurologic and radiologic examination.

MANAGEMENT

Ophthalmic Drugs

General Considerations Most ocular medications are administered as drops, which have the advantage of concentrating drug delivery to the anterior segment of the eye and reducing unwanted systemic side effects. Eye drops have the additional advantages of rapid absorption, brief effect, and minimal interference with the visual media.

Unfortunately, the eye only retains a small amount of the drug; the remainder is cleared by the rapid turnover of tears.

To improve absorption, patients who are taking more than one eye drop should wait 10 minutes between drops to prevent the second drop from washing out the first. Patients should apply digital pressure at the medial canthus of the eye to prevent drainage of drug via the nasolacrimal duct and keep their eyes closed for several minutes after instilling their drops to halt the lacrimal pumping mechanisms. Ointments increase the contact time of the medication with the anterior segment of the eye. Ointments provide a pleasant lubrication to the eye that has been traumatized and patched and do not seem to interfere with corneal wound healing.

Drug Classification

Box 66-1 provides a listing of the most commonly used agents in each of these categories.

Local anesthetics block neurotransmission along sensory nerve fibers. Ocular procedures facilitated by topical anesthetics include direct inspection, foreign body removal, irrigation, tonometry, and contact lens removal. Topical anesthetics inhibit wound healing, and severe keratopathy can result from indiscriminate use of topical anesthetics. Local anesthetic drops should never be prescribed as pain medicine for patient self-administration.

Antibiotics and antiviral agents are commonly prescribed. The choice of antibiotic agent should be guided by culture, Gram's stain, or suspected bacteria or virus. Antiviral agents are generally prescribed after consultation with an ophthalmologist.

Corticosteroids are used by ophthalmologists for many ocular conditions, but their use by emergency physicians should be limited. Corticosteroids can accelerate the activity of herpes simplex virus and should not be given to any patient when the diagnosis is uncertain. Posttraumatic iridocyclitis is one of the few conditions in which an emergency physician

Box 66-1 Commonly Used Ophthalmologic Medications

Anesthetics
- Proparacaine
- Tetracaine

Antibiotics
- Bacitracin
- Ciprofloxacin
- Erythromycin
- Gentamicin
- Neomycin/bacitracin/polymyxin B
- Norfloxacin
- Ofloxacin
- Polymyxin B/bacitracin
- Polymyxin B/trimethoprim
- Sulfacetamide
- Tobramycin

Antivirals
- Fomivirsen
- Trifluridine
- Vidarabine

Corticosteroids
- Dexamethasone
- Fluorometholone
- Loteprednol
- Prednisolone
- Rimexolone

Decongestants/Antiallergy
- Cromolyn sodium
- Levocabastine
- Lodoxamide tromethamine
- Naphazoline
- Naphazoline/pheniramine
- Olopatadine

Glaucoma: β-Blockers
- Betaxolol
- Carteolol
- Levobunolol
- Timolol

Glaucoma: Carbonic Anhydrase Inhibitors
- Acetazolamide
- Brinzolamide
- Dorzolamide

Glaucoma: Other
- Apraclonidine
- Brimonidine
- Cosopt
- Dipivefrin
- Echothiophate
- Latanoprost
- Pilocarpine

Mydriatics/Cycloplegics
- Atropine
- Cyclopentolate
- Homatropine
- Phenylephrine
- Tropicamide

Nonsteroidal
- Diclofenac
- Ketorolac

Other Medications
- Artificial tears

might consider prescribing a topical steroid agent, but close follow-up with an ophthalmologist is highly recommended.

Cycloplegics block the muscarinic receptors, producing paralysis of the ciliary muscle, which always causes mydriasis. Cycloplegics are useful in relieving pain and photophobia secondary to ciliary spasm related to corneal abrasion, ocular trauma, and iridocyclitis.[7] Mydriatics dilate the pupil, but not all mydriatics are cycloplegics. Mydriatics are contraindicated in any patient with a history of glaucoma, evidence of increased intraocular pressure, presence of a shallow anterior chamber, suspicion of a ruptured globe, or if a lens implant is present. Atropine has a long duration of action (1 to 2 weeks), and should only be prescribed by an ophthalmologist. Decongestants and antiallergy ocular medications are very commonly prescribed and lessen allergic ocular symptoms.

There are a number of glaucoma agents. It is important to know that these are absorbed, and can have systemic effects. For example, topical β blocker agents can result in increased bronchospasm in susceptible patients.

Nonsteroidal antiinflammatory agents are very useful in alleviating the symptoms of inflammation from a wide variety of ocular conditions.

Artificial tears relieve symptoms related to dry eyes and protect the corneas of unconscious patients as well patients suffering from Bell's palsy.

KEY CONCEPTS

- *Orbital floor fractures:* Surgical repair is only for persistent diplopia or cosmetic concerns and is generally not performed until swelling subsides in 7 to 10 days.
- *Retrobulbar hematoma:* When a retrobulbar hematoma compromises retinal circulation, immediate treatment of increased intraocular pressure includes carbonic anhydrase inhibitor, topical β blocker, and IV mannitol. A lateral canthotomy can be done in the ED as a temporizing measure before definitive decompression.
- *Corneal abrasions:* Data suggest that eye patching confers no benefit in healing small, uncomplicated corneal abrasions.
- *Globe rupture:* Treatment includes avoidance of further examination or manipulation and the placement of a protective metal eye shield to prevent accidental pressure on the globe. Antiemetics should be given if nausea is present. Broad-spectrum IV antibiotics should be instituted.
- *Retinal detachments:* Retinal tears or detachments do not cause pain. Examination may reveal the hazy gray membrane of the retina billowing forward but many tears are peripherally located and not seen with direct ophthalmoscopy. Visual acuity may be normal unless the macula is involved. Indirect ophthalmoscopy is warranted if historical clues to the presence of retinal tears are present.
- *Bacterial conjunctivitis:* In uncomplicated acute bacterial conjunctivitis, neomycin ophthalmic solutions should be avoided because of the high incidence of hypersensitivity reactions. Corticosteroids and eye patching should be avoided.
- *Glaucoma:* Attacks of primary angle closure glaucoma produce symptoms that are abrupt in onset and include severe eye pain, blurred vision, headache, nausea, vomiting, and occasionally abdominal pain. Signs include conjunctival injection and a cloudy (steamy) cornea with a mid to dilated pupil that is sluggish or fixed. Intraocular pressures will be markedly elevated.

REFERENCES

1. Department of Emergency Medicine, Hennepin County Medical Center, Emstat, 1999.
2. Baker SM, Hurwitz JJ: Sports and industrial ophthalmology: management of orbital and ocular adnexal trauma, *Ophth Clin North Am* 12:435-455, 1999.
3. O'Hare TH: Blowout fractures: a review, *J Emerg Med* 9:253, 1991.
4. Mathong RH: Management of orbital blowout fractures, *Otolaryngol Clin North Am* 24:79, 1991.
5. Spoor TC, Nesi FA: *Management of ocular, orbital, and adnexal trauma,* New York, 1988, Raven Press.
6. Birrer RB, Robinson T, Papachristos P: Orbital emphysema: how common, how significant? *Ann Emerg Med* 24:1115, 1994.
7. Dobler AA et al: A case of orbital emphysema as an ocular emergency, *Retina* 13:166, 1993.
8. Zimmer-Galler IE, Bartley GB: Orbital emphysema: case reports and review of the literature, *Mayo Clin Proc* 69:115, 1994.
9. Joondeph BC: Blunt ocular trauma, *Emerg Med Clin North Am* 6:147, 1988.
10. Murphy JC et al: Ocular irritancy responses to various pHs of acids and bases with and without irrigation, *Toxicology* 23:281, 1982.
11. Janda AM: Ocular trauma, *Postgrad Med* 90:51, 1991.
12. Dean BS: Cyanoacrylate and corneal abrasion, *Clin Toxicol* 27:169, 1989.
13. Leahey AB, Gottsch JD, Stark WJ: Clinical experience with N-butyl cyanoacrylate tissue adhesive, *Ophthalmol* 100:173, 1993.
14. Lubeck D, Greene JS: Corneal injuries, *Emerg Med Clin North Am* 6:73, 1988.
15. Rosenwasser GO et al: Topical anesthetic abuse, *Ophthalmol* 97:967, 1990.
16. Sklar DP, Lauth JE, Johnson DR: Topical anesthesia of the eye as a diagnostic test, *Ann Emerg Med* 18:1209, 1989.
17. Hulbert MF: Efficacy of eye pad in corneal healing after corneal foreign body removal, *Lancet* 337:643, 1991.
18. Roberts JR: Myths and misconceptions: an eye patch for simple corneal abrasions, *Emerg Med News,* Feb:4-14, 1995.
19. Hamill MB: Sports and industrial ophthalmology. Current concepts in the treatment of traumatic injury to the anterior segment. *Ophth Clin North Am* 12:457-464, 1999.
20. Safran MJ: Management of traumatic hyphema, *Hosp Physician* June:20-26, 1987.
21. Farber MD, Fiscella R, Goldberg MF: Aminocaproic acid versus prednisone for the treatment of traumatic hyphema: a randomized clinical trial. *Ophthalmol* 98:279, 1991.
22. Jackson J: Hyphema. *Optometry Clinics* 3:27, 1993.
23. Pavan-Langston D: *Manual of ocular diagnosis and therapy,* ed 3, Boston, 1991, Little, Brown.
24. Fong LP: Secondary hemorrhage in traumatic hyphema: predictive factors for selective prophylaxis, *Ophthalmol* 101:1583, 1994.
25. Charache S: Sickle cell disease: eye disease in sickling disorders, *Hematol/Oncol Clin North Am* 10:1357-1362, 1996.
26. Weisman RA, Savino PJ: Management of patients with facial trauma and associated ocular/orbital injuries, *Otolaryngol Clin North Am* 24:37, 1991.
27. Lubeck D: Penetrating ocular injuries, *Emerg Med Clin North Am* 6:127, 1988.
28. Shingleton BJ: Eye injuries, *N Engl J Med* 325:408, 1991.
29. Ferrari LR: Trauma. The injured eye, *Anesthesiol Clin North Am* 14:125-150, 1996.
30. Libonati MM, Leahy JJ, Ellison N: The use of succinylcholine in open eye surgery. *Anesthesiol* 62:637, 1985.
31. Reppucci VS, Movshovich A: Sports and industrial ophthalmology. Current concepts in the treatment of traumatic injury to the posterior segment. *Ophthalmol Clin North Am* 12:465-425A, 1999.
32. Solley WA, Broocker G: Ocular trauma. In Palay DA, Krachmer JH, editors: *Ophthalmology for the primary care physician,* St. Louis, 1997, Mosby.

33. Alfaro DV, Roth D, Liggett PE: Posttraumatic endophthalmitis. Causative organisms, treatment, and prevention, *Retina* 14:206, 1994.
34. Linden JA, Renner GS: Trauma to the globe, *Emerg Med Clin North Am* 13:581, 1995.
35. Diamant JI, Hwang DG: Ocular infections: update on therapy. Therapy for bacterial conjunctivitis, *Ophthalmol Clin North Am* 12:15-20, 1999.
36. Rhee DJ, Pyfer MF: Conjunctival/scleral/external disease. In Friedberg MA, Rapuano CJ, editors: *The Wills eye manual,* ed 3, Philadelphia, 1999, Lippincott Williams & Wilkins.
37. Treatment of sexually transmitted disease, *Med Lett* 32:5, 1990.
38. Barequet IS, O'Brien TP: Ocular infections: update on therapy. Therapy of herpes simplex viral keratitis, *Ophthalmol Clin North Am* 12:63-69, 1999.
39. Harding SSP: Management of ophthalmic zoster, *J Med Virol* 1 (Suppl):97, 1993.
40. Miedziak AI, O'Brien TP: Ocular infections: update of therapy. Therapy of varicella-zoster virus ocular infections. *Ophthalmol Clin North Am* 12:51-62, 1999.
41. Lederman C, Miller M: Hordeola and chalazia, *Pediatr Rev* 20:283-284, 1999.
42. Pederson JE: Glaucoma: a primer for primary care physicians, *Glaucoma* 90:41, 1991.
43. Shiose Y: Intraocular pressure: new perspectives, *Surv Ophthalmol* 34:413, 1990.
44. Beck AD: Glaucoma. In Palay DA, Krachmer JH, editors: *Ophthalmology for the primary care physician,* St. Louis, 1997, Mosby.
45. Urtti A, Salminen L: Minimizing systemic absorption of topically administered ophthalmic drugs, *Surv Ophthalmol* 37:435, 1993.
46. Fraunfelder FT: *Drug induced ocular side effects and drug interactions,* ed 3, Philadelphia, 1989, Lea & Febiger.
47. Kooner KS, Zimmermann TJ: Management of acute elevated intraocular pressure, I. Diagnosis, *Ann Ophthalmol* 20:46, 1988.
48. Yanofsky NN: The acute painful eye, *Emerg Med Clin North Am* 6:21, 1988.
49. Morgan A, Hemphill RR: The difficult diagnosis: acute visual change, *Emerg Med Clin North Am* 16:825-843, 1998.
50. Bertolini J, Pelucio M: The red eye, *Emerg Med Clin North Am* 13:561-579, 1995.
51. Delaney WV Jr: Ocular vascular disease: in-office primary care diagnosis, *Geriatrics* 48:60, 1993.
52. Sharma S, Brown M, Brown GC: Retinal vascular disorders: retinal artery occlusions, *Ophthalmol Clin North Am* 11:591-600, 1998.
53. Rassam SM, Patel V, Kohner EM: The effect of acetazolamide on the retinal circulation, *Eye* 7 (Pt 5):697, 1993.
54. Atebara N, Brown GC, Cater J: Efficacy of anterior chamber paracentesis and carbogen in treating nonarteritic central retinal artery occlusion, *Ophthalmol* 102:2029, 1995.
55. Hayreh SS: Retinal vascular disorders: central retinal vein occlusion, *Ophthalmol Clin North Am* 11:559-590, 1998.
56. Bolling JP, Hernan DC, Pach JM: Disorders of retina, vitreous, and choroid. Bartley GB, Liesegang TJ, editors: *Essentials of ophthalmology,* Philadelphia, 1992, JB Lippincott.
57. Hardy RA: Retina and intraocular tumors. In Vaughan D, Asbury T, Riordan EP, editors: *General ophthalmology,* ed 13, New York, 1992, Appleton & Lange.
58. O'Malley C: Vitreous. In Vaughan D, Asbury T, Riordan EP, editors: *General ophthalmology,* ed 13, New York, 1992, Appleton & Lange.
59. Alexander LJ: Age related macular degeneration: the current understanding of the status of clinicopathology, diagnosis and management, *J Am Optometric Assoc* 64:822, 1993.
60. Miller NR: *Walsh and Hoyt's clinical neuro-ophthalmology,* ed 4, Baltimore, 1991, Williams and Wilkins.
61. Optic Neuritis Study Group: The 5 year risk of MS after optic neuritis: experience of the optic neuritis treatment trial, *Neurology* 49:1404-1412, 1997.
62. Beck RW et al: The effect of corticosteroids for acute optic neuritis on the subsequent development of multiple sclerosis, *N Engl J Med* 329:1764, 1993.
63. Sellebjerg F et al: A randomized, controlled trial of oral high-dose methylprednisolone in acute optic neuritis, *Neurol* 52:1479-1484, 1999.
64. Weinberg DA et al: Giant cell arteritis: corticosteroids, temporal artery biopsy, and blindness, *Arch Family Med* 3:623, 1994.
65. Liu GT et al: Visual morbidity in giant cell arteritis: clinical characteristics and prognosis for vision, *Ophthalmol* 101:1779, 1994.
66. Wong RL: Temporal arteritis without an elevated erythrocyte sedimentation rate: case report and review of the literature, *Am J Med* 80:959, 1986.
67. Lam BL Thompson HS, Corbett JJ: The prevalence of simple anisocoria, *Am J Ophthalmol* 104:69, 1987.

67 Otolaryngology

James A. Pfaff
Gregory P. Moore

OTITIS MEDIA

Perspective

Background Otitis media (OM) is the most common diagnosis made by U.S. physicians for children less than 15 years of age.[1] Sixty percent of 877 children in the greater Boston area had at least one episode of acute otitis media (AOM) by 1 year of age; by 3 years of age, more than 80% had AOM, with 40% having more than three episodes.[2] The financial impact is enormous, with one estimate of $3.5 billion per year spent on the evaluation, treatment, and socioeconomic effects of this disease.[3]

Epidemiology The age at the first episode is an important predictor of recurrence or persistent middle ear effusion.[3,4] American Indians, Canadian Eskimos, Native Alaskans, and whites have a greater rate of OM and recurrence than do African-Americans.[5]

Male gender, day care attendance, parental smoking, and a family history of middle ear disease have been implicated to increase risk.[4,5] Children with anatomic abnormalities such as cleft palate and Down syndrome have a higher rate of OM, probably because of eustachian tube (Etb) abnormalities. Some immunocompromised patients, including those with human immunodeficiency virus (HIV), may have recurrent OM as an initial symptom of their underlying disease.[6] OM and upper respiratory infections both occur primarily in the winter. Breast feeding appears to be protective.

Definitions There are many classification schemes for OM, and the disease is often described as a continuum of pathology. In one common classification, OM is defined as inflammation of the middle ear and is classified into four entities.[7] Myringitis is inflammation of the tympanic membrane (TM). AOM has signs and symptoms of an acute infection, with evidence of effusion. This has also been called *acute suppurative* or *purulent otitis media.* Otitis media with effusion (OME) has effusion without signs or symptoms of an acute infection. Additional terms used to describe this include *serous, mucoid, nonsuppurative,* or *secretory* otitis media. OME is further classified into acute (< 3 weeks), subacute (3 weeks to 3 months), and chronic (> 3 months). Chronic otitis media, or chronic suppurative otitis media, refers to chronic discharge from the ear through perforation of an intact membrane. Recurrent otitis media is defined by three or more episodes over 6 months or four episodes in 1 year. For practical purposes, most authorities describe either AOM or OME in the literature.

Principles of Disease

Pathophysiology Etb dysfunction is the central theme to most theories of AOM pathogenesis. The Etb, between the middle ear cavity and the nasopharynx, ventilates the middle ear to equilibrate pressure, allow for middle ear drainage, and provide protection from nasopharyngeal secretions.[8] In children, it measures approximately 18 mm and is almost horizontal. As individuals age, the Etb widens, doubles in length, becomes more vertically oriented, and stiffens (which may explain the decreased incidence of AOM in adults). Normally, the tube is collapsed, but it opens during yawning, chewing, and swallowing.

The Etb may become either mechanically or functionally obstructed, decreasing middle ear ventilation. Examples of mechanical obstruction include inflammations from an upper respiratory infection, hypertrophied adenoids, and a cleft palate.[9] Functional obstruction from persistent tubal collapse occurs primarily in young children, who have less fibrocartilage support of the medial Etb than older children or adults.[9]

It has been postulated that this dysfunction results in negative middle ear cavity pressure, causing a transudate of fluid into the middle ear that combines with the reflux of nasopharyngeal secretions and bacteria. This provides a medium for bacterial proliferation and subsequent host inflammatory response.[9]

Etiology The most common bacterial causes are *Streptococcus pneumoniae, Haemophilus influenzae* (primarily nontypeable), and *Moraxella (Branhamella) catarrhalis. Streptococcus pyogenes* and *Staphylococcus aureus* are less common, although about one third of middle ear effusions are sterile.[10] Adult infection involves similar organisms.[11] In OME there is a greater proportion of *H. influenzae* and a higher percentage of sterile effusions.[12,13]

Viruses have also been found in the middle ear aspirates of children with OM. They are most likely a coinfectant with bacteria but have been a sole source in up to 13% of cases.[13] Respiratory syncytial virus (RSV) is the most common virus, followed by rhinovirus, influenzavirus, and adenovirus.[13] These viruses may be responsible for some of the treatment failures seen in AOM, possibly by interfering with eradication of bacterial pathogens.

In very young children, it was believed that gram-negative organisms and *S. aureus* were the causative factors. Although this may apply for intubated patients or those in the neonatal intensive care unit (NICU), healthy newborns tend to be infected by the same pathogens as normal children.[14] A special note should be made about bullous myringitis. Middle ear aspirates in this condition usually grow *S. pneumoniae* and *H. influenzae.*[15] *Mycoplasma pneumoniae* is uncommon.

Other, less likely, organisms that can cause AOM include *Mycobacterium tuberculosis* (primarily in children) and *Chlamydia trachomatis* (most commonly seen in children less than 6 months of age with pneumonia).[16]

Clinical Features

OM may be manifested by a multitude of symptoms, such as cough, poor appetite, diarrhea, vomiting, fever, and pulling at ears, all of which are nonspecific.[17,18] Older children may be able to verbalize pain, but otalgia is not universally present. In OM, pain often precedes otorrhea, unlike otitis externa, in which it accompanies the drainage. Children often have associated upper respiratory tract infections. Fever may be present, but in one large series, a temperature of 38.3° C or more was present in only 26% of the episodes, with only 4% having a fever of 40° C or higher.[19] Some authorities have modified the definition to include otoscopic findings of acute inflammation regardless of symptoms; with this definition, one third of cases will not initially be accompanied by acute symptoms.[20]

The auricle and external canal should be inspected for signs of erythema, discharge, or tenderness. If the canal is occluded with cerumen, an ear curet with direct visualization may be successful in clearing the canal. If not, the placement of 3% hydrogen peroxide or emulsifying drops, followed by gentle irrigation, may cleanse the canal.

The auricle should be pulled up and back to straighten the canal and ensure visualization. A dull gray or yellow color may signify edema or a middle ear effusion. The presence of erythema in itself is not indicative of infection because crying or fever may cause this, probably because of increased vascularity.

In OME the TMs will often be retracted, with the malleolus being particularly prominent. The landmarks may all be obscured in the presence of significant fluid. The emergency physician should observe for perforation. The lack of TM mobility is one of the most sensitive indicators of middle ear effusion.[21] Other physical signs of effusion include air-fluid levels, bubbles behind the TM, or any two of the following: decreased mobility, color change, or TM opacification.[22] A comparison examination of the other ear may be helpful in confirming suspected infection.

In neonates, the TM appears thickened and opaque normally in the first few weeks of life, and the TM is in a highly oblique position. With tympanostomy tubes, in the absence of infection, the TM may have decreased mobility, altered landmarks, opacity, or dullness.[23] If the tube is patent, erythema and discharge may indicate infection. If not, erythema, bulging of the TM, and immobility are indicative of AOM.[23]

In addition to pneumatic otoscopy, there are two other modalities for determining middle ear effusion. Tympanometry applies a continuous sound frequency in a closed space with the subsequent graphing of the eardrum movement and requires a tight seal in the canal and a cooperative patient. Its use in children less than 3 months of age is unreliable.[24] Normal tympanometry may be obtained in up to 15% of patients despite the presence of AOM.[24]

Acoustic reflectometry imparts intermittent sound waves into the ear canal and records the reflected sound from the TM. Acoustic reflectometry is not affected by crying or cerumen and does not require a tight seal, but it is sensitive to user technique. Its ease may make it useful for ED use.[25]

Complications Before the use of antibiotics, there was a 20% incidence of complications from AOM, with mastoiditis and otic meningitis relatively common.[26] Complications are generally considered either intratemporal or intracranial.

Intratemporal Hearing impairment is the most common complication in OM. Almost all children with OM will have a temporary conductive hearing loss; sensorineural deficit occurs less commonly, probably as a spread of infection through the round window. This may contribute to the association of OM with decreased or delayed speech, language, or cognitive development.[4,8]

TM perforation occurs most commonly at the pars tensa and usually resolves spontaneously. It may persist for a longer period, resulting in a chronic perforation.[16] Cholesteatoma is an accumulation of keratin-producing squamous epithelium in the middle ear and may result in erosion of bone within the middle ear cavity. It is seen most often in OME in which retraction of the TM is a common problem. Treatment is usually surgical.

Labyrinthitis occurs when infection spreads to the cochlear and vestibular apparatus, usually through the round or oval windows. Again, a variety of types are manifested by sensorineural hearing loss and vertigo. Treatment involves intravenous (IV) antibiotics and surgical drainage.

Facial nerve paralysis is a recognized complication in children with otitis. The facial nerve courses through the middle ear and may be affected by infection.[16] Treatment consist of IV antibiotics, myringotomy, and tube placement.

Infectious eczematoid dermatitis may result from the otorrhea of OM, with perforation or tympanostomy tubes infecting the external auditory canal. Treatment involves otic suspension (*not* solution). Although caution is urged with these products, the incidence of adverse effects is small.[27]

Intracranial Before antibiotics, intracranial complications occurred in 2.5% of patients. The incidence has significantly decreased and now they usually result from chronic middle ear disease.[16] Meningitis is the most common intracranial complication, more from hematogenous spread than direct invasion. The symptoms include headache, meningismus, fever, nausea, emesis, irritability, lethargy, and altered mental status. Meningitis is caused by the same organisms as AOM. Diagnosis is made by cerebrospinal fluid (CSF) analysis; treatment consists of IV antibiotics.

An extradural abscess may result from destruction of bone adjacent to the dura by cholesteatoma, infection, or both. Subdural empyema is a collection of fluid between the dura and arachnoid membrane as a result of infection or venous thrombophlebitis. Focal otic encephalitis is an edematous or inflamed area in the brain from a complication of OM, extradural abscess, or sinus dural thrombophlebitis.[28] It may be distinguished from brain abscess by a computed tomography (CT) scan. A brain abscess results from direct extension of the infection or follows the development of an adjacent infection such as lateral sinus thrombosis.[28] Organisms include *S. pyogenes, S. aureus,* and *S. pneumoniae.*[28,29] The treatment for these conditions includes IV antibiotics and surgical drainage.

Lateral venous sinus thrombosis occurs when the mastoid infection comes in contact with the sinus wall, which inflames the adventitia and penetrates the venous wall. Thrombosis and embolization both occur. It is rarely seen more often in adults with chronic ear disease than children.[30] Patients may have fever and chills, earache, headache, and mastoid and neck tenderness. Treatment involves IV antibiotics and surgical drainage.

Diagnostic Strategies

Tympanocentesis is aspiration of the middle ear effusion to identify causative organisms. Indications include patients with AOM who are seriously ill or toxic, are unresponsive to therapy, are less than 4 weeks old, are immunocompromised, are receiving antimicrobials, or have suppurative complications.[31]

Differential Considerations

OM usually does not cause a significantly high fever; in approaching a febrile, ill-appearing infant, the physician should seek other sources. If a child or adult complains of otalgia, additional considerations or possibilities include otitis externa, trauma, foreign bodies, and complications of OM such as mastoiditis. Ear pain may also be referred from the teeth, sinuses, throat, or temporomandibular joint.

Management

The need for antibiotics in OM is controversial. Some European countries have an observational period of 48 hours before starting treatment. Although 80% of cases of AOM resolve spontaneously, there is no way to predict which patients will improve without treatment. Because of this and the substantial decrease of complications from the preantibiotic era, most authorities in the United States still recommend antibiotic treatment.[32-34]

The most frequent outpatient use of antimicrobials in the United States is for OM, with the number of prescriptions increasing from 12 million in 1980 to more than 23.6 million in 1992.[35] This has led to concern for the increasing incidence of antimicrobial resistance, particularly of *S. pneumoniae.* There are now more than 16 antibiotics approved by the U.S. Food and Drug Administration (FDA) for treatment of OM.[34]

Although the incidence of β-lactamase resistance is significant in some areas, amoxicillin's cost, efficacy, safety profile, and palatability still make it a good first-line agent. In areas with β-lactamase resistance, trimethoprim-sulfamethoxazole (TMP-SMX) is often used as a first-line agent, with its twice-a-day dosing increasing compliance. TMP-SMX has potential sulfa sensitivity and should be avoided in children less than 2 months of age because of the potential for kernicterus. Some other commonly used antibiotics include erythromycin-sulfisoxazole, amoxicillin/clavulanate, azithromycin, clarithromycin, cefuroxime axetil, cefpodoxime, cefprozil, and cefixime. In patients with vomiting, a history of poor compliance, or lack of follow-up, a single dose of 50 mg/kg of intramuscular ceftriaxone is as effective as a 10-day course of amoxicillin.[36]

Patients should return if there is no improvement in 48 to 72 hours.[37] This could signal a lack of antibiotic concentration into the middle ear, poor patient compliance, or β-lactamase resistance. Treatment failures occur most often in children less than 18 months of age.[38] Changing to a β-lactamase–resistant antibiotic is a logical choice. The antibiotic treatment of AOM in adults is the same as children.

A recent Centers for Disease Control and Prevention (CDC) panel recommended the use of high dose (80-90 mg/kg/day up to 1.5 g) amoxicillin in patients at high risk for drug-resistant *S. pneumoniae.*[34] High-risk patients were defined as children younger than 2 years old, those going to day care, or those who have had antimicrobials in the preceding months.[34] Additional recommendations for treatment failures after 3 days include amoxicillin-clavulanate, oral cefuroxime axetil, and intramuscular ceftriaxone.[34]

Treatment historically involved a 10-day course. A number of studies have compared traditional management to shorter therapy, which is most appropriate for uncomplicated AOM.[39] Patients with TM perforations and those at high risk for treatment failures or with chronic or recurrent OM are probably more appropriately treated with a longer course.[39] Shorter courses also are not appropriate for children younger than 2 years of age, with some physicians recommending a full 10-day course in all children younger than 6.[40] The antibiotic treatment of AOM in adults is the same as in older children.

There is no indication for the use of antihistamines, decongestants, steroids, or tympanostomy tubes for an acute episode of AOM.[1,8,9,41] Benzocaine/antipyrine (Auralgan), a local anesthetic, may be helpful in some patients with an intact TM. If the TM perforates, the use of antibiotic suspension may be beneficial.

Recurrent AOM occurs primarily in the winter months, often in conjunction with upper respiratory infections. These individuals may benefit from prophylaxis with either amoxicillin 20 mg/kg or sulfisoxazole 50 mg/kg given at night.

Up to 50% of children may exhibit OME after a 10-day treatment with antibiotics, but 90% will resolve within 3 months.[42] The treatment of OME is controversial, but OME may interfere with hearing and subsequent development of speech and language. OME is by definition asymptomatic, and the effusion may be sterile or contain infectious agents. Clinical guidelines developed by the Agency for Health Care Policy recommend observation or the use of antibiotics in patients with acute or subacute OME, although some experts recommend observation alone given the increasing antibiotic resistance.[39] Antihistamines, decongestants, steroids, or surgical procedures are not beneficial in patients with acute or subacute OME.[42]

Myringotomy and tympanostomy tubes may be beneficial in children who have failed medical treatment, have had OME for 4 to 6 months, and have a greater than 20-db hearing loss.[1] Tonsillectomy is not beneficial, but adenoidectomy may be helpful in older children.[43]

Tympanostomy tubes have also been used in recurrent AOM unresponsive to prophylactic antibiotics; complications of AOM, including mastoiditis, meningitis, brain abscess, and facial nerve paralysis; and complications of ET dysfunction, including TM retraction with hearing loss, ossicular erosions, or retraction pocket formation.[42]

A newly developed conjugate pneumococcal vaccine has received an FDA advisory panel approval; this may markedly reduce the number of cases of OM.

Disposition

Children are normally seen in 10 to 14 days for follow up. This may not be necessary in children older than 2 years of age with resolution of symptoms and no recurrent risk factors.[44,45]

Infants less than 2 months of age with OM should be evaluated with blood, CSF, and urine cultures.[9] Anyone with complications needs ear, nose, and throat (ENT) referral.

Adults who have persistent OME need ENT referral to rule out nasopharyngeal carcinoma.[46]

EXTERNAL OTITIS

Principles of Disease

Anatomy and Physiology External otitis is an inflammation of the external auditory canal. The canal is lined with squamous epithelial cell and cerumen glands that provide a protective lipid layer.[47] This protective layer may be disrupted by high humidity, increased temperature, maceration of the skin after prolonged exposure to moisture, and local trauma (e.g., cotton swabs or the use of hearing aids), resulting in the introduction of bacteria.[48] The most common bacterial causes are *Pseudomonas aeruginosa* and *S. aureus.* Otitis externa occurs most often in the summer and is common in the tropics.

Clinical Features

The canal is initially pruritic and becomes erythematous and increasingly swollen. The diagnosis is made clinically with ear pain, erythema or edema of the canal, and reproduction of the discomfort with pulling on the auricle or tragus. Severe otitis externa is manifested by intense pain, canal occlusion, and conductive hearing loss.[47] Cultures are unnecessary.

The disease may progress to a chronic form with itching, eczema, and flaking of the epithelium, which may be from bacterial, fungal, or dermatologic conditions. In children it is usually secondary to OME.[49]

Differential Considerations

It may be difficult to distinguish otitis externa from OM, particularly in children. The TM may be erythematous in both, and the edema may preclude diagnosis. The discharge may be from otitis externa or a perforated TM, and in equivocal cases it is prudent to treat for both conditions.

Otomycosis or fungal infection can occur as a primary or secondary infection. Itching is the prominent symptom, often with minimal pain or otorrhea. Aspergillosis is the cause in most cases. Otomycosis appears most often in tropical climates, patients with diabetes, immunocompromised patients, or those on immunosuppressive therapy.[50] Treatment involves cleansing and acidifying and antifungal eardrops, such as thimerosal or gentian violet. Specific antifungal agents, such as clotrimazole and itraconazole, are also effective.[51]

Furunculosis is a small, erythematous, and well-circumscribed infection of the cartilaginous portions of the external canal, usually caused by *S. aureus.*[47] There is usually no drainage, and treatment involves incision, drainage, and an oral antistaphylococcal antibiotic. Cellulitis of the auricle and canal may cause erythema, induration, and other systemic signs. Again, treatment is with antibiotics directed at the offending organisms. Parenteral antistaphylococcal antibiotics (e.g., nafcillin) may be required in severe infections.

Herpes zoster oticus, also known as the *Ramsay Hunt syndrome,* is a viral manifestation of disease affecting the auricle, with resulting facial paralysis that may involve multiple cranial nerves. It initially causes pain, with erythema, swelling, and vesicles developing approximately 3 to 7 days later.[43] These patients need ENT referral. Treatment consists of analgesia, warm compresses, and acyclovir.[52]

Management

Initial management involves cleansing the external canal with a combination of gentle suctioning and irrigation. Cleansing solutions include tap water, sterile saline, 2% acetic acid, and Burow's solution. Acetic acid possesses antibacterial and antifungal properties that are more important than its acidifying properties.[49] The cleansing is followed by topical antibiotics (generally a compound of polymyxin, neomycin, and hydrocortisone) placed via 2 or 3 drops four times per day. In severe infections, a wick of cotton, gauze, or compressed hydroxycellulose will facilitate medication delivery.[49] The wick is placed 10 to 12 mm into the canal, moistened with antibiotic drops, and left in place for 2 to 3 days. The patient should return in 24 to 48 hours for a recheck. Cephalosporins and ciprofloxacin, among others, may be necessary in infections involving the skin and periauricular areas.[46] Opiate analgesia may be necessary. Patients with severe inflammation (fever, cervical lymphadenopathy, or periauricular nodes) need close follow-up and ENT referral.

NECROTIZING (MALIGNANT) EXTERNAL OTITIS

Previously known as malignant otitis externa because of its high mortality, necrotizing external otitis is an extremely aggressive form of otitis externa. It occurs primarily in adults with diabetes mellitus but has also been seen rarely in immunocompromised children.[53] *Pseudomonas* is the predominant pathogen, but *S. aureus, S. epidermidis, Proteus mirabilis, Klebsiella, Aspergillus,* and *Salmonella* have all been described.[54] The infection begins in the external canal, progressing through the periauricular tissue and cartilaginous bony junction of the external auditory meatus. It then spreads into the adjacent tissues along clefts in the floor of the meatus known as the *fissures of Santorini.*[55] It may then spread to the base of the skull at the temporal bone, with a resultant skull-base *osteomyelitis,* another term often used to describe this entity. The facial nerve is the first cranial nerve affected, but additional nerves may be involved as well. The pathogenesis is uncertain but may be related to vascular insufficiency or immune dysfunction.[53,56]

Clinical symptoms include pain, tenderness, and swelling around the periauricular area, headache, and otorrhea. It may be difficult to distinguish this entity from a severe external otitis, a further reason for close follow-up. Any persistent external otitis in an elderly person with diabetes with associated pain should be considered to be temporal bone osteomyelitis. The clinical finding characteristic for the disease is granulation tissue in the floor of the ear canal at the bony cartilaginous junction. Facial paralysis occurs when there is involvement of the styloid mastoid foramen, and further extension can result in cranial IX, X, and XI palsies as well.[57] Further complication include thrombosis of the sigmoid sinus and meningitis.

Bone scanning (^{99}technetium) and gallium are sensitive radiographic tests, but they are not specific for the disease. A CT scan is useful for detecting infratemporal spread of the disease and abscess formation,[55] which further defines the extent of the disease.[53]

Treatment includes an aminoglycoside and a semisynthetic penicillin. There has been excellent success with ciprofloxacin, and its oral availability makes it ideal.[58] Although extensive surgical debridement was previously used, its role is now limited. Hyperbaric oxygen has been used as an adjunct therapy.[47] Because of the incidence of external otitis in adults with diabetes, a blood glucose level should be obtained in all patients with severe external otitis.

MASTOIDITIS

The incidence of acute and chronic mastoiditis has decreased significantly since the advent of antibiotics. Although it is still primarily associated with OM, a number of patients do not have a recent episode of OM.[59,60] Mastoiditis has also been described as a complication of leukemia, mononucleosis, sarcoma of the temporal bone, and Kawasaki disease.[61]

Pathophysiology

Acute mastoiditis is a natural extension of middle ear infections because the mastoid air cells are generally inflamed during an episode of AOM. The aditus ad antrum is a narrow connection between the middle ear and mastoid air cells. If this connection becomes blocked, a closed space is formed, with the potential for abscess development and bone destruction. The infection may spread from the mastoid air cells by venous channels, resulting in inflammation of the overlying periosteum. Progression results in the destruction of the mastoid bone trabeculae and coalescence of the cells, resulting in acute mastoid osteitis or coalescent mastoiditis. The resulting pus may track through a number of routes: (1) through the aditus ad antrum with resultant spontaneous resolution; (2) lateral to the surface of the mastoid process, resulting in a subperiosteal abscess; (3) anteriorly, forming an abscess below the pinna or behind the sternocleidomastoid muscle of the neck, resulting in an abscess (often called a *Bezold abscess*); (4) medial to the petrous air cells of the temporal bone, resulting in a rare condition known as *petrositis;* and (5) posterior to the occipital bone, resulting in osteomyelitis of the calvarium or a Citelli abscess.[59-63]

Chronic mastoiditis is generally a complication of chronic otitis media. There may be extensive invasion of granulation tissue from the middle ear into the mastoid air cells. Another entity, latent or "masked" mastoiditis, has also been described. It is indolent in nature, with minimal signs and symptoms, little or no fever, and a history of otalgia. The TM may be intact or perforated. Suspicion should be raised in the presence of intracranial complications without an apparent source.[63] Patients at risk for this entity include newborns and immunosuppressed patients (recent chemotherapy, steroids, or diabetic or geriatric patients).[64]

Etiology

S. pneumoniae is the most common organism found in mastoiditis, but other organisms involved do not always mirror those of acute otitis.[59] Mixed cultures of aerobes and anaerobes are common. Common aerobes include group A streptococci, *S. aureus,* and *S. epidermidis.* Chronic mastoiditis will also often have mixed cultures, with *P. aeruginosa* as the predominant organism.

Diagnostic Findings

Clinical findings in acute mastoiditis include fever, headache, and erythema. Pain is universally present.[59] Physical findings include postauricular or supraauricular tenderness, with late edema. The TM is similar to AOM (erythema, bulging, and decreased mobility) but may be normal in up to 10% of the cases.[59] Suspicions should be heightened if symptoms of AOM have lasted longer than 2 weeks.[65,66]

In chronic mastoiditis, symptoms include persistent drainage through the perforated TM and may include redness, edema, and retroauricular sensitivity.[27]

Ancillary Testing

Radiographs of the mastoid area may be negative.[60,66] The CT scan is of greater value, especially when there is abscess formation.[67] A magnetic resonance imaging (MRI) scan may be more useful, particularly if there is evidence of intracranial complications.

Management

The diagnosis of mastoiditis requires admitting the patient for antibiotic therapy. Antibiotic choices include a semisynthetic penicillin combined with chloramphenicol, or a third-generation cephalosporin such as cefuroxime (50 to 150 mg/kg/day), or ceftriaxone (50 to 75 mg/kg/day), usually for 1 week.[61] Surgical procedures may range from myringotomy drainage and tympanostomy tube placement to mastoidectomy and drainage for more extensive disease progression. Mastoidectomy is required in approximately half of mastoiditis cases.[61]

Antibiotic choices for chronic mastoiditis are based on culture of the persistent drainage but often include medication to cover *Pseudomonas,* such as ticarcillin-clavulanate or ticarcillin alone. Local cleansing is also efficacious. Antibiotics may obviate the need for surgery, although mastoidectomy may be required in some cases.[66]

SUDDEN HEARING LOSS

Sudden hearing loss, although uncommon, may be of great concern to the patient. It may be gradually noticed or have a sudden onset. Although there is no accepted definition of sudden hearing loss, it is most often sensorineural in nature and occurs over a brief period, usually about 3 days.[68] The severity ranges from difficulty with conversation to complete hearing loss.

The speed of onset may give clues to its etiology (Box 67-1).[68-70] A sudden onset may be from trauma or a vascular complication; gradual hearing loss is suggestive of a tumor.[69] A history of trauma, medications, illnesses, physical activity at the time of the event, and unilateral or bilateral involvement are all helpful clues. The presence of tinnitus, vertigo, and neurologic symptoms ranging from cranial nerve abnormalities to brainstem or cerebellar dysfunction is helpful. In conductive hearing losses, such as otosclerosis, individuals hear better in noisy environments.[69]

Physical examination should include a thorough inspection of the external canal and tympanic membrane integrity. The Weber's test for hearing and the Rinne's test may help in distinguishing conductive versus sensorineural deficits. A comprehensive neurologic examination including cranial nerves and cerebellar testing may localize brainstem involvement. A CT scan may reveal trauma or tumors, and neurologic and chemical screening should be based on the history and physical findings.[70] Sudden sensorineural hearing loss is an otologic emergency.[68] Treatment is directed at the underlying causes.

Box 67-1 Causes of Sudden Hearing Loss

Infectious

Mumps
Measles
Influenza
Herpes simplex
Herpes zoster
Cytomegalovirus
Mononucleosis
Syphilis

Vascular

Macroglobulinemia
Sickle cell disease
Berger's disease
Leukemia
Polycythemia
Fat emboli
Hypercoagulable states

Metabolic

Diabetes
Pregnancy
Hyperlipoproteinemia

Conductive

Cerumen impaction
Foreign bodies
Otitis media
Otitis externa
Barotrauma
Trauma

Medications

Aminoglycosides (gentamicin, theomycin, vancomycin, kanamycin, streptomycin)
Loop diuretics (furosemide, ethacrynic acid)
Antineoplastics
Salicylates

Neoplasm

Acoustic neuroma

From Shikowitz MJ: *Med Clin North Am* 75:1239, 1991; Lawrence LJ, Brown CG: *Emerg Med Clin North Am* 5:193, 1987; and Nadol JB: *N Engl J Med* 329:1092, 1993.

EPISTAXIS

Perspective

Epidemiology Epistaxis is a common otolaryngologic problem, with 15 people per 10,000 requiring physician care annually and 1.6 per 10,000 requiring admission to the hospital.[71] Most cases occur under age 10, and the incidence decreases with age.[72] One survey of more than 6000 patients reports an 11% incidence of epistaxis.[73] It is more common in colder seasons and in northern climates because of decreased humidity and subsequent drying of the nasal mucosa. Epistaxis is a frightening condition for patients but is seldom life threatening. A solid understanding of physiology and treatment allows for prompt and efficient management of the disorder.

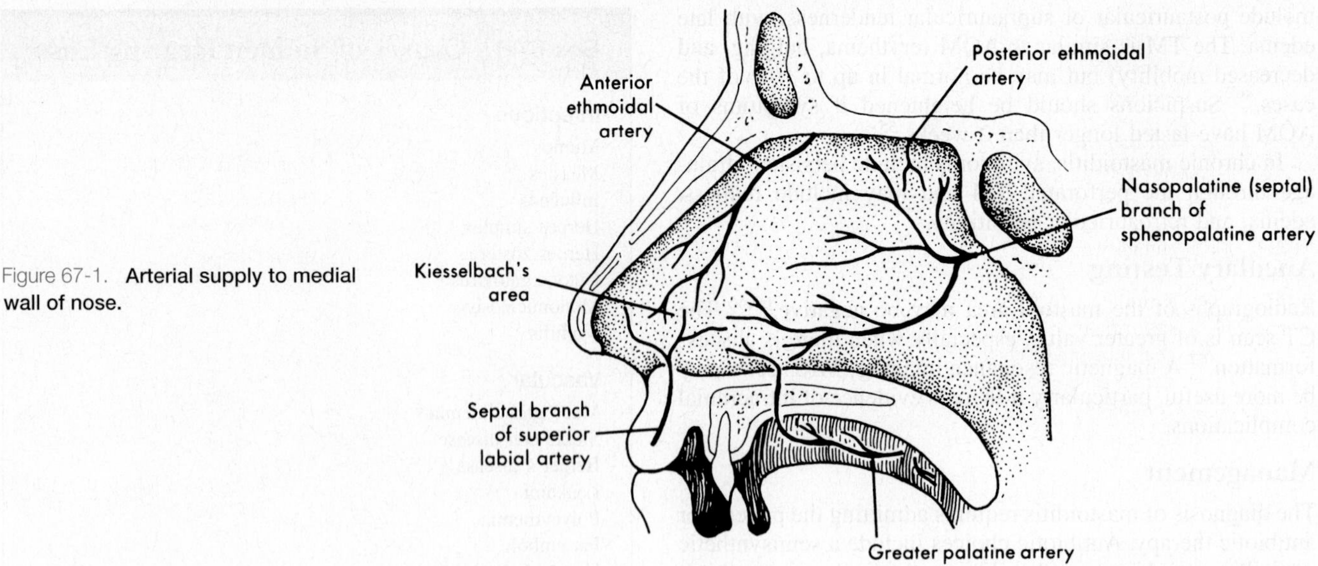

Figure 67-1. **Arterial supply to medial wall of nose.**

Definition Anterior epistaxis accounts for 90% of all nosebleeds and usually involves Kiesselbach's plexus on the anterior-inferior nasal septum.[72,73] Epistaxis is unilateral and can be controlled with anterior packing. Posterior epistaxis accounts for 10% of nosebleeds and usually arises from a posterior branch of the sphenopalatine artery.[72-74] It is not controlled with a well-placed anterior pack. Posterior bleeding is rare in children.[73]

Principles of Disease

Anatomy The nasal area is supplied by three arteries with anastomoses between them. The sphenopalatine artery supplies the turbinates and meatus laterally and the posterior and inferior septum medially. The anterior and posterior ethmoidal arteries from the ophthalmic branch of the internal carotid artery supply the superior mucosa both medially and laterally. The superior labial branch of the facial artery provides circulation to the anterior mucosal septum and anterior lateral mucosa (Figure 67-1).

Etiology There are many reasons for epistaxis, but the most common are upper respiratory infection with concomitant mucosal congestion and vasodilation and trauma, either accidental or iatrogenic (i.e., nose picking). See Box 67-2 for the causes of epistaxis.

Diagnostic Strategies

Patients should initially have their hemodynamic status evaluated, with resuscitation and laboratory studies performed as needed based on suspicion of possible etiologies mentioned in Box 67-2.[72,73] Patients often are anxious and hypertensive.[72] Elevated blood pressure is usually from stress and anxiety and resolves with treatment. Hypertension has never been clearly shown to cause epistaxis, although it can worsen the bleeding when present.[73,74] Sedation with benzodiazepines or narcotics may help these patients.[73]

The key to successful management is identifying the site of nasal bleeding and whether it is anterior or posterior.[72] If the nose is actively bleeding, the patient should clear clots by blowing his or her nose and then apply bilateral pressure on the nasal septum by compressing the cartilaginous part of the nose for 10 to 15 minutes. This simple maneuver also educates the patient on how to self-manage further episodes. During this time the emergency physician should assemble materials for illumination, suction, visualization, and treatment of the epistaxis. Discharge without identification and treatment of the bleeding site will often result in recurrences. Anterior clots and obstructions may give the appearance of a posterior epistaxis if the blood runs posteriorly. Persistent bleeding should be controlled with pledgets soaked in cocaine, lidocaine-epinephrine, or Neo-Synephrine to promote vasoconstriction and anesthesia.

Management

With an identified site of bleeding in anterior epistaxis, several treatments are available. Application of silver nitrate will chemically cauterize the area but will be unsuccessful during active bleeding. With 4 to 5 seconds of application, nitric acid is formed and coagulates tissue. It should never be maintained longer than 15 seconds because septal damage may occur.[72-74] The area should be cauterized peripherally to centrally and superior to inferior to avoid blood, which renders the sticks ineffectual. Bilateral usage of silver nitrate to the septum is contraindicated because it may deprive the septum of blood supply and lead to necrosis. Cautery should not be done in the face of a coagulopathy.[73,74] An alternative treatment is the application of topical agents such as Gelfoam and Surgicel with light packing, which induces coagulation at the site. Patients are instructed on compression techniques and to keep mucosa moist with antibiotic ointment. They should avoid closed-mouth sneezing, nose picking, coughing, nose blowing, and aspirin. If bleeding persists, anterior tamponade with a commercially available nasal tampon or balloon or a formal anterior nasal pack may be necessary. These work by three mechanisms: direct pressure is applied, resultant mucosal irritation from the foreign body decreases bleeding, and surrounding clot formation adds further pressure. Once placed, anterior packs should be left in place for at least 48 hours.[73] Their discomfort may require sedatives and narcotic pain medication. Bilateral packs are usually required to get adequate compression. Most emergency physicians place patients on antibiotics to prevent

Box 67-2 Etiology of Epistaxis

Local

Nasal or facial trauma
Upper respiratory tract infections
Nose picking
Allergies
Low home humidity
Nasal polyps
Foreign body in the nose
Environmental irritants
Nasopharyngeal mucormycosis
Traumatic internal carotid artery aneurysm
Chlamydial rhinitis neonatorum
Postoperative

Idiopathic

Habitual
Familial

Systemic

Atherosclerosis of nasal blood vessels
Hypertension (controversial)
Anticoagulant therapy
Pregnancy
Abrupt changes in barometric pressure
Hereditary hemorrhagic telangiectasia (Rendu-Osler-Weber disease)
Blood dyscrasias (e.g., hemophilia, leukemia, lymphoma, polycythemia vera, anemias, idiopathic thrombocytopenic purpura, granulocytosis, inherited platelet disorders, acquired platelet disorders [i.e., aspirin])
Hepatic disease
Rupture of internal carotid artery aneurysm
Diabetes mellitus
Alcoholism
Vitamin K deficiency
Folic acid deficiency
Chronic nephritis
Chemotherapy
Blood transfusion reactions
Migraine headache
Drug-induced thrombocytopenia

From Myers A, Kulig K: Epistaxis emergindex and Wurman LH et al: *Am J Otolaryngology* 13:193, 1992.

sinusitis from obstruction and toxic shock syndrome.[72-74] Recommended antibiotics are cephalexin 250 to 500 mg four times a day or amoxicillin-clavulanate potassium 250 to 500 mg three times daily (40 to 50 mg/kg/day divided three times daily in children).

Posterior epistaxis is identified when posterior bleeding occurs with a properly placed anterior nasal pack. A posterior pack is necessary in this case. A standard Foley catheter may be inserted into the posterior nares and inflated with water until the patient expresses discomfort. Slow increments in inflation are necessary for patient tolerance. Vaseline gauze should then be packed around the catheter anteriorly. Commercially available balloons such as the Nasostat and Epistat are more comfortable than the posterior pack. They are left in for 2 to 5 days, with antibiotic coverage as described previously. If these techniques do not provide successful control, ENT consultation is necessary. Definitive care may require internal maxillary artery ligation or embolization with Gelfoam or posterior endoscopic cautery.[73]

Patients with posterior nasal packs should be admitted to the hospital and may require sedation and supplemental oxygen. The Po_2 may drop 10 mm Hg, and Pco_2 may increase 10 mm Hg after posterior packing. This is thought to be secondary to a postulated nasopulmonary reflex.[72] Dysrhythmias, bradycardia, myocardial infarction, cerebrovascular accidents, and aspiration have also been reported after posterior nasal packing.[72]

SIALOLITHIASIS

Stones of the salivary glands occur in 1% of the population.[75] They are most commonly found between ages 30 and 50 years, although they are rarely reported in children. The most common gland affected is the submandibular (submaxillary) gland, accounting for 80% to 95% of cases. The patient has pain and swelling of the gland. Differential diagnosis includes infections, inflammation, and granulomatous and neoplastic processes. The most common viral pathogen is mumps. *Staphylococcus, Streptococcus viridans, S. pneumoniae,* and *H. influenzae* predominate in bacterial infections. Stones may be confirmed by palpation or purulent discharge from the glandular duct with massage. Radiography and ultrasonography are helpful imaging modalities, with the latter being capable of revealing diagnoses other than stones.[76] Treatment consists of antibiotics (covering penicillinase-resistant organisms), moist heat, massage, sialogogues (tart hard candies to promote glandular secretions), and sialolithotomy, if necessary, using probes or endoscopy.[77] Follow-up within 24 hours should be arranged for stones not removed in the ED and 4 to 5 days otherwise.

NECK MASSES

Perspective

Neck masses are a relatively common clinical finding and are usually the result of inflammation but may be an indicator of head and neck malignancy as well. Oral, head, and neck cancer accounts for 3% of all cancers in the United States and result in more than 8000 deaths annually.

An extensive discussion of head and neck cancer is beyond the scope of this chapter but some basics will be discussed. Children and young adults are more likely to have benign disorders such as inflammatory or developmental abnormalities, such as thyroglossal or brachial cleft cysts. Adult neck masses are more likely to be neoplastic. In general, 80% of nonthyroid neck masses in adults are neoplastic, of which 80% are malignant.[79] In children, however, more than 80% of neck masses are benign. This is often referred to as *the rule of 80* or *80% rule.*

Risk factors that may predispose patients to ENT malignancies include alcohol and tobacco use, viruses such as herpes virus, sunlight exposure, genetics, diet, exposure to dust, and inhalation exposures.[80]

Principles of Disease

It is critical for the clinician to be familiar with some basic anatomy of the neck. Identifying the location of the parotid and submandibular glands and thyroid cartilage and gland can help avoid confusion when evaluating the neck mass. In addition, knowing where the lymph nodes are can help distinguish lymph nodes from other types of masses.

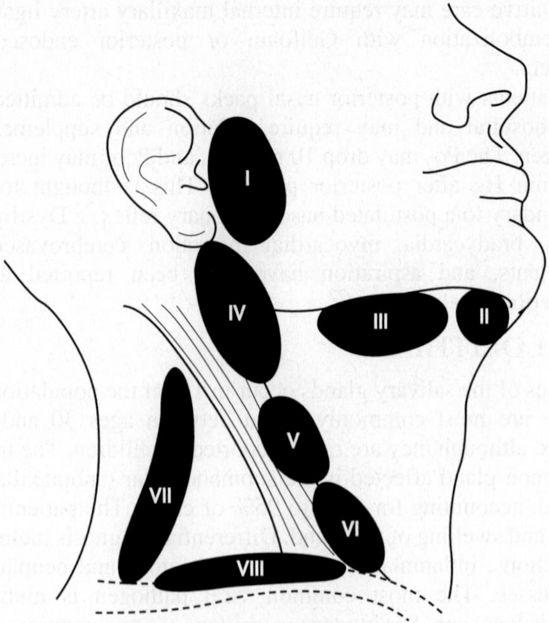

Figure 67-2. **Major lymph node groups in the head and neck: *I,* parotid nodes; *II,* submental nodes; *III,* submandibular nodes; *IV,* jugulodigastric nodes (superior jugular nodes); *V,* midjugular nodes; *VI,* lower jugular nodes; *VII,* spinal accessory nodes; and *VIII,* subclavian nodes. Groups VI and VII are often termed "scalene nodes."** ***Modified from Moloy PJ. In American Academy of Otolaryngology—Head and Neck Surgery Foundation:*** **Common problems of the head and neck region,** ***Philadelphia, 1995, WB Saunders.***

Figure 67-2 is an illustration of the primary lymph chains and their nomenclature.

Clinical Features

There are a number of symptoms that should be inquired about in head and neck disease. These include dysphagia, odynophagia, otalgia, stridor, speech disorders, and globus phenomena. *Dysphagia* is difficulty swallowing and may be caused by physical obstruction or neurologic disorders. *Odynophagia* is pain on swallowing and can be caused by a number of entities, such as tonsillitis or carcinoma of the pharynx. *Otalgia* is pain felt in the ear that may be referred from the larynx, pharynx, and cranial nerves V, IX, and X. Referred ear pain is considered an ominous sign in adults and should be presumed to be cancer until proven otherwise.[81] As mentioned in a previous section, unilateral OME in older adults should be considered nasopharyngeal carcinoma until proven otherwise. Stridor, specifically inspiratory stridor, is diagnostic of upper airway obstruction. It localizes a lesion to above or at the level of the larynx and, when present in adults with a neck mass, should increase the suspicion for carcinoma. Speech disorders, particularly that of hot potato speech, are suspicious for space-occupying lesions above the oropharynx, a classic example being peritonsillar abscess. The globus symptom is that of a lump in the throat. It has occurred in almost everyone at one time or another, is localized to the pharynx, and is often a functional complaint.[81] Hoarseness, the final symptom, is a fairly common complaint, with a myriad of etiologies ranging from viral pharyngitis to laryngeal cancer. Also, like the term *dizziness,* it has a number of descriptions to include breathiness, muffling, harshness, scratchiness, or unnatural deepening of the voice.[82] Hoarseness lasting longer than 2 weeks needs investigation.

Box 67-3 Differential Diagnosis of Neck Masses[83-85]

Inflammatory

Adenitis
- Bacterial (*Streptococcus, Staphylococcus*)
- Viral (HIV, EB-virus, HSV)
- Fungal (Coccidioidomycosis)
- Parasitic (Toxoplasmosis)

Cat scratch disease
Tularemia
Local cutaneous infections
Sialoadenitis (parotid and submaxillary glands)
Thyroiditis
Mycobacterium avium
Mycobacterium tuberculosis

Congenital/Developmental

Brachial cleft cyst
Thyroglossal duct cyst
Dermoid cyst
Cystic hydromas
Torticollis
Thymic masses
Teratomas
Ranula
Lymphangioma
Laryngocele

Neoplastic

Benign

Mesenchymal tumors (lipoma, fibroma, neural tumor)
Salivary gland masses
Vascular abnormalities (hemangiomas, AVM, lymphangiomas, aneurysm)

Malignant

Primary tumors
- Sarcoma
- Salivary gland tumor
- Thyroid or parathyroid tumors
- Lymphoma

Metastasis

From primary head and neck tumors
From infraclavicular primary tumors (such as lung or esophageal cancer)

From Armstrong WB, Giglio MF: *Postgrad Med* 104:63, 1998; McGuirt WF: *Med Clin North Am* 83:219, 1999; and Brown RL, Azizkhan RG: *Pediatric Clin North Am* 45:889, 1998.

Physical Examination

A thorough head and neck examination should be performed looking for masses, lesions, mucosal ulcerations or discolorations, and cranial nerve abnormalities. The mass itself should be palpated for location, size, and consistency. Lymph nodes are generally smaller than 1 to 1.5 cm, so any nodes larger than 1.5 cm should be considered abnormal.[83] Lymph nodes are also mobile, soft, and fleshy. Decreased mobility and/or firmness are warning signs of malignancy.[83]

Diagnostic Strategies

The diagnostic strategy should be tailored to results of the history and physical examination. Hoarseness for longer than 2 weeks should be investigated, generally with fiberoptic examination. Serologic and skin tests may be helpful in certain instances, but are best performed by the referring specialist. Chest radiography may identify lung carcinoma as the source of metastasis. Ultrasonography, CT, MRI, and, finally, needle biopsy can aid in the diagnosis, but usually are not required in the ED.

Differential Considerations

Box 67-3 lists some of the more common causes in the differential diagnosis of neck masses.[83-85]

Management and Disposition

Most masses in children are inflammatory; it is a reasonable strategy to start the patient on antibiotics with 2-week follow-up. If inflammation is considered in adults, a similar strategy can be used.[84] Adults generally will need ENT referral if the mass does not resolve in 2 weeks, the mass is enlarging, the mass is fixed, cervical lymph nodes are matted, or masses are noted in the parotid or thyroid gland.[83]

KEY CONCEPTS

- Amoxicillin is still the initial choice for treatment of AOM. Children younger than 2 years old, those at day care, or those receiving antimicrobials in preceding months may require 80 to 90 mg/kg/day.
- All neck masses that do not respond to antibiotics or persist for more than 2 weeks or hoarseness lasting for greater than 2 weeks need ENT referral.
- Consider necrotizing otitis externa in immunocompromised patients who have a persistent otitis externa.
- Patients with epistaxis with posterior nasal packing are most appropriately admitted and also started on antibiotic therapy.

REFERENCES

1. Stool SE et al: *Managing otitis media with effusion in young children: quick reference guide for clinicians,* AHCPR Pub 94-0623, Rockville, MD, 1994, Agency for Health Care Policy and Research, Public Health Service, US Dept of Health and Human Services.
2. Teele et al: Epidemiology of otitis media during the first seven years of life in children in greater Boston: a prospective cohort study, *J Infect Dis* 160:83, 1989.
3. Stool SE, Field MJ: The impact of otitis media, *Pediatr Infect Dis J* 8:S11, 1989.
4. Infante-Rivard C, Fernandez A: Otis media in children: frequency, risk factors and research avenues, *Epidemiol Rev* 15:444, 1993.
5. Daly K: Risk factors for otitis media sequelae and chronicity, *Ann Otol Rhinol Laryngol Suppl* 103:39, 1994.
6. Church JA: Recurrent otitis media as the presenting symptom in immune deficiency disorders, *Immunol Allergy Practice* 9:327, 1987.
7. Klein JO et al: Definition and classification, *Ann Otol Rhinol Laryngol* 98 (Suppl 139):10, 1989.
8. Bluestone CD, Kleine JO: Otitis media, atelectasis and eustachian tube dysfunction. In Bluestone CD, Stool SE, editors: *Pediatric otolaryngology,* Philadelphia, 1990, WB Saunders.
9. Bonadio WA: The evaluation and management of acute otitis media in children, *Am J Emerg Med* 12:193, 1994.
10. Swanson JA, Hoecher JL: Otitis media in young children, *Mayo Clin Proc* 71:179, 1996.
11. Celin SE et al: Bacteriology of acute otitis media in adults, *JAMA* 266:2249, 1991.
12. Bluestone CD et al: Ten-year review of otitis media pathogens, *Pediatr Infect Dis J* 11:S7, 1992.
13. Ruuskanen O, Heikkinen T: Otitis media: etiology and diagnosis, *Pediatr Infect Dis J* 13:S23, 1994.
14. Burton DM et al: Neonatal otitis media: an update, *Arch Otolaryngol Head Neck Surg* 119:672, 1993.
15. Roberts DB: The etiology of bullous myringitis and the role of mycoplasmas in ear disease: a review, *Pediatrics* 65:761, 1980.
16. Haddad J: Treatment of acute otitis media and its complications, *Otolaryngol Clin North Am* 27:431, 1994.
17. Niemela M et al: Lack of specific symptomatology in children with acute otitis media, *Pediatr Infect Dis J* 13:765, 1994.
18. Baker RD: Is ear pulling associated with ear infection? *Pediatrics* 90:1006, 1992.
19. Howie VM, Schwartz RH: Acute otitis media: a year in general practice, *Am J Dis Child* 137:155, 1983.
20. Berman S: Otitis media in children, *N Engl J Med* 332:1560-1565, 1995.
21. Karma PH et al: Otoscopic diagnosis of middle ear effusion in acute and nonacute otitis media: the value of different otoscopic findings, *Int J Pediatr Otorhinolaryngol* 17:37, 1989.
22. Paradise JL: On classifying otitis media as suppurative or nonsuppurative with a suggested clinical schema, *J Pediatr* 111:948, 1987.
23. Baker RC: Pitfalls in diagnosing acute otitis media, *Pediatr Ann* 20:591, 1991.
24. Combs JT: The diagnosis of otitis media: new technologies, *Pediatr Infect Dis J* 13:1039, 1994.
25. Jehle C, Cottington E: Acoustic otoscopy in the diagnosis of otitis media, *Ann Emerg Med* 18:396, 1989.
26. Giebin GS et al: Antimicrobial treatment of acute otitis media, *J Pediatr* 119:495, 1991.
27. Roland PS: Clinical ototoxicity of topical antibiotic drops, *Otolaryngol Head Neck Surg* 110:598, 1994.
28. Bluestone CD, Klein JO: Intracranial suppurative complications of otitis media and mastoiditis. In Bluestone CD, Stool SE, editors: *Pediatric otolaryngology,* Philadelphia, 1990, WB Saunders.
29. Fliss DM, Leiberman A, Dagan R: Medical sequelae and complications of acute otitis media, *Pediatr Infect Dis J* 13:S34, 1994.
30. Teichgraeber JF, Per-Lee JH, Turner JS: Lateral sinus thrombosis: a modern perspective, *Laryngoscope* 92:744, 1982.
31. Bluestone CD: Surgical management of otitis media: current indications and role related to increasing bacterial resistance, *Pediatr Infect Dis J* 13:1058, 1994.
32. Rosenfeld RM et al: Clinical efficacy of antimicrobial drugs for acute otitis media: metaanalysis of 5400 children from thirty three randomized trials, *J Pediatr* 124:355, 1994.
33. Canafax DM, Giebink GS: Antimicrobial treatment of acute otitis media, *Ann Otol Rhinol Laryngol* 103:11, 1994.
34. Dowell SF, Butler JC, Giebin GS, et al: Acute otitis media: management and surveillance in an era of pneumococcal resistance—a report from the drug resistant *S. pneumoniae* therapeutic working group, *Pediatr Infect Dis J* 18:1, 1999.
35. Culpepper L, Froom J: Routine antimicrobial treatment of acute otitis media: is it necessary? *JAMA* 278:1643-1647, 1997.
36. Green SM, Rothrock SG: Single dose intramuscular ceftriaxone for acute otitis media in children, *Pediatrics* 91:23, 1993.
37. Bluestone CD: Modern management of otitis media, *Pediatr Clin North Am* 36:1371, 1989.
38. Carlin SA et al: Host factors and early therapeutic response in acute otitis media, *J Pediatr* 118:178, 1991.
39. Dowell SF et al: Otitis media: principle of judicious use of antimicrobial agents, *Pediatrics* 101:165-171, 1998.
40. Paradise JL: Short course antimicrobial treatment for acute otitis media: not best for infants and young children, *JAMA* 278:1640, 1997.
41. Handler SD: Current indications for tympanostomy tubes, *Am J Otolaryngol* 15:103, 1994.
42. Rosenfeld RM: Comprehensive management of otitis media with effusion, *Otolaryngol Clin North Am* 27:443, 1994.
43. Gates GA et al: Effectiveness of adenoidectomy and tympanostomy tubes in the treatment of chronic otitis media with effusion, *N Engl J Med* 317:1444, 1987.

44. Hathaway TJ et al: Acute otitis media: who needs posttreatment follow up? *Pediatrics* 94:143, 1994.
45. Puczynske MS et al: Follow-up visit after acute otitis media, *Br J Clin Pract* 39:132, 1985.
46. Woolons AC, Morton RP: When does middle effusion signify nasopharyngeal cancer? *N Z Med J* 107:507, 1994.
47. Hirsch BE: Infections of the external ear, *Am J Otolaryngol* 13:145, 1992.
48. Hawke M et al: Clinical and microbiological features of otitis externa, *J Otolaryngol* 13:289, 1984.
49. Marcy SM: Infections of the external ear, *Pediatr Infect Dis J* 4:192, 1985.
50. Pelton SI, Klein JO: The draining ear: otitis media and externa, *Infect Dis Clin North Am* 2:117, 1988.
51. Bojrab DI et al: Otitis externa, *Otolaryngol Clin North Am* 29:761, 1996.
52. Dickin JRE et al: Herpes zoster oticus: treatment with intravenous acyclovir, *Laryngoscope* 98:776, 1988.
53. Rubin J, Yu VL: Malignant external otitis: insights into pathogenesis, clinical manifestations, diagnosis, and therapy, *Am J Med* 85:391, 1988.
54. Evan P, Hofman L: Malignant external otitis: a case report and review, *Amer Fam Phys* 49:427, 1994.
55. Guy RL et al: Computed tomography in malignant external otitis, *Clin Radiol* 43:166. 1991.
56. Rubin J et al: Malignant external otitis in children, *J Pediatr* 113:965, 1988.
57. Slattery WH, Brackman DE: Skull base osteomyelitis: malignant external otitis. *Otolaryngol Clin North Am* 21:795, 1996.
58. Sade J et al: Ciprofloxacin treatment of malignant external otitis, *Am J Med* 87 (Suppl 5A):138, 1989.
59. Gliklich RE et al: A contemporary analysis of acute mastoiditis, *Arch Otolaryngol Head Neck Surg* 122:135, 1996.
60. Hoppe JE et al: Acute mastoiditis: relevant once again, *Infection* 22:178, 1994.
61. Nadol JB, Eavery RD: Acute and chronic mastoiditis: clinical presentation, diagnosis, and management, *Curr Clin Topics Infect Dis* 15:204, 1995.
62. Bluestone CD, Klerrie JO: Intratemporal complications and sequelae of otitis media. In Bluestone CD, Stool SE, editors: *Pediatric otolaryngology,* Philadelphia, 1990, WB Saunders.
63. Martin-Hirsch DP et al: Latent mastoiditis: no room for complacency, *J Laryngol Otol* 102:115, 1991.
64. Holt GR, Gates GA: Masked mastoiditis, *Laryngoscope* 93:1034, 1983.
65. Myer CM: Diagnosis and management of mastoiditis in children, *Pediatr Ann* 20:622, 1991.
66. Ogle JW, Lauer B: Acute mastoiditis: diagnosis and complications, *Am J Dis Child* 140:1178, 1986.
67. Betar CN, Kluka EA, Steele RW: Mastoiditis in children, *Clin Pediatr* 35:391, 1996.
68. Shikowitz MJ: Sudden sensorineural hearing loss, *Med Clin North Am* 75:1239, 1991.
69. Lawrence LJ, Brown CG: Approach to decreased hearing, *Emerg Med Clin North Am* 5:193, 1987.
70. Nadol JB: Hearing loss, *N Engl J Med* 329:1092, 1993.
71. Josephson GD et al: Practical management of epistaxis, *Med Clin North Am* 75:1311, 1991.
72. Myers A, Kulig K: Epistaxis emergindex.
73. Wurman LH et al: The management of epistaxis, *Am J Otolaryngol* 13:193, 1992.
74. Ableson TI, Witt WJ: Otolaryngologic procedures. In Roberts J, Hedges J, editors: *Clinical procedures in emergency medicine,* Philadelphia, 1991, WB Saunders.
75. Pollack CV, Severance HW: Sialolithiasis: case studies and review, *J Emerg Med* 8:561, 1990.
76. Bruneton JN, Mourou MY: Ultrasound in salivary gland disease, *ORL J Otorhinolaryngol Relat Spec* 55:284, 1995.
77. Nahlieli O et al: Salivary gland endoscopy: a new technique for diagnosis and treatment of sialolithiasis, *J Oral Maxillofac Surg* 1994.
78. McGuff HS, Aufdemorte TB: Prognostic factors in oral, head and neck cancer, *Tex Dent J* 115:31, 1998.
79. Alvi A, Johnson JT: The neck mass: a challenging differential diagnosis, *Postgrad Med* 97:87, 1995.
80. Walton F, Masuredis C: The epidemiology of maxillofacial malignancy, *Oral Maxillofacial Surg Clin North Am* 5:189, 1993.
81. Moloy PJ: How to (and how not to) manage the patient with lump in the neck. In *Common problems of the head and neck region,* Philadelphia, 1995, WB Saunders.
82. Kenna MA: Hoarseness. *Pediatrics Review* 16:69, 1995.
83. Armstrong WB, Giglio MF: Is this lump in the neck anything to worry about? *Postgrad Med* 104:63, 1998.
84. McGuirt WF: The neck mass, *Med Clin North Am* 83:219, 1999.
85. Brown RL, Azizkhan RG: Pediatric head and neck lesions, *Pediatric Clin North Am* 45:889, 1998.

Section II PULMONARY SYSTEM

68 Asthma

Richard Nowak
Glenn Tokarski

PERSPECTIVE

Background

The word *asthma* is derived from the Greek ασυμα—signifying panting—and initially was used as a synonym for "breathlessness." In 1698 Floyer published "A Treatise of the Asthma" in which he attempted to define asthma more clearly and separate it from other pulmonary disorders. Subsequent definitions of asthma have highlighted concepts of airway hyperresponsiveness, bronchospasm, and reversible airway obstruction but failed to encompass the many facets of this disease.

In 1997 the National Heart, Lung and Blood Institute summarized our current understanding of asthma as ". . . a chronic inflammatory disorder of the airways in which many cells and cellular elements play a role . . . this inflammation causes recurrent episodes of wheezing, breathlessness, chest tightness, and coughing . . . episodes are usually associated with widespread but variable airflow obstruction that is often reversible either spontaneously or with treatment."[1] Asthma is thus a chronic inflammatory disease, and control of asthma symptoms is ultimately dependent on ameliorating the inflammatory reaction that produces alterations in airway function and structure.

EPIDEMIOLOGY

In the United States nearly 15 million people suffer from asthma. In 1995 asthma was responsible for more than 1.5 million ED visits, about 500,000 hospitalizations, and more

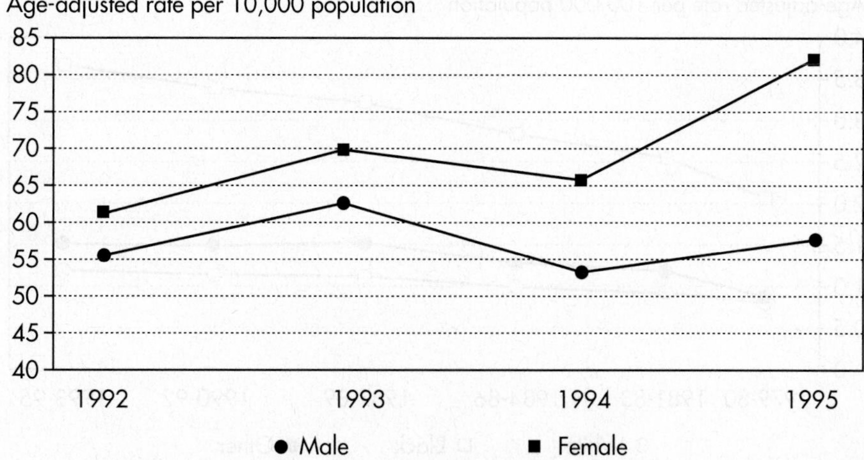

Figure 68-1. **Emergency department visits for asthma in the United States 1992-1995.** ***From the National Institutes of Health National Heart, Lung, and Blood Institute Data Fact Sheet, January 1999.***

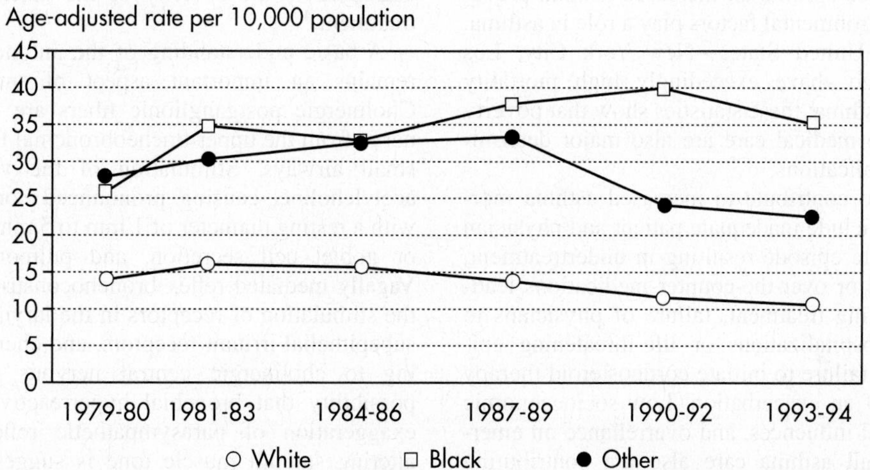

Figure 68-2. **Trends in hospitalization rates for asthma in the United States 1979-1994.** ***From the National Institutes of Health National Heart, Lung, and Blood Institute Data Fact Sheet, January 1999.***

than 5,500 deaths. The estimated direct and indirect costs of this disease in 1998 totaled $11.3 billion.[2] Nearly one third of these costs is attributable to hospitalization alone, and it is estimated that 20% of asthma patients account for 80% of the direct costs.[3] Asthma prevalence is higher among children than adults, in females than in males (except in children, where males have a higher prevalence), and in African Americans than in Caucasians. The prevalence of asthma increased in all age, sex, and racial groups from 1980 to 1994. During this time the overall age-adjusted prevalence increased by 75%, with the single greatest increase (160%) occurring in children ages 0 to 4 years.[2]

ED visits in the United States due to asthma increased from 1992 to 1995, with greater rates in females than males (Figure 68-1). The rate of hospitalization in 1995 was 3.5 times greater in African Americans than in Caucasians. Females had higher hospitalization rates and longer lengths of stay (4.1 versus 3.2 days) than males. Age-adjusted hospitalization rates appear to be declining among all races but the decline in African Americans, having its beginning in 1990-1992, lags approximately 10 years behind that of Caucasians (Figure 68-2).[2]

Disturbing increases in mortality resulting from asthma began to be reported in the 1980s, with a disproportionate number of deaths occurring in the 5 to 34 age range. In the United States, moderation in these trends was noted in the early 1990s and continued through the middle of the decade. Over the past 20 years the age-adjusted mortality rate increased nearly 50%. African Americans account for a disproportionate share of the increased mortality rate during this time (Figure 68-3).[2]

Reports of increased asthma prevalence, morbidity, and mortality are not limited to the United States. New Zealand, Australia, Great Britain, and Canada all reported increases in asthma prevalence, hospitalizations, and deaths during the 1980s with reversal of these trends during the early 1990s. Developed nations have higher rates of asthma, suggesting that urbanization and westernization are correlated with increased asthma prevalence. Interestingly, migrants who move from an area of low asthma prevalence to an area of

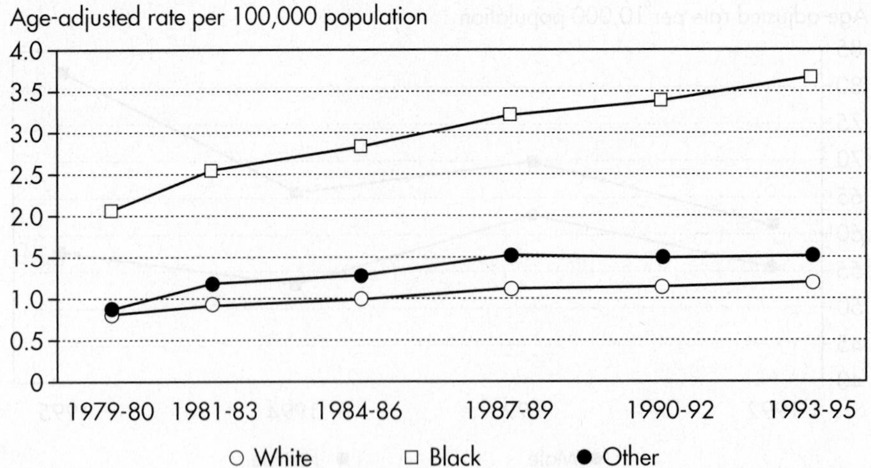

Figure 68-3. **Trends in mortality rates for asthma in the United States 1979-1995.** ***From the National Institutes of Health National Heart, Lung, and Blood Institute Data Fact Sheet, January 1999.***

high asthma prevalence assume an increased asthma prevalence, suggesting environmental factors play a role in asthma. Urban areas in the United States—New York City, Los Angeles, and Chicago—have exceedingly high mortality rates resulting from asthma; these statistics show that poverty and lack of access to medical care are also major determinants of asthma complications.

Factors believed to contribute to increased asthma morbidity and mortality include inadequate patient and physician assessment of an acute episode resulting in undertreatment, overuse of prescribed or over-the-counter medications leading to delays in seeking treatment, failure of physicians to consider previous hospitalizations or life-threatening episodes of asthma, and failure to initiate corticosteroid therapy early in the course of an exacerbation. Low socioeconomic factors, environmental influences, and overreliance on emergency facilities for all asthma care also are contributing factors. Recent initiatives to educate physicians and patients about asthma pathophysiology, monitoring, and therapy may in part be responsible for the moderation of asthma mortality.

PRINCIPLES OF DISEASE

Pathophysiology

Important advances in our understanding of the pathophysiology of asthma have occurred in the past 10 years. Although the concept of bronchial hyperreactivity is still applicable, understanding asthma is no longer limited to understanding smooth muscle dysfunction, airway obstruction, imbalances in adrenergic and cholinergic nervous systems, and immunoglobulin E (IgE) reactions. Rather, the inflammatory process occurring in the airways has now taken center stage and inflammatory cells (their messengers and metabolic products) and effector cells are now felt to be responsible for both acute and chronic asthma. Although still incomplete, our current understanding of the inflammatory process occurring in the airways now directs the therapeutic approach to asthma.

Bronchial reactivity describes the responsiveness of the airways to a bronchoconstricting stimulus (e.g., methacholine). Relative to normal patients, patients with asthma show bronchial hyperreactivity (also called hyperresponsiveness) in response to bronchoconstricting stimuli. This hyperresponsiveness of the airways is characteristic of asthma and correlates to the severity of the disease and the need for treatment.[4]

A basic understanding of the autonomic nervous system remains an important aspect of understanding asthma. Cholinergic postganglionic fibers are carried in the vagus nerve from the upper tracheobronchial tree to the level of the small airways. Stimulation of the vagus nerve releases acetylcholine, causing pronounced constriction of airways with a resting diameter of 1 mm to 5 mm, increased glandular or goblet cell secretion, and pulmonary vessel dilation. Vagally mediated reflex bronchoconstriction can result from the stimulation of receptors in the larynx and lower airways, subepithelial irritant receptors, and chemoreceptors responding to cholinergic central nervous system output. The possibility that bronchial hyperreactivity is caused by an exaggeration of parasympathetic reflex pathway activity altering smooth muscle tone is suggested by the fact that virtually all asthmatic patients have exaggerated bronchomotor sensitivity to muscarinic agonists and that muscarinic antagonists (e.g., atropine) are effective bronchodilators.[5]

Anatomic and physiologic studies of the adrenergic system reveal a sparsity of sympathetic neurons in the airways. Both α and β_2 receptors have been found in airway smooth muscle and on airway epithelial cells. The density of β_2 receptors increases as the airways become smaller.

Stimulation of β_2 receptors relaxes the smooth muscle in airways and bronchial and pulmonary vasculature, facilitates epithelial ion and water secretion, and may be involved in generating epithelial cell–derived relaxing factors.[6] β_2 receptors are also found on mast cells, eosinophils, and other inflammatory cells. Stimulation of α-adrenergic receptors in airway smooth muscle promotes bronchoconstriction, but significant contractile effects are not observed except with chronic bronchitis, bronchopneumonia, and conditions of β-adrenergic blockade.[7] The number of α receptors is thought to be small and it is doubtful that α receptor stimulation plays a significant role in bronchial hyperreactivity.

Nonadrenergic and noncholinergic (NANC) neurons have long been felt to play a role in asthma. Neuropeptides such as vasoactive intestinal peptide, substance P, and neurokinin may mediate bronchoconstriction and dilation. Tachykinins such as substance P are potent inducers of microvascular

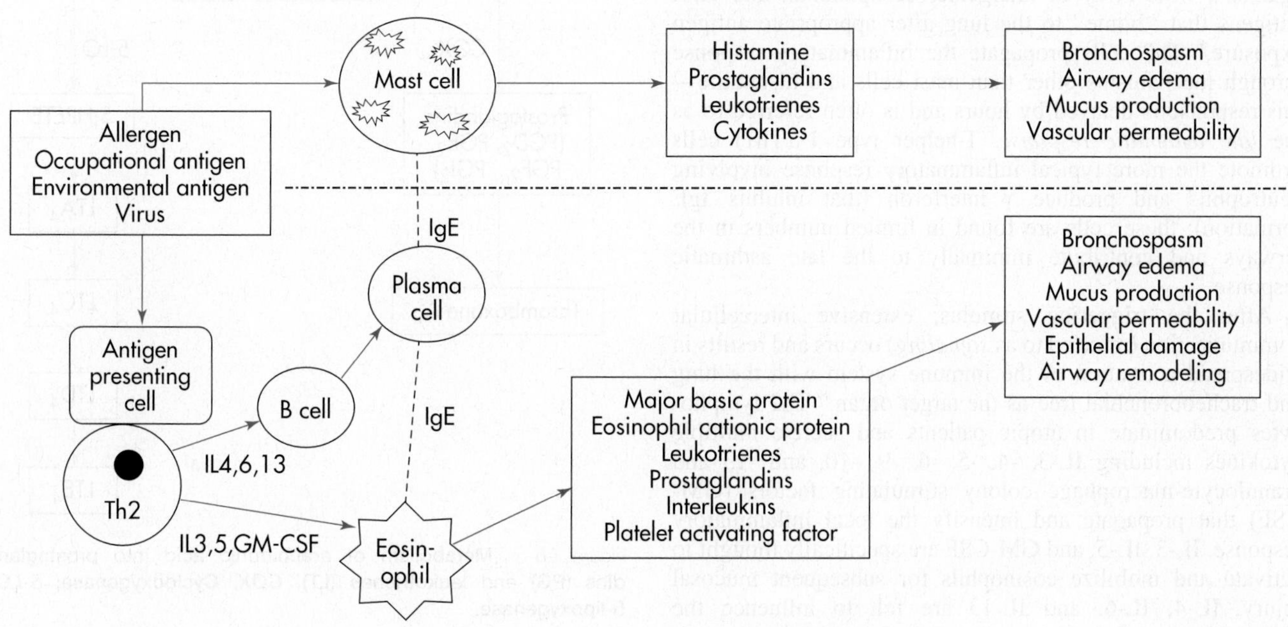

Figure 68-4. **Cellular mechanisms of the early and late asthmatic responses.**

leakage and mucus secretion. In animals, release of neuropeptides from sensory nerves in the airways may result in inflammation—a similar role in humans has not been described. There is compelling evidence that nitric oxide (NO) may also function as an NANC transmitter.[6] NO is a free radical gas produced in airway epithelial cells through the action of the enzyme nitric oxide synthase (NOS). NO is involved in mast cell activation, cell chemotaxis, and may be an endogenous suppressor of inflammation. NOS is stimulated by several inflammatory cytokines—exhaled NO levels are thus felt to be a simple noninvasive marker of airway inflammation, therefore having a possible impact on initiation of antiinflammatory therapy. At present, exhaled NO concentration measurements are not clinically useful and there is no evidence to suggest that modulation of NO production is useful therapeutically.[6]

The central role inflammation plays in asthma has become increasingly clear, and its importance now surpasses that of the autonomic nervous system. Through the mid-1980s the mast cell was felt to be pivotal in asthma. The "leaky" mast cell and its product histamine were felt to explain both extrinsic (atopic) and intrinsic (nonatopic) asthma.[8] Supporting this concept was the effectiveness of mast cell stabilizing agents such as cromolyn sodium in controlling asthma symptoms. Refuting the mast cell hypothesis was the fact that antihistamines had little therapeutic effect in asthma and that corticosteroids, an effective asthma therapy since the 1950s, had little effect on histamine release from mast cells in the lung. Furthermore, the fact that asthmatics continued to show bronchial hyperreactivity even between acute exacerbations led researchers to suspect that a chronic process was responsible. Studies using bronchial biopsy and bronchoalveolar lavage (BAL) findings identify inflammation in the airways of patients with all levels of disease—furthermore, the intensity of inflammation correlates well with the need for treatment. Techniques using electron microscopy, immunohistochemistry, and molecular biology have further advanced our knowledge about the inflammatory process and research is shifting toward antiinflammatory management. Research now focuses on lymphocytes, cytokines, eosinophils, eosinophil-generated mediators (leukotrienes and prostaglandins), and their relationships to asthma symptoms.

The first step of the airway inflammatory process is referred to as *triggering*[8,9] (Figure 68-4). Multiple triggers include allergens, environmental antigens (pollen, aspirin, dander, mites), occupational antigens, and viruses. After inhalation, these triggers may directly stimulate resident airway mast cells, causing cross linking of IgE on the mast cell surface, resulting in the release of preformed histamine and inducing the production of prostaglandins (PGs), leukotrienes (LTs), and enzymes such as tryptase, chymase, and carboxypeptidase. Simultaneously, mast cell–derived cytokines such as interleukin (IL)-4, -5, and -6 signal mast and other inflammatory cells and their mediators to the lung, whereas another cytokine (tumor necrosis factor α) initiates expression of cell adhesion molecules in pulmonary vascular endothelial cells.[10] These mast cell generated messengers thus amplify the initial mast cell reaction and localize further airway inflammation resulting in increased vascular permeability, mucus secretion, airway narrowing, limitation of airflow, bronchospasm, and wheezing. These events occur within minutes of antigen exposure and are referred to as the *early asthmatic response.* Prompt treatment with β_2 agonists is usually effective at this time.

Alternatively, triggers may be presented by macrophages or other antigen-presenting cells to activated T lymphocytes in the lung (see Figure 68-4). T-helper type 2 (Th2) cells are a specialized subset of chronically activated T cells sensitized against a wide array of allergenic, occupational, and viral antigens that "home" to the lung after appropriate antigen exposure.[8] Th2 cells propagate the inflammatory response through mechanisms other than mast cells and histamine—this response is delayed by hours and is often referred to as the *late asthmatic response.* T-helper type 1 (Th1) cells promote the more typical inflammatory response involving neutrophils and produce γ interferon (that inhibits IgE formation); these cells are found in limited numbers in the airways and contribute minimally to the late asthmatic response.

After the triggering stimulus, extensive intercellular communication (referred to as *signaling*) occurs and results in widespread activation of the immune system with the lung and tracheobronchial tree as the target organ.[8] Th2 lymphocytes predominate in atopic patients and secrete multiple cytokines including IL-3, -4, -5, -6, -9, -10, and -13 and granulocyte-macrophage colony stimulating factors (GM-CSF) that propagate and intensify the local inflammatory response. IL-3, IL-5, and GM-CSF are specifically thought to activate and mobilize eosinophils for subsequent mucosal injury. IL-4, IL-6, and IL-13 are felt to influence the differentiation of B lymphocytes into plasma cells that produce IgE specific for the antigenic stimulus.[11] This IgE subsequently binds to local mast cells and eosinophils—offending antigens then interact with the inflammatory cell-bound IgE, thereby propagating the inflammatory response. IL-4 also has a role in influencing the development of naïve T cell into Th2 cells.[12] Thus Th2 cells are capable of both regulating and propagating the inflammatory process. Mast cells, eosinophils, and airway epithelial cells also respond to Th2-derived ILs and produce their own cytokines and LTs, also amplifying the cellular response and intensifying the local inflammatory reaction.

Migration of inflammatory cells from the circulation into the pulmonary vasculature and then into the airway submucosa is likely controlled by cytokines and adhesion molecules. Eosinophils, basophils, mast cells, lymphocytes, and neutrophils are attracted to the airways. Exposure to the submucosa is thought in part to be the result of eosinophil-induced destruction of the airway epithelial barrier (resulting from eosinophilic mediators such as major basic protein and superoxide anions) and to the up-regulation of cell adhesion molecules (CAMs) on endothelial surfaces of the pulmonary vasculature and on eosinophils as well. Adhesion molecules (known as selectins) are responsible for initial "rolling" of inflammatory cells along the vascular walls, drawing them to the site of inflammation and slowing their transit time, thus allowing for maximum activation by local cytokines and LTs.[13] Firm attachment of the inflammatory cells to the vascular endothelium is mediated by other CAMs known as vascular cell adhesion molecules (VCAMs) and intercellular adhesion molecules (ICAMs). After firm attachment to the vascular endothelium, inflammatory cells, under the attraction of chemoattractants such as T cell cytokines, flatten and migrate (diapedesis) through the endothelial cell layer and into the extravascular and submucosal spaces.[14]

The presence of inflammatory cells in the airways is insufficient to produce asthma—inflammatory cells must first be *activated* before they can release their pathologic mediators. Activating substances found in the submucosal layers of the bronchi include GM-CSF, IL-3, and IL-5. Local

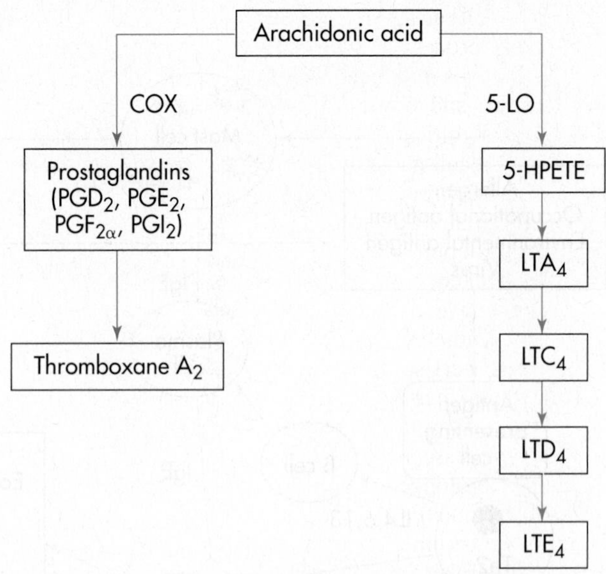

Figure 68-5. **Metabolism of arachidonic acid into prostaglandins (PG) and leukotrienes (LT). *COX,* Cyclooxygenase; *5-LO,* 5-lipoxygenase.**

production of these substances by Th2 cells not only activates eosinophils but also prolongs their survival in the lung.[13] Platelet activating factor produced by mast cells activates eosinophil oxidative and degranulatory pathways, stimulates eosinophils to produce cytokines, and enhances the production of arachidonic acid metabolites. Activation of the arachidonic acid pathway in several inflammatory cells (eosinophils, mast cells, T lymphocytes, endothelial cells) leads to the generation of LTs (Figure 68-5)[15]; modifying this pathway is an area of intense interest and may prove to be therapeutically beneficial. LT levels are increased in both the BAL fluid and urine of asthmatics, suggesting that LTs are activators of inflammatory cells as one of their multiple functions. Levels of eosinophilic cationic protein (a marker of eosinophil activation) are greater in asthmatics than in healthy subjects, and the increase in this marker correlates with disease severity. These activators stimulate the release of a multitude of substances from inflammatory cells (e.g., proteases, cationic proteins, superoxide radicals, and LTs) that precipitate, intensify, and prolong the symptoms of asthma.

Activated inflammatory cells and their mediators *produce tissue stimulation and damage.* The large number of eosinophils found in the airways of asthmatics implicates this cell line as a major effector of the late asthma response. Eosinophil-derived major basic protein causes bronchoconstriction of airway smooth muscle and desquamation of the airway epithelium, exposing nerve endings, providing submucosal access for inflammatory cells and mediators, and negating epithelial cell regulation of the inflammatory process. Eosinophil cationic protein increases airway mucus production and can cause histamine release from mast cells.

LTs are potent bronchoconstrictors produced by eosinophils that are more potent than methacholine.[16] LTs also promote the secretion of thick viscid mucus, leading to airway plugging, and enhance airway vascular permeability, leading to airway edema. Eosinophil produced ILs and GM-CSF stimulates eosinophil proliferation and enhances endothelial cell adhesion, serving to locally amplify the inflammatory process. Platelet activating factor, superoxides, and free radicals produced by eosinophils can also cause bronchospasm and bronchial tissue destruction.[13] Although debatable as significant as effector cells in the late asthmatic response, mast cell mediators such as histamine, tryptase, and chymase cause bronchoconstriction, vascular leakage, and damage to the airway basement membrane, possibly amplifying the eosinophil-induced alterations.

Left unchecked, chronic airway inflammation can result in airway connective tissue deposition, smooth muscle hypertrophy, and epithelial hyperplasia. In asthma the inflammatory response persists for indeterminate durations (possibly resulting from persistent exposure to triggers, lack of appropriate therapy, and impairment or destruction of cellular reparative processes). *Resolution* of inflammatory changes may thus be prolonged or not occur at all.

Airway remodeling occurs, consisting of airway wall thickening, subepithelial fibrosis, mucus gland metaplasia, increases in airway smooth muscle, myofibroblast hyperplasia and hypertrophy, and epithelial hypertrophy in the airways of asthmatics with prolonged disease.[17] There seems to be little doubt that airway remodeling is a feature distinctive to chronic asthma and that advanced airway remodeling is likely the result of repetitive or chronic airway inflammation. Changes such as basement membrane thickening may serve a protective function by preventing inflammatory cells and proteins from entering the airway submucosa through a damaged epithelium; simultaneously, they may be counterproductive because they reduce the elasticity of the small airways and lead to severe obstruction when mucosal swelling and smooth muscle contraction occur. Airway remodeling may explain the "resistance" to therapy observed in patients with prolonged asthma histories and be a future target for therapeutic interventions. Finally, there is evidence to suggest that if asthma is improperly treated, airway remodeling induced by chronic inflammation may lead to chronic, irreversible airflow limitation and a shortened life expectancy.[18]

The clinical implications of early and late asthmatic responses are crucial because therapy may be directed differently toward each phase. Mast cell stabilizers (e.g., β_2 agonists) are likely to be effective in the early asthmatic response but are of lesser use later in the course of an exacerbation. Antiinflammatory therapy (e.g., corticosteroids, LT antagonists) is more effective in the therapy of the late asthmatic response. Inhibition of T cell proliferation and cytokine activity are potential targets for future therapies. Suppression of chronic inflammation and modulation of airway remodeling are other potential avenues of therapy.

Miscellaneous Situations Many precipitants of asthma previously felt to be nonimmunologic ("intrinsic asthma") may be explained by the cellular mechanisms explained above. Thus asthma resulting from respiratory infections (viruses, Chlamydia), environmental precipitants (cigarette smoke), air pollution (ozone, sulfur dioxide), and occupational stimuli (byssinosis, latex) may reflect processing of antigenic stimuli by Th2 cells, the initiation of the late asthmatic response, chronic airway inflammation, and finally airway damage and remodeling. Aspirin-induced asthma (AIA) reflects arachidonic acid metabolism and leukotriene production. There remain a few types of asthma that have no identifiable antigenic stimulus (e.g., physical exertion–related asthma, menstrual-associated asthma, psychologic asthma) and whose mechanisms remain speculative.

Aspirin-Induced Asthma AIA was first described more than 100 years ago. The triad of aspirin sensitivity, asthma, and nasal polyps was first described in 1922 but was popularized by Sampter in 1968.[19] AIA affects about 10% of adult asthmatics. It occurs more often in women than men and rarely occurs in children. Nonsteroidal antiinflammatory drugs (NSAIDs) can also precipitate AIA. AIA is a common precipitant of life-threatening asthma; one survey found that 25% of asthmatics requiring mechanical ventilation were found to have AIA.[20]

Clinically, most patients with AIA have their first symptoms in their third decade, frequently after a viral respiratory illness. Over several months, chronic nasal congestion and rhinorrhea develop. Physical examination often reveals nasal polyps. Bronchial asthma and sensitivity to aspirin then develop. After ingestion of aspirin or a nonsteroidal drug, acute asthma symptoms occur within 3 hours, usually accompanied by profuse rhinorrhea, conjunctival injection, periorbital edema, and occasionally a scarlet flushing of the head and neck.

The pathogenesis of AIA was originally believed to be antigen-antibody mediated because, clinically, it appeared to be a hypersensitivity reaction. New evidence suggests that an immunologic explanation is unlikely. Metabolically, aspirin inhibits cyclooxygenase (COX). Two isoforms of COX are identified: COX 1 is present in almost all body tissues, whereas COX 2 is induced by inflammatory stimuli in pulmonary epithelial cells, alveolar macrophages, fibroblasts, and blood monocytes. Some investigators argue that aspirin inhibition of COX increases the production of LTs, some of which are potent bronchoconstrictors (see Figure 68-5). An alternate view is that LT production remains at basal levels, whereas there is a decrease in the COX-dependent production of PGE_2. PGE_2 modulates LT production by regulating the activity of 5-lipoxygenase and also prevents release of mast cell mediators—a decrease in the amount of PGE_2 removes the modulation of LT synthesis and decreases mast cell stability, resulting in asthma symptoms.[21]

Anti-LT drugs have been introduced as a treatment for AIA. These agents block synthesis of LTs (e.g., zileuton) or block specific LT receptors (e.g., zafirlukast). Most, but not all, patients with AIA seem to benefit from treatment with these agents. The β_2 agonist salbutamol also protects against AIA via a mechanism unrelated to its bronchodilator properties.[21]

Exercise-Induced Asthma Exercise-induced asthma (EIA) has been recognized since the first Olympic games. It is thought to occur in 70% to 90% of asthmatic patients and in 35% to 40% of atopic but nonasthmatic individuals.[22] Clinically, patients with EIA are usually able to complete an exercise task without difficulty, but within a few minutes of completion the symptoms of dyspnea and wheezing occur. Peak symptoms usually occur 5 to 10 minutes after exertion, then begin to spontaneously remit; recovery is usually complete within 60 to 90 minutes. Treatment is required only to abort the acute symptoms of bronchial narrowing and the patient will subsequently be free of symptoms.

The factors responsible for inducing EIA remain elusive. Airway heat flux and concomitant mucosal cooling associated with the increased minute ventilation of exercise are critical initial components of the process. Airway narrowing may be induced by hyperpnea-induced evaporation of periciliary fluid, resulting in increases in airway epithelial surface osmolality (dehydration) and subsequent mast cell degranulation.

Menstrual-Associated Asthma Menstrual-associated asthma is suggested by a higher incidence of hospital admissions in adult women and multiple reports of circa menstrual asthma. Fluctuations in estrogen levels and estradiol withdrawal are postulated as causal factors. Estradiol inhibits eosinophil degranulation and suppresses LT activity—estrogen withdrawal may enhance these actions. In animals, estrogen withdrawal down-regulates β receptors and increases cholinergic induced bronchoconstriction.[23]

Psychologic Factors Bronchospasm may be precipitated by psychologic factors. Associations between emotional states and asthma are described. Panic disorder may be between 2 and 8 times more common among asthmatics than the general population. An association between asthma and depression is noted in children. Mechanisms of bronchospasm associated with psychologic factors may be related to autonomic nervous system activation or hyperventilation; the influence of immunologic mediators is unknown. Relaxation as a therapy for asthma has inconsistent effects.[24] The actual influence of psychologic factors in the induction or continuation of an episode of asthma is unknown but probably varies from patient to patient and episode to episode.

Genetics and Asthma Identifying the genes predisposing an individual to asthma is complex. First, there is no gold standard for the diagnosis of asthma—thus identification of "true" asthmatics to study for genetic inheritance patterns is in many respects subjective. Second, environmental factors influence the phenotypic manifestations of many asthmatics, and the extent of exposure to environmental factors controls which patients develop or do not develop asthma. Finally, the inheritance of asthma does not seem to follow any classic Mendelian pattern.

The significance of genetic studies in asthma lies not only in knowing the basic molecular defects in asthma but also in developing a diagnostic test for asthma; thus, infants at high risk for asthma might be identified and subsequent allergen avoidance may modulate the development or the severity of asthma. The application of pharmacology to genetics has tremendous importance. Pharmacogenetics may allow therapy for asthma to be aimed at the genetic loci of mediators of this disease rather than at receptors or metabolic targets that current strategies employ.

Pathology

Airway morphology in asthmatics is principally described in patients dying of status asthmaticus. Grossly, the lungs are hyperinflated and may fail to collapse on opening of the pleural cavities.[25] Histologic examination reveals luminal plugs consisting of inflammatory cells, desquamated epithelial cells, and mucus. Marked thickening of the airway basement membrane, submucosal inflammatory cells, increased deposition of connective tissue, and hypertrophy of airway smooth muscle are also observed. Histopathologic examination of the airways in patients experiencing sudden-onset fatal asthma demonstrates less mucus in the airway lumens and an excess in the number of submucosal neutrophils compared to the number of submucosal eosinophils; an inverse relationship is noted in patients experiencing slow-onset fatal asthma, suggesting different mechanisms may be operable in these entities.[26]

Antemortem airway pathology in asthma has been traditionally reported by sputum analysis. In the late 1800s, Curschmann first described spiral mucoid casts of the airways in sputum and proposed that mucus plugs obstructed the airways in asthmatic patients. Sputum analysis after antigen challenge in asthmatics has revealed the presence of eosinophils and other inflammatory cells, whereas sputum obtained from patients presenting with spontaneous asthma exacerbations has a neutrophilic predominance.

Airway secretions are now evaluated by BAL in patients with mild to moderate asthma. Increased numbers of mast cells, eosinophils, T lymphocytes, and airway epithelial cells support the concept of chronic inflammation in the airways described previously. Correlation between indices of airway inflammation (as assessed by inflammatory cell counts) and indices of asthma severity are also reported.[27] Antemortem endobronchial biopsies demonstrate submucosal infiltration with eosinophils and other inflammatory cells along with epithelial cell denudation. Thickening of the airway basement membrane (termed subepithelial fibrosis) is observed in studies of asthmatics who have died from asthma as well as in those dying of non–asthma-related causes (suggesting a long-term attempt at repair of damaged respiratory epithelium). Although asthma is thought mainly to affect the large airways, the small airways also may be infiltrated by inflammatory cells, suggesting that inflammation (and possibly remodeling) occurs at this level as well.[28]

CLINICAL FEATURES

National and International Guidelines for the Diagnosis and Management of Asthma

In response to the increasing prevalence, morbidity, and mortality of asthma in the industrialized world, many guidelines have been created to improve the detection and treatment of this disease. Some of these, including the U.S. National Institutes of Health (NIH) Expert Panel Report 2 (EPR-2), have specific portions devoted to the management of acute exacerbations of asthma.[29] The NIH EPR-2 has been further condensed as a practical summary for emergency physicians[30] and critically analyzed regarding limitations and identifying areas for further study.[31] Although these guidelines are imperfect and often reflect multidisciplinary expert recommendations rather than graded evidence-based decisions, they do serve as a basis for education and provide a common set of recommendations for asthma management through which patient care can be audited and studied.

Emergency practice programs based on the ERP-2 improve acute asthma care[32] with effective resource utilization.[33] Many studies show suboptimal guideline implementation in chronic asthma management, especially in the use of antiinflammatory medications, resulting in more frequent ED and hospital use.[34,35] The chronic asthma management strategies in EPR-2 and the implementation of antiinflammatory therapy when appropriate on ED discharge can result in improved overall care.[35]

Symptoms

Most patients with acute asthma have a constellation of symptoms consisting of cough, dyspnea, and wheezing. Cough often begins early in the attack, may be the sole manifestation of the disease in cough-variant asthma and elderly patients, can be associated with sputum production, and is likely the result of subepithelial vagal stimulation. Nocturnal worsening is common, with most patients reporting cough or wheeze at least once per week and with a reported higher nighttime mortality than the general population. Although increased airway resistance, diminished flow rates, and increased bronchial hyperactivity are contributing factors, asthmatic patients who present nocturnally to the ED have similar disease severity as other asthmatics and are treated the same.[36] Up to 40% of asthmatic women suffer from premenstrual worsening of symptoms that peak at 2 to 3 days before menses and are associated with more severe disease[37] as reflected by increased ED visits during the perimenstrual interval.

There are interindividual differences in the dyspnea perceived by asthmatic subjects for the same level of airway narrowing. This results in poor correlation of symptoms to airway obstruction as determined by pulmonary function testing,[38] both chronically and on presentation to the ED. Importantly, patients with severe asthma, especially those with recurrent exacerbations, often have blunted perception of dyspnea (the "poor perceiver") and thus are at risk to underestimate the severity of an attack.[39]

The wheezing that develops depends on the air movement velocity and turbulence, and its intensity varies according to the radius of the bronchial tube. With severe airway obstruction it decreases or vanishes because there is insufficient air movement velocity to produce sound.

Many asthmatics report symptoms of gastroesophageal reflux (heartburn, regurgitation, and swallowing difficulties) that are thought to cause airway narrowing through a vagally mediated pathway or microaspiration. Proton pump inhibitor therapy decreases asthma symptoms in these patients. Approximately 80% of patients with asthma have symptoms of rhinitis. Approximately 5% to 15% of patients with perennial rhinitis have asthma, and control of sinonasal inflammation can lead to asthma improvement.

Lastly, as asthma can appear at any age, including the ninth decade, it is important to realize that the classic picture of wheezing and dyspnea may be ascribed by both patients and physicians to heart failure, bronchitis, occupational lung disease, or poor exercise capacity.

Historic Components

In the past, most asthma deaths followed a period of poor overall control, with increasing use of noneffective bronchodilator therapy, underestimation of symptom severity, and late arrival for care. It is now clear that a minority of patients suffer a predominately hyperacute, bronchospastic "sudden asphyxic asthma" that kills within hours. Studies of nonfatal, sudden, severe acute asthma show that these patients have less identifiable triggers but also have a rapid recovery.[40]

A brief asthma history is important to obtain as acute episodes in a patient tend to have similar courses and thus helps in decision-making concerning therapy and disposition. Risk factors for death from asthma are important to determine and are listed in Box 68-1.[1,41,42]

The brief history pertinent to the current exacerbation should include onset and possible triggers, severity of symptoms, other existing disease (especially those that may be aggravated by systemic corticosteroids such as diabetes, peptic ulcer, hypertension, and psychosis), all current asthma medications noting times and amounts recently used, and any potential asthma problem drugs used such as aspirin or NSAIDs, beta-blockers (including topical agents used for glaucoma), and angiotensin converting enzyme inhibitors.[43]

Box 68-1 Risk Factors for Death From Asthma

1. Past history of sudden severe exacerbations
2. Prior intubation for asthma
3. Prior asthma admission to an intensive care unit
4. Two or more hospitalizations for asthma in the past year
5. Three or more ED care visits for asthma in the past year
6. Hospitalization or an ED care visit for asthma within the past month
7. Use of >2 MDI short-acting β_2 agonist canisters per month
8. Current use of or recent withdrawal from systemic corticosteroids
9. Difficulty perceiving severity of airflow obstruction
10. Comorbidities such as cardiovascular diseases or other systemic problems
11. Serious psychiatric disease or psychosocial problems
12. Illicit drug use, especially inhaled cocaine and heroin

Physical Assessment

Adult women present more often than males to the ED and have higher hospitalization rates with longer stays, possibly due to hormonal, biochemical, or weight differences.

Although alterations in mentation or consciousness indicate severe asthma, restlessness and agitation are too nonspecific to always indicate hypoxia or hypercapnia. Diaphoretic patients who are sitting upright have severe airway obstruction but cyanosis is uncommon because of left shift of the oxyhemoglobin dissociation curve produced by respiratory alkalosis.

Vital signs usually display a tachycardia and tachypnea. A heart rate greater than 120 beats per minute is associated with severe obstruction, but a lesser or normal rate does not rule out severe asthma.[44] The respiratory rate poorly correlates to pulmonary function testing and indicates severe obstruction only if it is greater than 40 breaths per minute.[44]

A pulsus paradoxus or inspiratory fall in systolic blood pressure greater than 10 mm Hg usually signifies severe disease, but its absence does not rule it out and if present, it may disappear with minimal improvement in airflow through larger airways.[44] The same can be said for the presence or absence of the use of accessory muscles of respiration (sternocleidomastoid and scalenus muscles).

Wheezing does not designate the presence, severity, or duration of asthma. It correlates poorly with the degree of functional derangement and may be absent when maximal effort produces minimal airflow. Physical examination may help to identify the complications of asthma such as pneumonia, pneumothorax, or pneumomediastinum that may present atypically as subcutaneous emphysema or simulate upper airway obstruction.[45]

DIAGNOSTIC STRATEGIES

Pulmonary Function Studies

Because physicians tend to underestimate the degree of airway obstruction in acute asthma, particularly on initial assessment, routine pulmonary function testing (PFT) should be part of the ED assessment and monitoring of these patients.[46] The forced expiratory volume in 1 second from maximal inspiration (FEV_1) or the peak expiratory flow rate (PEFR) in liters per second starting with fully inflated lungs and sustained for at least 10 msec may be used in the ED. Both measurements require patient cooperation for maximal effort and whenever possible the best of three consecutive values should be recorded.

Most asthmatic assessments in the ED use portable peak flow meters because of ease of use. While recording valid values, there is wide limit of agreement between different devices and so different portable meters should not be used interchangeably.[47] Mechanical devices may lose accuracy with extensive use and require more frequent replacement. Lastly, although generally similar, the FEV_1 and PEFR measurements do not appear to be interchangeable in assessing acute airway obstruction, a fact that has not yet been addressed in all current management guidelines.[48]

Although absolute PFT measurements can be used,[49] percent predicted (% pred) values are better as they take into account the individual's age (now to age 85 years), sex, and height. More ideal recordings are the percent of the patient's personal best effort as this individualizes the assessment and treatment.

Arterial Blood Gas (ABG) Analysis

Assessment of oxygenation can be done quickly, continuously, and noninvasively in most patients using pulse oximetry, with changes in equilibration of oxygen saturation with supplemental oxygen occurring in 3 to 4 minutes. As airway obstruction increases, the partial pressure of carbon dioxide in arterial gas ($Paco_2$) normalizes (PFT 15% to 25% pred) and then increases (PFT $< 15\%$ pred) with worsening hypoxemia. Because neither pretreatment nor posttreatment ABGs correlate with PFTs or predict clinical outcome, ABG determination is rarely clinically useful in acute asthma exacerbations. ABG determination is of little value in determining the need for tracheal intubation. Clinical evaluation over time, particularly patient stamina, will guide the decision. Consideration for ABG sampling should be limited to a subset of patients with PFTs less than 30% pred, whose clinical course is perplexing. Occasionally, despite improving PFTs with bronchodilator therapy, some patients will have a transient fall in the partial pressure of oxygen in arterial gas (Pao_2) secondary to pulmonary vasodilation and worsening ventilation/perfusion mismatch.[50]

Other Blood Testing

Leukocytosis is common in patients with acute asthma exacerbation and has little meaning. A complete blood count may be appropriate in patients with fever or purulent sputum, realizing that modest leukocytosis is not of discriminatory value. Corticosteroid and epinephrine therapy demarginates polymorphonuclear leukocytes after 1 to 2 hours.

Serum electrolytes are likewise of little value unless the patient is taking corticosteroids or diuretics or has cardiovascular disease and is receiving aggressive β_2 agonist therapy. In theory, frequent albuterol treatments can cause transient hypokalemia, hypomagnesemia, and hypophosphatemia, but this is generally of no clinical significance.

A serum theophylline concentration should be measured in patients taking theophylline before presentation because there are no reliable clinical predictors of these levels, including those in the toxic range.

Radiology Studies

A chest radiograph should be obtained in patients suspected of a complicating cardiopulmonary process such as pneumonia, pneumothorax, pneumomediastinum, or congestive heart failure. Obtain a chest x-ray in those patients not responding to optimal therapy and who require hospital admission because they are at risk for unsuspected clinically significant pulmonary complications of asthma in 15% of cases.[51]

Electrocardiogram and Cardiac Monitoring

The electrocardiogram in patients with severe asthma may show a right ventricular strain pattern that reverses with improvement in airflow. Older patients, especially those with coexistent heart disease or with severe exacerbation, may require continuous cardiac monitoring to detect dysrhythmias.

Future Monitoring Strategies

Nasal capnography is a noninvasive and independent method of continuous, real-time monitoring of severity of bronchospasm. This technique will require further study before being routinely used in the ED.[52]

Noninvasive monitoring of bronchial inflammation may find a place in the ED assessment of acute asthma as a method of customizing care for individual patients. This may include measurement of cytokine profiles in the blood, evaluation of leukotriene E4 in the urine, and monitoring of pentane, hydrogen peroxide, nitric oxide, or carbon monoxide levels in exhaled breath.

Assessment Summary

The severity of airflow obstruction cannot be accurately judged when relying on patient symptoms, physical examination, and laboratory tests. Measurements of airflow obstruction (FEV_1 or PEFR) are key components of disease assessment and response to therapy. A more detailed comparison between commonly measured variables and PFTs is shown in Table 68-1.

DIFFERENTIAL CONSIDERATIONS (Box 68-2)

MANAGEMENT OF ACUTE EXACERBATIONS

Home Strategies

Patients ideally should know how to monitor their symptoms and PEFR to recognize early deterioration in their airflow and should have a written action plan to follow in the event of an exacerbation. This home management includes early use of oral corticosteroids, the increased use of inhaled β_2 agonists, and specific instructions on when to seek emergency care.[1]

Management of Acute Asthma in the ED

The main goal in the ED is to safely reverse the acute airflow obstruction, and the rapidity of this reversal is predictive of the outcome of the attack.[53] Effective bronchodilation often results in decreased need for hospitalization with significant cost savings.[54] Generally, as outlined in Table 68-2, the

Table 68-1. Objective Findings in Asthma Assessment

Factor	Severe asthma (FEV_1 <1.0 L)
Pulse rate (beats/min)	≥120, but may be less with equally severe asthma
Respiratory rate (breaths/min)	≥40, but most are >20, therefore nondiscriminating
Pulsus paradoxus (mm Hg)	≥10, but may be absent with equally severe asthma in 50% of cases
Pulse rate ≥120, respiratory rate ≥20, pulsus paradoxus ≥10	If all three abnormal, 90% with severe asthma, but only 40% with FEV_1 <1.0 L have all three abnormal
Use of accessory muscles of respiration	If present, may indicate severe asthma; if absent, may have equally severe asthma in 50% of cases
ABG analysis (mm Hg)	Pao_2 ≤60 or $Paco_2$ ≥42 indicates severe asthma; all other values difficult to interpret unless PEFR or FEV_1 known
Pulmonary function studies	PEFR and FEV_1 measure directly the degree of airflow obstruction; most useful in assessing severity and guiding treatment decisions

Box 68-2 The Differential Diagnosis of Asthma

Cardiac Conditions

Valvular heart disease
Congestive heart failure

COPD Exacerbation

Pulmonary Infection

Pneumonia
Allergic bronchopulmonary aspergillosis
Loeffler's syndrome
Chronic eosinophilic pneumonia

Upper Airway Obstruction

Laryngeal edema
Laryngeal neoplasm
Foreign body
Paradoxical vocal cord dysfunction

Endobronchial Disease

Neoplasm
Foreign body
Bronchial stenosis

Pulmonary Embolus

Carcinoid Tumor

Allergic/Anaphylactic Reaction

Miscellaneous Conditions

GERD
Noncardiogenic pulmonary edema
Addison's disease
Invasive worm infection

severity of attack as measured by PFTs determines the aggressiveness of the therapy.

Oxygen All patients should receive supplemental oxygen to maintain an arterial oxygen saturation greater than 90% (> 95% in pregnant women and those with coexistent heart disease). In addition give additional oxygen to those with PFTs less than 50% predicted. Continual oxygen saturation monitoring is essential during the acute phase.

Adrenergic Medications

Controversies in Use Epidemiologic studies report an association between death and near death from asthma and the use of inhaled β_2 agonists, with use of more than one cannister per month increasing this risk and it doubling for each additional monthly cannister used.[55] This relationship does not imply causality but may be a marker for more severe disease, particularly if antiinflammatory treatment is underused. Current recommendations for chronic use of inhaled β_2 agonists, however, allow for limited daily use in a rescue-only mode.[1]

The currently used form of albuterol is a racemic mixture of equal amounts of R and S isomers. Data from animal and human studies suggest that the S isomer, which contributes no bronchodilator activity, may induce bronchial hyperreactivity and explain the adverse effects of increased morbidity/mortality associated with regular or excessive use of this drug.[56]

Some investigations of the β adrenergic receptor polymorphisms show differential responsiveness to inhaled albuterol, a possible explanation for the varying responses seen clinically when treating patients with acute disease.[57]

Inhaled β_2 Agonist Choice/Dosing Schedule Albuterol (2.5 mg) is the main β_2 agonist used in the ED for treatment of acute asthma. It is more β_2 selective, longer acting, and with fewer side effects than other previously available drugs such as metaproterenol (15 mg) or isoetharine (5 mg). Other agents such as bitolterol and pirbuterol have not been studied in acute asthma. The amount and frequency of delivery of albuterol are dependent on the initial severity and response to therapy, as shown in Tables 68-2 and 68-3. Those patients with more severe obstruction on arrival to the ED with poor response to initial therapy should receive higher dosing schedules. Clinical trials of varying dosing approaches with albuterol for acute disease do not show significant airflow improvement with higher doses[58,59] as suggested by the guidelines, but one trial suggests that patients who are low responders to initial albuterol do better with more frequent treatments.[60] Thus, the optimal dosing regimen for acute asthma is not well established.

Levalbuterol (Xopenex), the R-isomer of racemic albuterol, is commercially available as a preservative-free nebulizer solution (unit doses of 0.63 or 1.25 mg) for prevention and treatment of bronchospasm. In chronic

Table 68-2. Initial Severity Assessments and Therapies in the ED

	Mild-moderate	Severe
FEV_1 or PEFR %	>50%	Unable or <50%
Oxygen	Maintain Sao_2 >90%	Maintain Sao_2 >90%
Inhaled β_2 agonists		
Nebulized solution (albuterol)	2.5 mg q 20-30 min × 3 doses	5.0 mg q 20-30 min × 3 doses Continuous for 1 hr if severe
MDI with spacer (albuterol, 90 μg/puff)	6-12 puffs q 20 min up to 4 hrs (with supervision)	May be unable to do
Inhaled anticholinergics		
Nebulized solution (ipratropium)	If known previous positive improvement	0.5 mg q 20-30 min × 3 doses (mix with β_2 agonist)
Systemic corticosteroids		
Oral (preferred)	40-60 mg prednisone	40-60 mg prednisone
IV (unable to take p.o. or has absorption problem)	60-125 mg methylprednisolone	60-125 mg methylprednisolone
Intravenous magnesium sulfate (possible intubation)	Not indicated	2-3 gm IV at rate of 1 gm/min

Table 68-3. Response to Initial Management Strategies*

	Moderate exacerbation	Severe exacerbation
FEV_1 or PEFR %	50-80%	<50%
Oxygen	Unnecessary	Maintain Sao_2 >90%
Inhaled β_2 agonists	Hourly for 1-3 hrs	Hourly or continuous
Inhaled anticholinergics	Unnecessary	Every 4-6 hrs
Corticosteroids	Every 6-8 hrs	Every 6-8 hrs

*Derived from the NIH guidelines.

asthma, levalbuterol seems to provide a better therapeutic index than the standard dose of racemic albuterol, further fueling the debate on the potential adverse effects of the S-isomer of β agonists.[61] Preliminary data obtained from levalbuterol therapy for acute asthma in the ED suggest that it is safe and effective at doses up to 15 mg in the first hour of treatment.[62]

Nebulizer versus Metered-Dose Inhaler and Spacer/Holding Chamber A metered-dose inhaler (MDI) plus spacer/holding chamber, used often and frequently (see Table 68-2), provides similar bronchodilation and side effects, even in severe asthma, when compared to wet nebulization.[63] This therapy requires more supervision because some patients will have difficulty firing the cannister before inhalation, inhaling slowly, and breath holding for 5 to 10 seconds. Wet nebulization via mouthpiece or mask requires no coordination and minimal cooperation.

Intravenous Use of Adrenergic Agonists Most international asthma guidelines, with the exception of those in the United States, recommend the use of intravenous β agonists for very severe and nonresponsive acute asthma. Albuterol is given as a load of 4 μg/kg for 2 to 5 minutes followed by an infusion of 0.1 to 0.2 μg/kg/min, with close cardiopulmonary monitoring.[29] Intravenous epinephrine can be given as 2 to 10 ml of a 1:10,000 solution over 5 minutes, repeated if necessary, and an infusion of 1 to 20 μg/min started if there is improvement with initial therapy.[64]

Others, however, observe that high-dose nebulized albuterol has greater efficacy with fewer side effects when compared to its intravenous use.

Subcutaneous Adrenergic Agents Epinephrine has been used in the treatment of asthma for almost 100 years. It has both α and β effects and can produce tachycardia, hypertension, dysrhythmias, and vasoconstriction, especially in older asthmatics with heart disease. Given the potential for increased side effects, it should be given subcutaneously (1:1,000 solution 0.2 to 0.5 ml q 20 to 30 minutes as needed for three doses) only to those asthmatics who are severely bronchospastic and not inhaling adequate albuterol.

Terbutaline is a longer-acting β_2 agonist with equivalent bronchodilating properties to epinephrine in acute asthma. It can cause skeletal muscle tremor and tachycardia. A 0.25 mg dose can be given subcutaneously every 20 minutes for three doses and, as with epinephrine, should only be used in those unable to adequately inhale bronchodilating drugs.

Long-Acting β_2 Agonists and Acute Disease Salmeterol (Serevent) is a long-acting (12 hours) β_2 agonist that is effective when used twice daily by MDI (two puffs) for management of daytime and nocturnal symptoms that are not adequately controlled by antiinflammatory medications. It has an onset of action of 20 minutes and thus is not indicated for the treatment of acute attacks. Patients regularly using salmeterol and with acute exacerbations of disease in the ED are not treated any differently, as it is unknown if they require specific care based on their use of long-acting β_2 agonists.

Formoterol is another long-acting β_2 agonist that has an onset of action within minutes (similar to albuterol) and maximal effect within 2 hours. This agent could evolve as a rescue medication with extended length of action (12 hours).

Corticosteroids Corticosteroids have been used to treat asthma for approximately 50 years and there is general agreement as to their effectiveness. Their main action in the airways is inhibition of recruitment of inflammatory cells and inhibition of release of proinflammatory mediators and cytokines from activated inflammatory and epithelial cells. Corticosteroids activate cytoplasmic glucocorticoid receptors to directly or indirectly regulate the transcription of certain target genes.

Despite this long history of corticosteroid use, the resolution of fundamental acute care issues remains uncertain. These include the types and quantities required to induce a rapid remission, the time needed for drug action, the route of administration, the existence of dose-response effects, and the determination of which patient populations will respond to this therapy.[65]

Systemic Corticosteroids in the ED These medications should be given promptly to patients with moderate to severe attacks or those experiencing incomplete response to initial β agonist therapy. In addition, consider systemic corticosteroids for patients who are taking oral or inhaled corticosteroids, have relapsed after a recent exacerbation, or have had prolonged symptoms. Generally 6 to 24 hours are required for steroids to initiate significant increases in pulmonary mechanics. Decisions to hospitalize patients are not affected by systemic steroid therapy.[65] Some data, however, suggest that the PEFR may improve within 2 hours of steroid therapy in those not responding to initial albuterol inhalation.[66]

Injectable preparations available include methylprednisolone and hydrocortisone. The former has 5 times more antiinflammatory effects, whereas the latter has marked mineralocorticoid effects resulting in sodium retention (thus making it unsuitable for some patients). Recommendations for ED intravenous methylprednisolone dosing are 60 to 125 mg and for hydrocortisone are 200 to 500 mg, each given every 6 to 8 hours until improvement, at which time frequency can be decreased.

Oral steroids used are prednisone or its active form, prednisolone (Medrol). Prednisone is commonly the agent of choice for oral therapy and is given in doses of 40 to 60 mg in the same regimen as the intravenous agents. No study demonstrates the superiority of intravenous corticosteroids over oral preparations. Oral steroid therapy is preferred unless the patient is very ill, is unable to swallow, or is suspected of having impaired gastrointestinal transit or absorption.

Side effects of short-term (hours or days) steroid use include reversible increases in glucose (important in diabetics) and decreases in potassium, fluid retention with weight gain, mood alterations including rare psychosis, hypertension, peptic ulcers, aseptic necrosis of the femur, and very rare allergic reactions to these agents.

Inhaled Corticosteroids in the ED Regular use of inhaled corticosteroids decreases airway hyperresponsiveness, reduces the frequency of exacerbations, improves PFTs and symptoms, and can decrease the need for systemic corticosteroids. The addition of these agents in treating acute attacks in the ED has shown no improvement in PFTs in 6 to 12 hours, but has shown a tendency for fewer admissions and medical management with no worsening of disease.[67] Thus, patients can safely continue their inhaled steroid regimens during exacerbations.

Corticosteroids and Discharged Patients Discharged patients who have received systemic corticosteroids in the ED should continue oral therapy for 3 to 10 days to control disease and prevent relapse, and the need for additional steroids should be determined at the patient's follow-up visit. An acceptable regimen is 40 to 60 mg of prednisone (or equivalent) per day in a single or divided dose. Dose tapering to prevent asthma rebound is unnecessary[68] unless the patient was already taking systemic steroids or a prolonged course of therapy is deemed necessary. An alternative approach, if compliance is an issue, is to give a single intramuscular 40 mg dose of triamcinolone diacetate before ED discharge, as this equally prevents relapse.[69]

Patients who present to the ED for acute exacerbations of asthma may be taking insufficient amounts of chronic controller medications based on their symptoms and excessive use of β_2 agonists.[1] If the patient is not on oral or inhaled steroids, then the addition of inhaled high dose budesonide (400 μg, two puffs twice per day) to their regular asthma medications on ED discharge improves symptoms and decreases relapse by approximately 50% in the ensuing 3 weeks.[70] Patients already inhaling steroids at low to medium doses may double the inhaled regimen until seen by their physician. These patients should use a spacer device and be reminded to rinse their mouth after steroid inhalation to decrease the side effects of dysphonia and oral or esophageal candidiasis.

Corticosteroid-Resistant Asthma Chronic asthma is considered a steroid-responsive disease. A small proportion of asthmatics fails to respond to even high doses of oral and inhaled glucocorticoids and these present considerable management problems. The mechanism of this steroid resistance may be related to abnormalities in the glucocorticoid receptor number or its binding properties. These patients present in the ED on alternative therapies such as cyclosporine, methotrexate, gold, or intravenous immune globulin.

Anticholinergic Agents The atropine-containing botanicals *Datura stramonium* (stinkweed or thorn apple) and *Atropa belladonna* (deadly nightshade) were smoked centuries ago in India for treatment of asthma. In the nineteenth century smoking leaves of the *Datura* species was common in England and by the middle of the last century Salter's treatise on asthma listed *Datura stramonium* as one of asthma's truly effective remedies. Atropine-containing cigarettes or powders smoked in pipes were available into the twentieth century, but their use faded after the introduction of the adrenergic agents.

The anticholinergic drugs available for inhalation therapy include atropine sulfate, atropine methylnitrate, glycopyrrolate, and ipratropium bromide. They all are bronchodilators that override the smooth muscle constrictor and secretory consequences of the parasympathetic nervous system, blocking reflex bronchoconstriction and reversing acute airway obstruction. As atropine use is associated with side effects and glycopyrrolate has not been well studied, the discussion will be limited to ipratropium bromide (Atrovent), a quaternary derivative of atropine that is poorly absorbed from the mucosal surfaces of the lung, resulting in decreased side effects.

The time to reach maximum effect with inhaled ipratropium is 30 to 120 minutes, with effect lasting for up to 6 hours. Its bronchodilating potency is lower and onset of action slower than that of the β_2 agonists and so it should not be used alone in patients with acute asthma. Meta-analyses of trials assessing the role of this drug in combination therapy with β_2 agonists for acute disease find that ipratropium provides a modest improvement in PFTs and a reduction in hospitalizations.[71,72] This benefit has been found to be higher in patients with more severe disease.[73] There is wide interpatient variability in response to anticholinergic therapy, implying that cholinergic mechanisms play a varied role in acute attacks. Accurate prediction of who the responders might be before therapy has not yet been established.

Current recommendations (see Table 68-2) are to add inhalation ipratropium (0.5 mg) to the first three β_2 agonists given to treat severe acute asthma (< 50% pred) and to continue this dose every 4 to 6 hours for those not responding to therapy for up to 36 hours. The equivalent MDI dose is approximately 10 to 20 puffs (18 μg/puff) in the acute setting. Ipratropium can be given to anyone, both acutely or on discharge, if they have had documented improvement with its use. There is evidence that ipratropium may be more effective in patients more than 40 years of age, should be used in reversing bronchospasm secondary to β blocking agents, and might help in those with psychologic factors contributing to their disease.

Magnesium Sulfate Magnesium relaxes bronchial smooth muscle *in vitro* and bronchodilates asthmatic airways *in vitro*. Mechanisms for this direct relaxing effect on bronchial smooth muscle include calcium channel blocking properties, inhibition of cholinergic neuromuscular transmission, stabilization of mast cells and T-lymphocytes, and stimulation of nitric oxide and prostacyclin. Intracellular magnesium levels are lower in asthmatics and the level correlates with airway reactivity.[74]

Magnesium has been reported to cause clinical bronchodilation since 1940, but its role in treating acute disease is becoming clarified. Aggressive intravenous magnesium therapy for severe attacks can obviate the need for intubation. Clinical trials and meta-analyses show that magnesium adjunctive administration in severe asthma attacks improves airflow obstruction and decreases the need for hospital admission.[75,76] Thus, in severe asthma it is reasonable to administer 2 to 3 gm of intravenous magnesium sulfate at a rate of 1 gm/min while continuing aggressive inhalation therapy. Clear evidence supporting the efficacy of magnesium is limited.

Side effects of magnesium infusion are dose related and include warmth, flushing, sweating, nausea and emesis, muscle weakness and loss of deep tendon reflexes, hypotension, and respiratory depression. These are relatively uncommon and manageable. Magnesium fatalities have occurred with massive dosage errors. Future use of inhalation magnesium in acute asthma may include its use as an isotonic vehicle for nebulized albuterol inhalation to improve the PFT response[77] or nebulized by itself for the significant bronchodilatory effect.[78]

Methylxanthines The naturally occurring methylxanthines caffeine and theobromine (in coffee and tea) have been used by asthmatics for hundreds of years to treat wheezing. Currently theophylline is the main oral methylxanthine used to treat asthma whereas aminophylline (80% theophylline by weight) is used intravenously. The mechanism for theophylline's bronchodilatory effects is unclear. It also enhances diuresis, cardiac output, mucociliary clearance, ventilatory drive, and contractility of the diaphragm while inhibiting the release of inflammatory mediators and suppressing microvascular permeability. A number of studies of chronic asthma demonstrate additional potential antiinflammatory and immunomodulatory activity of these drugs[79] and may explain the usefulness of theophylline in nocturnal asthma[80] and moderate asthma managed with inhaled corticosteroids.[81]

Table 68-4. Intravenous Dosage of Aminophylline

	Dosage
Loading dose (based on actual body weight)	5-6 mg/kg over 20 min, peripheral IV
Maintenance infusion (based on ideal body weight)	
Children to age 18	1.0 mg/kg/hr
Adult smokers under 50	0.9 mg/kg/hr
Adult nonsmokers under 50	0.5 mg/kg/hr
Adults over 50	0.4 mg/kg/hr
COPD, acute viral illness	0.6-0.7 mg/kg/hr
Congestive heart failure	0.35-0.68 mg/kg/hr
Liver dysfunction	0.25-0.45 mg/kg/hr

Many studies document the lack of clinical improvement in the first few hours of acute care when aminophylline is added to β_2 agonist therapy while side effects increase.[82] Nevertheless in a single study of hospitalized asthmatics the addition of aminophylline to standard care can result in greater improvement in PFTs using fewer albuterol inhalations. The true value of this therapy remains enigmatic, but in this group of nonresponding asthmatics, the optimization of serum theophylline may give some added benefit.[83]

Optimal serum theophylline levels are 5 to 15 μg/ml. It is important to measure this level in any asthmatic taking theophylline because there are no reliable clinical indicators. Guidelines for aminophylline loading are presented in Table 68-4, understanding that therapeutic levels can be achieved equally fast by the oral route using the alcohol-based elixir of theophylline. If theophylline levels need adjustment then every 1 mg/kg of aminophylline given will increase the serum level by approximately 2 μg/ml. A repeat theophylline level should be obtained 12 to 14 hours after maintenance therapy has been instituted and adjustments made if needed. Drugs that increase serum levels include ciprofloxacin, erythromycin, macrolide antibiotics, troleandomycin, cimetidine, allopurinol, propranolol, and influenza vaccine. Those that decrease levels include carbamazepine, phenobarbital, phenytoin, rifampin, and other drugs capable of inducing hepatic enzyme formation.

Theophylline has a narrow therapeutic window with many significant side effects. These include nervousness or agitation, nausea and vomiting, abdominal discomfort, headache, a variety of dysrhythmias, seizures, confusion, hyperglycemia, hypokalemia, hypophosphatemia, hypomagnesemia, leukocytosis, and respiratory alkalosis or metabolic acidosis.

Leukotriene Modifiers The cysteinyl leukotrienes (LTC4, LTD4, and LTE4) are highly potent mediators of inflammation thought to play a large role in the pathogenesis of asthma. Zafirlukast (Accolate, 20 mg bid) and montelukast (Singulair, 10 mg QD) are novel, rapid acting, safe, antiasthmatic drugs, taken orally, that are potent and highly selective antagonists of type 1 cysteinyl leukotriene receptors. These medications in a wide spectrum of chronic asthma severity as monotherapy or with inhaled steroids is increasing and their positioning in asthma management guidelines is being reassessed.

Asthmatics generally produce elevated levels of leukotrienes (LTs) and in acute attacks the levels in the urine can be markedly increased. LTs are potent bronchoconstrictors and both intravenous (7 mg) and oral (10 mg) montelukast provide mild to moderate non–β_2-mediated bronchodilation for up to 24 hours in patients who have stopped their regular asthma medications. Oral zafirlukast, when given as adjunctive therapy (20 or 160 mg) for acute asthma in the ED, improves PFTs and dyspnea with a strong tendency to decrease admissions to the hospital in the 160 mg group.[84]

The role of these agents in managing acute disease, preventing hospitalizations, reducing the length of hospital stay, and preventing the need for intubation and mechanical ventilation is evolving.

Other/Future Therapies In patients without signs of dehydration or hypovolemia, there is no evidence that vigorous administration of fluids will aid in clearing airway secretions. Mucolytics may worsen cough or airflow obstruction, and chest physical therapy in general is not beneficial. Sedatives are contraindicated in acute disease because of their respiratory depressant effect.

Bacterial, chlamydial, and mycoplasmal respiratory tract infections infrequently contribute to acute asthma. The decision to administer antibiotics should generally be reserved for those patients with fever, purulent sputum, pneumonia, or evidence of bacterial sinusitis.

Future asthma therapies may include the second-generation antihistamines, even though earlier compounds were considered contraindicated in the disease.[85] Neurokinin antagonists, inhaled loop diuretics (furosemide in acute attacks), and lidocaine may help in asthma through inhibition of neurogenic inflammation, and heparin may have a role in the inhibition of mast cell products. Lastly, specific cytokine antagonists, agonists, inhibitors of T cell function, selective inducible nitric oxide synthetase inhibitors, and possibly gene-directed therapies may become novel treatments for the disease.

Pregnancy and Acute Asthma The maternal and fetal risks of uncontrolled asthma are higher than those from using typical asthma medications to manage an attack, and so acute disease should be maximally treated.[86] Of note, pregnant asthmatics receive corticosteroid therapy in the ED less often than nonpregnant women, resulting in continued exacerbation at 2-week follow-up after discharge.[87]

Acute Severe, Near Fatal, and Fatal Asthma

Acute Severe Asthma Acute severe asthma is characterized by bronchospasm that is refractory to outpatient therapy.

Status Asthmaticus Status asthmaticus refers to severe bronchospasm that does not respond to aggressive therapies within 30 to 60 minutes.[88]

Near-Fatal Asthma Near-fatal asthma is identified by respiratory arrest or evidence of respiratory failure ($Paco_2 > 50$ mm Hg).

Fatal Asthma Fatal asthma occurs when patients succumb to asthma.[89]

Two types of fatal asthma are recognized. Slow-onset, near-fatal asthma typically reflects a gradual deterioration of asthma symptoms over several days usually superimposed on chronic poorly controlled asthma. Rapid-onset, near-fatal asthma is characterized by symptom onset and progression to life threatening status in 3 hours or less. Clinically, rapid-onset, near-fatal asthma is characterized by greater hypercapnia when compared to slow onset. Interestingly, the hypercapnia in rapid-onset, near-fatal asthma is rapidly reversible; these patients require shorter durations of mechanical ventilation. Deaths associated with the slow onset mechanism are felt to be preventable in many cases because the gradual progression of symptoms allows patients to seek medical evaluation before succumbing.

Risk factors for death from asthma are identified (see Box 68-1). Although a history of previous endotracheal intubation has been identified as a risk for fatal asthma,[89] lack of a history of previous endotracheal intubation better distinguishes fatal from near-fatal asthma (as patients with a history of asthma-related intubation receive prompt attention in most EDs).[90] Other risk factors linked to near fatal and fatal asthma include hospital admission for asthma treatment within the past 12 months, low socioeconomic status (related to increased allergen exposure and less access to health care), environmental exposures (air pollution, cigarette smoking), and psychosocial or emotional problems.[89] Patients with an episode of near-fatal asthma are also likely to depend on EDs for asthma crisis management.[91] Patients who succumb to fatal asthma commonly tend to be of African ancestry, live in inner city areas, and are between 15 and 34 years of age. Most deaths occur outside or on the way to the hospital, at night, and within 24 hours of the onset of symptoms.

Pathologic differences are noted in the airways of patients with rapid and slow-onset fatal asthma. At postmortem examination, the airways of rapid-onset fatal asthmatics are devoid of mucus and histologically have a neutrophilic predominance in the airway submucosa.[26] Conversely, slow-onset fatal asthmatic airways have a submucosal eosinophil predominance and an abundance of mucus,[92] suggesting different mechanisms may be operable in these clinical situations.

Clinical Approach to the Critically Ill Asthmatic The critically ill asthmatic appears agitated (hypoxemic), assumes an upright position, and appears in severe respiratory distress. Tachypnea, diaphoresis, and accessory muscle use are evident. Speech is fragmented into single or short bursts of syllables or words. Pulsus paradoxus is present. Absence of wheezing indicates severe expiratory obstruction and minimal air movement. Peak expiratory testing is difficult for the patient to perform, but when possible, indicates severe expiratory obstruction. Alterations in consciousness and bradypnea indicate hypercarbia and impending respiratory arrest.

There are no laboratory markers that identify patients with near-fatal asthma. In critically ill patients, elevated lactic acid levels reflect tissue hypoxemia and anaerobic metabolism; persistent elevations of arterial lactate levels are often associated with a poor prognosis. Patients with severe asthma typically have elevated lactate levels on admission—increases in the lactate levels occur even though clinical improvement is noted. The increase in lactate levels may be the result of respiratory muscle overproduction, decreased hepatic metabolism, or muscular "washout" after bronchodilation.[93] Nonetheless, hyperlactatemia is not predictive of respiratory failure in critically ill asthmatics, and blood lactate levels are not helpful.

Noninvasive Strategies Therapy must be initiated immediately (see Table 68-2). Patients should be administered high concentrations of supplemental oxygen. Attempts to abort the episode may be made by administration of high-dose frequent or continuously nebulized β_2 and anticholinergic agents. Simultaneous systemic therapy with subcutaneous terbutaline or epinephrine should be used. Intravenous use of magnesium sulfate or β_2 agonists (where available) may be of benefit. High-dose intravenous corticosteroids should be administered. The duration of this therapy depends on patient response.

Heliox (a mixture of 60% to 80% helium and 20% to 40% oxygen) improves PEFR and ABG results in nonintubated asthmatics and decreases peak airway pressures in ventilated asthmatics.[94,95] Helium is an inert gas with one eighth the density of nitrogen. When helium is blended with oxygen, the resulting gas mixture has a threefold reduction in density compared to air. Heliox reduces the resistance associated with gas flow through airways with nonlaminar flow (the upper and more proximal airways). This reduces respiratory muscle work and possibly improves gas exchange by improving ventilation perfusion relationships or distal gas mixing and diffusion.[94] Although Heliox is not intrinsically therapeutic, it may decrease the work of breathing long enough to abort intubation by allowing bronchodilators and antiinflammatory agents to achieve their effects. Heliox can be administered by face mask and may be an alternative strategy to mechanical ventilation in select asthmatics with evidence of early respiratory failure. Constant monitoring of oxygen saturation and frequent blood gas monitoring are recommended for patients receiving Heliox.

The use of noninvasive positive pressure ventilation in asthmatics is reported.[96,97] Theoretically, the use of positive pressure seems counterintuitive because these devices may worsen hyperinflation and air trapping, increase intrathoracic pressure resulting in decreased venous return, and contribute to barotrauma. Continuous positive airway pressure (CPAP) delivered via a face mask or nasal prongs is reported to be beneficial to asthmatics. Theoretically, CPAP improves oxygenation by increasing functional residual capacity and lung compliance. In addition, CPAP may supply some of the inflating pressure required during inspiration, thus reducing the use and fatigue of the respiratory muscles. Bilevel positive airway pressure (BLPAP) masks and nasal devices may be beneficial in some asthmatics. BLPAP provides CPAP but delivers higher pressure during inspiration than expiration. There are no controlled studies showing benefit in the treatment of acute asthma exacerbations with CPAP or BLPAP.

Ketamine, an intravenous dissociative anesthetic structurally similar to phencyclidine, may prevent the need for intubation and mechanical ventilation. Ketamine has bronchodilator effects[98] but may simultaneously increase airway secretions. Emergence reactions may also occur after ketamine use and may be prevented by the administration of benzodiazepines.[99]

Intubation and Ventilator Strategy With the exception of apnea or coma, there are no absolute indications for endotracheal intubation in the asthmatic patient. Persistent hypercarbia or normal or elevated Pa_{CO_2} values in a hyperventilating patient, exhaustion, and depression of mental status aid in decision making.

The bradypneic, somnolent asthmatic should be administered high concentrations of oxygen while immediate preparations for intubation are made. Time should not be wasted on trials of aerosolized, subcutaneous, or intravenous pharmacologic agents—respiratory arrest is imminent.

The technique of endotracheal intubation is operator dependent. Rapid-sequence intubation using muscle paralysis and induction agents is preferred. Lidocaine 1.5 mg/kg should be administered intravenously 3 minutes before the neuromuscular blocking agent, if possible. There is evidence that lidocaine may mitigate the reactive bronchospasm to intubation. Inhaled albuterol may also protect against intubation-induced bronchoconstriction in asthma.[100] Opioids further depress ventilatory drive in the patient with impending respiratory failure and may worsen oxygen delivery. After intubation, an opioid that does not release histamine, such as fentanyl, can be used to improve patient comfort on the ventilator.

Ketamine, a dissociative anesthetic, is the preferred agent for induction in this setting as it also causes bronchodilation. Succinylcholine or a competitive neuromuscular blocking agent, such as rocuronium, can be used for intubation paralysis. Rapacuronium, an ultra–short-acting competitive neuromuscular blocking agent, causes histamine release in a small number of patients, but may be an acceptable alternative to rocuronium when succinylcholine is contraindicated. After intubation, a benzodiazepine should be administered to keep the patient sedated and to prevent a ketamine emergence reaction. Ongoing neuromuscular blockade improves ventilator performance and pulmonary compliance. Muscle paralysis also decreases oxygen consumption and allows resting of the respiratory muscles while bronchospasm is being aggressively treated.

Nasotracheal intubation is an alternative approach, particularly if laryngoscopy or cricothyrotomy may be difficult. When the airway history or physical examination (atlantooccipital extension, thyromental distance, Mallampati criteria) suggests a difficult airway, nasotracheal intubation can be performed with the patient in a sitting and upright position.

After intubation has been accomplished, a ventilator strategy providing adequate oxygenation and ventilation while minimizing high airway pressures and barotrauma must be instituted. The technique of permissive hypercapnia (also called controlled hypoventilation) is common.[101] Oxygenation is maintained by using a high fraction of inspired oxygen; hypercarbia is tolerated and the respiratory acidosis and hypercarbia are slowly corrected to minimize ventilation pressures and barotrauma. Airway pressure is kept low by providing low tidal volumes (8-10 ml/kg) thus preventing excessive exacerbation of intrinsic peak end-expiratory pressure, stacking of ventilations, and barotrauma. Low ventilation rates ($\leq$ 10 breaths/min) and high inspiratory flow rates are also employed and provide prolonged time for expiration. Adjunctive therapies (in-line β_2 agonists and anticholinergics, intravenous corticosteroids, magnesium, theophylline) to decrease airway pressure and airway obstruction are delivered simultaneously.

Intubation and mechanical ventilation may be lifesaving for near-fatal asthma attacks. Although hazards of mechanical ventilation (nosocomial infection, barotrauma) may occur, the treatment of critically ill asthma with mechanical ventilation has demonstrated low or zero mortality and few complications. Most asthmatics requiring mechanical ventilation improve rapidly and require short intensive care unit stays.[102]

Complications of mechanical ventilation in the asthmatic patient include hypotension and barotrauma. Hypotension occurs almost uniformly secondary to increased intrathoracic pressure with a subsequent decrease in venous return and cardiac output. It is best managed by administration of intravenous fluids and maneuvers to reduce mean airway pressure. Pneumothorax should be suspected whenever sudden clinical deterioration occurs or when hypotension is accompanied by a significant rise in peak inspiratory ventilator pressures and falling oxygen saturation. When suspected, pneumothorax is treated with emergency tube thoracostomy, which may be indicated before confirmatory chest radiography.

Treatment of the Refractory Critically Ill Asthmatic

If the intubated critically ill asthmatic continues to have elevated airway pressures, persistent hypoxemia, and continued bronchospasm after the above agents and procedure have been employed, general anesthesia should be administered. This generally requires transfer to the operating room where anesthetic gases and scavenging systems are available. Isoflurane and halothane have similar bronchodilating efficacy but isoflurane has lower arrhythmogenic and hypotensive properties.[103]

External chest compression may be of assistance when patients cannot exhale.[104] Chest compression is delivered by bilateral squeezing of the lower chest walls immediately after end inspiration has occurred. Compression delivered too early (i.e., during inspiration) may increase airway pressure and result in barotrauma. In children, this technique has been reported to decrease peak airway pressure and partial pressure of carbon dioxide (Pco_2) and increase pH.[105]

Cardiopulmonary arrest may result from unrecognized barotrauma. Empiric bilateral tube thoracostomy should be performed if unexplained cardiac arrest occurs, especially in the context of dramatic increases in peak inspiratory pressure.[106] Intravenous epinephrine is a logical agent to use in the setting of cardiopulmonary arrest because it possesses both cardiostimulatory and bronchodilatory properties. Isoproterenol, a pure β agonist, may increase heart rate and provide bronchodilation but will decrease coronary perfusion pressure. Cardiopulmonary bypass and extracorporeal lung assist have also been used in the treatment of near fatal asthma.

DISPOSITION

Prediction of Relapse

Asthmatic patients discharged from the ED have reported rates of relapse (usually defined as any urgent treatment for asthma, regardless of location) that vary from 11% over 3 days to 45% at 8 weeks. In a multicenter study, the relapse rate was 17% in 2 weeks after ED discharge with increased risk for relapse in those with numerous asthma-related ED visits within the last year, on more outpatient medications, and with longer duration of symptoms before the ED visit.[107] Other studies have found similar out-of-control indices predicting relapse but have also included insufficient improvement in PFTs with hospital-based treatment for an attack.[108]

Inpatient versus Clinical Decision Unit (CDU)

Patients requiring extended care who are without life-threatening exacerbations, pregnancy, or complications of asthma can be generally managed in a CDU for 12 hours with 8-week outcomes equal to those managed in a hospital ward, but with significant cost savings.[109] The ability to predict discharge from the CDU can be assessed by the ED PEFR response to the third β_2 agonist treatment (PEFR > 40% predicted is often associated with successful CDU discharge).[110] Lastly, patients prefer CDU management of acute attacks over routine inpatient care when satisfaction and problems with care processes are assessed by standardized instrumentation.[111]

Table 68-5 summarizes disposition guidelines for asthmatics based upon their response to therapies in the ED.

Discharge Planning from the ED

An asthma exacerbation does not end on ED discharge; airway inflammation and peripheral obstruction may take hours to days to resolve. Patients will likely have need for some continued β_2 agonist rescue therapy during this time, and it is of paramount importance that they can demonstrate the correct use of their inhalers (Box 68-3). If the patient is having difficulty coordinating the cannister activation with inhalation, then a breath-activated inhaler (Maxair Autohaler) or spacer device can be prescribed. A patient using a portable, preloaded, multidose dry powder inhaler must inhale from the mouthpiece in a rapid and forceful inhalation to total lung capacity.

Patients receiving systemic corticosteroids in the ED must continue these orally for 3 to 5 days. Patients should also continue their regular asthma medications, but as most patients that come to the ED for acute care are somewhat out

Table 68-5. ED Disposition Decision-Making Guidelines

	Good response	Incomplete response	Poor response
FEV_1 or PEFR % (predicted/personal best)	>70%	>50% but <70%	<50%
Disposition site			
Home	Yes	Individualized decision (see text)	No, continue therapy
Clinical decision unit	No	Yes, if available	Yes, if available and appropriate
Hospital ward	No	Yes, if no CDU	Yes, if appropriate
Critical care unit	No	No	Yes, if with respiratory insufficiency/failure

Box 68-3 Instructions for Metered-Dose Inhaler Use

1. Remove cap from the MDI container.
2. Assemble the MDI and hold it upright.
3. Shake the canister.
4. Place the mouthpiece loosely between the teeth (or hold it 3 to 4 cm in front of the open mouth).
5. Exhale fully (to functional residual capacity).
6. Actuate the inhaler at the beginning of a slow and full inhalation (as if sipping hot soup) lasting 5 or 6 seconds.
7. Hold breath for at least 10 seconds.
8. Wait 1 minute before reuse.

of control, their controlling treatment regimen may be altered to prevent relapse. If the patient is not using inhaled steroids and with persistent disease, then high-dose inhaled steroids (1600 μg budesonide in divided doses) can be started. Another option is to prescribe a leukotriene antagonist (zafirlukast 20 mg bid) for discharged patients to decrease relapse and improve asthma control. Patients need to have an outpatient follow-up visit within the next 3 to 5 days. At this visit it can be decided if oral steroid therapy needs to be continued, if any ED adjustments to the control drug regimen are effective or require further changes, and a comprehensive asthma action plan made.

The ED can provide limited asthma education through written information about discharge medications, developing a simple action plan for medication adjustment if not improving, and the possible issuing of a peak flow meter with education on how to use it for daily measurements.

KEY CONCEPTS

- Inflammation of the airways is considered the major underlying problem in asthma, and current and future therapies to manage asthma are targeted to control the inflammatory response.
- Leukotriene antagonists (montelukast, zafirlukast) are new agents useful in the therapy of aspirin-induced asthma.
- The ED management of acute asthma is becoming longer in length (up to 24 hours) as more noncritically ill asthmatics are being managed in the clinical decision unit and discharged home.
- Integration of ED discharged acute asthmatics into chronic management strategies to prevent relapse requires ED physicians to be familiar with controlling medications such as inhaled corticosteroids and leukotriene modifiers.

REFERENCES

1. National Institutes of Health, National Heart, Lung, and Blood Institute: Expert panel report 2: Guidelines for the diagnosis and management of asthma. NIH Pub No 97-4051, 1997.
2. National Institutes of Health, National Heart, Lung, and Blood Institute: Data Fact Sheet: Asthma statistics. US Department of Health and Human Services: January 1999.
3. Smith D et al: A national estimate of the economic costs of asthma, *Am J Respir Crit Care Med* 156:787-793, 1997.
4. Barnes PJ: A new approach to the treatment of asthma, *N Engl J Med* 321:1517, 1989.
5. Barnes PJ: Overview of neural mechanisms in asthma, *Pulmonary Pharmacol* 8:151-159, 1995.
6. Berlyne G, Barnes N: No role for NO in asthma? *Lancet* 355:1029-1030, 2000.
7. Morrison KJ et al: β adrenoreceptors on smooth muscle, nerves and inflammatory cells, *Life Sciences* 52:2101, 1993.
8. Kay AB: Role of T cells in asthma. In MacDonald TT, editor: *Mucosal T cells in chem immunol,* Basel, 1998, Karger.
9. Wenzel SE: Arachidonic acid metabolites: mediators of inflammation in asthma, *Pharmacother* 17:3S-12S, 1997.
10. Bradding P, Holgate ST: The mast cell as a source of cytokines in asthma, *Ann NY Acad Sci* 796:272-281, 1996.
11. Kay AB: TH2-type cytokines in asthma, *Ann NY Acad Sci* 796:1-8, 1996.
12. Krug N, Frew AJ: The Th2 cell in asthma: initial expectations yet to be realized, *Clin Exper Allergy* 27:142-150, 1997.
13. Thomas LH, Warner JA: The eosinophil and its role in asthma, *Gen Pharmac* 27:593-597, 1996.
14. Nourshargh S: Adhesion molecules and asthma, *J Pharm Pharmacol* 49 (Suppl 3):33-38, 1997.
15. Pauwels GF et al: Leukotrienes as therapeutic target in asthma, *Allergy* 50:615-622,1995.
16. O'Byrne PM: Eicosanoids and asthma, *Ann NY Acad Sci* 796:251-261, 1996.
17. Elias JA et al: Airway remodeling in asthma, *J Clin Invest* 104:1001-1006, 1999.
18. Fabbri LM et al: Physiologic consequences of long-term inflammation, *Am J Respir Crit Care Med* 157:S195-S198, 1998.
19. Sampter M, Beers RF: Intolerance to aspirin. Clinical studies and consideration of its pathogenesis, *Ann Intern Med* 68:975-983, 1968.
20. Marquette CH et al: Long-term prognosis for near fatal asthma. A 6 year follow-up study of 145 asthmatic patients who underwent mechanical ventilation for near-fatal attack of asthma, *Am Rev Respir Dis* 146:76-81, 1992.
21. Szczeklik A, Stevenson DD: Aspirin-induced asthma: Advances in pathogenesis and management, *J Allergy Clin Immunol* 104:5-13, 1999.
22. McFadden ER, Gilbert IA: Exercise-induced asthma, *N Engl J Med* 330:1362-1367, 1994.
23. Skobeloff EM: Premenstrual asthma. In Kaliner MA, editor: *Emergency asthma.* New York, 1999, Marcel Dekker, Inc.
24. Lehrer PM: Emotionally triggered asthma: A review of research literature and some hypotheses for self-regulation therapies, *Appl Psychophysiol Biofeedback* 23:13-41, 1998.
25. Hogg JC: Pathology of asthma, *J Allergy Clin Immunol* 92:1, 1993.
26. Sur S et al: Sudden onset fatal asthma. A distinct entity with few eosinophils and relatively more neutrophils in the airway submucosa? *Am Rev Respir Dis* 148:713-719, 1993.
27. Fabbri LM et al: Physiologic consequences of long-term inflammation, *Am J Respir Crit Care Med* 157:S195-S198, 1998.
28. Roche WR: Inflammatory and structural changes in the small airways in bronchial asthma, *Am J Respir Crit Care Med* 157:S191-S194, 1998.
29. Nowak RM: National and international guidelines for the emergency management of adult asthma. In Brenner BE, editor: *Emergency asthma,* New York, 1999, Marcel Dekker, Inc.
30. Emond SD, Camargo CA, Nowak RM: 1997 national asthma education and prevention program guidelines: A practical summary for emergency physicians, *Ann Emerg Med* 31:579-589, 1998.
31. Emond SD, Camargo CA, Nowak RM: Advances, opportunities, and the new asthma guidelines, *Ann Emerg Med* 31:590-594, 1998.
32. Emond SD et al: Effect of an Emergency Department asthma program on acute asthma care, *Ann Emerg Med* 34:321-325, 1999.
33. Goldberg R et al: Critical pathway for the emergency department management of acute asthma: effect on resource utilization, *Ann Emerg Med* 31:562-567, 1998.
34. Doerschug KC et al: Asthma guidelines: an assessment of physician understanding and practice, *Am J Respir Crit Care Med* 159:1735-1741, 1999.
35. Akerman MJH, Sinet R: A successful effort to improve asthma care outcome in an inner-city emergency department, *J Asthma* 36:295-303, 1999.

36. Karras DJ, D'Alonzo GE, Heilpern KL: Is circadian variation in asthma severity relevant in the emergency department? *Ann Emerg Med* 26:558-562, 1995.
37. Shames RS et al: Clinical differences among women with and without self-reported perimenstrual asthma, *Ann Allergy Asthma Immunol* 81:65-72, 1998.
38. Teeter JG, Bleecker ER: Relationship between airway obstruction and respiratory symptoms in adult asthmatics, *Chest* 113:272-277, 1998.
39. In't Veen JCCM et al: Impaired perception of dyspnea in patients with severe asthma, *Am J Respir Crit Care Med* 158:1134-1141, 1998.
40. Woodruff PG et al: Sudden-onset severe acute asthma: Clinical features and response to therapy, *Acad Emerg Med* 5:695-791, 1998.
41. Osborn HH et al: New-onset bronchospasm or recrudescence of asthma associated with cocaine abuse, *Acad Emerg Med* 4:689-692, 1997.
42. Gaeta TJ et al: Association between substance abuse and acute exacerbation of bronchial asthma, *Acad Emerg Med* 3:1170-1172, 1996.
43. Craig T, Richardson HB, Moeckli J: Problem drugs for the patient with asthma, *Comprehen Ther* 22:339-344, 1996.
44. Carden DL, Nowak RM, Sarkar DD: Vital signs including pulsus paradoxus in the assessment of acute bronchial asthma, *Ann Emerg Med* 12:80, 1983.
45. Polosa R et al: Spontaneous pneumomediastinum with subcutaneous emphysema: Unusual presenting feature of a common condition, *Monaldi Arch Chest Dis* 54:330-331, 1999.
46. Emerman CL, Cydulka RK: Effect of pulmonary function testing on the management of acute asthma, *Arch Intern Med* 155:225-228, 1995.
47. Koyama H et al: Comparison of four types of portable peak flow meters (Mini-Wright, Assess, Pulmo-graph and Wright Pocket meters), *Resp Med* 92:505-511, 1998.
48. Giannini D et al: Comparison between peak expiratory volume in one second (FEV_1) during bronchoconstriction induced by different stimuli, *J Asthma* 34:105-111, 1997.
49. Nowak RM et al: Comparison of peak expiratory flow and FEV_1 admission criteria for acute bronchial asthma, *Ann Emerg Med* 11:64, 1982.
50. Nowak RM, Tomlanovich MC, Sarkar DD: Arterial blood gases and pulmonary function testing in acute bronchial asthma: Predicting patient outcomes, *JAMA* 249:2043, 1983.
51. Pickup CM, Nee PA, Randall PE: Radiographic features in 1016 adults admitted to hospital with acute asthma, *J Accid Emerg Med* 11:234-237, 1994.
52. Egleston CV, Aslam HB, Lambert MA: Capnography for monitoring non-intubated spontaneously breathing patients in an emergency room setting, *J Accid Emerg Med* 14:222-224, 1997.
53. Rodrigo G, Rodrigo C: Early prediction of poor response in acute asthma patients in the Emergency Department, *Chest* 114:1016-1021, 1998.
54. Stanford R, McLaughlin T, Okamoto LJ: The cost of asthma in the emergency department and hospital, *Am J Respir Crit Care Med* 160: 211-215, 1999.
55. Spitzer W et al: The use of beta-agonists and the risk of death and near death from asthma, *N Engl J Med* 326:501, 1993.
56. Lipworth BJ et al: Pharmacokinetics and extrapulmonary B2 adrenoreceptor activity of nebulized racemic salbutamol and its R and S isomers in healthy volunteers, *Thorax* 52:849-852, 1997.
57. Kotani Y et al: B2-adrenergic receptor polymorphisms affect airway responsiveness to salbutamol in asthmatics, *J Asthma* 36:583-590, 1999.
58. McFadden ER et al: Comparison of two dosage regimens of albuterol in acute asthma, *Am J Med* 105:12-17, 1998.
59. Emerman CL, Cydulka RK, McFadden ER: Comparison of 2.5 vs 7.5 mg of inhaled albuterol in the treatment of acute asthma, *Chest* 115:92-96, 1999.
60. Karpel JP et al: Emergency treatment of acute asthma with albuterol metered-dose inhaler plus holding chamber: how often should treatments be administered? *Chest* 112:348-356, 1997.
61. Jenne JW: The debate on S-enantiomers of B-agonists: tempest in a teapot or gathering storm? *J Allergy Clin Immunol* 102:893-895, 1998.
62. Nowak RM et al: Pilot study to determine the safety and efficacy of escalating doses of levalbuterol in the treatment of acute asthma in the emergency department (ED), *Acad Emerg Med* 7:433, 2000.
63. Idris AH et al: Emergency department treatment of severe asthma. Metered dose inhaler plus holding chamber is equivalent in effectiveness to nebulizer, *Chest* 103:665, 1993.
64. Bishop GF, Hillman KM: Acute severe asthma, *Int Care World* 10:166, 1993.
65. Rodrigo G, Rodrigo C: Corticosteroids in the emergency department therapy of acute adult asthma: an evidence-based evaluation, *Chest* 116:285-295, 1999.
66. Lin RY et al: Rapid improvement of peak flow in asthmatic patients treated with parenteral methylprednisolone in the emergency department: a randomized controlled study, *Ann Emerg Med* 33:487-494, 1999.
67. Afilalo M et al: Efficacy of inhaled steroids (beclomethasone dipropionate) for treatment of mild to moderately severe asthma in the emergency department: a randomized clinical trial, *Ann Emerg Med* 33:304-309, 1999.
68. Cydulka RK, Emerman CL: A pilot study of steroid therapy after emergency department treatment of acute asthma: is a taper needed? *J Emerg Med* 16:15-19, 1998.
69. Schuckman H et al: Comparison of intramuscular triamcinolone and oral prednisone in the outpatient treatment of acute asthma; a randomized controlled trial, *Ann Emerg Med* 31:333-338, 1998.
70. Rowe BH et al: Inhaled budesonide in addition to oral corticosteroids to prevent asthma relapse following discharge from the emergency department: a randomized controlled trial, *JAMA* 281:2119-2126, 1999.
71. Rodrigo G, Rodrigo C, Burschtin O: A meta-analysis of the effects of ipratropium bromide in adults with acute asthma, *Am J Med* 107:363-370, 1999.
72. Stoodley RG, Aaron SD, Dales RE: The role of ipratropium bromide in the emergency management of acute asthma exacerbation: a metaanalysis of randomized clinical trials, *Ann Emerg Med* 34:8-18, 1999.
73. Lin RY et al: Superiority of ipratropium plus albuterol over albuterol alone in the emergency department management of adult asthma: a randomized clinical trial, *Ann Emerg Med* 31:208-213, 1998.
74. Dominquez LJ, Barbagallo M, DiLorenzo G: Bronchial reactivity and intracellular magnesium: a possible mechanism for the bronchodilating effects of magnesium in asthma, *Clin Sci* 95:137-142, 1998.
75. Rowe BH et al: Intravenous magnesium sulfate in the treatment of severe asthma: A systematic review of the evidence, *Ann Emerg Med* 43:S85, 1999.
76. Alter HJ, Koepsell TD, Hilty WM: Intravenous magnesium sulfate as an effective adjunct in acute bronchospasm: a meta-analysis, *Acad Emerg Med* 6:521-522, 1999.
77. Nannini LJ et al: Magnesium sulfate as a vehicle for nebulized salbutamol in acute asthma, *Am J Med* 108:193-197, 2000.
78. Mangat HS, D'Souza GA, Jacob MS: Nebulized magnesium sulphate versus nebulized salbutamol in acute bronchial asthma: a clinical trial, *Eur Respir J* 12:341-344, 1998.
79. Spina D, Landells LJ, Page CP: The role of theophylline and phosphodiesterase isoenzyme inhibitors as anti-inflammatory drugs, *Clin Exper Allergy* 28 (Suppl 3):24-34, 1998.
80. Martin RJ: Nocturnal asthma and use of theophylline, *Clin Exper Allergy* 28 (Suppl 3):64-70, 1998.
81. Minoguchi K et al: Effect of theophylline withdrawal on airway inflammation in asthma, *Clin Exper Allergy* 28 (Suppl 3):57-63, 1998.
82. Rodrigo C, Rodrigo G: Treatment of acute asthma. Lack of therapeutic benefit and increase of the toxicity from aminophylline given in addition to high doses of salbutamol delivered by metered-dose inhaler with a spacer, *Chest* 106:1071, 1994.
83. Huang D et al: Does aminophylline benefit adults admitted to the hospital for an acute exacerbation of asthma? *Ann Intern Med* 289:1155, 1993.
84. Silverman RA et al: The Zafirlukast Acute Asthma Study Group: Zafirlukast improves emergency department outcomes after an acute asthma episode, *Ann Emerg Med* 35:S10, 2000.
85. Malick A, Grant JA: Antihistamines in the treatment of asthma, *Allergy* 52 (Suppl 34):55-66, 1997.

86. National Asthma Education Program Report of the Working Group on Asthma and Pregnancy: Management of Asthma During Pregnancy, NIH Publ No. 93-3279, 1993.
87. Cydulka RK et al: Acute asthma among pregnant women presenting to the emergency department, *Am J Respir Crit Care Med* 160:887-892, 1999.
88. Panacek EA, Pollack CV: Medical management of severe acute asthma. In Kaliner MA, editor: *Emergency asthma,* New York, 1999, Marcel Dekker, Inc.
89. Guishard K: Fatal asthma. In Kaliner MA, editor: *Emergency asthma,* New York, 1999, Marcel Dekker, Inc.
90. Strunk RC et al: Fatal and near-fatal asthma questionnaire: Prelude to a national registry, *J Allergy Clin Immunol* 104:763-768, 1999.
91. Turner MO et al.: Risk factors for near-fatal asthma. A case-control study in hospitalized patients with asthma, *Am J Respir Crit Care Med* 157:1804-1809, 1999.
92. Reid LM: The presence or absence of bronchial mucus in fatal asthma, *J Allergy Clin Immunol* 80:415-416, 1987.
93. Rabbat A et al: Hyperlactatemia during acute severe asthma, *Intensive Care Med* 24:304-312, 1998.
94. Manthous CA et al.: Heliox in the treatment of airflow obstruction: a critical review of the literature, *Respiratory Care* 42:1034-1042, 1997.
95. Kudukis TM et al: Inhaled helium-oxygen revisited: effect of inhaled helium-oxygen during the treatment of status asthmaticus in children, *J Ped* 130:217, 1997.
96. Shivaram U et al: Effects of continuous positive airway pressure in acute asthma, *Respiration* 52:157-162, 1987.
97. Lin HC et al: Effect of continuous positive airway pressure on methacholine-induced bronchospasm, *Respir Med* 89:121-128, 1995.
98. Sarma V: Ketamine and asthma. *Acta Scand* 36:1507-1510, 1992.
99. Green S, Johnson N: Ketamine sedation for pediatric procedures, 2. Review and implications, *Ann Emerg Med* 19:1033-1046, 1990.
100. Maslow AD et al: Inhaled albuterol, but not intravenous lidocaine, protects against intubation-induced bronchoconstriction in asthma, *Anesthesiol* 93:1198-1204, 2000.
101. Dries DJ: Permissive hypercapnia, *J Trauma: Injury, Infection Crit Care* 39:984-989, 1995.
102. Braman SS, Kaemmerlen JT: Intensive care of status asthmaticus, a 10 year experience, *JAMA* 264:366-368, 1990.
103. DeNicola LK et al: Inhalation anaesthetics as an adjunct to ventilator management in severe status asthmaticus, *Intensive Care World* 15:126-131, 1998.
104. Fisher M et al: External chest compression in acute asthma: a preliminary study, *Crit Care Med* 21:1824, 1993.
105. Weber JE, Goetting MG: Closed lung massage improves ventilation in status asthmaticus, *Acad Emerg Med* 1:A49, 1994.
106. Josephson EB, Goetting MG: Asthmatic cardiac arrest: an indication for empiric bilateral tube thoracostomies, *Ann Emerg Med* 18:457, 1989.
107. Emerman CL et al: Prospective multicenter study of relapse following treatment for acute asthma among adults presenting to the emergency department, *Chest* 115:919-927, 1999.
108. McCarren M et al: Prediction of relapse within eight weeks after an acute asthma exacerbation in adults, *J Clin Epidemiol* 51:107-118, 1998.
109. McDermott MF et al: A comparison between emergency diagnostic and treatment unit and inpatient care in the management of acute asthma, *Arch Intern Med* 157:2055-2062, 1997.
110. McCarren M et al: Predicting recovery from acute asthma in an emergency diagnostic and treatment unit, *Acad Emerg Med* 7:28-35, 2000.
111. Rydman RJ et al: Patient satisfaction with an emergency department asthma observation unit, *Acad Emerg Med* 6:178-183, 1999.

69 Chronic Obstructive Pulmonary Disease

Diku P. Mandavia
Robert H. Dailey

PERSPECTIVE

Chronic obstructive pulmonary diseases (COPDs) significantly afflict more than one fourth of all adults, account for an enormous number of days lost from work, cost billions of dollars a year for treatment,[1] and cause morbidity or mortality in more than 10% of our citizens.[2] COPDs are the fourth leading cause of death overall,[3] and, although mortality for men is leveling off, the rate for women is increasing.[2] COPDs are especially problematic for the emergency physician because of their intrinsic physiologic complexity, slow change over time, and undramatic response to therapy.

COPD is usually referred to in the singular sense, that is, disease instead of diseases. This usage is, paradoxically, both correct and misleading: correct in that a single common pathophysiologic determinant is operative (i.e., airway obstruction), yet misleading in the implication that only one disease process is present.[4] Indeed, COPD refers to a triad of distinct disease processes that, as a rule, coexist. The three disease processes are asthma (airway reaction), emphysema (airway collapse), and bronchitis (airway inflammation). These disease processes must be separated from numerous other nonobstructive chronic pulmonary diseases that are less commonly encountered (e.g., restrictive and infiltrative diseases).

PRINCIPLES OF DISEASE

Three-Component Division and Synthesis

Just as obstructive pulmonary diseases may coexist with other types of chronic pulmonary disease, so may the three component diseases of COPD coexist (Figure 69-1). A patient may have one, two, or three of these components and each in varying degrees. These concepts are illustrated in Figure 69-2, wherein open circle *A* represents asthma; *B,* bronchitis; and *E,* emphysema. The shaded circle represents an individual patient. Figure 69-2 would represent a patient with primarily bronchitis, a much lesser degree of reactive airway disease, and minimal emphysema—a mixed COPD picture. It is useful to consider each of the three components of COPD and then mixed COPD, using this scheme.[5] Although this classification facilitates a physiologic understanding, a re-

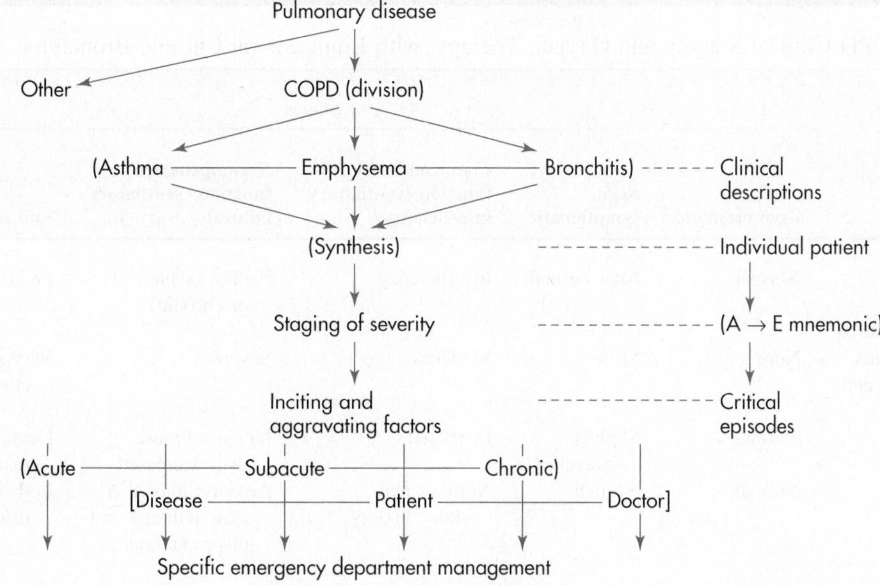

Figure 69-1. **Approach to COPD.**

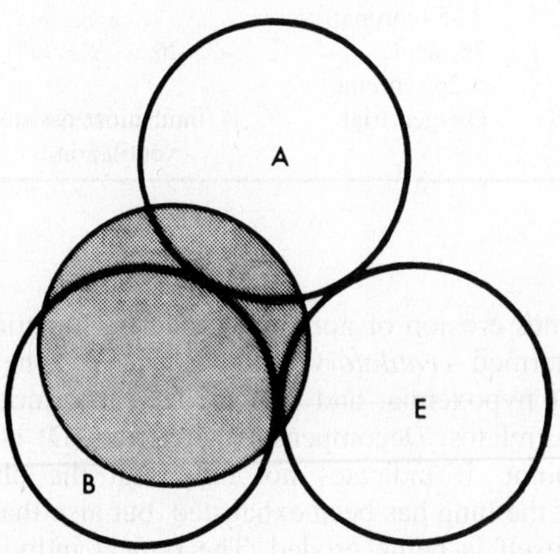

Figure 69-2. **Permutation of combinations of bronchitis (B), asthma (A), and emphysema (E).**

sponse to bronchodilators and steroids in the past provides a practical approach by delineating which patients have a more reactive airway component.

Pathophysiology

The two principal mechanisms of airway obstruction in asthma are bronchoconstriction and mucus plugging. Such variable obstruction of small airways results in uneven areas of air trapping and hyperinflation with right-to-left shunting and thus hypoxemia; if widespread and associated with respiratory exhaustion, hypercapnia ensues. Bronchoconstriction generally attracts the clinician's attention because it is usually suspected and diagnosed, is acute, and can directly and quickly respond to drug therapy. Mucus plugging of small bronchi and bronchioles is the "steady" component and, more important, the pathology found consistently in patients dying of asthma. It occurs over days and weeks and consists of inspissated mucus, edema, and cellular debris (bronchial epithelium, eosinophils, and polymorphonucleocytes). This process is less dramatic and is more difficult to diagnose than bronchospasm, and it is impossible to reverse quickly.

Two principal pathologic changes characterize emphysema: gradual destruction of alveolar septi and obliteration of the pulmonary capillary bed. Alveolar septi are responsible for support of the bronchial walls, and their destruction causes collapse of bronchi, producing significant obstruction to airflow on expiration. Obliteration of the pulmonary capillary bed is associated with decreased pulmonary capillary blood flow.

The most supportable theory for this parenchymal destruction is the elastase-antielastase hypothesis.[6,7] The enzyme elastase is implicated in lysis of pulmonary parenchyma. This enzyme is elaborated by polymorphonucleocytes and present in abundance in chronic smokers. Both $\alpha 1$ protease inhibitor and $\beta 2$ macroglobulin inactivate elastase and provide protection against elastolysis. A chronic imbalance of these systems leads to uncontrolled elastolytic damage to the pulmonary tree and clinical emphysema.

The pure emphysematous patient responds to this pulmonary destruction by increasing the ventilatory drive and is thus able to maintain a near normal Po_2, preventing any cyanosis. This tachypnea also causes a slightly low to normal Pco_2. With relatively normal blood gases, hypoxia-induced pulmonary hypertension and cor pulmonale do not occur; rather, a syndrome of pulmonary cachexia develops.

Chronic bronchitis affects both small and large bronchi. The endobronchial surface is grossly inflamed, edematous, and covered with secretions. Hypertrophy of goblet cells and submucosal glands contribute these secretions. Damage to endothelium impairs the mucociliary response that clears bacteria and mucus. Although most bouts of bronchitis are viral in origin, bacteria, including *Streptococcus pneumoniae, Haemophilus influenzae, Haemophilus parainfluenzae, Moraxella catarrhalis,* and *Neisseria* species flourish and probably contribute significantly to further inflammatory change.[8] It is inflammation and secretions that provide the obstructive component that so typifies chronic bronchitis.

Table 69-1. COPD Clinical Staging and Oxygen Therapy, with Emphasis on Chronic Bronchitis

	Stages				
	*A*symptomatic	*B*egin symptomatic	*C*ompromised function (ventilatory insufficiency)	*D*ecompensated function (ventilatory failure)	*E*nd stage
Ventilatory status	Normal	Near normal	Insufficiency	Failure (acute or chronic)	Failure (acute or chronic)
Bedside clinical evaluation					
Respiratory symptoms (cough, dyspnea, and wheezing)	None	Mild	Moderate	Severe	Very severe or quiet chest (!)
Respiratory effort	Normal	Slightly increased	Increased	Increased more than decreased	Decreased more than increased
Mental status	Normal	Normal	Normal; may show anxiety	Anxiety; may also slow lethargy and disorientation	Lethargy and sometimes disorientation
Laboratory studies					
ABG (sea level)					
Pao_2 (± 5)	80-100	60-80	50-60	< 50	< 50
$Paco_2$ (± 5)	40	40	< 40-40	40-60	> 60
pH (± 0.5)	7.40	7.40	> 7.40 (acute) 7.45 (chronic)	< 7.40 (acute) 7.35 (chronic)	< 7.30
Measured bicarbonate (carbon dioxide) (± 3)	26	26	26 (acute) < 26 (chronic)	26 (acute) > 26 (chronic)	> 26
Oxygen therapy	None	None	Unrestricted nasal oxygen	Oxygen trial	Intubation; assisted ventilation

Usually the pulmonary capillary bed is relatively undamaged in bronchitic, as opposed to emphysematous, patients. Variable emphysema occurs, but it is usually centrilobular as opposed to panlobular in pure emphysema.

Unable to meet the challenge of obstructive lung disease, the bronchitic person responds differently than the emphysematous patient. Arterial blood gases (ABGs) typically reveal severe hypoxia and hypercapnia. Respiratory acidosis supervenes in acute decompensation. Despite deranged blood gases, the pure bronchitic person fails to increase minute volume, and the chronic hypoxia leads to pulmonary hypertension with subsequent cor pulmonale and polycythemia.

Staging the Severity of Disease

Table 69-1 attempts a synthesis of the five stages of disease severity, based on classic terminology, describing deterioration in terms most consistent with the chronic bronchitis patient. The information in the table, of course, must be considerably modified if the major components are reactive airways disease or emphysema. Most COPD patients, however, show a mixed picture in the more advanced stages of disease.

*A*symptomatic is the term for the person in stage A COPD. This person has no respiratory symptoms, even on exertion, and minimal, if any, hypoxemia. *B*eginning symptomatic disease (B) has produced lung damage detectable to the person only when pulmonary function is stressed. This individual has mild symptoms and signs, and there is little, if any, disability. The individual demonstrates dyspnea only on exertion and has slight hypoxemia. *C*ompromised function (C) indicates erosion of normally used lung function, which may be termed *ventilatory insufficiency.* Dyspnea at rest, significant hypoxemia, and hypocarbia or normocarbia are clinical correlates. *D*ecompensated function (D) is a crucial turning point. It indicates not only that the physiologic reserve of the lung has been exhausted, but also that baseline function itself is being eroded. The typical individual with mixed COPD manifests chronic (with or without acute) ventilatory failure. Chronic ventilatory failure is either associated with, or soon eventuates, cor pulmonale. *E*nd-stage disease (E) indicates organ decompensation of a degree that the person will die without assisted ventilation (severe acute on chronic ventilatory failure).

Critical Episodes

Inciting or Aggravating Factors After assessing the types and severity of the three basic components of COPD, the emergency physician is ready to question what inciting or aggravating event has precipitated the critical episode. Clinical deterioration is classified here as the result of advancing disease or inappropriate patient or physician response to disease (Box 69-1).

Disease-Related Factors Disease-related factors are divided into acute, subacute, and chronic factors. Acute factors produce deterioration in a span of minutes. The "big three" (pneumothorax, pulmonary embolus, and lobar atelectasis) are relatively uncommon but often catastrophic.

Acute pneumothorax is both the most common and the most treatable catastrophe. In older patients with COPD, chest pain is often absent. A small pneumothorax cannot be

Box 69-1 Critical Episodes: Inciting or Aggravating Factors in COPD

I. Disease related
  A. Acute
    1. Pneumothorax
    2. Large pulmonary embolism
    3. Lobar atelectasis
  B. Subacute
    1. Acute bronchitis (allergic or infective)
    2. Pneumonia
    3. Small pulmonary emboli
    4. Pulmonary compression (e.g., obesity, ascites, gastric distention, pleural effusion)
    5. Segmental atelectasis
    6. Trauma (e.g., rib fractures, pulmonary contusion)
    7. Neuromuscular and metabolic diseases
  C. Chronic
    1. Cigarettes, air pollutants, childhood respiratory illnesses, α-antitrypsin deficiency
    2. Unrelated treatable chronic pulmonary disease (bronchiectasis, tuberculosis, sarcoidosis)
II. Patient related
  A. Noxious habits
  B. Noncompliance
III. Physician related (iatrogenic)
  A. Insufficient therapy
  B. Inappropriate therapy (e.g., deleterious drugs)

excluded by physical examination and is easily missed on inspiratory chest films, especially in patients with bullous emphysema.

Large pulmonary emboli constitute the second acute catastrophe. They must always be suspected in the individual with chronic bronchitis who deteriorates quickly with no other apparent cause. They have high blood viscosity, high peripheral venous pressure, and venous stasis. Unfortunately, diagnosis of pulmonary embolus in patients with COPD is extremely difficult.

The third catastrophe is acute lobar atelectasis. It occurs most commonly in patients with the combination of bronchopulmonary secretions, dehydration, and impaired cough. Impairment of the diaphragmatic motion secondary to quadriplegia, polio, or other neuromuscular disease provides the typical stage. A deviated trachea, unilateral decreased lung expansion, and decreased breath sounds typically occur, along with the subtle radiographic appearance of lobar collapse.

In contrast, subacute clinical deterioration occurs over hours or days, and it is this circumstance that probably most commonly draws the emergency physician's attention. Because subacute clinical deterioration is less dramatic than the big three, its causes demand special vigilance.

As chronic bronchitis is the most significant process of the three components of COPD, acute bronchitis is the most common aggravating cause. The term *acute bronchitis* refers to episodic cough and expectoration; fever and leukocytosis are ordinarily absent but can occasionally occur. Although inhalants and other factors may certainly contribute, the principal types of acute bronchitis are allergic and infective. The term *allergic bronchitis* is largely descriptive rather than diagnostic; it is characterized by predominantly eosinophilic expectoration that resolves with steroid treatment.

Although infective bronchitis is probably more common than allergic bronchitis, it is difficult to assess whether bacteria, viruses, or a combination are pathogenic in a given patient. Bronchial secretions distal to the carina almost invariably harbor *Haemophilus influenzae* and *Streptococcus pneumoniae,* but it is unclear whether these bacteria are primary invaders, secondary invaders, or relatively harmless commensals.[9]

Pneumonia is a common, devastating complication of COPD that causes death in many patients. Its appearance is more muted than the classic lobar pneumonia of young adults. The cough, fever, leukocytosis, and toxicity are less often seen than the more nonspecific and subtle symptoms of malaise, weakness, decreased activity, and anorexia. An infiltrate may or may not be seen, and correlation with previous x-ray studies is necessary.[10] The ABGs typically reveal worsening hypoxia.

Submassive pulmonary emboli play an uncertain role in deteriorating COPD. As mentioned, the patient with cor pulmonale is particularly prone to sustaining pulmonary emboli. In fact, worsening dyspnea, the most common symptom, is nonspecific and is present in almost all patients with COPD in the ED. Although a coexisting decrement in P_{CO_2} and P_{O_2} suggests pulmonary embolus in COPD patients, this finding is not sensitive. In most patients with COPD, ventilation-perfusion scanning results are intermediate, mandating further investigation.[11] Pulmonary angiography is invasive and has inherent risk, and the role of helical computed tomography is expanding.[12,13] Helical computed tomography can detect large central emboli but is currently much less sensitive in detecting small peripheral emboli. The identification of deep vein thrombosis of the legs with Doppler ultrasonography is a helpful strategy.

Pleural effusions compress the lung and enlarge the thoracic cage and can, respectively, worsen blood gases and decrease the mechanical advantage of respiratory muscles. Therefore, large pleural effusions should be treated by either diuresis or thoracentesis, depending on the cause and the acuity of the situation. Although plugging of terminal bronchioles by secretions and mucus is a particular problem in asthmatic patients, it may also occur in other COPD patients. The resulting segmental atelectasis may have few clinical manifestations, despite its large contribution to underventilated pulmonary segments. The chest film may show linear horizontal streaking or small flarelike shadows; more often, it may be normal. Hypoxemic reactive airway patients with a protracted wheezing course unresponsive to bronchodilators must be presumed to be atelectatic.

Rib fractures are particularly dangerous in patients with COPD. Splinting, stasis of secretions, and secondary pulmonary contusion or pneumothorax must be considered. They are, of course, most often secondary to trauma, but in patients receiving steroid therapy, they can be due to vigorous cough alone. Intercostal nerve block may relieve enough discomfort to restore baseline pulmonary function.

A final mix of subacute neuromuscular problems should be considered. Hypokalemia, hypomagnesemia, hypocalcemia, or hypophosphatemia may impair the contractility of muscles. In a similar manner, patients with paraplegia, polio, myasthenia, and other neuromuscular diseases may have either or both hypoventilation and impaired cough. The antibiotics neomycin and kanamycin interfere with motor end-plate function. As well, any conditions that embarrass diaphragmatic motion such as phrenic nerve injury, ascites, gastric distention, or massive obesity can produce hypoventilation.

The emergency physician seldom considers chronic disease processes that incite or aggravate COPD. Smoking and, on a broader scale, air pollution play a prominent role in COPD, and removal of the patient from such an environment may be necessary. Some chronic factors are quite beyond the control of the emergency physician. α1 Antitrypsin deficiency, especially in its homozygous state, produces devastating and relatively pure panlobular emphysema beginning in early adulthood.[14] Frequent childhood lower respiratory infections are particularly likely to produce chronic bronchitis and bronchiectasis.

There are other treatable chronic, nonobstructive pulmonary diseases. Bronchiectasis, mentioned previously, is an often overlooked cause of purulent expectoration. It may accompany and exacerbate the three components of COPD. Although its pathologic characteristic is dilation (not constriction) of airways and scarring, the secretions that accompany it certainly provide an obstructive component. Active tuberculosis must be considered in patients with infiltrates (not only apical), a chronic wasting course, and predisposing factors such as silicosis, subtotal gastrectomy, or human immunodeficiency virus (HIV) disease. A more unusual, treatable pulmonary disease is sarcoidosis. In addition, subacute left ventricular failure may produce the pulmonary picture of cough, dyspnea, wheezing, and rales that is termed *cardiac asthma*.

Patient-Related Factors The second major category of inciting and aggravating factors of COPD relates to the patient. Noncompliance with therapeutic regimens is common and problematic.[15] In many instances, it is due to inadequate instructions; in other instances, the patient disregards or misinterprets instructions.

Physician-Related Factors Finally, in addition to disease-related and patient-related factors, physician-related factors exist. Physicians may prescribe drugs that are either inappropriate or at improper doses. Many drugs may directly or indirectly produce bronchospasm (e.g., aspirin, propranolol, reserpine, cholinergics, opiates, and all drugs with prostaglandin-1 inhibiting action). A second generic group of potentially deleterious drugs are sedatives. Patients with chronic respiratory failure are abnormally sensitive to the respiratory depressant effect of such drugs, and, for those patients, even small doses may significantly worsen hypoventilation. Ethanol has multiple deleterious effects on both cardiac and pulmonary function, and the very frequency of its use may cause the unwary emergency physician to overlook it.[16] Finally, even though the mainstay of outpatient COPD therapy is metered dose inhalers, most patients do not understand their proper usage.

CLINICAL FEATURES

Asthma (Reactive Airways Disease)

This first of the three basic disease processes composing COPD usually presents no problem in diagnosis, its course is fairly predictable, and, most important, it usually occurs in a given patient without significant chronic bronchitis or emphysema. When it is the primary component of COPD, the term *asthma* is appropriate; however, when bronchoconstriction is of only secondary importance in a patient with primary chronic bronchitis or emphysema, it is preferable to use the term *reactive airways disease* because the typical natural history of asthma is lacking.

Clinical Manifestations Wheezing, of course, is the acknowledged classic sign of asthma; but cough, dyspnea, or chest pain may be predominant. Wheezing that is of rapid onset (minutes to hours), high pitched, and relieved by bronchodilators (with a greater than 25% increase in forced expiratory volume [FEV_1]) is most often due to bronchospasm. The clinician should conclude that there is mucus plugging when clinical deterioration occurs slowly over days and when wheezing is unrelieved by adequate bronchodilator dosing.

There are several bedside indicators of severe bronchoconstriction and diffuse mucus plugging. Clouding of consciousness with or without cyanosis should always suggest carbon dioxide narcosis and impending respiratory arrest. Because speech occurs on expiration, the number of words expressible at one time is an excellent measurement of FEV_1; a gasping answer of two or three words is worrisome, phrases are better, and short sentences are better still. Higher-pitched wheezes indicate more severe bronchoconstriction than lower-pitched wheezes; a silent chest to auscultation suggests little air exchange and is ominous. Diaphoresis, visible retractions, and accessory muscle use should concern the emergency physician, especially if persistent. The degree of tachycardia can be a useful parameter but may be related to β-agonist therapy. Many patients are able to assess their degree of airway obstruction better than their physicians can.

Natural History and Staging As opposed to the majority of asthmatic children who outgrow their asthma, the asthmatic adult is usually destined to a lifetime of gradually worsening disease (Figure 69-3). Only a minority of asthmatic adults begin their disease in childhood; most first manifest it in the third or fourth decades. In the first few years, stage B, the asthma is often mild and seasonal and may be related by the patient to specific environmental allergens. The wheezing comes in so-called attacks, is due primarily to bronchospasm, and is quite responsive to inhaled bronchodilators. If wheezing is not observed, or cough and dyspnea are not the primary complaints, the disease may be misdiagnosed as simple viral bronchitis or flu at this stage. It passes spontaneously, only to recur months later. As asthma becomes established, entering stage C, the attacks become more severe, prolonged, and persistent.

Unfortunately, adult asthma eventually becomes fixed as a year-round affair. A large percentage of such patients, despite vigilant care, experience critical episodes. These episodes are usually precipitated by acute bronchitis (viral or allergic bronchitis is more common than bacterial), last days to weeks, and are often associated with suboptimal medical attention and regimens. Frank acute respiratory failure commonly occurs, which characterizes stage D. Such patients cannot and do not have their wheezing broken in the ED because mucus plugging is an invariable part of their problem. They must be treated aggressively in an inpatient

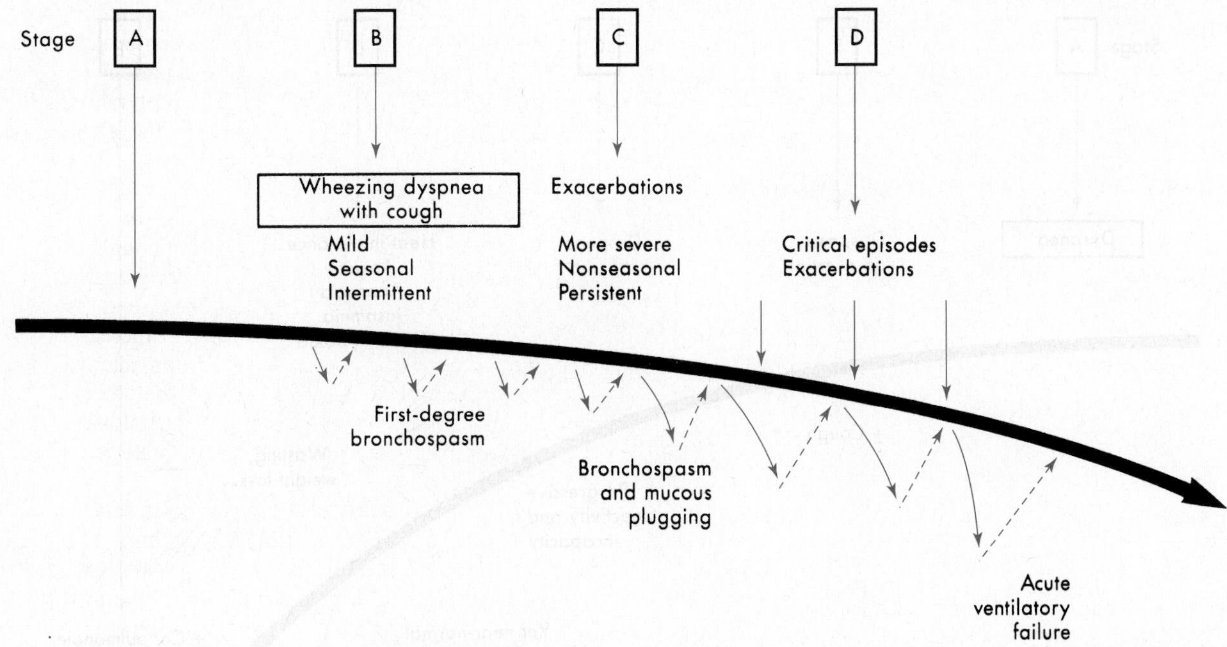

Figure 69-3. **Natural history of asthmatic adult.**

setting and, even then, return only slowly, over days to weeks, to baseline levels of pulmonary function. Even at stage D, in which such critical episodes occur with frequency, chronic respiratory failure does not supervene, underscoring the lack of significant associated chronic bronchitis and emphysema (the relative purity of disease and paucity of chronic parenchymal disease). This fact highlights the important concept that a stage E in typical adult asthmatics should rarely occur; prudent care should forestall death in this disease. That is, a given patient may expire acutely during a severe attack, but no chronic downhill path to death exists as in chronic bronchitis and emphysema.

The last two components of COPD, emphysema and chronic bronchitis, are examined in the model that emphasizes the phenotypic differences of the two types of patients, that is the emphysema patient and the chronic bronchitis patient. This model relies on the generally valid finding that each of these diseases, when in relatively pure form, has its own striking patient characteristics of body build, general appearance, and underlying disordered physiologic conditions.[17] These phenotypes can be especially helpful to the emergency physician because they are obvious at the bedside.

Emphysema (Airway Collapse)

This second of the three components of COPD is of less importance than asthma and chronic bronchitis because it is irreversible.

Clinical Manifestations The pure emphysema patient is typically thin, anxious, alert and oriented, dyspneic, and tachypneic. Dyspnea is the hallmark. Accessory muscles of breathing are used in the fight for breath. The pathognomonic posture of pursed lips on expiration (puffing) increases intraluminal bronchial pressure and supports bronchial walls internally that have lost their external support. The patient assumes a sedentary existence, chronically hunched forward. Supporting the torso with elbows on knees produces a subtle but characteristic sign: tanning and induration of the skin just proximal to the knees. Gross lung overinflation occurs, giving rise to low immobile diaphragms and increased anteroposterior diameter of the thorax with a large retrosternal airspace on lateral chest x-ray study. Percussion of the chest reveals hyperresonance, and auscultation demonstrates diminished breath sounds with faint end-expiratory rhonchi. Despite air hunger, the patient has good color (pink) and near-normal ABG levels. The heart is small and hypodynamic, the blood pressure low.

Natural History and Staging Because of the gradual progression of emphysema, the clinical course is slow and insidious (Figure 69-4). Patients may remain asymptomatic for many years by slowly limiting their activities in proportion to their pulmonary reserve (stage A). Dyspnea on exertion is the invariable initial symptom and may well not appear until the fifth or even sixth decade. When this occurs (stage B), the characteristic habitus is usually clinically evident. It is not long before the patient becomes truly incapacitated by dyspnea on minimal or no exertion (stage C). These patients are often discouraged; they are thin, anxious, chronically dyspneic, and often confined to bed or a chair. Decompensation (stage D) is manifested by profound muscle wasting and weight loss, which often prompts the clinician to seek an occult cancer or hyperthyroidism. Anorexia, insomnia, and heat intolerance become prominent symptoms. This determines the stage D label even though ventilatory failure per se has not occurred. Although the patient is susceptible to pneumonia at any stage, the lack of functional pulmonary reserve makes pneumonia a dreaded complication, often precipitating ventilatory failure. In the pure emphysematous patient, the emergence of cor pulmonale or chronic ventilatory failure is usually a preterminal event (stage E).

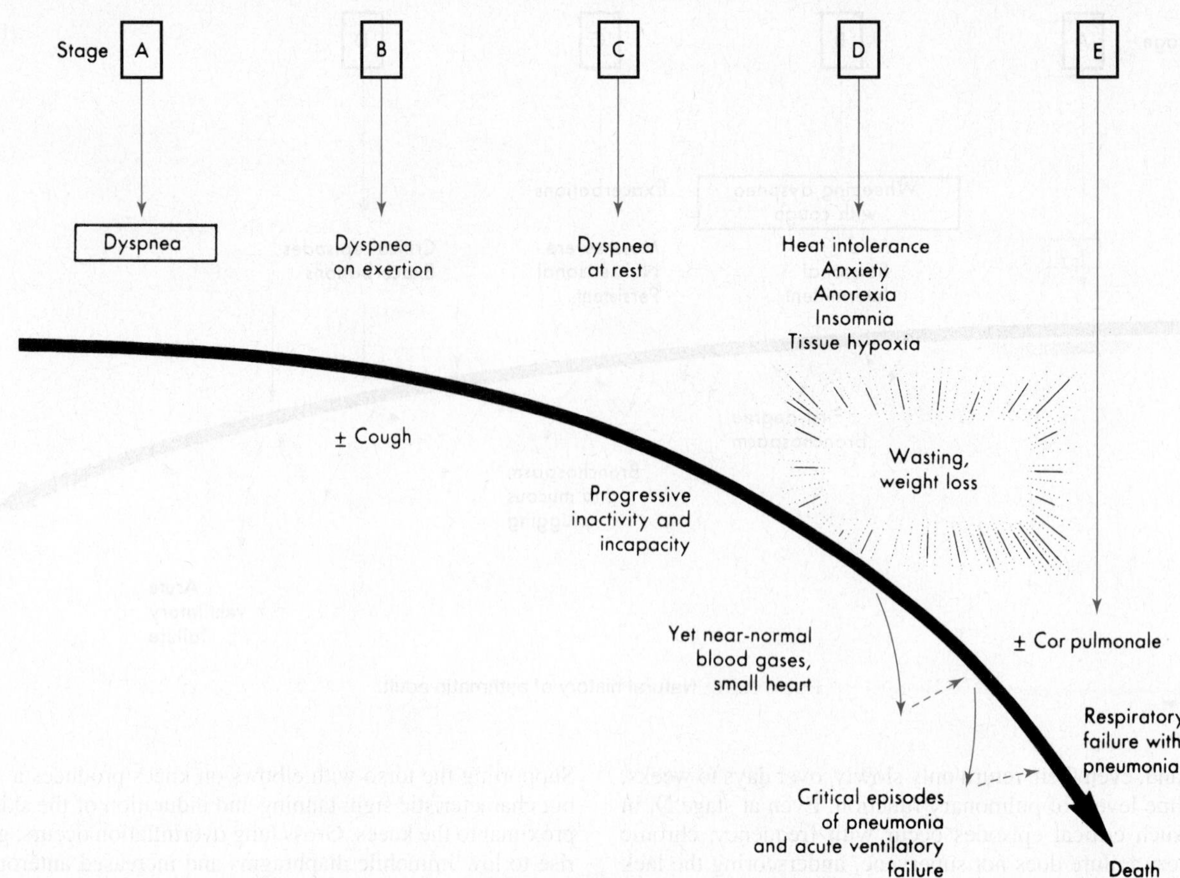

Figure 69-4. **Natural history of patient with emphysema.**

Chronic Bronchitis (Airway Inflammation and Secretions)

The third of the three components of COPD is of crucial importance. It is common, treatable, and reversible, and the clinical features of chronic ventilatory failure and secondary cardiac disease (cor pulmonale) are characteristic of many patients with mixed COPD.

Clinical Manifestations The fully developed, pure bronchitic patient eventually emerges when chronic respiratory failure and cor pulmonale supervene. Often little air hunger or anxiety is present, and the combination of polycythemia and hypoxemia accounts for the plethora and cyanosis. The chronic bronchitic does not hyperventilate. Cough, as the clinical hallmark of bronchitis, is prominent and, when vigorous, causes expectoration. If acute ventilatory failure is present, the patient's consciousness is clouded. This often can be described as "irritable somnolence," and asterixis may be present. If the patient is not comatose, activity is maintained at surprisingly normal levels. Compared with the pure emphysematous patient, tissue wasting is notably absent. Chronic ventilatory failure and cor pulmonale account for the prominent peripheral edema, anasarca, and chronic external jugular distention. Because little emphysema exists, the thoracic anteroposterior diameter is normal and diaphragms are not abnormally low. The presence of severe bronchopulmonary secretions is evidenced by scattered rhonchi and rales, especially at both lung bases posterolaterally. Cardiac examination is crucial to avoid overlooking cor pulmonale and coexisting left ventricular failure. A subxiphoid or retrosternal heave signifies chronic right ventricular hypertrophy, an S_4 suggests decreased left ventricular compliance, an S_3 indicates left ventricular failure, and a holosystolic blowing murmur of tricuspid insufficiency is secondary to right ventricular and tricuspid ring dilation.

Accentuation of the pulmonic component of the second-ary sound reflects pulmonary hypertension. Both pulmonary and cardiac findings are borne out on chest radiographs, which reveal normal lung volume, minimal or modest hyperaeration of upper lung fields, coarse reticulation of lower lung fields, slightly enlarged globular cardiac silhouette, and occasional pleural effusions. Most important, impingement on the retrosternal airspace by the enlarged right ventricle can be seen on the lateral film. Chronic visceral congestion causes hepatomegaly, hepatojugular reflex, and sometimes prominent abnormalities of liver function; it may also lead to marked digestive disturbances.

Natural History and Staging The bronchitic patient's disease course (Figure 69-5) begins with a mild, intermittent cough (morning or smokers' cough) (stage A). The patient is commonly unaware of the cough, and medical attention is not sought. After several years, this cough becomes chronic, occurring daily. In addition, the patient notes exacerbations productive of purulent sputum (stage B). These so-called chest colds sometimes prompt medical attention,

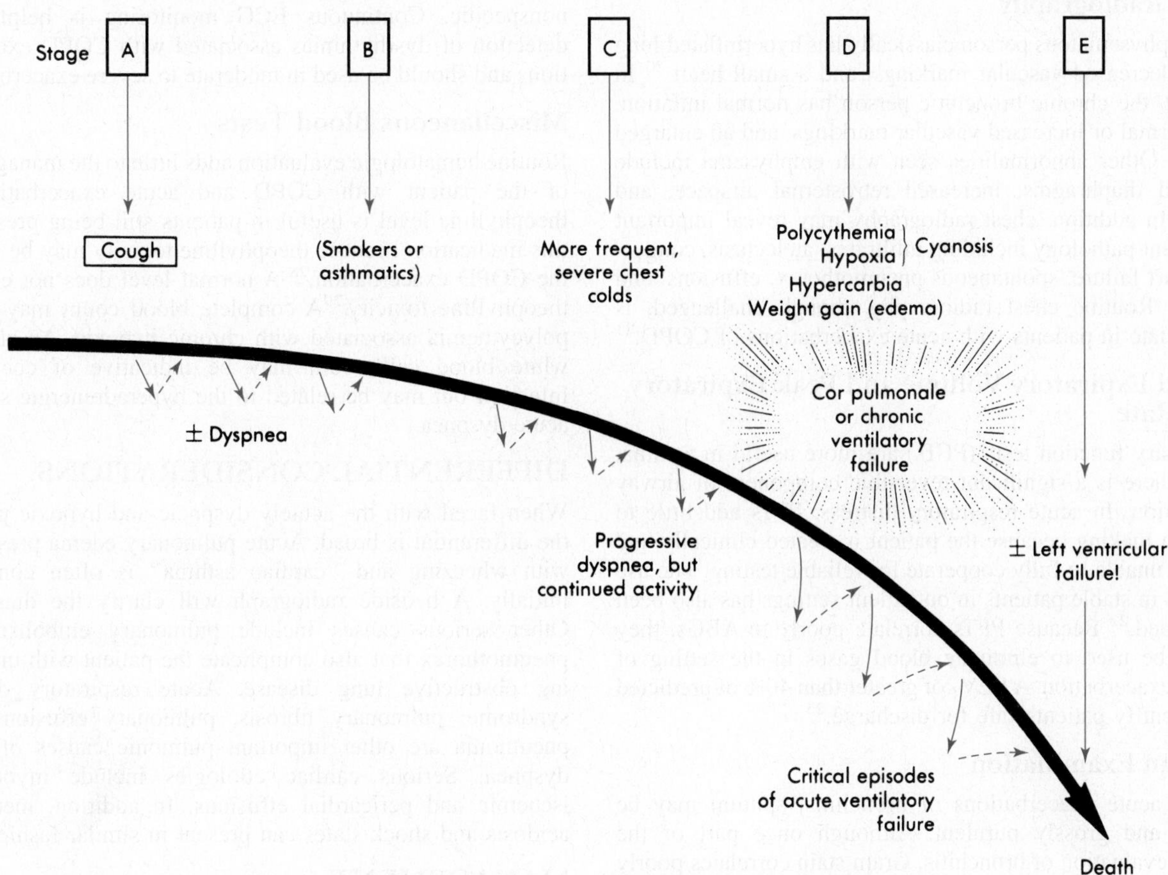

Figure 69-5. **Natural history of patients with chronic bronchitis (blue bloater).**

but the patient experiences little discomfort, disability, or dyspnea. Eventually, such episodes become prolonged, more severe, and associated with dyspnea on exertion and lead to lost workdays. A chronic cough, often paroxysmal, is obvious both to the one who is coughing and to surrounding persons.

Eventually during an exacerbation of these symptoms, laboratory and x-ray studies are performed. The patient is found to have significant hypoxemia, hypercarbia, polycythemia, and possibly even evidence of cor pulmonale (stage C). Despite continued activity and employment and despite the appearance of relative health, this patient's disease progresses (stage D). Commonly misdiagnosed as left ventricular failure, with the primary pulmonary nature of the disease unrecognized, this patient is at risk of inappropriate therapy and early demise. Correctly diagnosed and treated, the bronchitic patient with cor pulmonale may be eased through many crises to lead a productive and relatively comfortable life, despite decompensated disease.

DIAGNOSTIC STRATEGIES

Pulse Oximetry and ABG Analysis

Pulse oximetry has revolutionized noninvasive evaluation of critical patients and should be considered a fifth vital sign in the ED. It allows continuous monitoring of oxygenation and therefore should be part of the evaluation of every patient with a COPD exacerbation.[18] Hypoxia is present when the pulse oximetry reading is less than 95%, but low oxygen saturations are often baseline in many patients with COPD. Saturations less than 90% represent severe hypoxia in all patients. The change in pulse oximetry from baseline or in response to emergency therapy is generally more important than absolute levels.

The direct measurement of Pao_2, $Paco_2$, and pH by ABG is more reliable and sophisticated than the FEV_1.[19] pH and $Paco_2$ can be helpful when correlated to known baseline levels, but they add little to acute emergency management.

The A through E stages of COPD severity correlate well with ABG changes. Abnormal ventilation-perfusion relationships of COPD produce only modest decrements in Pao_2 in stages A (80 to 100 mm Hg) and B (60 to 80 mm Hg). But in stage C, *ventilatory insufficiency,* hypoxemia below 60 mm Hg stimulates respiratory centers, producing hyperventilation ($Paco_2 < 35$) and acute respiratory alkalosis. As pulmonary dysfunction progresses, the work of hyperventilation becomes cost ineffective; that is, more carbon dioxide is produced than cleared. Despite the body's mechanical hyperventilation, alveolar hypoventilation leads to CO_2 retention and acute respiratory acidosis. This characterizes stage D, *ventilatory failure.* With renal compensation through bicarbonate retention, the pH returns toward normal. Finally, in stage E, acute ventilatory failure is superimposed on the chronic ventilatory failure, producing a picture of elevated $Paco_2$, lowered pH, and elevated bicarbonate. Despite the additional information ABGs provide, it is important to acknowledge that immediate airway and ventilatory management depends on clinical findings in conjunction with pulse oximetry.

Chest Radiography

The emphysematous person classically has hyperinflated lung fields, decreased vascular markings, and a small heart.[20] In contrast, the chronic bronchitic person has normal inflation, with normal or increased vascular markings, and an enlarged heart.[20] Other abnormalities seen with emphysema include flattened diaphragms, increased retrosternal airspace, and bullae. In addition, chest radiography may reveal important coexistent pathology including infiltrates, atelectasis, congestive heart failure, spontaneous pneumothorax, effusions, and tumors. Routine chest radiography, though challenged, is appropriate in patients with acute exacerbations of COPD.[21]

Forced Expiratory Volume and Peak Expiratory Flow Rate

Pulmonary function tests (PFTs) are more useful in asthma, where there is a significant reversible component of airway obstruction. In acute respiratory distress, PFTs add little to decision making because the patient is treated clinically and is often unable to fully cooperate for reliable testing. The use of PFTs in stable patients in outpatient settings has also been questioned.[22] Because PFTs correlate poorly to ABGs, they cannot be used to eliminate blood gases in the setting of COPD exacerbation. A FEV_1 of greater than 40% of predicted may identify patients safe for discharge.[23]

Sputum Examination

During acute exacerbations of bronchitis, sputum may be thicker and grossly purulent. Although once part of the regular evaluation of bronchitis, Gram stain correlates poorly with cultures.[24] If the patient is acutely ill, has an infiltrate, and is being admitted, sputum culture is more appropriate. Sputum evaluation is diagnostic in certain pulmonary infections, including tuberculosis, *Legionella* organisms, and fungal and pneumocystis pneumonia.[25]

Electrocardiogram (ECG)

The finding of ECG criteria for right ventricular hypertrophy suggests the presence of established cor pulmonale; however, it unfortunately has low sensitivity and is unable to distinguish right ventricular from biventricular hypertrophy.[26,27] The finding of P pulmonale (peaked Ps in II, III, and aVF) suggests COPD; it may be chronic and stable but also may be present only with acute increases in right atrial pressure. The classic descriptions of low QRS voltage, clockwise rotation, and poor R wave progression are interesting correlates of COPD but are both insensitive and nonspecific. Continuous ECG monitoring is helpful for detection of dysrhythmias associated with COPD exacerbations and should be used in moderate to severe exacerbations.

Miscellaneous Blood Tests

Routine hematologic evaluation adds little to the management of the patient with COPD and acute exacerbation. A theophylline level is useful in patients still being prescribed this medication because theophylline toxicity may be part of the COPD exacerbation.[28] A normal level does not exclude theophylline toxicity.[29]A complete blood count may reveal polycythemia associated with chronic hypoxia. An elevated white blood cell count may be indicative of coexistent infection but may be related to the hyperadrenergic state of acute dyspnea.

DIFFERENTIAL CONSIDERATIONS

When faced with the acutely dyspneic and hypoxic patient, the differential is broad. Acute pulmonary edema presenting with wheezing and "cardiac asthma" is often confusing initially. A bedside radiograph will clarify the diagnosis. Other serious causes include pulmonary embolism and pneumothorax that also complicate the patient with underlying obstructive lung disease. Acute respiratory distress syndrome, pulmonary fibrosis, pulmonary effusions, and pneumonia are other important pulmonic causes of acute dyspnea. Serious cardiac etiologies include myocardial ischemia and pericardial effusions. In addition, metabolic acidosis and shock states can present in similar fashions.

MANAGEMENT

Successful management of patients with COPD demands a sophisticated understanding of disordered pulmonary function, an ability to make rapid and accurate clinical assessment, and skill in definitive aggressive airway and ventilation therapy. For each therapeutic modality, care will be discussed in decreasing order of acuity, that is, end-stage (E) first, asymptomatic (A) last. A complete summary of assessment and management is provided in Box 69-2.

Ventilation and Oxygenation

The *most important* consideration in emergency care of the COPD patient is the severity and acuity of ventilatory compromise, coupled with the patient's tolerance. Table 69-1 has clinical descriptions of the stages. All COPD patients in acute respiratory distress need continuous ECG and pulse oximetry monitoring.

Box 69-2 General Therapeutic Guidelines for COPD Exacerbations

Life-Threatening	Moderate/Severe	Mild
Address ABCs	Oxygen to maintain O_2 saturation 90%	Oxygen to maintain O_2 saturation 90%
Bag valve ventilation/preoxygenation	Nebulized β-agonist/anticholinergic	MDI or nebulized β-agonist/anticholinergic
Intubation +/− via rapid sequence intubation	Consider BLPAP ventilation if severe	Consider oral or IV corticosteroid
Inline β-agonist/anticholinergic	IV corticosteroid	Consider oral antibiotic on discharge
IV corticosteroids	IV antibiotic	
IV antibiotic		
+/− IV aminophylline		

It is important to consider an inciting or aggravating factor and provide specific therapy as discussed in text.
ABC, Airway, breathing, and circulation; *MDI,* metered dose inhaler; *BLPAP,* bilevel positive airway pressure.

The stage E patient in terminal ventilatory failure is cyanotic, speechless, lethargic, usually confused, and has gasping, ineffective respirations. For tracheal intubation. exhaustion may obviate the need for rapid sequence intubation. Initial ventilator settings should include an FIO_2 of 100%, tidal volume in the 6 to 8 ml/kg range, and respiratory rate of 8 to 10 breaths/min in an assist control mode with inspiratory flow of 80 to 100 L/min.[30] Permissive hypercapnia is essential to the ventilatory management of these patients, and subsequent normalization of pH and $Paco_2$ should be gradual over many hours. Low volume and rate settings will result in hypercapnia and respiratory acidosis, but this approach helps prevent associated barotrauma often seen in managing these patients.[31]

ABGs should be drawn after 15 to 20 minutes to ensure that ventilation is appropriate. Hyperventilation alkalosis must be scrupulously avoided, particularly because patients may have preexisting chronic metabolic alkalosis. This alkalosis can result in seizures and dysrhythmias, especially with coexisting hypokalemia.[32] Sedation and occasionally neuromuscular blockade are required to facilitate ventilation. Increased air trapping and resultant high intraalveolar pressures physiologically induce intrinsic positive end-expiratory pressure (iPEEP) that can cause barotrauma. In addition, increased intrathoracic pressure decreases cardiac filling and output; therefore, peak flow pressure and systemic blood pressure must be carefully monitored.

When the stage D patient has acute ventilatory failure superimposed on chronic ventilatory failure, delicate judgment is required to decide whether and when assisted ventilation is necessary. Noninvasive techniques can be highly effective in avoiding intubation in these patients.[33-35] Two of these techniques are nasal continuous positive airway pressure (CPAP)[36,37] and bilevel positive airway pressure (BLPAP).[38,39] Patients with COPD and respiratory distress have significant iPEEP, and this acts as an inspiratory threshold for the patient and increases the work of breathing.[40] Nasal CPAP helps counteract this iPEEP and decrease the work of breathing. Nasal CPAP is a simple technique, and 5 to 10 cm H_2O pressure is required.[36] When using BLPAP ventilation, expiratory positive airway pressure is usually kept at 2 to 4 cm H_2O and inspiratory positive airway pressure at 8 to 10 cm H_2O.[41] This technique is *not* for stage E patients, in whom orotracheal intubation is indicated.

A fundamental characteristic of these patients with respiratory distress is *hypoxia,* which needs to be treated immediately. An inherent anxiety exists among physicians to use oxygen therapy in these patients because of the fear of apnea by removing the hypoxic drive to breathe.[42] In fact although Pco_2 rises in response to oxygen therapy, minute ventilation changes little.[43,44] Patients with partial correction of hypoxia, who have mild respiratory acidosis, continue to have a high respiratory drive.[45] It is the patient who is breathing inappropriately *slowly* who is at highest risk of apnea with oxygen therapy.[46] The presence of tachypnea suggests that central chemoreceptors are receptive to CO_2 stimulus and respiratory drive will be maintained. High concentrations of oxygen are often unnecessary; the Fio_2 should be adjusted to maintain 90% saturation for most cases.[47]

If the patient experiences relief of dyspnea, has stronger respirations, and becomes more alert, intubation may be averted but diligent observation for deterioration must be maintained. Increasing respiratory rate, lethargy, exhaustion, speechlessness, paradoxical abdominal breathing movements, and falling oxygen saturation by oximetry despite therapy mandates assisted ventilation.

Care must be exercised in using ABGs to determine the necessity for intubation. *The most important factor in the decision to intubate is the patient's clinical status.* Even in the face of a significant rise in Pco_2 with oxygen administration, intubation may be unnecessary if the patient's clinical status has stabilized. Similarly, improving ABG values should not overrule the clinical impression of deterioration. Temporary improvement may be followed by exhaustion and respiratory failure.

The mixed COPD patient at stage C, although having respiratory insufficiency and significant compromise of function, has neither acute nor chronic ventilatory failure. Thus, chemoreceptor function is normal, respiratory acidosis is absent, and hypoxemia is of insufficient degree to cause significant tissue hypoxia. Although uncomfortable, the patient's life is not immediately threatened. Hypoxemia is partially compensated by hyperventilation. Administering oxygen by nasal cannula at 2 L/min raises the Fio_2 to approximately 28%. With this done, the dyspnea is relieved and the patient stops hyperventilating, thus reducing the work of breathing and oxygen consumption. It is important not to confuse hypoxic agitation with anxiety because the use of sedatives can lead to profound respiratory depression. The asymptomatic (A) patient or beginning symptomatic (B) patient has no significant hypoxemia and does not require oxygen administration.

General Drug Therapy

Four classes of drugs are commonly used in the ED management of patients with COPD: β-agonists, anticholinergics, corticosteroids, and methylxanthines.

β-Agonists β-Agonists form the mainstay of therapy, especially in patients with a significant bronchospastic component.[48,49] Although many choices are available, the most effective agents are those with selective β_2-receptor action because relaxation of bronchial smooth muscle is attained by stimulation of these receptors. The selective sympathomimetics have fewer cardiostimulatory side effects than are often seen with earlier generation β-agonists.[50,51] Although these drugs may be given through a variety of routes, inhalation is clearly the most effective with the least side effects and is the route of choice, provided the patient is able to comply.[52] Of the β_2-agonists, two drugs are most commonly used: albuterol and metaproterenol. The nebulization dose of albuterol is 2.5 to 5.0 mg (0.5 to 1.0 ml of 0.5% solution); the metaproterenol dose is 10 to 15 mg (0.2 to 0.3 ml of 5% solution).[53] Most patients are able to tolerate two to three rapid successive doses of oxygen-nebulized β-agonist with little problem. Therapy occasionally will need to be titrated if the side effects of tremor, tachycardia, or ventricular ectopy are significant. Subcutaneous administration of tertbutaline or epinephrine is only indicated in extremis. The COPD patient with a minor exacerbation may be able to receive the β-agonist by metered dose inhaler (MDI) protocol (see following). The intubated patient should receive in-line bronchodilator therapy.

Anticholinergics Nebulized anticholinergics are potent bronchodilators in COPD and should be used in conjunction with β_2-agonists as first-line therapy in acute exacerbations.[48,49] They block muscarinic receptors and prevent smooth muscle contraction while decreasing release of secretions from submucosal glands.[52] These agents are as effective as β_2-agonists in COPD and show synergism when given together.[54-57] Anticholinergics can be administered by nebulization or MDI and are effective in intubated patients. Atropine is the classic anticholinergic and is effective at doses of 0.5 to 2.5 mg. Unfortunately, it has significant systemic absorption, causing dry mouth, flushed skin, blurred vision, and tachycardia.[58] Ipratropium bromide, a quaternary ammonium compound, is extensively studied in COPD. It is virtually devoid of systemic effects, while having powerful bronchodilating properties.[59] It is available as a nebulization solution and is prepared in MDI form as well. The nebulization dosage is 0.5 mg every 4 hours.[53]

Bronchodilators are best administered by inhalation.[60] Studies demonstrate the efficacy and cost benefit of MDI over nebulization in acutely hospitalized patients. ED patients with mild to moderate exacerbations can also be candidates for MDI therapy with spacer.[61] Because of the smaller dose delivered with single MDI puffs, MDI protocols involve multiple puffs initially, followed by 1 puff every minute until clinical improvement occurs.[62] This mode of therapy should be considered only for stable cooperative emergency patients.

Corticosteroids The exact role of corticosteroids remains controversial, but their beneficial anti-inflammatory effects provide a strong rationale for their use in acutely ill patients with COPD.[7] Although steroids act too slowly to alter the immediate ED course, they do help decrease the relapse rate of acute exacerbations[63,64] and reduce treatment failures.[65,66] For severe exacerbations requiring admission, IV methylprednisolone is prudent, whereas a 2-week oral prednisone taper is appropriate for discharged patients.[67] Research demonstrates significant benefit from long-term inhaled corticosteroids.[68-70] In contrast to oral and IV corticosteroids, inhaled steroids have few adverse effects and should be considered for long-term therapy.[71]

Methylxanthines The use of aminophylline is surrounded by controversy. Proponents point to studies demonstrating efficacy: its multiple potentially beneficial modes of action (bronchodilatation, enhanced diaphragmatic contractility, stimulation of respiratory drive, inotropism, and improved mucociliary clearance) and its record of safety when properly used.[72-74] Research shows a synergism when used with β_2-agonists and ipratropium.[75] Theophylline withdrawal can worsen symptoms and lung function.[76] Opponents cite studies *not* demonstrating clinical efficacy, the need to monitor blood levels to avoid toxicity, and its side effects and cost.[77,78] These valid arguments have led to a decline in the use of this drug and thus this medication is recommended with reservation.

Acutely ill patients not previously taking aminophylline should receive approximately 5 mg/kg IV over 10 to 15 minutes to achieve the desired low therapeutic level of 10 μg/ml. To prevent possible toxicity, patients on oral aminophylline should await blood level results before IV doses. Administering 1 mg/kg results in approximately a 2 μg/ml increment in blood level. An adult with normal liver function should receive a maintenance infusion of about 0.5 mg/kg/hr. Alcoholism, old age, chronic liver disease, congestive heart failure, fever, and coadministration of erythromycin, ciprofloxacin, or H_2-blockers impair liver clearance and thus necessitate lower dosing.

Other Therapeutic Agents

Antibiotics Antibiotic therapy of acute bronchitis is controversial but may benefit COPD patients who have an increased sputum volume, sputum purulence, and dyspnea.[79] In these cases, antibiotic therapy decreases symptoms and improves respiratory function.[80,81] Furthermore some patients may have clinical pneumonia without radiographic evidence.[10] Since antibiotic therapy is generally benign and potentially beneficial, it makes sense to consider its use for acute bronchitis in this group of patients with significant morbidity.[82] Ideally, antibiotic therapy should be guided by sputum culture and sensitivity, but this is impractical for the acutely ill patient.

For outpatient therapy in acute bronchitis, macrolides (azithromycin, clarithromycin) and fluoroquinolones (e.g., levofloxacin, ciprofloxacin) have excellent monotherapy coverage.[83-85] Azithromycin has the added advantage of once-a-day doses for only 5 days.[53] Other good choices include amoxicillin/clavulanate or a second/third-generation cephalosporin.[84,86,87] Ampicillin alone is not recommended because of high bacterial resistance.[9]

Empiric antibiotic guidelines for pneumonia are outlined in Table 69-2.[88] For outpatient therapy, a macrolide, fluoroquinolone or doxycycline can be prescribed. Oral therapy should last for at least 10 days, with longer therapy (for 2 weeks) if mycoplasma or chlamydia is suspected. For inpatient therapy a combination of fluoroquinolone, β-lactam-β-lactamase inhibitor, macrolide, or third-generation cephalosporin provides the best antimicrobial coverage.

Mucokinetic Medications Because mucus production and cough are cardinal symptoms of COPD, a mucokinetic medication should in theory help symptoms. Unfortunately, little objective evidence exists that they are successful.

Table 69-2. Pneumonia Therapy in COPD Patients

Outpatient pneumonia therapy	Macrolide* Or Fluoroquinolone† Or Doxycycline
General inpatient pneumonia therapy	β-lactam‡ +/− Macrolide* Or Fluoroquinolone† alone
ICU inpatient pneumonia therapy	Erythromycin or Azithromycin or Fluoroquinolone† PLUS Cefotaxime or Ceftriaxone or β-lactam/β-lactamase inhibitor§

*Macrolide: azithromycin, clarithromycin, or erythromycin

†Fluoroquinolone: levofloxacin, sparfloxacin, grepafloxacin, or trovafloxacin

‡β-lactam: cefotaxime, ceftriaxone, or a ß-lactam/ß-lactamase inhibitor

§β-lactam/β-lactamase inhibitor: ampicillin/sulbactam, or ticarcillin/clavulanate, or piperacillin/tazobactam

Modified from Bartlett JG, et al: Community-acquired pneumonia in adults: guidelines for management. The Infectious Diseases Society of America, *Clin Infect Dis* 26:811-838, 1998.

Nebulized water and saline and the oral expectorants guaifenesin and saturated iodide are of no benefit.[89] Acetylcysteine may cause reflex bronchoconstriction. Research has demonstrated clinical improvement with oral iodinated glycerol, but this can cause thyroid dysfunction.[90,91] Simple oral hydration is likely the easiest and safest agent, if any is to be used.

Respiratory Stimulants Respiratory stimulants cannot be recommended for routine use in the ED. Agents studied include methylxanthines, narcotic antagonists, progesterone, acetazolamide, doxapram, and almitrine.[92,93] The most effective of these agents seems to be almitrine, which increases peripheral chemoreceptor sensitivity and improves ventilation-perfusion matching, but further work is needed to show its benefit in acute respiratory failure.[94]

DISPOSITION

Significant negative deviation from baseline is the general guideline for admission of patients with COPD. Important factors in the decision include coexisting pulmonary infection or other inciting factor, failed outpatient management for the current exacerbation, and lack of improvement while in the ED. Unlike asthma patients, COPD patients with an acute exacerbation often need a short stay admission. Attention should be directed to the following: vaccination history because influenza and pneumococcal vaccines are recommended, patient teaching on the proper technique of inhaler use, evaluation of support systems and appropriate referrals, and counseling on smoking cessation.[89,95,96]

KEY CONCEPTS

- COPD is a chronic disease with acute exacerbations, but in contrast to asthma, it has slow recovery periods and thus COPD patients do not usually show dramatic improvement after therapy.
- β-agonists, anticholinergics, and corticosteroids are the mainstay of drug therapy. Theophylline has a limited role in management. Therefore COPD is a frustrating disease for the emergency physician because therapeutic advances have not matched the severity of the disease.
- Noninvasive ventilation provides another therapeutic option in the COPD patient with respiratory failure. It has significant advantages over traditional mechanical ventilation and should be used whenever possible.
- Acute complications are common aggravating factors and need consideration during evaluation. These include pneumonia, pneumothorax, and pulmonary embolism.

REFERENCES

1. Sullivan SD, Ramsey SD, Lee TA: The economic burden of COPD, *Chest* 117:5S-9S, 2000.
2. Feinleib M et al: Trends in COPD morbidity and mortality in the United States, *Am Rev Respir Dis* 140:S9-18, 1989.
3. Hurd S: The impact of COPD on lung health worldwide: epidemiology and incidence, *Chest* 117:1S-4S, 2000.
4. Wedzicha JA: The heterogeneity of chronic obstructive pulmonary disease [editorial], *Thorax* 55:631-632, 2000.
5. Celli B, Benditt J, Albert R: Chronic obstructive pulmonary disease. In Albert R, Spiro S, Rett J, editors: *Comprehensive respiratory medicine*, St. Louis, 1999, Mosby.
6. Gurney JW: Pathophysiology of obstructive airways disease, *Radiol Clin North Am* 36:15-27, 1998.
7. Senior RM, Anthonisen NR: Chronic obstructive pulmonary disease (COPD), *Am J Respir Crit Care Med* 157:S139-147, 1998.
8. Chodosh S: Treatment of acute exacerbations of chronic bronchitis: state of the art, *Am J Med* 91:87S-92S, 1991.
9. Grossman RF: The value of antibiotics and the outcomes of antibiotic therapy in exacerbations of COPD, *Chest* 113:249S-255S, 1998.
10. Melbye H et al: Pneumonia—a clinical or radiographic diagnosis? Etiology and clinical features of lower respiratory tract infection in adults in general practice, *Scand J Infect Dis* 24:647-655, 1992.
11. Lesser BA et al: The diagnosis of acute pulmonary embolism in patients with chronic obstructive pulmonary disease [see comments], *Chest* 102:17-22, 1992.
12. Rathbun SW, Raskob GE, Whitsett TL: Sensitivity and specificity of helical computed tomography in the diagnosis of pulmonary embolism: a systematic review [see comments], *Ann Intern Med* 132:227-232, 2000.
13. Drucker EA et al: Acute pulmonary embolism: assessment of helical CT for diagnosis [see comments], *Radiology* 209:235-241, 1998.
14. Blank CA, Brantly M: Clinical features and molecular characteristics of alpha 1-antitrypsin deficiency [published erratum appears in *Ann Allergy* 72(4):305, 1994. *Ann Allergy* 72:105-120; quiz 120-122, 1994.
15. Dolce JJ et al: Medication adherence patterns in chronic obstructive pulmonary disease, *Chest* 99:837-841, 1991.
16. Dolly FR, Block AJ: Increased ventricular ectopy and sleep apnea following ethanol ingestion in COPD patients, *Chest* 83:469-472, 1983.
17. Staton G, Ingram R: Chronic obstructive diseases of the lung, *Sci Am Med* New York, 1995, Scientific American.
18. Hogan BM: Pulse oximetry for an adult with a pulmonary disorder, *Am J Occup Ther* 49:1062-1064, 1995.
19. Emerman CL et al: Relationship between arterial blood gases and spirometry in acute exacerbations of chronic obstructive pulmonary disease, *Ann Emerg Med* 18:523-527, 1989.
20. Takasugi JE, Godwin JD: Radiology of chronic obstructive pulmonary disease, *Radiol Clin North Am* 36:29-55, 1998.
21. Emerman CL, Cydulka RK: Evaluation of high-yield criteria for chest radiography in acute exacerbation of chronic obstructive pulmonary disease, *Ann Emerg Med* 22:680-684, 1993.
22. Casanova JE, Kaufman J: Utility of pulmonary function testing in the management of chronic obstructive pulmonary disease, *J Gen Intern Med* 8:448-450, 1993.
23. Emerman CL, Effron D, Lukens TW: Spirometric criteria for hospital admission of patients with acute exacerbation of COPD, *Chest* 99:595-599, 1991.
24. Minocha A, Moravec CL Jr: Gram's stain and culture of sputum in the routine management of pulmonary infection, *South Med J* 86:1225-1228, 1993.
25. Niederman MS et al: Guidelines for the initial management of adults with community-acquired pneumonia: diagnosis, assessment of severity, and initial antimicrobial therapy. American Thoracic Society. Medical Section of the American Lung Association, *Am Rev Respir Dis* 148:1418-1426, 1993.
26. Lehtonen J et al: Electrocardiographic criteria for the diagnosis of right ventricular hypertrophy verified at autopsy, *Chest* 93:839-842, 1988.
27. Klinger JR, Hill NS: Right ventricular dysfunction in chronic obstructive pulmonary disease. Evaluation and management, *Chest* 99:715-723, 1991.
28. Lubischer AV, Lucas LM: Monitoring theophylline therapy to prevent toxicity, *Am J Health Syst Pharm* 53:1292-1294, 1996.
29. Aitken ML, Martin TR: Life-threatening theophylline toxicity is not predictable by serum levels, *Chest* 91:10-14, 1987.
30. Jain S, Hanania NA, Guntupalli KK: Ventilation of patients with asthma and obstructive lung disease, *Crit Care Clin* 14:685-705, 1998.
31. Bidani A et al: Permissive hypercapnia in acute respiratory failure [see comments], *JAMA* 272:957-962, 1994.
32. Stogner S, George R: Steps to prevent cardiac arrhythmias in acute respiratory failure, *J Crit Ill* 9:1027, 1991.
33. Bardi G et al: Nasal ventilation in COPD exacerbations: early and late results of a prospective, controlled study, *Eur Respir J* 15:98-104, 2000.
34. Bott J et al: Randomised controlled trial of nasal ventilation in acute ventilatory failure due to chronic obstructive airways disease [see comments], *Lancet* 341:1555-1557, 1993.

35. Keenan SP et al: Effect of noninvasive positive pressure ventilation on mortality in patients admitted with acute respiratory failure: a meta-analysis [see comments], *Crit Care Med* 25:1685-1692, 1997.
36. Miro AM, Shivaram U, Hertig I: Continuous positive airway pressure in COPD patients in acute hypercapnic respiratory failure, *Chest* 103:266-268, 1993.
37. Goldberg P et al: Efficacy of noninvasive CPAP in COPD with acute respiratory failure, *Eur Respir J* 8:1894-1900, 1995.
38. Confalonieri M et al: Severe exacerbations of chronic obstructive pulmonary disease treated with BiPAP by nasal mask, *Respiration* 61:310-316, 1994.
39. Kramer N et al: Randomized, prospective trial of noninvasive positive pressure ventilation in acute respiratory failure [see comments], *Am J Respir Crit Care Med* 151:1799-1806, 1995.
40. Petrof BJ et al: Continuous positive airway pressure reduces work of breathing and dyspnea during weaning from mechanical ventilation in severe chronic obstructive pulmonary disease, *Am Rev Respir Dis* 141:281-289, 1990.
41. Meduri GU: Noninvasive positive-pressure ventilation in patients with acute respiratory failure, *Clin Chest Med* 17:513-553, 1996.
42. Hoyt JW: Debunking myths of chronic obstructive lung disease [editorial; comment], *Crit Care Med* 25:1450-1451, 1997.
43. Crossley DJ et al: Influence of inspired oxygen concentration on deadspace, respiratory drive, and Pa_{CO_2} in intubated patients with chronic obstructive pulmonary disease [see comments], *Crit Care Med* 25:1522-1526, 1997.
44. Dick CR et al: O_2-induced change in ventilation and ventilatory drive in COPD, *Am J Respir Crit Care Med* 155:609-614, 1997.
45. Erbland ML, Ebert RV, Snow SL: Interaction of hypoxia and hypercapnia on respiratory drive in patients with COPD, *Chest* 97:1289-1294, 1990.
46. Wasserman K: Uses of oxygen in the treatment of acute respiratory failure secondary to obstructive lung disease, *Monaldi Arch Chest Dis* 48:509-514, 1993.
47. Schmidt GA, Hall JB: Acute or chronic respiratory failure. Assessment and management of patients with COPD in the emergency setting [see comments], *JAMA* 261:3444-3453, 1989.
48. Ferguson GT: Recommendations for the management of COPD, *Chest* 117:2S-8S, 2000.
49. Laitinen LA, Koskela K: Chronic bronchitis and chronic obstructive pulmonary disease: Finnish National Guidelines for Prevention and Treatment 1998-2007, *Respir Med* 93:297-332, 1999.
50. Rossinen J et al: Salbutamol inhalation has no effect on myocardial ischaemia, arrhythmias and heart-rate variability in patients with coronary artery disease plus asthma or chronic obstructive pulmonary disease, *J Intern Med* 243:361-366, 1998.
51. Seider N, Abinader EG, Oliven A: Cardiac arrhythmias after inhaled bronchodilators in patients with COPD and ischemic heart disease, *Chest* 104:1070-1074, 1993.
52. Rosen RL, Bone RC: Treatment of acute exacerbations in chronic obstructive pulmonary disease, *Med Clin North Am* 74:691-700, 1990.
53. *Physicians desk reference,* ed 54, Montvale, NJ, 2000, Medical Economics Data Production.
54. Cydulka RK, Emerman CL: Effects of combined treatment with glycopyrrolate and albuterol in acute exacerbation of chronic obstructive pulmonary disease, *Ann Emerg Med* 25:470-473, 1995.
55. Campbell S: For COPD a combination of ipratropium bromide and albuterol sulfate is more effective than albuterol base [see comments], *Arch Intern Med* 159:156-160, 1999.
56. Routine nebulized ipratropium and albuterol together are better than either alone in COPD. The COMBIVENT Inhalation Solution Study Group, *Chest* 112:1514-1521, 1997.
57. Gross N et al: Inhalation by nebulization of albuterol-ipratropium combination (Dey combination) is superior to either agent alone in the treatment of chronic obstructive pulmonary disease. Dey Combination Solution Study Group, *Respiration* 65:354-362, 1998.
58. Ziment I: Pharmacologic therapy of obstructive airway disease, *Clin Chest Med* 11:461-486, 1990.
59. Cordova FC, Criner GJ: Management of advanced chronic obstructive pulmonary disease, *Compr Ther* 23:413-424, 1997.
60. Pauwels RA: National and international guidelines for COPD: the need for evidence, *Chest* 117:20S-22S, 2000.
61. Salzman GA et al: Aerosolized metaproterenol in the treatment of asthmatics with severe airflow obstruction. Comparison of two delivery methods, *Chest* 95:1017-1020, 1989.
62. Newhouse M, Dolovich M: Aerosol therapy: nebulizer vs metered dose inhaler [editorial], *Chest* 91:799-800, 1987.
63. Murata GH et al: Intravenous and oral corticosteroids for the prevention of relapse after treatment of decompensated COPD. Effect on patients with a history of multiple relapses [see comments], *Chest* 98:845-849, 1990.
64. Emerman CL et al: A randomized controlled trial of methylprednisolone in the emergency treatment of acute exacerbations of COPD, *Chest* 95:563-567, 1989.
65. Thompson WH et al: Controlled trial of oral prednisone in outpatients with acute COPD exacerbation, *Am J Respir Crit Care Med* 154:407-412, 1996.
66. Niewoehner DE et al: Effect of systemic glucocorticoids on exacerbations of chronic obstructive pulmonary disease. Department of Veterans Affairs Cooperative Study Group [see comments], *N Engl J Med* 340:1941-1947, 1999.
67. Hudson LD, Monti CM: Rationale and use of corticosteroids in chronic obstructive pulmonary disease, *Med Clin North Am* 74:661-690, 1990.
68. Dompeling E et al: Slowing the deterioration of asthma and chronic obstructive pulmonary disease observed during bronchodilator therapy by adding inhaled corticosteroids. A 4-year prospective study [see comments], *Ann Intern Med* 118:770-778, 1993.
69. Paggiaro PL et al: Multicentre randomised placebo-controlled trial of inhaled fluticasone propionate in patients with chronic obstructive pulmonary disease. International COPD Study Group [see comments] [published erratum appears in *Lancet* 1998 Jun 27;351(9120):1968], *Lancet* 351:773-780, 1998.
70. Barnes PJ: Chronic obstructive pulmonary disease, *N Engl J Med* 343:269-280, 2000.
71. McEvoy CE, Niewoehner DE: Adverse effects of corticosteroid therapy for COPD. A critical review [see comments], *Chest* 111:732-743, 1997.
72. Murciano D et al: A randomized, controlled trial of theophylline in patients with severe chronic obstructive pulmonary disease, *N Engl J Med* 320:1521-1525, 1989.
73. Vaz Fragoso CA, Miller MA: Review of the clinical efficacy of theophylline in the treatment of chronic obstructive pulmonary disease, *Am Rev Respir Dis* 147:S40-47, 1993.
74. Vassallo R, Lipsky JJ: Theophylline: recent advances in the understanding of its mode of action and uses in clinical practice, *Mayo Clin Proc* 73:346-354, 1998.
75. Karpel JP et al: A comparison of inhaled ipratropium, oral theophylline plus inhaled beta-agonist, and the combination of all three in patients with COPD, *Chest* 105:1089-1094, 1994.
76. Kirsten DK et al: Effects of theophylline withdrawal in severe chronic obstructive pulmonary disease [see comments] [published erratum appears in *Chest* 1994 Jul;106(1):328], *Chest* 104:1101-1107, 1993.
77. Bittar G, Friedman HS: The arrhythmogenicity of theophylline. A multivariate analysis of clinical determinants, *Chest* 99:1415-1420, 1991.
78. Lam A, Newhouse MT: Management of asthma and chronic airflow limitation. Are methylxanthines obsolete? [see comments], *Chest* 98:44-52, 1990.
79. Murphy TF, Sethi S, Niederman MS: The role of bacteria in exacerbations of COPD. A constructive view [comment], *Chest* 118:204-209, 2000.
80. Anthonisen NR et al: Antibiotic therapy in exacerbations of chronic obstructive pulmonary disease, *Ann Intern Med* 106:196-204, 1987.
81. Saint S et al: Antibiotics in chronic obstructive pulmonary disease exacerbations. A meta-analysis [see comments], *JAMA* 273:957-960, 1995.
82. Rodnick JE, Gude JK: The use of antibiotics in acute bronchitis and acute exacerbations of chronic bronchitis, *West J Med* 149:347-351, 1988.
83. Davies BI, Maesen FP: Clinical effectiveness of levofloxacin in patients with acute purulent exacerbations of chronic bronchitis: the relationship with in-vitro activity, *J Antimicrob Chemother* 43 Suppl C:83-90, 1999.
84. Shah PM et al: Levofloxacin versus cefuroxime axetil in the treatment of acute exacerbation of chronic bronchitis: results of a randomized, double- blind study, *J Antimicrob Chemother* 43:529-539, 1999.

85. Chodosh S et al: Randomized, double-blind study of ciprofloxacin and cefuroxime axetil for treatment of acute bacterial exacerbations of chronic bronchitis. The Bronchitis Study Group [see comments], *Clin Infect Dis* 27:722-729, 1998.
86. Beghi G et al: Efficacy and tolerability of azithromycin versus amoxicillin/clavulanic acid in acute purulent exacerbation of chronic bronchitis, *J Chemother* 7:146-152, 1995.
87. Henry D et al: Clinical comparison of cefuroxime axetil and amoxicillin/clavulanate in the treatment of patients with secondary bacterial infections of acute bronchitis, *Clin Ther* 17:861-874, 1995.
88. Bartlett JG et al: Community-acquired pneumonia in adults: guidelines for management. The Infectious Diseases Society of America. *Clin Infect Dis* 26:811-838, 1998.
89. Ferguson GT, Cherniack RM: Management of chronic obstructive pulmonary disease [see comments], *N Engl J Med* 328:1017-1022, 1993.
90. Repsher LH: Treatment of stable chronic bronchitis with iodinated glycerol: a double-blind, placebo-controlled trial, *J Clin Pharmacol* 33:856-860, 1993.
91. Becker CB, Gordon JM: Iodinated glycerol and thyroid dysfunction. Four cases and a review of the literature, *Chest* 103:188-192, 1993.
92. Bardsley PA: Chronic respiratory failure in COPD: is there a place for a respiratory stimulant? [editorial], *Thorax* 48:781-784, 1993.
93. Kerr HD: Doxapram in hypercapnic chronic obstructive pulmonary disease with respiratory failure, *J Emerg Med* 15:513-515, 1997.
94. Winkelmann BR et al: Low-dose almitrine bismesylate in the treatment of hypoxemia due to chronic obstructive pulmonary disease, *Chest* 105:1383-1391, 1994.
95. Borron W, deBoisblanc BP: Pharmacotherapy of chronic obstructive pulmonary disease, *J La State Med Soc* 150:596-600, 1998.
96. Celli BR: Standards for the optimal management of COPD: a summary, *Chest* 113:283S-287S, 1998.

70 Upper Respiratory Tract Infections

Frantz R. Melio

PHARYNGITIS (TONSILLOPHARYNGITIS)

Perspective

Tonsillopharyngitis (from this point on referred to as pharyngitis) is among the most common reasons for seeking medical attention.

Principles of Disease

Pharyngitis is an inflammatory syndrome of the oropharynx that is primarily caused by infections. Transmission is mainly through contact with respiratory secretions, but transmission through food and fomite contact is also possible. The infection tends to localize to lymphatic tissue, producing suppuration and swelling of the tonsils, tender cervical adenopathy, and fever. Occlusion of the eustachian tubes may result in secondary otitis media. Although most cases of pharyngitis are uncomplicated, the swelling may be of sufficient extent to threaten airway patency or preclude ingestion of adequate liquids, resulting in dehydration. Chronic pharyngitis differs from the acute infection. There appears to be inflammation and infection of the tonsillar crypts rather than the tonsils themselves.

Etiology

Viruses are responsible for most cases of pharyngitis. The etiology of bacterial pharyngitis in adults differs from that in children. Group A β-hemolytic streptococcus (GABHS) is the most common bacterial cause of pharyngitis in children, with peak incidence of 30%.[1,2] In adult patients, acute pharyngitis can be caused by β-hemolytic streptococcus (all groups 23%), *Mycoplasma pneumoniae* (9%), and *Chlamydia pneumoniae* (8%).[3,4]

Cultures obtained in cases of chronic or recurrent pharyngitis often grow mixed aerobic and anaerobic bacteria. Commonly isolated aerobic organisms include streptococcal species, *Staphylococcus aureus, Haemophilus influenzae,* and *Moraxella catarrhalis.* The anaerobic bacteria most commonly isolated include *Bacteroides,* anaerobic gram-positive cocci, and *Fusobacterium.* β-Lactamase production is extremely common in bacteria responsible for chronic pharyngitis. Epstein-Barr virus (EBV) and *Actinomyces* are also implicated as causes of chronic or recurrent pharyngitis.[3,5] Rare causes of bacterial pharyngitis include *Francisella tularensis* and *Yersinia enterocolitica.*[1]

Clinical Features

The most common symptom is pharyngeal pain that is aggravated by swallowing and may radiate to the ears. Examination usually reveals pharyngeal erythema, pharyngeal or tonsillar exudate, tonsillar enlargement, and tender cervical lymphadenopathy (Figure 70-1). Clinically differentiating the etiologic organisms is virtually impossible.[1,3,6,7]

Viral pharyngitis usually is seen in conjunction with cough, rhinorrhea, myalgia, headache, stomatitis, conjunctivitis, exanthem, and odynophagia. Low-grade fever and white pharyngeal exudates may be present. Cervical lymphadenopathy is usually absent.[7,8] Mild pharyngeal edema and erythema associated with a "scratchy" throat are present in 50% of patients with the common cold. Systemic viral infections including measles, cytomegalovirus, rubella, and human immunodeficiency virus (HIV) may present with mild pharyngitis.[1,7]

Influenza occurs in epidemics and is associated with high fever, myalgias, and headache. Whereas 50% to 80% of patients with influenza experience pharyngeal discomfort, pharyngeal exudate and cervical lymphadenopathy are rare. Adenovirus may cause severe pharyngitis similar to streptococcal pharyngitis. A total of 30% to 50% of adenovirus pharyngitis is associated with a follicular, usually unilateral, conjunctivitis.[7,9]

Pharyngitis is a common presentation of infectious mononucleosis (caused by EBV) in young adults.[7,9,10] Often a tonsillar exudate or membrane (which is cheesy or creamy white) is present. Generalized lymphadenopathy (90% to 100%) and splenomegaly (50%) are usually noted. Periorbital

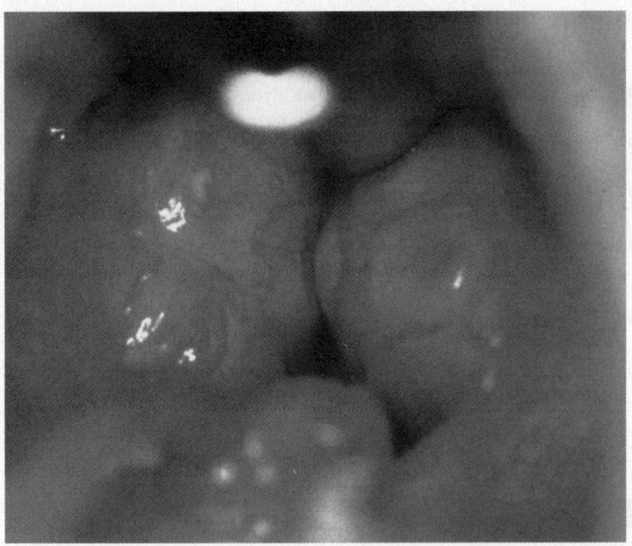

Figure 70-1. **Bilateral tonsillopharyngitis.**

edema and rash are rare findings. Up to 90% of patients with mononucleosis who are inadvertently given ampicillin or amoxicillin develop a diffuse macular rash that may be diagnosed as an allergic reaction.[7,9]

Herpes simplex also causes pharyngitis. These infections typically affect young adults. Herpes pharyngitis is characterized by painful superficial vesicles on an erythematous base. Ulcers may be present on the pharynx, lips, tongue, gums, and buccal mucosa. Pharyngeal erythema and exudate, fever, and tender lymphadenopathy are common for 1 to 2 weeks. In the immunocompromised host, large painful ulcers may be present. Herpes can be due to a primary infection or reactivation. Concomitant bacterial superinfection may occur.[7,8,10]

GABHS is primarily a disease of children 5 to 15 years old and in temperate climates occurs in winter and early spring.[1] It is responsible for less than 15% of pharyngitis in patients older than 15 years of age and rare in patients less than 3 years old. In epidemics, the incidence may double.[3,8,11] GABHS pharyngitis is associated with fever greater than 38.3° C (101° F), tonsillar exudates, palatal and uvular petechiae, uvular edema and erythema, and tender anterior cervical lymphadenopathy. Cough, rhinorrhea, coryza, or other viral symptoms are absent. GABHS pharyngitis associated with a fine sandpaper erythematous rash that subsequently desquamates is termed scarlet fever. These findings, however, cannot reliably diagnose or exclude streptococcal pharyngitis. Patients with recent exposure to others with GABHS pharyngitis are at increased risk of becoming infected.[1-3,12]

Diphtheria is a potentially lethal cause of pharyngitis that is uncommon in countries where adequate vaccinations are administered. US serologic surveys show that a large percentage of adults and adolescents lack immunity to diphtheria toxin.[13] Patients have a sore throat, fever, and dysphagia. Examination early in the disease process may reveal pharyngeal erythema and isolated spots of gray or white exudate that later coalesce to form a pseudomembrane. This gray-green pseudomembrane is usually well demarcated and covers the tonsils, pharyngeal mucosa, and occasionally, the uvula. The membrane may extend to involve the larynx and lead to hoarseness, cough, and stridor.

Tender, and at times painful, cervical lymphadenopathy may be found. Severe inflammation and edema can produce dysphonia and what is described as a "bull-neck" appearance. Some strains of *Corynebacterium diphtheriae* produce a systemic toxin that may cause myocarditis, polyneuritis (at first autonomic then peripheral), vascular collapse, diffuse focal organ necrosis, and death. Asymptomatic carriers may transmit the disease.[7,9,13]

Arcanobacterium hemolyticum (previously called *Corynebacterium hemolyticum*) typically affects the 10- to 30-year-old age group and can be indistinguishable from streptococcal pharyngitis. Most cases have an associated rash that may be scarlatiniform, urticarial, or erythema multiforme (occasionally skin manifestations may be the only complaint). Patients complain of moderately severe sore throats and are usually nontoxic and afebrile. *A. hemolyticum* may cause a membranous pharyngitis that strongly mimics diphtheria. *A. hemolyticum* is also associated with chronic tonsillitis.[7,14]

Anaerobic pharyngitis, or Vincent's angina, is characterized by superficial ulceration and necrosis that often results in the formation of a pseudomembrane. Foul-smelling breath, odynophagia, submandibular lymphadenopathy, and exudate are often present. Patients typically have poor oral hygiene.[5,7]

Gonococcal pharyngitis is a sexually transmitted disease that may occur independently of genital infection. The severity is variable and may result in an exudative or nonexudative pharyngitis. These differing presentations can be explained in part by the lack of symptoms during the latent period of infection. Asymptomatic carriers are described as are chronic and recurrent pharyngitis. Gonococcal pharyngitis is an important source of gonococcemia.[7,8,15] Syphilitic pharyngitis is a manifestation of primary or late (tertiary) syphilis and is seen as painless mucosal lesions.[8,9]

Tuberculosis pharyngitis usually occurs in patients with advanced disease. Symptoms and signs include hoarseness and dysphagia with pharyngeal ulcerations. Candidal pharyngitis is usually found in immunocompromised adults. Patients have dysphagia, odynophagia, and adherent white plaques with focal bleeding points.[8,9]

Mycoplasma pneumoniae infection usually causes a mild pharyngitis. Mycoplasma occurs in epidemics and in crowded conditions and can be responsible for approximately 10% of cases of adult pharyngitis.[3,4,7] Pharyngeal and tonsillar exudates, cervical lymphadenopathy, and hoarseness are common. Lower respiratory tract infection may also be present.[4]

Chlamydia pneumoniae pharyngitis resembles *M. pneumoniae* pharyngitis. It also occurs in epidemics or crowded conditions. Severe pharyngitis with laryngitis is suggestive of *C. pneumoniae* infection.[16] Swelling and pain of deep cervical lymph nodes may be prominent. Lower respiratory tract and concomitant sinusitis occur. The hallmarks of chlamydia pharyngitis are recurrence and persistence.[16,17]

In contrast to *C. pneumoniae, Chlamydia trachomatis* pharyngitis is a sexually transmitted disease. Similar to gonococcal infections, *C. trachomatis* pharyngitis is associated with orogenital sex. Urogenital culturing is necessary along with treatment of sexual contacts. Patients are usually asymptomatic or may have only mild symptoms.[3,8,18]

Diagnostic Strategies

Monospot tests are positive in up to 95% of adults, 90% of children more than 5 years of age, 75% of those 2 to 4 years old, and 30% of children 0 to 20 months with mononucleosis; but may be negative in the first week of illness. EBV capsid antigen immunoglobulin (Ig)M antibodies develop in 100% of cases. EBV nuclear antigens develop within 3 to 6 weeks and are useful if an initial negative test becomes positive at a later date. Peripheral blood smears demonstrate atypical mononuclear cells in 75% of patients, with the peak incidence in the second to third week of illness.[7-9] Herpes pharyngitis may be diagnosed by culture, cytopathologic tests of scrapings of lesions, and serologic tests. The diagnosis of GABHS infection is important to prevent complications, particularly rheumatic fever (RF). Even the most experienced practitioner has difficulty clinically diagnosing streptococcal pharyngitis.[1,7,11] Several authors propose scoring systems based on clinical findings, but these are complicated and inaccurate.[1,6,12] The only valid method of determining acute GABHS infection is by acute and convalescent ASO titers, which is not practical in the ED. A single throat culture has a sensitivity of 90% to 95% in detecting *Streptococcus pyogenes* in the pharynx. Variables that affect the accuracy of throat cultures include collection and culturing technique, as well as recent use of antibiotics.[1,7]

Rapid diagnostic tests for GABHS (listed in order of increasing sensitivity) detect streptococcal antigens by latex agglutination, enzyme-linked immunoassay (ELISA), optical immunoassay, or chemiluminescent DNA probes. Rapid strep tests (RST) have reported specificity of 70% to 100% (with most being > 95%) and sensitivity of 31% to 100% (with most being 60% to 95%). Sensitivity and specificity in actual practice are lower than in controlled trials.[1,7] A positive RST seems to reliably indicate the presence of *S. pyogenes* in the pharynx. Patients with positive cultures or RST may actually be carriers who may not need treatment and are at low risk for transmission and complications. Using RSTs only in patients with a clinical presentation consistent with GABHS may decrease false-positive results. On the other hand, RST are often negative in the setting of low bacterial count pharyngitis (these patients are still at risk for complications including RF). A negative RST must be followed by a confirmatory culture. Determination of the bacteriologic cause of pharyngitis in the adult by using methods for detecting only GABHS is insufficient. Pharyngitis caused by other treatable organisms is common and also associated with serious complications.[1,3,6-8,12,13]

Confirmation of diphtheria requires culturing on the proper media. Toxigenicity testing must also be performed.[9,13] The diagnosis of *A. hemolyticum* should be considered if pharyngitis is accompanied by a rash, including erythema multiforme. Vincent's angina is diagnosed based on clinical presentation and a Gram stain. Suspected gonococcal infection should be plated on Thayer-Martin agar. Tuberculosis pharyngitis is diagnosed by acid-fast staining. Syphilitic pharyngitis is diagnosed on dark-field microscopy, direct immunofluorescence, and serologic testing. Candidal pharyngitis is diagnosed by noting yeast on potassium hydroxide (KOH) preparation of throat swabs or Sabouraud's agar.[8,9] Diagnosis of mycoplasma can be confirmed serologically or by culture. Rapid antigen tests for mycoplasma are available.[4,7] Chlamydial pharyngitis can be diagnosed by serologic testing, by culture, or by antigen detection tests.[17] Studies on patients with chronic pharyngitis have found that surface cultures do not correlate well with the etiologic pathogens that are often concealed within the tonsillar crypts.[18]

Differential Considerations

The differential diagnosis of adult pharyngitis includes deep space infections, tumors, foreign bodies, pemphigus, Stevens-Johnson syndrome, drug reactions, allergic reactions, uvulitis, angioneurotic edema, chemical and thermal burns, esophagitis, gastroesophageal reflux disease, cricoarytenoid arthritis, thyroiditis, and epiglottitis.[7,8]

Management

Patients with pharyngitis should be treated symptomatically with warmed fluids, topical anesthetics (cepacol and others), and acetaminophen or ibuprofen (ibuprofen may be superior). Most cases of pharyngitis are self-limiting and follow a benign course.[1,2,7]

The treatment of infectious mononucleosis is supportive. Treatment consists of steroids, hydration, and supplemental oxygenation.[7,9] Patients should be advised to avoid contact sports for 6 to 8 weeks owing to the infrequent risk of splenic rupture.[7,9] Acyclovir or famciclovir is indicated in immunocompromised patients with herpetic pharyngitis.[7] The use of acyclovir or famciclovir in acute pharyngitis may be beneficial.[10]

Although many studies focus on GABHS pharyngitis, proper treatment of nonstreptococcal pharyngitis can also avoid serious complications. Because clinical judgment is insufficient and rapid diagnostic tests are not always accurate and diagnose only GABHS, this disease process is often treated empirically. The choice of antibiotic for the empiric treatment of adult pharyngitis is not fully elucidated. Some authors question whether antibiotics should be given in uncomplicated cases of non-GABHS pharyngitis. Antibiotics may shorten the course of the disease process, but are also associated with increased recurrences, increased bacterial drug resistance, decreased immune response, and patient expectation for antibiotics with subsequent episodes of pharyngitis.[1,2]

GABHS must be treated adequately (within 9 days) to prevent RF. The incidence of RF has markedly diminished with the use of antibiotics. The incidence of RF parallels that of GABHS, with the peak incidence in children 5 to 15 years old, less common in adults, and rare in children less than 3 years of age. Patients with mild cases of GABHS pharyngitis may contract RF. Current estimates show that RF complicates 0.3% of cases of GABHS pharyngitis, in epidemics this increases to 3%. More troubling has been a recent increase in sporadic outbreaks of RF.[7-9] The incidence and course of poststreptococcal glomerulonephritis that is caused by nephridogenic strains are unaffected by antibiotic therapy. Antibiotic therapy is extremely effective in eradicating GABHS and its other complications. Untreated, GABHS pharyngitis is a self-limiting illness that lasts 3 to 4 days. Early antibiotic treatment of streptococcal pharyngitis leads to a 13% earlier resolution of symptoms and shortens the course of illness by about 1 day. Antibiotic therapy decreases transmission. It is thought that patients no longer transmit GABHS after 24 hours of antibiotic treatment.[1,2,7,9]

There seems to be consensus that, in children, treatment of GABHS should be based on the evidence of infection (positive RST or culture).[1,2,7,19] Four ED strategies exist for the appropriate diagnosis and treatment of GABHS pharyngitis in adults. The first is to obtain throat cultures in all patients with pharyngitis and treat those who are culture positive for streptococcus. Disadvantages of throat cultures are cost, that only approximately 50% of those with positive throat cultures are infected (the others being incidental or chronic carriers), that waiting for culture results will delay treatment of symptoms and increase the risk of transmission, and that ED patients may not return as instructed (resulting in a missed opportunity to provide necessary therapy, increased incidence of complications and transmission, and obligating the ED staff to track down these noncompliant patients). The second strategy is to treat all patients, obtain a throat culture, and stop antibiotics if the culture is negative. This strategy is inefficient and not cost-effective. A third strategy is to perform an RST and treat those patients who test positive. The disadvantages of this method are that false-positive RST (positive tests in carriers) lead to overtreatment, and negative tests require confirmatory culture (leading to increased expense and other problems listed previously). A fourth strategy is to treat all patients with pharyngitis who clinically have a reasonable possibility of being infected with GABHS. This strategy is most attractive in the following situations: in areas where the incidence of streptococcal pharyngitis and its complications is high, in patients who are contacts of others with recently documented GABHS pharyngitis, in patients who present with presumed scarlet fever, and in areas lacking accessible laboratory facilities. This strategy leads to overtreatment of patients but avoids the disadvantages of testing. Several studies have attempted to determine the most cost-effective strategy. If the incidence of GABHS infection is high or the patient's clinical presentation is highly consistent with streptococcal pharyngitis, treatment should be given without testing. If the probability of streptococcal infection is low, treatment should be based on positive testing (culture or RST).[1,7,11,12]

At present, the antibiotic regimen of choice in adults for GABHS pharyngitis is either a single intramuscular injection of 1.2 million U of benzathine penicillin or a 10-day course of penicillin V, 250 mg orally three to four times a day. Some authors recommend oral dosage of 250 mg four times a day for 1 to 2 days, and the remainder of the course at 500 mg twice a day. Less frequent dosing is less effective in preventing RF.[1] Intramuscular penicillin may be more effective than oral penicillin and ensures compliance, but allergic reactions are more severe and treatment is more expensive. Penicillin failure is becoming more prevalent in the United States.[20] Penicillin failure is thought to be due to either noncompliance, reinfection, or the presence of β-lactamase producing organisms.[2] Erythromycin is recommended for patients who are allergic to penicillin. A 1 g total daily dose must be given for 10 days, but twice, three times, and four times a day dosing intervals are equally effective in preventing RF. Erythromycin resistance is rare in the United States (< 5%) versus 60% in Japan and Finland, areas where erythromycin is used more extensively to treat pharyngitis.[1,2,20]

Alternate regimens include cephalosporins, clindamycin, and the macrolide antibiotics. Oral cephalosporins may be more effective than penicillin in eradicating GABHS pharyngitis. Cure rates using 5-day therapy with oral cefpodoxime, cefixime, cefotiam, cefodroxil, and cefuroxime may prove to be more effective than 10 days of penicillin. Azithromycin is safe and effective and requires only 5 days of once daily therapy. Clarithromycin given twice a day is as effective as both penicillin and erythromycin and has fewer side effects than erythromycin. These alternative regimens should be reserved for the patient not responding to penicillin or unable to tolerate either penicillin or erythromycin.[1,2] Ampicillin, amoxicillin, and penicillinase-resistant penicillins generally offer no advantage in the treatment of uncomplicated streptococcal pharyngitis and are useful only when concomitant infections require additional coverage.[1]

When diphtheria is strongly suspected, based on clinical presentation, treatment must begin immediately. Airway collapse may occur suddenly and without warning. The mainstay of therapy is antitoxin (a horse serum product), which should be administered immediately on clinical suspicion of diphtheria. The dose of antitoxin varies widely based on the site of infection and the duration of symptoms. Specialty consultation is usually required. Antibiotics have little effect on the resolution of local infection and systemic toxicity but are useful in eradicating *C. diphtheriae* infection and preventing transmission. The antibiotic of choice is erythromycin, 500 mg four times a day for 10 days. A small percentage of patients require an additional 10-day course of erythromycin for persistent infection. Rifampin, 600 mg a day for 10 days, is also effective in eradicating this carrier state of *C. diphtheriae* and in treatment of erythromycin-resistant diphtheria.[9,13]

A. hemolyticum may be resistant to penicillin. Erythromycin, 250 mg orally four times a day for 10 days, is the treatment of choice.[14] Vincent's angina is treated with penicillin or clindamycin and oral oxidizing agent (hydrogen peroxide) rinses.[21] Gonococcal pharyngitis is often more difficult to eradicate than genital infections. Treatment is similar to that for gonococcal urethritis and consists of ceftriaxone, 125 mg intramuscularly, or single dose oral treatment with either ciprofloxacin 500 mg, ofloxacin 400 mg, or cefixime 400 mg. Concomitant treatment of chlamydia, with a single oral dose of 1 g of azithromycin or doxycycline 100 mg orally twice a day for 7 days, is also recommended.[21] Tuberculous pharyngitis is seen with disseminated disease. Patients should be isolated and treated with a multiple-drug regimen. Pharyngitis caused by primary syphilis is treated with 2.4 million U of benzathine penicillin (LA) with 14 days of tetracycline or doxycycline as an alternative. Candidal pharyngitis is treated with oral fluconazole or itraconazole. Alternate therapy includes nystatin (suspension or tablets) or oral clotrimazole for 14 days. Chronic suppression therapy with ketoconazole, clotrimazole, or fluconazole is usually required for HIV.[21]

M. pneumoniae is treated with erythromycin, tetracycline, or doxycycline for 7 to 14 days.[9,16] Chlamydial pharyngitis is treated with doxycycline, trimethoprim-sulfamethoxazole, or a macrolide antibiotic. *C. pneumoniae* pharyngitis should be treated for 7 to 10 days to prevent treatment failures and recurrence.[16] *C. trachomatis* pharyngitis may require prolonged or repeated courses of antibiotics.[17]

Treatment of recurrent or chronic tonsillitis should include β-lactamase–resistant antibiotics active against aerobic and anaerobic organisms. Choices include treatment with oral cephalosporins, amoxicillin-clavulanic acid, clindamycin, penicillin, rifampin, and metronidazole with a macrolide antibiotic.[1,3,20]

Steroids, given in conjunction with oral antibiotics in adults with acute pharyngitis, may significantly shorten the duration of symptoms and provide a greater degree of pain relief without increasing complications.[22]

Disposition

Although most cases of pharyngitis follow a benign course, life-threatening complications can occur. Complications often require specialty consultation and admission; airway compromise from tonsillar enlargement, local and distant spread of infection, deep neck abscesses, necrotizing fasciitis, sleep apnea, bacteremia, sepsis, and death are all reported.[23]

Infectious mononucleosis may lead to airway obstruction, tonsillar and peritonsillar abscess, lingual tonsillitis, necrotic epiglottitis, airway obstruction, hepatic dysfunction, splenic injury, neurologic disorders, pneumonitis, pericarditis, and hematologic disorders.[9] Herpetic pharyngitis may lead to necrotizing tonsillitis, epiglottitis, and recurrent disease. Complications of *A. hemolyticum* include peritonsillar abscess, sepsis, and airway obstruction.[13]

Complications of GABHS pharyngitis can be both suppurative and nonsuppurative. Suppurative complications include peritonsillar abscess, retropharyngeal and other deep space abscesses, suppurative cervical lymphadenitis, otitis media, sinusitis, and mastoiditis. In addition, bacteremia with subsequent sepsis, osteomyelitis, empyema, meningitis, or soft tissue infections are described. Nonsuppurative complications include scarlet fever, RF, poststreptococcal glomerulonephritis, nonrheumatic perimyocarditis, erythema nodosum, and streptococcal toxic shock syndrome. In contrast to RF, other complications of GABHS pharyngitis have increased in incidence and severity in the last decade. A chronic carrier state of streptococcal infection exists that can persist for several months regardless of whether antibiotics are given. These patients are asymptomatic, at low risk for RF, and not considered highly contagious. Non–group A streptococcal pharyngitis may be complicated by the same suppurative complications as group A infections. In addition, scarlet fever and acute glomerulonephritis are linked to group C and G pharyngitis.[1,2,23]

LINGUAL TONSILLITIS

Lingual tonsillitis (LT) is a rarely diagnosed cause of pharyngitis that usually occurs in patients who have had their palatine tonsils removed. The lingual tonsils are a collection of nonencapsulated lymphoid tissue most commonly (size and location are highly variable) located symmetrically on either side of the midline just below the inferior pole of the palatine tonsil and anterior to the vallecula at the base of the tongue. This lymphoid tissue may enlarge after puberty, repeated infections, and tonsillectomy.[24,25] Patients with LT have a sore throat that worsens with movement of the tongue (including tongue depression) and phonation. The patient may have a classic "hot potato" voice and complain of feeling a swelling in the throat. Dysphagia, fever, respiratory distress, and stridor may be present. Chronic or recurrent LT may also cause a chronic cough or sleep apnea. Physical findings are likely to show a normal appearing pharynx with mild hyperemia. Direct or indirect laryngoscopy reveals an edematous lingual tonsil covered with a purulent exudate. Diagnosis is aided by lateral soft tissue neck films. These films demonstrate a normal appearing epiglottis and aryepiglottic folds, with a scalloped appearance on the anterior surface of the vallecula caused by an enlarged lingual tonsil.[24,25]

Management includes maintenance of airway patency, antibiotics, and supportive therapy. Rarely, acute LT may be a life-threatening condition. Airway management includes warmed humidified oxygen, hydration, and corticosteroids. Nebulized epinephrine can successfully treat acute respiratory distress and stridor in this condition. Antibiotics of choice are similar to those used in the treatment of pharyngitis.[24,25]

LARYNGITIS

Laryngitis presents as hoarseness and aphonia. It is usually caused by viral upper respiratory tract infections. In up to 10% of cases, bacteria (including streptococcus and diphtheria) may be responsible. Other causes include tuberculosis, syphilis, leprosy, actinomycosis, and fungal infections.[7,9] These patients should be evaluated for epiglottitis. Antibiotics are not indicated unless signs of bacterial infection are present.[7] Steroids may aid in decreasing the time to resolution of symptoms.[26]

ADULT EPIGLOTTITIS

Perspective

Adult epiglottitis (AE) is a potentially life-threatening disease that can lead to rapid, unpredictable airway obstruction. AE was first described by LeMierre in 1936. Before the introduction of *H. influenzae* vaccine, epiglottitis was primarily a pediatric disease. In recent years the incidence of pediatric epiglottitis has diminished, and there has been an increase in the number of AE cases. Whether the increase of AE is due to increased recognition or prevalence is unknown.[5,27-29]

Principles of Disease

AE is a localized cellulitis involving the upper airway. There is marked involvement of the supraglottic structures including the base of the tongue, vallecula, aryepiglottic folds, arytenoid soft tissues, lingual tonsils, and the epiglottis itself. Inflammation does not extend to the infraglottic regions because the submucosa is so densely adherent to the mucosa below the vocal cords. Cases are reported of adults with a normal epiglottis in the setting of severe supraglottic involvement. These findings have led some authors to suggest that the term *supraglottitis* is a more accurate description of this disease process. Adults with epiglottic involvement are prone to develop epiglottic abscesses.[28-30]

The most commonly isolated bacterial pathogen causing AE is type b *H. influenzae.* Only a minority of patients, however, have *H. influenzae* isolated from epiglottic or blood cultures. *H. influenzae* infection is associated with a more aggressive disease course. In many cases, no organisms can be cultured from either the blood or the supraglottic structures. This suggests that respiratory viruses may play an important etiologic role. The predominant organisms isolated from epiglottic abscesses are *Streptococcus* and *Staphylococcus* species. AE may also result from thermal injury.[27-29,31]

Clinical Features

AE seems to have no age or seasonal prevalence. Males and smokers are more commonly affected. Adults with epiglottitis typically experience a prodrome that resembles that of a benign upper respiratory tract infection. The duration of the prodrome is usually 1 to 2 days but may be as long as 7 days or as short as several hours. Patients who have a rapid onset of their disease are more likely to require airway interventions.[28,29,32,33]

Patients usually have dysphagia, odynophagia, and a sore throat. Pharyngeal pain may be severe and is often disproportionate to the clinical findings. Dysphonia and a muffled voice are common. Hoarseness is usually not found. Fever is absent in up to 50% of cases and may develop only in the later stages of the disease. Tachycardia disproportionate to fever has been shown to correlate with severe disease. Tenderness to palpation of the anterior neck in the region of the hyoid and on moving the larynx side to side is a reliable finding in epiglottitis. Ear pain may be a manifestation of AE. Concomitant uvulitis, pharyngitis, tonsillitis, Ludwig's angina, peritonsillar abscess, and parotitis are reported; therefore these findings on pharyngeal examination do not exclude the diagnosis of epiglottitis. The symptoms and signs of imminent airway obstruction are respiratory difficulty, stridor, drooling, and aphonia. Patients who assume a classic sniffing position are prone to rapid airway obstruction and should not be laid flat or excessively agitated.[28-30]

Diagnostic Strategies

Although severe cases of AE are easily recognized, a large number of less severe cases are initially misdiagnosed. Up to one third of patients with AE are seen but not diagnosed as having epiglottitis within 48 hours of admission. The most common misdiagnosis is streptococcal pharyngitis.[5,27]

Adult patients without respiratory distress can safely undergo direct or indirect laryngoscopy. Flexible fiberoptic laryngoscopy has the advantage of providing direct visualization of the airway while serving as a guide for intubation. Laryngoscopy reveals a swollen epiglottis and surrounding structures (Figure 70-2). The epiglottis may appear "cherry red" but often is pale and edematous. In patients with respiratory distress, drooling, aphonia, or stridor, indirect laryngoscopy is contraindicated and direct laryngoscopy should be undertaken only when one is prepared to obtain definitive airway control.[27-29,30-33]

Lateral cervical soft tissue x-ray films have a sensitivity up to 90% compared with direct laryngoscopy; however, normal soft tissue x-ray films do not exclude AE. Patients with suspected AE and normal soft tissue x-ray films should undergo laryngoscopy. Radiologic findings include obliteration of the vallecula, swelling of the arytenoids and aryepiglottic folds, edema of the prevertebral and retropharyngeal soft tissues, and "ballooning" of the hypopharynx and mesopharynx. The edematous epiglottis appears enlarged and thumb-shaped (Figure 70-3). An epiglottic width of greater than 8 mm or an aryepiglottic fold width of greater than 7 mm is suggestive of epiglottitis.[34]

Differential Considerations

AE is often misdiagnosed as pharyngitis. Other entities that must be considered include mononucleosis, deep space abscesses, lingual tonsillitis, diphtheria, pertussis, and croup. Noninfectious considerations include angioedema, allergic reactions, foreign body aspiration, laryngospasm, tumors, toxic inhalation or aspiration, and laryngeal trauma.

Management

Adults with epiglottitis should be treated with extreme care because of the possibility of unpredictable sudden airway obstruction. The safety and efficacy of both orotracheal and laryngoscope-guided nasotracheal intubation are reported.[27,30-33] Blind nasotracheal intubation can lead to airway obstruction and is contraindicated in the setting of epiglottitis. Endotracheal intubation should always be performed under direct visualization. Intubation can be per-

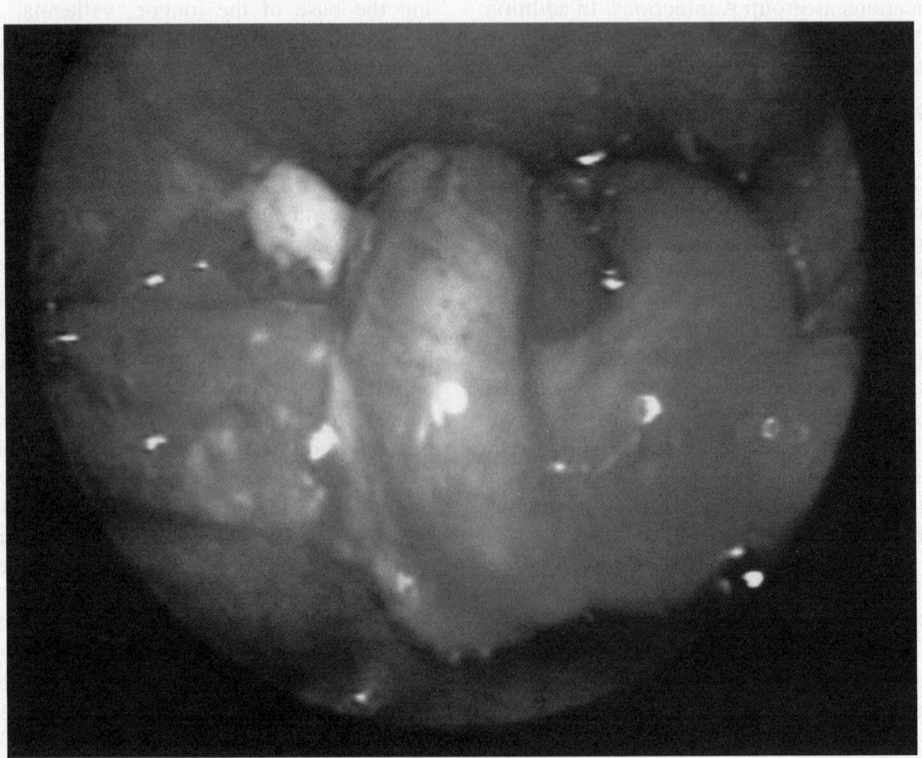

Figure 70-2. **Epiglottitis.**

formed over a fiberoptic laryngoscope with direct visualization of the vocal cords at the time of diagnosis. Be prepared for immediate cricothyrotomy when intubation is attempted. Whenever possible, definitive airway control should be performed in the operating room.[32]

Antibiotics should be initiated against *H. influenzae* and other likely bacterial pathogens. First-line agents pending cultures and sensitivities are cefotaxime and ceftriaxone. Alternative antibiotics include ampicillin-sulbactam and trimethoprim-sulfamethoxazole.[22] The role of steroids and racemic epinephrine is unresolved.[27-31]

Disposition

Stable patients without respiratory distress can be safely treated without intubation. Admission to an intensive care unit with continuous monitoring, medical therapy, and close observation is appropriate for mild cases. These include patients with mild swelling on laryngoscopy and without drooling, stridor, or dyspnea. Care should be taken with patients who have a rapidly progressive course, are immunocompromised, or have significant epiglottic enlargement on x-ray study or laryngoscopy.[28,29,35]

Extraepiglottic infections are less likely to occur in adults than in children. Meningitis, retropharyngeal abscess, pneumothorax, empyema, pneumonia, sepsis, adult respiratory distress syndrome, and pulmonary edema are reported in conjunction with epiglottitis.[30-32] Adults can develop epiglottitis after contact with children who have *Haemophilus B* meningitis. Mortality in adults is higher than in children, probably because of misdiagnosis and undertreatment.[28,29] With earlier recognition and treatment, the overall mortality is less than 7%.[27-29]

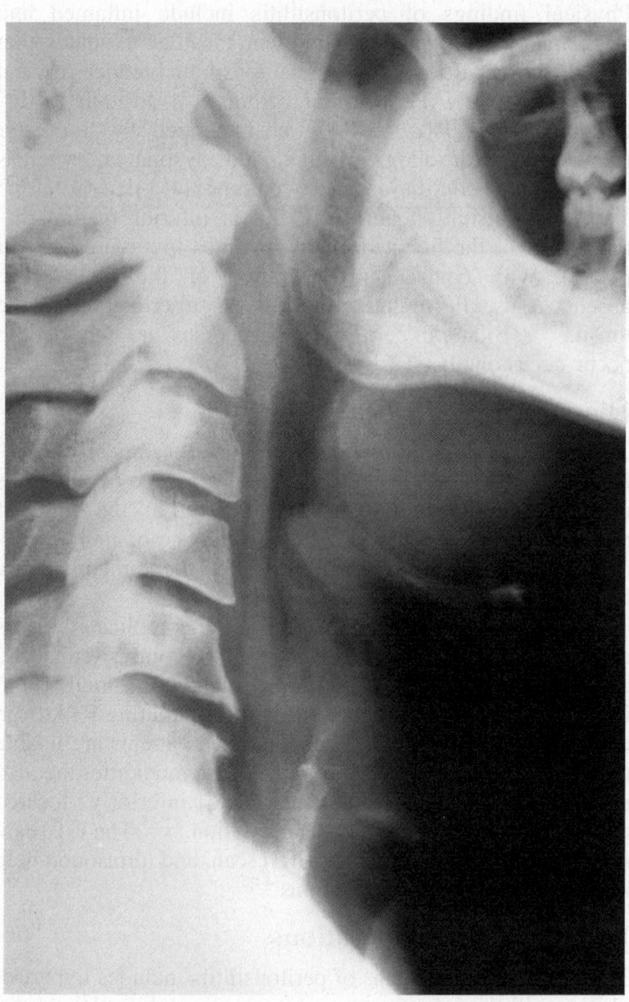

Figure 70-3. **Radiograph of epiglottitis.**

DEEP SPACE INFECTIONS OF THE LOWER FACE AND NECK (Figure 70-4)

Patients with deep space infections of the head and neck are in danger of rapid and fatal decompensation and must be treated aggressively with extreme care. The incidence and complications of deep space infections have decreased dramatically because of improved dental hygiene and the advent of antibiotics.[36,37] Airway distortion and trismus may complicate intubation attempts. Neuromuscular blockade may worsen the degree of airway obstruction by causing muscular laxity.[38] Fiberoptic-guided endoscopic intubation can be useful in this setting.[39] Blind tracheal intubation can cause abscess rupture, airway damage, and further compromise.[40,41]

The submandibular space is formed by the fasciae of the lower face. This space is a conglomerate of two spaces, the sublingual and submaxillary spaces. Clinically, these two spaces function as a single space. The submandibular space is involved in Ludwig's angina.[36,37,40] There are five main clinically relevant potential spaces in the neck: the peritonsillar, parapharyngeal, retropharyngeal, "danger," and prevertebral spaces. These spaces communicate freely with each other. The peritonsillar space is not a true space because it is not contained within fascial planes.[37] The parapharyngeal space contains the carotid artery, the jugular vein, the cervical sympathetic chain, and cranial nerves IX through XII. The retropharyngeal space lies in the midline (medial to the parapharyngeal space) and extends from the base of the skull to the superior mediastinum (at about the level of T2). The superior constrictor muscle adheres to the prevertebral fascia and forms a raphe in the medial aspect of the retropharyngeal space. Therefore retropharyngeal abscesses tend to occur lateral to the midline. Posterior to the retropharyngeal space lies the "danger space" that extends from the base of the skull to the diaphragm. The prevertebral space extends from the base of the skull to the coccyx. Danger space and prevertebral abscesses will be located in the midline. Retropharyngeal infections, danger space, and prevertebral space infections have easy access to the mediastinum.[36,37,42]

The primary pathologic process of deep space infection is a regional cellulitis. The fasciae may confine infections within their boundaries, leading to abscess formation. There is little resistance to the spread of infection within the fascial planes and spaces, allowing for rapid spread of infection.[36,43]

PERITONSILLITIS (PERITONSILLAR CELLULITIS AND PERITONSILLAR ABSCESS)

Perspective

Peritonsillar cellulitis and abscess should be regarded as the clinical continuum of peritonsillitis. Peritonsillar abscess (PTA), also termed *quinsy,* is the most common deep infection of the head and neck in the adult.

Principles of Disease

Peritonsillitis is thought to occur as a result of acute tonsillitis. Infection in either Weber's glands or the tonsillar

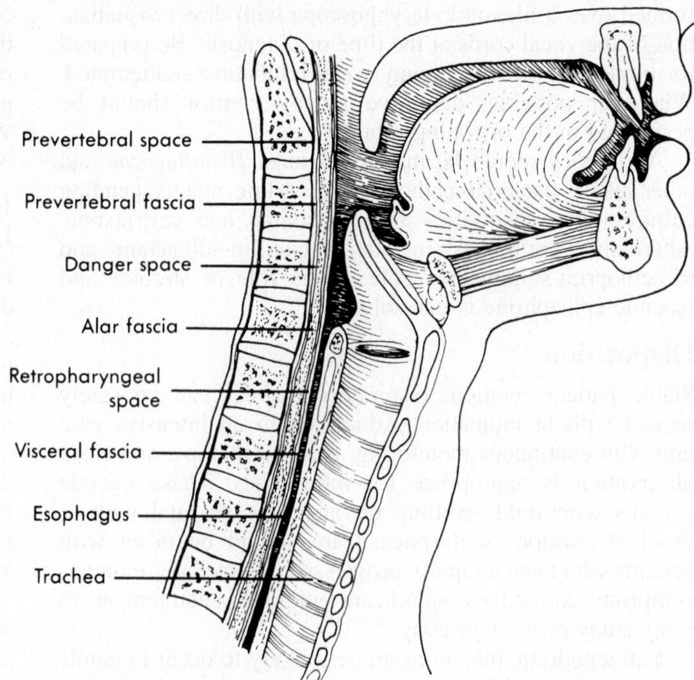

Figure 70-4. **Lateral view of neck showing relationship of fascia to prevertebral, "danger," retropharyngeal, and submandibular space.**

crypts invades the peritonsillar tissues, leading to a cellulitis that may progress to abscess formation.[43,44] Fibrous fascial septae divide the peritonsillar space into compartments and direct the infection anteriorly and superiorly.[45]

Chronic tonsillitis, infectious mononucleosis, smoking, chronic lymphocytic leukemia, and tonsilloliths are predisposing factors to the development of peritonsillitis.[45] Dental infection may also be a risk factor.[45,46] PTA is reported in patients who have undergone complete tonsillectomies and occurs in all age groups. Recurrence of peritonsillitis is reported to occur in up to 50% of patients, with the incidence of recurrent PTA approximately 10%.[45,46] The highest incidence of recurrence occurs in patients younger than 40 years of age and those with a history of chronic tonsillitis.[47,48]

Most PTAs are polymicrobial, with a mixture of aerobic and anaerobic organisms isolated. The etiologic agents are similar to those involved in pharyngitis. The most common aerobes cultured are *S. pyogenes* (GABHS), *Streptococcus milleri, H. influenzae,* and *Streptococcus viridans.* The most common anaerobic isolates are *Fusobacterium* sp, *Bacteroides* sp, *Peptostreptococcus* sp, and *Actinomyces* sp. In patients receiving antibiotics who develop PTAs, fewer aerobic bacteria are found, particularly streptococcal species, and more β-lactamase–producing organisms are isolated.[43,47,49-51]

Clinical Features

The symptoms and signs of peritonsillitis are both local and systemic. There is often a delay of an average of 2 to 5 days between abscess formation and the start of symptoms.[43] Symptoms include odynophagia, dysphagia, drooling, trismus, and referred otalgia. Patients may have a characteristic muffled, "hot potato" voice and rancid breath. Systemic signs include fever, malaise, and dehydration. Patients often relay a history of recurrent tonsillitis with multiple trials of antibiotics. A significant number of patients may currently be taking antibiotics without resolution of symptoms.[43-45,47]

Examination of the pharynx may be limited by trismus. Physical findings of peritonsillitis include inflamed and erythematous oral mucosa, purulent tonsillar exudates that may cover or partially obscure the tonsil, and tender cervical lymphadenopathy. Peritonsillar cellulitis is difficult to differentiate from PTA. PTA is characterized by a greater frequency of drooling, trismus, and dysphagia, whereas peritonsillar cellulitis is more commonly bilateral.[43,46,52] The distinguishing feature of PTA is inferior medial displacement of the infected tonsil (at times involving the soft palate), with contralateral deviation of the uvula. The abscess is usually unilateral and in the superior pole of the tonsil.[45,46] Bilateral peritonsillar abscesses are reported to occur occasionally.[49,50,53]

Diagnostic Strategies

The diagnosis of peritonsillitis is often made clinically.[43,48,54] Diagnosis of PTA is dependent on the presence of pus. This is frequently done by needle aspiration at the time of treatment. One study notes a 20% incidence of mononucleosis in a series of patients with PTA and recommends that a Monospot test be obtained.[53]

Roentgenographic examination in uncomplicated cases contributes little to the diagnosis. A contrast-enhanced computed tomography (CT) scan and ultrasound (both intraoral and transcutaneous) aid in differentiating PTA from cellulitis and are particularly useful when patients are unable to cooperate with needle aspiration. These modalities are also useful in diagnosing posteriorly and inferiorly located abscesses and in guiding needle aspiration.[52,55] The CT scan, magnetic resonance imaging (MRI) scan, and ultrasound help in the diagnosis of complications.[44,52]

Differential Considerations

The differential diagnosis of peritonsillitis includes hypertrophic tonsillitis, infectious mononucleosis, tubercular granuloma, diphtheria, other deep space infections of the neck, cervical adenitis, congenital or traumatic internal carotid artery aneurysms, foreign bodies, and neoplasms.[44]

Management

Emergency abscess aspiration may be necessary in cases of complete or impending airway obstruction. Peritonsillar cellulitis may be controlled by intravenous (IV) antibiotics alone. Penicillin is the antibiotic of choice, with erythromycin and other macrolides used in those patients with penicillin allergies.[48,51,54] The addition of metronidazole to penicillin may increase the success rate.[49] Other regimens include cefoxitin, amoxicillin-clavulanic acid, clindamycin, and the combination of penicillin and rifampin.[21] β-Lactamase–producing bacteria and poor penetration of antibiotics into the abscess limit the effectiveness of antibiotics in patients who have developed PTAs. Drainage of the abscess seems to be the most important factor in treating these patients. Patients with PTA who fail to improve with penicillin and proper drainage may benefit from a trial of a penicillinase-resistant antibiotic.[48,49,54]

Until recently, surgical treatment (immediate tonsillectomy or incision and drainage) was recommended for the treatment of PTA.[43,46,47,53] Several studies demonstrate the safety and cost-effectiveness of needle aspiration of PTAs by both emergency physicians and otolaryngologists (although false-negative aspirations occur in approximately 10% of cases, and another 10% may require repeated aspirations). Needle aspiration is diagnostic, less painful, safer, easier to perform, immediately relieves symptoms, and more cost-effective than incision and drainage.[43,47,48,54,55] Intraoral ultrasound-guided needle aspiration is a useful adjunct in the presence of trismus.[55] Immediate tonsillectomy under general anesthesia may be needed in the extremely young or uncooperative patient.[50]

Disposition

Admission is required for patients who have underlying disease, are dehydrated, are toxic appearing, are unable to tolerate oral fluids, are in severe pain, or have other complications. The most dangerous immediate complication of peritonsillitis is pharyngeal obstruction with upper airway compromise. Other complications include abscess rupture and pulmonary aspiration leading to pneumonia, empyema, and pulmonary abscess formation. Infection can spread contiguously to the parapharyngeal and retropharyngeal spaces. Ludwig's angina, mediastinal involvement (including mediastinitis, pneumonia, empyema, and pericarditis), myocarditis, carotid artery erosion, jugular vein thrombophlebitis, septic embolization, abscess formation, Lemierre's syndrome (postanginal septicemia), and cervicothoracic necrotizing fasciitis are reported to complicate peritonsillitis. Intracranial extension of peritonsillitis may result in meningitis, cavernous sinus thrombosis, and cerebral abscess. Systemic complications also include dehydration and sepsis.[44]

LUDWIG'S ANGINA

Perspective

Ludwig's angina (LA) is a cellulitis that was first described in 1836. LA is a potentially fulminant disease process that can lead to death within hours.[56,57] Modern dental care has markedly reduced the incidence of LA.

Principles of Disease

LA is a progressive cellulitis of the connective tissues of the floor of the mouth and neck that begins in the submandibular space. Dental disease is the most common cause of LA. An infected or recently extracted tooth is present in almost all affected patients.[56,57] The most commonly affected teeth are the lower second and third molars. Dentoalveolar abscesses may easily break through the relatively thin cortex of the mandible below the mylohyoid ridge and infect the submandibular space. Other causes of LA include a fractured mandible, foreign body or laceration to the floor of the mouth, tongue piercing, traumatic intubation and bronchoscopy, secondary infections of an oral malignancy, osteomyelitis, otitis media, submandibular sialoadenitis, peritonsillar abscess, a furuncle, infected thyroglossal cyst, and sepsis.[38,56,58]

LA is most commonly a polymicrobial disease of mixed aerobic-anaerobic bacteria of oral origin. The most commonly isolated organisms are streptococci, staphylococci, and *Bacteroides* sp. Other organisms include *H. influenzae, Pseudomonas aeruginosa, Klebsiella* sp, and *Candida albicans*.[38,56-61]

Clinical Features

Infection of the sublingual and submaxillary spaces leads to edema and soft tissue displacement, which may result in airway obstruction.[36,38,56,57] The most common symptoms of patients with LA include dysphagia, neck swelling, and neck pain.[57] Other symptoms include dysphonia, a "hot potato" voice, odynophagia, dysarthria, drooling, tongue swelling, pain in the floor of the mouth, restricted neck movement, and sore throat.[38,56,57] Patients should be questioned regarding recent dental extraction and disease. A foul taste in the patient's mouth, feeling air release at the time of extraction, the rapid development of crepitus, and unilateral pharyngitis in patients who have recently undergone tooth extraction may be early clues to the diagnosis of LA.

The most common physical findings in LA are bilateral submandibular swelling and elevation or protrusion of the tongue. Other findings include elevation of the floor of the mouth, posterior displacement of the tongue, and a "woody" consistency of the floor of the mouth. A tense edema and brawny induration of the neck above the hyoid may be present and is described as a "bull neck." Marked tenderness to palpation of the neck and subcutaneous emphysema may be noted. Trismus and fever are usually present, but usually no palpable fluctuance or cervical lymphadenopathy is present. Percussion tenderness may be elicited over the involved teeth.[38,56,57]

Diagnostic Strategies

The diagnosis of LA is usually made clinically according to five criteria: (1) cellulitis with little or no pus present in the submandibular space; (2) bilateral cellulitis; (3) gangrene present with serosanguinous, putrid fluid; (4) connective tissue, fascia, and muscles involved, but glandular tissue is spared; and (5) cellulitis spread by continuity and not by lymphatic vessels.[58]

Laboratory investigation is not overly useful. Gram stains with cultures and sensitivities of drained fluid and pus should be obtained. Soft tissue x-ray films of the neck may confirm the diagnosis by showing swelling of the affected area and airway narrowing and by identifying gas collections. Panorex and dental films may demonstrate associated periodontal abscess and other disease.[38,56] Chest radiography, CT, and MRI may aid in the diagnosis of mediastinitis and other thoracic complications. Ultrasonography is useful in diagnosing abscesses and edema in the setting of LA.[59]

Differential Considerations

The differential diagnosis includes deep cervical node suppuration, peritonsillar and other deep neck space abscess, parotid and submandibular gland abscess, oral carcinomas, angioedema, submandibular hematomas, and laryngeal diphtheria.

Management

Asphyxiation is the most common cause of death in patients with LA.[36,40,56,57] Patients without respiratory difficulty should be maintained in a sitting position. These patients should never be left unattended and should be continuously monitored. Airway impairment may occur suddenly. Stridor, tachypnea, dyspnea, inability to handle secretions, and agitation are all indicative of impending airway compromise. Fiberoptic-guided nasotracheal intubation is the preferred method of airway control. Endotracheal intubation may be difficult because of distortion of the upper airway, trismus, pooled secretions, and a tendency for the development of laryngospasm.[40,56,57] Cricothyrotomy may be difficult and opens tissue planes that increase the risk of spreading infection into the mediastinum.[39-41]

Antibiotic therapy must be started immediately. Appropriate antibiotic regimens include high-dose penicillin with metronidazole, or cefoxitin used alone. Alternately, clindamycin, ticarcillin-clavulanate, piperacillin-tazobactam, or ampicillin-sulbactam may be used.[21,40,59,60] The value of corticosteroids in the setting of LA is unclear.[61]

Surgical incision and drainage was the therapy of choice in the preantibiotic era. With the exception of dental extractions, surgery is reserved for those patients who do not respond to medical therapy and those with crepitus and purulent collections.[38-40,56,57]

Disposition

Mortality caused by LA is less than 10% with early aggressive antibiotic therapy and adequate protection of the airway.[38,56,57] Mortality is often due to complications and delays in diagnosis and treatment. Infection can easily spread into other deep spaces of the neck and into the thoracic cavity. Empyema, mediastinitis, mediastinal abscess, and pericarditis are all reported. Aspiration may lead to pneumonia and the formation of lung abscesses. Other reported complications are internal jugular vein thrombosis, carotid artery infection and erosion, bacteremia and sepsis, pneumoperitoneum, subphrenic abscess, cervicothoracic necrotizing fasciitis, and spontaneous pneumothorax.[57,60]

RETROPHARYNGEAL AND PREVERTEBRAL SPACE ABSCESSES

Perspective

Retropharyngeal swelling reflects expansion of either the retropharyngeal, danger, or prevertebral spaces. This discussion refers to infections in these spaces collectively as retropharyngeal abscesses (RPA).

Principles of Disease

RPA was previously a disease of childhood, with 96% of cases occurring in patients younger than 6 years old. Adults are now increasingly affected. Children less than 4 years old have prominent retropharyngeal lymph nodes that may become infected, leading to retropharyngeal cellulitis and abscess formation. The increased use of antibiotics to treat pharyngitis in children has led to the declining incidence of RPA in this age group. These retropharyngeal nodes atrophy after age 4 to 6 years, and thus the incidence and pathophysiology of this entity differ in adults.[62-64]

In adult patients, cellulitis develops in the retropharyngeal area.[62,65] Once the retropharyngeal space is involved, the infection spreads rapidly and an abscess may form. Nasopharyngitis, otitis media, parotitis, tonsillitis, peritonsillar abscess, dental infections and procedures, upper airway instrumentation, endoscopy, lateral pharyngeal space infection, and Ludwig's angina are all implicated in the development of RPA.[63,64,66] Other causes include blunt and penetrating (usually from foreign bodies, commonly fish bones) trauma, caustic ingestions, vertebral fractures, and hematologic spread from distant infections.[63,64,67,68] Vertebral osteomyelitis and diskitis may lead to infection of the prevertebral space. Danger space infections are caused by extension of infection from either the retropharyngeal or prevertebral spaces. Underlying systemic disorders (e.g., diabetes and depressed immune systems) may predispose individuals to developing retropharyngeal infections.[63,68]

Retropharyngeal abscesses are most commonly polymicrobial with a mixture of aerobes and anaerobes.[63,64] Although tuberculosis was the most common cause of RPAs in the past, it is now rarely reported in the United States.[69] *Staphylococcus* is currently the most common cause of pyogenic vertebral osteomyelitis leading to the formation of RPA.[70] Disseminated coccidiomycosis may also cause RPAs. The source is usually direct extension of vertebral body osteomyelitis that, unlike tuberculosis, spares the intervertebral disk.[71]

Clinical Features

Patients typically have a sore throat, dysphagia, odynophagia, drooling, muffled voice, neck stiffness, neck pain, and fever. Dysphonia is usually present and is described as a duck "quack" (*cri du canard*). Patients may complain of feeling a lump in their throat. Patients with RPAs may appear quite ill and will generally prefer to hold their necks extended and remain in the supine position. This position will keep the swollen posterior pharynx from compressing their upper airway. Forcing the patient to sit may lead to increased dyspnea.[63,67,68]

Physical examination may reveal tender cervical lymphadenopathy, tender cervical musculature, neck swelling, torticollis, and often a high fever. Trismus may be present, making visualization of the pharynx difficult. In cases of retropharyngeal cellulitis, diffuse edema and erythema of the posterior pharynx are present.[62-64,68] Once an abscess is present, palpation of the pharynx may demonstrate a unilateral mass if the retropharyngeal space is affected and a midline mass if the abscess is in the prevertebral or danger space. Palpation of a fluctuant mass is unreliable and carries a risk of inadvertent rupture of the abscess.[62,67] Tenderness on moving the larynx and trachea side to side (tracheal "rock"

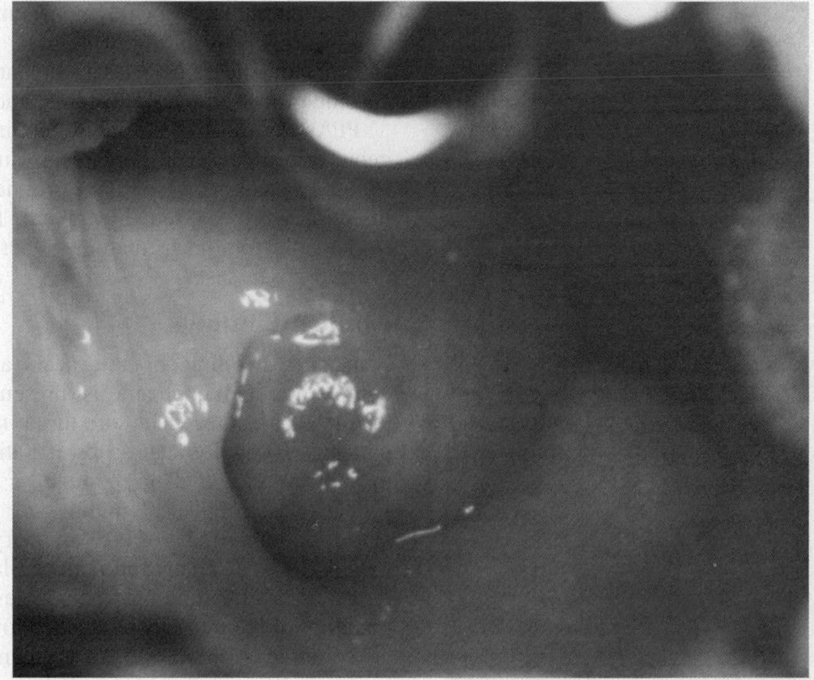

Figure 70-5. **Peritonsillar abscess with uvular displacement.**

sign) is commonly present. RPA may also be seen as pain in the back of the neck or shoulder precipitated by swallowing. Cold abscesses (caused by tuberculosis) are characterized by insidious onset, chronicity, constitutional symptoms, and less of a febrile response. Symptoms disproportionate to findings should prompt further evaluation.[68]

Diagnostic Strategies

Diagnosis rests on clinical presentation and lateral cervical radiographs (Figure 70-5). Inspiratory lateral neck films often demonstrate widening of the retropharyngeal soft tissues with forward displacement of the esophagus and trachea.[67] Soft tissue swelling may be diffuse in cases of cellulitis or more focal if an abscess cavity is present. A pathologic process should be suspected if: the retropharyngeal space on lateral neck films (measured from the anteroinferior aspect of the second vertebral body to the posterior pharyngeal wall) is wider than 7 mm in both children and adults, or the retrotracheal space (measured from the anteroinferior aspect of the sixth vertebral body to the posterior pharyngeal wall) is more than 14 mm in children and 22 mm in adults.[72] True lateral films with the neck fully extended during deep inspiration are the most reliable. Other radiographic findings include reversal of the normal lordosis of the cervical spine, air fluid levels in the abscess cavity, foreign bodies, and vertebral body destruction.[67] Chest radiographs should be obtained to determine whether mediastinal extension has occurred.

Plain films may not be sufficiently sensitive to diagnose RPA. A CT or MRI scan should be obtained in these instances. These studies will not only aid in the diagnosis and differentiation between cellulitis and abscess but will also determine the extent of the disease process and the presence of complications[63,64,70] (Figure 70-6). Ultrasonography is useful for differentiating retropharyngeal cellulitis from RPA.[62]

Differential Considerations

The differential diagnosis includes retropharyngeal tumors, foreign bodies, inflammation, hematoma, aneurysms, hemorrhage, lymphadenopathy, or edema. Other considerations include tendinitis of the longus colli muscle and retropharyngeal thyroid tissue.[69]

Management

Patients with retropharyngeal cellulitis are best treated with IV antibiotics.[65] Appropriate regimens are similar to those used for Ludwig's angina. Tuberculosis and fungal infections must also be considered. Resolution of retropharyngeal cellulitis is possible without surgical intervention in a small percentage of cases.[62,65,68]

RPA is treated with antibiotics given in conjunction with incision and drainage of the abscess by a specialist familiar with the procedure and complications. Cold abscesses should only be drained extraorally, unless the patient is in acute respiratory distress.[69]

Neck immobilization may be necessary in cases of vertebral body destruction caused by osteomyelitis or atlantoaxial separation.[73] These patients need neurosurgical or orthopedic evaluation and may require internal or external fixation.

Disposition

Patients with RPAs should be admitted to a monitored hospital bed or sent directly to the operating suite. Airway compromise can be caused by anterior displacement of the pharyngeal tissues. Pulmonary complications include abscess rupture with aspiration and subsequent pneumonia, empyema, and asphyxiation. Extension of the infection along tissue planes and through other deep spaces may lead to mediastinitis and mediastinal abscess formation, pericarditis, ple

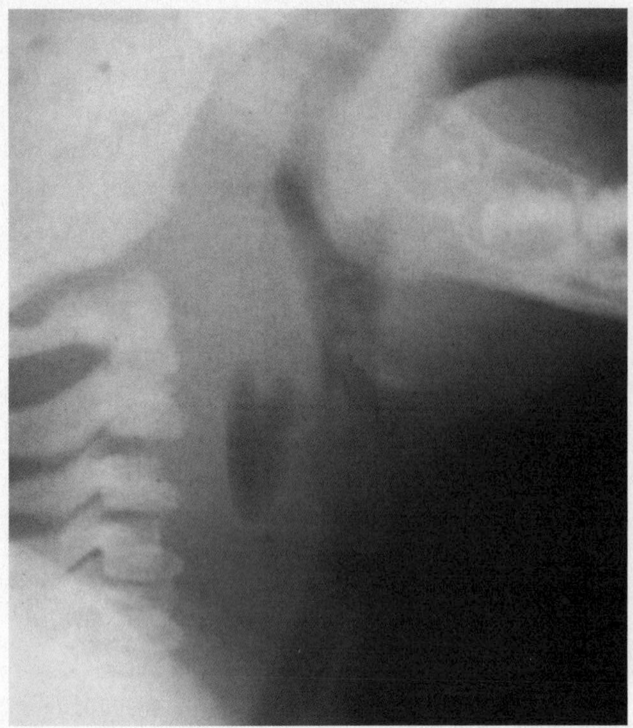

Figure 70-6. **Radiograph of retropharyngeal abscess demonstrating retropharyngeal soft-tissue swelling.**

ritis, and empyema.[63,68] In addition, abscesses may track into the back of the neck and into the axilla.[69,70] Vascular complications occur from the extension of the retropharyngeal abscess into the lateral pharyngeal space.[66,68] Atraumatic atlantoaxial separation is due to damage of the transverse ligament of the atlas by the abscess. These patients may have neurologic symptoms and a widened predental space on plain films. Diagnosis is made radiologically and may include a CT scan and flexion-extension plain films.[73] Acute transverse myelitis and epidural abscesses are also reported, both resulting in quadriplegia. Other complications include erosion into the esophagus and auditory canal, necrotizing fasciitis of the neck, acute respiratory distress syndrome, sepsis, and death.[67]

PARAPHARYNGEAL ABSCESS

Perspective

The parapharyngeal space, also known as the lateral pharyngeal and pharyngomaxillary space, is divided into two compartments by the styloid process. The anterior compartment contains connective tissue, muscle, and lymph nodes. The carotid sheath (which contains the carotid artery, internal jugular vein, vagus nerve, cranial nerves IX through XII, and the cervical sympathetic chain) runs in the posterior compartment.

Principles of Disease

Odontogenic and pharyngotonsillar infections are the most common causes of parapharyngeal space abscesses.[66,74] Parapharyngeal space infections can also arise from contiguous spreading from other surrounding deep neck space infections.[66,75,76] Other causes include parotitis, sinusitis, spread from infected neck tumors, infected branchial cleft cysts, suppuration of local lymphadenitis, iatrogenic introduction of organisms during mandibular nerve block or anesthesia for tonsillectomy, nasal intubation, tooth extractions, chronic otitis with cholesteatoma, and mastoiditis.[66,75,76]

PPAs are most often polymicrobial infections of odontogenic origin caused by organisms similar to those found in Ludwig's angina.[74,75] PPAs originating from pharyngeal infections are caused by mixed flora similar to those responsible for the formation of peritonsillar and retropharyngeal abscesses.[74]

Clinical Findings

Pain and swelling of the neck are the most common complaints. Odynophagia is present in most patients. A history of an antecedent sore throat may be elicited in some patients. Torticollis caused by irritation of the sternocleidomastoid muscle is also reported.[74,75]

The classic physical findings of infection involving the anterior compartment of the parapharyngeal space are medial tonsillar displacement and posterolateral pharyngeal wall bulge.[66,75] Other findings include fever, trismus (caused by irritation of the muscles of mastication), edema, and swelling at the angle of the jaw.[66] An erythematous, tender, nonfluctuant swelling at the angle of the mandible is a consistent finding in patients with anterior PPA.[74,75]

Posterior space involvement shows many of these same signs. If the anterior compartment is spared, however, little or no trismus occurs. Instead, posterior displacement of the tonsillar pillar and retropharyngeal swelling may be present.[66]

Diagnostic Strategies

The diagnosis of PPA is primarily made clinically. Blood cultures are usually sterile unless jugular vein thrombophlebitis is complicating the parapharyngeal space infection.[66,74] Lateral radiographs may show upper prevertebral soft tissue swelling but are often not helpful.[74,75] Ultrasonography, CT, and MRI scans are more useful in diagnosing PPA and its complications.[66,74-76] Angiography, Doppler flow studies, and MRI angiography may also be helpful in evaluating vascular complications.[74,76]

Differential Considerations

Differential diagnosis includes infections in other deep spaces of the neck, tumors and metastatic lymph nodes, thyroiditis, branchial cleft cyst, and carotid artery aneurysms.

Management

Treatment must be aggressive and consists of IV antibiotics and surgical drainage of the abscess cavity. Appropriate antibiotic regimens are discussed in the treatment of Ludwig's angina. IV antibiotics will cure 10% to 15% of parapharyngeal space infections and should be started emergently.[66,74,75] Successful resolution with high-dose IV antibiotics and repeated CT scan–guided aspirations is reported, although hospitalization is significantly prolonged compared with early surgical incision and drainage.[74,75]

Disposition

Complications of PPAs can be fatal. Local complications include airway obstruction and abscess rupture with subsequent aspiration, pneumonia, and empyema.[66] Infection can spread to surrounding spaces and into the mediastinum and pericardium.[66,74] This may lead to mediastinitis, mediastinal abscess, pericarditis, myocardial abscess, and empyema.[74] Other complications include osteomyelitis of the mandible, cervicothoracic necrotizing fasciitis, parotid abscess, cavernous sinus thrombosis, and meningitis.[5,66]

Posterior parapharyngeal space infections are particularly dangerous. These infections may affect the cervical sympathetic chain, carotid artery, or internal jugular vein. Ipsilateral Horner's syndrome and neuropathies of cranial nerves IX through XII may occur.[66] Carotid artery erosion may lead to hemorrhage and the formation of aneurysms. Oral, nasal, and aural warning bleeding is common with carotid artery erosion, aural bleeding being particularly ominous. Any unexplained bleeding associated with parapharyngeal or other deep neck space infection must be investigated thoroughly. Persistent peritonsillar swelling despite resolution of the PPA, or a tender unilateral pulsatile mass, may indicate arterial aneurysm. Aspiration or incision of a carotid artery aneurysm thought to be a PPA may have disastrous complications.[76]

Involvement of the internal jugular vein may lead to septic thrombosis and a Lemierre syndrome.[77] This entity, also called postanginal septicemia, affects primarily young healthy patients and is easily confused with right-sided endocarditis or aspiration pneumonia. The presentation is one of a pharyngitis that initially improves but then is followed by severe sepsis. It is thought that the pharyngeal infection spreads to the parapharyngeal space and causes a septic thrombophlebitis of the jugular vein. Patients are usually ill appearing and febrile. Metastatic infections involve primarily the lung and are manifest by bilateral nodular infiltrates, pleural effusions, and pneumothoraces. Septic arthritis, osteomyelitis, soft tissue cellulitis and abscesses, meningitis, and a vesiculopustular rash are also reported as a result of septic embolization. Leukocytosis and elevated bilirubin and liver function tests, with and without hepatomegaly and jaundice, are often present. Albuminuria, hematuria, and elevations of serum creatinine and blood urea nitrogen are reported. Patients rarely develop septic shock, although acute respiratory distress syndrome, transient coagulopathies, and hypotension commonly occur. The most common cause of this entity is *Fusobacterium* sp (primarily *F. necrophorum*), although *S. aureus* is the most common pathogen in intravenous drug users. Treatment consists of parenteral antibiotics. Jugular vein ligation and resection are necessary in cases of uncontrolled sepsis and respiratory failure caused by repeated septic pulmonary emboli. The value of anticoagulation is unknown.[76,77]

SINUSITIS

Perspective

Sinusitis ranks as one of the most common afflictions of Americans. It is estimated that 0.5% to 2% of viral upper respiratory tract infections are complicated by sinusitis.[78]

Principles of Disease

The paranasal sinuses (frontal, maxillary, ethmoid, and sphenoid) are named for the facial bones they occupy. Pneumatization may involve other bones but represents extension from the main sinus.[79] The maxillary sinus is triangular, with its base being the lateral nasal wall and apex extending into the zygoma. The ethmoid sinus, commonly divided into anterior and posterior, is composed of between two and eight anterior air cells and one to eight posterior cells. The blood supply to the ethmoid cells directly connects with the ophthalmic vessels and cavernous sinus. Infectious processes in this sinus are dangerous because of their ability to spread to the orbit or central nervous system.[79]

The frontal sinus has quite variable pneumatization, ranging from extensive to totally aplastic. Left and right frontal sinuses are separated by a bony septum. The paired sphenoid sinuses are also separated by a bony septum. The optic nerve and carotid artery occupy the lateral walls of the sphenoid sinus.[79] The maxillary, anterior ethmoid, and frontal sinuses drain into the medial meatus, located between the inferior and middle nasal turbinates. This area is named the ostiomeatal complex and is the focal point of sinus disease. The posterior ethmoid sinus drains into the superior meatus and the sphenoid sinus just above the superior turbinate.[80]

A healthy sinus depends on a patent ostia with free air exchange and mucus drainage. A healthy sinus is sterile and does not accumulate mucus. Viral upper respiratory tract infections and allergic rhinitis are the most common causes of ostial obstruction with resultant sinusitis. Ciliary abnormality or immobility inhibits drainage and is another important cause of sinusitis. Ciliary dysfunction can be temporary (e.g., upper respiratory infection) or permanent (e.g., syndromes associated with cilial structural abnormalities). Infection leads to increased mucus viscosity, further impeding drainage. Once drainage is compromised, resorption of air within the sinus lowers oxygen tension, and increased metabolism lowers the pH. Bacteria are introduced into the sinus by coughing and nose blowing. These processes lead to increased inflammation and bacterial overgrowth. Other factors predisposing to sinusitis include immunocompromised hosts, nasal septal deviation and other structural abnormalities, nasal polyps, nasal tumors, trauma and fractures, rhinitis medicamentosa, rhinitis caused by toxic mucosal exposure, barotrauma, foreign bodies, nasal cocaine abuse, and instrumentation (including nasogastric and nasotracheal intubation).[78]

It is important to distinguish infectious from allergic sinusitis. Allergic sinusitis is associated with sneezing, itchy eyes, allergen exposure, and prior episodes.[81] Approximately 90% of patients with colds have an element of viral sinusitis. Viral infection does play a role in acute sinusitis.[78] *S. pneumoniae,* nontypable *H. influenzae,* and *M. catarrhalis* are the primary pathogens responsible for acute bacterial sinusitis. Anaerobic bacteria, streptococcal species, and *S. aureus* are more prominent causes of chronic sinusitis.[82,83] *P. aeruginosa* is associated with sinusitis in the setting of HIV infection and cystic fibrosis. *Rhizopus, Aspergillus, Candida, Histoplasma, Blastomyces, Coccidioides,* and *Cryptococcus* species, as well as other fungi, may cause sinusitis, primarily in the immunocompromised host.[78,84]

Clinical Features

Acute sinusitis typically progresses over 7 to 10 days. During the first 5 to 7 days of illness, it may be difficult to differentiate viral from bacterial sinusitis. Bacterial disease is suggested by worsening symptoms after 5 days or persistent symptoms after 10 days, or "double sickening." This refers to patients with a cold who improve initially, only to have worsening sinus congestion and discomfort.[80] Patients may experience a variety of symptoms, including nasal congestion, mucopurulent nasal discharge, nasal obstruction, postnasal drip (that may lead to cough), pressure over the involved sinus, malaise, and fever.[85] Patients usually have facial pain or headache over the involved sinus. The exception to this is in cases of sphenoid sinusitis, which may present with vague headaches and focal points almost anywhere in the head. Maxillary sinusitis may be seen with pain over the zygoma, in the canine or bicuspid teeth, or periorbitally. Ethmoid sinusitis can cause medial canthal pain and periorbital or temporal headaches.[85]

Logistic regression analysis has shown five independent predictors of sinusitis: maxillary toothache, abnormal sinus transillumination (performed by an expert), poor response to nasal decongestants or antihistamines, colored nasal discharge, and mucopurulence seen during examination. Although no single variable is specific, the presence of four or more is highly predictive of sinusitis. The "overall clinical impression" of the emergency physician may be more accurate than any single finding.[85] Chronic sinusitis is slow in onset, prolonged in duration, and recurrent in frequency. Symptoms may be similar to acute disease, but may also include chronic cough, fetid breath, laryngitis, bronchitis, and worsening asthma.[80,81,86]

Physical examination is best performed after application of a topical decongestant. Mucosal erythema and edema are usually noted. Purulent discharge may be noted from the nasal meatus if the sinus ostia are not completely obstructed. Head positioning may be useful in differentiating the sinus involved. Pain caused by ethmoid, sphenoid, and frontal sinusitis is exacerbated by placing the patient supine and relieved by positioning the patient's head in an upright position. The reverse is generally seen in cases of maxillary sinusitis.

Invasive fungal sinusitis (mucormycosis) is an aggressive opportunistic rhinocerebral infection that affects immunocompromised hosts. Mucormycosis *(Rhizopus)* is usually associated with fever, localized nasal pain, and cloudy rhinorrhea. On examination, the affected tissue (usually the turbinates) appears gray, friable, anesthetic, and nonbleeding because of infarction caused by mucormycotic angioinvasion. In advanced cases the affected tissues are necrotic and black, and the infection spreads beyond the sinus.[82]

Diagnostic Strategies

Diagnosis is usually clinical. Both nasal and nasopharyngeal cultures correlate poorly with cultures of sinus aspirates and cultures obtained at the time of open antrostomy.[78,81] Culture and biopsy are indicated for chronic bacterial and fungal sinusitis. Radiographic examination should be limited to questionable diagnosis, to unresponsive disease, or to search for complications. The accuracy of plain films is much higher in cases of maxillary sinusitis compared with other sinuses. A Water's view alone can evaluate the maxillary sinus but runs the risk of missing pathologic conditions in other sinuses (Figure 70-7). Positive findings on plain films include sinus opacity, air-fluid level, or mucosal thickening of 6 mm or more. The diagnostic accuracy of plain films is limited in that opacity may represent other processes, including tumors. The gold standard of sinus imaging is axial and coronal CT scans. The CT scan findings suggestive of sinusitis include air-fluid levels, sinus opacification, sinus

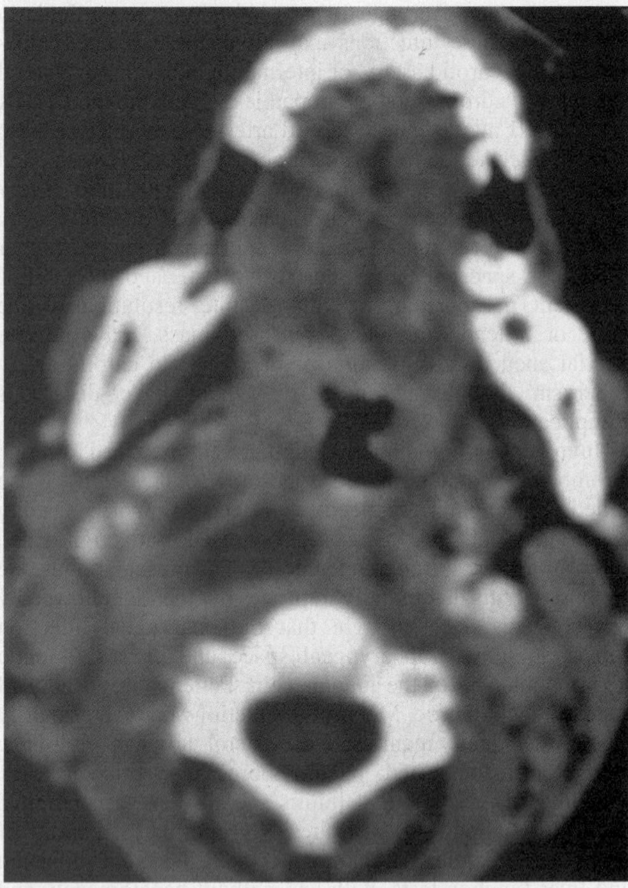

Figure 70-7. **CT scan demonstrating right-sided retropharyngeal abscess.**

wall displacement, and 4 mm or greater mucosal thickening (Figure 70-8). IV contrast may be required to evaluate central nervous system or orbital complications. In some centers, the CT scan with a limited number of cuts is used in place of plain films with little difference in cost or radiation exposure. The CT scan is sensitive, although not specific. Incidental sinus mucosal thickening is seen in about 40% of asymptomatic patients, and abnormal CT scan findings can also be noted in just over half the patients with seasonal allergies. An MRI scan is also helpful in distinguishing sinus disease and its complications, but at present has little role in the ED. Sinus endoscopy is useful for specialist evaluation of sinus pathology.[78,82,87]

Differential Considerations

Rhinitis can be differentiated from sinusitis by its increased response of nasal obstruction to treatment, clear nasal discharge, and the absence of pain. Rhinitis does not lead to ostial obstruction and thus patients will not complain of facial pain. Tension headaches, vascular headaches, foreign bodies, dental disease, brain abscesses, epidural abscesses, meningitis, and subdural empyema may also present in a manner similar to sinusitis.

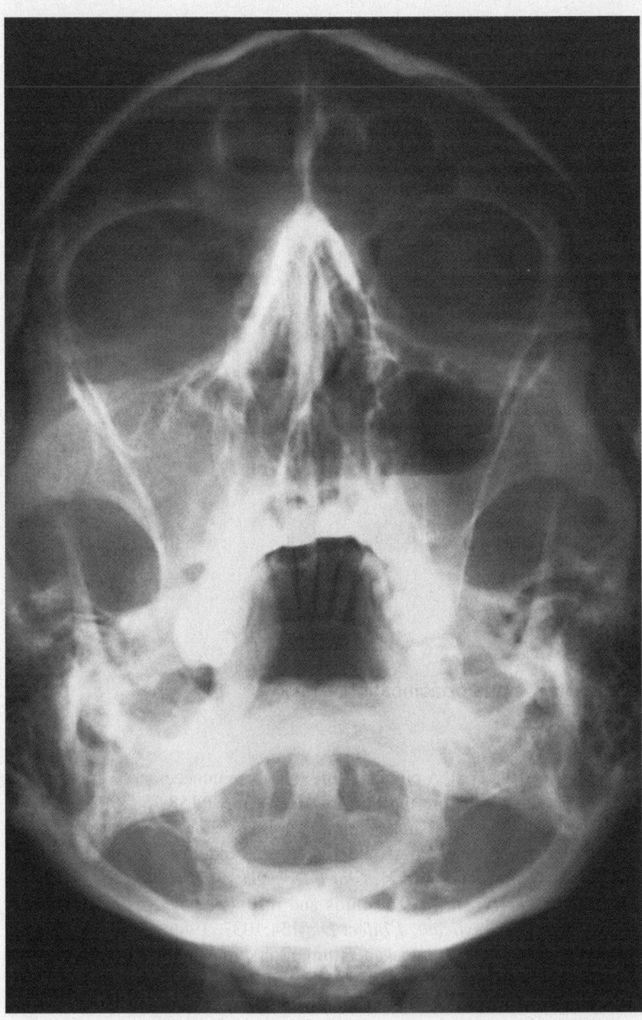

Figure 70-8. **Radiograph showing right maxillary sinus opacification and left maxillary sinus air-fluid level.**

Management

A large proportion of viral and bacterial sinusitis resolves spontaneously.[80,84] For this reason, the role of antibiotics in the treatment of uncomplicated sinusitis has been questioned. Current recommendations are that antibiotics should be started when one suspects bacterial disease (see previous discussion). The choice of antibiotics must consider β-lactamase–production and multiple-drug–resistant pneumococcus. Ten days of amoxicillin is still the first-line agent, but treatment failures occur in areas with a high percentage of β-lactamase–producing bacteria. Penicillin-allergic patients may be treated with trimethoprim-sulfamethoxazole. A 3-day course of trimethoprim-sulfamethoxazole or azithromycin and decongestants may be as effective as the standard 10-day antibiotic course.[88] Failure of symptoms to resolve after 7 days of therapy necessitates a change to a broader-spectrum antibiotic. Appropriate agents include a 10- to 14-day course of amoxicillin-clavulanate, cefuroxime axetil, other second- or third-generation cephalosporins, clindamycin alone or in combination with ciprofloxacin, sulfamethoxazole, azithromycin, clarithromycin, or one of the fluoroquinolones. Metronidazole may be added to any of these regimens to increase anaerobic activity. Antibiotics for chronic sinusitis should be effective against anaerobic and β-lactamase–producing bacteria. Treatment of life-threatening complications requires consultation, admission, and high-dose IV antibiotics, including cefuroxime, ceftriaxone, or ampicillin sulbactam.[21,80,82,83]

The goal of decongestant therapy is to reduce tissue edema, facilitate drainage, and maintain the patency of the sinus ostia. Although they are routinely recommended, there is no good scientific evidence that decongestants are effective. Decongestants are available in both topical and systemic preparations, both of which should be used simultaneously in conjunction with appropriate antibiotics. Local agents include phenylephrine hydrochloride 0.5% and oxymetazoline hydrochloride 0.05%. Topical agents should be used for only 3 to 5 days. Extended use results in rebound vasodilation and nasal obstruction, termed *rhinitis medicamentosa.* Systemic oral adrenergic agonists (e.g., phenylpropanolamine or pseudoephedrine) reduce nasal blood flow and congestion. These medications should be used cautiously in patients using tricyclic antidepressants, monoamine oxidase inhibitors, and nonselective β-adrenergic blockers.[78,82] Antihistamines should be reserved for the treatment of allergic sinusitis because these agents may impede sinus drainage. Topical steroids are indicated in cases of chronic and allergic sinusitis.[78,82]

Complications

Most cases of uncomplicated acute bacterial sinusitis can be treated on an outpatient basis with systemic decongestants, topical decongestants, and oral antibiotics. Failure of definitive antibiotic therapy suggests that the patient's sinusitis has extended to the chronic stage and requires referral to an otolaryngologist. Treatment of chronic sinusitis requires a prolonged (3 to 6 week) course of antibiotics.

Frontal or sphenoid sinusitis with air-fluid levels may require hospitalization. A previously healthy, nontoxic patient with good home support can be treated as an outpatient, but should return immediately for any signs or symptoms of complications, including severe headache, neurologic changes, or visual changes. Patients who are toxic, have a compromised immune system, or have poor home resources require admission and IV antibiotics.[84]

Sinusitis is associated with an increased incidence of bronchitis and asthma. Complications of sinusitis can be fulminant. Sinusitis may extend to involve the bones and soft tissues of the face and orbit. Facial cellulitis, periorbital cellulitis, periorbital abscess, optic neuritis, blindness, and orbital abscess may develop (Figure 70-9). Patients with orbital complications may have marked swelling, decreased ocular motility, and decreased visual acuity. Sinusitis may also lead to intracranial complications. Meningitis, cavernous sinus thrombosis, epidural or subdural empyema, and brain abscess are reported. Intracranial involvement may present with headache, decreased sensorium, or focal neurologic deficits and have a rapidly progressive course. Acute fulminant fungal sinusitis requires emergent consultation and admission for IV antifungal therapy and aggressive surgical debridement.[78,82,86] Complications of mucormycosis are directly related to delays in diagnosis and treatment. This opportunistic fungal infection rapidly progresses to involve the central nervous system and is associated with high morbidity and mortality.[78,82]

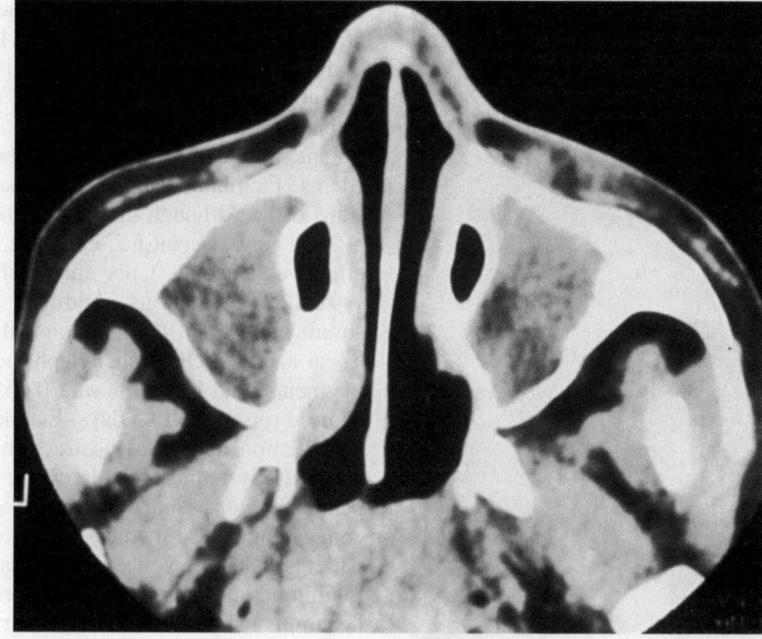

Figure 70-9. **CT scan showing bilateral maxillary sinus opacification.**

KEY CONCEPTS

- AE often presents with symptoms disproportionate to the clinical findings.
- Peritonsillar cellulitis is difficult to differentiate from PTA and may require needle aspiration.
- If a RPA is present, the mass is unilateral; in contrast, a midline mass suggests a prevertebral or danger space abscess.
- Posterior PPA may involve the cervical sympathetic chain, carotid artery, or internal jugular vein.
- Aspiration and incision of a carotid artery aneurysm thought to be a PPA may be disastrous.

REFERENCES

1. Bisno AL et al: Diagnosis and management of group A streptococcal pharyngitis: a practice guideline, *Clin Infect Dis* 25:574, 1997.
2. Pichichero ME, Cohen R: Shortened course of antibiotic therapy for acute otitis media, sinusitis, and tonsillopharyngitis, *Pediatr Infect Dis J* 16:680, 1997.
3. Huovinen P et al: Pharyngitis in adults: the presence and coexistence of viruses and bacterial organisms, *Ann Intern Med* 110:612, 1989.
4. Williams WC, Williamson HA, LeFevre ML: The prevalence of *Mycoplasma pneumoniae* in ambulatory patients with nonstreptococcal sore throat, *Fam Med* 23:117, 1991.
5. Finegold SM: Role of anaerobic bacteria in infections of the tonsils and adenoids. In Bluestone et al, editors: Workshop on role of anaerobic bacteria, *Ann Otol Rhinol Laryngol Suppl* 154:30, 1991.
6. Seppala H et al: Clinical scoring system in the evaluation of adult pharyngitis, *Arch Otolaryngol Head Neck Surg* 119:288, 1993.
7. Middleton DB: Pharyngitis, *Primary Care* 23:719, 1996.
8. Vukmir RB: Adult and pediatric pharyngitis: a review, *J Emerg Med* 10:607, 1992.
9. Isselbacher KJ et al, editors: *Harrison's principles of internal medicine,* ed 13, New York, 1994, McGraw-Hill.
10. McMillan JA et al: Pharyngitis associated with herpes simplex virus in college students, *Pediatr Infect Dis J* 12:280, 1993.
11. Cebul RD, Poses RM: The comparative cost-effectiveness of statistical decision rules and experienced physicians in pharyngitis management, *JAMA* 256:3353, 1986.
12. McIsaac WJ et al: A clinical score to reduce unnecessary antibiotic use in patients with sore throat, *Can Med Assoc J* 158:75, 1998.
13. Farizo KM et al: Fatal respiratory disease due to *Corynebacterium diphtheriae:* case report and review of guidelines for management, investigation, and control, *Clin Infect Dis* 16:59, 1993.
14. Banck G, Nyman M: Tonsillitis and rash associated with *Corynebacterium haemolyticum, J Infect Dis* 154:1037, 1986.
15. Wiesner PJ et al: Clinical spectrum of pharyngeal gonococcal infection, *N Engl J Med* 288:181, 1973.
16. Grayston JT et al: A new *Chlamydia* strain, TWAR, isolated in acute respiratory tract infections, *N Engl J Med* 315:161, 1986.
17. Ogawa H, Hashiguchi K, Kazuyama Y: Prolonged and recurrent tonsillitis associated with sexually transmitted *Chlamydia trachomatis, J Laryngol Otol* 107:27, 1993.
18. Uppal K, Bais AS: Tonsillar microflora-superficial surface vs deep, *J Laryngol Otol* 103:175, 1989.
19. Dowell SF et al: Appropriate use of antibiotics for URIs in children: Part II. Cough, pharyngitis and the common cold, *Am Fam Physician* 58:1335, 1998.
20. Coonan KM, Kaplan EL: In vitro susceptibility of recent North American group A streptococcal isolates to eleven oral antibiotics, *Pediatr Infect Dis J* 13:630, 1994.
21. Gilbert DN, Moellering RC, Sande MA: *The Sanford guide to antimicrobial therapy,* Hyde Park, 1999, Antimicrobial Therapy.
22. Marvez-Valls EG et al: The role of betamethasone in the treatment of acute exudative pharyngitis, *Acad Emerg Med* 5:567, 1998.
23. Shulman ST: Complications of streptococcal pharyngitis, *Pediatr Infect Dis J* 13(Suppl):S70, 1994.
24. Golding-Wood DG, Whittet HB: The lingual tonsil: a neglected symptomatic structure, *J Laryngol Otol* 103:922, 1989.
25. Allen DM, Hall KN, Barkman HW: Lingual tonsillitis: an uncommon cause of airway compromise responsive to epinephrine (letter), *Am J Emerg Med* 9:622, 1991.
26. Colton RH, Casper JK, editors: Understanding voice problems. A physiological perspective for diagnosis and treatment, ed 2, Baltimore, 1996, Williams & Wilkins.
27. Mayo Smith MF et al: Acute epiglottitis in adults: an eight-year experience in the state of Rhode Island, *N Engl J Med* 314:1133, 1986.
28. Mayo Smith MF et al: Acute epiglottitis: an 18 year experience in Rhode Island, *Chest* 108:1640, 1995.
29. Hebert PC et al: Adult epiglottitis in a Canadian setting, *Laryngoscope* 108:64, 1998.

30. Frantz TM, Rasgon BM, Quesenberry CP: Acute epiglottitis in adults: analysis of 129 cases, *JAMA* 272:1358, 1994.
31. Dort JC, Frohlich AM, Tate RB: Acute epiglottitis in adults: diagnosis and treatment in 43 patients, *J Otolaryngol* 23:281, 1994.
32. Deeb ZE et al: Acute epiglottitis in the adult, *Laryngoscope* 95:289, 1985.
33. Andreassen UK et al: Acute epiglottitis: 25 year experience with nasotracheal intubation, current management policy and future trends, *J Laryngol Otol* 106:1072, 1992.
34. Schumaker HM, Doris PE, Birnbaum G: Radiographic parameters in adult epiglottitis, *Ann Emerg Med* 13:588, 1984.
35. Rothstein SG et al: Epiglottitis in AIDS patients, *Laryngoscope* 99:389, 1989.
36. Lindner HH: The anatomy of the fasciae of the face and neck with particular reference to the spread and treatment of intraoral infections (Ludwig's) that have progressed into the adjacent fascial spaces, *Ann Surg* 204:705, 1986.
37. Levitt GW: Cervical fascia and deep neck infections, *Laryngoscope* 80:409, 1970.
38. Finch RG, Snider GE, Sprinkle PM: Ludwig's angina, *JAMA* 243:1171, 1980.
39. Dreyer AF, de Kock SE, Rantloane JL: Ludwig's angina: a case report and review, *J Dent Assoc So Afr* 45:397, 1990.
40. Allen D, Loughman TE, Ord RA: A re-evaluation of the role of tracheostomy in Ludwig's angina, *J Oral Maxillofac Surg* 43:436, 1985.
41. Feinberg SE, Peterson LJ: Use of cricothyroidostomy in oral and maxillofacial surgery, *J Oral Maxillofac Surg* 45:873, 1987.
42. Marra S, Hotaling AJ: Deep neck infections, *Am J Otolaryngol* 17:287, 1996.
43. Ophir D et al: Peritonsillar abscess: a prospective evaluation of outpatient management by needle aspiration, *Arch Otolaryngol Head Neck Surg* 114:661, 1988.
44. Petruzzelli GJ, Johnson JT: Peritonsillar abscess: why aggressive management is appropriate, *Postgrad Med* 88:99, 1990.
45. Ellsbury KE: Therapeutic alternatives and clinical outcomes in peritonsillitis, *J Fam Pract* 18:69, 1984.
46. Shoemaker M, Lampe RM, Weir MR: Peritonsillitis: abscess or cellulitis, *Pediatr Infect Dis* 5:435, 1986.
47. Savolainen S et al: Peritonsillar abscess: clinical and microbiological aspects and treatment regimens, *Arch Otolaryngol Head Neck Surg* 119:521, 1993.
48. Herzon FS: Peritonsillar abscess: incidence, current management practices, and a proposal for treatment guidelines, *Laryngoscope* 105:1, 1995.
49. Tuner K, Nord CE: Impact on peritonsillar infections and microflora of phenoxymethylpenicillin alone versus phenoxymethylpenicillin in combination with metronidazole, *Infection* 14:129, 1986.
50. Friedman NR et al: Peritonsillar abscess in early childhood, *Arch Otolaryngol Head Neck Surg* 123:630, 1997.
51. Kieff DA et al: Selection of antibiotics after incision and drainage of peritonsillar abscess, *Otolaryngol Head Neck Surg* 120:57, 1999.
52. Scott PM et al: Diagnosis of peritonsillar infections: a prospective study of ultrasound, computerized tomography and clinical diagnosis, *J Laryngol Otol* 113:229, 1999.
53. Harley EH: Quinsy tonsillectomy as the treatment of choice for peritonsillar abscess, *Ear Nose Throat J* 67:84, 1988.
54. Herzon FS, Nicklaus P: Pediatric peritonsillar abscess: management guidelines, *Curr Probl Pediatr* 26:270, 1996.
55. Haeggstrom A et al: Intraoral ultrasonography in the diagnosis of peritonsillar abscess, *Otolaryngol Head Neck Surg* 108:243, 1993.
56. Patterson HC, Kelly JH, Stome MM: Ludwig's angina: an update, *Laryngoscope* 92:370, 1982.
57. Moreland LW, Corey J, McKenzie R: Ludwig's angina: report of a case and review of the literature, *Arch Intern Med* 148:461, 1988.
58. Spitalnic SJ, Sucov A: Ludwig's angina: case report and review, *J Emerg Med* 13:499, 1995.
59. Hall SF: Ludwig's-like angina (pseudo-angina Ludovici), *J Otolaryngol* 13:321, 1984.
60. Schliamser SE, Berggren DV, Kercoff Y: Ludwig's angina and associated systemic complications, *Scand J Infect Dis* 18:477, 1986.
61. Freund B, Timon C: Ludwig's angina: a place for steroid therapy in its management?, *Oral Health* 82:23, 1992.
62. Ben-ami T, Yousefzadeh DK, Aramburo MJ: Pre-suppurative phase of retropharyngeal infection: contribution of ultrasonography in the diagnosis and treatment, *Pediatr Radiol* 21:23, 1990.
63. Sharma HS, Kurl DN, Hamzah M: Retropharyngeal abscess: recent trends, *Auris Nasus Larynx* 25:403, 1998.
64. Goldenberg D, Golz A, Joachims HZ: Retropharyngeal abscess: a clinical review, *J Laryngol Otol* 111:546, 1997.
65. Schlossberg D, Fugate JS: Retropharyngeal cellulitis, *Laryngoscope* 91:1738, 1981.
66. Dyzak WR, Zide MF: Diagnosis and treatment of lateral pharyngeal space infections, *J Oral Maxillofac Surg* 42:243, 1984.
67. Hamer R: Retropharyngeal abscess, *Ann Emerg Med* 11:549, 1982.
68. Tannebaum RD: Adult retropharyngeal abscess: a case report and review of the literature, *J Emerg Med* 14:147, 1996.
69. Arora VK, Bedi RS, Sharma ML: Unusual thoracic manifestation of retropharyngeal abscess, *Indian J Chest Dis Allied Sci* 29:60, 1987.
70. Bhargava SK, Gupta S: Large retropharyngeal cold abscess in an adult with respiratory distress, *J Laryngol Otol* 104:157, 1990.
71. Drutz DJ, Cantanzaro A: Coccidioidomycosis: part II, *Am Rev Respir Dis* 117:727, 1978.
72. Wholey MH, Bruwer AJ, Baker HL: The lateral roentgenogram of the neck, *Radiology* 71:350, 1958.
73. Robertson S, Pinstein ML, LaVelle DG: Non-traumatic atlantoaxial subluxation in an adult secondary to retropharyngeal abscess, *Orthopedics* 10:1545, 1987.
74. De Marie S et al: Clinical infections and nonsurgical treatment of parapharyngeal space infections complicating throat infections, *Rev Infect Dis* 11:975, 1989.
75. Sethi DS, Stanley RE: Parapharyngeal abscess, *J Laryngol Otol* 105:1025, 1991.
76. Gidley PW, Ghorayeb BY, Stiernberg CM: Contemporary management of deep neck space infections, *Otolaryngol Head Neck Surg* 116:16, 1997.
77. Weesner CL, Cisek JE: Lemierre syndrome: the forgotten disease, *Ann Emerg Med* 22:256, 1993.
78. Gwaltney JM: Acute community-acquired sinusitis, *Clin Infect Dis* 23:1209, 1996.
79. Wagenmann M, Naclerio RM: Anatomic and physiologic considerations in sinusitis, *J Allergy Clin Immunol* 90:419, 1992.
80. Poole MD: A focus on acute sinusitis in adults: changes in disease management, *Am J Med* 106:38S, 1999.
81. Josephson GD, Gross CW: Diagnosis and management of acute and chronic sinusitis, *Comp Ther* 23:708, 1997.
82. Kennedy DW, Gwaltney JM, Jones JG: Medical management of sinusitis: educational goals and management guidelines, *Ann Otolaryngol Rhinol Laryngol* 167:22, 1995.
83. Brook I et al: Microbiology and management of chronic maxillary sinusitis, *Arch Otolaryngol Head Neck Surg* 120:1317, 1994.
84. Rubin JS, Honigberg R: Sinusitis in patients with the acquired immunodeficiency syndrome, *Ear Nose Throat J* 69:460, 1990.
85. Williams JW, Simel DL: Does this patient have sinusitis? *JAMA* 270:1242, 1993.
86. Low DE et al: A practical guide for the diagnosis and treatment of acute sinusitis, *Can Med Assoc J* 156:S1, 1997.
87. Zinreich SJ: Imaging of chronic sinusitis in adults: x-rays, computed tomography, and magnetic resonance imaging, *J Allergy Clin Immunol* 90:445, 1992.
88. Williams JW et al: Randomized controlled trial of 3 vs 10 days of trimethoprim/sulfamethoxazole for acute maxillary sinusitis, *JAMA* 273:1015, 1995.

71 Pneumonia

Gregory J. Moran
David A. Talan

PERSPECTIVE

Pneumonia is the sixth leading cause of death, and the leading cause of death from infectious disease in the United States.[1] The annual incidence of community-acquired pneumonia in the United States ranges from 2 to 4 million, resulting in approximately 500,000 hospital admissions. The majority of cases of community-acquired pneumonia are managed in the outpatient setting and the mortality rate is low (< 1%), but pneumonia requiring hospitalization is associated with a much higher mortality rate, approximately 15%. Most deaths occur in the elderly or immunosuppressed, but pneumonia may develop in otherwise healthy persons as well, and may rarely be fatal in such patients. The evaluation and management of pneumonia remain challenging owing to a number of constantly changing factors, including an expanding spectrum of pathogens, changing antibiotic resistance patterns, the availability of newer antimicrobial agents, and increasing emphasis on cost-effectiveness and outpatient management.

The epidemiology of community-acquired pneumonia is changing. As the percentage of the population above age 65 continues to increase, the incidence of pneumonia can be expected to rise. Other factors are affecting the etiologic epidemiology of pneumonia. An increasing number of patients are taking immunosuppressive drugs related to treatment of malignancy, transplantation, or autoimmune disease, resulting in more cases of pneumonia caused by other opportunistic pathogens. With expanded travel and immigration, and increased prevalence of immunocompromising conditions, tuberculosis (TB) is increasingly recognized. In the 1980s, *Pneumocystis carinii* pneumonia (PCP) emerged in association with acquired immunodeficiency syndrome (AIDS). With the introduction of highly active antiretroviral therapy (HAART) in the 1990s, far fewer cases of advanced HIV infection and PCP now occur. Clinicians now must face the possibility of pneumonia caused by drug-resistant *Streptococcus pneumoniae,* and antibiotic resistance is becoming more widespread among other pathogens.

Although the morbidity and mortality of pneumonia may be significant, the outcome can be improved by prompt diagnosis and initiation of appropriate therapy.[2] Identification of a specific etiology of pneumonia is extremely difficult within the time frame of an ED visit. Even after a thorough inpatient evaluation, many patients with pneumonia will never have a specific pathogen identified. Once pneumonia is diagnosed, the priorities in the ED are to provide appropriate respiratory support, assess the severity of disease, recognize indications for hospitalization, and initiate appropriate empiric antibiotic therapy based on the most likely pathogens.

PRINCIPLES OF DISEASE

Despite the constant presence of potential pathogens in the respiratory tract, the lungs are remarkably resistant to infection. The alveolar surface of the lungs covers an area of approximately 140 m^2. Approximately 10,000 L of air pass through the respiratory tract each day, and typical ambient air can contain hundreds to thousands of microorganisms per cubic meter. Numerous potential respiratory tract pathogens may colonize the oropharynx and upper airways. Although the cough and laryngeal reflexes will keep most large particulate matter out of the lower respiratory tract, there is experimental evidence that aspiration of oropharyngeal contents may be a common occurrence during normal sleep.[3] Despite these hazards, the body is usually able to maintain a virtually sterile environment in healthy lungs.

The development of clinical pneumonia requires a defect in host defenses, the presence of a particularly virulent organism, or the introduction of a large inoculum of organisms. If the challenge of invading organisms overwhelms host defenses, then microbial proliferation will lead to inflammation, an immune response, and clinical pneumonia. If host defenses are weak, then a minimal challenge may lead to the development of pneumonia.

The mouth normally contains a large number of microorganisms. Saliva contains approximately 10^8 bacteria per milliliter, with anaerobic organisms predominating. *Bacteroides* and *Fusobacterium* spp are the most common anaerobic organisms. Streptococci are the most common aerobic organisms, but staphylococci, *Haemophilus* sp, *Moraxella catarrhalis,* and *Neisseria* sp are also found. The presence of these bacteria and their adherence to oral epithelium are important in maintaining the normal balance of oral flora. Various substances are present in mucus and saliva that control colonizing organisms, and many organisms that normally colonize the oropharynx produce products that inhibit the growth of other organisms. Anything that upsets the balance of normal oral flora may permit the growth of more virulent organisms. Systemic illness may alter epithelial binding of oral flora, leading to increased colonization with aerobic gram-negative bacilli. Antimicrobial therapy can also adversely alter normal oral flora.

The anatomy of the upper respiratory tract is such that larger particles are usually filtered out before reaching the alveoli. The gag reflex and closure of the epiglottis during normal swallowing protect against aspiration. Coughing is an effective means of expelling material from the larynx and central airways. Airflow in the trachea of about 250 m/sec during a cough creates a strong shear force to expel mucus and trapped particles. The sharp angles at which the central airways branch cause particles to impact on the mucosal surface where they are entrapped and removed by mucociliary clearance. Only small particles below 5 µm may reach the alveoli. At the alveoli a variety of substances such as immunoglobulin (Ig)G, complement, lysozyme, free fatty acids, and alveolar macrophages provide defense against infection.

Host defenses can be impaired in a number of ways. An altered level of consciousness of any cause (e.g., intoxication, stroke, seizures, anesthesia) can suppress the gag reflex and lead to aspiration of oropharyngeal contents into the lower respiratory tract. Interventions that bypass the usual defenses of the upper airways such as endotracheal intubation, nasogastric intubation, and respiratory therapy devices will predispose to infection. Cigarette smoking damages both mucociliary function and macrophage activity and is probably the most common cause of impaired respiratory tract defenses. Viral infections of the respiratory tract may destroy respiratory epithelium and predispose to bacterial infection. Increased risk of bacterial pneumonia after influenza or other viral respiratory infections is well described. The elderly appear to be at increased risk of pneumonia owing to decline of mucociliary clearance, elastic recoil of the lungs, and humoral and cellular immunity. HIV infection can impair both humoral and cellular immunity.

If an infectious organism is able to reach the alveoli and begin replicating, a series of host immune responses occurs that ultimately may lead to the development of clinical pneumonia. As antigens of the infecting organism are identified by the host, cytokines such as IL-1, IL-8, and tumor necrosis factor are produced that mediate the inflammatory response. Transudation of plasma fluids into the lung tissue allows entry of IgM and IgG for bacterial opsonization, complement activation, agglutination, and neutralization. Neutrophils are recruited into the lung to ingest and kill the infecting organisms. Cell-mediated immunity plays an important role in defense against certain pathogens such as viruses and intracellular organisms such as *Mycobacterium* sp and *Legionella* sp. As fluids and inflammatory cells enter the alveolar spaces to combat the infection, the patient develops the clinical and radiographic signs of pneumonia.

Etiologic Agents

The challenge in the evaluation of patients with pneumonia generally lies in identifying the etiologic agent rather than in diagnosis of pneumonia itself. It is extremely difficult to determine with a high degree of certainty the specific organism responsible for pneumonia, especially within the time frame of an ED evaluation. The physician must choose empiric therapy that will have activity against the spectrum of likely pathogens based on the overall clinical picture.

Difficulty in determining the specific etiology of pneumonia exists even with advanced microbiologic and serologic testing that is not generally available during an ED evaluation. In many studies of community-acquired pneumonia, a microbial etiology cannot be determined in one third to one half of cases even after thorough investigation. In a large multicenter study of hospitalized adults with community-acquired pneumonia, traditional pathogens such as *S. pneumoniae* and *H. influenzae* account for about one fourth of cases. *Legionella, Mycoplasma,* and *Chlamydia* spp together account for 15%.[4] Another large study including serologic testing for common viral agents revealed a viral etiology in about 17% of cases, with influenza and parainfluenza viruses being most common.[5] Studies of adults who require admission to the intensive care unit showed *S. pneumoniae* to be the most common pathogen, with a prevalence as high as 38%, and 50% or more of fatal cases. *Legionella, Staphylococcus aureus,* and aerobic gram-negative bacilli also appear to be relatively more common among adults with severe community-acquired pneumonia.[6,7] Atypical organisms such as *Mycoplasma* or viruses appear to account for a relatively higher proportion of pneumonias in those who have milder illness that is amenable to outpatient therapy.[8] Although the prevalence of various organisms can vary considerably in different settings, it is important to note the frequency with which atypical organisms are identified, even in patients with severe illness requiring hospitalization. Coinfection, such as with *Chlamydia pneumoniae* and *S. pneumoniae,* is also well recognized.

S. pneumoniae is a gram-positive coccus that is the single most common etiology of community-acquired pneumonia among adults. It is found in the nasopharynx of about 40% of healthy adults. Although this organism can cause pneumonia in healthy persons, those with a history of diabetes, cardiovascular disease, alcoholism, sickle cell disease, splenectomy, and malignancy or other immunosuppressive illness are at increased risk. A vaccine containing the 23 capsular polysaccharides of pneumococcal types most commonly associated with pneumonia reduces the likelihood of serious pneumococcal infection. It is recommended for persons at increased risk because of underlying illness or age > 65.[9] Many ED patients have not received pneumococcal vaccine, and vaccinating eligible patients in this setting appears to be feasible and effective.[10] A newer heptavalent protein-conjugate pneumococcal vaccine effectively reduces invasive pneumococcal disease, including pneumonia, in infants and young children.[11]

Haemophilus influenzae is a common pathogen in adults with chronic obstructive pulmonary disease (COPD), alcoholism, malnutrition, malignancy, or diabetes. The organism is a pleomorphic gram-negative rod that can be encapsulated and identified as serotypes a through f, with type b most commonly leading to serious illness with bacteremia. *H. influenzae* is the second most frequently isolated organism in community-acquired pneumonia among adults. Nontypeable strains of *H. influenzae* that were once thought to be benign are now recognized as a frequent cause of lower respiratory tract infection in patients with chronic lung disease.

Intravenous drug users may develop hematogenous spread of *S. aureus* that involves both lungs as multiple small infiltrates or abscesses (e.g., tricuspid endocarditis resulting in septic pulmonary emboli). *S. aureus* may also cause a primary bacterial pneumonia that may be clinically indistinguishable from other bacterial pneumonias, although organisms such as *S. pneumoniae* and *H. influenzae* are much more common. Staphylococcal pneumonias are often necrotizing, with cavitation and pneumatocele formation. An increased incidence of staphylococcal pneumonia is noted during epidemics of influenza.[12]

Other pyogenic bacterial etiologies include *M. catarrhalis,* a gram-negative diplococcus that can be associated with lower respiratory tract infections in patients with COPD. *Klebsiella pneumoniae* is a gram-negative rod that rarely causes disease in a normal host and accounts for a very small percentage of community-acquired pneumonias, but may cause severe pneumonia in debilitated patients with alcoholism, diabetes, or other chronic illness. Because the organism is often hospital-acquired, there is a high incidence of antibiotic resistance.

Mycoplasma pneumoniae is one of the most common causes of community-acquired pneumonia in previously healthy patients under the age of 40.[13] Another important organism in community-acquired pneumonia is *C. pneumoniae,* an intracellular parasite that is transmitted between humans by respiratory secretions or aerosols. Seroprevalence studies demonstrate that virtually everyone is infected with *C. pneumoniae* at some time, and that reinfection is common. *C. pneumoniae* has been found to be a relatively common etiology of community-acquired pneumonia, especially in older adults, accounting for at least 8% of cases, although this is likely an underestimate owing to difficulty in diagnosing infection with this organism.

At least 30 species of *Legionella* have been isolated since the 1976 outbreak in Philadelphia from which the organism derives its name, and at least 19 are known to be human pathogens. *Legionella* is an intracellular organism that lives in aquatic environments. There is no person-to-person transmission. Although it has often been implicated in point outbreaks related to cooling towers and similar aquatic sources, the organism also lives in ordinary tap water and has probably been underdiagnosed as an etiology of community-acquired pneumonia. Studies demonstrate that it may account for as much as 19% of community-acquired pneumonia cases, although the prevalence appears to vary greatly by region.[14]

Lower respiratory infections caused by anaerobic organisms generally result from the aspiration of oropharyngeal contents with large amounts of bacteria. These infections are typically polymicrobial, including *Peptostreptococcus* sp, *Bacteroides* sp, *Fusobacterium* sp, and *Prevotella* sp.[15] Presentation is often subacute or chronic, and may be difficult to distinguish clinically from other etiologies of pneumonia. Clinical factors that would suggest an anaerobic infection include risk factors for aspiration such as central nervous system depression or swallowing dysfunction, severe periodontal disease, fetid sputum, and the presence of a pulmonary abscess or empyema.

Viral pneumonias are common in infants and young children and are being recognized as an important cause of pneumonia in adults as well. Respiratory syncytial virus (RSV) and parainfluenza viruses are the most common causes of pneumonia in infants and small children, occurring mostly during autumn and winter. Influenza viruses are the most common cause of viral pneumonia in adults. Winter influenza outbreaks, usually caused by influenza type A, may cause as many as 40,000 deaths yearly in the United States, more than 90% of which occur in people age 65 or older.[16] Cytomegalovirus (CMV) primarily causes pneumonia in immunosuppressed patients such as transplant recipients. Varicella-zoster virus (VZV or chickenpox) may cause pneumonia that appears to be more common and more severe in adults, and is predisposed by factors such as smoking and pregnancy.

Fungal infections caused by organisms such as *Histoplasma capsulatum, Blastomyces dermatitides,* and *Coccidioides immitis* commonly present as pulmonary disease. These organisms are present in the soil in various geographic areas of the United States: *H. capsulatum* in the Mississippi and Ohio river valleys, *C. immitis* in desert areas of the southwest, and *B. dermatitides* in a poorly defined area extending beyond that of *H. capsulatum.* These infections should be considered in persons in appropriate geographic areas, especially in persons who are near activities that disturb the soil such as construction or dirt bike riding. Clinical presentation varies from an acute or chronic pneumonia to asymptomatic granulomas found on chest radiograph. Hilar adenopathy is frequently present.

PCP occurs in compromised hosts, principally persons with AIDS or malignancy. Although *P. carinii* has often been classified as a protozoan, biochemical evidence indicates that it is probably more closely related to fungi. PCP is one of the most common presentations leading to a diagnosis of HIV infection and AIDS. Patients who present with pulmonary complaints should be questioned about HIV risk factors, and clinicians should search for signs of HIV-related immunosuppression such as weight loss, lymphadenopathy, and oral thrush. PCP typically presents subacutely with fatigue, exertional dyspnea, nonproductive cough, pleuritic chest pain, and fever.

Another important consideration in patients with community-acquired pneumonia is TB. *Mycobacterium tuberculosis* is a slow-growing bacterium transmitted between persons by droplet nuclei produced from coughing and sneezing. *M. tuberculosis* survives within macrophages as a facultative intracellular parasite, and thus may remain dormant in the body for many years. Active TB develops within 2 years of infection in about 5%, and another 5% will develop reactivation disease at some later point over the course of a lifetime. Reactivation is more likely to occur in persons with impaired cell-mediated immunity, such as those with diabetes, renal failure, immunosuppressive therapy, malnutrition, or AIDS. The risk of developing active TB in HIV-infected persons with a positive tuberculin skin test is estimated to be 8% per year.[17]

TB causes more deaths worldwide than any other single infectious disease. It is estimated that about one third of the Earth's population is infected with *M. tuberculosis.* Approximately 8 million new cases of active disease develop annually, resulting in as many as 3 million deaths worldwide. An estimated 10 to 15 million persons in the United States (4% to 6% of the population) are infected with TB. The incidence of TB in the United States had decreased since the 1950s with the introduction of better public health measures and effective antituberculous drugs, but an increase in TB cases was noted after the mid 1980s, especially among the poor and ethnic minorities, as well as prison and homeless populations. Multidrug-resistant strains of *M. tuberculosis* (MDR-TB) are found in increasing numbers, especially among immigrants from Southeast Asia and AIDS patients. Increased efforts to control the disease in the United States have led to a decrease in TB cases in recent years.

Unusual Causes of Pneumonia Q fever is an acute febrile illness caused by the rickettsial organism *Coxiella burnetii* that may present as pneumonia. It is most common in persons with occupational exposure to cattle or sheep or parturient animals, including cats. Fever is present in all patients, and a severe headache occurs in approximately 75% of cases. This infection is rarely fatal. Other zoonotic pulmonary infections include *Rhodococcus equi* associated with exposure to horses and *Bordetella bronchosepticum* associated with exposure to ill dogs ("kennel cough").

Plague, caused by *Yersinia pestis,* is endemic in many parts of the world. It occurs in the southwestern states of the United States in persons bitten by fleas from infected rodents or carnivores. Hematogenous spread may lead to pneumonia that is highly contagious and has a high mortality rate. It typically presents with cough and chest pain with purulent sputum and hemoptysis associated with fever and adenopathy (i.e., a bubo).

Hantaviruses were previously known to be associated with hemorrhagic fever and with renal syndrome that occurs in Asia. They have also been found to be associated with a syndrome of severe respiratory distress and shock that has occurred in persons in several areas of the United States. Infection appears to occur from inhalation of aerosols of material contaminated with rodent urine and feces. Patients are typically healthy adults presenting with a prodrome of fever, myalgia, and malaise followed in several days by the onset of respiratory distress. Hypoxia may progress rapidly, requiring ventilatory support. Characteristic laboratory findings include thrombocytopenia, hemoconcentration, and leukocytosis with atypical lymphocytes. Chest radiographs demonstrate bilateral interstitial lung infiltrates that are more pronounced in dependent areas. Death typically occurs from depressed cardiac output and eventual cardiovascular collapse.[18]

Tularemia is a febrile illness caused by the bacterium *Francisella tularensis* that is spread by contact with body fluids of an infected mammal (especially rabbits) or the bite of an infected arthropod. Illness usually begins with an ulcerated skin lesion and painful regional lymphadenopathy. Some patients will have a typhoidal form with only fever, malaise, and weight loss. Pneumonia may occur with either form, presenting as a nonproductive cough and patchy infiltrates on chest radiograph.

Psittacosis can be spread to humans from birds infected with *Chlamydia psittaci.* It may occur in owners of pet birds, pet shop employees or others exposed to birds, or workers in poultry processing plants. Illness often begins rapidly with chills, high fever, myalgias, and malaise. Severe headache is often the major complaint. Cough is usually nonproductive. Splenomegaly is often present. Radiographic findings are variable, but patchy perihilar or lower lung field infiltrates are most common.

CLINICAL FEATURES

The ED evaluation should focus on establishing the diagnosis of pneumonia and determining the presence of epidemiologic and clinical features that will influence decisions regarding the need for hospitalization and choice of antibiotics. Key elements of patient history include the character and pattern of symptoms, the setting in which the pneumonia is acquired, geographic or animal exposures, and host factors that predispose to certain types of infections and are associated with patient outcome.

Pneumonia generally presents as a cough productive of purulent sputum, shortness of breath, and fever. In most healthy older children and adults, the diagnosis can be reasonably excluded on the basis of history and physical examination, with suspected cases confirmed by chest radiograph. Absence of any abnormalities in vital signs or chest auscultation substantially reduces the likelihood of pneumonia. No single clinical finding, however, is highly reliable in establishing or excluding a diagnosis of pneumonia.[19] Elderly or debilitated patients with pneumonia often present with nonspecific complaints and may not demonstrate the classic symptoms. Pneumonia commonly presents in the elderly as acute confusion or a deterioration of baseline function. Elderly patients are more likely to have advanced illness at the time of presentation, and may present with sepsis in the absence of a previous syndrome suggestive of pneumonia. Rarely, patients with lower lobe pneumonias present with a complaint of abdominal or back pain. The diagnosis of pneumonia may be more difficult in infants and small children who are unable to give an adequate history. Pneumonia may present in infants as a fever associated with irritability, tachypnea, tachycardia, intercostal retractions, nasal flaring, or grunting. Cough may be minimal or absent.

Pneumonia is often divided into "typical" pneumonia caused by pyogenic bacteria such as *S. pneumoniae* or *H. influenzae,* and "atypical" pneumonia caused by organisms such as *Mycoplasma* and *Chlamydia* sp. This division is somewhat artificial, and a clear differentiation between these two types of pneumonia on clinical grounds alone is impossible. Certain clinical factors are often said to be suggestive of atypical organisms. Factors studied prospectively and found *not* to be more frequent with atypical pneumonias than with pyogenic bacterial etiologies include gradual onset, viral prodrome, absence of rigors, nonproductive cough, lower degree of fever, absence of pleurisy, absence of consolidation, low leukocyte count, and an ill-defined infiltrate on chest radiograph.[4] Although it is impossible to determine with a high degree of certainty the specific etiology of pneumonia without results of microbiologic or serologic tests, certain clinical factors may suggest that a specific pathogen should be considered.

The classic presentation of pneumococcal pneumonia is the abrupt onset of a single shaking chill followed by fever, cough productive of rust-colored sputum, and pleuritic chest pain, but it is clear that many patients do not exhibit the classic pattern. Patients often have a preceding upper respiratory illness and the onset of pneumonia may be insidious, especially in the elderly or those with underlying lung disease. Patients with a history of asplenia, sickle cell disease, AIDS, multiple myeloma, or agammaglobulinemia are at increased risk of pneumococcal bacteremia and sepsis with high mortality rates. Extrapulmonary complications (e.g., meningitis, endocarditis, or arthritis) may rarely be present. Tachypnea and tachycardia are usually present. Examination of the chest may reveal signs of consolidation (dullness to percussion, coarse rales, bronchial breath sounds, or increased tactile fremitus).

Adults with chronic lung disease who develop pneumonia caused by *H. influenzae* typically present with an insidious worsening of baseline cough and sputum production, and bacteremia is rare.[20] *K. pneumoniae* may cause severe pneumonia in elderly or debilitated patients. Sputum is often described as "currant-jelly" because of the necrotizing, hemorrhagic nature of the infection. Abscess formation, empyema, and bacteremia are common with this organism and mortality is high.

The atypical pneumonia syndrome is caused by organisms such as *M. pneumoniae, C. pneumoniae,* viruses, *Legionella* sp, or rickettsiae such as *Coxiella burnetii. Mycoplasma* infection usually begins as a flulike illness with headache, malaise, and fever. Cough is usually nonproductive, but may sometimes produce clear or even purulent sputum. Skin lesions including maculopapular, vesicular, urticarial, or erythema multiforme type rashes are not uncommon, especially in younger patients.[21] Although bullous myringitis is sometimes described as a classic finding, it is not specific for mycoplasma infection, and is present in only a small minority of cases. Common physical findings include pharyngeal erythema, cervical adenopathy, and scattered rales and rhonchi. Rare extrapulmonary manifestations include pericarditis, glomerulonephritis, aseptic meningitis, and Guillain-Barré syndrome. Patients generally do not appear toxic, and the vast majority can be treated as outpatients. Although mucopurulent sputum generally indicates the presence of pyogenic bacterial pneumonia or bronchitis, it may also be present with mycoplasmal or viral pneumonia. Viral pneumonia in adults is often preceded by symptoms of upper respiratory infection such as rhinitis or sore throat. The onset of pneumonia may be insidious. Cough is usually nonproductive, and pleuritic chest pain is less common than with bacterial pneumonia. Chest examination often reveals scattered rhonchi or rales. Signs of consolidation are less common.

Most *C. pneumoniae* infections in young adults cause a minor, self-limited upper respiratory illness that is subacute in onset. This organism is also associated with bronchitis, wheezing, sinusitis, pharyngitis, and atherosclerosis.[22,23] Development of radiographically evident pneumonia is more common in the elderly, in contrast with the common perception that atypical pneumonias occur in the young.[24]

Some patients with *Legionella* infection will have a mild, self-limited atypical pneumonia presentation. Older patients, smokers, and those with chronic disease or immunosuppression are more prone to develop the more acute and severe manifestations of Legionnaire's disease. This infection presents as a severe systemic illness with malaise, lethargy, and high fever. Dry cough is usually present, accompanied by pleuritic chest pain in 25% to 30% of cases. Purulent sputum often develops later. Gastrointestinal symptoms such as diarrhea and abdominal cramping are sometimes prominent. Patients may appear quite toxic with high fever and altered mental status.

In addition to age, presence of underlying illness, and presenting symptoms, the setting of acquisition of pneumonia may provide clues to likely etiologies. Community-acquired pneumonia that occurs in otherwise healthy individuals is likely to be due to viruses, *Mycoplasma,* or *S. pneumoniae.* Patients in a nursing home setting are prone to influenza during outbreaks, and this may later be complicated with pneumonia caused by *S. aureus.* Hospitalized patients may develop pneumonia caused by agents that are uncommon in community-acquired pneumonia such as Enterobacteriaceae, *Pseudomonas aeruginosa,* and *S. aureus.* Healthy patients in an institutional setting such as a dormitory or military barracks are likely to have pneumonia caused by *Mycoplasma* or viruses.

Patients with underlying lung disease, especially COPD, constitute an important group likely to develop pneumonia. The lower respiratory tract of these patients is commonly colonized with organisms such *as S. pneumoniae, H. influenzae,* and *M. catarrhalis;* these are common causes of pneumonia in this group. Cystic fibrosis patients are prone to pneumonia caused by *P. aeruginosa* or *S. aureus.* Defective mucociliary clearance in both these groups make them highly susceptible to repeated episodes of pneumonia that may ultimately prove fatal.

Patients with immunosuppression resulting from hematologic malignancy, patients undergoing chemotherapy for malignancy, or transplant recipients are prone to pulmonary infections with a wide variety of organisms. In addition to the usual pathogens, these patients may develop pneumonia secondary to viruses such as CMV, varicella, or herpes simplex virus. They are also more likely to develop pneumonia from aerobic gram-negative bacilli, fungi such as *Candida* sp., or *Histoplasma capsulatum* and *P. carinii.*

DIAGNOSTIC STRATEGIES

The chest radiograph is generally the most important test to determine the presence of pneumonia. Although it is clear that many chest radiographs are performed unnecessarily on patients with upper respiratory tract infections or bronchitis, it is difficult to identify a set of specific criteria to direct test ordering that is better than the clinical judgment of an experienced physician.[25] A routine chest radiograph for all patients who present with cough is not necessary, but may be reserved for those without a history of asthma who have other suggestive findings (e.g., fever, tachycardia, or an abnormal lung examination).[26] Among patients suspected of pneumonia, these clinical findings are prospectively validated and are better predictors of a radiographic infiltrate than physician judgment.[27] Patients with serious underlying disease, severe sepsis, or shock, and those in whom hospitalization is considered should have a chest radiograph performed. Young healthy adults who will be treated as outpatients may have a chest radiograph deferred unless there is a suspicion of immunocompromise or other unusual features of disease. A chest radiograph should be performed subsequently if there is a poor initial response to treatment. Routine performance of a chest radiograph for patients with exacerbation of chronic bronchitis or COPD is of low yield, and may be limited to those with other signs of infection or congestive failure.[28] Studies of infants with fever show that a routine chest radiograph is of very low yield in the absence of other symptoms or signs of lower respiratory tract infection (e.g., cough, rales, elevated respiratory rate).[29,30] Some studies suggest that leukocytosis is associated with occult pneumonia in children,[31] but it is not clear that identifying these cases has any clinical significance.[32]

Although the causative agent cannot be determined solely by the results of chest radiography, certain radiographic patterns may suggest the possibility of specific pathogens. In pyogenic bacterial pneumonias, radiographs usually show an area of segmental or subsegmental infiltration and air bronchograms (Figure 71-1). Lobar consolidation is present in a minority of cases of bacterial pneumonia, often due to pneumococcus or *Klebsiella.* A dense lobar infiltrate with a bulging fissure appearance on chest radiograph is often described with pneumonia caused by *Klebsiella,* but this finding is nonspecific and most cases present as a more subtle bronchopneumonia. Pneumonia resulting from spread of infection along the intralobular airway results in fluffy or patchy infiltrates in the involved areas of the lung. A wide variety of bacteria may cause this pattern, as well as agents such as *Chlamydia, Mycoplasma, Legionella,* viruses, and fungi.

An interstitial pattern on chest radiograph (Figure 71-2) is typically caused by *Mycoplasma,* viruses, or *P. carinii.* Tiny nodules disseminated throughout both lungs represent a miliary pattern typical of granulomatous pneumonias such as tuberculosis or fungal disease. The location of infiltrates may also give a clue to the etiology. Aspiration pneumonia occurs

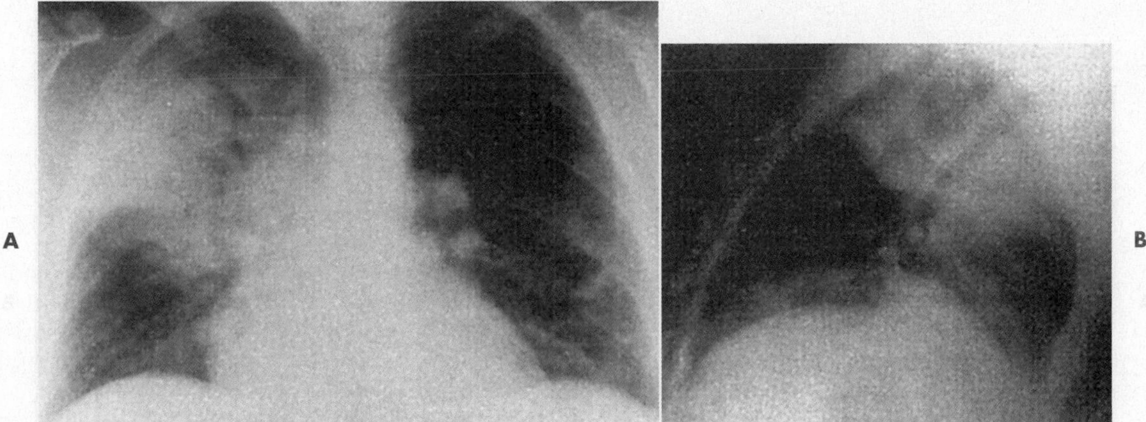

Figure 71-1. Posteroanterior (A) and lateral (B) chest radiographs reveal a right upper lobe pneumonia as well as a patchy left lower lobe infiltrate. A variety of organisms can produce this pattern, including *S. pneumoniae, H. influenzae, Legionella* sp., *Chlamydia pneumoniae*, gram-negative bacilli, and even *Mycoplasma* or viruses.

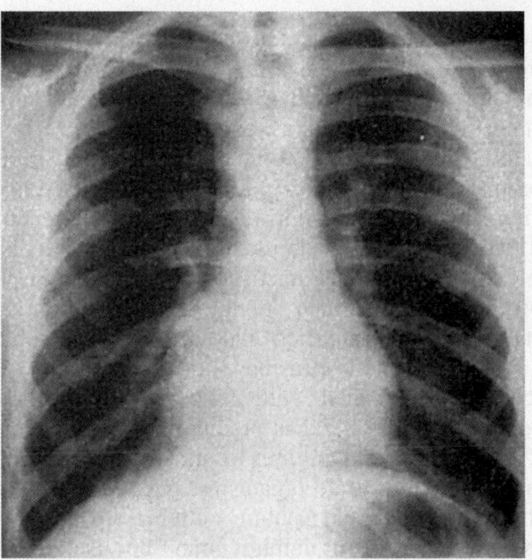

Figure 71-2. Posteroanterior chest radiograph reveals a diffuse interstitial infiltrate. Viruses or *Mycoplasma* are the most likely etiologies in an otherwise healthy patient, but a number of bacterial organisms may also give this pattern.

in dependent areas of the lung, most commonly the superior segments of the lower lobes or posterior segments of the upper lobes. Pneumonias produced by hematogenous spread (e.g., *S. aureus*) tend to be peripheral. Apical infiltrates suggest TB.

The presence of additional radiographic features in association with infiltrates may suggest a specific etiology. An infiltrate associated with hilar or mediastinal adenopathy suggests the presence of tuberculosis or fungal disease, or may indicate pneumonia associated with a neoplasm. Bacteria most likely to be associated with cavitation (Figure 71-3) are anaerobes, aerobic gram-negative bacilli, and *S. aureus.* Cavitation may also be present in fungal disease or tuberculosis and with noninfectious processes (e.g., malignancy and pulmonary vascular disease). Pneumatoceles or spontaneous pneumothorax may be seen in AIDS patients with *P. carinii* pneumonia. Pleural effusions can be seen with a wide variety of organisms, including many types of pyogenic bacterial pneumonias, *Chlamydia, Legionella,* and tuberculosis. Anaerobic infections associated with an effusion are especially prone to development of empyema. The diagnosis and aspiration of pleural effusions can be aided by use of ED bedside ultrasonography.

It should be emphasized that radiographic findings are nonspecific for predicting a particular infectious etiology. For example, *Mycoplasma* pneumonia may present as a dense infiltrate, or pneumococcal pneumonia may present as a diffuse interstitial infiltrate. Immunocompromised patients are particularly prone to having atypical radiographic appearances. Rarely, patients with a clinical picture strongly suggestive of pneumonia will have a normal chest radiograph, and some will be found to have an infiltrate noted within the next 24 to 48 hours. The absence of findings on chest radiograph should not preclude the use of antimicrobial therapy in appropriate patients with a clinical diagnosis of pneumonia.[33] Whether the state of hydration can affect the radiographic appearance of pneumonia is controversial. Although severe dehydration could theoretically result in a diminished exudative response by decreasing blood volume and hydrostatic pressure, this is not demonstrated experimentally.[34,35]

Laboratory studies are also nonspecific for identifying the etiology of pneumonia. Although the finding of a white blood cell count (WBC) of > 15,000/mm^3 increases the probability that the patient has a pyogenic bacterial etiology rather than a viral or atypical etiology, this finding is of limited value when used to make decisions regarding individual therapy. A WBC count may be helpful if it yields evidence of immunosuppression such as neutropenia or if it reveals lymphopenia that may indicate immunosuppression from AIDS. Serum chemistry studies may be helpful in identifying patients with renal or hepatic dysfunction associated with sepsis or with underlying disease. Such findings may assist in predicting a complicated course and will influence decisions regarding disposition, choice of antimicrobial agents, and dosages.

Assessment of respiratory function with arterial blood gas measurements or pulse oximetry is important in the evaluation of patients with pneumonia. Because clinical assessment of oxygenation can be inaccurate,[36] a pulse oximetry reading

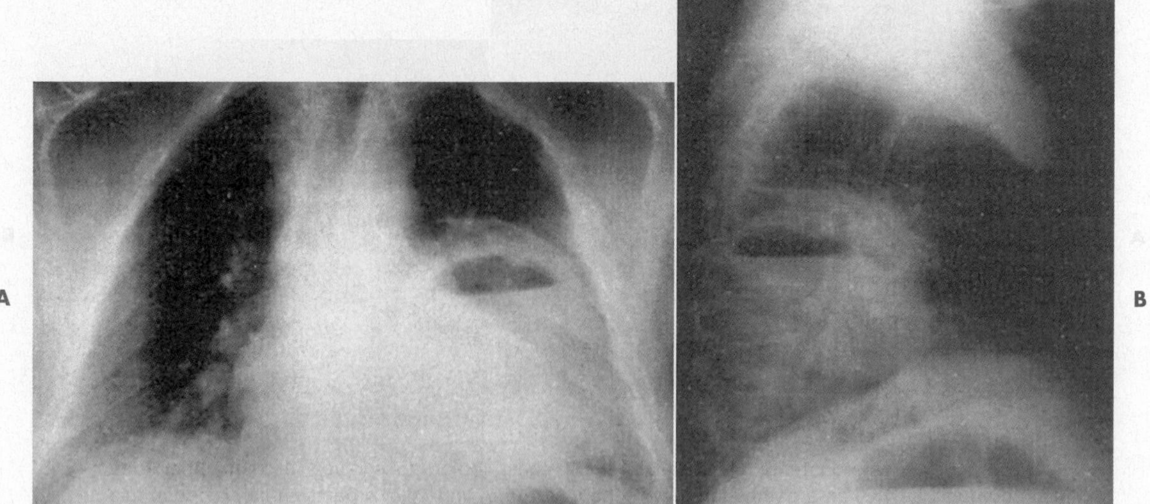

Figure 71-3. **Posteroanterior (A) and lateral (B) chest radiographs reveal a lung abscess in the left lower lobe with a distinct air-fluid level.**

should be obtained in any patient suspected of pneumonia in the ED. Respiratory failure caused by pneumonia is common in elderly patients and may require intubation and mechanical ventilation.

Sputum Gram stain is often recommended as a means to determine the presence of a bacterial pathogen, allowing more specific antimicrobial therapy. Community-acquired pneumonia guidelines by the American Thoracic Society (ATS) and the Infectious Diseases Society of America (IDSA) vary in their recommendations regarding the use of this test. IDSA guidelines recommend more aggressive attempts at etiologic diagnosis to provide pathogen-specific therapy.[1] ATS guidelines recommend a more empirical approach to therapy, reserving more aggressive diagnostic testing for those with more severe illness or those who fail to respond to therapy.[37] It is reasonable to target Gram stain and culture for the subset of patients with more serious illness (e.g., admitted to the ICU), in whom bacteriologic diagnosis and pneumococcal etiology are most likely, and for whom the outcome may be most dependent on optimal antimicrobial therapy.

The use of sputum Gram stain as a basis for empiric therapy in the ED can be problematic for several reasons. A large number of patients will not be able to provide an adequate sputum specimen. Induction of sputum without adequate isolation facilities can put patients and staff at risk if sputum is induced from persons with unrecognized TB. Correlation between identification of pneumococcus on Gram stain and sputum culture results is poor, even when commonly used criteria for an adequate sputum specimen (< 5 squamous epithelial cells and > 25 WBC/hpf) are applied. Gram stains are even less likely to demonstrate gram-negative pathogens such as *H. influenzae* and should not be relied on to rule out a gram-negative etiology. Sputum Gram stains are less accurate when done by less experienced physicians outside the microbiology laboratory and may lead to erroneous conclusions regarding which pathogens are present.[38] Fortunately, empiric antimicrobial agents can be clinically effective if well chosen based on clinical information even if sputum Gram stain is not done.[39]

Blood cultures should be obtained in seriously ill patients, preferably before the initiation of antibiotics (although antibiotics should not be delayed for this reason). Blood culture results will not be helpful to the emergency physician, but may be valuable later in the course of the patient's care. When positive, blood cultures reflect the etiologic agent more accurately than sputum cultures. Bacteremia occurs in approximately 25% to 30% of hospitalized pneumococcal pneumonia cases. Although IDSA guidelines recommend blood cultures for all admitted pneumonia patients,[1] the cost-effectiveness of this practice is questionable in patients without risk factors such as immunosuppression, recent hospitalization, or suspected endovascular infection.[40] Patients with a pleural effusion should have a diagnostic thoracentesis performed with fluid sent for cell count, differential, pH (pH < 7.2 is predictive of a need for chest tube), Gram stain, and culture. Routine bacterial cultures of sputum may demonstrate organisms, but the sensitivity and specificity are poor and sputum cultures are not routinely recommended. Sputum cultures may be useful if drug-resistant *S. pneumoniae* is suspected or if an organism that is never part of normal respiratory flora, such as *M. tuberculosis, Legionella* sp, or endemic fungi, is suspected.

Serologic tests are available for the diagnosis of a number of organisms, including *Chlamydia pneumoniae, Legionella* sp, and fungi. The use of serologic tests to determine the etiology of pneumonia may be helpful retrospectively, but they usually require acute and convalescent serum titers and are therefore of little use to the emergency physician. *Mycoplasma* pneumonia is associated with the presence of serum cold hemagglutinins in up to 60% of cases, but they may also be present in a number of viral infections. Diagnosis of the exact etiology of viral pneumonia is made difficult by the nonspecificity of presentation and the lack of widely available rapid tests. Rapid diagnostic tests for viral antigens are available for several viruses including RSV, influenza, and CMV. Rapid testing for influenza A and B is available. Although the specificity of these tests appears to exceed 90%, sensitivity is lower, thus making it difficult to exclude this infection on the basis of a negative result in a high-risk patient.[41] These tests may be most useful to document the existence of an influenza outbreak in a community at the beginning of an epidemic. Also, testing of admitted pneumonia patients during an influenza outbreak may be a reasonable indication for early adjunctive antiviral therapy. Developments in rapid testing using technology such as urine antigen tests or polymerase chain reaction may provide emergency physicians with a reliable method to determine the specific etiology of pneumonia.

Pneumonia Associated with HIV Infection

The AIDS epidemic has greatly changed the spectrum of pulmonary infections seen in many communities. The approach to an HIV-infected patient with pulmonary complaints must consider the likelihood of opportunistic lung infections. Although the use of highly active antiretroviral therapy (HAART) is decreasing opportunistic infections among HIV-infected patients, those who are not under regular care will often present to EDs. In the setting of a patient with risk factors for HIV but an unknown serologic status, a decision must be made as to the likelihood of AIDS and the need to aggressively search for opportunistic pathogens.

Respiratory infections are the most common type of opportunistic infection in AIDS patients. *Pneumocystis carinii* is the most common cause of pneumonia in AIDS patients, but there is also an increased incidence of pneumonia caused by *M. tuberculosis* and common bacterial pathogens such as *S. pneumoniae* and *H. influenzae*. The incidence of pneumococcal pneumonia is 7 to 10 times higher in HIV-infected persons, and the incidence of *H. influenzae* pneumonia is about 100 times higher than in non–HIV-infected individuals.[42,43] Other less important causes of pneumonia in HIV-infected patients include *Mycobacterium avium* complex, CMV, aerobic gram-negative bacilli, *Cryptococcus neoformans,* and *Rhodococcus equi*.

Before antimicrobial prophylaxis for PCP became widespread in AIDS patients, PCP was the initial opportunistic infection in more than 60% of the patients with AIDS reported to the Centers for Disease Control and Prevention.[44] An additional 20% of AIDS patients developed PCP later in the course of their illness.[45] The incidence of AIDS in general, and PCP in AIDS patients, specifically has decreased as a result of the use of HAART and routine PCP prophylaxis.

Although some patients have known HIV infection or AIDS, many patients are unaware of their HIV status, and many are reluctant to volunteer that they may have risk factors for HIV. The first crucial step in the diagnosis of PCP is the recognition that a patient may be at risk. If the possibility of HIV infection is established, then the likelihood of immunosuppression must be determined. The potential for opportunistic pulmonary infection can be predicted by a recent absolute CD4 lymphocyte count $< 200/mm^3$. This is often known by patients with recognized HIV infection who are followed closely by their physicians, or may be surmised by a peripheral total lymphocyte count below 1000.[46,47] In those patients who do not know their HIV status, the presence of findings such as weight loss, hairy leukoplakia, and oral candidiasis strongly suggests immunosuppression.

Although patients with PCP may present with typical features of subacute onset of nonproductive cough, fever, shortness of breath, diffuse interstitial infiltrates on chest radiograph, and arterial hypoxemia, as many as 10% to 20% of patients subsequently proven to have PCP lack these findings.[48] PCP usually has a subacute presentation characterized by nonproductive cough, exertional dyspnea, and weight loss. Tachypnea and tachycardia are usually present.

The classic radiographic findings in PCP are bilateral interstitial infiltrates that begin in the perihilar region. Radiographic manifestations of PCP, however, can vary considerably, ranging from a normal appearance to dense consolidation. Lobar infiltrates, pleural effusions, hilar adenopathy, parenchymal nodules, and cavitary disease are also described. Apical infiltrates, spontaneous pneumothoraces, and extrapulmonary PCP are more common in patients receiving inhaled aerosolized pentamidine for PCP prophylaxis. Hypoxemia, hypocapnea, and an increased arterial-alveolar oxygenation gradient are usually present.[49] Serum lactate dehydrogenase (LDH) is significantly elevated in AIDS patients with PCP compared to those with non-PCP pneumonia.[50,51] The demonstration of oxygen desaturation with mild exercise may be helpful in patients with more subtle presentations.[52,53]

Confirmation of the diagnosis of PCP requires sputum induction and staining, and in some cases further invasive procedures such as bronchoscopy with bronchoalveolar lavage or biopsy. In most settings this includes admission to the hospital with presumptive therapy against PCP while diagnostic testing is done.

AIDS patients are also predisposed to developing life-threatening bacterial pneumonias that may mimic or coexist with PCP. The bacterial pathogens most commonly responsible for pneumonia in these patients are those most frequently encountered in immunocompetent individuals with community-acquired pneumonia.[54] Typical pyogenic pneumonia may have atypical radiographic presentation in these abnormal hosts. In studies of AIDS patients with pneumonia caused by pathogens such as *S. pneumoniae* and *H. influenzae,* more than half have diffuse infiltrates.[54,55]

There is a broad differential diagnosis for pulmonary infiltrates in the AIDS patient population (Figure 71-4). Because AIDS patients with pulmonary TB cannot be reliably distinguished from those with other pulmonary infections at presentation, it is important to consider TB in all HIV-infected patients with respiratory complaints and to place these patients in respiratory isolation. AIDS patients are also at risk for pneumonia caused by other mycobacterial species (e.g., *M. avium* complex), although the finding of acid-fast bacilli in the sputum should prompt empiric therapy against *M. tuberculosis* unless another mycobacterial species is definitively identified. They are also at increased risk for pneumonia caused by *C. neoformans* or other fungi associated with geographic exposure. Viral pneumonia caused by CMV usually presents as a systemic illness and often coexists with PCP in end-stage AIDS patients. Kaposi's sarcoma also may present with pulmonary infiltrates.

DIFFERENTIAL DIAGNOSIS CONSIDERATIONS

At times, the differentiation between upper and lower respiratory tract infections may be difficult. A chest radiograph is helpful to differentiate between upper respiratory tract infection or bronchitis and pneumonia, but is probably not necessary for all patients with cough and sputum production unless other factors are present that would suggest the possibility of pneumonia or would obscure its clinical diagnosis (e.g., toxic appearance, extremes of age, underlying illness, abnormal chest examination).

A number of noninfectious etiologies may result in inflammatory lung processes including exposure to mineral

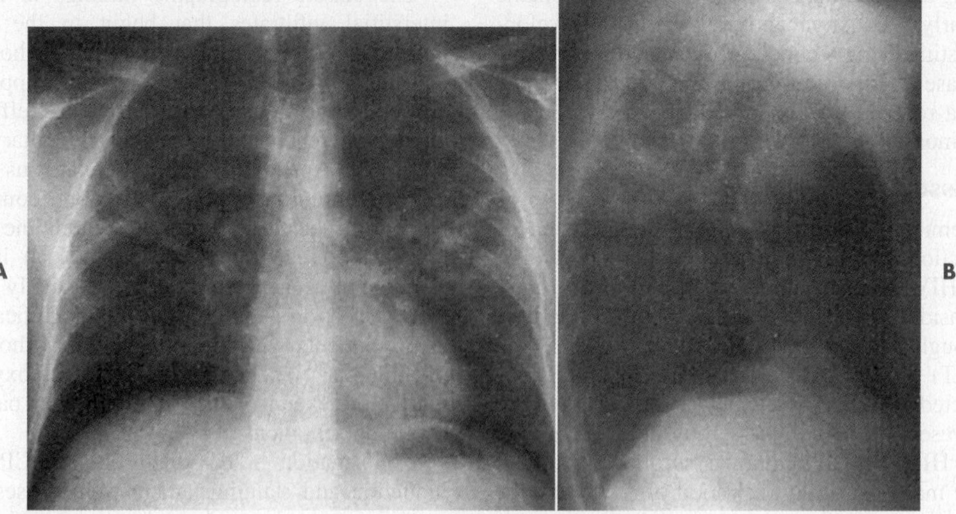

Figure 71-4. **Posteroanterior (A) and lateral (B) chest radiographs of an HIV-infected patient reveal interstitial disease mixed with patchy alveolar infiltrates. *P. carinii* is the most common etiology, but bacterial pathogens and TB must also be considered.**

dusts (e.g., silicosis), chemical fumes (e.g., chlorine, ammonia), toxic drugs (e.g., bleomycin), radiation, thermal injury, or oxygen toxicity. Immunologic diseases (e.g., sarcoidosis, Goodpasture's syndrome, collagen vascular disease), or hypersensitivity to environmental agents (e.g. farmer's lung disease) may also result in pneumonia. Tumors may be confused with pneumonia radiographically or may present initially as a postobstructive infection or adenopathy with peripheral infiltrates. Lymphangitic spread of lung malignancy may resemble interstitial pneumonia.

Aspiration

It is important to recognize the distinction between the acute aspiration of gastric contents or other liquids and bacterial pneumonia that may later develop as a complication of aspiration. Aspiration of liquids into the lung disrupts surfactant and causes an inflammatory response that may lead to hypoxia and respiratory failure. Aspiration of acidic gastric contents is particularly damaging to lungs, and is common in patients who are unconscious from intoxication or anesthesia or who have neurologic deficits. Patients may present initially with coughing or shortness of breath or may appear well initially and then develop respiratory dysfunction over the next several hours. Patients who aspirate while unconscious are sometimes unrecognized until respiratory insufficiency develops.

Acute aspiration of acidic fluid into the lungs may produce fever, leukocytosis, purulent sputum, and radiographic infiltrates that mimic bacterial pneumonia. Although many of these patients will go on to develop bacterial pneumonia, prophylactic administration of antibiotics is controversial. Some studies indicate that prophylactic antibiotics do not appear to be of benefit and may select for resistant organisms.[56] Antibiotics should be initiated if the patient develops signs of bacterial pneumonia including new fever, expanding infiltrate appearing more than 36 hours after aspiration, or unexplained deterioration. Studies of systemic corticosteroids for acute aspiration have yielded inconsistent results, and corticosteroids are not recommended.

Management

As with any seriously ill ED patient, initial attention should focus on ensuring adequate ventilation, oxygenation, and perfusion. Patients with underlying asthma or COPD who present with wheezing may benefit from bronchodilator therapy and corticosteroids. Seriously ill patients who present with volume depletion or septic shock will require fluid resuscitation and vasopressors.

In the ED, consider the possibility of communicable disease. Patients suspected of possible pulmonary TB because of a history of TB exposure, suggestive symptoms (e.g., persistent cough, weight loss, night sweats, hemoptysis), or belonging to a group at high risk for TB (e.g., homeless, intravenous drug user, alcoholic, HIV risk, immigrant from high-risk area) should immediately be placed into respiratory isolation until active TB can be ruled out by further evaluation, including chest radiograph.[57] EDs that frequently care for patients with TB or at risk for TB should consider triage protocols to rapidly identify these individuals before patients or staff are unnecessarily exposed.[58]

It is usually necessary to begin empiric antimicrobial therapy for pneumonia before a definite microbiologic etiology is established. Because timely antimicrobial treatment for community-acquired pneumonia is associated with improved patient outcomes for patients requiring hospital admission,[2] this therapy should be started in the ED. The antibiotics chosen must provide coverage of the likely etiologies based on clinical, laboratory, radiologic, and epidemiologic information.

The prevalence of drug-resistant *S. pneumoniae* (DRSP) has increased steadily over the past decade. In the United States, among outpatient pneumococcal sputum isolates collected between 1997 and 1998, approximately 30% were resistant to penicillin, with 12% high-level resistance.[59] Isolates that are resistant to penicillin are also very likely to be resistant to other β-lactams, as well as macrolides, tetracyclines, and trimethoprim/sulfamethoxazole (TMP/SMX). A number of extended spectrum or "respiratory" fluoroquinolones are available, such as levofloxacin, moxifloxacin, and

Table 71-1. Community-Acquired Pneumonia in Older Children and Adults: Outpatient Treatment

Clinical setting	Antibiotic regimen	Comments
Age < 60, otherwise healthy (atypical pathogens likely)	Erythromycin	Poor activity vs. *H. influenzae*, GI upset common.
	Doxycycline	Preferred for adolescent/young adult when likelihood of mycoplasma is high; variable activity vs. *S. pneumoniae*.
	Clarithromycin	Treats common typical bacterial and atypical pathogens.
	Azithromycin	5-day course, treats common typical bacterial and atypical pathogens.
	Extended spectrum fluoroquinolone	Treats common typical bacterial and atypical pathogens; active vs. DRSP.
Age ≥ 60, COPD, purulent sputum (pyogenic bacterial etiology likely)	Second- or third-generation cephalosporin (e.g., cefuroxime axetil, cefpodoxime, cefprozil)	No activity vs. atypical pathogens or some resistant *S. pneumoniae*.
	Amoxicillin/clavulanate	Better activity vs. anaerobes; frequent diarrhea. No activity vs. atypical pathogens or some resistant *S. pneumoniae*.
	Extended spectrum fluoroquinolone	Treats common typical bacterial and atypical pathogens; active vs. DRSP.

GI, Gastrointestinal; *DRSP,* drug-resistant *S. pneumoniae; COPD,* chronic obstructive pulmonary disease.

gatifloxacin. These agents have activity against DRSP as well as other typical and atypical pneumonia pathogens. Because oral bioavailability of fluoroquinolones is high, oral therapy provides serum and tissue levels essentially equivalent to parenteral therapy as long as there is adequate absorption. These fluoroquinolones are recommended instead of vancomycin if DRSP is a concern. It is not clear, however, whether in vitro resistance, and what level of resistance, is related to adverse clinical outcome to treatment drugs given at conventional doses. In one study, patients infected with resistant pneumococcal isolates (mostly intermediate level) had no greater mortality than those with susceptible organisms, even when treated with antibiotics to which the organism was resistant.[60] Other studies suggest that high-level resistance may be associated with increased mortality.[61]

Appropriate agents for outpatient treatment of adults with community-acquired pneumonia include macrolides, doxycycline, and fluoroquinolones with enhanced activity against *S. pneumoniae*[1,37] (Table 71-1). Alternative options that would be appropriate in those patients with a higher likelihood of a "typical" bacterial etiology include amoxicillin/clavulanate or an oral cephalosporin such as cefuroxime axetil, cefpodoxime, or cefprozil. These ß-lactam agents do not have activity against atypical pathogens, thus, except in patients who cannot take fluoroquinolones (e.g., children), these agents would not be preferred. In patients properly identified at low risk for complications and who are evaluated for careful outpatient follow-up, use of a macrolide or doxycycline is reasonable. Extended spectrum fluoroquinolones should be considered for patients with a higher likelihood of DRSP (e.g., patients with more severe illness, underlying disease, or recent exposure to antibiotics).[62] Use of ampicillin or amoxicillin is not generally recommended owing to the high prevalence of β-lactamase–producing pneumonia pathogens, although these have been used successfully for this condition in higher doses (e.g., amoxicillin 1 g three times a day) in countries with a high prevalence of DRSP. Trimethoprim/sulfamethoxazole has also been largely abandoned for treatment of pneumonia because of concern about increasing resistance. Except for the administration of fluoroquinolones, these recommendations also apply to school-aged children and adolescents in whom *Mycoplasma* is common. Also, new ketolides, related to macrolides, with enhanced activity against DRSP are expected to be approved soon.

For patients whose illness is severe enough to require hospital admission and parenteral antibiotics, options include a combination of a third-generation cephalosporin (e.g., ceftriaxone or cefotaxime) and a macrolide (e.g., intravenous erythromycin or azithromycin, or oral azithromycin), or an extended spectrum fluoroquinolone alone. These regimens have been associated with lower mortality in elderly patients hospitalized for community-acquired pneumonia compared with monotherapy with a third-generation cephalosporin for the treatment of the most common bacterial pathogens such as *S. pneumoniae, M. catarrhalis,* and *H. influenzae* as well as atypical pathogens such as *Mycoplasma, Chlamydia,* and *Legionella.*[63] Intravenous azithromycin alone is another option, although this drug does not achieve significant serum levels and lacks significant activity against many aerobic gram-negative bacilli and DRSP. Azithromycin alone might be an appropriate choice for persons with milder illness who are less likely to be bacteremic. If anaerobic organisms are suspected (e.g., aspiration), then clindamycin or metronidazole could be added to the regimen or a β-lactam/β-lactamase inhibitor antibiotic such as ampicillin/sulbactam or piperacillin/tazobactam can be used. Some quinolones such as moxifloxacin and gatifloxacin are also active against anaerobes. Recommendations for initial inpatient empiric therapy for community-acquired pneumonia are summarized in Table 71-2.

Table 71-2. Community-Acquired Pneumonia in Older Children and Adults: Inpatient Antimicrobial Treatment

Clinical setting	Antibiotic regimen	Comments
Community-acquired, nonimmunocompromised	Third-generation cephalosporin + macrolide	Third-generation cephalosporin more likely than second-generation to be active against DRSP. Macrolide should be added to treat atypical pathogens.
	Extended spectrum fluoroquinolone (e.g., levofloxacin, gatifloxacin, moxifloxacin)	Treats most common bacterial as well as atypical pathogens. Active vs. DRSP.
	Azithromycin (alone)	Treats most common typical as well as atypical pathogens. High tissue levels, but low serum levels and poor CSF penetration. Not active against gram-negative bacilli.
	β-lactam/β-lactamase inhibitor (e.g., ampicillin-sulbactam) + macrolide	Superior activity vs. anaerobes. Piperacillin-tazobactam more active vs. gram-negative pathogens, including *P. aeruginosa*.
Suspected aspiration	Cefoxitin or cefotetan	Best anaerobic activity among cephalosporins
	β-lactam/β-lactamase inhibitor	
	Clindamycin ± aminoglycoside	
	Metronidazole + second-/third-generation cephalosporin	
Severe pneumonia (ICU)	Cefotaxime, ceftriaxone, cefepime, or β-lactam/β-lactamase inhibitor plus fluoroquinolone	Consider adding aminoglycoside if septic shock is present.
Severe pneumonia with neutropenia, bronchiectasis, or recent hospitalization	Antipseudomonal β-lactam (e.g., cefepime, piperacillin, imipenem) + ciprofloxacin (high-dose) or aminoglycoside + macrolide	Add aminoglycoside if neutropenic or in septic shock. Choice of antipseudomonal aminoglycoside is based on local antibiotic resistance patterns.
AIDS	Trimethoprim/sulfamethoxazole	Alternatives for sulfa allergy include: Pentamidine + third-generation cephalosporin, or clindamycin + primaquine

DRSP, Drug-resistant *S. pneumoniae; CSF,* cerebrospinal fluid.

Severely ill and compromised patients are at relatively greater risk of infection from *S. pneumoniae,* aerobic gram-negative bacilli, *S. aureus,* and in some areas *Legionella* spp. For pneumonia patients admitted to an intensive care unit, adequate activity against DRSP may be more important. A third-generation cephalosporin or β-lactam/β-lactamase inhibitor combination can be combined with a fluoroquinolone. Addition of an aminoglycoside should be considered if septic shock is present. Those with recent hospitalization, neutropenia, or underlying bronchiectasis are at increased risk of infection with *Pseudomonas aeruginosa.* Empirical therapy should include two drugs with extended gram-negative activity including *P. aeruginosa.* Empirical regimens include cefepime, a carbepenem, or piperacillin/tazobactam, *plus* either ciprofloxacin (high dose), or an aminoglycoside and a macrolide.

For patients with AIDS, it is important to treat *P. carinii* as well as bacterial pathogens such as *S. pneumoniae.* Trimethoprim/sulfamethoxazole is the treatment of choice; the usual regimen is 20 mg/kg of trimethoprim and 100 mg/kg of sulfamethoxazole in four divided doses, to be continued for 21 days.[64] For most adult patients a regimen of three ampules (80 mg TMP, 400 mg SMX per ampule) every 6 hours is appropriate. For patients allergic to sulfa, pentamidine can be given 4 mg/kg over 1 hour. Toxicities of pentamidine include acute hypotension and hypoglycemia. Because pentamidine has no activity against *S. pneumoniae* or other bacterial pathogens, it is important to add a cephalosporin or other antibacterial agent to the initial empiric regimen. Other options include clindamycin, 900 mg IV every 8 hours, plus primaquine, 15 mg given orally daily, trimethoprim plus dapsone, atovaquone, or trimetrexate. The addition of steroids (prednisone, 40 mg given orally twice a day) reduces mortality and clinical deterioration in patients with $PaO_2 < 70$ or A-a gradient > 35.[65] *Mycoplasma, Legionella,* and *Chlamydia* are uncommon etiologies of severe pneumonia in AIDS patients, so empiric therapy with erythromycin or doxycycline is not routinely recommended.

Many EDs initiate outpatient therapy in moderately ill patients, who previously might have been hospitalized, with an initial parenteral dose of a long-acting antibiotic such as ceftriaxone and observe for an extended period (e.g., 12 to 24 hours) while administering supportive care such as hydration, antipyretics, and bronchodilators before discharge on an oral regimen. Certain patients may also be brought back to the ED for follow-up evaluation in 24 hours and receive a second parenteral or observed oral dose of antibiotics. An extended spectrum fluoroquinolone (oral or parenteral) is another option that may be advantageous owing to additional activity against atypical pathogens and DRSP.

There is little experimental evidence that directly addresses the question of duration of therapy for pneumonia. Outpatient treatment for pneumonia is generally given for 10 to 14 days. Shorter treatment courses are possible with azithromycin owing to its long tissue half-life. Outpatient trials comparing azithromycin for 5 days versus erythromycin for 10 days suggest that the shorter course is equally effective.[66]

The antiviral agents amantidine and rimantidine (active against influenza A) and newer neuraminidase inhibitors zanamavir and oseltamavir (active against influenza A and B) can decrease the duration and severity of influenza if started within 48 hours of symptom onset.[67] They may also be useful as prophylaxis to control outbreaks within families or group settings such as nursing homes, but should not be regarded as a substitute for immunization. The newer agents appear to cause less adverse effects than amantadine and rimantadine. Because they are not effective against other respiratory viruses, they should be used only if influenza virus is confirmed with a rapid test or is highly likely based on the clinical findings (e.g., presence of fever) and epidemiology (i.e., documented influenza outbreak in the community).

DISPOSITION

The decision to hospitalize a patient with pneumonia is not necessarily a commitment to prolonged inpatient care. Observation for 12 to 24 hours in the ED or hospital ward may allow the early discharge of certain moderate-risk patients. Inpatient treatment of pneumonia is 15 to 20 times more expensive per patient than outpatient treatment, and most patients are more comfortable in a home environment.[68]

Although no firm guidelines exist regarding hospital admission, a number of well-recognized risk factors are associated with an increased risk of death or a complicated clinical course.[37,69,70] A prospectively validated predictive rule for mortality among immunocompetent adults with community-acquired pneumonia suggests a two-step approach to assess risk.[71] Patients in the lowest risk class who are recommended for outpatient management are those less than age 50, without significant comorbid conditions (neoplasm, congestive heart failure, cerebrovascular disease, renal disease, liver disease, and HIV), and without the following findings on physical examination: altered mental status, pulse ≥ 125/min, respiratory rate ≥ 30/min, systolic blood pressure < 90, and temperature < 35° C or ≥ 40° C. Patients who do not fit the lowest risk category are classified into categories based on a scoring system that accounts for age, comorbid illness, physical examination findings, and laboratory abnormalities (Table 71-3). Hospitalization is recommended for those with a score > 91, and brief admission or observation may be considered for those with a score of 71 to 90. Although this method of assessing the likelihood of successful outpatient management is helpful in establishing general guidelines, it can be cumbersome to use, has not been modeled to predict acute life-threatening events, does not take into account dynamic evaluation over time, and has many important exceptions (e.g., an otherwise low-risk patient with severe hypoxia would be discharged by strict interpretation of this rule). Good clinical judgment should supersede a strict interpretation of this scoring system. A study in which physicians were educated and provided the patient's risk score, however, revealed a significantly lower overall admission rate, cost-savings, and similar quality of life scores compared with patients conventionally managed by their physicians.[72] Additional discharge criteria could include improving and stable vital signs over a several-hour observation period, ability to take oral medications, an ambulatory pulse oximetry greater than 90%, home support, and ability to follow up.

The disposition of HIV-infected patients with possible *P. carinii* pneumonia is dictated by the likelihood of progression to severe disease and by the feasibility of close outpatient follow-up. Factors associated with decreased survival in AIDS patients with PCP include history of prior PCP, an elevated respiratory rate, an abnormal chest examination, WBC count > 10,300/mm^3, elevated LDH, hypoxemia, hypoalbuminemia, or an abnormal chest radiograph.[73,74] Patients without multiple poor prognostic factors may be discharged from the ED with close outpatient follow-up, ideally within 2 to 3 days. Because of the potential toxicity of TMP/SMX, empiric treatment with this agent for well-appearing patients with a low probability of disease is generally not recommended. An empiric trial of a macrolide may be indicated for treatment of bronchitis or mild community-acquired pneumonia in a patient at low risk for PCP (e.g., recent CD4 count above 350/mm^3). Any deterioration on outpatient oral antibiotics should prompt admission for a more extensive evaluation. Some clinicians will initiate oral outpatient therapy with TMP/SMX or an alternate drug for those with a high probability of PCP and favorable clinical parameters, but this should be done only if the patient can be followed closely for continued diagnostic workup and observation for toxicity.

Most patients with community-acquired pneumonia do not need respiratory isolation. Those who are suspected of having an etiology of pneumonia that could pose a threat of transmission to other patients (e.g., influenza, varicella, TB, plague) should be isolated. Neutropenic patients are generally placed in reverse isolation. HIV-infected patients who present with pneumonia ideally should be isolated until TB can be evaluated by sputum acid-fast bacillus (AFB) smears, particularly those with other risk factors for TB. The chest radiograph cannot be relied on to exclude TB in AIDS

Table 71-3. Scoring System for Pneumonia Mortality Prediction

Patient characteristics	Points
Demographic factor	
Age	
Male	No. years of age
Female	No. years of age − 10
Nursing home resident	10
Comorbid illness	
Neoplastic disease	30
Liver disease	20
Congestive heart failure	10
Cerebrovascular disease	10
Renal disease	10
Physical examination finding	
Altered mental status	20
Respiratory rate > 30	20
Systolic blood pressure < 90	20
Temperature < 35° C or > 40° C	15
Pulse > 125	10
Laboratory or radiographic finding	
Arterial pH < 7.35	30
Blood urea nitrogen > 30 mg/dl	20
Sodium < 130 mEq/L	20
Glucose > 250 mg/dl	10
Hematocrit < 30%	10
Arterial Po_2 < 60 mm Hg	10
Pleural effusion	10

Adapted from Bartlett JG et al: *Clin Infect Dis* 31:347-382, 2000.

patients because it often does not have the typical appearance of TB. Isolation should be strongly considered for others at high risk for TB such as inner-city homeless persons or IV drug users.

ACUTE RESPIRATORY DISTRESS SYNDROME

The acute respiratory distress syndrome (ARDS) is a form of noncardiogenic pulmonary edema that is a result of the nonspecific response of the lung to a variety of insults. ARDS is defined as respiratory failure indicated by a requirement for mechanical ventilation and PaO_2/FiO_2 ratio ≤ 200, in the appropriate clinical setting with one or more recognized risk factors. This is accompanied by new, bilateral, diffuse, patchy or homogeneous pulmonary infiltrates on chest radiograph, with no clinical evidence of heart failure, fluid overload, or chronic lung disease (pulmonary artery occlusion pressure ≤ 18 mm Hg).[75]

Respiratory failure results from damage to the region of alveolar-capillary oxygen exchange with increased permeability to plasma fluid and protein. ARDS can be caused by either a direct injury to the lungs (e.g., aspiration of liquids or inhaled toxins) or may result from circulating inflammatory mediators associated with multisystem trauma, sepsis, or drugs such as aspirin or opiates. Conditions associated with ARDS are summarized in Box 71-1. A variety of mediators are implicated in the development of ARDS, including neutrophil production of proteases and oxygen radicals, interleukins and other cytokines, tumor necrosis factor, and complement factors.[76] This syndrome most often develops in patients already seriously ill in the hospital, but these patients may rarely present to the ED.

Treatment of ARDS is primarily supportive. High inspiratory pressures and positive end expiratory pressure are often required to maintain oxygenation, so it is difficult to avoid barotrauma. Peak airway pressures should be kept < 35 cm H_2O if possible. Outcome is improved with use of reduced tidal volumes, allowing $Paco_2$ to rise.[77] Inverse-ratio ventilation with prolonged inspiratory time may also be beneficial. Fluid balance must be carefully managed to avoid increased pulmonary capillary pressure while maintaining organ perfusion. Prone positioning during ventilation may improve distribution of perfusion to ventilated lung regions, but improvement in oxygenation is variable. Inhaled nitric oxide is an endogenous vasodilator used in ARDS, although the clinical response is variable and may not be sustained.[78] Drugs such as N-acetylcysteine, prostaglandin E_1, ketoconazole, and nonsteroidal antiinflammatory drugs have been studied for ARDS, but results have been disappointing.[79] Corticosteroids do not reduce mortality in early ARDS, but may have benefit in the late fibroproliferative phase. Although mortality is high in ARDS, most survivors recover normal or near-normal lung function. Current research is focusing on preventive measures for ARDS that may someday be used in the ED for patients at risk. Agents being studied include aerosolized surfactant, free radical scavengers, prostaglandin inhibitors, and agents that can modify interleukins and other inflammatory mediators.

Box 71-1 Conditions Associated with ARDS

Sepsis
Shock
Toxic gas or smoke inhalation
Aspiration
- Gastric contents
- Near drowning
- Hydrocarbons/solvents

Pneumonia
Drug reaction
- Salicylates
- Opiates
- Tricyclic antidepressants
- Cyclosporin
- Amiodarone
- Cancer chemotherapeutic agents (e.g., bleomycin)
- Hydrochlorothiazide
- Many others

Trauma
Burns
Transfusion reaction
Radiation injury
Pancreatitis
Thromboembolism
Fat embolism
Air embolism
Amniotic fluid embolism
Eclampsia
Neurogenic (e.g., subarachnoid hemorrhage, head trauma)
Disseminated intravascular coagulation
High altitude exposure
Oxygen toxicity
Cardiopulmonary bypass

KEY CONCEPTS

- Empiric antimicrobial therapy should be started in the ED for patients admitted with pneumonia. Empirical therapy should treat the most likely pathogens, including *S. pneumoniae, H. influenzae, M. pneumoniae,* and *C. pneumoniae*.
- HIV or other immunosuppression should be considered in all patients in whom pneumonia is suspected.
- Respiratory function should be assessed in patients with pneumonia using pulse oximetry or other means.
- Tuberculosis should be considered, and respiratory isolation initiated, for patients with HIV or other risk factors for TB.
- The disposition of patients with pneumonia is dictated by the patient's underlying medical conditions, the severity of illness and likelihood of clinical deterioration, and the feasibility of home care and outpatient follow-up monitoring.

REFERENCES

1. Bartlett JG et al: Practice guidelines for the management of community-acquired pneumonia in adults, *Clin Infect Dis* 31:347-382, 2000.
2. Meehan TP et al: Quality of care, process, and outcomes in elderly patients with pneumonia, *JAMA* 278:2080-2084, 1997.
3. Huxley EJ et al: Pharyngeal aspiration in normal adults and patients with depressed consciousness, *Am J Med* 64:564-568, 1978.
4. Fang GD et al: New and emerging etiologies for community-acquired pneumonia with implications for therapy: a prospective multicenter study of 359 cases, *Medicine* 69:307-316, 1990.

5. Marrie TJ, Durant H, Yates L: Community-acquired pneumonia requiring hospitalization: 5-year prospective study, *Rev Infect Dis* 11:586-599, 1989.
6. Potgieter PD, Hammond JM: Etiology and diagnosis of pneumonia requiring ICU admission, *Chest* 101:199-203, 1992.
7. Pachon J et al: Severe community-acquired pneumonia: etiology, prognosis, and treatment, *Am Rev Respir Dis* 142:369-373, 1990.
8. Berntsson E et al: Etiology of community-acquired pneumonia in outpatients, *Eur J Clin Microbiol* 5:446-447, 1986.
9. Ortiz CR, LaForce FM: Prevention of community-acquired pneumonia, *Med Clin North Am* 78:1173-1198, 1994.
10. Stack SJ, Martin DR, Plouffe JF: An emergency department-based pneumococcal vaccination program could save money and lives, *Ann Emerg Med* 33:299-303, 1999.
11. American Academy of Pediatrics, Committee on Infectious Diseases: Policy statement: recommendations for the prevention of pneumococcal infections including the use of pneumococcal conjugate vaccine (Prevnar), pneumococcal polysaccharide vaccine, and antibiotic prophylaxis, *Pediatrics* 106:362-366, 2000.
12. Martin CM et al: Severe staphylococcal pneumonia complicating influenza, *Arch Intern Med* 103:532-542, 1959.
13. Mansel JK et al: *Mycoplasma pneumoniae* pneumonia, *Chest* 95:639-646, 1989.
14. Bates JH et al: Microbial etiology of acute pneumonia in hospitalized patients, *Chest* 101:1005-1012, 1992.
15. Barlett JG: Anaerobic bacterial infections of the lung and pleural space, *Clin Infect Dis* 16(Suppl 4):S248-S255, 1993.
16. Centers for Disease Control and Prevention: Prevention and control of influenza: recommendations of the Immunization Practices Advisory Committee (ACIP), *MMWR* 49:1-38, 2000.
17. Centers for Disease Control and Prevention: Prevention and treatment of tuberculosis among patients infected with human immunodeficiency virus: principles of therapy and revised recommendations, *MMWR* 47:1-51, 1998.
18. Butler JC, Peters CJ: Hantaviruses and hantavirus pulmonary syndrome, *Clin Infect Dis* 19:387-395, 1994.
19. Metlay JP, Kapoor WN, Fine MJ: Does this patient have community-acquired pneumonia? *JAMA* 278:1440-1445, 1997.
20. Griffith DE: Pneumonia in chronic obstructive lung disease, *Infect Dis Clin North Am* 5:467-484, 1991.
21. Murray HW et al: The protean manifestations of *Mycoplasma pneumoniae* infection in adults, *Am J Med* 58:229-242, 1975.
22. Hahn DL, Dodge RW, Golubjatnikov R: Association of *Chlamydia pneumoniae* (Strain TWAR) infection with wheezing, asthmatic bronchitis, and adult-onset asthma, *JAMA* 266:225-230, 1991.
23. Grayston JT: Background and current knowledge of *Chlamydia pneumoniae* and athersclerosis, *J Infect Dis* 181:S402-410, 2000.
24. Grayston JT: Infections caused by *Chlamydia pneumoniae* Strain TWAR, *Clin Infect Dis* 15:757-763, 1992.
25. Singal BM, Hedges JR, Radack KL: Decision rules and clinical prediction of pneumonia: evaluation of low yield criteria, *Ann Emerg Med* 18:13, 1989.
26. Heckerling PS et al: Clinical prediction rule for pulmonary infiltrates, *Ann Intern Med* 113:664-670, 1990.
27. Emerman CL et al: Comparison of physician judgment and decision aids for ordering chest radiographs for pneumonia in outpatients, *Ann Emerg Med* 20:1215-1219, 1991.
28. Sherman S, Skoney JA, Ravikrishman KP: Routine chest radiographs in exacerbations of chronic obstructive pulmonary disease: diagnostic value, *Arch Intern Med* 149:2493-2496, 1989.
29. Bramson RT et al: The futility of the chest radiograph in the febrile infant without respiratory symptoms, *Pediatrics* 92:524-526, 1993.
30. Baraff LJ et al: Practice guideline for the management of infants and children 0 to 36 months of age with fever without source, *Ann Emerg Med* 22:1198-1210, 1993.
31. Bachur R, Perry H, Harper MB: Occult pneumonias: empiric chest radiographs in febrile children with leukocytosis, *Ann Emerg Med* 33:166-173, 1999.
32. Green SM, Rothrock SG: Evaluation styles for well-appearing febrile children: are you a "risk-minimizer" or a "test-minimizer"? *Ann Emerg Med* 33:211-214, 1999.
33. Melbye H et al: Pneumonia: a clinical or radiographic diagnosis? *Scand J Infect Dis* 24:647-655, 1992.
34. Hall FM, Simon M: Occult pneumonia associated with dehydration: myth or reality? *Am J Radiol* 148:853-854, 1987.
35. Caldwell A et al: The effects of dehydration on the radiologic and pathologic appearance of experimental canine segmental pneumonia, *Am Rev Respir Dis* 112:651-656, 1975.
36. Mower WR et al: A comparison of pulse oximetry and respiratory rate in patient screening, *Respir Med* 90:593-599, 1996.
37. Niderman MS et al: Guidelines for the initial management of adults with community-acquired pneumonia: diagnosis, assessment of severity, and initial antimicrobial therapy, *Am Rev Respir Dis* 148:1418-1426, 1993.
38. Fine MJ et al: Evaluation of housestaff physicians' preparation and interpretation of sputum Gram stains for community-acquired pneumonia, *J Gen Intern Med* 6:189-198, 1991.
39. Brown RB et al: Management of pneumonia by emergency department physicians, *Curr Ther Res* 49:651-658, 1991.
40. Chalasani NP et al: Clinical utility of blood cultures in adult patients with community-acquired pneumonia without defined underlying risks, *Chest* 108:932-936, 1995.
41. Landry ML, Cohen S, Ferguson D: Impact of sample type on rapid detection of influenza virus A by cytospin-enhanced immunofluorescence and membrane-linked immunosorbent assay, *J Clin Microbiol* 38:429-430, 2000.
42. Garcia-Leoni ME et al: Pneumococcal pneumonia: adult hospitalized patients infected with the human immunodeficiency virus, *Arch Intern Med* 152:1808-1812, 1992.
43. Steinhart R et al: Invasive *Haemophilus influenzae* infection in men with HIV infection, *JAMA* 268:3350-3352, 1992.
44. Glatt AE, Chirgwin K: *Pneumocystis carinii* pneumonia in human immunodeficiency virus infected patients, *Arch Intern Med* 150:271-279, 1990.
45. Silik RM, Starcher ET, Curran JW: Opportunistic diseases reported in AIDS patients: frequencies, associations, and trends, *AIDS* 1:175-182, 1987.
46. Kennedy CA, Goetz MB, Mathisen GE: Absolute CD4 lymphocyte counts and the risk of opportunistic pulmonary infection, *Rev Infect Dis* 12:561-562, 1990.
47. Blatt SP et al: Total lymphocyte count as a predictor of absolute CD4+ count and CD4+ percentage in HIV-infected persons, *JAMA* 269:622-626, 1993.
48. Goodman JL, Tashkin DP: *Pneumocystis* with normal chest x-ray film and arterial oxygen tension, *Arch Intern Med* 143:1981-1982, 1983.
49. Hopewell PC: *Pneumocystis carinii* pneumonia: diagnosis, *J Infect Dis* 157:1115-1119, 1988.
50. Kagawa FT et al: Serum lactate dehydrogenase activity in patients with AIDS and *Pneumocystis carinii* pneumonia: an adjunct to diagnosis, *Chest* 94:1031-1033, 1988.
51. Katz MH, Baron RB, Grady DB: Risk stratification of ambulatory patients suspected of *Pneumocystis* pneumonia, *Arch Intern Med* 151:105-110, 1991.
52. Stover DE, Greeno RA, Gagliardi AJ: The use of a simple exercise test for the diagnosis of *Pneumocystis carinii* pneumonia in patients with AIDS, *Am Rev Respir Dis* 139:1343-1346, 1989.
53. Smith DE: Diagnosis of *Pneumocystis carinii* pneumonia in HIV antibody positive patients by simple outpatient assessments, *Thorax* 47:1005, 1992.
54. Magnenat JL et al: Mode of presentation and diagnosis of bacterial pneumonia in human immunodeficiency virus–infected patients, *Am Rev Respir Dis* 144:917, 1991.
55. Polsky B et al: Bacterial pneumonia in patients with the acquired immunodeficiency syndrome, *Ann Intern Med* 104:38-41, 1986.
56. Tietjen PA, Kaner RJ, Quinn CE: Aspiration emergencies, *Clin Chest Med* 15:117-135, 1994.
57. Centers for Disease Control and Prevention: Guidelines for preventing the transmission of *Mycobacterium tuberculosis* in health-care facilities, 1994, *MMWR* 43:1-132, 1994.
58. Moran GJ et al: Delayed recognition and infection control for tuberculosis patients in the emergency department, *Ann Emerg Med* 26:290-295, 1995.

59. Doern GV et al: Antimicrobial resistance with *Streptococcus pneumoniae* in the United States, 1997-98, *Emerg Infect Dis* 5:757-765, 1999.
60. Pallares R et al: Resistance to penicillin and cephalosporin and mortality from severe pneumococcal pneumonia in Barcelona, Spain, *N Engl J Med* 333:474-480, 1995.
61. Feikin DR et al: Mortality from invasive pneumococcal pneumonia in the era of antibiotic resistance, 1995-1997, *Am J Public Health* 90:223-229, 2000.
62. Heffelfinger JD et al: Management of community-acquired pneumonia in the era of pneumococcal resistance, *Arch Intern Med* 160:1399-1408, 2000.
63. Gleason PP et al: Associations between initial antimicrobial therapy and medical outcomes for hospitalized elderly patients with pneumonia, *Arch Intern Med* 159:2562-2572, 1999.
64. Masur H: Prevention and treatment of *Pneumocystis* pneumonia, *N Engl J Med* 327:1853-1860, 1992.
65. The NIH-University of California Expert Panel for Corticosteroids as Adjunctive Therapy for *Pneumocystis* Pneumonia, *N Engl J Med* 323:1500-1504, 1990.
66. Schonwald S et al: Comparison of azithromycin and erythromycin in the treatment of atypical pneumonias, *J Antimicrob Chemother* 25(Suppl A):123-126, 1990.
67. Centers for Disease Control and Prevention: Neuraminidase inhibitors for treatment of influenzae A and B infections, *MMWR* 48:1-9, 1999.
68. Pomilla PV, Brown RB: Outpatient treatment of community-acquired pneumonia in adults, *Arch Intern Med* 154:1793-1802, 1994.
69. Fine MJ, Smith DN, Singer DE: Hospitalization decision in patients with community-acquired pneumonia: a prospective cohort study, *Am J Med* 89:713-721, 1990.
70. Black ER et al: Predicting the need for hospitalization of ambulatory patients with pneumonia, *J Gen Intern Med* 6:394-440, 1991.
71. Fine MJ et al: A prediction rule to identify low-risk patients with community-acquired pneumonia, *N Engl J Med* 336:243-250, 1997.
72. Marrie TJ et al: A controlled trial of a critical pathway for treatment of community-acquired pneumonia, *JAMA* 283:749-755, 2000.
73. Brenner M et al: Prognostic factors and life expectancy of patients with acquired immunodeficiency syndrome and *Pneumocystis carinii* pneumonia, *Am Rev Respir Dis* 136:1199-1206, 1987.
74. Kales CP et al: Early predictors of in-hospital mortality for *Pneumocystis carinii* pneumonia in the acquired immunodeficiency syndrome, *Arch Intern Med* 147:1413-1417, 1987.
75. Ware LB, Matthay MA: The acute respiratory distress syndrome, *N Engl J Med* 342:1334-1339, 2000.
76. Martin TR: Lung cytokines and ARDS, *Chest* 116:2S-8S, 1999.
77. The Acute Respiratory Distress Syndrome Network: Ventilation with lower tidal volumes as compared with traditional tidal volumes for acute lung injury and the acute respiratory distress syndrome, *N Engl J Med* 342:1301-1308, 2000.
78. Rossaint R et al: Inhaled nitric oxide for the adult respiratory distress syndrome, *N Engl J Med* 328:399-405, 1993.
79. Wyncoll DLA, Evans TW: Acute respiratory distress syndrome, *Lancet* 354:497-501, 1999.

72 Pleural Disease

Joshua M. Kosowsky

Pleural disease is commonly encountered in the ED. Presentations range in severity from asymptomatic pleural effusion to tension pneumothorax. This chapter reviews the two most common nontraumatic pleural problems seen in the ED: spontaneous pneumothorax and pleural inflammation and effusion. Pleural space problems associated with trauma are discussed in Chapter 38 (see Chapter 18 for the approach to a patient presenting with pleuritic chest pain).

SPONTANEOUS PNEUMOTHORAX

Perspective

Under normal conditions, the visceral and parietal pleura lie in close apposition, with only a potential space between them. *Pneumothorax* implies the presence of free air in the intrapleural space. A *spontaneous pneumothorax* is not caused by any external precipitating factor, either traumatic or iatrogenic. *Primary spontaneous pneumothorax* occurs in individuals without clinically apparent lung disease. *Secondary spontaneous pneumothorax* arises in the context of an underlying pulmonary disease process.

The pathophysiology of pneumothorax was described in 1747 by Combulsier as compression of the lung caused by air in the pleural space.[1] The term *pneumothorax* was first coined by Itard in 1803, and the clinical features were described in detail by Laennec in 1819.[2] Most cases of spontaneous pneumothorax were regarded as being secondary to pulmonary tuberculosis until 1932, when Kjaergaard described primary spontaneous pneumothorax as a distinct entity arising in previously healthy adults.[3]

The incidence of primary spontaneous pneumothorax is estimated at approximately 15 cases per 100,000 population per year among men, and 5 cases per 100,000 population per year among women.[4] Primary spontaneous pneumothorax typically occurs in healthy young men of taller than average height.[5]

Factors associated with primary spontaneous pneumothorax include cigarette smoking and changes in ambient atmospheric pressure.[6,7] Physical exertion does not appear to be a precipitating factor.[8] Familial patterns suggest an inherited propensity in some cases of primary spontaneous pneumothorax.[9] Mitral valve prolapse and Marfan's syndrome are associated with spontaneous pneumothorax in the absence of clinically apparent lung disease.[10,11]

Approximately one third of spontaneous pneumothoraces occur in the context of underlying pulmonary disease (Box 72-1). The incidence of secondary spontaneous pneumothorax is six cases per 100,000 population per year among men and two cases per 100,000 population per year among women.[4] The most common condition associated with secondary spontaneous pneumothorax is chronic obstructive pulmonary disease (COPD). The overall incidence is approximately 26 per 100,000 patients with COPD per year.[12] Patients with severe COPD (e.g., with forced expiratory volume in one second of less than 1 L) are at highest risk. The incidence of spontaneous pneumothorax among patients hospitalized for emphysema is 0.8% and for asthma 0.3%.[13,14]

In some urban settings, patients with acquired immune deficiency syndrome (AIDS) constitute the majority of cases

Box 72-1 Causes of Secondary Spontaneous Pneumothorax

Airway Disease

Chronic obstructive pulmonary disease
Asthma
Cystic fibrosis

Infections

Necrotizing bacterial pneumonia/lung abscess
Pneumocystis carinii pneumonia
Tuberculosis

Interstitial Lung Disease

Sarcoidosis
Idiopathic pulmonary fibrosis
Lymphangiomyomatosis
Tuberous sclerosis
Pneumoconioses

Neoplasms

Primary lung cancers
Pulmonary/pleural metastases

Miscellaneous

Connective tissue diseases
Pulmonary infarction
Endometriosis/catamenial pneumothorax

of secondary spontaneous pneumothorax.[15] Spontaneous pneumothorax occurs in approximately 2% of patients with AIDS, almost always in the setting of *Pneumocystis carinii* pneumonia (PCP).[16] Bilateral pneumothoraces are common with PCP, as are problems with delayed reexpansion and recurrences. Mortality in this group of patients is high.[17]

Malignancy is another common etiology of secondary spontaneous pneumothorax. The occurrence of spontaneous pneumothorax in a patient with known malignancy should prompt a search for lung metastases. In developing countries, tuberculosis and lung abscess remain leading causes of secondary spontaneous pneumothorax.

Catamenial pneumothorax is a rare condition in which recurrent spontaneous pneumothorax occurs in association with menses (typically within 72 hours of onset).[18] Although it has been termed *thoracic endometriosis syndrome,* and often responds to ovulation-suppressing medications, the exact etiology of catamenial pneumothorax remains uncertain.

Pathophysiologic Principles

Normally, intrapleural pressure is negative (less than atmospheric), fluctuating from ×10 to ×12 mm Hg during inspiration to approximately ×4 mm Hg during expiration. Intrabronchial and intraalveolar pressures are negative during inspiration (×1 to ×3 mm Hg) and positive during expiration (+1 to +3 mm Hg). The alveolar walls and visceral pleura form a barrier that separates the intrapleural and intraalveolar spaces and maintains the pressure gradient. If a defect occurs in this barrier, air enters the pleural space until either the pressures equalize or the communication seals.

With the loss of negative intrapleural pressure in one hemithorax, the ipsilateral lung collapses. A large pneumothorax results in a restrictive ventilation impairment, with reduced vital capacity, functional residual capacity, and total lung capacity. Shunting of blood through nonventilated lung tissue may result in acute hypoxemia, although over time this effect is mitigated by compensatory vasoconstriction in the collapsed lung. In tension pneumothorax, the alveolar-pleural defect acts as a one-way valve, allowing air to pass into the pleural space during inspiration and trapping it there during expiration (Figure 72-1). This leads to progressive accumulation of intrapleural air, and increasingly positive intrapleural pressure causing compression of the contralateral lung with asphyxia and worsening hypoxia. Intrapleural pressure exceeding 15 to 20 mm Hg impairs venous return to the heart. If allowed to progress, cardiovascular collapse and death ensue.

In primary spontaneous pneumothorax, disruption of the alveolar-pleural barrier is thought to occur when a subpleural bulla (or bleb), typically located at the lung apex, ruptures into the pleural space. Subpleural bullae are found in almost all patients who undergo surgical treatment for primary spontaneous pneumothorax, and can be identified on computed tomography of the chest in up to 90% of cases.[19,20] The etiology of these bullae is unclear, but is thought to be related to degradation of elastic fibers within the lung and an imbalance in the protease-antiprotease and oxidant-antioxidant systems.[21]

In the case of secondary spontaneous pneumothorax, it is the underlying lung disease that weakens the alveolar-pleural barrier. In patients with PCP, for example, the cytotoxic effects of repeated episodes of inflammation lead to bullous and cystic changes. In patients with COPD, chronic exposure to cigarette smoke results in the development of large, thin-walled bullae that are at an increased risk of rupture. Other factors, including increased intrabronchial and intraalveolar pressures generated by bronchospasm and coughing, probably also play a role.

Clinical Features

Symptoms of primary spontaneous pneumothorax typically begin suddenly while at rest. Ipsilateral chest pain and dyspnea are the most common symptoms. At the outset, the pain is typically "pleuritic" in nature (i.e., often described as sharp and made worse with deep inspiration), but it often evolves over time into a dull, steady ache. While patients frequently describe shortness of breath, extreme dyspnea is uncommon in the absence of underlying lung disease or tension pneumothorax. Cough is present in a minority of individuals. Occasionally, patients will be asymptomatic or have only nonspecific complaints. Patients may wait several days before they seek medical attention, and a significant number (up to 18% in one study) delay presentation for a week or more.[22] Without treatment, symptoms often resolve spontaneously within 24 to 72 hours, even though the pneumothorax is still present.

Physical findings tend to correlate with the degree of symptoms. A mild sinus tachycardia is the most common physical finding. With a large pneumothorax, decreased or absent breath sounds with hyperresonance to percussion may be present. Other classic signs include unilateral enlargement of the hemithorax, decreased excursion with respirations, absent tactile fremitus, and inferior displacement of the liver or spleen. Absence of any or all of these findings does not exclude pneumothorax, however, and a chest radiograph should be obtained when pneumothorax is suspected.

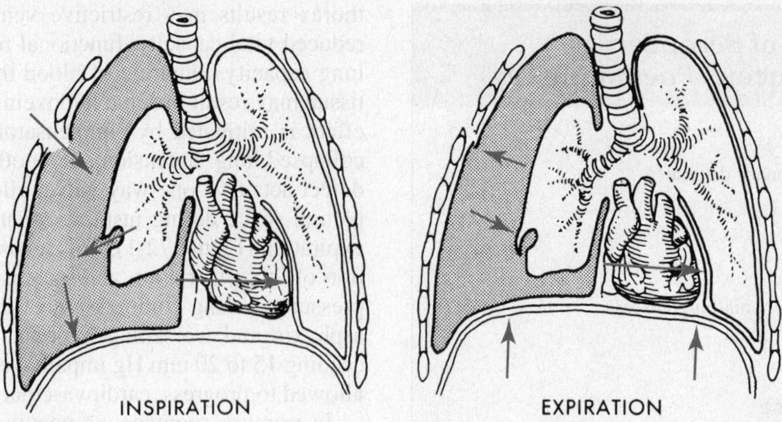

Figure 72-1. **Tension pneumothorax with total collapse of right lung and shift of mediastinal structures to left. Air is forced into pleural space during expiration and cannot escape during inspiration.**

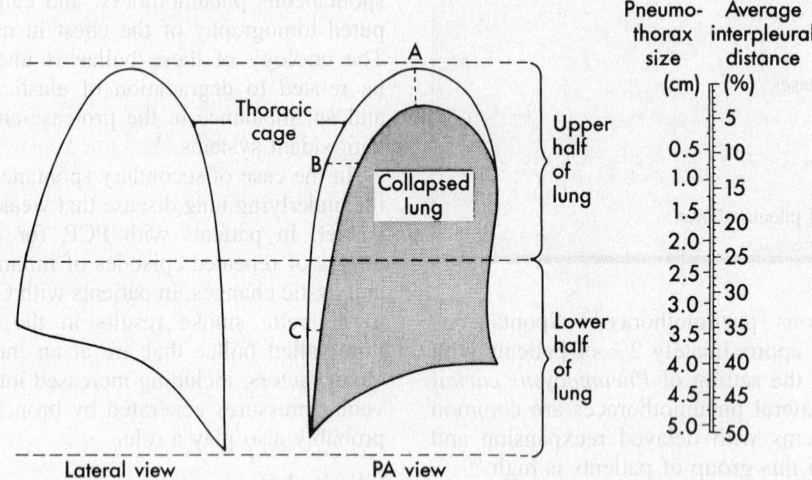

Figure 72-2. **Determining size of pneumothorax. Calculation of average interpleural distance to predict pneumothorax size.**

With tension pneumothorax, signs of asphyxia and decreased cardiac output develop. Tachycardia (often exceeding 120 beats/min) and hypoxia are common. Hypotension is a late and ominous finding. Distention of the jugular veins is common, but may be difficult to detect. Displacement of the trachea to the contralateral side is classically described, but is a rare, late finding. Its absence should not be considered evidence that a tension phenomenon is not present.[23]

In patients with significant underlying lung disease, pneumothorax presents differently. Because of poor pulmonary reserve, dyspnea is nearly universal, even when the pneumothorax is small, and symptoms tend not to resolve on their own.[24,25] Physical findings, such as hyperexpansion and distant breath sounds, often overlap considerably with the underlying lung disease, making the clinical diagnosis difficult. For this reason, the diagnosis of pneumothorax should be considered whenever a patient with COPD presents with an exacerbation of dyspnea.

Although suggested by the patient's history and physical examination, the diagnosis of pneumothorax is generally made with the chest radiograph. The classic radiographic appearance is that of a thin, visceral pleural line lying parallel to the chest wall, separated by a radiolucent band devoid of lung markings. The average width of this band can be used to estimate the size of the pneumothorax with a fair degree of accuracy (Figure 72-2).[26] The estimated size of the pneumothorax and the patient's clinical status can be useful in guiding management decisions.

Tension pneumothorax is a clinical diagnosis, and delaying treatment to obtain radiographic confirmation is inadvisable. When the diagnosis of tension pneumothorax is not apparent clinically, and a chest radiograph is obtained, the classic appearance is one of complete lung collapse with gross distention of the thoracic cavity on the affected side and shift of mediastinal structures across the midline (Figure 72-3). In patients with underlying pulmonary disease, however, pleural adhesions and lack of lung elasticity may mask the fact that a pneumothorax is under significant positive pressure.

When pneumothorax is suspected but not seen on a standard chest radiograph, an expiratory film may be obtained. Theoretically, the volumes of both the lungs and the chest cavity are reduced during expiration, so that the relative size of the pneumothorax is enhanced. Although occasionally helpful in identifying a small apical pneumothorax, routine

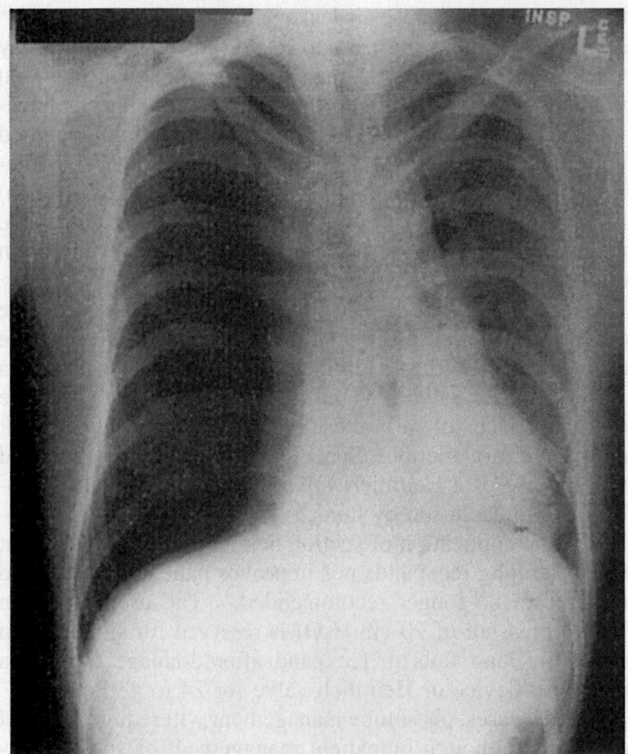

Figure 72-3. **Radiograph of tension pneumothorax with mediastinal shift to left.**

use of expiratory films does not improve diagnostic yield.[27,28] In some cases, a lateral decubitus film (with the suspected hemithorax up) allows visualization of a small amount of intrapleural air along the lateral chest wall. In critically ill patients for whom only a supine chest radiograph can be obtained, the finding of a "deep sulcus," that is, a deep lateral costophrenic angle, can suggest the presence of pneumothorax on that side.[29]

Special care should be taken when viewing the chest radiographs of patients with underlying lung disease. In patients with COPD, for example, the relative paucity of lung markings makes pneumothorax more difficult to detect. At the same time, giant bullae may simulate the radiographic appearance of pneumothorax. A clue to differentiating a pneumothorax from a giant bulla is that the former tends to run parallel to the chest wall, while the latter tends to have a more concave appearance. When the diagnosis is unclear, a radiograph obtained in a different position (e.g., decubitus) or computed tomography can be used to differentiate between the two entities.[30]

The differential diagnosis of pneumothorax includes numerous conditions associated with chest pain and dyspnea. The most important of these is acute pulmonary embolism, which may present in identical fashion but without confirmatory radiographic findings of pneumothorax. Acute or chronic pulmonary embolism should especially be considered in patients with COPD exacerbation that is not typical for them. Pleural irritation caused by inflammation may also mimic pneumothorax. Often, the pain of the pleural irritation creates a sensation of shortness of breath, even when true dyspnea and hypoxemia are absent. Most pleural based processes (pneumonia, embolism, tumor) have corresponding findings on chest radiograph.

Pneumothorax can mimic an acute myocardial infarction with electrocardiographic (ECG) changes simulating an acute injury pattern.[31] ECG changes, including axis deviation, decreased QRS voltage, and T-wave inversions, may occur as a consequence of mechanical displacement of the heart, increased intrathoracic air, acute right ventricular overload, or hypoxia resulting in myocardial ischemia.

Spontaneous pneumomediastinum is a closely related clinical entity, diagnosed by presence of subcutaneous emphysema and the finding of mediastinal air on chest radiograph. In contrast to spontaneous pneumothorax, spontaneous pneumomediastinum typically occurs during exertion, particularly after a strenuous Valsalva maneuver. Most cases of spontaneous pneumomediastinum occur in the absence of known underlying disease and have a benign course. Secondary causes of pneumomediastinum (such as Boerhaave's syndrome) are more serious, and treatment is aimed at the underlying disorder.[32]

Spontaneous hemopneumothorax is a rare but potentially serious condition that occurs when collapse of the lung is associated with rupture of a vessel in a parietopleural adhesion. The clinical presentation is similar to that of spontaneous pneumothorax, but may be accompanied by symptoms and signs of hemorrhagic shock. Treatment entails large-caliber tube thoracostomy, to evacuate the pleural space, reexpand the lung, and tamponade bleeding.

Fortunately, pneumothorax has a readily available, highly reliable confirmatory diagnostic test (i.e., chest radiography). Absence of a pneumothorax on chest radiograph should prompt a search for an alternate diagnosis.

Management

In the prehospital setting, the approach to the patient with spontaneous pneumothorax is generally supportive unless tension pneumothorax is suspected. Supplemental oxygen should be administered, intravenous access obtained, and transport to definitive care expedited. If a patient with pneumothorax is markedly hemodynamically unstable or requires positive pressure ventilation, the pleural space should be decompressed to prevent development or worsening of tension pneumothorax. Similarly, if air transfer is necessary, decompression of the pleural space should be considered to prevent expansion of the pneumothorax under the reduced atmospheric pressure at altitude.

Whether in the field or in the ED, if the clinical circumstances suggest tension pneumothorax, treatment should not be delayed awaiting further evidence of cardiovascular compromise or definitive diagnosis by chest radiograph. As soon as tension pneumothorax is suspected, the pleural space should be decompressed. This may be accomplished by insertion of an intravenous catheter or by immediate tube thoracostomy, depending on the availability of equipment and the expertise of the providers. The diagnosis is confirmed by the hiss of air escaping under positive pressure as the needle or chest tube enters the pleural space. Needle decompression is only a temporizing procedure, and definitive management requires tube thoracostomy as soon as possible.

In general, management of spontaneous pneumothorax has two goals: (1) to evacuate air from the pleural space and (2) to prevent recurrence. Pursuit of the latter goal extends well beyond the realm of the ED, but often influences the initial decision making as well. Therapeutic approaches to pneumothorax range from simple observation or aspiration with a catheter to video-assisted thoracoscopic surgery or thoracotomy. Decisions must be individualized and take into consideration several factors, including size of the pneumothorax, severity of signs, presence of underlying pulmonary disease, other comorbidities, history of previous pneumothoraces, patient reliability, degree and persistence of the air leak, and available follow-up monitoring.

For otherwise healthy, young patients with a small primary spontaneous pneumothorax (i.e., < 20% of the hemithorax) observation alone may be appropriate. The intrinsic reabsorption rate is in the range of 1% to 2% a day, a rate that is accelerated by a factor of 4 with the administration of 100% oxygen.[33,34] By lowering the alveolar partial pressure of nitrogen, supplemental oxygen increases the rate at which air diffuses across the pleural-alveolar barrier. The disposition of patients managed noninterventionally for a small pneumothorax varies by institution. Most physicians admit these patients for at least 6 hours of observation, often in an ED-based observation unit. A repeat chest radiograph can be obtained before discharge to document that there is no increase in the size of the pneumothorax. Discharged patients must be able to obtain emergency medical services quickly and should have definitive follow-up evaluation in 24 hours. Air travel and underwater diving must be avoided until the pneumothorax has completely resolved. Unreliable patients are not candidates for this approach.

For primary spontaneous pneumothoraces that are larger in size (i.e., ≥ 20% of the hemithorax), aspiration with an intravenous catheter may be attempted. Other than to provide relief of symptoms, however, there is little evidence that simple aspiration provides any outcome benefit over observation alone. If the chest radiograph 6 hours after aspiration shows no reaccumulation of the pneumothorax, the catheter is removed and the patient can be discharged home, with the same caveats that apply to patients managed with observation alone.

Advantages of simple aspiration include low morbidity, lack of invasiveness, and overall cost savings. Reported rates of successful outcome range from 45% to 71%.[35-38] Success is less likely when the patient is over age 50 or the volume of air aspirated exceeds 2.5 L, suggesting a continuing air leak. If aspiration fails to fully reexpand the lung, the catheter can be attached to a water-seal device or to a one-way Heimlich valve and managed like a small-caliber chest tube (see later).

Although the trend for the last two decades has been toward less invasive approaches, tube thoracostomy remains widely used, and is the treatment of choice in a number of clinical circumstances. Most secondary spontaneous pneumothoraces should be managed with tube thoracostomy because less invasive approaches (i.e., observation or simple aspiration) are associated with significantly lower success rates.[38] Patients who present with respiratory distress, have tension pneumothorax, or are likely to require mechanical ventilation should undergo tube thoracostomy to definitively reexpand the lung. If there is detectable pleural fluid (hemothorax or hydrothorax), tube thoracostomy is also required. Finally, tube thoracostomy may be considered in uncomplicated cases of primary spontaneous pneumothorax either as a first-line intervention or after a less invasive approach (i.e., observation or simple aspiration) has failed.

For most primary spontaneous pneumothoraces, placement of a small-caliber (7 to 14 French) tube is generally all that is required, because air leakage tends to be minimal.[39,40] Small-caliber tubes are easy to insert, are well tolerated by patients, and leave only a small scar after removal. Potential problems with small-caliber tubes include kinking, malposition, inadvertent removal, occlusion by pleural fluid or clotted blood, and large persistent air leaks. For secondary spontaneous pneumothorax, a standard size (20 to 28 French) thoracostomy tube is recommended. When there is detectable pleural fluid or an anticipated need for mechanical ventilation a larger tube size (≥ 28 French) is required.

Once inserted, the tube is attached to a water-seal device and left in place until the lung has reexpanded fully and the air leak has ceased. A Heimlich valve, which consists of a one-way flutter valve covered in transparent plastic, can be used in place of a water-seal device and allows for unhindered ambulation. Specific complications associated with the use of a Heimlich valve include accidental disconnection and occlusion by fluid.

Routine application of suction neither increases the rate at which the lung reexpands nor improves patient outcome and is therefore no longer recommended.[41] The use of suction (with a pressure of 20 cm H_2O) is reserved for situations in which the lung fails to reexpand after drainage through a water-seal device or Heimlich valve for 24 to 48 hours.

In most cases, chest tube management will require hospital admission, although outpatient management of spontaneous pneumothorax with a small-caliber tube and Heimlich device is described.[42]

Common complications of chest tube placement include incorrect placement, pleural infection, and prolonged pain. Reexpansion pulmonary edema and reexpansion hypotension are rare occurrences after rapid evacuation of large pneumothoraces.[43,44]

Outcome

The majority of spontaneous pneumothoraces resolve within 7 days of tube thoracostomy.[45] Air leaks that persist for longer than 2 days are less likely to resolve on their own.[46] If an air leak persists beyond 4 to 7 days, tube thoracostomy is considered to have failed, and surgical intervention is generally recommended.

Failure of tube thoracostomy is more common with secondary spontaneous pneumothoraces because these tend to be associated with larger and more persistent air leaks.[46] In the setting of COPD, healing of the alveolar-pleural barrier may be impaired by chronic inflammatory changes and loss of vascularity in pulmonary tissue. The success rate also decreases substantially with recurrent episodes of pneumothorax, declining from 91% for treatment of a first pneumothorax to 52% for treatment of a first recurrence and to 15% for treatment of a second recurrence.[47]

Recurrences of spontaneous pneumothorax are common. The risk of recurrence after a primary spontaneous pneumothorax is approximately 1 in 3, with studies reporting a range of rates between 16% and 50%.[48] Younger age, lower weight/height ratio, and history of smoking are associated with an increased rate of recurrence. Recurrence rates after a secondary spontaneous pneumothorax range slightly higher, from 39% to 47%.[21]

Because recurrences may be life threatening for patients with serious underlying lung disease, intervention is advocated to prevent recurrence as part of the initial approach to secondary spontaneous pneumothorax.[21] In contrast, for patients with primary spontaneous pneumothorax, interventions are typically not considered until after a second ipsilateral pneumothorax. Preventive treatment is also recommended for patients who plan to continue activities such as flying or diving that increase the risk of serious complications if a pneumothorax recurs. Computed tomography can be used in primary spontaneous pneumothorax to detect emphysematous changes, predict the likelihood of recurrence, and thereby guide decisions with respect to intervention.[49]

A variety of operative and nonoperative interventions prevent recurrences.[21] One strategy promotes adherence of parietal and visceral pleura, which obliterates the pleural space. Pleurodesis can be accomplished by mechanical pleural abrasion or by instillation of sclerosing agents. Another strategy involves resection of apical bullae or other lesions at risk for causing recurrences. Often, the two strategies are combined. Minimally invasive procedures such as video-assisted thoracoscopic surgery allow for both resection of bullae and pleurodesis.[50] On the other hand, patients with extensive bullae may require thoracotomy for wider visualization of lesions. There are limited data comparing the various interventions to prevent recurrences.[21] Success rates are generally quite good, ranging from 86% to 100%.

PLEURAL INFLAMMATION AND EFFUSION

Perspective

Under normal circumstances, a thin layer of fluid lies between the visceral and parietal pleura. Pleural effusion implies the presence of an abnormally large amount of fluid in the pleural space. Pleural effusions are relatively common, with an incidence in the United States estimated to be at least 800,000 cases per year.[51]

The most common cause of pleural effusions in Western countries is congestive heart failure, followed by malignancy, bacterial pneumonia, and pulmonary embolism.[51] In developing countries, tuberculosis remains the leading etiology of pleural effusions.[52] Other conditions commonly associated with pleural effusions include viral infections of the lung parenchyma or pleura, uremia, myxedema, cirrhosis, the nephrotic syndrome, collagen vascular diseases (e.g., systemic lupus erythematosus, rheumatoid arthritis), and intraabdominal processes (e.g., acute pancreatitis, subphrenic abscess, ascites). Esophageal perforation is a rare but uniquely morbid cause of a pleural effusion.

Pleuritis is a nonspecific term denoting inflammation of the pleura. Pleuritis (also referred to as pleurisy) can occur without significant exudation of fluid into the pleural space (e.g., epidemic pleurodynia). Commonly there is an associated pleural effusion at some point in time.

A pleural effusion associated with bacterial pneumonia, bronchiectasis, or lung abscess is called a parapneumonic effusion. The term *complicated parapneumonic effusion* refers to those parapneumonic effusions that require tube thoracostomy for their resolution. Empyema (or pus in the pleural space) implies the presence of bacteria on Gram stain of the pleural fluid.

When fluid is anatomically confined and not freely flowing in the pleural space, a loculated effusion is said to be present. Loculated effusions occur when there are adhesions between the visceral and parietal pleura.

Hemothorax (i.e., blood in the pleural space) and chylothorax (i.e., from rupture of the thoracic duct) are special instances of pleural effusion and are approached separately.

Pathophysiologic Principles

Pleural fluid is produced from systemic capillaries at the parietal pleural surface and absorbed into pulmonary capillaries at the visceral pleural surface. Lymphatics also play an important role in removing pleural fluid. Movement of fluid across the pleural surfaces is governed by Starling's law, so that under normal circumstances the direction of pleural fluid flow is largely governed by the difference in hydrostatic pressure between the systemic and pulmonary circulations (Figure 72-4). Pleural fluid exists in a dynamic equilibrium in which influx equals efflux, with approximately 1 L of fluid traversing the pleural space in 24 hours. Under normal

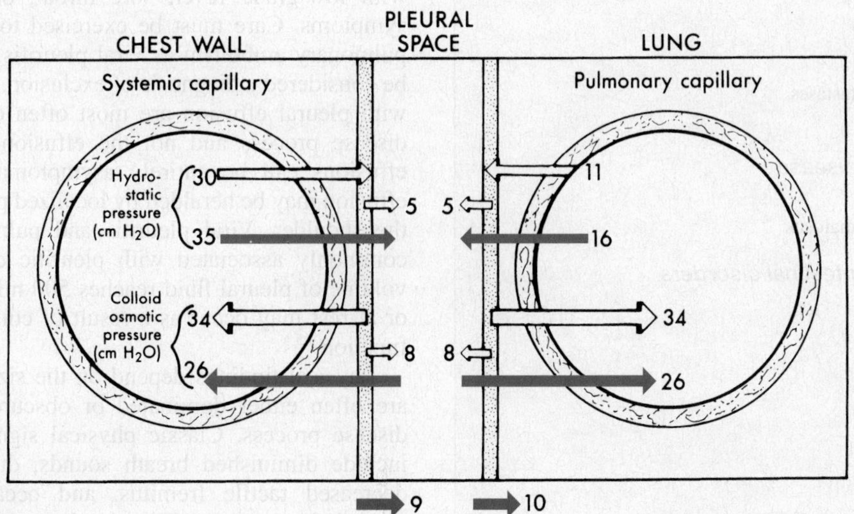

Figure 72-4. **Diagram representing pressures involved in formation and absorption of pleural fluid.** ***Modified from Fraser RG et al:*** **Diagnosis of diseases of the chest, *ed 3, Philadelphia, 1988, WB Saunders.***

conditions, the amount of fluid that remains in the pleural space is very small (approximately 0.1 to 0.2 mL/kg body weight) and undetectable either clinically or radiographically.

Pleural effusion develops whenever influx of fluid into the pleural space exceeds efflux of fluid from the pleural space. A vast number of disorders can lead to formation of a pleural effusion. Pleural effusions are classically divided into two groups—*transudates* and *exudates*—according to the composition of the pleural fluid present (Box 72-2).

Transudates are essentially ultrafiltrates of plasma, containing very little protein. A *transudative effusion* develops when there is an increase in the hydrostatic pressure or decrease in the oncotic pressure within pleural microvessels. The primary cause of increased hydrostatic pressure is congestive heart failure, which is responsible for about 90% of transudative effusions. In hepatic cirrhosis and nephrotic syndrome, increased hydrostatic pressure is combined with loss of plasma oncotic pressure because of significant decreases in serum albumin. Patients with severe malnutrition may develop transudative effusions resulting from severe hypoalbuminemia alone.

Exudates contain relatively high amounts of protein, reflecting an abnormality of the pleura itself. An *exudative effusion* is the result of increased membrane permeability or defective lymphatic drainage. Any pulmonary or pleural process associated with inflammation can result in an exudative effusion. The most common form of exudative effusion is a parapneumonic effusion, in which infection of the adjacent lung elicits an intense inflammatory response in pleura, disrupting normal membrane permeability. Malignant effusions are the second most common form of exudative effusion, and often reflect alterations in pleural permeability as well as problems with lymphatic drainage. Exudative effusions may also arise in response to inflammatory abdominal processes such as pancreatitis or subphrenic abscess, presumably owing to altered permeability of the diaphragm itself. Exudative effusions may be reabsorbed or organize into fibrous tissue, resulting in pleural adhesions.

Some pleural effusions can present as either transudates or exudates or may have characteristics of both. In the case of pulmonary embolism, for example, the pathogenesis of pleural effusion is often multifactorial, reflecting increased pulmonary vascular pressure (a transudative process) as well as ischemia and breakdown of the pleural membrane (an exudative process).

Massive effusions (larger than 1.5 to 2 L) are most commonly associated with malignancy but can also arise in the setting of congestive heart failure, cirrhosis, and other conditions. Massive effusions may restrict respiratory movement, compress the lungs, and result in intrapulmonary shunting. In extremely rare cases, tension hydrothorax can develop, with mediastinal shift and circulatory embarrassment.[53]

Box 72-2 Causes of Pleural Effusion

Transudates

- Congestive heart failure
- Cirrhosis with ascites
- Nephrotic syndrome
- Hypoalbuminemia
- Myxedema
- Peritoneal dialysis
- Glomerulonephritis
- Superior vena cava obstruction
- Pulmonary embolism

Exudates

Infections

- Bacterial pneumonia
- Bronchiectasis
- Lung abscess
- Tuberculosis
- Viral illness
- Neoplasms
- Primary lung cancer
- Mesothelioma
- Pulmonary/pleural metastases
- Lymphoma

Connective tissue disease

- Rheumatoid arthritis
- Systemic lupus erythematosus

Abdominal/gastrointestinal disorders

- Pancreatitis
- Subphrenic abscess
- Esophageal rupture
- Abdominal surgery

Miscellaneous

- Pulmonary infarction
- Uremia
- Drug reactions
- Postpartum
- Cylothorax

Clinical Features

History is important in establishing the diagnosis for pleural effusion or pleural inflammation. A history of congestive heart failure, liver disease, uremia, or malignancy may direct subsequent evaluation. The pain of viral pleuritis is typically preceded by several days of a typical viral prodrome, often with low-grade fever, sore throat, or other constitutional symptoms. Care must be exercised to avoid misdiagnosing pulmonary embolism as viral pleuritis, and the latter should be considered a diagnosis of exclusion. Symptoms associated with pleural effusion are most often due to the underlying disease process and not the effusion itself. Small pleural effusions can be entirely asymptomatic.[54] A new pleural effusion may be heralded by localized pain or pain referred to the shoulder. Viral pleuritis and pulmonary infarction are commonly associated with pleuritic chest pain. When the volume of pleural fluid reaches 500 ml, dyspnea on exertion or at rest may occur as a result of compromised pulmonary function.[55]

Physical findings depend on the size of the effusion, but are often either dominated or obscured by the underlying disease process. Classic physical signs of pleural effusion include diminished breath sounds, dullness to percussion, decreased tactile fremitus, and occasionally a localized pleural friction rub. The simple technique of auscultatory percussion (i.e., percussing the chest while listening for a dullness with the stethoscope) may be even more sensitive and specific for the physical diagnosis of pleural effusion.[56]

Egophony and enhanced breath sounds can often be appreciated at the superior border of the effusion because of underlying atelectatic lung tissue. In the setting of pleuritis, a pleural friction rub may be appreciated. With massive effusions signs of mediastinal shift may be present. In general, concordance among observers is quite high (> 75%) for these physical signs.[57]

Chest radiography confirms the clinical suspicion of pleural effusion and occasionally reveals a pleural effusion as an incidental or unexpected finding. The classic radiographic appearance of a pleural effusion is blunting of the costophrenic angle on the upright chest radiograph. On a frontal (anteroposterior or posteroanterior) projection, a volume of 250 to 500 ml of pleural fluid is required before radiographic demonstration is possible. A lesser amount of fluid may be visible in the posterior costophrenic gutter on a lateral projection.[58] With larger effusions, the hemidiaphragm is obscured and an upwardly concave meniscus may be seen, as pleural fluid has a tendency to layer higher laterally than centrally. Pleural fluid can extend up a major fissure and appear as a homogeneous density in the lower two thirds of the lung field. Massive pleural effusion can appear as a totally opacified hemithorax.

In the recumbent patient, free pleural fluid gravitates superiorly, laterally, and posteriorly and may not be clearly discernible on a supine radiograph. If the effusion is large enough, diffuse haziness or partial opacification of a hemithorax may be seen.[59] Other findings on the supine radiograph may include apical capping, obliteration of the hemidiaphragm, and a widened minor fissure. A cross-table lateral radiograph obtained in the supine position can be used to demonstrate posterior layering of a pleural effusion, but a lateral decubitus radiograph (with the involved side down) is better for detection of small amounts of fluid. When combined with slight Trendelenburg positioning, the lateral decubitus view can detect as little as 5 to 15 ml of pleural fluid.[60] A lateral decubitus film can also be used to confirm the layering nature of free pleural fluid. For example, on an upright chest radiograph pleural thickening may blunt the costophrenic angle and simulate a small pleural effusion. On the lateral decubitus radiograph, however, thickened pleura does not change in configuration as does free pleural fluid, which will seek a new position. Likewise, a loculated pleural effusion will not freely layer on a lateral decubitus film. Ipsilateral and contralateral decubitus views may also allow visualization of the underlying lung and demonstrate the underlying cause of the effusion.[61]

The radiographic appearance of pleural effusions can sometimes be confusing. Subpulmonic effusions (fluid collections between the lung base and the diaphragm) can be difficult to diagnose, often simulating an elevated hemidiaphragm. Clues to the presence of a subpulmonic effusion include shifting of the apparent dome of the diaphragm toward the lateral chest wall and, when located on the left side, an increase in the distance between the gastric bubble and aerated lung. Fluid that loculates in a fissure may take on a fusiform appearance and can simulate a mass (Figure 72-5). Such "fluid pseudotumors" are common in patients with congestive heart failure.

Other imaging techniques such as ultrasound, computed tomography, and magnetic resonance imaging may be helpful in localizing effusions, distinguishing transudates from exudates, and characterizing underlying lung processes.[62] Ultrasound can be used to guide thoracentesis and decrease the risk of complications, particularly in the case of small or loculated effusions.[63]

Pulmonary embolism is the most commonly overlooked disorder in the workup of patients with pleural effusions.[64] Ventilation-perfusion ($\dot{V}/\dot{Q}$) scanning, helical computed tomography, or pulmonary angiography should be considered for any pleural effusion of uncertain etiology if pulmonary embolism is a diagnostic consideration.

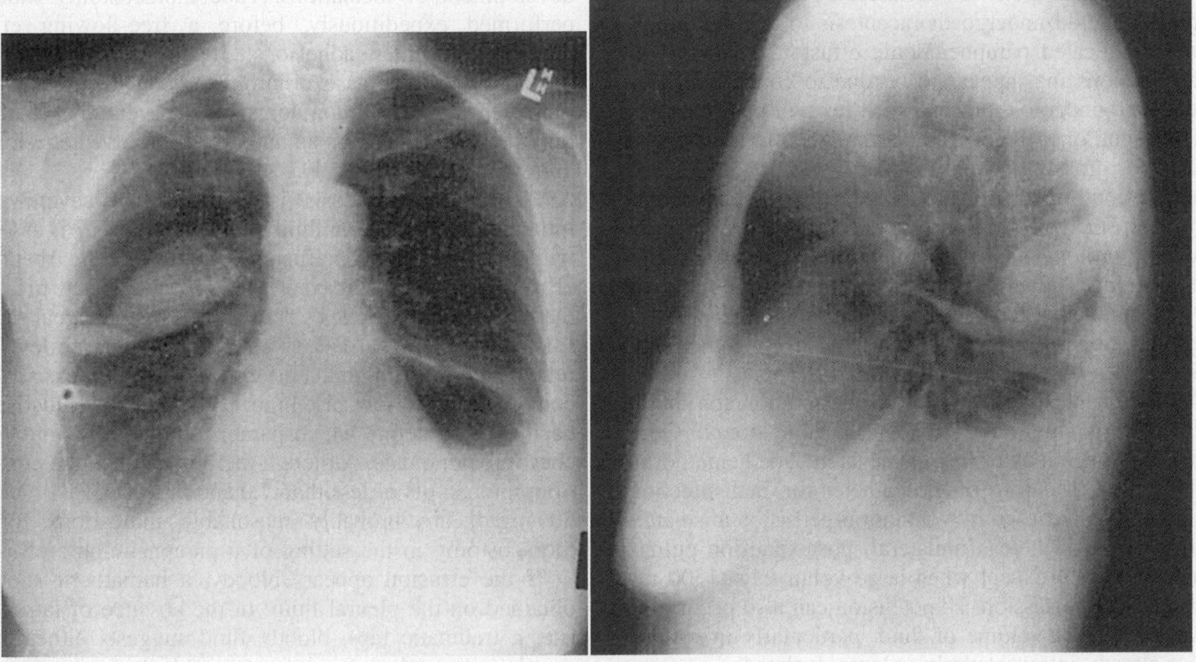

Figure 72-5. **Radiograph of pleural effusion along major and minor fissures.**

Laboratory studies, such as serum lactate dehydrogenase (LDH), can be used to help determine the characteristics of obtained pleural fluid. Serum electrolytes may confirm uremia. Complete blood counts and specifically leukocyte counts are too insensitive and nonspecific to be of discriminatory diagnostic value.

Management

For the most part, the ED management of pleural effusion centers on the underlying disease process. Treatment of serious conditions such as pulmonary edema or pneumonia should be initiated without delay.

Pain relief is an important consideration in the management of patients with pleuritis, which may have a significant inflammatory component. Nonsteroidal antiinflammatory drugs (NSAIDs) are used with relatively good success in treating pleural pain.[65] Opioid analgesia is safe and effective, but care should be exercised in debilitated patients or those with severe lung disease because of potential for respiratory depression.

The decision to proceed with thoracentesis in the ED, for either diagnostic or therapeutic purposes, must be individualized. Unless thoracentesis is necessary for stabilization of the patient's respiratory or circulatory status, it is appropriately deferred until the patient is admitted to the hospital. Relatively asymptomatic pleural effusions of clear etiology may not require any further attention. In general, any unexplained pleural effusion requires further investigation.

Diagnostic thoracentesis in the ED is indicated to rule out immediately life-threatening conditions such as empyema or esophageal rupture in a patient who appears toxic. Thoracentesis is sometimes undertaken in the ED for patients with known, recurrent malignant effusion, in whom the symptomatic relief obtained may permit discharge home. In most other cases, if thoracentesis is performed in the ED, hospital admission is required to treat the underlying illness and to observe for any complications of the procedure.

Patients with pneumonia and significant pleural effusion on chest radiograph (i.e., > 10 mm wide on a lateral decubitus radiograph) should undergo thoracentesis to rule out empyema or complicated parapneumonic effusion. Patients with pleural effusions that appear to be due to congestive heart failure should undergo thoracentesis if fever or pleuritic chest pain is present, or if the effusion is unilateral (particularly if left-sided) or grossly unequal in size.

Relative contraindications to thoracentesis include coagulopathy and other bleeding disorders. Thoracentesis may be safe with a prolonged prothrombin time in the absence of active bleeding.[66] Pleural adhesions, suggested by a prior history of empyema, represent a relative contraindication to thoracentesis because of the high risk of pneumothorax associated with blind needle insertion.

After thoracentesis is completed a chest radiograph should be obtained to rule out iatrogenic pneumothorax. Other potential complications of thoracentesis include hemothorax, lung laceration, shearing of the catheter tip, and infection. Transient hypoxia caused by ventilation-perfusion mismatching often occurs, whereas unilateral, postexpansion pulmonary edema is rare except when large volumes (> 1500 ml) are drained in one session. Hypotension can also occur after removal of a large volume of fluid, particularly in patients who are already intravascularly volume depleted.

The primary goal of pleural fluid analysis is to distinguish between transudative and exudative effusions. The presence of a transudate directs attention toward treatment of the underlying process (e.g., congestive heart failure, nephrotic syndrome), whereas the presence of an exudate indicates the need for a more extensive diagnostic evaluation.

Although numerous alternative measurements are proposed, Light's criteria still remain a widely accepted means of differentiating transudates and exudates.[67] By these criteria, pleural fluid is considered an exudate if one or more of the following hold true:

1. Pleural fluid protein divided by serum protein is greater than 0.5.
2. Pleural fluid LDH divided by serum LDH is greater than 0.6.
3. Pleural fluid LDH is greater than two-thirds the upper limit of normal for the serum LDH.

Light's criteria have high sensitivity (98%) for the diagnosis of an exudative effusion, but occasionally misclassify a transudative process as exudative.[68] Some investigators recommend turning to the serum-effusion albumin gradient in such cases.[69] If the serum albumin minus the pleural fluid albumin is greater than 1.2 g/dl, the patient in all probability has a transudative effusion and Light's criteria can be ignored.[68]

In the presence of an exudative effusion, additional pleural fluid analyses further classify the effusion for both diagnostic and therapeutic purposes.

The visual appearance and odor of an exudative effusion may or may not be diagnostic of empyema. Regardless, pleural fluid from any patient with an undiagnosed exudative pleural effusion should undergo Gram stain and culture for bacteria (aerobic and anaerobic), mycobacteria, and fungi. (Routine staining for mycobacteria and fungi has a low yield.)

The presence of empyema on the basis of either visual appearance or Gram staining mandates insertion of a chest tube to adequately drain the pleural space and prevent the development of loculations. Tube thoracostomy should be performed expeditiously, before a free-flowing effusion develops fibrinous adhesions. If an effusion is already loculated, streptokinase or urokinase can be injected by a thoracic surgeon, pulmonologist, or interventional radiologist into the pleural space in an attempt to dissolve adhesions and allow fluid to drain freely.

Pleural fluid acidosis is a marker of severe pleural inflammation. A pleural fluid pH of less than 7.3 is associated with parapneumonic effusions, malignancies, rheumatoid effusions, tuberculosis, and systemic acidosis. A pH of less than 7.0 strongly suggests empyema (or esophageal rupture). Like low pH, high LDH levels and low glucose levels also reflect an active inflammatory process. On this basis, various combinations of low pH, high LDH, and low glucose have been used to define which parapneumonic effusions require chest tube drainage. Although there is no absolute consensus of opinion, a pH of less than 7.0 and/or a glucose of less than 50 mg/dl are probably reasonable indications for tube thoracostomy in the setting of a parapneumonic effusion.[68]

If the effusion appears bloody, a hematocrit should be obtained on the pleural fluid. In the absence of iatrogenesis (i.e, a traumatic tap), bloody fluid suggests either trauma, neoplasm, or pulmonary infarction.[68] If the hematocrit of the pleural fluid is more than 50% that of the peripheral blood, the effusion is, by definition, a hemothorax. Atraumatic hemothorax is relatively rare, but can occur with spontaneous rupture of a tumor or blood vessel (e.g., ruptured aortic aneurysm). Hemothorax should be treated with tube thoracostomy to evacuate the pleural space, allow quantification of bleeding, and bring about apposition of the two pleural surfaces to tamponade hemorrhage. If bleeding exceeds 200 ml/hr, thoracotomy should be considered.

A pleural fluid cell count can sometimes be of use. Normal pleural fluid contains less than 1,000 white blood cells (WBCs)/mm^3; exudative pleural fluid may contain 10,000 or more WBCs/mm^3. While the absolute cell count has limited diagnostic value, the differential cell count can be helpful.[70] A predominance of neutrophils suggests an acute process such as pneumonia, pulmonary embolus, or acute tuberculous pleuritis. A predominance of monocytes or lymphocytes suggests a more chronic process such as malignancy or established tuberculosis.

Additional pleural fluid analyses may be indicated depending on the clinical circumstances. For example, an elevated pleural fluid amylase is highly sensitive for effusions caused by pancreatic disease or esophageal rupture. Pleural fluid amylase level is also elevated in approximately 10% of malignant effusions. Bacterial antigen testing may provide for rapid identification of the pathogen responsible for a parapneumonic effusion. A pleural fluid adenosine deaminase (ADA) level above 45 IU/L or a γ interferon level (IFN) level above 3.7 U/ml is strongly suggestive of a tuberculous effusion.[71,72]

If the diagnosis of a malignant pleural effusion is being considered, at least 50 ml of pleural fluid should be submitted for cytologic examination. Cytologic analysis will provide the diagnosis of cancer in 40% to 87% of malignant effusions.[68]

Outcomes

The clinical course of a pleural effusion depends on the underlying disease process responsible for its presence.

Some pleural effusions carry little or no clinical significance. For example, pleural effusions are a common finding in the postpartum state.[73] Small pleural effusions are also common after abdominal surgery, most resolving spontaneously within a few days.[74] Effusions associated with viral pleuritis are generally self-limited and resolve without specific treatment

For patients with congestive heart failure, pleural effusions generally respond well to diuretic therapy. If an effusion persists despite several days of aggressive diuresis, a diagnostic thoracentesis should be considered to rule out an alternative diagnosis.

Pleural effusions associated with malignancy carry a poor prognosis and are a significant cause of morbidity in patients with advanced cancer. The presence of a malignant effusion indicates disseminated disease, and most of the malignancies that cause pleural effusions—lung carcinoma, breast carcinoma, and lymphoma comprising the vast majority—are not curable by this stage. Therapeutic thoracentesis can relieve dyspnea in the short term, but malignant effusions tend to be recurrent, often rapidly so. Management strategies include chemical or mechanical pleurodesis to obliterate the pleural space, or placement of a pleuroperitoneal shunt to provide continual drainage. Control of pleural effusions can reduce morbidity and improve quality of life in these patients.[75]

Parapneumonic effusions contribute significantly to the morbidity and mortality of pneumonia.[76] For this reason alone, the presence of a parapneumonic effusion factors into the decision to hospitalize a patient with community-acquired pneumonia.[77] Empyema can be expected in 5% to 10% of patients with a parapneumonic effusion.[76] In most cases, empyema can be adequately treated with parenteral antibiotics and pleural drainage. When a loculated empyema cannot be drained, surgical or thorascopic decortication may be required.

Pulmonary embolism with associated pleural effusion is treated no differently than pulmonary embolism without pleural effusion. Typically the pleural effusion resolves within a few days after instituting anticoagulation therapy.

In nearly 20% of pleural effusions, no definitive diagnosis can be established even after extensive investigation.[78] It is believed that a sizeable percentage of these effusions are due to viral infections. Most of these effusions resolve spontaneously without sequelae.

KEY CONCEPTS

- For healthy, young patients with a small (< 20%) primary spontaneous pneumothorax, observation alone is an appropriate treatment option.
- In most cases of secondary spontaneous pneumothorax, tube thoracostomy should be considered, because less invasive approaches are associated with lower rates of success.
- Tension pneumothorax is a clinical diagnosis, and life-saving treatment should not be delayed to obtain radiographic confirmation.
- The most common cause of pleural effusions in Western countries is congestive heart failure, followed by malignancy and bacterial pneumonia; however, the diagnosis of pulmonary embolism should not be overlooked with a pleural effusion of uncertain etiology.
- In the ED, therapeutic thoracentesis is indicated for the relief of acute respiratory or cardiovascular compromise.
- The clearest indication for diagnostic thoracentesis in the ED is to diagnose immediately life-threatening conditions such as empyema or esophageal rupture in a patient who appears toxic; in most other cases, diagnostic thoracentesis to distinguish between transudative and exudative processes can be deferred to the inpatient unit.

REFERENCES

1. Withers JN et al: Spontaneous pneumothorax: suggested etiology and comparison of treatment methods, *Am J Surg* 108:772-776, 1964.
2. Laennec RTH: Traite de l'auscultation mediate et des maladies des poumons et du coeur, Tome Second, Paris 1819.
3. Kjaergaard H: Spontaneous pneumothorax in the apparently healthy, *Acta Med Scand Suppl* 43:1, 1932.
4. Melton LJ, Hepper NGG, Offord KP: Incidence of spontaneous pneumothorax in Olmstead County, Minnesota: 1950-1974, *Am Rev Respir Dis* 120:1379, 1979.
5. Voge VM et al: Spontaneous pneumothorax in the USAF aircrew population: a retrospective study, *Aviat Space Environ Med* 57:939, 1986.
6. Bense L et al: Smoking and the increased risk of contracting spontaneous pneumothorax, *Chest* 92:1009, 1987.

7. Scott GC, Berger R, McKean HE: The role of atmospheric pressure variation in the development of spontaneous pneumothoraces, *Am Rev Respir Dis* 139:659, 1989.
8. Bense L, Wiman LG, Hedenstierna G: Onset of symptoms in spontaneous pneumothorax: correlations to physical activity, *Eur J Respir Dis* 71:181, 1987.
9. Abolnik IZ: On the inheritance of primary spontaneous pneumothorax, *Am J Med Genet* 40:155, 1991.
10. Margaliot S et al: Spontaneous pneumothorax and mitral valve prolapse, *Chest* 89:93, 1986.
11. Sensenig DM, LaMarche P: Marfan's syndrome and spontaneous pneumothorax, *Am J Surg* 139:602-604, 1980.
12. Dines DE, Clagett OT, Payne WS: Spontaneous pneumothorax in emphysema. *Mayo Clin Proc* 45:481-487, 1970.
13. Cabiran LR, Ziskina MM: Spontaneous pneumothorax in pulmonary emphysema, *Dis Chest* 46:571, 1964.
14. Burke GJ: Pneumothorax complicating acute asthma, *GJ Afr Med J* 55:508-510, 1979.
15. Sassoon CS: The etiology and treatment of spontaneous pneumothorax, *Curr Opin Pulm Med* 1:331-338, 1995.
16. McClellan MD et al: Pneumothorax with *Pneumocystis carinii* pneumonia in AIDS. Incidence and clinical characteristics, *Chest* 100:1224-1228, 1991.
17. Ingram RJ et al: Management and outcome of pneumothoraces in patients infected with human immunodeficiency virus, *Clin Infect Dis* 23:624-627, 1996.
18. Carter EJ, Ettensohn DB: Catamenial pneumothorax, *Chest* 98:713-716, 1990.
19. Inderbitzi RG et al: Three years' experience in video-assisted thoracic surgery (VATS) for spontaneous pneumothorax, *J Thorac Cardiovasc Surg* 107:1410-1415, 1994.
20. Mitlehner W, Friedrich M, Dissmann W: Value of computer tomography in the detection of bullae and blebs in patients with primary spontaneous pneumothorax, *Respiration* 59:221-227, 1992.
21. Sahn SA, Heffner JE: Spontaneous pneumothorax, *N Engl J Med* 342:868-874, 2000.
22. Seremetis MG: The management of spontaneous pneumothorax, *Chest* 57:65, 1970.
23. Holloway VJ, Harris JK: Spontaneous pneumothorax: is it under tension? *J Accid Emerg Med* 17:222-223, 2000.
24. Dines DE, Clagett OT, Payne WS: Spontaneous pneumothorax in emphysema, *Mayo Clin Proc* 45:481-487, 1970.
25. Tanaka F et al: Secondary spontaneous pneumothorax, *Ann Thorac Surg* 55:372-376, 1966.
26. Rhea JT, Deluca SA, Greene RE: Determining the size of pneumothorax in the upright patient, *Radiology* 144:733, 1982.
27. Bradley M, Williams C, Walshaw MJ: The value of routine expiratory chest films in the diagnosis of pneumothorax, *Arch Emerg Med* 8:115-116, 1991.
28. Seow A et al: Comparison of upright inspiratory and expiratory chest radiographs for detecting pneumothoraces, *AJR* 166:313-316, 1996.
29. Gordon R: The deep sulcus sign, *Radiology* 136:25, 1980.
30. Bourgouin P et al: Computed tomography used to exclude pneumothorax in bullous lung disease, *J Can Assoc Radiol* 36:341-342, 1985.
31. Werne CS, Sands MJ: Left tension pneumothorax masquerading as anterior myocardial infarction, *Ann Emerg Med* 14:164, 1985.
32. Panacek EA et al: Spontaneous pneumomediastinum: clinical and natural history, *Ann Emerg Med* 21:1222, 1992.
33. Kircher LT Jr, Swartzel RL: Spontaneous pneumothorax and its treatment, *JAMA* 155:24, 1954.
34. Northfield TC: Oxygen therapy for spontaneous pneumothorax, *BMJ* 4:86, 1971.
35. Delius RE et al: Catheter aspiration for simple pneumothorax, *Arch Surg* 124:833, 1989.
36. Talbot-Stern J et al: Catheter aspiration for simple pneumothorax, *J Emerg Med* 4:437, 1986.
37. Vallee P et al: Sequential treatment of a simple pneumothorax, *Ann Emerg Med* 5:45, 1988.
38. Soulsby T: British Thoracic Society guidelines for the management of spontaneous pneumothorax: do we comply with them and do they work? *J Accid Emerg Med* 15:317-321. 1998.
39. Martin T et al: Use of pleural catheter for the management of simple pneumothorax, *Chest* 110:1169-1172, 1996.
40. Conces DJ Jr et al: Treatment of pneumothoraces utilizing small caliber chest tubes, *Chest* 94:55-57, 1988.
41. So SY, Yu DYC: Catheter drainage of spontaneous pneumothorax: suction or no suction, early or late removal? *Thorax* 37:46, 1982.
42. Campisi, P, Voitk AJ: Outpatient treatment of spontaneous pneumothorax in a community hospital using a Heimlich flutter valve: a case series, *J Emerg Med* 15:115-119, 1997.
43. Pavlin DJ et al: Reexpansion hypotension: a complication of rapid evacuation of prolonged pneumothorax, *Chest* 89:70-74, 1986.
44. Rozenman J et al: Re-expansion pulmonary edema following spontaneous pneumothorax, *Respir Med* 90:235-238, 1996.
45. Chee CB et al: Persistent air-leak in spontaneous pneumothorax: clinical course and outcome, *Respir Med* 92:757-761, 1998.
46. Schoenenberger RA et al: Timing of invasive procedures in therapy for primary and secondary spontaneous pneumothorax, *Arch Surg* 125: 764-766, 1991.
47. Jain SK, Al-Kattan KM, Hamdy MG: Spontaneous pneumothorax: determinants of surgical intervention, *J Cardiovasc Surg* (Torino) 39:107-111, 1998.
48. Schramel FM, Postmus PE, Vanderschueren RG: Current aspects of spontaneous pneumothorax, *Eur Respir J* 10:1372-1379, 1997.
49. Warner BW, Bailey WW, Shipley RT: Value of computed tomography of the lung in the management of primary spontaneous pneumothorax, *Am J Surg* 162:39-42, 1991.
50. Massard G, Thomas P, Wihlm JM: Minimally invasive management for first and recurrent pneumothorax, *Ann Thorac Surg* 66:592-599, 1998.
51. Marel M et al: The incidence of pleural effusion in a well-defined region: epidemiologic study in central Bohemia, *Chest* 104:1486-1489, 1993.
52. Al-Qorain A et al: Pattern of pleural effusion in eastern province of Saudi Arabia: a prospective study, *East Afr Med J* 71:246-249, 1994.
53. Negus RA, Chachkes JS, Wrenn K: Tension hydrothorax and shock in a patient with a malignant pleural effusion, *Am J Emerg Med* 8:205-207, 1990.
54. Smyrnios NA, Jederlinic PJ, Irwin RS: Pleural effusion in an asymptomatic patient, *Chest* 97:192-196. 1990.
55. Altschule MD: Some neglected aspects of respiratory function in pleural effusions, *Chest* 89:602, 1986.
56. Guarino JR, Guarino JC: Auscultatory percussion: a simple method to detect pleural effusion, *J Gen Intern Med* 9:71-74, 1994.
57. Bhalla A et al: Interobserver variations in clinical signs for diagnosis of pleuritis, *Indian J Med Sci* 51:303-307, 1997.
58. Collins JD et al: Minimum detectable pleural effusion: a roentgen pathology model, *Radiology* 105:51, 1972.
59. Woodring JH: Recognition of pleural effusion on supine radiograph: how much fluid is required? *AJR* 142:59-64, 1984.
60. Henschke CI et al: Pleural effusions: pathogenesis, radiologic evaluation, and therapy, *J Thorac Imag* 4:49, 1989.
61. Hollerman JJ, Simms SM: The contralateral decubitus chest film, *Ann Emerg Med* 15:198, 1986.
62. McCloud TC, Fowler CD: Imaging the pleura: sonography, CT, MR imaging, *AJR* 156:145, 1991.
63. Yu CJ et al: Diagnostic and therapeutic uses of chest sonography: value in critically ill patients, *AJR* 159:695, 1992.
64. Brown SE, Light RW: Pleural effusion associated with pulmonary embolization, *Clin Chest Med* 6:77-81, 1985.
65. Klein RC: Effects of indomethacin on pleural pain, *South Med J* 77:1253, 1984.
66. McVay PA, Toy PT: Lack of increased bleeding after paracentesis and thoracentesis in patients with mild coagulation abnormalities, *Transfusion* 31:164, 1991.
67. Light RW et al: Pleural effusions: the diagnostic separation of transudates and exudates, *Ann Intern Med* 77:507-513, 1972.
68. Light RW: Useful tests on the pleural fluid in the management of patients with pleural effusions, *Curr Opin Pulm Med* 6:245-249, 1999.
69. Roth BJ, O'Meara TF, Cragun WH: The serum-effusion albumin gradient in the evaluation of pleural effusions, *Chest* 98:546-549, 1990.
70. Light RW, Erozan YS, Ball WC: Cells in the pleural fluid: their value in differential diagnosis, *Arch Intern Med* 132:854-880, 1973.
71. Valdes L et al: Tuberculous pleurisy: a study of 254 patients, *Arch Intern Med* 158:2017-2021, 1998.

72. Villena V et al: Interferon-gamma in 388 immunocompromised and immunocompetent patients for diagnosing pleural tuberculosis, *Eur Resp J* 9:2635-2639, 1996.
73. Gourgoulianis KI et al: Benign postpartum pleural effusion, *Eur Respir J* 8:1748-1750, 1995.
74. Light RW, George RB: Incidence and significance of pleural effusion after abdominal surgery, *Chest* 69:621-625, 1976.
75. Ruckdeschel JC: Management of malignant pleural effusion: an overview, *Semin Oncol* 15:24-28, 1988.
76. Teixeira LR, Villarino MA: Antibiotic treatment of patients with pneumonia and pleural effusion, *Curr Opin Pulm Med* 4:230-234, 1998.
77. Fine MJ et al: A prediction rule to identify low-risk patients with community-acquired pneumonia, *N Engl J Med.* 336:243-250, 1997.
78. Storey DD, Dines DE, Coles DT: Pleural effusion: a diagnostic dilemma, *JAMA* 236:2183-2186, 1976.

Section III CARDIAC SYSTEM

73 Acute Ischemic Coronary Syndromes

Tom P. Aufderheide
William J. Brady
W. Brian Gibler

PERSPECTIVE

Although angina pectoris was clearly described in the eighteenth century by Heberden, acute myocardial infarction (AMI) went unrecognized until the early twentieth century. Herrick is generally credited with delineating the clinical features of acute coronary thrombosis by reporting the first case of nonfatal AMI in the United States in 1912. Herrick's important observations attracted little attention until physicians had an objective means of demonstrating that a patient's chest discomfort and associated symptoms were unequivocally cardiac in origin. Einthoven first described the string galvanometer in 1901, and the first electrocardiogram (ECG) was introduced in the United States by Cohn in 1909. The introduction of electrocardiographic precordial leads in 1932 by Wolferth and Wood was a major advance in the electrocardiographic diagnosis of ischemic syndromes. Through the next half century, ischemic heart disease (IHD) was increasingly recognized, but the management of patients with ischemic syndromes changed relatively little. Treatment consisted of pain relief, absolute bed rest for 6 to 8 weeks, prevention of thromboembolism, and treatment of congestive heart failure (CHF). Victims of cardiopulmonary arrest were virtually never resuscitated; cardiopulmonary arrest was viewed as an irreversible event.

Several advances in the 1950s and 1960s drastically changed the strategy for acute coronary care and, subsequently, for emergency medical care. During the 1950s, the development of external defibrillators and cardiac pacemakers by Zoll and others provided physicians with an effective mechanical approach to the treatment of life-threatening dysrhythmias. The introduction of selective coronary arteriography by Sones in 1959 revolutionized the evaluation and management of patients with known or suspected coronary artery disease (CAD). In 1960 Kouwenhoven and colleagues published their method of external cardiac massage, which inaugurated the modern era of cardiopulmonary resuscitation (CPR). Advances in the pharmacologic treatment of dysrhythmias were reported as well.

With the availability of effective treatment for the dysrhythmias that cause high periinfarct mortality came recognition that the time between the onset of life-threatening dysrhythmias and the initiation of therapy was critical. This realization led Day to organize a cardiac arrest team in 1960 and to establish the first coronary care unit (CCU) 2 years later. After the initial year of operation, the mortality rate for AMI was reduced by 50%. Application of the newly introduced mechanical and pharmacologic advances by other coronary units resulted in similar mortality rate reductions.

In recent decades, some pathologists began to question whether thrombotic occlusion of an atherosclerotic coronary artery was the causative factor in AMI. In the 1980s, DeWood et al performed coronary angiography early in the course of AMI and demonstrated that approximately 90% of those patients studied within 4 hours of the onset of symptoms had total coronary occlusion in the infarct-related artery. This report and the early experience of Rentrop with the intracoronary administration of streptokinase in AMI ushered in the era of thrombolytic therapy. Additional experience with primary percutaneous transluminal coronary angioplasty (PTCA) with various pharmacologic agents and intracoronary stenting has only improved the physician's ability to care for the patient with acute ischemic coronary syndrome (AICS) with high degrees of success.

As many as two thirds of sudden deaths from IHD occurred outside the hospital. It became apparent that established effective therapies must be initiated before hypoperfusion and hypoxemia led to irreversible cardiac or cerebral ischemia and death. In 1969, advanced prehospital cardiac care was initiated in Belfast, Ireland, with the use of Pantridge's mobile CCUs. In 1970, Nagel et al reported the successful use and benefits of prehospital telemetry in the emergency medical system of Miami. Single-lead telemetry with online medical control provided the technologic basis for prehospital emergency cardiac care and advanced cardiac life support (ACLS) in patients experiencing dysrhythmias or sudden cardiac death. The success of this approach led to the Emergency Medical Service (EMS) Systems Acts of 1973 and 1976, which provided funding for the national development of EMS systems.

Although single-lead telemetry is diagnostic for dysrhythmia identification, it provides no information on the other two major clinical syndromes of CAD, unstable angina pectoris (USAP) and AMI. In 1986, the introduction of portable prehospital 12-lead ECGs made field diagnosis of ischemic syndromes possible prior to ED arrival. European physician-staffed mobile intensive care units were the first to apply this technology. Similar protocols in the United States have also demonstrated that trained paramedics can accurately and successfully implement prehospital 12-lead ECGs under remote supervision of a physician.

Important changes have occurred in the recent past concerning the diagnosis and treatment of patients with AICS—USAP and AMI. In the 1970s, patients with USAP, suspected AMI, or confirmed AMI were admitted to a CCU for observation and palliative therapy such as nitroglycerin and morphine. Thrombolytic therapy and interventional techniques such as PTCA revolutionized treatment of patients with ST segment elevation (STE) AMI during the 1980s. This revolution in acute reperfusion therapy has made early diagnosis and rapid treatment a substantial challenge for the clinician.

During the past 10 years, considerable effort has been made to improve the diagnostic evaluation of patients with AMI who present with nondiagnostic ECGs, USAP, and the complaint of acute chest pain. Additional investigation, currently in progress, will only improve the diagnostic and therapeutic tools available to the clinician. Diagnostically, much information is still contained within the ECG; among other techniques, computer-assisted interpretations will improve the clinician's ability to manage patients appropriately. Serum markers, alone and in combination with other diagnostic modalities, not only establish the diagnosis but also predict risk and outcome. The chest pain center (CPC), no longer an investigational entity, enables the clinician to effectively and safely evaluate and treat the patient with chest pain and possible AICS using additional tools such as echocardiography, exercise stress testing, and nuclear imaging and electrocardiographic monitoring. The most recent area of activity concerning treatment involves the combination of various reperfusion strategies in addition to various antiplatelet and antithrombotic agents.

Epidemiology

IHD continues to be the leading cause of death among adults in the United States. It accounts for nearly 1 million deaths in the United States annually (nearly 50% of deaths from all causes), including approximately 500,000 deaths from CAD, most of which are sudden deaths. More than 160,000 of these deaths occur before the age of 65 years, and more than one half of all deaths from cardiovascular disease occur in women. Coronary artery heart disease is a major cause of morbidity and mortality in women beyond their middle to late fifties. It has been estimated that more than 5 million years of potential life are lost annually in the United States due to cardiovascular disease.

A significant reduction in age-adjusted mortality from CAD has been noted in the United States over the past 40 years.[1,2] In large part, the decline in death rate from CAD has been accompanied by a diminished mortality from AMI. This fall in the mortality appears to be caused by two new factors: a reduction in the incidence of AMI by 25% and a similarly sharp drop in the case fatality rate once an AMI has occurred. The reasons for this decline in mortality are multiple. According to some estimates, more healthful lifestyles have undoubtedly played a role, along with significant advances in medical treatment including prehospital resuscitation, CCUs, improved treatment of left ventricular failure and shock, and the advent of thrombolytic therapy.

Despite advances, there is still much room for progress. In the 1990s, 3.6 million people were hospitalized with an initial discharge diagnosis of heart disease and approximately 675,000 with a diagnosis of AMI. Forty-five percent of all AMIs occur in people under 65 years of age. Based on 1989 statistics, an estimated 6.2 million Americans have significant CAD. Many of these people are at increased risk for sudden death or AMI. Approximately two thirds of sudden deaths from CAD take place outside the hospital and usually occur within 2 hours after onset of symptoms. It is possible that a large number of these deaths can be prevented by improving the ability to provide rapid entry into the EMS system, prompt provision of CPR, early defibrillation, and rapid treatment with reperfusion therapy when appropriate.

PRINCIPLES OF DISEASE

Physiology

AICSs can be defined as the spectrum of myocardial ischemia through myocardial necrosis, including stable angina, USAP, and AMI. Stable angina pectoris is defined as transient, episodic chest discomfort resulting from myocardial ischemia. This discomfort is typically predictable and reproducible, with the frequency of attacks constant over time. Physical exercise or intense emotional periods may provoke an attack of angina that resolves over a certain, predictable period spontaneously, with rest, or with nitroglycerin. Fixed, stenotic atherosclerotic coronary artery lesions are believed to be responsible for these symptoms, because a reduction in usual coronary artery blood flow results in chest discomfort. The Canadian Cardiovascular Society Classification for angina is defined as follows: Class I–ordinary physical activity; Class II–slight limitation of normal activity: angina occurs with walking, climbing stairs, or emotional stress; Class III–severe limitation of ordinary physical activity: angina occurs on walking one or two blocks on a level surface or climbing one flight of stairs in normal conditions; and Class IV–inability to carry on any physical activity without discomfort: anginal symptoms may be present at rest.

USAP is broadly defined from the perspective of the following features: development (i.e., new-onset event or recurrence of past issue), duration, provocation, pattern, and magnitude. Rest angina is defined as angina occurring at rest, lasting longer than 20 minutes, and occurring within 1 week of the ED visit. New-onset angina is angina of at least class III severity with onset during the last 2 months. Increasing or progressive angina is diagnosed when it becomes more frequent, longer in duration, or increased by one class within the last 2 months and is of at least class III severity. Symptoms that last longer than 20 minutes are consistent with unstable angina. USAP has also been termed crescendo angina, preinfarction angina, intermediate coronary syndrome, and preocclusive syndrome. USAP should be considered the harbinger of AMI, and hence should be treated and evaluated aggressively. If a patient with a diagnosis of angina comes to the ED, the presumption of USAP should be made by the clinician until a thorough clinical history and examination by the emergency physician reliably determines otherwise.

Variant angina, or Prinzmetal's angina, is caused by coronary artery vasospasm at rest with minimal CAD; it can sometimes be relieved by exercise or nitroglycerin. The ECG will reveal STE that is impossible to discern from AMI electrocardiographically and, at times, clinically.

AMI is defined as myocardial necrosis. Consideration for the diagnosis of AMI requires two of the following three World Health Organization (WHO) criteria: clinical history (usually more than 20 minutes of chest discomfort or equivalent symptom consistent with ischemia), electrocardiographic changes, and/or positive myocardial serum testing.[3] AMI may present electrocardiographically with both STE (the so-called *STE AMI*) and other electrocardiographic abnormalities, such as T wave inversion and ST segment depression (the so-called *non-STE AMI*). In the recent past, AMI was separated into Q wave and non-Q wave events. The former was felt to involve a transmural process that initially caused STE and resulted in significant myocardial necrosis if the process was unchecked. The latter was defined as a nontransmural, or subendocardial, process that manifested electrocardiographic changes other than STE and resulted in smaller portions of infarcted myocardium; the diagnosis of the non-Q wave AMI was made by positive serum markers. More recent research has suggested that the descriptors transmural and Q wave are misnomers in that they fail to adequately describe the coronary event, related pathophysiology, electrocardiographic findings, and pathologic outcome. The terms STE and non-STE AMI are best used today. This phraseology defines the process more appropriately from the clinician's perspective, particularly so when one considers therapeutic indications of the various reperfusion and adjunctive strategies available to the clinician.

Pathophysiology

Thrombus formation is considered an integral factor in all forms of AICS, including USAP, non-STE AMI, and STE AMI. All of these syndromes are initiated by endothelial damage, usually by atherosclerotic plaque disruption, which leads to platelet aggregation and thrombus formation. The resulting thrombus can occlude more than 50% of the vessel lumen. Vessel occlusion can lead to myocardial ischemia, hypoxia, acidosis, and eventually infarction. The consequences of the occlusion depend on the extent of the thrombotic process, the characteristics of the preexisting plaque, and the availability of collateral circulation. Coronary arteries of patients with AICS tend to have eccentric, ragged, irregular walls and nearly occluded lumens. The wide variety of clinical pictures of patients with complete coronary artery occlusion suggests marked differences in the rate of development of total occlusion, the amount of collateral circulation, or both.

Another important aspect of AICS is vasospasm. After significant thrombotic occlusion, local mediators induce vasospasm, which further compromises blood flow. Central and sympathetic nervous system input increases as α-receptors proliferate within minutes of the occlusion. Unopposed α-sympathetic stimulation can result in more coronary vasospasm. Coronary artery spasm with subsequent thrombus formation and without significant underlying CAD is involved in approximately 10% of AMIs and can precipitate sudden cardiac death. This mechanism may be more prevalent during USAP and other coronary syndromes that do not result in infarction. Sympathetic stimulation by endogenous hormones such as epinephrine and serotonin may also result in increased platelet aggregation and neutrophil-mediated vasoconstriction.

Further myocardial injury at the cellular level occurs during the reperfusion phase, either by spontaneous or therapeutically induced thrombolysis. In particular, the introduction of calcium, oxygen, and cellular elements into ischemic myocardium can lead to irreversible myocardial damage that causes reperfusion injury, prolonged ventricular dysfunction (known as *myocardial stunning*), or reperfusion dysrhythmias. Neutrophils probably play an important role in reperfusion injury by occluding capillary lumens, decreasing blood flow, accelerating the inflammatory response, and resulting in the production of chemoattractants, proteolytic enzymes, and reactive oxygen species.

CLINICAL FEATURES

Prehospital Evaluation

Prehospital patients with a history consistent with AICS should be assumed to be having an AMI until proven otherwise. Chest pain itself is a poor predictor of the prehospital diagnosis of AMI; diaphoresis in the patient with chest pain, however, is very suggestive of AMI.[4] Also, the presence of complete heart block on prehospital rhythm strips is strongly associated with AMI.[5] Traditional EMS protocols for management of patients with chest pain include immediate vital signs, a brief history and physical examination, administration of oxygen, establishment of an intravenous line, and initiation of cardiac monitoring. Persistent chest pain should be treated with either nitroglycerin (0.2 mg SL) or morphine sulfate (2 to 4 mg IV) if the systolic blood pressure is greater than 90 mm Hg. Oral aspirin therapy is also recommended in the prehospital patient with possible AICS. Additional prehospital therapies for the complications of AICS, including dysrhythmia, are discussed elsewhere.

Recognizing the importance of rapid identification and treatment of AMI and advances in technology have influenced prehospital emergency cardiac care. Prehospital 12-lead ECG is one important new development. Although patients having AMIs delay an average of 2 to 6 hours before seeking health care, patients who use the EMS system represent a subgroup who obtain care quickly (median time 60 minutes). Paramedics can accurately identify thrombolytic candidates with a 12-lead ECG in an average of 3 to 5 minutes' addition to the scene time, which provides a diagnosis 47 minutes earlier than for patients diagnosed in the ED.[6] Other studies have shown that when 12-lead ECGs are transmitted prior to arrival at the hospital, thrombolytic treatment is initiated up to 55 minutes earlier, highlighting the interaction of prehospital and ED care.

Emergency Department

The history remains the cornerstone in the assessment of the patient with suspected myocardial ischemia. Many studies have shown that patients with classic features for ischemia, such as pressure-like discomfort, radiation of discomfort, diaphoresis, and male gender, have a high likelihood for AICS despite an initially normal or nondiagnostic 12-lead ECG.[7,8] Advances in cardiovascular diagnostic testing, therefore, continue to remain adjuncts to a carefully acquired history. In fact, the history and the clinician's interpretation of this history should be prioritized and primarily guide the physician's clinical decision making. The clinician should obtain information regarding the onset and evolution of symptoms (their location, quality, intensity, duration, and precipitating and alleviating factors), associated symptoms, and response to any therapeutic interventions. A carefully acquired and valuable history takes time; no other technique is as important as taking whatever time is necessary to establish a firm clinical impression, an impression that will minimize the need for ancillary testing and reliably guide the clinician with continued diagnostic evaluation and patient disposition.

Personal habits such as cigarette smoking, alcohol intake, and use of illicit drugs such as cocaine should be ascertained. Risk factors that increase the likelihood for atherosclerosis and IHD—family history, cigarette smoking, hypertension, hypercholesterolemia, and diabetes mellitus (DM)—should be sought. There has been controversy over whether the so-called *"coronary risk factors"* (e.g., hypertension, hypercholesterolemia, smoking, DM, male gender, age) should be weighed significantly in the emergency physician's triage decisions. An early report[9] suggested that such factors, which were initially derived because of their ability to predict the development of coronary atherosclerosis and its complications over decades, have minimal predictive value as to whether a patient who comes to the ED will develop an AMI and its complications over the next several days. However, this study included the ECG in the multiple regression analysis. The power of an abnormal ECG in effect overwhelmed any measurable short-term predictive value of the risk factors. More recent analysis done on patients coming to the ED with signs or symptoms suggesting AICS but with a normal or nondiagnostic ECG indicates that the coronary risk factors, in fact, do have significant predictive value and should be considered in the decision-making process.[10]

Artificial or early menopause and the use of contraceptive pills may increase the likelihood of IHD in women. A history of AMI or chronic IHD, along with previous cardiac testing such as 12-lead ECGs, treadmill test, radionuclide study, or cardiac catheterization, should be obtained. If a patient already carries a known diagnosis of IHD, a risk factor analysis is unnecessary because the risk is known to be 100%.

Angina pectoris by definition includes a sense of choking, strangulation, or constriction. Common descriptions of the discomfort, therefore, usually include not pain but sensations of pressure, squeezing, fullness, burning, or heaviness "like someone is sitting on my chest." In fact, the patient may actually deny the presence of pain but, *when asked by the clinician,* will relate a history of pressure or tightness. If the sensation is described as pain, its character is usually dull or aching rather than sharp or stabbing. Caution is advised with the interpretation of the descriptor "sharp." Certain geographic and ethnic groups use the word sharp to denote a rapid onset of the pain or a severe nature of the discomfort; most clinicians equate sharp with a pleuritic pain syndrome. In some patients, the symptoms are perceived as gastrointestinal and are reported as "gas" or "indigestion." The classic location for angina is substernal and in the left chest. The discomfort often occurs concurrently in or radiates to the shoulders, neck, mandible, and arms. The left side is more commonly involved, particularly the ulnar aspect of the left arm; patients with USAP and AMI may also complain of pain in the right chest radiating to the right shoulder and arm. Many patients experience associated symptoms such as dyspnea, diaphoresis, nausea, vomiting, dizziness, and anxiety during an anginal attack. See Table 73-1 for the clinical characteristics of angina.

The quality of chest discomfort has been variably reported as correlating with angina pectoris and AMI. One study of adult patients with chest pain in the ED notes that "crushing, pressure, tightness, heaviness, or similar discomfort" is frequently associated with acute coronary ischemic events; in fact, 24% of these patients had AMI and another 30% had USAP.[11] Of patients who described chest discomfort as "burning or indigestion," 23% had AMI, and another 21% had USAP.[11] Of those who described a "chest ache," 13% had an infarction. Five percent of patients who described a "sharp or stabbing" discomfort ultimately were diagnosed with AMI, while another 17% of patients using the same descriptors had USAP.[11] Others report that 54% of adult patients with AMI complained of a "dull, pressure-like" discomfort, whereas 19% of patients with an infarction had a "sharp or pleuritic" discomfort.[12]

Because angina is a visceral sensation that is poorly defined and localized, some patients may have an anginal equivalent syndrome. Patients experiencing myocardial ischemia may complain only of dyspnea and associated discomfort limited to areas of secondary radiation such as the ulnar aspect of the left arm, lower jaw, teeth, neck, or shoulders; the development of gas and belching, nausea, indigestion, dizziness, weakness, or diaphoresis may also be encountered. The pattern and presence of exacerbating and relieving factors are the same for anginal equivalents as for angina. Patients with altered cardiac pain perception (e.g., the elderly or patients with long-standing DM) are at risk to have anginal equivalent syndromes or even asymptomatic "silent ischemia."

The duration of chest pain or discomfort is important in determining its cause. Angina pectoris generally lasts from several to 15 minutes. Patients with AMIs generally experience more than 15 to 20 minutes of discomfort. Intermittent, sharp, lancinating, localized chest discomfort lasting less than several seconds usually is not coronary in origin. Chest discomfort lasting for hours may be seen with AMI, pericarditis, aortic dissection, esophageal disease, musculoskeletal chest wall pain, herpes zoster, or functional chest pain.

Table 73-1. Clinical Characteristics of Angina

Characteristic	More likely to be angina	Less likely to be angina
Type of pain	Dull, pressure	Sharp, stabbing
Duration	2 to 5 min, always <15-20 min	Seconds or hours
Onset	Gradual	Rapid
Location	Substernal	Lateral chest wall, back
Reproducible	With exertion	With inspiration
Associated symptoms	Present	Absent
Palpation of chest wall	Not painful	Painful, exactly reproduces pain complaint

Modified from Zink BJ: Angina and unstable angina. In Gibler WB, Aufderheide TP, editors: *Emergency cardiac care,* St Louis, 1994, Mosby.

Angina pectoris is classically precipitated by exertion, a large meal, a cold environment, or emotional stress. An exception is Prinzmetal's variant angina, which characteristically occurs at rest. The pattern of symptoms should also be explored carefully. A history that reveals symptoms precipitated by decreasing levels of exertion, increased frequency of symptoms, greater intensity or duration of symptoms, or onset of symptoms at rest is consistent with AICS. Patients with known CAD may have ischemic symptoms precipitated by use of illicit drugs such as cocaine or the development of hypoxic conditions such as pneumonia or pulmonary embolism.

Symptoms classically associated with myocardial ischemia or infarction include nausea, vomiting, diaphoresis, and shortness of breath. Nausea, vomiting, and diaphoresis result from significant sympathetic stimulation caused by the severe pain usually associated with USAP and AMI. Dyspnea is an uncomfortable sensation of air hunger, which occurs at rest or at a level of physical activity not expected to cause this symptom. In patients with large AMIs, dyspnea is the clinical expression of pulmonary venous and capillary engorgement resulting from variable decreases in left ventricular output. Although dyspnea may occur suddenly with acute onset of left ventricular dysfunction, sudden development of dyspnea may also result from pulmonary embolism, pneumothorax, chronic obstructive pulmonary disease (COPD) exacerbation, pneumonia, CHF, or airway obstruction. Patients may have no chest discomfort, noting only an anginal equivalent complaint such as nausea, vomiting, diaphoresis, and dyspnea; these symptoms, rather than chest pain, are felt to represent angina—hence the term *anginal equivalent complaint.* In a recent large survey of 434,877 confirmed AMIs, a significant minority of these individuals (approximately 30%) lacked chest pain, noting only the anginal equivalent complaint of dyspnea.[13]

The symptoms of angina pectoris usually improve dramatically within 2 to 5 minutes after rest or nitroglycerin. If more than 10 minutes transpire before relief, the diagnosis of angina is suspect and consideration of USAP, AMI, or a noncardiac diagnosis should be considered. Although nitroglycerin usually relieves the discomfort of stable angina, it also relieves symptoms of diffuse esophageal spasm and other esophageal disorders. Caution is also advised in the patient with chest pain who appears to respond to antacid administration; over-reliance on this response as a major reason in "ruling out" AICS is not encouraged.

Physical Examination The physical examination, although crucial to many life-threatening disease processes, is often not helpful in diagnosing AICS unless the patient has frank cardiac dysfunction—manifested by acute CHF with or without cardiogenic shock. Change in mental status, poor peripheral perfusion, diaphoresis, rales, jugular venous distention, and S_3 and S_4 heart sounds often provide evidence of significant myocardial dysfunction in AMI. Investigators have noted rales in 38% and a third heart sound in 17% of patients with AMI. These physical findings, however, are noted in patients without acute coronary events; for example, one large study noted rales in 18% and a third heart sound in 5% of patients without infarction.[12] Patients in the ED with evidence of myocardial dysfunction including S_3 heart sound, S_4 heart sound, or rales are at much greater risk for adverse cardiovascular events, including nonfatal AMI, death, stroke with deficit, life-threatening dysrhythmia, and the requirement for cardiac surgery.

Caution should be exercised when attributing a chest wall source for pain based on palpation or movement. To safely relate the chest discomfort to a chest wall problem, the pain must be described as sharp or stabbing (i.e., pleuritic in nature) and be completely reproducible by palpation.[11] Up to 15% of patients with AMI have tenderness on chest wall palpation.[12] Careful questioning of the patient may reveal that the pain caused by chest wall palpation is different than the sensation that caused the patient to come to the hospital.

Atypical Features of AMI

Atypical features of AMI are encountered in approximately 10% to 30% of AMI cases[13-18]; the factors contributing to this diagnostic challenge include patient age, alternate chief complaints, atypical discomfort, and certain comorbid states. See Table 73-2 for a listing of the various symptoms of AMI.

Non-Chest Pain Chief Complaint Anginal equivalent complaints, which occur in the setting of the painless AMI, classically include dyspnea, diaphoresis, nausea, and emesis. Other anginal equivalent symptoms to consider are cough, palpitations, and anxiety. The most frequently encountered anginal equivalent chief complaint is dyspnea, which is found in 10% to 30% of patients with AMI, often due to pulmonary edema.[13-15] Isolated emesis and diaphoresis are quite rare.[14,15] The geriatric patient may also have an atypical clinical picture with acute weakness (3% to 8%) and syncope (3% to 5%).[16] Unexplained sinus tachycardia, bronchospasm resulting from cardiogenic asthma, and new-onset lower extremity edema have all been reported as anginal equivalent symptoms for AMI, particularly in older individuals. Anginal equivalent syndromes typically involve neurologic problems with acute mental status abnormalities and stroke among the very elderly. From the perspective of acute delirium, less than 1% of such patients in an ED population with altered mentation will be found to have AMI. Less pronounced mental status abnormalities, including both confusion and lethargy, are classically reported findings in the elderly patient with AMI and are described in approximately 5% of cases. AMI associated with acute stroke is noted in approximately 5% to 9% of patients, usually over age 60 years.[16]

Atypical Pain Syndromes When discomfort or another painful sensation is noted as the complaint resulting from AMI, it may be atypical from a number of different perspectives. The patient may complain of epigastric, jaw, neck, arm, or back discomfort—pain in an atypical location. Further, the unpleasant feeling may be perceived as a sharp sensation or have a burning quality, representing an atypical description of discomfort. Lastly, the discomfort may be reproducible on palpation, illustrating an atypical examination. The discomfort may be located in non-chest portions of the body. In certain cases, the discomfort is experienced only in the epigastric, anterior neck, jaw, or left upper extremity area. While not the classic clinical picture of an AICS, these symptoms usually do not challenge the clinician's diagnostic ability; in the appropriate patient, such pain distributions are suggestive of AICS. The discomfort may be located in the back, posterior neck, and right arm in the rare patient, potentially suggesting another explanation for the unpleasant

Table 73-2. Symptoms of Acute Myocardial Infarctions

Symptom	Bayer et al[a,b]	Tinker[c]	Uretsky et al[d]	Pathy[e]
Typical				
Chest pain	515	51	75	75
Atypical				
Dyspnea	118	19	14	77
Syncope	72	4	1	27
Confusion	46	1		51
Stroke	32	6		26
Fatigue	36	2	4	10
Nausea/emesis	28		1	10
Sudden death				31
Giddiness	18	3		22
Diaphoresis	18			2
Arterial embolus	3			19
Palpitation	4			14
Renal failure				11
Pulmonary embolus				8
Restlessness				4
Abdominal pain			5	
Arm pain only			1	
Cough			1	
Silent				
No symptoms	17	1		
Total	**777[a]**	**87[f]**	**102[g]**	**387[f]**

Modified from Scott PA et al: *Am J Emerg Med* 9:547, 1991.
[a]Patients able to report multiple symptoms; therefore, total exceeds 777.
[b]Bayer AJ et al: *J Am Geriatr Soc* 34:263, 1986.
[c]Tinker GM: *Age Ageing* 10:237, 1981.
[d]Uretsky BF et al: *Am J Cardiol* 40:498, 1977.
[e]Pathy MS: *Br Heart J* 29:190, 1967.
[f]Patients classified by principal symptom although all patients with complaint of chest or epigastric discomfort were placed in typical group.
[g]Same as [f] except patients with epigastric complaints were placed in atypical group.

sensation; other highly unusual clinical pictures include cephalalgia as well as hip and lower back pain.

The actual description of the chest discomfort ranges from the classic "crushing, heaviness, pressure-like" to the atypical "sharp, knife-like." If one considers all patients entering the ED with typical complaints such as crushing or pressure-like, only slightly more than half experience AICS (of those, approximately 50% are having AMIs and 50% USAP).[11] The remainder of patients are found to have gastrointestinal, pulmonary, and musculoskeletal diagnoses. Chest discomfort is described as "burning" or "indigestion-like" in an adult ED population with chest pain found to have AMI in 23% and USAP in 21%.[11] Interestingly, patients may relate a favorable response to the infamous "GI cocktail" in a minority of cases of AMI who complain of a burning chest discomfort; caution is advised in using the response to antacid as sole datum for ruling out AICS. Patients note "sharp," "knife-like," or pleuritic pain in a small minority of instances due to AICS.[12] During the physical examination, which frequently is unremarkable in patients with AMI, chest wall tenderness may lead the clinician away from the true diagnosis in up to 15% of confirmed cases.[11,12]

The Young Patient The clinician may feel that the patient is too young to be experiencing AMI. While most AMIs occur in patients over age 40 years, a not insignificant minority of them are encountered in this relatively young group. The vast majority of patients will manifest typical features of AMI and exhibit similar rates of both diagnostic and nondiagnostic ECGs. The young adult cocaine abuser may complain of chest discomfort and deny illicit substance use; clearly, such a patient with an atypical chest complaint, a normal examination, and an unremarkable ECG may be inadvertently discharged from the ED with ultimate AMI. The primary point here is that AMI does strike the young patient; the physician must not rule out the possibility prior to a thorough, reasoned evaluation—i.e., a history, physical examination, and 12-lead ECG.

The Elderly Patient Advanced age almost always impacts the clinician's ability to evaluate the patient and assess for the potential of AMI. For example, in one large autopsy series of elderly patients, the correct diagnosis of AMI was made in fewer than one half of the patients prior to death; the very elderly constituted a large portion of this group of patients with the postmortem diagnosis of myocardial infarction. As a patient ages, a multitude of factors—including autonomic neuropathy, injury to cardiac sensory afferent nerves due to past IHD, cortical failure resulting from cerebrovascular or other CNS disease, extensive comorbidity, higher pain thresholds, and pre-existing mental status abnormalities—all contribute to a higher rate of atypical symptoms and medically unrecognized AMI. These various factors combine and cause clinically an increased prevalence among the geriatric populace of anginal equivalent chief complaints, "silent" myocardial infarction, and a preponderance of neurologic syndromes.

The clinical picture of AMI in the elderly is frequently nonclassical; atypical symptoms are encountered with increasing frequency in sequentially older populations.[16] In elderly patients less than age 85 years, chest pain becomes less frequent while equivalent complaints are noted more often. Stroke, weakness, and altered mentation became more common with increasing age, frequently without chest discomfort. Chest pain and typical findings, however, are nonetheless found in the majority of cases in the "younger" elderly population (i.e., less than age 85 years). Over age 85 years, atypical features are the norm and should be anticipated. The incidence of painless AMI increases dramatically with age in that 60% to 70% of elderly infarct patients over age 85 years will arrive in the ED with an anginal equivalent complaint or syndrome, most often with a change in the mental status. The elderly also seek treatment frequently for complications of AMI rather than the actual symptoms of the acute ischemic event. For example, very elderly patients seen for new-onset, unexplained CHF should be screened for acute ischemia. Similarly, the elderly patient who suffers from malignant bradycardia, atrioventricular (AV) block, or ventricular dysrhythmia should be assessed for AMI while appropriate therapies and other evaluations are performed.[16]

The Diabetic Patient Patients with DM suffer AMI more often than the general population; they also experience AMI at an earlier age with both more frequent atypical manifestations and the more common unrecognized AMI—unrecognized by patients, family members, and health care providers. Medically unrecognized AMI is felt to occur in approximately 40% of patients with DM compared to the 25% rate for the nondiabetic population.[17] Autopsy studies have demonstrated that myocardial scar without an antemortem diagnosis of AMI—indicative of the medically unattended, past infarct—is three times more frequent in the diabetic than the nondiabetic population. The medical and legal literature discussing the missed AMI frequently cites a history of DM as a risk factor for an unrecognized event; in fact, DM is often implicated in legal cases as a medical factor leading to the error in diagnosis. As with the elderly patient, numerous factors contribute to atypical manifestations of acute IHD in the diabetic patient, including polyneuropathy, altered perception of cardiac pain, and extensive comorbidity.

The diabetic patient's abnormal perception of myocardial infarction may lead to atypical or less impressive symptoms of AMI. Accurate diagnosis based on history, the primary tool available to the clinician, is therefore made much more difficult. Atypical symptoms such as dyspnea, confusion, fatigue, and emesis may be the initial complaint in up to 40% of diabetics having an AMI. The diabetic may also experience more frequently the less-than-classic pain syndromes, including discomfort in unusual locations and with abnormal descriptions. All of the features mentioned reduce numbers of patients who receive adequate medical care. The patient may believe that the pain or the abnormal sensation likely results from some other malady, and therefore may not consult a physician at all or until later in the event. Or, if the patient does seek medical attention, the complaint may be such that the physician is unaware of the actual diagnosis, leading to an inappropriate disposition and therapies.

Outcome of Patients with Atypical Presentations The prognosis for patients with AMI having atypical presentations is typically worse than for patients with classic, typical symptoms. A threefold increased mortality for patients with atypical complaints is seen; a 50% mortality rate in the patient with atypical AMI is noted compared to an 18% rate in those with classical descriptions of chest discomfort; cardiogenic shock is the chief cause of death in these patients with unusual AMI symptoms, followed by myocardial rupture and dysrhythmias.[15] A large survey of patients with AMI without chest pain reported that they were often diagnosed at a later time and less often received early reperfusion therapy; their medical outcome, understandably, was less favorable than that of those patients who had chest pain.[13] Advanced age with associated comorbidity is considered a contributing factor for the increased mortality of the group with atypical clinical pictures in this study. In addition, failure to seek immediate treatment and delayed diagnosis can reduce the use of thrombolytic therapy for these individuals, which will also increase mortality.[13,15] These patients less often receive other important, mortality reducing adjunctive therapies as well—aspirin, heparin, and β-blockade. The Framingham study demonstrates an increased long-term mortality rate for unrecognized infarctions; a 10-year 45% mortality rate was observed for patients with unrecognized infarctions, and individuals with symptoms had a 39% mortality rate.

The characteristics of patients with AICS who are released from the ED and subsequently progress to AMI are of great interest. Multiple studies document that 2% to 10% of patients with chest discomfort and AMI are unintentionally released from the ED.[19,20] Based on an estimate of 800,000 patients admitted with AMI each year in the United States and a 5% unintentional release rate, approximately 40,000 patients will be released from the ED with undiagnosed AMI. These patients represent considerable risk for potential liability; it has been estimated that approximately 20% of the malpractice dollars awarded for emergency care in the United States are related to the emergent diagnosis and treatment of acute ischemic coronary disease.

In one study group, 4% of patients with undiagnosed AMI released from the ED were significantly younger, had atypical symptomatology, and were less likely than a control group of patients with AMI to have electrocardiographic evidence of ischemia or infarction.[21] Mortality for the group released from the ED tended to be higher than for those admitted, postulated to be due to a return to normal activity rather than bed rest. In this study, improved ECG reading skills and the admission to the CCU of patients with obvious ischemic pain at rest could have correctly diagnosed 49% of the patients with missed AMI.[21]

From another study population with a 9% release rate for AMI, three of five patients released from the ED were young men between 30 and 45 years of age with nonspecific clinical and electrocardiographic findings. A large multicenter study finds a 2.9% release rate from the ED for patients with AMI. Improved ECG reading skills would have decreased the number of patients with AMI released from the ED.[19] A recently published large investigation reported a 2.1% rate of unintentional ED release of patients with AMI and a similar rate of 2.3% for those with USAP.[20] Factors associated with unrecognized AICS were female gender below age 55 years, nonwhite race, and either a normal or nondiagnostic ECG. Patients with AICS who were inadvertently discharged from the ED had considerably higher rates of poor outcome compared to admitted patients. As with other studies, misinterpretation of the patient's history and of the ECG contributed heavily to the misdiagnosis.

A review of closed-claim data from two insurance companies revealed a study group of 65 patients with AMI undiagnosed in the ED.[22] Per patient insurance losses averaged $113,806 with a standard deviation of $178,330. Study patients compared with concurrent controls are younger, have atypical symptoms, and have fewer ECGs diagnostic for AMI. Physicians responsible for the care of these patients have less experience in the ED, tend to document histories less clearly, admit fewer patients to the hospital, and have difficulty interpreting ECGs.

DIAGNOSTIC STRATEGIES

Electrocardiogram

The electrocardiogram is used to establish the diagnosis of AICS or other noncoronary ailment, select appropriate therapy, determine the response to ED-delivered treatments, determine the correct inpatient disposition location, and predict risk of cardiovascular complications and death. In the case of AMI with STE, reperfusion treatments and other therapies must be considered urgently. Conversely, in the instance of the patient with chest pain demonstrating STE resulting from a noninfarction syndrome, the correct diagnosis must be made not only to offer appropriate management for that particular illness but to avoid the incorrect application of potentially dangerous therapies such as thrombolysis. The clinician may also use the ECG to monitor the response to treatment in the patient with acute ischemic coronary syndromes. For example, thrombolytic therapy has been reported to cause more rapid resolution of STE.

The initial ED 12-lead ECG may be a helpful guide for determination of cardiovascular risk and, as such, the choice of in-hospital admission location. Brush et al[23] have classified initial ECGs into high- and low-risk groups. The low-risk electrocardiographic group had absolutely normal ECGs, nonspecific ST segment–T wave (NSSTTW) changes, or no change when compared with a previous ECG. High-risk ECGs had significant abnormality or confounding pattern—such as pathologic Q waves, ischemic ST segment or T wave changes, left ventricular hypertrophy (LVH), left bundle branch block (LBBB), or ventricular paced rhythm (VPR). Patients with initial ECGs classified as low risk have a 14% incidence of AMI, 0.6% incidence of life-threatening complications, and a 0% mortality rate. Patients with initial ECGs classified as high risk have a 42% incidence of AMI, 14% life-threatening complications, and 10% mortality rate. Another approach to risk prediction involves a simple calculation of the number of electrocardiographic leads with ST segment deviation (elevation or depression), with an increasing number of abnormal leads being associated with higher risk. Along similar lines, the clinician is also able to qualitatively predict risk with a summation of the total millivolts of ST segment deviation; once again, higher totals are associated with greater risk.

Limitations of Electrocardiogram From the perspective of the electrocardiographic diagnosis of AMI, the ECG has numerous shortcomings, including the "normal" and "nondiagnostic" interpretations, confounding and evolving AMI patterns, the non-STE AMI, confounding and mimicking patterns, and the isolated acute posterior wall AMI. The ECG that provides clear evidence of acute ischemia without obvious infarct—clearly not a diagnostic dilemma—is encountered in approximately 50% of patients found to have AMI. The remaining patients represent the potential electrocardiographic diagnostic dilemma group. Within this segment of patients, the ECG may be entirely normal, nonspecifically abnormal, or clearly abnormal yet without pathologic STE indicative of AMI. Refer to Table 73-3 for a review of the electrocardiographic findings in the patient with chest pain and the association with ultimate diagnosis.

In a classic study of adult patients with chest pain managed in the ED, Lee and colleagues[11] found that approximately 20% of such patients had an absolutely normal 12-lead electrocardiogram. The description "absolutely normal" translates into the absence of NSSTTW, AV block, intraventricular conduction delay, repolarization changes, and rhythms other than sinus rhythm. The final hospital diagnoses of this group of patients with chest pain and a normal 12-lead ECG in the ED included numerous gastrointestinal, musculoskeletal, and pulmonary syndromes, as expected; this group also included a minority of patients with the final hospital diagnoses of USAP (4%) and AMI (1%). A not insignificant minority of patients with chest pain and an absolutely normal ECG were ultimately found to have AICS. Similar issues have been reported[7] demonstrating that patients with a normal ECG and classic symptoms of angina are at risk of AICS, with 3% of patients having a final hospital diagnosis of AMI. The clinical history must be relied upon heavily in patients with either normal or nonspecifically abnormal ECGs

Table 73-3. ECG Findings in Adult Patient with Chest Pain: Association with Ischemic Events

Interpretation	Total	MI	USAP	Other
		Number of patients* (%)		
Normal (95)	114	1 (1)	5 (4)	108
Nonspecific ST or T wave changes (75)	150	4 (3)	34 (23)	112
Abnormal but not diagnostic of ischemia	72	3 (4)	15 (21)	54 (75)
Ischemia, strain, or infarction, but changes known to be old	60	4 (7)	29 (48)	27 (45)
Ischemia or strain not known to be old	114	29 (25)	49 (43)	36 (32)
Probable MI	86	63 (73)	11 (13)	12 (14)
Total	**596**	**104**	**143**	**349**

Modified from Aufderheide TP, Brady WJ: Electrocardiography in the patient with myocardial ischemia or infarction. In Gibler WB, Aufderheide TP, editors: *Emergency cardiac care,* St Louis, 1994, Mosby; and Lee TH et al: *Arch Intern Med* 145:65, 1985.
*$p < .001$.

and a convincing description of ischemic chest discomfort. Management and disposition decisions must be made based upon the history and not on the nondiagnostic study.

The ECG may be described as "nondiagnostic" if NSSTTW changes are noted. These nonspecific changes are defined as less than 1 millimeter of ST segment depression (STD) or STE with or without abnormal morphology, and blunted, flattened, or biphasic T waves without obvious inversion or hyperacuity. Other electrocardiographic abnormalities that may produce nondiagnostic changes are sinus tachycardia and bradycardia, or artifact such as a wandering or irregular baseline. Lee et al[11] noted that adult patients with chest pain and nonspecific or other nondiagnostic electrocardiographic features had a relatively low risk of AMI ranging from 3% to 4%, but a significant risk of USAP, which occurred in approximately one fifth of all such cases. Other investigators have found that approximately 6% of patients with AMI demonstrate a "nonspecifically abnormal" initial ECG.

Additionally, it has been shown that over-reliance on a normal or nonspecifically abnormal ECG in a patient with anginal chest pain who is currently pain free—due either to spontaneous resolution or medical therapy—should be avoided. Patients with an initially nondiagnostic ECG who later develop AMI during that hospitalization more often are pain free or minimally uncomfortable when they arrive; these patients frequently lack a history of IHD. Further, the total elapsed time from chest pain onset in patients with normal ECGs does not assist in ruling out the possibility of AMI with a single electrocardiographic observation. Although the negative predictive value is quite high, it is not 100% even up to 12 hours after the onset of chest discomfort.[24] Once again, the patient's history of the event is more helpful in determining ED disposition, particularly if pain is absent when the ECG is obtained.

Alternatively, in a somewhat different application of the term, the nondiagnostic ECG is initially encountered in approximately 50% of patients ultimately found to have experienced AMI. With this use of the descriptor nondiagnostic, the clinician is referring to the lack of pathologic STE noted on the ECG. Significant STD or T wave changes may be seen in these situations, findings certainly suggestive of an active coronary ischemic event.

The electrocardiographic abnormalities associated with AMI may be masked by the altered patterns of ventricular conduction encountered in patients with confounding patterns; classically these patterns include LBBB, VPR, and LVH. These patterns may obscure or mimic the typical electrocardiographic findings of AMI. Common medical opinion holds that the electrocardiographic diagnosis of AMI is difficult to impossible in the presence of such findings when, in fact, this diagnosis is at times straightforward when the physician is aware of the characteristics of these patterns.

Electrocardiographic Abnormalities of Acute Ischemic Coronary Syndromes The earliest electrocardiographic finding resulting from AMI is the hyperacute T wave, which may appear minutes after the interruption of blood flow; the R wave also increases in amplitude at this stage. The hyperacute T wave, a short-lived structure that evolves rapidly to STE over a 5- to 30-minute period, is often asymmetric with a broad base; these T waves are also associated not infrequently with reciprocal STD in other electrocardiographic leads. Such a finding on the ECG is transient in the patient with AMI; progressive STE is usually encountered. The differential diagnosis of the hyperacute T wave includes transmural AMI, hyperkalemia, benign early repolarization (BER), acute pericarditis, and LVH. See Figure 73-1 for a representative example of the hyperacute T wave associated with AMI.

As the infarction progresses, the hyperacute T wave evolves into STE with the ST segment assuming a more easily recognized morphology. The initial upsloping portion of the ST segment usually is either convex or flat; if the STE is flat, it may be horizontally or obliquely so. An analysis of the ST segment waveform may be particularly helpful in distinguishing among the various causes of STE and identifying the AMI case. This technique uses the morphology of the initial portion of the ST segment–T wave, defined as beginning at the J (junction) point and ending at the apex of the T wave. Patients with noninfarctional STE (i.e., early repolarization or LVH-related change) tend to have a concave morphology of the waveform. Conversely, patients with STE due to AMI have either obliquely flat or convex waveforms. The use of this STE waveform analysis in the ED may increase the sensitivity for the correct electrocardiographic diagnosis of AMI. This morphologic observation should be used only as a guideline. As with most guidelines, it is not infallible. The electrocardiographic differential diagnosis of STE is broad, including AMI, bundle branch block, LVH, VPRs, pericarditis, and LVA, among many other entities. Refer to Figure 73-2 for depictions of STE morphology in AMI and non-AMI syndromes.

STD is generally considered to represent subendocardial, noninfarctional ischemia, although STD may be the initial electrocardiographic finding in the non-STE AMI. The morphology of subendocardial ischemic STD is classically horizontal or downsloping; upsloping STD is also seen, yet is less often associated with acute ischemia. With subendocardial ischemia, the STD is often diffuse and can be located in both the anterior and inferior leads. STD also occurs with non-STE AMI and transmural AMI associated with primary STE and reciprocal STD; also, STD in the right precordial leads may represent posterior wall AMI. Nonischemic causes of STD include hyperventilation, LVH with strain, digitalis effect, and hypokalemia. Refer to Figures 73-3 and 73-4 for depictions of STD.

Reciprocal STD, also known as *reciprocal change,* is defined as STD in leads separate and distinct from leads reflecting STE. The STD is either horizontal or downsloping (Figure 73-4). Reciprocal change in the setting of transmural AMI identifies a patient with increased chance of poor

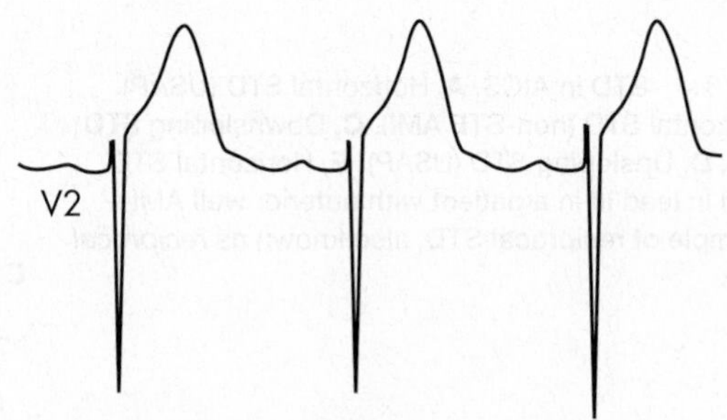

Figure 73-1. **Hyperacute T wave of AMI. Hyperacute T waves of early AMI are often asymmetric with a broad base as seen here in lead V_2 of a patient with early anterior wall infarction.**

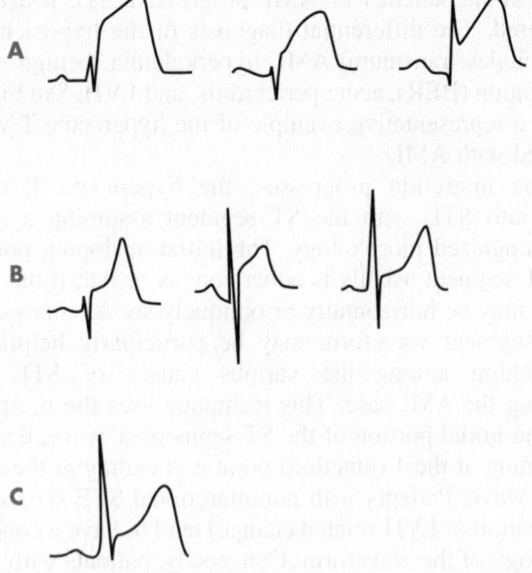

Figure 73-2. **An analysis of the ST segment–T wave morphology (from the beginning at the J point to the end at the apex of the T wave) may be particularly helpful in distinguishing among the various causes of STE and identifying the AMI case. A, The initial upsloping portion of the ST segment usually is either flat (horizontally or obliquely) or convex in the patient with AMI. This morphologic observation, however, should only be used as a guideline—it is not infallible. B, Non-AMI causes of STE are seen here with concavity of the ST segment–T wave (left BER, middle pericarditis, right BER). C, Patients with ST segment elevation due to AMI may demonstrate concavity of this portion of the waveform.**

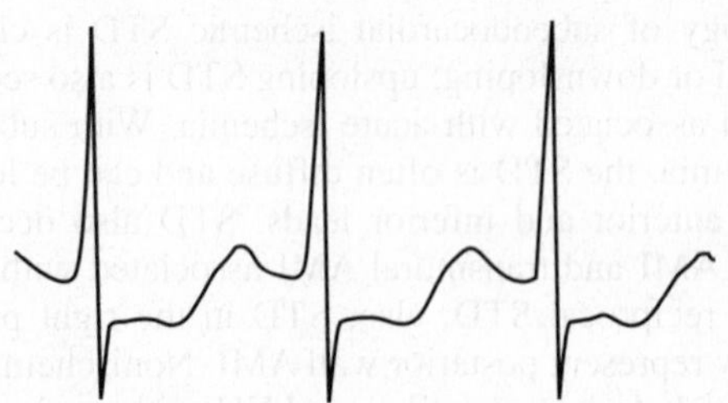

Figure 73-3. **Horizontal STD as seen in lead V_3 in a patient with USAP.**

outcome and, therefore, an individual who may benefit from a more aggressive approach in the ED. Furthermore, its presence on the ECG supports the diagnosis of AMI with very high sensitivity and positive predictive values greater than 90%. The use of reciprocal change in both prehospital and ED patients with chest pain increases the diagnostic accuracy in the electrocardiographic recognition of AMI.[25] Reciprocal change is seen in approximately 75% of inferior wall AMIs and much less often in anterior wall AMIs—30%.

Inverted T waves (Figure 73-5) produced by myocardial ischemia are classically narrow and symmetric. T wave inversion associated with AICS is morphologically characterized by an isoelectric ST segment that is usually bowed upward (i.e., concave) and followed by a sharp symmetric downstroke. The terms *coronary T wave* and *coved T wave* have been used to describe these T wave inversions. Prominent, deeply inverted, and widely splayed T waves are more characteristic of the noninfarctional, nonischemic conditions such as cerebrovascular accident. Noninfarctional causes of T wave inversion include juvenile T wave patterns, LVH, acute myocarditis, Wolff-Parkinson-White (WPW) syndrome, acute pulmonary embolism, cerebrovascular accident, and later stages of pericarditis.

An important subgroup of patients with USAP often have deep T wave inversions (Figure 73-5) in the precordial leads (V_1 through V_4); the T wave may also be biphasic in this same distribution. The syndrome is important to recognize because it is highly specific for stenosis of the left anterior descending (LAD) coronary artery with anterior wall AMI as the natural history. This has been termed the LAD T wave, or Wellen's syndrome. T wave inversion may also be caused by non-STE infarction and evolving states of STE AMI.

In general, Q waves represent established myocardial necrosis. Q waves alone are rarely the sole manifestation of AMI. Pathologic Q waves may be caused by a prior infarction, or conversely, a prior infarction may mask ischemic extension in the same anatomic location. Twelve percent of healthy young men have Q waves in the inferior leads. Q waves usually develop within 8 to 12 hours after a transmural AMI, yet they may be noted as early as 1 to 2 hours after the onset of complete coronary occlusion. As such, the simultaneous presence of Q waves and STE does not preclude consideration of thrombolytic therapy.

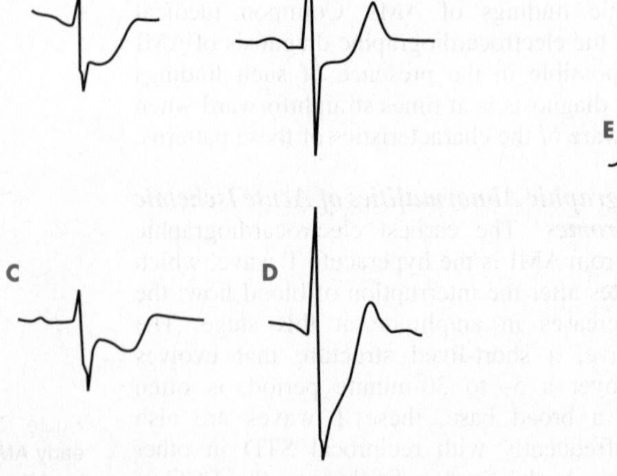

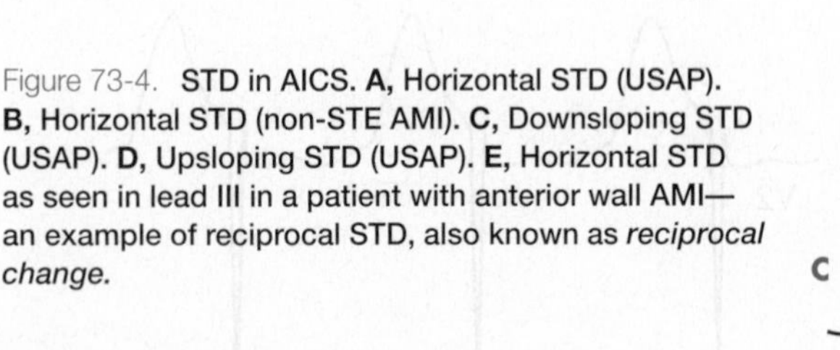

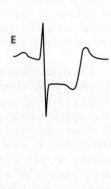

Figure 73-4. **STD in AICS. A, Horizontal STD (USAP). B, Horizontal STD (non-STE AMI). C, Downsloping STD (USAP). D, Upsloping STD (USAP). E, Horizontal STD as seen in lead III in a patient with anterior wall AMI—an example of reciprocal STD, also known as *reciprocal change*.**

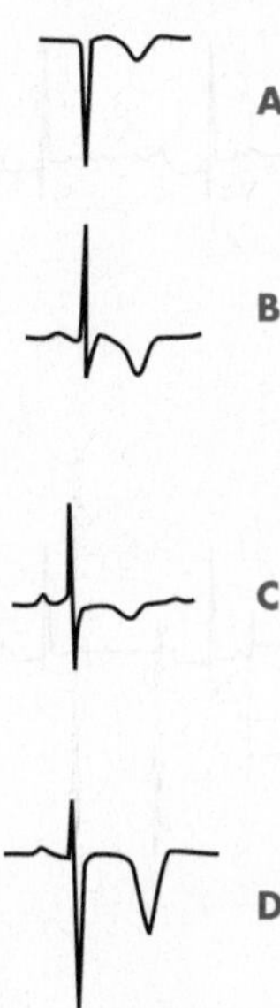

Figure 73-5. **T Wave inversions of AICS. A and B, T wave inversions in patients with AICS. C, T wave inversion in a patient with non-STE AMI. D, Deeply inverted T waves in a patient with proximal LAD stenosis—Wellen's syndrome.**

Anatomic Location of AMI It is important to identify the anatomic location of an AMI to estimate the amount of jeopardized myocardium and to determine the relative risk of morbidity and mortality. The extent of myocardial necrosis varies greatly with the site of occlusion and presence of collateral circulation. See Table 73-4 for a listing of electrocardiographic leads, ST segment finding, and involved anatomic segment of the infarcting heart. Proximal occlusion of the LAD artery results in more extensive anterior wall myocardial necrosis than midartery occlusion. Electrocardiographic identification of anterior wall AMI is made using the standard precordial leads V_1 through V_4. If STE occurs in one or more of leads V_1 through V_4 only, it is termed either anterior or anteroseptal. Extension to the lateral wall (anterolateral AMI) results in additional STE located in leads I, aV_L, V_5, or V_6.

The lateral wall of the left ventricle is variably supplied by the left circumflex coronary artery, the LAD coronary artery, or a branch of the right coronary artery. Isolated lateral wall infarctions usually involve occlusion of the circumflex artery. More commonly, the lateral wall is involved with proximal occlusion of the LAD artery (anterolateral AMI) or a branch of the right coronary artery (inferolateral AMI).

The right coronary artery supplies the AV node and inferior wall of the left ventricle in 90% of patients. The left circumflex artery performs this function in the 10% of patients with a dominant left coronary artery. Inferior AMIs are characterized by STE in at least two of the inferior leads (II, III, and aV_F). Patients with inferior wall AMI with electrocardiographic evidence of more extensive infarction, such as reciprocal changes in the anterior precordium, lateral extension with STE in leads V_5 and V_6, or right ventricular infarction identified by STE in the right precordial lead V_{4R}, are at risk for in-hospital mortality.

The term *posterior myocardial infarction (PMI)* refers to infarction involving the posterior wall of the left ventricle, resulting from occlusion of either the right coronary artery, its posterior descending branch, or less commonly the circumflex artery. Posterior wall involvement occurs in 15% to 21% of all AMIs, usually in conjunction with inferior or lateral infarction. PMI can occur as an isolated phenomenon (Figure 73-6), but the incidence is probably low. Patients experiencing acute inferior wall AMI with either right precordial STD or posterior lead STE, in general, have larger-sized myocardial infarctions with lower resultant ejection fractions and higher rates of acute cardiovascular complications and death compared to patients with inferior AMI without such changes.[26]

Table 73-4. Acute Myocardial Infarction Location and Reflecting Leads

Location	Leads	ST segment
Anterior wall MI	V_1 through V_4	Elevation
Lateral wall MI	I, aV_L, V_5, and V_6	Elevation
Inferior wall MI	II, III, and aV_F	Elevation
Right ventricular wall MI	V_{4R}	Elevation
Posterior wall MI	V_8 and V_9	Elevation
	V_1 through V_3	Depression

Modified from Aufderheide TP, Brady WJ: Electrocardiography in the patient with myocardial ischemia or infarction. In Gibler WB, Aufderheide TP, editors: *Emergency cardiac care*, St Louis, 1994, Mosby.

As the standard 12-lead ECG does not include posterior leads, changes associated with necrosis in this region are reflected in the anterior chest leads. These electrodes are opposite rather than adjacent to the site of damage, and the changes seen are the reverse of what one would normally expect (Figure 73-7). Thus, the STE that occurs with PMI becomes STD in the right precordial leads, V_1 through V_3. Abnormalities are most frequently detected in leads V_1 and V_2, to a lesser extent in lead V_3. Electrocardiographic abnormalities noted on the standard 12-lead ECG suggestive of acute PMI (Figures 73-6, 73-8, and 73-9) include the following (in leads V_1, V_2, or V_3): (1) horizontal STD; (2) a tall, upright T wave; (3) a tall, wide R wave; and (4) an R/S wave ratio greater than or equal to 1.0. Further, the combination of horizontal STD with an upright T wave increases the diagnostic accuracy of these two separate electrocardiographic findings. It must be remembered that a dominant R wave, which is in fact an evolving Q wave, takes a number of hours to develop and therefore is not frequently seen on the initial ECG. The use of the additional posterior leads, V_8 and V_9 (Figure 73-9), may well confirm the presence of a PMI and is felt to be superior to the findings noted in leads V_1 through V_3.

Right ventricular infarction occurs in the setting of 25% to 40% of inferior wall AMIs. Right ventricular involvement usually occurs as a result of occlusion of the right coronary artery proximal to the right ventricular branch, with associated acute inferior wall infarction; less commonly, right ventricular infarction results from occlusion of a dominant circumflex artery in the setting of acute lateral wall myocardial infarction. In the setting of inferior wall AMI, the clinical findings of hypotension and raised jugular venous pressure are highly suggestive of right ventricular infarction. It has also been suggested that nitrate-induced hypotension is suggestive of right ventricular infarction. It is important to

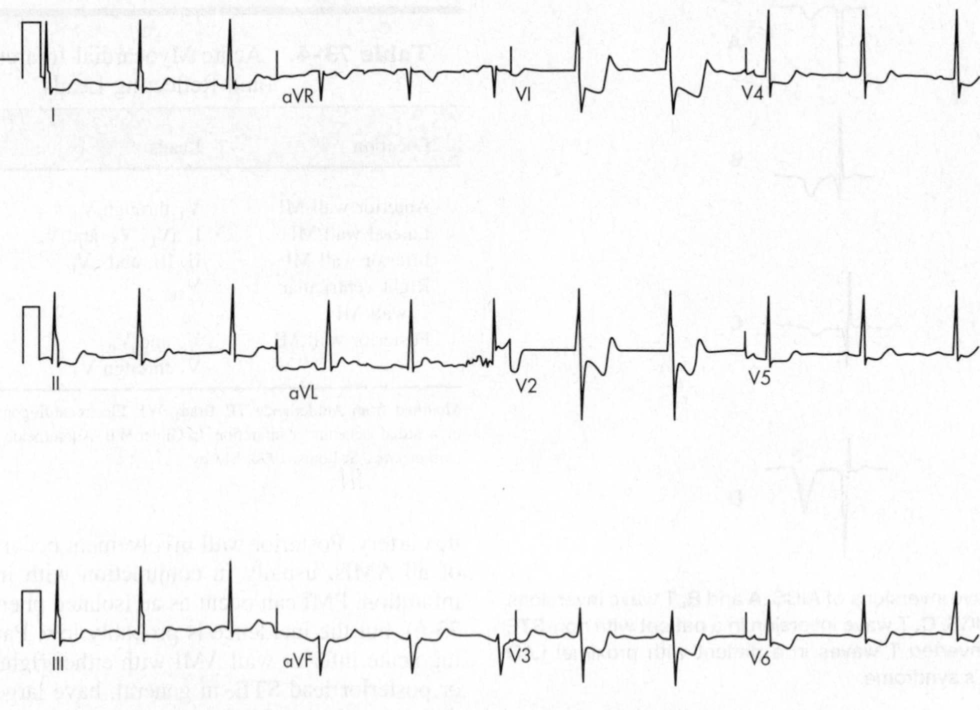

Figure 73-6. **Isolated posterior wall AMI. Note the prominent R wave with downsloping STD and upright T waves in leads V_1 to V_3.**

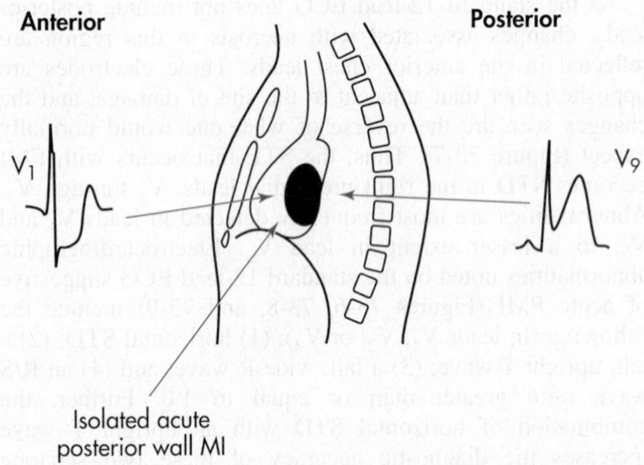

Figure 73-7. **Isolated posterior wall AMI. The standard electrocardiographic precordial (anterior) leads image the posterior wall of the left ventricle from the anterior perspective of the thorax. Acute infarction of this region will manifest electrocardiographic changes that are frequently the reverse of the typical abnormalities of AMI. In this schematic example, lead V_1 reveals STD with upright T wave and prominent R wave. Use of the posterior lead V_9 demonstrates STE, consistent with AMI.**

diagnose right ventricular infarction, since the associated hypotension will likely respond to intravenous fluid administration whereas diuretic agents, morphine, and nitrates may further complicate the situation. Patients with inferior wall AMI with coexistent right ventricular infarction have larger-sized infarcts and experience more in-hospital complications and higher cardiac mortality rates.[27]

The standard 12-lead electrocardiographic findings for right ventricular infarction include STE in the inferior distribution as well as in the right precordial chest leads, particularly V_1, perhaps the only lead on the standard ECG that reflects changes in the right ventricle. In the setting of inferior wall AMI, if the degree of STE is disproportionately greater in lead II relative to the other inferior leads, right ventricular infarction is also suggested. At times, coexisting acute posterior wall AMI may obscure the STE resulting from right ventricular infarction in lead V_1, as seen in the patient with the acute inferoposterior myocardial infarction with right ventricular involvement. Recordings from leads placed on the right side of the chest are much more sensitive and specific in detecting the changes of right ventricular infarction. The right-sided precordial electrodes are placed across the right side of the chest in a mirror image of the standard left-sided leads and are labeled V_{1R} to V_{6R}—RV_1 to RV_6 is another commonly used nomenclature for this lead distribution. The clinician may use either the entire right-sided leads V_{1R} to V_{6R} or the single lead V_{4R}. Lead V_{4R} (right 5th intercostal space at the mid-clavicular line) is the most useful lead for detecting STE associated with right ventricular infarction and may be used solely in the evaluation of the possible right ventricular infarction (Figure 73-10). The STE that occurs in association with right ventricular infarction is frequently quite subtle, reflecting the relatively small muscle mass of the right ventricle; at other times, the STE is quite prominent, similar in appearance to the ST segment changes seen in the standard 12 leads.

Additional-Lead Electrocardiograms It has been suggested that the sensitivity of the 12-lead ECG may be improved if three additional body surface leads are employed in selected individuals. Acute posterior and right ventricular myocardial infarctions are likely to be underdiagnosed, as the standard lead placement of the 12-lead ECG does not allow these areas to be assessed directly. Additional leads frequently

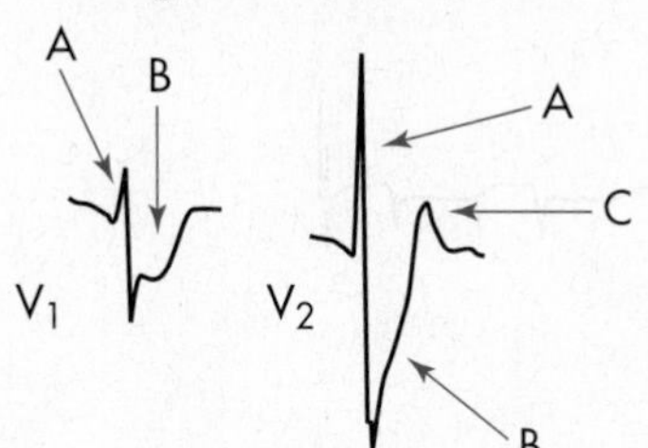

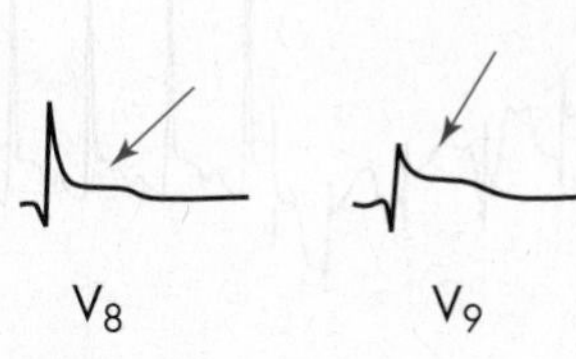

Figure 73-8. **Isolated posterior wall AMI. The right precordial leads V_1 and V_2 reveal typical findings of PMI with prominent R wave (A), STD (B), and upright T wave (C). The posterior leads V_8 and V_9 in this same case demonstrate STE *(arrows)*, confirming isolated PMI.**

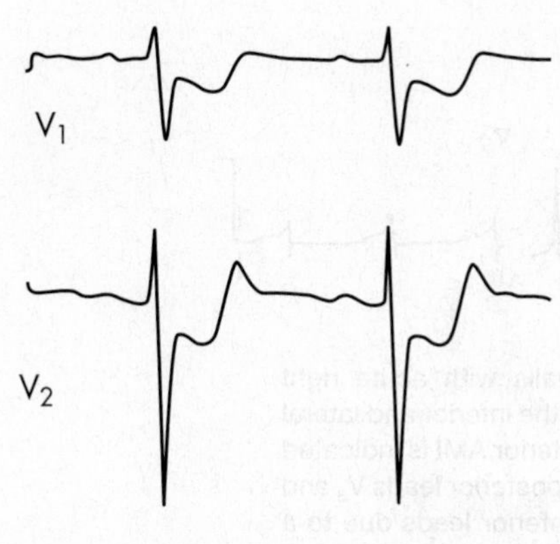

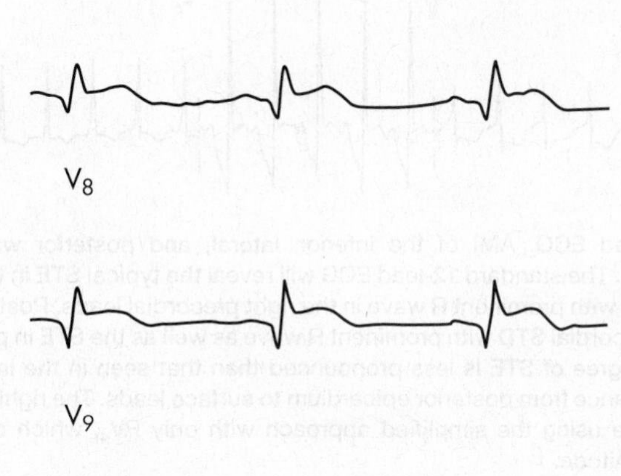

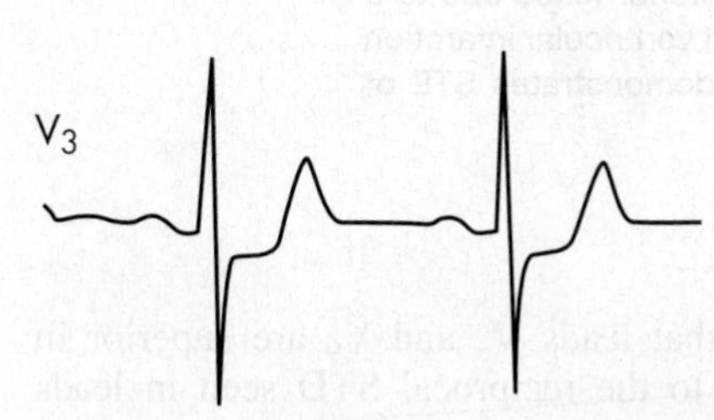

Figure 73-9. **Isolated posterior wall AMI. Use of the additional leads V_8 and V_9 confirms the presence of PMI in this patient who has chest pain with right precordial electrocardiographic abnormality as seen here in leads V_1 through V_3.**

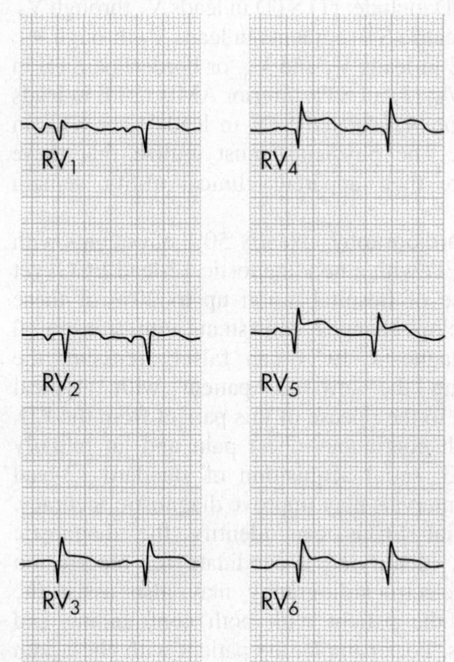

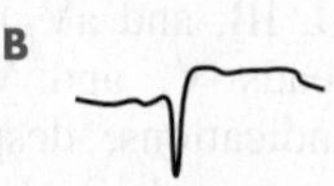

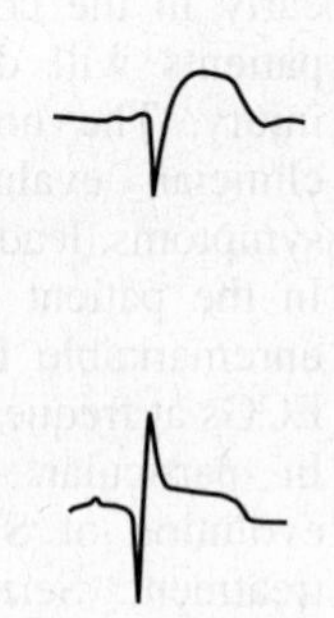

Figure 73-10. **Right ventricular infarction. A, Leads RV_1-RV_6 reveal STE, consistent with acute right ventricular infarction. Note that the degree of STE is less pronounced than that usually encountered in the patient with AMI. This diminution of the STE is due to the smaller muscle mass of the right ventricle. B, Alternatively, a single right-sided lead, lead RV_4, may be used to evaluate the right ventricular for infarction. Here are three examples of lead RV_4 in patients with acute right ventricular myocardial infarction.**

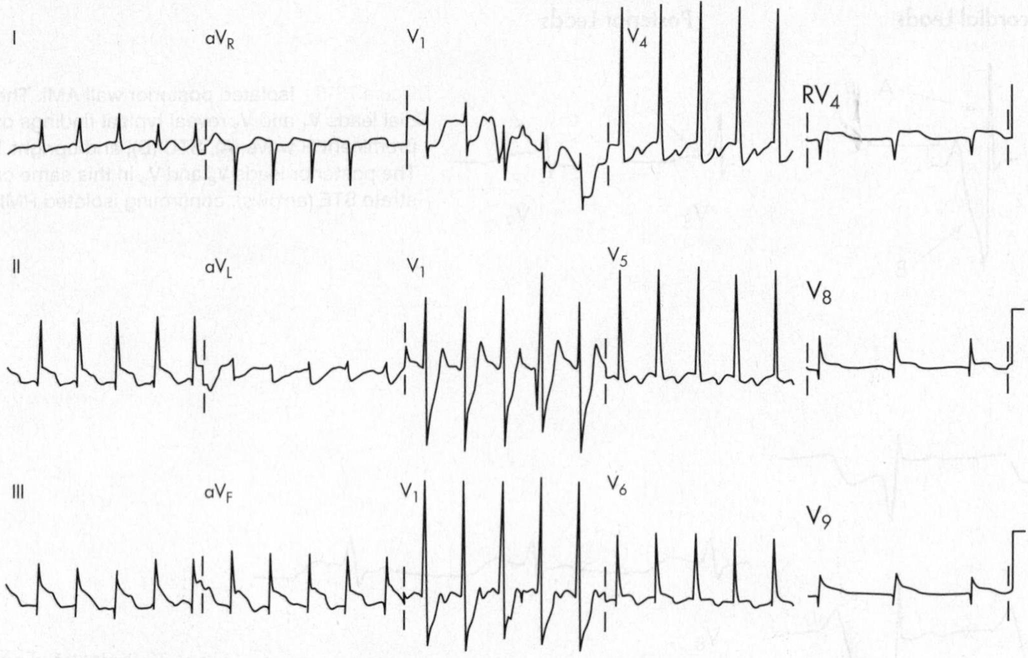

Figure 73-11. **15-lead ECG. AMI of the inferior, lateral, and posterior walls with acute right ventricular infarction. The standard 12-lead ECG will reveal the typical STE in the inferior and lateral leads as well as STD with prominent R wave in the right precordial leads. Posterior AMI is indicated by both the right precordial STD with prominent R wave as well as the STE in posterior leads V_8 and V_9. Note that the degree of STE is less pronounced than that seen in the inferior leads due to a relatively longer distance from posterior epicardium to surface leads. The right ventricular infarction is noted in this case using the simplified approach with only RV_4, which demonstrates STE of relatively small magnitude.**

used include leads V_8 and V_9, which image the posterior wall of the left ventricle, and lead V_{4R}, which reflects the status of the right ventricle. The standard ECG coupled with these additional leads constitutes the 15-lead ECG, the most frequently employed extra-lead ECG in clinical practice. Without doubt, a more detailed description of the extent of the myocardial injury may be obtained if additional leads are used to augment the standard 12-lead ECG in selected patients. The use of the additional leads may confirm the presence of AMI and alter treatment decisions. See Figure 73-11 for a representative example of a 15-lead ECG in a patient with AMI of the inferior, posterior, and lateral walls, and of the right ventricle.

In a study of all ED patients with chest pain, Brady et al reported that the 15-lead ECG provided a more accurate description of myocardial injury in those patients with AMI, yet failed to alter rates of diagnosis, the use of reperfusion therapies, or disposition locations.[28] Looking at a more select population of ED patients, Zalenski et al investigated the use of the 15-lead ECG in those with chest pain who had a high or moderate-to-high pretest probability of AMI and were already identified as candidates for hospital admission.[29] In this 15-lead ECG study, the authors reported an 11.7% increase in sensitivity with no loss of specificity (i.e., no increase in false-positive findings for the diagnosis of STE AMI).[29] They concluded that "the findings of ST elevation by use of these extra leads can strengthen the ED diagnosis of acute myocardial infarction on the initial tracing and may provide an indication for thrombolytic treatment."[29] They further suggest that leads V_8 and V_9 are superior in the diagnosis of PMI to the reciprocal STD seen in leads V_1 to V_3.[29]

Additional-lead ECGs may produce valuable information about injury, necrosis, and ischemia in carefully selected cases.[28,29] Indications to obtain 15-lead ECGs in patients with suspected acute IHD include: (1) STD in leads V_1 through V_3, or suspicious isoelectric ST segments in leads V_1 through V_3; (2) borderline STE in leads V_5 and V_6, or borderline STE in leads II, III, and aV_F; (3) all STE inferior AMIs (STE in leads II, III, and aV_F); or (4) isolated STE in lead V_1 or STE in leads V_1 and V_2. The physician must realize that these indications, despite their apparent clinical utility, remain unproved.

Serial Electrocardiography Nearly 50% of patients with AMI come to the ED with a nondiagnostic 12-lead ECG, yet early in the course of hospitalization up to 20% of these patients will develop changes consistent with transmural injury. The nondiagnostic ECG can falsely reassure the clinician evaluating the low-risk patient with atypical symptoms, leading to the release of this patient from the ED. In the patient with continuous chest pain and an initially unremarkable ECG, serial acquisition of standard 12-lead ECGs at frequent intervals may improve diagnostic accuracy. In particular, serial ECGs can identify the diagnostic evolution of STE, identifying a candidate for reperfusion treatment. Serial electrocardiography may also assist the physician treating the patient with both confounding and mimicking patterns. For example, the patient with chest pain

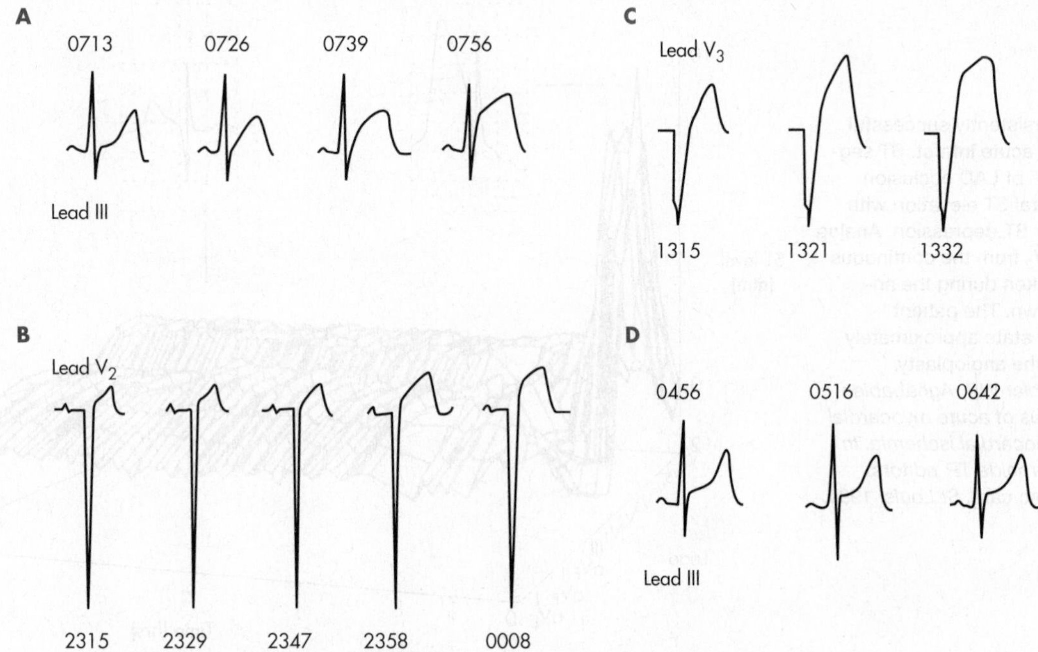

Figure 73-12. **Serial electrocardiography. A, Representative example of lead III in a patient with chest pain and an initially nondiagnostic ECG depicting the evolution of STE AMI. B, Representative example of lead V_2 in a patient with the LVH pattern. Serial sampling of this patient with ongoing chest pain and a confounding electrocardiographic pattern reveals the progression to STE AMI. C, Representative example of lead V_3 in a patient with LBBB and evolving AMI. D, Representative examples of lead III in a patient with chest pain and noninfarctional STE; note the lack of change (degree of elevation as well as morphology of elevation) over time in this patient with BER.**

and electrocardiographic LVH will manifest STE; initial diagnostic uncertainly can be addressed using serial electrocardiography. The patient with STE AMI will likely demonstrate progression of the elevation while the individual who lacks ischemia will reveal a static pattern over the short term in the ED. The technique of serial electrocardiography may be accomplished using frequent applications of the standard 12-lead ECG or computer-assisted ST segment trend monitoring.

Potentially, serial ECGs may provide electrocardiographic surveillance of patients coming to the ED with chest pain and who have an initial nondiagnostic ECG.[30,31] In the CCU setting, ST segment monitoring applied during the first few hours after admission reportedly provided important, additional information not noted on the initial ECG in the ED.[32] In fact, 17% of such patients demonstrated dynamic electrocardiographic changes during the first 6 hours of CCU monitoring. Such ST segment trend monitoring may provide the earliest evidence of coronary occlusion in patients with preinfarction angina. In addition, such evaluation may provide evidence of painless or silent ischemia. Scientific support for ST segment trend monitoring in the ED is sparse. Fesmire et al[33] applied this technique to 1000 ED patients with chest pain; serial ST segment monitoring identified an additional 16.2% patients with myocardial injury who were not identified on the initial ECG. The patient with the confounding ECG may also benefit from this diagnostic technique. The LBBB pattern, a classic confounder to the electrocardiographic diagnosis of AMI, may be further investigated with serial electrocardiography. Fesmire encountered five patients with final diagnosis of AMI in the presence of LBBB who demonstrated significant electrocardiographic changes during the early phase of ED care and surveillance using frequent serial ECGs.[34]

Serial 12-lead ECG tracings obtained every 20 seconds, with computer interpretation and comparison, have been developed for the continuous monitoring of the ST segment in patients receiving thrombolytic therapy for AMI. Three-dimensional computer representations show graphic images of initial occlusion in patients with AMI and subsequent reperfusion. In one series, Krucoff et al note that angiographically proven reperfusion is detected with a sensitivity of 89% using serial ST segment trend monitoring, with a corresponding specificity of 82%.[35] In multiple investigations ST segment trend monitoring has proved to be an effective method for noninvasive evaluation of reperfusion after delivery of thrombolytic therapy.

Refer to Figures 73-12 and 73-13 for examples of serial ECGs and ST segment trend monitoring in patients with chest pain.

Confounding Electrocardiographic Patterns

Left Bundle Branch Block LBBB markedly reduces the diagnostic power of the ECG. Common medical opinion holds that the electrocardiographic diagnosis of AMI is impossible in the presence of LBBB when, in fact, this diagnosis is often straightforward and considered "disarmingly easy" by others.

In the patient with LBBB,[36] the anticipated or expected ST segment–T wave configurations are discordant, directed

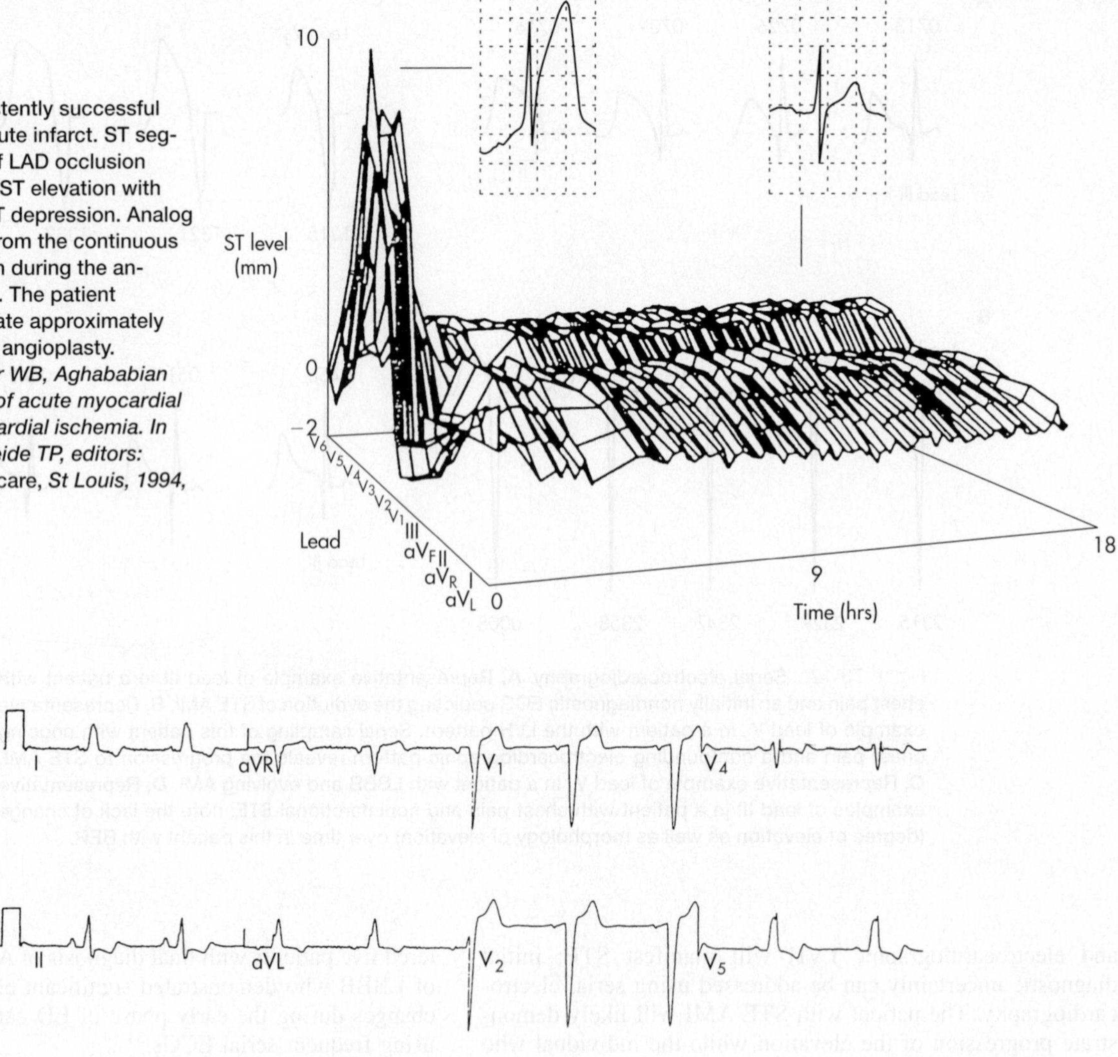

Figure 73-13. **Persistently successful reperfusion of an acute infarct. ST segment "fingerprint" of LAD occlusion shows anterolateral ST elevation with reciprocal inferior ST depression. Analog beats from lead V_2 from the continuous ECG recording taken during the angioplasty are shown. The patient reached a steady state approximately 20 minutes after the angioplasty.** ***Modified from Gibler WB, Aghababian RV: Early diagnosis of acute myocardial infarction and myocardial ischemia. In Gibler WB, Aufderheide TP, editors:*** **Emergency cardiac care, *St Louis, 1994, Mosby.***

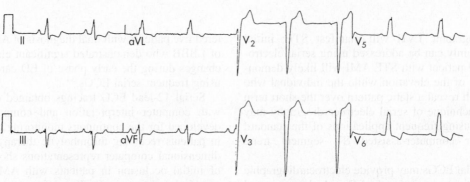

Figure 73-14. **Representative example of uncomplicated LBBB. The ST segments and T wave morphologies are appropriate for this form of altered intraventricular conduction.** ***Modified from Aufderheide TP, Brady WJ: Electrocardiography in the patient with myocardial ischemia or infarction. In Gibler WB, Aufderheide TP, editors:*** **Emergency cardiac care, *St Louis, 1994, Mosby.***

opposite from the terminal portion of the QRS complex and called *QRS complex–T wave axes discordance* (Figure 73-14). As such, inferior and right precordial leads with either QS or rS complexes may have markedly elevated ST segments, mimicking acute myocardial infarction. The lateral leads, with the large monophasic R wave, demonstrate STD. The T wave, especially in the right to mid-precordial leads, has a convex upward shape or a tall vaulting appearance, similar to the hyperacute T wave of early myocardial infarction. The T waves in leads with the monophasic R wave are frequently inverted. Loss of this normal QRS complex–T wave axes discordance in patients with LBBB may imply an acute process, such as AMI. An inspection of the ECG in patients with LBBB must be performed, looking for a loss of this QRS complex-ST segment–T wave axes discordance. See Figures 73-15 and 73-16 for an example of a LBBB pattern with expected ST segment–T wave configurations.

A clinical rule has been developed to assist in the ECG diagnosis of AMI in the presence of LBBB using specific electrocardiographic findings.[37] Sgarbossa et al analyzed the numerous electrocardiographic abnormalities previously reported to be suspicious or diagnostic for AMI in patients with LBBB and identified three criteria suggestive of acute infarction. This rule, developed from 131 patients with LBBB and enzymatically proven AMI who were enrolled in the GUSTO-I trial,[37] reported that three specific ECG criteria

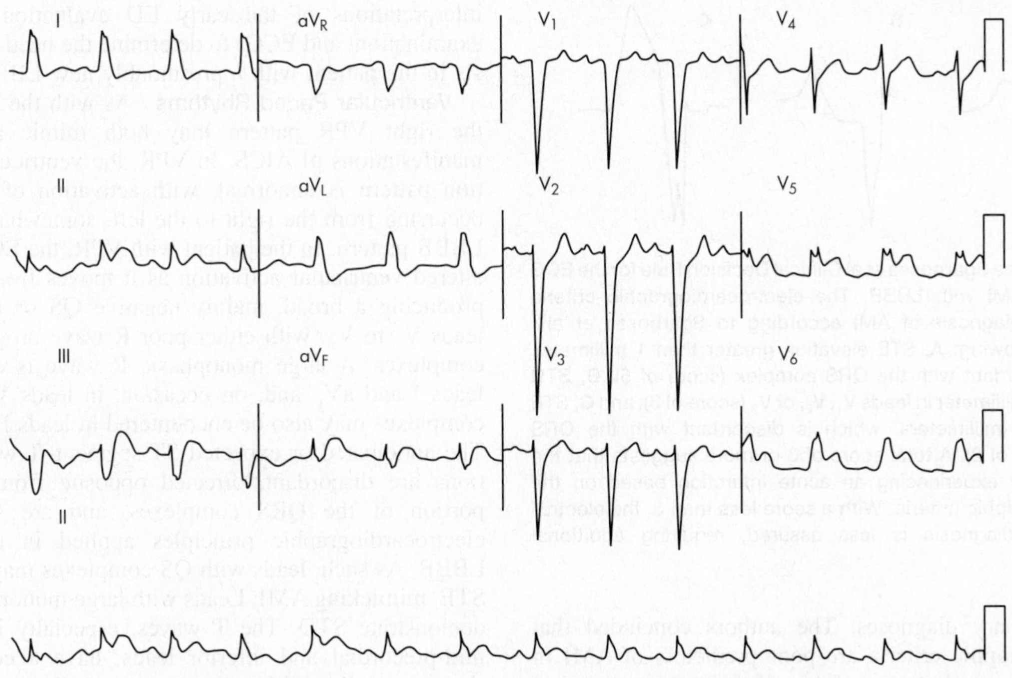

Figure 73-15. **LBBB pattern with AMI. LBBB pattern with abnormal findings, diagnostic for AMI, including concordant STE in leads II, V_5, and V_6. Also, although not diagnostic of AMI yet suggestive of acute abnormality in the appropriate chest pain patient, concordant STD is seen in lead V_2. The patient was in the early stage of anterolateral AMI with a pre-existing LBBB.**

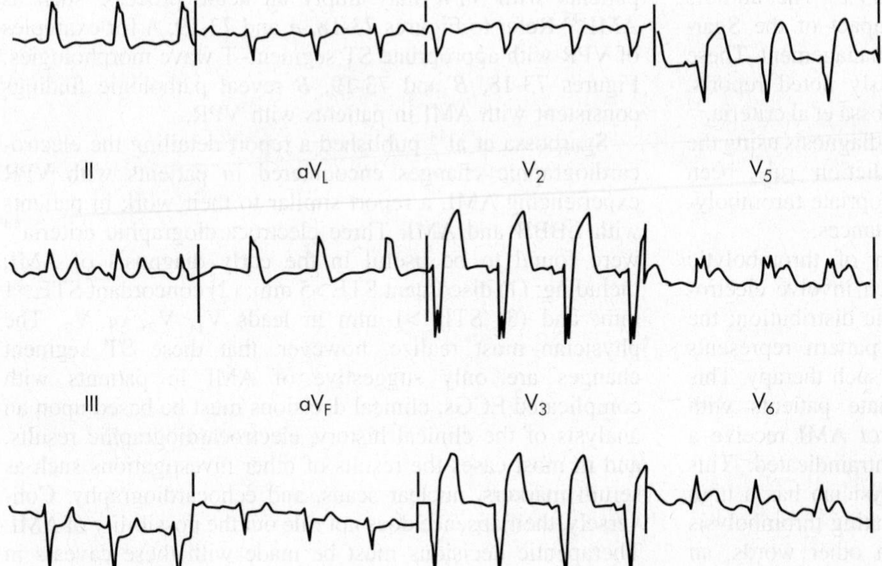

Figure 73-16. **LBBB pattern with AMI. LBBB pattern with abnormal findings, diagnostic for AMI, including concordant STE in leads V_5 and V_6. Also, though not diagnostic of AMI yet suggestive of acute abnormality in the appropriate patient with chest pain, other findings include: excessive discordant STE seen in leads V_2, V_3, and V_4 and concordant STD in leads III and aV_F. The patient ruled in for an anterolateral AMI with past LBBB.**

were independent predictors of myocardial infarction. The ECG criteria (Figure 73-17) suggesting a diagnosis of AMI, ranked with a scoring system based on the probability of such a diagnosis, include (1) STE greater than 1 millimeter, which was concordant with the QRS complex (Figure 73-17, *A,* a score of 5); (2) STD greater than 1 millimeter in leads V_1, V_2, or V_3 (Figure 73-17, *B,* a score of 3); and (3) STE greater than 5 millimeters, which is discordant with the QRS complex (Figure 73-17, *C,* score of 2). A total score of 3 or more suggests that the patient is likely experiencing an AMI based on the electrocardiographic criteria. With a score less than 3, the electrocardiographic diagnosis is less assured, requiring additional evaluation.

Subsequent literature[38,39] has suggested that the Sgarbossa et al[37] clinical prediction rule is less useful than reported. The first such investigation,[38] which applied the Sgarbossa et al[37] criteria to patients with chest pain and LBBB in the ED of a North American hospital, found much less promising results—a very low sensitivity coupled with poor interobserver reliability. A second study[39] investigated the diagnostic and therapeutic impact of these criteria; none effectively distinguished the patients who had AMI from those patients

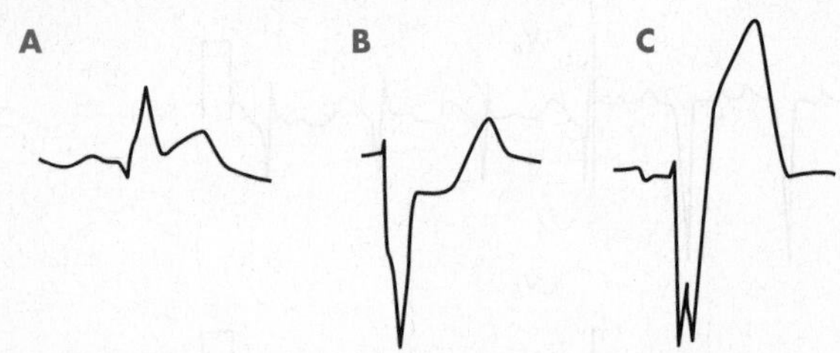

Figure 73-17. **The Sgarbossa et al Clinical Decision Rule for the ECG Diagnosis of AMI with LBBB. The electrocardiographic criteria suggesting a diagnosis of AMI according to Sgarbossa et al[37] include the following: A, STE elevation greater than 1 millimeter, which is concordant with the QRS complex (score of 5); B, STD greater than 1 millimeter in leads V_1, V_2, or V_3 (score of 3); and C, STE greater than 5 millimeters, which is discordant with the QRS complex (score of 2). A total score of 3 or more suggests that the patient is likely experiencing an acute infarction based on the electrocardiographic criteria. With a score less than 3, the electrocardiographic diagnosis is less assured, requiring additional evaluation.**

with noncoronary diagnoses. The authors concluded that electrocardiographic criteria are poor predictors of AMI in LBBB situations and suggested that all patients suspected of AMI with LBBB should be considered for thrombolysis. A third investigation[40] followed just this recommendation—using a thrombolytic agent in all patients with LBBB presumed to have AMI; they also reported an alarmingly high rate of inappropriate thrombolysis in patients with chest pain who had LBBB and presumed AMI—49%. The authors also[40] retrospectively investigated the impact of the Sgarbossa et al[37] criteria on the diagnosis and management. These investigators, in contrast to the previously noted reports, found significant accuracy using the Sgarbossa et al criteria,[37] noting an approximate 80% rate of correct diagnosis using the prediction rule. Had the clinical prediction rule been employed, the authors suggest that inappropriate thrombolysis would have been avoided in many instances.

Traditional criteria for administration of thrombolytic agents in the patient with AMI most often involve electrocardiographic STE situated in an anatomic distribution; the presence of a presumably new LBBB pattern represents another electrocardiographic criterion for such therapy. This second criterion suggests that appropriate patients with LBBB pattern and a history suggestive of AMI receive a thrombolytic agent if not otherwise contraindicated. This approach is perhaps reasonable if the physician has a high suspicion of AMI and is comfortable initiating thrombolysis based solely on clinical information—in other words, an analysis of the patient's history and physical examination. Physicians, however, may be uncomfortable administering a thrombolytic agent under such circumstances; in fact, patients with electrocardiographic LBBB and AMI less often receive thrombolysis despite an increased risk of poor outcome[37,41] and the potential for significant benefit.[42] The clinician must realize that of all patients with chest pain, electrocardiographic LBBB pattern without obvious infarction, and clinically presumed AMI, only a minority will actually be experiencing AMI.[37] Treating all such patients with LBBB and presumed AMI will subject a number of patients without infarction to the not insignificant risks and expense of thrombolysis as seen in the Edhouse et al study.[40] Ultimately in this complicated scenario, clinicians must rely on their interpretations of the early ED evaluation (i.e., history, examination, and ECG) to determine the need for thrombolysis in the patient with a presumably new LBBB pattern.

Ventricular Paced Rhythms As with the LBBB pattern, the right VPR pattern may both mimic and mask the manifestations of AICS. In VPR, the ventricular depolarization pattern is abnormal, with activation of the ventricles occurring from the right to the left, somewhat resembling a LBBB pattern. In the patient with VPR, the ECG records the altered ventricular activation as it moves from right to left, producing a broad, mainly negative QS or rS complex in leads V_1 to V_6, with either poor R wave progression or QS complexes. A large monophasic R wave is encountered in leads I and aV_L and, on occasion, in leads V_5 and V_6. QS complexes may also be encountered in leads II, III, and aV_F. The anticipated or expected ST segment–T wave configurations are discordant, directed opposite from the terminal portion of the QRS complexes, and are similar to the electrocardiographic principles applied in the setting of LBBB. As such, leads with QS complexes may have marked STE, mimicking AMI. Leads with large monophasic R waves demonstrate STD. The T waves, especially in the right to mid-precordial and inferior leads, have a convex upward shape or a tall, vaulting appearance, similar to the hyperacute T waves of early AMI. The T waves in leads with the monophasic R wave are frequently inverted. An inspection of the ECG in patients with VPR must be performed, looking for a loss of this QRS complex–T wave axes discordance. Loss of this normal QRS complex–T wave axes discordance in patients with VPR may imply an acute process, such as AMI.[43] Refer to Figures 73-18, *A* and 73-19, *A* for examples of VPR with appropriate ST segment–T wave morphologies; Figures 73-18, *B* and 73-19, *B* reveal pathologic findings consistent with AMI in patients with VPR.

Sgarbossa et al[44] published a report detailing the electrocardiographic changes encountered in patients with VPR experiencing AMI, a report similar to their work in patients with LBBB and AMI. Three electrocardiographic criteria[44] were found to be useful in the early diagnosis of AMI, including: (1) discordant STE >5 mm; (2) concordant STE >1 mm; and (3) STD >1 mm in leads V_1, V_2, or V_3. The physician must realize, however, that these ST segment changes are only suggestive of AMI in patients with complicated ECGs; clinical decisions must be based upon an analysis of the clinical history, electrocardiographic results, and in most cases the results of other investigations such as serum markers, nuclear scans, and echocardiography. Conversely, their absence does not rule out the possibility of AMI. Therapeutic decisions must be made with these caveats in mind. Of course, serial ECGs and/or past ECGs may be of value in the electrocardiographic examination of these patients.

Left Ventricular Hypertrophy Electrocardiographic signs of LVH and the related repolarization changes are not uncommonly encountered in the ED patient experiencing chest pain. Their presence on the ECG, particularly the repolarization changes that alter the morphology of the ST segment or the T wave, may confound the early ED evaluation. In patients with LVH, ST segment–T wave changes are encountered in approximately 70% of cases; these changes result from altered repolarization of the ventricular myocardium[45] and represent the new normal for the patient with electrocardiographic LVH. These changes

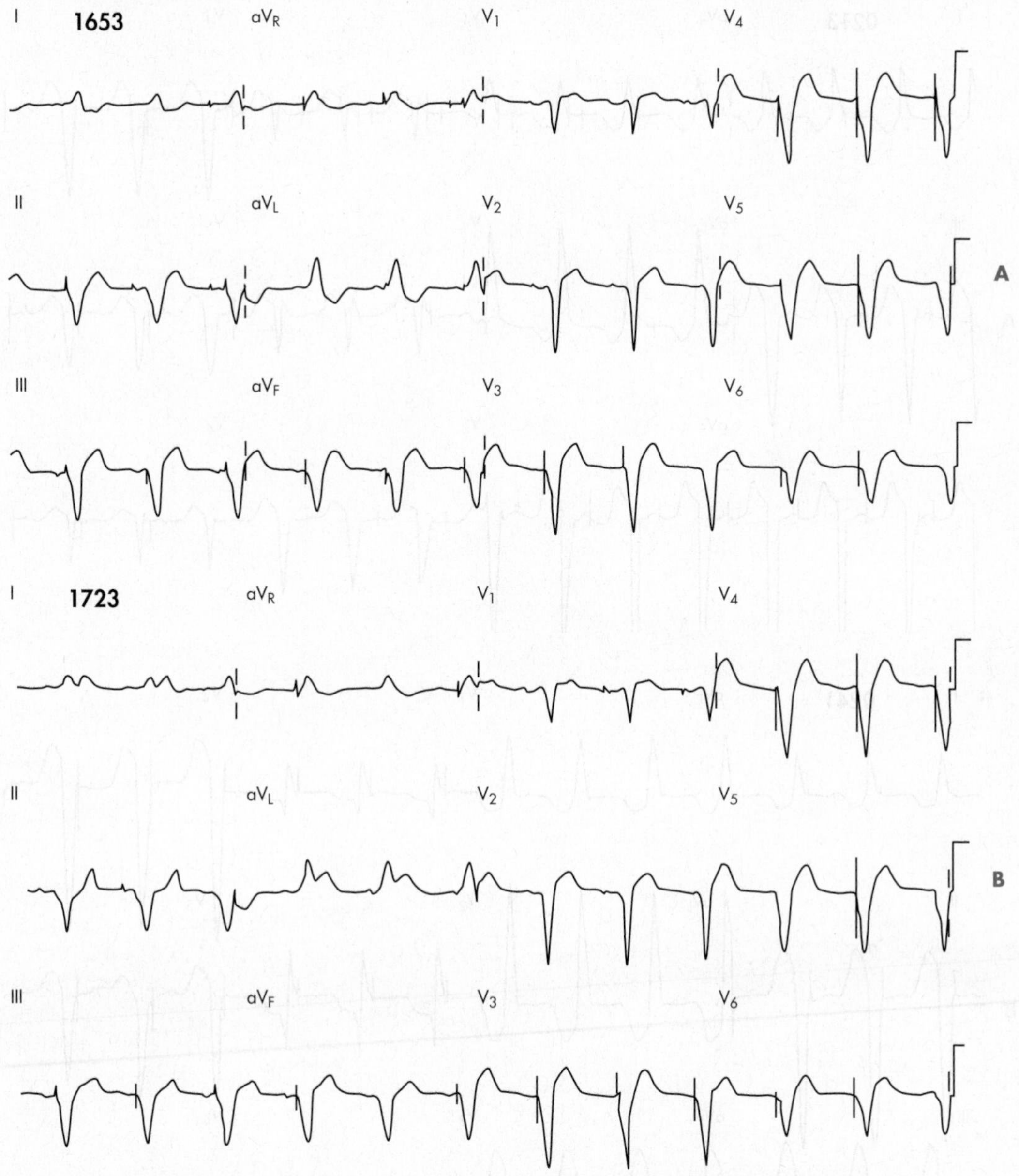

Figure 73-18. **Ventricular paced rhythm. A, Appropriate ST segment–T wave findings in the patient with a paced rhythm. B, Serial ECG from the patient in A, revealing evolution of changes worrisome for AMI, including concordant STE in leads I and aV_L consistent with lateral wall AMI.**

may mask or mimic the early findings consistent with acute coronary ischemia; this effect, however, occurs to a lesser extent than that encountered in the LBBB and VPR situations. LVH is associated with poor R wave progression and loss of the septal R wave in the right to mid-precordial leads, most commonly producing a QS pattern. In general, these QS complexes are located in leads V_1 and V_2, rarely extending beyond lead V_3. As predicted by the concept of appropriate discordance, STE is encountered in this distribution along with prominent, hyperacute T waves. The STE seen in this distribution may be greater than 5 mm in height and is difficult to distinguish from that associated with AMI. The initial, upsloping portion of the ST segment–T wave complex is frequently concave in LVH compared to the flattened or convex pattern observed in the patient with AMI. This morphologic feature is not diagnostic; early AMI may reveal such a concave feature. See Figure 73-20 for an example of LVH and Figure 73-12, *B* for AMI with an LVH pattern.

Non-STE AMI It has been reported that total occlusion of the infarct-related artery is uncommon in the early hours after non-STE AMI (formerly designated the non-Q wave infarction). When total occlusion is present, perfusion is maintained by collateral vessels. These anatomic findings support the contention that the non-STE infarction often indicates an incomplete ischemic event, with additional myocardium at risk. Patients with non-STE infarction may have transient and nonspecific findings, such as STD or T wave abnormalities in any of the anatomic leads of the 12-lead ECG. Symmetric convex downward STD or inverted or biphasic T waves are characteristically seen. Differentiating non-STE anterior AMI from posterior AMI can be

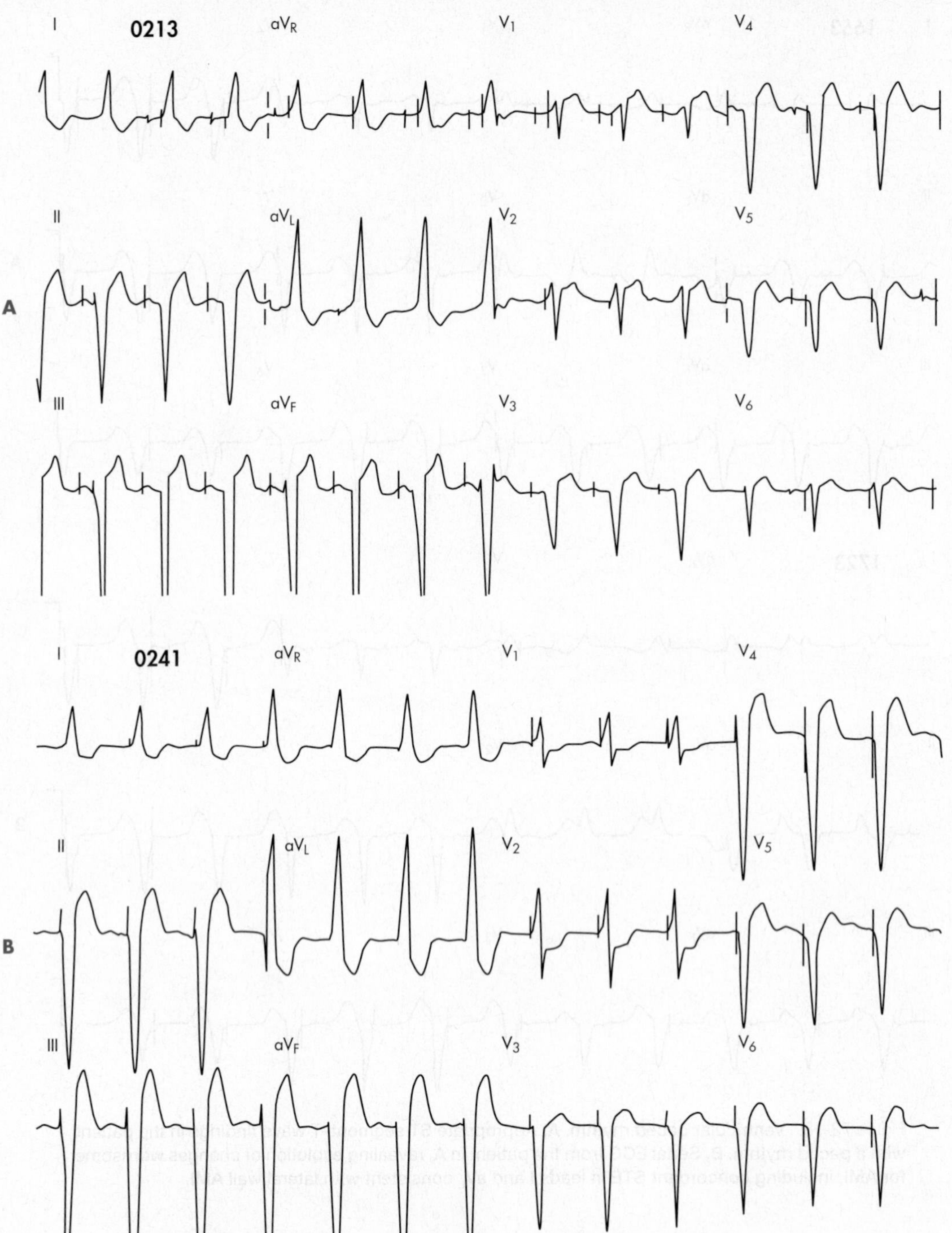

Figure 73-19. **Ventricular paced rhythm. A, Appropriate ST segment–T wave findings in the patient with a paced rhythm. B, Serial ECG from the patient in A, revealing evolution of changes worrisome for AMI, including progressive discordant STE in leads II, III and aV$_F$. These particular findings, although not diagnostic of an AMI, are very suggestive of acute infarction in this ill-appearing patient with chest pain unresponsive to aggressive antianginal therapy.**

difficult. The additional leads V_8 and V_9 may further assist this differentiation.

Patterns that Resemble AICS Unfortunately, STE is a not uncommon finding on the ECG of the ED patient with chest pain; its cause infrequently is AMI. The occurrence of numerous other noninfarctional STE syndromes only reinforces the point that STE is an insensitive marker of AMI.[46] One prehospital study of adult patients with chest pain demonstrated that the majority of those manifesting STE on the ECG did not have AMI as a final hospital diagnosis; rather, LVH and LBBB accounted for the majority of the cases.[25] Further, in a review of adult ED patients who had chest pain associated with STE on the ECG, STE was the result of AMI in only 15%. LVH, seen in 30% of this population, was the most frequent cause of STE.[47] These

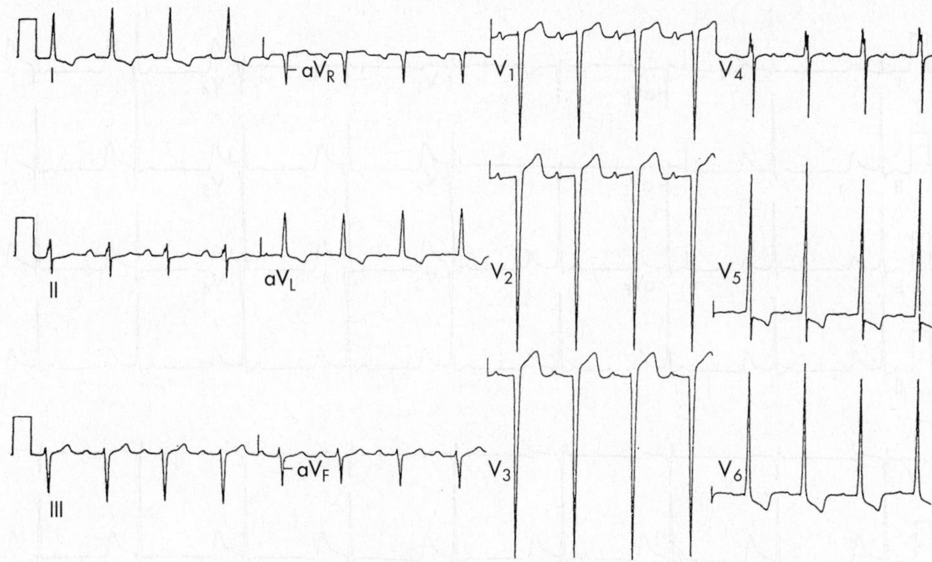

Figure 73-20. **Example of LVH.** ***Modified from Aufderheide TP, Brady WJ: Electrocardiography in the patient with myocardial ischemia or infarction. In Gibler WB, Aufderheide TP, editors:*** **Emergency cardiac care, *St Louis, 1994, Mosby.***

noninfarct STE syndromes are not infrequently misdiagnosed as acute infarction, and the patient may then be subjected to unnecessary and potentially dangerous therapies and procedures. For example, a report by Sharkey et al[48] noted that 11% of patients receiving thrombolytic agents were not experiencing AMI. The electrocardiographic syndromes producing this pseudo-infarct STE included BER (30%), LVH (30%), and various intraventricular conduction abnormalities (30%).[48]

LVH, LBBB, and VPR, which also must be considered in the electrocardiographic differential diagnosis of STE, have been discussed in the section of this chapter concerning confounding patterns. Other such mimicking patterns include BER, acute pericarditis, and left ventricular aneurysm (LVA).

The syndrome of BER is felt to be a normal variant, not indicative of underlying cardiac disease. The electrocardiographic definition of BER includes the following characteristics: (1) STE; (2) upward concavity of the initial portion of the ST segment; (3) notching or slurring of the terminal QRS complex; (4) symmetric, concordant T waves of large amplitude; (5) widespread or diffuse distribution of STE on the ECG; and (6) relative temporal stability.[36] See Figures 73-21, *A* and 73-22 for examples of BER.

The STE begins at the J point, the portion of the electrocardiographic cycle where the QRS complex ends and the ST segment begins. The degree of J point elevation is usually less than 3.5 mm. This STE appears as if the ST segment has been evenly lifted upward from the isoelectric baseline at the J point. This elevation results in a preservation of the normal concavity of the initial, upsloping portion of the ST segment–T wave complex, a very important electrocardiographic feature used to distinguish BER-related STE from STE associated with AMI. The STE elevation encountered in BER is usually less than 2 mm but may approach 5 mm in certain individuals. Eighty to ninety percent of individuals demonstrate STE less than 2 mm in the precordial leads and less than 0.5 mm in the limb leads; only 2% of cases of BER manifest STE greater than 5 mm. The degree of STE related to BER is usually greatest in the mid- to left precordial leads

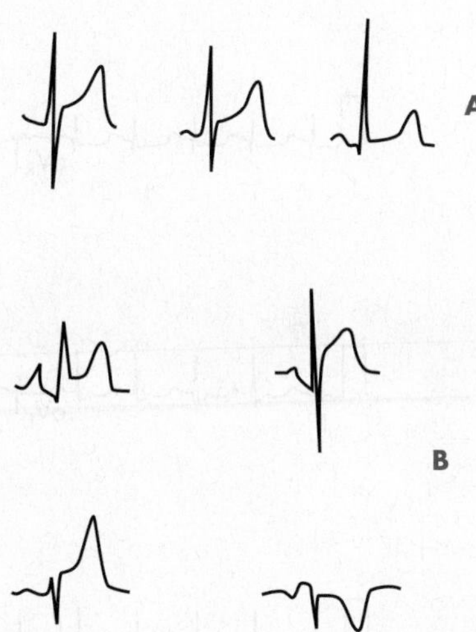

Figure 73-21. **Noninfarctional ST segment elevation. A, Benign early repolarization with concave STE. B, Acute pericarditis with concave STE and PR segment depression (upper two examples); concave STE without PR segment abnormalities (lower left example); and "reciprocal" STD and PR segment elevation in lead aV_r (lower right example).**

(leads V_2 through V_5). The ST segments of the remaining electrocardiographic leads are less often elevated to the extent observed in leads V_2 through V_5. The limb leads (I, II, III, aV_L, and aV_F) are less often observed to demonstrate STE; one large series reported that the limb leads revealed STE in only 45% of cases of BER. "Isolated" BER in the limb leads—i.e., no precordial STE—is a very rare finding. Such "isolated" STE in the inferior (II, III, and aV_F) or lateral (I and aV_L) leads should prompt consideration of another explanation for the observed ST segment abnormality.

Acute pericarditis produces diffuse inflammation of the superficial epicardium, resulting in a current of injury that is manifested by electrocardiographic STE (Figures 73-21, *B*

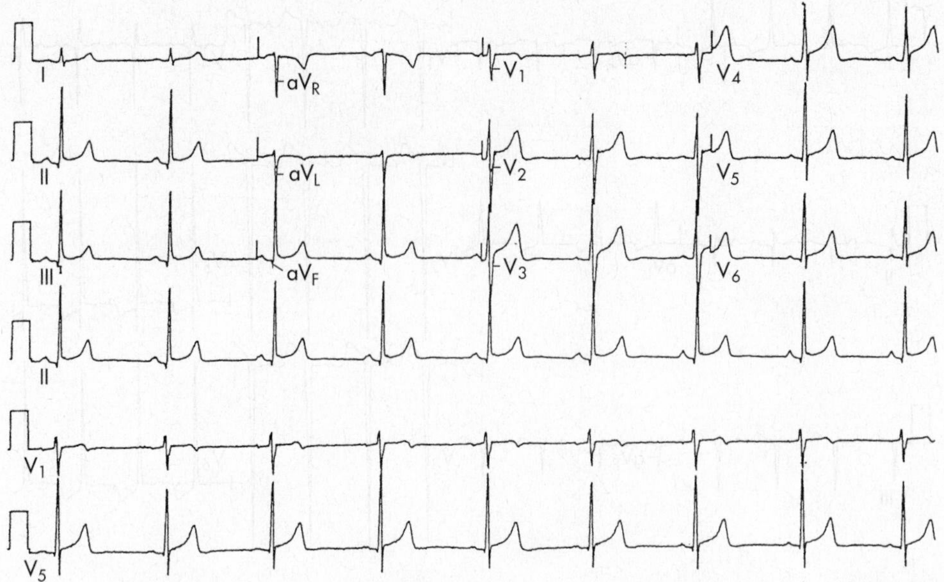

Figure 73-22. **Example of benign early repolarization.** ***Modified from Aufderheide TP, Brady WJ: Electrocardiography in the patient with myocardial ischemia or infarction. In Gibler WB, Aufderheide TP, editors:*** **Emergency cardiac care,** ***St Louis, 1994, Mosby.***

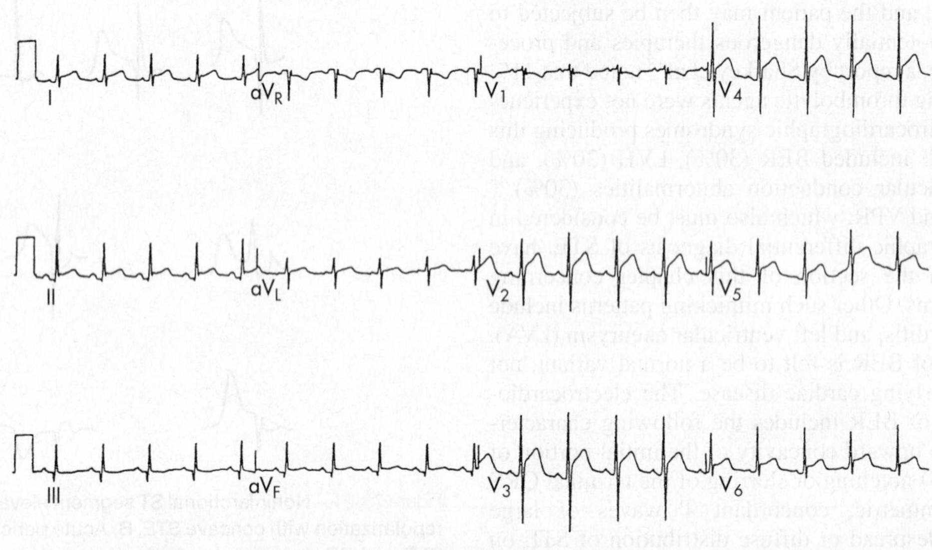

Figure 73-23. **Representative example of 12-lead ECG in patient with acute pericarditis. Note diffuse STE in leads I, II, aV$_F$, and V$_2$ through V$_6$. PR segment depression is best seen in lead V$_6$ and II.** ***Modified from Aufderheide TP, Brady WJ: Electrocardiography in the patient with myocardial ischemia or infarction. In Gibler WB, Aufderheide TP, editors:*** **Emergency cardiac care,** ***St Louis, 1994, Mosby.***

and 73-23). STE is usually less than 5 mm in height, observed in numerous leads, and characterized by a concavity to its initial upsloping portion. In some instances, the STE may actually be obliquely flat; convexity of the STE, however, strongly suggests AMI. The STE due to acute pericarditis is usually noted in the following electrocardiographic leads: I, II, III, aV$_L$, aV$_F$, and V$_2$ through V$_6$ (essentially, all leads except V$_1$); reciprocal STD is also seen in lead aV$_R$ and occasionally in lead V$_1$. The STE is most often seen in many leads simultaneously, although it may be limited to a specific anatomic segment. If the process is focal, the inferior wall is often involved, with leads II, III, and aV$_F$ commonly affected. PR segment depression associated with pericarditis is the most helpful feature in arriving at the correct electrocardiographic diagnosis; such a finding has been described as "almost diagnostic" for acute pericarditis and is best seen in lead V$_6$ and the inferior leads. Reciprocal PR segment elevation is seen in lead aV$_R$.

LVA is defined as a localized area of infarcted myocardium that bulges outward during both systole and diastole. LVAs most often are noted after large anterior wall events but may also be encountered status post inferior and posterior wall

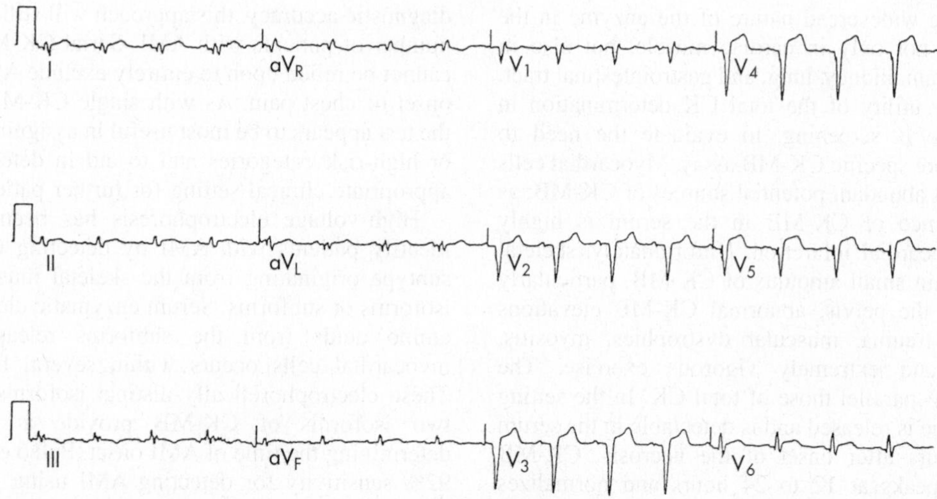

Figure 73-24. **Representative example of 12-lead ECG from patient with anterior LVA. Note well-developed, completed Q waves in leads V_2 through V_5 and absence of reciprocal changes in contralateral leads.** *Modified from Aufderheide TP, Brady WJ: Electrocardiography in the patient with myocardial ischemia or infarction. In Gibler WB, Aufderheide TP, editors:* Emergency cardiac care, *St Louis, 1994, Mosby.*

AMIs. In most cases, the LVA is manifested electrocardiographically by varying degrees of STE that may be difficult to distinguish from ST segment changes due to AMI, particularly in the patient with chest pain and known past myocardial infarction.[36] LVA is characterized electrocardiographically by persistent STE seen several weeks after AMI. Because of the frequent anterior location of LVA, STE is most often observed in leads I, aV_L, and V_1 through V_6. Of course, the inferior wall LVA would be manifested on the surface ECG by STE in the inferior leads; such STE, however, is usually less pronounced than the ST segment changes seen in the anterior leads. The actual ST segment abnormality due to the LVA may be seen with varying morphologies, ranging from obvious, convex STE to minimal, concave elevations. The distinction from STE in the patient with AMI may be difficult. Refer to Figure 73-24 for an example of electrocardiographic changes seen in the LVA pattern.

Serum Markers

The elevation of cardiac markers in the serum over several days of hospitalization has been the standard method for diagnosing AMI over the last 30 years. Creatinine phosphokinase-MB fraction (CK-MB) once was the typical marker used by most clinical laboratories to indicate myocardial necrosis. The troponins are now the most commonly used serologic tests. In the past, detection of AMI by characteristic enzyme elevations over 48 to 72 hours was sufficient to establish the diagnosis of AMI. Because of the evolution of thrombolytic therapy and acute intervention, significant pressure now exists to identify patients with AMI for early intervention. In patients coming to the ED with a nondiagnostic ECG, early serum markers of myocardial cell necrosis have the potential to alter the diagnostic course, treatment plans, and disposition location. Caution is advised, however, when interpreting the results of serum marker

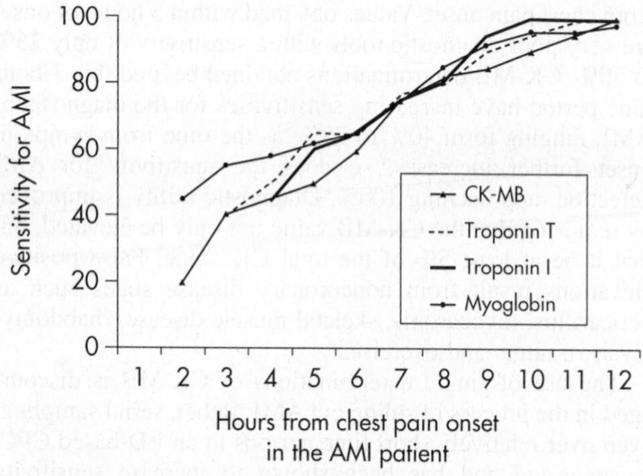

Figure 73-25. **Serum marker sensitivity relative to the time of onset of chest pain in the patient with AMI.** *Data obtained from the medical literature.*

determinations. Patient history remains the most vital portion of the diagnostic evaluation of the patient with chest pain and potential AICS. Refer to Figure 73-25 for a depiction of the sensitivities for AMI diagnosis relative to the time from chest pain onset for CK-MB, the troponins, and myoglobin.

Creatine Kinase Creatine kinase (CK) is an enzyme found in large quantities in cardiac and skeletal muscle. Following AMI, increases in serum CK are detectable within 3 to 8 hours with a peak at 12 to 24 hours after injury; assuming a single, one-time event, the levels will normalize within 3 to 4 days. Total CK values obtained at the time of ED arrival show a sensitivity of 40% and a specificity of 80% for the diagnosis of AMI; measurements taken as late as 12 hours after the onset of chest pain have a marginally improved sensitivity approaching 50%.

The major problem that reduces the total CK's clinical utility involves the widespread nature of the enzyme in the body; it is found not only in cardiac muscle, but also in skeletal muscle, brain, kidney, lung, and gastrointestinal tract. The current major utility of the total CK determination in acute cardiac care is screening, to evaluate the need to perform the far more specific CK-MB assay. Myocardial cells are by far the most abundant potential sources of CK-MB; as such, the appearance of CK-MB in the serum is highly suggestive of myocardial infarction. Unfortunately, skeletal muscle does contain small amounts of CK-MB, particularly the muscle about the pelvis; abnormal CK-MB elevations may be seen in trauma, muscular dystrophies, myositis, rhabdomyolysis, and extremely vigorous exercise. The kinetics of CK-MB parallel those of total CK. In the setting of AMI, the enzyme is released and is detectable in the serum as early as 3 hours after onset of the necrosis. CK-MB characteristically peaks at 12 to 24 hours and normalizes within 2 to 3 days following injury. Elevated CK-MB values identify a patient at considerable risk for poor outcome. As with total CK measurement, however, the peak CK-MB value does not correlate well with infarct size; in fact, studies demonstrate that an elevated CK-MB is associated with a poor prognosis, regardless of the magnitude of the elevation.

The sensitivity of a single CK-MB determination in diagnosing AMI is entirely dependent upon the elapsed time from chest pain onset. Values obtained within 3 hours of onset are very poor diagnostic tools with a sensitivity of only 25% to 50%. CK-MB determinations obtained beyond this 3-hour time period have increasing sensitivities for the diagnosis of AMI, ranging form 40% to 75%; as the time from symptom onset further increases, so does the sensitivity for AMI detection, approaching 100%. Diagnostic utility is improved by requiring that the CK-MB value not only be elevated, but that it be at least 5% of the total CK value. False positive elevations result from noncoronary disease states such as pericarditis, myocarditis, skeletal muscle disease, rhabdomyolysis, trauma, and exercise.

The use of single determinations of CK-MB is discouraged in the process of ruling out AMI; rather, serial sampling, even over relatively short time periods in an ED-based CPC, is suggested and has been shown to increase sensitivity considerably. CK-MB values rise quickly following an AMI, typically doubling within 3 to 6 hours of the event. Two studies illustrate the use of serial CK-MB sampling in the ED. In the first investigation,[49] patients who complained of chest pain had serial CK-MB samples drawn on ED arrival and a second set 3 hours later. One hundred eighty-three patients were evaluated, with 31 patients having AMI diagnosed by WHO criteria; all were detected by this serial testing approach within 3 hours of ED arrival. In the second study,[50] 313 patients who came to an ED with complaints of acute chest pain had serum samples obtained for CK-MB at arrival and then hourly for 3 hours, a total of 4 samples. Infarction was present in 70 patients (22%). Sensitivity and specificity for detection of infarction were 76% and 72%, respectively, as determined from the initial CK-MB values only and increased with each additional sample to a maximum of 92% and 96%, respectively, in all four samples. Other investigators have reported that an increase in the CK-MB of at least 1.5 ng/ml over a 2-hour period had an 88% sensitivity in diagnosing AMI; such CK-MB increases over a specific time interval indicated AMI more accurately than did troponin I. While serial CK-MB measurements increase the test's diagnostic accuracy, this approach will still miss a significant number of patients with AMI. Serial CK-MB sampling thus cannot be relied upon to entirely exclude AICS soon after the onset of chest pain. As with single CK-MB determinations, the test appears to be most useful in assigning patients to low- or high-risk categories and to aid in determining the most appropriate clinical setting for further patient evaluation.

High-voltage electrophoresis has been used to rapidly identify patients with AMI by detecting CK-MM (the CK subtype originating from the skeletal muscle) and CK-MB isoforms or subforms. Serum enzymatic cleavage of terminal amino acids from the subforms released by infarcted myocardial cells occurs within several hours after onset. These electrophoretically distinct isoforms of CK-MM and two isoforms of CK-MB provide a "fingerprint" for determining the time of AMI onset. Puleo et al demonstrate a 92% sensitivity for detecting AMI using CK-MB isoforms within 4 to 6 hours after symptom onset and 100% sensitivity within 6 to 8 hours after symptom onset.[51] In a fashion similar to immunochemical testing for CK-MB, such isoform analysis can provide the clinician with valuable information for diagnosis, treatment, and disposition of the patient with AMI who has a nondiagnostic ECG.

Clinicians must recognize the limitations of the various CK-MB determinations when making clinical decisions based on such laboratory results. A positive CK-MB in the appropriate patient strongly suggests AMI; such patients should be admitted to the CCU. A negative test, in the form of either a single determination or serial measurement, does not reliably exclude AMI. A single negative result in the patient suspected of AICS suggests only that a non-CCU admission disposition is appropriate. In an ED-based observation unit, an otherwise low-risk patient who has unremarkable serial testing results and a normal to minimally abnormal ECG may be safely evaluated as an outpatient. Single CK-MB determinations should not be used as the sole diagnostic test in determining an outpatient disposition.

Troponins Two myocardial-specific proteins, troponin T (TnT) and troponin I (TnI), have early release kinetics similar to CK-MB. Troponin T (molecular weight approximately 38,000 daltons) and troponin I (molecular weight approximately 22,000 daltons) appear to slightly precede the release of CK-MB into the serum. The cardiac troponins are genetically distinct from those forms found in skeletal muscle, making them highly cardiac-specific markers. Monoclonal antibodies have been developed with little cross-reactivity to troponins from skeletal muscle. The cardiac troponins are not found in the serum of healthy individuals—a significant distinction from the CK and CK-MB characteristics.

The biokinetics of troponin release are related to the location of the protein within the cell. Normally, small quantities of troponins are free in the cytosol, while the majority is entwined in the muscle fiber. Following injury, a biphasic rise in serum troponins corresponding to early release of the free cytoplasmic proteins is followed by a slower and greatly prolonged rise with breakdown of the actual muscle fiber; the slow destruction of the myocardial cell contractile proteins provides a sustained release of the troponins for 5 to 7 days. Serum troponin concentrations begin to rise measurably in the serum at about the same time as CK-MB elevations become detectable—as early as 3 hours after onset—but troponin levels remain elevated for a week or more. The cardiac-specific troponins are highly sensitive for the early detection of myocardial injury in AICS. A positive test is associated with significant risk while a negative study (i.e., serial troponins) predicts low risk.[52]

Troponin T, an approximately 38,000-dalton protein, is found in the serum of patients with AICS and in the serum of individuals with skeletal muscle disease and renal failure. Following AICS, TnT rises as early as 3 to 4 hours, although elevations may not be detected until 10 hours after symptom onset in some patients. Serum levels remain elevated for 4 to 8 days after AMI.

Regarding the use of TnT in the diagnosis of AMI, sensitivity of TnT approaches 50% within 3 to 4 hours of the event. The test is positive in about 75% at 6 hours after onset of symptoms; at 12 hours, the test is almost 100% sensitive. The relatively slow appearance of TnT in the serum following an acute cardiac event severely limits the utility of this test by emergency physicians in excluding AMI.

TnT has actually outperformed the existing "gold standard" serum marker (CK-MB) in the diagnosis of AMI. In fact, TnT determinations may return positive in a patient with chest pain and normal CK-MB values. Authorities have not yet agreed on the nomenclature of such a scenario—a severe form of USAP or a non-STE AMI? For the clinician, such rhetorical debates are meaningless. It is known that AICS patients with nondiagnostic ECGs, positive TnT values, and negative CK-MB values have poor prognoses—not dissimilar to patients with STE AMIs.[53,54] The probability of cardiac complications in patients with elevated TnT values who don't meet standard criteria for diagnosis of AMI actually appears to be equal to that of patients diagnosed with AMI.[53,54] Furthermore, the risk of such complications is proportional to the concentration of TnT in the serum. The likely explanation for this pattern of serum marker results is that TnT is released by *reversibly injured* myocardium—i.e., the patients have USAP. The presence of TnT in the serum thus serves more as a marker of a significant AICS episode rather than a specific marker of AMI. Patients with abnormal TnT levels at 3 or more hours following arrival in the ED have a much higher rate of cardiac complications within 2 to 6 months. Thus elevated TnT values appear to be excellent indicators of risk of death, AMI, and acute cardiovascular complications—in all AICS patients, even those who do not meet traditional criteria for AMI. A negative test result, however, does not necessarily imply a favorable prognosis.

Troponin I, an approximate 22,000-dalton protein, is found only in the serum of patients with significant AICS, and in contrast to TnT is not found in the presence of other muscular diseases. Following AICS, TnI levels rise within 3 to 6 hours of chest pain onset, peaking at 12 to 18 hours and remaining elevated for 5 to 7 days—longer than CK-MB yet not as long as TnT.

The diagnostic utility of TnI is very similar to the features encountered with TnT. The test has little sensitivity within 3 hours of chest pain onset; TnI assays are likely to be positive in patients within 6 hours of onset. In clinical comparisons of the cardiac troponins, TnI may be the slightly better marker of AICS, ultimately having 100% sensitivity for AMI and 36% sensitivity for USAP, although the differences likely do not have clinical significance. As with TnT, elevations in TnI are seen in a substantial minority of patients ultimately diagnosed with non-AMI AICS events; such patients have a much higher rate of cardiac complications, AMI, and death than those without abnormal TnI values.

Myoglobin Myoglobin is attractive as an indicator for myocardial injury. It is small, with a molecular weight of 17,000 daltons. Myoglobin levels are elevated in the serum within 1 to 2 hours after symptom onset, peaking 4 to 5 hours after AMI in patients coming to the ED with AMI.[55] Sensitivity improves from 62% on ED arrival to 100% 3 hours later, compared with 50% and 95%, respectively, for immunochemical CK-MB analyses. Myoglobin has a 100% negative predictive value for AMI—*not AICS*.[55] Myocardial myoglobin, however, is not currently distinguishable immunologically from skeletal muscle myoglobin, reducing its specificity to approximately 80% compared with 94% for immunochemical CK-MB determination 3 hours after ED admission.[55] Myoglobin is elevated in patients with renal failure because of reduced clearance, making this marker less useful in a patient population that tends to be at risk for AICS. It also will be elevated in any clinical situation involving the skeletal muscle, such as trauma, exercise, and significant systemic illness.

Serial determinations markedly improve the myoglobin assay's diagnostic power. Using a doubling of serum myoglobin values within 2 hours of arrival as a marker of AMI, serial determinations have been found to have a sensitivity and specificity approaching 95%. Serial myoglobin determinations, therefore, appear to be useful in the evaluation of the patient with AICS soon after symptom onset; in fact, they may be more sensitive early on than CK-MB or serial CK-MB assays. The serial testing strategy, however, still fails to detect up to 10% of AMIs. Myoglobin may also be used in a prognostic, rather than diagnostic, sense in the AICS patient; a positive determination is associated with an increased risk of poor outcome.

Theoretically, the addition of carbonic anhydrase determination to myoglobin testing would increase myoglobin's utility, because carbonic anhydrase is found in skeletal and striated muscle—but not in myocardial tissue. With skeletal muscle injury, carbonic anhydrase is released into the serum in a fixed ratio with myoglobin. In that carbonic anhydrase is not released in the setting of myocardial injury, measurement of a myoglobin/carbonic anhydrase ratio may therefore distinguish elevations in serum myoglobin concentration due to myocardial infarction from non–cardiac muscle injury. While attractive theoretically, this biochemical property has not yielded overly promising clinical results. The ratio determination was found to be more reliable than CK-MB determination at 3 hours[56]; the sensitivity, however, dropped to less than 50% at the 6-hour mark. At times greater than 6 hours, the assay was inferior to CK-MB testing.

Echocardiography

Two-dimensional echocardiography has been demonstrated to be an effective tool for detecting regional wall motion abnormality associated with AICS in the emergency setting. Impaired myocardial contractility can be observed echocardiographically in patients with AICS, often following a progressive course from hypokinesis to akinesis. Impaired myocardial relaxation during diastole results in decreased ventricular distensibility. After AMI, paradoxical wall motion observed during systole indicates the subsequent loss of muscle tone from necrosis. Decreased ejection fraction may result from these ventricular wall motion abnormalities.

Studies evaluating patients coming to the ED with chest pain have correlated regional wall motion abnormality with the presence of myocardial ischemia and AMI, assisting in the diagnostic process particularly in those individuals who have nondiagnostic ECGs.[57-59] With the demonstration of regional wall motion abnormality in patients with chest pain, sensitivities for AMI detection range from 88% to 94% with specificities of 50% to 75% in patients treated within 12 hours after symptom onset in a CCU.[57] Technical limitations restrict the use of echocardiography in the emergent diagnosis of AMI and myocardial ischemia. These limitations include the quality of the study, which is proportional to the experience of the operator, and the expertise of the reader interpreting the study at the patient's bedside. In addition, the usefulness of the two-dimensional echocardiogram is further limited by its inability to distinguish between ischemia, AMI, old infarction, and the potential absence of wall motion abnormality in nontransmural infarctions. Echocardiography is typically less expensive than radionuclide ventriculography, however, and offers more anatomic detail while avoiding the use of radionuclides. Echocardiography can also be performed rapidly in the acute care setting.

Radionuclide Scanning

Nuclear scintigraphy is useful in detecting AICS in selected ED patients who complain of chest pain. Two of the common isotopes used are thallium-201 and technetium-99. The first isotope used was thallium-201, a potassium analogue that relies on uptake by viable myocardium. Technetium-99 is a lipophilic monovalent cation that relies on the negatively charged mitochondrial membrane for uptake; technetium provides important information about myocardial perfusion at the time of injection. Nuclear scintigraphy has promising positive and negative predictive values for cardiac events with a high sensitivity and a good specificity for CAD.

Multiple studies have been performed in ED patients with ongoing chest pain or in those with recent chest pain. These studies revealed an annual major cardiac event rate (cardiac death or nonfatal MI) of less than 1% in patients with scans showing normal perfusion. For example, in a study by Hilton et al,[60] 150 ED patients underwent single photon emission computed tomography (SPECT) imaging with technetium-99 if they had typical chest pain with either a normal or nondiagnostic ECG. This particular group had a 10% to 20% risk for nonfatal AMI based on typical chest pain and a normal or nondiagnostic ECG. At 90 days postscan, no patient with a normal scan had a cardiac event or experienced death. Multiple studies have found a relatively high incidence of cardiac events after a nuclear scan showed abnormal perfusion. The probability of a cardiac event was tenfold higher in patients with abnormal scan results than in those patients whose results were normal. The incidence of cardiac events after a normal scan was 1% or less per year. For example, Kontos et al[61] investigated the efficacy of early perfusion imaging using technetium-99m sestamibi to predict adverse cardiac outcomes in patients with possible AICS who had nondiagnostic ECGs. After a brief ED evaluation, patients underwent rapid sestamibi injection. A total of 532 consecutive patients underwent serial myocardial marker analysis and rest perfusion imaging. Of these patients, perfusion imaging was abnormal in 171 (32%); imaging that showed abnormal perfusion was highly associated with AMI (93% sensitivity) and the need for revascularization. Perfusion imaging accurately identified patients at high risk for adverse cardiac outcomes, and negative perfusion imaging (normal perfusion) identified a low-risk patient group.

Radionuclide studies are difficult to perform in the very early period after patient arrival in the ED. Radioisotopes and the personnel to administer them may not be immediately available; furthermore, in most centers physician reader availability is quite variable.

Graded Exercise Testing

An awareness of the limitations of exercise stress testing for detecting significant underlying CAD is a must if the clinician employs such evaluations in the ED or interprets the results of past studies when patients have chest discomfort. Graded exercise testing in the general population has a sensitivity of 60% to 70% for identifying patients with exercise-induced ischemia and underlying CAD. As with any diagnostic test, the pretest probability of disease in the population studied must be considered. In view of this, the clinician will find that a negative stress test result in a patient with a high pretest probability for CAD is likely to be a false-negative result, whereas a positive stress test result in a patient with a low pretest probability will likely be a false-positive result. The specificity of the test is decreased in the face of underlying electrocardiographic abnormalities secondary to medications, electrolyte abnormalities, LVH, or artifact, along with numerous other causes. A false positive stress test result may be due to aortic stenosis or insufficiency, hypertrophic cardiomyopathy, hypertension, arteriovenous fistula, anemia, hemoglobinopathies, low cardiac output states, COPD, digitalis, toxic states, LVH, hyperventilation, mitral valve prolapse, and bundle branch blocks. False-positive test results in women, a more common situation in the female patient, tend to decrease the usefulness of graded exercise testing in the younger female patient.

The use of a CPC-based mandatory exercise stress testing evaluation in an ED chest pain population was investigated by one study group. The authors[62] reported on their experience with the portion of the ED population felt to be at intermediate risk for AICS. They employed an abbreviated ED-based CPC "rule-out MI" protocol followed by mandatory stress testing. Of the 477 patients in the study, 67 patients (13%) were admitted to the hospital from the CPC, of whom 44 (66%) had a final diagnosis of CAD or IHD. Twenty-four patients with such diagnoses were identified only with stress testing; the remaining admitted patients had abnormal ECGs, positive serum markers, or other clinical findings suggestive of AICS. Four hundred ten patients (86%) were discharged home from the CPC after the complete evaluation; these patients were alive and well 5 months later without having suffered AMIs. In this ED study population, the cost of mandatory stress testing to identify one patient with IHD after AMI was ruled out was $3125. An average cost-per-case savings of 62% was achieved for each patient managed as such who would otherwise have been hospitalized.

The use of immediate stress testing (i.e., without the "rule-out MI" evaluation) has been suggested to be safe and cost effective in low-risk patients suspected of having AICS. Investigators[63] attempted to determine the safety and utility of *immediate* exercise testing in the evaluation of low-risk patients presenting to the ED with chest pain; this investigation tested the accuracy and safety of early exercise testing in the very heterogeneous ED patient population. Immediate exercise testing was performed; screening history, physical examination, and resting ECGs were performed prior to exercise testing. A total of 212 patients (121 men and 91 women) underwent exercise testing with no adverse effects. Twenty-eight (13%) patients had positive results on exercise ECGs, with 23 of these individuals demonstrating abnormalities strongly suggestive of significant, multivessel CAD on subsequent evaluation. One hundred twenty-five patients (59%) had negative exercise test results while 59 patients (28%) had nondiagnostic results. All patients with negative test results and 93% with nondiagnostic test results were discharged directly from the ED. Thirty-day follow-up was achieved in 201 (95%) patients and revealed no mortality in any of the patients in the three groups. One patient with a positive exercise test result returned to the ED within 30 days with mild CHF.

Computer-Aided Decision Making

Computer-assisted diagnostic algorithms provide an interesting approach to evaluating the patient with chest pain and possible AICS. Improving physician risk estimates for patients with chest discomfort coming to the ED will increase the detection rates of AICS. This in turn will ultimately increase the prevalence of appropriate admission to the hospital while decreasing the likelihood of inappropriate release from the ED.

Several reports indicate that retrospectively validated computer programs can prospectively match the sensitivity and specificity demonstrated by the physician. Using recursive partitioning analysis, Goldman et al attempted to define a high-risk group for AMI of 7% or greater.[64] Initial data suggest a protocol sensitivity of 92% and specificity of 70%, which is equivalent to the accuracy found in clinicians not using the protocol. In revising the initial protocol, the algorithm was used prospectively on 4770 patients with chest pain at the six study hospitals.[65] Although sensitivity did not increase beyond the clinicians' impressions, 88% based on CCU admission of patients with AMI, specificity was significantly better when using the algorithm (74% versus 71%). If used by the physicians it would have reduced CCU admissions by 11.5% in patients without AMI while admitting the same number of patients with AMI.

An innovative software approach for detecting AICS describes the training of a neural network. A neural network differs from conventional software analysis in that the network consists of a neuron-like system that has the ability to sum inhibitory and excitatory stimuli to produce a discrete output, which in turn may synapse with other similar outputs. The network can also be "taught" to make informed decisions by providing it with sets of input data and pairing these input data with their associated outputs. Over time, the discriminatory capability of a neural network should improve. The neural network is considered free of the many biases and random errors that may influence the busy clinician.

The neural network has been prospectively validated in a trial of 331 consecutive ED patients with the chief complaint of anterior chest pain.[66] Thirty-six of these patients were ultimately diagnosed as having AMI. The network performed with a sensitivity of 97.2% and a specificity of 96.2% in this patient cohort. The physicians caring for the study patients performed with a sensitivity of 77.7% and a specificity of 84.7%.

CPCs—Specialized ED-based Evaluation and Treatment Units

Multiple objectives must be attained if clinicians are to improve efficiency and rapidity in the diagnosis and treatment of patients with chest pain while controlling costs and reducing unnecessary hospital admissions. The National Heart Attack Alert Program (NHAAP) of the National Heart, Lung, and Blood Institute (NHLBI) has challenged clinicians to provide care for ED patients with clear signs and symptoms of AMI within 30 minutes after ED arrival. Despite findings from multiple studies that demonstrate that very early administration of thrombolytic therapy to patients with AMI significantly reduces mortality, most treatment is initiated after this important time window in many U.S. hospitals. Substantial effort will be required in most U.S. hospitals to meet this challenge.

The care of patients with chest pain and possible AICS can be approached in a protocol-driven fashion in a CPC—where urgent evaluation and treatment may occur in addition to prolonged observation with abbreviated "rule-out MI" programs. A CPC protocol should rapidly direct patients with possible AICS into a high-level treatment area in the ED. With an ECG and clinical examination obtained within the first 10 minutes after ED arrival, patients with STE AMI requiring immediate reperfusion therapy or patients having clinical syndromes consistent with USAP in need of further intervention can be identified quickly. Identifying AMI and obvious USAP in ED patients can be combined with an efficient ED evaluation of patients with low to moderate risk for AICS. The greatest medical benefit from the CPC likely will be the early identification and treatment of patients with AMI and USAP; the most significant financial impact will probably be its potential for reducing the number of hospital admissions—and financial cost—for noncardiac chest pain.

CPCs must have procedures established to achieve a target "door-to-drug" time of 30 minutes (or less) or a door-to-balloon-inflation (where PTCA is available) time of 90 (± 30) minutes (or less) for patients with typical features of AMI with STE. In a position paper[67] the NHAAP has recommended: (1) a specific area of the ED equipped for assessing and monitoring patients potentially having ischemia, including standing orders for initial diagnostic and therapeutic actions; (2) a standing protocol with inclusion and exclusion criteria for reperfusion therapies, including language authorizing the physician to administer thrombolytic therapy or to mobilize the catheterization lab for prespecified cases; (3) a clear demarcation of responsibilities for all members of the reperfusion team; and (4) policies and procedures for the treatment and possible transfer of patients with STE AMI who are ineligible for thrombolytic therapy. The ED should also have a procedure in place for the treatment of patients with non-AMI AICS.

The CPC can serve as both an acute evaluation section of the ED and an observation unit. In the first instance, the CPC has assigned nursing personnel who rapidly evaluate the patient having chest pain with a 12-lead ECG, vital signs screening, and cardiac monitoring. The physician is informed of patients with significant ST segment changes. Appropriate therapy is then initiated in expeditious fashion; urgent cardiology consultation is also possible. This role of the CPC is referred to as a *heart attack program* for the rapid treatment of AICS, particularly the STE AMI. The CPC may also be used as an observation unit in which patients with chest pain and low-to-intermediate clinical likelihood of AICS can be monitored with electrocardiography, ST segment trending, serial 12-lead ECGs, and sequential serum markers; these tools compose the accelerated "rule-out MI" protocol. During the period of monitoring, the patient's status is closely scrutinized; the development of any life threat, including sudden cardiac death, is rapidly identified and aggressively managed. This function of the CPC is described as a diagnostic (observational) program. Evaluation of such protocols has been proven medically effective and safe with follow-up obtained on patients within 48 hours and 30 days after evaluation. Significant cost savings have also been demonstrated. Typical charges and actual costs range from 20% to 50% of the usual 2-day or less inpatient diagnostic approach to possible AICS.

The Chest Pain Evaluation in the Emergency Room (CHEER) investigators performed a prospective, randomized trial of chest pain unit (CPU) evaluation compared to the traditional hospital admission for "rule-out MI" in patients with chest pain.[68] Over a 16-month period, adult patients with chest pain were evaluated initially with a history, physical examination, and ECG; based on the results, the eligible patients (determined to be at intermediate risk) were then randomized to either CPC or hospital admission for additional evaluation for AMI. Exclusion criteria included ST segment abnormalities (elevation or depression), obvious noncardiac etiology, coexisting issues requiring hospitalization, and high-risk issues predictive of cardiac events. CPC patients then underwent serial serum marker and ECG determinations over a minimum of 6 hours; aspirin and heparin (selected cases) were administered. If test results were negative and the course uncomplicated, patients then underwent further evaluation with exercise stress test, nuclear stress test, or stress echocardiography—interpreted by a cardiologist. If the results of further evaluation were positive, the patient was referred to a cardiologist; if negative, the patient was discharged with cardiology follow-up scheduled within 72 hours. The 6-month end points were cardiac event (primary) and the need for coronary revascularization, additional cardiac investigation, or admission for cardiac reasons (secondary). Initially 2517 patients were evaluated for this study, and of those, 424 (17%) were enrolled. The rate of primary cardiac events was not significantly different between the two groups: 15 events for admitted patients (13 AMI, two CHF) and seven events for the CPC group (five AMI, one CHF, one death). Among CPC patients with a negative evaluation, no cardiac events occurred after ED discharge; these events occurred in the 114 patients admitted to the hospital from the CPC because of a positive evaluation. For a 6-month period after discharge, cardiac investigations and therapies were greater among patients in the admitted group. Admissions to the hospital were reduced by 45.8% during the study. The authors concluded that for patients with chest pain that was likely to represent USAP and who were at intermediate risk for acute cardiac complications, an ED-based CPC evaluation was safe, effective, and cost-efficient.

Gibler et al[69] evaluated a comprehensive diagnostic 9-hour evaluation (Heart ER Program) for patients with chest pain and possible AICS. A total of 1010 consecutive patients with those symptoms were enrolled in the Heart ER Program over 32 months. Patients with history of CAD, hemodynamic instability, acute ST changes, or a clinical syndrome consistent with USAP were admitted directly to the hospital. All patients underwent serial testing with the following: CK-MB on arrival and at 3, 6, and 9 hours, continuous 12-lead ECGs, and serial ST segment trend monitoring. Two-dimensional echocardiography and graded exercise testing were performed in the ED after the 9-hour evaluation. Of 1010 patients, 829 (82.1%) were released from the ED; 153 (15.1%) required admission for further cardiac evaluation. Fifty-two of 153 (33.9%) admitted patients were found to have a cardiac cause for their symptoms: 43 had AICS (12 AMI and 31 USAP). Such a program provided an effective method for evaluating low- to moderate-risk patients with possible AICS in the ED setting. This study once again suggests that the CPC approach is safe and effective. The resources required for a successful operation, however, are considerable; many institutions may not be able to replicate such a successful program.

As seen in the above two investigations, the medical literature suggests that a "rule-out MI" protocol that does not involve hospital admission is feasible, accurate, and may be cost effective. For patients with chest pain or related symptoms without STE, the rapid exclusion of AICS is accomplished via serial testing and aggressive, continuous monitoring over a relatively short period. In fact, the medical literature indicates that approximately 80% of patients with chest pain can be safely and effectively evaluated in the ED with ultimate discharge to home. An overall perspective of CPC resource utilization and associated costs was recently provided by a multicenter study of ED observation units. The authors found that the presence of a CPC increased the number of patients who underwent "rule-out MI" evaluation instead of being discharged home directly after the ED clinical evaluation; simultaneously, patients admitted to the hospital decreased by the same number. This study suggests that in appropriately selected patients, outpatient evaluation may contribute to the goal of high detection rates for patients with AICS at a lower cost. Anecdotal reports also, however, suggest that physicians may overuse the CPC "rule-out MI" approach in patients that they otherwise would have discharged from the ED.

Patients appear satisfied with "rule-out MI" care rendered in CPCs. A survey was performed investigating their level of satisfaction with CPC versus in-hospital stay for the "rule-out MI" evaluation. The survey was distributed via U.S. mail to patients who underwent the evaluation. They were randomly chosen from the rosters of a university hospital and its ED. The rates of positive feedback were greater than 80% in all areas of comfort, safety, and satisfaction for both groups. CPC and hospitalized patients demonstrated statistically similar rates of satisfaction concerning feelings of medical safety, nurse and physician evaluation and monitoring, comfort, and degree of disruption in daily schedule. This survey demonstrates that the ED-based CPC offers the patient an equally satisfying place of observation when compared to the traditional admission.[69a]

With the mandate for a more efficient yet safe method for evaluating patients with low to intermediate risk for AICS, the CPC may offer a reasonable alternative to the traditional 48-hour inpatient admission. It is estimated that approximately 20% of hospital EDs in the United States now employ the CPC approach. Issues to consider prior to developing such a unit include patient entry criteria; the resources, abilities, and desires of the ED staff; the availability of cardiac diagnostic testing; support from the local cardiology groups; and the impact on the primary care physician. The appropriate patient—low- to intermediate-risk—must be chosen for such an evaluation. The ED must also have a dedicated area for aggressive cardiac monitoring with dedicated nursing staff and resources, timely return of serum marker values, and knowledgeable, motivated physicians. Support from the cardiologist is vital in the form of cardiac diagnostic testing availability 7 days a week, 24 hours a day, and timely outpatient follow-up. Without such continuous support from the hospital and the cardiologist, the CPC approach is not recommended. Many hospitals can provide diagnostic testing only on a limited basis; without complete risk evaluation prior to discharge from the ED, the patient and physician are placed at risk. The primary care physician must also be considered in this process in terms of financial issues, referral, and resource utilization concerns.

MANAGEMENT

The pathophysiology of USAP is presumed similar to AMI, representing thrombus formation in the lumen of a coronary artery, which occurs after atherosclerotic plaque rupture and platelet aggregation. The following steps occur in an episode of myocardial ischemia: (1) endothelial damage through plaque disruption, irregular luminal lesions, shear injury; (2) platelet aggregation; (3) thrombus formation causing partial or total lumen occlusion; (4) coronary artery vasospasm; and (5) reperfusion injury caused by oxygen free radicals, calcium, and neutrophils. In patients with USAP, spontaneous thrombolysis occurs rapidly, minimizing ischemic insult. Persistence of the occlusive luminal thrombus for 60 to 90 minutes before spontaneous lysis of the clot results in a non-STE AMI. STE AMI occurs when the thrombus occlusion lasts for 2 to 3 hours or longer.

Treatment of patients with USAP and AMI follows the same five basic approaches: (1) increase myocardial oxygen supply through supplemental inhaled oxygen and thrombolytic therapy, which restores coronary blood flow; (2) use ß-adrenergic blockade to decrease the force of myocardial contraction and therefore oxygen demand; (3) increase metabolic substrate availability to the myocardium through nitroglycerin, morphine, thrombolytic agents, and PTCA; (4) protect injured myocardial cell function by decreasing inflammation or toxic injury through antiinflammatory drugs and perfluorochemicals; and (5) prevent reocclusion of the coronary artery through inhibition of platelet aggregation and thrombus formation through the use of antiplatelet agents such as aspirin and antithrombins, including heparin.

Relationship of Time to Treatment on Outcome

Both experimental observations and clinical trials support the concept that the beneficial effect of reperfusion is a function of the length of time between symptom onset and treatment. Reimer et al described the wavefront phenomenon of ischemic cell death in 1977. In the canine infarct model, myocardial necrosis progresses from the subendocardium to the epicardium after an experimental coronary occlusion. Release of the occlusion after variable periods demonstrates that the early release produces a smaller infarct characterized by less transmural progression of the necrosis. In human clinical studies, the 40% to 50% reduction in mortality observed in patients treated within the first hour and the overall 25% to 30% mortality reduction seen in randomized clinical trials also support this hypothesis. The relationship between time to reperfusion versus benefit is shown in Figure 73-26.

Early patency resulting in myocardial salvage is the key benefit of thrombolytic therapy. The angiographic substudy of 2431 GUSTO (Global Utilization of Streptokinase & t-PA for Occluded Coronary Arteries) patients corroborates the findings of these animal and human studies.[70] Preserved left ventricular function and associated significantly lower mortality at both the 24-hour and the 30-day end points are related to angiographic patency at 90 minutes.[70] Thrombolytic therapy of patients with AMI has significantly greater benefit for those treated within the first or second hours than for those treated later. The MITI trial demonstrates that the mortality rate among patients treated within 70 minutes is 1.3% compared with 8.7% in those treated later.[71] Conversely, there appears to be a modest but significant benefit for patients treated between 6 and 12 hours after the onset of symptoms than if they were not treated. A unifying hypothesis that explains the clinical data requires the assumption that reperfusion therapy improves survival by

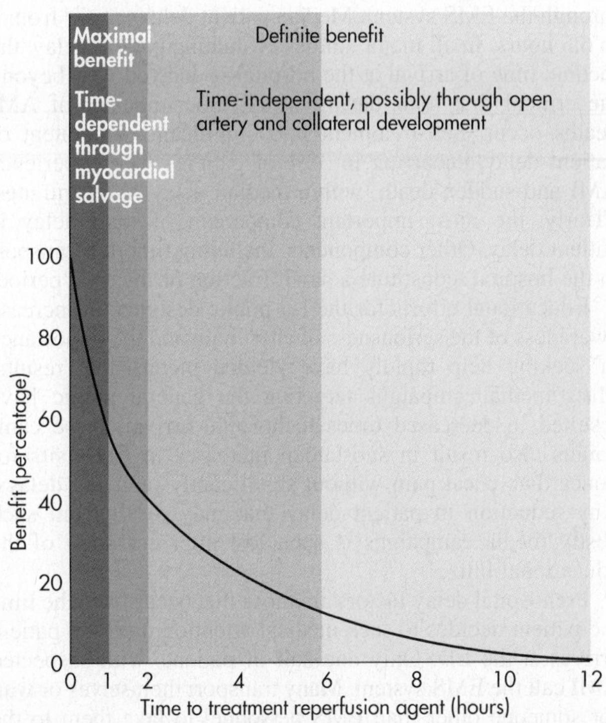

Figure 73-26. **This figure depicts combined human and animal data and represents the time-dependent benefit anticipated, depending on the length of the interval between coronary artery occlusion and reperfusion.** ***Modified from Tiefenbrunn AJ, Sobel BE: Circulation 85(6):2311, 1992; © 1992 American Heart Association. Reproduced from US Department of Health and Human Services, Public Health Service, National Institutes of Health, National Heart, Lung, and Blood Institute, NIH Publication No. 93-3278, p. 8, September 1993.***

several mechanisms. Treatment within the first several hours after symptom onset may result in substantial myocardial salvage that is time-dependent and affects both survival and left ventricular function. Treatment from 2 to 12 hours later may result in a modest benefit after completion of myocardial necrosis by opening the occluded artery and resulting in less adverse ventricular remodeling, reduced occurrence of ventricular aneurysm, increased blood flow to myocardium still in jeopardy, and improved electrophysiologic stability. These mechanisms are assumed to be more time-independent.

It is now well established that substantial delays occur between symptom onset and hospital-based initiation of thrombolytic therapy. From 26% to 44% of patients having an AMI delay more than 4 hours before seeking medical care. There are often delays associated with transport to the hospital. Further delays occur between the patient's arrival at the hospital and administration of the thrombolytic agent. These data support the following conclusions: (1) time is critical to an optimal outcome for patients with AMI; (2) major trials of thrombolytic therapy document that maximum treatment benefit occurs during the first 1 to 2 hours following symptom onset; and (3) a small percentage of patients with AMI receive treatment within 1 hour of onset of symptoms.

In 1991, the NHLBI launched the NHAAP to promote the rapid identification and treatment of AMI, with the goal of reducing AMI morbidity and mortality. The factors responsible for delay in the care of patients having AMIs have been grouped by the NHAAP into three phases: patient/bystander, prehospital, and hospital. Patient/bystander factors are those that keep the patient from seeking immediate medical care through the EMS system. Median patient delays range from 2 to 6.5 hours. In all major studies evaluating patient delay, the median time of arrival at the hospital is delayed well beyond the critical first hour during which time one half of AMI deaths occur. Self-treatment is a significant component of patient delay, occurring in 32% of patients who experience AMI and sudden death, with a median delay of 59 minutes. Clearly, the most important component of total delay is patient delay. Other components, including time for transport to the hospital, constitute a small fraction of the total period.

Educational efforts for the lay public designed to increase awareness of the seriousness of chest pain and the importance of seeking help rapidly have yielded inconsistent results. Mass media campaigns targeting the general public have resulted in decreased times to hospital arrival; these campaigns also result in substantial increases in ED visits for noncardiac chest pain without significantly reducing delays. Any reduction in patient delay that may result from such costly media campaigns is soon lost after cessation of the educational blitz.

Prehospital delay factors are those that occur from the time the patient decides to seek medical attention until the patient arrives at the ED. Only one half of patients with suspected AMI call the EMS system. Many transport themselves or wait for someone other than EMS personnel to take them to the hospital, increasing patient risk and delay. Other patients far removed from an emergency facility spend considerable time being transported to a hospital. Further complicating prehospital issues is the lack of universal enhanced 911 capabilities and wide variations in availability and quality of emergency medical systems throughout the United States. If patients with chest pain are to be encouraged to enter the EMS system rapidly, improvements in access, dispatch, transportation, communication, training, and levels of service must be achieved.

Substantial further delays can occur between the time a patient arrives in the hospital and initiation of thrombolytic therapy. Overall, the average time that elapses during this interval ranges from 60 to 90 minutes, although shorter times have been reported. The GUSTO trial demonstrates a median time from hospital arrival to treatment with thrombolytic therapy of 70 minutes.[70] The American Heart Association (AHA) recommends that all heart attack patients who are to receive thrombolytic therapy get the treatment within 30 to 60 minutes of arrival in the ED. Patients with AMI who are to undergo primary PTCA should undergo the procedure no later than 90 minutes after arrival.[72,73]

Patients with AMI who receive hospital-based reperfusion therapies (thrombolytic agent or primary PTCA) progress through a sequence of steps that can be used to define process time points. Figure 73-27 shows the time points and intervals. Within each interval, various barriers and impediments to timely care can occur. Identifying the causes for delays in evaluation and treatment, and adopting interventions to minimize these delays, will improve overall care of the patient having AMI. Reducing delay times is applicable to all time points in the ED by addressing the four Ds: door (events prior to arrival at the ED), data (obtaining the ECG), decision (arriving at the diagnosis of AMI and deciding upon therapy), and drug (administering the thrombolytic drug or passing the catheter across the culprit lesion for PTCA candidates).

Prehospital care providers may alert the ED to the impending arrival of a patient with a suspected AMI, allowing preparation that will speed time to treatment. A 12-lead ECG acquired in the field may assist the ED in making a more rapid diagnosis and decrease the time to administration of thrombolytic therapy. In fact, the major lasting effect of the prehospital thrombolysis trials was the recognition that an ECG obtained in the out-of-hospital

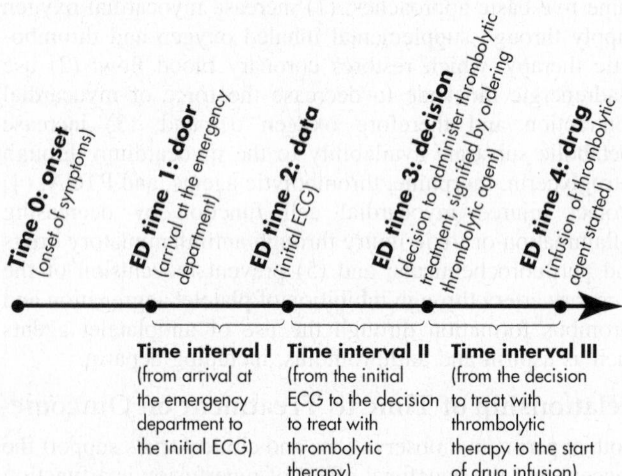

Figure 73-27. **Process time points and intervals through which the patient with AMI passes until treatment in the ED.** ***Reproduced from US Department of Health and Human Services, Public Health Service, National Institutes of Health, National Heart, Lung, and Blood Institute, NIH Publication No. 93-3278, p. 10, September 1993.***

setting markedly reduced the time to ED-based thrombolytic administration. Walk-in patients with a chief complaint of chest pain should be evaluated by a triage nurse immediately. A nurse's identification of a potential AMI should be communicated immediately to the emergency physician.

A 12-lead ECG on patients with a suspected AMI should be considered part of the patient's vital signs assessment. Furthermore, ED nurses should be trained to recognize electrocardiographic changes indicative of AMI. The 12-lead ECG should be given to the emergency physician immediately for interpretation. In addition to obtaining vital signs and an ECG, emergency nurses should act on standing orders to initiate the following interventions for patients with suspected AMI or myocardial ischemia: (1) administration of aspirin for possible AICS, (2) cardiac monitor, (3) oxygen therapy, (4) intravenous access, (5) laboratory tests, and (6) administration of nitrates.

Development of protocols for identifying and rapidly treating patients will reduce the amount of time to treatment. Checklists of inclusion and exclusion criteria for thrombolytic therapy and lists of absolute and relative contraindications should be available. Physical examinations should be brief and focused. In cases of uncomplicated AMI, the emergency physician should activate the hospital-based system for reperfusion. In cases where the hospital is able to offer primary PTCA, then immediate consultation with the cardiologist is a must. If the patient is scheduled for primary PTCA, then the cardiology team must rapidly mobilize with the plan of placing the PTCA catheter across the culprit lesion within 90 minutes of ED arrival. If such is not possible and the patient is a thrombolytic candidate, then thrombolytic therapy must be administered in timely fashion—optimally, less than 30 minutes after ED arrival. Communication with family physicians, internists, or cardiologists may result in unnecessary delays.

Thrombolytic agents should be stored in the ED to avoid delays. Treatment should be administered in the ED and not delayed by transporting the patient to another area of the hospital. Standard protocols for administering thrombolytic and other drugs should be available to facilitate ordering and use of these agents. In hospitals offering primary PTCA, catheterization laboratory personnel must be ready to respond immediately. Delays beyond 90 minutes to definitive catheter placement are absolutely unacceptable in the patient who is a thrombolytic candidate. The interhospital transfer of patients with AMI for PTCA—those who are candidates also for thrombolysis—must be discouraged in most instances without administering the thrombolytic agent prior to transfer; the exception involves the transfer to another hospital's interventional suite so that catheter placement across the lesion can occur within 90 minutes of arrival from entry into the medical system (i.e., the initial health care facility).

Nitroglycerin

Nitrates provide substantial benefit to patients with AICS by decreasing myocardial preload and, to a lesser extent, afterload. Nitrates increase venous capacitance, inducing venous pooling, which decreases preload and myocardial oxygen demand. Direct vasodilation of coronary arteries may increase collateral blood flow to ischemic myocardium. Most studies of intravenous nitroglycerin (NTG) administration in the setting of AMI are from the prethrombolytic era. A meta-analysis of multiple small trials notes a 35% mortality reduction with the use of intravenous NTG.[74]

In the emergency setting, patients with possible AICS and a systolic blood pressure greater than 90 mm Hg should receive a sublingual NTG tablet (0.4 mg) upon arrival. If symptoms are not fully relieved with three sublingual tablets, the patient should be started on intravenous NTG. Care must be exercised in patients with bradycardia, hypotension, inferior wall AMI, and right ventricular infarction when administering NTG, because a sudden decrease in preload associated with NTG use can result in profound hypotension. Initial infusion rates should start at 10 µg/min with titration to a pain free state. The clinician should increase the infusion at regular intervals, allowing for a 10% reduction in the mean arterial pressure if normotensive and a 20% to 30% reduction if hypertensive. Maximal benefit is likely achieved at 200 µg/min, although certain patients may receive additional benefit at higher infusion rates.

Morphine

The use of morphine sulfate for the treatment of USAP has not been evaluated in large, randomized trials. Morphine is a potent analgesic and has anxiolytic effects, both of which can be beneficial in the treatment of patients with AICS. If a patient with possible AICS is unresponsive to NTG or has recurrent symptoms despite maximal antiischemic therapy, administration of morphine sulfate is appropriate. The relief of pain and anxiety decreases oxygen consumption and myocardial work. Some vasodilatory effects also occur that can decrease preload to the heart. Standard doses of morphine sulfate are 2 to 5 mg delivered intravenously, repeated every 5 to 30 minutes as necessary. In addition to allergic reactions, the most significant adverse effect of morphine sulfate administration is hypotension, which is managed with intravenous fluid in bolus fashion.

β-Adrenergic Blockers

β-Adrenergic blocking agents are effective in ameliorating catechol-induced tachycardia, increased contractility, and myocardial oxygen demand. β_1-receptors, located in the myocardium, also increase sinoatrial (SA) node rate and AV nodal conduction velocity when stimulated. β_2-receptors are located primarily in vascular smooth muscle and the lungs. β-blockade has been demonstrated effective in decreasing mortality for patients with AMI. Although the impact of β-adrenergic blockade in treating USAP is less well studied, a meta-analysis shows a 13% reduction in the risk of subsequent AMI.

Intravenous metoprolol can be given in 5 mg increments by slow infusion over 1 to 2 minutes, with repeat doses of 5 mg given at 5-minute intervals for a total of 15 mg. Alternatively, atenolol, esmolol, and propranolol can be administered. Atenolol is the longest-acting agent. Esmolol is an ultra–short-acting β-blocker that can be given to patients who potentially will not tolerate β-adrenergic antagonism, such as patients with mild CHF or COPD. Contraindications to β-adrenergic blockade include pulmonary edema or other manifestations of acute CHF, COPD, asthma, AV nodal blockade, bradycardia, and systemic hypotension.

Despite the potentially beneficial effects of this treatment in the early phase of management of the patient with AICS, clinicians appear to use this medication less often than is possible. Physicians must consider the use of β-adrenergic blockade in all such patients.

Calcium Channel Blockers

The primary benefit of calcium channel blockers appears to be symptom resolution, similar to the effect of β-blockade. Unfortunately, these agents may be accompanied by a significant vasodilatory effect, resulting in hypotension and therefore the potentiation of the coronary ischemic process. As with β-blocking agents, calcium channel blockers have substantial negative inotropic effect, further compromising perfusion. AV nodal blockade is also a significant side effect that may be exacerbated in patients previously treated with ß-blockers or those with ischemia-related conduction disturbance. In most instances of AICS, calcium channel blocker agents are not recommended.

Antiplatelet Therapy

Platelets play a major role in the thrombotic response to rupture of coronary artery plaque; platelets, in aggregate form, are integrally involved in the pathophysiology of AMI. Platelet-rich thrombi are also more resistant to thrombolysis than are fibrin and erythrocyte-rich thrombi. In USAP patients, dramatic reductions in the progression to AMI have been noted with aggressive antiplatelet therapy; furthermore, patients in the acute phase of myocardial infarction also experience significant benefit with antiplatelet therapy, with mortality reductions ranging from 25% to 50%. Thus there is a sound scientific basis for recommending administration of antiplatelet therapy in the ED for *all* patients with AMI—both with and without STE *and* irrespective of whether thrombolytic therapy is administered.

Aspirin Aspirin, the standard antiplatelet agent, represents the most cost-effective treatment available for patients with AICS; it should be administered early in all patients suspected of AICS who do not have allergy or significant gastrointestinal bleeding. It irreversibly acetylates platelet cyclooxygenase, thereby removing all cyclooxygenase activity for the life span of the platelet (8 to 10 days). Thus aspirin stops the production of proaggregatory thromboxane A_2 and is also an indirect antithrombotic agent. Aspirin also has important nonplatelet effects because it likewise inactivates cyclooxygenase in the vascular endothelium and thereby diminishes formation of antiaggregatory prostacyclin.

The ISIS-2 trial provides the strongest evidence that aspirin independently reduces the mortality of patients with AMI without thrombolytic therapy (overall 23% reduction) and is synergistic when used with thrombolytic therapy (42% reduction in mortality).[42] Standard doses range from 160 to 324 mg given orally. Minimal side effects are noted, particularly with the 160 mg dose. Administration of aspirin in the ED is strongly recommended for all patients with suspected AMI or USAP; it should be administered to all patients with AICS unless significant allergy or life-threatening hemorrhage contradicts its use.

Glycoprotein IIb-IIIa Receptor Inhibitors During platelet damage, several receptors are activated, most notably the membrane glycoprotein IIb-IIIa receptors. Once activated, these receptors allow macromolecules, such as the circulating von Willebrand factor and fibrinogen, to link receptors together in a chain, resulting in platelet adhesion. The glycoprotein IIb-IIIa receptors represent the final common pathway for platelet activation and aggregation. For these reasons, inhibition of IIb-IIIa receptors more effectively inhibits platelet function than that achieved with aspirin.

Approximately 10 drugs in this broad class are currently under investigation; three parenteral agents are available for clinical use today: abciximab, eptifibatide, and tirofiban. The first platelet IIb-IIIa antagonists to be developed were murine monoclonal antibodies; these antibodies completely inhibit platelet aggregation, prevent thrombosis, and augment activity of thrombolytic agents. Abciximab was the first such glycoprotein receptor inhibitor to have undergone large clinical trials. As a monoclonal antibody specific for the glycoprotein IIb-IIIa receptor, it provides prolonged inhibition of platelet aggregation even after cessation of drug infusion. Abciximab is highly effective in preventing thrombosis in stenosed coronary arteries and provides better protection against ischemic complications than other antiplatelet agents.

The EPIC trial[75] investigated the effect of the drug in high-risk patients with USAP and AMI scheduled to undergo coronary angioplasty or atherectomy. This study demonstrated a 35% reduction in mortality rate, nonfatal AMI, unplanned surgical revascularization, unplanned repeat PTCA, and the use of stents or intraaortic balloon pumps for treatment of refractory ischemia. Bleeding episodes and transfusions, however, were more common in patients treated with abciximab. The EPILOG trial[76] further evaluated the effect of abciximab in high- and low-risk patients with USAP or AMI undergoing a variety of invasive coronary interventions. A significant 68% reduction in death or nonfatal AMI was noted, coupled with a lower incidence of major bleeding among treated patients compared with the EPIC trial. A meta-analysis of studies of abciximab and other platelet IIb-IIIa inhibitors showed that the effects of treatment with these agents are uniformly positive, regardless of the characteristics of the study population or the types of coronary intervention.

In the CAPTURE trial,[77] investigators introduced the glycoprotein inhibitor to patients with USAP who failed standard medical stabilization and were scheduled for PTCA; of note, these patients had well defined coronary anatomy that appeared amenable to angioplasty—clearly, a population unlike those patients seen in the ED. The abciximab group had a significantly lower rate of AMI prior to angioplasty and a reduction in the primary end point (death, AMI, or urgent revascularization) at 1 month. In the GRAPE study,[78] abciximab was administered to ED patients scheduled for urgent catheterization with possible PTCA. Increased rates of TIMI grade 3 flow were noted in the abciximab group.

Eptifibatide, a synthetic peptide, prevents binding of fibrinogen to the glycoprotein IIb-IIIa receptor, blocking platelet aggregation and subsequent thrombus formation. The IMPACT-AMI investigators[79] reported the results of a trial in patients with AMI receiving tissue plasminogen activator (t-PA) and aspirin with varying doses of eptifibatide. The primary end point was Thrombolysis in Myocardial Infarction (TIMI) grade 3 flow at 90 minutes; secondary end points were time to ST segment recovery, an in-hospital composite (death, reinfarction, stroke, revascularization procedures, new heart failure, or pulmonary edema), and bleeding. They found considerably higher rates of reaching the primary end points as well as more rapid ST segment resolution in the treatment group compared to the placebo group; they found similar rates of secondary end point issues. In the IMPACT-II trial,[80] patients with AICS who were candidates for PTCA were assigned a placebo or eptifibatide (low- and high-dose). A modest reduction in the rate of revascularization, AMI, or death at 30 days was seen; any differences in the groups were lost, however, at 6 months. The PURSUIT trial investigators[81] used eptifibatide in patients with non-AMI AICS. Patients admitted with recent or ongoing ischemic chest pain and electrocardiographic changes indicative of ischemia (excluding STE) were enrolled in the study comparing eptifibatide to placebo; additionally, all patients received standard medical therapy for ischemic chest pain. In 10,948 patients, the eptifibatide group had a significant reduction in the incidence of the primary end point (a composite of death and nonfatal AMI occurring up to 30 days); this reduction, however, was demonstrated only in patients receiving PTCA (patients were not randomized to receive this intervention). Bleeding was more common in the eptifibatide group, although there was no increase in the incidence of hemorrhagic stroke.

Tirofiban is also a synthetic, shorter acting agent; it acts similarly to eptifibatide but is a nonpeptide compound. In the Platelet Receptor Inhibition in Ischemic Syndrome Management (PRISM) study[82] investigators studied patients with USAP who were already taking aspirin, and compared the effects of adding intravenous tirofiban versus heparin for 48 hours. Tirofiban reduced ischemic events for the initial 48 hours, but did not result in reduced ischemia or AMI at 30 days. The PRISM-PLUS trial[83] compared tirofiban versus placebo in 1915 patients with either USAP or non-STE AMI; heparin was used in all patients. The combination of tirofiban plus heparin significantly reduced the intracoronary thrombus burden of the culprit lesions (primary end point), improved the perfusion grade (secondary end point), and decreased the severity of the obstruction.

Several unanswered questions remain with regard to these agents. Perhaps the most pressing question for the clinician involves the ED indications for such treatment. Certainly, the patient with AICS who is bound for the catheterization laboratory is a reasonable candidate; their efficacy in conjunction with interventional revascularization procedures such as PTCA with stenting seems sound. Another patient group who likely will benefit are AICS patients with ongoing ischemia and electrocardiographic abnormality who have not responded to initial aggressive therapy; the successful use of these agents in this subgroup of AICS patients, however, remains unproved. The use in combination with lower dose thrombolytic agents in the treatment of AMI may also introduce an area for the ED use of these drugs. Lastly, the thrombolytic-ineligible patient who is transferred to another institution for primary coronary angioplasty may benefit from a glycoprotein IIb-IIIa receptor antagonist prior to and during transfer.

Other Antiplatelet Agents Ticlopidine inhibits the transformation of the glycoprotein IIb-IIIa receptor into its high-affinity ligand-binding state. This irreversibly inhibits platelet aggregation and lasts for the duration of the life of the platelet. Ticlopidine has nonlinear kinetics and, after repeated dosing, reaches a maximal effect after 8 to 11 days of dosage. In patients with USAP, a significant reduction in total coronary events is noted; this drug may be considered if aspirin is thought to be inadequate or ineffective. Because of the time delay to the onset of action, ticlopidine's use in the ED is limited; it is not suited for use at the onset of AMI and cannot replace aspirin during the acute phase. Furthermore, ticlopidine is associated with a risk of neutropenia and agranulocytosis. It should therefore be reserved for patients who are intolerant of aspirin therapy but need an antiplatelet agent as prophylaxis for AMI. The standard dosage of ticlopidine is 250 mg twice daily taken with food (to lessen gastric intolerance).

Clopidogrel is a ticlopidine analog. Its advantages are a rapid onset of action and an intravenous route of administration. It also prevents the transformation of the glycoprotein IIb-IIIa receptor into its high-affinity state. It also appears to promote formation of platelet cAMP and therefore lowers platelet calcium. While its use in the hospitalized coronary stent population is reasonably well defined, information regarding acute treatment in the ED patient with AICS is lacking.

Unfractionated Heparin

The term *heparin* refers not to a single structure but rather to a family of mucopolysaccharide chains of varying lengths and composition—unfractionated—with pronounced antithrombotic properties. Unfractionated heparin is composed of a mixture of polysaccharide chains with varying molecular weights. At standard doses, unfractionated heparin binds to antithrombin III, forming a complex that then is able to inactivate factor II (thrombin) and activated factor X. This prevents the conversion of fibrinogen to fibrin, thus preventing clot formation. Heparin by itself has no anticoagulant property. This indirect effect on thrombin inhibits clot propagation; however, it prevents heparin from having any effect on bound thrombin in a thrombus. Unfractionated heparin also assists in the inactivation of factors XIa and IXa via antithrombin, and interacts with platelets.

Heparin has been shown to have a profound synergistic effect with aspirin in preventing death, AMI, and refractory USAP. Heparin should be administered early in patients with AICS. The initial dose is 60 U/kg by intravenous bolus, followed by a maintenance infusion of 12 U/kg/hr. The activated partial thromboplastin time (aPTT) should be titrated to 1.5 to 2.5 times control using the maintenance infusion. Contraindications to heparin therapy include active ongoing life-threatening hemorrhage or predisposition to such hemorrhage.

Low Molecular Weight Heparin

The low molecular weight (LMW) heparins inhibit the coagulation system in a similar fashion to that of unfractionated heparin. LMW heparins constitute approximately one third of the molecular weight of heparin and are less heterogeneous in size. Approximately 25% to 30% of the molecules bind to both antithrombin III and thrombin. The remaining molecules of LMW heparin bind only to factor Xa. The variable efficacy has been found among the LMW heparins, which has been attributed to differing ratios of antifactor Xa to antifactor IIa. High-ratio preparations appear to demonstrate a clear advantage over standard heparin; enoxaparin has the highest ratio of the currently available LMW heparins. LMW heparin was designed based on the hypothesis that inhibition of earlier steps in the blood coagulation system would be associated with a more potent antithrombotic effect than inhibiting subsequent steps. This effect is felt to result from the amplification process inherent in the coagulation cascade; that is, a single factor Xa molecule can lead to the generation of multiple thrombin molecules.

The advantages of LMW heparin over unfractionated heparin are numerous. LMW heparin inactivates factor Xa, which is resistant to inactivation by unfractionated heparin. LMW heparins have lesser binding characteristics to coagulation factors such as platelet factor IV, other plasma proteins, and endothelial cells, resulting in higher bioavailability. LMW heparin has a longer half-life and less individual variability of the anticoagulant response when compared with unfractionated heparin. They have lower affinity for von Willebrand factor, increased vascular permeability, and a weak effect on platelet function. These differences could explain why LMW heparin produces less bleeding than unfractionated heparin with equivalent or higher antithrombotic effects. The long half-life of LMW heparins and their predictable anticoagulant response to weight-adjusted doses allow once-daily subcutaneous administration without laboratory monitoring. LMW heparins are the agents of choice when heparin is contraindicated by unavailability of aPTT measurements, but the disadvantage is expense.

The FRISC trial[84] established that the combination of aspirin, ß-blocker, and LMW heparin (dalteparin) significantly decreased the rate of nonfatal AMI or death after 1 week of therapy, with a less pronounced effect at 40 to 150 days and an increased number of minor bleeding episodes. The FRIC study[85] investigated the use of dalteparin compared to unfractionated heparin in patients with unstable coronary disease (USAP and non-STE AMI). The rates of death, recurrent angina, and AMI, and the need for revascularization procedures were similar at 1 week and at 45 days. In this study, both forms of heparin provided similar benefit in these unstable coronary patients. In the ESSENCE study,[86] a benefit was found with LMW heparin at 30 days; the risk of minor bleeding was higher.

In general, it appears that the LMW heparin, particularly enoxaparin with its favorable antifactor Xa/antifactor IIa ratio, offers a short-term benefit in the unstable coronary patient that lessens significantly beyond the first week of treatment. It may be administered in a twice daily regimen subcutaneously at a dose of 1 mg/kg; doses should be reduced for patients with pronounced renal insufficiency.

Hirudin, Hirulog, and Argatroban

Hirudin, hirulog, and argatroban are potent antithrombin anticoagulants providing significant theoretical advantages over heparin. Hirudin is an amino acid peptide derived from the leech salivary gland but is also synthesized as recombinant hirudin. It binds directly with high affinity to thrombin and can inactivate thrombin already bound to fibrin (clot-bound thrombin), which unfractionated heparin cannot do as effectively. Hirudin does not require endogenous cofactors such as antithrombin III for its activity. Also, unlike heparin, hirudin can inhibit thrombin-induced platelet aggregation. Unlike LMW and unfractionated heparin, hirudin has not been associated with drug-induced thrombocytopenia.

In the OASIS-2 trial,[87] patients with USAP or suspected non-STE AMI were randomly assigned to receive intravenous heparin or hirudin with the primary outcome measure being cardiovascular death or recurrent AMI within 1 week. Patients in both groups experienced the same rate of death and recurrent AMI, yet symptomatic angina was noted less often in the hirudin group. Of concern, patients in the hirudin group more often experienced major bleeding requiring transfusion. The HIT-4 trial[88] investigated the use of hirudin as an adjunct to thrombolysis in patients with AMI. In a randomized trial, patients with AMI who were treated with streptokinase received either hirudin or heparin; the study end points included the restoration of coronary flow at 90 minutes and the time to normalization of STE. No significant difference was noted between groups regarding coronary flow, yet STE resolution occurred more rapidly in the hirudin segment. No major differences were noted in other outcome parameters including death, recurrent acute coronary ischemia, major bleeding, and stroke.

Hirulog is a bifunctional 20-amino acid peptide designed on the structure of hirudin. It has similar properties to hirudin, but in addition interacts with the catalytic site of thrombin. In the HERO trial,[89] patients with AMI treated with streptokinase and aspirin were randomized to receive either heparin or hirulog with a primary outcome measurement of achieving TIMI grade 3 flow at 90 to 120 minutes. TIMI grade III flow was reached more often in the hirulog-treated patients; furthermore, death, cardiogenic shock, recurrent infarction, major bleeding, and stroke were less often encountered in this group. Hirulog appeared to be more effective than heparin in producing early patency in patients treated with aspirin and streptokinase, without increasing the risk of adverse outcome including death.

Argatroban is an arginine derivative that binds to thrombin with intermediate affinity and is a competitive antagonist inhibiting fibrinogen cleavage and platelet activation by thrombin. Compared with heparin, argatroban is significantly more effective in the prevention of platelet-rich thrombi after vascular injury. The MINT trial[90] examined the effect of argatroban on reperfusion produced by t-PA in AMI. The study randomized 125 patients with AMI to heparin, low-dose argatroban, or high-dose argatroban in addition to t-PA. The primary end point was the rate of TIMI grade 3 flow at 90 minutes, which was achieved more often in the argatroban-treated patients. Major bleeding was observed more often in the heparin-managed patients. A composite of death, recurrent AMI, cardiogenic shock, and revascularization at 30 days occurred but was not significantly different in the three treatment groups. Argatroban appears to enhance reperfusion with thrombolysis in patients with AMI, particularly in those patients with delayed treatment, with fewer side effects.

Reperfusion Therapies

Thrombolytic Therapy Re-establishing perfusion in the infarct-related coronary artery with the use of thrombolytic therapy, in essence reopening the infarct-related artery, increases the opportunity for salvage of the ischemic myocardium and, consequently, reduces morbidity and mortality. The contention that rapid, complete, and sustained recanalization will have the greatest benefit in terms of infarct size limitation and patient survival has been termed the open-artery hypothesis. Thrombolytic therapy unequivocally improves survival in patients who have STE AMI. Numerous large thrombolytic investigations have supported this statement. For instance, a meta-analysis of nine major investigations of thrombolytic therapy in patients with AMI demonstrated an approximate 20% reduction in short-term mortality with the use of such agents compared to placebo. When all patient groups were pooled, a reduction of 18 deaths per 1000 patients treated was found.

Thrombolytic Agent Selection Three megatrials comparing tissue plasminogen activator (t-PA) to streptokinase have been published. The GISSI-2 trial[91] and the closely related International Study[92] compared a 100 mg infusion of t-PA over 3 hours to streptokinase with or without heparin. The GISSI-2 was the first of the large-scale mortality trials directly comparing t-PA and streptokinase in patients with AMI. The investigators found no difference in mortality between the two treatment groups. More strokes were reported with t-PA than with streptokinase (1.3% versus 1%) in the International Study, yet the frequency of confirmed hemorrhagic stroke was similar for both agents. Similar results were found in the ISIS-3 trial,[93] the next thrombolytic megatrial, which compared t-PA, streptokinase, and anisoylated plasminogen streptokinase activator complex (anistreplase or APSAC) in approximately 40,000 patients. In marked contrast to current practice, the inclusion criteria allowed entry up to 24 hours after symptom onset and did not require diagnostic electrocardiographic change. All patients received adjunctive aspirin therapy and approximately one half of the patients were given delayed, unmonitored subcutaneous heparin. A significant difference in both 35-day mortality and ICH was not found. The results of the ISIS-3 study[93] proved controversial again because of the unmonitored, delayed subcutaneous heparin protocol, particularly with studies now proving improved infarct artery patency using early therapeutic intravenous doses of heparin. Current thrombolytic practice was highly affected by the results of the Global Use of Streptokinase and t-PA for Occluded coronary arteries (GUSTO-I) trial.[70] The purpose of the GUSTO-I trial was to test the hypothesis that early and sustained infarct vessel patency was associated with better survival rates in patients with AMI.[70] More than 41,000 patients were randomized to four different thrombolytic strategies—accelerated t-PA given over 90 minutes plus intravenous heparin, a combination of streptokinase plus a reduced dose of t-PA along with intravenous heparin, and two control groups (streptokinase plus subcutaneous heparin and streptokinase plus intravenous heparin). Unlike previous trials, t-PA was given in a more aggressive, front-loaded 90-minute infusion (referred to as "accelerated" t-PA). In addition to a primary end point of 30-day mortality, the GUSTO investigators explored coronary artery patency and degree of normalization of flow in an angiographic substudy; this portion of the larger trial was designed to determine the relationship between early coronary artery patency and outcome. In this trial, accelerated t-PA, administered with intravenous heparin, was shown to significantly reduce 30-day mortality by 15% as compared to streptokinase with either form of heparin, or the combination of t-PA and streptokinase with intravenous heparin. The benefit was highly consistent across virtually all subgroups, including the elderly, location of AMI, and time from symptom onset. These differences remained significant at 1 year of follow-up. The angiographic substudy demonstrated a strong relationship between TIMI flow and outcome. Patients with strong forward flow (i.e., TIMI grade 3 flow) at 90 minutes had significantly lower mortality rates compared with patients with little to no flow. The mechanism for this benefit was found to be earlier, more complete infarct vessel patency with accelerated t-PA; this early t-PA patency advantage over other agents was lost by 180 minutes after symptom onset. As would be expected, the patients with higher risk derived the most substantial benefit with accelerated t-PA compared to streptokinase in this large study. Patients who received accelerated t-PA did suffer more hemorrhagic strokes compared to those who received streptokinase, but the combined end point of death and disabling stroke still favored the accelerated t-PA regimen.

Another recent addition to the thrombolytic agent literature base includes the GUSTO-III investigation.[94] This study compared accelerated t-PA to r-PA. In this very large trial, r-PA was found to be equivalent to accelerated t-PA, and the overall results were nearly identical for the two drugs. The one exception is in patients who seek treatment more than 4 hours after onset of symptoms—a significant number of patients in many institutions. In this group of patients, accelerated t-PA may be superior to r-PA, because of its greater fibrin specificity.[94] r-PA is a mutant form of t-PA that allows it to be administered in a fixed double-bolus dose, with no adjustment required for weight, thus simplifying administration.

The recently reported ASSENT-2 trial investigated the use of tenecteplase (TNK), another mutant of wild-type t-PA. TNK has several interesting characteristics and associated potential benefits: (1) its longer half-life allows it to be administered as a single bolus; (2) it is 14 times more fibrin-specific than t-PA and even more so than r-PA; and (3) it is 80 times more resistant to plasminogen activator inhibitor-1 (PAI-1) than t-PA. The ASSENT-2 trial[95] randomized approximately 17,000 patients with AMI to single-bolus TNK (30 to 50 mg based upon body weight) or accelerated t-PA (100 mg total infusion); the primary outcome variable was 30-day all-cause mortality. The investigators found no differences in mortality or ICH.[95] In subgroup analysis, however, significantly lower 30-day mortality was noted among patients who came to the hospital more than 4 hours after onset of symptoms; furthermore, fewer nonintracranial major bleeding episodes were encountered in the TNK group. Based on these results, it was concluded that TNK was equally or minimally more effective, particularly in patients who sought treatment late. Concerning adverse reactions, TNK also appeared to be modestly safer than accelerated t-PA. Lastly, due to its single bolus administration, TNK is markedly easier to use in the ED and in other settings, such as the air and ground prehospital environments.

Eligibility Criteria for Thrombolytic Agent Therapy

The 12-lead electrocardiogram Combined with the patient's history and physical examination, the 12-lead ECG is the key determinant of eligibility for thrombolysis. The electrocardiographic findings include two basic issues: (1) STE of 1 mm or more in two or more anatomically contiguous *standard limb* leads and 2 mm or more elevation in two or more contiguous *precordial* leads; or (2) new or presumed new LBBB. No evidence of benefit from thrombolytic therapy is found in patients with ischemic chest pain who lack either appropriate STE or the new development of LBBB.

Patients with LBBB and AMI are at an increased risk of experiencing a poor outcome; these patients should be rapidly and aggressively managed in the ED with appropriate reperfusion therapies.[37,96] This observation was noted prior to the introduction of thrombolytic agents and continues to be true today. In patients with AMI, new-onset LBBB is a clinical marker for a significantly worse prognosis in terms of higher mortality, lower left ventricular ejection fraction, and increased incidence of cardiovascular complications.[37,96] The new development of LBBB in the setting of AMI suggests proximal occlusion of the LAD artery; such an obstruction places a significant portion of the left ventricle in ischemic jeopardy. Despite this increased risk of poor outcome, patients with LBBB less often receive thrombolytic agents. These same patients show significant benefit when treated with thrombolytic therapy.[96]

Patients with AMI in anterior, inferior, or lateral anatomic locations benefit from administration of thrombolytic therapy. The relatively favorable prognosis associated with inferior infarction without thrombolytic therapy requires larger sample sizes to detect a significant survival benefit. The large ISIS-2 trial[42] demonstrated a statistically significant mortality benefit for thrombolytic therapy in patients with inferior AMI: the mortality at 5 weeks is 6.5% for those treated with streptokinase plus aspirin versus 10.2% when placebo is given. Patients with inferior AMI and coexisting right ventricular infarctions, as detected by additional-lead ECGs, are likely to benefit because of the large amount of jeopardized myocardium. Acute, isolated posterior wall AMI, diagnosed by posterior leads, may represent yet another electrocardiographic indication for thrombolysis. Though unproved in large thrombolytic agent trials, isolated patients with posterior AMI may be considered for possible candidacy for reperfusion therapy.

In general, the larger the myocardial infarct, the greater the mortality reduction with thrombolytic therapy. The size of AMI—and therefore the associated risk of cardiovascular complications and death—is reflected by either the absolute number of leads showing STE on the ECG or a summation of the total ST segment deviation from the baseline (i.e., both ST segment depressions and elevations).

The current evidence strongly indicates that thrombolytic therapy should not be used routinely in patients with STD only on the 12-lead ECG. Mortality rate may actually be increased by administration of thrombolytics in this patient subgroup. The TIMI-3 trial[97] demonstrated a significant difference in outcome in thrombolytic-treated patients with only STD—7.4% incidence of death compared with 4.9% in the placebo group. These findings are further supported in the Fibrinolytic Therapy Trialists (FTT) meta-analysis, which demonstrated that the mortality rate among patients with STD who received thrombolytic therapy is 15.2% compared with 13.8% among controls.[96]

Patient age Past trials do not provide evidence to support withholding thrombolytic therapy on the basis of the patient's age. In fact, the FTT Collaborative Group[96] concluded that "clearly, age alone should no longer be considered a contraindication to thrombolytic therapy." At the same time, it must be recognized that patients over 75 years of age do have a higher incidence of hemorrhagic stroke than younger patients.

Time from symptom onset The generally accepted therapeutic window for administration of a thrombolytic agent after the onset of STE AMI is 12 hours. Considerable data support this time period.[42,70,71,91-96] Certainly, the earlier the treatment is initiated, the greater the likelihood that the patient will experience a good outcome. Such is the case in patients within the first 6 hours of AMI. Later administrations, occurring from 6 to 12 hours after AMI onset, also confer benefit though of a lesser magnitude.[98] The Late Assessment of Thrombolytic Efficiency (LATE) trial, which compared thrombolytic therapy with placebo, finds a significant 26% decrease in 35-day mortality in patients treated with t-PA, heparin, and aspirin 6 to 12 hours after the onset of symptoms.[99] There is no significant decrease in mortality among patients treated 12 to 24 hours after symptom onset. These studies, then, clearly establish benefit from 0 to 12 hours in patients who are otherwise appropriate candidates for thrombolytic therapy. Treatment beyond that time is not supported by results of currently available trials. The single exception may be a patient with a "stuttering" nature of chest pain between 12 and 24 hours after symptom onset—once again emphasizing the importance of an adequate history. With evidence of marked STE on the 12-lead ECG, the patient should be considered as a potential thrombolytic candidate.

Blood pressure extremes Current evidence indicates that patients with a history of chronic hypertension should not be excluded from thrombolytic therapy if their blood pressure is under control or can be lowered to acceptable levels using standard therapy for ischemic chest pain. The admission blood pressure is also an important indicator of risk of intracerebral hemorrhage. The FTT meta-analysis[96] demonstrates that the risk of cerebral hemorrhage increases with systolic blood pressure greater than 150 mm Hg on admission and further increases when systolic blood pressure is 175 mm Hg or greater. Despite an increased mortality rate during days 0 and 1, the FTT meta-analysis demonstrates an overall long-term benefit of 15 lives saved per 1000 for patients with systolic blood pressures greater than 150 mm Hg and 11 lives saved per 100 for patients with systolic blood pressures 175 mm Hg or greater.[96] Although the FTT meta-analysis appears to indicate an acceptable risk-benefit ratio for patients with substantially increased systolic blood pressure, a persistent blood pressure greater than 200/120 mm Hg is generally considered to be an absolute contraindication to thrombolytic therapy.

The benefit of thrombolytic therapy in patients with hypotension remains controversial. The GISSI-1 and GISSI-2 trials show no apparent reduction of mortality rate with thrombolytic therapy among patients classified in either Killip class III or IV.[91,100] These findings have led to the previous suggestion that primary angioplasty, not thrombolytic therapy, should be used in patients with cardiogenic shock. The FTT meta-analysis, however, does not support this hypothesis.[96] In this meta-analysis, patients with an initial systolic blood pressure less than 100 mm Hg who were not treated with thrombolytic therapy had a very high risk of death (35.1%), and those who were treated with thrombolytic therapy had the largest absolute benefit (60 lives saved per 1000 patients).[96] Based on this evidence, the FTT Collaborative Group suggests that hypotension, heart failure, and perhaps even shock should not be contraindications to thrombolytic therapy.[96] These data support immediate treatment followed by diagnostic angiography and further intervention as indicated.

Retinopathy Active diabetic hemorrhagic retinopathy is a strong *relative* contraindication to thrombolytic therapy because of the potential for permanent blindness caused by intraocular bleeding. Current data, however, indicate that there is no reason to withhold a thrombolytic agent in a diabetic patient with evidence of simple background retinopathy. Patients with DM who sustain an AMI have an almost doubled incidence of mortality.

Cardiopulmonary resuscitation CPR is not a contraindication to thrombolytic therapy unless CPR has been prolonged, i.e., greater than 10 minutes, or extensive chest trauma from manual compression is evident.[101] Although the in-hospital mortality rate is higher in patients with AMI who experience cardiac arrest and then receive ED-based thrombolytic agents, no difference is found in the rates of bleeding complications. No hemothorax or cardiac tamponade occurred with cardiac arrest in those patients receiving thrombolytics.[101]

Previous stroke or transient ischemic attack A history of stroke or transient ischemic attack (TIA) is a major risk factor for hemorrhagic stroke after treatment with thrombolytic therapy. A history of ischemic stroke should be considered a strong relative contraindication to thrombolytic therapy. A history of hemorrhagic stroke is an absolute contraindication.

Previous myocardial infarction or coronary artery bypass graft In the setting of AMI, a previous MI should not preclude consideration for treatment with thrombolytic agents.[96] Without treatment, there is a potential for greater loss of function in the newly infarcting region of the myocardium. Although the GISSI-1 trial[100] showed no treatment benefits for patients with previous infarctions, the ISIS-2 trial demonstrated a 26% relative mortality rate reduction for patients with previous myocardial infarctions treated with thrombolytic therapy.[42] The FTT meta-analysis further demonstrates that patients with a history of AMI who receive thrombolytic therapy for recurrent acute infarction have a mortality rate of 12.5% compared with 14.1% among control patients.[96]

Many studies report successful thrombolysis in patients with AMI and prior coronary artery bypass graft (CABG). Complete thrombotic occlusion of the bypass graft is the cause of AMI in approximately 75% of cases, as opposed to native vessel occlusion. It has been suggested that because of the large mass of thrombus and absent flow in the graft, conventional thrombolytic therapy may be inadequate to restore flow. Patients who have undergone CABG may be relatively resistant to thrombolytic therapy, so they should be considered for direct angioplasty or combined thrombolysis and rescue angioplasty.[102]

Recent surgery or trauma Recent surgery or trauma is considered a relative contraindication to thrombolytic therapy. The term *recent* has been variably interpreted, however, in thrombolytic therapy trials. In the GISSI-1 trial,[100] patients were excluded if they had surgery or trauma within the previous 10 days. In the ASSET trial, patients were excluded for surgery or trauma within the previous 6 weeks.[103] Other thrombolytic therapy trials have not defined "recent surgery or trauma." It is prudent to consider alternative interventions such as angioplasty—if available—in patients with AMI within 10 days of surgery or significant trauma.

Menstruating women There has been concern regarding whether menstruating women with AMI should be considered candidates for thrombolytic therapy. Because natural estrogen is cardioprotective, there has been little experience with thrombolysis among premenopausal women. Significant adverse effects, however, have not been reported by clinicians who administer thrombolytic therapy to such patients. Gynecologists indicate that any excessive vaginal bleeding that may occur after receiving thrombolytic therapy should be readily controllable by vaginal packing and therefore can be considered a compressible site of bleeding.

Contraindications A list of absolute and relative contraindications is shown in Box 73-1.

Percutaneous Transluminal Coronary Angioplasty

Primary Angioplasty Although thrombolysis has widespread availability and a proven ability to improve coronary flow, limit infarct size, and improve survival in patients with AMI, many individuals with acute infarction are not considered suitable candidates for such treatment. Patients with absolute contraindications to thrombolytic therapy, certain relative contraindications, cardiogenic shock, and USAP may be ineligible to receive thrombolytic therapy. The requirement of administering prompt reperfusion therapy to these patients, as well as the other limitations of thrombolytic therapy, has led many clinicians to advocate PTCA, also known as *percutaneous coronary intervention (PCI),* as the primary therapy and treatment of choice for AMI. Primary PTCA has many theoretical advantages over thrombolysis, including an increased number of eligible patients, a lower risk of intracranial bleeding, a significantly higher initial reperfusion rate, and an earlier definition of coronary anatomy, which results in more rapid triage to

Box 73-1 Contraindications for Thrombolytic Therapy in the Patient with AMI

- Recent (within 10 days) major surgery (e.g., coronary artery bypass graft, obstetric delivery, organ biopsy, previous puncture of noncompressible vessels)
- Cerebrovascular disease
- Recent gastrointestinal or genitourinary bleeding (within 10 days)
- Recent trauma (within 10 days)
- Hypertension: systolic BP ≥180 mm Hg or diastolic BP ≥110 mm Hg
- High likelihood of left heart thrombus (e.g., mitral stenosis with atrial fibrillation)
- Acute pericarditis
- Subacute bacterial endocarditis
- Hemostatic defects, including those secondary to severe hepatic or renal disease
- Significant liver dysfunction
- Diabetic hemorrhagic retinopathy or other hemorrhagic ophthalmic condition
- Septic thrombophlebitis or occluded AV cannula at seriously infected site
- Advanced age (over 75 years of age)
- Patients currently receiving oral anticoagulants (e.g., warfarin sodium)
- Any other condition in which bleeding constitutes a significant hazard or would be particularly difficult to manage because of its location

Modified from *Physicians' Desk Reference,* ed 50, Montvale, NJ, 1996, Medical Economics.

surgical intervention and risk stratification, allowing safe, early hospital discharge.

Several trials of varying sizes comparing primary PTCA with thrombolysis have been reported in the past 10 years. Interventions in the early trials were performed using PTCA, prior to the current widespread use of coronary stents. Despite a clear and consistent benefit of primary PTCA in restoring patency of the infarct-related artery, differences in mortality in the individual trials were difficult to evaluate due to the smaller sample sizes in the studies.

The PAMI trial[104] enrolled 395 patients who were randomly assigned to undergo primary PTCA or to receive t-PA. Compared with standard-dose t-PA, primary PTCA reduced the combined occurrence of nonfatal reinfarction or death, was associated with a lower rate of intracranial hemorrhage, and resulted in a similar left ventricular function. The results of the Netherlands trial indicate that primary angioplasty was associated with a higher rate of patency of the infarct-related artery, a less severe residual stenotic lesion, better left ventricular function, and less recurrent myocardial ischemia and infarction than was streptokinase infusion.[105]

In a substudy of the GUSTO-IIb trial,[106] the authors randomly assigned 1138 patients with AMI to either primary PTCA or accelerated t-PA. The composite end point of the study included death, nonfatal reinfarction, and nonfatal disabling stroke, all occurring within 30 days of the AMI. Of those patients assigned to primary PTCA therapy, 83% were candidates for such treatment and underwent angioplasty 1.9 hours after ED arrival for a total elapsed time from chest pain onset to therapy of 3.8 hours. Ninety-eight percent of the patients assigned to thrombolytic therapy received t-PA 1.2 hours after hospital arrival. The occurrence of the composite end point was encountered significantly less often in the PTCA group (9.6%) compared to the t-PA group (13.7%) at 30 days. When the individual components of the composite end point at 30 days were considered separately, the incidence of death (5.7% versus 7%), infarction (4.5% versus 6.5%), and stroke (0.2% versus 0.9%) occurred at statistically similar rates for both treatment groups—PTCA and t-PA, respectively. Additional work in the form of a meta-analysis by Weaver et al[107] reviewed 10 major studies comparing thrombolysis versus primary PTCA in more than 2600 patients. The 30-day mortality was found to be significantly lower in the PTCA group, 4.4% versus 6.5% in the patients treated with thrombolytics. Primary PTCA was also associated with a significant reduction in strokes, both total and hemorrhagic.

The longer term results of primary PTCA, however, are less clear. The GUSTO-IIb study[106] showed no overall mortality advantage of primary PTCA at 6 months; conversely, 2-year follow-up from the PAMI trial[104] found a significant reduction in hospital readmission, recurrent ischemia, target vessel revascularization, and reinfarction, with a trend toward a reduction in mortality in the PTCA group, compared to treatment with thrombolysis. Much of the literature comparing the acute reperfusion therapies in the patient with AMI does not include the use of coronary stenting during PTCA. The introduction of intracoronary stenting likely will favorably alter the outcomes of patients with AMI, making PTCA with stent placement a superior method of management.

Rescue Angioplasty Current information suggests that rescue angioplasty may be advantageous in patients whose infarct-related arteries fail to reperfuse after thrombolytic therapy.[108] Some centers routinely catheterize patients after thrombolytic therapy to determine whether successful reperfusion has occurred, and to perform angioplasty if necessary and anatomically feasible. Other centers catheterize patients after thrombolytic therapy only if there is clinical evidence that the infarct-related artery has failed to open, such as continued chest pain or persistent STE.

Reperfusion Therapy Method Choice: Considerations for the Emergency Physician

It is widely accepted that the early restoration of perfusion in the patient with AMI limits myocardial damage, preserves left ventricular function, and reduces mortality. Such restoration may be accomplished by either administration of a thrombolytic agent or performance of PTCA. In the rare case, emergent CABG placement is a third revascularization method. The rapid application of reperfusion therapy is a must in the patient with STE AMI. Many factors must be considered by clinicians regarding the early reperfusion treatment decisions when managing the patient with AMI. While primary angioplasty may offer improved outcome over thrombolysis, PTCA must be applied without prolonged delay. Should catheterization laboratory activation delay be anticipated or actually occur, the treating physician must proceed with thrombolysis, assuming the patient is an appropriate candidate. Prior agreement between the ED and the cardiovascular physicians at institutions with angioplasty capability must be obtained such that PTCA consideration will not introduce further delays in thrombolytic drug administration; such cooperation has been shown to limit additional delays in the administration of thrombolytic agents in patients who are considered for PTCA for AMI.

If applied without delay in experienced hands, PTCA may improve outcome in the urgent treatment of AMI. It must be stressed that although PTCA is felt to be superior in the treatment of AMI, it must be initiated within 90 minutes of arrival at the hospital ED.[72,73] If the time required to mobilize staff and arrange for PTCA is prolonged (i.e., greater than approximately 90 minutes to balloon catheter inflation across the culprit coronary lesion), then thrombolysis is preferred. Delays beyond this time period are unacceptable if the patient originally was a thrombolytic candidate. These various time limits are suggestions; individual patient and system issues must be considered in the treatment decisions.

Several related issues must be considered by the clinician. First, the literature base to answer this question is somewhat heterogeneous in construction (e.g., differing therapies, study sites, outcome measures, etc.), making absolute, all-encompassing recommendations impossible and thus providing fuel for further debate. Second, the question of technical expertise should be considered. In the GUSTO-IIb trial,[106] the vast majority of physicians performed at least 75 procedures per year; these results may not generalize to smaller-volume centers with less-experienced operators (i.e., fewer than 50 cases per year). Third, another systems issue regarding time-to-arrival in the catheterization laboratory must be considered. In certain centers PTCA may not be available, necessitating rapid transfer to another facility; alternatively, in centers with PTCA capability, the catheterization laboratory may not be in operation at the time of the patient's arrival, particularly a consideration at night and during weekends.

Reperfusion Therapy in Cardiogenic Shock

Patients with AMI who are in cardiogenic shock, which occurs in up to 10% of cases, demand special consideration due to a mortality rate approaching 80%. Thrombolysis is not effective in these ill patients likely due to a significantly lower coronary perfusion pressure; it is felt that in the shock state the occlusive thrombus is not exposed to the thrombolytic agent, resulting in clinical failure of the drug. In reviewing large thrombolytic trials such as GISSI-1[100] and ISIS-2,[42] patients with AMI in cardiogenic shock did not benefit from thrombolysis. Conversely, primary PTCA has been investigated in over 600 such patients in several small studies; a cumulative analysis of the data revealed a significantly lower mortality rate (45%) compared to placebo and historical controls.[109]

The SHOCK trial[110] compared the outcomes of patients with AMI in cardiogenic shock; patients were randomly assigned to emergency revascularization (primary PTCA or emergent CABG) or initial medical stabilization including thrombolysis. The primary end point was mortality from all causes at 30 days; 6-month survival was the secondary end point. Overall mortality at 30 days did not differ significantly between the revascularization and medical therapy groups (46.7% versus 56%, respectively). Six-month mortality was lower in the revascularization group than in the medical therapy group. The authors concluded that in patients with AMI and cardiogenic shock, emergency revascularization did not significantly reduce overall mortality at 30 days. After 6 months, however, there was a significant survival benefit. The prespecified subgroup analysis of patients less than 75 years of age showed an absolute reduction of 15.4% in 30-day mortality and 21.4% in 6-month mortality in the revascularization group. Thus, when catheterization facilities are not available, thrombolytic therapy should be given to eligible patients, and urgent transfer to an interventional facility should be strongly considered.[110]

Combination Therapies in the Reperfusion-Treated Patient

The above discussion has focused on the use of either primary PTCA or thrombolysis in the patient with AMI. Recent research, however, has focused on the use of therapeutic combinations, including glycoprotein inhibition with both PTCA and thrombolysis, low-dose thrombolysis followed by primary angioplasty, and stent placement during PCI.

Reperfusion with primary PTCA has been improved with the use of glycoprotein IIb-IIIa inhibitors. Abciximab with stenting in AMI has been studied in the RAPPORT,[111] the ADMIRAL,[112] and the CADILLAC trials.[112a] In the RAPPORT trial,[111] a significant reduction in the combined end point of death, recurrent AMI, and urgent need for revascularization was noted at 30 days; no significant differences, however, were seen at 6 months. An increase in major bleeding episodes and the need for transfusions were encountered in the abciximab group likely due to high-dose heparin therapy. The ADMIRAL trial[112] reported a significantly lower rate of occurrence of the combined end point of death, recurrent AMI, and target vessel revascularization at 30 days in the treatment group. In addition, lower doses of heparin were given to patients in the abciximab group, and no increase in major bleeding was observed. The CADILLAC trial randomized primary PTCA patients with AMI to stenting and abciximab versus placebo. Preliminary results suggest that the abciximab-treated patients appeared to have had a modest reduction in acute events. The use of glycoprotein inhibitors in the setting of AMI treated with primary angioplasty appears to benefit the patient. The clinician should consider their use in the patient with AMI bound for the catheterization laboratory as long as attention is paid to heparin dosing to minimize bleeding risk.

For the clinician, perhaps the most interesting area of "combination therapy" approach to the patient with AMI involves the use of a thrombolytic agent and a glycoprotein inhibitor. The IMPACT-AMI study[79] examined patients with AMI and randomly assigned them to receive either eptifibatide or placebo. In addition, patients received aspirin, heparin, and t-PA. Thus, this study looked at the role of a glycoprotein IIb-IIIa inhibitor (eptifibatide) in conjunction with a thrombolytic agent in AMI—a departure from studies of USAP with or without catheter-mediated revascularization. The highest dose of eptifibatide studied achieved higher 90 minute patency rates than placebo, but similar rates of in-hospital death, stroke, reinfarction, vascular procedures, and new heart failure. The PARADIGM trial[113] was designed to assess the safety and efficacy of combination therapy involving the platelet glycoprotein IIb-IIIa inhibitor lamifiban when given with thrombolytic agents (t-PA or streptokinase) to patients with STE AMI. A composite of angiographic, continuous electrocardiographic, and clinical markers of reperfusion was the primary efficacy end point; bleeding was the primary safety end point. Lamifiban induced more rapid reperfusion, although a higher rate of bleeding was noted (transfusions in 16.1% lamifiban-treated versus 10.3% placebo-treated patients). This trial, while small, suggests that such combination therapy may hasten clinical improvement and favorably alter outcome; additional large trials are required to further explore this issue.

The use of a reduced-dose thrombolytic agent in the patient with AMI who is a candidate for primary PTCA has also been explored. The PACT trial[114] randomized patients in the ED to either reduced-dose t-PA (50 mg) or placebo in preparation for primary angioplasty. Thrombolytic-managed patients demonstrated higher rates of infarct vessel patency and TIMI grade 3 flow with similar rates of adverse effect, suggesting that reperfusion can be enhanced prior to immediate PTCA. This approach, called *"facilitated PCI,"* suggests that early reperfusion therapy prior to catheterization is not only safe but also effective.

A significant development in the use of PTCA in the treatment of AMI involves coronary stents. In the recent past, early use of stenting in the patient with AMI was considered problematic due to the real possibility of stent thrombosis. With the introduction of aggressive antiplatelet therapy using aspirin, ticlopidine, or clopidogrel, the rates of stent thrombosis have significantly decreased. Exploring early stent placement in the patient with AMI, the PAMI-stent trial[115] compared urgent treatment with PTCA with or without stenting in 900 patients. Stenting significantly reduced both stenosis and reocclusion at 6 months. No differences in death, reinfarction, or stroke at 6 months, however, were noted.

Thus, it appears that in selected patients with AMI, primary stenting can be applied safely and effectively, resulting in a lower incidence of recurrent infarction and a significant reduction in the need for subsequent target-vessel revascularization compared with balloon angioplasty.

Patient Transfer

Indications for transfer of a patient with AMI to a regional tertiary care facility with angioplasty and cardiovascular surgery capability include patients with thrombolytic therapy contraindications who may benefit from PTCA or CABG, persistent hemodynamic instability, persistent ventricular dysrhythmias, or postinfarction or postreperfusion ischemia. Hospital transfer for primary PTCA is required in patients with thrombolytic agent contraindications. The urgent transfer of a thrombolytic-eligible patient to another institution for primary PTCA is not recommended until thrombolytic therapy is initiated; the delay in restoring perfusion in such a patient is not acceptable in most instances. If the patient is an acceptable candidate, the thrombolytic agent should be started before or during transport to the receiving hospital.

KEY CONCEPTS

- The ECG is diagnostic for AMI in only 50% of patients ultimately diagnosed with acute infarction. The remainder of these patients demonstrate normal, nonspecifically abnormal, and confounding patterns.
- Serum markers of myocardial injury are of value in ruling out AMI only when used in serial fashion. In most cases, isolated determinations are of little clinical value.
- Aspirin is the most cost effective agent available in the treatment of acute coronary ischemic events; its use either alone or in conjunction with other therapies dramatically reduces mortality.
- Acute reperfusion therapies in the patient with AMI include both thrombolysis and primary angioplasty. Primary angioplasty, if performed within 90 minutes of ED arrival, likely produces a better outcome. If primary angioplasty is not immediately available and the patient is a candidate for thrombolysis, the clinician should consider treatment with a thrombolytic agent.
- Atypical symptoms of AMI are seen in up to 30% of infarct patients. The rate of atypical clinical pictures is highest among the very elderly in whom mental status change, syncope, and other nonspecific symptom-sign complexes are seen.
- The simultaneous presence of STE and pathologic Q waves in the patient who has chest pain and suspected AMI does not preclude consideration for acute reperfusion therapies. Q waves may appear as early as 2 hours after the onset of AMI.

REFERENCES

1. Hunink MGM et al: The recent decline in mortality from coronary heart disease, 1980-1990. The effect of secular trends in risk factors and treatment, *JAMA* 227:535, 1997.
2. Rosamond WD et al: Trends in the incidence of myocardial infarction and in mortality due to coronary heart disease, 1987 to 1994, *N Engl J Med* 339:861, 1998.
3. World Health Organization, Ischaemic heart disease registers: Report of the Fifth Working Group, Copenhagen, 1971, World Health Organization.
4. Hargarten KM et al: Limitation of prehospital predictors of acute myocardial infarction and unstable angina, *Ann Emerg Med* 16:1325, 1987.
5. Swart G et al: Acute myocardial infarction complicated by hemodynamically unstable bradyarrhythmia: prehospital and emergency department treatment with atropine, *Am J Emerg Med* 17:647, 1999.
6. Aufderheide TP et al: The diagnostic impact of prehospital 12-lead electrocardiography, *Ann Emerg Med* 19:1280, 1990.
7. Rouan GW et al: Clinical characteristics of patients with acute myocardial infarction and nonspecific electrocardiograms, *Clin Res* 35:360A, 1987.
8. Tierney WM et al: Predictors of myocardial infarction in emergency room patients, *Crit Care Med* 13:526, 1985.
9. Jayes RL et al: Do patients' coronary risk factor reports predict acute cardiac ischemia in the emergency department? A multicenter study, *J Clin Epidemiol* 45:621, 1992.
10. Ornato JP et al: Value of coronary artery disease risk factors in judging whether chest pain accompanied by a normal or nondiagnostic ECG in the emergency department is due to acute cardiac ischemia, *J Am Coll Cardiol* 27:31A, 1996.
11. Lee T et al: Acute chest pain in the emergency room: identification and examination of low risk patients, *Arch Intern Med* 145:65, 1985.
12. Tierney WM et al: Physicians' estimates of the probability of myocardial infarction in emergency room patients with chest pain, *Med Decis Making* 6:12, 1986.
13. Canto JG et al: Prevalence, clinical characteristics, and mortality among patients with acute myocardial infarction presenting without chest pain, *JAMA* 283:3223, 2000.
14. Lusiani L et al: Prevalence, clinical features, and acute course of atypical myocardial infarction, *Angiology* 45:49, 1994.
15. Uretski B et al: Symptomatic myocardial infarction without chest pain: prevalence and clinical course, *Am J Cardiol* 40:498, 1977.
16. Bayer AJ et al: Changing presentation of myocardial infarction with increasing old age, *J Am Geriatr Soc* 34:263, 1986.
17. Jacoby RM, Nesto RW: Acute myocardial infarction in the diabetic patient: pathophysiology, clinical course, and prognosis, *J Am Coll Cardiol* 20:736, 1992.
18. Bertolet BD, Hill JA: Unrecognized myocardial infarction, *Cardiovasc Clin* 20:173, 1989.
19. McCarthy BD et al: Missed diagnoses of acute myocardial infarction in the emergency department: results from a multicenter study, *Ann Emerg Med* 22:579, 1993.
20. Pope JH et al: Missed diagnosis of acute cardiac ischemia in the emergency department, *N Engl J Med* 342:1163, 2000.
21. Lee TH et al: Clinical characteristics and natural history of patients with acute myocardial infarction sent home from the emergency room, *Am J Cardiol* 60:219, 1987.
22. Rusnak RA et al: Litigation against the emergency physician: common features in cases of missed myocardial infarction, *Ann Emerg Med* 18:1029, 1989.
23. Brush JE et al: Use of the initial electrocardiogram to predict in-hospital complications of acute myocardial infarction, *N Engl J Med* 312:1137, 1985.
24. Singer AJ et al: Effect of duration from symptom onset on the negative predictive value of a normal ECG for exclusion of acute myocardial infarction, *Ann Emerg Med* 29:575, 1997.
25. Otto LA, Aufderheide TP: Evaluation of ST segment elevation criteria for the prehospital electrocardiographic diagnosis of acute myocardial infarction, *Ann Emerg Med* 23:17, 1994.
26. Matetzky S et al: Significance of ST segment elevations in posterior chest leads (V_7 to V_9) in patients with acute inferior myocardial infarction: application for thrombolytic therapy, *J Am Coll Cardiol* 31:506, 1998.
27. Zeymer U et al: Effects of thrombolytic therapy in acute myocardial infarction with or without right ventricular involvement, *J Am Coll Cardiol* 2:876, 1998.
28. Brady WJ et al: A comparison of the 12-lead ECG to the 15-lead ECG in emergency department chest pain patients: impact on diagnosis, therapy, and disposition, *Am J Emerg Med* 18:239, 2000.
29. Zalenski RJ et al: Assessing the diagnostic value of an ECG containing leads V_{4R}, V_8, and V_9: the 15-lead ECG, *Ann Emerg Med* 22:786, 1993.

30. Fesmire FM, Smith EE: Continuous 12-lead electrocardiograph monitoring in the emergency department, *Am J Emerg Med* 11:54, 1993.
31. Gibler WB et al: Serial 12-lead electrocardiographic monitoring in patients presenting to the emergency department with chest pain, *J Electrocardiol* 26(Suppl):238, 1994.
32. Jernberg T et al: ST-segment monitoring with continuous 12-lead ECG improves early risk stratification in patients with chest pain and ECG nondiagnostic of acute myocardial infarction, *J Am Coll Cardiol* 34:1413, 1999.
33. Fesmire FM et al: Usefulness of automated serial 12-lead ECG monitoring during the initial emergency department evaluation of patients with chest pain, *Ann Emerg Med* 31:3, 1998.
34. Fesmire FM: ECG diagnosis of acute myocardial infarction in the presence of left bundle branch block in patients undergoing continuous ECG monitoring, *Ann Emerg Med* 26:69, 1995.
35. Krucoff MW et al: Noninvasive detection of coronary artery patency using continuous ST-segment monitoring, *Am J Cardiol* 57:916, 1986.
36. Aufderheide TP, Brady WJ: Electrocardiography in the patient with myocardial ischemia or infarction. In Gibler WB, Aufderheide TP, editors: *Emergency cardiac care,* ed 1, St. Louis, Mosby, 1994.
37. Sgarbossa EB et al: Electrocardiographic diagnosis of evolving acute myocardial infarction in the presence of left bundle branch block, *N Engl J Med* 334:481, 1996.
38. Shapiro NI et al: Validation of electrocardiographic criteria for diagnosing acute myocardial infarction in the presence of left bundle branch block, *Acad Emerg Med* 5:508, 1998.
39. Shlipak MG et al: Should the electrocardiogram be used to guide therapy for patients with left bundle branch block and suspected acute myocardial infarction? *JAMA* 281:714, 1999.
40. Edhouse JA et al: Suspected myocardial infarction and left bundle branch block: electrocardiographic indicators of acute ischaemia, *J Accid Emerg Med* 16:331, 1999.
41. Rogers WJ et al: Treatment of myocardial infarction in the United States (1990 to 1993): observations from the National Registry of Myocardial Infarction, *Circulation* 90:2103, 1994.
42. ISIS-2 (Second International Study of Infarct Survival) Collaborative Group: Randomized trial of intravenous streptokinase, oral aspirin, both, or neither amount 17,187 cases of suspected acute myocardial infarction: ISIS-2, *Lancet* 2:349, 1988.
43. Kozlowski FH et al: The electrocardiographic diagnosis of acute myocardial infarction in patients with ventricular paced rhythms, *Acad Emerg Med* 5:52, 1998.
44. Sgarbossa EB et al: Early electrocardiographic diagnosis of acute myocardial infarction in the presence of ventricular paced rhythm, *Am J Cardiol* 77:423, 1996.
45. Huwez FU et al: Variable patterns of ST-T abnormalities in patients with left ventricular hypertrophy and normal coronary arteries, *Br Heart J* 67:304, 1992.
46. Rude RE et al: Electrocardiographic and clinical criteria for recognition of acute myocardial infarction based on analysis of 3697 patients, *Am J Cardiol* 52:936, 1983.
47. Brady WJ: ST segment elevation: causes and diagnostic accuracy, *J Emerg Med* 16:797, 1998.
48. Sharkey SW et al: Impact of the electrocardiogram on the delivery of thrombolytic therapy for acute myocardial infarction, *Am J Cardiol* 73:550, 1994.
49. Gibler WB et al: Early detection of acute myocardial infarction in patients presenting with chest pain and nondiagnostic ECGs: serial CK-MB sampling in the emergency department, *Ann Emerg Med* 19:1359, 1990.
50. Marin MM, Teichman SL: Use of rapid serial sampling of creatine kinase MB for early detection of myocardial infarction in patients with acute chest pain, *Am Heart J* 123:354, 1992.
51. Puleo PR et al: Early diagnosis of acute myocardial infarction based on assay for subforms of creatine kinase-MB, *Circulation* 82:759, 1990.
52. Hamm CW et al: Emergency room triage of patients with acute chest pain by means of rapid testing for cardiac troponin T or troponin I, *N Engl J Med* 337:1648, 1997.
53. Antman EM et al: Cardiac-specific troponin I levels to predict the risk of mortality in patients with acute coronary syndromes, *N Engl J Med* 335:134, 1996.
54. Ohman EM et al: Cardiac troponin T levels for risk stratification in acute myocardial ischemia, *N Engl J Med* 335:1333, 1996.
55. Gibler WB et al: Myoglobin as an early indicator of acute myocardial infarction, *Ann Emerg Med* 16:851, 1987.
56. Brogan GX et al: Improved specificity of myoglobin plus carbonic anhydrase assay versus that of creatine kinase-MB for early diagnosis of acute myocardial infarction, *Ann Emerg Med* 27:22, 1996.
57. Horowitz RS et al: Immediate diagnosis of acute myocardial infarction by two-dimensional echocardiography, *Circulation* 65:323, 1982.
58. Peels CH et al: Usefulness of two-dimensional echocardiography for immediate detection of myocardial ischemia in the emergency room, *Am J Cardiol* 65:687, 1990.
59. Sabia P et al: Importance of two-dimensional echocardiographic assessment of left ventricular systolic function in patients presenting to the emergency room with cardiac-related symptoms, *Circulation* 84:1615, 1991.
60. Hilton TC et al: Technetium-99m sestamibi myocardial perfusion imaging in the emergency room evaluation of chest pain, *J Am Coll Cardiol* 23:1016, 1994.
61. Kontos MC et al: Value of acute rest sestamibi perfusion imaging for evaluation of patients admitted to the emergency department with chest pain, *J Am Coll Cardiol* 30:976, 1997.
62. Mikhail MG et al: Cost-effectiveness of mandatory stress testing in chest pain center patients, *Ann Emerg Med* 29:88, 1997.
63. Kirk JD et al: Evaluation of chest pain in low-risk patients presenting to the emergency department: the role of immediate exercise testing, *Ann Emerg Med* 32:1, 1998.
64. Goldman L et al: A computer-delivered protocol to aid in the diagnosis of emergency room patients with acute chest pain *N Engl J Med* 307:588, 1982.
65. Goldman L et al: A computer protocol to predict myocardial infarction in emergency department patients with chest pain, *N Engl J Med* 318:797, 1988.
66. Baxt WB: Use of an artificial neural network for the diagnosis of myocardial infarction, *Ann Intern Med* 115:906, 1991.
67. Zalenski RJ, et al: National Heart Attack Alert Program position paper: Chest pain centers and programs for the evaluation of acute cardiac ischemia. Ann Emerg Med 35:462, 2000.
68. Farkouh ME et al: A clinical trial of a chest-pain observation unit for patients with unstable angina. Chest Pain Evaluation in the Emergency Room (CHEER) Investigators, *N Engl J Med* 339:1882, 1998.
69. Gibler WB et al: A rapid diagnostic and treatment center for patients with chest pain in the emergency department, *Ann Emerg Med* 25:1, 1995.

69a. W Brady: Unpublished information, University of Virginia, Charlottesville, Va., 2000.

70. The GUSTO Angiographic Investigators: The effects of tissue plasminogen activator, streptokinase, or both on coronary-artery patency, ventricular function, and survival after acute myocardial infarction, *N Engl J Med* 329:1615, 1993.
71. Weaver WD et al (for the Myocardial Infarction Triage and Intervention Project Group): Prehospital-initiated vs hospital-initiated thrombolytic therapy: the myocardial infarction triage and intervention trial, *JAMA* 270:1211, 1993.
72. Ryan TJ et al: 1999 Update: ACC/AHA guidelines for the management of patients with acute myocardial infarction, *J Am Coll Cardiol* 34:890, 1999.
73. Ryan TJ et al: ACC/AHA: ACC/AHA guidelines for the management of patients with acute myocardial infarction: executive summary, *Circulation* 94:2341, 1996.
74. Yusuf S et al: Effect of intravenous nitrates on mortality in acute myocardial infarction: an overview of the randomized trials, *Lancet* I (8594):1088, 1988.
75. The EPIC Investigators: Use of a monoclonal antibody directed against the platelet glycoprotein IIb/IIIa receptor in high-risk coronary angioplasty, *N Engl J Med* 330:956, 1994.
76. The Epilog Investigators: Platelet glycoprotein IIb/IIIa receptor blockade and low-dose heparin during percutaneous coronary revascularization, *N Engl J Med* 336:1689, 1997.
77. The CAPTURE Investigators: Randomized placebo-controlled trial of abciximab before and during coronary intervention in refractory unstable angina: the CAPTURE study, *Lancet* 349:1429, 1997.

78. Lambert F et al: Abciximab in the treatment of acute myocardial infarction eligible for primary percutaneous transluminal coronary angioplasty, *J Am Coll Cardiol* 33:1528, 1999.
79. Ohman EM et al: Combined accelerated tissue-plasminogen activator and platelet glycoprotein IIb/IIIa integrin receptor blockade with Integrilin in acute myocardial infarction. Results of a randomized, placebo-controlled, dose-ranging trial. The IMPACT-AMI Investigators. *Circulation* 95:846, 1997.
80. The IMPACT-II Investigators: Randomized placebo-controlled trial of effect of eptifibatide on complications of percutaneous coronary intervention: IMPACT II. Integrilin to minimize platelet aggregation and coronary thrombosis-II, *Lancet* 349:1422, 1997.
81. Anonymous: Inhibition of platelet glycoprotein IIb/IIIa with eptifibatide in patients with acute coronary syndromes. The PURSUIT Trial Investigators. Platelet glycoprotein IIb/IIIa in unstable angina: receptor suppression using Integrilin therapy, *N Engl J Med* 339:436, 1998.
82. The Platelet Receptor Inhibition in Ischemic Syndrome Management (PRISM) Study Investigators: A comparison of aspirin plus tirofiban with aspirin plus heparin for unstable angina, *N Engl J Med* 338:1498, 1998.
83. Zhao XQ et al: Intracoronary thrombus and platelet glycoprotein IIb/IIIa receptor blockade with tirofiban in unstable angina or non-Q-wave myocardial infarction. Angiographic results from the PRISM-PLUS trial (Platelet receptor inhibition for ischemic syndrome management in patients limited by unstable signs and symptoms). PRISM-PLUS Investigators, *Circulation* 100:1609, 1999.
84. Wallentin L et al for the FRISC group: Low molecular weight heparin during instability in coronary artery disease, *Lancet* 347:561, 1996.
85. Klein W et al: Comparison of low-molecular-weight heparin with unfractionated heparin acutely and with placebo for 6 weeks in the management of unstable coronary artery disease. Fragmin in unstable coronary artery disease study (FRIC), *Circulation* 96:61, 1997.
86. Cohen M et al: A comparison of low-molecular-weight heparin with unfractionated heparin for unstable coronary artery disease. Efficacy and safety of subcutaneous enoxaparin in Non-Q-Wave Coronary Events Study Group, *N Engl J Med* 337:447, 1997.
87. Anonymous: Effects of recombinant hirudin (lepirudin) compared with heparin on death, myocardial infarction, refractory angina, and revascularisation procedures in patients with acute myocardial ischaemia without ST elevation: a randomised trial. Organisation to Assess Strategies for Ischemic Syndromes (OASIS-2) Investigators, *Lancet* 353:429, 1999.
88. Neuhaus KL et al: Recombinant hirudin (lepirudin) for the improvement of thrombolysis with streptokinase in patients with acute myocardial infarction: Results of the HIT-4 trial, *J Am Coll Cardiol* 32:876, 1998.
89. White HD et al: Randomized, double-blind comparison of hirulog versus heparin in patients receiving streptokinase and aspirin for acute myocardial infarction (HERO). Hirulog Early Reperfusion/Occlusion (HERO) Trial Investigators, *Circulation* 96:2155, 1997.
90. Jang IK et al: A multicenter, randomized study of argatroban versus heparin as adjunct to tissue plasminogen activator (TPA) in acute myocardial infarction: myocardial infarction with novastan and TPA (MINT) study, *J Am Coll Cardiol* 33:1879, 1999.
91. GISSI-2: A factorial randomised trial of alteplase versus streptokinase and heparin versus no heparin among 12,490 patients with acute myocardial infarction, *Lancet* 336:65, 1990.
92. The International Study Group: In-hospital mortality and clinical course of 20,891 patients with suspected acute myocardial infarction randomized between alteplase and streptokinase with or without heparin, *Lancet* 336:71, 1990.
93. ISIS-3: A randomised comparison of streptokinase vs tissue plasminogen activator vs anistreplase and or aspirin plus heparin vs aspirin alone among 41,299 cases of suspected acute myocardial infarction, *Lancet* 339:753, 1992.
94. The GUSTO-III Investigators: An international, multicenter, randomized comparison of reteplase with alteplase for acute myocardial infarction, *N Engl J Med* 337:1118, 1997.
95. Single-bolus tenecteplase compared with front-loaded alteplase in acute myocardial infarction: the ASSENT-2 double-blind randomized trial, *Lancet* 354:716, 1999.
96. Fibrinolytic Therapy Trialists' (FTT) Collaborative Group: Indications for fibrinolytic therapy in suspected acute myocardial infarction: collaborative overview of early mortality and major morbidity results from all randomised trials of more than 1000 patients, *Lancet* 343:311, 1994.
97. The TIMI-IIIB Investigators: Effects of tissue plasminogen activator and a comparison of early invasive and conservative strategies in unstable angina and non-Q-wave myocardial infarction: results of the TIMI-IIIB trial, *Circulation* 89:1545, 1994.
98. Estudio Multicentrico Estreptoquinas Republicas de America del Sur (EMERAS) Collective Group: Randomised trial of late thrombolysis in patients with suspected acute myocardial infarction: EMERAS, *Lancet* 342:767, 1993.
99. LATE Study Group: Late assessment of thrombolytic efficacy (LATE) study with alteplase 6-24 hours after onset of acute myocardial infarction, *Lancet* 342:759, 1993.
100. Gruppo Italiano per lo Studio della Streptochinasi nell'Infarto Miocardico (GISSI): Effectiveness of intravenous thrombolytic treatment in acute myocardial infarction, *Lancet* 1:397, 1986.
101. Tenaglia AN et al: Thrombolytic therapy in patients requiring cardiopulmonary resuscitation, *Am J Cardiol* 68:1015, 1991.
102. Grines CL et al: A comparison of immediate angioplasty with thrombolytic therapy for acute myocardial infarction, *N Engl J Med* 328:673, 1993.
103. Wilcox RG et al for the ASSET Study Group: Trial of tissue plasminogen activator for mortality reduction in acute myocardial infarction: the Anglo-Scandinavian Study of Early Thrombolysis (ASSET), *Lancet* 2:525, 1988.
104. Grines CL et al: A comparison of immediate angioplasty with thrombolytic therapy for acute myocardial infarction, *N Engl J Med* 328:673, 1993.
105. Zijlstra F et al: A comparison of immediate coronary angioplasty with intravenous streptokinase in acute myocardial infarction, *N Engl J Med* 328:680, 1993.
106. The GUSTO IIb Angioplasty Substudy Investigators: A clinical trial comparing primary coronary angioplasty with tissue plasminogen activator for acute myocardial infarction, *N Engl J Med* 336:1621, 1997.
107. Weaver WD et al: Comparison of primary coronary angioplasty and intravenous thrombolytic therapy for acute myocardial infarction: a quantitative review, *JAMA* 278:2093, 1997.
108. Califf RM et al: Evaluation of combination thrombolytic therapy and timing of cardiac catheterization in acute myocardial infarction: results of thrombolysis and angioplasty in myocardial infarction phase 5 randomized trial, *Circulation* 83:1543, 1991.
109. Goldberg RJ et al: Cardiogenic shock after acute myocardial infarction: incidence and mortality from a community-wide perspective, 1975 to 1988, *N Engl J Med* 325:1117, 1991.
110. Hochman JS et al: Early revascularization in acute myocardial infarction complicated by cardiogenic shock, *N Engl J Med* 341:625, 1999.
111. Brener SJ et al: Randomized, placebo-controlled trial of platelet glycoprotein IIb/IIIa blockade with primary angioplasty for acute myocardial infarction. ReoPro and Primary PTCA Organization and Randomized Trial (RAPPORT) Investigators, *Circulation* 98:734, 1998.
112. Montalescot G et al: Abciximab associated with primary angioplasty and stenting in acute myocardial infarction: the ADMIRAL study, 30 day final results, *Circulation* 100:I-87, 1999.
112a. Stone GW: CADILLAC Trial. Presented at the American Heart Association's 72nd Scientific Sessions, Atlanta, November 9, 1999.
113. Anonymous. Combining thrombolysis with the platelet glycoprotein IIb/IIIa inhibitor lamifiban: results of the Platelet Aggregation Receptor Antagonist Dose Investigation and Reperfusion Gain in Myocardial Infarction (PARADIGM) trial, *J Am Coll Cardiol* 32:2003-2010, 1998.
114. Ross AM et al: A randomized trial comparing primary angioplasty with a strategy of short-acting thrombolysis and immediate planned rescue angioplasty in acute myocardial infarction: the PACT trial, *J Am Coll Cardiol* 34:1954, 1999.
115. Suryapranata H et al: Randomized comparison of coronary stenting with balloon angioplasty in selected patients with acute myocardial infarction, *Circulation* 97:2502, 1998.

74 Dysrhythmias

Donald M. Yealy
Theodore R. Delbridge

PRINCIPLES OF DISEASE

Cardiac Cellular Electrophysiology

Although controversy over nomenclature exists, the term *dysrhythmia* (as opposed to *arrhythmia*) is used to denote any abnormality in cardiac rhythm. The function of individual cells in the conductive and contractile tissues of the heart depends on an intact resting membrane potential. Na^+, K^+, and Ca^{++} ions create the membrane potential and regulate conduction and contraction. The membrane potential is the result of a differential concentration of Na^+ and K^+ on each side of the cell membrane; the potential measures approximately 90 mV in normal resting nonpacemaker cells, with a relative net negative intracellular charge (Figure 74-1). This electrical gradient is created and maintained mainly by the sodium-potassium exchange pump and by the natural concentration-dependent flow of K^+ out of the cell. A Na^+-Ca^{++} exchange also exists, regulating the intracellular concentration of Ca^{++}. Although this latter exchange mechanism contributes little to the resting membrane potential, it does influence myofibril contractility.

The sodium-potassium pump depends on adenosine triphosphate (ATP) for energy to transport Na^+ out to the extracellular fluid. The energy generation process for this pump requires ATPase and Mg^{++}. During normal pump function, three Na^+ ions are transported out of the cell in exchange for two K^+ ions, generating a 10-mV potential across the membrane (see Figure 74-1). This process creates an osmotic gradient, allowing Ca^{++} to be exchanged for Na^+ without energy expenditure. Disturbances in intracellular and extracellular ion concentrations from ischemia, electrolyte and metabolic derangements, or drugs can alter the membrane potential and produce abnormalities of impulse generation, conduction, and myofibril contraction.

The remainder of the resting membrane potential is generated from the flow of K^+ down a concentration gradient toward the extracellular fluid (see Figure 74-1). The cell membrane is far more permeable to potassium ions than sodium ions, resulting in a greater loss of intracellular positive charge. Abnormalities in the K^+ gradient can interfere with normal impulse formation and conduction.

In normal nonpacemaker cells, the application of an electrical stimulus causes the membrane potential to become less negative, termed *depolarization*. When the membrane potential reaches –70mV, specialized channels for Na^+ entry open, causing a rapid influx of positive charge into the cell. This "fast" channel activity further decreases the membrane potential and is augmented at approximately –30 to –40 mV by a second "slow" channel that allows Ca^{++} influx. When channels close, the resting potential is restored by the sodium-potassium pump and the K^+ concentration gradient, an event known as repolarization.

The electrical activity of a myocardial cell membrane can be traced with a microelectrode and is called the *action potential* (Figure 74-2). Phase 4 represents electrical diastole, with the normal cell membrane at a resting potential of –90mV. Nonpacemaker cells maintain this potential until an electrical stimulus arrives. When a stimulus arrives, abrupt membrane depolarization occurs (phase 0). Phase 1 is a short period of membrane repolarization, caused by the closure of the fast Na^+ channels and transient K^+ efflux from the cell. Phase 2 is the plateau phase of the action potential, where the slow Ca^{++} channels remain open, maintaining a near balance between ion influx and efflux. During this phase, an increase in the cytosol Ca^{++} concentration occurs as both the extracellular and intracellular (within the sarcoplasmic reticulum) stores are mobilized. This increase in intracellular Ca^{++} concentration facilitates mechanical coupling and myofibril contraction. Phase 3 represents the rapid membrane repolarization period as the slow channels close and K^+ flows down the concentration gradient. The ATP-driven pump exchanges Na^+ and K^+ until the phase 4 resting potential is reached.

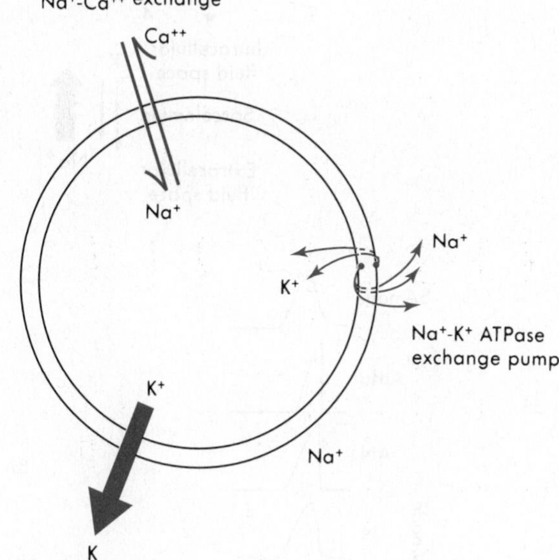

Figure 74-1. **Flow of various ions across myocardial cell membrane. Na^+-K^+ pump exchanges three Na^+ ions for each two K^+ ions, generating a net negative flow of 10 mV. The flow of K^+ down the concentration gradient *(dark arrow)* generates another 80 mV of current. The Na^+-Ca^{++} exchange adds little to the resting potential.** *From Marriott HJL, Conover MB:* **Advanced concepts in arrhythmias,** *ed 2, St Louis, 1989, Mosby.*

In nonpacemaker cells, additional depolarization from a second electrical stimulus is not possible when the membrane

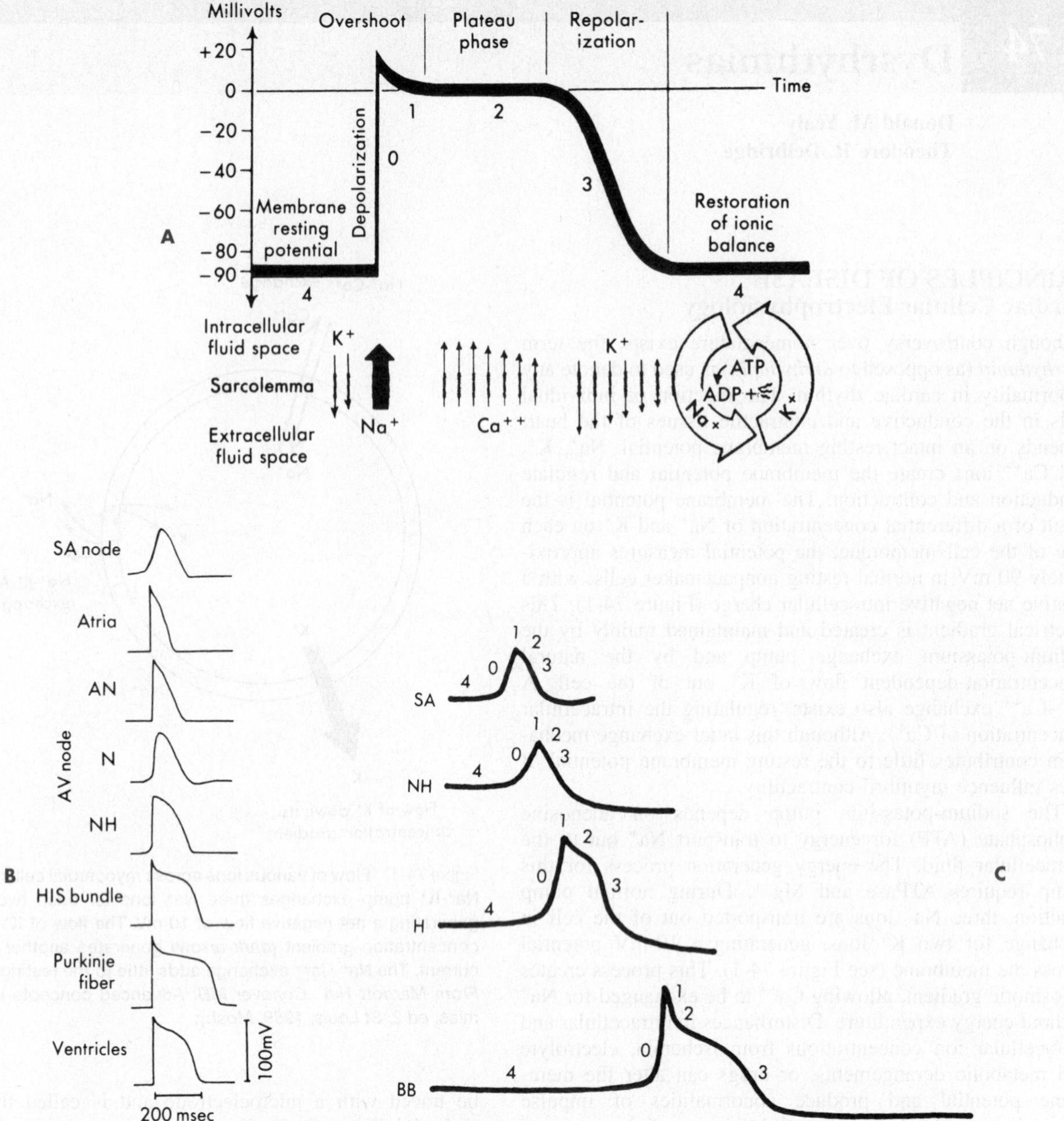

Figure 74-2. **A, Action potential of a myocardial cell and its relation to ion flow. B, Action potentials of various myocardial tissues. C, Action potentials of various pacemaker cells. Note that phase 4 becomes flatter as location becomes more distal.** ***SA,*** **Sinoatrial;** ***NH,*** **nodal-His;** ***H,*** **His bundle;** ***BB,*** **bundle branch fascicles.** ***A and B, from*** **Calcium in cardiac metabolism,** ***New Jersey, 1980, Knoll Pharmaceutical*** **Co;** ***C, from Conover M:*** **Understanding electrocardiography,** ***ed 5, St Louis, 1988, Mosby.***

potential is more positive than –60mV (initially achieved during phase 0 and maintained until phase 3) irrespective of impulse strength. This period is termed the *effective refractory period* (Figure 74-3). At a membrane potential of –60 to –70 mV, a strong impulse can cause a response that is likely to be propagated, although abnormally; this response represents the *relative refractory period* (see Figure 74-3). At a membrane potential of –70mV or less, virtually all fast channels are ready for activity if properly stimulated.

Pacemaker cells differ from non-impulse-generating cells in two ways: the resting membrane potential is less negative and they can exhibit spontaneous depolarization during phase 4 (see Figure 74-2). Pacemaker cells are found within the sinoatrial (SA) and atrioventricular (AV) nodes, as well as on the atrial surfaces of the AV valves and within the His-Purkinje system. The spontaneous depolarization is the result of slow Na^+ influx. When the membrane threshold is reached, further depolarization in pacemaker cells occurs largely from activation of the slow Ca^{++} channels. Nonpacemaker cells may develop altered resting potentials and undergo spontaneous depolarization under pathologic conditions, especially during ischemia.

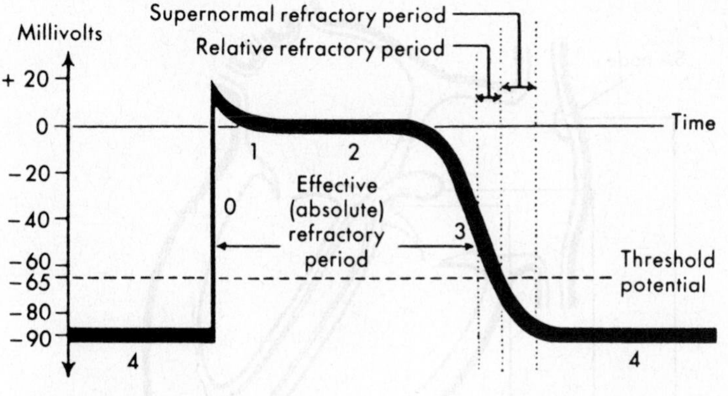

Figure 74-3. **Action potential showing various refractory periods.** *From* **Calcium in cardiac metabolism,** *New Jersey, 1980, Knoll Pharmaceutical Co.*

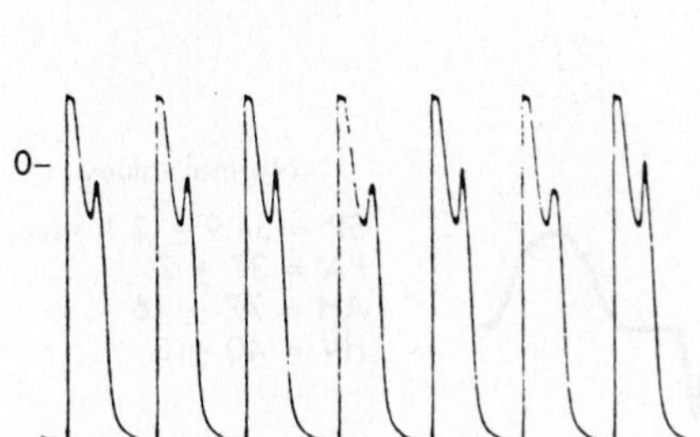

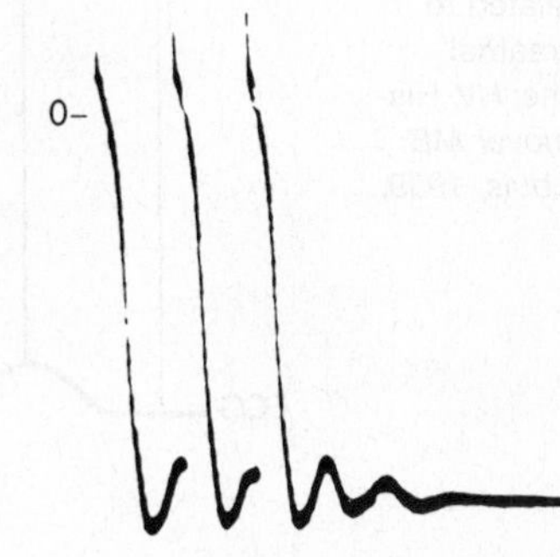

Figure 74-4. **Early afterdepolarizations** *(left)* **compared with delayed afterdepolarizations** *(right).* *From Marriott HJL, Conover MB:* **Advanced concepts in arrhythmias,** *ed 2, St Louis, 1989, Mosby.*

Afterdepolarizations are fluctuations in membrane potential that occur as the resting potential is approached; these fluctuations may precipitate another depolarization (Figure 74-4). Afterdepolarizations can occur just before full resting potential (early afterdepolarizations) or after full resting potential (delayed afterdepolarizations) is reached. Delayed afterdepolarizations are associated with ischemia, pump failure, catecholamine excess, and electrolyte disturbances (especially K^+, Mg^{++}, and Ca^{++}) and are enhanced by faster heart rates. Early afterdepolarizations are associated with high resting membrane potentials and are enhanced by slower heart rates.

Basic Anatomy and Conduction

The SA node is located at the junction of the right atrium and the superior vena cava. It is supplied by the right coronary artery (RCA) in 55% and the left circumflex artery (LCA) in 45% of subjects. The normal SA node produces spontaneous depolarizations at a faster rate than other pacemakers and thus functions as the dominant pacemaker. When the SA node is injured or when other pacemakers generate impulses at a faster rate, nonsinus cardiac rhythms are observed. The SA node is normally under a slight parasympathetic dominance, keeping the resting heart rate between 60 and 90 beats/min in most adults. Hypothermia and increased relative vagal stimulation slow the rate of SA node impulse formation, whereas hyperthermia and increased relative sympathetic stimulation can increase the rate. Other pacemaker sites may be similarly affected by temperature and autonomic tone.

Figure 74-5 correlates the normal surface electrocardiographic (ECG) events to those occurring at the electrophysiologic level. The impulse generated from within the SA node, imperceptible on the surface ECG, is propagated through the atrial tissue to the AV node. The atrial depolarization wave is characterized by the P wave on the surface ECG. The AV node is supplied by a branch of the RCA in 90% of subjects (termed *right dominant circulation*) and by the LCA in the remaining 10% of patients (*left dominant circulation*). Transport of the impulse within the AV node is slower than other areas of the conducting system (Table 74-1) because of the dependence on slow-channel ion influx to depolarize the cell membranes. This delay limits the ventricular rate and allows complete atrial emptying, providing a greater ventricular diastolic volume and increased stroke volume. The two functionally distinct pathways within the AV node are termed α and β. The α pathway has relatively slow conduction and a short refractory period, and the β pathway exhibits faster conduction and a longer refractory period. These paths can be important in sustaining a reentrant tachycardia (see later discussion). The PR interval (normally 0.10 to 0.20 second) represents the time needed for conducting of a sinus impulse through the atria and AV node. Impulses originating in the low atrial tissues, the AV junction, or other infranodal tissues are associated with a shortened PR interval, along with impulses conducted to the ventricles by accessory pathways. PR prolongation usually results from nodal or supranodal conduction system disease.

After entry into the AV node, the impulse is carried down through the His bundle to the three main bundle branch fascicles. The His bundle is the distal-most portion of the AV node and derives its blood supply from the RCA and left anterior descending (LAD) artery. The bundle branch fascicles beyond the His area supply the right (RBB), left anterior-superior (LASB), and left posterior-inferior (LPIB) ventricular myocardium. Before separating into the three fascicles, His bundle fibers assume a topographic distribution. The appearance of a specific bundle branch pattern on the ECG can be the result of injury within a specific bundle

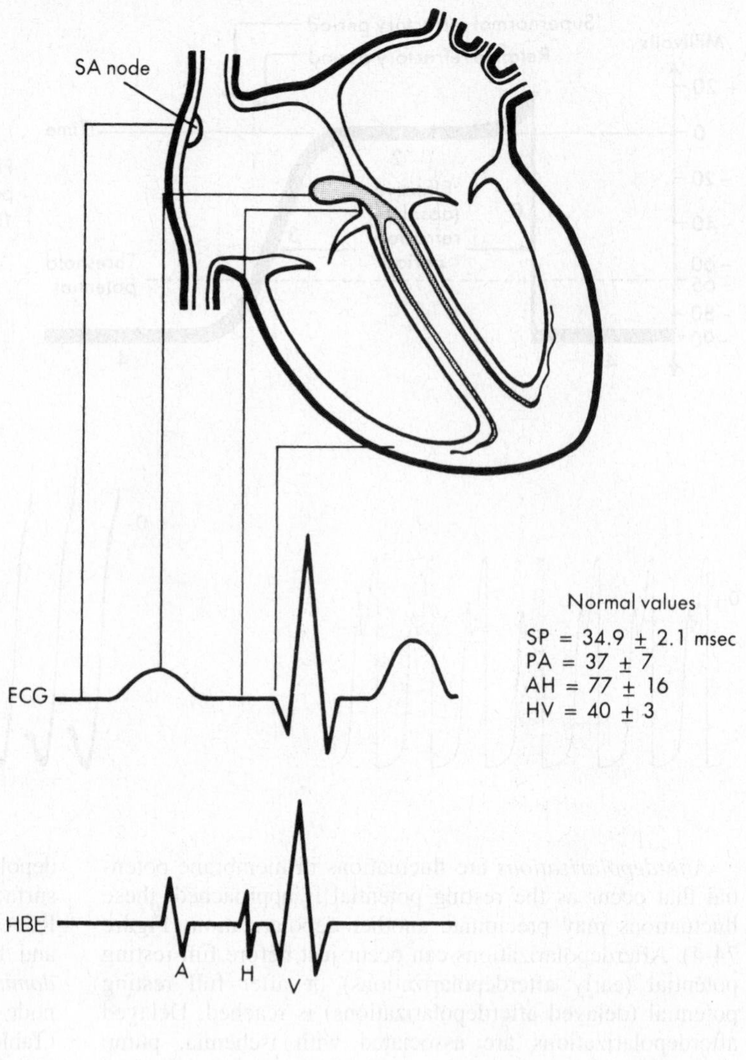

Figure 74-5. **Electrical events in heart related to surface ECG and His bundle electrogram *(HBE).* Approximate relationship of sinus node discharge is also related to surface ECG. *SP,* SA conduction time; *PA,* intraatrial conduction time; *AH,* AV nodal conduction time; *HV,* His-Purkinje conduction.** ***From Marriott HJL, Conover MB:*** **Advanced concepts in arrhythmias, *ed 2, St Louis, 1989, Mosby.***

Table 74-1. Conduction Velocities in Various Heart Tissues

Tissue	Velocity (m/sec)
Atrium	1000
AV node	200
His-Purkinje system	4000
Ventricles	400

branch fascicle or a lesion within the main His bundle. The RBB and LASB are supplied by the LAD, and the LPIB can be supplied by either the RCA or the LCA. Occlusion of these vessels can cause a variety of conduction abnormalities; commonly, RCA occlusion causes AV node block, whereas LAD occlusion usually causes infranodal (bundle branch) block.

After conduction down the three main bundle branches, each impulse is delivered to the Purkinje fibers. These fibers carry the impulse to the ventricular myocardial tissues in a rapid and orderly fashion, stimulating contraction and ejection of the ventricular contents. The QRS complex (normally < 0.10 second) represents ventricular depolarization, and the T wave reflects repolarization. The total time of ventricular depolarization and repolarization is represented by the QT interval; the normal duration of QT interval must be corrected for age, sex, and heart rate.

The time required for complete conduction system repolarization is a function of the preceding cardiac cycle length. Shorter cycle lengths, represented as shorter preceding RR intervals (i.e., faster heart rates), beget a shorter repolarization time. Conversely, longer cardiac cycles (slower heart rates) are associated with longer repolarization times. If an underlying slow sinus rhythm is present and an ectopic atrial impulse arrives between sinus impulses, the ectopic impulse may be conducted aberrantly (if bundles are relatively refractory), or they may be blocked (if the bundles are completely refractory). The preceding cycle is called the *setup cycle* because it dictates the refractory time of the infranodal conducting tissues. The *Ashman phenomenon* refers to aberrant ventricular conduction of an atrial extrasystole after a long setup cycle, which can occur in any irregular atrial dysrhythmia. Classically, the Ashman phenomenon is seen in atrial fibrillation, in which long-short cycle sequences are often seen as a result of the chaotic rhythm. In normal subjects the right bundle branch is the last part of the infranodal system to completely repolarize. Thus aberrantly conducted impulses in the Ashman phenomenon usually assume a right bundle branch appearance on the ECG.

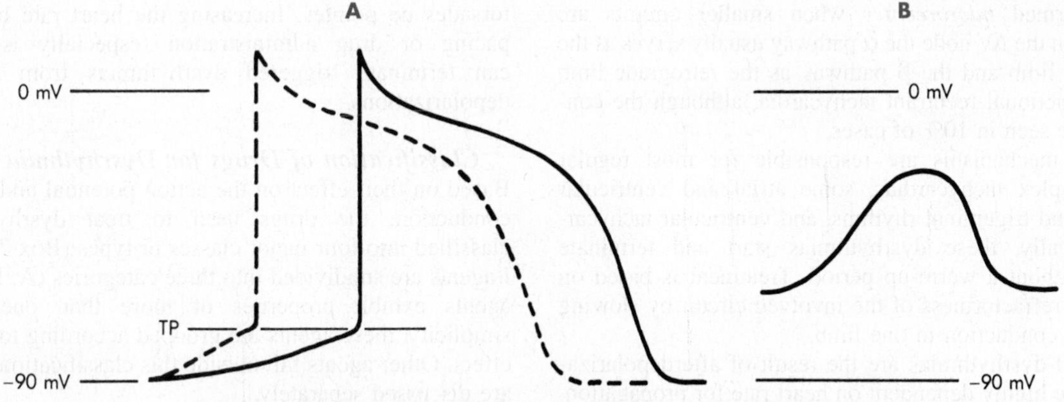

Figure 74-6. **A, Enhanced normal automaticity *(dashed line)*. B, Abnormal automaticity.** ***From Marriott HJL, Conover MB:*** **Advanced concepts in arrhythmias, *ed 2, St Louis, 1989, Mosby.***

Normally the AV node is the preferred path for impulse delivery to the infranodal conducting system. In some patients, pathologic accessory pathways connecting atrial, infranodal conducting, and ventricular myocardial cells may exist. These accessory pathways do not share the normal conduction delay of the AV node and may allow a rapid ventricular response rate and subsequent reduced cardiac output when supplanting the normal conduction system. *Preexcitation* refers to the early depolarization of ventricular myocardium when accessory paths are employed instead of the normal conduction system (discussed later.)

The AV node may serve as a subsidiary pacemaker in the absence of normal SA node activity; this node has an intrinsic impulse formation rate of 45 to 60 beats/min. Infranodal pacemakers, found within the His bundle, bundle branches, and the Purkinje system, usually function at a rate of 30 to 45 beats/min. These rates may vary widely based on the underlying pathologic process present. Additionally, as a result of ischemia or drug effect, atrial and ventricular nonpacemaker myocardial cells may become pacemakers.

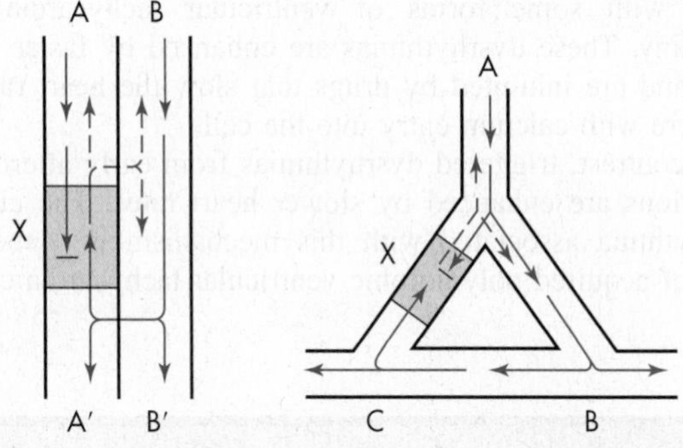

Figure 74-7. **Mechanism of reentry.**

Physiology

Mechanisms for Dysrhythmia Formation There are three accepted theories of dysrhythmia formation: altered automaticity, reentry, and triggered mechanisms. The history and surface ECG may differentiate these mechanisms.

Altered automaticity can result from spontaneous phase 4 depolarization in nonpacemaker cells (abnormal automaticity) or an increase in the slope of depolarization in cells that normally undergo phase 4 depolarization (enhanced automaticity) (Figure 74-6). Both types of altered automaticity can occur in the setting of ischemia, electrolyte disturbances, and drug therapy.

Dysrhythmias caused by altered automaticity usually require a warm-up period; clinically a patient may report a gradual increase in palpitations as opposed to an abrupt onset. A similar gradual increase in abnormal impulses should accompany these symptoms on the ECG. These dysrhythmias tend also to terminate in a gradual fashion. Ventricular tachycardia within the first 24 hours after myocardial infarction is often the result of abnormal automaticity.

Enhanced automaticity occurs when catecholamine excess stimulates a non-SA nodal pacemaker source to become the dominant pacemaker. A typical enhanced automatic dysrhythmia is an idioventricular rhythm (from increased depolarization of the Purkinje fiber) after myocardial infarction. Another enhanced automatic dysrhythmia is atrial or junctional tachycardia with digitalis toxicity. In this setting, digitalis interferes with SA node impulse conduction and increases phase 4 depolarization in other myocardial cells, resulting in the above dysrhythmia.

Reentry mechanisms are a common cause of narrow-complex tachydysrhythmias, accounting for 50% to 80% of these rhythms. For reentry to occur, three conditions must exist: two paths (or a circuit) must be available for a given impulse to travel through, unequal responsiveness of each limb of the circuit must be present, and slowed conduction must exist in one limb. Reentry dysrhythmias are the result of abnormal conduction, as opposed to the abnormal impulse formation that occurs with altered automatic dysrhythmias (Figure 74-7).

In a reentrant dysrhythmia, an impulse reaching a circuit finds one of the two limbs refractory. The impulse is conducted down the nonrefractory limb to the distal tissues. If the initial refractory limb has recovered during the time required for the impulse to traverse the other limb, the impulse can then enter the distal end of the latter limb and travel in a retrograde direction. This unequal responsiveness of the limbs creates a functional unidirectional block of one limb. When the impulse exits the second (retrograde conducting) limb, it may then reenter the first limb. Each cycle can be repeated, creating a self-sustaining, or circus movement, tachycardia. These cycles can be ordered or disordered (i.e., fibrillatory) and are termed *microreentry* when smaller circuits are employed. In the AV node the α pathway usually serves as the anterograde limb and the β pathway as the retrograde limb during a junctional reentrant tachycardia, although the converse can be seen in 10% of cases.

Reentry mechanisms are responsible for most regular narrow-complex tachycardias, some atrial and ventricular bigeminal and trigeminal rhythms, and ventricular tachycardias. Clinically, these dysrhythmias start and terminate abruptly, without a warm-up period. Treatment is based on altering the refractoriness of the involved circuit by slowing or speeding conduction in one limb.

Triggered dysrhythmias are the result of afterdepolarizations and are highly dependent on heart rate for propagation. Triggered dysrhythmias secondary to delayed afterdepolarizations are associated with an intracellular Ca^{++} overload and can occur during reperfusion therapy in myocardial infarction and with digitalis toxicity. Ectopic atrial and junctional rhythms are often the result of this mechanism, along with some forms of ventricular tachycardia and bigeminy. These dysrhythmias are enhanced by faster heart rates and are inhibited by drugs that slow the heart rate or interfere with calcium entry into the cell.

In contrast, triggered dysrhythmias from early afterdepolarizations are enhanced by slower heart rates. The classic dysrhythmia associated with this mechanism is a specific form of acquired polymorphic ventricular tachycardia called torsades de pointes. Increasing the heart rate by overdrive pacing or drug administration (especially isoproterenol) can terminate triggered dysrhythmias from early afterdepolarizations.

Classification of Drugs for Dysrhythmia Treatment

Based on their effect on the action potential and on impulse conduction, the drugs used to treat dysrhythmias are classified into four major classes or types (Box 74-1).[1] Class I agents are subdivided into three categories (A, B, C). Some agents exhibit properties of more than one class; for simplicity, these agents are grouped according to their major effect. Other agents fall outside this classification system and are discussed separately.

Class I agents exert their major effect on the fast Na^+ channels, resulting in slowed conduction and membrane stabilization. The subclasses are based on specific effects on action potential duration and conduction. Class IA agents moderately slow depolarization, prolong repolarization and action potential duration, and slow conduction. Class IB agents cause minimal slowing of depolarization and conduction and shorten repolarization and action potential duration. Class IC agents markedly slow depolarization and conduction and prolong repolarization and action potential duration.

Class II agents are the β-adrenergic antagonists (blockers); these agents slow the SA node rate and AV node conduction. β-Blockers also prolong the action potential and can depress

Box 74-1 Classification/Types of Antidysrhythmic Drugs

Class I

Sodium (fast) channel blockers. Slow depolarization with varying effects on repolarization. Called "membrane-stabilizing" drugs and have prominent antiectopic effects.

IA

Moderate slowing of depolarization and conduction. Prolong repolarization and action potential duration.

Quinidine
Procainamide
Disopyramide

IB

Minimally slow depolarization and conduction. Shorten repolarization and action potential duration.

Lidocaine
Phenytoin
Tocainide
Mexiletine
Moricizine*
Aprindine

IC

Markedly slow depolarization and conduction. Prolong repolarization and action potential duration.

Flecainide
Encainide
Lorcainide
Propafenone*

Class II

Adrenergic blockers
Propranolol
Esmolol
Acebutolol
Nadolol
Metoprolol

Class III

Antifibrillatory agents. Prolong action potential duration and refractory period duration with antifibrillatory properties.

Bretylium
Amiodarone
Dofetilide
Ibutilide†
Sotalol†

Class IV

Calcium (slow) channel blockers.

Verapamil
Diltiazem

Miscellaneous

Digitalis
Magnesium sulfate
Adenosine

*Shares effects with class IA agents.
†Shares activity with class II agents.

conduction in ischemic myocardial tissues, although the normal His-Purkinje system is unaffected. Class III agents prolong the action potential and refractory period duration, thus exhibiting a clinical antifibrillatory effect. Class IV agents are the slow Ca^{++} channel entry antagonists, causing a depression of anterograde conduction through the AV node and suppression of other calcium-dependent dysrhythmias. Miscellaneous agents important in the emergency treatment of dysrhythmias include magnesium sulfate, digitalis, and adenosine.

Although the drugs mentioned here are used as antidysrhythmics, they are also associated with prodysrhythmic effects.[2] This term refers to the exacerbation of an underlying dysrhythmia or to the provocation of a new dysrhythmia after institution of drug therapy. In general, the class IB agents have the least frequent prodysrhythmic effect (< 2% incidence), class IA intermediate (2% to 5%), and the class IC the most prominent (5% to 15%). The most feared rhythm induced is ventricular tachycardia, especially polymorphic, which may lead to syncope or sudden death. For the class II and IV agents, the prodysrhythmic effects are primarily an extension of the electrophysiologic actions (i.e., bradycardia and increasing AV nodal block).

Class IA Agents All class IA agents slow conduction through the atria, AV node, and His-Purkinje system directly, and decrease conduction in accessory pathways. Class IA agents also exhibit anticholinergic and negative inotropic effects, with disopyramide displaying the most prominent and procainamide the least effect on contractility. Both procainamide and quinidine have peripheral vasodilatory actions (from α-adrenergic blockage) that also contribute to hypotension after administration. Disopyramide has vasoconstrictor properties, which together with its marked negative inotropic effects limits its use for acute dysrhythmia treatment.

Each class IA agent has high oral bioavailability after an oral dose. This subclass of drugs, particularly quinidine and procainamide, is associated with prolonged ventricular repolarization and a lengthened QT interval on the surface ECG. These changes mirror an increased risk of acquired polymorphic ventricular tachycardia in some patients treated with these agents.[2,3] The aggregate incidence of prodysrhythmic effects appears to be approximately 5% in this class.

Procainamide Procainamide is the most commonly used class IA agent in the emergency treatment of ventricular and supraventricular dysrhythmias.[4-7] Intravenous procainamide is administered at a rate of 20 to 30 mg/min until the dysrhythmia is terminated, hypotension occurs (defined as a drop in the mean blood pressure of 15% or greater of the pretreatment value, or to a systolic pressure below 90 mm Hg), the QRS complex widens (to greater than 50% of the pretreatment width), or a total dose of 17 mg/kg is administered (or 12 mg/kg if congestive heart failure is present). The arbitrary limiting of the total dose to 1 g may interfere with the success of this agent. Intravenous procainamide can cause a transient increase in heart rate when used to treat a supraventricular dysrhythmia as a result of its anticholinergic properties. A decrease in heart rate from its direct effect on AV nodal conduction and depolarization, however, may also occur and force the termination of its use because of bradycardia. If successful, intravenous maintenance therapy can be instituted at a rate of 1 to 4 mg/min, with the lower rate suggested for elderly patients, patients with congestive heart failure, and patients with renal failure. Oral therapy can be started at 2 g daily in divided doses (depending on the preparation) and titrated to effects and serum levels of procainamide and n-acetylprocainamide (an active metabolite). In addition to prodysrhythmia, other complications that can occur with prolonged use are heart block, orthostasis, abnormal liver function tests, and a "lupuslike" automimmune syndrome that clears on cessation.

Quinidine and disopyramide Quinidine and disopyramide can be used for emergent rhythm control, but are better suited for long-term oral therapy.[8,9] Intravenous quinidine is not indicated in the ED because better agents are available.

Oral quinidine is well absorbed and is eliminated primarily by hepatic metabolism (50% to 80%), with some renal excretion. The initial daily oral dose for adults is 150 to 300 mg every 6 hours, with serum levels of 3 to 8 μg/ml considered therapeutic. Oral quinidine can also be used in the pharmacologic conversion of atrial fibrillation in the ED but requires extended (2 to 6 hours) observation (see Box 74-1). Sustained-release preparations are best used after successful titration with short-acting preparations.

Intravenous disopyramide is not approved for use in the United States. Oral doses are well absorbed (80% to 95%) by the gastrointestinal tract and are eliminated by hepatic metabolism (50%) and renal excretion. Treatment is begun with 400 to 800 mg/day in four divided doses, and the therapeutic serum level during long-term use is 2 to 4 μg/ml. Approximately 15% to 20% of patients treated with disopyramide develop new or increased clinical signs of congestive heart failure, limiting its long-term use.

Class IB Agents Of all the class I agents, class IB agents slow conduction and depolarization the least, and they shorten repolarization and action potential duration instead of the prolongation seen with the class IA and IC agents. These agents have little effect on accessory pathway conduction. The class IB most commonly administered in the ED are phenytoin and lidocaine. Until recently, lidocaine has been the drug of choice in the initial prehospital and ED treatment of most ventricular dysrhythmias, but recent evidence has suggested an expanded role for amiodarone instead of lidocaine for all ventricular dysrhythmias, especially pulseless ventricular tachycardia and ventricular fibrillation.

Lidocaine Lidocaine is rapidly absorbed by the gastrointestinal tract but largely inactivated by first-pass hepatic metabolism, limiting oral utility. Lidocaine can suppress dysrhythmias secondary to enhanced automaticity, although it has little effect on abnormal automatic rhythms. When used for ventricular dysrhythmias, lidocaine will be successful in terminating 60% to 90%, depending on the specific rhythm encountered and the dose used.[10-12] Lidocaine can also depress SA and AV node conduction and slow the ventricular rate, usually in the presence of myocardial ischemia. In atrial fibrillation or flutter, lidocaine may cause a transient increase in conduction and heart rate; otherwise, it is usually devoid of effects on autonomic and vascular tone, myocardial contractility, and the surface ECG in therapeutic doses.

Although still a useful agent in prophylaxis from ventricular tachycardia and ventricular fibrillation (especially in selected cases where acute myocardial ischemia exists), lidocaine is less favored now in the treatment of ventricular tachycardia. The recent American Heart Association guidelines have universally downplayed the role of lidocaine outside of prophylaxis, noting the limited supporting data.[13]

However, there are just as limited data suggesting the improved effectiveness of the alternative agents outside of cardiac arrest. Thus, we still believe lidocaine is one of the first line drugs in many nonarrest ventricular rhythms. It is easy to quickly administer and often effective, but may produce lower rates of dysrhythmia termination. Lidocaine (in both prophylactic and treatment settings, especially if hyperkalemia exists) may rarely be associated with asystole,[14,15] but the relative rates compared to amiodarone, procainamide, and other agents are not known.

Phenytoin Phenytoin is used for the treatment of generalized seizures, but it also has antidysrhythmic properties.[16] Currently, phenytoin has a limited role in the emergency treatment of dysrhythmias, primarily in the rare situation of the need to concurrently treat both generalized seizures and a ventricular dysrhythmia or as a third line agent for polymorphic ventricular tachycardia.

Phenytoin is 70% to 90% protein bound and is eliminated primarily by hepatic metabolism, with only 5% excreted by the kidneys. Often during long-term outpatient use, the daily dose must be lowered as metabolism slows. Many drugs increase or decrease phenytoin levels from their effects on protein binding and metabolism (Box 74-2).

Intravenous phenytoin should be started at a rate no greater than 50 mg/min (25 mg/min in those with heart failure); this dose is given by intermittent bolus or by continuous infusion in a non-dextrose-containing solution (usually normal saline) with ECG monitoring. In therapeutic doses phenytoin has little effect on the ECG aside from mild shortening of the PR and QT intervals. Intravenous loading should be discontinued if the dysrhythmia is controlled, if hypotension or conduction delays develop (as outlined previously), or after a total dose of 18 mg/kg has been administered. Although serum phenytoin levels between 10 and 20 µg/ml are considered therapeutic for seizure prophylaxis, these targets are often not applicable in the rare case where this drug is used for rhythm control.

Box 74-2 Drugs Affecting Phenytoin Levels

Increase Level

Sulfonamides
Cimetidine
Trazodone
Isoniazid
Warfarin (Coumadin)
Chloramphenicol
Halothane
Disulfiram
Ethanol (acute)
Salicylates

Increase or Decrease Level (By Effects on Hepatic Metabolism)

Phenobarbital
Valproic acid/sodium valproate

Decrease Level

Ethanol (long term)
Calcium-containing preparation (especially antacids)
Carbamazepine
Reserpine

Other Class IB Agents Mexiletine and tocainide are sometimes used in the outpatient treatment of ventricular dysrhythmias[17-19] but are more commonly used in neuropathic pain syndromes. A positive response to intravenous lidocaine predicts successful dysrhythmia control with either of these agents.

Treatment with mexiletine starts with 400 to 600 mg/day in three to four doses. Tocainide is usually given as an initial 800-mg dose in adults, followed by 1200 to 1800 mg/day in two or three doses. Their side effects are similar to those seen with lidocaine, although the reported incidence of dizziness and paresthesia is slightly greater. Neither agent has a significant effect on the ECG in therapeutic doses. There is an additive side-effect risk when lidocaine is used in patients maintained on either of these two agents.[19]

Moricizine hydrochloride is a phenothiazine derivative that shares activity with Class IA, IB, and IC agents. The usual dosage is 200 mg orally every 8 hours initially. Moricizine currently has no role in the initial management of ventricular dysrhythmias, although it is useful in the outpatient management of select refractory ventricular dysrhythmias.

Class IC Agents The class IC agents profoundly slow depolarization and conduction and are associated with significant antidysrhythmic properties.[20-22] Debate continues about the true incidence of prodysrhythmic effects in this class, as these agents are used primarily in patients refractory to more conventional therapies, creating a potential magnification of the effect. Up to 15% of patients treated with class IC experience new or increased ventricular dysrhythmias and 5% develop polymorphic or sustained monomorphic ventricular tachycardia. The incidence of prodysrhythmia, especially polymorphic ventricular tachycardia, is highest when IC agents are used in patients with a persistent ventricular tachycardia or decreased ejection fraction. The total morbidity and mortality associated with any cardiac-related event (including dysrhythmias and shock) is also relatively high when these agents are used long term, even in those patients being treated for mildly symptomatic cases of ventricular dysrhythmias.[20]

Currently, only oral IC agents are approved for use in the United States. Because of this, these drugs have a limited role in the initial management of dysrhythmias, serving primarily as third-line agents in refractory cases of intermittent ventricular tachycardia or atrial fibrillation. In Europe, these agents are used for emergent intravenous dysrhythmia treatment. Each can cause an increase in the PR, QRS, and QT intervals on the surface ECG, although the ECG does not reliably predict the risk of polymorphic ventricular tachycardia.

Flecainide Flecainide, in addition to the electrophysiologic effects shared with all class IC agents, also increases the refractory period in most accessory pathways. It has a mild negative inotropic effect, with up to 4% of treated patients experiencing increased heart failure. Flecainide is well absorbed from the gastrointestinal tract, with 30% excreted unchanged in the urine and 70% metabolized by the liver. The mean serum half-life is 14 hours, although this time may vary widely in a given patient.

Flecainide will control 60% to 90% of all ventricular dysrhythmias and between 40% and 100% of supraventricular dysrhythmias. Side effects may occur in up to 40% of treated patients, but are usually minor. These include visual disturbances, dizziness, paresthesia, headache, and nausea and are treated by decreasing the dose. An increase in ventricular rate may occur in 10% and hypotension in another 10% of treated patients in addition to the previously mentioned risk of heart failure. Because of these latter risks, and the risk of prodysrhythmic effects, oral therapy must be done with caution and closely monitored.

Encainide Encainide has an electrophysiologic profile similar to flecainide, with the advantage of a less negative inotropic effect.[20,23] It is well absorbed from the gastrointestinal tract, with extensive hepatic metabolism forming two active metabolites. The serum half-life of all active forms is 3 to 12 hours. Treatment is usually begun with 75 mg/day in three dosages and increased every 3 to 5 days based on response and side effects to a maximal daily dose of 300 mg. Although not approved for intravenous use, a dosage of 0.6 to 1 mg/kg over 15 minutes has been effective in treating ventricular and supraventricular dysrhythmias. The side effects and success rates are similar to those seen with flecainide.

Propafenone This agent shares properties with IA and IC agents, with effects intermediary with respect to sodium channels.[24] Propafenone also posseses some β-adrenergic and calcium channel blocking properties. It is not available for intravenous use, but is available for the oral treatment of ventricular dysrhythmias. Propafenone will convert and maintain sinus rhythm in 40% to 60% of patients with atrial fibrillation and flutter. Compared with other class IC agents, propafenone has a lower observed prodysrhythmic rate in therapeutic doses. Its side effects are usually related to conduction disturbances on the ECG, dizziness, taste alteration, or blurred vision.

Class II Agents In general, class II agents (β-blockers) are better suited to control ventricular response rates and break a reentrant circuit in a supraventricular dysrhythmia than to treat a ventricular dysrhythmia. In the setting of acute myocardial infarction, however, ventricular dysrhythmia and reinfarction prophylaxis are important indications for β-blockers, especially metoprolol.

All β-blockers are active at both β-1 and β-2 receptors (Table 74-2) to varying degrees; those with more prominent β-1 effects are termed selective. Through their effects on β-1 receptors, all class II agents slow SA node impulse formation and depress myocardial contractility to varying degrees. β-1 selectivity also lowers (not eliminates) the frequency of bronchospasm with therapeutic doses. The usual effect of class II agents on the ECG is slowing of the heart rate and PR prolongation, with no effect on QRS and QT duration.

Relative contraindications to the use of β-blockers include asthma or chronic obstructive lung disease, severe congestive heart failure, and third-trimester pregnancy. Long-term use of β-blockers in patients with diabetes mellitus is not recommended, although their use to terminate a dysrhythmia is acceptable. β-blockers should not be used in patients with bradycardia or greater than first-degree heart block. Although often used together during long-term oral therapy, intravenous β-blockers should be given with great caution after recent intravenous calcium channel antagonist (class IV) use because of the increased risk of hemodynamic side effects, including high grade AV block. Acute side effects of β-blockers include bronchospasm, heart failure, excessive bradycardia, hypotension, and vasospasm (especially if the Raynaud syndrome is present).

Propranolol Propranolol is nonselective and well absorbed by the gastrointestinal tract. It undergoes extensive first-pass liver metabolism after oral intake, requiring a much higher dose via this route than an equipotent intravenous dose. The serum half-life is 3 to 6 hours, allowing for a four times a day dosing regimen. Therapy is usually monitored by rhythm control and side effects. Oral dosages begin at 80 mg/day of a short-acting preparation in divided doses. Oral propranolol is better suited for maintenance therapy than for acute dysrhythmia treatment. Intravenous propranolol is given in 0.5 to 1 mg dosages over 60 to 120 seconds every 15 minutes until a therapeutic effect is seen, side effects occur, or a total dose of 0.2 mg/kg has been given.[25,26]

Propranolol terminates 30% to 80% of reentrant supraventricular tachycardias, depending on the pathway, especially if the rhythm is catecholamine induced. Because of its long effect, it is not commonly used in emergent settings. Its use in other rhythms is associated with a lower success rate and increased side effects compared with class I agents.

Esmolol Esmolol is an attractive β-blocker in the emergency treatment of supraventricular tachydysrhythmias. It is β-1 selective with a rapid onset of action and a 5- to 10-minute duration of effect.[25,26] The brief clinical effect is the result of its short elimination half-life (9½ minutes) because of metabolism by plasma cholinesterase. Esmolol is given as an intravenous bolus of 500 μg/kg, followed by a continuous infusion starting at 50 μg/kg/min; if side effects are seen, stopping the infusion will result in a rapid decrease in therapeutic and toxic effects. If the dysrhythmia persists after the initial bolus and infusion, a repeat loading dose should be given and the infusion rate increased in increments

Table 74-2. Cardiac and Respiratory β-Adrenergic Receptors and Responses to Pharmacologic Manipulation

Receptors	Location	Response to: Stimulation	Response to: Antagonism
β_1	Heart	Increased heart rate and ectopy Increased contractility	Decreased heart rate and ectopy Decreased contractility
β_2	Airway (smooth muscle) Peripheral vasculature	Decreased tone (relaxation) Decreased tone (relaxation)	Increased tone (contraction) Increased tone (contraction)

of 50 μg/kg/min. Usually an infusion rate of 200 μg/kg/min or less is effective, and the maximal recommended rate is 300 μg/kg/min.

Metoprolol Another β-1 selective agent, metoprolol, is available in oral and intravenous preparations. Although currently unapproved for dysrhythmia treatment in the United States, metoprolol (5 to 10 mg intravenously every 10 to 15 minutes) is effective in the treatment of narrow-complex tachycardias, with response patterns similar to that seen with verapamil. Its familiarity to emergency physicians makes it an attractive alternative to propranolol bolus doses and esmolol infusions.

Nadolol and acebutolol Nadolol and acebutolol are used for oral dysrhythmia treatment but are not currently approved for intravenous use. The effectiveness and side-effect profile of each are similar to propranolol and metoprolol, aside from a lowered risk of bronchospasm with acebutolol.

Class III Agents Currently, four class III agents are available in the United States: bretylium, amiodarone, ibutilide, and dofetilide. Another agent, sotalol, has a structure similar to class II agents and effects similar to class III agents. All class III agents prolong the refractory period and action potential duration, and can prolong the QT interval in addition to having profound antifibrillatory properties. In general, class III agents share a first- or second-line role with the class I agents for the treatment of ventricular dysrhythmias outside of cardiac arrest, with amiodarone assuming a higher priority in treating pulseless ventricular tachycardia and ventricular fibrillation.

Bretylium Until the emergence of amiodarone, bretylium was the most commonly used class III agent. Because of its profound hemodynamic effects, it is rarely used outside of cardiac arrest. Its sympathetic release features were believed (but not proven) to be useful in cardiac arrest, although outside of this setting sympathetic block dominates, resulting in frequent hypotension. Because of its side effect profile, and the emergence of amiodarone, bretylium has little role in acute dysrhythmia management now.

Amiodarone Amiodarone is approved for the treatment of both ventricular and supraventricular dysrhythmias, including atrial fibrillation/flutter and accessory pathway syndromes.[27-37] It prolongs the action potential duration and refractory period, slows automaticity in pacemaker cells, and slows conduction in the AV node. It also displays a noncompetitive blockade of adrenergic receptors and causes smooth muscle relaxation. When given intravenously, amiodarone may cause a mild drop in blood pressure and heart rate along with a slight decrease in contractility. Recent data suggest that return of spontaneous circulation is more frequent with combined early epinephrine and amiodarone compared with placebo plus epinephrine in pulseless ventricular tachycardia and ventricular fibrillation, although ultimate outcome is unaffected. This has prompted a challenge to the historical role of lidocaine after epinephrine in these patients.

After an oral dose, amiodarone absorption is slow and erratic, varying widely among subjects. The serum half-life is about 50 days during long-term oral use and approximately 25 hours after a single intravenous dose. Because of the unusual pharmacokinetics, oral dosing regimens vary widely, starting at 600 to 1000 mg/day initially for up to 7 days followed by 400 to 800 mg/day for a maintenance dosage. The recommended intravenous dose is 5 mg/kg (or 300 mg in average size adults), as a rapid push in arrest and over 10 minutes in other settings.

Acute side effects of amiodarone are primarily limited to hypotension, bradycardia, and heart failure (Box 74-3). Long-term use is associated with a long list of side effects, with many patients requiring tapering or discontinuation of treatment after 1 to 2 years. Because of the high risk of pulmonary toxicity, this agent should be used with extreme caution in patients with underlying pulmonary disease. Amiodarone also causes an increase in the serum level of many agents and can cause an additive risk of bradycardia and hypotension when used in conjunction with calcium channel or β-adrenergic blockers.

Ibutilide This agent is approved in the United States for intravenous use only. When given in a dose of 0.015 to 0.02 mg/kg, approximately 50% to 65% of patients converted from atrial fibrillation or flutter to a sinus rhythm, usually within 20 minutes.[38] Prodysrhythmia is infrequent (approximately 4% of patients) and is unrelated to serum levels, with few other side effects yet reported. This drug is an alternative to intravenous procainamide and amiodarone for pharmacologic conversion of atrial fibrillation and flutter in the ED, with easier use and good safety profile being balanced by higher current cost.

Dofetilide Recently approved for oral use, this new agent shares similar electrophysiologic properties with others in this class. It is approved for the conversion of atrial fibrillation, although this usually requires 24 to 48 hours and inpatient monitoring. The usual dose is 500 μg twice a day, decreased in those patients with renal failure. The QT interval must be monitored closely, with therapy withheld in those with prolonged intervals.

Sotalol Sotalol has an emerging role in the short-term management of dysrhythmias, now serving as a second- or

Box 74-3 Adverse Effects of Amiodarone

Acute

Hypotension
Slowing of heart rate
Decreased contractility

Long-Term

Common

Corneal deposits
Photosensitivity
Gastrointestinal intolerance

Less Common

Hyperthyroidism
Heart failure
Pulmonary toxicity
Hypothyroidism
Bradycardia
Prodysrhythmic effect

Drug Interactions

Increases levels

Quinidine
Phenytoin
Procainamide
Warfarin
Digoxin
Flecainide

third-line agent in atrial fibrillation, accessory pathway tachycardias, and recurrent ventricular tachycardia.[39,40] Sotalol is associated with a higher incidence of prodysrhythmia (especially polymorphic ventricular tachycardia) than other class III agents, primarily when used for longer intervals. Intravenous sotalol should be given over 10 minutes at a dose of 1 to 1.5 mg/kg. Like its Class II and III relatives, sotalol can acutely cause bradycardia, hypotension, conduction interferences (including QT interval prolongation), and prodysrhythmia. The latter is rare in patients treated acutely unless a preexisting QT prolongation exists.

Class IV Agents The major action of the class IV agents is to block the slow calcium channels in both the myocardial and vascular smooth muscle cells.[41-44] Each agent exhibits activity at both the myocardial and peripheral vascular levels, with specificity for particular areas within the group. Verapamil and diltiazem exhibit the most potent effects on myocardial cell calcium entry and hence conduction and contractility; verapamil has the least effect on peripheral vascular tone, and diltiazem has an effect intermediary between verapamil and nifedipine, although all can cause hypotension.

Verapamil Verapamil is an alternative first-line agent to treat narrow-complex tachycardia and rapid atrial flutter or fibrillation, terminating or controlling the ventricular response rate in 80% to 90% of cases.[41,42] Verapamil has little direct effect on accessory pathways and is used in these syndromes only when anterograde conduction through the AV node alone exists.

Verapamil slows conduction within the AV node (primarily at the atrial-His level) more than it does within the SA node. These actions are only partially reversed by atropine. In diseased ventricular tissues, particularly during acute ischemia, verapamil can diminish the conduction of reentrant impulses, but conduction within the normal His-Purkinje system is unaffected by this agent. After an intravenous dose, the surface ECG usually is unchanged aside from a slower heart rate and prolonged PR interval. Because of its effects on conduction, intravenous verapamil should not be used in patients with second- or third-degree AV block and should be used with close monitoring in those with first-degree block.

Verapamil has negative inotropic and mild peripheral vasodilatory properties. Reflex increases in sympathetic tone usually maintain cardiac output and blood pressure, but elderly patients, those with sepsis or hypovolemia, and those using adrenergic blocking or other negative inotropic drugs may be prone to heart failure or significant hypotension. In particular, intravenous verapamil should be used with great caution after intravenous administration of any class II agent (aside from esmolol after an appropriate "washout" period). Most evidence suggests that in the absence of hypovolemia, heart block, hypotension, or left ventricular dysfunction, verapamil can also be used safely in infants.[43,44]

The usual intravenous verapamil dose is 0.1 mg/kg over 1 to 2 minutes; for the average healthy adult, this translates to a dose of 5 to 10 mg. Repeat doses should be given every 10 minutes based on response; use of a longer dosing interval, especially if more than 30 minutes, may interfere with successful treatment of a dysrhythmia. Hypotension in supraventricular tachycardia is often a direct effect of the excessive ventricular rate; it is usually not worsened and may be reversed when verapamil is used in these doses.[45] Nonetheless, the emergence of adenosine has limited the need to use verapamil in those with hypotension. In elderly patients or those with borderline hypotension (systolic blood pressure of 90 to 110 mm Hg), a smaller dose (0.05 mg/kg, or 2.5 mg increments) should be used. Another regimen, using 25 mg of verapamil in 50 ml of crystalloid infused at a rate of 1 mg/min (120 ml/hr), will successfully and safely treat more than 80% of patients with a narrow-complex tachycardia within a mean time of 20 minutes.

Calcium chloride, 500 to 1,000 mg (5 to 10 ml of a 10% solution), can limit or reverse some cases of verapamil-induced hypotension.[42,46] Calcium salts attenuate the peripheral vasodilatory actions without altering the chronotropic (antidysrhythmic) effects of verapamil. If hypotension persists after calcium administration and intravenous fluids, administer a direct-acting vasopressor and seek an alternate explanation for the hypotension (e.g., myocardial ischemia, hypovolemia, or sepsis). Aside from AV block, hypotension, and congestive heart failure, verapamil can cause other side effects, including nausea, vomiting, constipation, dizziness, nervousness, and pruritus.

Verapamil is rapidly absorbed from the gastrointestinal tract, but undergoes such extensive first-pass liver metabolism that only 25% to 30% of an oral dose is biologically available. As with propranolol, this low availability results in a much larger oral dosing requirement compared with an equipotent intravenous dose. The drug is 90% protein bound and is eliminated primarily by renal excretion. After an oral dose, the duration of effect is 4 to 6 hours, with a total elimination half-life of 3 to 12 hours. Daily maintenance with 120 to 720 mg of a short-acting preparation in four divided doses is recommended for prophylaxis from recurrent dysrhythmias. A long-acting preparation of verapamil is available, but it is not currently approved for the treatment of dysrhythmias.

Diltiazem Like verapamil, diltiazem prolongs AV conduction and is an alternative first-line agent in the treatment of narrow complex tachycardias and atrial fibrillation/flutter. Enteral doses are rapidly absorbed, although a significant first-pass effect is seen. Intravenous diltiazem (0.25 mg/kg over 2 minutes, followed by 0.35 mg/kg if the first dosage is unsuccessful but tolerated) will control the ventricular response rate in up to 93% of patients with atrial fibrillation and atrial flutter and is associated with minimal hypotension.[47,48] If the intravenous bolus is successful, a continuous infusion (10 to 15 mg/hr) or an oral dose (60 to 90 mg initially) can be started and titrated based on the response. Although laboratory data suggest that diltiazem causes less diminution in myocardial contractility than verapamil, clinical experience suggests that the relative difference in practice of induced hypotension or heart failure when comparing these two agents is modest,[49] if it exists at all.

Miscellaneous Agents

Digitalis Digoxin is the main form of digitalis used in the emergent and outpatient treatment of cardiac dysrhythmias. In addition to their positive inotropic effects, digitalis compounds have variable electrophysiologic effects on myocardial cells (Table 74-3). These effects can be divided into excitant and depressant actions. Digitalis excitant effects are manifested as an increase in altered automatic and triggered ectopic impulses, particularly in toxic doses. Digitalis also depresses conduction and lengthens refractoriness in the AV node in therapeutic doses, with toxic dysrhythmias the result of either or both of these mecha-

Table 74-3. Effects of Digitalis on Heart Tissues

Tissue and property	Direct therapeutic effect*	Direct toxic effect	Indirect effect†
SA node automaticity	0	D	D
Atrial conduction	0	I	D
Atrial refractoriness	I (small)	I	D
AV node refractoriness and conduction	I (small)	I	I
Purkinje fibers			
Automaticity and conduction	I (small)	I	0
Refractoriness	I (small)	D	0
Conduction	0	I	I
Refractoriness	I (small)	D	0

*I, Increases; D, decreases; 0, minimal effect.
†Indirect autonomic effects (vagotonic and sympatholytic).

nisms, whereas the therapeutic effects are the result primarily of the depressive actions.

Digitalis inhibits the membrane-bound enzyme ATPase, impairing the active transport of Na^+ out of and K^+ into the cell. Aside from increasing intracellular Na^+ concentration and decreasing intracellular K^+ concentration, the disruption of the pump indirectly causes a mild increase in intracellular Ca^{++} concentration, which accounts for the positive inotropic effects of digitalis. In therapeutic doses, many of the observed clinical effects of digitalis are a result of indirect effects on the autonomic nervous system (Box 74-4). On the surface ECG, digitalis usually slows the heart rate and decreases the QT interval slightly in therapeutic doses. Also, characteristic ST segment depression and shortening and T-wave inversion are seen during digoxin therapy.

Digoxin is often used as a positive inotropic agent in congestive heart failure, with therapeutic target serum levels between 0.8 and 2 ng/ml. When digoxin is used as an antidysrhythmic, similar serum levels are often sought, but higher levels may be necessary. Digitalis controls the ventricular rate in narrow-complex tachycardias, including atrial fibrillation, atrial flutter, and paroxysmal supraventricular tachycardia. Because of its relatively slow onset of action and narrow therapeutic window, digitalis is not a first-line agent for emergency therapy, but is a good choice in the outpatient management of these rhythms, particularly when underlying heart failure is present.

Digoxin is given in an initial intravenous dose of 0.5 mg in adults. A clinical effect may be seen within 30 minutes, but the peak effect does not occur until 1½ to 2 hours. Because of this, repeat dosages are given every 1 to 2 hours when used for rate control and every 4 to 6 hours when used for inotropic effect. These repeat dosages are administered in 0.25-mg increments until the rate is controlled or the dysrhythmia terminated, side effects occur, or the total dose reaches 1.5 mg. The latter ceiling is controversial, because some patients may require a higher dose to control rate, but risk increased side effects.

Digoxin is excreted 50% to 75% unchanged in the urine and is 25% protein bound with a large volume of distribution.

Box 74-4 Adverse Effects of Digitalis

Common

Gastrointestinal intolerance (nausea, vomiting, abdominal pain, diarrhea, anorexia)
Fatigue
Drowsiness
Visual disturbances
Headache
Depression
Apathy

Less Common

Psychosis
Cardiac symptoms
Heart block
Increased ectopy
Combined block and ectopy (multifocal atrial tachycardia with block or complete AV-block with accelerated junctional rhythm)
Ventricular tachycardia

The serum half-life is 24 to 48 hours, allowing for a daily or every other day maintenance regimen. Effects of digoxin are listed in Box 74-4 and are enhanced by hypokalemia, hypercalcemia, hypomagnesemia, increased catecholamines, and severe acid-base disturbances. The concomitant use of quinidine can increase the serum levels of digoxin by interfering with renal and nonrenal elimination. Finally, digoxin overdose can cause systemic hyperkalemia because of its effect on the Na^{++}/K^+ pump.

Two misconceptions about digoxin use persist. Often it is used in atrial fibrillation because of a belief that spontaneous conversion to a sinus rhythm will be more likely than after the use of other rate-controlling agents.[50,51] Objective data do not confirm this perception. Furthermore, β-adrenergic and calcium channel blockers are often better tolerated and effective much more quickly (minutes compared with 6 to 12 hours) than digoxin when attempting to control the ventricular rate in the absence of ventricular dysfunction. Another concern has been the safety of cardioversion during digoxin therapy and the possible development of ventricular dysrhythmias. If no clinical or laboratory evidence of toxicity is present, cardioversion of atrial fibrillation or flutter is safe, with little added risk of precipitating ventricular dysrhythmias compared with patients not receiving digoxin.[52]

Magnesium Magnesium has been used for 40 years as an antidysrhythmic, but is often forgotten by practicing physicians. It may control the ventricular response rate in a variety of narrow-complex tachycardias, including atrial fibrillation, multifocal atrial tachycardia, and reentrant supraventricular tachycardia.[53-55] Unfortunately, magnesium has not been subjected to rigorous studies comparable to the other antidysrhythmics, so much of the information is anecdotal or difficult to assess compared with other agents. Magnesium (2 to 4 g as a slow IV bolus) can terminate ventricular tachycardia, including digoxin-induced and polymorphic ventricular tachycardia (especially torsades de pointes). Aside from the latter rhythm, magnesium is generally a second-or third-line agent.

Adenosine Adenosine is a naturally occurring purine nucleoside used as a first-line agent (along with class IV drugs) for the intravenous treatment of narrow-complex tachydysrhythmias. It causes a concentration-dependent slowing of AV conduction and a slowing of conduction in both anterograde and retrograde paths of a reentrant circuit.[56,57] This agent shortens the action potential duration and is essentially devoid of effects on ventricular contractility. Adenosine hyperpolarizes atrial myocardial cells and can cause a decrease in atrial contractility. It also reduces cyclic AMP levels and attenuates presynaptic norepinephrine release. In extremely low doses, adenosine causes selective coronary vasodilation; as the dose is increased to the level needed for a maximal antidysrhythmic effect, peripheral vasodilation occurs.[57]

After an intravenous dose, adenosine has an onset of action of 5 to 20 seconds, with a duration of effect of 30 to 40 seconds. It is eliminated primarily by deamination in endothelial and blood cells, with a 10-second serum half-life. Aside from a decreasing heart rate and an increasing AV block, adenosine has little effect on the ECG. Except in rare cases of catecholamine-induced ventricular dysrhythmias,[58] adenosine has little effect on infranodal conduction.

Currently, an initial dose of 6 mg as a rapid bolus for adults weighing 50 kg or greater is recommended. If no response is seen within 1 to 2 minutes, the dose is doubled (12 mg) and repeated. If no effect is seen after a third dose, the rhythm should be reassessed and another agent used. Pediatric doses of 0.05 mg/kg initially are suggested at similar intervals to a total dose of 0.25 mg/kg.[59]

Side effects coincide with the onset of clinical effects and occur in up to a third of patients but are usually minor. These include flushing, dyspnea, chest pressure, nausea, headache, and dizziness, with hypotension seen rarely as a result of its vasodilatory properties. All rapidly resolve without treatment, although many patients will be intensely uncomfortable for a short period. Aminophylline and methylxanthines (including caffeine) antagonize the effects of adenosine, and dipyridamole and carbamazepine potentiate its effects. Digitalis, calcium channel blockers, and benzodiazepines can all augment the activity of adenosine.

In comparative studies of patients with narrow-complex tachydysrhythmias, adenosine has response rates equivalent to verapamil (85% to 90%) with fewer serious side effects.[60-62] Recurrence of the tachycardia after adenosine occurs in 10% to 58% (mean of approximately 25%) of patients. For this reason, adenosine is not a definitive therapeutic agent for atrial fibrillation or flutter and nonreentrant rhythms, although its effects on conduction can help unmask these rhythms when they are not apparent on the initial ECG. Similarly, adenosine should not replace a careful search for a ventricular source or the rare but potentially lethal combination of atrial fibrillation with an accessory pathway. Use of any drug that depresses the AV node primarily in these settings (including adenosine, calcium channel or β-blockers) can result in precipitous hemodynamic collapse.[63] Finally, adenosine often "fails" in practice because it is used for the wrong reason, especially unrecognized atrial fibrillation or ventricular tachycardia.

CLINICAL FEATURES AND MANAGEMENT

General Approach

Dysrhythmias can be classified according to their electrophysiologic origin, ECG appearance, and the underlying ventricular rate. The following five categories are presented in this chapter, although overlap exists between categories:

- Bradycardias, sinus and atrial rhythms, SA and AV block
- Extrasystoles and parasystoles
- Narrow-complex (QRS < 0.12 seconds) tachycardias
- Preexcitation and accessory pathway syndromes
- Wide-complex (QRS 0.12 seconds or greater) tachycardias

Treatment of specific dysrhythmias can also be divided into two broad categories based on clinical stability, which is a continuum. Unstable patients are defined as those with evidence of end-organ hypoperfusion as a direct result of the dysrhythmia. The specific signs and symptoms of unstable rhythms follow:

- Hypotension
- Chest pain suggestive of myocardial ischemia
- Dyspnea or pulmonary edema
- Altered sensorium (from mild changes to coma)

Skin changes of hypovolemia or early shock (coolness, clammy or pale appearance) are sensitive and should be sought but are not specific. Similarly, blood pressure alone can be difficult to interpret, although extreme changes offer little challenge. For example, a patient with chronic hypertension who has a blood pressure of 110/60 and crushing chest pain with a wide-complex tachycardia at a rate of 180 beats/min is "more unstable" than a young woman with a similar rhythm and a blood pressure of 88/50 without other symptoms. Patients with an unstable rhythm deserve rapid pharmacologic or electrical therapy after a focused assessment, whereas stable patients can tolerate a more detailed and lengthy evaluation. In general, patients with rapid unstable dysrhythmias aside from sinus tachycardia require sedation and cardioversion, especially when more than one sign or symptom of instability is present. Patients with slow unstable dysrhythmias require a temporary pacemaker, although atropine can be used while preparing for pacing.

The Initial Approach to Stable Patients

The approach to the patient with a stable dysrhythmia is based on an orderly attempt to gather subjective and objective data concerning the underlying rhythm. The following data should be gathered by the physician or prehospital care personnel:

- Directed history
- Physical examination
- ECG recording of the rhythm
- Diagnostic and therapeutic interventions

Often these steps are taken concurrently to facilitate a rapid assessment and improve data collection. *In the face of clear or profound instability, treatment with electricity—pacing or countershock—should quickly follow brief assessment and ECG analysis.*

The exact subjective nature of any symptoms and the timing and velocity (gradual or abrupt) of symptom onset must be elicited. Palpitations, dizziness, chest pain, dyspnea, or syncope should be specifically sought. The previous history, especially of heart disease or dysrhythmias, and current medications are important, as both may offer a clue about the underlying rhythm in a patient. For example, a 22-year-old man treated with propranolol for "palpitations," who seeks treatment for abrupt onset of a regular tachycardia with a QRS duration of 0.12 second at a rate of 200 beats/min, is more likely to have a reentrant supraventricular tachycardia with aberrant conduction or an accessory pathway syndrome than ventricular tachycardia. Conversely, a 55-year-old man with a history of a previous myocardial infarction and "extra heart beats," who takes nitroglycerin and procainamide and has palpitations and chest pain and a similar wide-complex regular tachycardia, is more likely by history to have ventricular tachycardia

On physical examination, evidence of end-organ hypoperfusion should be sought. Alteration in cognitive function (from mild excitation to depressed consciousness), as well as clammy or dusky skin, suggest hypoperfusion. Certain clinical toxidromes, such as organophosphate, anticholinergic, and cyclic antidepressant ingestion, have prominent features on physical examination.

The surface ECG is the central objective tool diagnosing and treating a dysrhythmia (Box 74-5). Diagnosis using a single lead is often successful, but in selected cases, multiple leads are needed to accurately define the dysrhythmia. Although lead II is usually chosen, at least two other leads should be examined. Occasionally, an apparently narrow-complex rhythm is discovered to be a wide-complex rhythm when a different lead is examined. The paddles from a defibrillator and monitor unit can be helpful for short periods, as a modified chest lead can be created to optimize the appearance of the P wave and QRS complexes. Long-term monitoring using paddles is impractical; often leads V_1 or V_2 can be substituted to provide data that lead II does not. Vagal maneuvers are often overlooked because of the ease of adenosine use and because of their frequent failure, which is often due to poor performance. Even with the availability of adenosine, carotid massage (in the absence of a bruit) or a Valsalva maneuver, each done with the patient supine, can help identify supraventricular causes and terminate a rhythm on occasion with little cost or risk of harm. Finally, the most useful information about paroxysmal dysrhythmias occurs at the onset and termination of the rhythm. On the ECG these areas should be carefully analyzed.

A long rhythm strip (up to a minute) may be needed to define a dysrhythmia. Other adjuncts to standard ECG monitoring include increasing the paper speed and the use of esophageal electrodes. Normally, a paper speed of 25 mm/sec is used; when the speed is increased to 50 to 100 mm/sec, the relationship of the P wave to the QRS complex may be better defined (Figure 74-8). Esophageal leads can also help better define the P-QRS relationship (Figure 74-9). A pill electrode is available for virtually painless recording of esophageal tracings and can be helpful in determining the source of a dysrhythmia.

Box 74-5 Basic ECG Observations During Dysrhythmia Analysis

1. Ventricular rate: Fast (>100 beats/min), slow (<60 beats/min), or normal (60 to 100 beats/min).
2. Rhythm: Regular, completely irregular (chaotic), regular with occasional irregularities, or grouped impulses. Calipers and long strips are recommended to detect subtle irregularities.
3. QRS width: Prolonged (>0.12 sec), borderline (0.09 to 0.12 sec), or normal. If done without ECG physically present (e.g., prehospital radio medical command), ask for QRS duration in number of small boxes from printed rhythm strip (each box equals 0.04 sec) to ensure accuracy.
4. P-wave presence and relationship to QRS complexes may require mapping of P-waves with calipers to detect those falling within QRS complex or T-wave.
5. Rhythm changes: Examine these areas closely for clues.
6. Multiple leads, especially chest leads or esophageal lead if difficulties with no. 4.
7. Compare with previous tracing (if available).

Pseudodysrhythmias

Occasionally an artifact on the surface ECG can produce an apparent dysrhythmia. Muscle contraction or movement (especially shivering), loose leads, and stray external signals from other electrical equipment and monitoring devices can produce these artifacts, called *pseudodysrhythmias* (Figure 74-10). Often these findings may be mistaken for serious ventricular dysrhythmias, including ventricular fibrillation. The importance of pseudodysrhythmias lies in the need to avoid treating the ECG; a close evaluation of the clinical setting, monitoring strips, and leads usually uncovers the problem.

Specific Dysrhythmias

Bradycardia and Sinoatrial and Atrioventricular Block Bradycardia, variably defined as a heart rate of less than 50 to 60 beats/min, can be normal in well-conditioned subjects or the result of two basic disturbances.[64] Depression of the dominant pacemaker, usually the sinus node, can cause clinical bradycardia. Another cause is conduction system block, where the normal sinus node impulses are incompletely carried to the AV node and ventricular tissues. In both situations, a subsidiary pacemaker may assume the dominant role, with heart rates of 30 to 60 beats/min commonly seen, depending on their location. The rhythms seen with subsidiary pacemakers during SA and AV nodal block are called "escape" rhythms, as they provide a physiologic escape from no impulse generation (asystole).

Treatment of bradydysrhythmias is based on the underlying cause and symptoms. The two basic therapies are intravenous atropine (0.5 to 1 mg for adults) and a temporary pacemaker, either transcutaneous or transvenous. Isoproterenol, a nonselective β-agonist, can also increase the heart rate but may cause hypotension (from vasodilation) and ventricular dysrhythmias. Because of these undesirable effects and the wide availability of transcutaneous pacemakers, isoproterenol has a limited role in the treatment of bradydysrhythmias. These rhythms require emergent treatment only when the rate is less than 50 beats/min with evidence of hypoperfusion or if the rhythm carries a high risk of progression to complete block. Patients with the latter rhythm may be observed closely, with a transcutaneous pacemaker readily available if needed.

Sinus Bradycardia Sinus bradycardia appears on the surface ECG as a regular rhythm at a rate of fewer than 50 to 60 beats/min with a normal consistent P-wave morphology and PR-interval duration (Figure 74-11). This pattern may be found in healthy adults or during sleep and periods of fright. Other causes include hypothermia, excessive parasympathetic or diminished sympathetic stimulation (often from drug therapy), and carotid sinus hypersensitivity. The last can be manifested as bradycardia or syncope from wearing a tight shirt collar. Sinus bradycardia may be seen in the early stages of an acute inferior wall myocardial infarction, when it is believed to result from parasympathetic stimulation. Gener-

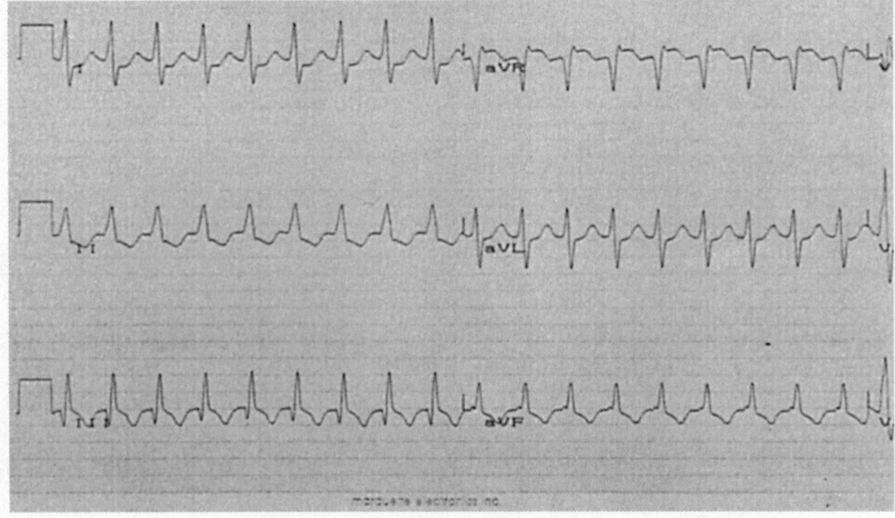

Figure 74-8. **Note the P waves before the QRS complexes in lead aVF.**

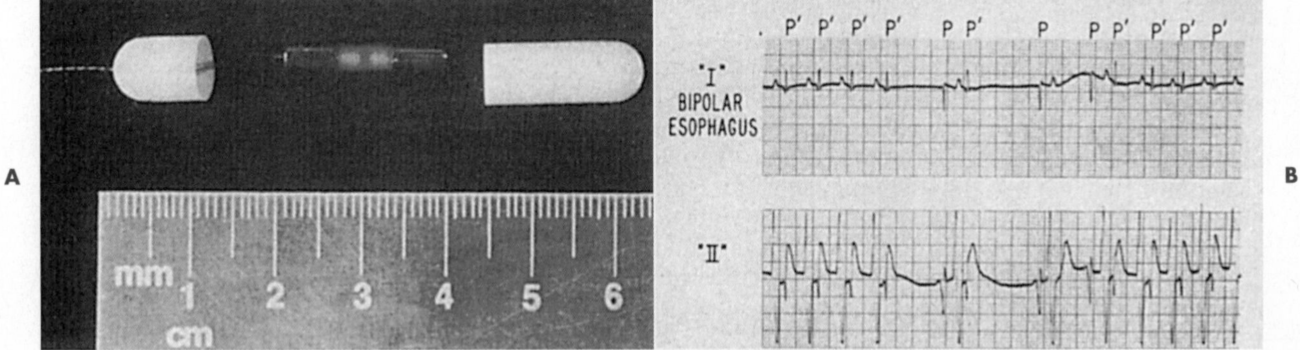

Figure 74-9. **An esophageal pill electrode (A) and a representative tracing of an AV nodal reentrant tachycardia with retrograde (P′) depolarization not appreciated on the simultaneously recorded lead II strip (B).** ***From Hammill SC, Pritichett ELC. In Campbell R, Murray A, editors:*** **Dynamic electrocardiography,** ***Edinburgh, 1985, Churchill Livingstone.***

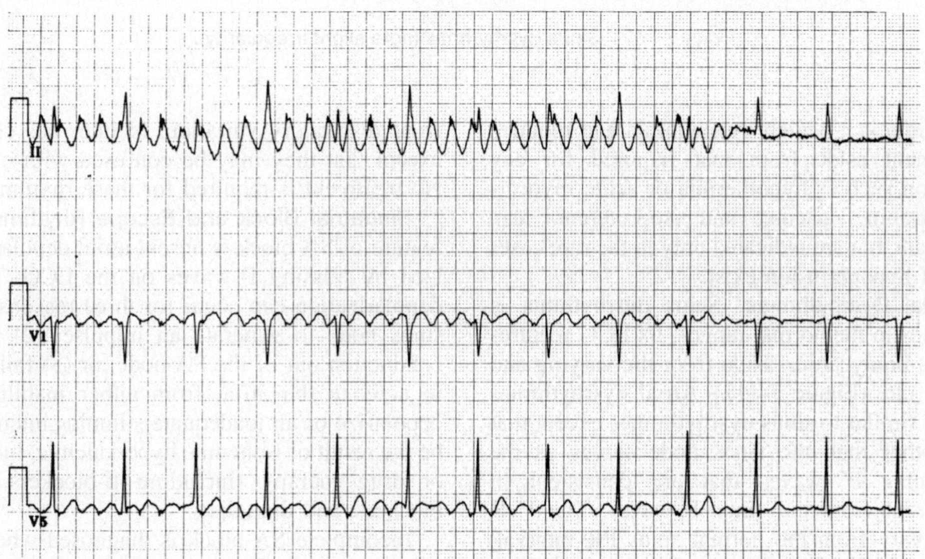

Figure 74-10. **Pseudodysrhythmia. In this case, atrial flutter waves appear to be present but are recognized as an artifact when examining the patient and the right side of the electrocardiogram.**

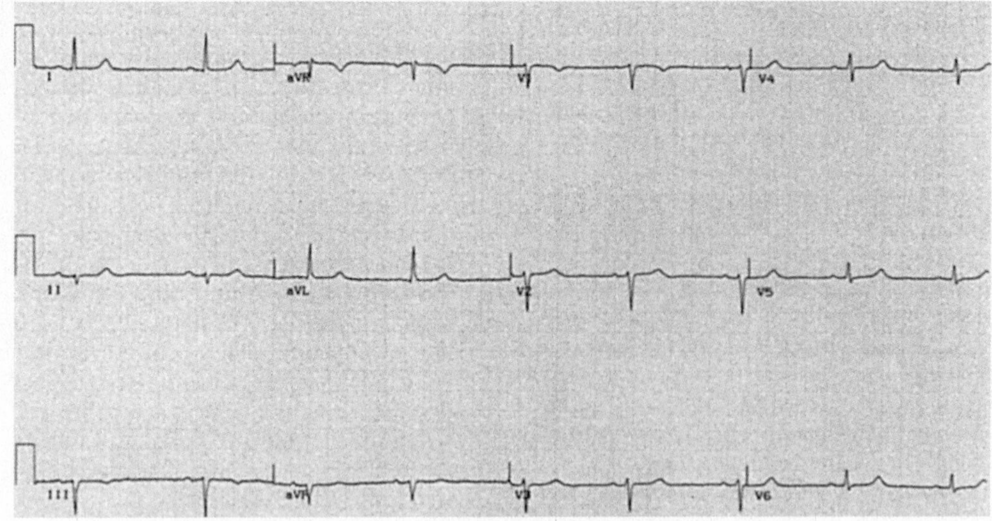

Figure 74-11. **Sinus bradycardia.**

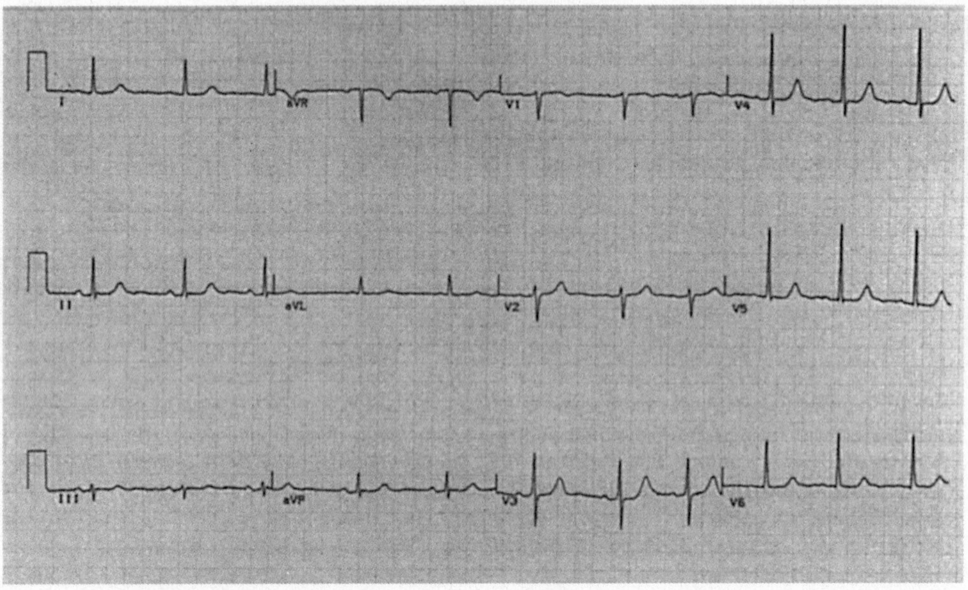

Figure 74-12. **Sinus dysrhythmia (note slight irregularity).**

ally, sinus bradycardia is a benign dysrhythmia and requires no specific treatment aside from that required for any underlying condition such as hypothermia or acute myocardial ischemia. Atropine, pacing, and isoproterenol can increase the heart rate, but are indicated only in the rare cases when symptoms of hypoperfusion exist.

Sinus and Atrial Dysrhythmias Sinus dysrhythmia is seen at variable rates in the normal ranges. Its ECG features are similar to sinus bradycardia, aside from the varying and normal ventricular rate (Figure 74-12). Atrial dysrhythmias have ECG features similar to sinus dysrhythmias, except that an atrial source other than the sinus node serves as the pacemaker, producing P′ waves that are consistent in structure yet different from the sinus P waves. The P′-R interval may also vary from the normal sinus PR interval, helping to distinguish these rhythms. Both dysrhythmias may be normal variants, with sinus dysrhythmias often resulting from respiratory variation. Neither has clinical significance except that they may be confused with other dysrhythmias. No treatment is required for these rhythms.

Sinoatrial Block and Escape Rhythms The underlying feature of SA block is absent atrial depolarization, characterized by missing P waves on the ECG. This lack of atrial depolarization can occur for three reasons: (1) failure of the sinus node to generate an impulse, (2) failure of impulse conduction out of the SA node, or (3) failure of the impulse to activate the atria, from either inability of the atria to depolarize or an inadequate stimulus intensity. SA block can be the result of ischemia, hyperkalemia, increased vagal tone, or drug therapy (including β-blockers, calcium channel blockers, and digitalis).

Incomplete SA block is diagnosed when an occasional P wave is dropped from the normal P-QRS-T sequence on the ECG. Complete SA block (or sinus arrest) manifests as no

P waves on the surface ECG (Figure 74-13). Usually, a lower pacemaker will assume control in complete SA block; if this pacemaker is within the AV node, the QRS complex will be narrow, and an "idiojunctional" escape rhythm at a rate of 45 to 60 beats/min is seen. Pacemakers within the His-Purkinje system usually result in a wide-complex "idioventricular" escape rhythm at a rate of 30 to 45 beats/min.

Treatment of SA block in the field or ED is based on symptoms, with atropine (aside from the setting of digitalis toxicity) and temporary pacing used if needed. Those patients without evidence of hypoperfusion should be observed without treatment. Class I agents should be avoided, as they may extinguish an escape rhythm.

Sinus Node Dysfunction ("Sick Sinus Syndrome") This syndrome refers to a myriad of overlapping pathologic states, from frequent sinus pauses and bradycardia to the tachycardia-bradycardia syndrome.[65] The latter represents bursts of an atrial tachydysrhythmia, usually atrial fibrillation, alternating with periods of sinus or atrial bradycardia. The tachycardia-bradycardia syndrome usually occurs in the elderly, but has also been associated with ischemia, inflammatory diseases, cardiomyopathy, connective tissue diseases, and drug therapy (especially β-blockers, calcium channel blockers, digitalis, and quinidine).

The diagnosis is made when symptoms, such as palpitations or syncope, are correlated with the bradycardia or tachycardia. This correlation often is made with outpatient Holter monitoring. The ECG manifestations vary, depending on the rhythm seen at the time of presentation. Emergency treatment consists of rate stimulation with atropine or a pacemaker or rate control with calcium channel blockers, β-blockers, or digitalis when symptoms of hypoperfusion coexist. Either modality should be attempted with caution, as excessive bradycardia or tachycardia may result, although generally the response is blunted (i.e., the heart rate increases to ≤90 beats/min after 1 mg of atropine). Recognition and referral are the mainstays of ED management. Long-term management often is accomplished by a combination of an antidysrhythmic to suppress the tachycardia and a demand pacemaker to provide a "floor" against excessive bradycardia.

Atrioventricular (AV) Block AV block is the result of impaired conduction through the atria, AV node, or proximal His-Purkinje system. Although electrophysiologic studies using His bundle tracings can pinpoint the area of conduction disturbance, the surface ECG can provide information and guide clinical decision making. AV block is divided into three grades, based on the ECG and clinical characteristics. First- and second-degree AV block represent an incomplete conduction disturbance, whereas third-degree block indicates complete AV conduction interruption.

First-Degree Atrioventricular Block First-degree AV block is defined as prolonged conduction of atrial impulses without the loss of any single impulse. This can occur at the level of the atria, AV node (most common), or His-Purkinje system (least common). On the surface ECG, a regular narrow-complex rhythm at slow (40 to 60 beats/min) to normal ventricular rates with a prolonged PR interval (> 0.20 second) is seen (Figure 74-14). First-degree AV block is often a normal variant without clinical significance, occurring in 1.6% of healthy young adults. This variant requires no specific treatment.

Second-Degree Atrioventricular Block Second-degree AV block is an intermediate step between every impulse being conducted (albeit slowly) to no impulses being conducted.[64] On the ECG this type of block is manifested as one or more sinus impulses failing to reach the ventricles. The "conduction ratio" in all types of incomplete AV block is described as the ratio of the number of P waves to the number of QRS complexes (3:2, 4:3, etc). Second-degree AV block can be divided into two types, based on the ECG appearance and clinical characteristics (Table 74-4).

Type I second-degree atrioventricular block Type I second-degree AV block, also called Wenckebach or Mobitz I AV block, is associated with a conduction deficit within the AV node. On the surface ECG, a narrow-complex rhythm with the following three basic characteristics is seen (Figure 74-15):

- Grouped beating (especially pairs or trios, but occasionally larger groups)
- Progressive lengthening of the PR interval until an impulse is not conducted ("dropped beat")
- The longest cycle (of the dropped beat) is less than twice the length of the shortest (usually the impulse after the dropped beat).

The progressive lengthening of the PR interval gives the appearance of successive P waves retreating into the preceding QRS complexes. This highlights another feature of type I block, the concept of *RP/PR reciprocity.* This means that as the interval between the preceding R wave and the next P wave gets shorter, the PR interval of the next cycle gets longer until an impulse is dropped.

Type I second-degree AV block occurs in a variety of acute and chronic conditions (see Table 74-4) and usually requires no treatment. In the setting of acute myocardial infarction, this type of AV block is associated with inferior wall ischemia and a good outcome. Children with asymptomatic type I second-degree AV block may eventually develop complete heart block, but usually remain asymptomatic because of adequate subsidiary pacemaker function. Carotid massage and increased vagal tone worsen type I block, whereas atropine and isoproterenol improve conduction.

The Wenckebach phenomenon can occur in other conduction disturbances, including SA block, producing grouped impulses. Grouped impulses should always raise the question "Is a Wenckebach mechanism present?" (Box 74-6).

Type II second-degree atrioventricular block Type II second-degree AV block, or *Mobitz II block,* is never a normal variant and implies a conduction block below the level of the AV node, usually in the His-Purkinje system. On the surface ECG, intermittent conduction of atrial impulses occurs without changes in the PR interval (Figure 74-16). The QRS complex of conducted beats is often narrow, but wide-complex beats may result if infranodal conduction disturbances such as bundle branch block or escape impulses are present. Type II second-degree AV block is associated with a variety of acute and chronic diseases (see Table 74-4). Compared with type I second-degree AV block, type II block carries a worse prognosis. In acute myocardial infarction, type II AV block is associated with anterior wall ischemia and often progresses to complete AV block. This variety of block is further complicated by poor subsidiary pacemaker function and mandates that temporary pacing be readily available to ensure an adequate heart rate.

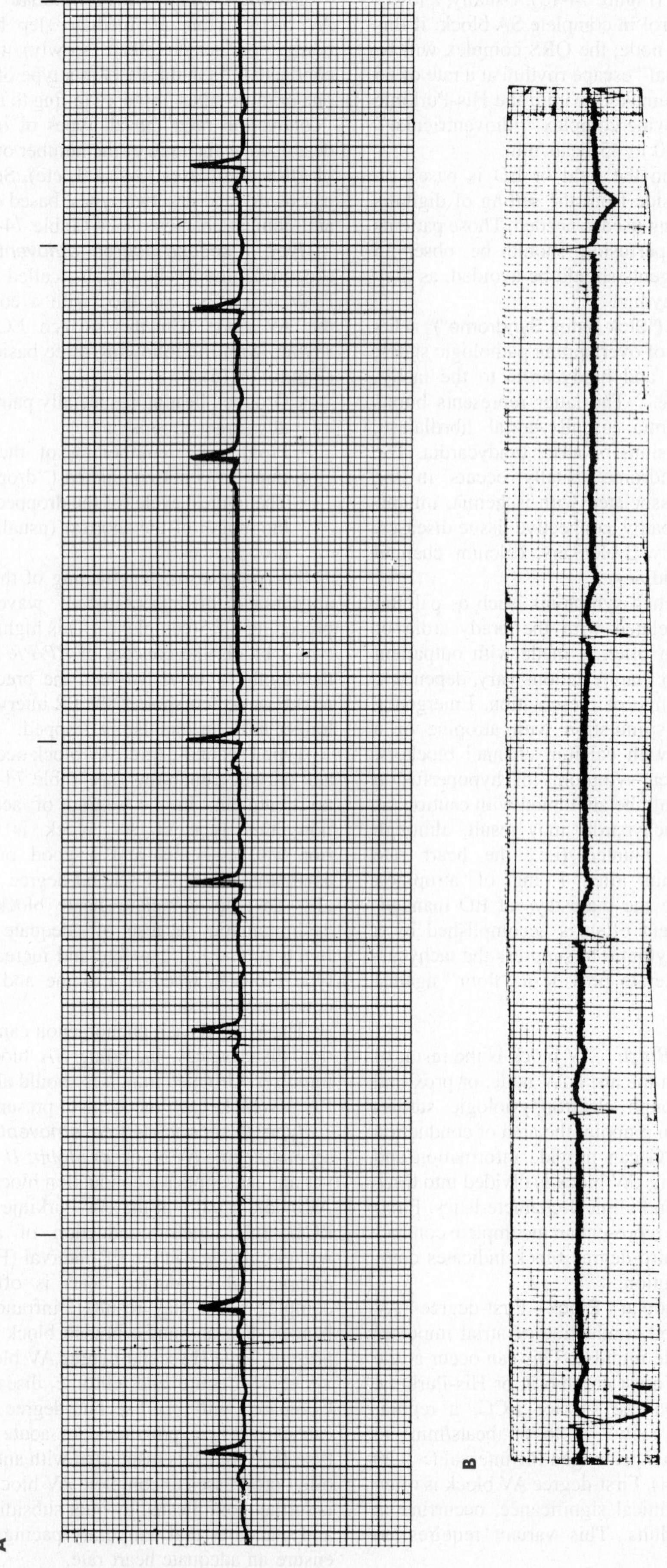

Figure 74-13. **A,** Incomplete sinus block (sinus arrest). **B,** Complete sinus block (sinus arrest) with ventricular escape rhythm.

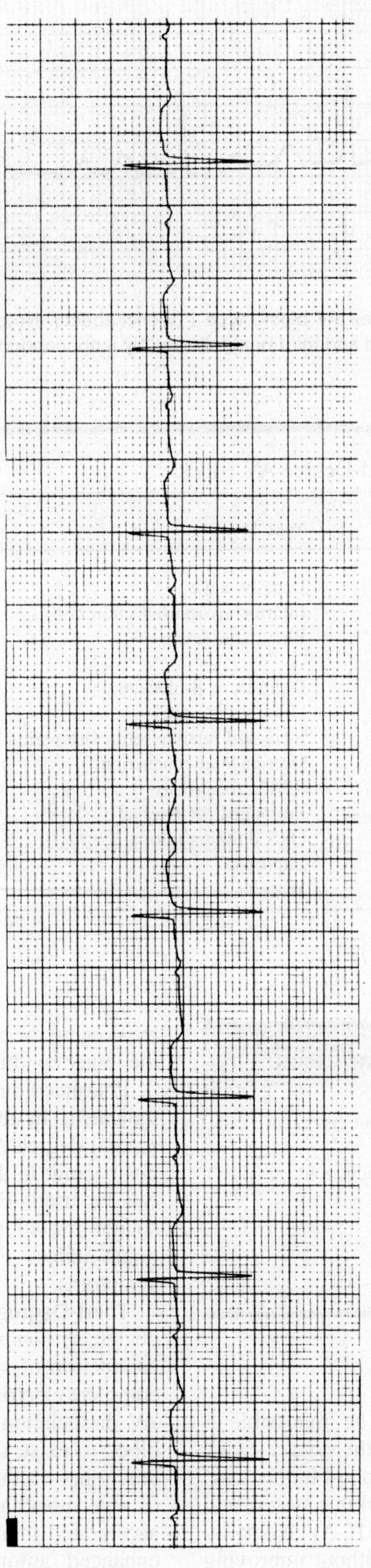

Figure 74-14. **First-degree AV block.**

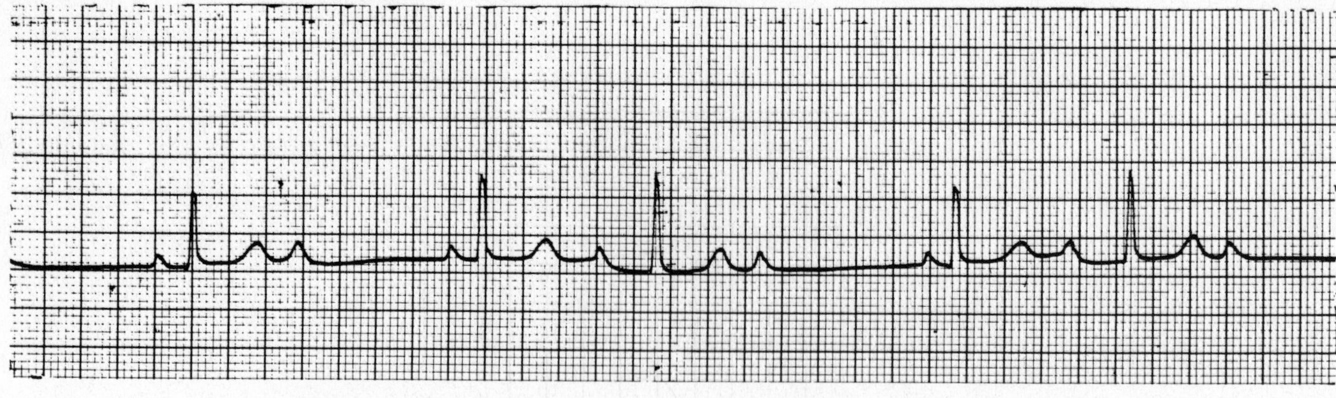

Figure 74-15. **Second-degree AV block, type I (Wenckebach). Note the prolongation of the PR interval between the second and third beat followed by a nonconducted atrial impulse.**

Table 74-4. Characteristics of Second-Degree AV Block

Feature	Type I	Type II
Clinical	Usually acute	Often chronic
	Inferior myocardial infarction	Anteroseptal
	Rheumatic fever	Lenegre disease
		Lev disease
	Digitalis or β-blockers	Cardiomyopathy
Anatomic	Usually AV node	Infranodal
Electrophysiology	Increased relative refractory period	No relative refractory period
	Decremental conduction	All-or-none conduction
ECG features	RP/PR reciprocity	PR interval stable
	Prolonged PR interval	PR interval usually normal
	QRS duration normal	QRS duration prolonged
Response to atropine and exercise	Improves	Worsens
Response to carotid massage	Worsens	Improves*

*Primarily refers to conduction ratio.

Box 74-6 Causes of Grouped Impulses

- Wenckebach mechanism (usually at AV node, but can occur elsewhere)
- Atrial tachycardia or flutter with alternating conduction (e.g., 2:1 with 3:2 or 4:1)
- Frequent extrasystoles (two or more impulses)
- Nonconducted atrial trigeminy
- Concealed or interpolated extrasystoles

When the conduction ratio is 2:1, it may be impossible to distinguish type I from type II AV block on the surface ECG. The response to autonomic manipulation can aid in this task. Atropine usually has no effect on the His-Purkinje system and may worsen the conduction ratio in type II AV block by increasing the number of atrial impulses without improving conduction (although clinical deterioration is not likely). Carotid sinus massage may transiently improve the conduction ratio (but not the overall condition) in type II AV block by slowing the conduction in the proximal AV node, allowing the lower conductive tissues to recover and be less refractory.

Pharmacologic treatment of type II AV block is not indicated. In the prehospital setting, symptomatic type II second-degree AV block should be treated with transcutaneous pacing; in the ED, transcutaneous or transvenous pacing can be used. Emergent cardiology consultation should be sought for all patients, and none should be discharged to home unless the condition is chronic and without new symptoms.

Third-Degree (Complete) Atrioventricular Block Third-degree, or *complete,* AV block is characterized by the absent conduction of all atrial impulses (Figure 74-17) resulting in complete electrical and mechanical AV dissociation.[64] Not all AV dissociation is complete heart block; for complete heart block to exist, the rate of the underlying supraventricular or junctional rhythm must be sufficient to overcome the action of any subsidiary infranodal pacemakers. For example, an accelerated junctional focus at 80 beats/min (as a result of enhanced automaticity from catecholamine excess) may usurp the sinus node and become the dominant pacemaker. In this situation, the underlying sinus rhythm of less than 80 beats/min would be manifest as regular P waves unrelated

A

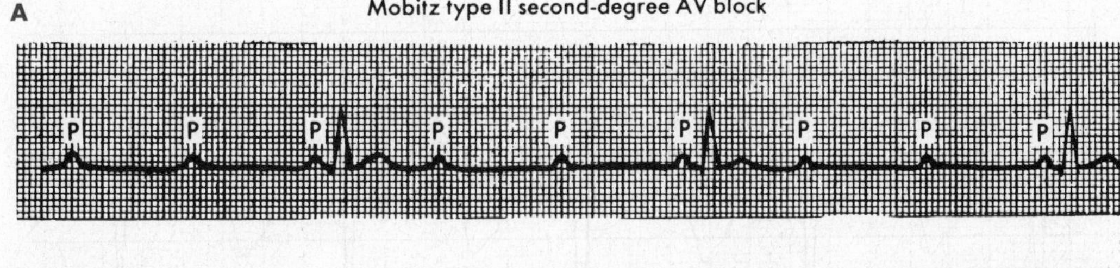

B

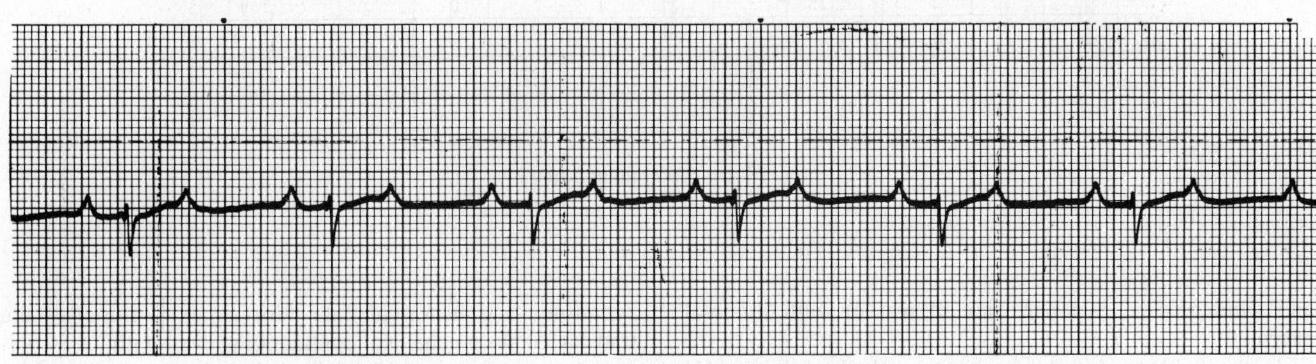

Figure 74-16. **A, Second-degree AV block, type II. In this example, 3:1 conduction is seen. B, Second-degree AV block with 2:1 conduction. From the rhythm strip alone, it is difficult to categorize this as a type I or II block.** ***A, from Goldberger AL, Goldberger E:*** **Clinical electrocardiography, *ed 2, St Louis, 1981, Mosby.***

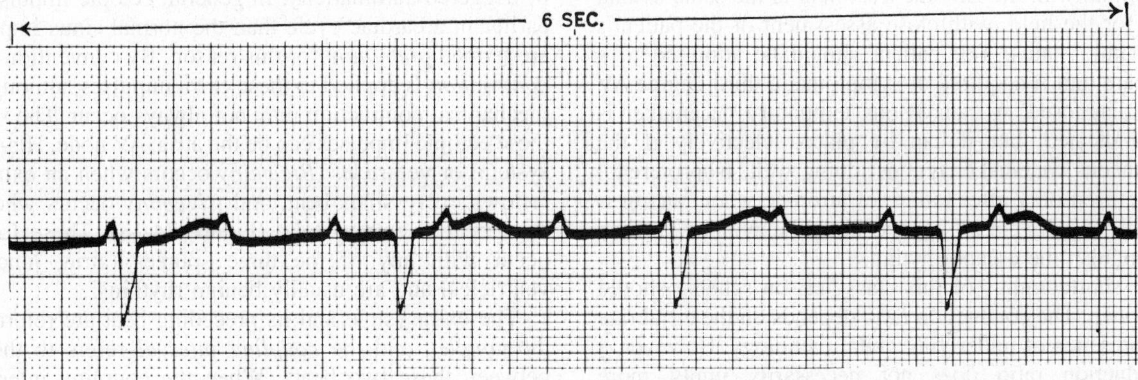

Figure 74-17. **Complete (third-degree) AV block. Note that there is no constant relationship of P waves to QRS complexes, even though some are noted in close proximity.**

to the source of ventricular depolarization, the junctional rhythm. This junctional rhythm is not complete heart block, because no underlying AV nodal conduction disorder is present. In a similar fashion, complete SA block coupled with a junctional or ventricular escape rhythm can be misidentified as complete AV block (see Figure 74-13).

During complete heart block, the P waves and QRS complexes are present but are unrelated and occur at different rates. When the atrial and escape rates are similar, the situation is referred to as *isorhythmic AV dissociation,* and it can be difficult to appreciate unless a long rhythm strip is examined and the P waves and QRS complexes are closely tracked. The duration of the QRS complex depends on the site of the escape rhythm pacemaker. Those pacemakers above the His bundle produce a narrow complex, whereas pacemakers at or below the His bundle produce a wide-complex rhythm. The narrow-complex rhythms usually operate at a faster rate (45 to 60 beats/min) and respond to atropine and isoproterenol, whereas the wide-complex escape rhythms are slower (30 to 45 beats/min) and are unaffected by autonomic drugs. When atrial P or fibrillatory waves are coupled with a slow and completely regular ventricular response, atrial tachycardia or fibrillation with third-degree heart block and a junctional rhythm should be suspected; this combination commonly is the result of digitalis toxicity.

Third-degree AV block can be congenital or acquired.[64] In general, congenital third-degree AV block is associated with a narrow-complex escape rhythm and minimal symptoms. The fixed rate of the subsidiary pacemaker limits the ability to increase cardiac output, with exercise intolerance of varying degrees resulting. Acquired third-degree block is often associated with a wide-complex escape rhythm

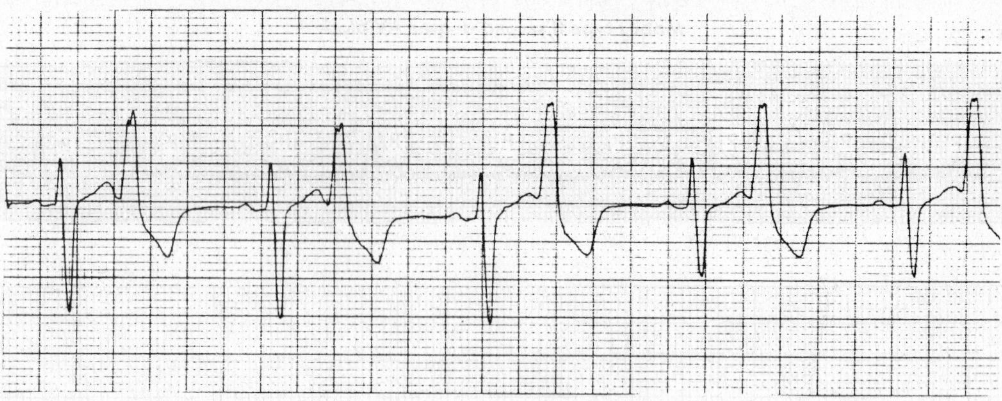

Figure 74-18. **Ventricular bigeminy.**

and symptoms of hypoperfusion at rest or with minimal exertion.

In the field, treatment of patients with third-degree AV block depends on the symptoms. Patients with clinical evidence of hypoperfusion can receive atropine but are better treated with transcutaneous pacing. Asymptomatic patients should be rapidly transported, with the preceding therapies readily available, and care should be taken to avoid maneuvers that increase vagal tone (e.g., Valsalva maneuver, painful stimuli). In the ED, the treatment is the same as that outlined for the field, with close assessment of the patient's hemodynamic status. The patient should be admitted to a cardiac care unit if acquired or symptomatic third-degree AV block is diagnosed. A transvenous temporary pacemaker is usually indicated, but it can be placed electively if the transcutaneous pacemaker is functioning well. Isoproterenol should be used only after failure of atropine when pacing is unavailable. Again, class I agents should be avoided, as they may extinguish the escape rhythm.

A few shortcomings of this classification scheme should be mentioned. The conduction ratio depends on the atrial rate and the presence of underlying nodal pathology. However, a 2:1 conduction ratio does not necessarily imply more conduction system disease than a 3:2 ratio, and all 2:1 conduction is not pathologic. The following two examples of 2:1 AV conduction can help illustrate the latter point. An atrial impulse rate of 300 beats/min (as seen in atrial flutter) presented to the AV node usually results in conduction of half the impulses, producing a ventricular rate of 150 beats/min; this conduction ratio does not represent significant AV block, as the AV node is responding normally and preventing excessive ventricular stimulation. Conversely, a sinus rhythm at a rate of 70 beats/min paired with a similar conduction ratio produces a ventricular rate of 35 beats/min; this ratio clearly represents significant second-degree AV block. The term *high-grade second-degree block* should be applied to conduction disturbances that prevent physiologic ventricular response rates and not solely to higher conduction ratios.

Extrasystoles and Parasystole *Extrasystoles,* defined as ectopic impulses that occur in addition to the underlying normal sinus rhythm, are present in most individuals when monitored closely. Certain specific extrasystoles may help identify patients with a poor prognosis when coupled with symptoms and historical data. Not all extra impulses are translated into mechanical contractions; even without associated contractions, nonconducted impulses can trigger a secondary irregularity of the pulse by interfering with conduction. In fact, the most common cause of a pause on the ECG is a nonconducted atrial extrasystole that resets the SA node.

The mechanism responsible for most extrasystoles is abnormal automaticity, although some can result from reentry or triggered automaticity. In general, ectopic impulses occur earlier in a cardiac cycle than the normal sinus impulse and are termed *premature* for this reason. By convention the term *contraction* is applied to these extra impulses, although a true mechanical contraction may not always occur. The source of these ectopic impulses can be the atria, AV node, His-Purkinje system, or ventricles. *Bigeminy* occurs when an extrasystole follows every sinus beat, and *trigeminy* occurs when every third beat is extrasystolic (Figure 74-18). These forms can occur with any of the three sources (atria, junction, or ventricles) and are usually benign rhythms.

The extrasystole and its preceding beat are referred to as the *couplet,* and the *coupling interval* refers to the period between these two beats. When the coupling interval in a given rhythm is constant (or fixed), a single focus is believed to be responsible for the extrasystoles. Although fixed coupling was previously considered to be solely the result of reentry, data suggest that it does not reliably define the mechanism of ectopic impulse formation. The three basic extrasystolic foci are discussed next, along with a specific form of abnormal impulse generation and propagation called *parasystole.*

Premature Atrial Contractions Premature atrial contractions (PACs) are often the precipitating event for a variety of dysrhythmias, including atrial fibrillation, atrial flutter, and supraventricular tachycardia. Abnormal automaticity and atrial or AV nodal reentry are the most common causes of PACs. The diagnosis of PACs is made from the ECG, where an abnormal P′ wave is seen early within a cardiac cycle (Figure 74-19). The P′ wave may be difficult to see if it is buried within the preceding T wave, although increasing the paper speed and use of an esophageal lead can help. Inverted P′ waves suggest an atrial source near the AV junction, where nearly normal P′ waves imply a focus near the SA node. If the P′ waves, P′R intervals, and coupling intervals are constant,

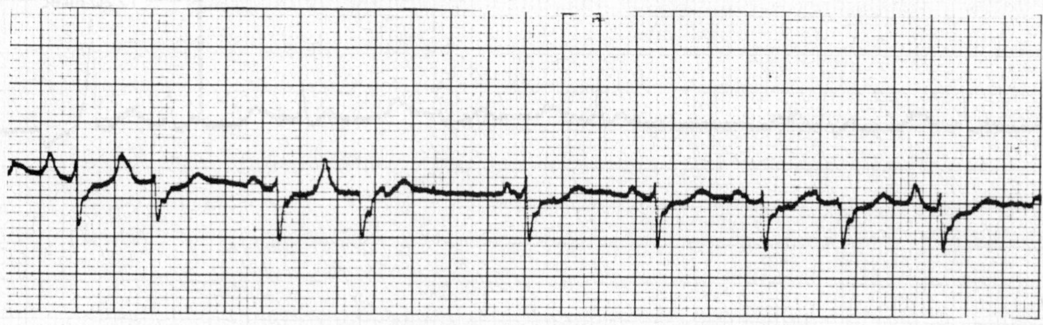

Figure 74-19. **Premature atrial contractions.**

Table 74-5. Features to Distinguish Premature Atrial Contractions with Abnormal Conduction from Premature Ventricular Contractions

Premature atrial contractions	Premature ventricular contractions
No compensatory pause	Fully compensatory pause (unless interpolated)
Preceding P wave (different from sinus P wave; occasionally buried in T wave)	No preceding P waves (although retrograde atrial conduction can cause inverted P wave after QRS)
Usually classic right bundle branch block pattern (especially if long-short cycle sequence appears)	Left bundle branch block, right bundle branch block, or hybrid pattern
Initial QRS deflection identical to sinus QRS	Bizarre QRS structure
QRS axis normal or near normal	Frequently bizarre QRS axis
QRS rarely > 0.14 sec	QRS often > 0.14 sec

a single focus is likely. Variations in these three characteristics are consistent with multiple foci. Either the left or right atrium can be the source of PACs.

Most PACs depolarize the sinus node, resulting in the intrinsic sinus node rate being reset. On the ECG, the PP interval after a conducted PAC is equal to the PP interval of the cycle preceding the PAC. Because of this adjustment of the sinus cycle, the RR interval surrounding the ectopic beat is less than twice the intrinsic RR cycle length (see Figure 74-19). This is referred to as a *noncompensatory pause,* a hallmark of PACs. Occasionally, PACs do not depolarize the sinus node, and a compensatory pause may result. Fully compensatory pauses are more commonly seen with premature ventricular complexes (PVCs). Table 74-5 lists ECG features to help distinguish PACs from PVCs.

If it is conducted to the ventricles, a PAC results in a QRS complex occurring earlier than the expected sinus QRS complex. The QRS complex from a PAC is narrow and identical to the sinus rhythm complex unless aberrant conduction occurs (Figure 74-20). Aberrancy is likely to occur if a PAC arrives early within the cardiac cycle, with a right bundle branch block pattern commonly seen on the ECG. In a similar fashion, a PAC that follows a long cardiac cycle (reflected as a preceding long RR interval) may also be aberrantly conducted, because the bundles require more time to repolarize. In this latter setting, aberrant conduction occurs because of the relative early arrival of the PAC for the given cycle length. This aberrant conduction is called the *Ashman phenomenon* (see p. 1056) and can occur with any irregular atrial rhythm, including PACs and atrial fibrillation.

A PAC is the most common cause of a pause on the ECG. Although the source of this type of pause can be obvious when a PAC is conducted, nonconducted PACs are frequently responsible for pauses. In this situation, the sinus node is depolarized by the PAC, causing an interruption and resetting of the regular rhythm. If this same extrasystolic impulse reaches the AV node or infranodal conducting system during the refractory period, no ventricular depolarization is possible. This combined sinus node reset with a nonconducted atrial extrasystole creates the pause seen on the ECG. Often the PAC responsible for a pause falls within the previous T wave and is not visible on the surface ECG.

On rare occasions an extremely late PAC can cause atrial depolarization in combination with the sinus node impulse. The P′ waves in these cases represent a *fusion complex* and carry qualities of both impulses.

Management of PACs is based on recognition, with no need for specific therapy. Underlying causes, such as catecholamine excess, hypoxia/hypoxemia, myocardial ischemia, congestive heart failure, or acid-base and electrolyte imbalance, should be sought and treated if symptomatic or frequent PACs occur. If caused by a reentrant mechanism,

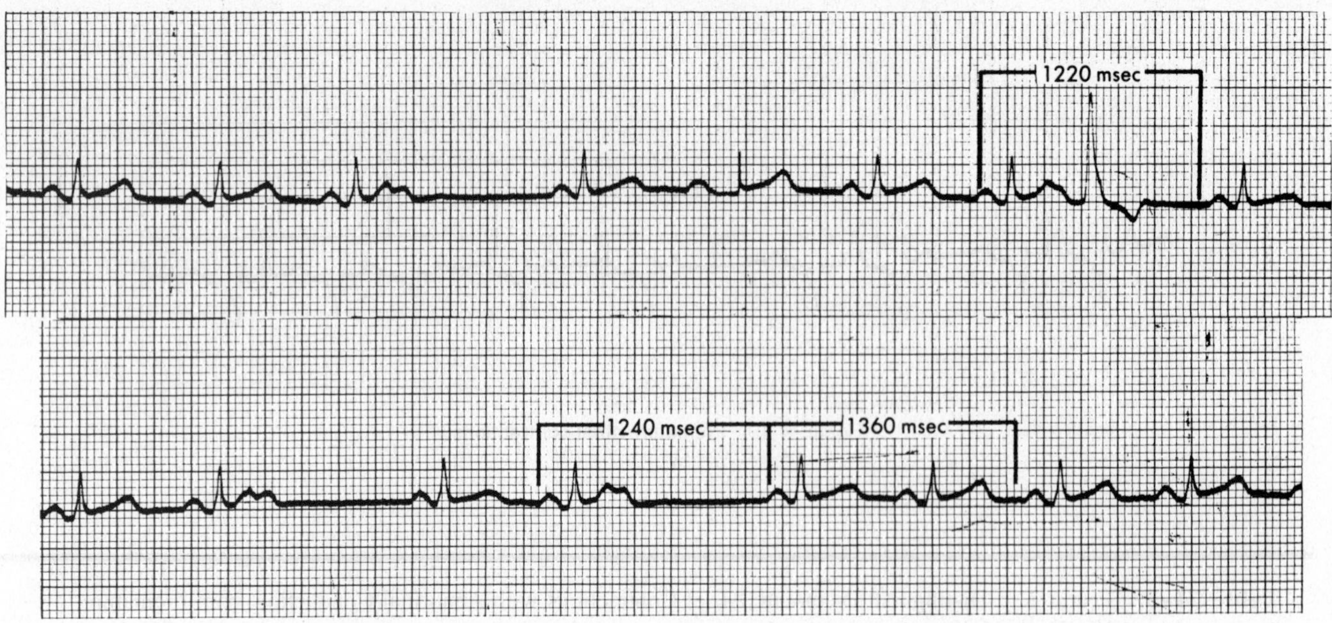

Figure 74-20. **Premature atrial contractions with noncompensatory pauses and one aberrantly conducted impulse *(upper strip).* Note that both conducted and nonconducted PACs reset the sinus node, with the latter creating a pause.**

frequent PACs can be terminated with a calcium channel blocker, a β-adrenergic blocker, or magnesium; however, this treatment is rarely needed.

Premature Junctional Contractions Premature junctional contractions (PJCs) are the result of either altered automaticity or nodal microreentry. On the surface ECG, a P′ wave from retrograde atrial depolarization is buried within the QRS complex, and the extrasystole appears as a lone additional QRS complex (from a high nodal focus) may be seen as a result of retrograde conduction to the atria. If seen, the P′ waves from PJCs are usually inverted because of the opposite direction of the depolarization wave compared with the normal sinus impulses and can be difficult to distinguish from PACs emanating from a low atrial source. If a high nodal focus is involved, the QRS complex is narrow; wide QRS complexes imply a lower His source or abnormal infranodal conduction (bundle branch block).

Fully compensatory pauses and aberrant conduction occur more often with PJCs than with PACs. The causes and treatment of PJCs are the same as those of PACs.

Premature Ventricular Contractions Premature ventricular contractions (PVCs) can occur in a variety of pathologic and nonpathologic states. Their major importance is not the symptoms caused but the clinical scenario accompanying their presence and the risk of more serious ventricular dysrhythmias (i.e., ventricular tachycardia and fibrillation).[66] Extrasystoles that occur during ventricular repolarization (the "R-on-T phenomenon") are believed to carry a higher risk of precipitating ventricular tachycardia, although the magnitude of this effect is debated. Other data suggest that PVCs occurring during the next atrial depolarization (the "R-on-P phenomenon") carry as high or a higher risk of precipitating serious ventricular dysrhythmias as R-on-T PVCs.

PVCs can be caused by varying mechanisms (Box 74-7), including reentry, abnormal automaticity, and triggered afterdepolarizations. Classically, PVCs appear on the ECG as wide QRS complex extrasystoles (> 0.12 second) unassociated with a preceding P wave (Figure 74-21). In a single lead a PVC may appear as a narrow QRS complex. This narrow complex occurs if the wave of depolarization is traveling directly perpendicular to the ECG lead and underscores the need to examine multiple leads to accurately identify PVCs. Although P waves from nonconducted sinus impulses may be seen on

Box 74-7 Causes of Premature Ventricular Contractions and Ventricular Tachycardia

Acute myocardial infarction
Hypokalemia
Hypoxemia
Ischemic heart disease
Valvular disease
Catecholamine excess*
Other drug intoxications
Idiopathic causes†
Digitalis toxicity
Hypomagnesemia
Hypercapnia
Type I agents
Alcohol
Myocardial contusion (especially cyclic antidepressants)
Cardiomyopathy
Acidosis
Alkalosis
Methylxanthine toxicity

*Relative increase in sympathetic tone from drugs (direct or indirect) or conditions that augment catecholamine release or decrease parasympathetic tone.
†Isolated PVCs can occur in up to 50% of young subjects without obvious cardiac or noncardiac disease; however, multiform and repetitive PVCs and ventricular tachycardia are rarely seen in this population.

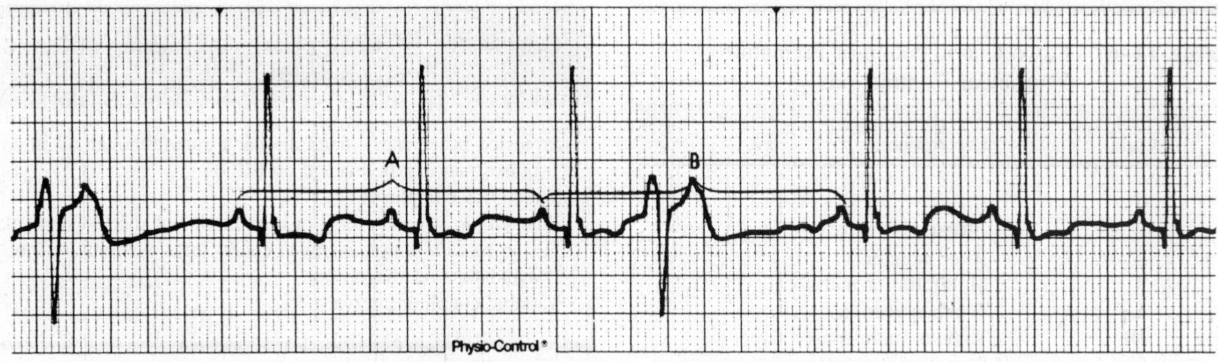

Figure 74-21. **Premature ventricular contraction with compensatory pause. Note that a sinus P wave can be seen in the T wave of the extrasystolic beat. Also note the secondary T-wave changes in beats 1 and 4 (T wave is opposite the main deflection of the QRS complex).**

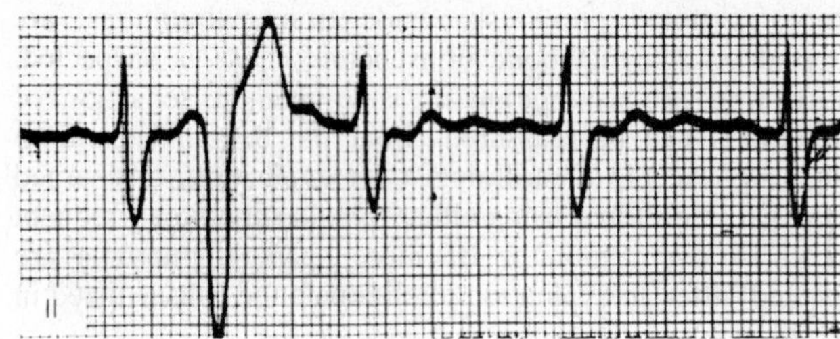

Figure 74-22. **Interpolated premature ventricular contraction.**

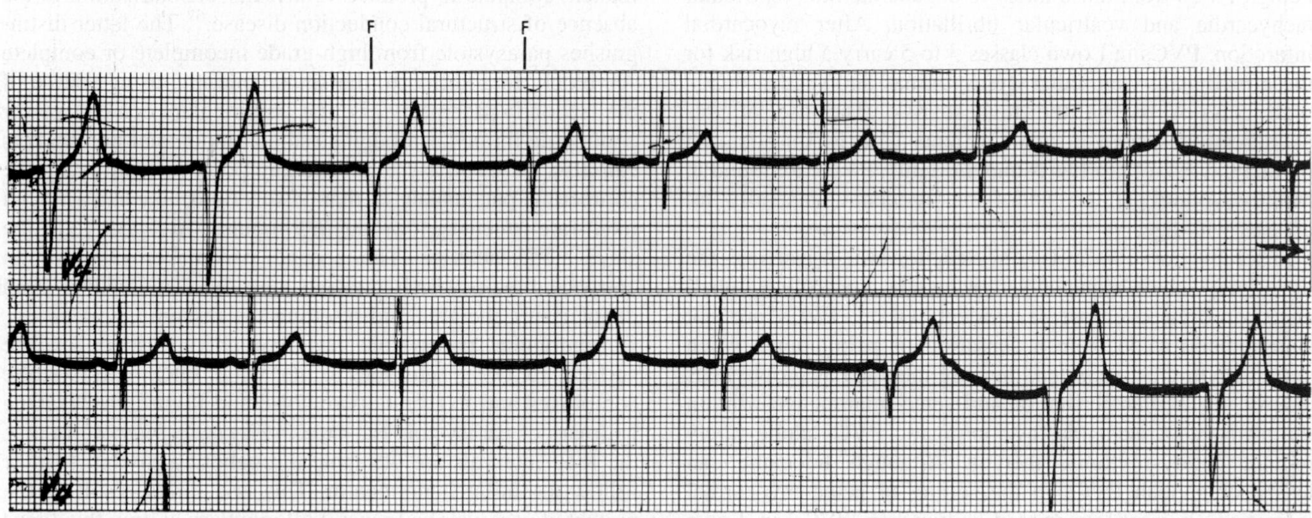

Figure 74-23. **Sinus rhythm with run of accelerated idioventricular rhythm. Note fusion beats *(F)* displaying hybrid appearance of both morphologies.**

the ECG, they should have no consistent relationship with the QRS complexes from the PVCs. Retrograde conduction of PVCs can produce an inverted P′ wave after each QRS complex. PVCs usually cause a fully compensatory pause, with the resulting RR interval encompassing the PVC equal to twice the intrinsic RR-interval length (see Figure 74-21). Rarely, noncompensatory or subcompensatory pauses can be seen with PVCs and are associated with retrograde conduction and sinus node depolarization. *Interpolated PVCs* refer to another rare instance when the underlying sinus rhythm is unaffected by a PVC (Figure 74-22).

The structure of the QRS complexes depends on the origin of the impulse. PVCs with a left bundle branch appearance result from a wave of depolarization beginning in a right ventricular source and vice versa. Multiform (or multifocal) PVCs refer to ventricular extrasystoles from more than one source and appear as varying QRS complex structures. When a PVC depolarizes the ventricles at a similar time as a conducted atrial beat, a *fusion QRS complex* is seen (Figure 74-23). Identification of fusion QRS beats indicates the presence of PVCs.

PVCs produce abnormal repolarization as a direct result of the abnormal depolarization of the ventricles. *Secondary T-wave abnormalities* refer to those repolarization changes

Table 74-6. Lown Classification of Premature Ventricular Contractions

Class	Description
0	None
1	<30/hr
2	30 or more/hr
3	Multiform (or multifocal)
4A	Two consecutive
4B	Three or more consecutive
5	R on T phenomenon

Box 74-8 ECG Features of Ventricular Parasystole

Protected pacemaker—fixed discharge rate (although all impulses may not be evident on ECG)
Wide QRS complexes
Interectopic intervals fixed or in multiples of shortest interval
Fusion beats if simultaneous to conducted sinus impulse (not mandatory for diagnosis)
Variable coupling intervals

seen as a result of pathologic depolarization and are seen with PVCs along with bundle branch blocks and left ventricular hypertrophy. These secondary T-wave changes consist of widening and deflection opposite the main QRS deflection (see Figure 74-21). *Primary T-wave abnormalities* refer to changes in ventricular repolarization caused by underlying cardiac disease (such as ischemia) and are not solely the result of depolarization abnormalities. Primary T-wave changes often consist of T-wave deflection in the same direction as the main QRS vector.

The pattern of PVCs is commonly classified by the Lown criteria (Table 74-6). These criteria are intended to distinguish benign PVCs from those likely to degenerate into ventricular tachycardia and ventricular fibrillation. After myocardial infarction, PVCs in Lown classes 3 to 5 carry a high risk for these malignant ventricular dysrhythmias and sudden death, with class 4 having the highest risk. The use of this classification system in other patients with PVCs does not predict the risk of morbidity and mortality. PVCs are found in healthy young patients and their frequency generally increases with age.

Therapy for PVCs is directed toward correcting the underlying cause, especially if ischemia, electrolyte imbalance, or drug overdose is evident. Often, PVCs are not symptomatic aside from a sensation of palpitations; when antidysrhythmics are given, they are intended as prophylaxis against ventricular fibrillation and ventricular tachycardia. In the absence of ischemia, asymptomatic PVCs alone rarely require antidysrhythmic therapy. Although lidocaine can lessen or abolish PVCs in the setting of acute myocardial infarction, it is recommended only when PVCs in Lown classes 3 to 5 are present or when close monitoring and rapid defibrillation capabilities are not readily available. Routine lidocaine use outside of the higher risk setting noted, even with concurrent acute myocardial ischemia, may result in more frequent bouts of asystole. Procainamide and amiodarone are alternative first-line choices to treat PVCs. The difficulty of delivery limits the use of all class I agents except lidocaine in the field. In selected cases, β-blockers (e.g., catecholamine-induced PVCs and those occurring after myocardial infarction) and calcium channel blockers (after reperfusion therapy) can diminish PVC frequency and decrease the risk of ventricular fibrillation and ventricular tachycardia. Magnesium sulfate (2 to 4 g IV over 10 to 20 minutes) can also diminish the frequency of PVCs, particularly in the setting of acute myocardial ischemia.

Patients with syncope, presyncope, dyspnea, chest pain, or frequent palpitations associated with PVCs should be monitored. This is done on an inpatient basis if any of the symptoms noted previously, aside from palpitations, are reported or if a metabolic or ischemic cause is suspected. Those who are asymptomatic aside from a sensation of palpitations can be reassured about the benign short-term course, referred to a cardiologist for evaluation, discharged home, and monitored using either a Holter monitor (frequent PVCs) or event monitor (if more sparse symptoms are expected) after an evaluation to eliminate the causes listed in Box 74-7.

Parasystole Parasystole occurs when two separate pacemakers compete to produce ventricular depolarization in the absence of structural conduction disease.[67] The latter distinguishes parasystole from high-grade incomplete or complete AV block. In addition to the sinus node, the usual source of the second pacemaker is the ventricular conductive or contractile tissues, although atrial and junctional pacemakers can also cause parasystole. The key point in identifying the competing pacemaker is that it functions like an artificial fixed-rate pacemaker, producing impulses irrespective of the sinus node activity. The second pacemaker displays an entrance block, which prevents any outside impulse from depolarizing the area and resetting the rhythm.

Ventricular parasystole has five characteristics on the surface ECG in addition to its wide QRS extrasystolic complexes and fixed rate (Box 74-8 and Figure 74-24). One hallmark of parasystole is a *fixed interectopic interval.* In this, the R′R′ intervals are the same throughout a rhythm strip or follow a similar denominator. This is a direct result of the protected parasystolic focus; if all impulses exiting this focus find the conducting system nonrefractory, a fixed interectopic interval is observed. If the conducting tissues are refractory (usually from recent conduction of a sinus impulse), no ventricular depolarization is seen on the ECG, yet the protected parasystolic focus continues to fire at the same rate. If the next impulse from the parasystolic focus finds nonrefractory conducting tissues, the interectopic interval will be equal to two times the basic cycle length. If the first and second parasystolic impulses are not conducted, but the third in a series finds nonrefractory tissues, the interectopic interval will be three times the basic cycle length, and so on. For example, based on a 1-second interval, ventricular parasystole may have R′R′ intervals in multiples of this interval (e.g., impulses seen 1, 2, or 3 seconds apart at various times).

Ventricular parasystole is usually the result of an altered

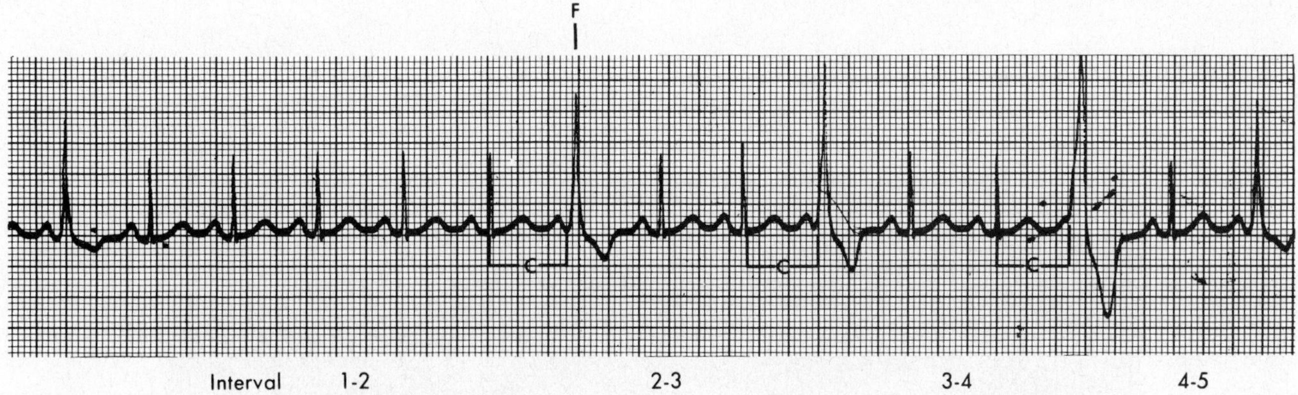

Figure 74-24. **Ventricular parasystole. Fusion *(F)* beats are seen, and coupling intervals *(C)* vary. Interectopic intervals are all based on a common denominator (0.4 second).**

automatic mechanism and does not have the serious implications that frequent PVCs have even when an R-on-T phenomenon is seen. Ventricular parasystole may be difficult to distinguish from frequent PVCs in the field, as it requires close observation of a prolonged rhythm strip with multiple leads. Fusion QRS complexes may be seen but are not essential to the diagnosis. Ventricular parasystole is usually a benign rhythm, with treatment similar to that of nonischemia-related PVCs.

Box 74-9 Causes of Completely Irregular (Chaotic) Rhythms

Atrial fibrillation
Atrial tachycardia or flutter with varying conduction
Multifocal atrial tachycardia
Multiple extrasystoles
Wandering pacemaker (usually atrial)
Parasystole

Narrow Complex Tachycardia *Narrow-complex tachycardias* are defined as rhythms with a QRS complex duration of less than 0.12 second and a ventricular rate of greater than 100 beats/min.[68] Although virtually all narrow-complex tachydysrhythmias originate from a focus above the ventricles (with the rare exception of a very high His bundle rhythm), the term *supraventricular tachycardia* is conventionally used to denote those rhythms aside from sinus tachycardia, atrial tachycardia, atrial fibrillation, and atrial flutter. The atrial depolarization waves may be difficult to appreciate on the surface ECG, especially if the ventricular response rate is more than 150 beats/min. The use of multiple-surface leads, increased paper speed, an esophageal lead, or vagal maneuvers can help identify the atrial depolarization waves and diagnose the source of the dysrhythmia. Also, atrial or junctional parasystole can create a narrow-complex tachycardia termed *pseudotachycardia,* as neither focus has a rate greater than 100 beats/min.

One ECG feature that can help distinguish the source of a tachydysrhythmia is the location of the P waves and the regularity of the QRS complexes. If near-normal-appearing atrial depolarization waves precede each QRS complex and the underlying pattern is regular, a sinus rhythm, atrial flutter, or single-focus atrial tachycardia is commonly present. If a completely irregular (or chaotic) pattern of QRS complexes is seen, atrial fibrillation, multifocal atrial tachycardia, or one of the preceding rhythms with varying conduction is possible (Box 74-9). Identification of atrial depolarization waves and the appearance of irregularity or regularity can be deceiving within any short rhythm strip, and the general categories described here are not completely exclusive.

Treatment of each narrow-complex tachycardia is based on the specific rhythm and symptoms. In general, adenosine, class II, and class IV agents are used to slow AV nodal conduction, although these agents may terminate certain dysrhythmias (especially nodal reentry). Class IA and IC agents are useful in converting other narrow-complex tachycardias (e.g., atrial flutter and fibrillation) to a sinus rhythm. Finally, cholinesterase inhibitors such as edrophonium or neostigmine slow AV conduction, but are associated with frequent side effects such as nausea, vomiting, and bronchospasm. As a result, these latter agents have little role in the current treatment of narrow-complex tachycardias.

After identifying the specific dysrhythmia during an episode, the underlying cause of the tachycardia should be sought while treatment is begun. Hypovolemia should always be considered as a possible cause of a narrow-complex tachycardia, especially in the young. Fever, anemia, hypoxemia or impaired oxygen delivery (including abnormal hemoglobin states), relative sympathetic excess, drug intoxication, endocrinologic disease (especially thyroid), metabolic derangements, ischemia, infections, and inflammatory causes (including myocarditis and pericarditis) should also be considered.

Sinus Tachycardia Sinus tachycardia is characterized by a narrow-complex regular rhythm at a rate greater than 100 beats/min. The P waves are upright in all leads, but aVR and the appearance of each is consistent (Figure 74-25). The PR and PP intervals are usually constant, but both may shorten as the rate increases. Increasing vagal or decreasing sympathetic tone decreases the rate of impulse formation and conduction in a graded continuous manner. Conversely, sinus tachycardia can result from increased catecholamine tone or decreased vagal stimulation.

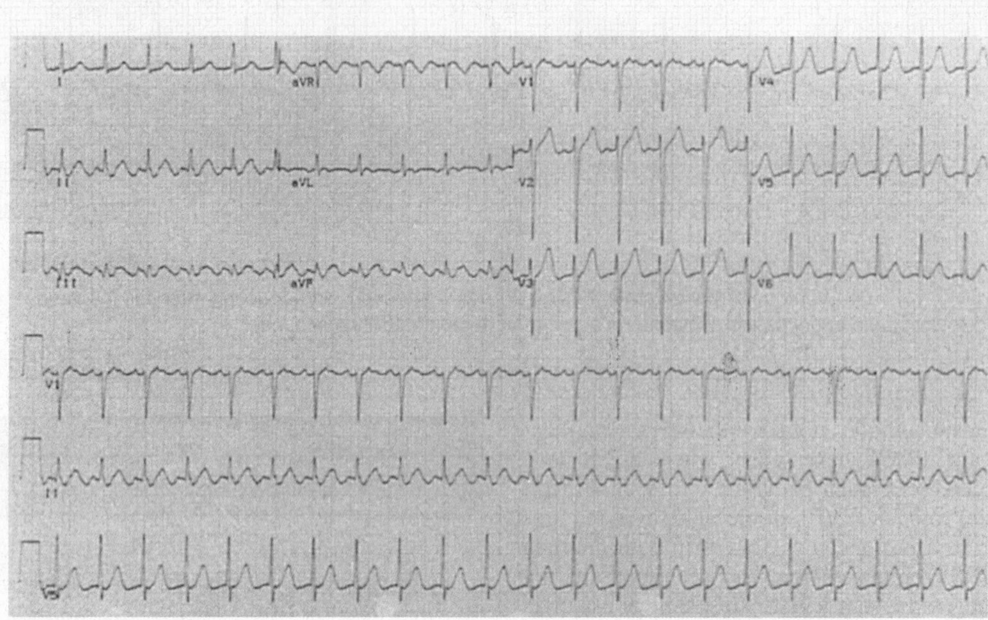

Figure 74-25. **Sinus tachycardia.**

Functionally, sinus tachycardia is a response to physiologic stress and is intended to increase cardiac output. This response can be compensatory for a relative lack of perfusion or oxygen delivery (e.g., congestive heart failure, pulmonary embolism, hypovolemia, anemia, or sepsis) or can occur in nonhypoperfusion states when a relative sympathetic excess exists. Treatment is based on the recognition and treatment of the underlying cause. Although anxiety or pain can cause sinus tachycardia in patients, this is a diagnosis of exclusion after a careful search for evidence of the aforementioned physiologic causes of tachycardia.

Sinus tachycardia can be easily mistaken for other causes of a regular narrow-complex tachycardia, especially in young patients. Infants and young children can easily attain ventricular rates of 170 to 225 beats/min with an episode of hypovolemia-induced sinus tachycardia, which may be mistaken for a paroxysmal atrial or junctional tachycardia,[69] with disastrous consequences if a rate-controlling drug is given. It is rare for an adult to sustain a rate above 160 to 170/min due to the "braking" properties of the AV node.

Specific antidysrhythmic therapy for sinus tachycardia is almost never indicated. If the patient is symptomatic or if the risk of precipitating myocardial ischemia is high, the use of a β-blocker is warranted only after all possible primary causes are treated or eliminated from consideration.

Atrial Tachycardia and Multifocal Atrial Tachycardia Atrial tachycardia refers to any rapid dysrhythmia from a nonsinus focus above the AV node. Atrial tachycardia can be gradual in onset (suggesting an abnormal automatic mechanism) or abrupt (suggesting a reentrant mechanism). The hallmark of this dysrhythmia on the surface ECG is a narrow-complex tachycardia at a rate above 100 beats/min, with each QRS complex preceded by a P′ wave that is morphologically different from the sinus P wave (Figure 74-26). If the P′ wave is inverted, a low atrial source is likely. The P′R interval can be normal or abnormal and is usually constant unless more than one focus is involved. Generally, the conduction ratio is 1:1, but it can vary, especially as the atrial rate increases. If no ECG tracing of the normal sinus rhythm is available, single-focus atrial tachycardia can be indistinguishable from sinus tachycardia.

Paroxysmal atrial tachycardia (PAT) is an intermittent dysrhythmia with an abrupt onset and termination and is often seen in children and young adults without concomitant SA node disease. PAT is usually reentrant in origin, as opposed to nonparoxysmal (sustained) atrial tachycardia (NPAT), which is often automatic in nature. PAT can be precipitated by a PAC (or rarely by a PVC) and often originates and terminates abruptly. Other causes of PAT and NPAT include electrolyte and acid-base disturbances, drug toxicity, fever, and hypoxemia. NPAT with varying or complete AV block is classically seen in digitalis toxicity.

Multifocal atrial tachycardia (MAT) is a subset of atrial tachycardia, with more than two foci of impulse formation.[70] On the ECG, at least three distinctly different P waves with varying P′R, RR, and P′P′ intervals are seen (Figure 74-27). Debate exists as to whether the sinus P wave can be included to satisfy the criteria needed to diagnose MAT. Strictly defined, MAT requires three or more nonsinus foci, but distinguishing the sinus P wave from nonsinus P′ waves can be difficult. In addition to the causes just listed for PAT, MAT is often associated with pulmonary disease and hypoxemia, either directly from these conditions or as a result of β-adrenergic agonist or methylxanthine treatment. MAT often resolves when hypoxemia is resolved with supplemental therapy and when other therapies are optimized.

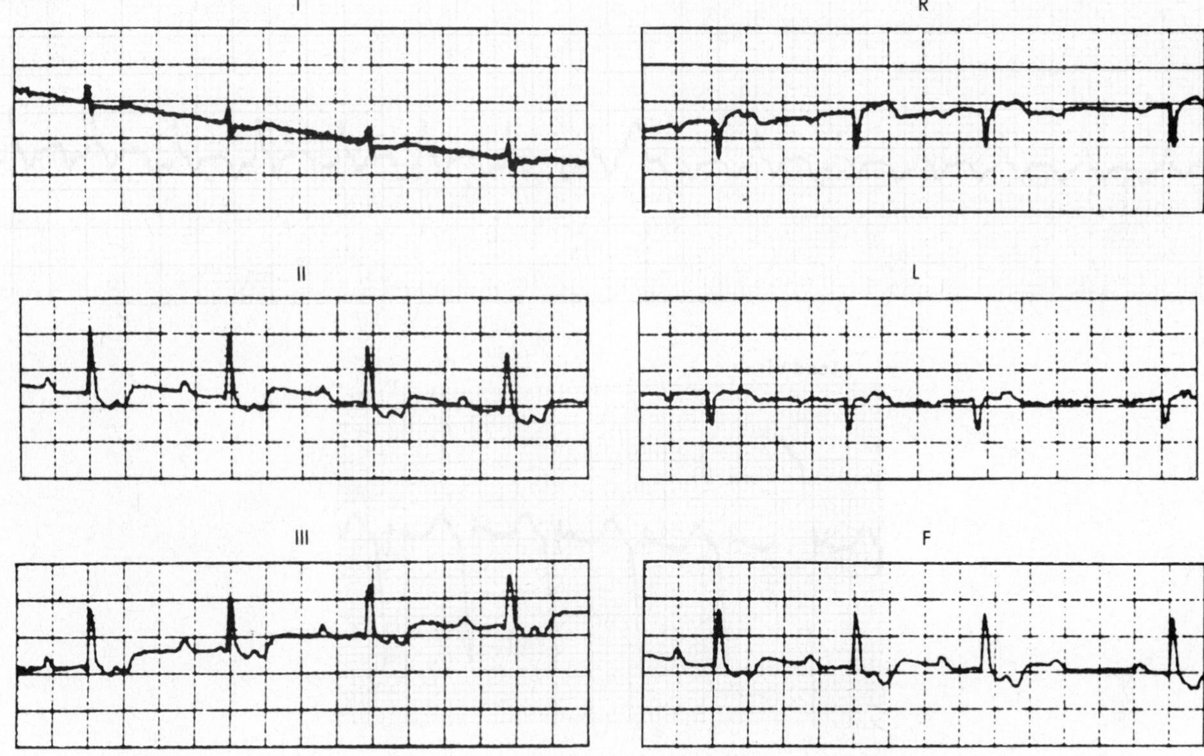

Figure 74-26. **Atrial tachycardia (with 2:1 conduction) in patient with digitalis toxicity.** *From Marriott HIL, Conover MB:* **Advanced concepts in arrhythmias,** *ed 2, St Louis, 1989, Mosby.*

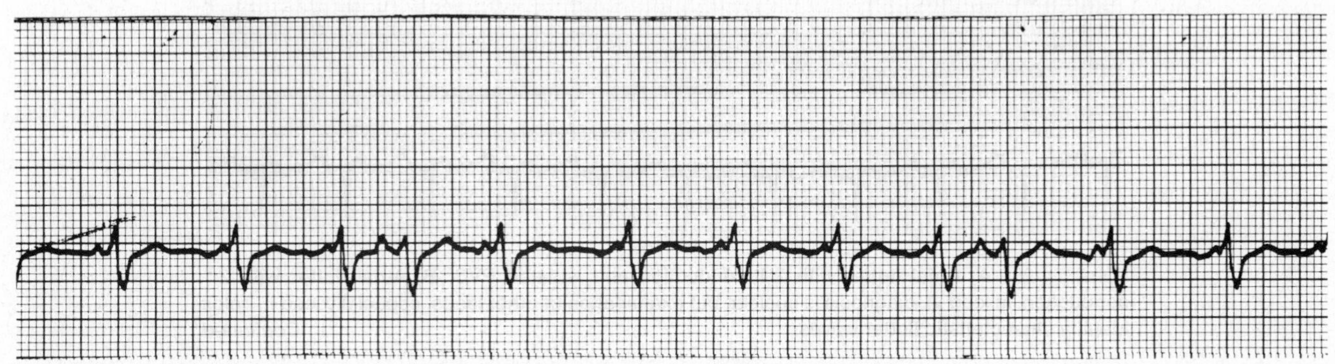

Figure 74-27. **Multifocal atrial tachycardia. Note that although the rhythm is irregular, at least three distinct P-wave morphologies are present.**

PAT, NPAT, and MAT are usually treated by correcting the underlying primary disturbance. If the patient is symptomatic and without evidence of instability or if concerns about precipitating myocardial ischemia are present, emergent treatment with a β-blocker or calcium channel blocker (verapamil or diltiazem) can be begun in the absence of hypotension.[42,90] Magnesium (2 to 4 g IV) is a third-line agent for PAT and MAT.[53] Although adenosine may slow the ventricular rate or extinguish atrial tachycardias, these rhythms often recur because of the short therapeutic effect of this drug. Procainamide, amiodarone, and digitalis are used as second-line agents or for outpatient maintenance therapy. Overdrive transvenous atrial pacing can be used if a reentrant mechanism is suspected and drug treatment fails.

In general, electrical treatment is rarely needed in PAT and MAT. If hypotension or other manifestations of instability exist, synchronized cardioversion with sedation at 50 to 100 J can be performed. Cardioversion is not useful in refractory cases of MAT, as the dysrhythmia is likely to recur if no other treatment is used. When the result of digitalis toxicity, PAT and MAT should be treated by correcting hypokalemia if it exists followed by administration of magnesium and digitalis antibody fragments. Emergency cardioversion should be avoided if possible in this setting.

A

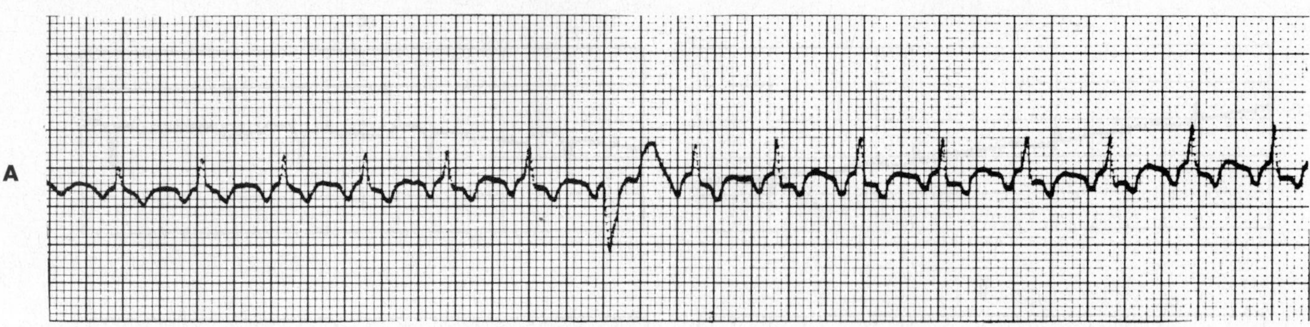

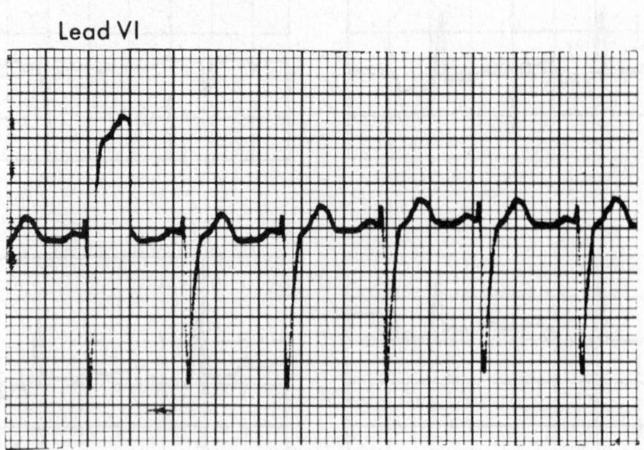

B

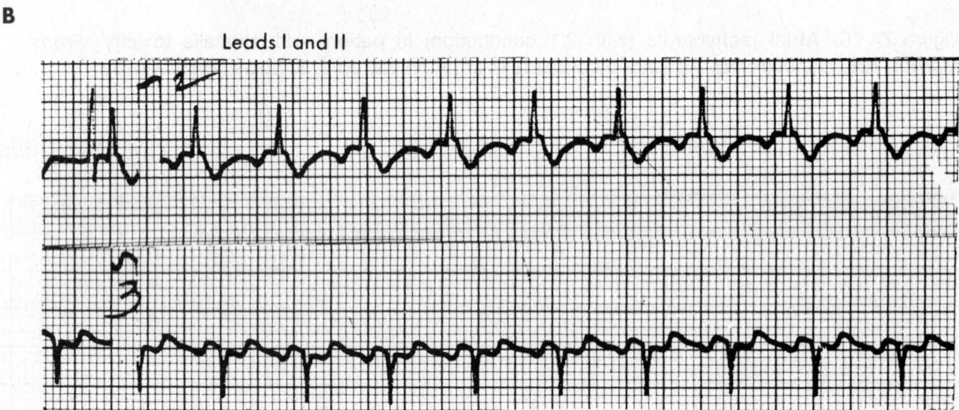

Figure 74-28. **A, Atrial flutter with 2:1 conduction and isolated PVC. B, Atrial flutter with 2:1 conduction. In lead VI, diagnosis is unclear, but examination of other leads, especially lead II, helps identify characteristic flutter waves.** *Continued*

Atrial Flutter Although atrial flutter has been recognized for more than 100 years, its precise definition still varies among authors. The most accepted characteristics of atrial flutter are the following[71] (Figure 74-28):

- A regular atrial depolarization rate of 250 to 350 beats/min, with a rate of 300 beats/min considered classic, although commonly this is not present.
- Distinct ECG manifestations of abnormal atrial depolarizations in a "sawtooth appearance." These are referred to as *flutter waves* and are best seen in leads II, III, aVF, and V_{1-2}.
- Common association with a 2:1 or 4:1 AV conduction ratio, although any conduction ratio may be seen. The 2:1 ratio accounts for the classic (although not exclusive) ECG appearance of atrial flutter as a narrow-complex tachycardia with a regular ventricular rate of 150 beats/min.

Most experimental data suggest a reentrant mechanism for atrial flutter, although some patients may display an abnormal automatic mechanism. In the ED, it is easy to mistake atrial flutter for sinus tachycardia, especially if the flutter waves resemble normal P waves or if a nonclassic ventricular rate is present.

Atrial flutter is often associated with underlying heart disease, congestive heart failure, valvular dysfunction (especially mitral), or metabolic derangements. The clinical importance of atrial flutter is primarily the result of its association with cardiac pathology and the symptoms caused by the ventricular response rate, including palpitations, syncope, presyncope, hypotension, chest pain, and heart failure. Varying AV conduction and the presence of a Wenckebach mechanism can produce an irregular ventricular response rate. Rarely, high-grade AV conduction block can result in a slow response rate and clinical bradycardia.

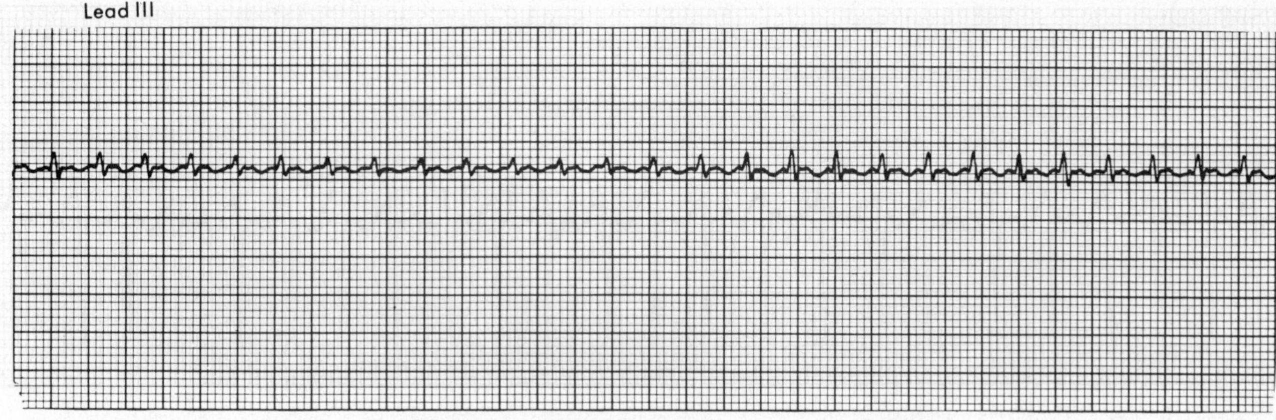

C

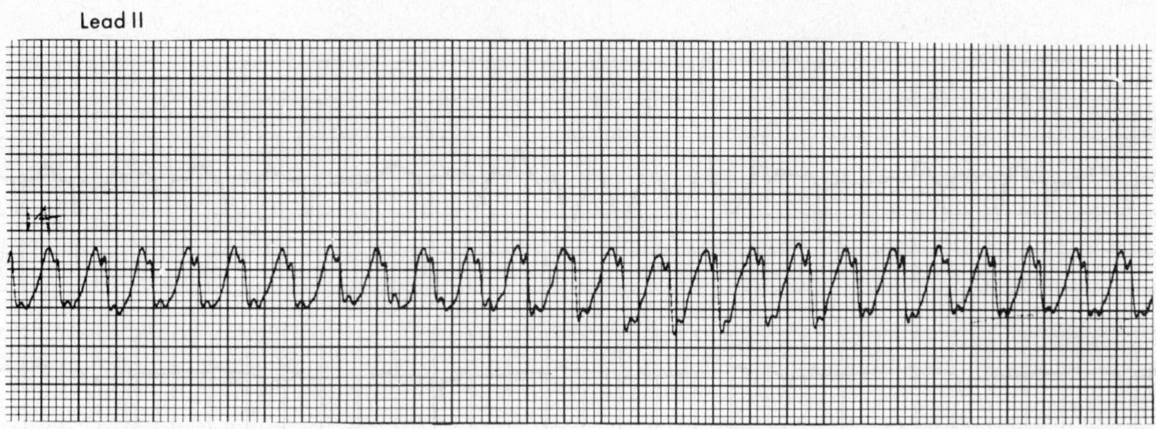

Figure 74-28, cont'd. **C, Atrial flutter with 1:1 conduction. This is rare and can be mistaken for ventricular tachycardia (lead II).**

In stable patients, ventricular response rates can be controlled with a calcium channel blocker (verapamil or diltiazem) or a β-adrenergic blocker. Diltiazem is touted as a better choice in atrial flutter and fibrillation because of laboratory and limited clinical data suggesting less evidence of negative inotropic effect and resultant hypotension. In practice, there is little difference in the effects and complication rates between equipotent doses of verapamil and diltiazem in patients without overt ventricular failure. Digitalis can be used as a second-line agent or in those with mild tachycardia and preexisting congestive heart failure. Magnesium (2 to 4 g IV) can be used as an adjunctive or third-line therapy to control the ventricular response rate. The major value of adenosine may be in unmasking flutter waves in a narrow-complex tachydysrhythmia, helping to correctly identify the underlying rhythm.

All AV nodal conduction slowing agents, including calcium channel blockers, β-adrenergic blockers, adenosine, and digitalis, should be avoided in patients with atrial flutter and a suspected accessory pathway, as these agents primarily block AV nodal conduction and may enhance anterograde conduction in the accessory path. Rapid ventricular response rates (especially > 200 beats/min) are a tip to the possibility of an accessory pathway because normal AV nodal tissues rarely allow a ventricular response rate of more than 150 to 165 beats/min. *The use of any predominately AV nodal blocking agent in the presence of an accessory pathway and atrial flutter or fibrillation may allow for unbridled rapid ventricular response rates and precipitate ventricular fibrillation.*

Class IA (especially procainamide) or III agents (ibutilide, amiodarone, or sotalol) can be used to convert atrial flutter if the previously mentioned drugs fail, or they may be used to prevent recurrence in an outpatient setting. Finally, synchronized electrical cardioversion with sedation, beginning at 25 to 50 J, is effective in terminating atrial flutter in refractory or unstable patients. If electrical therapy is successful but atrial flutter recurs, a type IA agent should be used before repeat electrical cardioversion is attempted to help prevent recurrence.

Atrial Fibrillation Atrial fibrillation is the result of chaotic depolarization of atrial tissues. This chaotic activity can lead to reduced cardiac output from a loss of coordinated atrial contractions and a rapid ventricular rate, both of which may limit the diastolic filling and stroke volume of the ventricles. Atrial fibrillation may be paroxysmal or chronic; the paroxysms may last for minutes to days. On the ECG, fibrillatory waves are seen and accompanied by an irregular QRS pattern (Figure 74-29). These fibrillatory waves are best seen in the inferior leads or lead V_1 and are described as "fine" to "coarse" based on their amplitude. Atrial fibrillation is the result of multiple microreentry circuits, creating 300 to 600 impulses/min.

The QRS complexes are usually narrow, unless an underlying bundle branch block is present. The previously mentioned *Ashman phenomenon* can cause isolated or

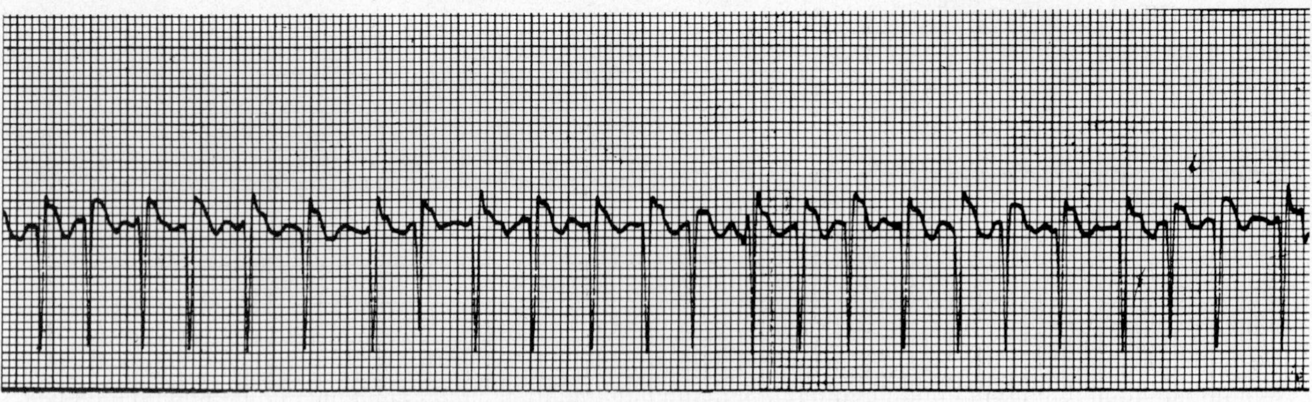

Figure 74-29. **Atrial fibrillation with rapid ventricular response.**

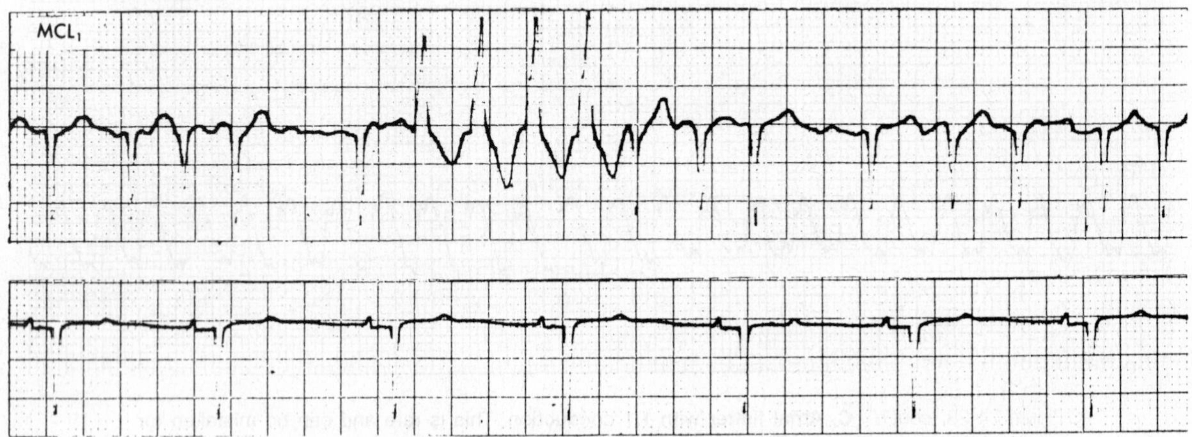

Figure 74-30. **Atrial fibrillation with classic Ashman phenomenon series of beats. Note long-short cycle before aberrantly conducted impulses.** *From Marriott HJL, Conover MB:* **Advanced concepts in arrhythmias,** *ed 2, St Louis, 1989, Mosby.*

repeated aberrant ventricular conduction, usually in a right bundle branch block pattern (Figure 74-30). These Ashman beats can be mistaken for PVCs if the long-short cycle sequence is not recognized. The ventricular response rate depends on the conduction path and ratio, with the normal AV node maximal response rate being no greater than 160 to 170 beats/min. As noted with atrial flutter, the presence of a chaotic rhythm (irrespective of the QRS duration) at a rate of more than 200 beats/min strongly suggests atrial fibrillation coupled with conduction down an accessory pathway. This rhythm is prone to deteriorating to ventricular fibrillation, especially if the rate reaches 250/min or greater or if an AV nodal blocking agent is administered.

Atrial fibrillation is associated with a variety of underlying diseases (Box 74-10) One etiology that may be seen in patients brought to the ED with new-onset atrial fibrillation is the "holiday heart syndrome," which is seen after an ethanol binge, producing atrial fibrillation, atrial flutter, or atrial tachycardia. These rhythms usually spontaneously revert to a sinus rhythm after 24 to 48 hours.

Atrial fibrillation may also result from the degeneration of atrial flutter, irrespective of the cause. In this case, an intermediary condition called *atrial fibrillation-flutter* is described by some, in which the surface ECG shows characteristics of both rhythms. This may be manifested as fine fibrillatory waves with irregular QRS complexes intermixed with flutter waves and a stretch of regular QRS complexes. Rapid atrial fibrillation followed by sinus bradycardia in an elderly patient suggests the aforementioned *bradycardia-tachycardia syndrome.* Finally, irregular atrial fibrillatory waves coupled with regular narrow or wide QRS complexes may represent atrial fibrillation coupled with complete heart block and an accelerated junctional or ventricular rhythm; this syndrome strongly suggests digitalis toxicity.

Treatment of atrial fibrillation is based on distinguishing it from other chaotic rhythms (Box 74-11) and the recognition of any underlying causes and symptoms. Asymptomatic atrial fibrillation at a rate of 120 beats/min or less requires no specific emergency therapy. Patients who are unstable from acute rapid atrial fibrillation should receive sedation and synchronized cardioversion starting at 50 to 100 J. Electrical cardioversion is not associated with an increased risk of malignant ventricular dysrhythmias in patients receiving digitalis unless clinical or laboratory evidence of toxicity coexists.

In the ED, the therapeutic course chosen depends on the aforementioned principles plus the duration of the dysrhyth-

Box 74-10 Causes of Atrial Fibrillation

Ischemic heart disease*
Valvular disease (especially mitral)*
Pericarditis
Hyperthyroidism
Sick sinus syndrome
Myocardial contusion
Acute ethanol intoxication (holiday heart syndrome)
Idiopathic
Hypertensive heart disease*
Cardiomyopathy*
Cardiac surgery
Catecholamine excess
Pulmonary embolism
Congestive heart failure*†
Accessory pathway (Wolff-Parkinson-White) syndrome‡

*Related to increased left atrial size.
†Can also be a result of atrial fibrillation.
‡Especially in patients with a ventricular response rate >200 beats/min.

Box 74-11 Pharmacologic Approach to Atrial Fibrillation Conversion

Intravenous procainamide, 50 mg/min, up to a total dose of 18 mg/kg (12 mg/kg in patients with congestive heart failure) or until conversion or side effects occur

or

Ibutilide, 0.015 to 0.02 mg/kg IV, over 10 minutes (conversion usually occurs within 20 minutes if successful)

or

Amiodarone, 5 mg/kg IV, over 10 to 15 minutes

or

Dofetilide 500 μg every 12 hours (decrease if renal failure present)

or

Oral quinidine sulfate, 200 to 300 mg initially, then 200 to 300 mg every hour until conversion, side effects, or a total dose of 1000 mg has been administered.

If needed:

A calcium channel blocker (verapamil, 40 to 80 mg orally or 5 to 10 mg IV, or diltiazem, 60 to 120 mg orally or 20 to 25 mg IV) can be given before the type IA agent (if no contraindications are present) to lower the ventricular response rate to <120 beats/min and to attenuate further tachycardia from the vagolytic effects of these agents.

mia. Both chronic and paroxysmal atrial fibrillation are associated with atrial thrombus formation and embolic events. Acute paroxysmal atrial fibrillation lasting longer than 72 hours is best treated initially by rate control if needed, as conversion to a sinus rhythm may be associated with an increased risk of embolic phenomenon within the first hours to days. The latter is especially true the longer atrial fibrillation has been present or when underlying valvular disease or chamber enlargement is present. In stable patients with new-onset atrial fibrillation of 48 hours or less duration, ventricular rate control and cardioversion can be attempted.[72] Patients with atrial fibrillation lasting longer than 48 hours should receive systemic anticoagulation for 1 to 3 weeks before attempts at conversion to decrease the risk of an embolic event. The longer duration of fibrillation predisposes to atrial clot formation; this clot can develop during fibrillation and after, the latter owing to "stunned myocardium" that can last for days after restoration of a sinus rhythm. Currently studies are underway to evaluate the role of transesophageal echocardiography in selecting patients at low risk for clot presence to shorten or eliminate the need for anticoagulation before cardioversion.

Emergency control of rapid ventricular response rates in symptomatic atrial fibrillation is best done with intravenous calcium channel blockers (verapamil or diltiazem) or β-adrenergic blockers, as both decrease AV nodal conduction and may interrupt the microreentry circuits responsible for the dysrhythmia. As noted earlier with atrial flutter, the relative effectiveness and complication rates in clinical practice between verapamil and diltiazem are similar in the absence of overt heart failure. Careful titration of either agent is appropriate; verapamil is less expensive.

β-adrenergic blockers are particularly effective in atrial fibrillation secondary to hyperthyroidism or catecholamine excess. Digitalis is a second- or third-line agent for ventricular rate control because of its relatively slow onset of action. Calcium channel and β-adrenergic blockers, adenosine, and digitalis should not be administered in patients with atrial fibrillation and an accessory pathway because of the risk of precipitating ventricular fibrillation.

Intravenous magnesium sulfate (2 g over 2 minutes) can serve as a third-line or adjunctive therapy to decrease the ventricular response rate. Similar to its use in atrial flutter, adenosine is not indicated as a primary therapy because of its short duration of effect. For outpatient rate control, calcium channel and β-adrenergic blockers are preferred over digitalis in those patients without contraindications.

Pharmacologic cardioversion of atrial fibrillation is best accomplished with a type IA or III agent.[6,7,27-30,38,40,73,74] If pharmacologic cardioversion is attempted, a calcium channel blocker or β-adrenergic blocker should be given before a type IA agent to control the ventricular rate, with a target of 100 to 120 beats/min before administering the type IA agent (see Box 74-11). This approach may also prevent or attenuate any increase in the ventricular rate from the type IA agent. In general, procainamide is preferred, as it is easier to administer in a timely fashion. Irrespective of the route and specific agents chosen, pharmacologic cardioversion requires close monitoring and extended observation; the latter may limit the use of this procedure in a busy ED. Other class III agents including ibutilide, amiodarone, and sotalol are alternatives to procainamide. Oral propafenone is another option, but is associated with longer conversion times without improved effect or safety compared with the previous agents noted.

Other type IC agents are not available for IV use in the United States (but are used in Europe for this indication) and therefore not currently indicated in the emergency management of atrial fibrillation. Electrical cardioversion (with 50 to 100 J) may be indicated if the previously described measures fail to convert symptomatic atrial fibrillation or in unstable patients. Although a synchronized countershock is recommended, the irregularity may require delivery of an unsynchronized countershock.

Admission criteria for a patient with atrial fibrillation include symptoms of instability or myocardial ischemia,

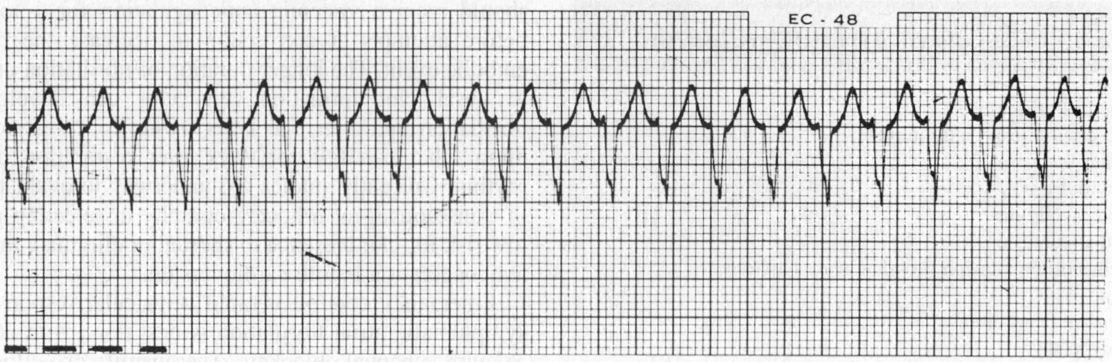

Figure 74-31. **Paroxysmal supraventricular tachycardia. Note the narrow, regular QRS complexes.**

symptomatic recurrence in the ED, or the need to electrically cardiovert. Traditionally, all patients with new-onset atrial fibrillation have been admitted to the hospital, irrespective of symptoms, to "rule out" causes such as occult myocardial ischemia or infarction and pulmonary embolism. These diagnoses are rarely occult, however, and selective discharge of patients in the absence of clinical evidence of acute coronary ischemia, new valve dysfunction, acute lung illness (including pulmonary embolism), or thyroid disease may be acceptable if close follow-up monitoring can be arranged after conversion to sinus rhythm.[75] Simply put, when precipitated by myocardial ischemia or pulmonary embolism, atrial fibrillation is usually accompanied by other signs or symptoms, so admission to "rule out MI or PE" in the absence of these signs or symptoms is not needed.

Junctional (Atrioventricular Nodal) Tachycardia The identification of paroxysmal junctional tachycardia (PJT) on the surface ECG is based on the presence of a narrow-complex regular tachycardia without preceding atrial depolarization waves (Figure 74-31). PJTs often produce retrograde atrial depolarization and a P′ wave, but these P′ waves are usually buried within the QRS complex. However, P′ waves may be located anywhere in relation to the QRS complex and assume either a normal or abnormal structure. The location of the P′ waves can be useful in defining the electrophysiologic source of a PJT and help distinguish it from other causes of a regular narrow-complex tachycardia (Figure 74-32).

Of all patients with a regular paroxysmal supraventricular tachycardia, reentrant PJT (also termed *AV nodal reentry*) is the most common cause.[68] The α-pathway within the AV node is used for anterograde conduction in 90% of cases of sustained PJT and accounts for the common finding of P waves buried within the QRS complexes (see Figure 74-32). Clinically, patients experience the abrupt onset of a regular tachycardia at a rate of 120 to 200 beats/min. A PJC or PAC often initiates PJT. Termination is also abrupt, from increased vagal tone, drug therapy, or spontaneous conversion. PJTs at a rate more than 200 beats/min are rare and when seen suggest an accessory pathway syndrome. As noted previously, sinus tachycardia may be easily mistaken for PJT in infants and young children.[69]

Nonparoxysmal (or sustained) junctional tachycardia (NPJT) is usually the result of an automatic mechanism, with gradual onset and termination and rarely exceeding a rate of 130 beats/min. Compared with PJT, NPJT is more often associated with underlying heart disease, electrolyte imbalance, or excess catecholamine states.

Asymptomatic junctional tachycardia at a rate less than 120 beats/min does not require specific therapy aside from correcting any underlying abnormalities, although outpatient treatment may be started. Stable symptomatic patients can be successfully treated in 85% to 90% of cases with a calcium channel blocker or a β-adrenergic blocker (see previous dosing regimens in pharmacology section) if PJT persists after vagal maneuvers.[76,77] Typically the tachycardia slows with treatment before abrupt conversion to a sinus rhythm; this slowing is the result of increasing block within the reentrant circuit. Adenosine is another first-line option for emergent therapy, giving initial success rates similar to those seen with verapamil but higher recurrence rates because of the short therapeutic effect.[59-61] Calcium channel blockers and adenosine have been studied in the prehospital treatment of PJTs, with both considered safe and effective in the presence of strong medical control.[78,79]

Synchronized cardioversion with 50 to 100 J should be performed in unstable patients with PJT or NPJT. Refractory but stable patients can be treated with procainamide or amiodarone.

Many adult patients can be discharged to home if the PJT is terminated. Oral therapy with a class II or IV agent should be considered for those with frequent symptomatic episodes of PJT. Those patients with underlying serious medical illnesses, recurrent symptoms, or any evidence of instability should be admitted. Most patients requiring electrical cardioversion should be admitted, although an otherwise healthy patient who is easily cardioverted without recurrence may be considered for discharge with close outpatient follow-up monitoring. Referral for ambulatory Holter monitoring and electrophysiology studies/interventions should be considered for anyone discharged to home who has not previously been evaluated, particularly if recurrent or associated with profound symptoms.

Preexcitation and Accessory Pathway Syndromes

Preexcitation refers to depolarization of the ventricular myocardium earlier than would occur by conduction of an impulse through the AV node. This implies the existence of a pathway from the atria to the ventricular myocardium in addition to the AV node, hence the term *accessory pathway.* These terms are related but not interchangeable, as not all accessory paths are used to activate the ventricles early.

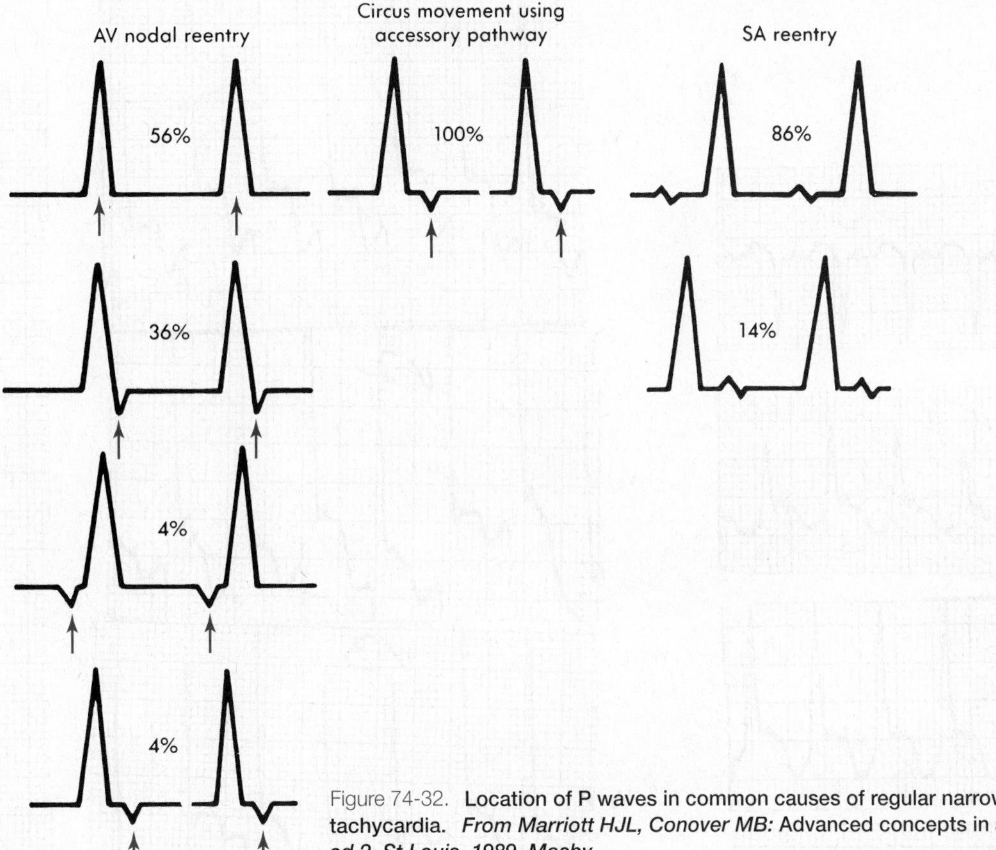

Figure 74-32. **Location of P waves in common causes of regular narrow-complex tachycardia.** ***From Marriott HJL, Conover MB:*** **Advanced concepts in arrhythmias, *ed 2, St Louis, 1989, Mosby.***

The Wolff-Parkinson-White (WPW) syndrome is the most common accessory pathway syndrome, although it likely represents a group of pathologic conditions.[80] The clinical hallmark of this syndrome is paroxysmal tachycardia at a rate of 150 to 300 beats/min, the direct result of the loss of the normal AV node conduction restraint. Any tachycardia in an adult at a rate greater than 200 beats/min should raise the suspicion of an accessory pathway syndrome.

The classic WPW syndrome consists of tachycardia with the following three features (Figure 74-33):

- A short PR interval (<0.12 second)
- QRS duration greater than 0.10 second
- A slurred upstroke to the QRS complex, referred to as a *delta wave*

The short PR interval is the result of the absent AV node conduction delay, and the delta wave occurs because of early activation of the ventricular myocardium. Although the WPW syndrome typically has a prolonged QRS duration as a result of the delta wave, the QRS duration commonly varies based on the location and conduction direction of the accessory pathway. Those pathways inserting into infranodal conducting tissues can produce a near-normal QRS complex, whereas those inserting in the nonconductive tissues produce a wide QRS complex with an abnormal structure. If this classic triad is present, secondary T-wave changes (a deflection opposite the main QRS vector) are seen.

The accessory path(s) can participate in a reentry circuit that produces or sustains the tachycardia. The AV node often makes up one limb of these circuits. When the QRS complex is narrow and a delta wave is absent, the AV node is being used for anterograde conduction to the ventricles and the accessory path is used for retrograde conduction; this is termed an *orthodromic tachycardia.* Conversely, if the QRS complex is wide and a delta wave is present, the accessory pathway is being used as the anterograde limb and the AV node the retrograde limb of the reentry circuit; this is termed an *antidromic tachycardia.* The majority of symptomatic patients with the WPW syndrome have a regular orthodromic tachycardia.[80] However, the asymptomatic WPW syndrome is usually discovered when a delta wave(s) is seen on the ECG during sinus rhythm (Figure 74-34).

Patients with the WPW syndrome often have one or more of the classic features missing on the surface ECG, especially if a sinus rhythm is present at the time of evaluation. In these times, the presence of the pathway is concealed, and the normal sinus impulse is carried to the ventricles through the AV node. A PAC, PJC, or PVC can serve to initiate a tachycardia. The WPW syndrome is present in 0.1% to 0.3% of the population, with males affected twice as often as females. Based on this prevalence, it is estimated that only 25% to 50% of patients with the WPW syndrome become symptomatic. The WPW syndrome is associated with a variety of conditions, although up to 70% of patients have no underlying heart disease (Box 74-12). In those without underlying heart disease, especially if the WPW syndrome is discovered in the absence of symptoms, the prognosis is excellent, with an extremely low risk of sudden death. It is postulated that most patients with asymptomatic delta waves eventually lose the ability to conduct through the accessory pathway.

The presenting rhythm in symptomatic patients with the WPW syndrome is usually a reentrant tachycardia (70% to

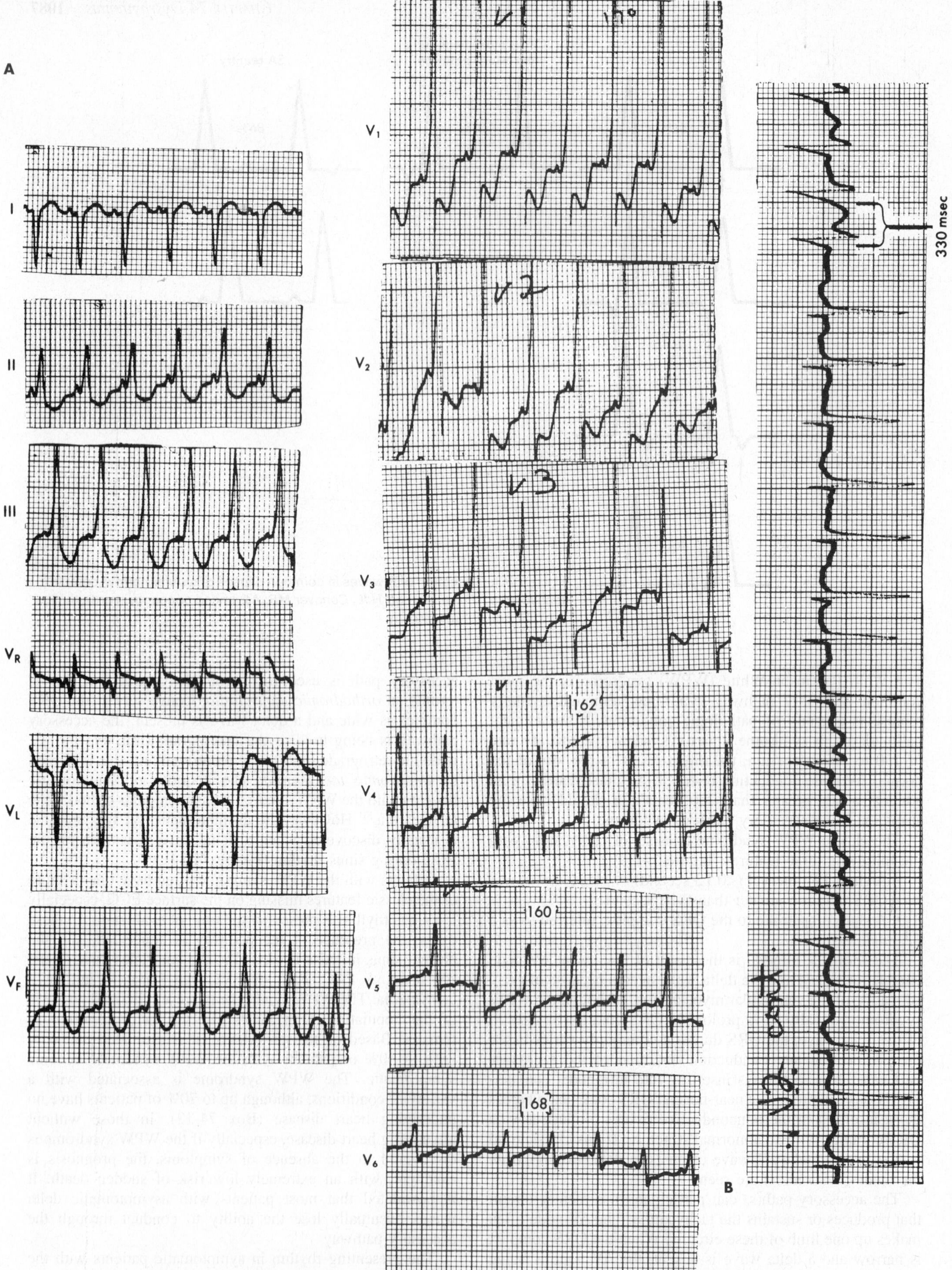

Figure 74-33. **A, Wolff-Parkinson-White (WPW) syndrome. B, WPW syndrome with atrial fibrillation. Note short refractory period (330 msec).** *A, from Watanabe Y, Dreifus LS:* Cardiac arrhythmias, *New York, 1977, Grune & Stratton.*

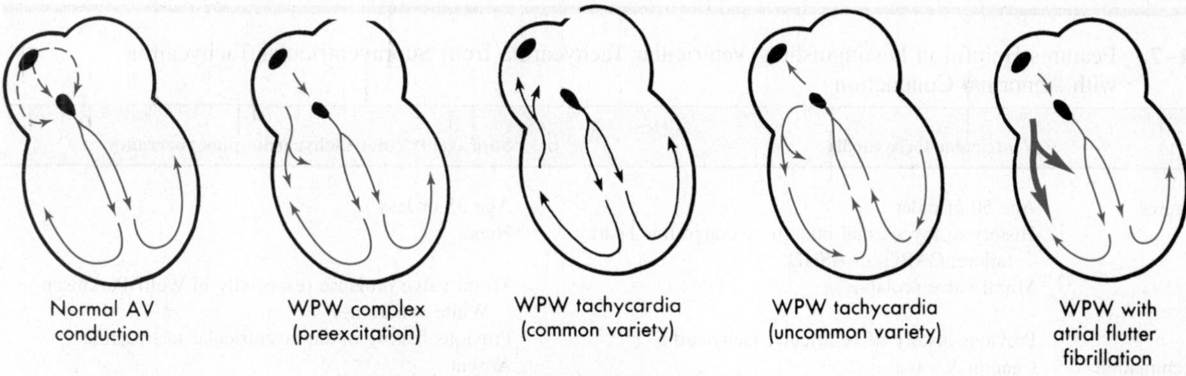

Figure 74-34. **WPW paths and associated rhythms.** *From Watanabe Y, Dreifus LS:* **Cardiac arrhythmias,** *New York, 1977, Grune & Stratton.*

Box 74-12 Diseases Associated with Wolff-Parkinson-White Syndrome

Idiopathic*
Cardiomyopathy (especially hypertrophic)
Transposition of great vessels
Endocardial fibroelastosis
Mitral valve prolapse
Tricuspid atresia
Ebstein disease

*Most common.

80%), although atrial fibrillation can be seen in 10% to 30% of patients.[80,81] Emergency treatment depends on the following three observations:

- Symptoms of instability
- Prolonged QRS duration or delta-wave presence (see Figure 74-33)
- QRS regularity or irregularity (see Figure 74-33)

Unstable patients, irrespective of the QRS duration or regularity, should be cardioverted (synchronized preferred) with 50 to 100 J (0.5 to 2 J/kg for children) after sedation if time permits.

A regular orthodromic (narrow QRS complex) tachycardia is the single most common presentation of the WPW syndrome and is treated the same as PJT. Calcium channel blockers, β-adrenergic blockers, adenosine, procainamide, and amiodarone are all suitable for first-line therapy if vagal maneuvers fail. We prefer to use procainamide or amiodarone as the primary therapy for all stable patients with the WPW syndrome and tachycardia because of their effectiveness and safety irrespective of the conduction pathway. Digitalis or class IC agents are alternative therapies for orthodromic (narrow QRS complex) regular tachycardias. All of these drugs except adenosine are suitable for outpatient prophylaxis after termination of the tachycardia in the ED. Lidocaine is unlikely to have any effect on orthodromic WPW-related tachycardia,[82] and magnesium is not well studied in this syndrome.

Symptomatic patients with an antidromic (wide QRS complex) regular tachycardia or any irregular tachycardia (irrespective of QRS duration) have a more serious prognosis because of the high risk of ventricular fibrillation, especially when the RR interval is less than 0.20 second. In these situations, *all AV nodal blocking drugs (especially calcium channel and β-adrenergic blockers, but also digoxin and adenosine) are contraindicated.*[63,80,83-85] These agents may create a faster ventricular response rate from unopposed and potentially enhanced conduction through the accessory path. The rapid rates are associated with a high risk of degeneration into intractable ventricular fibrillation. It is important to emphasize that irregularity can be difficult to detect at extremely fast rates and must be carefully sought. A wide-complex irregular tachycardia at a rate of 250 beats/min or greater is highly suggestive of atrial fibrillation and the WPW syndrome.

Procainamide or amiodarone are the drugs of choice in all antidromic or irregular WPW-related tachycardias.[32,86] Electrical cardioversion should be considered any time the ventricular rate is 250 beats/min or greater, or if clinical deterioration is noted during drug therapy. The other class IA and IC agents are second-line drugs, but the latter are not currently available for intravenous use. Lidocaine has unclear utility in antidromic or irregular accessory pathway syndromes; it usually has little effect on conduction, although isolated reports of both decreased and enhanced conduction through the accessory pathway have been published.[82-87] For these reasons, lidocaine is not recommended for antidromic or irregular accessory pathway syndromes.

All patients requiring electrical cardioversion should be observed for an extended period or admitted to the hospital, as should patients who experience recurrence in the ED and those with underlying complicating diseases or symptoms such as chest pain, congestive heart failure, and electrolyte imbalance. Those easily terminated without the aforementioned features can be discharged and referred for electrophysiologic studies to map the location of the pathway. These studies are not indicated in the asymptomatic patient, although exercise ECG testing may be used to determine the true latency of the pathway.

The Lown-Ganong-Levine syndrome is a rare accessory pathway syndrome associated with paroxysmal tachycardia, a short PR interval, and a normal QRS complex. The syndrome is believed to be the result of an intranodal bypass tract. Patients usually have a paroxysmal reentrant narrow-complex tachycardia initially, but occasionally ventricular tachycardia is seen. The treatment parallels that for the WPW syndrome.

Table 74-7. Features Helpful in Distinguishing Ventricular Tachycardia from Supraventricular Tachycardia with Abnormal Conduction

	Ventricular tachycardia	Supraventricular tachycardia plus aberrancy
Clinical features	Age 50 or older	Age 35 or less
	History of myocardial infarction, congestive heart failure, CABG, or ASHD	None
	Mitral valve prolapse	Mitral valve prolapse (especially in Wolff-Parkinson-White syndrome)
	Previous history of ventricular tachycardia	Previous history of supraventricular tachycardia
Physical examination	Cannon A waves	Absent
	Variation in arterial pulse	Absence of variability
	Variable first heart sound	Absence of variability
ECG	Fusion beats	None
	AV dissociation	Preceding P waves with QRS complexes
	QRS > 0.14 sec	QRS usually < 0.14 sec
	Extreme LAD (<−30 degrees)	Axis normal or slightly abnormal
	No response to vagal maneuvers	Slow or terminate with vagal maneuvers
Specific QRS patterns	V_1: R, qR, or RS	V1: rsR′
	V_6: S, rS, or qR	V6: qRs
	Identical to previous ventricular tachycardia tracing*	Identical to previous supraventricular tachycardia tracing*
	Concordance of positivity or negativity†	

*If proven by electrophysiologic studies or by a preponderance of evidence.
†Main deflection of QRS complex either positive or negative in every precordial lead.
CABG, Coronary artery bypass graft; *ASHD,* arteriosclerotic heart disease; *LAD,* left anterior descending artery.

Wide-Complex Tachycardias *Wide-complex tachycardia* refers to dysrhythmias greater than 100 beats/min associated with a QRS duration of 0.12 second or more.[88,89] Wide-complex tachycardia can be divided into two broad categories, based on whether the initiating focus is supraventricular or ventricular. Supraventricular foci can produce a wide-complex tachycardia if a conduction abnormality exists. The widened QRS can occur with a preexisting bundle branch block, with an acquired bundle branch block (often related to fast or irregular heart rates and ischemia), or from conduction through an accessory pathway. A focus below the level of the AV node results in ventricular tachycardia. The treatment of wide-complex tachycardia is based on the ability to distinguish ventricular tachycardia from supraventricular tachycardia with abnormal conduction.

The approach to the differential diagnosis of a wide-complex tachycardia is based on systemic evaluation of evidence gained from a focused history, physical examination, and ECG tracing. The Wellens criteria (Table 74-7)[88-89] are based on multiple, unordered clinical data points to help estimate the likelihood of a ventricular or supraventricular source. As an improvement, the Brugada criteria[90-91] use the ECG principles encased in the Wellens approach, surrounded in a 4-step decision tree approach (Figure 74-35).

No single criterion or system that helps distinguish a supraventricular from a ventricular source is infallible. A careful collection of multiple data points, however, will usually lead to the correct diagnosis. *The treating physician should always initially assume that any new onset symptomatic wide-complex tachycardia is ventricular tachycardia until proven.* When in doubt, choose an agent safe and effective for any cause of wide complex tachycardia; procainamide or amiodarone is ideal in this setting. Lidocaine is usually safe unless concomitant hyperkalemia exists (which may precipitate asystole[15]), but has no consistent effect on supraventricular rhythms.

Patients with a history of a previous myocardial infarction are far more likely to have ventricular tachycardia than supraventricular tachycardia with abnormal conduction.[92,93] This point, coupled with the onset of a dysrhythmia after the infarction, strongly suggests the diagnosis of ventricular tachycardia. Other historical features more frequently associated with ventricular tachycardia are an age of 50 years or older, known ischemic heart disease, congestive heart failure, and a previous history of ventricular dysrhythmias. Conversely, younger patients (< 35 years) and those with a history of supraventricular tachycardia are more likely to have a supraventricular source with abnormal conduction.

During the physical examination, clues about the source of a wide-complex tachycardia can be gleaned from careful inspection, auscultation, and specific maneuvers. Evidence of AV dissociation (variation in the first heart sound or in the systolic blood pressure beat to beat, or cannon jugular waves) suggests a ventricular origin. The absence of these findings, however, does not imply a supraventricular source. Slowing or termination of a wide-complex tachycardia in response to carotid sinus massage, Valsalva maneuvers, or other techniques of increasing vagal tone suggests a supraventricular source.

One common error in the differential diagnosis of wide-complex tachycardia is the belief that the blood pressure and level of consciousness can be used to distinguish ventricular tachycardia from supraventricular tachycardia with abnormal conduction. Although ventricular tachycardia is more often associated with reduced cardiac output, hypotension, and a depressed sensorium, the absolute blood pressure and level of consciousness are not useful in discriminating ventricular tachycardia from supraventricular tachycardia with abnormal conduction.[92-94] Many patients with ventricular tachycardia tolerate the dysrhythmia well, with few subjective complaints.

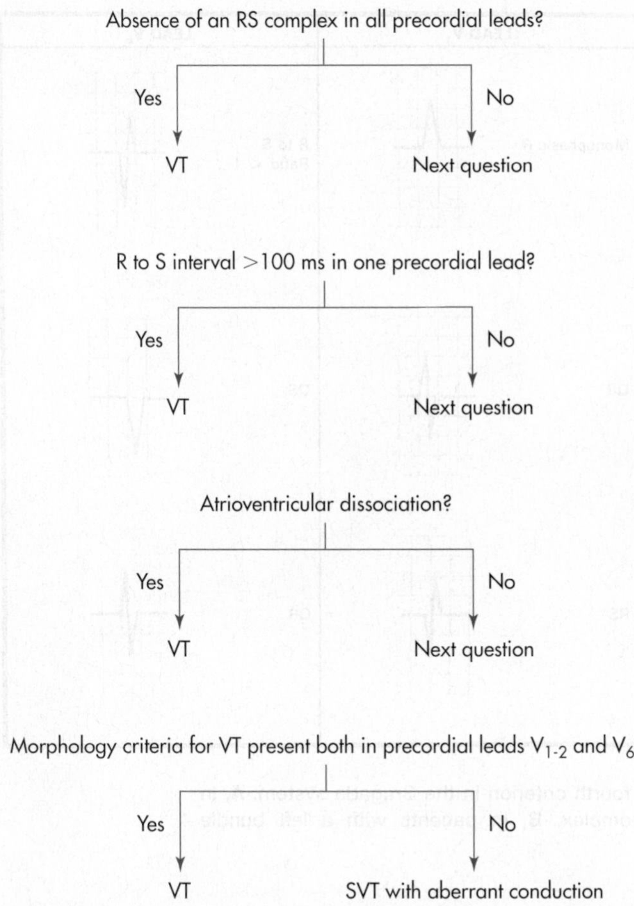

Figure 74-35. **Four-step approach for differentiating ventricular tachycardia and wide QRS SVT. Only when a negative response to all four questions occurs is a supraventricular rhythm with abnormal conduction diagnosed. As soon as a single "yes" answer is noted, ventricular tachycardia is diagnosed.** ***Modified from Brugada P et al:* Circulation *83:1649, 1991, American Heart Association.***

ECG clues to the origin of a wide-complex tachycardia can be distilled into a few simple rules (see Table 74-7 and Figure 74-35). *Evidence of AV dissociation strongly suggests a ventricular source for a wide-complex tachycardia.* Retrograde conduction to the atria during ventricular tachycardia, however, can occasionally produce a consistent P′ wave after the QRS complex, creating the appearance of AV association (though the P waves should look abnormal). Another strong indicator that ventricular tachycardia is present are "fusion beats," which occur when an atrial impulse reaches the AV node and infranodal conduction system at the same time as the ventricular impulse, creating a hybrid QRS complex. This hybrid fusion QRS complex is often intermediate in duration and structure between the narrow atrial impulse and the wide ventricular impulse.

The appearance of specific QRS patterns in the precordial leads, especially leads V_1 and V_6, can also help identify the origin of a wide-complex tachycardia (see Table 74-7). A QRS duration of greater than 0.14 second is more commonly associated with ventricular tachycardia, especially when coupled with a history of previous myocardial infarction. A bizarre QRS axis, manifested as an extreme left-axis deviation, also suggests ventricular tachycardia. Finally, a previous ECG tracing can be helpful; QRS complexes that are identical to those seen on an old ECG strongly suggest the same source. If the QRS morphology during a wide-complex tachycardia is the same as the morphology of sinus rhythm with bundle branch block, then it is more likely that the wide-complex tachycardia is supraventricular with aberration, rather than ventricular tachycardia. This indicator is not without pitfalls; subtle changes in QRS morphology or duration can be difficult to see, but may be important clues in separating ventricular tachycardia from supraventricular tachycardia with abnormal conduction.[95]

The Brugada ECG-based criteria search for four pieces of evidence of ventricular tachycardia from among those listed previously[90,91] (Figure 74-36); as soon as one is found, the diagnosis is made. *The rhythm must be regular to use these criteria* (irregularity or chaos suggests atrial fibrillation with altered conduction). The sequential criteria are shown in Figure 74-35. Only in the absence of all of the is a supraventricular etiology diagnosed. Although the original authors found excellent sensitivity (98.7%) and specificity (96.5%) in detecting VT, follow-up investigations did not duplicate this level of accuracy in ED patients, with nonagreement between emergency physicians seen in 22% of cases. Also, it is clear that in patients receiving class I agents the Brugada criteria are less reliable.

Most episodes of ventricular tachycardia and supraventricular tachycardia with abnormal conduction are completely or predominately regular, although some irregularity can be seen with both, limiting the usefulness of this finding. *A wide-complex tachycardia with an underlying chaotic rhythm (irregularly irregular) should raise the suspicion of atrial fibrillation with abnormal conduction.* The conduction abnormality can result from a preexisting bundle branch block, an acquired bundle branch block (often in a right bundle branch block appearance), or an accessory pathway syndrome. The last should be suspected whenever a chaotic rhythm at a rate of 200 beats/min or greater is seen, irrespective of the QRS duration.

Unstable patients with a wide-complex tachycardia should be treated as if ventricular tachycardia is present. For unstable patients with a wide-complex tachycardia and a palpable pulse, cardioversion with 50 to 100 J initially (with sedation if time permits) is recommended. If the initial countershock(s) is unsuccessful, repeat attempts with increased doses in 50 to 100 J increments (up to a maximum of 360 to 400 J) should be administered. Although a synchronized countershock is preferred, unsynchronized countershock of ventricular tachycardia is acceptable and is not associated with an increased risk of postcardioversion ventricular fibrillation (occurring at an incidence of 5% with both methods).

If the patient is "borderline unstable" (only one nonextreme symptom or sign present) or if the patient is stable but the source of the wide-complex tachycardia is unclear, treatment should proceed on the assumption that ventricular tachycardia is present. Pharmacologic agents such as amiodarone, procainamide, or lidocaine can be used. Lidocaine can be given rapidly and will terminate many cases of ventricular tachycardia, although its overall success rate may be lower than the other first-line drugs.[5,10-13,15,31,34-36] Lidocaine is unlikely to have an appreciable effect on a supraventricular tachycardia with abnormal conduction, but will cause no harm. Many authors prefer procainamide or amiodarone as the initial agent in patients with a wide-

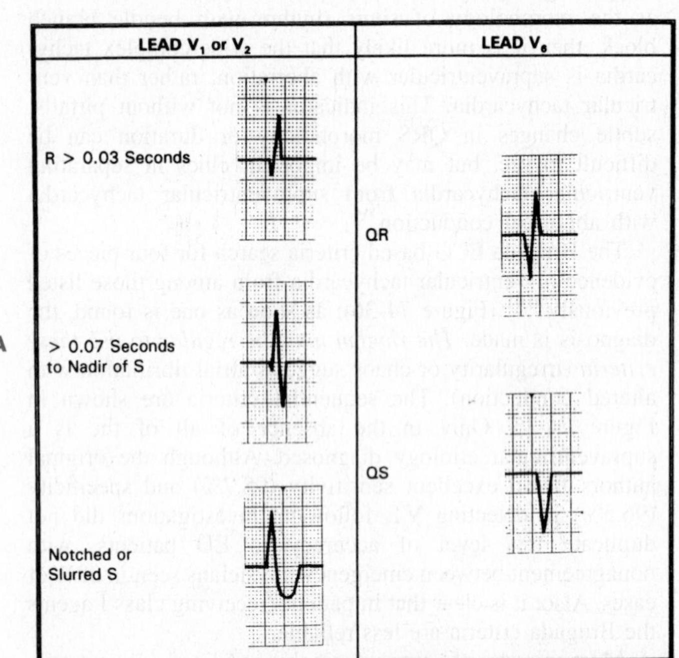

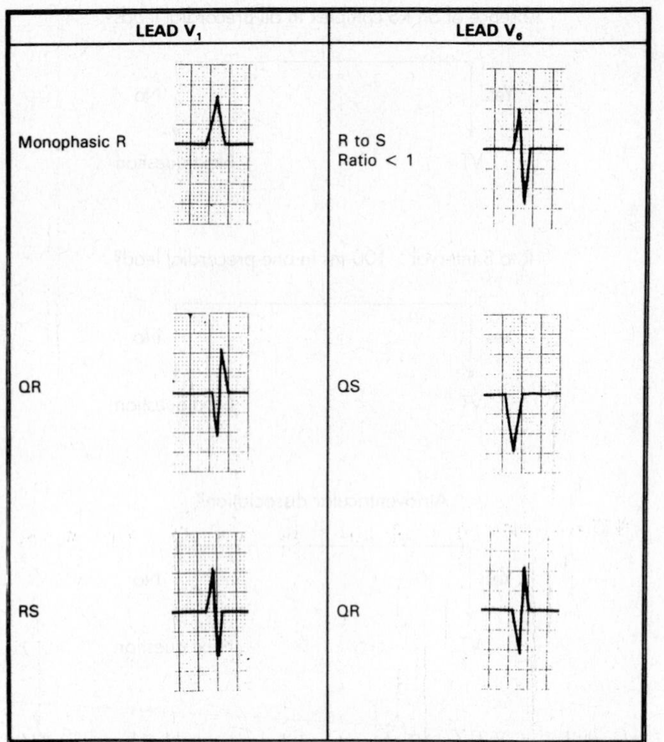

Figure 74-36. **The morphology associated with the fourth criterion in the Brugada system. A, In patients with a right bundle branch-appearing complex. B, In patients with a left bundle branch-appearing complex.**

complex tachycardia of uncertain origin, as they can convert both supraventricular tachycardia (including those associated with accessory pathways) and ventricular tachycardia. Electrical cardioversion remains an option in "borderline" or stable patients if pharmacologic treatment fails.

Because ventricular tachycardia rarely responds to adenosine (approximately 5% to 10% of cases)[95] and because most supraventricular tachycardias are terminated or temporarily slowed, it has been suggested that this agent be used to help in the differential diagnosis of wide-complex tachycardia. Overall, this approach is relatively safe, although case reports of poorly defined hemodynamic collapse after adenosine administration in wide-complex tachycardia exist, tempering the widespread enthusiasm associated with this approach.[63] *The evaluation of clinical and ECG data should not be replaced with indiscriminate adenosine (or other drug) therapy.* This parallels (albeit to a much lessor magnitude) the experience with calcium channel blockers, which were previously believed to be useful as a diagnostic measure for similar reasons. It is now clear that calcium channel blockers are contraindicated in the initial treatment of wide-complex tachycardia.[70] Although calcium channel blockers have little direct effect on most forms of ventricular tachycardia, many patients with this rhythm experience immediate cardiovascular collapse from the vasodilatory effects of these drugs. When a supraventricular source for a wide-complex tachycardia has been verified, the principles of treatment parallel those outlined for narrow-complex tachycardia.

Ventricular sources of wide-complex tachycardia can be divided into three categories: ventricular fibrillation and flutter, paced ventricular rhythms, and ventricular tachycardia.

Ventricular Tachycardia Ventricular tachycardia is the result of a dysrhythmia originating within or below the termination of the His bundle.[88] On the ECG, a minimum of three consecutive wide QRS complex beats is necessary to diagnose ventricular tachycardia. *Nonsustained* refers to short episodes (seconds) that spontaneously revert, whereas the term *sustained ventricular tachycardia* refers to more prolonged episodes. Reentry mechanisms are the most common cause of ventricular tachycardia, although automatic and triggered mechanisms also occur. Ventricular tachycardia can be precipitated by any extrasystole, with PVCs being the most common inciting stimulus. Extrasystoles that occur during ventricular repolarization (the R-on-T phenomenon) are commonly believed to carry a high risk of precipitating ventricular tachycardia, although the magnitude of this risk is debated. Most patients with ventricular tachycardia have underlying heart disease, although other conditions can be responsible.

Several groups of ventricular tachycardia can be identified based on the ECG pattern and history.[88,96] *Monomorphic ventricular tachycardia* can occur in the presence or absence of ischemic heart disease and appears as morphologically consistent QRS complexes, usually in a regular pattern and at a rate of 150 to 200 beats/min (Figures 74-37 and 74-38). An irregular rhythm and a rate greater than 200 beats/min or less than 150 beats/min may be seen in some cases of

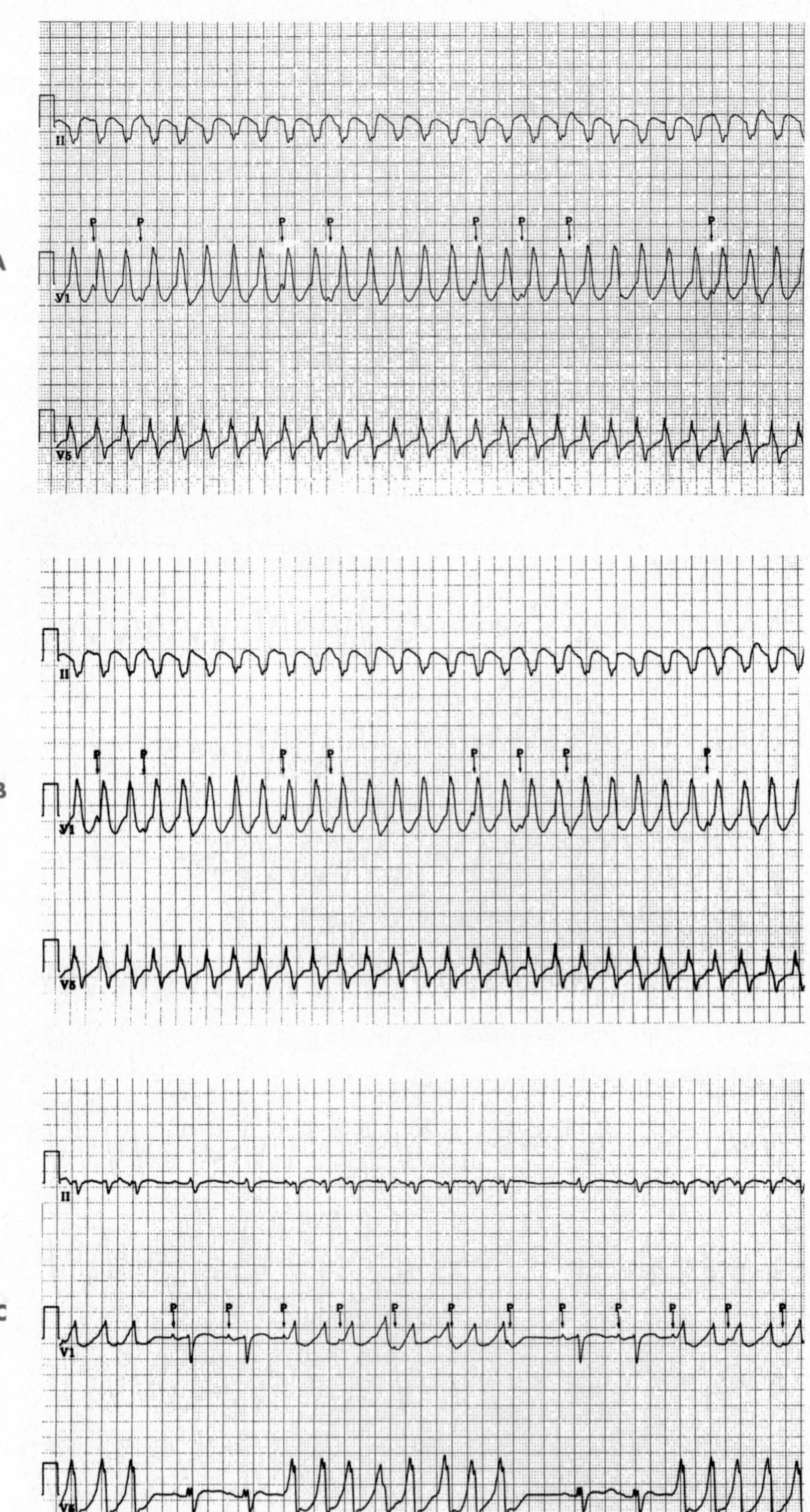

Figure 74-37. **A and B, Ventricular tachycardia. Note atrioventricular dissociation. C, Intermittent, nonsustained ventricular tachycardia. Atrioventricular dissociation is evident.** *Courtesy Edward Curtis, MD.*

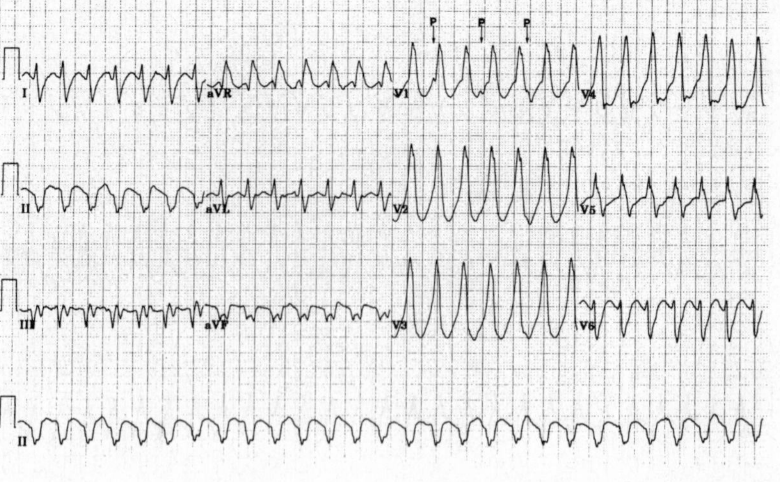

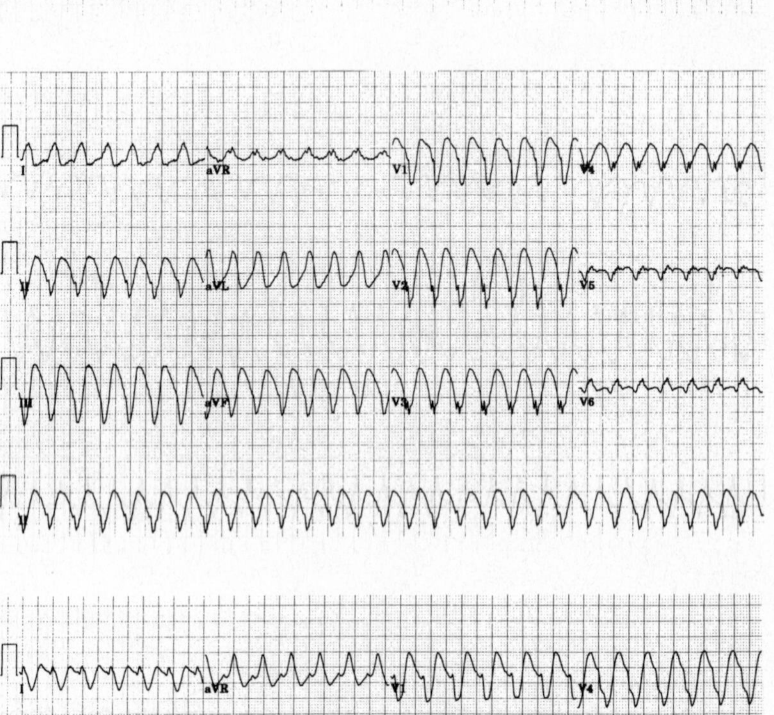

C

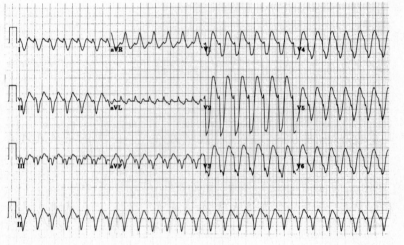

Figure 74-38. **Ventricular tachycardia. A, RS complexes are present in chest leads, but RS duration is >100 ms. Although Brugada criteria indicate that no further analysis is necessary, atrioventricular dissociation is also evident and QRS morphology (R:S ratio < 1 in lead V_6) is consistent with ventricular tachycardia. B, Some RS complexes are present, RS duration is not >100 ms, and AV dissociation is difficult to appreciate; morphologic criteria for ventricular tachycardia are fulfilled because S is notched in V_1 and QR is present in V_6. C, Diagnosis is based on morphologic criteria because S is notched or slurred in V_1 and V_2 and QS is present in V_6.** *Courtesy Edward Curtis, MD.*

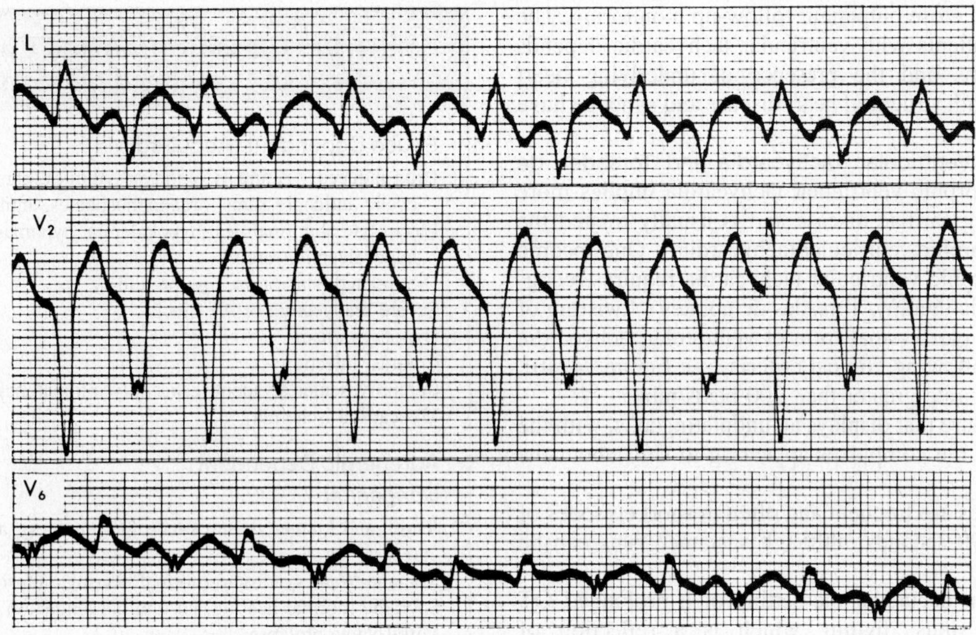

Figure 74-39. **Bidirectional ventricular tachycardia in a patient with digitalis toxicity.** *From Marriott HJL, Conover MB:* Advanced concepts in arrhythmias, *ed 2, St Louis, 1989, Mosby.*

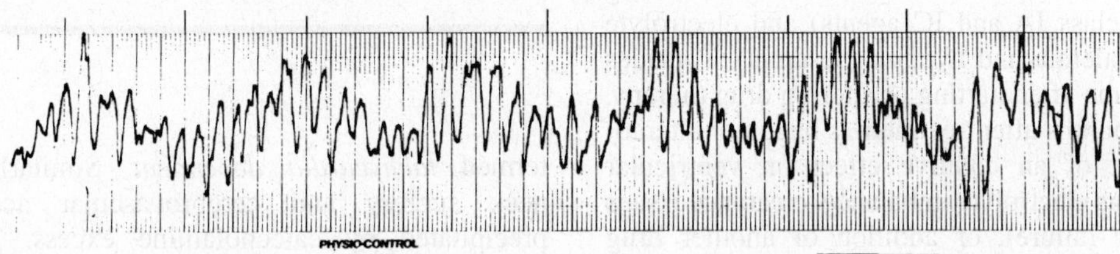

Figure 74-40. **Torsades de pointes with classic spiraling of QRS complexes around baseline.**

monomorphic ventricular tachycardia. Monomorphic ventricular tachycardia associated with chronic coronary artery disease is the single most common form of ventricular tachycardia.

Polymorphic ventricular tachycardia is manifested as QRS complexes that vary in structure or duration and is associated with more severe underlying disease[97] (Figures 74-39 and 74-40). *Torsades de pointes* is a specific form of polymorphic ventricular tachycardia. *Bidirectional* (or *alternating*) *ventricular tachycardia* occurs most frequently in digitalis intoxication and appears as a ventricular tachycardia with a QRS structure and an axis that change periodically (see Figure 74-39). During all forms of ventricular tachycardia, the main vectors of the ST segment and T wave are usually in an opposite direction from the terminal portion of the QRS complex; this phenomenon is termed a *secondary repolarization abnormality*.

Treatment of stable monomorphic ventricular tachycardia is based on correcting any underlying cause (especially electrolyte imbalance, hypoxemia or hypercapnia, and myocardial ischemia) and pharmacologically intervening to terminate the dysrhythmia. Amiodarone (5 mg/kg or 300 mg), procainamide (up to 18 mg/kg over 30 minutes), or lidocaine (1.0 to 1.5 mg/kg bolus, up to 3 mg/kg maximum) remain the drugs of choice initially, with up to 90% of episodes successfully terminated. Sotalol (1.5 mg/kg over 10 minutes) is a second-line option. Magnesium sulfate (2 to 4 g IV as a slow bolus) is another option in the treatment of ventricular tachycardia, especially in the setting of ischemia, although most data supporting it are anecdotal or from small case series. Unstable patients or those refractory to drug therapy should be cardioverted with 50 to 100 J initially, with maximal doses of 360 J in 50 to 100 J increments.

In the rare cases of ventricular tachycardia caused solely by catecholamine excess, β-adrenergic blockers may be useful in the primary treatment; otherwise, these agents are best suited for prophylaxis. Calcium channel blockers may prevent ventricular tachycardia associated with reperfusion, but are not indicated for the treatment of ventricular tachycardia. These two classes of agents are also useful in young patients without underlying structural heart disease who have monomorphic ventricular tachycardia and a classic right bundle branch block (calcium channel blockers) or left bundle branch block (β-blockers) pattern.

All patients with symptomatic ventricular tachycardia, new-onset ventricular tachycardia, or ventricular tachycardia requiring electrical therapy should be admitted. The only patients eligible for discharge are those with chronic ventricular tachycardia who have no change in symptoms or acute ischemia. These patients should be released after consultation with close outpatient follow-up monitoring. The prognosis for patients with ventricular tachycardia depends on the symptoms and the presence of underlying heart disease. Those with structural heart disease and syncope have a poor prognosis.

Polymorphic Ventricular Tachycardia and Torsades de Pointes Polymorphic ventricular tachycardia implies more severe underlying cardiac disease and is usually treated the same as monomorphic ventricular tachycardia.[97] One specific form of polymorphic ventricular tachycardia requires recognition and specific therapy. Torsades de pointes ("twisting of the points") is a paroxysmal form of ventricular tachycardia that meets the following clinical criteria (see Figure 74-40):

1. Ventricular rate greater than 200 beats/min.
2. QRS structure that displays an undulating axis, with the polarity of the complexes appearing to shift about the baseline.
3. Occurrences are frequent and often in short episodes of less than 90 seconds, although sustained runs can be seen.

Torsades often occurs in the setting of a prolonged QT interval during sinus rhythm, which is a reflection of abnormal ventricular repolarization. The true normal ranges for QT duration are debated and must be corrected for age, sex, and heart rate. This repolarization abnormality can be congenital or acquired; the latter is more common. Acquired QT prolongation and torsades are often the result of drug therapy (especially class IA and IC agents) and electrolyte disturbances (hypokalemia and hypomagnesemia). Torsades can be seen at any time after starting or altering drug therapy. Delayed episodes (months after treatment is begun or altered) are often the result of an additive effect on ventricular repolarization, such as electrolyte imbalance, clearance issues (e.g., renal or liver failure), or addition of another drug implicated in this syndrome.

The majority of adult cases of torsades are *pause dependent* and are associated with an acquired QT prolongation (Box 74-13). These episodes of torsades are precipitated by a slow heart rate. Treatment is based on correcting any underlying metabolic or electrolyte abnormalities and increasing the heart rate to shorten ventricular repolarization. The latter can be done with isoproterenol or overdrive pacing (external or transvenous) to a ventricular rate of 100 to 120 beats/min. Intravenous magnesium sulfate (2 to 4g IV) may terminate or prevent paroxysmal torsades.[98] Little data exist regarding the use of other drugs. The class IB agents (including lidocaine and phenytoin) shorten repolarization, but the overall success rate is unclear and seemingly low.[99] Class IA and IC agents are contraindicated, as they may aggravate the dysrhythmia by further prolonging repolarization. Little data exist regarding the usefulness of the class III agents in polymorphic ventricular tachycardia, although their properties frequently induce this condition. Sustained torsades should be treated with cardioversion as outlined in the treatment of ventricular tachycardia.

Unsynchronized countershocks (50 to 100 J) initially up to a maximal dose of 360 J will usually be needed because of the varying R-wave structures. Torsades related to class III agents may not be associated with QT prolongation but is otherwise treated the same as already described.

In contrast, torsades de pointes associated with a congenital QT prolongation syndrome is rare and usually presents in childhood or early adulthood. This form is precipitated by catecholamine excess (e.g., exercise or medications) and termed *tachycardia dependent.* Similarly, torsades after neck surgery and cerebrovascular accidents may be precipitated by catecholamine excess. Treatment of all forms of catecholamine-induced torsades is based on slowing the heart rate, usually with β-adrenergic blockers.

Box 74-13 Classification and Causes of Prolonged QT Syndromes

Pause Dependent (Acquired)

Drug induced: 1A and 1C antidysrhythmics, phenothiazines, cyclic antidepressants, organophosphates, antihistamines.
Electrolyte abnormalities: hypokalemia, hypomagnesemia, hypocalcemia (rarely)
Diet related: starvation, low protein
Severe bradycardia or AV block
Hypothyroidism
Contrast injection
Cerebrovascular accident (especially intraparenchymal)
Myocardial ischemia

Adrenergic Dependent

Congenital

Jervell and Lange-Nielsen syndrome (deafness, autosomal recessive)
Romano-Ward syndrome (normal hearing, autosomal dominant)
Sporadic (normal hearing, no familial tendency)
Mitral valve prolapse

Acquired

Cerebrovascular disease (especially subarachnoid hemorrhage)
Autonomic aurgery: radical neck dissection, carotid endarterectomy, truncal vagotomy

KEY CONCEPTS

- Unstable patients with a new dysrhythmia deserve a very focused examination, brief ECG analysis, and prompt electrical therapy (pacing for slow rates, countershock at 100 J for most fast rates).
- Digoxin is not an emergent intervention in dysrhythmia treatment.
- New-onset wide-complex tachycardia with symptoms is ventricular tachycardia until proven otherwise; the fatal mistakes a physician can make come from assuming a supraventricular source is present. Procainamide and amiodarone are good choices if uncertainty exists. Adenosine is recommended in patients in whom a supraventricular source is suspected and not as a "blind" diagnostic/therapeutic agent.
- All ECG criteria that differentiate ventricular tachycardia from supraventricular tachycardia are fallible, although some (e.g., AV dissociation, previous tracing identical) are less so.
- Admission decisions are generally based on the cause, end-organ manifestations, or recurrence/persistence of a rhythm rather than the presence of a specific rhythm.
- Very fast heart rates (> 250/min) usually are the result of an accessory pathway syndrome coupled with atrial fibrillation or flutter; these deteriorate rapidly and deserve countershock. Irregularity may be hard to appreciate at these rates.

- Accessory pathway or prolonged QT interval syndromes should be suspected in young patients with syncope, especially if palpitations were noted.
- Antidysrhythmics both treat and cause rhythm disturbances, especially in patients receiving high doses, multiple drugs, or with underlying structural heart disease.
- Lidocaine has a long history of use in dysrhythmia treatment, although comparative data supporting it over other drugs are lacking. It is still helpful in the prophylaxis from VT/VF in select high-risk patients suffering acute myocardial ischemia. Outside of this indication, it now plays a more limited role, especially in cardiac arrest, being supplanted by amiodarone. However, for VT accompanied by pulses, it is easy to give, inexpensive, and often effective outside of arrest.

REFERENCES

1. Vaughan Williams EM: A classification of antiarrhythmic actions reassessed after a decade of experience, *J Clin Pharmacol* 24:129, 1984.
2. Roden DM: Risks and benefits of antiarrhythmic therapy, *N Engl J Med* 331:785, 1994.
3. Nygaard TW et al: Adverse reactions to antiarrhythmic drugs during therapy for ventricular arrhythmias, *JAMA* 256:55, 1986.
4. Wyse DG, McAnulty JH, Rahimtoola SH: Influence of plasma drug level and the presence of conduction disease on the electrophysiologic effects of procainamide, *Am J Cardiol* 43:619, 1979.
5. Callans DJ, Marchlinski FE: Dissociation of termination and prevention of inducibility of sustained ventricular tachycardia with infusion of procainamide: evidence for distinct mechanisms, *J Am Coll Cardiol* 19:111, 1992.
6. Mattioli AV et al: Propafenone versus procainamide for conversion of atrial fibrillation to sinus rhythm, *Clin Cardiol* 21:763, 1998.
7. Kochiadakis GE et al: Conversion of atrial fibrillation to sinus rhythm using acute intravenous procainamide infusion, *Cardiovasc Drugs Ther* 12:75, 1998.
8. Morady F, Scheinman MM, Desai J: Disopyramide, *Ann Intern Med* 96:337, 1982.
9. Coplen SE et al: Efficacy and safety of quinidine therapy for maintenance of sinus rhythm after cardioversion, *Circulation* 82:1106, 1990.
10. Griffith MJ et al: Relative efficacy and safety of intravenous drugs for termination of sustained ventricular tachycardia, *Lancet* 336:670, 1990.
11. Armengol RE et al: Lack of effectiveness of lidocaine for sustained, wide QRS complex tachycardia, *Ann Emerg Med* 18:254, 1989.
12. Gorgels AP et al: Comparison of procainamide and lidocaine in terminating sustained monomorphic ventricular tachycardia, *Am J Cardiol* 78:43, 1996.
13. Advanced cardiovascular life support Section 5: Pharmacology I: Agents for arrhythmias. *Resuscitation* 46:135, 2000.
14. Hine LK et al: Meta-analytic evidence against prophylactic use of lidocaine in acute myocardial infarction, *Arch Intern Med* 149:2694, 1989.
15. McLean SA, Paul ID, Spector PS: Lidocaine-induced conduction disturbance in patients with systemic hyperkalemia, Ann Emerg Med 36:615, 2000.
16. Cranford RE et al: Intravenous phenytoin: clinical and pharmacokinetic aspects, *Neurology* 28:874, 1978.
17. Campbell RWF: Drug therapy: mexiletine, *N Engl J Med* 316:29, 1987.
18. Roden DM, Woosley RL: Drug therapy: tocainide, *N Engl J Med* 315:41, 1986.
19. Shuster MR et al: Effect on seizure threshold in dogs of tocainide/lidocaine administration, *Ann Emerg Med* 16:749, 1987.
20. Echt DS et al: Mortality and morbidity in patients receiving encainide, flecainide, or placebo. The cardiac arrhythmia suppression trial, *N Engl J Med* 324:781, 1991.
21. Roden DM, Woosley RL: Drug therapy: flecainide, *N Engl J Med* 315:36, 1986.
22. Berns E et al: Efficacy and safety of flecainide acetate for atrial tachycardia or fibrillation, *Am J Cardiol* 59:1337, 1987.
23. Horowitz LN: Encainide in lethal ventricular arrhythmias evaluated by electrophysiologic tests and decrease in symptoms, *Am J Cardiol* 58:83C, 1986.
24. Funck-Bretano C et al: Propafenone, *N Engl J Med* 322:518, 1990.
25. Venditti FJ, Garan H, Ruskin JN: Electrophysiologic effects of beta blockers in ventricular arrhythmias, *Am J Cardiol* 60:3D, 1987.
26. Abrams J et al: Efficacy and safety of esmolol vs propranolol in the treatment of supraventricular tachyarrhythmias: a multicenter double blind trial, *Am Heart J* 110:913, 1985.
27. Noc M, Stajer D, Horvat M: Intravenous amiodarone versus verapamil for acute conversion of paroxysmal atrial fibrillation to sinus rhythm, *Am J Cardiol* 65:679, 1990.
28. Galve E et al: Intravenous amiodarone in treatment of recent-onset atrial fibrillation: results of a randomized, controlled study, *J Am Coll Cardiol* 27:1079, 1996.
29. Clemo HF et al: Intravenous amiodarone for acute heart rate control in the critically ill patient with atrial tachyarrhythmias, *Am J Cardiol* 81:594, 1998.
30. Cybulski J et al: Intravenous amiodarone is safe and seems to be effective in termination of paroxysmal supraventricular tachyarrhythmias, *Clin Cardiol* 19:563, 1996.
31. Leak D: Intravenous amiodarone in the treatment of refractory life-threatening cardiac arrhythmias in the critically ill patient, *Am Heart J* 111:456, 1986.
32. Kuga K, Yamaguchi I, Sugishita Y: Effect of intravenous amiodarone on electrophysiologic variables and on the modes of termination of atrioventricular reciprocating tachycardia in Wolff-Parkinson-White syndrome, *Jpn Circ J* 63:189, 1999.
33. Kudenchuk PJ et al: Amiodarone for resuscitation after out-of-hospital cardiac arrest due to ventricular fibrillation, *N Engl J Med* 341:871, 1999.
34. Scheinman MM et al: Dose-ranging study of intravenous amiodarone in patients with life-threatening ventricular tachyarrhythmias, *Circulation* 92:3264, 1995.
35. Levine JH et al: Intravenous amiodarone for recurrent sustained hypotensive ventricular tachyarrhythmias, *J Am Coll Cardiol* 27:67, 1996.
36. Kowey PR et al: Randomized, double-blind comparison of intravenous amiodarone and bretylium in the treatment of patients with recurrent, hemodynamically destabilizing ventricular tachycardia or fibrillation, *Circulation* 92:3255, 1995.
37. Larbuisson R, Venneman I, Stiels B: The efficacy and safety of intravenous propafenone versus intravenous amiodarone in the conversion of atrial fibrillation or flutter after cardiac surgery, *J Cardiothorac Vasc Anesth* 10:229, 1996.
38. Ellenbogen KA et al: Efficacy of intravenous ibutilide for rapid termination of atrial fibrillation and atrial flutter: a dose-response study, *J Am Coll Cardiol* 28:130, 1996.
39. Anderson JL, Prystowsky EN: Sotalol: an important new antiarrhythmic, *Am Heart J* 137:388, 1999.
40. Hohnoser SH, Woosley RL: Sotalol, *N Engl J Med* 331:31, 1994.
41. Tommaso C et al: Atrial fibrillation and flutter: immediate control and conversion with intravenously administered verapamil, *Arch Intern Med* 143:877, 1983.
42. Salerno DM et al: Intravenous verapamil for treatment of multifocal atrial tachycardia with and without calcium pretreatment, *Ann Intern Med* 107:623, 1987.
43. Porter CJ, Garson A, Fillette PC: Verapamil: an effective calcium blocking agent for pediatric patients, *Pediatrics* 71:748, 1983.
44. Epstein ML, Kiel EA, Victoria BE: Cardiac decompensation following verapamil therapy in infants with supraventricular tachycardia, *Pediatrics* 75:737,1985.
45. Haynes BE, Niemann JT, Hanyes KS: Supraventricular tachyarrhythmias and rate-related hypotension: cardiovascular effects and efficacy of intravenous verapamil, *Ann Emerg Med* 19:861, 1990.
46. Haft JI, Habbab MA: Treatment of atrial arrhythmias: effectiveness of verapamil when preceded by calcium infusion, *Arch Intern Med* 146:1085, 1986.
47. Schreck DM, Rivera AR, Tricarico VJ: Emergency management of atrial fibrillation and flutter: intravenous diltiazem versus intravenous digoxin, *Ann Emerg Med* 29:135, 1997.
48. Ellenbogen KA et al: Safety and efficacy of intravenous diltiazem in atrial fibrillation or atrial flutter, *Am J Cardiol* 75:45, 1995.

49. Phillips BG et al: Comparison of intravenous diltiazem and verapamil for the acute treatment of atrial fibrillation and atrial flutter, *Pharmacotherapy* 17:1238, 1997.
50. Falk RH et al: Digoxin for converting recent-onset atrial fibrillation to sinus rhythm: a randomized double-blinded trial, *Ann Intern Med* 106:503, 1987.
51. Jordaens L et al: Conversion of atrial fibrillation to sinus rhythm and rate control by digoxin in comparison to placebo, *Eur Heart J* 18:643, 1997.
52. Mann DL, Maisei AS, Atwood JE: Absence of cardioversion-induced ventricular arrhythmias in patients with therapeutic digoxin levels, *J Am Coll Cardiol* 5:822, 1985.
53. Iseri LT et al: Magnesium and potassium therapy in multifocal atrial tachycardia, *Am Heart J* 110:789, 1985.
54. Iseri LT, Chung P, Tobis J: Magnesium therapy for intractable ventricular tachyarrhythmias in normomagnesemic patients, *West J Med* 138:832, 1983.
55. Cohen L, Kitzes R: Magnesium sulfate and digitalis-toxic arrhythmias, *JAMA* 249:2808, 1983.
56. Belardinelli L, Linden J, Berne RM: The cardiac effects of adenosine, *Prog Cardiovasc Dis* 32:73, 1989.
57. Wilson RF et al: Effects of adenosine on human coronary arterial circulation, *Circulation* 82:1595, 1990.
58. Lerman BB et al: Adenosine-sensitive ventricular tachycardia: evidence suggesting cyclic AMP-mediated triggered activity, *Circulation* 74:270, 1986.
59. Clarke B et al: Rapid and safe termination of spontaneous supraventricular tachycardia in children by adenosine, *Lancet* 1:299, 1987.
60. Garratt C et al: Comparison of adenosine and verapamil for termination of paroxysmal tachycardia, *Am J Cardiol* 64:1310, 1989.
61. DiMarco JP et al: Adenosine for paroxysmal supraventricular tachycardia: dose ranging and comparison with verapamil, *Ann Intern Med* 113:104, 1990.
62. Cairns CB, Niemann JT: IV adenosine for the emergency department management of PSVT: just a pharmacologic vagal maneuver? *Ann Emerg Med* 19:957, 1990.
63. Exner DV, Muzyka T, Gillis AM: Proarrhythmia in patients with the Wolff-Parkinson-White syndrome after standard doses of intravenous adenosine, *Ann Intern Med* 122:351, 1995.
64. Mangrum JM, DiMarco JP: The evaluation and management of bradycardia, *N Engl J Med* 342:703, 2000.
65. Brower PJ: Sick sinus syndrome, *Arch Intern Med* 138:133, 1978.
66. Horan MJ, Kennedy HL: Ventricular ectopy. History, epidemiology, and clinical implications, *JAMA* 251:380, 1984.
67. Glass L, Goldberger AL, Belair J: Dynamics of pure parasystole, *Am J Physiol* 251:H481, 1986.
68. Klein GJ et al: Classification of supraventricular tachycardias, *Am J Cardiol* 60:27D, 1987.
69. Binder LS, Beoche R, Atkinson D: Evaluation and management of supraventricular tachycardia in children, *Ann Emerg Med* 20:51, 1991.
70. Kastor JA: Multifocal atrial tachycardia, *N Engl J Med* 322:1713, 1990.
71. Boineu JP: Atrial flutter: a synthesis of concepts, *Circulation* 72:249, 1985.
72. Kadish SL, Lazar EJ, Frishman WH: Anticoagulation in patients with valvular heart disease, atrial fibrillation, or both, *Cardiol Clin* 5:591, 1987.
73. Joseph AP, Ward MR: A prospective, randomized controlled trial comparing the efficacy and safety of sotalol, amiodarone, and digoxin for the reversion of new-onset atrial fibrillation, *Ann Emerg Med* 36:1, 2000.
74. Volgman AS et al: Conversion efficacy and safety of intravenous ibutilide compared with intravenous procainamide in patients with atrial flutter or fibrillation, *J Am Coll Cardiol* 31:1414, 1998.
75. Mulcahy B et al: New-onset atrial fibrillation: when is admission medically justified? *Acad Emerg Med* 3:114, 1996.
76. Esmolol Research Group: Intravenous esmolol for the treatment of supraventricular tachyarrhythmias: results of a multicenter baseline controlled safety and efficacy study in 160 patients, *Am Heart J* 112:498, 1986.
77. Anderson S et al: Comparison of the efficacy and safety of esmolol, a short acting beta blocker, with placebo in the treatment of supraventricular tachycardias, *Am Heart J* 111:42, 1986.
78. O'Toole KS et al: Intravenous verapamil in the prehospital treatment of paroxysmal supraventricular tachycardia, *Ann Emerg Med* 19:291, 1990.
79. McCabe JL et al: Intravenous adenosine in the prehospital treatment of supraventricular tachycardia, *Ann Emerg Med* 20:445, 1991.
80. Wellens HJJ, Brugada P, Penn OC: The management of preexcitation syndromes, *JAMA* 57:2325, 1987.
81. Schatz I et al: Wolff-Parkinson-White syndrome presenting in atrial fibrillation, *Ann Emerg Med* 16:574, 1987.
82. Barrett PA et al: The electrophysiologic effects of intravenous lidocaine in the Wolff-Parkinson-White syndrome, *Am Heart J* 100:23, 1980.
83. McGovern B, Garan H, Ruskin JN: Precipitation of cardiac arrest by verapamil in patients with Wolff-Parkinson-White syndrome, *Ann Intern Med* 104:791, 1986.
84. Garratt C et al: Misuse of verapamil in pre-excited atrial fibrillation, *Lancet* 1:367, 1989.
85. Brodsky MA et al: Life-threatening alterations in heart rate after the use of adenosine in atrial flutter, *Am Heart J* 130:564, 1995.
86. Leitch JW et al: Differential effect of intravenous procainamide on anterograde and retrograde accessory pathway refractoriness, *J Am Coll Cardiol* 19:118, 1992.
87. Akhtar M, Gilbert CJ, Shenasa M: Effect of lidocaine on atrioventricular response via the accessory pathway in patients with Wolff-Parkinson-White syndrome, *Circulation* 63:435, 1981.
88. Wellens HJJ, Bar F, Lie KI: The value of the electrocardiogram in the differential diagnosis of tachycardia with a widened QRS complex, *Am J Med* 64:27, 1978.
89. Isenhour JL et al: Wide-complex tachycardia: continued evaluation of diagnostic criteria, *Acad Emerg Med* 7:769, 2000.
90. Brugada P et al: A new approach to the differential diagnosis of a regular tachycardia with a wide QRS complex, *Circulation* 83:1649, 1991.
91. Herbert ME et al: Failure to agree on the electrocardiographic diagnosis on ventricular tachycardia, *Ann Emerg Med* 27:35, 1996.
92. Tchou P et al: Useful clinical criteria for the diagnosis of ventricular tachycardia, *Am J Med* 84:53, 1988.
93. Baerman M et al: Differentiation of ventricular tachycardia from supraventricular tachycardia with aberration: value of the clinical history, *Ann Emerg Med* 16:40, 1987.
94. Steinman RT et al: Wide QRS tachycardia in the conscious adult: ventricular tachycardia is the most frequent cause, *JAMA* 261:1013, 1989.
95. Halperin BD et al: Misdiagnosing ventricular in patients with underlying conduction disease and similar sinus and tachycardia morphologies, *West J Med* 152:677, 1990.
96. Stewart RD, Bardy GH, Greent H: Wide complex tachycardia: misdiagnosis and outcome after emergent therapy, *Ann Intern Med* 104:766, 1986.
97. Akhtar M: Clinical spectrum of ventricular tachycardia, *Circulation* 82:1561, 1990.
98. Peticone F, Adinolfi L, Bonaduce D: Efficacy of magnesium sulfate in the treatment of torsades de pointes, *Am Heart J* 112:847, 1986.
99. Vukmir RB, Stein KL: Torsades de pointes therapy with phenytoin, *Ann Emerg Med* 20:198, 1991.

75 Implantable Cardiac Devices

James T. Niemann

PERSPECTIVE

Electrical cardiac pacing for the management of bradyarrhythmias was first described in 1952, and permanent transvenous pacing devices were introduced into clinical practice in the early 1960s.[1] The first devices for endocardial defibrillation were implanted in surviving victims of sudden cardiac death in 1980.[2] Currently implanted electrical devices for the management of cardiac dysrhythmias have changed rapidly over recent years with both increasing complexity and miniaturization. In 1991, it was estimated that 1 million patients in the United States had permanent pacemakers, and survey data from 1993 indicate that about 425 new pacemakers per million of the population were implanted annually in the United States.[3,4] New indications for the use of permanent pacemakers in the management of congenital and acquired heart disease are being defined.[5]

As of 1996, the number of implanted endocardial defibrillation devices approximated 45,000.[2] Since 1996, large clinical trials comparing implantable cardioverter-defibrillators (ICDs) to antiarrhythmic drugs for the prevention or recurrence of sudden cardiac death resulting from ventricular dysrhythmias indicate that ICDs significantly improve survival.[6,7] Hence, the number of ICDs currently in use has continued to increase. The widespread use of these devices ensures that the emergency physician will frequently encounter such patients, often with symptoms that may be related to malfunction of the pacemaker or ICD.

This chapter reviews the basic concepts of pacemaker and ICD technology and therapy and provides an ED approach for recognizing malfunction of these devices.

INDICATIONS FOR PERMANENT PACEMAKERS AND ANTIARRHYTHMIA DEVICES

Guidelines for the implantation of these devices have been developed by a joint task force of the American Heart Association and the American College of Cardiology (AHA/ACC) and are periodically reviewed and updated.[8] Using an evidence-based approach, recommendations are categorized as Class I, II, or III. Class I includes conditions for which there is general agreement that a device should be implanted. A Class II recommendation includes conditions for which these devices are frequently used but for which there is disagreement about their need or benefit. Class III is reserved for conditions for which there is general agreement that a device is not needed.

In the case of pacemaker therapy, additional factors are considered when selecting the mode of pacing (see later) and include, but are not limited to, overall health, lifestyle, and occupation of the patient. Class I indications for a permanent pacemaker or ICD are listed in Boxes 75-1 and 75-2. In general, pacing is recommended for patients with symptomatic heart block, symptomatic sinus bradycardia, and atrial

Box 75-1 Class I Indications for Permanent Pacing in Adults

1. Third-degree AV block at any anatomic level associated with any of the following:
   - Symptomatic bradycardia presumed secondary to AV block
   - Symptomatic bradycardia secondary to drugs required for dysrhythmia management or other medical condition
   - Documented periods of asystole lasting more than 3 seconds or an escape rate of less than 40 beats in an awake, asymptomatic patient
   - After catheter ablation of the AV node
   - Postoperative AV block that is not expected to resolve
   - Neuromuscular disease with AV block (e.g., the muscular dystrophies)
2. Symptomatic bradycardia resulting from second-degree AV block regardless of type or site of block.
3. Chronic bifascicular or trifascicular block with intermittent third-degree AV block or type II second-degree AV block
4. After acute myocardial infarction with any of the following conditions:
   - Persistent second-degree AV block at the His-Purkinje level with bilateral bundle-branch block or third-degree AV block at the level of or below the His-Purkinje system
   - Transient second- or third-degree infranodal AV block and associated bundle-branch block
   - Symptomatic, persistent second- or third-degree AV block
5. Sinus node dysfunction with symptomatic bradycardia (including sinus pauses) or chronotropic incompetence
6. Recurrent syncope caused by carotid sinus stimulation

Box 75-2 Class I Indications for ICD Therapy

1. Cardiac arrest resulting from VF or VT not caused by a transient or reversible event
2. Spontaneous sustained VT
3. Syncope of undetermined origin with clinically relevant, hemodynamically significant sustained VT or VF induced at electrophysiologic study when drug therapy is ineffective, not tolerated, or not preferred.
4. Nonsustained VT with coronary artery disease, prior myocardial infarction, left ventricular dysfunction, and inducible VF or sustained VT at electrophysiologic study that is not suppressible by a Class I antiarrhythmic drug

fibrillation with a symptomatic bradycardia (low ventricular response rate) in the absence of medications that affect atrioventricular (AV) conduction. Controversial indications include pacing in patients with syncope, heart block, or fatigue in the presence of some conduction disease or bradycardia. The likelihood of patient improvement after pacing can be assumed only if the symptoms can be closely correlated with inadequate rate.

PACEMAKER TERMINOLOGY

A letter code, initially established in 1974 and since revised as technology has advanced, standardizes nomenclature for pacemakers.[9] Table 75-1 includes an explanation of the five-letter code scheme and the standard abbreviations in each category. The first three code letters are used most commonly. Using this table, one should be able to understand the features of any pacing mode. For example, a VDD pacemaker is

Table 75-1. 5-Letter Pacemaker Code

Letter 1	Letter 2	Letter 3	Letter 4	Letter 5
Chamber Paced	Chamber Sensed	Sensing Response	Programmability	Antitachycardia Functions
A = atrium	A = atrium	T = triggered*	P = simple	P = pacing
V = ventricle	V = ventricle	I = inhibited	M = multiprogrammable	S = shock
D = dual	D = dual	D = dual (A and V inhibited)	R = rate adaptive	D = dual (shock + pace)
O = none	O = none	O = none	C = communicating	
			O = none	

*In the triggered response mode, the pacemaker discharges or fires when it recognizes an intrinsic depolarization. As a result, pacemaker spikes occur during inscription of the QRS complex. Because this mode results in high-energy consumption and a shortened battery life and because the sensing response can be misinterpreted as pacemaker malfunction, this sensing mode is not used with modern pacemakers.

Table 75-2. Common Permanent Pacemakers

Code	Indication	Advantages	Disadvantages
VVI	Intermittent back-up pacing; inactive patient	Simplicity; low cost	Fixed rate; risk of pacemaker syndrome
VVIR	Atrial fibrillation	Rate responsive	Requires advanced programming
DDD	Complete heart block	Atrial tracking restores normal physiology	No rate responsiveness; requires two leads and advanced programming
DDDR	Sinus node dysfunction; AV block and need for rate responsiveness	Universal pacer; all options available by programming	Complexity, cost, programming, and follow-up evaluation

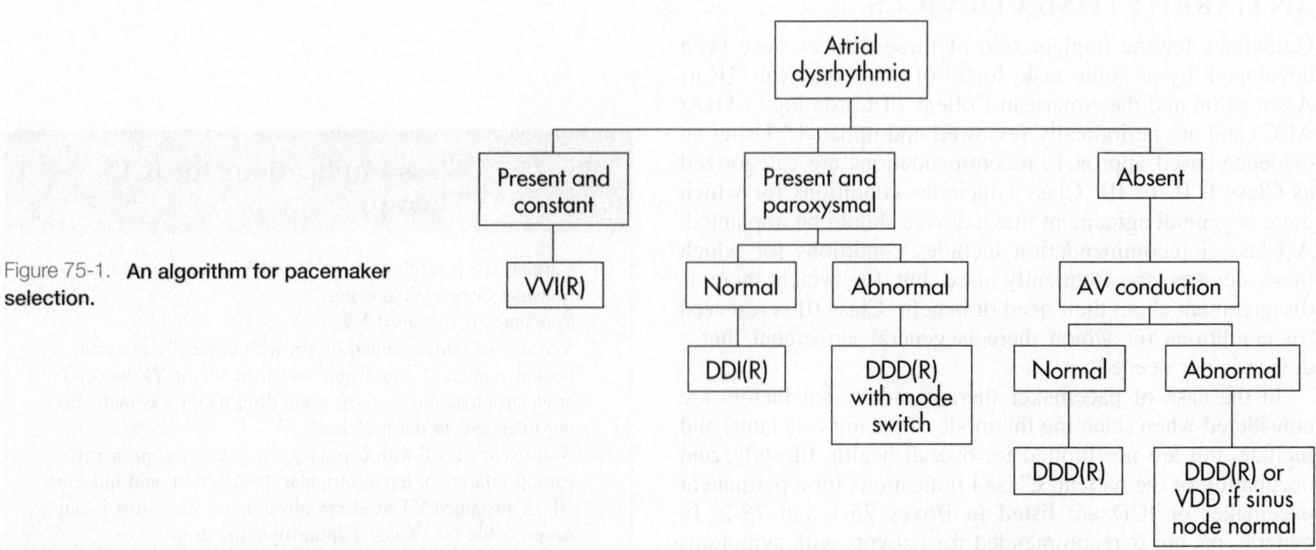

Figure 75-1. **An algorithm for pacemaker selection.**

capable of pacing only the ventricle, sensing both atrial and ventricular intrinsic depolarization, and responding by dual inhibition of both ventricular pacing if intrinsic ventricular depolarization occurs and triggering a paced ventricular beat in response to a sensed intrinsic atrial depolarization. The codes of permanent pacemaker that are used most frequently and the indications, advantages, and disadvantages of each are listed in Table 75-2. An algorithm that summarizes a selection process for optimal pacing for an individual patient is shown in Figure 75-1. More detailed algorithms for matching a patient with a pacemaker have been developed.[8] The majority of permanent pacemakers are now dual chamber and often rate-adaptive.[10]

PACEMAKER COMPONENTS

All pacemaker systems are composed of three basic components: the pulse generator, which houses the power source (battery); the electronic circuitry; and the lead system, which connects the pulse generator to the endocardium.

Nearly all currently implanted pacemakers are lithium powered. Lithium-powered pulse generators function normally for 4 to 10 or more years, depending on the pacemaker "features" such as single versus dual chamber, pacing threshold, and rate adaptiveness. This long "battery life," and the fact that the output voltage of the lithium-iodine cell decreases gradually rather than abruptly as occurred with the early mercury-zinc cell, make sudden pulse generator failure an unlikely cause of pacemaker malfunction.[1]

Current permanent pacemakers use endocardial leads that are positioned in contact with the endocardium of the right ventricle and, in the case of a dual chamber device, the right atrium using a subclavian or cephalic vein approach for insertion. On occasion, an epicardial lead may be implanted during open-heart surgery performed for another indication such as prosthetic valve insertion or correction of a congenital cardiac defect. Pacemaker leads, like power sources, continue to undergo major technical improvements.[1] Innovations include the resilient plastic insulation surrounding the electrodes that reduces the chance of complete lead disruption or breakage (resulting in failure to pace or sense) or the chance of partial fracture (resulting in a "make or break contact" with intermittent failure to sense or pace). The expected incidence of lead disruption is approximately 2% per patient-year.[11] Endocardial leads are designed to "actively" fix to the atrial and ventricular endocardium using tined or "screw in" tips. The expected incidence of lead displacement is about 2% for ventricular leads and 5% for atrial leads, whether actively or passively fixed to the endocardium.[11] A lead capable of active fixation is more commonly used in patients with cardiomyopathies and right ventricular dilation complicated by tricuspid regurgitation.

Pacemaker leads may be either bipolar or unipolar in configuration. A bipolar endocardial lead has both the negative (distal) and positive (proximal) electrodes, separated by about 1 cm, within the heart. A unipolar lead has the negative electrode in contact with the endocardial surface, and the positive pole is the metallic casing of the pulse generator. Each lead system has potential advantages and disadvantages.[10] The unipolar configuration is not compatible with ICD systems, is prone to oversensing of myopotentials and electromagnetic interference, but is of smaller diameter and less susceptible to fracture. The bipolar configuration is compatible with ICD systems, but is larger and more prone to lead fractures; however, oversensing is rarely a problem. The selection of lead configuration usually depends on the experience and preference of the operator.

THE STANDARD ELECTROCARDIOGRAM DURING NORMAL CARDIAC PACING

The modern pacemaker has two basic functions: to electrically stimulate the heart and to sense intrinsic cardiac electrical activity. Additional functions are available and noted in the pacemaker code system (letters 4 and 5, Table 75-1). The pacemaker delivers an electrical stimulus to either the atrium or ventricle if it does not recognize (sense) any intrinsic electrical activity from that chamber after a selected time interval. This interval is usually programmed at the time of implantation and can be changed noninvasively at a later time, if necessary, using a programming and "interrogating" device provided by the pacemaker manufacturer. If the pacemaker recognizes or senses an intrinsic atrial depolarization (P wave) or ventricular depolarization (QRS complex), the pacemaker inhibits or resets its output to prevent "competition" with the underlying intrinsic rhythm. The stimulus intensity and sensing threshold (amplitude of electrical activity that is detected as being intrinsic) are typically set at the time of implantation but can also be reprogrammed later.

The two basic functions of a pacemaker can be easily recognized and confirmed on a standard 12-lead electrocardiogram or rhythm strip. The normal function of a single chamber VVI pacemaker is most easily recognized (Figure 75-2). After a programmed interval is surpassed during which time intrinsic ventricular activity does not occur, a "pacer spike" or stimulus artifact appears. The "pacer spike" is a narrow deflection that is usually less than 5 mm in amplitude with a bipolar lead configuration, and usually 20 mm or more in amplitude with a unipolar lead. A wide QRS complex appears immediately after the stimulus artifact. Depolarization begins in the right ventricular apex and the spread of excitation does not follow normal conduction pathways. Characteristically, a left bundle branch block conduction pattern is seen. A right bundle branch pattern is abnormal and suggests lead displacement. In VVI pacing, the paced QRS complexes occur independent of intrinsic atrial depolarization if present (AV dissociation).

The recognition of normal dual chamber pacing is more complex owing to the interactive sensing and pacing of the right atrium and ventricle (Figure 75-3).[12] Pacing intervals are preprogrammed, may be changed noninvasively at a later time, and are generally specific to the patient's needs. Pacing rates and delay intervals typically vary from patient to patient. Dual chamber devices are typically used in patients with nonfibrillating atria coupled with intact AV conduction (Figure 75-1). A normal appearing QRS complex may follow an intrinsic "p" wave, owing to normal sinoatrial node discharge, if the intrinsic atrial depolarization is conducted to the ventricles. The intrinsic "p" wave and QRS complex will inhibit the atrial and ventricular circuitry. A normal QRS complex will follow a paced "p" wave if the paced atrial beat is conducted through the AV node and the programmed AV delay period is not exceeded. If it is not conducted to the ventricles (AV delay period exceeded), the pacemaker will stimulate the ventricle, resulting in a paced "p" wave and a

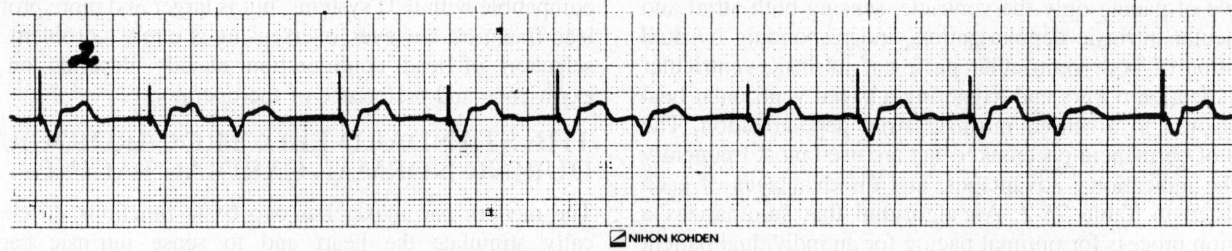

Figure 75-2. **Normal VVI pacemaker (rhythm strip). This rhythm strip was recorded in a patient with a VVI pacemaker implanted for the treatment of symptomatic complete heart block. The pacing rate is approximately 75 beats/min (determined by measuring the time between consecutive pacemaker spikes). Each pacemaker spike is followed by a paced QRS complex. The third QRS from the left has a slightly different morphology than the paced QRS complexes. It is an intrinsic QRS complex that is sensed by the pacemaker, and a paced beat does not occur again until the programmed rate of the pacemaker is exceeded. The time interval between the spontaneous QRS and the next paced beat is about the same as the interval between consecutive pacemaker spikes. This sequence is subsequently repeated twice on this strip.**

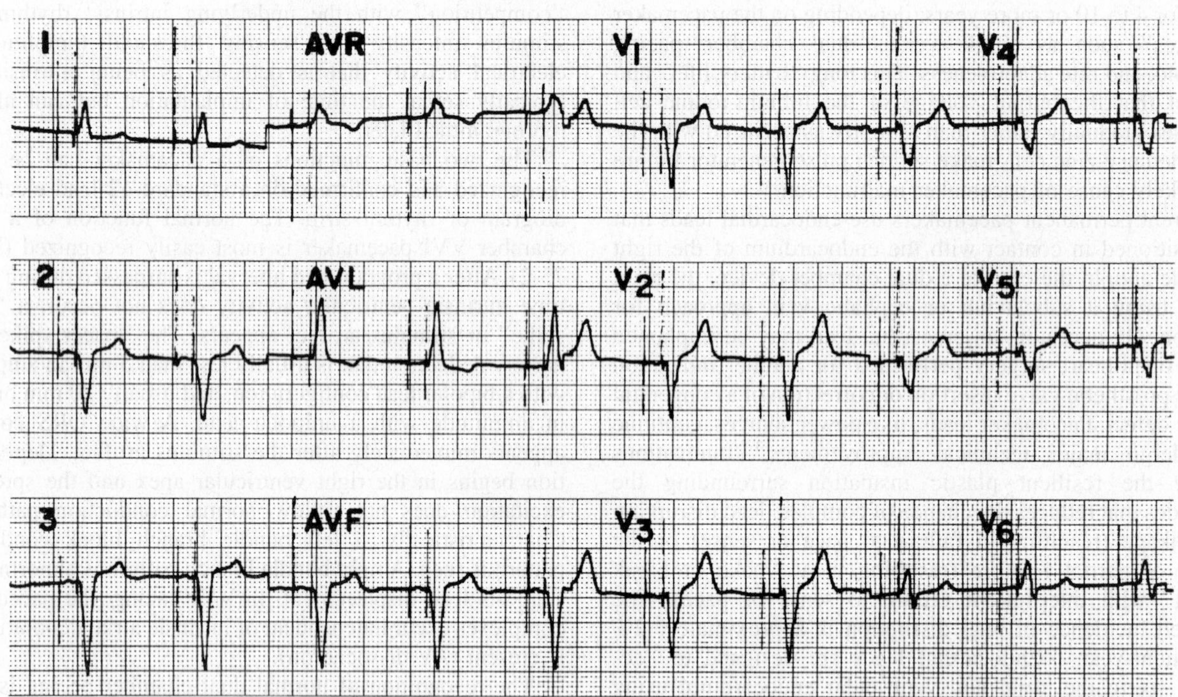

Figure 75-3. **Normal DDD pacemaker (12-lead ECG). Each QRS complex is preceded by two pacemaker spikes. The first spike results in atrial depolarization, and the second produces a wide QRS complex. The QRS complex is conducted with a left bundle branch morphology, which is expected with endocardial pacing at the right ventricular apex.**

wide, paced QRS complex with left bundle branch block configuration. Recognition of the interactivity of the paced chambers is important. A paced "p" wave may be mistaken for failure to sense or pace, and malfunction may be diagnosed when it is not present (pseudomalfunction). In addition, if the programmed rate of the pacemaker approximates the patient's intrinsic heart rate, fusion of paced and native beats may occur and represents another common type of pseudomalfunction (Figure 75-4).

COMPLICATIONS OF PACEMAKER IMPLANTATION

Infection

Pacemaker implantation is a surgical procedure and, like all surgery, carries a risk of infection, and the presence of a foreign body enhances this risk. In recent series, the incidence of infection is small—about 2% for wound and subcutaneous pacemaker "pocket" infection, and about 1% for bacteremia with sepsis.[13] The presence of a foreign body complicates

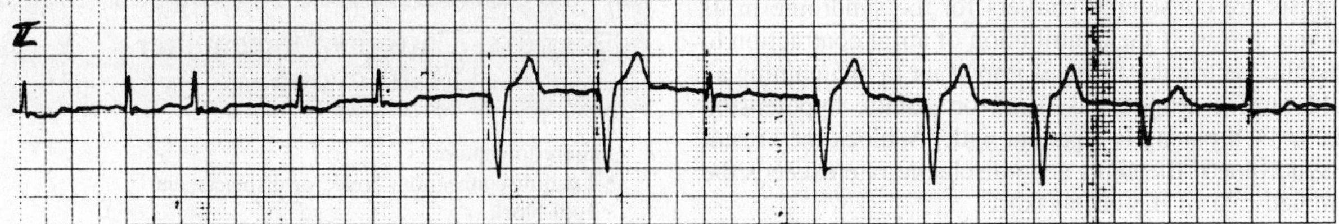

Figure 75-4. **VVI pacemaker with fusion beats (pseudomalfunction). This VVI pacemaker was implanted in a patient with atrial fibrillation and intermittent symptomatic complete heart block. In the lead II rhythm strip, the first five QRS complexes are normal in morphology and irregular, as would be expected in atrial fibrillation. The next two QRS complexes are wide and preceded by a pacemaker spike. This represents normal sensing and pacing. The eighth QRS complex is narrow but preceded by a pacemaker spike. The spikes occur at a fixed and regular interval. In this instance, spontaneous ventricular depolarization had begun at about the time the pacemaker discharged. The twelfth QRS complex in the sequence represents a fusion beat. Within the QRS complex of the thirteenth beat, a pacemaker spike is visible. Again, this represents nearly simultaneous conduction of a supraventricular beat and pacemaker electrical discharge. At first glance, this may appear to be failure to sense; however, the pacemaker is functioning normally and competing with the underlying rhythm.**

management, and few cases of bacteremia that develop after implantation can be managed with antibiotics alone. In most instances, reimplantation and replacement of the lead system are necessary.

Pain and local inflammation at the site of the pacemaker are the first manifestations of a wound infection, cellulitis, or pocket infection. Approximately 20% to 25% of patients with a local infection have positive blood cultures. Bacteremia may occur in the absence of a focal infection and may present with the typical manifestations of the systemic inflammatory response syndrome or sepsis. A hematoma of the pacemaker pocket may mimic a wound or pocket infection. Needle aspiration of the pocket, if performed, should be done with extreme caution, preferably under fluoroscopy, because the needle may cut the insulation surrounding the pulse generator or that portion of the pacemaker lead that lies within the pacemaker pocket.

When a local infection or bacteremia is suspected, blood cultures should be obtained and intravenous antibiotic therapy initiated. *Staphylococcus aureus* and *Staphylococcus epidermidis* are the organisms isolated in approximately 60% to 70% of cases. Empiric antibiotic therapy should include vancomycin pending culture and sensitivity data. If blood cultures are positive, the pulse generator and pacemaker lead are usually removed, temporary transvenous pacing performed, and intravenous antibiotic therapy continued for 4 to 6 weeks. The permanent pacemaker and lead are subsequently reimplanted.[14]

Thrombophlebitis

The incidence of venous obstruction associated with permanent transvenous pacemakers ranges from 30% to 50%, with about one third of patients having complete venous occlusion. Thrombosis of varying degrees can involve the axillary, subclavian, and innominate veins or the superior vena cava (SVC). The site of insertion does not appear to affect the incidence of this complication. Chronic thrombosis of the veins of the upper arm is common and usually asymptomatic owing to extensive venous collateral circulation.

Because of extensive collateralization, only about 0.5% to 3.5% of patients develop symptoms usually indicative of acute thrombosis.[15] These patients typically present with edema, pain, and venous engorgement of the arm ipsilateral to the site of lead insertion. Although rare, SVC syndrome resulting from pacemaker lead-induced thrombosis is reported. The signs and symptoms of lead-induced SVC syndrome are identical to those described in patients with SVC syndrome and malignancy. Whether pulmonary embolism is associated with pacemaker therapy and thrombosis is controversial.[15]

Although symptoms might suggest thrombosis, definitive diagnosis of acute thrombosis usually requires duplex sonography of the jugular venous system, conventional venography, or contrast-enhanced computed tomography. The symptoms typically respond to intravenous heparin therapy followed by long-term warfarin administration. Thrombolytic therapy is most effective if used early in management (within 7 to 10 days).

The "Pacemaker Syndrome"

After pacemaker implantation, a patient may present with new complaints or report a worsening of the symptoms that prompted evaluation and eventual pacemaker therapy. Such complaints often include syncope or near syncope, orthostatic dizziness, fatigue, exercise intolerance, weakness, lethargy, chest fullness or pain, cough, uncomfortable pulsations in the neck or abdomen, right upper quadrant pain, and other nonspecific symptoms.

These symptoms have been referred to as the "pacemaker syndrome."[10,16] The etiology of this syndrome is the loss of AV synchrony and the presence of ventriculoatrial (VA) conduction, and it is most commonly encountered in the setting of VVI pacing but has been described with the DDI mode. With VVI pacing, the ventricle is electrically stimulated and depolarized, resulting in ventricular systole. If sinus node function is intact, the atria can be depolarized by a sinus impulse and contract when the tricuspid and mitral valves are closed. This contractile asynchrony results in an increase in jugular and pulmonary venous pressures and may produce symptoms of congestive heart failure. Atrial distention can result in reflex vasodepressor effects mediated by the central nervous system. Elevated levels of atrial natriuretic peptide and diuresis are considered markers for the syndrome in its more severe forms. If the contribution of atrial contraction to late diastolic ventricular filling is important in maintaining an adequate cardiac output, basal and orthostatic hypotension may occur. DDI pacing in a patient with AV block may result in this syndrome if the sinus node discharge rate exceeds the programmed rate of the pacemaker.

Approximately 20% of patients report symptoms suggesting the pacemaker syndrome after pacemaker insertion. In most instances, symptoms are mild and patients adapt to them. In about one third of these patients, symptoms are severe. Treatment usually requires replacing a VVI pacemaker with a dual chamber pacemaker or lowering the pacing rate of the VVI unit. If symptoms occur in a patient paced in the DDI mode, optimizing the timing of atrial and ventricular pacing is usually required. Patients appear to prefer dual chamber pacing to the VVI modality.[17,18]

Although the pacemaker syndrome may be suspected in the ED in the patient with suggestive symptoms shortly after pacemaker implantation, consultation with a cardiologist is recommended. The same symptoms may be observed in patients with true pacemaker malfunction, which may necessitate pacemaker reprogramming or replacement of the pulse generator or pacemaker lead.

PACEMAKER MALFUNCTION

The term *pacemaker malfunction* refers specifically to problems with the circuitry or power source of the pulse generator, the pacemaker lead (most commonly displacement or fracture), or the interface between the pacing electrode and the myocardium (pacing or sensing threshold). In addition, environmental factors such as extracardiac or extracorporeal electrical signals may interfere with normal pacemaker function. Using the standard electrocardiogram, pacemaker malfunction can be separated into three broad categories: (1) failure to capture (no pacemaker spikes or spikes not followed by an atrial or ventricular complex), (2) inappropriate sensing (oversensing or undersensing—spikes occur prematurely or do not occur even though the programmed interval is exceeded), or (3) inappropriate pacemaker rate. Symptomatic pacemaker malfunction after implantation occurs in less than 5% of patients and is rarely immediately life threatening. Malfunction is most commonly due to inappropriate sensing, followed by failure to capture.[11] Typical presentations and etiologies of pacemaker malfunction are listed in Box 75-3.

When the emergency physician suspects pacemaker malfunction, knowledge of the pacing modalities (Table 75-1) and what is normal for a given pacing modality is critical when reviewing the electrocardiogram. Fortunately, patients are provided with important identifying information, usually in the form of a wallet card, after pacemaker implantation. The most important information for the emergency physician is provided in the 5-letter code. If this information is not available, a standard posteroanterior (PA) and lateral chest radiograph can provide critical information. A single lead in the apex of the right ventricle will be a VVI pacemaker. With VVI pacing, only one stimulus artifact or spike is seen with each stimulated ventricular depolarization (Figure 75-2). If sinus node activity is present, paced QRS complex is dissociated from the intrinsic "p" waves. If separate leads are identified in the right atrium and right ventricle, the pacing modality is most often DDD or DVI, and paced "p" waves

Box 75-3 Causes of Pacemaker Malfunction

Failure to capture
- Lead disconnection, break, or displacement
- Exit block
- Battery depletion

Undersensing
- Lead displacement
- Inadequate endocardial lead contact
- Low voltage intracardiac p waves and QRS complexes
- Lead fracture

Oversensing
- Sensing extracardiac signals: myopotentials
- T wave sensing

Inappropriate rate
- Battery depletion
- VA conduction with pacemaker-mediated tachycardia
- 1:1 response to atrial dysrhythmias

and QRS complexes (two spikes for each QRS complex) are seen (Figure 75-3). However, although DDD and DVI units are capable of pacing both the right atrium and ventricle, only one spike may be seen (Figure 75-5). Failure to identify two spikes with a DDD or DVI unit can represent normal pacemaker function.

A magnet placed externally over the pulse generator is frequently used in the assessment of pacemaker function. The effect of such an intervention on pacemaker function, however, is often misunderstood by the noncardiologist. Magnet application does not inhibit or turn off a pacemaker. It does result in closure of a reed switch present within the pacemaker circuitry and converts the pacemaker to an asynchronous or fixed-rate pacing mode, and the pacemaker is no longer inhibited by the patient's intrinsic electrical activity. The technique is most commonly used when the patient's intrinsic heart rate exceeds the pacemaker's set rate and pacemaker function is inhibited. Magnet application then allows pacing to occur, and pacing rate and the presence of capture can be determined. Magnets are usually manufacturer specific as are available external reprogramming devices.

Failure to Capture

Failure to capture may range from the complete absence of pacemaker spikes to spikes not followed by a stimulus-induced complex (Figure 75-6). A complete absence of pacemaker spikes may result from complete battery depletion, complete fracture of the pacemaker lead, or disconnection of the lead from the pulse generator unit.

Compared with the earlier mercury-zinc cells, the current lithium iodine batteries are not prone to abrupt failure.[1,11] This power source displays typical end-of-life functional changes over a period of months and usually up to a year before complete depletion. Usually the first sign of voltage depletion is a decrease in the programmed pacing rate. This change is gradual and should be noticed during the 1- to 3-month follow-up evaluations that pacemaker patients receive. When voltage output falls to a critical level, stimulus strength falls below the required threshold and failure to capture or intermittent failure to capture may be observed late

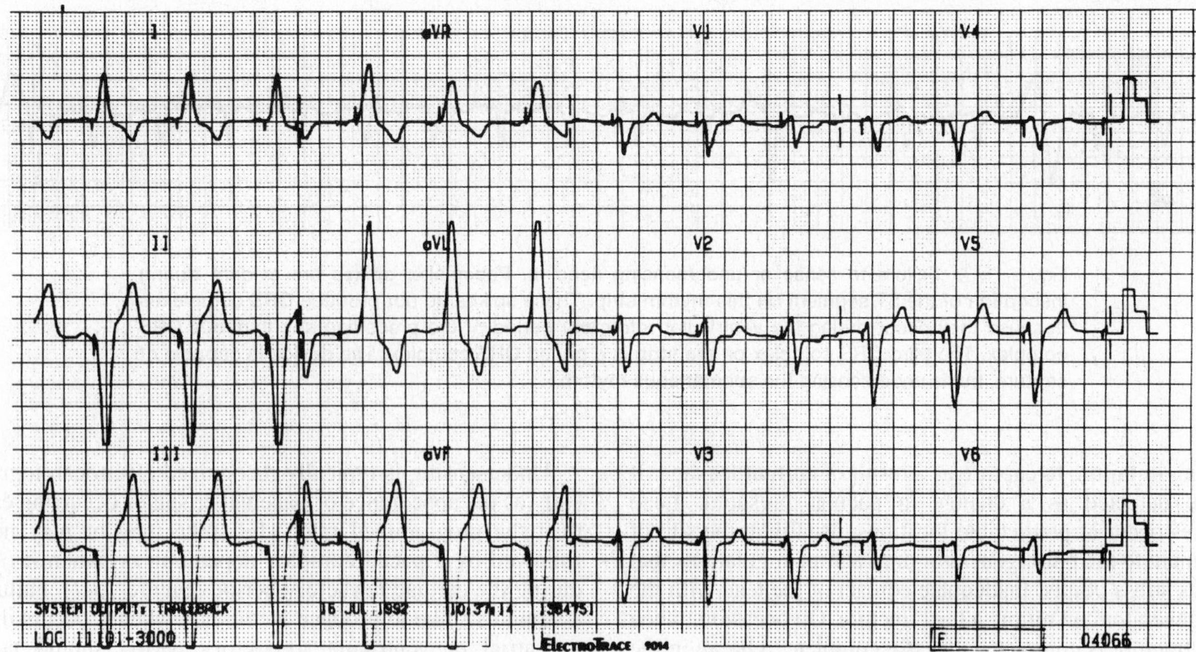

Figure 75-5. **Normal DDD pacemaker (half-standard 12-lead ECG). Three paced QRS complexes preceded by a stimulus artifact or spike are evident in leads I, II, and III. Paced QRS complexes occur after spontaneous or intrinsic p waves are sensed and AV conduction delay exceeds the pacemaker's programmed AV interval. The first QRS complex in the augmented leads, best seen in lead aVF, demonstrates both a paced p wave and a paced QRS complex. Although a dual chamber device, two spikes may not always be seen preceding every QRS complex and the presence of only one spike, or no spikes, should not be interpreted as evidence of pacemaker malfunction. Also evident on this ECG are the different amplitudes of the pacer spikes from lead to lead. When a single lead rhythm strip is recorded, the selected lead should be the one in which the pacemaker spikes are most easily identified.**

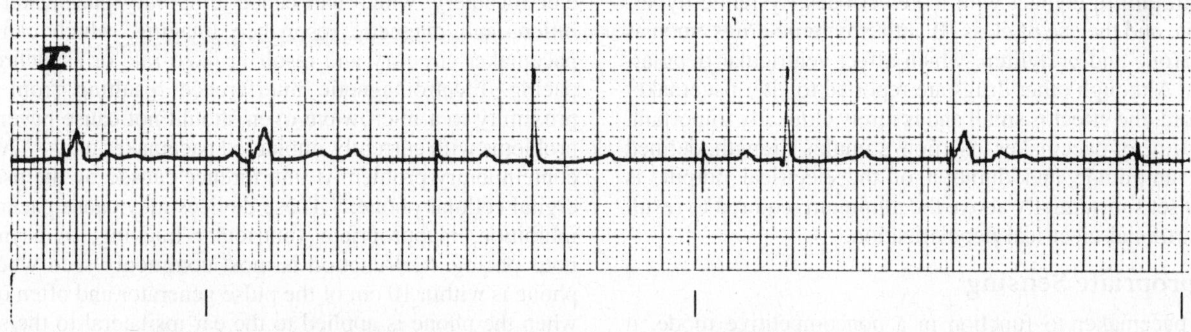

Figure 75-6. **Intermittent failure to capture and slow pacing rate (lead I). This lead I rhythm strip demonstrates intermittent failure to capture of a VVI pacemaker. The first and second pacemaker spikes are followed by wide-paced QRS complexes; the third and fourth spikes are not. The pacemaker spikes occur at a rate of approximately 50/min. The device was programmed to pace at a rate of 75/min. This is a typical example of "end-of-life" pacing characteristics of a depleted battery.**

in battery life. As a result, urgent or emergent battery replacement is rare.

Failure to capture, which may be complete or intermittent, is most commonly a lead problem. Lead displacement is the most common cause and is most likely to occur within the first month of pacemaker insertion. The chest radiograph may demonstrate the tip of the pacing catheter displaced from the right ventricular apex. The catheter tip is commonly found in the pulmonary outflow tract where it may have intermittent contact with endocardium, resulting in intermittent failure to pace and sense. The atrial leads of dual chamber devices are commonly displaced into the body of the right atrium, resulting in loss of contact between the pacing lead and the atrial endocardium.

Lead fracture, which is uncommon with the current polyurethane lead coating,[1] produces an insulation break,

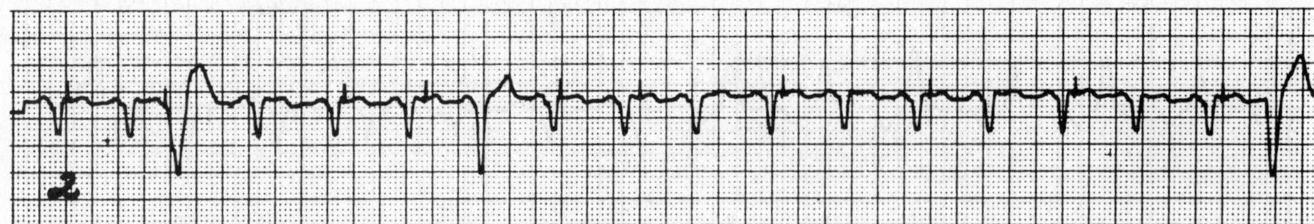

Figure 75-7. **Failure to sense or undersensing (lead II). Pacemaker spikes are evident during inscription of the ST segment on this rhythm strip. These spikes do not produce QRS complexes because they occur during the ventricular refractory period of the preceding spontaneous QRS complex. The third QRS complex on the strip is a paced QRS complex. The device is capable of capture, but is undersensing the spontaneous rhythm.**

resulting in failure to capture as a result of current leakage. It can be detected as a change in pacing threshold. Lead fractures occur at predictable locations, usually at the site of attachment to the pulse generator or at abrupt angulations that serve as stress points. Inadequate contact of the lead with the pulse generator can mimic a lead fracture. On occasion, when a lead fracture is complete or nearly complete, a break in the catheter or its insulation can be detected on an overpenetrated PA chest radiograph. Loss of lead-pulse generator contact can be detected on the chest radiograph with close inspection of the pulse generator.

Exit block (the failure of an adequate stimulus to depolarize the paced chamber) can also result in failure to pace. Exit block should be considered when the preprogrammed pacing stimulus output fails to result in capture in the presence of a normally functioning pulse generator and an intact lead system. This problem is most commonly due to changes in the endocardium in contact with the pacing system. Etiologies include ischemia or infarction of the endocardium in contact with the electrodes, systemic hyperkalemia, and the use of class III antiarrhythmic drugs, such as amiodarone and bretylium, which affect ventricular depolarization. Although other drugs are reported to alter pacemaker threshold, the effect is small and is rarely clinically important. At the time of pacemaker insertion, stimulus strength, defined as the amplitude and duration of the electrical output, is always set substantially above the minimum required to result in an artificial electrical depolarization.

Inappropriate Sensing

For a pacemaker to function in a noncompetitive mode, it must be capable of sensing the intrinsic or "native" electrical activity of the heart. The electrical activity that is sensed is determined by the pacing modality (Table 75-1). Sensing parameters are determined at the time of pacemaker insertion based on signal size of the intracardiac ECG and can be changed or "fine tuned" externally at a later time if needed.

Undersensing

Failure to sense may be complete or intermittent. It may result from a change in the sensing parameters selected at the time of insertion. This is most commonly encountered after acute right ventricular infarction or during the progressive fibrosis that accompanies many cardiomyopathies, causing intracardiac signals to decrease in amplitude. Lead displacement, fracture, and poor contact with the endocardium may also cause undersensing.

Undersensing is typically recognized electrocardiographically as the appearance of pacemaker spikes occurring earlier than the programmed rate. The spike may or may not be followed by a paced complex depending on when it occurs during the cardiac refractory period (Figure 75-7). Failure of a stimulus spike to produce a complex when it occurs during the atrial or ventricular refractory period should not be interpreted as failure to pace.

Oversensing

In rare instances, the pacemaker may detect electrical activity that is not of cardiac origin. The result may be intermittent, irregular pacing or an apparent complete absence of pacemaker function. Myopotentials produced by the pectoralis muscular (Figure 75-8) and extracorporeal electrical signals are frequently oversensed when a unipolar lead system is used. T waves following an intrinsic ventricular depolarization are the most common oversensed cardiac signals. Common medical sources of electrical interference include electrocautery, which can cause temporary pacemaker inhibition, and magnetic resonance imaging, which can alter pacemaker circuitry and result in fixed-rate or asynchronous pacing. Electromagnetic interference resulting from close proximity to a microwave oven should not cause pacemaker problems with currently implanted pacemaker units.[11] A more contemporary problem is interference caused by the use of a digital cellular phone.[19] These devices may cause pacemaker inhibition, inappropriate ventricular tracking, or asynchronous pacing. Malfunction is most commonly seen when the phone is within 10 cm of the pulse generator and often occurs when the phone is applied to the ear ipsilateral to the site of the pacemaker pocket.

Inappropriate Pacemaker Rate

A pacing rate below the programmed rate is a typical finding in pulse generator depletion and does not occur abruptly with lithium iodine batteries. An extreme increase in pacing rate, the so-called run-away pacemaker,[20] can cause profound hypotension and cardiovascular collapse and is a true pacemaker emergency. It is rarely, if ever, encountered with current pacemaker technology and circuitry in which upper rate limits are set (typically < 140/min). An "endless loop tachycardia" may develop during dual chamber pacing when ventriculoatrial conduction occurs and the resulting retrograde atrial depolarization results in a stimulated or paced ventricular depolarization.[21] If atrial flutter develops during dual chamber pacing, flutter waves may be sensed and

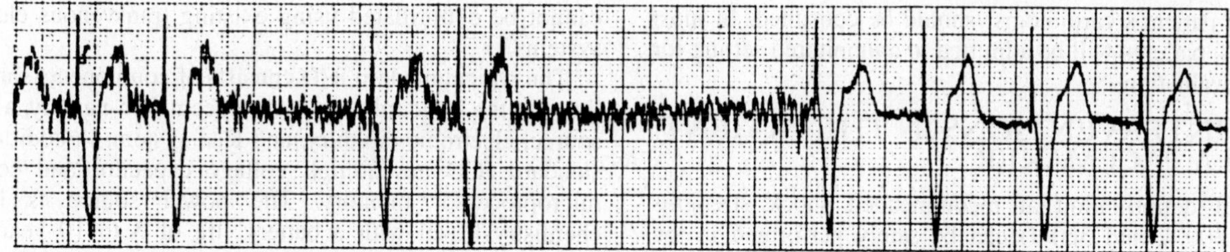

Figure 75-8. **Oversensing (lead II). This VVI unipolar lead pacemaker is oversensing myopotentials produced by contraction of the pectoralis major. Myopotentials result in the undulating and irregular baseline seen in the middle of the strip. After muscular contraction ceases, normal pacing resumes (last four complexes on the strip).**

tracked, resulting in a rapid, paced ventricular rate. In both instances, the ventricular rate will not exceed its set upper limit. Patients with such rhythms may complain only of palpitations or symptoms of hemodynamic compromise. When such rhythms are detected, magnet application usually converts the pacemaker to a fixed rate in a competitive mode and terminates the tachyarrhythmia.

MANAGEMENT

History

The patient should always be asked for the pacemaker identification card. The information on the card explains why a pacemaker was placed and the pacing modality used.

Most patients with pacemaker malfunction present with symptoms reminiscent of those that prompted pacemaker therapy: syncope, near syncope, orthostatic dizziness, lightheadedness, dyspnea, or palpitations.

The majority of pacemaker complications and most instances of pacemaker malfunction occur within the first few weeks or months of pacemaker implantation. After wound healing, palpation of the pulse generator site should not elicit tenderness. A wound infection or pocket infection typically presents with localized pain. Bacteremia secondary to infection of the pacing catheter, however, may present only with fever and without other manifestations of the systemic inflammatory response syndrome. Pain in the arm ipsilateral to the site of insertion should suggest acute thrombophlebitis.

Patients who develop the pacemaker syndrome secondary to the loss of AV synchrony may present with nonspecific complaints of easy fatigability, generalized weakness, dyspnea, or an uncomfortable fluttering or "pounding" sensation in the neck or abdomen. Syncope or near syncope may also occur, but these complaints should prompt an evaluation for true pacemaker malfunction. The pacemaker syndrome should be a diagnosis of exclusion.

Physical Examination

A pacemaker infection should always be suspected in the presence of fever, even if another potential source of infection can be identified. Extremely low (<60) or high pulse rates (>100 in the resting patient) are suggestive of altered pacing parameters (battery depletion or pacemaker mediated tachycardias). Hypotension may be present in either instance. Cannon "a" waves on inspection of the jugular venous pulse wave indicate AV asynchrony. Auscultation of lungs may reveal normal or nonspecific findings. On occasion, bibasilar rales may be heard if congestive heart failure is present.

During pacing, the first heart sound may vary in intensity as a result of AV dissociation (VVI mode), and the second heart sound may be paradoxically split when ventricular pacing occurs (the right ventricle is activated first).[22] The latter is observed clinically in about 25% of patients. A pericardial friction rub may also be heard if the tip of the pacing catheter has perforated the wall of the right ventricle. Perforation, however, usually occurs at the time of pacemaker implantation and is usually recognized at that time. Although the pacing catheter traverses the tricuspid valve, tricuspid regurgitation is rarely heard unless there is myocardial disease such as right ventricular dilation that is common in the cardiomyopathies. Pedal edema may be present and is important if it is a new symptom or if chronic edema has recently worsened.

Chest Radiograph

A chest radiograph should be obtained to define pacing catheter tip position and to determine the number of pacing leads unless this information is available from another source. A ventricular pacing catheter tip in the right ventricular outflow tract or an atrial catheter tip in the superior vena cava or right ventricle is always abnormal. The pulse generator site should also be examined on the radiograph. On occasion, disconnection of the lead from the pulse generator may be observed. In some cases, this is due to patient manipulation of the pulse generator ("twiddler's syndrome").[23]

12-lead Electrocardiogram

A standard electrocardiogram and a long rhythm strip should be obtained in all patients. With bipolar pacing systems, the stimulus artifact may be extremely small and difficult to recognize in some leads (Figure 75-5). Inspection of the rhythm strip may reveal failure to sense or pace, a low pacing rate, or an abnormally rapid rhythm, suggesting a pacemaker-mediated tachycardia.

DISPOSITION OF THE ED PATIENT WITH A PACEMAKER

As a result of the current design of modern pacemakers and the frequent follow-up evaluation of pacemaker patients, life-threatening emergencies resulting from pacemaker malfunction requiring immediate ED intervention are rare. Most instances of malfunction are subtle and difficult to recognize without "interrogation" of the pacemaker using manufacturer-specific devices by someone skilled in the technique. In all instances of suspected pacemaker malfunction, the patient's cardiologist should be consulted. In most instances, patients will be admitted to a monitored setting for further evaluation.

ACLS INTERVENTIONS IN THE PATIENT WITH A PACEMAKER

Electrical defibrillation at recommended shock strengths (200 J, 300 J, and 360 J) can be safely performed in the patient with a pacemaker.[24] If the sternal paddle is placed adjacent to the sternum, it will be at a safe distance (≥10 cm) from the pulse generator. Alternatively, defibrillation electrodes can be placed in an anteroposterior configuration. A cardiologist should check the pacing parameters of the unit if the resuscitation is successful. A chest radiograph should also be obtained after resuscitation to ensure that the pacing catheter was not displaced during chest compression, although this is an extremely uncommon occurrence.

Immediate return of pacing (capture) may not occur after defibrillation; this is more commonly the result of global myocardial ischemia and increased pacing threshold, rather than an indication of pacemaker malfunction. Temporary transcutaneous pacing may be needed. Transcutaneous pacing can also be safely used because the anterior and posterior pacing electrodes, if properly positioned, are distant from the pulse generator. Attempting temporary transvenous pacing is usually not necessary and is unlikely to be successful, especially if undertaken without fluoroscopic guidance. Chronic venous thrombosis, which is common and most often asymptomatic after pacemaker insertion, may preclude temporary catheter insertion via the neck veins. Insertion via the femoral vein is also difficult because the permanently implanted catheter may prevent entry into the right ventricle. Blind insertion may also dislodge the permanent catheter.

IMPLANTABLE CARDIOVERTER-DEFIBRILLATORS

The ICD was first used clinically in 1980. During the last 20 years, technical refinements in this modality for treating ventricular dysrhythmias have progressed even more rapidly than refinements in the less complex standard pacemaker. Recent estimates are that more than 200,000 ICD implants have been performed worldwide.[25] A surge in the use of ICDs has followed the publication of several studies that indicate improved survival with ICDs versus antiarrhythmic therapy in patients at risk for sudden death resulting from ventricular dysrhythmias.[6,7] Additional trials, designed to determine the benefit in patients with nonischemic cardiomyopathies, are in progress. Although some disparity in study results has been noted, differences may be related to the study design inclusion criteria. Generally accepted indications for ICD implantation are noted in Box 75-2. Many patients still require drug therapy after ICD implantation to suppress ventricular dysrhythmias, minimize the frequency of ICD shocks, improve patient tolerance, and decrease energy use that prolongs ICD life.

ICD TERMINOLOGY AND COMPONENTS

The majority of ICDs are now placed percutaneously in a manner similar to that of the standard pacemaker.[2] A transvenous electrode system has largely replaced epicardial lead placement, which required thoracotomy. An epicardial defibrillation lead may, on occasion, still be placed during coronary artery bypass surgery or in a few patients who cannot be defibrillated using existing transvenous electrode systems.

The typical modern ICD consists of components similar to those in the standard permanent pacemaker, namely, a power source, electronic circuitry, and lead system. In addition, the standard ICD has a high voltage capacitor and complex microprocessor memory. The power source is lithium chemistry based with a battery life of 5 to 10 years. The longevity is largely determined by the frequency of shocks. All ICDs are also ventricular pacemakers, providing pacing for bradyarrhythmias. More complex pacing functions can also be incorporated if indicated. The lead system is implanted in a fashion similar to that described previously for pacemakers.

The right ventricular lead is used for sensing and pacing, and shocks are typically delivered between a coil in the right ventricular lead and the pulse generator. If dual chamber pacing is required, a second lead is placed in contact with the endocardium of the right atrium. A biphasic waveform is currently the preferred waveform for internal defibrillation. The shape and characteristics of the shock waveform vary among manufacturers. The biphasic waveform is more effective at lower energies than earlier monophasic waveforms and allows a smaller capacitor to be used, thereby reducing the size and increasing the comfort of the ICD unit.

The diagnostic and treatment functions of the ICD are determined at the time of implantation.[2] In most instances, the cardioversion and defibrillation thresholds are determined at the time of ICD insertion by inducing ventricular tachycardia and fibrillation and adjusting the shock strength at a level above the minimum required to terminate the induced rhythm. Optimally, the required shock strength for defibrillation is less than half the maximum output (approximately 30 J) of the device. Ventricular tachycardia is typically managed using either low energy shocks or programmed pacing that interrupts the ventricular tachycardia reentrant circuit. Programmed pacing is less likely to have proarrhythmic effects and requires less energy, thereby extending battery life. In the setting of VF, ICDs are capable of delivering up to five additional discharges if the first shock fails.

Close follow-up monitoring by a cardiologist familiar with ICD programming is essential for the ICD patient. It allows the cardiologist to determine the frequency of ICD activation (programmed antitachycardia pacing or shocks) and to confirm the programmed functions of the device. The majority of patients with ICDs have underlying heart disease, most commonly extensive atherosclerotic coronary artery disease, that is complicated by a low ejection fraction and congestive heart failure. The patient's medications and metabolic status, such as electrolyte disorders that accompany diuretic usage, may also affect ICD function.

COMPLICATIONS OF ICD IMPLANTATION

Complications of ICD implantation are nearly identical in type and frequency to those of permanent pacemaker implantation. They include infection of the wound, the subcutaneous pouch fashioned for the device, and the lead system, as well as acute thrombophlebitis and chronic thrombosis of the veins traversed for lead insertion.[26,27] Management of these complications is similar to that for patients with permanent pacemakers.

Box 75-4 Causes of ICD Malfunction

Increase or abrupt change in shock frequency
- Increased frequency of VF or VT (consider ischemia, electrolyte disorder, or drug effect)
- Displacement or break in ventricular lead
- Recurrent nonsustained VT
- Sensing and shock of supraventricular tachyarrhythmias
- Oversensing of T waves
- Sensing noncardiac signals

Syncope, near syncope, dizziness
- Recurrent VT with low shock strength (lead problem, change in defibrillation threshold)
- Hemodynamically significant supraventricular tachyarrhythmias
- Inadequate back-up pacing for bradyarrhythmias (spontaneous or drug induced)

Cardiac arrest
- Assume malfunction, but probably due to VF that failed to respond to programmed shock parameters

ICD MALFUNCTION

Patients with ICD malfunction usually present to the ED with a limited number of specific symptoms (Box 75-4).

In contrast to patients with a permanent pacemaker, ICD patients are aware of when the ICD discharges to terminate ventricular tachycardia or VF. The most common complaint of ICD patients is the occurrence of frequent shocks (i.e., occurring at a rate greater than what they are accustomed to).[2,25] Increasing shock rate may be appropriate and not indicative of ICD malfunction if the patient is experiencing an increase in the frequency of ventricular tachycardia (VT) or VF episodes. This may occur in the setting of hypokalemia, hypomagnesium, ischemia (with or without infarction) related to underlying coronary artery disease, or the proarrhythmic effect of drugs administered to decrease the frequency of ventricular tachyarrhythmias.

An increase in the shock frequency is a manifestation of ICD sensing malfunction if (1) a supraventricular tachyarrhythmia is inappropriately sensed as ventricular tachycardia, (2) shocks are delivered for nonsustained ventricular tachycardia, or (3) intracardiac T waves detected by the ICD system are sensed as QRS complexes and the ICD interprets this as an increased heart rate. Temporary ICD deactivation with magnet application may be necessary if oversensing is the problem. Syncope, near syncope, dizziness, or lightheadedness in the patient with an ICD may indicate undersensing of sustained ventricular tachycardia or inappropriately low shock strength to terminate the rhythm.

ACLS INTERVENTIONS IN THE PATIENT WITH AN ICD

An ICD will not prevent sudden death in all patients at risk, and a patient with an ICD may present in cardiac arrest (2% annual incidence in implanted patients). Cardiac arrest is not necessarily an indication of ICD malfunction. Appropriate repeated shocks may have been delivered but were ineffectual. Alternatively, the ICD may not have sensed VF or the ventricular ectopic activity that typically precedes VF. Resuscitation efforts in the patient with an ICD should be undertaken in accordance with current recommendations. Transthoracic defibrillation can be performed in the standard fashion with a stacked sequence of shocks (200 J, 300 J, 360 J) if VF is the arrest rhythm. The sternal electrode or paddle should be placed in a parasternal location about 10 cm from the ICD subcutaneous pouch if the device has been implanted in the right deltopectoral area. If it has been implanted in the left deltopectoral region, this recommended safety distance is usually exceeded.

If the ICD discharges during manual chest compressions, the rescuer may feel a weak shock. There have been no reports of injury to rescuers from such discharges during resuscitation efforts. The device can be deactivated with magnetic application during resuscitation efforts. Deactivation is probably more important in the immediate postresuscitation period because recurrent ventricular dysrhythmias are common at this time owing to prolonged global myocardial ischemia during the arrest period, reperfusion, and the hyperadrenergic state worsened by the use of intravenous epinephrine during resuscitation efforts. ICD malfunction should be assumed and these postresuscitation rhythms treated with standard pharmacologic agents (lidocaine, amiodarone, bretylium). Although Class 1 antidysrhythmic agents may raise the defibrillation threshold of the ICD, their impact on the defibrillation threshold during transthoracic countershock is clinically inconsequential owing to the high shock strengths that are used.

DISPOSITION OF THE ED PATIENT WITH AN ICD

As a result of the difficulty in documenting or excluding ICD malfunction in the patient with transient symptoms, the emergency physician should consult the patient's cardiologist regarding evaluation and therapy. In almost all instances, admission to a monitored setting with extended telemetric observation will be necessary. ICD "interrogation" allows assessment of ICD function and preceding dysrhythmia episodes. Reprogramming may be necessary. If a lead problem is detected, reimplantation is required.

KEY CONCEPTS

- Pacemaker malfunction soon after implantation (within 6 to 8 weeks) is usually due to a lead problem, such as a lead displacement, or to pacemaker programming failure, such as a pacing rate too slow for the patient's needs.
- Pacemaker malfunction presents in a limited number of ways: failure to pace, oversensing, undersensing, and pacing at an inappropriate rate (too fast or too slow).
- In the modern era of technology, abrupt battery failure is an unlikely cause of pacemaker malfunction.
- If a patient with a pacemaker presents with a fever of unclear etiology, pacemaker lead infection and endocarditis must be considered.
- Because paced ventricular complexes are conducted with a left bundle branch block pattern, a paced rhythm will obscure the ECG diagnosis of acute myocardial infarction.
- Magnet application does not turn off a pacemaker. It does convert an inhibited or noncompetitive pacemaker to one that is not inhibited. Fixed rate pacing and competition with the pacing underlying rhythm will occur.
- Defibrillation is safe in patients with a pacemaker or

ICD if paddles are placed at least 10 cm from the subcutaneous implant site of the device. Alternatively, anteroposterior defibrillation with adhesive defibrillation electrodes can be performed.

REFERENCES

1. Jeffrey K, Parsonnet V: Cardiac pacing, 1960-1985. A quarter century of medical and industrial innovation, *Circulation* 97:1978-1991, 1998.
2. O'Callaghan PA, Ruskin JN: Current status of implantable cardioverter-defibrillators, *Curr Probl Cardiol* 22:645-707, 1997.
3. Buckingham TA, Volgman AS, Wimer E: Trends in pacemaker use: results of a multicenter registry, *PACE* 14:1437-1439, 1991.
4. Bernstein AD, Parsonnet V: Survey of cardiac pacing in the United States in 1989, *Am J Cardiol* 69:331-338, 1992.
5. Glikson M, Espinosa RE, Hayes DL: Expanding indications for permanent pacemakers, *Ann Intern Med* 123:443-451, 1995.
6. The Antiarrhythmic versus Implantable Defibrillators (AVID) Investigators: a comparison of antiarrhythmic drug therapy with implantable defibrillators in patients resuscitated from near fatal ventricular arrhythmias, *N Engl J Med* 337:1576-1583, 1997.
7. Moss AJ et al, for the Multicenter Automatic Defibrillator Implantation Trial (MADIT) Investigators: improved survival with an implanted defibrillator in patients with coronary artery disease at high risk for ventricular arrhythmias, *N Engl J Med* 335:1933-1940, 1996.
8. Gregoratos G et al: ACC/AHA guidelines for implantation of cardiac pacemakers and antiarrhythmia devices: a Report of the American College of Cardiology/American Heart Association Task Force on Practice Guidelines (Committee on Pacemaker Implantation), *J Am Coll Cardiol* 31:1175-209, 1998.
9. Bernstein AD et al: The NASPE/BPEG generic pacemaker code for antibradyarrhythmia and adaptive rate pacing and antitachyarrhythmia devices, *PACE* 10:794-799, 1987.
10. Mitrani RD et al: Cardiac pacemakers: current and future status, *Curr Probl Cardiol* 24:341-420, 1999.
11. Hayes DL, Vlietstra RE: Pacemaker malfunction, *Ann Intern Med* 119:828-835, 1993.
12. Kusumoto FM, Goldschlager N: Cardiac pacing, *N Engl J Med* 334:89-98, 1996.
13. Da Costa A et al: Secondary infection after pacemaker implantation, *Rev Med Intern* 21:256-265, 2000.
14. Arber et al: Pacemaker endocarditis. Report of 44 cases and review of the literature, *Medicine* 73:299-305, 1994.
15. Barakat K, Robinson NM, Spurrell RA: Transvenous pacing lead-induced thrombosis: a series of cases with a review of the literature, *Cardiology* 93:142-148, 2000.
16. Ausubel K, Furman S: The pacemaker syndrome, *Ann Intern Med* 103:420-429, 1985.
17. Connolly SJ et al: Dual-chamber versus ventricular pacing: critical appraisal of current data, *Circulation* 94:578-583, 1996.
18. Ovsyshcher IE, Hayes DL, Furman S: Dual-chamber pacing is superior to ventricular pacing. Fact or controversy? *Circulation* 97:2368-2370, 1998.
19. Hayes DL et al: Interference with cardiac pacemakers by cellular telephones, *N Engl J Med* 336:1473-1479, 1997.
20. Mickley H, Anderson C, Nielsen IH: Runaway pacemaker: a still existing complication and therapeutic guidelines, *Clin Cardiol* 12:412-416, 1989.
21. Greenberg RM et al: Pacemaker-mediated tachycardia: a complication of atrioventricular universal (DDD) pacemakers, *Arch Intern Med* 144:1061, 1984.
22. Misra KP et al: Auscultatory findings in patients with cardiac pacemakers, *Ann Intern Med* 74:245-250, 1971.
23. Lal RB, Avery RD: Aggressive pacemaker twiddler's syndrome. Dislodgement of an active fixation ventricular pacing electrode, *Chest* 97:756-758, 1990.
24. Kerber RE, Roberston CE: Transthoracic defibrillation. In Paradis NA, Halperin HR, Nowak RM, editors: *Cardiac arrest. The science and practice of resuscitation medicine,* Baltimore, 1996, Williams & Wilkins.
25. Pinski SL, Fahy GJ: Implantable cardioverter-defibrillators, *Am J Med* 106:446-458, 1999.
26. Pfeiffer D et al: Complications of pacemaker-defibrillator devices: diagnosis and management, *Am Heart J* 127:1073-1080, 1994.
27. Smith PN et al: Infections with nonthoracotomy implantable cardioverter-defibrillators: can these be prevented? *PACE* 19:2156-2157, 1998.

76 Heart Failure

Jay L. Falk
John F. O'Brien
Robert Shesser

Heart failure may be defined as the pathophysiologic state in which, *at normal filling volumes,* the heart is incapable of pumping a sufficient supply of blood to meet metabolic requirements. Filling volumes must be normal because a failing heart may continue to maintain systemic perfusion by using the compensatory Frank-Starling mechanism of preload reserve that results in the maintenance of normal stroke volume despite reduced ejection fraction. Conversely, low filling volumes indicate a pump priming problem distinct from cardiac disease.

A complex regulatory system exists between the heart and multiple organ systems. Feedback loops mediated through a variety of vasoactive substances secreted by the kidneys, autonomic nervous system, adrenals, lungs, and vascular endothelium are most important. Accordingly, the cardiovascular system must be viewed as dynamic, continually adapting to optimize organ perfusion. Dysfunction of the heart or any component of the system results in hormonal and other compensatory responses. Some of these compensatory mechanisms are not precisely titrated and may themselves be maladaptive over time. In many circumstances, heart failure occurs as a consequence of pathologic conditions involving the renal, peripheral vascular, neurohormonal, and pulmonary systems. The degree of myocardial dysfunction may be dependent not only on the amount of primary myocardial disease but the functional status of these other organ systems.

EPIDEMIOLOGY

Heart failure represents the only significant cardiovascular disease that is increasing in prevalence in our society. Nearly 5 million people in the United States have been diagnosed with heart failure, and approximately 75% of them are older than 65 years of age.[1] The prevalence of heart failure increases directly with age to 4% to 6% for those over 65 years old.[2] Heart failure is more common in men than women.

Congestive heart failure (CHF) represents the most common reason for hospital admission in patients over 65 years of age, accounting for 900,000 hospitalizations each year.[3] The aging population, coupled with improvements in the medical therapy of heart failure, contributes to current expectations that the prevalence of this disease will continue to increase.[4]

The Framingham Heart Study demonstrates the lethality of heart failure, which has a 5-year mortality rate of approximately 50%. Half of those patients with the most severe disease die within the first year after diagnosis.[5] More recent survival data in patients with CHF continue to demonstrate the lethality of this syndrome.[6] Progressive hemodynamic deterioration accounts for approximately 50% of the deaths, and sudden death resulting from malignant ventricular dysrhythmias occurs in 40% of patients. Current medical therapy has not been successful in reducing the frequency of sudden dysrhythmic deaths but has improved overall outcome from pump failure. Angiotensin-converting enzyme (ACE) inhibitors as well as β-blockers decrease the death rate among heart failure patients by both improving functional status and slowing the rate of progression of pump dysfunction. Hospital survival across all age groups has improved steadily over the last 15 years.[4]

The prognosis in patients with CHF can be related to a number of factors, including age, ejection fraction, exercise tolerance, plasma norepinephrine levels, cardiothoracic ratio on chest radiograph, and the presence of ventricular dysrhythmias.[7] Ventricular ejection fraction is the most precise independent predictor of mortality in patients with heart failure.[8,9] Its correlation with functional capacity is less consistent.

CELLULAR MECHANISMS

The heart is composed of a mass of individual striated muscle cells (myocytes) that form a branching syncytium. Each myocyte contains a central nucleus, mitochondria, an intracellular tubular system known as the *sarcoplasmic reticulum*, and numerous cross-banded strands called *myofibrils* that traverse the length of the myocyte. The myofibrils, in turn, contain multiple subunits called *sarcomeres*. They form the basic functional unit of myocardial contraction and are arranged in series. Sarcomeres occupy approximately 50% of the mass of myocardial cells and are composed of the contractile proteins actin and myosin along with the regulatory proteins troponin and tropomyosin. These proteins are surrounded by invaginations of the myocardial cell membrane (sarcolemma) and the sarcoplasmic reticulum.

The sarcomere ranges in length from 1.6 to 2.2 μm, depending in part on the tension exerted on the muscle before contraction (preload). Sarcomere contraction occurs when the thin, double-helix actin is exposed to the thick myofilament myosin in the presence of Mg^{++} and adenosine triphosphate (ATP). This interaction, and thus myocyte contraction as well as relaxation, is controlled by the intracellular Ca^{++} level. When Ca^{++} is increased, it binds to the contraction regulatory protein troponin, which causes a conformational change in tropomyosin that exposes actin to myosin. In the presence of ATP, linkages are rapidly made and broken between actin and myosin, causing the actin to slide along the myosin filaments. This process generates muscle tension and ultimately myocyte contraction. A drop in intracellular Ca^{++} level reconforms the troponin-tropomyosin complex in such a way that myosin and actin linkages are broken, allowing for sarcomere relaxation. Intracellular ionic calcium is the principal mediator of the inotropic state of the heart. Most positive inotropic agents, including digitalis and catecholamines, act by increasing the availability of intracellular calcium in the vicinity of the myofibrils. Calcium levels are primarily regulated by sarcoplasmic reticulum membrane proteins, which respond to a variety of stimuli.

The normal cardiac index is 2.5 to 4.0 L/min/m^2 at rest. It is determined by the preload, afterload, heart rate, and contractility. In normal hearts, the collective force of contraction of the cardiac chamber is the sum of the forces generated by the individual myocytes. Myocyte force is in turn a function of the ability of the contractile proteins to generate power (inotropic state or contractility), as well as the degree of sarcomere stretch at the start of contraction (preload). Stretching the sarcomere progressively toward its optimum length of 2.2 μm increases the force of contraction by allowing the maximum number of actin-myosin myofilament interactions. This forms the basis of the Frank-Starling relation, which states that within physiologic limits, the force of ventricular contraction is directly related to the end-diastolic length of cardiac muscle.

Preload is the amount of force stretching the myofibril before contraction. In the intact ventricle, preload is produced by the venous return into the chamber resulting in stretch of the myofibrils comprising the chamber walls. The volume filling the chamber also results in the development of pressure that can be measured clinically in either ventricle. Pressure measured within a chamber is determined by both the volume stretching the chamber wall and the compliance characteristics of the muscle. For this reason, pressure is only an indirect reflection of the preload. Changes in compliance may occur acutely (ischemia) or chronically (hypertrophy) and may substantially alter the relationship between chamber volume, pressure, and preload (Figure 76-1). These considerations notwithstanding, the bedside measurement of the pulmonary artery occlusion pressure (PAOP) via a balloon flotation pulmonary artery catheter remains a useful clinical tool in estimating preload of the left heart.

Optimum preload is the filling pressure that maximally stretches ventricular myofibrils and leads to the greatest stroke output per contraction. The actual optimum PAOP must be individualized for each patient because it will be affected by the loading conditions and compliance characteristics of that patient. Patients with acute myocardial infarction tend to have stiffer, less compliant left ventricles. In these patients, optimum PAOP ranges are higher, usually in the range of 20 to 22 mm Hg, whereas patients in septic shock tend to have more compliant hearts, with optimum PAOP in the 12 to 15 mm Hg range. Irrespective of the inotropic state of the ventricle, optimizing preload results in the maximum stroke output for that ventricle (Figure 76-2).

Ventricles possessing normal compliance accommodate

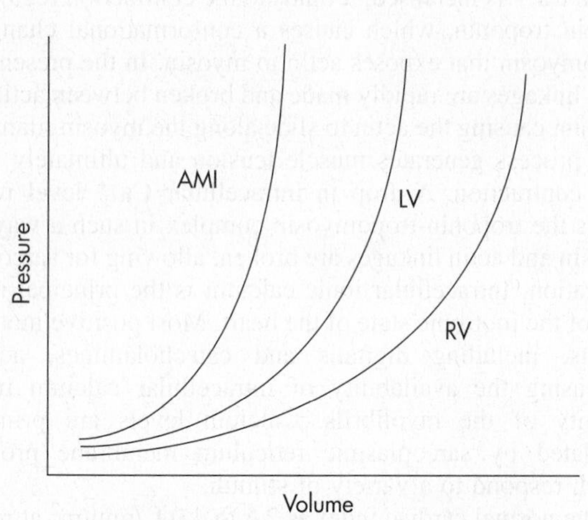

Figure 76-1. **The end-diastolic pressure of the chamber is determined by the filling volume and the compliance characteristics of the chamber. The right ventricle (RV) is more compliant than the more muscular left ventricle (LV), which becomes stiffer still under conditions of ischemia or acute myocardial infarction (AMI).**

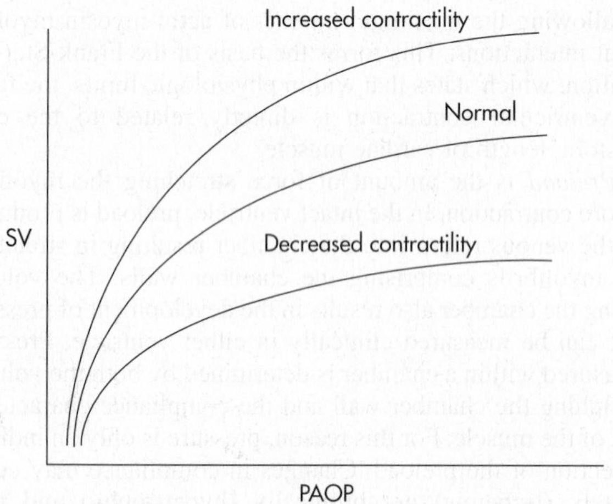

Figure 76-2. **Increased preload, represented as pulmonary artery occlusion pressure (PAOP), results in increased stroke volume (SV) irrespective of the contractile state of the ventricle. At any level of contractility, an optimum PAOP is reached beyond which further increases in pressure may result in increased risk of pulmonary edema, with minimal incremental increase in SV.**

larger volumes before the chamber pressure rises. Accordingly, if pressure is used to estimate preload, the normal ventricle will have more dramatic increases in stroke output for similar increases in filling pressure (steeper Starling curve). The risk of pulmonary edema increases when PAOP rises above normal ranges (15 mm Hg). In patients with low colloid osmotic pressures secondary to hypoalbuminemia, pulmonary edema may occur at even lower filling pressures. This risk must be considered when titrating therapy.

Afterload represents the mural tension acting on myocardial cells during contraction. It is determined by the total

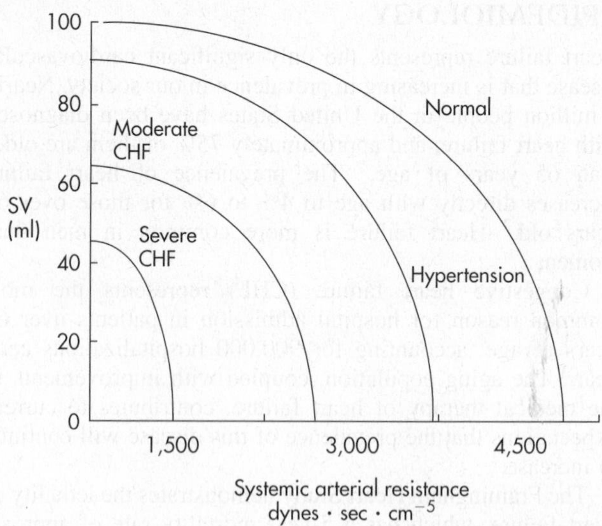

Figure 76-3. **Normal hearts can perform pressure work against high peripheral resistance, maintaining cardiac output even in the face of very high SAR. Failing hearts are more afterload sensitive and exhibit decreased stroke volume (SV) when confronted with high or high-normal resistances.** ***Modified from Weil et al. In Braunwald E, editor:*** **Heart disease: a textbook of cardiovascular medicine,** ***ed 4, Boston, 1992, WB Saunders.***

peripheral vascular resistance and the cardiac chamber size. The peripheral resistance is affected by the total cross-sectional area of the circulation, the blood viscosity, and other factors. The arterioles are the major resistance vessels in the circulation. Flow is directly proportional to the fourth power of the vessel radius (Poiseuille's law). Pulsatile blood flow is converted to more continuous flow by the elastic aorta and major arteries, but most of the pressure drop in the system occurs at the arterioles. The larger the ventricular cavity, the greater the mural tension and thus myocardial work that is required during contraction (law of LaPlace). Failing ventricles cannot overcome increases in peripheral resistance to eject blood (Figure 76-3). In the face of "afterload mismatch," these ventricles dilate further, increasing their end diastolic volumes such that stroke volume is maintained, even in the face of decreasing ejection fraction ("preload reserve"). Failing hearts are, therefore, extremely "afterload sensitive."

For clinical purposes, afterload can be thought of as the pressure against which the heart must pump to eject blood. Blood pressure (BP) is determined by the product of the resistance and flow (BP = SVR × CO). Patients with heart failure and low cardiac output (CO) tend to maintain BP by peripheral vasoconstriction mediated via endogenous catecholamines and the renin-angiotensin system. Afterload reduction may be beneficial for these patients because it allows the conversion of pressure work into flow work (Figure 76-4). When BP is decreased, the isovolumetric phase of contraction is shortened and the ejection phase is lengthened such that CO increases. Because flow work is proportionally less oxygen demanding, afterload reduction therapy has the additional benefit of decreasing myocardial oxygen demands.

Heart rate and rhythmic contraction are important determinants of optimal CO. As heart rate increases to the range of 150 to 160 beats/min in the adult, output increases progres-

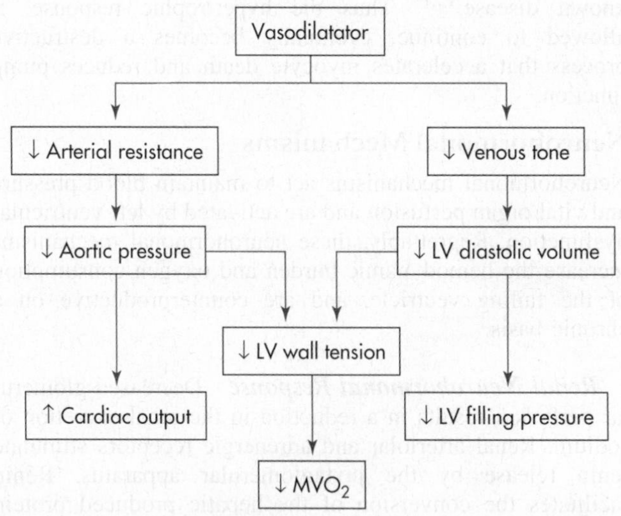

Figure 76-4. **Arterial dilators decrease arterial resistance and result in increased cardiac output. Venodilators decrease venous return to the heart and relieve pulmonary congestion. Balanced agents (nitroprusside, ACE inhibitors) do both. Decreased mural tension reduces myocardial oxygen demands (MVO_2) and may relieve ischemia.**

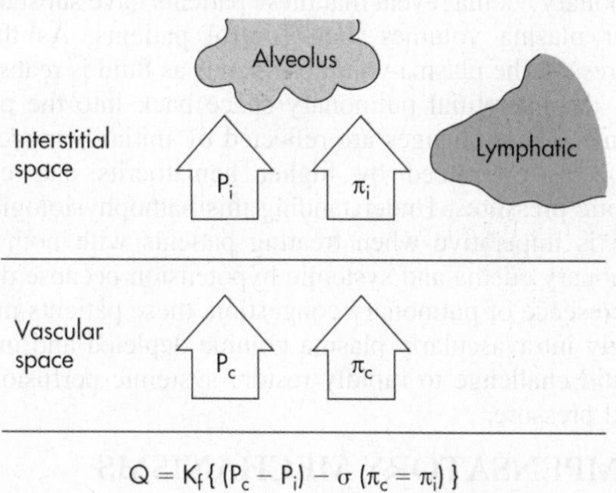

$$Q = K_f\{(P_c - P_i) - \sigma(\pi_c = \pi_i)\}$$

Figure 76-5. **The Starling equation defines fluid flux across the pulmonary capillary membrane. The pulmonary capillary pressure (P_c) is the principal Starling force driving fluid out of the vascular space. The interstitial hydrostatic pressure (P_i) and interstitial colloid osmotic pressure (π_i) both act to draw fluid out of the vascular space as well, but are clinically less important than Pc (measured as PAOP). The plasma colloid osmotic pressure (π_c) is the only Starling force tending to retain fluid in the vascular space. Fluid entering the interstitial space is cleared via lymphatics.**

sively. Tachycardia above this level compromises diastolic filling time and leads to decreased CO. Myocardial perfusion, which occurs during diastole, also becomes impaired by severe tachycardia. Stroke volume is maximized when atrial contraction "primes" the ventricular pumps before they contract. Accordingly, any derangement of intracardiac conduction or dysrhythmia can reduce stroke output. Loss of atrial priming can lead to marked deterioration in cardiac index, especially in diseased, stiffer hearts that require high filling pressures to optimize preload.

Contractility is directly related to intracellular Ca^{++} concentrations and may be affected by a host of factors. Multiple physiologic depressants (hypoxia, hypercarbia, acidosis, ischemia) and pharmacologic depressants (e.g., many cardiac antidysrhythmic agents, calcium antagonists, β-blockers, barbiturates, alcohol) decrease myocardial contractility. Correcting physiologic myocardial depressant factors and discontinuing certain medications with negative inotropic properties are important first steps in managing heart failure patients. Inotropic agents enhance contractility and may improve hemodynamics both acutely (catecholamines) and chronically (cardiac glycosides).

PATHOPHYSIOLOGY OF ACUTE PULMONARY EDEMA

Pulmonary edema is classified clinically into cardiogenic and noncardiogenic forms. Most patients seen in the emergency setting with acute pulmonary edema have the acute cardiogenic variety. Cardiogenic pulmonary edema results from elevated pulmonary capillary hydrostatic pressures. Most commonly cardiogenic pulmonary edema is seen in patients with acute myocardial ischemia or infarction, cardiomyopathies, valvular heart disease, and hypertensive emergencies. In contradistinction, noncardiogenic pulmonary edema generally results from an alteration in the permeability characteristics of the pulmonary capillary membrane. This may result from such diverse causes as systemic sepsis or septic shock, inhalation injuries, drugs and toxins, aspiration syndromes, the fat emboli syndrome, neurogenic causes, and high altitude (Figure 76-5).

Cardiogenic pulmonary edema results primarily from increases in pulmonary capillary hydrostatic pressure that forces a protein sparse plasma ultrafiltrate across the pulmonary capillary membrane into the pulmonary interstitium. As in all forms of pulmonary congestion, this increase in fluid flux immediately results in an increase in the lymphatic drainage of fluid from the lung. These compensatory mechanisms, however, may quickly become overwhelmed as large amounts of edema begin to accumulate in the pulmonary interstitium, ultimately leading to alveolar flooding. The increase in left ventricular end-diastolic pressure that causes the rise in capillary or pulmonary artery occlusion pressure may result from a variety of causes. Increases in left ventricular end-diastolic pressures do not always reflect increases in plasma volume. Although this is generally the case in patients with chronic CHF, in those who present with the acute onset of cardiogenic pulmonary edema (as may result from acute myocardial ischemia, infarction, or other abrupt increases in afterload), plasma volume is generally not expanded and may be contracted. In this scenario, the acute onset of ischemia, infarction, or an abrupt afterload challenge to a ventricle with minimal reserve results in an abrupt shift of the pressure volume curve up and to the left (Figure 76-1). This immediate change in ventricular compliance (diastolic dysfunction) results in the generation of tremendously high left ventricular pressures despite there being no change in volume.[10] The pressures are reflected backward to the pulmonary capillaries, forcing a protein sparse fluid from the plasma into the pulmonary interstitium.

Volumes as large as 1 to 2 L may leave the plasma over a short time and create serious respiratory compromise.

Plasma volume studies in patients with acute cardiogenic pulmonary edema reveal that these patients have substantially lower plasma volumes than control patients. As therapy progresses, the plasma volume expands as fluid is reabsorbed from the interstitial pulmonary space back into the plasma volume. These changes are reflected by initial hemoconcentration as evidenced by higher hematocrits and colloid osmotic pressures. Understanding this pathophysiologic scenario is imperative when treating patients with both acute pulmonary edema and systemic hypotension because despite the presence of pulmonary congestion, these patients may be acutely intravascularly plasma volume depleted and in need of fluid challenge to rapidly restore systemic perfusion and blood pressure.

COMPENSATORY MECHANISMS

Multiple compensatory mechanisms aid the heart in maintaining perfusion in response to an imposed hemodynamic burden or when significant numbers of myocytes are lost because of disease. These adaptive mechanisms include the following.

Increase in Stroke Volume

Increased stroke volume occurs in response to an increase in preload (the Frank-Starling mechanism). This compensatory mechanism is immediate and effective in improving CO in response to acute cardiac demands. It is a limited response, however, because myofibril stretch to a sarcomere length beyond 2.2 μm does not further increase and may actually reduce stroke output.

Increase in Systemic Vascular Resistance

Increased systemic vascular resistance results in redistribution of a subnormal CO away from skin, skeletal muscles, and kidneys to maintain normal blood flow to the brain and heart.

Cardiac Hypertrophy

Development of cardiac hypertrophy is the primary mechanism of the heart to compensate for pump failure. This hypertrophy occurs mainly by increasing the number of myofibrils per cell, as the heart has very limited ability to produce new cells (hyperplasia). New myofibrils arrange in series in response to an increased chamber volume (leading to dilation over time) and in parallel when responding to higher pressure loads (leading to increased chamber wall thickness).[11] In addition to myofibril hypertrophy, mitochondrial mass also expands, leading to adequate ATP provision for the expanded myofibril mass. Initially, hypertrophy leads to improved function of each myocardial cell, but at a higher energy cost. Unfortunately, capillary mass may not increase significantly in response to myocyte hypertrophy. In addition, hypertrophy is associated with myosin isoform synthesis shifts, with related slowing of the rate of contraction, prolongation of the time to peak tension, and reduced rate of relaxation. With the continued influence of volume overload, myofibril mass expands more than mitochondrial mass and relative capillary blood flow is reduced, leading to progressive myocyte death (apoptosis) with fibrosis and increased stress on the remaining myocytes. This appears to be a particular problem with aging, where substantial diffuse loss of myocytes, increased fibrosis, and reactive hypertrophy of remaining myocytes are demonstrated even in hearts without known disease.[12,13] Thus the hypertrophic response, if allowed to continue, eventually becomes a destructive process that accelerates myocyte death and reduces pump function.

Neurohormonal Mechanisms

Neurohormonal mechanisms act to maintain blood pressure and vital organ perfusion and are activated by left ventricular dysfunction. Regrettably, these neurohormonal mechanisms increase the hemodynamic burden and oxygen consumption of the failing ventricle, and are counterproductive on a chronic basis.

Renal Neurohormonal Response Decreased glomerular perfusion results in a reduction in the renal excretion of sodium. Renal arteriolar and adrenergic receptors stimulate renin release by the juxtaglomerular apparatus. Renin facilitates the conversion of the hepatic produced protein angiotensinogen to angiotensin I, which is further converted to angiotensin II by ACE. Angiotensin II is a potent vasoconstrictor and also an important stimulus for aldosterone release by the adrenal cortex. Aldosterone increases renal sodium retention.

With long-standing heart failure, renal adaptation to hypoperfusion occurs, mainly through production of vasodilatory hormones such as prostacyclin, along with prostaglandins PGI_2 and PGE_2. Aspirin and other nonsteroidal anti-inflammatory agents (NSAIDs) interfere with prostaglandin synthesis by inhibiting cyclooxygenase. Accordingly, their use optimally should be avoided in patients with chronic heart failure because they may precipitate acute renal insufficiency with concomitant salt and water retention.

Central and Autonomic Nervous System Neurohormonal Response The heart and great vessels contain sensory receptors that detect changes in perfusion. Metabolic receptors in muscles also exert inhibitory and excitatory influences on brainstem vasomotor neurons. Heart failure results in a generalized stimulation of sympathetic activity and inhibition of parasympathetic tone. Arginine vasopressin (antidiuretic hormone [ADH]) is released from the pituitary gland, promoting mild vasoconstriction and renal water retention. ADH secretion contributes to water retention and may be a significant cause of hyponatremia in patients with severe heart failure.

Increased sympathetic outflow results in the release of increased epinephrine and norepinephrine from the adrenal glands, and norepinephrine at peripheral sympathetic nerve endings. These elevated catecholamine levels stimulate surface receptors in the heart and blood vessels, increasing cardiac contractility, heart rate, and vascular tone. The resulting increased venous tone is thought to improve blood return to the heart and augment preload, which tends to maintain stroke output (preload reserve).

Increased arterial smooth muscle tone increases afterload. This mechanism presumably evolved to maintain adequate blood pressure in the face of hypovolemia. Increased afterload is deleterious to the failing ventricle that is incapable of maintaining stroke output against this resistance to flow. This adaptive mechanism therefore exacerbates myocardial dysfunction. Afterload reduction can permit improved stroke output as pressure work is converted to flow work (Figure 76-4). Care must be taken to maintain adequate preload to achieve optimum benefit. Acutely, arterial blood pressure is improved and CO increased by the positive inotropic catecholamines, but chronically, a decrease in the number and affinity of surface catecholamine receptors occurs in myocardial tissue, reducing responsiveness to epinephrine and norepinephrine.

Cardiac Neurohormonal Response Increases in atrial chamber volume activate the release of at least three types of atrial natriuretic peptide (ANP), the main two from cardiac tissue.[14] A variety of ANP receptors exist on endothelial cells, vascular smooth muscle cells, and renal epithelial cells, and in the myocardium as well.[15] ANP serves to inhibit activation of the renin-angiotensin-aldosterone system. It is an effective vasodilating agent, and it contributes to improved sodium homeostasis by enabling salt wasting. Circulating ANP is greatly increased in CHF as a result of increased synthesis. In early heart failure, it may play a key role in compensation for left ventricular dysfunction. Unfortunately, a progressive attenuation of renal response to ANP occurs as heart failure progresses, probably because of multiple factors including decreased renal perfusion pressure, ANP receptor downregulation, and increase in activity of functional antagonists to ANP including circulating norepinephrine and the renin-angiotensin-aldosterone system. Research focuses on inhibition of degradation of ANP by the ectoenzyme neutral endopeptidase 24, with favorable hemodynamic responses.[13,16]

MYOCARDIAL PATHOPHYSIOLOGY

Heart failure can result from primary disease of the coronary arteries, myocardium, cardiac valves, pericardium, peripheral vessels, or lungs. Commonly, recognition of the underlying disease process is impossible late in the course of heart failure; however, early recognition in many situations can lead to appropriate interventions that may improve the clinical condition, such as valvular repair for progressive aortic stenosis.

Coronary Artery Disease

In developed countries, atherosclerotic coronary artery disease remains the leading cause of heart failure. Acute coronary thrombosis in vessels compromised by atheromatous plaques leads to focal myocardial necrosis with resultant myocardial fibrosis and scarring. This process leads to areas of dyskinesis that result in decreased ejection fraction. When 40% of the left ventricular muscle mass is infarcted, the pump can no longer support the circulation and cardiogenic shock ensues. Abnormal dilation of infarcted areas with paradoxical motion during systole may disproportionately decrease ejection fraction. Surgical repair may be beneficial in selected cases. Transient loss of contractile function may result from episodes of myocardial ischemia that do not cause frank necrosis or from an ischemic zone surrounding an infarct. This so-called *myocardial stunning* may persist for several days.[17]

Chronic coronary insufficiency leads to a more diffuse myocardial fibrosis, sometimes called *ischemic cardiomyopathy.* Revascularization of ischemic but not infarcted myocardial tissue provides a clear survival benefit in patients with CHF resulting from ischemic left ventricular systolic dysfunction. Diseases affecting the coronary microcirculation (e.g., vasoocclusive sickle cell anemia and diabetes mellitus) result in similar pathology. Compensatory mechanisms may occur after large myocardial infarction and progressive cardiac disease, which are collectively termed ventricular remodeling. They include cardiac dilation, reactive hypertrophy, and changes in wall conformation that may result from elevated chamber filling pressures as well as neurohumoral factors.

Cardiomyopathies

The cardiomyopathies refer to a group of disease processes that affect the myocardium primarily. Myocardial disease resulting from coronary, valvular, and pericardial pathologies is excluded. Cardiomyopathies are categorized as primary, in which case the cause is unknown, or secondary to some identifiable cause or systemic illness (Box 76-1). Clinically, patients with cardiomyopathy tend to present in three forms: dilated, hypertrophic, or restrictive. In reality, there may be

Box 76-1 Etiologic Classification of Cardiomyopathies

I. Primary myocardial involvement
   A. Idiopathic (D,R,H)
   B. Familial (D,H)
   C. Endomyocardial fibrosis (R)
II. Secondary myocardial involvement
   A. Infective (D)
      1. Viral myocarditis
      2. Bacterial myocarditis
      3. Fungal myocarditis
      4. Protozoal myocarditis
      5. Metazoal myocarditis
   B. Metabolic (D)
   C. Familial storage disease (D,R)
      1. Glycogen storage disease
      2. Mucopolysaccharidosis
   D. Deficiency (D)
      1. Electrolytes
      2. Nutritional
   E. Connective tissue disorders (D)
      1. Systemic lupus erythematosus
      2. Polyarteritis nodosa
      3. Rheumatoid arthritis
      4. Progressive systemic sclerosis
      5. Dermatomyositis
   F. Infiltrations and granulomas (R,D)
      1. Amyloidosis
      2. Sarcoidosis
      3. Malignancy
      4. Hemochromatosis
   G. Neuromuscular (D)
      1. Muscular dystrophy
      2. Myotonic dystrophy
      3. Friedreich's ataxia (H,D)
      4. Refsum's disease
   H. Sensitivity and toxic reactions (D)
      1. Alcohol
      2. Radiation
      3. Drugs
   I. Peripartum heart disease (D)
   J. Endocardial fibroelastosis (R)

Modified from the WHO/ISFC task force report on the definition and classification of cardiomyopathies, 1980. From *Harrison's principles of internal medicine,* ed 12, New York, 1991, McGraw-Hill.

The principal clinical manifestations of each etiologic grouping are denoted by D (dilated), R (restrictive), or H (hypertrophic) cardiomyopathy.

substantial overlap among these categories. In addition, patients with acute myocarditis may have the precipitous onset of heart failure.

Dilated Cardiomyopathy Dilated cardiomyopathy is the most common form of cardiomyopathy. In most cases no definitive cause is identified. Rather, a variety of infectious, toxic, and metabolic agents probably contribute to the myocardial damage. Some are thought to be postviral in origin with secondary immunologic mechanisms resulting in progressive myocardial damage. Heavy alcohol consumption over years may be contributory in many cases. Cocaine use is a more recently recognized cause. A familial disease is present in less than 20% of patients with dilated cardiomyopathy, with autosomal dominant inheritance in many cases.[18,19]

Dilated cardiomyopathy is characterized by four-chamber cardiac enlargement, often with mural thrombi. Pump dysfunction is primarily systolic. CO may be normal at rest, but it does not adequately increase with exertion. Patients have typical symptoms of CHF. Histologic examination reveals interstitial and perivascular fibrosis with minimal necrosis or cellular infiltration.

Hypertrophic Cardiomyopathy Hypertrophic cardiomyopathy refers specifically to a form of hypertrophy that is not secondary to a hemodynamic load as may be imposed by conditions such as hypertension or valvular aortic stenosis. Approximately half of all cases of hypertrophic cardiomyopathy are familially linked. One third of the first-degree relatives of patients with hypertrophic cardiomyopathy have evidence of the disease, although many have only mild, asymptomatic cases. This disease is characterized by left ventricular hypertrophy, typically without chamber enlargement, but with common and characteristic excessive thickening of the upper left ventricular septum. There is abnormal systolic anterior motion of the anterior mitral valve leaflet that may result in a dynamic outflow obstruction to left ventricular ejection, but causes a significant pressure gradient in only approximately one fourth of the patients. Diastolic dysfunction is the main pathologic abnormality. Increased stiffness of the hypertrophied cardiac muscle results primarily from elevated intracellular calcium levels.

Hypertrophic cardiomyopathy is often clinically silent but is a common cause of sudden death in young adults, which often occurs during or just after exertion. Dyspnea on exertion is the most common complaint among symptomatic patients. Exertional syncope is another common presentation. Symptoms are not always related to the severity of the outflow gradient. The classic physical examination finding in hypertrophic cardiomyopathy is a harsh systolic murmur heard best at the lower left sternal border and increased by maneuvers that decrease preload (e.g., Valsalva maneuver), decrease afterload (e.g., vasodilator therapy), or increase inotropicity (e.g., exercise). Young patients with syncope or dyspnea with suggestive clinical findings should undergo urgent echocardiography, the easiest means of confirming the diagnosis. Patients with suspected or diagnosed hypertrophic cardiomyopathy should be cautioned to avoid strenuous exercise. β-Blockers, amiodarone, and calcium channel blockers are used successfully in these patients. Digitalis, diuretics, nitrates, and β-agonists should in general be avoided in hypertrophic cardiomyopathy.

Restrictive Cardiomyopathy Restrictive cardiomyopathy, the least common type of cardiomyopathy, occurs when cardiac muscle is infiltrated by other substances such as iron (hemochromatosis), protein (amyloidosis), granulomas (sarcoidosis), or fibrotic tissue. The chambers are stiff. Abnormalities in diastolic relaxation predominate, but systolic function is generally well preserved. Clinically, patients have sequelae of chronically elevated venous pressure such as peripheral edema, ascites, and congestive hepatomegaly.

Myocarditis

Myocarditis is defined as an acute inflammatory reaction of the myocardium. It may precipitate heart failure. Most cases of myocarditis go clinically unrecognized. In mild cases, nonspecific complaints of fatigue and dyspnea resolve after a short period of illness. Most commonly the result of a viral infectious process, myocarditis may also be caused by various other infectious agents, toxins, autoimmune disorders, and some physical agents. A small number of patients with acute myocarditis develop life-threatening dysrhythmias or progressive heart failure. Others may transiently recover only to develop a dilated cardiomyopathy after a latent period of weeks to years.

The clinical presentation of patients with myocarditis is generally nonspecific. Complaints of chest discomfort are often pleuritic and suggest associated pericarditis. Unexplained sinus tachycardia and nonspecific ST-segment and T-wave changes on the electrocardiogram (ECG) may be present. In some patients, acute myocarditis may simulate myocardial infarction with chest pain, ECG changes, and elevated cardiac enzyme levels. Chest radiography may show an enlarged heart and echocardiography may reveal diffuse wall motion abnormalities and chamber dilation.

Valvular Heart Disease

Cardiac valvular disease is the third leading cause of heart failure, after ischemic heart disease and dilated cardiomyopathy. Acute valvular dysfunction may precipitate fulminant heart failure. This includes acute mitral regurgitation secondary to papillary muscle rupture in acute myocardial infarction or acute aortic insufficiency secondary to acute bacterial endocarditis or aortic dissection. Most acute valvular dysfunction involves either the mitral or aortic valves. Acute valvular failure usually results in fulminant regurgitant lesions. Acutely stenotic lesions are predominantly restricted to mechanical catastrophes of prosthetic valves. Typical murmurs may be difficult to appreciate in acute valvular insufficiency because of early equilibration of pressures across the defective valve. Accordingly, patients may present in extremis with fulminant pulmonary edema predominating the clinical picture.

Acute mitral regurgitation commonly occurs as a result of dysfunction of the valvular supporting apparatus, the papillary muscles, and chordae tendineae, which connect the valve leaflets to the papillary muscles. Infectious endocarditis and myxomatous degeneration are common causes of chordae tendineae rupture. Any cause of acute left ventricular dilation may cause functional mitral regurgitation. Papillary muscle dysfunction most commonly occurs as a result of acute myocardial ischemia. Transient dysfunction may occur during episodes of angina pectoris, whereas permanent dysfunction and even papillary muscle rupture may occur early in the course of myocardial infarction. Papillary muscle failure days to weeks after infarction may lead to delayed cardiac decompensation.

Aortic dissection and infectious endocarditis are the most common causes of acute aortic regurgitation. Type A aortic dissection (involving the aortic arch) commonly disrupts the annulus of the aortic valve and may precipitate acute aortic insufficiency. This is identified clinically by hypotension, fulminant pulmonary edema, and an aortic diastolic murmur in a patient with a widened mediastinum on chest radiograph. Rapid surgical correction affords the only chance for survival. Type A dissections may also precipitate pericardial tamponade. Failure to recognize this clinical entity may cause a fatal therapeutic misadventure if thrombolytic therapy is used because aortic dissection may present with severe chest pain along with coronary osteal occlusion. Patients with infectious endocarditis may have fever, stigmata of intravenous (IV) drug use, and evidence of heart block from infectious involvement of myocardial conduction tissue surrounding the valve.

Acute endocarditis may cause valvular obstruction as a result of large vegetations. Outflow obstruction may also be seen with the rare conditions of atrial myxoma or air embolism. With the increasing prevalence of prosthetic heart valves more patients will present with acute mechanical failure not only because of structural problems, but more commonly because of occlusion by thrombus or pannus. These cases often present as acutely stenotic lesions with syncope or obstructive shock. An important new adage is that acute heart failure in any patient with a prosthetic cardiac valve requires immediate evaluation to demonstrate that the valve is operating normally.

Chronic Valvular Disease

Among the chronic valvular lesions, mitral insufficiency and aortic stenosis are most commonly associated with CHF. Often, more than one valvular lesion may be present, leading to complex clinical presentations. Acute decompensation usually has some recognizable precipitating cause. The precise valvular derangement may not typically be definable by clinical examination alone, but suggestive cardiac murmurs in the appropriate clinical setting should prompt echocardiographic or more invasive evaluation.

Knowing the precise valvular pathology may have important implications for emergency therapy of patients with heart failure. For example, patients with decompensated aortic stenosis should not receive vasodilator agents. These patients cannot increase flow across their fixed obstruction and therefore may become hypotensive if given this therapy. On the other hand, patients with mitral regurgitation benefit greatly from vasodilators, which improve antegrade flow by reducing systemic afterload.

Pericardial Diseases

Pericardial diseases may significantly affect cardiac performance, causing both decreased CO and increased intracardiac pressures. Accumulation of fluid in the pericardial sac surrounding the heart may occur acutely in such conditions as blunt or penetrating trauma, acute pericarditis, uremia, or malignancy. The pericardium cannot stretch acutely. Accordingly, fluid accumulation of as little as 100 ml may compromise cardiac filling and decrease CO. The presence of elevated venous pressures, pulsus paradoxus, hypoperfusion, and tachycardia should prompt a rapid evaluation for the presence of cardiac tamponade in the appropriate clinical setting. Echocardiography shows the presence of pericardial fluid and compromised ventricular filling. An alternative approach is bedside right heart catheterization, which demonstrates increased and equal diastolic pressures in all chambers with low cardiac output.

Constrictive pericarditis is a rare clinical entity that restricts diastolic filling of all cardiac chambers because of a thickened and sometimes calcified pericardial sac. Symptoms are related to low cardiac output, often with a prominent finding of right heart failure. This clinical condition is difficult to distinguish from restrictive cardiomyopathy. It should be considered in all low CO states.

Pulmonary Disease

Pulmonary dysfunction causing hypoxia reduces myocardial oxygen supply while increasing CO demand by perfusing all tissues with suboptimally oxygenated blood. Hypoxia leads to pulmonary arteriolar vasoconstriction, and along with various destructive processes such as emphysema and pulmonary fibrosis, which reduce lung vascular bed area, causes elevation of pulmonary artery pressures. Chronic increases in pulmonary arterial pressure lead to right ventricular hypertrophy and dilation. When compensatory mechanisms fail, the patient develops clinical evidence of right heart failure (cor pulmonale), usually with left ventricular output preserved, at least at rest. Causes of acute cor pulmonale (e.g., a large pulmonary embolus) may precipitate sudden systemic hypotension and even death caused by decreased left ventricular priming.

Distinguishing primary pulmonary disease causing predominantly right-sided heart failure from left ventricular failure with secondary right-sided dysfunction is sometimes clinically challenging. Both entities may present primarily with wheezing or rhonchi on physical examination. The chest radiograph may be difficult to interpret because both disease types cause interstitial changes. Hyperinflation depresses the diaphragm, which elongates the cardiac silhouette and may mask cardiomegaly.

CLASSIFICATION OF HEART FAILURE

Many different methods of classifying heart failure exist. Late in the disease process these distinctions become blurred and somewhat artificial. Early in the course of heart failure they may be useful clinical descriptors suggesting particular causes and treatment strategies.

High Output versus Low Output Failure

High output failure is nonintuitive, but refers to patients who are in a hyperdynamic state with supranormal CO and low arteriovenous oxygen difference (decreased oxygen extraction ratio). They concurrently experience pulmonary congestion and peripheral edema as a consequence of elevated diastolic pressures. Diastolic dysfunction and circulatory overload contribute to the congestive symptoms. As the condition progresses, systolic myocardial dysfunction is superimposed, symptoms progress, and at this point normal or even low cardiac outputs are present. Ultimately, untreated patients have classic CHF clinically indistinguishable from other end-stage cardiomyopathies.

A persistent hyperdynamic state resulting in myocardial damage over time is consistent with animal models of hyperdynamic, pacemaker-induced tachycardia that invariably results in overt heart failure.[20,21] The hyperdynamic state may result from increased preload (e.g., renal retention of salt and water, mineralocorticoids), decreased systemic vascular resistance (e.g., arteriovenous fistulas, pregnancy, cirrhosis, severe anemia, beriberi, thyrotoxicosis, Paget's disease, vasodilator medications), increased β-sympathetic activity, or persistent tachycardia. Early identification of the hyperdynamic state may result in effective therapy of the underlying condition, thus avoiding the development of heart failure.

Low output failure is the more typical variety of heart failure and occurs as the result of entities such as ischemic heart disease, dilated cardiomyopathy, valvular disease, and chronic hypertension. Low CO (systolic dysfunction), high filling pressures (diastolic dysfunction), and increased systemic oxygen extraction ratio (widened arteriovenous oxygen content difference) characterize this more commonly encountered classic form of heart failure.

Acute versus Chronic Heart Failure

The prototypical case of acute heart failure is in the healthy person who develops a large myocardial infarction or acute valvular dysfunction. Chronic heart failure is best characterized by a disease state such as dilated cardiomyopathy, with gradual deterioration of cardiac function. In acute heart failure, the early presentation may be due to systolic dysfunction and hypoperfusion, often with acute pulmonary edema resulting from the sudden reduction in chamber compliance (diastolic dysfunction) that accompanies acute ischemia or infarction. Chronic heart failure usually presents with symptoms related to fluid retention, with compensatory mechanisms adjusted so that normal perfusion exists, at least in the resting state. In chronic heart failure, treatment must be directed at not only the failing pump but also the compensatory mechanisms that result in peripheral vasoconstriction as well as salt and water retention.[22]

Right-Sided versus Left-Sided Heart Failure

The notion that one of the cardiac chambers can fail independently of the other is somewhat artificial. The right and left circulations are connected, and over time output from the two chambers must be equal. Furthermore, the right and left ventricles share an interventricular septum. Acute right-sided heart failure from pulmonary hypertension secondary to acute respiratory failure causes bulging of the interventricular septum into the left ventricular chamber. This so-called *septal shift* results in decreased left ventricular preload and low CO that is volume responsive. In addition, cardiac biochemical changes such as abnormal catecholamine response affect all chambers. Chronic left-sided heart failure leads to pulmonary hypertension with resultant right-sided heart failure. Nonetheless, the terms have some usefulness in identifying the predominant clinical presentation. Fluid accumulation "behind" the involved ventricle is responsible for many of the clinical manifestations of heart failure. For example, left ventricular failure leads primarily to pulmonary congestion with symptoms mostly of dyspnea and orthopnea. Right-sided heart failure presents with symptoms of systemic venous congestion such as pedal edema and hepatomegaly.

In the ED when patients who were previously normal have acute pathology, the concept of left- versus right-sided heart failure may be useful clinically. Patients with acute myocardial infarction of the anterior wall may present in acute pulmonary edema with pulmonary crackles on auscultation and an S_3 gallop. Yet, unlike patients with chronic heart failure, they will generally not have jugular venous distention or pedal edema because the central venous pressure remains normal. Chest radiograph reveals evidence of pulmonary venous congestion (cephalization), interstitial edema (Kerley's A and B lines), and in fulminant cases, alveolar edema. Because there has not yet been time for cardiac dilation, the size of the cardiac shadow is normal.

Patients with acute right ventricular infarction typically have jugular venous distention and hypotension but often without pulmonary crackles. Bulging of the interventricular septum into the left ventricular chamber results in decreased left ventricular preload. The low CO and hypotension are, in many cases, responsive to fluid challenge.[23] Jugular venous distention is a sign of acute right heart diastolic dysfunction. Failure to recognize this sign results in the withholding of a therapeutic fluid challenge if the distended neck veins are interpreted simply as a sign of heart failure.

Forward versus Backward Heart Failure

Forward failure refers to inadequate systemic perfusion resulting from low CO. Symptoms of forward failure include weakness, fatigue, oliguria, prerenal azotemia, and in advanced cases hypotension and cardiogenic shock. Backward failure refers to symptoms referable to the back pressure that builds up "behind" a failing chamber. Pulmonary edema, hepatomegaly, and pedal edema represent backward failure symptoms.

Systolic versus Diastolic Dysfunction

The classification of systolic and diastolic dysfunction requires precise thinking regarding pathophysiology and allows for specific treatment strategies (Figure 76-6).[24] Systolic dysfunction refers to impairment of contractility. Stroke output is reduced and forward flow is compromised. Systolic dysfunction is typically caused by myocyte destruction as occurs in myocardial infarction or acute myocarditis. Diastolic dysfunction indicates a primary problem with the ability of the ventricles to relax and fill normally. In many cases, normal or even supernormal systolic function is preserved.

Echocardiographic and nuclear imaging techniques demonstrate that approximately 40% of patients with congestive symptoms have normal ejection fractions.[25] Diastolic dysfunction is the predominant pathophysiologic problem in hypertrophic and restrictive cardiomyopathies, chronic hypertension, valvular aortic stenosis, and other conditions. Diastolic dysfunction predominately occurs as a result of one of three mechanisms: impaired ventricular relaxation, increased ventricular wall thickness, or accumulation of myocardial interstitial collagen.[26,27] Impaired relaxation capacity of the myocardium leads to higher ventricular filling pressure, which results in congestive symptoms. Myocardial relaxation is an active, energy-requiring process. Failure of myocytes to relax may be secondary to low intracellular energy stores.

Most patients with heart failure have components of both systolic and diastolic dysfunction. Patients with predominantly diastolic dysfunction, however, have an advantage in having intact myocardial contractile function. This may allow for the safe administration of therapeutic interventions such as β-blocker therapy that may improve diastolic dysfunction by reducing myocardial oxygen demands. The negative

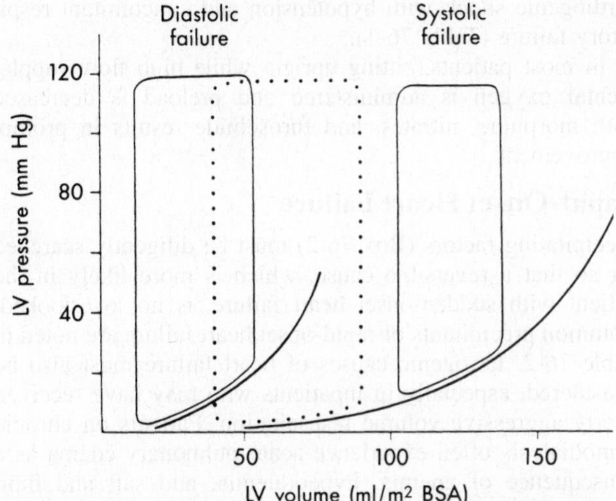

Figure 76-6. **Schematic diagram of left ventricular pressure-volume loops in diastolic and systolic failure. The dotted line represents a normal loop. In diastolic failure, the chamber volume is normal or decreased, the systolic ejection fraction is normal or above normal, and the chamber stiffness is increased. Because of the increased stiffness, end-diastolic pressure is elevated. In systolic failure, the chamber is dilated and the systolic ejection fraction is low. The end-diastolic pressure may or may not be increased.** *From Stauffer JC, Gaasch WH:* **Prog Cardiovasc Dis** *32:319, 1990.*

inotropic effects should be well tolerated in this group of patients with normal contractility; however, caution in the treatment of diastolic dysfunction is also important. These stiffer hearts have steep pressure volume curves, so small reductions in diastolic filling volume, as may occur with aggressive diuretic therapy, may markedly decrease ventricular filling (see Figure 76-1). This preload deficiency may compromise stroke output.

CLINICAL EVALUATION OF PATIENTS WITH SUSPECTED HEART FAILURE

The presentation of patients in heart failure varies with the stage of the disease at the time of presentation. Careful consideration of the differential diagnosis is symptom based. The most common manifestation of acute heart failure is acute respiratory distress caused by pulmonary edema. Accordingly, the differential diagnosis includes exacerbation of chronic obstructive pulmonary disease or asthma, pulmonary embolus, pneumonia, anaphylaxis, and other causes of acute respiratory distress. Hypoperfusion may be caused by some of these, as well as by sepsis syndrome, hypovolemia, hemorrhage, cardiac tamponade, tension pneumothorax, and other disease processes.

Precipitating Causes

Stresses that may result in the acute decompensation are noted in Box 76-2. The presence and character of chest pain, previous heart disease, cardiac catheterization, surgery, and cardiac history all must be explored.

Orthopnea, breathlessness that occurs in recumbency, is a type of dyspnea seen among patients with heart failure. The supine position enhances venous return to the heart, precipitating increases in diastolic cardiac pressure. The symptoms abate when the patient sits up and venous return decreases.

Box 76-2 Common Precipitating Causes of Acute Heart Failure

- Systemic hypertension
- Myocardial infarction/ischemia
- Dysrhythmia
- Systemic infection
- Anemia
- Dietary, physical, environmental, and emotional excesses
- Pregnancy
- Thyrotoxicosis
- Acute myocarditis
- Acute valvular dysfunction
- Pulmonary embolus
- Pharmacologic complications

Paroxysmal nocturnal dyspnea (PND) is breathlessness that awakens the patient from sleep. It results from pulmonary congestion precipitated by plasma volume expansion that occurs as interstitial edema fluid is reabsorbed into the circulation because venous hydrostatic pressures in the legs decrease during recumbency. Nocturia, frequent urination interrupting sleep, results from the same pathophysiologic process.

Physical Examination

Clammy, vasoconstricted patients with thready pulse and delayed capillary refill may have systemic hypoperfusion despite adequate blood pressure (maintained by intense vasoconstriction). Frankly hypotensive patients require intraarterial pressure monitoring. Noninvasive assessment of blood pressure in the vasoconstricted patient with low CO is inaccurate.[28] Cuff pressures in these patients typically reflect mean rather than systolic arterial pressure. Obtaining true intraarterial pressure may make a substantial difference in the choice of therapeutic agent. For example, a patient with a cuff pressure of 80 mm Hg might receive a catecholamine vasoconstrictor to maintain coronary perfusion pressure despite the negative impact of these drugs on afterload and ischemia. If it were known that the mean intraarterial pressure was 80 mm Hg, that same patient might more appropriately receive carefully titrated venodilators (nitroglycerin).

Severe hypoperfusion to the brain often results in mental confusion, and hypoperfusion to the kidneys significantly reduces urine output. Hypertension in the setting of heart failure allows liberal use of vasodilators. Because elevated afterload impairs ventricular ejection and places high oxygen demands on the myocardium, hypertension should be aggressively treated in patients with heart failure. This is critically important in patients who have active ongoing myocardial ischemia or infarction.

Physical examination in patients with acute pulmonary edema resulting from acute myocardial infarction includes a search for surgically correctable lesions such as mitral regurgitation and ventricular septal defect. Patients with pulmonary congestion secondary to heart failure develop interstitial and alveolar pulmonary edema, causing reduced pulmonary compliance and decreased functional residual capacity. These factors result in decreased tidal volumes and tachypnea. Inspiratory crackles reflect alveolar flooding and are present in patients with pulmonary edema. Wheezing may also be a prominent finding in patients with pulmonary edema, which may be mistaken for bronchospastic airway disease. Unfortunately, relief obtained from bronchodilators tends to be short lived in patients with pulmonary edema, and the β effect of tachycardia may be deleterious, especially to ischemic hearts. The upright chest radiograph may be the most useful tool to distinguish cardiogenic pulmonary edema from other causes of dyspnea.

TREATMENT OF HEART FAILURE

The immediate therapeutic goals in treating heart failure patients are to improve respiratory gas exchange and maintain adequate arterial saturation (PAO_2 >60 mm Hg or 90% saturation), and to decrease pulmonary artery occlusion pressure while maintaining adequate cardiac and systemic perfusion. The acute congestive state may be controlled by (1) reducing the cardiac workload by decreasing both preload and afterload, (2) controlling excessive retention of salt and water, and (3) improving cardiac contractility. Patients may have a wide spectrum of symptoms and signs ranging from mild dyspnea on exertion or orthopnea to full-blown cardiogenic shock with hypotension and concomitant respiratory failure (Table 76-1).

In most patients, sitting upright while high flow supplemental oxygen is administered and preload is decreased with morphine, nitrates, and furosemide results in prompt improvement.

Rapid-Onset Heart Failure

Precipitating factors (Box 76-2) must be diligently searched for so that a reversible cause, which is more likely in the patient with sudden-onset heart failure, is not overlooked. Common precipitants of rapid-onset heart failure are noted in Table 76-2. Iatrogenic causes of heart failure must also be considered, especially in inpatients who may have received overly aggressive volume resuscitation. Patients on chronic hemodialysis often experience acute pulmonary edema as a consequence of anemia, hyperkalemia, and salt and fluid overload and will require acute hemodialysis.

Acute Pulmonary Edema

The ability of the left ventricle to generate systolic pressures above 160 mm Hg in some patients with acute pulmonary

Table 76-1. Agents Useful in the Treatment of Heart Failure

			Action				
Agent	**Route**	**Mechanism**	**PAOP**	**CI**	**BP**	**HR**	**Comment**
Morphine	IV	Sympatholytic	↓↓↓	–	↓	↓	Excellent in APE avoid in COPD
Nitroglycerin	Sublingual Transmucosal Transcutaneous	Direct smooth muscle dilator	↓↓	–	– or ↓	–	Venodilator or relieves ischemia
Nitroglycerin	IV		↓↓↓↓	↑	↓	–	Venodilator or vasodilator in larger doses tachyphylaxis
Furosemide	Oral IV	Loop diuretic venodilator	↓↓	–	– or ↓	–	Electrolyte abnormalities
ACE inhibitors	Oral IV	Angiotensin coronary enzyme inhibition	↓↓	↑↑	↓↓	– or ↓	Improves outcome in chronic CHF antihypertension
Nitroprusside	IV	Direct smooth muscle dilator	↓↓↓↓	↑↑↑	↓↓↓	– or ↓	Intraarterial monitoring required Thiocyanate and cyanide toxicity
Digoxin	Oral IV	Increased Ca^+ availability	↓	↑	–	↓	Most effective in a-fib with chronic CHF
Dobutamine	IV	β-Agonist	↓↓	↑↑	– or ↓	– or ↑	Safest catecholamine inotrope May cause hypotension
Dopamine	IV	β-, β-dopaminergic agonist	–	↑↑	↑↑	↑	Effects differ with dose range
Levarterenol	IV	α-Agonist	↑	↑	↑↑↑↑	↑	Most effective vasopressor
Epinephrine	IV	α- and β-agonist	–	↑↑↑	↑↑↑	↑↑↑	High potential to induce ischemia
Amrinone	IV	Phosphodiesterase inhibitor	↓↓	↑↑	↓	↓	Nontitratable inotropic vasodilator
β-Blockers	Oral IV	Beta blockade	↑↑	↓↓	↓↓	↓↓	May be useful chronically to treat diastolic dysfunction

APE, Acute pulmonary edema; *CHF,* congestive heart failure; *CI,* cardiac index; *COPD,* chronic obstructive pulmonary disease; *IV,* intravenous.

edema indicates the presence of considerable myocardial reserve and is associated with a better prognosis than that seen in normotensive or hypotensive patients.[29] This group must be quickly distinguished from patients with pulmonary edema with evidence of hypoperfusion (cold, clammy skin and altered mental status) who present a greater therapeutic challenge.[29] Patients with hypertensive pulmonary edema are easier to manage because afterload reduction with the use of vasodilators is extremely effective and well tolerated in this group.

Most patients with acute pulmonary edema are diaphoretic because of intense sympathetic activation. Typical pulmonary findings include crackles or wheezes, although both may be absent with decreased ventilation in more agonal patients. Jugular venous distention is present in approximately 50%, and one third of patients have peripheral edema.[29] An S_3 gallop may be present in up to 25% but is often difficult to appreciate in this clinical setting. An enlarged cardiac silhouette is seen on chest radiograph in 70% of cases. These common clinical findings of chronic CHF are prevalent among patients with acute pulmonary edema because most patients have acute exacerbations superimposed on chronic underlying disease. The absence of jugular venous distention, pedal edema, and cardiomegaly is the rule rather than the exception in previously healthy individuals with pulmonary edema resulting from an initial episode of acute myocardial infarction or unstable angina. Accordingly, a normal-size heart on chest x-ray study may be consistent with acute cardiogenic pulmonary edema. In addition, this finding should suggest the possibility of diastolic dysfunction, chronic obstructive pulmonary disease (COPD), or noncardiogenic pulmonary edema.

Supplemental oxygen should be administered immediately via high-flow face mask in spontaneously breathing patients. Hypoxia causes pulmonary artery constriction, increases CO requirements, increases the risk of dysrhythmias, and may exacerbate metabolic acidosis.

Most patients with fulminant acute pulmonary edema have lactic acidosis resulting from the combination of decreased systemic perfusion and the increased muscular work of breathing.[30] Most patients have concomitant respiratory alkalosis resulting from the tachypnea stimulated by metabolic acidosis, hypoxemia, and decreased pulmonary compliance. A substantial minority of these patients present with respiratory acidosis. This may manifest either in the form of inadequate respiratory compensation for the metabolic acidosis (P_{CO_2} <40 mm Hg but pH <7.35) or frank carbon dioxide retention (P_{CO_2} >45 mm Hg). Underlying chronic lung disease need not be present for CO_2 retention to be manifest. Dead space to total ventilation ratio (VD/VT) may be significantly increased from the pulmonary edema itself. Respiratory muscle fatigue may supervene in the most serious cases and result in frank hypoventilation. Endotracheal intubation at presentation is reserved for apneic patients or those with agonal respirations. Most spontaneously breathing patients respond rapidly to medical therapy. Even hypercarbic patients can be managed without mechanical ventilation in most instances.[30]

Two noninvasive respiratory therapy techniques show promise in treating severely compromised but not agonal acute pulmonary edema patients. Continuous positive airway pressure (CPAP) applied by tight fitting facemask and biphasic positive airway pressure applied via a plastic molded nasal mask increase functional residual capacity, improve oxygenation, reduce the work of breathing, and result in decreased left ventricular preload and afterload (by raising intrathoracic pressure) (Figure 76-7). These techniques result in more rapid restoration of normal vital signs and oxygenation than supplemental oxygen alone. Moreover, fewer patients required endotracheal intubation when these techniques were used.[31-33] Adding pressure support to CPAP via facemask has now been termed noninvasive positive pressure ventilation. This combines the beneficial effects of CPAP, with even further reductions in the work of breathing resulting from the inspiratory pressure support phase.

Table 76-2. Precipitating Causes of Acute Cardiogenic Pulmonary Edema (APE)

Cause	Incidence (%)
Worsening heart failure	26
Coronary insufficiency	21
Subendocardial infarction	16
Transmural infarction	10
Acute dysrhythmia	9
Medication noncompliance	7
Dietary indiscretion	3
Valvular insufficiency	3
Other	5

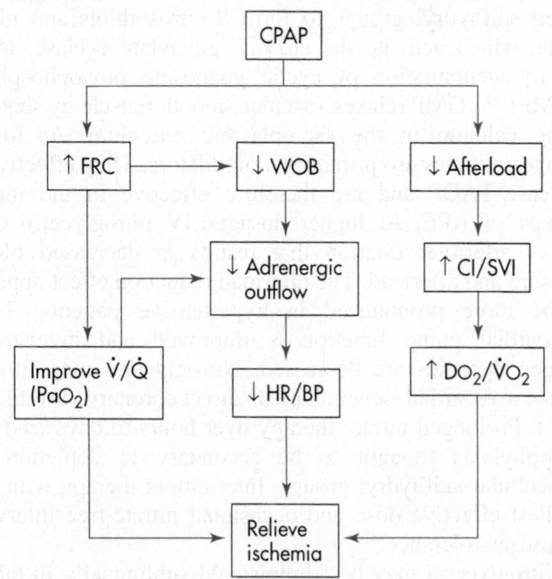

Figure 76-7. **Continuous positive airway pressure (CPAP) recruits collapsed alveoli and increases functional residual capacity (FRC), which improves oxygenation and reduces work of breathing (WOB). These factors tend to reduce sympathetic tone, heart rate (HR), and blood pressure (BP), relieving myocardial ischemia. CPAP also acts as an afterload-reducing agent, which tends to directly improve cardiac index (CI) and systemic oxygen delivery (DO_2) and consumption (VO_2).**

Acute Pulmonary Edema with Adequate Perfusion

Adequately perfused patients with acute pulmonary edema (APE) are recognized by the presence of normal or elevated blood pressure, a normal mental status, and the ability to make adequate amounts of urine. Therapeutic interventions should be directed at decreasing both preload and afterload. Optimal agents are short acting, titratable, and have minimal side effects. Excessive preload reduction may result in an abrupt decrease in CO, which could cause hypotension. This occurs more readily in patients with less compliant hearts (e.g., those with diastolic dysfunction, aortic stenosis, or acute myocardial infarction). Fluid challenge generally restores blood pressure quickly in these patients. In general, three categories of drugs should be used initially: morphine sulfate, nitrates, and diuretics.

Morphine Sulfate This narcotic reduces pulmonary congestion through a central sympatholytic effect that causes peripheral vasodilation. This decreases central venous return and reduces preload, lowering PAOP. In addition, through reduced systemic catecholamines, morphine decreases heart rate, blood pressure, cardiac contractility, and myocardial oxygen consumption. Patients with APE tend to be agitated as a result of their air hunger. The calming effect of morphine is therefore advantageous in this setting. Morphine is administered in repetitive 2 to 5 mg IV doses titrated to effect. Should oversedation result in hypoventilation, gentle stimulation will effectively restore ventilatory effort. In APE, mild CO_2 retention is not a contraindication to the use of morphine because it results from acute alveolar flooding.[30] Patients who are obtunded at presentation are not given morphine unless airway support is accomplished.

Nitrates Organic nitrates react with intracellular reduced sulfhydryl groups to form S-nitrosothiols and nitric oxide, which activate the enzyme guanylate cyclase, leading to accumulation of cyclic guanosine monophosphate (cGMP).[34] cGMP relaxes vascular smooth muscle by sequestering calcium in the sarcoplasmic reticulum. At lower dosages, nitrates are primarily venodilators. They effectively decrease PAOP and are therefore effective in the initial therapy of APE. At higher dosages IV nitroglycerin also causes arteriolar dilation that results in decreased blood pressure and afterload. The afterload reduction effect appears to be more pronounced in hypertensive patients. Thus myocardial pump function is improved and myocardial oxygen demands are decreased. Nitroglycerin may further reduce myocardial ischemia by its direct coronary vasodilator effect. Prolonged nitrate therapy over hours to days leads to tachyphylaxis thought to be secondary to depletion of intracellular sulfhydryl groups. Intermittent therapy with the smallest effective dose and occasional nitrate-free intervals minimizes tolerance.[35]

Nitroglycerin may be administered sublingually in tablet or spray forms, transcutaneously, or intravenously by continuous infusion. Therapy may be initiated most expeditiously via the sublingual route even before IV access is established. Hypotension from excessive preload reduction or vagally mediated idiosyncratic reactions may occur.[36] IV access allows immediate fluid challenge to restore blood pressure in these patients. Sublingual tablets (0.4 mg) or transmucosal sprays have their onset of action within 2 minutes. The effect of the tablets lasts approximately 20 minutes, and the effects of the sprays last 2 hours. Repeated dosing is reasonable if blood pressure is maintained.

Topical nitroglycerin may be used in well-perfused patients. Patients with APE are often diaphoretic with poor skin perfusion, making the cutaneous route less attractive in this setting. Absorption may be erratic, and earlier applied ointment might be absorbed later in the course when skin perfusion is improved, resulting in "unexplained" hypotension. Cutaneous nitroglycerin patches may ignite during defibrillation. On balance, these factors mitigate against the use of cutaneous nitroglycerin in patients with APE.

IV nitroglycerin is a titratable agent with rapid onset and offset of action. Dosing begins at 10 to 20 µg/min via infusion pump with frequent clinical assessment and vital sign monitoring. The dosage may be rapidly titrated upward in 5 to 10 µg/min increments every 3 to 5 minutes. Dosages of 50 to 80 µg/min provide antianginal effect and decreased preload in most cases. Dosages as high as 200 to 300 µg/min may be needed for maximal antihypertensive effect.

Loop Diuretics Loop diuretics (furosemide, bumetanide) work primarily through inhibition of sodium resorption from the renal filtrate in the ascending limb of Henle's loop in the medulla. This action leads to significant increases in renal salt and water excretion. In patients with volume overload, this diuretic action lowers plasma volume, decreasing preload and pulmonary congestion.

Although intravenously administered loop diuretics have a rapid onset of action (5 to 10 minutes), symptom relief in patients with APE occurs much faster than can be explained by the diuretic effect alone. These improvements are probably the result of diuretic-induced neurohumoral changes. Furosemide is both a vasodilator (promotes both renal prostaglandin E_2 and ANP secretion) and a vasoconstrictor (stimulates renin release).[37]

Patients with abrupt-onset APE who do not have underlying chronic CHF may have low plasma volumes at presentation. Diuresis in this group of patients may be unnecessary. Patients who fail to respond to loop diuretic administration may have severely compromised renal perfusion. Invasive hemodynamic monitoring may be beneficial in these patients. Diuretic therapy causes depletion of the important cations K^+ and Mg^{++}, which may be significant in patients already depleted by chronic diuretic therapy or other agents.

Nitroprusside Nitroprusside is a potent titratable direct smooth muscle relaxing agent administered by continuous infusion. Continuous pressure monitoring is mandatory to avoid dangerous levels of hypotension that can occur precipitously. Nitroprusside is a balanced vasodilating agent that results in both preload and afterload reduction (Figures 76-4 and 76-8). It is the drug of choice in the therapy of patients in hypertensive crisis with pulmonary edema. Patients with acute myocardial ischemia or infarction, however, are better served using high-dose nitroglycerin therapy to avoid the potential for "coronary steal" syndrome in which less diseased vessels dilate and "steal" flow from more diseased vessels. These patients are also particularly vulnerable to unintended hypotension, an event much more likely to occur with nitroprusside than with nitroglycerin. Patients with renal failure may experience thiocyanate

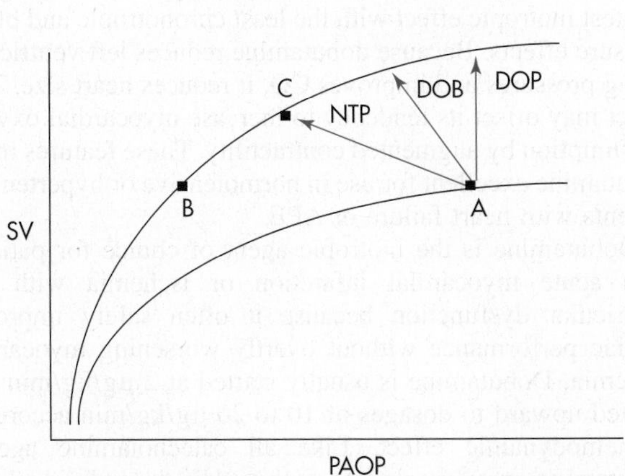

Figure 76-8. **Treatment of patients with severe left ventricular (LV) dysfunction is determined by multiple clinical factors. Hypotensive patients benefit from dopamine (DOP), which tends to increase blood pressure and cardiac output, with little effect on LV pressure (PAOP). Dobutamine (DOB), an inotropic vasodilator, increases cardiac output and decreases PAOP. It may lower blood pressure. Patients with high peripheral resistance and hypertension may show marked improvement with nitroprusside (NTP). Care must be taken not to go from point A to point B (preload overly reduced). Fluid challenge may be needed to return to point C.**

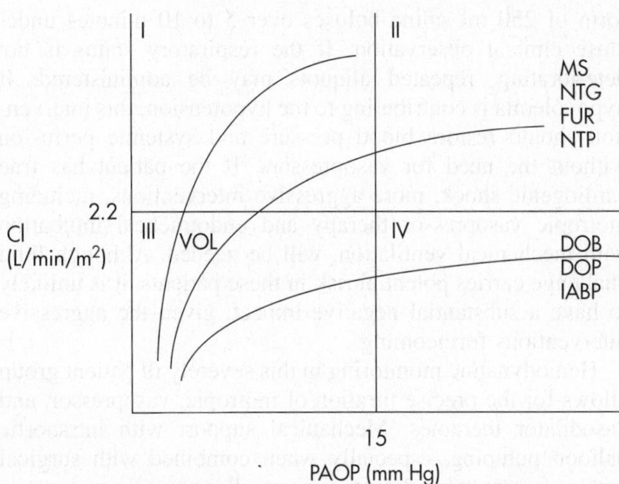

Figure 76-9. **Patients with heart failure may be managed according to their hemodynamic subset. Subset I patients have normal Starling curves and require no treatment. Subset II patients have adequate cardiac index (CI) but high pulmonary artery occlusion pressures (PAOP) and pulmonary edema. They may be treated with venodilators such as morphine (MS), nitroglycerin (NTG), furosemide (FUR), or if hypertensive, nitroprusside (NTP). Subset III patients are both hypoperfused and hypovolemic and may benefit from fluid challenge (Vol). Subset IV patients are most severely compromised. They are hypoperfused and may be hypotensive while PAOP is high and pulmonary edema is present. They require inotropic, vasopressor support and may need intraaortic balloon pumping (IABP). Subset IV patients often require endotracheal intubation and mechanical ventilation.** *Modified from Forrester JS et al:* N Engl J Med *295:1356, 1976.*

toxicity from high-dose infusions. Accordingly, levels should be monitored in these patients. Cyanide toxicity, recognized clinically by the presence of agitation and lactic acidosis, may occur in individuals with genetic predisposition.

Other Therapies Most patients with APE and adequate systemic perfusion respond promptly to treatment with oxygen, morphine, nitrates, and diuretics. Other previously applied therapies (e.g., rotating tourniquets, phlebotomy, and aminophylline) have no demonstrated efficacy in APE. In particular, rotating tourniquets may be deleterious because the minimal reduction in preload they may achieve is more than offset by increased afterload with corresponding reduction in CO.[38]

Treatment of Acute Pulmonary Congestion in Hypotensive Patients

Patients with acute cardiogenic pulmonary edema and apparent systemic hypotension present a therapeutic dilemma. Coronary perfusion in patients with coronary artery disease depends on the pressure gradient between the aorta and left ventricular chamber in diastole. The combination of hypotension and elevated left-sided filling pressure dramatically decreases coronary perfusion and leads to further impairment of contractility from increased ischemia. Accordingly, vasopressor administration to maintain coronary perfusion pressure would be necessary if this set of conditions truly existed. Vasopressor therapy, however, has the potential to increase afterload, decrease CO, increase myocardial oxygen demands, exacerbate ischemia, and precipitate dysrhythmias.

Patients with this clinical condition uniformly have low CO and intense peripheral vasoconstriction. Under these conditions, noninvasive assessment of arterial pressure is notoriously unreliable.[28] Gradients of 60 mm Hg between cuff systolic and true intraarterial systolic pressures are common in this clinical setting. Intraarterial pressure monitoring should be instituted as soon as possible in these patients. This maneuver may allow the judicious use of effective and myocardium-sparing venodilator agents and avoid the use of potentially dangerous vasopressors.

If the patient is truly hypotensive, aggressive measures to raise the blood pressure must be undertaken to maintain or restore coronary perfusion pressure. In this setting the patient is either in true cardiogenic shock (pulmonary congestion, hypotension, and decreased peripheral perfusion) or is volume depleted. Patients in true cardiogenic shock have lost as much as 40% of their ventricular muscle mass and have an in-hospital mortality rate of more than 80%. They have both low cardiac index (<2.2 L/min/m^2) and high left-sided filling pressures (PAOP >15 mm Hg). Patients with depressed contractility and APE may also be plasma volume depleted, with cardiac index less than 2.2 L/min/m^2 and PAOP less than 15 mm Hg (Figure 76-9). It is *impossible* to distinguish between these two subsets of patients by physical examination alone because they both have signs of systemic hypoperfusion and pulmonary edema. Pulmonary artery catheterization is needed to accurately assess the hemodynamic status of these individuals.

In patients with acute myocardial infarction and clinical evidence of systemic hypoperfusion, nearly 25% will have low PAOP, indicating the presence of hypovolemia. Fluid challenge alone in these patients results in restoration of hemodynamic stability in half the cases. Hypotensive patients with APE should receive a judicious fluid challenge in the form of 250 ml saline boluses over 5 to 10 minutes under close clinical observation. If the respiratory status is not deteriorating, repeated aliquots may be administered. If hypovolemia is contributing to the hypotension, this intervention should restore blood pressure and systemic perfusion without the need for vasopressors. If the patient has true cardiogenic shock, more aggressive interventions, including inotropic vasopressor therapy and endotracheal intubation with mechanical ventilation, will be needed. Although fluid challenge carries potential risk in these patients, it is unlikely to have a substantial negative impact, given the aggressive interventions forthcoming.

Hemodynamic monitoring in this severely ill patient group allows for the precise titration of inotropic, vasopressor, and vasodilator therapies. Mechanical support with intraaortic balloon pumping, especially when combined with surgical repair of correctable defects (i.e., papillary muscle rupture) or coronary revascularization, may be life saving.

Dopamine Dopamine is a naturally occurring catecholamine and a norepinephrine precursor. It has a dose-dependent effect on peripheral vascular tone and acts in a dose-dependent fashion as a positive inotropic and chronotropic agent. At a starting dosage of 2 to 5 μg/kg/min, it stimulates primarily dopaminergic receptors in renal and mesenteric vessels. This selective vasodilator effect increases renal perfusion, enhancing urine output. At dosages of approximately 5 to 15 μg/kg/min, the β-adrenergic effects of dopamine predominate, resulting in increased cardiac contractility and heart rate. In this dosage range, PAOP may decrease because of improved ejection fraction and peripheral vasodilation. At dosages greater than 15 μg/kg/min, dopamine acts to vasoconstrict all vascular beds in a manner similar to norepinephrine.[39] Accordingly at higher dosages, dopamine is essentially a vasopressor that can effectively maintain blood pressure. The increased afterload, contractility, and heart rate seen with dopamine in vasopressor dose ranges may precipitate myocardial ischemia and dysrhythmias. Venoconstriction in this dose range may increase PAOP, tending to exacerbate pulmonary edema, an effect that may be ameliorated with the concomitant administration of a venodilator such as nitroglycerin. Dopamine use in patients with APE is reserved for persistently oliguric patients (dopaminergic dosages of 2 to 5 μg/kg/min) or hypotensive patients failing to respond to fluid challenge (pressor dosages 10 to 20 μg/kg/min) to maintain dopaminergic doses of dopamine and add levarterenol as the pressor agent in profoundly hypotensive patients (Figure 76-8).

Dobutamine Dobutamine is a synthetic catecholamine structurally related to isoproterenol. Dobutamine is mainly a β_1-receptor agonist with some β_2- and β-agonist activity. It is an inotropic vasodilator at therapeutic dosages ranging from 5 to 25 μg/kg/min. Accordingly, it increases CO and decreases PAOP.[39] If CO increases, blood pressure is generally maintained. If CO does not increase, the vasodilator effect may precipitate hypotension. Accordingly, dobutamine must be used with caution in patients with borderline hypotension. It cannot be used alone in hypotensive patients, but it may be added to a vasopressor after blood pressure is restored. Dobutamine is reputed to result in less tachycardia for given increases in CO than other catecholamines. This may be related to the fact that it does not result in norepinephrine release from nerve endings. It is currently the most attractive inotropic catecholamine agent, producing the greatest inotropic effect with the least chronotropic and blood pressure effects. Because dobutamine reduces left ventricular filling pressures and improves CO, it reduces heart size. This effect may offset its tendency to increase myocardial oxygen consumption by augmented contractility. These features make dobutamine excellent for use in normotensive or hypertensive patients with heart failure or APE.

Dobutamine is the inotropic agent of choice for patients with acute myocardial infarction or ischemia with left ventricular dysfunction because it often safely improves cardiac performance without overtly worsening myocardial ischemia. Dobutamine is usually started at 2 μg/kg/min and titrated upward to dosages of 10 to 20 μg/kg/min according to hemodynamic effect. Like all catecholamine agents, dobutamine may precipitate tachycardia in individual patients. Patients should be closely monitored and dosages reduced if tachycardia develops. Dobutamine infusions of 24 to 48 hours duration result in sustained benefit in chronic CHF patients refractory to traditional chronic therapies.[40]

Other Catecholamines Norepinephrine is the most potent α-vasopressor agent with only modest β effect. Accordingly, it is the pressor agent of choice for volume repleted, profoundly hypotensive patients. Dopaminergic doses of dopamine may be added to overcome renal vasoconstriction and preserve renal perfusion and urine output. Dobutamine may be added to increase CO once blood pressure is restored. In cardiogenic shock, norepinephrine administration should be viewed as a necessary temporizing maneuver to maintain coronary perfusion pressure while other rescue strategies such as angioplasty, intraaortic balloon pumping, or cardiac surgery are planned.

Epinephrine is a potent α and β agent that maintains blood pressure and increases CO. It is used primarily in cardiac surgery patients to combat the effects of myocardial "stunning" after operations using cardiopulmonary bypass. Isoproterenol is a potent β-agonist that causes profound tachycardia and vasodilation, making it dangerous to use. It should be avoided if more attractive options are available.

Digitalis The cardiac glycosides act by inhibiting the ATPase-dependent sodium potassium pump in the cell membrane of the cardiac myocyte. This ultimately increases the availability of calcium to contractile proteins in myocardial cells, increasing the force of myocardial contraction; however, the expected hemodynamic improvement from this positive inotropic agent appears to be modest. In the setting of acute myocardial infarction with pulmonary congestion, it has minimal potency in improving hemodynamics compared with dobutamine. Digitalis preparations have little role in acute heart failure. Evidence that they improve abnormal baroreceptor responsiveness and decrease sympathetic outflow in chronic heart failure makes them standard agents in this setting.[41]

Nondigitalis, Noncatecholamine Cardiotonic Agents Amrinone is the prototype of phosphodiesterase type III inhibitors, which produce increased levels of cyclic adenosine monophosphate (cAMP) in the myocardium and peripheral smooth muscle. Other agents in this class include milrinone, enoximone, vesnarinone, and pimobendan. Only

IV forms of amrinone and milrinone are approved by the FDA for use in heart failure. These vasodilating inotropic agents increase CO and reduce left ventricular pressures without producing significant changes in heart rate and blood pressure.

The positive inotropic effects of dobutamine and amrinone are additive, and concomitant use of both drugs appears to be better tolerated than aggressive dosing of dobutamine alone, with lower metabolic costs.[42] Nevertheless, long-term use of orally administered milrinone has been shown to reduce survival in CHF in functional NYHA classes III and IV.[43] These agents appear to be prodysrhythmic. They may be useful on a short-term basis, for example, as in patients awaiting heart transplantation. Amrinone's relatively long half-life makes its use somewhat risky in the ED, especially if invasive hemodynamic monitoring is not in place.

Treatment of Heart Failure Without Pulmonary Congestion

On occasion, heart failure may lead to hypoperfusion without significant pulmonary congestion. For example, patients with dysfunction because of congestive cardiomyopathy may have been overly diuresed or developed a dysrhythmia that has negatively impacted pump function without creating pulmonary edema. When presented with a hypotensive patient, the emergency physician must differentiate among a myriad of clinical possibilities, including septic shock and massive pulmonary embolus. Hypotension in this situation may not be pathologic because chronic adaptive changes and medical therapies may leave patients with a low blood pressure that is well tolerated. Clammy, cyanotic extremities, altered mental status, metabolic acidosis, and decreased urine output are some of the important findings that help define significant hypoperfusion. If hypoperfusion is present, cautious volume challenge with isotonic crystalloid should be instituted. Invasive hemodynamic monitoring is indicated in this clinical setting because chamber filling pressures will help define the particular cardiovascular pathology.

Acute right ventricular infarction is one important cause of acute hypoperfusion with jugular venous distention and absent pulmonary congestion. Approximately one third of patients with acute inferior infarction have right ventricular involvement, which leads to inadequate pulmonary perfusion and low left ventricular priming. These patients have hypotension that is often symptomatic. Jugular venous distention is prominent, but pedal edema is usually absent. These patients often have evidence of ST-segment elevation or depression in the V_1 lead. Right-sided leads may provide further evidence of right ventricular infarction. Large volume fluid resuscitation along with inotropic support may be required to provide adequate preload to the left ventricle and restore blood pressure.

Treatment of Chronic Heart Failure

Patients with chronic heart failure often have complex multiorgan dysfunction and polydrug medical regimens. Any therapeutic intervention in this clinical setting needs to occur with the consideration of its potential impact on the entire spectrum of disease and compensatory mechanisms. For example, adding an NSAID to the medical regimen of a patient with chronic heart failure may negatively affect renovascular function and precipitate increased fluid retention and pulmonary edema. Chronic heart failure often involves a much more gradual onset of symptoms, with a gradual increase in dyspnea with minimal exertion, progressive orthopnea, fatigue, and other symptoms. The New York Heart Association classification is a time-honored classification system for patients with chronic heart failure (Box 76-3). Depending on the severity of illness, the physical examination may reveal only subtle findings of pulmonary congestion, displaced apical impulse, S_3 gallop (left-sided) or peripheral edema, jugular venous distention, hepatomegaly, and ascites (right-sided heart failure).

Box 76-3 Classification System for Chronic Heart Failure: New York Heart Association Functional Classes

I. Asymptomatic on ordinary physical activity
II. Symptomatic on ordinary physical activity
III. Symptomatic on less than ordinary physical activity
IV. Symptomatic at rest

Frequent precipitating factors of chronic heart failure include medication noncompliance or toxicity; ongoing myocardial ischemia; cardiac dysrhythmia; dietary indiscretion; increased physical, emotional, or metabolic stress; and any systemic disease that increases myocardial workload. In general, exacerbations of chronic heart failure require admission if the cause of the exacerbation cannot be readily recognized and corrected, if the disease process is unstable because of increased ischemia or new dysrhythmia, or if clinical deterioration of the patient appears likely.

Vasodilator Therapy The mainstay of early treatment of chronic heart failure as well as asymptomatic left ventricular dysfunction is vasodilator therapy, which benefits pump function by reducing both afterload and preload. The most important vasodilators for heart failure are ACE inhibitors, angiotensin II receptor antagonists, nitrates, and calcium channel blocking agents (Figure 76-4 and Table 76-1).

Angiotensin-Converting Enzyme Inhibitors ACE inhibitors provide the most effective therapy for left ventricular dysfunction. They bind to a zinc moiety on ACE, inactivating the enzyme, and thus reducing angiotensin II and aldosterone production. ACE inhibitors increase survival for all classes of chronic heart failure and also prevent the development of heart failure in patients with myocardial infarction and asymptomatic left ventricular dysfunction.[44-47]

The actions of ACE inhibitors appear to be related to their ability to inhibit production of angiotensin II, thereby producing direct vasodilation in addition to a natriuretic effect mediated via inhibition of aldosterone secretion. Additional pathways for ACE inhibitor effects include inhibition of the degradation of bradykinin and a reduction of intrinsic endothelium-dependent vasoconstriction.[48] ACE inhibitors are therefore natriuretic vasodilators that reduce diuretic and potassium supplement requirements. Unlike other vasodilators, they do not induce reflex tachycardia. The main side effects of ACE inhibitors are hypotension and deterioration of renal function, which can in general be avoided by careful drug titration. Chronic cough secondary to bronchospasm as well as upper airway angioedema are reported. These complications may abate at lower dosages but may require discontinuation of the drug. Optimal ACE inhibitor dosing appears to be neglected in many CHF patients, particularly the elderly.[49,50]

Angiotensin II Receptor Blockade Bronchospasm induction presenting as chronic cough and angioedema are the main reasons many patients with heart failure do not tolerate ACE inhibitors. In addition, ACE inhibition incompletely suppresses angiotensin II formation and also leads to accumulation of bradykinin. Furthermore, there is evidence that alternate pathways of conversion of angiotensin I to angiotensin II, including a chymase pathway, may restore angiotensin II levels despite ACE inhibition. Type I angiotensin II receptors (AT_1) appear to promote the deleterious effects of angiotensin II. In heart failure patients intolerant to ACE inhibitors, AT_1 receptor blockers may have utility. AT_1 receptor blockers appear to avoid the side effects of cough and bradykinin accumulation. Two studies comparing AT_1 receptor antagonists with ACE inhibitors in symptomatic heart failure failed to conclude that one drug type had a clear advantage in this clinical setting.[51-53] Addition of AT_1 receptor antagonists to maximally tolerated doses of ACE inhibitors improved hemodynamic features in chronic heart failure patients[54] and enhanced peak exercise capacity while alleviating symptoms in these patients.[55] Large scale studies are required to better understand the relative utility of AT_1 receptor antagonists compared with ACE inhibitors in chronic heart failure, as well as the optimal agents and dosing for combination therapy.

Nitrates Nitrate therapy, by virtue of its direct venodilator effect, improves exercise tolerance in chronic heart failure. In combination with the arteriolar dilator hydralazine, it also prolongs survival in patients with CHF.[56] ACE inhibitors are more efficacious than combination therapy with nitrates and hydralazine in reducing mortality from CHF.[57] Nitrate therapy appears to offer a potential for hemodynamic improvement in patients already taking ACE inhibitors.[58] The main problem with nitrate therapy is rapid drug tolerance, which can be partially addressed by daily nitrate drug-free intervals.[59-61]

Calcium Channel Blockers These compounds are effective vasodilators. Their negative inotropic effect limits their usefulness in patients with CHF. First-generation calcium channel blockers (verapamil, diltiazem, and nifedipine) do not improve survival in chronic heart failure. Their use may precipitate clinical deterioration.[62] Second-generation dihydropyrimidines (nicardipine, amlodipine) may have more moderate negative inotropic effects. Amlodipine reduces fatal and nonfatal cardiac events in nonischemic but not ischemic heart disease.[63] There is no compelling evidence for the utility of calcium channel blockers in heart failure. Calcium channel blockers are indicated for the treatment of hypertension, angina, and dysrhythmias but should be used with caution in patients with associated chronic heart failure.

Diuretics Diuretic therapy remains a standard treatment modality for chronic heart failure. Patients with chronic heart failure exhibit a reduced ability to excrete a sodium and water load, with abnormal cardiac and hemodynamic adaptations to salt excess.[64,65] Loop diuretics remain the most commonly used natriuretic agents in heart failure. They are associated with significant side effects, including hypovolemia, electrolyte disturbances (low K^+, Mg^{++}, and Na^+), hyperuricemia, and metabolic alkalosis. The hypokalemia and hypomagnesemia secondary to diuretic therapy may be prodysrhythmic.[66]

Spironolactone directly antagonizes aldosterone and is traditionally relegated to the treatment of cirrhosis. A landmark study in patients with severe heart failure (ejection fraction <35%) who were already being treated with an ACE inhibitor, a loop diuretic, and in most cases digoxin was discontinued early due to a striking 30% reduction in the risk of death among patients in the spironolactone group.[67] In addition, chronic heart failure patients receiving spironolactone had a significant improvement in symptoms as defined by New York Heart Association functional class.

Spironolactone may lead to serious hyperkalemia in the face of significant renal insufficiency or in patients taking supplemental potassium. Spironolactone may be efficacious in patients refractory to loop diuretics and ACE inhibitors alone. Spironolactone is now a mandatory component of CHF treatment regimens unless contraindicated.

Inotropic Agents

Cardiac Glycosides Digoxin remains the most commonly used cardiac glycoside. Although it engenders significant controversy, digoxin is of benefit in patients with CHF.[68,69] Digoxin is useful for rate control in chronic atrial flutter and fibrillation, but its ability to effect conversion to normal sinus rhythm remains in question. Overall, digoxin improves left ventricular ejection fraction and increases exercise capacity in CHF. Its effects on mortality are unclear,[70] although digoxin appears to reduce the rate of hospitalization in chronic heart failure. In the studies demonstrating improved survival from ACE inhibitors, most of the patients were already receiving and continued to receive digoxin and diuretics.

Digitalis therapy is an option in patients with heart failure who exhibit atrial fibrillation with a rapid ventricular response or left ventricular hypertrophy with diastolic dysfunction. Digitalis has numerous favorable effects on neurohumoral responses to heart failure. The IV loading dose of digoxin is 0.5 mg repeated in 0.25 mg dosages every 30 minutes to a maximum of 1.5 mg. Some patients will require more. In acute situations, this may be administered aggressively, whereas in less urgent situations, digitalis is given over several hours. Maintenance therapy is 0.25 mg/day and should be reduced or avoided in the setting of renal insufficiency. Digitalis toxicity manifests by various dysrhythmias and is increased by hypokalemia, hypercalcemia, hypoxia, and systemic acidosis.

Phosphodiesterase Inhibitors Amrinone and milrinone therapy, when given on a long-term basis, appear to increase morbidity and mortality in patients with severe chronic heart failure.[71] Other agents in this class (enoximone, imazodan) along with the partial β-adrenergic agonist xamoterol demonstrate limited efficacy with potential for increased mortality in small studies.[72-74] These effects may be due to acceleration of the progression of the underlying disease and provocation of the development of serious ventricular dysrhythmias. Vesnarinone is a newer agent in this class, which in long-term treatment modestly raises inotropic state with reduced afterload, but also increases mortality.[75]

β-Blocker Therapy Despite the apparent paradox of using agents that reduce myocardial contractility in the setting of heart failure, carefully titrated β-adrenergic blocking agents have significant efficacy in chronic heart failure.[76-79] Long-term activation of the sympathetic nervous system in heart failure, including vasoconstriction, activation of the renin-angiotensin system, myocardial β-adrenergic receptor downregulation, and direct cardiotoxicity because of elevated norepinephrine levels, is associated with adverse effects. Inhibition of these effects by β-blockers appears to explain their efficacy. A meta-analysis of β-adrenergic blockade in chronic heart failure revealed β-blockers increase the ejection fraction by 29% and reduce the combined risk of death or hospitalization for heart failure by 37%.[80]

β-Blocker therapy should not normally be initiated in acute heart failure. Its use in chronic heart failure requires careful titration and is most useful in heart failure associated with other conditions in which there are indications for β-blocker therapy, including hypertension, angina pectoris, and significant dysrhythmias. Interestingly, the mortality risk is reduced most by nonselective β-blockers compared with β-selective agents.[80] Carvedilol, a third-generation α- and β-blocker with antioxidant properties, may be a particularly effective agent in chronic heart failure.[81] β-Blockers with intrinsic sympathomimetic activity should be avoided.

Glucagon Glucagon, a naturally occurring polypeptide hormone, acts as a positive inotropic and chronotropic agent. Its use in the ED is reserved for the treatment of acute β-blocker or calcium channel blocker overdose with hemodynamic compromise. Its mechanism of action is via a glucagon-specific membrane receptor on cardiac myocytes that is not blocked by these agents. Bolus IV therapy with 0.05 mg/kg is titrated to effect.[82]

Other Therapeutic Interventions in Chronic Heart Failure

Ultrafiltration and Renal Dialysis The use of ultrafiltration reduces volume overload in chronic heart failure and is an effective therapeutic intervention when diuretic therapy is inadequate.[83-85] Renal dialysis may be important for effective therapy of heart failure in end-stage renal disease. Potential complications of renal disease that may require special consideration include fluid overload, severe hyperkalemia, iatrogenic hypermagnesemia, uremia-pericardial effusion with possible tamponade, and drug toxicity (especially digitalis).

Antidysrhythmic Therapy Ventricular dysrhythmias are common in patients with heart failure. Most patients with cardiomyopathy and CHF have frequent premature ventricular beats and 40% to 80% will manifest runs of nonsustained ventricular tachycardia.[86,87] There is an associated increased risk of sudden death in these patients.[88] Unfortunately, neither electrophysiologic testing nor signal-averaged ECGs identify individuals at risk. Most antidysrhythmic drugs are not effective at preventing sudden death in this setting.

A meta-analysis of postmyocardial infarction and CHF patients randomized to amiodarone versus placebo showed a 15% reduction in total mortality by amiodarone, with arrhythmic sudden death reduced by 29%.[89] In chronic heart failure, amiodarone prevented the development of atrial fibrillation and converted significantly more patients with atrial fibrillation to sinus rhythm compared with placebo, but did not affect overall mortality.[90] Unfortunately this as well as all the other antidysrhythmic agents have significant toxicities and may be prodysrhythmic.

Alternate approaches to dysrhythmias in chronic heart failure are electrical. The impact of implantable cardiac defibrillators (ICD) in prevention of sudden cardiac death continues to be evaluated. MADIT,[91] the first prospective randomized trial of ICDs for prevention of sudden death in post–myocardial infarction patients with ejection fraction below 35%, nonsustained ventricular tachycardia, and inducible VT not suppressible by procainamide, was recently completed.[91] In this group, where the 2-year mortality rate of the conventionally treated group was 32%, ICD implantation reduced the risk of death by 54%. The Coronary Artery Bypass Graft (CABG)-Patch trial looked at 900 patients with left ventricular ejection fraction < 36% and abnormal signal-averaged ECG, who were randomized to implantation of an epicardial ICD during CABG surgery.[92] During a 3-year follow-up period, there was no mortality advantage to ICD implantation. Thus, the advantage of ICD use in reducing mortality in chronic heart failure without ECG documentation or symptoms of life-threatening arrhythmias requires further study.

The Antiarrhythmic Versus Implantable Defibrillator Trial (AVID)[93] involved 1,016 patients (mean ejection fraction, 32%) with documented symptomatic VT or VF and compared ICD implantation to antidysrhythmic drug therapy (almost exclusively amiodarone). The 2-year mortality rate in the antidysrhythmic drug group was 25% and was reduced by 39% in the ICD group at year 1 and by 27% and 31% after 2 and 3 years, respectively. Other studies have confirmed that ICDs have a mortality advantage over antidysrhythmics in chronic heart failure.[94,95]

In addition, patients with severe CHF with aberrant ventricular conduction benefit from atrioventricular (AV) sequential pacing with improved cardiac output.[96,97] Also, ventricular pacing after AV node ablation appears more effective than pharmacologic therapy for CHF with chronic atrial fibrillation.[98]

Left Ventriculoplasty and Ventricular Assist Devices Batista et al[99] stunned the medical community in 1996 by reporting the utility of partial left ventriculoplasty (PLV) in the treatment of chronic heart failure. The surgery is a mechanical method of reducing left ventricular chamber size, which by Laplace's law should make the residual myocardium more efficient by reducing left ventricular workload. A meta-analysis looked at more than 600 patients who have undergone PLV since 1985.[100] Improvement in average New York Heart Association class occurred in 80% to 85% of hospital survivors.

Multiple totally implantable left ventricular assist devices are in various trial stages. They show promise to revolutionize cardiac surgery for chronic heart failure, not only in their recent use as a bridge to transplantation, but also as a surgical alternative to chronic medical management.[101,102] Although cardiac transplantation has an 84% survival at 1 year and 74.5% survival at 3 years in the United States,[103] the limited availability of heart transplant donors makes alternative surgical techniques tempting to use in end-stage heart failure. Further research in this area is required.

SUMMARY

Diagnosis and management of patients with CHF remain important and challenging aspects of emergency medicine. Recent advances in the chronic medical management of CHF include the routine use (unless contraindicated) of digoxin, diuretics, ACE inhibitors, β-blockers, and spironolactone. Deliberate consideration of all differential diagnostic entities, careful physical examination, and utilization of the diagnostic tools available in the ED, combined with a sound understanding of the pathophysiology and pharmacotherapy, can produce rewarding results when caring for this frequently encountered, and ever challenging, diverse patient group.

KEY CONCEPTS

- Patients with both acute pulmonary edema and systemic hypotension may have acute intravascular plasma volume depletion and require a fluid challenge.
- Failure to recognize type A aortic dissection may cause a fatal therapeutic misadventure if thrombolytic therapy is used.
- In heart failure, patients with decompensated aortic stenosis should not receive vasodilator agents; in contrast, patients with mitral regurgitation benefit greatly.
- Patients with acute right ventricular infarction may present with distended neck veins, yet require a fluid challenge.
- Patients with acute cardiogenic pulmonary edema have low cardiac output and intense peripheral vasoconstriction. Noninvasive assessment of arterial pressure is notoriously unreliable.
- Dobutamine is the inotropic agent of choice with acute myocardial ischemia or infarction.

REFERENCES

1. Croft JB et al: Heart failure survival among older adults in the United States: a poor prognosis for an emerging epidemic in the Medicare population, *Arch Intern Med* 159:505, 1999.
2. Cleland JGF, Clark A: Has the survival of the heart failure population changed? Lessons from trials, *Am J Cardiol* 83:112D, 1999.
3. Kannel WB, Belanger AJ: Epidemiology of heart failure, *Am Heart J* 121:951, 1991.
4. Haldeman GA et al: Hospitalization of patients with heart failure: National Hospital Discharge Survey, 1985 to 1995, *Am Heart J* 137:352, 1999.
5. Schocken DD et al: Prevalence and mortality rate of congestive heart failure in the United States, *J Am Coll Cardiol* 20:301, 1992.
6. Ho KKL et al: Survival after the onset of congestive heart failure in Framingham heart study subjects, *Circulation* 88:107, 1993.
7. Cohn JN et al: Ejection fraction, peak exercise oxygen consumption, cardiothoracic ratio, ventricular arrhythmias, and plasma norepinephrine as determinants of prognosis in heart failure, *Circulation* 87:VI-5, 1993.
8. Gradman A et al: Predictors of total mortality and sudden death in mild to moderate heart failure, *J Am Coll Cardiol* 14:564, 1989.
9. Cohn JN et al: Effect of vasodilator therapy on mortality in chronic congestive heart failure, *N Engl J Med* 314:1547, 1986.
10. Gilbert JC, Glantz SA: Determinants of left ventricular filling and of the diastolic pressure-volume relation, *Circ Res* 64:827, 1989.
11. Morgan HE, Baker KM: Cardiac hypertrophy: mechanical, neural and endocrine dependence, *Circulation* 83:13, 1991.
12. Wei JY: Age and the cardiovascular system, *N Engl J Med* 327:1732, 1992.
13. Olivetti G et al: Cardiomyopathy of the aging human heart: myocyte loss and reactive cellular hypertrophy, *Circ Res* 68:1560, 1991.
14. Brandt RR et al: Atrial natriuretic peptide in heart failure, *J Am Coll Cardiol* 22:86A, 1993.
15. Nurez DJR, Dickson MC, Brown MJ: Natriuretic peptide receptor mRNA's in the rat and human heart, *J Clin Invest* 90:1966, 1992.
16. Elsner D et al: Effectiveness of endopeptidase inhibition (candoxatril) in congestive heart failure, *Am J Cardiol* 70:494, 1992.
17. Bolli R: Mechanisms of myocardial stunning, *Circulation* 82:723, 1990.
18. Baig MK et al: Familial dilated cardiomyopathy: cardiac abnormalities are common in asymptomatic relatives and may represent early disease, *J Am Coll Cardiol* 31:195, 1998.
19. Grunig E et al: Frequency and phenotypes of familial dilated cardiomyopathy, *J Am Coll Cardiol* 31:186, 1998.
20. Morgan ED et al: Evaluation of ventricular contractility indexes in the dog with left ventricular dysfunction induced by rapid atrial pacing, *J Am Coll Cardiol* 14:489, 1989.
21. Vaitkus PT et al: Incessant atrial tachycardia and heart failure, *Heart Failure* 6:183, 1990.
22. Chatterjee K: Chronic congestive heart failure. In Hurst JW, editor: *Current therapy in cardiovascular disease,* St Louis, 1994, Mosby.
23. Roberts N et al: Right ventricular infarction with shock but without significant left ventricular infarction: a new clinical syndrome, *Am Heart J* 110:1047, 1985.
24. Sheldon EL, Grossman W: Diastolic dysfunction as a cause of heart failure, *J Am Coll Cardiol* 22:49A, 1993.
25. Soufer R, Wohlgelernter D, Vita NA: Intact systolic function in clinical congestive heart failure, *Am J Cardiol* 55:1032, 1985.
26. Brutsuert DL, Sys SU, Gillebert TC: Diastolic failure: pathophysiology and therapeutic implications, *J Am Coll Cardiol* 22:318, 1993.
27. Goldsmith SR, Dick C: Differentiating systolic from diastolic heart failure: pathophysiologic and therapeutic considerations, *Am J Med* 95:645, 1993.
28. Cohn JN: Blood pressure measurement in shock: mechanisms of inaccuracy of auscultatory and palpatory methods, *JAMA* 199:118, 1967.
29. Goldberger JJ et al: Prognostic factors in acute pulmonary edema, *Arch Intern Med* 146:489, 1986.
30. Aberman A, Fulop M: The metabolic and respiratory acidosis of acute pulmonary edema, *Ann Intern Med* 76:173, 1972.
31. Bersten AD et al: Treatment of severe cardiogenic pulmonary edema with continuous positive airway pressure delivered by face mask, *N Engl J Med* 325:1825, 1991.
32. Baratz DM et al: Effect of nasal continuous positive airway pressure on cardiac output and oxygen delivery in patients with congestive heart failure, *Chest* 102:1397, 1992.
33. Bradley TD et al: Cardiac output response to continuous positive airway pressure in congestive heart failure, *Am Rev Respir Dis* 145:377, 1992.
34. Kukovetz WR, Holzmann S: Mechanisms of nitrate-induced vasodilation and tolerance, *Eur J Clin Pharmacol* 38:9, 1990.
35. Elkayam U: Tolerance to organic nitrates: evidence, mechanisms, clinical relevance, and strategies for prevention, *Ann Intern Med* 114:667, 1991.
36. Come PC, Pitt B: Nitroglycerin-induced severe hypotension and bradycardia in patients with acute myocardial infarction, *Circulation* 54:624, 1976.
37. Packer M: Neurohormonal interactions and adaptations in congestive heart failure, *Circulation* 77:721, 1988.
38. Klein HO et al: The effect of venous occlusion with tourniquets on peripheral blood pooling and ventricular function, *Chest* 103:521, 1993.
39. Calvin JE: Inotropic therapy for the failed heart: picking the right drug for the job. In Kaplan J, editor: *Cardiothoracic and vascular anesthesia update,* Philadelphia, 1991, WB Saunders.
40. Oliva F et al: Intermittent 6-month low-dose dobutamine infusion in severe heart failure: DICE Multicenter Trial, *Am Heart J* 138:247, 1999.
41. Hirsch AT, Dzau VJ, Creager MA: Baroreceptor function in congestive heart failure: effect on neurohormonal activation and regional vascular resistance, *Circulation* 75:36, 1987.
42. Gage J et al: Additive effects of dobutamine and amrinone on myocardial contractility and ventricular performance in patients with severe heart failure, *Circulation* 74:367, 1986.

43. Packer M et al for the PROMISE Study Research Group: Effect of oral milrinone on mortality in severe chronic heart failure, *N Engl J Med* 325:1468, 1991.
44. Pfeffer MA: Angiotensin-converting enzyme inhibition in congestive heart failure: benefit and perspective, *Am Heart J* 126:789, 1993.
45. Paul SD et al: Costs and effectiveness of angiotensin converting enzyme inhibition in patients with congestive heart failure, *Arch Intern Med* 154:1143, 1994.
46. Pitt B: Use of converting enzyme inhibitors in patients with asymptomatic left ventricular dysfunction, *J Am Coll Cardiol* 22:158A, 1993.
47. Pfeffer MA et al: The effect of captopril on mortality in patients with left ventricular dysfunction following myocardial infarction: results of the Survival and Ventricular Enlargement (SAVE) trial, *N Engl J Med* 327:669, 1992.
48. Nakamura M et al: Effect of angiotensin-converting enzyme inhibitors on endothelium-dependent peripheral vasodilation in patients with chronic heart failure, *J Am Coll Cardiol* 24:1321, 1994.
49. Gattis et al: Is optimal angiotensin-converting enzyme inhibitor dosing neglected in elderly patients with heart failure? *Am Heart J* 136:43, 1998.
50. Van Veldhuisen DJ et al: High- versus low-dose ACE inhibition in chronic heart failure: a double-blind placebo-controlled study of imidapril, *J Am Coll Cardiol* 32:1811, 1998.
51. Brunner-LaRocca HP, Vaddadi G, Esler MD: Recent insight into therapy of congestive heart failure: focus on ACE inhibition and angiotensin-II antagonism, *J Am Coll Cardiol* 33:1163, 1999.
52. Pitt B, Chang P, Timmermans PB: Angiotensin II receptor antagonists in heart failure: rationale and design of the evaluation of losartan in the elderly (ELITE) trial, *Cardiovasc Drugs Ther* 9:693, 1995.
53. Mazayex VP et al: Valsartan in heart failure patients previously untreated with an ACE inhibitor, *Int J Cardiol* 65:239, 1999.
54. Baruch L et al: Augmented short- and long-term hemodynamic and hormonal effects of an angiotensin receptor blocker added to angiotensin converting enzyme inhibitor therapy in patients with heart failure, *Circulation* 99:2658, 1999.
55. Hamroff G et al: Addition of angiotensin II receptor blockade to maximal angiotensin-converting enzyme inhibition improves exercise capacity in patients with severe congestive heart failure, *Circulation* 99:990, 1999.
56. Cohn JN et al: Effect of vasodilator therapy on mortality in chronic congestive heart failure: results of a Veterans Administration Cooperative Study, *N Engl J Med* 314:1547, 1986.
57. Cohen JJ et al: A comparison of enalapril with hydralazine-isosorbide dinitrate in the treatment of chronic congestive heart failure, *N Engl J Med* 325:303, 1991.
58. Mehra A et al: Persistent hemodynamic improvement with short-term nitrate therapy in patients with chronic congestive heart failure already treated with captopril, *Am J Cardiol* 70:1310, 1992.
59. Cohn JN: Mechanisms of action and efficacy of nitrates in heart failure, *Am J Cardiol* 70:88B, 1992.
60. Elkayam U et al: Nitrate resistance and tolerance: potential limitations in the treatment of congestive heart failure, *Am J Cardiol* 70:98B, 1992.
61. Elkayam U et al: The role of organic nitrates in the treatment of heart failure, *Prog Cardiovasc Dis* 41:255, 1999.
62. Elkayam U et al: Calcium channel blockers in heart failure, *J Am Coll Cardiol* 22(Suppl A):139A, 1993.
63. Follath F et al: Etiology and response to drug treatment in heart failure, *J Am Coll Cardiol* 32:1167, 1998.
64. Volpe M et al: Abnormalities of sodium handling and of cardiovascular adaptations during high salt diet in patients with mild heart failure, *Circulation* 88:1620, 1993.
65. Cody RJ: Clinical trials of diuretic therapy in heart failure: research directions and clinical considerations, *J Am Coll Cardiol* 22(Suppl A):165A, 1993.
66. Dyckner T: Relation of cardiovascular disease to potassium and magnesium deficiencies, *Am J Cardiol* 65:44K, 1990.
67. Pitt B et al: The effect of spironolactone on morbidity and mortality in patients with severe heart failure, *N Engl J Med* 341:709, 1999.
68. Uretsky BF et al: Randomized patients with mild to moderate chronic congestive heart failure: results of the PROVED trial, *J Am Coll Cardiol* 22:955, 1993.
69. Packer M et al: Withdrawal of digoxin from patients with chronic heart failure treated with angiotensin-converting enzyme inhibitors, *N Engl J Med* 329:1, 1993.
70. The Digitalis Investigation Group: The effect of digoxin on mortality and morbidity in patients with heart failure, *N Engl J Med* 336:525, 1997.
71. Packer M: The development of positive inotropic agents for chronic heart failure: how have we gone astray? *J Am Coll Cardiol* 22:119A, 1993.
72. Dec GW et al: Long-term outcome of enoximone therapy in patients with refractory heart failure, *Am Heart J* 125:423, 1993.
73. Goldberg AD, Nicklas N, Goldstein S for the Imazodan Research Group: Effectiveness of imazodan for treatment of chronic congestive heart failure, *Am J Cardiol* 68:631, 1991.
74. Cruickshank JM: The xamoterol experience in the treatment of heart failure, *Am J Cardiol* 71:61C, 1993.
75. Kass DA et al: Dose dependence of chronic positive inotropic effect of vesnarinone in patients with congestive heart failure due to idiopathic or ischemic cardiomyopathy, *Am J Cardiol* 78:652, 1996.
76. Anderson JL et al: Long-term beneficial effects of beta-adrenergic blockade with bucindolol in patients with idiopathic dilated cardiomyopathy, *J Am Coll Cardiol* 17:1373, 1991.
77. Fowler MG: Controlled trials with beta blockers in heart failure: metoprolol as the prototype, *Am J Cardiol* 71:45C, 1993.
78. Eichhorn EJ: The paradox of beta-adrenergic blockade for the management of congestive heart failure, *Am J Med* 92:527, 1992.
79. CIBIS-II Investigators and Committees: The cardiac insufficiency bisoprolol study II (CIBIS-II): a randomised trial, *Lancet* 353:9, 1999.
80. Lechat P et al: Clinical effects of ß-adrenergic blockade in chronic heart failure: a meta-analysis of double-blind, placebo-controlled, randomized trials, *Circulation* 98:1184, 1998.
81. Di Lenarda A et al: Long-term effects of carvedilol in idiopathic dilated cardiomyopathy with persistent left ventricular dysfunction despite chronic metoprolol, *J Am Coll Cardiol* 33:1926, 1999.
82. Weinstein RS: Recognition and management of poisoning with beta-adrenergic blocking agents, *Ann Emerg Med* 13:1123, 1984.
83. Agostoni P et al: Sustained improvement in functional capacity after removal of body fluid with isolated ultrafiltration in chronic cardiac insufficiency: failure of furosemide to provide the same result, *Am J Med* 96:191, 1994.
84. Agostoni PG et al: Isolated ultrafiltration in moderate congestive heart failure, *J Am Coll Cardiol* 21:424, 1993.
85. Marenzi G et al: Interrelation of humoral factors, hemodynamics, and fluid and salt metabolism in congestive heart failure: effects of extracorporeal ultrafiltration, *Am J Med* 94:49, 1993.
86. Gorgels APM et al: Ventricular arrhythmias in heart failure, *Am J Cardiol* 70:37C, 1992.
87. Francis GS: Development of arrhythmias in the patient with congestive heart failure: pathophysiology, prevalence and prognosis, *Am J Cardiol* 57:3B, 1986.
88. Massie BM, Conway M: Survival of patients with congestive heart failure: past, present and future prospects, *Circulation* 75(Suppl IV):11, 1987.
89. Amiodarone Trials Meta-Analysis Investigators: Effect of prophylactic amiodarone on mortality after acute myocardial infarction and in congestive heart failure: meta-analysis of individual data from 6500 patients in randomized trials, *Lancet* 350:1417, 1997.
90. Deedwania PC et al: Spontaneous conversion and maintenance of sinus rhythm by amiodarone in patients with heart failure and atrial fibrillation: observations from the Veterans Affairs Congestive Heart Failure Survival Trial of Antiarrhythmic Therapy (CHF-STAT), *Circulation* 98:2574, 1998.
91. Moss AJ, MADIT Investigators: Improved survival with an implanted defibrillator in patients with coronary disease at high risk for ventricular arrhythmia, *N Engl J Med* 335:1933, 1996.
92. Bigger JT Jr, Coronary Artery Bypass Graft (CABG) Patch Trial Investigators: Prophylactic use of implanted cardiac defibrillators in patients at high risk for ventricular arrhythmias after coronary-artery bypass graft surgery, *N Engl J Med* 337:1569, 1997.
93. The Antiarrhythmics versus Implantable Defibrillators (AVID) Investigators: A comparison of antiarrhythmic-drug therapy with implantable defibrillators in patients resuscitated from near-fatal ventricular arrhythmias, *N Engl J Med* 337:1576, 1997.

94. Kuck KH, ACC NewsOnline: CASH, 1998.
95. Connolly SJ, ACC NewsOnline: CIDS, 1998.
96. Auricchio A et al: Effect of pacing chamber and atrioventricular delay on acute systolic function of paced patients with congestive heart failure, *Circulation* 99:2993, 1999.
97. Leclercq C et al: Acute hemodynamic effects of biventricular DDD pacing in patients with end-stage heart failure, *J Am Coll Cardiol* 32:1825, 1998.
98. Brignole M et al: Assessment of atrioventricular junction ablation and VVIR pacemaker versus pharmacological treatment in patients with heart failure and chronic atrial fibrillation: a randomized, controlled study, *Circulation* 98:953, 1998.
99. Batista RJV et al: Partial left ventriculectomy to improve left ventricular function in end-stage heart disease, *J Card Surg* 11:96, 1996.
100. Acker MA: Dynamic cardiomyoplasty: at the crossroads, *Ann Thoracic Surg* 68:750, 1999.
101. Sun et al: 100 long-term implantable left ventricular assist devices: the Columbia Presbyterian interim experience, *Ann Thoracic Surg* 68:688, 1999.
102. Pennington DG, Oaks TE, Lohmann DP: Permanent ventricular assist device support versus cardiac transplantation, *Ann Thoracic Surg* 68:729, 1999.
103. Keck BM et al: Worldwide thoracic organ transplantation: a report from the UNOS/ISHLT International Registry for Thoracic Organ Transplantation, *Clin Transpl* 31,1996.

77 Pericardial and Myocardial Disease

Nicholas J. Jouriles

PERICARDIAL DISEASE (PERICARDITIS)

Perspective

Our understanding of pericardial function and disease has increased greatly since Hippocrates described the pericardium in 460 BC as "a smooth tunic which envelops the heart and contains a small amount of fluid resembling urine." Galen provided the first description of a pericardial effusion and performed the first pericardial resection.[1] Lancisi first described the appearance of constrictive pericarditis at autopsy in 1728. Also in the eighteenth century, Laennec said, "There are few diseases attended by more variable symptoms and more difficult to diagnose than [pericarditis]."[1] This is still true today.

During the 1930s, Claude Beck researched and developed the practice of cardiac surgery. He is credited with first describing the clinical presentation of cardiac tamponade, which today is known as Beck's triad (i.e., hypotension, jugular venous distention, and muffled heart sounds).[2]

Etiology

The causes of acute and chronic pericardial disease are numerous (Box 77-1). Each of the disorders listed in Box 77-1 can produce acute pericarditis, with or without pericardial effusion. In addition, most of these disorders can progress to cardiac tamponade or constrictive pericarditis, although infrequently.

Most cases of pericarditis are idiopathic. Even exhaustive clinical testing identifies a specific etiology in only approximately 22% of patients, with the remainder being considered idiopathic.[3]

Epidemiology

Acute pericarditis is a syndrome caused by inflammation of the pericardium. Although the exact incidence is unknown, autopsy series have shown an incidence of pericarditis ranging from 2% to 6%. Pericarditis accounts for approximately 1 of 1000 hospital admissions. It is more prevalent in men than in women, and in adults more than children. There is no information available about the epidemiology of pericarditis in the ED.

Principles of Disease

Pericardial Anatomy The normal pericardium consists of parietal and visceral layers, with a narrow potential space between them. The thin visceral pericardium is closely applied to the epicardium of the heart and merges with the adventitia of the great arteries and veins at their attachment points, where it is also reflected to form the parietal layer. The parietal pericardium consists of a dense layer of collagen, approximately 1 mm thick, containing sparse elastic fibers. The position of the heart within the chest is stabilized by the attachment of the parietal pericardium to the manubrium and xiphoid anteriorly, to the diaphragm inferiorly, and to the vertebral column posteriorly.[4,5] The phrenic nerves traverse the parietal pericardium laterally and are thus at risk of being damaged when the pericardial sac is opened.

Pericardial Physiology Between 15 and 60 ml of fluid, an ultrafiltrate of plasma, is normally contained in the pericardial space. Abnormal amounts of pericardial fluid can accumulate when the venous or lymphatic drainage of the heart is obstructed.[4]

Several functions of the pericardium are proposed: maintain the heart's position, lubricate the heart's surface, prevent the spread of infection or adhesion formation from adjacent thoracic structures, prevent cardiac overdilation, augment atrial filling, and maintain the normal pressure-volume relationships of the cardiac chambers. Despite these suggested functions, patients with congenital absence (or surgical removal) of the pericardium show few, if any, problems.[4]

Box 77-1 Etiology of Pericarditis*

I. Trauma
  A. Pericardiotomy
  B. Indirect trauma to chest
  C. Transseptal catheterization
  D. Pressure injection of contrast media
  E. Perforation of right ventricle by indwelling catheter
  F. Implantation of epicardial pacemaker
  G. Blow to chest
  H. Perforation of right ventricle with catheter for parenteral nutrition
II. Viral infections
  A. Coxsackie B5, B6
  B. Echovirus
  C. Adenovirus
  D. Infectious mononucleosis
  E. Influenza
  F. Lymphogranuloma venereum
  G. Chickenpox
  H. *Mycoplasma pneumoniae*
  I. Acquired immunodeficiency syndrome (AIDS)
III. Bacterial infections
  A. Staphylococci
  B. Pneumococci
  C. Meningococci
  D. Streptococci
  E. *Haemophilus influenzae*
  F. Psittacosis
  G. *Salmonella*
  H. Tuberculosis
IV. Amebiasis
V. Echinococcus cysts
VI. Fungus infections—histoplasmosis, aspergillosis, blastomycosis, coccidioidomycosis
VII. Rickettsia
VIII. Radiation
IX. Amyloidosis
X. Tumors
  A. Primary
    1. Mesothelioma
      a. Rhabdomyosarcoma
      b. Teratoma
      c. Fibroma
      d. Leiomyofibroma
      e. Lipoma
      f. Angioma
    2. Metastatic
      a. Bronchogenic carcinoma
      b. Carcinoma of breast
      c. Lymphoma
      d. Leukemia
      e. Melanoma
  B. Sarcoid
    1. Collagen disease
      a. Rheumatoid fever
      b. Lupus erythematosus
      c. Rheumatoid arthritis
      d. Vasculitis
      e. Polyarteritis nodosa
      f. Scleroderma
      g. Dermatomyositis
XI. Anticoagulants
  A. Heparin
  B. Warfarin
XII. Myocardial infarction—post–myocardial infarction pericarditis (Dressler's syndrome)
XIII. Idiopathic thrombocytopenic purpura
XIV. Drugs
  A. Procainamide
  B. Cromolyn sodium
  C. Hydralazine
  D. Dantrolene
  E. Methysergide
XV. Dissecting aneurysm
XVI. Infective endocarditis (SBE) with valve ring abscess
XVII. Thymic cyst

From Shabetai R: Pericardial disease. In Hurst JW, Schlant RC, editors: *The heart,* ed 7, New York, 1990, McGraw-Hill.

*Principal causes of pericardial disease and pericardial heart disease. Most can cause pericardial effusion, cardiac tamponade, or constrictive pericarditis. The more common causes of these syndromes are mentioned under the syndromes and under specific disorders.

Idiopathic Pericarditis

Clinical Features

Symptoms and Signs The classic description of pericarditis includes chest pain, a pericardial friction rub, and electrocardiographic abnormalities. A prodrome of fever and myalgias may occur.

Pericarditis chest pain is usually substernal and varies with respiration. It is classically sharp or pleuritic in character, but need not be. It is typically relieved by sitting forward and worsened by lying down or swallowing. It may mimic myocardial infarction (MI) pain. Although pericarditis pain does not radiate to the arms, it often does radiate to the trapezius muscles and may present as isolated shoulder pain.

True dyspnea is rare with pericarditis, but breathing may be shallow because of the respirophasic nature of the pain. Other common symptoms include anxiety and anorexia.

The physical examination hallmark of acute pericarditis is the pericardial friction rub. The rub may be caused by friction between inflamed or scarred visceral and parietal pericardium or may result from friction between the parietal pericardium and adjacent pleura. It may be audible anywhere over the precordium but is best heard at the lower left sternal border. Friction rubs are best heard using the diaphragm of the stethoscope, with the patient in the sitting position holding his or her breath. The rub characteristically sounds "scratchy," "creaky," or "Velcro-like." The classic biphasic "to and fro" rub occurs in approximately 25% of cases. Unlike murmurs, pericardial friction rubs tend to be intermittent and migratory. They also vary with respiration, being loudest when the patient is sitting forward. The incidence of ED patients with pericarditis who have rubs is unknown.

Other parts of the physical examination, including vital signs and heart rate, are nonspecific for pericarditis.

Diagnostic Strategies The electrocardiogram (ECG) typically evolves through four stages. These four stages occur over time, however, and the emergency physician rarely has the luxury of performing serial tracings. Stage 1, occurring in the first hours to days of illness, includes diffuse ST-segment elevation seen in leads I, II, III, aVL, aVF, and V_2 through V_6, as well as reciprocal ST depression in aVR and V_1. Most patients with acute pericarditis will have concurrent PR-segment depression during stage 1 (Figure 77-1). In stage 2, the ST and PR segments normalize, but the T waves flatten. The characteristic finding of stage 3 is deep, symmetric T-wave inversion. In stage 4, the ECG reverts to normal, though the T-wave inversions may become permanent.[6]

The early ECG findings of acute pericarditis may be difficult to distinguish from those of acute MI, coronary artery spasm, or benign early repolarization. It is very important to be able to differentiate acute MI (AMI) from acute pericarditis because thrombolytic therapy is contraindicated in pericarditis because its use may precipitate hemorrhagic cardiac tamponade.

Unlike the ECG in AMI, the ST elevations in stage 1 acute pericarditis are concave upward rather than convex upward, and simultaneous T-wave inversions are not seen. Subsequent tracings do not evolve through a typical MI pattern, and Q waves do not appear.

There is a virtual absence of ventricular dysrhythmias in pericardial disease. Therefore patients with pericarditis who have ventricular dysrhythmias should be presumed to have underlying cardiac disease or have been misdiagnosed.[7]

Definitive diagnosis of pericarditis with effusion is made by echocardiography. In addition, cardiac tamponade, increased pericardial thickness, pericardial tumors and cysts, constrictive pericarditis, and the congenital absence of the pericardium can all be diagnosed by echocardiography.[8]

Some patients with acute pericarditis have an elevated CK-MB or troponin enzyme. This may be caused by myopericarditis, myocarditis, or ischemia. The white blood cell (WBC) count and erythrocyte sedimentation rate (ESR)

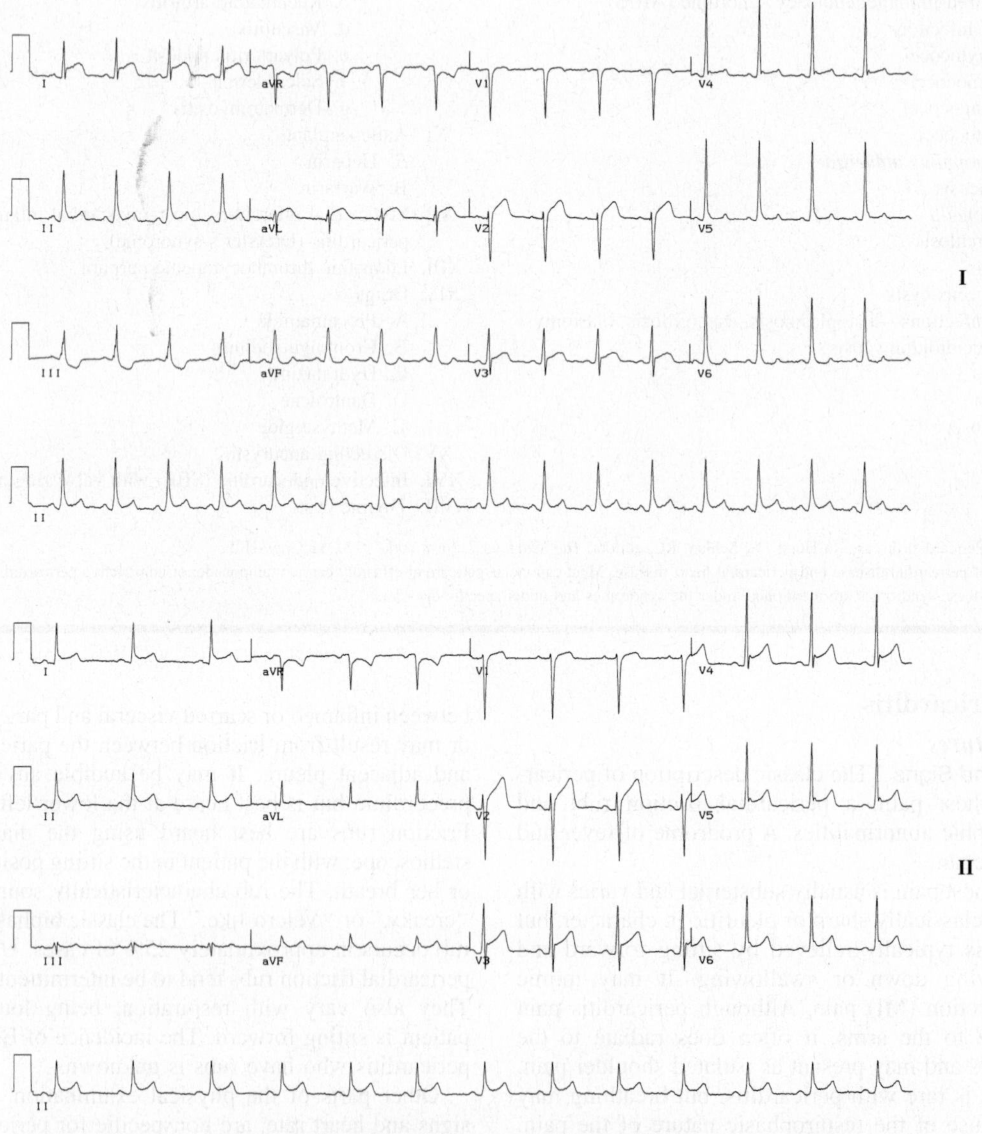

Figure 77-1. **These two ECGs, obtained 11 hours apart, show diffuse ST-T changes and minimal PR depression characteristic of pericarditis.** ***Courtesy of Stephen W. Meldon, MD, MetroHealth Medical Center, Case Western Reserve University, Cleveland, Ohio.***

may be elevated but are nonspecific. Other laboratory studies should be directed at determining nonidiopathic causes of pericarditis.

Management Patients with a known etiology for their pericarditis should have therapy for that disease.

Therapy of acute idiopathic pericarditis is aimed at relief of symptoms. Analgesia can usually be obtained with a nonsteroidal antiinflammatory drug (NSAID) regimen. Aspirin, ibuprofen, and indomethacin are all excellent choices. Oral prednisone is the mainstay of therapy for chronic pericarditis. Methylprednisolone and colchicine are also effective for recurrent pericarditis.[9]

Disposition In the ED, pericarditis should be considered only after other life-threatening conditions have been excluded. Patients with severe or intractable pain, or with new or changing pericardial effusion, should be placed in observation or hospitalized. Also, patients in whom the emergency physician cannot exclude MI, pulmonary embolus, or other life-threatening processes should be admitted.

Complications The clinical course of pericarditis is variable; one study showed that 60% of patients have complete recovery within 1 week, and 18% have complete recovery within 3 weeks.[10] Only 3% have a prolonged course with symptoms for more than 3 weeks before complete resolution. Sixteen percent have recurrent symptoms within the first year, and 3% have recurrent symptoms beyond the first year.[10] Patients with recurrent pericarditis should be referred for follow up, including echocardiography to rule out effusion or tumor.[11]

Uremic Pericardial Disease

Perspective

Etiology Pericarditis was first recognized as a complication of uremia in 1936. It may occur secondary to end-stage renal disease (ESRD) itself or may be associated with chronic hemodialysis. It is clinically detected in up to 20% of uremic patients.[12] The etiology is unknown, but several mechanisms have been proposed, including toxic metabolites, bleeding diathesis of uremia, an infectious process, and immunologic mechanisms. Because renal failure causes immune suppression, the evaluation of a patient with chronic renal disease who has signs of pericarditis requires a diligent search for viral, bacterial, and tuberculous causes.

Clinical Features and Diagnostic Strategies Patients with uremic pericarditis present with chest pain, unexplained fever, and a coarse friction rub. They may also have significant effusions bordering on tamponade.

The ECG in uremic pericarditis is often normal because little epicardial inflammation occurs. In a dialysis patient, cardiac enlargement on chest radiograph in the absence of signs of volume overload or congestive heart failure (CHF) should be considered to represent pericarditis or pericardial effusion until proven otherwise. An echocardiogram will confirm the presence of pericardial effusion. Uremic pericarditis has an effusion that is fibrinous and often grossly bloody. Diagnostic pericardiocentesis is indicated to rule out infection.

Management Uremic pericarditis causing pericardial effusion without hemodynamic compromise is initially treated with a 2- to 6-week course of intensive dialysis, including daily treatments, if necessary. NSAIDs should be used cautiously and probably in consultation with the primary nephrologist because of the risk of exacerbating the bleeding tendency of uremia and their tendency to decrease glomerular filtration rate (in patients with some function). Systemic steroids have been used but require 1 to 2 weeks of therapy to produce a response.

Complications Uremic pericardial effusions are among the most common causes of cardiac tamponade. When hemodynamic compromise is present, pericardial fluid must be drained urgently. Uremic pericardial effusions may be locular and difficult to fully drain with a catheter. Therapeutic options in this situation include pericardiocentesis, pericardial window, or pericardiectomy. Pericardiocentesis is usually not definitive.

Post–Myocardial Infarction Pericarditis

Approximately 20% of patients with transmural infarctions experience a new and different quality of chest pain between 2 and 4 days after infarction. Such patients may also develop low-grade fever and have a transient pericardial friction rub. This often requires careful and frequent auscultation for detection. The diffuse ST-segment elevations typical of pericarditis are rarely seen, and a substantial pericardial effusion is unusual. Early post-MI pericarditis is generally short-lived and disappears with 1 to 3 days of NSAID therapy.

The ECG changes of pericarditis are usually masked by the AMI changes. Patients with post-MI pericarditis have more dysrhythmias and heart failure. This suggests that pericarditis in AMI may be an indicator of greater myocardial damage and therefore of poorer outcome.[13]

In 1956 Dressler reported a syndrome of fever, pleuritis, leukocytosis, pericardial friction rub, and chest radiograph evidence of new pericardial or pleural effusions in 10 post-MI patients. Frequent relapses and a high incidence of friction rubs (8 of 10 patients) led Dressler to describe this syndrome as a delayed complication of MI in contrast to the well-known syndrome of early post-MI pericarditis.[14] The etiology is unknown but thought to be autoimmune. It may also be seen with pulmonary embolus and postpericardotomy. Anticoagulants should be discontinued to reduce the risk of hemorrhagic effusion.

Post-MI pericarditis, early and delayed, is treated with NSAID medications. Aspirin and steroids are alternatives.

Posttraumatic Pericarditis

Perspective Postcardiac injury syndrome (PCIS) is defined as pericarditis after MI, cardiac surgery, or trauma.[15] The exact etiology is unknown. The incidence ranges from approximately 5% after MI to 30% after thoracic surgery or trauma.

Pericarditis will develop in as many as 22% of patients with a penetrating cardiac injury, few of whom will have cardiac tamponade.[16]

Principles of Disease Injury to the pericardium in blunt trauma may range from contusion to laceration or rupture. Some degree of traumatic pericarditis is found at autopsy or operation in many patients sustaining severe blunt trauma of the chest.

Penetrating wounds to the heart usually cause laceration of both the pericardium and the myocardium, with secondary pericarditis and pericardial infections. Although the exact incidence is unknown, infection, tamponade, myocarditis, and inflammatory pericarditis may occur.

An immune pathogenesis is suggested by the development of cardiac autoantibodies, although these autoantibodies are common after injury, even in patients who do not develop pericarditis.[17]

Constrictive pericarditis secondary to trauma occurs. It may be due to pericardial blood, possibly secondary to the decreased resorptive power of damaged pericardium, with secondary fibrosis and constriction.[18]

Clinical Features Signs and symptoms of PCIS include pericardial rub, fever, leukocytosis, high ESR, and chest pain. Although the diagnosis is usually established on clinical grounds, confirmation by echocardiography is helpful.[15] The time between injury and the onset of the pericarditis varies from 4 to 12 days.[15] During hospitalization, purulent pericarditis should be considered as a possible source of sepsis in a trauma patient with multisystem organ failure.[19]

Management and Disposition Most patients respond to aspirin or NSAIDs. The use of steroids has not been shown to cause adverse effects in large studies.

Uncomplicated pericarditis secondary to blunt trauma usually resolves. The patient should be observed until other life-threatening disease processes are excluded.

Neoplastic Pericardial Disease

Perspective Malignant pericardial tumors typically present late, which makes diagnosis and treatment difficult. Malignant involvement of the pericardium is observed in 3.4% of general autopsies and from 2% to 31% of cancer autopsies. The most common causes are lung cancer (30%), breast (23%), leukemia (9%), non-Hodgkin's lymphoma (9%), or Hodgkin's disease (8%).[20]

Primary malignancies of the pericardium are rare (calculated at an annual incidence of 1 in 41 million in Canada) and include mesothelioma, fibrosarcoma, angiosarcoma, malignant teratoma, and primary liposarcoma.[21]

Principles of Disease

Pathophysiology The pattern of cardiac involvement by a malignant tumor is determined by the heart's lymphatic drainage system. A subendocardial plexus of small lymphatics coalesces into a few vessels, which perforate the myocardium and drain into an epicardial plexus. The epicardial lymphatics drain in turn into larger vessels, which accompany the coronary arteries to the aortic root. There they empty into the cardiac lymph nodes in the mediastinum between the innominate artery and the superior vena cava. The route of metastasis is usually retrograde from involved mediastinal lymph nodes to the relatively narrow passage at the root of the aorta. This is where obstruction to cardiac lymphatic drainage occurs.[8]

Malignant pericardial effusions contribute directly to the patient's demise in up to 85% of cases. The large volume of the effusion and the tendency for rapid fluid accumulation frequently cause cardiac tamponade. Although the underlying disease process is often irreversible when tamponade develops, prolongation of the patient's life can be achieved if tamponade is recognized and treated promptly.

Clinical Features Primary cardiac neoplasms such as angiosarcoma and teratoma can present initially with symptoms consistent with benign, idiopathic pericarditis.[22] The typical course is that of an acute pericarditis that resolves and then subsequently recurs.

Malignant pericardial disease is difficult to diagnose. Most patients are asymptomatic or have nonspecific symptoms such as shortness of breath, cough, palpitations, ill-defined chest pain, weakness, dizziness, hiccups, or fatigue. Malignant pericardial effusion should be suspected in any cancer patient with a change in cardiorespiratory symptoms.[4]

Diagnostic Strategies The diagnostic workup for a malignant pericardial effusion includes a strong clinical suspicion and an echocardiogram, computed tomography (CT), or magnetic resonance imaging (MRI) when clinically indicated. When a pericardial effusion is identified, pericardial fluid cytology is recommended. Cytologic analysis of pericardial fluid is 80% to 90% sensitive for detecting malignant cells and more sensitive than pericardial biopsy.[23]

Management Treatment strategies for malignant pericardial effusion include therapeutic pericardiocentesis, pericardiocentesis with instillation of sclerosing or chemotherapeutic agents, systemic chemotherapy, cardiac irradiation, surgical stripping of the pericardium, or construction of a pericardial window. The method chosen depends on the site and susceptibility of the primary tumor, the patient's expected length of survival, the availability of local expertise for each method, and the presence or absence of cardiac tamponade.[4]

Disposition The prognosis for patients with malignant pericardial disease depends on the type and extent of cancer. The outlook is generally poor but is better for breast cancer and lymphoma patients than for those with lung cancer. Patients with a tumor diagnosed in the ED should be considered for admission, as should all patients who are compromised or symptomatic.

Radiation-Induced Pericarditis

Fewer than 5% of patients treated with radiation therapy develop pericarditis. The actual incidence has decreased over the last 25 years with the advent of modern radiation therapy techniques. The percentage of pericardial volume irradiated, dose, and fractionation help determine which patients will develop pericarditis.[24] Radiation-induced pericarditis is most commonly seen in patients with breast cancer and Hodgkin's lymphoma. In general, patients with Hodgkin's disease are younger and have high survival rates. They constitute the majority of patients who develop radiation pericarditis. Pericardial effusion and constrictive pericarditis are common forms of radiation pericarditis. Tumor recurrence should be considered. The clinical presentation, diagnostic studies, and management are similar to other forms of pericarditis.

Pericardial Disease Related to Systemic Connective Tissue Disorders

Rheumatoid Arthritis Pericarditis occurs in approximately one third of patients with rheumatoid arthritis (RA) at some point during the course of their disease. Approximately 20% of patients develop pericarditis within 3 years of their initial diagnosis of RA.[25]

Rheumatoid pericardial disease is rarely clinically significant. Occasional patients develop chronic locular effusions, constrictive pericarditis, or cardiac tamponade; these patients usually have rheumatoid nodules, elevated circulating rheumatoid factor levels, and valvular heart disease. Pericardial involvement should be suspected in any RA patient who experiences the onset of signs of right-sided CHF. There are no suggestive ECG or chest radiograph findings. Pericardiocentesis is indicated in symptomatic RA patients with echocardiographic-proven effusion. Elevated pericardial fluid, LDH, and gamma globulin levels; rheumatoid factor; and low glucose level support the diagnosis. Corticosteroid treatment is useful in symptomatic cases.

Systemic Lupus Erythematosus Pericarditis is found in more than 50% of patients with systemic lupus erythematosus (SLE) at autopsy. The effusion is usually thick and fibrinous. Either cardiac tamponade or constrictive pericarditis may develop. Lupus erythematosus cells may be identified in pericardial fluid specimens. Corticosteroid therapy is indicated for pericardial involvement in SLE.[26]

Other Approximately 33% of patients with Sjögren's syndrome will show evidence of pericarditis.[27] Giant cell arteritis is known to produce granulomatous myocarditis and, on rare occasions, pericarditis that responds to methylprednisolone.[28] Cardiac abnormalities are seen in a substantial number of patients with mixed connective tissue disease (MCTD), with pericarditis being the most common cardiac abnormality.[29] Other connective tissue diseases that may cause pericarditis include ankylosing spondylitis, Reiter's syndrome, Behçet's disease, systemic sclerosis, and polyarteritis nodosa.

Miscellaneous Infectious Causes of Pericarditis

Other etiologies of pericarditis include *Rickettsia conorii,* which causes Mediterranean spotted fever (treated with doxycycline), *Mycoplasma pneumoniae, Nocardia asteroides* (treated with pericardiectomy and long-term use of antibiotics such as sulfisoxazole), *Chlamydia trachomatis,* Epstein-Barr virus, cytomegalovirus (CMV) infection, *Haemophilus actinomycetemcomitans* (treatment with chloramphenicol has been successful), and coccidioidomycosis (endemic in the southwestern United States).

Viral and bacterial causes of pericarditis can coexist, such as varicella-zoster infection subsequently becoming superinfected with *Staphylococcus aureus.* Bacterial superinfections associated with varicella are more common in children.

Pericardial Effusion

Etiology of Pericardial Effusion The most common causes of pericardial effusion are viral or idiopathic pericarditis, malignancy, uremia, trauma, and radiation therapy. Drug reactions and autoimmune diseases are less common causes.

Clinical Features Pericardial effusion is often asymptomatic. It should be suspected in patients with the presence of known associated conditions (e.g., cancer or renal failure) who present with cough, fever, chest pain, or dyspnea.

Diagnostic Strategies Pericardial effusion presents with an enlarged cardiac silhouette on chest radiograph, usually with normal pulmonary vascularity. A minimum of 200 to 250 ml of pericardial fluid is usually necessary to produce cardiomegaly on chest radiograph. Other radiographic signs suggestive of pericardial effusion are a rapid change in heart size, splaying of the subcarinal angle to more than 80 degrees (normal range 45 to 70 degrees), and displacement of the subepicardial fat line from the anterior chest wall on the lateral radiograph.

Echocardiography is the diagnostic modality of choice for detection of pericardial effusion. It easily distinguishes cardiomegaly caused by pericardial fluid from that caused by cardiac chamber enlargement. It can also provide information about the quality of myocardial wall motion. An echocardiogram should be obtained for the initial diagnosis of pericardial effusion or if hemodynamic changes are present.

CT scan may be useful in diagnosing pericardial effusion when the echocardiogram is technically unsatisfactory. MRI can also be diagnostic. Nuclear scans may be useful in detecting purulent pericardial effusions.

Pericardiocentesis may be performed for either diagnostic or therapeutic purposes. Diagnostic pericardiocentesis is indicated in cancer patients (in whom differentiation of malignant effusion from postradiation pericarditis may be necessary) for failure to respond to usual treatment or when bacterial pericarditis is suspected.

Pericardiocentesis is a risky procedure. Common complications are induction of cardiac dysrhythmias, pneumothorax, perforation of myocardium, laceration of coronary or internal mammary arteries, and liver laceration. Echocardiographic-guided pericardiocentesis is much safer than blind or ECG-guided pericardiocentesis and should be the procedure of choice when available.

Pericardial fluid should be analyzed for protein, glucose, specific gravity, cell count and differential, hematocrit, cytology, Gram's and acid-fast stains, fungal smear, and corresponding cultures.

The gross appearance of the pericardial fluid provides a clue to the cause of the effusion. Serosanguineous effusions are most commonly associated with neoplasms, tuberculosis, uremia, and radiation-induced and idiopathic pericarditis. Grossly bloody effusions are always ominous and are caused by blunt or penetrating thoracic trauma, postinfarction myocardial rupture, aortic dissection, coagulopathies, and iatrogenic cardiac perforation during catheterization procedures. Purulent pericardial fluid is seen with pneumonia, empyema, or bacterial endocarditis.

Pericardial effusions that are transudates (protein <3.0 g/100 ml and specific gravity <1.015) are usually due to systemic disorders such as volume overload, CHF, or hypoproteinemia. Exudative effusions (protein content >3.0 g/100 ml and specific gravity >1.015) are generally caused by pericardial injury from malignancy or infection.[4]

Cardiac Tamponade

Etiology As many as 10% of all patients with cancer develop cardiac tamponade.[30] All patients with penetrating chest wounds should be suspected to have tamponade.

Pathophysiology Cardiac tamponade is the result of compression of the myocardium by the contents of the pericardium. This is usually caused by fluid, but may be gas, pus, blood, or a combination of factors.[30]

Cardiac tamponade is a physiologic continuum reflecting the amount of fluid, the rate of accumulation, and the nature of the heart. The three stages necessary for tamponade to develop include fluid filling the recesses of the parietal pericardium, fluid accumulating faster than the rate of the parietal pericardium's ability to stretch, and fluid accumulating faster than the body's ability to increase blood volume to support right ventricle filling pressure. The final result is increased pericardial pressure, which causes decreased cardiac compliance and decreased flow of blood into the heart, which leads to decreased cardiac output.[30]

Symptoms and Signs Cardiac tamponade symptoms are nonspecific. The patient may complain of chest pain, cough, or dyspnea.

The classic triad of cardiac tamponade signs described by Beck is hypotension, distended neck veins, and muffled heart sounds. There is also pulsus paradoxus. These signs may not be present if tamponade develops quickly.

Diagnostic Strategies The chest radiograph will show cardiomegaly only if there is a large accumulation of fluid (200 to 250 ml). The ECG classically shows decreasing voltage or electrical alternans, but the latter is rare. Echocardiography confirms the diagnosis when an effusion and paradoxical systolic wall motion are seen. Thermodilution catheters can also be diagnostic, showing equalization of right and left ventricular pressures.

Management and Prognosis Initial treatment includes intravenous fluids. This adds volume to the right ventricle and increases the filling pressure in an effort to overcome pericardial constriction pressure.

Pericardiocentesis, preferably ultrasound guided, is the treatment of choice. Enough fluid should be withdrawn to hemodynamically stabilize the patient. If tamponade recurs, pericardiocentesis may be repeated, or a drainage catheter may be left in the pericardial space. A pericardotomy may ultimately be necessary.

Cardiac tamponade has a very high mortality that depends on the severity and nature of the underlying disease, the time course of onset, and the rapidity of ED diagnosis and intervention.

Purulent Pericarditis

Epidemiology and Etiology Purulent pericarditis is an acute and catastrophic illness. In the pre-antibiotic era, purulent pericarditis accounted for approximately 40% of all cases of pericarditis and was responsible for 1% of all deaths. Despite the use of antibiotics, it is still a life-threatening process and is most commonly seen in patients with systemic illnesses who develop sepsis. It can occur in any age group.[31]

Etiologic organisms commonly include streptococcus, staphylococcus, Haemophilus, Pseudomonas, Klebsiella, *Escherichia coli,* meningococcus, legionella, Nocardia, *Salmonella typhimurium, Salmonella enteritidis,* and *Clostridium septicum. S. aureus,* group B streptococcus (*Streptococcus agalactiae*), and pneumococcal pericarditis usually are caused by direct extension from a pneumonia or empyema.[31]

Fungal etiologies of purulent pericarditis include *Candida,* Aspergillus, and Histoplasma. *Candida* pericarditis is found in three groups of patients: after cardiac surgery, those with impaired host defenses, and those with severe debilitating underlying diseases.[32] Histoplasma infection of the pericardium occurs in patients from the Ohio and Mississippi river valleys. The organism is rarely seen in pericardial fluid and is difficult to culture.

Principles of Disease

Pathophysiology Purulent pericarditis occurs by several mechanisms: (1) spread from an adjacent infection such as pneumonia or empyema, (2) hematogenous spread from a distant site, (3) direct inoculation of bacteria (trauma or procedure), and (4) spread from an intracardiac source.[31] The most common mechanism is spread from a distant site.

Clinical Features Purulent pericarditis usually presents as a febrile illness lasting 2 to 3 days. Common presenting signs include tachycardia, dyspnea, hepatomegaly, elevated central venous pressure (CVP), chest pain, friction rub, and a leukocytosis.

The most common presentation is a patient with a serious underlying disease who initially improves after treatment of the primary process, but later develops fever, dyspnea, and chest pain.

The key to successfully diagnosing purulent pericarditis is to consider the diagnosis early in the patient's course. The diagnosis should be suspected in any febrile patient with multisystem illness who has a pericardial effusion.

Diagnostic Strategies Pericardiocentesis is necessary to establish the diagnosis, to obtain fluid for microbiologic studies, and to relieve cardiac tamponade.

Management The treatment of purulent pericarditis is controversial. Although purulent pericarditis has been traditionally treated by pericardiectomy, placement of an indwelling catheter, coupled with lavage and drainage, may avoid the need for surgical drainage.[33] For either approach, use of intravenous (IV) antibiotics or antifungals is mandatory.

Disposition Those patients not in an intensive care setting should be admitted there.

The overall survival rate for purulent pericarditis is approximately 30% with antibiotic therapy alone, and 50% when combined with early complete surgical drainage, either open or percutaneous.[34]

In addition to the initial complications related to sepsis and tamponade, there can be long-term sequelae of purulent pericarditis, such as the development of constrictive pericarditis.

Tuberculous Pericarditis

Epidemiology and Etiology Tuberculous pericarditis is estimated to occur in 1% to 2% of patients with pulmonary tuberculosis.[35] Tuberculous pericarditis is more common in patients who are socioeconomically deprived or who have acquired immunodeficiency syndrome (AIDS) or another immunodeficiency state. Although rare, isolated tuberculous pericarditis still exists. It is a known complication of tuberculosis and presents in patients with, or at risk for, tuberculosis.

Principles of Disease Tuberculous pericarditis most commonly spreads to the pericardium by direct extension from the tracheobronchial tree, mediastinal or hilar lymph nodes, sternum, or spine.

Clinical Features and Diagnostic Strategies The most common physical findings are those of tuberculosis and pericarditis.

In many patients, the chest radiograph shows an enlarged cardiac silhouette, but a pulmonary infiltrate is often absent. Pericardial fluid aspirates will reveal acid-fast bacilli by smear or culture (which may require 4 to 6 weeks to become positive) in approximately 50% of all cases.[35] Because of this, pericardial biopsy can be an important diagnostic tool.

Diagnostic workup should include assessment for human immunodeficiency virus (HIV). The diagnosis of tuberculous pericarditis may be difficult in AIDS patients because negative tuberculin skin tests are common.

Management and Disposition Patients with tuberculous pericarditis should be hospitalized and observed for evidence of cardiac tamponade. Triple drug therapy should be started in the hospital and continued for at least 9 months.[35] In addition, the patient should be placed in protective isolation, which should be initiated in the ED at the earliest suspicion of possible tuberculosis infection.

Patients with chronic pericardial effusions may benefit from oral prednisone therapy. Patients with evidence of pericardial thickening, constrictive pericarditis, or hemodynamic compromise should be referred for surgical treatment. Pericardiocentesis may be a temporary measure until surgical treatment is available.

Complications and Prognosis Complications of tuberculous pericarditis include constrictive pericarditis, myocarditis, and impaired cardiac function, either directly or by tamponade.[35]

Before the introduction of antituberculosis medications, tuberculous pericarditis was usually fatal. When treated with medication and surgery, the current mortality rate is approximately 20%.[35]

Other Causes

Amyloid deposition can cause either restrictive cardiomyopathy or constrictive pericarditis. Pericarditis can occur on rare occasions as an extraintestinal complication of inflammatory bowel disease (IBD). Pericardial complications of IBD are independent of the clinical course of the gut disorder.[36]

Iatrogenic pericarditis can also be seen as a complication of an implantable defibrillator or an atrial lead of a permanent pacemaker. A polymicrobial bacterial pericarditis can occur after transbronchial needle aspiration, or as a complication of endoscopic variceal sclerotherapy.

Rarely, pericarditis can also be caused by erosion through the esophagus into the pericardium of a foreign body, such as a sewing needle or toothpick.

Medications that have been reported to cause pericarditis are listed in Box 77-1.

Pericarditis and Acquired Immunodeficiency Syndrome

Epidemiology and Etiology Progressive dysfunction of multiple organ systems occurs in AIDS. Pericarditis is usually nonspecific in origin, but can be associated with Kaposi's sarcoma, lymphoma, or any infectious pathogen. Infectious etiologies may include *Mycobacterium tuberculosis, Cryptococcus, S. aureus,* CMV, herpes simplex, *N. asteroides,* pneumococcus, and *Listeria monocytogenes.*[37]

Less than 1% of patients with HIV develop acute pericarditis, but up to 40% have asymptomatic pericardial effusion. In 33% of these patients, the effusion is moderate or large in size. Pericardial effusion is more frequent in patients in the more advanced stages of HIV infection and is an independent predictor of decreased survival.[38,39]

Clinical Features and Diagnostic Strategies Although the etiology may differ, the clinical features and diagnostic evaluation of patients with AIDS-related pericarditis are the same as in patients without AIDS. Pericarditis should be suspected in HIV-positive (and HIV-negative) patients who have signs of pulmonary infection, particularly those with empyema.

Management Treatment is the same as for patients without AIDS.

Pericardial Disease and Pregnancy

Pericardial effusion and pericarditis both occur rarely during pregnancy, usually during the third trimester. Both are usually asymptomatic. If the effusion enlarges, pericardial drainage and possibly pericardiotomy may be necessary. If constrictive pericarditis develops, cardiovascular complications may prevent the patient from carrying the pregnancy to term.[40]

Pneumopericardium

Perspective and Etiology Pneumopericardium and pyopneumopericardium are both rare. In most patients, pyopneumopericardium results from trauma, aspiration or ingestion of a foreign body, ingestion of caustic substances, or invasive procedures (e.g., esophagoscopy, thoracentesis, endotracheal intubation). Pneumopericardium may also be caused by diseases that can lead to formation of fistulous communications between the pericardial space and pleural space, bronchial tree, or upper gastrointestinal tract (e.g., peptic ulcer disease, carcinoma of the esophagus or stomach, esophageal diverticulum, bronchial carcinoma), infection with gas-producing microorganisms, or it can be idiopathic. Spontaneous pneumopericardium may complicate asthma, labor, barotrauma from positive pressure ventilation, or Valsalva maneuvers, such as might occur during weightlifting. Cocaine inhalation from positive pressure devices can also cause pneumopericardium.[41]

Pneumopericardium can resolve spontaneously or on rare occasions can lead to tension pneumopericardium.

Principles of Disease

Pathophysiology Pneumopericardium is most commonly caused by a rise in intraalveolar pressure above atmospheric pressure, resulting in rupture of alveoli. This allows air to dissect into the hilum and mediastinum, through the pericardial reflection on the pulmonary vessels, and into the pericardium.[42]

Clinical Features and Diagnostic Strategies Findings on physical examination depend on the quantity of fluid and gas in the pericardial space. Heart sounds can be of variable intensity, can vary depending on body position, and sometimes have a metallic quality that may be accompanied by splashing sounds. *Hamman's sign,* and *mediastinal crunch* are the terms used for a loud, crunching sound associated with pneumopericardium or pneumomediastinum. This sound is best heard at the precordium with the patient in a left lateral recumbent position and is diagnostic for the presence of mediastinal air. The diagnosis of pneumopericardium is confirmed by chest radiograph, CT scan, or echocardiography.

Tension pneumopericardium presents with clinical findings of acute cardiac tamponade.

Management Stable patients with uncomplicated spontaneous pneumopericardium can usually be observed and discharged from the ED. In the rare patient with pneumopericardium who is stable after penetrating chest injury, once all other life-threatening injuries and complications are excluded, prolonged observation is indicated with no expected long-term sequelae.[43] Tension pneumopericardium should be treated with emergency pericardiocentesis. Surgical intervention may also be needed. Antibiotics are indicated for infectious etiologies.

Constrictive Pericarditis

Perspective and Etiology Tuberculosis is still the leading cause of constrictive pericarditis in developing countries, but accounts for only a minority of cases in western cultures. Many postulate that constrictive pericarditis is a late consequence of viral pericarditis.[44] There is an increased incidence of constrictive pericarditis complicating uremic pericardial disease as the result of improved survival of patients with chronic renal disease. Other predisposing conditions include previous mediastinal irradiation, cardiac trauma, purulent pericarditis, cardiac actinomycosis, and postpericardiotomy adhesions.[34]

Principles of Disease

Pathophysiology Constrictive pericarditis is characterized by impaired diastolic filling from external cardiac compression caused by a thickened pericardium. In advanced cases, the visceral and parietal pericardial layers may be adherent, completely obliterating the normal pericardial space.[5] Unlike the pericardial fluid collection in tamponade, however, the constricted pericardium does not transmit the respiratory variation in intrathoracic pressure, so no inspiratory increase in venous return and right-side volumes occurs. Consequently, pulsus paradoxus is a rare finding in constrictive pericarditis.

Because the pericardium limits volume, ventricular filling is rapid and completed within the first one third of diastole, after which left ventricular (LV) volume and pressure remain unchanged. Early ventricular filling followed by a period of unchanging pressure yields a corresponding dip and plateau pattern or square root sign on the LV diastolic pressure curve.

Clinical Features The symptoms and signs of constrictive pericarditis are virtually indistinguishable from those of CHF. Dyspnea, fatigue, and weight gain are the most common complaints. Hepatomegaly, marked pitting lower-extremity edema, and ascites are seen on physical examination.[44] Pulsus paradoxus is absent, in contrast to cardiac tamponade. The presence of jugular venous distention differentiates this from liver disease. The characteristic auscultatory finding of constrictive pericarditis is a pericardial knock in early diastole, corresponding to the abrupt halt in ventricular filling. A friction rub may also be audible.

Diagnostic Strategies Heart size on the chest radiograph is typically small but may be increased in the presence of atrial enlargement or marked pericardial thickening. Pericardial calcification is a helpful sign when present. Liver function tests are consistent with passive congestion.[44] ECG findings include low QRS voltage, nonspecific ST-T–wave abnormalities, and atrial dysrhythmias.

Echocardiography may be helpful in differentiating constrictive pericarditis from restrictive cardiomyopathy or cardiac tamponade, especially Doppler echocardiography.

Cardiac catheterization and simultaneous measurement of right ventricular (RV) and LV end-diastolic pressures or endomyocardial biopsy may be necessary to make the diagnosis.

Differential Considerations Constrictive pericarditis is most often confused with CHF because of the presence in both conditions of shortness of breath, elevated jugular venous pressure, hepatomegaly, and edema. A history of viral or bacterial pericarditis, radiation therapy, tuberculosis, chest trauma, or cardiac surgery should lead to consideration of constrictive pericarditis. The diagnosis should also be considered with signs of elevated venous pressure but no history of myocardial dysfunction. Patients with cirrhosis may have ascites and liver enlargement, but they do not have jugular venous distention. RV infarction causes a hemodynamic picture similar to that of constriction, but the echocardiogram reveals abnormal RV function and wall motion.[5]

The hemodynamic picture in restrictive cardiomyopathy is virtually identical to that of constrictive pericarditis; both are associated with signs of elevated venous pressure and small heart size. The echocardiogram may reveal the presence of infiltrative myocardial disease in patients with restrictive cardiomyopathy.

Management Pericardiectomy is the therapy of choice for constrictive pericarditis. It often causes dramatic symptomatic improvement. Because the disease process progresses slowly, surgery can often be delayed in patients who are hemodynamically stable.[45]

MYOCARDIAL DISEASE (MYOCARDITIS)

Perspective

The term *myocarditis* was used initially by Sobernheim in 1837. Romberg reported the association with scarlet fever and typhus in 1891, and "isolated idiopathic interstitial myocarditis" was described by Fiedler in 1899. In 1941, Saphir proposed one of the first classification systems.[46]

Myocarditis is not common, but can be devastating and remains an important diagnosis for the emergency physician.

Epidemiology and Etiology

Myocarditis is detected in almost 10% of routine autopsies but often is not recognized clinically.[17] The overall incidence is unknown. The enteroviruses, especially the Coxsackie B virus, predominate as causative agents. Coxsackie B virus usually causes infection during the summer months, but outbreaks do not occur every year. Other organisms that may cause myocarditis include adenovirus, influenza A and B, streptococcus, mononucleosis, chlamydia, mycoplasma, parainfluenza, mumps, CMV, rubeola, rubella, rabies, lymphocytic choriomeningitis virus, hepatitis A and B, and varicella-zoster.[47]

CMV and *Toxoplasma gondii* have emerged as potential causes of myocarditis in cardiac transplant patients. Fifty-two percent of patients dying of AIDS have myocarditis on autopsy. Worldwide, Chagas' disease is a leading cause of myocarditis, especially in South America.[48]

Principles of Disease

Pathophysiology Myocardial injury from myocarditis presumably occurs by one or more of the following mechanisms: (a) necrosis from direct invasion of an offending infectious agent and its replication within or near myocytes; (b) destruction of cardiac tissue from infiltration of host cellular immune components or from cytotoxic effect of activated host humoral defenses or both, initiated by the infectious agent; or (c) the toxic effect of exogenous chemicals or endotoxins produced by a systemic pathogen.[49]

Enteroviruses are thought to be associated with most cases of myocarditis in humans. In neonates the pathologic changes appear to be more related to direct viral damage, whereas adults appear more susceptible to immunologic damage.[47]

Myocarditis is linked to the development of dilated cardiomyopathy. Autoantigens are present after myocarditis. This leads to the hypothesis that idiopathic dilated cardiomyopathy after myocarditis is predominately autoimmune in origin, resulting from either shared antigens or molecular mimicry.[50] The amino acid sequences of the Coxsackie B virus and beta myosin heavy chain protein are more than 50% similar. An immune response to the former yields damage to the latter (molecular mimicry). There is also a higher concentration of IgG anti-alpha-myosin antibodies in patients with myocarditis and dilated cardiomyopathy than in controls.[51]

There is a clinicopathologic description of myocarditis based on endomyocardial biopsy. Myocarditis is classified as fulminant, acute, chronic active, or chronic persistent. This categorization system parallels that used with other viruses such as hepatitis.[52]

Clinical Features

Flulike complaints, including fever, fatigue, myalgias, vomiting, and diarrhea are usually the first symptoms and signs of myocarditis. Altered vital signs include fever, tachycardia, tachypnea, and uncommonly, hypotension. A tachycardia disproportionate to the temperature or apparent toxicity is a clinical clue. Cardiac examination is often unremarkable. CHF and dysrhythmias also occur. Unexplained CHF is a common manifestation of myocarditis. Approximately 12% of patients suffer from chest pain. As a result, myocarditis is frequently a diagnosis of exclusion.[49]

In children, prominent physical findings include grunting respirations and intercostal retractions. Although most patients will have clear lungs on auscultation, approximately 10% to 15% of patients will have wheezing. Infants often have a fulminant syndrome characterized by fever, cyanosis, respiratory distress, tachycardia, and cardiac failure. When children have ventricular dysrhythmias, myocarditis and idiopathic dilated cardiomyopathy are commonly seen on endomyocardial biopsy, despite findings of structurally normal hearts by noninvasive studies.[53]

Diagnostic Strategies

Common ECG changes include sinus tachycardia and low electrical activity. The ECG can also show a prolonged corrected QT interval, atrioventricular (AV) block, or AMI pattern with abnormalities, ST-segment depression, and T-wave inversion.[54]

Cardiac enzymes are frequently elevated. The WBC count and ESR are both nonspecific. The echocardiographic features of myocarditis are polymorphous and nonspecific, but can show multichamber dysfunction (e.g., reduced LV ejection fraction, global hypokinesis, and regional wall motion abnormalities). CT and MRI scans may also be diagnostic.

Indium-111 antimyosin antibodies bind specifically to exposed myosin in damaged myocardial cells, thereby providing a noninvasive approach for the diagnosis of myocardial necrosis.[55] They may also be used to detect ongoing myocyte necrosis in myocarditis, AMI, dilated cardiomyopathy, and cardiac transplant rejection.[56]

Viral titers are helpful, but the yield is low. Few patients show a significant rise in titers for Coxsackie B3 virus. A fourfold rise in viral titers or a high titer of viral specific immunoglobulin M (IgM) may help establish a viral etiology.

Endocardial biopsy, the gold standard, has variable specificity and sensitivity.[57] Histologic criteria for myocarditis are present in only 5% to 30% of patients with clinically suspected myocarditis, 41% of patients with acutely dilated cardiomyopathy, and up to 63% of patients with chronic dilated cardiomyopathy. Molecular genetic probes, such as polymerase chain reaction (PCR), are used to supplement standard histologic analysis. Patients with virus present on biopsy tissue have a much worse clinical course.[58]

Differential Diagnosis

Myocarditis can masquerade as AMI because patients with either may have severe chest pain, ECG changes, elevated serum levels of creatine kinase, and heart failure. Patients with myocarditis are usually young (usually <35 years of age) and have few risk factors for coronary artery disease. ECG abnormalities may be present beyond a single coronary artery distribution, or there are global, rather than segmental, wall motion abnormalities on echocardiography.[59] The diagnosis of myocarditis also should be considered in an otherwise healthy patient who has symptoms and signs of CHF or atrial dysrhythmias.[57]

In myocarditis, chest pain continues with no further evolution of the ECG to indicate ischemia. Coronary arteriography is usually normal, which should prompt consideration of endomyocardial biopsy. Myocarditis can be found in over 30% of patients with AMI symptoms and normal coronary arteries.[59]

Echocardiography in myocarditis shows global dysfunction that does not correspond to coronary artery distribution, but it also may show segmental ventricular wall motion abnormalities similar to those seen in MI.[8]

With antimyosin scintigraphy, myocarditis is usually characterized by a diffuse, faint, heterogeneous uptake of antimyosin antibody because myocyte necrosis is typically widespread. AMI is almost always characterized by an intense, localized uptake of antibody in the region of the occluded coronary artery. A normal antimyosin scan excludes both AMI and myocarditis.[55]

Management

The current treatment for myocarditis is supportive therapy. Only bed rest is uniformly accepted as being of benefit.[47] Patients with a fulminant clinical course require cardiac transplantation.

The demonstration of replicating enterovirus RNA in myocarditis leads some authors to postulate that the first phase of myocarditis may be treated with antiviral agents in addition to supportive care.[60,61]

The latter phases of myocarditis may be immune-mediated and may respond to immunosuppressive therapy. There are reports of success in uncontrolled studies using immunosuppressive therapy, but the National Institutes of Health (NIH)–sponsored multicenter trial for myocarditis treatment did not establish the efficacy of immunosuppressive therapy.[61-63] These data are being reviewed to identify patient and treatment subsets in which immunosuppressive therapy may be of benefit.

Because myocardial damage in myocarditis may be mediated by immunologic mechanisms, high-dose gamma globulin (IVIG) therapy has been studied in a pediatric population. High-dose IVIG may be associated with improved recovery of LV function and better survival during the first year after presentation.[64]

In some cases of myocarditis, the deterioration of cardiac function is reversible if the patient can survive the critical care phase with the aid of a cardiopulmonary support system. These devices have been used successfully over extended periods (up to 70 days). They should be considered a treatment option in patients with fulminant myocarditis, and this therapy may be tried before transplantation.[65]

Disposition All patients with myocarditis should be admitted, usually to a monitored setting. Those with hemodynamic instability require admission to the intensive care unit. Complications of myocarditis include ventricular dysrhythmias, LV aneurysm, and cardiac failure.

In the NIH myocarditis trial, the mortality rate was 20% at 1 year and 56% at 4.3 years of follow-up, despite optimal medical management. Ejection fraction and RV function 1 year after initial presentation may be the best predictors of subsequent survival.[48,66] The long-term prognosis in patients who do not die is variable.

Patients who undergo transplantation because of heart failure caused by myocarditis have decreased 1-year survival compared with patients transplanted for other reasons (58% versus 82%) and have allograft rejection rates more than twice that of other recipients. This rejection often occurs within 2 weeks of transplantation.[67]

Chagas' Disease

Chagas' disease is one of the leading causes of death in many countries in Latin America, particularly in Central America. It is caused by the protozoan *Trypanosoma cruzi*. Transmission to humans is by insect vector. The exact pathogenesis is unknown.[68]

Approximately three fourths of seropositive patients with Chagas' disease never have cardiac symptoms. One fourth have angina-like chest pain, dysrhythmias, embolic episodes, heart failure, conduction abnormalities (bundle branch block, left anterior hemiblock, first degree or higher AV block), multifocal ventricular premature contractions, and abnormal ST-segment and T-wave abnormalities in the precordial leads.[69] Ventricular tachycardia, sustained or nonsustained, is also common. Syncopal or near-syncopal episodes occur in nearly two thirds of patients.[69]

The diagnosis is established by demonstrating serum parasites. It should be suspected in ED patients with new cardiac symptoms and a Latin America travel history.

In more than half of the patients who die of chronic Chagas' disease, autopsy reveals a unique LV apical aneurysm or scar, which is a reliable marker of the disease.[69] Echocardiography may also show this. The extent of tissue damage correlates with the amount of parasites, which can also be found in histologic sections of infected tissues.

Chagas' disease can be treated with the antitrypanosomal drug nifurtimox. Amiodarone may be useful to treat ventricular tachycardia.

Trichinosis

Trichinosis is caused by ingestion of the cysts of *Trichinella spiralis* in undercooked meat. In the United States, the meat involved has traditionally been pork, but today it is more likely to be wild game such as bear or cougar. Larvae may be deposited in the myocardium, where their presence incites an eosinophilic inflammatory reaction and necrosis of muscle fibers. The acute illness consists of fever, myalgias, muscle tenderness, neck stiffness, and a characteristic periorbital edema.

Myocardial involvement is present in approximately 20% of clinically diagnosed cases and appears in the second or third week of illness, a time when other symptoms are declining. Cardiac manifestations include precordial pain, dyspnea, cardiomegaly, dysrhythmias, or CHF. ECG findings such as nonspecific ST-T–wave abnormalities, dysrhythmias, and conduction blocks may appear transiently, even in the absence of cardiac symptoms. Peripheral eosinophilia and an elevated ESR are common.

The diagnosis is usually made by serologic studies or by biopsy of any symptomatic muscle group. Treatment usually involves corticosteroids and antihelmintic drugs such as thiabendazole or albendazole. The prognosis for full recovery is good, with spontaneous remission of myocarditis in most patients. Myocardial involvement is the most common cause of death from trichinosis and is present in 94% of autopsies of fatal cases.[70]

Diphtheria

Diphtheria is rare in the United States, with only 41 cases reported to the Centers for Disease Control and Prevention (CDC) between 1980 and 1995. It is more common outside the United States. It is still fatal, with up to 10% of all infected patients in the United States dying. Those at risk include the nonimmunized (the CDC reports as many as 60% of adults in the United States older than 20 are not immunized) and those with contact with farm animals and unpasteurized dairy products.

Diphtheria is caused by the toxin of the gram-positive organism *Corynebacterium diphtheriae*. The principal manifestations of the illness are nasopharyngitis with membrane formation and respiratory obstruction, myocarditis, and polyneuritis. Myocardial involvement is clinically evident in 10% to 25% of cases and is the major cause of death. Early signs of myocarditis are tachycardia and faint heart sounds; this progresses to CHF in some cases. Cardiac enzymes are often elevated. Prolongation of the PR interval and ST-T–wave abnormalities occur within the first 2 weeks of onset. Other ECG abnormalities, such as bundle branch block or complete heart block, precede total circulatory collapse and are associated with an extremely poor prognosis.

Hospitalization with monitoring in an intensive care unit is mandatory in suspected cases. In addition to supportive treatment, specific therapy involves high-dose penicillin and diphtheria antitoxin. Treatment with oral carnitine, a cofactor in the transport of fatty acids to mitochondria, is associated with a lower incidence of heart failure, severe conduction blocks, and decreased mortality.

Lyme Disease

Epidemiology and Clinical Features Lyme disease is caused by infection with the spirochete *Borrelia burgdorferi* and is discussed in Chapter 128.

Lyme disease–related carditis occurs a median of 21 days after the onset of erythema migrans.[71] Cardiac complications occur in 4% to 10% of patients, including conduction disturbances; bundle branch block; first-, second-, and third-degree heart block; cardiac arrest; dysrhythmias; and LV dysfunction.

Diagnostic Strategies Patients with Lyme disease present with fever, myalgias, arthralgias, headache, adenopathy, and fatigue. A characteristic skin eruption, erythema chronicum migrans, develops at the site of the tick bite in 89% of cases. Lyme disease–related carditis should be suspected in otherwise healthy persons who have unexplained heart block and a history of potential exposure to ticks in an endemic area.

Lyme disease is diagnosed by identification of the spirochete in blood, skin, or cerebrospinal fluid (CSF), or by serologic testing. Silver staining of endomyocardial biopsy demonstrates the spirochete. A screening ECG should be performed whenever the diagnosis of Lyme disease is suspected.

Management and Disposition Atropine or isoproterenol may be used to treat first- or second-degree heart block or third-degree block that is hemodynamically stable. Placement of a temporary pacemaker is often required in unstable patients.

Antibiotic therapy with IV penicillin G (20 million U/day) or oral tetracycline (250 mg qid) for 10 to 20 days is effective and can reverse AV block. Erythromycin should be prescribed in place of tetracycline in young children. Ceftriaxone is also effective. The role of antibiotics in preventing Lyme disease–related carditis is unknown. Prednisone (40-60 mg/day in divided doses, tapered by 5 to 10 mg/week) for the treatment of patients with Lyme disease–related carditis and conduction delays may prove useful. Patients with Lyme disease–related carditis require hospitalization and cardiac monitoring.[71]

Acquired Immunodeficiency Syndrome–Related Myocardial Disease

Epidemiology The cardiac manifestations of AIDS are diverse and are thought to be the cause of death in at least 6% of patients with HIV.[72] The prevalence of LV dysfunction in adult AIDS patients is approximately 20%. Myocarditis has been described in approximately 46% of AIDS patients undergoing postmortem examination. Most AIDS patients demonstrate cardiac involvement as their underlying disease worsens.[73]

Etiology The pathogenesis of HIV-related heart muscle disease is probably multifactorial. The direct etiologic role of HIV infection in cardiomyopathy is controversial.[73]

CMV infection is a major cause of morbidity in AIDS and can cause myocarditis, as can infection with Toxoplasma. Of AIDS patients with toxoplasmosis, 28% initially have cardiac symptoms such as cardiomegaly, CHF, dysrhythmias, pericarditis, pericardial tamponade, or chest pain.[74] *Mycobacterium tuberculosis, Aspergillus fumigatus,* Coxsackie B virus, and cryptococcal and Histoplasma myocarditis also occur.

Kaposi's sarcoma is the most common neoplasm found in AIDS patients and may involve the heart. Cardiac B-cell lymphoma can also occur and may cause tamponade, CHF, or conduction abnormalities.

HIV disease treatment may also lead to cardiac toxicity. Pentamidine, which is structurally similar to procainamide, can cause torsades de pointes ventricular tachycardia.[72] Both zidovudine and dideoxyinosine can also lead to cardiac dysfunction.

Other Causes of Myocarditis

Cardiac involvement of *Legionella pneumophila* occurs uncommonly. Clinical symptoms are the same as those of pericarditis and myocarditis. Dysrhythmias and conduction blocks occur. After treatment with erythromycin, normal cardiac function may return. In some cases, the myocardium may be the only affected organ.

Cardiac toxoplasma infection may lead to clinically significant disease. It occurs in patients with acute lymphocytic leukemia or lymphoma who are receiving chemotherapy. It is well described in recipients of bone marrow and cardiac transplantation. Immunocompromised patients with toxoplasmic myocarditis may have CHF, pericarditis, and dysrhythmias (including bundle branch block) as a result of lesions in the conducting system. Untreated toxoplasmic myocarditis is fatal.[75]

Myocarditis associated with *M. pneumoniae* infection may be caused by either direct invasion of the myocardium, an autoimmune mechanism, or an increased tendency for intravascular coagulation.[76]

Miliary tuberculosis, including tuberculosis myocarditis, can lead to sudden death.[77] Granulomas within the myocardial conduction system can precipitate fatal dysrhythmias.

Sudden death can occur secondary to *Chlamydia pneumoniae* myocarditis.[78] Antibodies are present in the serum, and the heart shows small foci of lymphocytic infiltrates and degenerative changes within the myocytes.

Myocarditis, presumably mediated by exotoxin, is associated with shigella infection.

Cardiac involvement of the conduction system and the pericardium may also occur in dermatomyositis and polymyositis. Patients are usually asymptomatic, but pericarditis, myocarditis, and dysrhythmias can occur.[79]

Doxorubicin (Adriamycin) Cardiotoxicity

Both acute and chronic cardiotoxicity occur secondary to the use of doxorubicin.[80] Manifestations of acute cardiotoxicity include dysrhythmias, pericarditis-myocarditis, and LV dysfunction.

Cocaine

The earliest report of cocaine damaging the heart was in 1911. Price and Leaky reported that cocaine use for local dental anesthesia could induce severe myocardial damage leading to death.[81] Cocaine has various effects on the heart, including myocarditis and dilated cardiomyopathy.

Myocarditis is a common autopsy finding in patients who died of cocaine abuse. The mechanism responsible for the cardiotoxic effects of cocaine remains largely unknown.

Theories include: (1) cocaine may have a direct effect on lymphocyte activity; (2) IV cocaine can increase natural killer cell activity in blood, which may be cytotoxic to myocardial cells; (3) there is a cocaine-related eosinophilic infiltrate that suggests a hypersensitivity reaction; and (4) catecholamine administration can induce a focal myocarditis.[82] Cocaine users are at increased risk for infection, and concomitant viral infection causing myocarditis is possible. Cocaine has a direct, negative inotropic effect on cardiac muscle.

Autopsy studies show that patients who die with detectable cocaine levels have myocarditis and myocardial contraction bands more often than controls. The severity of contraction-band necrosis correlates with the serum and urine concentrations of cocaine. It is postulated that catecholamine excess caused by cocaine use contributes to contraction-band necrosis, which may supply the anatomic substrate for ventricular dysrhythmias.[83]

In summary, there appears to be a transient toxic cardiomyopathy associated with cocaine use. Autopsy studies support the concept that cocaine may induce scattered foci of necrosis and myocarditis independent of coronary artery disease or clinically documented AMI.

Kawasaki Disease

Kawasaki disease, which is of unknown etiology, primarily affects children. The diagnosis is made based on clinical criteria. As many as 25% of all patients develop coronary artery abnormalities, usually several weeks after symptom onset. These are usually reversible, but may lead to aneurysm formation or secondary thrombosis and myocardial ischemia. Myocarditis occurs during the initial phase of the disease in up to 50% of all patients. Rarely, this leads to cardiogenic shock or CHF. Pericarditis also occurs in up to 25% of patients.[84,85]

CARDIOMYOPATHIES AND SPECIFIC HEART MUSCLE DISEASE

Cardiomyopathies are diseases of the heart in which the dominant feature is involvement of the heart muscle itself. The exact incidence is unknown. Cardiomyopathies are defined and classified into three categories according to the World Health Organization (WHO): (1) *dilated,* with ventricular dilation, contractile dysfunction, and CHF symptoms; (2) *hypertrophic,* with LV hypertrophy (LVH) and asymmetric septum involvement, and preserved contraction; and (3) *restrictive,* with impaired diastolic filling.

Dilated Cardiomyopathy

Epidemiology and Etiology Idiopathic dilated cardiomyopathy (IDC) is a spectrum of disorders that have in common a dilated and failing heart for which no cause can be established. The diagnosis therefore is one of exclusion. The incidence of dilated cardiomyopathy is estimated to be 7.5 cases per 100,000 persons per year.[86] The true incidence is probably underestimated because many asymptomatic cases remain undiagnosed.[87] The etiology is unknown. One of the current theories is that approximately 30% of cases are of infectious etiology.

Dilated cardiomyopathy affects men more often than women and may occur in any age group, with middle age (ages 40 to 65) being the most common. Risk factors include ethanol and tobacco abuse, pregnancy, hypertension, and infection.

Table 77-1. Etiologies of Idiopathic Dilated Cardiomyopathy

Etiology	Percentage (%)
Idiopathic	47
Myocarditis	12
Coronary artery disease	11
Postpartum cardiomyopathy	5
Human immunodeficiency virus	5
Ethanol	3
Drug induced*	3
Connective tissue diseases	2
Amyloidosis	2
Hypertension	2
Familial	2
Miscellaneous	6

From Kasper EK et al: *J Am Coll Cardiol* 23:586, 1994.
*Drug-induced etiology included Adriamycin, lithium, interleukin-2, and prednisone.

Despite extensive evaluations, almost half of all patients with CHF caused by dilated cardiomyopathy will ultimately be considered idiopathic (Table 77-1).[88]

Clinical Features Symptoms of IDC are of insidious onset. Left-sided heart failure occurs as the initial manifestation of IDC in 75% to 85% of patients, with dyspnea (usually with exertion or while supine) the major symptom. Exacerbation of heart or renal disease, dietary indiscretion, and medication error or noncompliance are the key contributors to the exacerbation. Chest pain on exertion is the initial symptom in 8% to 20% of patients, and systemic or pulmonary emboli are the initial manifestation in 4%. Right-sided heart failure is a late and ominous sign.[87]

Diagnostic Strategies The chest radiograph reveals cardiomegaly. ECG findings are nonspecific. There may be poor R-wave progression, intraventricular conduction delay, or left bundle branch block pattern. Holter monitoring may show frequent premature ventricular contractions (PVCs) and occasional ventricular tachycardia, which is nonsustained. Sudden death (SD) is uncommon.[87]

Echocardiography shows LV dilation, reduced systolic function, and variable wall motion abnormalities.[8] Abnormal ventricular contractility defines IDC, and an ejection fraction below 45% is generally required for diagnosis. End-diastolic and systolic volumes are increased, as is pulmonary capillary wedge pressure and CVP.[87]

Endomyocardial biopsy may also be necessary. New histochemical, immunologic, and molecular biologic techniques may improve the diagnostic yield of biopsy tissue.

Management Therapy includes supportive measures, such as adequate rest, weight control, abstaining from tobacco, moderation in alcohol consumption, and reduced physical activity during periods of decompensation. Medical treatment includes those measures that treat CHF and include preload and afterload reduction.

Because presentation to the ED usually includes pulmonary edema, ED treatment includes diuretics, oxygen, vasodilators, and other measures.

Angiotensin-converting enzyme inhibitors are the treatment of choice. Other afterload reducing agents, such as hydralazine and isosorbide dinitrate, also prolong survival in patients with mild, moderate, and severe heart failure. Vasodilator therapy may be used for any patient with symptomatic LV dysfunction. Antidysrhythmic treatment and anticoagulation have both been used, but their use is not proven to be efficacious.[87] There have been mixed results with the use of positive inotropic agents. Digoxin may not alter mortality, but may lead to decreased symptoms and hospitalizations.[89] Calcium channel blockers, such as amlodipine, may be effective, particularly if the etiology is microvascular spasm secondary to infection.[90]

Circulating catecholamines increase in patients with heart failure in proportion to the severity of disease. This fact leads to the hypothesis that sympathetic activation plays an important part in heart failure. Though previously thought to be contraindicated, controlled trials with several different beta blockers have shown that these drugs can reduce symptoms and improve left ventricular function and functional capacity.[91]

Anticoagulation is controversial. The incidence of systemic thromboembolism is about 2% per year. A prospective study has not been performed to document efficacy of anticoagulation in preventing these events in the setting of IDC. Trials in patients with low ejection fractions after MI show a decreased number of strokes in patients on Coumadin.[92]

Because medical therapy usually fails, IDC is the leading indication for heart transplantation in both adults and children.

Disposition Patients with impaired oxygenation, circulation, or problems with their cardiac or renal status should be admitted to the hospital. There is a growing body of evidence that protocol-driven care in an ED observation unit can be equally effective as or beneficial to hospital admission.[93]

Outcome Patients with IDC show progressive deterioration, with 75% of patients dying within 5 years of diagnosis.

The clinical course for children is variable, with a 1-year mortality rate of 21% and a 5-year mortality of 36%.[94] There is a better prognosis in young children, with most deaths occurring within the first 2 years. Some children show late, spontaneous, and unexplained improvement.

Hypertrophic Cardiomyopathy

Perspective Although this condition has been known as idiopathic hypertrophic subaortic stenosis (IHSS), obstructive cardiomyopathy, or hypertrophic obstructive cardiomyopathy (HOCM), the currently accepted name is *hypertrophic cardiomyopathy (HCM).*

The prevalence of HCM is estimated to be 0.1% to 0.2% of the general population. This is probably an underestimate because many patients are asymptomatic.[95] HCM may be somewhat more common in men than women and in African-Americans than Caucasians, but this is disputed.

Principles of Disease

Anatomy HCM is a disease involving abnormalities of heart muscle at anatomic, cellular, and genetic levels. The defining anatomic feature of HCM is a hypertrophied, nondilated LV in the absence of another cause of LV hypertrophy. The thickening is usually asymmetric, involving the septum to a greater extent than the free ventricular wall. The extent of hypertrophy at any given site can vary greatly and bears importantly on the manifestation of the disease.[96]

The dimensions of both the LV and RV cavities are small or normal. Atrial dilation is another universal feature. The mitral valve is thickened in 95% of cases. An endocardial plaque, or area of fibrous thickening on the endocardial surface of the LV outflow tract, occurs in 75% of cases.[97] Ventricular aneurysm formation also occurs. There is an associated resting pressure gradient across the LV outflow tract in only 25% of cases.

Histologically, individual muscle cells are hypertrophied, showing a disorganized, characteristic whorled pattern. Sarcomere disarray is the histologic hallmark of HCM. In addition, abnormal fibrous tissue is often found in the LV. The scarring mimics a healed MI. This abnormality may be visible as a perfusion defect on thallium scan.[97]

A few patients with HCM progress to a late, "burned-out" phase characterized by ventricular wall thinning, cavity dilation, and poor contractility resembling IDC. This phase is usually associated with severe congestive symptoms.[98]

Pathophysiology HCM is caused by mutations in genes that encode for sarcomere contractile proteins.[95] More than 100 different mutations have been identified.[99] These mutations have been shown at the muscle fiber level to cause differences in force stiffness ratio, maximum shortening velocity, and power.[95]

Mutations of the beta-myosin heavy chain (BMHC) gene appear to be the most significant. At least 36 BMHC mutations have been shown to be responsible for HCM. BMHC is a contractile protein with enzyme activity responsible for hydrolyzing ATP. It makes up approximately 30% of the myocardial protein.[100]

Cardiac troponin-T comprises approximately 5% of the total myofibrillar protein and is involved in regulation of calcium. A decreased quantity of stable cardiac troponin-T alters the stoichiometry of the sarcomere.[100] Alpha-tropomyosin protein comprises 5% of the total myofibrillar protein. It bridges the binding of troponin protein complex to thin actin filament. Mutations for both these proteins have been discovered in patients with HCM. Also, familial HCM with Wolff-Parkinson-White (WPW) syndrome maps to a locus on chromosome 7q3.[96]

In addition, genetic studies of families with HCM identify specific mutations that correlate with sudden cardiac death, intermediate risk for sudden cardiac death, and near normal life expectancy.[100] For example, the Arg403Gln mutation appears to be associated with markedly reduced survival. In families with this mutation, less than half of affected family members survive past 45 years of age.[101]

Genetics alone does not account for HCM. Even within the same family, the phenotypic expression among affected individuals sharing the same mutation varies markedly, indicating a role for environmental factors and possibly other factors.[100]

Individuals with the same HCM genotype have a broad spectrum of echocardiographic findings. The presence and extent of hypertrophy on echocardiogram reflect clinical severity.[100]

The hypertrophy in HCM may be a compensatory response to the cardiac protein abnormalities.[96] In vitro studies show that mutant BMHC protein exhibits impaired contractility and disrupts formation of the normal sarcomere. This leads to increased stress for the nonaffected contractile fibers. The heart's usual response to physiologic stress is hypertrophy, dilation, or a combination of both.[100] The theory is that a gene mutation leads to mutant protein that leads to impaired cellular structure and function. This causes compensatory tissue hypertrophy that is manifest clinically as the disease known as HCM.

Clinical Features HCM occurs in all ages. The average age at diagnosis is between 30 and 40 years. Approximately 2% of cases are diagnosed in children under 5 years of age and 7% before 10 years of age.

The presentation of HCM varies widely. There usually are no presenting symptoms, although it may be discovered through screening relatives of patients who have HCM.

In many patients, the initial sign is sudden death, which usually occurs during exertion. Ninety percent of patients have shortness of breath. Other symptoms in decreasing order of frequency include chest pain, syncope, near-syncope, and palpitations. The severity of symptoms correlates roughly with the degree of hypertrophy and is independent of a systolic gradient.[98]

Physical examination reveals a loud S_4 gallop and a harsh crescendo-decrescendo midsystolic murmur. This murmur is made louder by Valsalva's maneuvers or by standing. It becomes quieter when the patient lies down, squats, or does isometric exercises, such as those using hand grips. The changes in the murmur reflect LV end-diastolic volume.

Other physical findings may include a bifid arterial pulse, a double systolic or triple apex beat, reversed splitting of the second heart sound, and, rarely, a mitral leaflet septal contact sound.[96]

Many dysrhythmias are seen in HCM, including premature atrial and ventricular contractions, multifocal ventricular ectopy, and ventricular and supraventricular tachydysrhythmias.

In the ED, the diagnosis should be suspected in anyone with a family history, characteristic murmur, and cardiopulmonary symptoms (i.e., chest pain, dyspnea, dysrhythmia) not explained by other life-threatening conditions. HCM should be suspected whenever a patient complains of ischemic chest pain but has normal coronary arteries at cardiac catheterization.

Diagnostic Strategies Patients with suspected HCM should have an ECG, chest radiograph, and echocardiogram. The ECG is abnormal in approximately 90% of patients and shows a variety of patterns. The most common abnormalities are LV hypertrophy, ST-segment alterations, T-wave inversion, left atrial enlargement, abnormal Q waves, and diminished or absent R waves in the lateral leads. Chest radiographs may be normal or show LV or either atrial enlargement.[102]

Echocardiography is the most important diagnostic strategy. Findings include LVH, LV outflow tract narrowing, a small LV cavity, or reduced septal motion.[96] It is the dynamic characteristic of HCM that distinguishes it from the discrete forms of obstruction to ventricular flow. Doppler techniques are helpful in assessing the severity of this obstruction at rest and with provocative maneuvers.[8]

Nuclear studies can be used to assess both systolic and diastolic ventricular function. Electrophysiologic studies may be helpful to determine dysrhythmias. Genetic screening may be helpful to predict other family members at risk.[96]

Differential Diagnosis HCM mimics many disorders. In individuals who have a gradient and a loud systolic murmur, HCM may be confused with aortic stenosis, pulmonic stenosis, ventricular septal defect, or mitral regurgitation. In the absence of a murmur, symptoms may suggest mitral valve prolapse, left atrial myxoma, primary pulmonary hypertension, or coronary artery disease. ECG changes, such as severe LVH, deeply inverted T waves, or Q waves in the inferior and chest leads without a history of preceding MI, should suggest HCM as well, although coronary artery disease and HCM coexist in 10% to 15% of cases. Echocardiography may be helpful, but ultimately cardiac catheterization may be necessary to confirm the diagnosis.

Management Beta blockers are the mainstay of therapy. The beneficial effects on symptoms (primarily dyspnea and chest pain) and exercise tolerance appear to be due largely to a decrease in the heart rate with a consequent prolongation of diastole and increased passive ventricular filling. Beta blockers may also reduce inotropic response and lessen myocardial oxygen demand.[101] Beta-blocker therapy should be used to slow the heart rate to 60 to 65 beats per minute.[96]

Calcium channel blockers, particularly verapamil, are also useful. Verapamil reduces obstruction in patients with a gradient by decreasing contractility and improving diastolic relaxation and filling. It improves exercise capacity in individuals both with and without obstruction, and its negative effects on heart rate and blood pressure decrease oxygen consumption and the incidence of angina. Verapamil is contraindicated when conduction blocks are present but should be considered when there is no response to beta blockers.

Nitrates, the traditional initial ED management for chest pain, are not indicated in HCM-associated chest pain because they decrease ventricular volume and outflow-tract dimensions.

Amiodarone is the drug of choice for treatment of ventricular dysrhythmias in HCM and is also used when treatment with beta blockers or calcium blockers fails. Automatic implantable defibrillators are also effective. Pharmacologic agents such as amiodarone or sotalol may be tried for atrial fibrillation.[96]

Because 5% of patients with HCM develop subacute bacterial endocarditis, patients with HCM should receive antibiotic prophylaxis before undergoing diagnostic or therapeutic procedures. Dual-chamber pacing has been advocated to decrease outflow gradient and improve symptoms, but this is controversial.[101]

Surgical treatment is reserved for patients with very large (>50 mm Hg) systolic gradients, severe symptoms, and poor quality of life who do not respond to drug therapy. The most common procedure is septal myomectomy, in which a portion of the basal septum is resected via an aortic incision. Success rates as high as 95% are reported, with improvement in symptoms and quality of life despite the lack of any effect on diastolic dysfunction or the other components of HCM.[98]

Disposition The natural history of HCM is variable and probably reflects the many different genetic etiologies. The annual mortality rate of HCM is 1%.[96] The annual incidence of sudden cardiac death is higher in young patients with HCM (6%) than in the elderly (1%).[100] The risk of cardiac death is 0.7% per year.[103]

The onset of atrial fibrillation in a patient with HCM is a medical emergency. It often precipitates marked hemodynamic compromise and severe CHF. Immediate systemic heparinization and cardioversion to restore sinus rhythm are indicated; anticoagulation should be continued in patients with HCM once atrial fibrillation is identified, regardless of whether it responds to attempts at cardioversion. Rate control and anticoagulation to prevent thromboembolism are the hallmarks of therapy for chronic atrial fibrillation. Embolic phenomena can also occur in HCM from bacterial endocarditis, which most commonly affects the mitral valve.[101]

The best predictor of outcome may be the genetic defect. At present, clinical risk factors for sudden death are young age, syncope, malignant family history, myocardial ischemia (particularly in the young), outflow obstruction, sustained ventricular tachycardia on electrophysiologic testing, and ventricular tachycardia on ambulatory monitoring.[96] Syncope is an ominous sign in children. Symptomatic patients should have 48-hour ambulatory Holter monitoring, exercise thallium scintigraphy, and a combined cardiac catheterization and electrophysiologic study.[95]

Sudden death usually occurs with exercise. Patients with HCM who do not have the above risk factors may engage in low-intensity sports. Patients with HCM initially diagnosed in the ED should have strenuous physical activity specifically proscribed until cleared by their cardiologist.

In the ED, patients with HCM who have angina, syncope, near syncope, dysrhythmias, and abrupt changes in their cardiopulmonary status should be hospitalized.

Restrictive Cardiomyopathy

Perspective The hallmark of restrictive (obliterative) cardiomyopathy is a gradual and progressive limitation of ventricular filling secondary to endocardial or myocardial lesions. Restrictive cardiomyopathy is the least common type of cardiomyopathy in developed countries where the most common etiology is amyloidosis. Other etiologies include sarcoidosis, hemochromatosis, scleroderma, neoplastic cardiac infiltration, radiation heart disease, glycogen storage disorders, Fabry's disease, and Gaucher's disease.

The most common cause of restrictive cardiomyopathy worldwide is tropical endomyocardial fibrosis (EMF). EMF is endemic to India, Africa, and Latin America. Symptoms include an initial viral-like illness followed by persistent fever, malaise, and the development of severe right-sided heart failure. Both infectious and immunologic causes are proposed.

Principles of Disease Restriction of ventricular filling results in low end-diastolic ventricular volumes, high end-diastolic ventricular pressures, and decreased cardiac output. Systolic function is maintained. Grossly, there is atrial enlargement with nondilated ventricles. As the disease progresses, the ventricular cavities may become obliterated by fibrous tissue, scarring, or thrombus.

Clinical Features Symptoms include exercise intolerance (cardiac output cannot be increased because ventricular filling is compromised), elevated central venous pressure (CVP), peripheral edema, and S_3 and S_4 gallops on auscultation.

Diagnostic Strategies Differentiation from constrictive pericarditis requires CT, MRI, or Doppler echocardiography. On occasion, pericardial calcification can be seen on chest radiographs. This would favor a diagnosis of constrictive pericarditis over the diagnosis of restrictive cardiomyopathy.

Echocardiography shows a thickened LV and no change in the LV isovolumic relaxation time with respirations, as occurs with restrictive pericarditis. Atrial dimensions are often increased, which is rarely true in constrictive pericarditis.[104]

Biopsy is the gold standard for making the diagnosis and can rule out treatable causes. Because some genetically transmitted diseases cause restrictive cardiomyopathy, genetic counseling may be helpful.[104]

Management and Disposition With few exceptions (e.g., hemochromatosis), there is no specific treatment for restrictive cardiomyopathy. Treatment is symptomatic. Patients presenting to the ED with a suspected diagnosis of restrictive cardiomyopathy should be admitted for confirmatory testing, including possible endocardial biopsy. Close management is important because restrictive cardiomyopathy has a relentless progression, with 90% of patients dying within 10 years of diagnosis.

Peripartum Cardiomyopathy

Perspective Peripartum cardiomyopathy (PPCM) is uncommon. It represents less than 1% of the cardiovascular problems associated with pregnancy.

PPCM is a form of dilated cardiomyopathy, with symptoms and signs of heart failure as a result of LV systolic dysfunction that becomes manifest for the first time in the peripartum period. PPCM usually occurs during the last 3 months of pregnancy or the first 6 months postpartum.

Etiology The etiology of PPCM is unknown. One theory is that PPCM is the result of a pregnancy cardiovascular stressor, such as preeclampsia or Cesarean section, superimposed on an underlying (and probably not-yet diagnosed) cardiovascular disorder. Other proposed etiologies include myocarditis, nutrition, viral agents, or immunologic factors.[105]

Epidemiology The incidence is approximately 28 cases of PPCM per 100,000 pregnancies and is greater in women who are multiparous, have twin pregnancies, are over 30 years old, or are African-American.

Clinical Features and Diagnostic Strategies Patients usually have symptoms of CHF, chest pain, palpitations, and occasionally thromboembolism. Physical examination often reveals tachycardia, tachypnea, pulmonary rales, an enlarged heart, and an S_3 heart sound.[105]

The ECG may show LVH and nonspecific ST-T changes. On echocardiography, all four chambers are enlarged, with marked reduction in LV systolic function. A small to moderate pericardial effusion may be found. The hemodynamic changes are indistinguishable from those of other forms of dilated cardiomyopathy. Endomyocardial biopsy should be considered to exclude myocarditis.

Management and Disposition Treatment of PPCM includes limitation of physical activity, alteration of preload with diuretics, increase in ventricular contractility using agents such as digitalis, and most important, afterload reduction.[105] Hydralazine is an effective and safe afterload reducing agent during pregnancy. Angiotensin-converting enzyme inhibitors may be used in the postpartum period. Because the risk of associated thromboembolic phenomenon is very high, anticoagulation prophylaxis should be used.

As many as a third of patients with PPCM may die. Of survivors, half show complete or near-complete recovery of cardiac function within the first 6 months. Patients who do not recover completely show either continuous clinical deterioration or persistent LV dysfunction. Subsequent pregnancies are often associated with relapses and a high risk of maternal mortality.

In the ED, patients with signs of hemodynamic instability or failure to maintain oxygenation should be admitted. Because testing of fetal oxygenation is difficult, observation with fetal monitoring should be used routinely.

Specific Heart Muscle Diseases

Amyloidosis Disorders of amyloid deposition are divided into two categories: primary (associated with a high incidence of cardiac involvement) and amyloidosis secondary to multiple myeloma, RA, tuberculosis, or lymphoma, in which the heart is involved in approximately 50% of cases.

Cardiac amyloidosis is a disease of the immune system in which cells of the reticuloendothelial system are stimulated to deposit amorphous material in the ventricle, coronary arteries, or valves. Massive amyloid deposition results in an increased cardiac weight and the diastolic dysfunction of restrictive cardiomyopathy.

CHF occurs in 85% of cases of cardiac amyloidosis, as do mitral or tricuspid regurgitation. Hypotension and a narrow pulse pressure may also be present; cardiac amyloidosis is one of the few causes of spontaneous reversal of arterial hypertension. Involvement of the conduction system produces AV or intraventricular blocks, axis deviation, and various dysrhythmias. Sudden death is common.

The chest radiograph reveals either a normal heart size or atrial dilation, with evidence of pulmonary vascular congestion. The ECG is always abnormal in later stages of cardiac amyloidosis. Echocardiography shows unexpectedly normal chamber dimensions, with poor wall movement. Biopsy of the endomyocardium, tongue, or mucous membranes should be diagnostic.[106]

Standard CHF and antidysrhythmic therapy is indicated, although the dysrhythmias in amyloid heart disease are often refractory to treatment. The presence of high-grade AV block may require pacemaker insertion. The prognosis is poor, with death often resulting from progressive heart failure within 1 year of symptom onset.[106]

Sarcoidosis Cardiac granulomas are reported in approximately 25% of cases of systemic sarcoidosis at autopsy, usually involving small microscopic areas of myocardium. Granulomas are preferentially located in the basilar septum (where they cause severe conduction defects, especially complete heart block), in the papillary muscles (causing mitral regurgitation), and in the ventricular walls (producing scarring and wall motion abnormalities). Cardiac involvement is clinically unrecognized in one third of these cases, while in the remaining two thirds it is manifested as dysrhythmias, conduction defects, or CHF.

Symptoms of cardiac sarcoidosis include dyspnea, palpitations, atypical chest pain, or Stokes-Adams attacks. Signs of systemic sarcoidosis accompanied by CHF, a mitral regurgitation murmur, or an abnormal ECG with dysrhythmias or AV block should suggest cardiac involvement. Q waves resembling those from healed MI may appear after steroid treatment. Complete heart block is the most common conduction block and is associated with a high risk of sudden death. Ventricular dysrhythmias also predispose to sudden death and are often refractory to therapy.

Myocardial involvement in sarcoidosis is an indication for systemic corticosteroid therapy. Steroids heal granulomas by a process that may produce scarring and ventricular aneurysms. Steroid therapy may resolve AV block and dysrhythmias. Antidysrhythmic therapy may also be needed. Refractory cardiac failure or dysrhythmias are indications for heart transplantation.[107]

Connective Tissue Disorders and Disease of the Myocardium Myocarditis associated with various connective tissue diseases occurs more often than is recognized clinically. Cardiac abnormalities occur in RA, juvenile RA (Still's disease), MCTD, and primary Sjögren's syndrome.

Systemic Lupus Erythematosus SLE is the connective tissue disease most commonly associated with cardiac abnormalities. Cardiac involvement in SLE includes pericarditis, endocarditis, and myocarditis. Postmortem examination demonstrates pericarditis in approximately 80% of cases, with approximately 50% of patients having had symptoms at some time during their disease.[49]

Scleroderma Primary myocardial involvement is a major complication of diffuse scleroderma and develops as scleroderma worsens. Estimates of the frequency of myocardial involvement in scleroderma vary widely. Presentation includes CHF, angina, and dysrhythmias. Pericardial disease can also occur. Azathioprine may be a beneficial adjunct to steroid therapy.[108]

Sudden Death Sudden death in patients less than 21 years of age can be attributed to disease of the myocardium approximately 25% of the time. Cardiac etiologies include myocarditis, HCM, and anomalous coronary artery circulation. In patients with sudden death attributed to cardiac etiologies, prodromal symptoms are reported in over half of the patients, most commonly chest pain (25%) in patients over 20 years of age and dizziness (16%) in those less than 20 years of age.[109]

The distribution of sudden death etiologies by age is as follows:

- Age less than 20 years: myocarditis 22% and HCM 22%
- Age 20 to 29 years: myocarditis 22% and HCM 13%
- Age 30 to 39 years: myocarditis 11% and HCM 2%

Coronary artery disease becomes the leading cardiac etiology (58%) in sudden death in those ages 30 to 39 years.[109] HCM is the cardiac disease most commonly found

Box 77-2 Specific Heart Muscle Diseases

Nutritional

Beriberi (vitamin B_1 deficiency), pellagra (vitamin B_6 deficiency), scurvy (vitamin C deficiency), hypervitaminosis D, kwashiorkor

Metabolic

Amyloidosis, glycogen storage disease type II (Pompe disease), McArdle's syndrome, carnitine deficiency, hemochromatosis, acquired hemosiderosis, Fabry's disease, Tay-Sachs disease, Sandhoff's disease, GM1, gangliosidosis, Niemann-Pick disease, Gaucher's disease, cardiac lipidosis, porphyria, Hurler's syndrome, other mucopolysaccharidoses, type II hyperlipoproteinemia (familial xanthomatosis), Hand-Schüller-Christian disease, gout, oxalosis, alkaptonuria, uremia

Hematologic

Leukemia, myeloma, sickle cell disease, sickle cell trait, thrombotic thrombocytopenic purpura, hereditary hemorrhagic telangiectasia, Henoch-Schönlein purpura

Neuromuscular

Duchenne muscular dystrophy, Erb (limb-girdle) muscular dystrophy, facioscapulohumeral muscular dystrophy, Friedreich's ataxia, myotonic dystrophy, myasthenia gravis, tuberous sclerosis

Toxic/hypersensitivity

Ethanol, cobalt (beer-drinker's cardiomyopathy) emetine, chloroquine, phenothiazines, lithium, tricyclic antidepressants, methysergide, cyclophosphamide, daunorubicin, Adriamycin (doxorubicin), heavy metals (arsenic, antimony fluoride, mercury, lead), phosphorus, carbon monoxide, catecholamines, dextroamphetamine, phenylpropanolamine, venoms (scorpion, black widow, snake, wasp), tick paralysis

Physical

Radiation, hypothermia, electric shock, trauma, heat stroke

Miscellaneous

Sarcoidosis, rheumatoid arthritis, Reiter syndrome, Behçet's syndrome, transplant rejection, Noonan's syndrome, Wegener's granulomatosis, Reye's syndrome, mulibrey nanism, inflammatory bowel disease, acquired immunodeficiency syndrome

Modified from Wenger NK, Ablemann WH, Robert WC: Cardiomyopathy and specific heart muscle disease. In Hurst JW, Schlant RC: *The heart,* ed 7, New York, 1990, McGraw-Hill.

on postmortem diagnosis of athletes with sudden death. HCM and anomalous coronary arteries are more often seen in sports-related deaths than in deaths not related to sports.

Other Specific Heart Muscle Diseases Box 77-2 lists the numerous other conditions associated with myocardial dysfunction.

KEY CONCEPTS

- Pericarditis must be differentiated from AMI. Thrombolytic therapy is contraindicated in pericarditis because of the potential for hemorrhagic pericarditis or tamponade.
- Cardiac tamponade must be suspected (distended neck veins, hypotension, and muffled heart sounds), diagnosed (echocardiography), and treated (pericardiocentesis) quickly. If echocardiography is not readily available and the patient is unstable, pericardiocentesis may be both diagnostic and therapeutic.
- Purulent pericarditis should be suspected when multiorgan system failure, a pericardial effusion, and fever are present.
- Dilated cardiomyopathy is common. Symptoms, signs, and treatment are the same as those of CHF.
- Myocarditis should be considered in any patient with the combination of viral illness symptoms and signs of cardiac disease.
- Hypertrophic cardiomyopathy is a genetic-based disease with anatomic manifestations. It frequently presents as sudden death, especially during exercise in young, seemingly healthy individuals.

REFERENCES

1. Spodick DH: Medical history of the pericardium, *Am J Cardiol* 26:447, 1970.
2. Beck CS: Two cardiac compression triads, *JAMA* 104:714, 1935.
3. Zayas R et al: Incidence of specific etiology and role of methods for specific etiologic diagnosis of primary acute pericarditis, *Am J Cardiol* 75:378, 1995.
4. McKenna RJ Jr et al: Pleural and pericardial effusions in cancer patients, *Curr Probl Cancer* 9:1, 1985.
5. Boltwood CM Jr, Shah PM: The pericardium in health and disease, *Curr Probl Cardiol* 9:1, 1984.
6. Chan T, Brady WJ, Pollack M: Electrocardiographic manifestations: acute myopericarditis. *J Emerg Med* 17:864, 1999.
7. Spodick DH: Macrophysiology, microphysiology, and anatomy of the pericardium: a synopsis, *Am Heart J* 124:1046, 1992.
8. ACC/AHA guidelines for the clinical application of echocardiography: a report of the American College of Cardiology/American Heart Association Task Force on Assessment of Diagnostic and Therapeutic Cardiovascular Procedures, *J Am Coll Cardiol* 16:1505, 1990.
9. Melchior TM et al: Recurrent acute idiopathic pericarditis treated with intravenous methylprednisolone given as pulse therapy, *Am J Heart* 123:1086, 1992.
10. Mast HL et al: Pericardial effusion and its relationship to cardiac disease in children with acquired immunodeficiency syndrome, *Pediatr Radiol* 22:548, 1992.
11. Galve E et al: Self limited acute pericarditis as initial manifestation of primary cardiac tumor, *Am Heart J* 123:1690, 1992.
12. Smith SH: Uremic pericarditis in chronic renal failure: nursing implications, *ANNA J* 20:432, 1993.
13. Correale E et al: Pericardial involvement in acute myocardial infarction in the post-thrombolytic era: clinical meaning and value, *Clin Cardiol* 20:327, 1997.
14. Dressler W: A post-myocardial infarction syndrome, *JAMA* 160:1379, 1956.
15. Kahn AH: The postcardiac injury syndromes, *Clin Cardiol* 15:67, 1992.
16. Bellanger D et al: Delayed posttraumatic tamponade, *South Med J* 89:1197, 1996.
17. Ledford DK: Immunologic aspects of cardiovascular disease, *JAMA* 268:2923, 1992.
18. Wolfenden H, Newman DC: Constrictive pericarditis associated with trauma and pectus excavatum, *Aust N Z J Surg* 62:750, 1992.
19. Van Vooren JP, Thys JP, Vanderhoeft P: Purulent pericarditis resulting from blunt chest trauma, *J Thorac Cardiovasc Surg* 100:932, 1990.
20. Wilkes JD et al: Malignancy-related pericardial effusion: 127 cases from the Roswell Park Cancer Institute, *Cancer* 76:1377, 1995.
21. Lionarons RJ, van Baarlen J, Hitchcock JR: Constrictive pericarditis caused by primary liposarcoma, *Thorax* 45:566, 1990.
22. Galve E et al: Self-limited acute pericarditis as initial manifestation of primary cardiac tumor, *Am Heart J* 123:1690, 1992.

23. Meyers DG, Bouska DJ: Diagnostic usefulness of pericardial fluid cytology, *Chest* 95:1142, 1989.
24. Schultz-Hector S: Radiation-induced heart disease: review of experimental data on dose response and pathogenesis, *Int J Radiat Biol* 61:149, 1992.
25. Hara KS et al: Rheumatoid pericarditis: clinical features and survival, *Medicine* 69:81, 1990.
26. Moder KG, Miller TD, Tazelaar HD: Cardiac involvement in systemic lupus erythematosus, *Mayo Clin Proc* 74:275, 1999.
27. Rantapaa-Dahlqvist S et al: Echocardiographic findings in patients with primary Sjögren's syndrome, *Clin Rheumatol* 12:214, 1993.
28. Guillaume M, Vachiery F, Cogan E: Pericarditis: an unusual manifestation of giant cell arteritis, *Am J Med* 91:662, 1991.
29. Beier JM, Nielsen HL, Nielsen D: Pleuritis-pericarditis: an unusual initial manifestation of mixed connective tissue disease, *Eur Heart J* 13:859, 1992.
30. Spodick DH: Pathophysiology of cardiac tamponade, *Chest* 113:1372, 1998.
31. Park S, Bayer AS: Purulent pericarditis, *Curr Clin Top Infect Dis* 12:56, 1992.
32. Kraus WE, Valenstein PN, Corey GR: Purulent pericarditis caused by candida: report of three cases and identification of high risk populations as an aid to early diagnosis, *Rev Infect Dis* 10:35, 1988.
33. Thavendrarajah V et al: Catheter lavage and drainage of pneumococcal pericarditis, *Cathet Cardiovasc Diagn* 29:322, 1993.
34. Defouilloy C et al: Intrapericardial fibrinolysis: a useful treatment in the management of purulent pericarditis, *Intensive Care Medicine* 23:117, 1997.
35. Fowler NO: Tuberculous pericarditis, *JAMA* 266:99, 1991.
36. Abid MA, Gitlin N: Pericarditis: an extraintestinal complication of inflammatory bowel disease, *West J Med* 153:314, 1990.
37. Acierno LJ: Cardiac complications in acquired immunodeficiency syndrome (AIDS): a review, *J Am Coll Cardiol* 13:1144, 1989.
38. Silva-Cardoso J et al: Pericardial involvement in human immunodeficiency virus infection, *Chest* 115:418, 1999.
39. Chen Y et al: Human immunodeficiency virus–associated pericardial effusion: report of 40 cases and review of the literature, *Am Heart J* 137:516, 1999.
40. Bakri YN et al: Pregnancy complicating irradiation-induced constrictive pericarditis, *Acta Obstet Gynecol Scand* 71:143, 1992.
41. Ivey MJ, Gross BH: Back pain and fever in an elderly patient, *Chest* 103:1851, 1993.
42. Katzir D et al: Spontaneous pneumopericardium: case report and review of the literature, *Cardiology* 76:305, 1989.
43. Demetriades D et al: Pneumopericardium following penetrating chest injuries, *Arch Surg* 125:1187, 1990.
44. Osterberg L, Vagelos R, Atwood JE: Case presentation and review: constrictive pericarditis, *West J Med* 169:232, 1998.
45. Astudillo R, Ivert T: Late results after pericardiectomy for constrictive pericarditis via left thoracotomy, *Scand J Thorac Cardiovasc Surg* 23:115, 1989.
46. Lieberman EB, Hutchins GM, Herskowitz A: Clinicopathologic description of myocarditis, *J Am Coll Cardiol* 18:1617, 1991.
47. See DM, Tilles JG: Viral myocarditis, *Rev Infect Dis* 13:951, 1991.
48. Liu P et al: Viral myocarditis: balance between viral infection and immune response, *Can J Cardiol* 12:935, 1996.
49. Olinde KD, O'Connell JB: Inflammatory heart disease: pathogenesis, clinical manifestations, and treatment of myocarditis, *Annu Rev Med* 45:481, 1994.
50. Sole MJ, Liu P: Viral myocarditis: a paradigm for understanding the pathogenesis and treatment of dilated cardiomyopathy, *J Am Coll Cardiol* 22:99A, 1993.
51. Caforio A et al: Circulating cardiac-specific autoantibodies as markers of autoimmunity in clinical and biopsy-proven myocarditis, *Eur Heart J* 18:270, 1997.
52. Lieberman EB et al: A clinicopathologic description of myocarditis, *Clin Immunol Immunopathol* 68:191, 1993.
53. Singer JI, Isaacman DJ, Bell LM: The wheezer that wasn't, *Pediatr Emerg Care* 8:107, 1992.
54. Wiles HB et al: Cardiomyopathy and myocarditis in children with ventricular ectopic rhythm, *J Am Coll Cardiol* 20:359, 1992.
55. Narula J et al: Brief report: recognition of acute myocarditis masquerading as acute myocardial infarction, *N Engl J Med* 328:100, 1993.
56. Matsuura H et al: Intraventricular conduction abnormalities in patients with clinically suspected myocarditis are associated with myocardial necrosis, *Am Heart J* 127:1290, 1994.
57. Lambert K, Isaac D, Hendel R: Myocarditis masquerading as ischemic heart disease: the diagnostic utility of antimyosin imaging, *Cardiology* 82:415, 1993.
58. Why HJ et al: Clinical and prognostic significance of detection of enteroviral RNA in the myocardium of patients with myocarditis of dilated cardiomyopathy, *Circulation* 89:2582, 1994.
59. Dec GW et al: Viral myocarditis mimicking acute myocardial infarction, *J Am Coll Cardiol* 20:85, 1992.
60. Kandolf R et al: Molecular studies on enteroviral heart disease: patterns of acute and persistent infections, *Eur Heart J* 12:49, 1991.
61. Rose NR, Neumann DA, Herskowitz A: Autoimmune myocarditis: concepts and questions, *Immunol Today* 12:253, 1991.
62. Mason JW et al: A clinical trial of immunosuppressive therapy for myocarditis, *N Engl J Med* 333:269, 1995.
63. Talwar KK, Goswami KC, Chopra P: Immunosuppressive therapy in inflammatory myocarditis: long-term follow-up, *Int J Cardiol* 34:157, 1992.
64. Drucker NA et al: Gammaglobulin treatment of acute myocarditis in the pediatric population, *Circulation* 89:252, 1994.
65. Morishima I et al: A case of fulminant myocarditis rescued by long-term percutaneous cardiopulmonary support, *Jpn Circ J* 58:433, 1994.
66. Mendes LA et al: Right ventricular dysfunction: an independent predictor of adverse outcome in patients with myocarditis, *Am Heart J* 128:301, 1994.
67. Brown CA, O'Connell JB: Myocarditis and idiopathic dilated cardiomyopathy, *Am J Med* 99:309, 1999.
68. Mengel JO, Rossi MA: Chronic chagasic myocarditis pathogenesis: dependence on autoimmune and microvascular factors, *Am Heart J* 124:1052, 1992.
69. Case records of the Massachusetts General Hospital: weekly clinicopathological exercises. Case 32-1993. A native of El Salvador with tachycardia and syncope, *N Engl J Med* 329:488, 1993.
70. Compton SJ et al: Trichinosis with ventilatory failure and persistent myocarditis, *Clin Infect Dis* 16:500, 1993.
71. Nagi K, Joshi R, Thakur R: Cardiac manifestations of Lyme disease: a review, *Can J Cardiol* 12:503, 1996.
72. Currie PF, Boon NA: Cardiac involvement in human immunodeficiency virus infection, *QJM* 86:751, 1993.
73. DeCastro S et al: Heart involvement in AIDS: a prospective study during various stages of the disease, *Eur Heart J* 13:1452, 1992.
74. Hofman P et al: Prevalence of toxoplasma myocarditis in patients with the acquired immunodeficiency syndrome, *Br Heart J* 70:376, 1993.
75. Israelski DM, Remington JS: Toxoplasmosis in the non-AIDS immunocompromised host, *Curr Clin Top Infect Dis* 13:322, 1993.
76. Agarwala BN, Ruschhaupt DG: Complete heart block from *Mycoplasma pneumoniae* infection, *Pediatr Cardiol* 12:233, 1991.
77. Chan AC, Dickens P: Tuberculous myocarditis presenting as sudden cardiac death, *Forensic Sci Int* 57:45, 1992.
78. Wesslen L et al: Myocarditis caused by *Chlamydia pneumoniae* (TWAR) and sudden unexpected death in a Swedish elite orienteer (letter), *Lancet* 340:427, 1992.
79. Tami LF, Bhasin S: Polymorphism of the cardiac manifestations in dermatomyositis, *Clin Cardiol* 16:260, 1993.
80. Gaudin PB et al: Myocarditis associated with doxorubicin cardiotoxicity, *Am J Clin Pathol* 100:158, 1993.
81. Price FW, Leaky AB: Grave and prolonged cardiac failure following the use of cocaine in dental surgery, *Lancet* 1:797, 1911.
82. Cregler LL: Cocaine: the newest risk factor for cardiovascular disease, *Clin Cardiol* 14:449, 1991.
83. Virmane R et al: Cardiovascular effects of cocaine: an autopsy study of 40 patients, *Am Heart J* 115:1068, 1988.
84. Rowley AH, Shulamn ST: Kawasaki's syndrome, *Pediatr Clin North Am* 46:313, 1999.
85. Barron KS et al: Report of the National Institute of Health Workshop on Kawasaki Disease, *J Rheumatol* 26:170, 1999.

86. Edwards WD: Cardiomyopathies, *Hum Pathol* 18:625, 1987.
87. Dec GW, Fuster V: Idiopathic dilated cardiomyopathy, *N Engl J Med* 331:1564, 1994.
88. Kasper EK et al: The causes of dilated cardiomyopathy: a clinicopathologic review of 673 consecutive patients, *J Am Coll Cardiol* 16:260, 1994.
89. Garg R et al: The Digitalis Investigation Group: The effect of digoxin on mortality and morbidity in patients with heart failure, *N Engl J Med* 336:525, 1997.
90. Packer M et al: Effect of amlodipine on morbidity and mortality in severe chronic heart failure, *N Engl J Med* 335:1107, 1996.
91. Packer M, Bristow M, Cohn J: The effect of carvedilol on morbidity and mortality in patients with chronic heart failure, *N Engl J Med* 334:1349, 1996.
92. Borrowman T, Love R, Mason JW: Dilated cardiomyopathy: problems in diagnosis and management, *Chest* 115:569, 1999.
93. Peacock WF, Albert NM: Observation unit management of heart failure, *Emerg Clin North Am* 19:209, 2001.
94. Ciszewski A et al: Dilated cardiomyopathy in children: clinical course and prognosis, *Pediatr Cardiol* 15:121, 1994.
95. Fananapazir L: Advances in molecular genetics and management of hypertrophic cardiomyopathy, *JAMA* 281:1746, 1999.
96. Wigle E et al: Hypertrophic cardiomyopathy: clinical spectrum and treatment. *Circulation* 92:1680, 1995.
97. Maron BJ et al: Hypertrophic cardiomyopathy: interrelation of clinical manifestations, pathophysiology, and therapy (part 1), *N Engl J Med* 316:780, 1987.
98. Maron BJ et al: Hypertrophic cardiomyopathy: interrelations of clinical manifestations, pathophysiology, and therapy (part 2), *N Engl J Med* 316:844, 1987.
99. Sangwatanaroj S et al: Mutations in the gene for cardiac myosin-binding protein C and late-onset familial hypertrophic cardiomyopathy, *N Engl J Med* 338:1245, 1998.
100. Roberts M, Roberts R: Recent advances in the molecular genetics of hypertrophic cardiomyopathy, *Circulation* 92:136, 1995.
101. Spirito P et al: The management of hypertrophic cardiomyopathy, *N Engl J Med* 336:775, 1997.
102. Lerakis S, Sheahan R, Stouffer G: Hypertrophic cardiomyopathy: presentation and pathophysiology, *Am J Med Sci* 314:324, 1997.
103. Cannan C et al: Natural history of hypertrophic cardiomyopathy: a population-based study, 1976 through 1990, *Circulation* 92:2488, 1995.
104. Wilmshurst PT, Karitsis D: Restrictive cardiomyopathy, *Br Heart J* 63:323, 1990.
105. Lee W: Clinical management of gravid women with peripartum cardiomyopathy, *Obstet Gynecol Clin North Am* 18:257, 1991.
106. Roberts WC, Waller BF: Cardiac amyloidosis causing cardiac dysfunction: analysis of 54 necropsy patients, *Am J Cardiol* 52:137, 1983.
107. Valantine H et al: Sarcoidosis: a pattern of clinical and morphological presentation, *Br Heart J* 57:256, 1987.
108. Follansbee WP, Zerbe TR, Medsger TA Jr: Cardiac and skeletal muscle disease in systemic sclerosis (scleroderma): a high risk association, *Am Heart J* 125:194, 1993.
109. Drory Y et al: Sudden unexpected death in persons less than 40 years of age, *Am J Cardiol* 68:1388, 1991.

78 Infective Endocarditis and Valvular Heart Disease

Susan M. Dunmire

INFECTIVE ENDOCARDITIS

Perspective

Infective endocarditis was described as early as the late seventeenth century in the medical literature. The term *endocarditis* was introduced by Bouillaud in 1825. In 1846 Ruldolf Virchow described a valvular vegetation and was one of the first physicians to demonstrate bacteria in vegetations. The treatment of infective endocarditis remained supportive until the discovery of the sulfanilamides in 1932 and penicillin and streptomycin in the 1940s.

Infective endocarditis is a challenging diagnosis. Although bacteria remain the most common cause, virtually all organisms (including viruses, fungi, and rickettsiae) cause endocarditis. The traditional classification of infective endocarditis as acute, subacute, and chronic has become less meaningful since the development of antibiotics. Early diagnosis of endocarditis and identification of the causative organism play a significant role in the clinical outcome of this potentially life-threatening disease.

Principles of Disease

Although the average age of patients with infective endocarditis was less than 39 years before the antibiotic era, over the past 3 decades the mean age has increased to 55 years.[1] This is due to an increase in the average age of patients, as well as an increase in the incidence of prosthetic cardiac valves.

Most patients with bacterial endocarditis have one of the following predisposing factors: rheumatic or congenital heart disease, calcific degenerative valve disease, prosthetic heart valve(s), mitral valve prolapse (MVP), a history of intravenous (IV) drug use, or a history of endocarditis. Although the incidence of rheumatic heart disease has decreased, it remains an important predisposing factor for endocarditis, with the mitral valve as the most common site of infection.

Congenital cardiac lesions involving high pressure gradients (e.g., ventricular septal defects, pulmonary stenosis, tetralogy of Fallot) will place a patient at increased risk for infective endocarditis. Calcific or degenerative disease of both the aortic and mitral valves is now recognized (due to increased use of echocardiography) as being an extremely common entity in the elderly patient.

Prosthetic valve endocarditis is a devastating complication of valve replacement. The incidence of endocarditis in prosthetic valve recipients ranges from 0.5% to 4% per year.[2] Mitral valve prolapse is a particularly important and common predisposing factor for infective endocarditis. Clearly the risk is greatest when regurgitant flow is demonstrated by echocardiography or in the presence of a murmur.

IV drug use is a major risk factor for infective endocarditis. Although any valve can be affected, IV drug use is the most common cause of right-sided endocarditis. The recurrence rate of endocarditis in IV drug users is approximately 41%, in contrast to a recurrence rate of less than 20% in other patients.[3,4] Endocarditis is a major risk factor for recurrence because infected valves heal with irregularities that become sites for future vegetations.

Pathophysiology

The classic lesion of endocarditis is the vegetation. It originates as a sterile thrombus on which microorganisms adhere and colonize. The initial thrombus may form at a site of trauma, inflammation, or abnormal turbulence induced by mechanical damage. In IV drug users, contaminants such as talc can injure the previously normal valve leaflets and produce a site for bacterial implantation.

A subclinical bacteremia usually precedes the onset of symptoms of bacterial endocarditis by approximately 1 week. A variety of surgical procedures result in transient bacteremia, including dental procedures, cystoscopy, urethral dilatation, endoscopic retrograde cholangiopancreatography (ERCP), and esophageal dilation.[5,6]

The infective organism responsible depends on the predisposing factor for endocarditis. Streptococci are common pathogens for left-sided endocarditis in patients with congenital valvular disease or MVP. *Streptococcus viridans* remains the most common organism. Less common species include non–group A ß-hemolytic (groups B, C, and G) and members of the *Streptococcus milleri* group. There is an association between *Streptococcus bovis* endocarditis and coexisting gastrointestinal malignancy. Staphylococcus accounts for approximately 10% to 30% of native valve endocarditis; conversely it is the causative agent in over 80% of cases of bacterial endocarditis in patients with a history of IV drug abuse.[7] Coagulase-negative staphylococcus is the most common infecting organism in prosthetic valve endocarditis. *Staphylococcus lugdunensis* is emerging as a virulent coagulase-negative staphylococcus that is implicated in bacterial endocarditis infecting native valves and resulting in rapid valve destruction and paravalvular abscess formation.[8,9]

The HACEK group (*Haemophilus aphrophilus, Actinobacillus, Cardiobacterium hominis, Eikenella corrodens,* and *Kingella kingae*) are fastidious gram-negative bacilli that can cause culture-negative (due to fastidious nature and slow multiplication) endocarditis.[10] These organisms are known to result in large-vessel septic thrombi. The fastidious Bartonella species of bacteria are implicated in endocarditis, particularly at the aortic valve site, and are more common in disadvantaged or homeless individuals.[11]

Candida and Aspergillus species account for most cases of fungal endocarditis. Predisposing factors for fungal endocarditis include patients with long-term indwelling IV catheters; patients who are immunosuppressed because of malignancy, AIDS, or organ transplantation; and IV drug users. The large fungal vegetations often embolize, lodging in arteries. Because these patients usually have negative blood cultures, histologic study of these emboli may be the first clue to the presence of fungal endocarditis.

Clinical Features

Symptoms associated with infective endocarditis are nonspecific and diverse. Many patients present early during the bacteremic phase of the illness, do not have a cardiac murmur, and are indistinguishable from the large population of patients who present to the ED with acute viral illness. It is often only when the symptoms persist, or the illness does not follow a typical course for viremia, that the diagnosis of infective endocarditis can be made. The classic triad of fever, anemia, and a heart murmur should suggest the presence of infective endocarditis. The most common symptoms are intermittent fever (85%) and malaise (95%). Fever is a more common finding in the IV drug user with endocarditis (98%). Other symptoms (e.g., weakness, myalgias, dyspnea, chest pain, cough, headaches, and anorexia) vary widely in their incidence and are nonspecific. Thirty to forty percent of patients have neurologic symptoms or signs such as confusion, personality changes, decreased level of consciousness, or focal motor deficits. These symptoms are most commonly caused by embolization.

Almost all patients with infective endocarditis have a cardiac murmur at some time during the course of their illness. The murmur may be absent in up to 15% of patients at the time of presentation, and in even greater numbers earlier in their course. The most common murmurs are those of aortic, mitral, or tricuspid regurgitation. Conversely, fewer than 35% of IV drug users with endocarditis have a murmur on initial presentation.[12] This is most likely because most endocarditis associated with IV drug use is right sided and, consequently, the murmur is much more difficult to elicit on physical examination.

Over 50% of patients will have some form of vasculitic lesion, including petechiae, splinter hemorrhages, Osler's nodes, and Janeway lesions. Petechiae may be present on either a mucosal surface or the skin. Often the petechiae on mucous membranes or the conjunctivae will have a pale center. These petechiae are nontender and do not blanch with pressure. Splinter hemorrhages may be found under the nails but are nonspecific and can commonly be due to minor trauma to the nail. Osler's nodes are painful, tender, erythematous nodules on the palmar surface of the fingertip. Janeway lesions are nontender, erythematous, flat, macular lesions on the palms and soles that blanch with pressure. Approximately 30% of patients have splenomegaly. Several ocular findings are associated with infective endocarditis, including conjunctival or retinal hemorrhages. Retinal hemorrhages may simply be flame shaped or may have a pale center surrounded by a red halo (Roth's spots).

Diagnostic Strategies

Laboratory findings in bacterial endocarditis are nonspecific. A leukocytosis with polymorphonuclear predominance is only present in approximately 50% of cases, and its absence does not rule out infective endocarditis. An elevated erythrocyte sedimentation rate (ESR) and/or C-reactive protein level may be present. Most patients have a mild anemia, and over 50% have microscopic hematuria as a result of embolic lesions of the kidney. Three or four blood cultures should be obtained on all patients with suspected endocarditis, with the first and last culture being drawn at least 1 hour apart. Patients are then admitted for treatment with IV antibiotics until blood cultures and echocardiogram exclude the diagnosis. An electrocardiogram (ECG) may demonstrate conduction abnormalities if an abscess has formed in the myocardium. Transesophageal echocardiography (TEE) is an essential early diagnostic test in the evaluation of infective

Box 78-1 The Duke Criteria for Diagnosis of Infective Endocarditis

Clinical diagnosis requires the following:
- Two major criteria
- *or*
- One major and three minor criteria
- *or*
- Five minor criteria

Major Criteria

Positive blood cultures (of typical pathogens) from at least two separate cultures

Evidence of endocardial involvement by echocardiography, such as the following:
- Endocardial vegetation
- Paravalvular abscess
- New partial dehiscence of prosthetic valve
- New valvular regurgitation

Minor Criteria

Predisposition: Predisposing heart condition or IV drug use

Fever: Greater than or equal to 38° C

Vascular phenomena: Arterial emboli, septic pulmonary infarcts, mycotic aneurysm, conjunctival hemorrhages, or Janeway lesions

Immunologic phenomena: Osler's nodes, Roth's spots, and rheumatoid factor

Microbiologic evidence: Single positive blood culture (except for coagulase negative staphylococcus, or an organism that does not cause endocarditis

Echocardiographic findings: Consistent with endocarditis, but do not meet major criteria

Box 78-2 Initial Therapy for Bacterial Endocarditis

Vancomycin
- Initial dose for adults: 15 mg/kg
- Initial dose for children: 10 mg/kg
- Subsequent dose for adults: 500 mg q 6 hr
- Subsequent dose for children: 10 mg/kg q 6 hr

Plus

Gentamicin
- Initial dose 1-3 mg/kg (subsequent dose 1 mg/kg q 8 hr)

Or

Ceftriaxone
- Adults: 1-2 g q 12 hr
- Children: 50-75 mg/kg q day

Plus

Gentamicin
- Initial dose 1-3 mg/kg (subsequent dose 1 mg/kg q 8 hr)

Box 78-3 Moderate to High Risk Conditions for Bacterial Endocarditis

Prosthetic heart valve

History of endocarditis

Congenital cardiac malformations, particularly cyanotic lesions (e.g., tetralogy of Fallot, transposition of great vessels)

Rheumatic heart disease

Mitral valve prolapse with regurgitation

Hypertrophic cardiomyopathy

endocarditis. Multiple studies demonstrate its superiority to transthoracic echocardiography (TTE).[13,14] Visualization of a vegetation on a prosthetic valve and prosthetic valve insufficiency is superior via TEE, with a sensitivity and a specificity of around 90%.[15,16] The negative predictive value of TEE for infective endocarditis is 95%.

The Duke criteria stratify patients with suspected bacterial endocarditis into three distinct categories: definite, possible, and rejected (Box 78-1).[17] There are proposed modifications to the Duke criteria that expand the minor criteria to include an elevated C-reactive protein level or ESR, new splenomegaly, splinter hemorrhages, or hematuria.[18] These modifications also propose that a patient must have either one major criterion or three minor criteria to qualify for the "possible" category. The specificity and sensitivity of the Duke criteria are validated by many studies and are estimated to be approximately 99% and 95%, respectively.[19-22]

Management

Appropriate antibiotics must be selected before the causative organism is known or before the diagnosis is proven. Box 78-2 provides guidelines for empiric therapy. In most cases, if the patient does not appear acutely ill and vital signs are stable, it is helpful to obtain all necessary blood cultures before starting antibiotics. Patients who are IV drug users or have a prosthetic heart valve and are febrile should be admitted for evaluation of bacteremia and the possibility of endocarditis.[23] An exception would be a transient fever in the IV drug user that resolves spontaneously in the ED and is thought to be a result of an injected contaminant.

Acute valve replacement is rarely necessary during the active episode of infective endocarditis. Indications for surgery include severe congestive heart failure (CHF) resulting from valvular incompetence, paravalvular leak around a prosthetic valve, fungal endocarditis, and persistent bacteremia despite antibiotics.

With proper antibiotic therapy, patients will defervesce within 1 week. The 5-year mortality rate for native valve endocarditis is 20%, but in the presence of a prosthetic valve it rises to 20% to 60%.[24,25]

Prophylaxis

Antibiotic prophylaxis in patients undergoing procedures in the ED is important for those with prosthetic heart valves, a history of endocarditis, or congenital cardiac malformations. Antibiotics are thought to prevent infective endocarditis by decreasing the degree of bacteremia and reducing the ability of bacteria to adhere to the valve surface. Box 78-3 lists those individuals thought to be at high enough risk of endocarditis to warrant prophylaxis. Common procedures for which prophylaxis is recommended are listed in Box 78-4.[26]

Table 78-1. Prophylactic Regimens for Bacterial Endocarditis

Dental procedures	Agent	Regimen
Standard oral prophylaxis	Amoxicillin	*Adults:* 2.0 g 1 hr before procedure *Children:* 50 mg/kg 1 hr before procedure
Unable to take oral medication	Ampicillin	*Adults:* 2.0 g IM or IV 30 min before procedure *Children:* 50 mg/kg 30 min before procedure
Allergic to penicillin	Clindamycin	*Adults:* 600 mg orally 1 hr before procedure *or* 600 mg IV 30 min before *Children:* 20 mg/kg orally 1 hr before procedure or IV 30 minutes before
	Azithromycin or clarithromycin	*Adults:* 500 mg orally 1 hr before procedure *Children:* 15 mg/kg orally 1 hr before procedure

From Dajani AS et al: *JAMA* 277:1794, 1997.

Box 78-4 Indications for Endocarditis Prophylaxis

Prophylaxis Recommended

Prophylactic cleaning of teeth
Bronchoscopy (with rigid bronchoscope only)
Endoscopic retrograde cholangiopancreatography (ERCP)
Cystoscopy
Urethral dilation

Prophylaxis Not Recommended

Local anesthetic injections (nonintraligamentary)
Endotracheal intubation
Tympanostomy tube insertion
Transesophageal echocardiography
Endoscopy
Vaginal delivery
Urethral catheterization
Uterine dilation and curettage
Insertion or removal of an intrauterine device

From Dajani AS et al: *JAMA* 227:1794, 1997.

Relatively clean procedures, such as suturing of clean lacerations, endotracheal intubation, or the placement of a central venous catheter, probably do not require prophylaxis. Table 78-1 summarizes recommendations for prophylaxis against bacterial endocarditis.

RHEUMATIC FEVER

Perspective

From 1920 to 1950 acute rheumatic fever was the leading cause of death in American children and the most common cause of heart disease in individuals under the age of 40. During the 1960s and 1970s the incidence of this disease in developed countries declined dramatically because of widespread antibiotic use to treat streptococcal infections, declining prevalence of the more virulent strains of group A streptococci, and improved living conditions. In the mid-1980s a resurgence of rheumatic fever occurred in several areas of the United States.[27,28] This was thought to be caused by the emergence of a more virulent strain of group A streptococcus.[29] The incidence of rheumatic fever during epidemics of streptococcal pharyngitis is 3%, although sporadic cases of streptococcal sore throat rarely result in this disease. Children between the ages of 4 and 18 years are at greatest risk of developing rheumatic fever. In many developing nations, rheumatic fever continues to be a leading cause of death in infants and adolescents.

Principles of Disease

Although the exact pathogenesis of rheumatic fever remains unclear, all affected individuals demonstrate an antibody response indicating a recent infection with group A β-hemolytic streptococcus. The most popular theory is that rheumatic fever results from an abnormal immunologic response to group A streptococcus, resulting in antibodies that cross-react with certain tissues within the heart, joints, skin, and central nervous system.

Clinical Features

Up to one third of patients with rheumatic fever do not remember having pharyngitis in the preceding month. The average latent period between pharyngitis and rheumatic fever is 18 days, but the period ranges from 1 to 5 weeks. In 1944 Jones formulated major and minor criteria for the diagnosis of rheumatic fever. Revised in 1965 and further modified in 1984 and 1992, the Jones criteria remain the diagnostic basis for this disease (Box 78-5).[30,31] The diagnosis of rheumatic fever requires evidence of an antecedent streptococcal infection plus at least one major and two minor, or two major manifestations from the Jones criteria.

A migratory polyarthritis is the most common symptom of rheumatic fever. This often affects larger joints such as the knees, ankles, elbows, and wrists, and the pain is usually much more severe than physical findings suggest. Arthritis occurs early in the course of rheumatic fever and often coincides with a rising titer of streptococcal antibodies.

Up to 40% of patients with rheumatic fever have a pancarditis manifested by a heart murmur, cardiomegaly, pericardial effusion, and occasionally CHF. The mitral valve is by far the most common valve affected by rheumatic fever, often resulting in mitral regurgitation and its classically high-pitched blowing systolic murmur.

Chorea (Sydenham's chorea, St. Vitus' dance) consists of

Box 78-5 The Jones Criteria (Revised) for the Diagnosis of Rheumatic Fever

Major Manifestations

Carditis
Polyarteritis
Chorea
Erythema marginatum
Subcutaneous nodules

Minor Manifestations

Arthralgias
Fever
Increased erythrocyte sedimentation rate or C-reactive protein
Prolonged PR interval

random, rapid, purposeless movements, usually of the upper extremities and face. It is a rare manifestation of rheumatic fever. Chorea may coexist with carditis, but it never occurs simultaneously with arthritis. If chorea is the only finding, diagnosis may become difficult because all other clinical and laboratory signs may be absent.

Erythema marginata and subcutaneous nodules are found in fewer than 10% of cases of acute rheumatic fever; however, their presence should immediately suggest the diagnosis. Erythema marginatum is a nonpruritic, painless, evanescent "smoke ring" of erythema that commonly appears on the trunk and proximal extremities. Subcutaneous nodules are pea sized, nontender, and usually appear over the extensor surfaces of the wrists, elbows, knees, and occasionally the spine.

Fever is present during the acute phase of rheumatic fever. It rarely lasts more than 2 weeks and has no characteristic pattern.

Diagnostic Strategies

In diagnosing rheumatic fever, it is helpful to document a recent streptococcal infection. Although throat cultures are usually negative at the time of clinical onset of rheumatic fever, antistreptococcal antibodies (ASA) titers remain positive for 4 to 6 weeks after the streptococcal infection. The ESR and C-reactive protein level are typically elevated. Approximately 50% of patients will have mild proteinuria or casts in their urine. There are no ECG findings pathognomonic of rheumatic fever, although a prolonged PR interval is common and suggestive.

Management

Acute rheumatic fever can be prevented by appropriate treatment of streptococcal pharyngitis. This can be accomplished by early treatment of pharyngitis with either a single injection of benzathine penicillin (600,000 U in children under 25 kg and 1.2 million U in adults) or a 10-day course of oral penicillin or erythromycin. If the oral route is chosen, it is important that a 10-day course be completed to eradicate the presence of streptococcus in the pharynx.

Management of acute rheumatic fever consists of treating the group A streptococcus infection, reducing inflammation, and evaluating for CHF. Patients with acute rheumatic fever must receive prophylaxis against streptococcal infections for at least 5 years. This is accomplished by treatment with penicillin or erythromycin twice daily or an injection of benzathine penicillin once a month. Inflammation is very responsive to salicylates and other antiinflammatory agents. Corticosteroids are not indicated for treatment of arthritis; however, they are effective in treating carditis.

VALVULAR HEART DISEASE

Principles of Disease

Of the four heart valves, three (tricuspid, pulmonic, and aortic) are composed of three cusps, whereas the mitral valve has only two. Each cusp is a double layer of endocardium that is attached at its base to the fibrous skeleton of the heart. The margins of the cusps are attached to muscular projections from the ventricles (papillary muscles) via tendinous cords (chordae tendineae). Contraction of the ventricle, and consequently the papillary muscle, results in the opening or closing of the valve, depending on its location.

Mitral Valve Prolapse

Congenital MVP is an extremely common valvulopathy, affecting up to 10% of the population.[32,33] Young women constitute the majority of patients affected. Although this is usually an asymptomatic disorder discovered by routine physical examination or echocardiography, occasionally the patient may experience palpitations and chest pain. Rare complications of MVP include endocarditis, malignant dysrhythmias, and sudden death.

Patients with MVP may be encountered in a variety of clinical scenarios. Patients may have symptoms of palpitations or chest pain that may be related to the previously diagnosed MVP, or auscultation may reveal a new click or murmur.

Pathophysiology Structurally, myxomatous proliferation of the spongiosa layer within the valve causes focal interruption of the fibrosa layer and allows abnormal stretching of the valve leaflet during systole. The posterior leaflet alone most commonly prolapses, and regurgitation does not occur. If both leaflets prolapse, regurgitation may occur. MVP is commonly associated with other connective tissue disorders such as Marfan syndrome, Ehlers-Danlos syndrome, and skeletal abnormalities such as pectus excavatum, a straight back, and severe scoliosis.

Clinical Features The most common symptoms associated with MVP are palpitations and chest pain. Palpitations are most often caused by premature ventricular contractions (PVCs); however, paroxysmal reentry supraventricular tachycardia and, very rarely, ventricular tachycardia are reported.[34,35] The chest pain associated with MVP usually differs from angina pectoris in that it is sharp, localized, of variable duration, and nonexertional. Rarely, the patient will have pain mimicking angina that may respond to nitroglycerine. Theories regarding the etiology of this pain include localized ischemia secondary to stretching of the papillary muscles and coronary artery spasm.[36]

Fatigue, lightheadedness, and shortness of breath are other symptoms commonly associated with MVP. Exercise testing of these individuals usually is normal. Generalized anxiety, panic attacks, and eating disorders are commonly described as part of the MVP syndrome. The psychiatric literature on this subject is divided, and anxiety disorders may not be more prevalent in patients with MVP than they are in the general population.[37]

The patient with MVP may demonstrate a wide variety of clicks and murmurs on cardiac auscultation. These vary widely among patients and tend to disappear and reappear at different times in an individual patient. Approximately 20% of patients with MVP have the classic midsystolic click followed by a late systolic crescendo murmur heard best between the apex and left sternal border, with the patient in the left lateral decubitus position. Any diagnostic maneuver that reduces end-diastolic ventricular volume, such as having the patient stand or perform Valsalva's maneuver, will move the click closer to S_1 and may bring out a previously unheard click. This click is thought to result from snapping of the chordae tendineae during the prolapse of the valve.

Diagnostic Strategies Diagnosis of MVP depends on detecting the typical auscultatory findings and is confirmed by echocardiography. In most patients, a thorough history and physical examination are sufficient to make the diagnosis. Echocardiography can be helpful in the patient suspected of MVP with normal auscultatory findings. The ECG can have a variety of abnormalities in MVP, including ST segment depression in leads II, III, and aVF consistent with inferior ischemia, QT interval prolongation, and premature atrial and ventricular contractions.[38]

Complications There are a variety of complications that can occur with MVP. Individuals with MVP and associated mitral regurgitation are at an increased risk of infective endocarditis.[39] MVP is associated with a variety of neurologic abnormalities, including migraine headaches and cerebrovascular events ranging from transient ischemic attacks to cerebrovascular accidents (CVAs).[40-42] Cerebral ischemic events may be secondary to sterile emboli from platelet and fibrin deposits on the defective mitral valve.

Very rarely, malignant ventricular dysrhythmias are associated with MVP and result in sudden death. In a review of patients with sudden death related to MVP, risk factors include a history of syncope or near syncope, a click and a late systolic or pansystolic murmur, ST-T segment abnormalities in the inferior or lateral leads, and multiple PVCs.[43]

Management Propranolol or other β-blockers may control symptoms such as palpitations, chest pain, and anxiety. Often, quiet reassurance and explanation of the disease entity will suffice. Patients with severe mitral regurgitation or life-threatening dysrhythmias unresponsive to drug therapy may require valve replacement.

Mitral Stenosis

The most common cause of mitral stenosis is rheumatic heart disease. There usually is a latency period of approximately 20 years between rheumatic fever and the onset of symptoms from mitral stenosis. Without surgical intervention, steady deterioration will occur, resulting in an 85% mortality rate 20 years after the onset of symptoms. Other less common causes of mitral stenosis are congenital mitral stenosis, atrial myxoma, thrombus, and calcification of the mitral annulus and leaflets.

Pathophysiology The stenosis of the mitral valve impedes flow from the left atrium to the left ventricle, resulting in left atrial hypertension and eventually left ventricular failure and pulmonary edema. As the disease progresses, some patients develop severe pulmonary hypertension, which leads to right ventricular failure.

Clinical Features Patients with hemodynamically significant mitral stenosis often complain of dyspnea on exertion, orthopnea, and hemoptysis. These symptoms are a result of left ventricular failure and pulmonary hypertension. The physician should specifically examine the patient for mitral stenosis in the setting of new-onset CHF. The following findings are suggestive of mitral stenosis: a palpable diastolic thrill over the apex, a loud S_1, and an opening snap of the mitral valve in early diastole and a low-pitched, rumbling diastolic murmur heard best at the apex.

Although the chest radiograph may be normal, in more advanced cases left atrial enlargement is present and results in straightening of the left heart border. Calcification of the mitral orifice occasionally can be seen.

The most common ECG abnormalities include atrial fibrillation and evidence of left atrial enlargement (a notched P wave in lead II and a negative terminal deflection of the P wave in lead V_1).

Complications Atrial fibrillation is the most common complication of mitral stenosis; the incidence may be as high as 40% and depends on left atrial size. The sudden onset of atrial fibrillation can cause severe heart failure when accompanied by a rapid ventricular response. Embolic events are a serious complication of mitral stenosis. The incidence of embolism may be as high as 20%, with approximately 75% of these affecting the brain.[44] Patients with right ventricular failure are prone to recurrent pulmonary emboli.

Other complications are frequent respiratory infections and, occasionally, massive pulmonary hemorrhage from rupture of pulmonary bronchial venous connections. Infective endocarditis is rare with isolated mitral stenosis.

Mitral Regurgitation

Acute and chronic mitral regurgitation are two distinct disease entities. Acute mitral regurgitation is usually a catastrophic event resulting from the rupture of chordae tendineae or papillary muscle or perforation of the valve leaflet. Common causes include acute myocardial infarction (MI), bacterial endocarditis, and trauma. Chronic mitral regurgitation is most commonly a result of rheumatic heart disease and often coexists with mitral stenosis. Other causes of chronic mitral regurgitation include MVP and connective tissue disorders such as Marfan syndrome and Ehlers-Danlos syndrome.

Pathophysiology In acute mitral regurgitation, the regurgitant volume can be three to four times the forward flow, resulting in pulmonary edema and peripheral vascular collapse.

In chronic mitral regurgitation, the left ventricle compensates by increasing stroke volume and maintaining cardiac output. Symptoms related to low output state, including fatigue and dyspnea on exertion, only occur late in the disease, and patients commonly remain asymptomatic for their lifetime. Most patients eventually develop atrial fibrillation; however, CHF is uncommon.

Clinical Features The clinical picture of acute mitral regurgitation is one of fulminant pulmonary edema. This often occurs in the setting of an acute MI. The carotid pulse rises rapidly but is poorly sustained. Atrial and ventricular gallops are frequently present. The murmur of acute mitral regurgitation is a loud crescendo-decrescendo murmur ending before S_2 and heard best at the apex. The ECG in acute mitral regurgitation is notable for the absence of left atrial and ventricular hypertrophy. The chest radiograph usually reveals pulmonary edema and a normal cardiac silhouette.

Characteristic findings in chronic mitral regurgitation include a palpable left ventricular heave and thrill. The murmur is high-pitched, holosystolic, and heard best at the apex, radiating to the axilla. The ECG usually reflects left atrial and ventricular hypertrophy. Atrial fibrillation is a common rhythm. Left atrial enlargement is commonly seen on the chest radiograph.

Management When the diagnosis of acute mitral regurgitation is suspected, emergency echocardiography and/or cardiac catheterization is indicated to assess the degree of regurgitation and determine whether emergent surgery is indicated. Initial stabilization of the patient should include treatment of the pulmonary edema with nitrates, nitroprusside, morphine, and diuretics. In the hypotensive patient, an intraaortic balloon pump may provide temporary stabilization before surgery.

Chronic mitral regurgitation is medically managed with diuretics, salt restriction, and digoxin. If the degree of regurgitation becomes debilitating and the symptoms cannot be controlled by medications, surgery is indicated.

Aortic Stenosis

The cause of aortic stenosis (AS) varies according to the age of the patient. In individuals less than 65 years, the most common cause is a congenital bicuspid valve, whereas in those older than 65 years stenosis is usually a result of calcific degeneration of the valve cusp. Rheumatic heart disease is the second most common cause of AS in patients under age 65. In these patients, the mitral valve is usually also affected.

Pathophysiology Significant obstruction of the left ventricular outflow tract is thought to occur when the valve orifice becomes less than 1.0 cm or when a pressure gradient across the valve exceeds 50 mm Hg. Compensatory left ventricular hypertrophy maintains stroke volume and cardiac output until the stenosis becomes critical, which is why symptoms appear only late in the disease.

Clinical Features The classic triad of symptoms from AS are (1) dyspnea on exertion from left ventricular failure, (2) angina, and (3) exertional syncope. Syncope is a result of either inadequate cerebral perfusion or occasional dysrhythmias. Once symptoms occur, the life expectancy averages 5 years without operative intervention. Once symptoms of heart failure occur, the life expectancy is less than 2 years.

The classic auscultatory finding in AS is a low-pitched, rasping systolic crescendo-decrescendo murmur heard best at the base and radiating into the carotids. Often, the carotid pulse is diminished in intensity (parvus) and slow rising (tardus). The left ventricle is often hyperdynamic, with a palpable heave. Although the pulse pressure may be reduced in AS, this is not a constant finding.

The ECG usually reveals left ventricular hypertrophy. Left ventricular enlargement may be seen on chest radiographs late in the disease.

Management Once symptoms occur in patients with AS, medical management has a limited role. These patients are at significant risk of sudden death and should be referred for valve replacement. The patient with critical AS maintains a delicate balance between preload and afterload. The addition of any medication that alters either of these parameters can lead to acute decompensation. Patients who have decompensated from AS most commonly are hypotensive. This usually can be treated with gentle fluid resuscitation; however, inotropic agents occasionally are necessary. An intraaortic balloon pump can be used as a temporizing measure until the valve is replaced.

Aortic Regurgitation

Aortic regurgitation may be a chronic disease process evolving slowly over years, or it may occur acutely, presenting as fulminant heart failure. The most common cause of chronic aortic regurgitation is rheumatic heart disease. Acute aortic regurgitation is most commonly associated with fulminant endocarditis, aortic dissection, or trauma. A variety of connective tissue diseases such as Marfan syndrome, ankylosing spondylitis, rheumatoid arthritis, Takayasu's arteritis, and syphilitic aortitis can predispose a patient to develop acute or chronic aortic regurgitation.

Pathophysiology During acute aortic regurgitation, left ventricular diastolic pressure rises rapidly, resulting in left ventricular failure and fulminant pulmonary edema. In chronic aortic regurgitation, the left ventricle hypertrophies and dilates, allowing the heart to maintain cardiac output despite significant regurgitation.

Clinical Features Patients with acute aortic regurgitation have severe CHF, with symptoms of dyspnea, tachypnea, and occasionally chest pain. Decreased cardiac output results in cool, pale extremities and a resting tachycardia. The systolic and diastolic pressures are normal or low, and the pulse pressure is not widened. The first heart sound is diminished or absent because of early closure of the mitral valve. A short, soft diastolic murmur (regurgitation) and a midsystolic flow murmur may be present. The diagnosis of acute aortic regurgitation can be difficult because of the lack of physical findings. Consider acute mitral and aortic regurgitation in any patient presenting with new-onset CHF. Because therapy for acute or chronic aortic regurgitation is quite similar, differentiating between these two entities can await stabilization. The diagnosis can be made definitively by echocardiography.

In chronic aortic regurgitation, physical examination reveals a rapidly rising and falling carotid pulse (water-hammer, or Corrigan's pulse). Other physical signs include nail pulsations (Quincke's sign), a to-and-fro murmur over the femoral artery (Duroziez's murmur), and head bobbing in severe cases. The pulse pressure is almost always widened. A high-pitched, blowing diastolic murmur at the left sternal border is characteristic. The Austin Flint murmur, a soft diastolic rumble caused by the regurgitant stream hitting the mitral valve, may also be present.

Management Acute aortic regurgitation is a surgical emergency requiring immediate valve replacement. Medical stabilization should be attempted with the use of afterload reducers, diuretics, and, if necessary, an intraaortic balloon pump while awaiting surgical therapy. In those cases in which bacterial endocarditis is the cause of acute aortic regurgitation, the timing of surgery is controversial. The CHF of chronic aortic regurgitation can be managed with afterload reducers, nitrates, and digoxin. Aortic valve replacement should be considered once left ventricular failure occurs.

Tricuspid Stenosis/Regurgitation

Pathophysiology Tricuspid stenosis is almost always rheumatic in origin and commonly coexists with mitral and aortic disease. Patients often complain of fatigue and symptoms related to increased venous congestion such as edema, ascites, and hepatosplenomegaly. Left ventricular failure is rare and occurs only with associated aortic or mitral stenosis.

Tricuspid regurgitation is most commonly the result of pulmonary hypertension; however, it can also be caused by rheumatic fever, right-sided endocarditis, and occasionally trauma.

Clinical Features In tricuspid stenosis, physical examination reveals a prominent jugular venous "A" wave and a high-pitched diastolic murmur along the left sternal border that increases with inspiration. Hepatosplenomegaly usually is present.

Signs and symptoms of tricuspid regurgitation include dyspnea, painful hepatomegaly, ascites, and peripheral edema, reflecting associated pulmonary hypertension and right ventricular failure. On physical examination a right ventricular heave is commonly present. The murmur is high-pitched, pansystolic, and best heard at the fourth intercostal space parasternally. A prominent P_2 and S_3 are often heard on auscultation. A right bundle branch block or atrial fibrillation may be present on ECG.

Management Initial treatment of tricuspid stenosis and tricuspid regurgitation consists of fluid and salt restriction but may eventually require valve replacement.

Complications of Prosthetic Valves

Since 1960 more than 1 million prosthetic valves have been placed. Artificial heart valves are implanted in over 40,000 patients per year in the United States. Prosthetic heart valves are separated into two groups: mechanical valves consisting of synthetic materials, and bioprosthetic, or tissue, valves made with either porcine or bovine tissue cusps. The original mechanical valve, the Starr-Edwards caged-ball prosthesis, was first implanted in 1960. Since that time, many other designs for mechanical valves have been introduced, with the most common being the caged ball, the tilting disk, and the bileaflet hinged-disk prostheses. Dissatisfaction with the need for lifelong anticoagulation led to the development of bioprosthetic valves. Tissue valves are most commonly porcine, but rarely may be made of hand-sewn human tissue. Although these valves offer the advantage of optional anticoagulation, they are much less durable than their mechanical counterparts. To properly evaluate a patient with a prosthetic valve, it is necessary to know the type, location, and age of the prosthesis. All patients are provided with a card containing this information at the time of their surgery.

All mechanical prostheses have a prominent metallic closure sound and a softer metallic opening click. Bioprostheses, on the other hand, have opening and closing sounds similar to the native valve. Almost all prostheses result in some obstruction to flow, and, when in the aortic position, a systolic ejection murmur is normal.

A PA and lateral chest radiograph is helpful in determining the position of the prosthesis and evaluating the presence or absence of vascular congestion that may accompany valve dysfunction. A decreasing hematocrit level may be a result of significant hemolysis, indicating paravalvular leak or primary failure of the prosthesis. Coagulation studies are helpful only in the setting of suspected valve thrombosis, embolism, or hemorrhage and to check for adequate anticoagulation.

Early complications from prosthetic heart valves are often surgically related, whereas later complications include embolization, valve obstruction from thrombus formation, endocarditis, hemolytic anemia, and primary failure of the valve.

Thromboembolic events are the most serious complication of prosthetic valves. Thrombus formation can result in obstruction of the valve outlet or dislodgment of emboli into the systemic circulation. The risk of thrombus formation depends on the type and location of the prosthesis. Mechanical valves have a much higher incidence of thrombus formation than bioprosthetic valves. Patients with a thrombosed mechanical heart valve usually have an acute onset of hypotension, CHF, and an absent or muted metallic closure sound. Thrombosis may also develop subacutely with gradually worsening symptoms over periods as long as 6 months. Patients with mechanical valves usually require lifelong anticoagulation with warfarin plus or minus aspirin or dipyridamole. The international normalized ratio (INR) in these patients should be maintained in the range of 2.5 to 3.5. Patients with bioprosthetic valves usually require only aspirin. If the left atrium is dilated, however, warfarin may be recommended for mitral valve bioprostheses.

The incidence of infective endocarditis in patients with prosthetic valves is approximately 0.5% per patient year. During the first two postoperative months, *Staphylococcus epidermidis* and other hospital-acquired organisms predominate. After the initial 2 months, the causative organisms are similar to those causing native valve endocarditis.

Chronic hemolysis from the turbulence of blood flow past the prosthetic valve occurs in up to 70% of patients. The hemolysis is usually low grade in nature and responds well to iron therapy. The hemolysis occasionally can be severe, suggesting the possibility of a paravalvular leak or primary valve failure, both of which may require valve replacement. This chronic hemolysis may predispose the patient to cholelithiasis.

Primary valve failure in patients with prosthetic heart valves can lead to regurgitant blood flow, acute valvular occlusion, embolism of a piece of the prosthesis, or severe hemolysis. In bioprosthetic valves, primary tissue failure results from cuspal tears and perforations, calcification, and loss of pliability of the leaflets. Approximately 30% of aortic and mitral bioprosthetic valves have tissue failure at 10 years, necessitating replacement. Although mechanical valves are extremely durable, structural failures are reported. The Björk-Shiley 60- and 70-degree convexoconcave valves were withdrawn from the market in 1985 and 1983, respectively, because of a high incidence of strut fracture and resultant embolization of the tilting disk.[45] By 1985 over 80,000 convexoconcave valves had been placed, and over 4000 of them were the 70-degree model.[46] There is still a significant population with these prostheses in place who are at risk of strut fracture and disk escape. These patients experience the dramatic onset of CHF and hypotension. On physical examination, there is absence of the metallic closure sound and a regurgitant murmur. The murmur may be the only finding that differentiates this from valve thrombosis. A chest radiograph will reveal the disk to be dislodged or absent.

KEY CONCEPTS

- Most patients with bacterial endocarditis have one of the following predisposing factors:
  1. Rheumatic or congenital heart disease
  2. Calcific degenerative valve disease
  3. Prosthetic heart valve
  4. History of intravenous drug use
  5. History of endocarditis
  6. MVP with regurgitant flow
- *Streptococcus viridans* is the most common cause of infective endocarditis in patients with congenital valvular disease or MVP, whereas Staphylococcus is most common in patients with a history of IV drug use and/or prosthetic valves.
- Fewer than 35% of IV drug users with infective endocarditis have a murmur on initial presentation.
- Transesophageal echocardiography is the diagnostic test of choice for infective endocarditis. Rheumatic fever most commonly affects the mitral valve.
- The classic findings of chronic aortic regurgitation, including Corrigan's pulse, Quinke's sign, Duroziez's murmur, are absent in acute aortic regurgitation.
- Absence of auscultated metallic closure sounds in a mechanical valve prosthesis should raise the suspicion of valve dysfunction (dislodgment or thrombosis).

REFERENCES

1. Verheul HA et al: Effects of change in management of active infective endocarditis on outcome in a 25-year period, *Am J Cardiol* 72:682, 1993.
2. Ghann JW, Cobbs CG: Infections of prosthetic valves and intravascular devices. In Mandel GI, editor: *Principles and practices of infectious disease,* New York, 1985, John Wiley and Sons.
3. Pelletier LL, Petersdorf RG: Infective endocarditis: a review of 125 cases from the University of Washington Hospitals, 1963-1972, *Medicine* 56:287, 1977.
4. Welton DE et al: Recurrent infective endocarditis: analysis of predisposing factors and clinical features, *Am J Med* 66:932, 1979.
5. Dajani AS et al: Prevention of bacterial endocarditis, *JAMA* 227:1797, 1997.
6. Hoesley CJ, Cobbs G : Endocarditis at the millennium, *J Infect Dis* 179(suppl 2):S360, 1999.
7. Hecht SR, Berger M: Right-sided endocarditis in intravenous drug users: prognostic features in 102 episodes, *Ann Intern Med* 117:560, 1992.
8. Lessing MA et al: Native-valve endocarditis caused by *Staphylococcus lugdunensis, Q J Med* 89:855, 1996.
9. Vagdenesch F et al: Endocarditis due to *Staphylococcus lugdunensis:* report of 11 cases and review, *Clin Infect Dis* 17:871, 1993.
10. Wilson WR et al: Antibiotic treatment of adults with infective endocarditis due to streptococci, enterococci, staphylococci, and HACEK microorganisms: American Heart Association, *JAMA* 274: 1706, 1995.
11. Spach D et al: Bartonella (Rochalimaea) species as a cause of apparent "culture negative" endocarditis, *Clin Infect Dis* 20:1044, 1995.
12. Delaney KA: The double challenge of endocarditis, *Emerg Med* 22:53, 1990.
13. Shively BK et al: Diagnostic value of transesophageal compared with transthoracic echocardiography in infective endocarditis, *J Am Coll Cardiol* 18:391, 1991.
14. Shapiro SM et al: Transesophageal echocardiography in diagnosis of infective endocarditis, *Chest* 105:377, 1994.
15. Daniel WG et al: Comparison of transthoracic and transesophageal echocardiography for detection of abnormalities of prosthetic and bioprosthetic valves in the mitral and aortic positions, *Am J Cardiol* 71:210, 1993.
16. Birmingham GD, Rahko PS, Ballantyne F: Improved detection of infective endocarditis with transesophageal echocardiography, *Am Heart J* 123:774, 1992.
17. Durack DT, Lukes AS, Bright DK: New criteria for diagnosis of infective endocarditis: utilization of specific echocardiographic findings: Duke Endocarditis Service, *Am J Med* 96:200, 1994.
18. Lamas CC, Eykyn SJ: Suggested modifications to the Duke criteria for the clinical diagnosis of native valve and prosthetic valve endocarditis: analysis of 118 pathologically proven cases, *Clin Infect Dis* 25:713, 1997.
19. Heiro M et al: Diagnosis of infective endocarditis: sensitivity of the Duke vs. von Reyn criteria, *Arch Intern Med* 158:18, 1998.
20. Nettles RE et al: An evaluation of the Duke criteria in 25 pathologically confirmed cases of prosthetic valve infective endocarditis, *Clin Infect Dis* 25:1401, 1997.
21. Hoen B et al: The Duke criteria for diagnosing infective endocarditis are specific: analysis of 100 patients with acute fever or fever of unknown origin, *Clin Infect Dis* 23:298, 1996.
22. Dodds GA et al: Negative predictive value of the Duke criteria for infective endocarditis, *Am J Cardiol* 77:403, 1996.
23. Weisse AB et al: The febrile parenteral drug abuser: a prospective study of 121 patients, *Am J Med* 94:274, 1993.
24. Verheul HA et al: Effects of changes in management of active infective endocarditis on outcome in a 25-year period, *Am J Cardiol* 72:682, 1993.
25. Martin JM, Neches WH, Wald ER: Infectious endocarditis: 35 years of experience at a children's hospital, *Clin Infect Dis* 24:669, 1997.
26. Dajani AS et al: Prevention of bacterial endocarditis: recommendations by the American Heart Association, *JAMA* 277:1794, 1997.
27. Veasy LG et al: Resurgence of acute rheumatic fever in the intermountain area of the United States, *N Engl J Med* 316:421, 1987.
28. Hosier D et al: Resurgence of rheumatic fever, *N Engl J Med* 316:421, 1987.
29. Kaplan EL, Johnson DR, Cleary PP: Group A streptococcal serotypes isolated from patients and sibling contacts during the resurgence of rheumatic fever in the United States in the mid-1980s, *J Infect Dis* 159:101, 1989.
30. Committee on the Prevention of Rheumatic Fever and Bacterial Endocarditis of the American Heart Association: The Jones criteria (revised), *Circulation* 78:1082, 1988.
31. Committee on Rheumatic Fever, Endocarditis, and Kawasaki Disease of the Council on Cardiovascular Disease in the Young, American Heart Association: Prevention of bacterial endocarditis, *JAMA* 264: 2919, 1990.
32. Cheitlin MD, Byrd RC: Prolapsed mitral valve: the commonest disease? *Curr Probl Cardiol* 8:1, 1984.
33. Fontana ME et al: Mitral valve prolapse and the mitral valve prolapse syndrome, *Curr Probl Cardiol* 16:315, 1991.
34. Mason DT et al: Arrhythmias in patients with mitral valve prolapse, *Med Clin North Am* 68:1039, 1984.
35. Savage DD et al: Mitral valve prolapse in the general population. Part 3. Dysrhythmia: the Framingham study, *Am Heart J* 106:582, 1983.
36. Mautner RK et al: Coronary artery spasm: a mechanism for chest pain in selected patients with the mitral valve prolapse syndrome, *Chest* 79:449, 1981.
37. Mazza DL et al: Prevalence of anxiety disorders in patients with mitral valve prolapse, *Am J Psychiatry* 143:349, 1986.
38. Bhutto ZR et al: Electrocardiographic abnormalities in mitral valve prolapse, *Am J Cardiol* 70:265, 1992.
39. Corrigall D et al: Mitral valve prolapse and infective endocarditis, *Am J Med* 63:215, 1977.
40. Litman GI, Friedman HM: Migraine and the mitral valve prolapse syndrome, *Am Heart J* 96:610, 1978.

41. Jackson AC et al: Mitral valve prolapse and cerebral ischemic events in young patients, *Neurology* 34:784, 1984.
42. Kouvaras G et al: Association of mitral valve leaflet prolapse and cerebral ischaemic events in the young and early middle-aged patient, *Q J Med* 56:387, 1986.
43. Jeresaty RM: Sudden death in the mitral valve prolapse-click syndrome, *Am J Cardiol* 37:317, 1976.
44. Aberrantly WS, Willis PW III: Thromboembolic complications of rheumatic heart disease, *Cardiovasc Clin* 5:131, 1973.
45. Hendel PN: Björk-Shiley strut fracture and disc escape: literature review and a method of disc retrieval, *Ann Thorac Surg* 47:436, 1989.
46. Ostermeyer J et al: The Björk-Shiley 70-degree convexoconcave prosthesis strut fracture problem (present state of information), *Thorac Cardiovasc Surg* 35:71, 1987.

Section IV VASCULAR SYSTEM

79 Hypertension

Richard O. Gray, James J. Mathews

PERSPECTIVE

With as many as 50 million hypertensive people in the United States, hypertension represents a serious health problem.[1] Hypertension was not even recognized as a major cause of serious medical problems until relatively recently. Effective means of blood pressure (BP) measurement were developed in the late nineteenth century. For most of the twentieth century, however, elevated BP readings were thought to be associated with, but not causing, morbidity and mortality. Not until the large population-based studies in the 1960s, such as the Framingham study, did physicians began to focus on hypertension as a treatable risk factor of stroke (cerebrovascular accident), myocardial infarction (MI), peripheral vascular disease, congestive heart failure, and renal disease. The general public's knowledge and awareness of hypertension have increased greatly. Patients are now much more apt to seek medical attention for hypertension and to follow medical advice about therapy. This has resulted in a 50% reduction in stroke mortality on an age-adjusted basis and has probably been responsible in part for the recent decline in mortality from coronary artery disease. As a matter of public health, however, much remains to be done in the treatment of hypertension. Although approximately 75% of patients with chronically elevated BP are aware of their disease, as few as one half to one quarter of these patients are adequately treated. Although hypertension may be epidemic in the United States, it rarely represents an emergency condition for the individual patient. In the absence of acute end-organ damage, it is rarely, if ever, necessary to lower a patient's BP acutely in the ED.

Hypertension is frequently encountered in the ED, where many factors can cause elevated BP. Anxiety and pain often cause transient hypertension, but the EP still must carefully evaluate the patient with elevated BP for evidence of acute end-organ ischemia. Most patients, even those with an exacerbation of chronically elevated BP, will show a substantial decrease in pressure without intervention during a short observation period in the ED.[2,3] Even if the patient's BP does remain elevated without end-organ damage, urgent treatment is rarely beneficial, and an appropriate referral should be made (Table 79-1).

Table 79-1. Recommendations for Follow-up Based on Initial Blood Pressure (BP) Measurements for Adults

Initial BP (mm Hg)*		
Systolic	**Diastolic**	**Follow-up recommended†**
<130	<85	Recheck in 2 years
130-139	85-89	Recheck in 1 year‡
140-159	90-99	Confirm within 2 months‡
160-179	100-109	Evaluate or refer to source of care within 1 month
≥180	≥110	Evaluate or refer to source of care immediately or within 1 week depending on clinical situation

Modified from the Sixth Report of the Joint National Committee on Prevention, Detection, Evaluation, and Treatment of High Blood Pressure, *Arch Intern Med* 157:2413, 1997.

*If systolic and diastolic BPs are different, follow recommendations for shorter time follow-up (e.g., patient within BP of 160/86 mm Hg should be evaluated or referred to source of care within 1 month).

†Modify scheduling of follow-up according to reliable information about past BP measurements, other cardiovascular risk factors, or target organ disease.

‡Provide advice about lifestyle modifications.

PRINCIPLES OF DISEASE

Definition and Determination of Hypertension

Within the population, as the baseline BP increases, the risk of cardiovascular complications also increases. As such, the definition of hypertension is somewhat arbitrary. In adults, a systolic pressure less than 140 mm Hg and a diastolic pressure less than 90 mm Hg are considered normal. If the systolic pressure is between 140 and 159 mm Hg, or if the diastolic pressure is between 90 and 95 mm Hg, the term *borderline hypertension* is applied. The patient with a systolic pressure of 160 mm Hg or greater or a diastolic pressure over 95 mm Hg is considered to be hypertensive. If hypertension, as defined by these arbitrary values, is not controlled, the patient is at great risk of long-term morbidity and mortality.[4,5]

In patients less than 45 years of age, the diastolic pressure is the primary determinant of future cardiovascular risk. Even isolated systolic hypertension in elderly patients is a significant risk factor for cardiovascular disease, especially when combined with other risk factors. In older patients, an elevated pulse pressure (determined by subtracting diastolic from systolic pressure) is an equally significant risk factor for stroke and MI.[6-8]

Proper technique is required to obtain accurate BP readings, with special attention to the cuff size used. In patients with larger extremities, use of a standard-size cuff may result in a falsely elevated BP. Using a larger cuff corrects this error, and these cuffs should be readily available in the ED. The cuff should be deflated slowly, since with rapid deflation the inertia of the mercury column causes a gap between the actual pressure in the cuff and the measured pressure on the gauge. This may lead to falsely elevated levels. It is much easier to obtain an accurate reading with a slowly falling column of mercury. Aneroid instruments are somewhat less susceptible to this problem, but in general they are not as accurate. The systolic pressure should be recorded when the first tapping sound is heard as the cuff is deflated. Although several endpoints have been used to define diastolic pressure, the most widely accepted is the total disappearance of sound. In patients who do not have complete disappearance of these sounds, the point of distinct muffling should be recorded as the diastolic pressure.

A single elevated BP does not necessarily mean that the patient has hypertension. This is especially true in children.[9] BP measurement should be repeated after the patient is in a reclining position for at least 10 minutes and should be checked in both arms. If this second reading is also elevated or close to the hypertensive range, the patient should be advised of the potential for hypertension and referred for follow-up.

Pathophysiology

Hypertension is not a distinct disease but rather the result of a number of disease processes. By far the most common category is *essential hypertension.* No specific cause of essential hypertension has been identified, although a mosaic of factors, including heredity, age, race, obesity, and the amount of sodium ingested, may contribute to the elevated BP.[10] The patient group with borderline hypertension has been intensely studied because those who later become hypertensive may provide clues about the changes in physiologic conditions that eventually produce a fixed elevation of BP. Two major theories exist: (1) hypertension results from alterations in the contractile properties of smooth muscle in arterial walls and (2) alterations of arterial smooth muscle are a response to chronically elevated BP resulting from a primary failure of normal autoregulatory mechanisms. More recent research has focused on the role of calcium ions in vascular smooth muscle.[11] Vascular tone depends on a transmembranous supply of calcium ions, and calcium antagonists suppress virtually all vasoconstrictive responses of vascular smooth muscles, including the peripheral resistance vessels.

Most patients with established hypertension have elevated peripheral arterial resistance and normal cardiac output. The findings are similar in the majority of borderline hypertensive individuals, many of whom have decreased plasma volume and elevated heart rate. This tachycardia seems to be caused not by an increased sympathetic tone but by a decreased parasympathetic tone. Autoregulatory mechanisms are blunted, and pharmacologic autonomic blockade has minimal effect on BP.

Many borderline hypertensive patients and some patients with mild to moderate hypertension have a very different circulatory status with an elevated cardiac output and hyperkinetic circulation. The increase in cardiac output results from an increase in both heart rate and stroke volume. There appears to be a large sympathetic component with an increase in both cardiac β-adrenergic and α-adrenergic tone. Autonomic blockade returns the BP readings to normal.

Renin and Angiotensin The role of renin and angiotensin as a cause of essential hypertension is not clear. Renin is an enzyme produced by the kidney that splits off angiotensin I from a plasma globulin precursor.[12] Angiotensin I is acted on by a converting enzyme in the lung to produce angiotensin II. Angiotensin II is a potent vasoconstrictor and it also stimulates aldosterone production in the adrenal gland. Figure 79-1 summarizes the factors that control renin inhibition and release. Patients with hypertension may be divided into clinical groups according to renin levels. Determining the renin-sodium profile, which is the plasma renin activity measured against the 24-hour urine sodium content, is especially useful in making this division.

In normal individuals, angiotensin effects depend on sodium levels. Inhibition of angiotensin-converting enzyme (ACE) has some effect on BP in normotensive individuals with normal total body sodium but greatly reduces BP in those with sodium depletion. When administered to patients with hypertension, the acute effect of ACE inhibitors on BP is closely related to the plasma renin activity. With chronic administration, however, the effect of ACE inhibitors on BP no longer correlates with pretreatment plasma renin activity.[13] Elevated renin and angiotensin levels are responsible for the hypertension seen in ischemic renal disease, and angiotensin is a major contributor to maintaining the progressive rise of BP in accelerated hypertension. In the latter condition, renin and angiotensin levels are increased because of areas of renal ischemia secondary to arteriolar necrosis. ACE inhibitors or angiotensin blockers are clearly the drugs of choice in hypertensive patients with diabetes and/or decreased left ventricular function.

Renal Disease Although most cases of hypertension are considered to be essential hypertension, several specific causes do exist. Early identification of secondary hypertension is important because it may lead to cure or at least to a specific and much easier treatment regimen. Of these other causes, renal disease is the most prevalent. All types of renal disease have been associated with hypertension, although a direct relationship can be demonstrated only in cases of unilateral renal disease in which the removal of the affected kidney cures the hypertension. This is clearly demonstrated in cases of unilateral renal arteriostenosis. The pathophysiology of *renovascular hypertension* is overproduction of renin induced by ischemia secondary to reduced blood flow through the stenotic renal artery. The increased levels of renin lead to activation of the angiotensin pathway and resultant hypertension. The response to surgery can best be predicted by determining renin levels in selective renal veins. If the renin level in the affected kidney is more than 50% higher than the level in the normal kidney, a complete or partial cure of the hypertension can be anticipated.

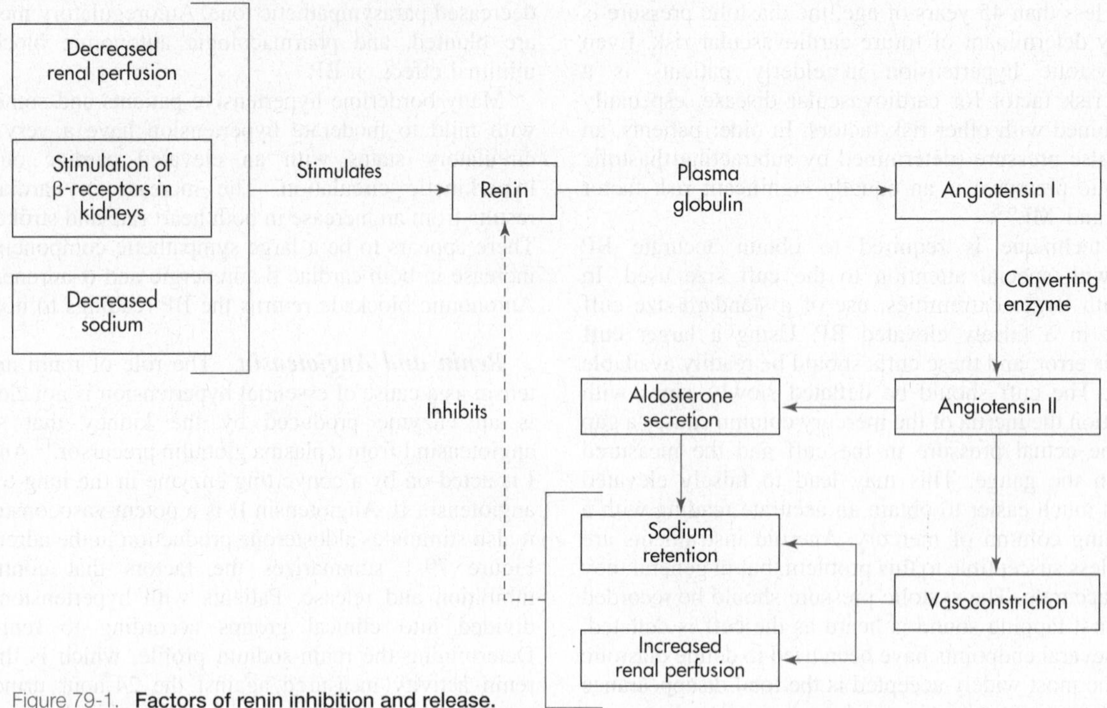

Figure 79-1. **Factors of renin inhibition and release.**

Another vascular lesion associated with arterial stenosis and hypertension is fibromuscular dysplasia of the renal arteries.[14,15] This disease is predominant in young white women, and flank bruits are often present. The various types affect different areas of the renal arteries. The result is progressive hypertension. Neither pharmacologic therapy nor surgical revision offers a cure, but both treatments reduce the progress of the disease process and help preserve functional renal mass.

Primary renal disease can produce hypertension, but the exact mechanism remains unknown. Up to 70% of patients with chronic pyelonephritis have elevated BP. Local ischemia within the kidney is suspected as the cause of hypertension. Hypertension in patients with nonspecific glomerulonephritis may result from arteriolar lesions producing ischemia at the level of the individual nephron. With the exception of renin-secreting renal tumors, the exact cause of hypertension associated with the various nephropathies has not been determined.

Arterial Disease Abnormalities of the large arteries can also produce hypertension. Although not common, coarctation of the aorta is an important cause of secondary hypertension, since early surgical intervention can greatly improve the patient's prognosis.[16] Coarctation may be suggested on the basis of the physical findings. The triad of upper extremity hypertension, a systolic murmur best heard over the back, and delayed femoral pulses should alert the examiner to the diagnosis of coarctation. Hypertension associated with coarctation appears to result from the combined effects of mechanical obstruction and activation of the renin-angiotensin system.[17] Early diagnosis of coarctation is important in that long-term follow-up after surgical repair has demonstrated a consistent and sustained lowering of BP.

Loss of elasticity in the larger arteries associated with the aging process produces systolic hypertension. Until recently, elevated systolic pressure was not considered significant and frequently was not treated. The current literature strongly suggests that isolated systolic hypertension is associated with an increased risk of stroke, heart disease, and renal failure and should be treated. The cause of reduced elasticity in the arteries associated with isolated systolic hypertension has not been fully determined. Increased intracellular calcium in arterial smooth muscle appears to be associated with early atherosclerosis. The amount of calcium in arterial smooth muscle increases with natural senescence and with other risk factors for atherosclerosis (e.g., nicotine use, diabetes, hypertension). Calcium channel blockers may help prevent this rise in intracellular calcium levels.

Glucocorticoids Excessive glucocorticoids are associated with hypertension. The most common cause of this problem is iatrogenic steroid therapy. Endogenous overproduction is uncommon and occurs from excessive adrenocorticotropic hormone (ACTH) production by a pituitary tumor, ectopic ACTH production by a nonpituitary tumor, or glucocorticoid production by tumors of the adrenal cortex. These patients show other signs and symptoms of excessive glucocorticoids, including centripetal fat distribution, striae, easy bruising, muscular weakness, and poor healing. The hypertension associated with hyperadrenalism usually is not severe and can be controlled by treating the underlying disease process. Spontaneous hypokalemia in a patient with hypertension should suggest primary aldosteronism. Catecholamine levels may also be abnormal. Primary aldosteronism is confirmed by a failure to inhibit aldosterone levels in the urine or plasma with sodium loading.

Pheochromocytoma Pheochromocytomas are responsible for less than 1% of cases of hypertension. More than 90% of these patients are curable with early diagnosis. Pheochromocytomas produce catecholamines and arise from cells of the sympathetic nervous system. The most common site is the adrenal medulla. Patients with neurofibromatosis (von Recklinghausen's disease) have an increased incidence of pheochromocytoma. Pheochromocytoma, medullary carcinoma of the thyroid, and parathyroid adenomas form the triad of multiple endocrine neoplasia (adenomatosis), type II.

The characteristic feature of pheochromocytoma is paroxysms of hypertension associated with palpitations, tachycardia, malaise, apprehension, and sweating. Many patients have a persistently elevated BP interspersed with episodes of greater hypertension that occur sporadically and vary greatly in severity, frequency, and duration. These episodes may be related to physical and emotional stress, eating, position, or even micturition. A prodrome of apprehension and nonspecific abdominal pain progressing to headache, palpitations, and angina may be seen. Because of the episodic nature of this syndrome, the patient is often labeled "psychoneurotic," and a diagnosis of hyperventilation syndrome or anxiety attack is made. An excessively elevated BP associated with these symptoms is enough to suggest a pheochromocytoma. Patients may also display increased BP when treated with beta-blocking agents (β-blockers).

The diagnosis of this tumor is confirmed by demonstrating elevated urinary levels of catecholamines, metanephrines, and vanillylmandelic acid.[18] Usually in pheochromocytoma, all parameters are increased to more than twice the normal levels. Provocative pharmacologic testing to diagnose pheochromocytoma is no longer indicated and has been replaced by the widespread availability of these biochemical tests. Treatment of hypertension associated with pheochromocytoma consists of alpha blockade to control hypertension and subsequent beta blockade for the control of cardiac dysrhythmias. After the hypertension is adequately controlled, the tumor should be surgically removed.

Other Agents The ingestion of foods containing large amounts of *tyramine* can cause hypertension (Box 79-1). Tyramine causes release of norepinephrine stored in nerve endings. This normally is a transient response; tyramine is rapidly destroyed by monoamine oxidase. Problems arise if a patient is being treated with a monoamine oxidase inhibitor (MAOI), which protects tyramine from destruction. Relatively small amounts of tyramine can cause severe and prolonged hypertension (see Chapter 146). A number of therapeutic agents can also induce a hypertensive crisis in patients taking MAOIs. These include meperidine, the amphetamines, ephedrine, reserpine, guanethidine, and the tricyclic antidepressants. The control of hypertension can be obtained by using an alpha-blocking agent (α-blocker) such as phentolamine.

Excess catecholamine effect can result from the acute withdrawal of clonidine or β-blocker therapy.[19] *Clonidine* acts centrally as an α-adrenoreceptor agonist. The sudden withdrawal of this agent may result in catecholamine excess and severe hypertension 16 to 48 hours later. Many of the symptoms associated with clonidine withdrawal are similar to those of pheochromocytoma, including anxiety, tremor, palpitations, and severe headache. Urinary catecholamine levels are markedly elevated. Treatment consists of either restarting clonidine therapy or using α-blockers. This characteristic limits clonidine's usefulness as an antihypertensive agent in noncompliant patients.

Box 79-1 Foods and Drugs Causing Hypertensive Crisis in Patients Taking Monoamine Oxidase Inhibitors

Foods*

Natural or aged cheeses
Pickled herring
Chicken liver
Coffee in large amounts
Chocolate
Broad beans
Beer, wine
Snails
Yeast
Citrus fruits
Cream

Drugs

Sympathomimetic amines (e.g., amphetamines)
Methyldopa
Dopamine
Tryptophan
Reserpine
Guanethidine
Tricyclic antidepressant

*All contain significant amounts of tyramine except for broad beans, which contain dopamine.

Emergency Department Presentation Hypertension presents in the ED in the following four general ways:

1. "Hypertensive emergency" or "hypertensive crisis" with acute end-organ ischemia
2. "Hypertensive urgency" or significantly elevated blood pressure with nonspecific symptoms
3. Mild hypertension without end-organ ischemia
4. Transient hypertension related to anxiety or the primary complaint

CLINICAL PRESENTATION OF HYPERTENSIVE EMERGENCIES

A small number of hypertensive patients may present with a true hypertensive emergency. In these patients blood pressure is usually markedly elevated and there is evidence of *acute* dysfunction in the cardiovascular, neurologic, or renal organ system (Box 79-2).

These conditions are true medical emergencies and, when diagnosed, mandate immediate reduction of BP within 1 hour.[4,20] In the past the range of hypertensive emergencies included patients who presented with any emergent condition associated with a marked elevation of BP and patients without end-organ damage. The elevated BP in these patients is often a physiologic response to an acute condition, and aggressive treatment for hypertension may actually *increase* morbidity and mortality. This is especially true for those patients with acute intracranial events.[21]

Hypertensive Encephalopathy

Throughout the normal range of BP, cerebral blood flow is maintained by fluctuations in the vascular tone of the cerebral

Box 79-2 Conditions Defining Hypertensive Crisis

Accelerated or Malignant Hypertension

Hypertensive encephalopathy
Microangiopathic hemolytic anemia
Acute renal failure

Aortic Dissection

Eclampsia/Preeclampsia

Severe Hypertension in the Setting of:

Myocardial ischemia
Left ventricular failure
Uncontrolled hemorrhage
Systemic reperfusion therapy for stroke or myocardial infarction

resistance vessels. This phenomenon is known as *autoregulation* and occurs to some degree in all vascular beds. Hypertensive encephalopathy is an uncommon syndrome resulting from an abrupt, sustained rise of BP that exceeds the limits of cerebral autoregulation of the small resistance arteries in the brain. Above a mean arterial pressure (MAP) of approximately 160 mm Hg, autoregulation may be unable to control cerebral blood flow. Marked vasospasm may occur, with ischemia, increased vascular permeability, punctate hemorrhages, and resultant brain edema. Immediate reduction of BP by 30% to 40% will reverse the vasospasm. *Excessive reduction of blood pressure must be avoided* to prevent the increased cerebral ischemia that results if the pressure falls below the lower level of cerebral autoregulation. In normal humans, this is set at an MAP of about 60 mm Hg. In patients with uncontrolled hypertension, however, the level of autoregulation is elevated, and cerebral ischemia may occur at a much higher MAP. BP below this level will result in cerebral ischemia.

Hypertensive encephalopathy is (1) acute in onset and (2) reversible. Patients often present with severe headaches, vomiting, drowsiness, and confusion. Seizures, blindness, focal neurologic deficits, or coma may occur. Papilledema is usually present, along with significant hypertensive retinopathy. Differential diagnosis includes all types of strokes and intracranial bleeds, meningoencephalitis, brain tumors, and metabolic coma. Careful neurologic examination is mandatory and often differentiates between a space-occupying lesion and hypertensive encephalopathy; focal deficits secondary to hypertensive encephalopathy usually do not follow a singular anatomic pattern. They may occur on opposite sides of the body or may have a patchy distribution. Systemic signs of infection associated with meningitis are absent. Metabolic causes of coma can be ruled out by serum chemistry testing. Computed tomography is usually normal, and the electroencephalogram shows only nonspecific abnormalities. The cerebrospinal fluid is clear, with an increased opening pressure and normal or increased protein.

Hypertensive encephalopathy is a true medical emergency; untreated patients develop increasing coma, and death may ensue within a few hours. The rapid *measured* reduction of BP is mandatory. The standard treatment regimen is intravenous (IV) nitroprusside with the careful reduction of the MAP by 25% over an hour, with a minimum diastolic pressure of 110 mm Hg. Use of an oral or nontitratable agent may result in an excessive reduction of BP and irreversible cerebral ischemia. The standard agent in the United States has long been sodium nitroprusside, but fenoldopam mesylate and labetalol are now widely used, with nicardipine and enalaprilat gaining favor in some circles (see later discussions). Although fast-acting nifedipine has been widely used in the past for symptomatic hypertension, numerous serious adverse effects related to uncontrolled hypotension and sympathetic release have been reported, and its use in acute hypertension is contraindicated.[22-24]

All patients with hypertensive encephalopathy should be hospitalized, and invasive BP monitoring may be preferable.

Malignant Hypertension

Malignant (*accelerated*) hypertension is defined as severe hypertension associated with evidence of acute and progressive damage to end organs. This syndrome can occur at any time in the clinical course of hypertension. The diastolic BP is usually greater than 130 mm Hg. Readings below this level are seldom associated with either malignant hypertension or hypertensive encephalopathy, although rarely either can occur with diastolic pressures as low as 110 mm Hg. *Most patients with diastolic pressures above 130 mm Hg do not develop either of these clinical syndromes.* Malignant hypertension only affects 1% of the hypertensive population.[20]

The pathologic change responsible for end-organ damage is fibrinoid necrosis of small arterioles. This process begins when a rapid, sustained rise in BP overwhelms the high-pressure autoregulatory mechanism, causing the small arterioles to dilate. As these vessels dilate, pressure in the proximal capillary beds increases, and fluid leaks into the tissues. The arterioles may rupture and leak plasma and blood, resulting in fibrin deposition into their walls. This combination of necrosis of myofibrils in smooth muscle cells, leaking of plasma, and fibrin deposition in the walls of arterioles is *fibrinoid necrosis.* These changes within the small arterioles are directly visible in the retina as linear hemorrhages dissecting along nerve fibers. The disruption of the arteriolar wall causes the obstruction of the vessel and ischemia downstream. In the retina this produces a cotton-wool spot that consists of swollen, ischemic axons. The aggregation of materials within the ischemic axons produces a nuclear-like structure termed the *cytoid body.* Hard exudates, which consist of lipid deposits located deep in the retina, are also a common finding. These fine, punctate, shiny lesions can be distinguished from cotton-wool spots, which are larger and have blurred edges and a more diffuse appearance.

Patients with malignant hypertension appear ill and often present with complaints of severe headache, blurred vision, dyspnea, and chest pain or with symptoms of uremia. Malignant hypertension is a medical emergency. If untreated, it may result in acute renal failure, severe cardiac decompensation, MI, hypertensive cerebral hemorrhage, or hypertensive encephalopathy.

The diagnosis of malignant hypertension cannot be made on the basis of BP readings alone. In addition to elevated BP, these patients must demonstrate evidence of acute end-organ damage as a result of the hypertension. The physical examination may reveal an enlarged left ventricle and rales at the lung bases. Marked retinal findings are often present, including linear hemorrhages and cotton-wool patches. Acute elevation of blood urea nitrogen (BUN) and serum creatinine or the presence of hematuria indicates involvement of the kidneys. Rarely the blood smear reveals red cell fragments, and fibrin degradation products are elevated, giving a clinical picture compatible with microangiopathic hemolytic anemia. Left ventricular hypertrophy and strain are usually seen on the electrocardiogram (ECG). The chest radiograph may reveal cardiomegaly and evidence of congestive heart failure.

The treatment of malignant hypertension consists of the judicious lowering of MAP to 25% of pretreatment levels over the initial minutes to hours of treatment, then toward 160/100 over 2 to 6 hours, avoiding excessive falls in pressure that may precipitate renal, cerebral, or coronary ischemia.[4,20,25]

As in the treatment of hypertensive encephalopathy, all patients with malignant hypertension should be hospitalized, and invasive BP monitoring may be preferable. An easily titratable agent is used, most often sodium nitroprusside, to avoid any episodes of hypotension.

Stroke Syndromes

Hypertension is often associated with stroke syndromes.[26] In most of these patients, elevated BP is the result of the physiologic response to the stroke itself and is not the immediate cause. About 85% of strokes are nonhemorrhagic, and most patients who have embolic or thrombotic strokes without an associated hemorrhage do not sustain substantially elevated BP. These patients have mild to moderate hypertension that has little effect on the clinical course. Again, in patients with longstanding hypertension, rapid reduction of the BP may further reduce cerebral blood flow and cause increased ischemia.

In most cases, antihypertensive therapy is unnecessary and may be harmful. An exception is stroke secondary to aortic dissection. Some have recommended careful antihypertensive treatment for patients with persistent, extreme elevations of BP after a stroke (e.g., diastolic pressure >140 or MAP >130 mm Hg), but data are lacking. The EP must consider BP in treatment of stroke patients with systemic reperfusion therapy. Significant elevations of BP greatly increase the risk of secondary intracranial hemorrhage (ICH) with reperfusion therapy.[23] Patients with persistent pressures greater than 185/110 should not receive thrombolytic therapy.

Patients with ICH often have a profound, reactive elevation of BP. In most patients with ICH, hypertension is transitory and is secondary to the increased intracranial pressure (ICP) and to irritation of the autonomic nervous system. This type of hypertension often disappears rapidly and has little effect on clinical outcome. Data to support the pharmacologic lowering of BP in patients with ICH are lacking.[26] Persistent hypertension is associated with a poorer functional outcome after ICH, and traditionally, many centers treat hypertension after ICH. Because cerebral perfusion pressure (CPP) depends on systemic pressure, this practice may not be beneficial. Deterioration in most patients with ICH results from hemorrhagic enlargement or edema. Although no conclusive evidence indicates that treating hypertension in the acute period after ICH is beneficial, modest reductions in BP (e.g., 20% reduction in MAP) have not been clearly associated with a worse outcome.

If BP reduction is pursued in these patients, vasodilating agents such as nitroprusside or nitroglycerin should *not* be the first-line agents. Vasodilators increase ICP, impair cerebrovascular reactivity to changes in carbon dioxide partial pressure (P_{CO_2}), and exacerbate any decrease in CPP for a given level of BP reduction. Labetalol is probably the agent of choice in this setting. Labetalol and the other adrenergic blockers shift cerebral autoregulation to lower pressures in patients with intracranial mass lesions. This shift preserves cerebral blood flow at lower pressures. Adrenergic blockers also preserve reactivity to P_{CO_2}.[26] ACE inhibitors also shift autoregulation but have not been extensively studied in patients with ICH or elevated ICP.

Pulmonary Edema

Most patients with congestive heart failure have some degree of increased peripheral vascular resistance (PVR) and resultant hypertension; this is a normal response. The degree of BP elevation is moderate and does not represent a medical emergency. When poorly controlled, however, longstanding hypertension produces myocardial hypertrophy, which continues until the hypertrophy can no longer overcome the increased PVR; then the left ventricle begins to fail and dilates.

In most patients with this combination the hypertension results from increased PVR caused by elevated catecholamines associated with the stress of pulmonary edema. With standard treatment of pulmonary edema, including morphine, nitrates, oxygen, and furosemide, catecholamine levels fall and BP returns rapidly toward normal. In a small number of patients, pulmonary edema results from an abrupt, severe elevation of BP that precipitates acute left ventricular failure. The BP must be lowered to reverse this process. Nitroglycerin is usually the first drug used, but if it does not adequately reduce BP, nitroprusside should be the next choice. Nitroprusside does not cause sodium retention; it improves cardiac function, especially in the failing heart, and can be carefully titrated and rapidly reversed. ACE inhibition has also been used successfully as an adjunct in the acute treatment of pulmonary edema.[27,28] Although pressure often falls significantly with treatment of congestive heart failure, stroke syndromes can occur as a consequence of hypotension occurring during the treatment of acute pulmonary edema.[29]

Cardiac Ischemia

Hypertension and angina are often found together. If severe hypertension is present with concurrent angina, immediate lowering of BP is indicated to prevent myocardial damage. In most of these patients, nitroglycerin is the agent of choice. Patients with extremely elevated BP generally do not have adequate pressure reduction with nitrate therapy alone and may require the addition of a β-blocker. ACE inhibitors may be a useful adjunct and have also been shown to reduce mortality in patients with MI. Calcium channel blockers may be a useful alternative for patients unable to tolerate β-adrenergic blockade because of bronchospasm. Nitroprusside may induce a reflex tachycardia and must be used with caution in patients with cardiac ischemia. When considering systemic reperfusion therapy for MI, the same considerations apply regarding the risk of ICH as with stroke, and BP should be aggressively controlled.[30]

Renal Failure

The most important cardiovascular complication of chronic renal failure (CRF) is hypertension.[31,32] Uncontrolled hypertension accelerates the development of cardiovascular problems, which are the most common cause of death in both dialysis and transplant patients. Hypertension also causes further damage to diseased kidneys. Hypertension may appear at any time during the course of CRF and occurs in more than 80% of patients with advanced renal failure. Glomerular disease is associated with a higher incidence of hypertension than is tubulointerstitial disease. In the absence of hypertension, CRF worsens more slowly, and if hypertension is present but controlled, the progression of CRF can be delayed. Patients with renal failure secondary to malignant hypertension often demonstrate a transient worsening of renal function during their initial treatment period. After this initial period, renal function will improve.

The primary cause of hypertension for patients with CRF is an actual or relative increase in extracellular volume secondary to sodium retention, as well as activation of the renin-angiotensin system in diseased kidneys. Glomerular disease is associated with greater sodium retention than is tubulointerstitial disease. Diuretics to improve fluid balance and ACE inhibitors or calcium channel blockers should be the first-line agents to control hypertension in patients with renal failure.[33] Patients with CRF are frequently seen in the ED. If their BP is significantly elevated, the managing physician should be contacted and the antihypertensive regimen adjusted.

Severe elevation of BP may lead to acute renal failure or may exacerbate CRF. This requires immediate reduction of BP. Nitroprusside is the drug of choice, although the IV calcium channel blocker nicardipine is a reasonable alternative.[22]

Pregnancy

Hypertension is one of the most common complications of pregnancy, involving 5% to 10% of all pregnancies at some time during gestation (see Chapters 173 and 174). Antihypertensive agents may be needed but in most patients can be delayed until hospital admission. The exceptions are those women with severe preeclampsia or eclampsia, both of which represent hypertensive emergencies and can occur without an extreme elevation of BP. Any acute elevation of the diastolic BP above 100 mm Hg in the pregnant patient represents a true hypertensive emergency. The treatment of hypertensive emergencies of pregnancy should include reduction of BP, prevention and control of seizures, and early obstetric consultation. Although it may cause tachycardia and hypotension, the antihypertensive agent of choice in preeclampsia has classically been IV hydralazine.[34] Alternative antihypertensives include labetalol, nicardipine, and occasionally nitroprusside. Nitroprusside is relatively contraindicated because of the potential for accumulation of cyanide in utero. Because of this potential complication, nitroprusside should be reserved for those patients in whom other agents have failed.

Aortic Dissection

Aortic dissection is associated with a history of hypertension (see Chapter 80). Medical therapy consists of reducing BP to limit the extent of the dissection. The goals of medical therapy are to lower the BP to a systolic level of 100 to 120 mm Hg and to reduce the ejection force of the heart; using a vasodilator as a single agent is therefore contraindicated. The drugs of choice for reducing BP in patients with aortic dissection are a β-blocker to control tachycardia and a vasodilator such as nicardipine, nitroprusside, or fenoldopam. The ganglionic blocker trimethaphan camsylate (Arfonad) and the combined α/β-blocker labetalol have been used successfully in these patients.[20,22]

MANAGEMENT

Vasodilators

Sodium Nitroprusside Nitroprusside (Nipride, Nitropress) is a powerful vasodilator, with a direct effect on the smooth muscle of both resistance and capacitance vessels. Nitroprusside is considered the agent of choice for most hypertensive emergencies (Table 79-2). Its rate of onset is extremely rapid, and its duration of action is very short. Nitroprusside does not worsen angina. The cardiac response depends on the state of myocardial function. Because of the reduction of preload by venous dilation, the cardiac output often improves if congestive heart failure or borderline myocardial function is present. Because nitroprusside is a cerebral vasodilator, it may increase ICP secondary to increased cerebral blood flow. Nitroprusside is metabolized to thiocyanate and is excreted slowly by the kidneys. Cyanide is an intermediate metabolite, but cyanide toxicity is extremely rare. In the presence of renal failure or during prolonged nitroprusside therapy, the thiocyanate concentration may

Table 79-2. Drugs Used in Treatment of Hypertensive Emergencies

Emergency	Drug(s) of choice	Alternative or second-line drug(s)
Accelerated hypertension, hypertensive encephalopathy	Nitroprusside, fenoldopam	Labetalol, nicardipine
Intracranial hemorrhage	Labetalol	Nitroprusside, nicardipine
Acute pulmonary edema	Nitroglycerin, nitroprusside	Fenoldopam, ACE inhibitor
Cardiac ischemia	Nitroglycerin, β-blockers	Nitroprusside, labetalol
Aortic dissection	Nitroprusside + β-blockers	Labetalol, trimethaphan
Adrenergic crises	Phentolamine; nitroprusside + β-blockers	Labetalol
Eclampsia, preeclampsia	Labetalol	Nicardipine, hydralazine

reach toxic levels of 10 mg/dl, and a clinical picture of weakness, hypoxia, nausea, tinnitus, muscle spasm, disorientation, and psychosis may develop. The prolonged use of nitroprusside may produce hypothyroidism by inhibition of iodine transport, and methemoglobinemia has occurred.

Nitroprusside must be used as an IV solution. As capacitance vessels dilate, the patient must be kept recumbent to prevent profound orthostatic hypotension. Because of nitroprusside's short half-life, stopping the infusion returns the BP to pretreatment levels within 1 to 10 minutes. The amount of BP reduction is dose related. Elderly patients and those receiving antihypertensive medications are more sensitive to nitroprusside's effects. In all patients the starting dose should be 0.25 to 1.0 μg/kg body weight/min. The average dose required for the control of hypertension is 3.0 μg/kg/min. Dosages greater than 800 μg/min are seldom required and should not be used for long periods because of the accumulation of cyanide and thiocyanate. Patients treated with nitroprusside should be admitted to the intensive care unit (ICU) for close monitoring of BP, preferably by an intraarterial line. The drug should be diluted and given by an automatic infusion device. Nitroprusside is unstable in ultraviolet light, and the IV bag should be wrapped in opaque material. Only fresh solutions of nitroprusside less than 4 hours old should be used.

No type of hypertension has been found to be refractory to nitroprusside, although certain patients may not have an adequate response. Side effects are directly related to excessive vasodilation and resultant hypotension and can be avoided by careful monitoring of BP and regulation of infusion rate. Extreme caution must be taken to avoid the extravasation of nitroprusside because local necrosis can be severe. Nitroprusside has not been proven to be safe during pregnancy and should be avoided because of the potential effect of thiocyanate on fetal thyroid tissue, the risk of cyanide poisoning to the fetus, and the possibility of fetal methemoglobinemia.

Fenoldopam Fenoldopam (Corlopam) is a peripheral dopamine-1-receptor agonist approved for the treatment of hypertensive emergencies. Dopamine-1 receptors are located postsynaptically in the systemic and renal vasculature and mediate systemic, renal, and mesenteric vasodilation as well as natruresis. In contrast to treatment with nitroprusside, renal function in patients with malignant hypertension improves acutely with fenoldopam therapy.[35] Fenoldopam does not cross the blood-brain barrier, has a rapid onset of action, and has an elimination half-life of 9 minutes.[36-38] Reflex tachycardia, flushing, and headache may be observed but hypotension occurs less often than with nitroprusside therapy.

The initial dose of fenoldopam is 0.1 μg/kg/min, and the dose is titrated in 0.1 μg/kg/min increments every 15 minutes until the desired effect is seen. The maximum recommended dose is 1.6 μg/kg/min. Fenoldopam represents a reasonable alternative to nitroprusside in the treatment of hypertensive emergencies without the concerns of light sensitivity and cyanide or thiocyanate toxicity and with a lower incidence of hypotensive episodes.

Nitroglycerin Nitroglycerin is a vasodilating agent that acts predominantly on the venous system, decreasing left ventricular end-diastolic pressure. At normal doses, nitroglycerin has little effect on arterial vascular tone and reduces BP by reducing preload and cardiac output. These effects may be undesirable in patients with impaired cerebral and renal perfusion. Nitroglycerin use should be limited to patients with cardiac ischemia or pulmonary edema. Nitroglycerin may be administered either sublingually or intravenously (IV). Care must be exercised in patients with right ventricular dysfunction to avoid hypotension, which may exacerbate cardiac ischemia.

Hydralazine Hydralazine (Apresoline) is a direct arteriolar vasodilator that was widely used in the past for the treatment of hypertensive emergencies of pregnancy. Recent studies, however, have shown that nicardipine and labetalol are superior agents in this setting.[39] The usual starting dose of hydralazine is 5 mg IV, with repeat doses of 5 to 10 mg every 20 minutes as needed to keep the diastolic pressure below 110 mm Hg. Typically a latent period of 5 to 15 minutes is followed by a progressive and at times precipitous fall in BP lasting for up to 12 hours.[22] Hydralazine is also associated with significant reflex tachycardia, which may provoke angina in patients with coronary artery disease. Other common side effects are flushing, nausea, and headache. Chronic use is associated with a lupuslike syndrome that usually resolves with discontinuation of the medication.

β-Blockers

Labetalol Labetalol (Trandate, Normodyne) is a selective α_1-blocker and nonselective β-blocker with a ratio of α/β-blockade between 1:3 and 1:7. It can be given orally or IV. Labetalol lowers BP by blockade of the α_1-receptors in vascular smooth muscle and the cardiac β-receptors. Because of the simultaneous β-receptor blockade, the usual reflex tachycardia associated with vasodilators does not occur. Labetalol does not cause the significant drop in cardiac output associated with other β-blockers. Although the oral administration of labetalol is less likely to produce orthostatic hypotension, IV use is marked by profound orthostatic changes. After IV labetalol the patient should be kept in the supine position for several hours. Labetalol does not affect cerebral blood flow or renal function.[22,26] With IV labetalol, BP generally falls within 5 to 10 minutes, with maximum effect in 30 minutes.

The initial dose of labetalol is 20 mg infused over 2 minutes. The BP should be rechecked every 5 minutes, and if only minimal change occurs, an additional dose is given every 10 minutes in increments of 20, 40, or 80 mg, to a total of 300 mg of labetalol, depending on BP response. Alternatively, after the initial loading dose an infusion may be started at 1 to 2 mg/min and titrated upward.[40,41] When given in this manner, labetalol appears to be a safe agent, with minimal adverse reactions. Because labetalol is a β-blocker, it is contraindicated in patients with congestive heart failure, heart block, and asthma. Labetalol also appears to be contraindicated for treatment of hypertension secondary to pheochromocytoma because it may result in paradoxical hypertension.

Labetalol therapy cannot be as closely controlled or as quickly reversed as nitroprusside therapy. However, use of labetalol may not require admission to an ICU. Labetalol does not appear to exacerbate coronary artery disease or cause uncontrolled drops in BP.

The transition to oral therapy is smooth. After initial control of BP with IV labetalol, oral labetalol should be started when diastolic pressure rises 10 mm Hg. Labetalol is an excellent alternative to nitroprusside when constant BP monitoring is not feasible. Labetalol is superior as a single agent in patients who have aortic dissection or cardiac ischemia with intact left ventricular function.

Esmolol Esmolol (Brevibloc) is an ultrashort-acting, selective β_1-blocker without intrinsic sympathomimetic activity. It typically has little effect on BP in normal individuals but may be very useful to control the reflex tachycardia seen with vasodilating agents such as nitroprusside. Esmolol is initiated with a loading dose of 500 μg/kg over 1 minute, followed by an infusion of 50 to 100 μg/kg/min. Maximal effect occurs in 5 minutes. If necessary, the patient receives another bolus of 500 μg/kg, and the drip is increased by 50 μg/kg/min. This cycle may be repeated every 5 minutes until the desired heart rate response is seen, up to a maximum dose of 300 μg/kg/min. The elimination half-life of esmolol is 9 minutes, so any effect will resolve within 30 minutes of discontinuing the infusion, with substantial recovery from β-blockade in 10 to 20 minutes. Contraindications are similar to those with labetalol, including cocaine overdose, pheochromocytoma, congestive heart failure, heart block, and reactive airway disease. Esmolol also causes tissue necrosis when extravasated into the soft tissue and may cause thrombophlebitis when infused into small veins.

α-Blockers

Phentolamine (Regitine) is an α-blocking agent used for the management of catecholamine-induced hypertensive crises (e.g., pheochromocytoma, MAOI crisis, cocaine overdose). Phentolamine is usually given IV in 1-mg to 5-mg boluses, although it may be given as an infusion at a rate of 5 to 10 μg/kg/min.[22,25] The effect is immediate and may last up to 15 minutes. Reflex tachycardia may be seen. Once the BP is under control, oral *phenoxybenzamine,* a long-acting α-blocker, may be used.

Ganglionic Blocker

Trimethaphan (Arfonad) is a nondepolarizing cholinergic blocking agent that acts at both the sympathetic and the parasympathetic ganglia. This blockade interrupts the adrenergic control of arterioles, resulting in vasodilation, improved blood flow to some vascular beds, and decreased BP. The therapeutic effect of trimethaphan is limited by the rapid development of decreasing responsiveness, or tachyphylaxis. Side effects include bladder atony, ileus, gastric atony, cycloplegia, and severe postural hypotension from blockade of circulatory reflex pathways. The heart rate may rise in response to the decrease in peripheral resistance. When trimethaphan is used in hypertensive patients, cardiac output, stroke volume, and left ventricular work decrease. Its effect on the blood flow to different tissues is variable.

Trimethaphan is given by an IV drip at the rate of 0.3 to 3 mg/min. This agent has a rapid onset of action, and its effects are of short duration. Trimethaphan is seldom used today for the treatment of hypertensive emergencies, although it was used in the past as a first-line agent for the treatment of aortic dissection (see Chapter 80).

Newer Agents

Nicardipine Nicardipine (Cardene) is a parenteral dihydropyridine calcium channel blocker that has become very popular in the treatment of postoperative hypertension. Nicardipine is titratable, is less negatively inotropic, and induces less tachycardia than nifedipine. Nicardipine acts predominantly as a vasodilator, but as with other calcium channel blockers, caution must be used when administered to patients with left ventricular failure. Nicardipine is administered as an infusion beginning at 5 mg/hr, increasing the infusion rate every 15 minutes until the desired reduction of BP has been achieved, to a maximum dose of 15 mg/hr. Onset of action is 5 to 15 minutes and duration of action 4 to 6 hours. As with labetalol, an oral form may facilitate the transition from acute to chronic therapy.

Nicardipine is heavily metabolized in the liver, so caution must be used in patients with cirrhosis. Nicardipine decreases the glomerular filtration rate in patients with compromised renal function, a trait shared by nitroprusside. Similar to the other vasodilators, headache, flushing, and tachycardia are the most common adverse reactions seen with nicardipine. Nicardipine has been best studied in pregnant patients and the settings of postoperative and malignant hypertension, where it appears to be a less toxic alternative to nitroprusside.[22,24]

Enalaprilat/Enalapril Enalaprilat (Vasotec) is a parenteral active metabolite of the ACE inhibitor enalapril. This drug has been studied in limited numbers of patients with true hypertensive emergencies. Hypotension has not been frequently reported with the use of enalaprilat, but caution should be used in patients who may be volume depleted. The acute dose is 0.625 to 5 mg administered as a single bolus. Peak effects generally occur in 15 minutes but may be delayed for hours. The response is not dose related, and one study showed an average drop in MAP of 35% at all doses and a 60% response rate.[43] Although no adverse effects were seen in the study, which excluded patients older than 80 and with known renovascular disease, such a significant drop in MAP might exceed the limits of vascular autoregulation in some patients. In fact, azotemia has been reported among older patients in studies of ACE inhibition after MI.[44]

Adverse effects that may be seen with ACE inhibitors such as enalaprilat include idiopathic angioedema, cough, and renal failure. Renal failure has been classically described in patients with bilateral renovascular disease. ACE inhibitors are considered toxic in the first trimester of pregnancy.

HYPERTENSIVE URGENCIES

Elevated BP without evidence of progressive end-organ involvement rarely mandates urgent antihypertensive therapy.[4] These patients appear to do well with a gradual lowering of BP, without the inherent risks of cerebral and myocardial ischemia seen with acute reduction. It is unnecessary to lower BP acutely in patients with so-called hypertensive urgencies, and a growing body of literature suggests that this practice may actually cause increased risk to the patient.[45]

Patients with elevated BP who are asymptomatic or have nonspecific symptoms require an appropriate evaluation to rule out progressive end-organ disease, including a thorough history and physical examination paying special attention to the cardiovascular, funduscopic, and neurologic systems. Requisite laboratory testing includes a urinalysis to evaluate renal function and with an abnormality an electrolyte panel, BUN, and creatinine. A chest radiograph and ECG are obtained to evaluate any patient with chest pain or symptoms of cardiac dysfunction. If this initial evaluation fails to show any acute end-organ damage, the patient may be promptly

Table 79-3. Risk Stratification and Treatment*

Blood pressure stages (mm Hg)	Risk group A (no risk factors; no TOD/CCD)†	Risk group B (at least 1 risk factor, not including diabetes; no TOD/CCD)	Risk group C (TOD/CCD and/or diabetes, with or without other risk factors)
High-normal (130-139/85-89)	Lifestyle modification	Lifestyle modification	Drug therapy§
Stage 1 (140-159/90-99)	Lifestyle modification (up to 12 months)	Lifestyle modification‡ (up to 6 months)	Drug therapy
Stages 2 and 3 (≥160/≥100)	Drug therapy	Drug therapy	Drug therapy

For example, a patient with diabetes and a blood pressure of 142/94 mm Hg plus left ventricular hypertrophy should be classified as having stage 1 hypertension with target organ disease (left ventricular hypertrophy) and with another major risk factor (diabetes). This patient would be categorized as stage 1, risk group C, and recommended for immediate initiation of pharmacologic treatment.

Modified from the Sixth Report of the Joint National Committee on Prevention, Detection, Evaluation, and Treatment of High Blood Pressure, *Arch Intern Med* 157:2413, 1997.
*Lifestyle modification should be adjunctive therapy for all patients recommended for pharmacologic therapy.
†TOD/CCD, Target organ disease/clinical cardiovascular disease.
‡For patients with multiple risk factors, clinicians should consider drugs as initial therapy plus lifestyle modifications.
§For those with heart failure, renal insufficiency, or diabetes.

referred. In some patients it will be evident that ongoing chronic pharmacologic therapy is indicated, and the EP may initiate an appropriate oral regimen before follow-up. It is not generally necessary to document an acute change in BP before discharge.

In special situations (e.g., sympathomimetic overdose, clonidine or β-blocker withdrawal, postoperative hypertension) and in some patients with extremely elevated BP, the EP may choose to institute "urgent" therapy for patients without end-organ ischemia. Clonidine is probably the agent of choice, at an initial oral dose of 0.1 to 0.2 mg, with maximum effects after 60 minutes. If required, additional 0.1-mg doses of clonidine may be given hourly until the diastolic pressure is reduced either by no more than 20% from pretreatment levels or to a level of 110 mm Hg. The patient with chronic hypertension is then started on outpatient antihypertensive therapy with an appropriate agent.

Clonidine usually produces a smooth, predictable fall in BP. Sublingual captopril as well as oral and parenteral β-blockers have also been used in this setting. Whenever oral agents are used to lower BP acutely, patients should be observed until maximum effect has developed before any further treatment or discharge. Short-acting dihydropyridine calcium channel blockers should be avoided. If any evidence of progressive end-organ disease is present, hypertensive patients should be considered emergent and admitted to the hospital.

Ambulatory Treatment

In the ambulatory setting the decision to initiate pharmacologic therapy for well-documented hypertension is based on the degree of hypertension, the presence of other cardiovascular risk factors, or chronic target organ damage (Table 79-3). The treatment of hypertension on an outpatient basis is usually not the responsibility of the EP. This is a chronic problem, and once it is diagnosed, the patient must have a lifelong commitment to treatment. An established patient-physician relationship will greatly enhance the successful management of hypertension. Lack of patient adherence is the most common cause of treatment failure.

In certain situations, however, the EP may choose to initiate or substantially modify the outpatient treatment of hypertension by arranging appropriate follow-up and, if possible, discussing the treatment plan with the patient's physician. Patient education should be started and the importance of ongoing management stressed. Numerous agents are available for the treatment of hypertension (Table 79-4). Other available agents contain drugs from two or more drug classes. The initial agent should be easy to take, well tolerated, and affordable for the patient and should have good efficacy. Because these factors may vary from patient to patient, accurate prediction of results is impossible. Ideally, BP may be controlled with a single agent, although this may not be possible for all patients. The choice of initial therapy is primarily empiric, but general guidelines exist. Individuals with low levels of plasma renin do not respond to monotherapy with β-blockers or ACE inhibitors as do other patients. African-Americans tend to have low renin levels and have an excellent response to diuretic monotherapy. A similar profile occurs in older patients, and diuretics are a good initial choice. Other patients may merit a trial of diuretic monotherapy because it is well tolerated and inexpensive. β-blockers should probably be the second choice unless contraindicated.[4,8,46]

The best agent for uncomplicated hypertension remains unknown and is an object of intense study. For patients with other health problems, specific classes of drugs have been shown to be particularly beneficial; the comorbid conditions should guide antihypertensive therapy. For patients with intact left ventricular function and a history of MI, a β-blocker is the agent of choice. Based on evidence of increased mortality, such patients should not be treated with immediate-release dihydropyridine calcium channel blockers.[47] For patients with diabetes, ACE inhibitors have benefits with respect to the preservation of renal function beyond that seen with BP control alone. In diabetic patients, as well as in those with a history of left ventricular failure, an ACE inhibitor should be the drug of choice. Elderly patients with isolated systolic hypertension may benefit from the addition of a long-acting calcium channel blocker when diuretic monotherapy fails. Patients with prostatism or dyslipidemia may benefit from α-blocker therapy, although a recent report from a large prospective trial comparing the thiazide diuretic chlorthalidone with three other types of therapy showed an increased incidence of congestive heart failure and stroke in the group treated with the α-blocker doxazosin.[48]

Table 79-4. Antihypertensive Drugs

Drug	Trade name	Usual dose range (total mg/day and interval)	Common side effects and comments
Diuretics (common)			Short term: increases cholesterol and glucose levels; biochemical abnormalities: decreases potassium, sodium, and magnesium levels, increases uric acid and calcium levels; rare: blood dyscrasias, photosensitivity, pancreatitis, hyponatremia
Thiazides			
Chlorthalidone	Hygroton	12.5-50 qd	
Hydrochlorothiazide	HydroDiuril, Microzide, Esidrix	12.5-50 qd	
Indapamide	Lozol	1.25-5 qd	
Metolazone	Mykrox	0.5-1 (b-tid)	
	Zaroxolyn	2.5-10 (b-tid)	
Loop diuretics			
Bumetanide	Bumex	0.5-4 b-tid	
Ethacrynic acid	Edecrin	25-100 b-tid	
Furosemide	Lasix	40-240 b-tid	
Torsemide	Demadex	3-100 q-bid	
Potassium-sparing agents			Hyperkalemia may occur
Amiloride	Midamor	5-10 qd	
Spironolactone	Aldactone	25-100 qd	
Triamterene	Dyrenium	25-100 qd	
Adrenergic inhibitors			Postural hypotension
Peripheral agents			
Guanadrel	Hylorel	10-75 bid	
Guanethidine	Ismelin	10-150 qd	
Reserpine	Serpasil	0.05-0.25 qd	
Central α-agonists			Sedation, dry mouth, bradycardia, withdrawal hypertension
Clonidine	Catapres	0.2-1.2 b-tid	
Guanabenz	Wytensin	8-32 bid	
Guanfacine	Tenex	1-3 qd	
Methyldopa	Aldomet	500-3000 bid	Hepatitis, lupuslike syndrome
α-Blockers			Postural hypotension
Doxazosin	Cardura	1-16 qd	
Prazosin	Minipress	2-30 b-tid	
Terazosin	Hytrin	1-20 qd	
β-Blockers			Bronchospasm, bradycardia, heart failure, may mask insulin-induced hypoglycemia; less serious: impaired peripheral circulation, insomnia, fatigue, decreased exercise tolerance, hypertriglyceridemia (except agents with intrinsic sympathomimetic activity)
Acebutolol[1,2]	Sectral	200-800 qd	
Atenolol[1]	Tenormin	25-100 q-bid	
Betaxolol[1]	Kerlone	5-20 qd	
Bisoprolol[1]	Zebeta	2.5-10 qd	[1]β_1-selective
Carteolol[2]	Cartrol	2.5-10 qd	[2]Intrinsic sympathomimetic activity
Metoprolol tartrate[1]	Lopressor	50-300 bid	
Metoprolol succinate[1]	Toprol XL	50-300 qd	
Nadolol	Corgard	40-320 qd	
Penbutolol[2]	Levatol	10-20 qd	
Pindolol[2]	Visken	10-60 bid	
Propranolol	Inderal	40-480 bid	
	Inderal LA	40-480 qd	
Timolol	Blocadren	20-60 bid	

Table 79-4. Antihypertensive Drugs—cont'd

Drug	Trade name	Usual dose range (total mg/day and interval)	Common side effects and comments
Combined α- and β-blockers			Postural hypotension, bronchospasm
Carvedilol	Coreg	12.5-50 bid	
Labetalol	Normodyne, Trandate	200-1200 bid	
Direct vasodilators			Headaches, fluid retention, tachycardia
Hydralazine	Apresoline	50-300 bid	Lupuslike syndrome
Minoxidil	Loniten	5-100 qd	Hirsutism
Calcium antagonists			Conduction defects, worsening of systolic dysfunction, gingival hypertrophy
Nondihydropyridines			
Diltiazem	Cardizem SR	50-300 bid	
	Cardizem CD, Dilacor XR, Tiazac	5-100 qd	
Verapamil	Isoptin SR, Calan SR	90-480 bid	Constipation
	Verelan, Covera HS	120-480 qd	
Dihydropyridines			Pedal edema, flushing, headache, gingival hypertrophy
Amlodipine	Norvasc	2.5-10 qd	
Felodipine	Plendil	2.5-20 qd	
Isradipine	DynaCirc	5-20 bid	
Nicardipine	DynaCirc CR	5-20 qd	
	Cardene SR	60-90 bid	
Nifedipine	Procardia XL, Adalat CC	30-120 qd	
Nisoldipine	Sular	20-60 qd	
ACE inhibitors			Common: cough; rare: angioedema, hyperkalemia, rash, loss of taste, leukopenia
Benazepril	Lotensin	5-40 q-bid	
Captopril	Capoten	25-150 b-tid	
Enalapril/enalaprilat	Vasotec	5-40 q-bid	
Fosinopril	Monopril	10-40 q-bid	
Lisinopril	Prinivil, Zestril	5-40 qd	
Moexipril	Univasc	7.5-15 q-bid	
Quinapril	Accupril	5-80 q-bid	
Ramipril	Altace	1.25-20 q-bid	
Trandolapril	Mavik	1-4 qd	
Angiotensin II receptor blockers			Angioedema (very rare), hyperkalemia
Irbesartan	Avapro	150-300 qd	
Losartan	Cozaar	25-100 q-bid	
Valsartan	Diovan	80-320 qd	

Mild or Transient Hypertension

A vast percentage of the hypertension encountered in the ED is either transient or mild. The most common causes of transient hypertension are pain and anxiety. In these patients, end-organ ischemia is highly unlikely, and treatment of the primary process results in prompt resolution of their acute hypertension. For this reason, all patients without evident complications should be allowed to rest for 60 minutes and have their pressure reassessed. Most patients, even those with poorly treated chronic hypertension, will show an improvement in their BP with watchful waiting.[3] During this period of observation, a search for acute end-organ ischemia may be undertaken. Definitive diagnosis of hypertension is rarely if ever made in the ED without acute or chronic evidence of target organ damage (e.g., retinopathy, left ventricular hypertrophy, nephropathy). For patients with mild to moderate elevation of BP, a diagnosis of hypertension should not be made until three consecutive elevated readings are obtained. This diagnosis may have a profound effect on the patient's life, especially with regard to employment, insurability, and general sense of well-being. Patients with mild or transient hypertension rarely require specific intervention beyond close follow-up.

KEY CONCEPTS

- The presence or absence of acute target organ damage determines whether a hypertensive emergency exists.
- All patients with persistent elevations in blood pressure should be carefully evaluated for the presence of acute end-organ ischemia.
- The EP should be familiar with the agents of choice in specific hypertensive emergencies.
- The therapeutic goal for treatment of the majority of hypertensive emergencies is careful reduction of the blood pressure with a titratable agent. Mean arterial pressure should be reduced by no more than 20% to 25% over minutes to hours. The diastolic pressure generally should not fall below 100 to 110 mm Hg. The exceptions to these rules may be patients with hypertensive complications of pregnancy, hypertensive emergencies of the pediatric population, and patients with aortic dissection.
- Patients without acute end-organ ischemia rarely require urgent management of their blood pressure and may be safely referred for close follow-up.

REFERENCES

1. Burt V et al: Prevalence of hypertension in the U.S. adult population: results from the Third National Health and Nutrition Examination Survey, 1988-1991, *Hypertension* 25:303, 1995.
2. Chiang WEA: Asymptomatic hypertension in the ED, *Am J Emerg Med* 16:1701, 1998.
3. Pitts SR: Emergency department hypertension and regression to the mean, *Ann Emerg Med* 31:214, 1998.
4. Sixth Report of the Joint National Committee on Prevention, Detection, Evaluation, and Treatment of High Blood Pressure, *Arch Intern Med* 157:2413, 1997.
5. Kannel WB, Schwartz MJ, McNamara PM: Blood pressure and risk of coronary heart disease: the Framingham study, *Dis Chest* 56:43, 1969.
6. Cushman WC: The clinical significance of systolic hypertension, *Am J Hypertens* 11:182S, 1998.
7. He J, Whelton PK: Elevated systolic blood pressure and risk of cardiovascular and renal disease: overview of evidence from observational epidemiologic studies and randomized controlled trials, *Am Heart J* 138:211, 1999.
8. Abate G et al: Treatment of hypertension in the elderly, *Cardiologia* 44:427, 1999.
9. Bartosh SM: Childhood hypertension: an update on etiology, diagnosis, and treatment, *Pediatr Clin North Am* 46:235, 1999.
10. Kornitzer M, Dramaix M, De Backer G: Epidemiology of risk factors for hypertension: implications for prevention and therapy, *Drugs* 57: 695, 1999.
11. Triggle DJ: The pharmacology of ion channels: with particular reference to voltage-gated Ca^{2+} channels, *Eur J Pharmacol* 375:311, 1999.
12. Allikmets K, Parik T, Viigimaa M: The renin-angiotensin system in essential hypertension: associations with cardiovascular risk, *Blood Press* 8:70, 1999.
13. Brown NJ, Vaughan DE: Angiotensin-converting enzyme inhibitors, *Circulation* 97:1411, 1998.
14. Youngberg SP, Sheps SG, Strong CG: Fibromuscular disease of the renal arteries, *Med Clin North Am* 61:623, 1977.
15. Kloner RA, Friedewald VE Jr: Case 6: renovascular hypertension, *Am J Cardiol* 86:368, 2000.
16. Cheitlin MD: Coarctation of the aorta, *Med Clin North Am* 61:655, 1977.
17. Lipke DW et al: Coarctation induces alterations in basement membranes in the cardiovascular system, *Hypertension* 22:743, 1993.
18. Graves JW: Management of difficult to control hypertension, *Mayo Clinic Proc* 75:278, 2000.
19. Geyskes GG, Boer P, Dorhout Mees EJ: Clonidine withdrawal: mechanism and frequency of rebound hypertension, *Br J Clin Pharmacol* 7:55, 1979.
20. Kitiyakara C, Guzman NJ: Malignant hypertension and hypertensive emergencies, *J Am Soc Nephrol* 9:133, 1998.
21. Barry DI: Cerebrovascular aspects of antihypertensive treatment, *Am J Cardiol* 63:14C, 1989.
22. Varon J, Marik P: The diagnosis and management of hypertensive crises, *Chest* 118:214, 2000.
23. American Heart Association, International Liaison Committee on Resuscitation: Guidelines 2000 for cardiopulmonary resuscitation and emergency cardiovascular care. Part 7. The era of reperfusion. Section 2. Acute stroke, *Circulation* 102(suppl 8):I204, 2000.
24. Grossman E et al: Should a moratorium be placed on sublingual nifedipine capsules given for hypertensive emergencies and pseudo-emergencies? *JAMA* 276:1328, 1996.
25. Vaughan CJ, Delanty N: Hypertensive emergencies, *Lancet* 356:411, 2000.
26. Adams RE, Powers WJ: Management of hypertension in acute intracerebral hemorrhage, *Crit Care Clin* 13:131, 1997.
27. Hamilton RJ, Carter WA, Gallagher EJ: Rapid improvement of acute pulmonary edema with sublingual captopril, *Acad Emerg Med* 3:205, 1996.
28. Sacchetti AR et al: ICU use in acute pulmonary edema: does ED management matter? *Ann Emerg Med* 30:430, 1997.
29. Hoshide S et al: Hemodynamic cerebral infarction triggered by excessive blood pressure reduction in hypertensive emergencies, *J Am Geriatr Soc* 46:1179, 1998 (letter).
30. American Heart Association, International Liaison Committee on Resuscitation: Guidelines 2000 for cardiopulmonary resuscitation and emergency cardiovascular care. Part 7. The era of reperfusion. Section 1. Acute coronary syndromes (acute myocardial infarction), *Circulation* 102(suppl 8):I172, 2000.
31. Zanchetti A: Impact of hypertension and antihypertensive treatment on organ damage, *Am J Cardiol* 84:18K, 1999.
32. Salvetti A, Mattei P, Sudano I: Renal protection and antihypertensive drugs: current status, *Drugs* 57:665, 1999.
33. McCarthy JT: A practical approach to the management of patients with chronic renal failure, *Mayo Clin Proc* 74:269, 1999.
34. Hypertension in pregnancy, *J Am Soc Nephrol* 9:314, 1998.
35. Shusterman NH, Elliott WJ, White WB: Fenoldopam, but not nitroprusside, improves renal function in severely hypertensive patients with impaired renal function, *Am J Med* 95:161, 1993.
36. Oparil S et al: Fenoldopam: a new parenteral antihypertensive: consensus roundtable on the management of perioperative hypertension and hypertensive crises, *Am J Hypertens* 12:653, 1999.

37. Panacek EA, Fenoldopam Study Group: Randomized, prospective trial of fenoldopam vs. sodium nitroprusside in the treatment of acute severe hypertension, *Acad Emerg Med* 2:959, 1995.
38. Post JB, Frishman WH: Fenoldopam: a new dopamine agonist for the treatment of hypertensive urgencies and emergencies, *J Clin Pharmacol* 38:2, 1998.
39. Walker JJ: Severe pre-eclampsia and eclampsia, *Baillieres Clin Obstet Gynaecol* 14:57, 2000.
40. Lebel M et al: Labetalol infusion in hypertensive emergencies, *Clin Pharmacol Ther* 37:615, 1985.
41. Cressman MD et al: Intravenous labetalol in the management of severe hypertension and hypertensive emergencies, *Am Heart J* 107:980, 1984.
42. Wallin JD et al: Intravenous nicardipine for the treatment of severe hypertension: a double-blind, placebo-controlled multicenter trial, *Arch Intern Med* 149:2662, 1989.
43. Hirschl MM et al: Clinical evaluation of different doses of intravenous enalaprilat in patients with hypertensive crises, *Arch Intern Med* 155:2217, 1995.
44. Swedberg K et al: Effects of the early administration of enalapril on mortality in patients with acute myocardial infarction: results of the Cooperative New Scandinavian Enalapril Survival Study II (CONSENSUS II), *N Engl J Med* 327:678, 1992.
45. Zeller KR, Von Kuhnert L, Matthews C: Rapid reduction of severe asymptomatic hypertension: a prospective, controlled trial, *Arch Intern Med* 149:2186, 1989.
46. Ramsay LE et al: The rationale for differing national recommendations for the treatment of hypertension, *Am J Hypertens* 11:79S, 1998.
47. Kostis JB et al: Association of calcium channel blocker use with increased rate of acute myocardial infarction in patients with left ventricular dysfunction, *Am Heart J* 133:550, 1997.
48. ALLHAT Collaborative Research Group: Major cardiovascular events in hypertensive patients randomized to doxazosin vs. chlorthalidone: the Antihypertensive and Lipid-Lowering Treatment to Prevent Heart Attack Trial (ALLHAT), *JAMA* 283:1967, 2000.

80 Aortic Dissection

Felix Ankel

PERSPECTIVE

Aortic dissection is a longitudinal cleavage of the aortic media created by a dissecting column of blood. The term "dissecting aortic aneurysm" has been inaccurately applied to this entity since 1819, when Laennec first used the term *aneurysme dissequant.* The term *aortic dissection* is preferred to dissecting aortic aneurysm because the affected aorta is infrequently aneurysmal.[1] In 1955, DeBakey outlined the principles that remain the basis for the surgical treatment of this entity. Medical treatment of aortic dissection was first advocated in the 1960s and is indicated for certain types of dissections.

Epidemiology

Aortic dissection occurs more often in men and increases with age.[2-7] The incidence and prevalence are difficult to determine because of underreporting of this condition.[8] Mortality is 1 to 5 per 100,000 population per year.[6,7] Hypertension is the most common risk factor associated with aortic dissection and is seen in most patients.[2-5,9] A history of cardiac surgery is present in about 18%[2] and a bicuspid aortic valve in 14% of all patients with aortic dissections, but more often in proximal dissections.[9,10] Atherosclerosis is rarely involved at the site of dissection.[10]

Aortic dissection is uncommon before age 40 except in association with congenital heart disease, Ehlers-Danlos or Marfan syndrome, giant cell arteritis,[11] and possibly pregnancy.[12] As many as 44% of patients with Marfan syndrome develop aortic dissection and account for 6% of such cases.[2,9,10] Women with Marfan syndrome are at particular risk during pregnancy.[13] Dissection also occurs with stimulant use[14] and trauma.[15] It may also be seen in patients who undergo cardiac surgery[2] or intraaortic balloon pump insertion.[16]

Blunt trauma from a high-speed deceleration injury usually causes traumatic aortic rupture, which is an entity distinct from aortic dissection.

PRINCIPLES OF DISEASE

Anatomy and Physiology

With each contraction, the heart swings side to side, resulting in flexion of both the ascending aorta and descending aorta. The descending aorta flexes just distal to the left subclavian artery, where the mobile aorta is tethered. At an average of 70 heartbeats per minute, this sequence occurs about 37 million times a year, causing a repetitive stress on the aorta.[17]

The aortic wall has three distinct layers: the intima, the media, and the adventitia. The *media* is comprised of elastic tissue and smooth muscle. Dissection occurs through a degeneration of the media characterized by loss of smooth muscle cells and elastic tissue, accompanied by scarring, fibrosis, and hyalin-like changes. Pathologic studies show that this process is neither cystic nor necrotic; therefore the term "cystic medial necrosis" is no longer used.[18,19]

Pathophysiology

Medial degeneration, previously thought to be specific for aortic dissection, is now considered to be part of normal aging, although it is augmented by hypertension and with aortic dissection. The anatomic differences between the "normal" aorta and a dissection are typically *quantitative* rather than qualitative.[18,19]

The repetitive hydrodynamic forces produced by the ejection of blood into the aorta with each cardiac cycle contribute to weakening of the aortic intima and worsening of medial degeneration. These hydrodynamic forces primarily affect the ascending aorta. Sustained hypertension intensifies these forces and results in an increase in medial degeneration. A bicuspid aortic valve may disrupt laminar flow and reorient the flow of blood toward the aortic wall, producing local injury. The hemodynamic changes that occur in pregnancy—increases in cardiac output, blood volume, and stroke output—may contribute to the increased incidence of aortic dissection. In Marfan and Ehlers-Danlos syndromes, normal hydrodynamic forces act on an aortic media that is already weakened.

As a result of medial degeneration and repeat flexion of the aorta, hydrodynamic stress tears the aortic intima, and a column of blood gains access into the aortic media. An alternate theory suggests that these forces damage the vasa vasorum of the aorta, which rupture and hemorrhage into the aortic media,[20] which explains the absence of an intimal tear in some cases of dissection.[10] Regardless of which of these theories is correct, the depth of penetration into the media and the distance and direction of dissection are at least partially determined by the degree of medial degeneration.

Once a dissecting hematoma is established in the media, migration of the hematoma occurs in an antegrade or retrograde fashion, or both, forming a "false lumen." The false lumen forms in the outer half of the media, and propagates until it ruptures back into the "true lumen" of the aorta, resulting in a rare "spontaneous cure," or out of the adventitia and into the pericardial sac or pleural cavity. Because the outer wall of the aorta that contains the hematoma is thin, rupture is much more likely to occur to the outside. The most important factors favoring continued dissection of the aorta are (1) the degree of elevation of blood pressure and (2) the steepness (slope) of the pulse wave (dP/dt). Both these hemodynamic factors must be controlled to halt migration of the hematoma.

Classification

Anatomic classification is important for diagnosis and therapy. The DeBakey and the Stanford classifications are both widely used. The *DeBakey classification* assigns aortic dissection into three types: type I dissections involve the ascending aorta, the aortic arch, and the descending aorta; type II dissections are confined to the ascending aorta; and type III dissections are confined to the descending aorta distal to the left subclavian artery. Type III can be subdivided into those that stay above the diaphragm (type IIIA) and those that propagate below it (type IIIB).

The *Stanford classification* is based on the involvement of the ascending aorta. Type A dissections involve the ascending aorta; type B dissections do not. Dissections that involve the ascending aorta are much more lethal than those limited to the distal aorta and have a different therapeutic approach. Type A dissections are more common than type B dissections.[2] Patients with distal dissections tend to be older, heavy smokers with chronic lung disease and more often with generalized atherosclerosis and hypertension compared with patients who have proximal aortic dissections.

A dissection is *acute* if less than 2 weeks in duration and *chronic* if present for more than 2 weeks. Approximately 75% of patients with untreated aortic dissection die within 2 weeks of the onset of symptoms.

CLINICAL FEATURES

History

Pain is by far the most common presenting complaint, affecting more than 90% of patients.[9] Most cases of painless aortic dissection are chronic in nature.[9] The pain is usually excruciating, occurs abruptly, is most severe at onset, and is typically described as "sharp"[2] more often than "tearing" or "ripping."[21]

The location of the pain may help localize the dissection. Anterior chest pain is associated with the ascending aorta, neck and jaw pain with the aortic arch, pain in the interscapular area with the descending thoracic aorta, and pain in the lumbar area or abdomen with involvement below the diaphragm. Migration of pain consistent with propagation of the dissection suggests aortic dissection but occurs in only 16% of cases.[2] The onset of aortic dissection is often accompanied by vasovagal symptoms, such as diaphoresis, nausea, vomiting, lightheadedness, and severe apprehension.

Syncope occurs early in aortic dissection in approximately 9% of cases and may be the sole presentation in some patients.[2] It most often heralds dissection into the pericardium, causing pericardial tamponade, but may occur from interruption of blood flow to the cerebral vasculature. Other causes of syncope secondary to aortic dissection are hypovolemia, excessive vagal tone, and cardiac conduction abnormalities. Neurologic symptoms such as focal weakness or change in mental status occur in up to 6% of cases.[2,9]

Physical Examination

Generally the patient appears apprehensive. Most of the patients have a history of chronic hypertension that may be exacerbated by a catecholamine release related to the acute event. Severe hypertension refractory to medical therapy may occur if the dissection involves the renal arteries with subsequent renin release. If hypotension is present, either the dissection has progressed back into the pericardium, with resulting pericardial tamponade, or hypovolemia has occurred from rupture through the adventitia. *Pseudohypotension,* a condition where the blood pressure in the arms is low or unobtainable and the central arterial pressure is normal or high, may be present. This results from the interruption of blood flow to the subclavian arteries.

Aortic regurgitation occurs in up to 31% of patients and is more common with type A dissections.[2,9] The murmur of aortic insufficiency may have a musical, vibrating quality with variable intensity, and congestive heart failure may develop. The patient with presumed aortic dissection should be examined carefully for findings that suggest hemorrhage into the pericardium or tamponade, such as jugular venous distention, muffled heart sounds, tachycardia, and hypotension.

When the integrity of one of the branches of the aorta is compromised, the expected ischemic findings occur. Pulse deficits and discrepancies in blood pressure between limbs can be helpful if present, occurring in up to 24% of patients with aortic dissection.[2,9,22] Usually these are present in the upper extremities and result from involvement of one or both of the subclavian arteries. Obstruction of one or both common iliac or superficial femoral arteries may produce pulse deficits in the lower extremities. Arterial obstruction may occur by either of two mechanisms. An intimal flap produced by the dissection may cover the true lumen of a branch vessel, or the dissecting hematoma may compress an adjacent true lumen. Frequent reexamination may detect transient pulse deficits.

Neurologic findings relate to the site of blood flow interruption. Proximal dissections are a more frequent cause of strokes (cerebrovascular accidents) or coma. Stroke treatment with thrombolytics in the patient with aortic dissection occurs rarely but can be fatal.[23] Distal dissections occluding the anterior spinal artery often cause ischemic paraparesis or ischemic peripheral neuropathy.[9]

In less than 1% of cases a proximal dissection can dissect into the ostium of a coronary artery, most frequently the right coronary artery, and can cause an acute myocardial infarction (MI), usually inferoposterior. Incorrect administration of thrombolytics in patients with aortic dissection occurs in about 0.1% to 0.2% of MIs.[24,25] Distal extension of aortic dissections into the abdomen can cause mesenteric ischemia, renal failure, femoral pulse deficits, and lower extremity ischemia.[22,26]

DIAGNOSTIC STRATEGIES

Routine laboratory tests are of little value in the diagnosis of aortic dissection. Unless massive hemorrhage has occurred, the hemoglobin is normal or only modestly reduced. The leukocyte count typically is mildly elevated.

Electrocardiography

The electrocardiogram (ECG) is often useful in excluding MI; however, many patients with aortic dissection may have ECG abnormalities suggesting ischemia.[2,27] Proximal dissections that involve the right coronary artery may show an inferior wall MI.[3] The ECG typically shows left ventricular hypertrophy, reflecting long-standing hypertension. Other findings include nonspecific ST-segment–T-wave changes and prior Q-wave infarction.[2,3]

Chest Radiography

Routine chest x-ray studies will be abnormal in 80% to 90% of patients, but the abnormalities are nonspecific and rarely diagnostic.[2,9] Mediastinal widening occurs in more than 75% of cases,[9] may occur in the ascending aorta, aortic arch, or the descending portion of the thoracic aorta, and may be difficult to differentiate from the aortic tortuosity that is associated with chronic hypertension. A plain chest radiograph is inadequate to rule out aortic dissection. Up to 12% of patients with aortic dissection have a normal chest film.[2]

The "calcium sign" is an uncommon radiographic manifestation of aortic dissection. Ordinarily, when intimal calcification is visible on a radiograph, it is butted up against the outer border of the aorta. With dissection of the aortic media, the calcium deposit becomes separated from the outermost portion of the aorta by more than 5 mm.

Other helpful radiographic signs include a double-density appearance of the aorta suggesting true and false channels, a localized bulge along a normally smooth aortic contour, a disparity in the caliber between the descending and ascending aorta, obliteration of the aortic knob, and displacement of the trachea or nasogastric tube to the right by the dissection. Previous chest radiographs, when available, are useful for comparison.

Echocardiography

Transthoracic echocardiography (TTE) has not been a useful tool in the detection and delineation of aortic dissection because wave transmission is hindered by overlying sternum, ribs, and lungs.[28] In an unstable patient, however, emergent bedside transthoracic ultrasonography can help determine whether cardiac tamponade is the cause of hypotension in a patient with aortic dissection.

Transesophageal echocardiography (TEE) has improved the quality of echocardiography in the diagnosis of aortic dissection.[29] The proximity of the esophagus to the aorta and the ability to use higher transducer frequencies help to better delineate the aorta. TEE is highly sensitive[30-32] but less specific[30] (Table 80-1). TEE is excellent at detecting pericardial effusion and aortic regurgitation.[30] TEE can be quickly performed at the patient's bedside under sedation or light anesthesia and requires no radiation or contrast injection. Evaluating the ascending aorta and proximal arch may be difficult because of the interposition of the air-filled trachea and left mainstem bronchus. Evaluation of this "blind spot" has been aided by biplanar and multiplanar probes.[32]

Table 80-1. Sensitivities and Specificities of Imaging Modalities for Diagnosing Aortic Dissection

Test	Sensitivity (%)	Specificity (%)
TEE	98	77
CT	94	87
MRI	98	98

Data from Nienaber CA: *N Engl J Med* 328:1, 1993.

The use of TEE is institution specific and is dependent on the experience and availability of the echocardiographer. It is the primary diagnostic method in many institutions for detecting aortic dissection[2] and is the procedure of choice in unstable patients.[33]

Computed Tomography

Computed tomography (CT) scan is a reliable test for diagnosing aortic dissection[30] (Table 80-1) and is the primary diagnostic test of choice in most institutions.[2] Findings suggestive of aortic dissection include dilation of the aorta, identification of an intimal flap, and the clear demonstration of both the false and the true lumina.[28] Dynamic scanning, in which rapid scans are obtained at multiple levels immediately after a bolus injection of intravenous (IV) contrast, improves the accuracy of the CT scan in the diagnosis of aortic dissection by allowing detection of differential filling rates in the true and false lumina.[34] Dynamic scanning performed with helical CT improves sensitivity and specificity.[35]

Aortography

Historically, aortography was the gold standard against which other modalities were measured. With the advent of TEE and CT scanning, however, aortography is rarely used as the initial diagnostic modality.[2] The findings of aortic dissection typically seen at angiography include (1) filling of a false channel or channels with or without an intervening intimal flap, (2) distortion of the true lumen by either a patent or a thrombosed false lumen, (3) thickening of the aortic wall by more than 5 to 6 mm from a thrombosed false lumen, and (4) displaced intimal calcification. Aortography is accurate for determining the site of the intimal tear and the extent of the dissection. Aortic regurgitation is easily demonstrated with aortography and demonstrates the extent and location of dissection into aortic side branches.

With the use of other diagnostic modalities, the sensitivity of aortography has been shown to be as low as 77%.[36] Misdiagnoses occur in one of several situations. The intimal flap may not be visualized when it is located in a plane tangential to the x-ray beam. Thrombosis of the false channel may prevent visualization of either the intimal flap or a double lumen. The true and false lumina may opacify simultaneously and therefore may not be clearly delineated from one another.

Magnetic Resonance Imaging

Magnetic resonance imaging (MRI) is an appealing option in the detection of aortic dissection.[37] Sensitivity and specificity are excellent[30,38] (see Table 80-1). The MRI scan shows the site of intimal tear, type and extent of dissection, presence of aortic insufficiency, and differential flow velocities in the true and false channels and in the aortic side branches. It requires no contrast media or ionizing radiation and is noninvasive. It is particularly useful in the evaluation of chronic aortic dissection, in the follow-up of postoperative patients, and for monitoring nonoperative patients for progression of the dissection.

Choice of Diagnostic Test

Although aortic dissection can be suspected on the basis of history and physical examination, diagnostic imaging is necessary to establish the diagnosis. The EP should have a clear and efficient imaging strategy.[39] The clinical services within the hospital involved in the diagnosis and treatment of patients with aortic dissection should prospectively agree on a strategy. This strategy should consider (1) the available technology at the institution, (2) the institution-specific sensitivities and specificities for the diagnostic tests, (3) the benefits of diagnosing nondissecting causes of chest pain, and (4) the ease of obtaining each test, especially "after hours." Some tests (e.g., CT, MRI, aortography) may require moving a potentially unstable patient outside of the care of the ED.

DIFFERENTIAL CONSIDERATIONS

The differential diagnosis for the patient with symptoms suggestive of aortic dissection is extensive. Signs and symptoms associated with aortic dissection are variable and depend on the extent of aortic and branch vessel involvement. Patients with the ultimate diagnosis of aortic dissection are often initially thought to have other conditions such as myocardial ischemia, congestive heart failure, or pulmonary embolus (PE).[3,9] Several clinical syndromes are particularly suggestive of aortic dissection: pain that progresses over hours or days from chest to neck to arms to abdomen, chest pain with concomitant neurologic deficits, and chest pain with pulse deficits.

Although chest pain is the most common symptom of aortic dissection, it is also the most common presenting complaint of at least three other serious and more common clinical entities: acute MI, PE, and pericarditis. An ECG can be helpful in excluding MI, although aortic dissection and MI may coexist as a result of the dissection proceeding retrograde down a coronary artery and causing infarction. In cases where aortic dissection is excluded, a CT scan may reveal other abnormalities that explain a patient's presentation (e.g., PE).[40] TEE is helpful in identifying alternate etiologies of chest pain other than aortic dissection (e.g., cardiac ischemia).[41]

When the initial presentation of the aortic dissection is pain or dysfunction in an extremity from disruption of the blood supply, peripheral neurologic diagnoses should be included in the differential diagnosis. An aortic dissection may involve the carotid artery, with the initial presentation mimicking a primary central nervous system lesion such as a stroke. The diagnosis of aortic dissection should be considered in any patient with a new diagnosis of pericardial effusion, pericardial tamponade, or aortic insufficiency.

Two other aortic conditions are closely related to aortic dissection: penetrating aortic ulcer[42] and intramural hemorrhage without an intimal flap.[43] Both groups of patients have similar clinical symptoms and management recommendations as patients with aortic dissection. *Penetrating atherosclerotic ulcers* of the aorta occur in older hypertensive patients with evidence of coronary artery disease.[42] CT shows a focal ulceration without dissection, most often in the distal descending aorta.[44] The progression of penetrating ulcers results in progressive aortic enlargement with saccular and fusiform aneurysm formation. An *intramural hemorrhage* is a contained hematoma within the aortic wall and occurs in about 10% of aortic dissections.[2] Rupture of the vasa vasorum is believed to be the initial event.[45]

MANAGEMENT

Emergency Department

Early therapy for aortic dissection is critical and should be initiated while diagnostic tests are being performed. Opioids should be administered in adequate amounts for pain control and to decrease sympathetic tone. Patients with aortic dissections typically are hypertensive. The two goals of medical management are to (1) reduce blood pressure and (2) decrease of the rate of the arterial pulse increase (dP/dt) to diminish shearing forces.[46] *Sodium nitroprusside* should be titrated to maintain the systolic blood pressure at 100 to 120 mm Hg or at the lowest level to maintain vital organ perfusion. Nitroprusside, 50 mg, is mixed in 500 ml of 5% dextrose in water (D5W) and initially infused at a rate of 0.3 to 5.0 μg/kg/min.

The use of beta-adrenergic blockers (β-blockers) is the cornerstone of aortic dissection management. Because nitroprusside increases the heart rate and may also increase the dP/dt, a β-blocker must be started before or in conjunction with sodium nitroprusside to lower the dP/dt. *Esmolol* is an ultrashort-acting β-blocker that is easily titrated. After mixing 5 g in 500 ml D5W, an initial bolus of 500 μg/kg is given, followed by an infusion of 50 to 200 μg/kg/min. *Labetalol* has both α-blocking and β-blocking activity and can be used as monotherapy. A suggested dose is an initial 20 mg IV bolus every 5 to 10 minutes, incrementally increased to 80 mg until a target heart rate has been reached or a total of 300 mg is given. A maintenance dose of labetalol is then given at 1 to 2 mg/hr. A target heart rate should be between 60 and 80 beats/min. If a patient is normotensive, a β-blocker should still be used to lower the dP/dt. In patients with a history of chronic obstructive pulmonary disease or at risk for bronchospasm, a selective β-blocker such as metoprolol or atenolol should be considered (see Chapter 79).

When contraindications to the use of β-blockers exist,

such as second-degree or third-degree heart block or congestive heart failure, an alternative can be used. *Trimethaphan* is mixed as a solution of 500 mg in 500 ml D5W and is infused at a rate of 1 to 2 mg/min. Trimethaphan is a ganglionic blocker that reduces both arterial pressure and its rate of increase, thus not requiring the use of concomitant β-blockade. It is more difficult, however, to titrate trimethaphan than to titrate nitroprusside, and tachyphylaxis frequently occurs after 24 to 48 hours.[46] Additionally, the frequency and severity of side effects (e.g., respiratory depression, nausea, urinary retention) limit the use of trimethaphan.

The calcium channel blocker *nifedipine* was used to treat aortic dissection but is no longer recommended. Nifedipine has minimal inotropic or chronotropic effects and may reflexively stimulate sympathetic activity and increase shear stress on the aortic wall.[46] IV *nitroglycerin* is often used initially in patients with hypertensive chest pain and suspected but uncertain aortic dissection. Nitroglycerin is a less effective arterial dilator than nitroprusside and less desirable than nitroprusside for the treatment of patients with aortic dissection.

Patients presenting with hypotension secondary to aortic rupture or pericardial tamponade should be resuscitated with IV fluids. Care should be taken that this hypotension is not a pseudohypotension caused by an intimal flap obstructing the extremity in which the blood pressure is measured. In patients with electromechanical dissociation or marked hypotension, the EP should consider pericardiocentesis to raise the blood pressure to the lowest acceptable level while awaiting definitive surgery.

Surgery

Type A acute aortic dissections require prompt surgical treatment.[8] The aortic segment containing the original intimal tear is resected when possible, with graft replacement of the ascending aorta to redirect blood into the true lumen. If aortic insufficiency is present, it can be corrected through aortic valve resuspension or replacement.

Definitive treatment of type B acute aortic dissections is less clear.[47] These patients in general tend to be worse surgical risks. Uncomplicated distal dissections have traditionally been treated with blood pressure control, and surgery has been reserved for those patients who have persistent pain, uncontrolled hypertension, occlusion of a major arterial trunk, frank aortic leaking or rupture, or development of a localized aneurysm. As surgical management for these patients improves, however, medical therapy may be replaced by operative treatment as the preferred definitive approach. Emergence of newer endovascular stenting techniques may also become more common in patients with distal dissections.[48-50]

DISPOSITION

Patients who present with chronic aortic dissection have already survived their period of greatest mortality risk and are usually treated by blood pressure control and close monitoring unless complications mandate surgery. All patients who have sustained and survived an aortic dissection, regardless of the type of definitive therapy used, require careful long-term management. Major complications that may occur with time are redissection, development of a localized aneurysm, and progressive aortic insufficiency.

KEY CONCEPTS

- Risks factors for aortic dissection include advanced age, hypertension, and connective tissue disorders such as Marfan or Ehlers-Danlos syndrome.
- Most patients with aortic dissection have chest pain, described as sudden onset, sharp, and migratory. Chest pain associated with neurologic symptoms or syncope should heighten the suspicion of aortic dissection.
- Physical examination findings may include pulse deficit, aortic insufficiency murmur, or neurologic findings.
- Diagnosis is difficult using only the history, physical examination, and chest radiograph. Computed tomography and transesophageal echocardiography are the confirmatory tests used most often.
- Treatment of type A proximal dissection is surgical. Treatment of uncomplicated type B distal dissection is usually medical, with a β-blocker and nitroprusside to control blood pressure and dP/dt shearing forces.

REFERENCES

1. Dmowski AT, Carey MJ: Aortic dissection, *Am J Emerg Med* 17:372, 1999.
2. Hagan PG et al: The International Registry of Acute Aortic Dissection (IRAD): new insights into an old disease, *JAMA* 283:897, 2000.
3. Sullivan PR et al: Diagnosis of acute thoracic aortic dissection in the emergency department, *Am J Emerg Med* 18:46, 2000.
4. Torossov M, Singh A, Fein SA: Clinical presentation, diagnosis, and hospital outcome of patients with documented aortic dissection: the Albany Medical Center experience, 1986 to 1996, *Am Heart J* 137:154, 1999.
5. Meszaros I et al: Epidemiology and clinicopathology of aortic dissection, *Chest* 117:1271, 2000.
6. Lilienfeld DE et al: Epidemiology of aortic aneurysms. I. Mortality trends in the United States, 1951 to 1981, *Arteriosclerosis* 7:637, 1987.
7. Johansson G, Markstrom U, Swedenborg J: Ruptured thoracic aortic aneurysms: a study of incidence and mortality rates, *J Vasc Surg* 21:985, 1995.
8. Kouchoukos NT, Dougenis D: Surgery of the thoracic aorta, *N Engl J Med* 336:1876, 1997.
9. Spittell PC et al: Clinical features and differential diagnosis of aortic dissection: experience with 236 cases (1980 through 1990), *Mayo Clin Proc* 68:642, 1993.
10. Larson EW, Edwards WD: Risk factors for aortic dissection: a necropsy study of 161 cases, *Am J Cardiol* 53:849, 1984.
11. Evans JM et al: Thoracic aortic aneurysm and rupture in giant cell arteritis: a descriptive study of 41 cases, *Arthritis Rheum* 37:1539, 1994.
12. Oskoui R, Lindsay JJ: Aortic dissection in women <40 years of age and the unimportance of pregnancy, *Am J Cardiol* 73:821, 1994.
13. Elkayam U et al: Cardiovascular problems in pregnant women with the Marfan syndrome, *Ann Intern Med* 123:117, 1995.
14. Swalwell CI, Davis GG: Methamphetamine as a risk factor for acute aortic dissection, *J Forensic Sci* 44:23, 1999.
15. Rogers FB, Osler TM, Shackford SR: Aortic dissection after trauma: case report and review of the literature, *J Trauma* 41:906, 1996.
16. Jacobs LE et al: Aortic dissection following intraaortic balloon insertion: recognition by transesophageal echocardiography, *Am Heart J* 124:536, 1992.
17. Wheat MW Jr: Fundamentals of clinical cardiology. Acute dissecting aneurysms of the aorta: diagnosis and treatment—1979, *Am Heart J* 99:373, 1980.
18. Schlatmann TJM, Becker AE: Histologic changes in the normal aging aorta: implications for dissecting aortic aneurysm, *Am J Cardiol* 39:13, 1977.
19. Schlatmann TJM, Becker AE: Pathogenesis of dissecting aneurysm of aorta: comparative histopathologic study of significance of medical changes, *Am J Cardiol* 39:21, 1977.
20. Lui RC, Menkis AH, McKenzie FN: Aortic dissection without intimal rupture: diagnosis and management, *Ann Thorac Surg* 53:886, 1992.

21. Wooley CF, Sparks EH, Boudoulas H: Aortic pain, *Prog Cardiovasc Dis* 40:563, 1998.
22. Fann JI et al: Treatment of patients with aortic dissection presenting with peripheral vascular complications, *Ann Surg* 212:705, 1990.
23. Fessler AJ, Alberts MJ: Stroke treatment with tissue plasminogen activator in the setting of aortic dissection, *Neurology* 54:1010, 2000.
24. European Myocardial Infarction Project Group: Prehospital thrombolytic therapy in patients with suspected myocardial infarction, *N Engl J Med* 329:383, 1993.
25. Kamp TJ et al: Myocardial infarction, aortic dissection, and thrombolytic therapy, *Am Heart J* 128:1234, 1994.
26. Pacifico L, Spodick D: ILEAD—ischemia of the lower extremities due to aortic dissection: the isolated presentation, *Clin Cardiol* 22:353, 1999.
27. Hirata K, Kyushima M, Asato H: Electrocardiographic abnormalities in patients with acute aortic dissection, *Am J Cardiol* 76:1207, 1995.
28. Cigarroa JE et al: Diagnostic imaging in the evaluation of suspected aortic dissection: old standards and new directions, *N Engl J Med* 328:35, 1993.
29. Willens HJ, Kessler KM: Transesophageal echocardiography in the diagnosis of diseases of the thoracic aorta. Part 1. Aortic dissection, aortic intramural hematoma, and penetrating atherosclerotic ulcer of the aorta, *Chest* 116:1772, 1999.
30. Nienaber CA et al: The diagnosis of thoracic aortic dissection by noninvasive imaging procedures, *N Engl J Med* 328:1, 1993.
31. Evangelista A et al: Diagnosis of ascending aortic dissection by transesophageal echocardiography: utility of M-mode in recognizing artifacts, *J Am Coll Cardiol* 27:102, 1996.
32. Keren A et al: Accuracy of biplane and multiplane transesophageal echocardiography in diagnosis of typical acute aortic dissection and intramural hematoma, *J Am Coll Cardiol* 28:627, 1996.
33. Rizzo RJ et al: Rapid noninvasive diagnosis and surgical repair of acute ascending aortic dissection: improved survival with less angiography, *J Thorac Cardiovasc Surg* 108:567, 1994.
34. Hamada S et al: Type A aortic dissection: evaluation with ultrafast CT, *Radiology* 183:155, 1992.
35. Sommer T et al: Aortic dissection: a comparative study of diagnosis with spiral CT, multiplanar transesophageal echocardiography, and MR imaging, *Radiology* 199:347, 1996.
36. Bansal RC et al: Frequency and explanation of false negative diagnosis of aortic dissection by aortography and transesophageal echocardiography, *J Am Coll Cardiol* 25:1393, 1995.
37. Fattori R, Nienaber CA: MRI of acute and chronic aortic pathology: pre-operative and postoperative evaluation, *J Magn Reson Imaging* 10:741, 1999.
38. Laissy JP et al: Thoracic aortic dissection: diagnosis with transesophageal echocardiography versus MR imaging, *Radiology* 194:331, 1995.
39. Sarasin FP et al: Detecting acute thoracic aortic dissection in the emergency department: time constraints and choice of the optimal diagnostic test, *Ann Emerg Med* 28:278, 1996.
40. Oliver TB, Murchison JT, Reid JH: Spiral CT in acute non-cardiac chest pain, *Clin Radiol* 54:38, 1999.
41. Armstrong WF et al: Clinical and echocardiographic findings in patients with suspected acute aortic dissection, *Am Heart J* 136:1051, 1998.
42. Harris JA et al: Penetrating atherosclerotic ulcers of the aorta, *J Vasc Surg* 19:90, 1994.
43. O'Gara PT, DeSanctis RW: Acute aortic dissection and its variants: toward a common diagnostic and therapeutic approach, *Circulation* 92:1376, 1995.
44. Kazerooni EA, Bree RL, Williams DM: Penetrating atherosclerotic ulcers of the descending thoracic aorta: evaluation with CT and distinction from aortic dissection, *Radiology* 183:759, 1992.
45. Mohr-Kahaly S et al: Aortic intramural hemorrhage visualized by transesophageal echocardiography: findings and prognostic implications, *J Am Coll Cardiol* 23:658, 1994.
46. Grossman E, Ironi AN, Messerli FH: Comparative tolerability profile of hypertensive crisis treatments, *Drug Saf* 19:99, 1998.
47. Elefteriades JA et al: Management of descending aortic dissection, *Ann Thorac Surg* 67:2002, 1999.
48. Nienaber CA et al: Nonsurgical reconstruction of thoracic aortic dissection by stent-graft placement, *N Engl J Med* 340:1539, 1999.
49. Dake MD et al: Endovascular stent-graft placement for the treatment of acute aortic dissection, *N Engl J Med* 340:1546, 1999.
50. Grabenwoger M et al: Thoracic aortic aneurysms: treatment with endovascular self-expandable stent grafts, *Ann Thorac Surg* 69:441, 2000.

81 Abdominal Aortic Aneurysm

Howard A. Bessen

PERSPECTIVE

Most abdominal aortic aneurysms (AAAs) are *true aneurysms.* A true aortic aneurysm is a localized dilation of the aorta caused by weakening of its wall; it involves all three layers (intima, media, and adventitia) of the arterial wall (Figure 81-1). AAAs should not be confused with *aortic dissections,* which are sometimes called "dissecting aortic aneurysms." In aortic dissections, blood enters the media of the aorta and splits (dissects) the aortic wall (see Chapter 80). True aortic aneurysms and aortic dissections are very different diseases, with different complications, clinical presentations, diagnostic methods, and treatments.

A *pseudoaneurysm* (false aneurysm) is a collection of flowing blood that communicates with the arterial lumen but is not enclosed by the normal vessel wall; it is contained only by the adventitia or surrounding soft tissue. Pseudoaneurysms can arise from a defect in the arterial wall, or a leaking anastomosis as a complication of AAA repair.

Aneurysms can develop in any segment of the aorta, but most involve the aorta below the renal arteries. The diameter of the normal adult infrarenal aorta is approximately 2 cm. The aorta is slightly larger in men than in women and enlarges gradually with increasing age.

An infrarenal aortic diameter of 3 cm or more can be used to define an AAA.[1] Rupture can occur once a diameter of 3 cm has been reached but almost never before then.[2,3]

Epidemiology

AAA is a disease of aging, and the prevalence of AAAs is expected to increase as the population of elderly patients grows. AAAs are rare before age 50 years but are found in 2% to 4% of the population older than 50.[3,4] The average age at

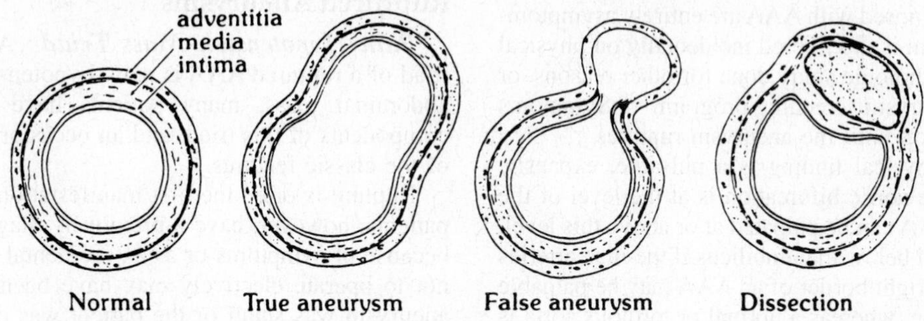

Figure 81-1. Types of aortic aneurysms. *Modified from LaRoy LL et al:* AJR Am J Roentgenol *152:785, 1989.*

Table 81-1. Prevalence of Abdominal Aortic Aneurysms in Selected Risk Groups

Group	Incidence (%)
Autopsy subjects aged 50 or older[3,4]	2-4
Men aged 65 or older[1,7]	5-10
Patients with occlusive peripheral vascular disease[8]	10-15
Brothers of patients with AAAs[9]	20-25
Patients with femoral or popliteal artery aneurysms[10,11]	35-40

the time of diagnosis is 65 to 70, and men are affected much more often than women.[5,6] The patient often has atherosclerotic occlusive disease that involves the coronary, carotid, or peripheral vessels, which may influence the clinical presentations, complications, and management.[5]

Certain groups are at greatest risk for AAAs (Table 81-1). An AAA can be found in 5% to 10% of elderly men who are screened with ultrasound and in an even higher percentage of patients with peripheral vascular disease. A family history of an AAA is a very strong risk factor; those with an affected first-degree relative have a tenfold to twentyfold increased risk of an AAA developing.[12] Awareness of these high-risk groups may speed the recognition of AAAs in these patients.

PRINCIPLES OF DISEASE

Pathophysiology

AAAs have traditionally been attributed to atherosclerosis, but other factors probably contribute to their formation. Most patients with advanced atherosclerosis have occlusive disease, not aneurysms. Biochemical abnormalities leading to the loss of elastin and collagen, the major structural components of the aortic wall, have been identified in patients with AAAs.[13] The propensity to form aneurysms may have a genetic basis, but the exact mode of inheritance is uncertain. The Society for Vascular Surgery has recommended labeling the typical degenerative AAA as nonspecific, rather than "atherosclerotic," to reflect this uncertain cause.[14]

AAAs sometimes result from specific causes, such as infection, trauma, connective tissue diseases, and arteritis. Such aneurysms are rare compared with nonspecific, degenerative aneurysms.

Natural History

AAAs progressively enlarge, ultimately resulting in rupture of the aneurysm and fatal hemorrhage. Although other potential complications are possible, by far the most common and most important is rupture.

The most important factor determining the risk of rupture is the size of the aneurysm.[3,15] The rupture risk increases dramatically with increased aneurysm size, and most ruptured AAAs have diameters greater than 5 cm. However, no "safe" size exists, and small aneurysms can rupture at any time.[2,3,15]

In a symptomatic patient, the finding that the aneurysm is small should not be considered reassuring. Any aneurysm can rupture and may be the source of the symptoms causing the patient's ED presentation.

Rupture of an AAA usually occurs into the retroperitoneum, where hemorrhage may be temporarily limited by clotting and tamponade at the rupture site. Of patients with ruptures, 10% to 30% have free intraperitoneal rupture, which is often rapidly fatal.[3,16,17] Occasionally, rupture occurs into the gastrointestinal (GI) tract or the inferior vena cava.

Complications can also arise from intact AAAs. The walls of AAAs are often lined with clot and atheromatous material, which can embolize and occlude distal vessels. Aortic thrombosis may occur rarely. Patients may also have complications caused by impingement on adjacent structures.

In approximately 5% of AAAs, a dense inflammatory and fibrotic reaction develops in the aneurysm wall and adjacent retroperitoneal tissue.[5,18] In these "inflammatory" AAAs, the periaortic fibrosis may incorporate and obstruct adjacent structures, such as the ureters.

The overwhelming concern in the patient with an AAA is the potential for rupture of the aneurysm. The natural history of expansion and rupture can be interrupted only by timely surgical repair.

CLINICAL FEATURES

Unruptured Aneurysms

The prevalence of symptoms in patients with unruptured AAAs is unknown. Patients may have symptoms that lead to the aneurysm's discovery and are believed to be caused by the aneurysm. These symptoms can include pain in the abdomen, back, or flank; an awareness of an abdominal mass or fullness; or a sensation of abdominal pulsations.[19]

The pain associated with stable, intact aneurysms has a gradual onset and a vague, dull quality. It is usually constant but may be described as throbbing or colicky. Acute or severe pain is an ominous symptom that suggests imminent or actual aortic rupture.

Most patients diagnosed with AAA are entirely asymptomatic, and the aneurysm is discovered incidentally on physical examination, on a radiologic study done for other reasons, or in an ultrasound aneurysm screening program.[5,20] Symptoms usually do not develop until the aneurysm ruptures.

The diagnostic physical finding is a pulsatile, expansile abdominal mass. The aortic bifurcation is at the level of the umbilicus, and an AAA can be palpated at or above this level. The mass may extend below the umbilicus if the iliac arteries are aneurysmal. The right border of an AAA may be palpable to the right of midline, whereas a normal or tortuous aorta is usually not. Most intact AAAs are nontender; tenderness suggests aneurysm expansion or rupture.[19]

Symptomatic aneurysms are usually fairly large and are often palpable. Likewise, the patient with an aneurysm large enough to warrant elective repair often has a palpable abdominal mass.[19] However, an AAA may be difficult to palpate if the aneurysm is small or the patient is obese. Approximately 30% of nonruptured aneurysms measuring 3.0 to 3.9 cm by ultrasound can be detected by abdominal palpation; 50% of aneurysms measuring 4.0 to 4.9 cm and 75% of aneurysms 5 cm or larger can be palpated.[21] There is virtually no risk of causing aneurysm rupture by abdominal palpation.

When the physical examination is suspicious for an AAA, the aorta often proves to be of normal size.[22] A tortuous aorta may appear enlarged, and prominent aortic pulsations, especially in a thin patient, may simulate an aneurysm. Aortic pulsations may be transmitted to an adjacent mass. Nonetheless, clinical suspicion of an AAA warrants further investigation.

An abdominal bruit is found in only 5% to 10% of patients with AAAs.[19,23] The presence of a bruit is a nonspecific finding because bruits may also originate in a stenotic renal, iliac, or mesenteric artery. A loud continuous bruit suggests the diagnosis of aortovenous fistula.

Perfusion distal to an AAA is usually well maintained, and most patients have normal femoral pulses.[19,23] Diminished femoral pulses may result from iliofemoral occlusive disease or from hypotension in the patient with a ruptured aneurysm.

Thromboembolic complications can occur spontaneously or when atheromatous plaques are disrupted during invasive procedures such as angiography.[24] Large emboli can acutely occlude major vessels such as the iliac, femoral, or popliteal artery, causing acute painful lower extremity ischemia with absent distal pulses. Rarely, the aneurysm itself can thrombose, rendering both lower extremities acutely ischemic.

More often, microemboli consisting of cholesterol crystals or clot obstruct small distal vessels, such as the digital arteries of the toes and arterioles and capillaries of the skin. These patients have livedo reticularis; one or more cool, painful, cyanotic toes; and palpable pedal pulses. This constellation of findings, often called the blue toe syndrome, is highly suggestive of a proximal source of emboli (see Figure 82-3). When an AAA is the source, the aneurysm is often too small to palpate and may only be discovered after radiologic investigation.[24]

Rarely, an intact AAA causes symptoms by compressing adjacent structures. Large, long-standing aneurysms can cause vertebral body erosion and severe back pain. Compression of the duodenum between the superior mesenteric artery and an AAA can cause duodenal obstruction, vomiting, and weight loss.[25] Obstruction of the ureters in the patient with an inflammatory aneurysm can cause ureteral colic.[18]

Ruptured Aneurysms

Pain-Hypotension-Mass Triad Although the classic triad of a ruptured AAA is pain, hypotension, and a pulsatile abdominal mass, many patients have only one or two components of this triad, and an occasional patient has none of the classic features.

Rupture is often the first manifestation of an AAA. Some patients, however, have a previously diagnosed AAA, either because of symptoms or as an incidental finding. A decision not to operate electively may have been made because the aneurysm was small or the patient was considered too high risk. If such a patient has acute symptoms, the presumptive diagnosis is aneurysm rupture.

Most patients with a ruptured AAA experience pain in the abdomen, back, or flank.[16,19] Pain is usually acute, severe, and constant and may radiate to the chest, thigh, inguinal area, or scrotum. The history of pain may be unobtainable if the patient's mental status is compromised by severe hypotension.

The mechanism of the pain associated with aneurysm rupture is poorly understood. It may be caused by expansion of the aortic wall or by stimulation of sensory nerves in the retroperitoneum. Identical pain can occur with intact but acutely expanding aneurysms, which may be impossible to differentiate clinically from ruptured aneurysms.[26,27] Acute pain in the patient with an AAA should be considered a symptom of rupture or impending rupture.

The duration of symptoms before presentation varies greatly. Some patients are seen shortly after severe pain and hypotension develop. In others, rupture is initially contained in the retroperitoneum, blood loss is small, and the presentation is delayed. The patient with a ruptured AAA occasionally has symptoms for several days or even weeks before seeking medical attention.[28,29] A long duration of symptoms does not exclude the diagnosis of ruptured AAA.

Rupture of an AAA may be accompanied by nausea and vomiting, and sudden hemorrhage can cause syncope or near-syncope.[17,19,30] Compensatory hemodynamic mechanisms may then return the blood pressure and cerebral perfusion to normal. Transient improvement in symptoms is fairly common but will be followed by hemodynamic deterioration if diagnosis and treatment are delayed.[30,31]

Ruptured AAAs are often large, and most patients have palpable abdominal masses.[17,19,29] As with intact aneurysms, a ruptured AAA may not be palpable if the aneurysm is small or the patient is obese. The examination may be difficult if abdominal guarding is present or if an ileus causes significant distention. Aortic pulsations may not be prominent if the blood pressure is low. When a mass is not palpable, the diagnosis is often delayed.[31]

Hypotension is the least consistent part of the triad, occurring in only half to two thirds of patients,[16,17] and is often a late finding. When the initial blood loss is minor, vital signs are often normal. The patient with initially normal vital signs may deteriorate and become hypotensive suddenly and unpredictably.

Occasionally, rupture into the retroperitoneum is sealed and contained for many weeks or months.[32] These patients develop abdominal or back pain, presumably at the time of aneurysm leakage, that subsequently diminishes or resolves completely. If the diagnosis is made, evidence of chronic rupture (organized hematoma) is found at surgery. These patients can have chronic pain and may progress to free rupture and subsequent massive hemorrhage at any time.[32]

Aortoenteric Fistula An AAA may rupture into the GI tract (aortoenteric fistula) or inferior vena cava (aortocaval fistula). A *primary* aortoenteric fistula (AEF) is formed when an AAA erodes into the GI tract, usually the third or fourth portion of the duodenum.[33] A *secondary* AEF, a communication between the site of previous aortic surgery and the GI tract, may occur as a late complication of AAA repair.

Early in the formation of a primary AEF, the bowel wall is eroded from the outside by the adjacent AAA. This can lead to the leakage of intestinal contents, with local infection and sometimes abscess formation. Eventually, breakdown of the aortic wall leads to an AEF and GI bleeding.

The patient with an AEF may have abdominal or back pain, fever, or other signs of intraabdominal infection or GI bleeding. Because most of these fistulas are into the duodenum, hemorrhage usually manifests as hematemesis or melena. The initial bleeding results from erosion of vessels in the bowel wall and is often minor. Later, often after several days to a week or longer, massive bleeding results from rupture into the intestinal lumen.

The possibility of a primary AEF should be considered in any patient older than 50 years with unexplained GI bleeding. If an AAA is diagnosed by history, physical examination, or any other modality, the patient should be presumed to have an AEF until proven otherwise.

Aortovenous (Aortocaval) Fistula An aortovenous (usually aortocaval) fistula arises when periaortic inflammation causes adherence of the aorta to an adjacent vein, with pressure on the vessel walls causing the development of an arteriovenous (AV) communication. If concomitant extravasation of blood into the retroperitoneum occurs, the clinical presentation is similar to that of other patients with ruptured AAAs, often with hypovolemic shock. More often the aneurysm ruptures into the vena cava without leaking externally, and the signs and symptoms of a large AV fistula dominate the clinical picture.[34,35]

Shunting of blood from the arterial to the venous system increases venous pressure, venous volume, and venous return to the heart. Total peripheral vascular resistance is decreased, leading to hyperdynamic circulation with tachycardia, wide pulse pressure, and increased cardiac output. The increase in cardiac work leads to dilation of cardiac chambers and eventually to decompensation and high-output cardiac failure.

As in other patients with AAAs, a patient with an aortovenous fistula may have abdominal or back pain. An aneurysm that becomes fistulous with the vena cava is usually large, and 80% to 90% are palpable. A continuous abdominal bruit can be auscultated in approximately 75% of patients with aortovenous fistulas, and 25% of patients have a palpable abdominal thrill.[34,35]

Signs and symptoms of high-output congestive heart failure (dyspnea, jugular venous distention, pulmonary edema) are often present, and half the patients have signs of regional venous hypertension distal to the fistula.[34,35] The increased venous volume and pressure can cause lower extremity edema or cyanosis, and dilated superficial veins may be seen on the legs or abdominal wall. Distention and rupture of veins in the bladder mucosa may cause gross or microscopic hematuria; rectal bleeding may occur for similar reasons. Because of shunting of arterial blood into the venous system, the lower extremities may be cool with diminished pulses.

The patient with an aortovenous fistula often has renal insufficiency caused by decreased renal perfusion accompanying high-output congestive heart failure and by increased renal venous pressure. Hematuria in these patients may originate from the kidneys or the bladder.[36] Hematuria is common when an aortovenous fistula is present but not in other patients with AAAs.[34-36] With an AAA and hematuria, aortography may be indicated to rule out aortovenous fistula formation.[36]

DIAGNOSTIC STRATEGIES

Abdominal Radiographs

Signs of AAA large enough to cause symptoms are seen on plain abdominal radiographs in two thirds to three fourths of patients.[17,37] Thus a normal plain radiograph does not exclude this diagnosis. The most common findings are curvilinear calcification of the aortic wall (Figure 81-2) or a paravertebral soft tissue mass. Rarely, with longstanding aneurysms, erosion of one or more vertebral bodies may be seen. With rupture the psoas or renal outlines may be obscured, although rupture cannot be reliably confirmed or excluded with plain films.

AAA can be seen on both anteroposterior (AP) and lateral radiographs. A lateral lumbar spine film (or cross-table lateral of the lumbar spine area) is often the easiest to evaluate because the right border of the aneurysm may overlie the spine on the AP view. In many cases, enough calcium is present in both lateral walls (on an AP view) or in the anterior and posterior walls (on a lateral view) to measure the aortic diameter and diagnose the presence of an aneurysm. If only the anterior wall is calcified (on the lateral view), the distance from the anterior wall calcification to the front of the vertebral bodies correlates well with the true aortic size.

Although plain film radiographs cannot be used to exclude the presence of an AAA, they are readily obtained and may allow rapid diagnosis of an AAA without the need for more sophisticated (and sometimes time-consuming) tests. In the proper clinical setting, they can provide strong evidence that a patient's symptoms are caused by a ruptured aneurysm, allowing prompt mobilization of the surgical team.

Ultrasound

Ultrasound (US) is virtually 100% sensitive in detecting AAA (Figure 81-3), provided that a technically adequate study can be obtained.[38,39] Measurements of aortic diameter are very accurate. Because it is relatively inexpensive and requires no contrast agents or radiation exposure, US is often chosen for nonemergency aneurysm diagnosis and used to follow patients with known aneurysms.

US has distinct advantages in the emergency evaluation of a patient with a suspected ruptured AAA. It can be performed very rapidly at the patient's bedside, obviating the need to take a potentially unstable patient to the radiology suite. If US is immediately available, it can be used to evaluate the aorta more quickly than abdominal radiography, and US is much more sensitive in detecting an AAA. If an aorta with a normal diameter through its entire abdominal course is visualized, the patient's symptoms are not caused by an AAA. US sometimes provides alternative explanations for the patient's pain by revealing conditions such as acute cholecystitis.[39]

Ultrasonography has certain limitations. It is more operator dependent than other diagnostic modalities and may be prone to technical or interpretive error. Even with elective studies, the aorta is sometimes not well visualized because of

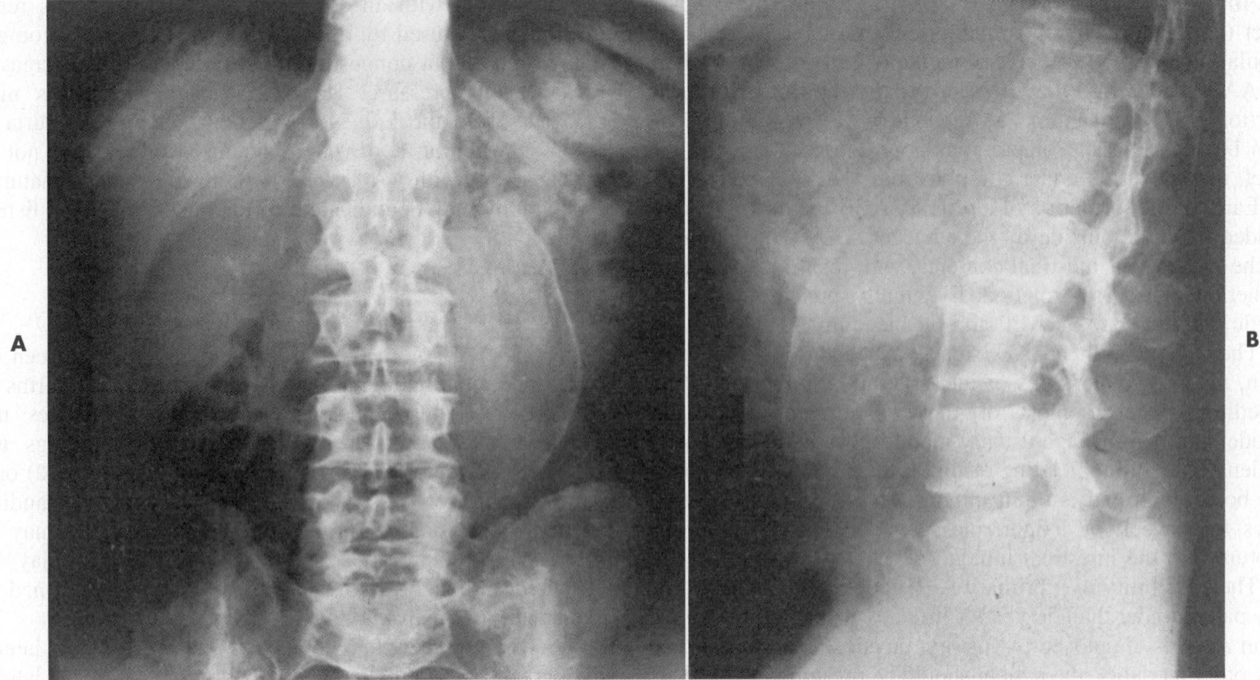

Figure 81-2. **Anteroposterior (A) and lateral (B) views of large AAA with calcification of aortic wall.** ***From Juergens JL, Spittell JA Jr, Fairbairn JF II: Peripheral vascular diseases, ed 5, Philadelphia, 1980, WB Saunders; by permission of the Mayo Foundation.***

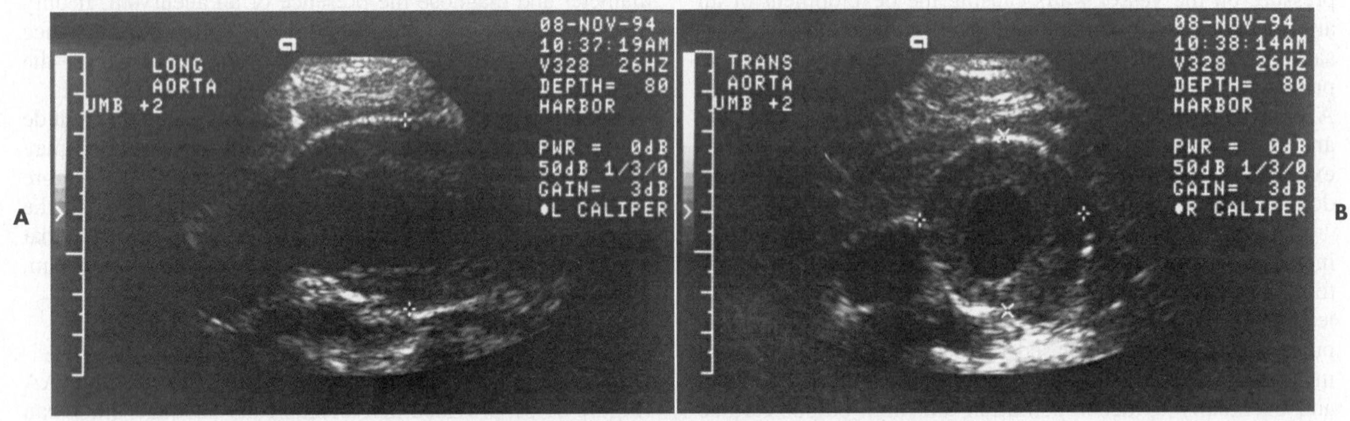

Figure 81-3. **Longitudinal (A) and transverse (B) sonograms of AAA. Markers denote outside of aneurysm wall. Central patent lumen is surrounded by echogenic mural thrombus.** ***Courtesy Richard Renslo, MD.***

obesity or excess bowel gas.[1,38] In many settings, US is not immediately available and requires waiting for the arrival of a radiologist or technologist. Importantly, although US is extremely sensitive in demonstrating the presence of an AAA, it cannot be used to determine reliably whether an AAA has ruptured.

Rupture can be confirmed if free intraperitoneal or retroperitoneal blood is seen in the presence of an AAA. However, the sensitivity of emergency US in detecting extraluminal blood is very low.[39] The purpose of the study is to confirm or exclude the presence of an aneurysm; clinical information (or a CT scan) must be used to determine the likelihood of rupture. If US reveals AAA in an unstable patient, the EP must presume aneurysm rupture, and the patient requires immediate surgery.

Computed Tomography

As with ultrasound, the abdominal computed tomography (CT) scan is virtually 100% accurate in determining the presence or absence of an AAA and provides accurate measurements of the aortic diameter.[38,40] The CT scan is less subject to technical problems and interpretation errors than US. CT is often used to help plan elective procedures because it can demonstrate the proximal and distal extent of the aneurysm, the status of the renal and visceral arteries, and unsuspected pathologic conditions that may influence operative management.[40]

Intravenous (IV) contrast is usually administered in elective studies but is not essential in emergency situations.[38,40] IV contrast will opacify the aortic lumen and distinguish patent lumen from mural thrombus. It can

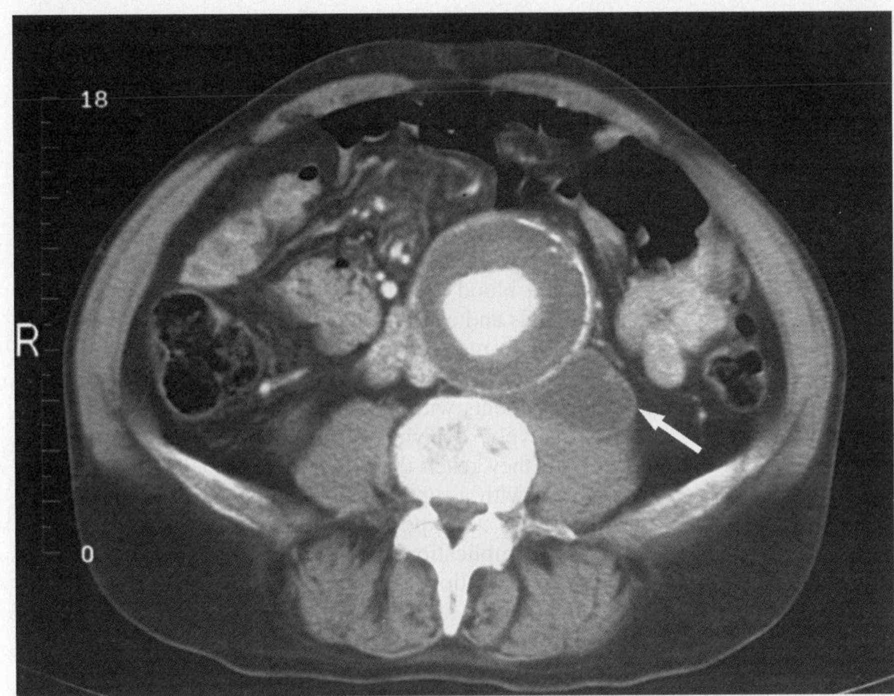

Figure 81-4. **CT scan of ruptured AAA, with calcification of aortic wall and intraluminal thrombus. The patent lumen enhances with contrast but the periaortic hematoma (*arrow*) does not.** *Courtesy Richard Renslo, MD.*

demonstrate periaortic fibrosis because the soft tissue surrounding an inflammatory AAA often enhances.[40] IV contrast is not necessary to identify the aneurysm, however, and acute hemorrhage is well visualized on scans done without contrast.[38,40]

When evaluating a patient with a suspected ruptured AAA, a normal aortic diameter on CT scan excludes an AAA as the cause of the patient's symptoms. CT scans provide more information than US about other retroperitoneal or intraperitoneal disorders and may reveal diagnoses such as ureterolithiasis, pancreatitis, or diverticulitis.[26,41] However, CT scans take longer to perform than ultrasound and require moving the patient out of the ED. Therefore obtaining a CT scan is appropriate only in hemodynamically stable patients.

The CT scan is much more sensitive than US in detecting the retroperitoneal hemorrhage associated with aneurysm rupture. The reported sensitivity ranges from 77% to 100%.[26,41,42] Blood is seen as a retroperitoneal fluid collection adjacent to the aneurysm, often tracking into the perinephric space or along the psoas muscle (Figure 81-4).

Although CT scans are sensitive in detecting retroperitoneal blood, the scan results are sometimes misleading. Rarely, the CT scan is falsely positive for rupture and an intact aneurysm is found at surgery. This can occur when tumor, lymph nodes, inflammatory soft tissue, or bowel loops adjacent to the aorta are identified as blood.[40,41] False-negative scans are more serious; in these cases, an aneurysm is seen on the CT scan, but there is no evidence of hemorrhage. Typically, hemodynamic deterioration occurs a short time later, and a ruptured aneurysm is found at surgery.[42,43]

This situation can occur if hemorrhage is missed on the CT scan, or if rupture occurs shortly after the scan is completed. A CT scan cannot determine whether an AAA is the cause of the patient's pain or whether rupture of the aneurysm is imminent. Another cause of pain can be diagnosed only if the CT scan shows no aneurysm or shows an intact aneurysm and clearly demonstrates an alternative explanation for the patient's symptoms.

Other Diagnostic Modalities

Although *angiography* is helpful in establishing the diagnosis of aortic dissection, it has no place in the emergent evaluation of the suspected ruptured AAA. Most AAAs contain significant amounts of mural thrombus, and the patent lumen may be only slightly enlarged or even normal in caliber. Because contrast opacifies only the patent lumen, angiography often underestimates aneurysm size and can miss the aneurysm entirely.[40] In addition, angiography is time-consuming and performed away from the ED. Its use in the patient with an AAA is limited to helping plan elective surgery.

Magnetic resonance imaging (MRI) and *magnetic resonance angiography* (MRA) can also be used for elective preoperative assessment, but not for the evaluation of possible aortic rupture.[44] Acutely hemorrhaged blood can be difficult to identify with MRI, and the necessary monitoring equipment cannot be used.[40]

DIFFERENTIAL CONSIDERATIONS

Because the patient with a ruptured AAA usually has abdominal, back, or flank pain, with or without hypotension, common misdiagnoses are other disease processes causing these symptoms (Box 81-1). The sudden onset of pain often leads to the clinical suspicion of renal colic. Abdominal pain and tenderness may suggest pancreatitis, intestinal ischemia, or other intraabdominal disorders. The diagnosis of musculoskeletal back pain is especially dangerous because such patients are often discharged from the ED.

Presentation with epigastric pain and hypotension may lead to an admission diagnosis of acute myocardial infarction. Because the patient with a ruptured AAA often has coexistent coronary artery disease, blood loss from a ruptured aneurysm may diminish coronary perfusion and cause chest pain or

Box 81-1 Common Misdiagnoses in Patients with Ruptured AAAs

Renal colic
"Acute abdomen"
- Pancreatitis
- Intestinal ischemia
- Diverticulitis
- Cholecystitis
- Appendicitis
- Perforated viscus
- Bowel obstruction

Musculoskeletal back pain
Acute myocardial infarction

electrocardiographic changes consistent with cardiac ischemia. These findings do not rule out the presence of a ruptured AAA.

To avoid missing the diagnosis, ruptured AAA should be considered in middle-age or elderly patients with any part of the classic triad. The diagnosis of ruptured AAA should also be considered when making the diagnoses listed in Box 81-1, especially when the diagnosis is not clear-cut or the patient is at high risk for an AAA.

MANAGEMENT

Ruptured Aneurysms

The patient with a ruptured AAA is *unstable* until the aorta is cross-clamped in the operating room (OR). No patient with a known or suspected aortic rupture should be considered stable, regardless of the initial vital signs or initial hematocrit.

When the patient arrives at the ED, large-bore IV access should be established with at least two lines and blood sent for crossmatching. (See following discussion for initial fluid administration rates.) At least 10 units of blood should be made available because patients with ruptured AAAs have large transfusion requirements.[16,45] The surgical team should be notified immediately. Further management depends on hemodynamic stability and diagnostic certainty.

The hemodynamically unstable patient in whom a ruptured AAA has been diagnosed or is strongly suspected should be taken to the OR as soon as possible. Diagnostic testing should be kept to a minimum. The diagnosis can often be made from the clinical presentation and abdominal examination, and bedside US can quickly confirm or exclude the presence of an aneurysm. If US is unavailable, abdominal radiographs may help confirm the diagnosis. More time-consuming tests inappropriately delay definitive therapy and increase the risk of exsanguination. Hypotensive patients may have to be taken to the OR based on a strong clinical presumption of the diagnosis, without definitive diagnostic imaging. Some of these patients will not have ruptured aneurysms, but they usually have other acute abdominal conditions requiring laparotomy.[46]

Attempts to resuscitate these patients fully in the ED and normalize the vital signs should be avoided. Hypotensive patients need to be taken to the OR so that the aorta can be clamped and hemorrhage stopped. Attempts to stabilize the patient in the ED are often fruitless and waste valuable time.

Fluid Resuscitation The appropriate degree of preoperative volume resuscitation is controversial. Preoperative hypotension is the strongest predictor of mortality in the patient with a ruptured AAA.[16,17,45] However, correcting the hypotension before clamping the aorta may not improve mortality and may even be harmful.

It has been argued that hypotension slows bleeding in patients with AAA and allows local clot formation and tamponade of the rupture site. Raising the intravascular volume and blood pressure before clamping the aorta may dislodge clots and cause further bleeding.[47,48] Large volumes of crystalloid may contribute to bleeding by causing a dilutional coagulopathy. These concerns are similar to those in trauma patients with uncontrolled hemorrhage.

Alternatively, delaying resuscitation of hypotensive patients until they reach the OR may have deleterious effects. The patient with a ruptured AAA often survives the surgery but dies in the early postoperative period. These deaths are caused by complications of prolonged hypotension, such as myocardial infarction, respiratory failure, and renal failure. The patient with a ruptured AAA is usually elderly, often has coexisting conditions, and tolerates hypovolemia and hypotension poorly.

No prospective studies have compared different preoperative fluid regimens in hypotensive patients with ruptured AAAs, and the optimal resuscitation strategy has not been determined. The priority in these patients is expeditious transportation to the OR for definitive control of aortic hemorrhage. In the prehospital setting and in the ED before the availability of the surgeon and the OR, the blood pressure should be raised with crystalloid or blood products to a level that maintains adequate cerebral and myocardial perfusion.[47,48] The goal is to prevent irreversible end-organ damage. An arbitrary blood pressure goal cannot be specified because the blood pressure necessary for vital organ perfusion varies among patients, but a reasonable target is 90 to 100 mm Hg systolic.

Aortic Clamping Cross-clamping the aorta through a left lateral thoracotomy is sometimes performed in the OR for severely hypotensive patients.[16] Thoracic aortic clamping adds the morbidity of a thoracotomy and may cause ischemic damage to the spinal cord and intraabdominal organs. ED thoracotomy may be appropriate, however, when a patient with severe hemodynamic compromise or cardiac arrest fails to respond to standard resuscitative measures and cannot be taken quickly to the OR.

Diagnostic Confirmation In the patient with acute abdominal or back pain but without hypotension, more time can be taken to confirm the presence of an AAA. If an AAA can be diagnosed with bedside testing (abdominal examination, plain radiographs, or US), the surgeon will often proceed immediately to the OR with a clinical diagnosis of aneurysm rupture, because a delay in surgery places the patient with a ruptured AAA at risk for sudden and unpredictable hemodynamic deterioration. If an AAA cannot be identified with bedside testing and the patient remains hemodynamically stable, an abdominal CT scan can be obtained to confirm or exclude the presence of an aneurysm. The patient who is sent for a CT scan must be monitored closely and taken to the OR immediately if hemodynamic deterioration occurs.

The CT scan can also identify the retroperitoneal

hemorrhage associated with rupture and confirm the need for an emergency procedure. The surgeon may want confirmation of rupture to avoid the problems of performing emergency surgery with an intact aneurysm. With emergency surgery, detailed anatomic evaluation and careful preoperative planning are often impossible, evaluation and optimization of the patient's cardiopulmonary and renal function may be precluded, and invasive hemodynamic monitoring may be unavailable. For these reasons, patients who are taken for emergency surgery and found to have intact, symptomatic aneurysms have a significantly higher mortality rate (20% to 25%) than patients having elective aneurysm repair (5% or less).[19,27,49]

Once an AAA has been diagnosed, the decision to obtain a CT scan to distinguish a ruptured from an unruptured aneurysm should be made very cautiously and in close consultation with a surgeon. If a CT scan demonstrates an intact AAA and the decision is made to delay surgery, the patient must be closely observed for signs of rupture in an intensive care setting.

Patients may be hypertensive on admission because of pain or underlying chronic hypertension. Unlike the situation with aortic dissection, no evidence exists that lowering the blood pressure is beneficial in the patient with a ruptured AAA, and these patients are at risk of developing precipitous hypotension.

Surgery and Mortality Ruptured AAA is uniformly fatal unless treated surgically. Thus, once this diagnosis is made, operative repair should be attempted in almost all patients.[16] Attempts have been made to identify patients with a very low likelihood of survival, and it has been suggested that surgery may be withheld in patients with prehospital or ED cardiac arrest.[45] Survival has been reported in up to 25% of patients with preoperative cardiac arrest, however, and no variables that can be assessed in the ED are universally predictive of a fatal outcome.[6,16] Surgery is indicated unless the patient's life expectancy is very short because of underlying illnesses or the patient's quality of life is so poor that surgery is considered unreasonable.[49]

Surgical mortality in patients with ruptured AAAs is approximately 50% and has shown little improvement in the past two decades.[47,49,50] Hypotension is the most important factor predicting a poor outcome; a low initial hematocrit also increases the likelihood of perioperative death.[16,17,45,48]

Operative mortality rates significantly underestimate the true lethality of the ruptured AAA. The patient with a ruptured AAA may die at home or may reach the hospital but die before surgery. When patients who do not reach the OR are considered, the overall mortality rate is 80% to 90%.[51,52]

Intact, Asymptomatic Aneurysms

An incidental diagnosis of AAA may be made in the ED, or a patient with a known AAA may present to the ED. Therefore the EP must understand the mangement principles for intact, asymptomatic AAA.

The decision to repair an asymptomatic aneurysm depends on the risk of aneurysm rupture, the patient's life expectancy and likelihood of dying from other causes, and the surgical risk. The latter factors are determined by the patient's age and coexisting illnesses. The risk of rupture is largely a function of aneurysm size.

Two general approaches to these patients have been taken. Some favor *early repair* of small aneurysms soon after diagnosis, as long as the patient is otherwise in good health.[49,53] The bases of this approach are that (1) small aneurysms may rupture, (2) they often enlarge with time and eventually require surgery, and (3) the risk of elective surgery often increases as the patient ages.

Alternatively, a strategy of *selective management* may be used. Small aneurysms are followed with serial US or CT scans, and surgery is performed only if symptoms develop, rapid expansion is documented, or a threshold size (usually 5 to 6 cm) is reached.[54,55] This approach is often chosen when the risk of elective surgery is considered high because of underlying medical problems.

The relative merits of the two approaches are being evaluated in clinical trials. In these studies, patients with small AAAs are randomized to early surgery or selective management.[55,56] Data from the United Kingdom show equivalent mortality rates with these two strategies.[55] The "watchful waiting" approach is only appropriate for asymptomatic aneurysms, and the presence of the AAA must be strongly considered when evaluating any symptoms in these patients.

Traditional Repair The conventional technique for repair of AAAs is an open approach with a laparotomy. The aneurysm is opened longitudinally and repaired from within (Figure 81-5). A graft is inserted inside the aneurysm and anastomosed to uninvolved vessels above and below. When possible, a straight graft is used between the infrarenal and distal aorta. If the aneurysm involves the aortic bifurcation, or if iliac artery aneurysmal or occlusive disease is present, a bifurcation graft is used, with the distal anastomosis to the iliac or femoral arteries. The aneurysm wall is then closed around the graft to help separate it from adjacent structures.

Newer Technique A method of repairing AAAs without laparotomy has been developed for select patients.[57-59] A stent graft is placed into the femoral artery through a groin incision and is advanced under fluoroscopic guidance to a position that spans the aneurysm (Figure 81-6). Depending on the anatomy of the aneurysm, a tube or bifurcated graft may be chosen; several anchoring methods have been employed.

This technique avoids the morbidity of a laparotomy. It also may allow the repair of AAAs in some high-risk patients who might not tolerate conventional aneurysm surgery. Detailed preoperative imaging and planning are required, and the technique is generally not applicable to the patient with a ruptured aneurysm.[59]

Survival The mortality rate of elective AAA repair is now less than 5%, in stark contrast to the results with ruptured aneurysms.[47,49,50] Patients who survive the operation have an excellent prognosis, with a long-term survival close to that of the general population.[60] After repair of the aneurysm, long-term survival is primarily limited by associated cardiac disease.

LATE COMPLICATIONS OF REPAIR

Graft infection, AEF formation, and anastomotic aneurysm (pseudoaneurysm) formation can occur at any time from weeks to many years after the surgery.[61-65] These complications often occur together, their clinical presentations overlap, and they are diagnosed by similar means. A unique

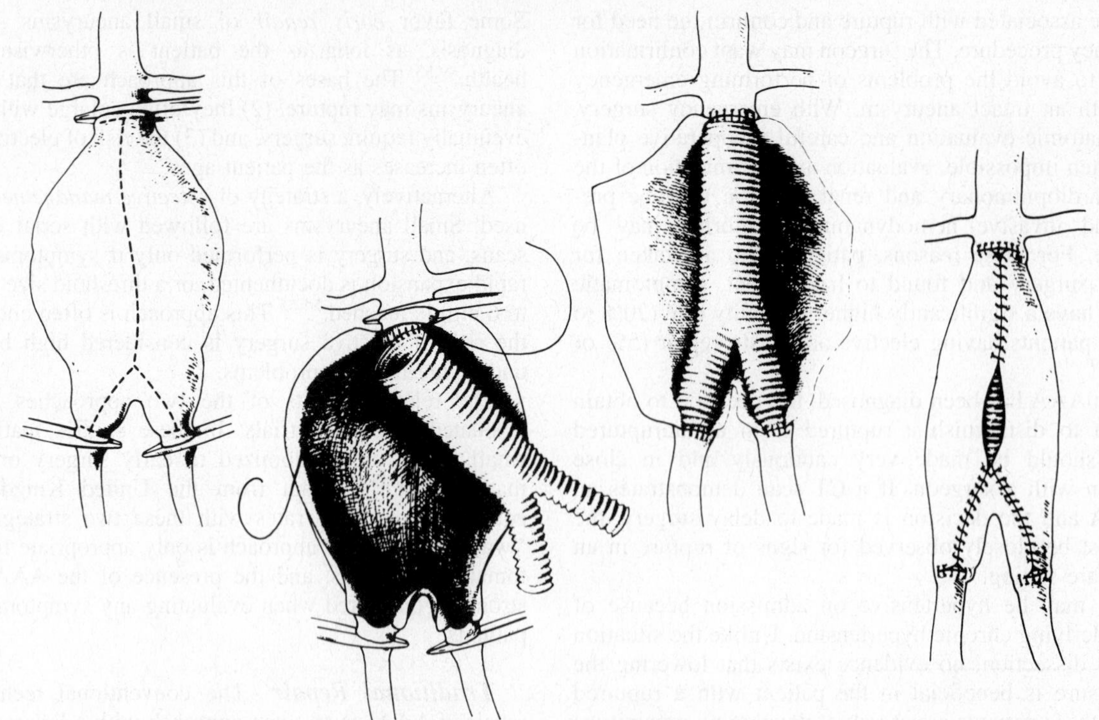

Figure 81-5. **Steps in repair of abdominal aortic aneurysm. See text for details.** *From Kent KC, Boyce SW, Skillman J. In Lindsay J Jr, editor:* Diseases of the aorta, *Philadelphia, 1994, Lea & Febiger.*

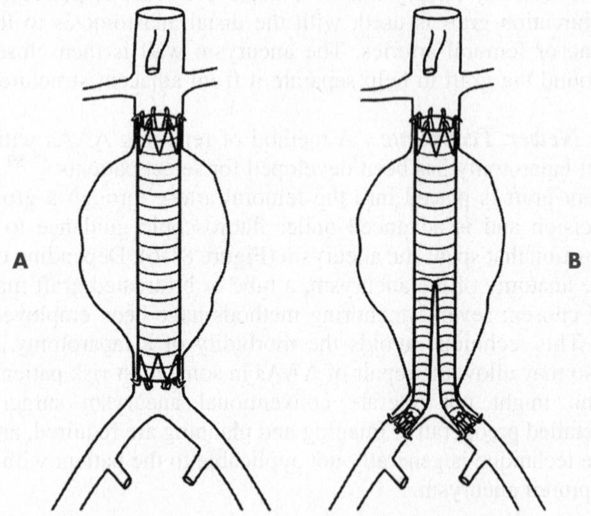

Figure 81-6. **Endovascular stent grafts positioned in aorta. A, Tube graft. B, Bifurcated graft.** *From Moore WS et al:* Ann Surg *230:298, 1999.*

complication of endovascular repair of an AAA is the development of an internal leak (endoleak).

Graft Infection

Graft infection may result from contamination of the graft at surgery, spread of a contiguous infection, or hematogenous seeding. Infection can disrupt the anastomosis between native artery and graft, leading to leakage of blood and pseudoaneurysm formation. The infection may be localized to a portion of the graft, most often the inguinal portion of an aortofemoral graft, or may involve the entire graft.[63]

Infection of the distal limb of an aortofemoral graft may be clinically evident, with local signs of infection or a palpable false aneurysm. Intraabdominal graft infection is often subtle, with low-grade fever and vague abdominal or back pain.[61,63] Abdominal tenderness or a palpable mass may be present at the leaking anastomosis. A CT scan should be obtained to evaluate suspected graft infection.[40,66] Collections of fluid or gas around the graft provide evidence of infection, although false-negative studies occasionally occur.[61,66]

Aortoenteric Fistula

Graft infection may lead to secondary AEF formation. These fistulas, which are much more common than primary AEFs, can develop years after AAA repair or after aortoiliac or aortofemoral bypass surgery for peripheral vascular disease. Secondary AEFs usually form between the proximal aortic anastomosis and the distal duodenum. However, they can occur anywhere in the GI tract and may cause upper or lower GI bleeding.[33,65]

The clinical presentation of the patient with a secondary AEF may be identical to that of a patient with graft infection alone, with fever and other signs of infection. More often, however, the patient with an AEF has GI bleeding.[64,65] The bleeding can be acute or chronic, and its severity ranges from minor to massive.

An AEF must be considered in any patient with GI bleeding and a history of abdominal aortic surgery. Most of these patients, however, ultimately prove to have other, more common causes of GI bleeding.[67] The diagnostic approach depends on the patient's hemodynamic stability.

If the patient with a suspected AEF is unstable with massive bleeding, diagnostic testing may be dangerously time-consuming. In these patients, emergency laparotomy may be necessary to control hemorrhage and diagnose or exclude the presence of an AEF.[65,67] Stable patients can be evaluated with endoscopy or a CT scan.

Upper GI endoscopy is often recommended as the initial diagnostic test.[64,65] Direct visualization of the fistula into the distal duodenum is sometimes possible. However, endoscopy cannot be relied on to identify an AEF, and its main value is in establishing another diagnosis. If an active bleeding site other than an AEF is clearly seen, emergency surgery may be avoided.

An abdominal CT scan can also be used to evaluate a suspected AEF.[40,66] Although imaging of the fistula is often impossible, graft infection is almost invariably present in patients with secondary AEFs, and the CT scan can demonstrate the associated infection. Radiographically distinguishing an AEF from intraabdominal graft infection alone may be difficult, but the distinction is not crucial because both need surgical management.[64,66]

Pseudoaneurysm (Anastomotic Aneurysm)

Pseudoaneurysms can arise at the site of a leaking anastomosis.[68,69] They may be associated with graft infection or AEF formation but more often result from degeneration of the native vessel.[69]

The patient with an anastomotic aneurysm may have pain or a pulsatile mass in the abdomen or groin. The aneurysm may give rise to distal emboli or may rupture and cause life-threatening hemorrhage. Suspected pseudoaneurysms can be evaluated with angiography, CT scans, or ultrasound.[68,69]

Endoleak

After endovascular AAA repair, leakage of blood outside of the graft lumen but within the aneurysm sac is termed an endoleak.[58,59,70] These leaks may develop shortly after the procedure or much later. They may resolve spontaneously or may require secondary endovascular procedures or surgical intervention. With persistent leakage of blood into the aneurysm sac, the patient is at risk for rupture of the aneurysm.[58,59,70]

Surgeon's Role

The management of late complications of AAA repair depends on the type, site, and extent of the lesion and will be determined by the consulting surgeon.

DISPOSITION

A patient with an acutely symptomatic AAA requires hospital admission and urgent or emergency surgical repair. A patient whose aneurysm is asymptomatic and discovered incidentally must be referred for consideration of elective repair. The patient with an AAA should be referred for an outpatient workup only if it is clear that the symptoms prompting the ED visit are unrelated to the aneurysm. If the patient is discharged, instructions should be given to seek medical attention immediately if abdominal, back, or flank pain develops.

In the patient who has had an AAA repaired, unexplained fever, abdominal pain, or GI bleeding suggests the presence of a graft-related complication and the need for inpatient evaluation.

KEY CONCEPTS

- A ruptured AAA should be considered in any patient older than 50 who presents with abdominal or back pain. The complete triad of pain, hypotension, and a pulsatile mass is often not present.
- The risk of rupture increases with aneurysm size, but even small aneurysms can rupture at any time.
- In the patient with an AAA and acute symptoms, rupture is imminent or has already occurred.
- The patient with a ruptured AAA who is initially hemodynamically stable may suddenly deteriorate at any time.
- The patient with a ruptured AAA should be moved expeditiously to the operating room, bypassing complete resuscitation and time-consuming imaging.

REFERENCES

1. Scott RAP, Ashton HA, Kay DN: Abdominal aortic aneurysm in 4237 screened patients: prevalence, development and management over 6 years, *Br J Surg* 78:1122, 1991.
2. Ouriel K et al: An evaluation of new methods of expressing aortic aneurysm size: relationship to rupture, *J Vasc Surg* 15:12, 1992.
3. Darling RC et al: Autopsy study of unoperated abdominal aortic aneurysms: the case for early resection, *Circulation* 56(suppl 2):161, 1977.
4. Bengtsson H, Bergqvist D, Sternby NH: Increasing prevalence of abdominal aortic aneurysms: a necropsy study, *Eur J Surg* 158:19, 1992.
5. Johnston KW, Scobie TK: Multicenter prospective study of nonruptured abdominal aortic aneurysms. I. Population and operative management, *J Vasc Surg* 7:69, 1988.
6. Chen JC et al: Predictors of death in nonruptured and ruptured abdominal aortic aneurysms, *J Vasc Surg* 24:614, 1996.
7. Wilmink ABM, Quick CRG: Epidemiology and potential for prevention of abdominal aortic aneurysm, *Br J Surg* 85:155, 1998.
8. Galland RB, Simmons MJ, Torrie EPH: Prevalence of abdominal aortic aneurysm in patients with occlusive peripheral vascular disease, *Br J Surg* 78:1259, 1991.
9. Webster MW et al: Ultrasound screening of first-degree relatives of patients with an abdominal aortic aneurysm, *J Vasc Surg* 13:9, 1991.
10. Vermilion BD et al: A review of one hundred forty-seven popliteal aneurysms with long-term follow-up, *Surgery* 90:1009, 1981.
11. Graham LM et al: Clinical significance of atherosclerotic femoral artery aneurysms, *Arch Surg* 115:502, 1980.
12. Johansen K, Koepsell T: Familial tendency for abdominal aortic aneurysms, *JAMA* 256:1934, 1986.
13. MacSweeney STR, Powell JT, Greenhalgh RM: Pathogenesis of abdominal aortic aneurysm, *Br J Surg* 81:935, 1994.
14. Johnston KW et al: Suggested standards for reporting on arterial aneurysms, *J Vasc Surg* 13:452, 1991.
15. Sterpetti AV et al: Factors influencing the rupture of abdominal aortic aneurysms, *Surg Gynecol Obstet* 173:175, 1991.
16. Gloviczki P et al: Ruptured abdominal aortic aneurysms: repair should not be denied, *J Vasc Surg* 15:851, 1992.
17. Donaldson MC, Rosenberg JM, Bucknam CA: Factors affecting survival after ruptured abdominal aortic aneurysm, *J Vasc Surg* 2:564, 1985.
18. Boontje AH, van den Dungen JJAM, Blanksma C: Inflammatory abdominal aortic aneurysms, *J Cardiovasc Surg* 31:611, 1990.
19. Vohra R et al: Long-term survival in patients undergoing resection of abdominal aortic aneurysm, *Ann Vasc Surg* 4:460, 1990.
20. Chervu A et al: Role of physical examination in detection of abdominal aortic aneurysms, *Surgery* 117:454, 1995.
21. Lederle FA, Simel DL: Does this patient have abdominal aortic aneurysm? *JAMA* 281:77, 1999.
22. Beede SD et al: Positive predictive value of clinical suspicion of abdominal aortic aneurysm: implications for efficient use of abdominal ultrasonography, *Arch Intern Med* 150:549, 1990.

23. Lederle FA, Walker JM, Reinke DB: Selective screening for abdominal aortic aneurysms with physical examination and ultrasound, *Arch Intern Med* 148:1753, 1988.
24. Baxter BT et al: Distal embolization as a presenting symptom of aortic aneurysms, *Am J Surg* 160:197, 1990.
25. Sostek M, Fine SN, Harris TL: Duodenal obstruction by abdominal aortic aneurysm, *Am J Med* 94:220, 1993.
26. Kvilekval KHV et al: The value of computed tomography in the management of symptomatic abdominal aortic aneurysms, *J Vasc Surg* 12:28, 1990.
27. Sullivan CA, Rohrer MJ, Cutler BS: Clinical management of the symptomatic but unruptured abdominal aortic aneurysm, *J Vasc Surg* 11:799, 1990.
28. Harris LM et al: Ruptured abdominal aortic aneurysms: factors affecting mortality rates, *J Vasc Surg* 14:812, 1991.
29. Akkersdijk GJM, van Bockel JH: Ruptured abdominal aortic aneurysm: initial misdiagnosis and the effect on treatment, *Eur J Surg* 164:29, 1998.
30. Lederle FA, Parenti CM, Chute EP: Ruptured abdominal aortic aneurysm: the internist as diagnostician, *Am J Med* 96:163, 1994.
31. Marston WA et al: Misdiagnosis of ruptured abdominal aortic aneurysms, *J Vasc Surg* 16:17, 1992.
32. Sterpetti AV et al: Sealed rupture of abdominal aortic aneurysms, *J Vasc Surg* 11:430, 1990.
33. Bessen HA: Aortoenteric fistula, *J Emerg Med* 3:195, 1985.
34. Potyk DK, Guthrie CR: Spontaneous aortocaval fistula, *Ann Emerg Med* 25:424, 1995.
35. Gilling-Smith GL, Mansfield AO: Spontaneous abdominal arteriovenous fistulae: report of eight cases and review of the literature, *Br J Surg* 78:421, 1991.
36. Salo JA et al: Hematuria is an indication of rupture of an abdominal aortic aneurysm into the vena cava, *J Vasc Surg* 12:41, 1990.
37. Loughran CF: A review of the plain abdominal radiograph in acute rupture of abdominal aortic aneurysms, *Clin Radiol* 37:383, 1986.
38. LaRoy LL et al: Imaging of abdominal aortic aneurysms, *AJR Am J Roentgenol* 152:785, 1989.
39. Shuman WP et al: Suspected leaking abdominal aortic aneurysm: use of sonography in the emergency room, *Radiology* 168:117, 1988.
40. Siegel CL, Cohan RH: CT of abdominal aortic aneurysms, *AJR Am J Roentgenol* 163:17, 1994.
41. Johnson WC et al: The role of computed tomography in symptomatic aortic aneurysms, *Surg Gynecol Obset* 162:49, 1986.
42. Weinbaum FI et al: The accuracy of computed tomography in the diagnosis of retroperitoneal blood in the presence of abdominal aortic aneurysm, *J Vasc Surg* 6:11, 1987.
43. Greatorex RA et al: Limitations of computed tomography in leaking abdominal aortic aneurysms, *BMJ* 297:284, 1988.
44. Durham JR et al: Magnetic resonance angiography in the preoperative evaluation of abdominal aortic aneurysms, *Am J Surg* 166:173, 1993.
45. Johansen K et al: Ruptured abdominal aortic aneurysm: the Harborview experience, *J Vasc Surg* 13:240, 1991.
46. Valentine RJ et al: Nonvascular emergencies presenting as ruptured abdominal aortic aneurysms, *Surgery* 113:286, 1993.
47. Ernst CB: Abdominal aortic aneurysm, *N Engl J Med* 328:1167, 1993.
48. Brimacombe J, Berry A: A review of anaesthesia for ruptured abdominal aortic aneurysm with special emphasis on preclamping fluid resuscitation, *Anaesth Intensive Care* 2:311, 1993.
49. Hollier LH, Taylor LM, Ochsner J: Recommended indications for operative treatment of abdominal aortic aneurysms: report of a subcommittee of the Joint Council of the Society for Vascular Surgery and the North American Chapter of the International Society for Cardiovascular Surgery, *J Vasc Surg* 15:1046, 1992.
50. Kazmers A et al: Abdominal aortic aneurysm repair in Veterans Affairs medical centers, *J Vasc Surg* 23:191, 1996.
51. Bengtsson H, Bergqvist D: Ruptured abdominal aortic aneurysm: a population-based study, *J Vasc Surg* 18:74, 1993.
52. Choksy SA, Wilmink ABM, Quick CR: Ruptured abdominal aortic aneurysm in the Huntingdon district: a 10-year experience, *Ann R Coll Surg Engl* 81:27, 1999.
53. Katz DA, Littenberg B, Cronenwett JL: Management of small abdominal aortic aneurysms: early surgery vs. watchful waiting, *JAMA* 268:2678, 1992.
54. Scott RAP et al: A 14-year experience with 6 cm as a criterion for surgical treatment of abdominal aortic aneurysm, *Br J Surg* 86:1317, 1999.
55. UK Small Aneurysm Trial Participants: Mortality results for randomised controlled trial of early elective surgery or ultrasonographic surveillance for small abdominal aortic aneurysms, *Lancet* 352:1649, 1998.
56. Lederle FA et al: Design of the Abdominal Aortic Aneurysm Detection and Management Study, *J Vasc Surg* 20:296, 1994.
57. Blum U et al: Endoluminal stent-grafts for infrarenal abdominal aortic aneurysms, *N Engl J Med* 336:13, 1997.
58. Moore WS et al: Abdominal aortic aneurysm: a 6-year comparison of endovascular versus transabdominal repair, *Ann Surg* 230:298, 1999.
59. Zarins CK et al: AneuRx stent graft versus open surgical repair of abdominal aortic aneurysms: multicenter prospective clinical trial, *J Vasc Surg* 29:292, 1999.
60. Norman PE et al: Long term relative survival after surgery for abdominal aortic aneurysm in Western Australia: population based study, *BMJ* 317:852, 1998.
61. McCann RL, Schwartz LB, Georgiade GS: Management of abdominal aortic graft complications, *Ann Surg* 217:729, 1993.
62. Hallett JW et al: Graft-related complications after abdominal aortic aneurysm repair: reassurance from a 36-year population-based experience, *J Vasc Surg* 25:277, 1997.
63. Goldstone J: The infected infra-renal aortic graft, *Acta Chir Scand* 538:72, 1987.
64. Goldstone J, Cunningham CC: Diagnosis, treatment and prevention of aorto-enteric fistulas, *Acta Chir Scand Suppl* 555:165, 1990.
65. Peck JJ, Eidemiller LR: Aortoenteric fistulas, *Arch Surg* 127:1191, 1992.
66. Low RN et al: Aortoenteric fistula and perigraft infection: evaluation with CT, *Radiology* 175:157, 1990.
67. Pabst TS et al: Gastrointestinal bleeding after aortic surgery: the role of laparotomy to rule out aortoenteric fistula, *J Vasc Surg* 8:280, 1988.
68. Allen RC et al: Paraanastomotic aneurysms of the abdominal aorta, *J Vasc Surg* 18:424, 1993.
69. Dennis JW et al: Anastomotic pseudoaneurysms: a continuing late complication of vascular reconstructive procedures, *Arch Surg* 121: 314, 1986.
70. Schurink GWH, Aarts NJM, von Bockel JH: Endoleak after stent-graft treatment of abdominal aortic aneurysm: a meta-analysis of clinical studies, *Br J Surg* 86:581, 1999.

82 Peripheral Arteriovascular Disease

Tom P. Aufderheide

PERSPECTIVE

Treatments for peripheral arterial disease date from the late eighteenth century. In 1785, Hunter demonstrated complete thrombosis of an aneurysmal sac with a ligature proximal to a popliteal aneurysm.[1] In 1877, Eck reported the first successful anastomosis between two vessels, the portal vein and the inferior vena cava. In 1963, surgical embolectomy became widely established by the introduction of the Fogarty balloon catheter. Recent advances in noninvasive hemodynamic testing, imaging techniques, interventional devices, and chronic indwelling catheters present the EP with a wide range of new diagnostic and therapeutic challenges.

Arteries are classified into three categories on the basis of their size and histologic features: (1) large or elastic arteries (the aorta and its immediate proximal, larger branches, including the innominate, subclavian, common carotid, and pulmonary arteries), (2) medium-size or muscular arteries (located just distal to elastic arteries, including the common femoral, axillary, and carotid arteries), and (3) small arteries (usually <2 mm in diameter) that course in the substance of tissues and organs. This chapter considers disease manifestations in medium and small arteries.

PRINCIPLES OF DISEASE

Arterial Anatomy

All arteries possess three layers: the tunica intima, tunica media, and tunica adventitia. As peripheral arteries diminish in caliber, these three layers become progressively indistinct and are no longer identifiable at the level of the arteriole (precapillary vessel containing smooth muscle).

The *tunica intima* has an inner lining of endothelial cells surrounded by subendothelial connective tissue. The outer limit of the tunica intima is demarcated by a longitudinally dispersed layer of elastic fibers known as the internal elastic lamina. The single layer of continuous endothelium is a unique thromboresistant layer between blood and the potentially thrombogenic subendothelial tissues. The integrity of the endothelium is a fundamental requirement for maintenance of normal structure and function of the entire vessel wall. Endothelial injury can result in intraluminal thrombosis and may contribute to the initiation of atherosclerosis.

The *tunica media* is made up primarily of circular or spiral smooth muscle cells arranged in concentric layers. The outer limit of this layer is marked by a well-defined, external elastic membrane. The elastic content of the tunica media gives resilience to medium-size arteries. In the aging process the elastic fibers deteriorate and are replaced by fibrous tissue. This loss of elasticity results in stretching and elongation and accounts for the progressive tortuosity and development of arterial aneurysms with aging. Vascular smooth muscle cells are capable of many metabolic functions, may be important in lipid accumulation in the vessel wall during atherosclerosis, and participate in vasoconstriction and dilation.

The *tunica adventitia* is a poorly defined layer of connective tissue in which nerve fibers and small, thin-walled nutrient vessels (vasa vasorum) are dispersed. Medium-size arteries contain more nerve fibers than larger vessels, reflecting the importance of their role in the autonomic regulation of blood flow.

The peripheral arterial vascular system is a single end organ subject to a variety of pathologic conditions. This chapter describes eight basic pathophysiologic processes: atherosclerosis, aneurysm, embolism, thrombosis, inflammation, trauma, vasospasm, and arteriovenous fistula. Most peripheral arterial problems are caused by two of the eight pathologic processes: atherosclerosis and thrombosis.

Pathophysiology

Atherosclerosis Atherosclerosis is a disease of large and medium-size muscular arteries. The basic lesion, the *atheroma* or fibrofatty plaque, is a raised focal plaque within the intima; it has a lipid core (mainly cholesterol, usually complexed to proteins and cholesterol esters) covered by a fibrous cap. As the plaques increase in size and number, they progressively encroach on the lumen of the artery and the adjacent media. Atheromas have two main effects: compromising arterial blood flow and weakening walls of the affected arteries.

The distribution of atherosclerotic plaques is rather constant. The abdominal aorta has more atherosclerotic disease than the thoracic aorta, and aortic lesions tend to be much more common and prominent around the ostia of major branches. Other vessels greatly affected by atherosclerosis are the aortoiliac, femoral, and popliteal arteries; the descending thoracic aorta; the coronary arteries; the internal carotid arteries; and the circle of Willis. Vessels of the upper extremities are usually spared.

As atherosclerosis progresses, atheromas almost always undergo calcification, resulting in hard, brittle vessels. Ulceration of the luminal surface and rupture of the atheromatous plaques may result in discharge of the debris into the bloodstream, producing atheroemboli (cholesterol emboli). Fissured or ulcerated lesions can produce in situ thrombosis, causing acute intraluminal occlusion.

Hemorrhage into the plaque may further compromise the arterial lumen. Although atherosclerosis primarily affects the intima, in severe cases the tunica media undergoes pressure atrophy and loss of elastic tissue, with sufficient weakening to create aneurysmal dilation.

Aneurysms A *true aneurysm* is an abnormal localized dilation of the intact vessel wall. In a *pseudoaneurysm* the entire wall perforates or ruptures, and the extravasated blood is contained by the surrounding tissues, eventually forming a fibrous sac that communicates with the artery.

Mural and mechanical factors contribute to true aneurysm formation.[2] The major cause of aneurysms is a weakness or defect in the integrity of the arterial wall. The only aneurysms that develop in a normal arterial segment are *poststenotic aneurysms,* such as with coarctation. Acceleration of flow past a narrow point creates slower flow beyond the stenosis lateral to the jet stream, producing increased lateral pressure. Aneurysmal dilation accelerates, increasing the risk of rupture as diameter increases; Laplace's law states that the tension (lateral pressure) in the wall of a hollow viscus varies directly with its radius (T = Pr).

The most common cause of aneurysms is severe atherosclerosis resulting from thinning and destruction of the tunica media. Atheromatous ulcers covered by mural thrombi are common within an aneurysm. Such mural thrombi can form emboli that lodge in distal vessels. When an entire aneurysm is filled with thrombus material, arterial occlusion results.

Aneurysms cause clinical symptoms through (1) rupture with subsequent hemorrhage, (2) impingement on adjacent structures, (3) occlusion of a vessel by either direct pressure or mural thrombus formation, (4) embolism from mural thrombus, and (5) presentation as a pulsatile mass.

Arterial Embolism An embolus is a blood clot or other foreign body that is carried by the blood to a site distant from its point of origin. Most emboli are the result of detached thrombus formation (thromboembolism). Less common sources include debris from ruptured atherosclerotic plaques, tumor debris, or foreign bodies. Unless otherwise specified, the term *embolus* in this chapter is defined as *thromboembolus.*

Thromboembolism Most arterial emboli (85%) originate in thrombus formation in the heart. Left ventricular thrombus formation resulting from myocardial infarction (MI) accounts for nearly 60% to 70% of arterial emboli. Atrial thrombi associated with mitral stenosis and rheumatic heart disease account for only 5% to 10% of arterial embolism.[3] Coexisting atrial fibrillation, often without mitral stenosis, is present in 60% to 75% of peripheral arterial embolic events, since atrial fibrillation itself may predispose patients to intracardiac clotting.[4]

Acute arterial emboli often cause distal tissue infarction. Clinical outcome depends most on the amount of collateral circulation present, but also on the size of the vessel and the degree of obstruction. Patients with longstanding atherosclerosis have well-developed collateral circulation, whereas sudden occlusion of a normal artery without collateral pathways results in severe ischemia. After acute obstruction the embolus can propagate proximally or distally, fragment and embolize further to distal vessels, or precipitate associated venous thrombosis by initiating a localized inflammatory reaction.

Because vessel diameters change most abruptly at branch points, embolic occlusion most often occurs at major arterial bifurcations. The bifurcation of the common femoral artery is the most frequent site of arterial embolism, accounting for 35% to 50% of all cases.[3] The smaller femoral and popliteal arteries are involved twice as often as the larger aortic and iliac vessels, reflecting the small size of most emboli.

Cell death from arterial ischemia can produce high concentrations of potassium, lactic acid, and myoglobin in the extremity distal to an arterial occlusion. Their sudden release after revascularization can produce life-threatening hyperkalemia, metabolic acidosis, and myoglobinuria. This myonephropathic-metabolic syndrome accounts for approximately one third of the deaths from arterial embolism after revascularization.[5]

Atheroembolism Atheroembolism refers to microemboli consisting of cholesterol, calcium, and platelet aggregates dislodged from proximal complicated atherosclerotic plaques that lodge in distal end arteries. In the central nervous system (CNS), atheroemboli cause transient ischemic attacks (TIAs) and strokes (cerebrovascular accidents). In the peripheral vascular system, atheroemboli characteristically present with cool, painful, and cyanotic toes, or the blue toe syndrome.[6]

Atheroemboli are caused by a proximally located arterial lesion, usually atherosclerotic plaques or aneurysms. Bilateral distal extremity involvement usually implies an aortic source, whereas unilateral atheroemboli usually arise from sites distal to the aorta. Distal lesions are most common in the femoropopliteal arteries (60%) and the aortoiliac arteries (40%). Aortic lesions (e.g., aneurysms, polytetrafluoroethylene grafts) are a less common source of microemboli.[6]

Atheroemboli tend to lodge in arteries 100 to 200 μm in size, such as the digital arteries. Single atheroembolic events seldom result in tissue loss, but atheroemboli tend to cluster. If unrecognized, repeated events ultimately result in loss of collateral circulation, progressive symptoms, and extensive tissue infarction.[6]

Infectious emboli from bacterial endocarditis can produce septic infarcts that may convert to large abscesses. Rarely, cardiac and noncardiac tumors or foreign bodies may gain access to the arterial circulation and embolize. Primary or metastatic lung neoplasms, malignant melanoma, and bullet emboli have been reported. In patients with cyanotic congenital heart disease (e.g., patent foramen ovale), venous emboli may pass directly to the arterial circulation ("paradoxical" emboli). Although rare, this possibility should be considered in any patient with simultaneous arterial and venous emboli, particularly if a source of the arterial embolus is not evident.

Arterial Thrombosis Thrombosis is the in situ formation of a blood clot within the noninterrupted arterial vascular system. Complicated atherosclerotic plaques are usually responsible for the two major factors that cause in situ thrombosis: (1) endothelial injury and (2) alterations in normal blood flow. Less common causes include acute vasculitis and trauma. Thrombosis is rare in normal arteries.[7]

Peripheral arterial thrombi are usually occlusive, although they may be limited to one wall (mural) in larger vessels. Peripheral arterial thrombi are usually firmly attached to the damaged arterial wall and infrequently embolize. The clot may propogate proximally and distally, which intensifies the ischemia.

Inflammation Inflammatory arterial injury can be caused by drugs, irradiation, mechanical trauma, or bacterial invasion. The major cause of arteritis is noninfectious systemic necrotizing vasculitis (see Chapter 112). Most cases of infectious arteritis are caused by direct invasion of the arterial wall. Septicemia, intravenous (IV) drug abuse, or infective endocarditis is most often responsible. Certain fungal infections, particularly aspergillosis and mucormycosis, are frequently associated with vasculitis and thrombosis.

Trauma Different types of vascular injury result in characteristic pathologic syndromes.[8] Partial arterial lacerations continue to bleed because the intact portion of the vessel wall prevents retraction and closure of the arterial wound. This may form an expanding hematoma, causing progressive deformity, pain, and nerve compression. Complete arterial transection usually has only moderate or insignificant bleeding because of arterial spasm of the transected ends of the artery and the formation of a temporary thrombus. Delayed hemorrhage in completely transected arteries may result from relaxation of arterial spasm, eventual liquefaction of the thrombus, or displacement of the thrombus by arterial pressure. Blunt injury may produce partial or complete intimal disruption. Dissection of the distal intima can lead to progressive obstruction and thrombosis. Complete occlusion may not occur for hours or days after injury. Vasospasm can accompany injuries that are adjacent to blood vessels; spontaneous resolution always occurs in the absence of arterial disruption or intimal injury.

Vasospasm Vasospastic disorders (Raynaud's disease, Raynaud's phenomenon, livedo reticularis, acrocyanosis, erythromelalgia) produce an abnormal vasomotor response in distal small arteries. The exact cause of these disorders is unknown but is thought to be related to hyperlability of the autonomic innervation of the peripheral arterioles. The vasospastic disorders are characterized by the presence of ischemic symptoms and the absence of tissue loss. True organic changes within the arterial wall are absent. In contrast, patients with digital ulceration and gangrene always have fixed arterial occlusions in the distal extremity arteries.

Arteriovenous Fistulas Abnormal communication between arteries and veins may result from congenital defects, rupture of an arterial aneurysm into an adjacent vein, penetrating injuries, and inflammatory necrosis associated with neoplasms or infection. Arteriovenous (AV) fistulas can occur in any region of the body. The artery proximal to the fistula becomes distended, tortuous, and aneurysmal. Similar changes occur in the venous side of the fistula. Proximal and distal veins respond to alterations in hemodynamics with intimal proliferation and fibrosis, followed by a decrease in the internal elastic lamina, resulting in distention, tortuosity, and aneurysm formation. The resultant chronic venous hypertension may cause dermatitis and ulceration of overlying skin. The size of the opening between artery and vein generally increases with time.

Approximately 60% of AV fistulas are associated with a false aneurysm.[9] False aneurysm formation can occur as part of the fistulous tract or as the result of arterial or venous dilation.[9]

The increase in cardiac output that occurs when blood switches from the arterial to the venous system can result in a widened pulse pressure or high-output cardiac failure.

CLINICAL FEATURES

History

Patients with peripheral arterial disease have pain, tissue loss (ulceration or gangrene), or a change in sensation or appearance (swelling, discoloration, or temperature change). Because the primary cause of peripheral arterial disease is atherosclerosis, related conditions that constitute secondary evidence of atherosclerosis are cardiac disease, MI, cardiac dysrhythmias (e.g., atrial fibrillation), stroke, TIAs, and renal disease. Factors that increase the likelihood of atherosclerosis are cigarette smoking, diabetes, hypercholesterolemia, and hypertension.

Risk factors not related to atherosclerosis include prior injuries or surgeries, major illnesses, a history of phlebitis or pulmonary embolism, the presence of autoimmune disease or arthritis, and a history of prior coagulation abnormalities. IV drug use can lead to arterial injury. Aortoiliac obstruction can cause sexual impotence in men (Leriche's syndrome).

Acute Arterial Occlusion The patient with acute arterial occlusion usually exhibits some variant of the "five Ps": pain, pallor, pulselessness, paresthesias, and paralysis. Paresthesias and paralysis indicate limb-threatening ischemia that requires emergency surgical intervention regardless of the cause. In patients with non-limb-threatening ischemia, accurate differentiation between embolism and in situ thrombosis as the cause of acute arterial occlusion determines patient management. Arterial embolism is best managed by emergency Fogarty catheter embolectomy. Non-limb-threatening ischemia from in situ thrombosis is often aggravated by emergency surgical intervention and is therefore initially best managed nonoperatively, if possible (Figure 82-1). Acute arterial embolus usually occurs in patients without significant peripheral atherosclerosis and without well-developed collateral circulation. For this reason, acute embolus usually presents as sudden limb-threatening ischemia. Patients describe a sensation of the leg's being "struck" by a severe shocking pain. Often the patient may have to sit or fall to the ground during the event.

In situ thrombosis usually occurs in patients who have longstanding significant peripheral atherosclerosis and well-developed collateral circulation. For this reason, in situ thrombosis often is seen subacutely with non-limb-threatening ischemia. A history of claudication is common with in situ thrombosis and rare in patients with arterial embolus.

Chronic Arterial Insufficiency Chronic arterial insufficiency causes two characteristic types of pain: intermittent claudication and ischemic pain at rest. The level of arterial occlusion and the location of intermittent claudication are closely correlated. Calf claudication is associated with femoral and popliteal disease. Patients complain of a cramping pain, reliably reproduced by the same degree of exercise and completely relieved by rest (usually 1 to 5 minutes). Aortoiliac occlusive disease typically causes claudication in the buttocks and hips, as well as the calves. The calf pain in aortoiliac disease is generally more severe than the buttock and thigh pain, which is more often described as an aching, discomfort, or weakness. Some patients even deny pain, complaining only that the thigh or hip "gives out" with exercise. Aortoiliac occlusive disease severe enough to produce bilateral claudication is almost always associated with impotence in men (Leriche's syndrome). Even in the absence of impotency, bilateral hip or thigh pain in a man should indicate the possibility of aortoiliac occlusive disease.

Chronic arterial insufficiency may progress so that ischemic pain occurs at rest. Rest pain often begins in the feet and typically involves the foot distal to the metatarsals, awakening the patient from sleep. Ischemic rest pain is a severe, unrelenting pain aggravated by elevation and unrelieved by analgesics. Typically, patients sleep with the leg dangling over the side of the bed or sleep in a chair to

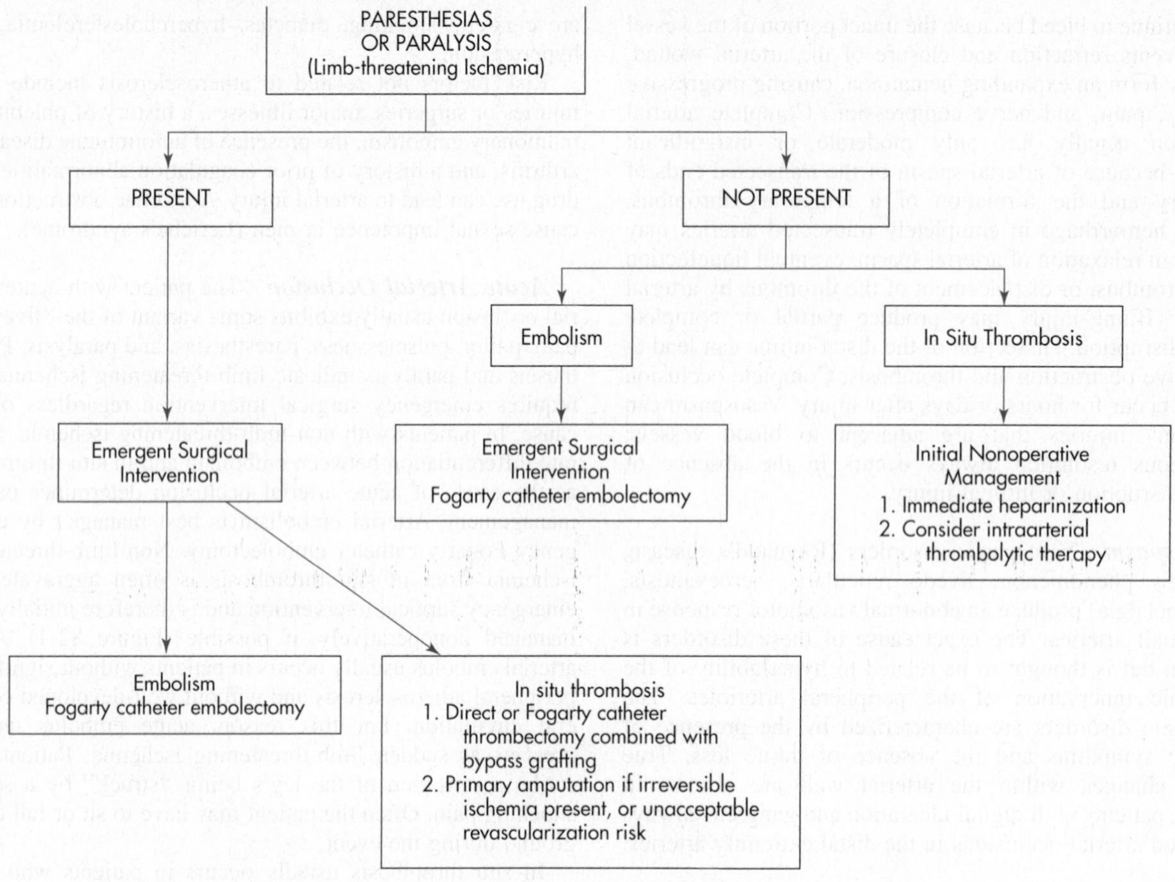

Figure 82-1. **Clinical presentation and management of acute arterial occlusion.**

improve perfusion pressure to the distal tissues. Patients have prompt relief of pain by any activity that involves a standing position.

Physical Examination

A systematic assessment of the peripheral vascular system is imperative. Palpation of the pulse volume in the pairs of brachial, radial, femoral, posterior tibial, and dorsalis pedis arteries should be performed and documented on a 0 to 4+ scale. Carotid arteries should be gently palpated singly and findings similarly documented.

Approximately 10% of the population do not have one of the dorsalis pedis pulses.[10] The lower extremities should be examined for signs of chronic and advanced ischemia. Muscular atrophy, particularly in the lower extremities, and loss of hair growth over the dorsum of the toes and foot with thickening of the toenails resulting from slowness of nail growth are common signs of arterial insufficiency. As ischemia becomes more advanced, the skin becomes shiny, scaly, and "skeletonized" from atrophy of the skin, subcutaneous tissue, and muscle.

Any area in which ischemia is suspected can be tested by blanching with finger pressure; a delay in return of normal color on relieving the pressure (compared with that of the nonaffected extremity) implies reduced perfusion.

Buerger's sign provides reliable evidence of severe advanced ischemia. With the patient supine, the patient's feet are elevated more than 12 inches above the estimated level of the right atrium, and any change in the color of the feet is noted. If the color does not change, the patient dorsiflexes the feet five or six times; latent color changes induced by exercise are noted. With the patient sitting, the feet are then allowed to hang down over the side of the stretcher; the time of normal color return is recorded. Normal color should return within 10 seconds, and the veins should fill within 15 seconds. If the veins require more than 20 seconds to become distended, advanced ischemia is present.

With severely restricted arterial inflow and chronic dilation of the peripheral vascular bed, the foot turns chalk white on elevation and intensely hyperemic after 1 minute of dependency. Localized pallor or cyanosis associated with poor capillary filling is usually a prelude to ischemic gangrene or ulceration.

Doppler ultrasound should be used in the ED in all patients with questionable or absent pulses. Doppler testing is more sensitive than palpation in detecting peripheral pulses. An estimate of blood flow to the lower extremities can be made by measuring the systolic blood pressure at the level of the ankle and comparing it to the brachial systolic pressure. With the patient supine, a blood pressure cuff is applied just proximal to the malleolus, inflated above brachial systolic pressure, and then deflated slowly. Ankle systolic pressure can be accurately measured with a Doppler probe placed over the dorsalis pedis or posterior tibial arteries. This pressure is normally 90% or more of the brachial systolic pressure; with mild arterial insufficiency, it is between 70% and 90%;

Table 82-1. Differentiation of Embolus from Thrombosis

	Embolus	Thrombosis
Identifiable source for embolus	Usual, particularly atrial fibrillation	Less common
History of claudication	Rare	Common
Physical findings suggestive of occlusive disease	Few; proximal and contralateral limb pulses normal	Often present; proximal or contralateral limb pulses diminished or absent
Demarcation of ischemia	Sharp	Diffuse
Arteriography	Minimal atherosclerosis; sharp cutoff; few collaterals	Diffuse atherosclerosis, tapered, irregular cutoff; well-developed collaterals

From Brewster DC, Chin AK, Fogarty TJ: *Vascular surgery,* Philadelphia, 1990, WB Saunders.

with moderate insufficiency, between 50% and 70%; and with severe insufficiency, less than 50%.

Allen's test is helpful in assessing patency of the radial or ulnar artery distal to the wrist. The patient initially opens and closes the hand and then clenches the fist to expel as much blood from the hand as possible; the examiner then compresses the radial and ulnar arteries. When the patient opens the fist, the hand is pale. The examiner then releases pressure from the radial artery but maintains it on the ulnar artery. If the radial artery distal to the wrist is patent, the hand becomes pink rapidly; if it is occluded, the hand remains pale. The maneuver is then repeated by maintaining pressure on the radial artery while releasing the ulnar artery. A comparison can be made with the opposite hand.

Arterial Embolism The physical examination can assist in differentiating between arterial embolism and in situ thrombosis in patients who have acute arterial occlusion. The sudden loss of a previously present pulse is the hallmark of arterial embolus. It is difficult, however, to recognize this finding if the prior pulse status of the limb is unknown or is abnormal as the result of associated atherosclerosis. A bounding pulse may be felt initially at the location of an embolus as a result of transmitted pulsations through the fresh clot. In general, patients with arterial embolus have few physical findings suggestive of longstanding peripheral vascular disease with normal, proximal, and contralateral limb pulses. Occasional tenderness to palpation can be noted at the site of an embolic occlusion.

If arterial embolus is suspected, the physical examination should be directed to identify its source. The two most common sites are (1) left ventricular mural thrombus secondary to a prior MI and (2) left atrial thrombus in a patient with mitral valve disease. Coexistent atrial fibrillation is common.

The limb distal to an embolic occlusion is initially chalk white. Because of absence of blood from the venules of the subcapillary layer, the demarcation between ischemic and nonischemic tissue is sharp. With time, cyanosis may appear, indicating desaturation of blood with continued ongoing ischemia. Paresthesia or paralysis indicates limb-threatening ischemia. The presence of sensitivity to light touch is often the best guide to viability of the tissue. Complete anesthesia demands immediate surgical intervention. Paralysis represents severe skeletal muscle and neural ischemia and may be associated with irreversibility. Involuntary muscle contracture with woody hardness represents irreversible ischemia.

Arterial Thrombosis Physical findings of in situ thrombosis are often accompanied by evidence of atherosclerotic occlusive disease. Proximal or contralateral limb pulses are usually diminished or absent. An identifiable source of an embolus, such as mitral valve disease or atrial fibrillation, is usually not present. Because of collateral circulation, demarcation of limb ischemia is less well defined in these patients (Table 82-1).

Carotid and femoral arteries may have bruits, and there may be evidence of abdominal aortic aneurysm or renal arterial bruits. If an occlusion of the upper extremity vessels is suspected, the subclavian artery should be evaluated by palpating for thrills and listening for bruits in the supraclavicular fossa.

A funduscopic examination allows direct visualization of retinal arterioles that may yield evidence of arteriosclerosis or hypertension. Hollenhorst plaques (atheromatous emboli containing cholesterol crystals in the retinal arterioles) may be detected. Roth's spots (round or oval white spots seen near the optic disk) may be present in infective endocarditis.

Embolic phenomenon can cause diverse end-organ damage: hemiplegia from cerebral emboli, flank pain with hematuria from renal emboli, left upper quadrant abdominal pain from splenic infarcts, and pleuritic pain with hemoptysis from pulmonary emboli. Septic pulmonary emboli from right-sided endocarditis may be confused with pneumonia.

Inflammation Inflammatory vascular disease manifests primarily as skin involvement. Skin lesions typically appear as palpable purpura; other cutaneous manifestations of vasculitis include macules, papules, vesicles, bullae, subcutaneous nodules, ulcers, and recurrent or chronic urticaria. The skin lesions may be pruritic or even painful, with a burning or stinging sensation. Lesions more often occur in dependent areas: in the lower extremities in ambulatory patients or in the sacral area in bedridden patients. Edema may accompany some lesions, and hyperpigmentation often occurs in the areas of recurrent or chronic lesions.

Vasospasm Vasospastic disorders cause a sharp border between ischemic and normal tissue. *Raynaud's disease* is characterized by intermittent attacks of triphasic color changes: pallor, cyanosis, and then rubor.[11] The most important element is pallor, during which the digits turn chalk white. Attacks generally last 15 to 60 minutes, and rewarming the hands restores normal color and sensation. Color changes do not occur above the metacarpophalangeal joints and rarely involve the thumb.

Two other vasospastic disorders have a characteristic appearance. *Livedo reticularis* is characterized by a persistent cyanotic mottling of the skin that has a typical fishnet appearance and may involve all parts of the extremities and trunk. *Acrocyanosis* is the least common vasospastic disorder and is characterized by persistent, painless, diffuse cyanosis of the fingers, hands, toes, and feet. Cyanosis usually intensifies with exposure to cold and decreases with warming. The involved parts are nearly always cold, exhibit excessive perspiration, and have normal arterial pulses.

Arteriovenous Fistulas AV malformations and fistulas, although rare, must be distinguished from vascular bruits or aneurysms. True aneurysms and arterial stenoses are associated with a systolic murmur. Pseudoaneurysms generally have a loud systolic and sometimes a separate faint diastolic murmur. AV fistulas have a constant systolic and diastolic (to-and-fro) murmur heard best directly over the lesion and often associated with a palpable thrill. Unless congenital, AV fistulas occur at prior operative or trauma sites. The skin overlying the lesion may be warm, but distally the temperature is often decreased. Veins peripheral to the fistula are usually distended and varicose. Large and longstanding AV fistulas produce high cardiac output and widened pulse pressure. Tachycardia in these patients may suddenly decrease when the artery leading to the fistula or the fistula itself is occluded (Branham's sign).

DIAGNOSTIC STRATEGIES

An accurate diagnosis of peripheral arterial occlusive disease can be achieved in most patients by careful history and physical examination supplemented by bedside testing.

Noninvasive Assessment

Doppler ultrasonography (ultrasound, US) measures blood flow velocity by detecting the frequency shift of sound waves reflected from red blood cells that move toward and away from the Doppler probe. The Doppler signal can be processed to generate a normal triphasic-velocity waveform for recording and analysis. Progressive arterial narrowing alters the triphasic waveform to biphasic and finally monophasic shape. Such Doppler US waveform analysis can detect significant arterial occlusive disease, although it is less accurate in determining exact location.

Real-time B-mode US imaging uses differences in sound wave reflection from the interfaces between tissues with different acoustic impedances to provide anatomic detail of underlying structures. US imaging is useful in detecting and evaluating atherosclerotic plaques and mural thrombi and in sizing aneurysms of the abdominal aorta, iliac, femoral, and popliteal arteries. B-mode US is noninvasive, painless, less expensive than other modalities, and universally available. EPs can scan and interpret bedside US studies, which can lead to rapid diagnosis of life-threatening conditions as well as reduce the number of delayed or invasive diagnostic procedures.[12] B-mode US imaging is the diagnostic procedure of choice for the initial evaluation and determination of the size of peripheral artery aneurysms.

Duplex scanning combines the image of B-mode US and sophisticated on-line computer analysis of accurately sampled Doppler waveforms to allow simultaneous acquisition of both the image of a vascular structure and the characteristics of blood flow velocity within it. Duplex scanning permits noninvasive and accurate diagnosis of peripheral vascular, cerebrovascular, and venous disease.

Color imaging of blood flow has been combined with duplex scanning and is known as color-coded Doppler, Doppler angiography, or angiodynography. Color flow imaging is achieved by assignment of colors to the direction of blood flow detected by Doppler waveform signals. Red represents flow away from the US probe, and blue represents flow toward the probe. Color-coded Doppler, the procedure of choice for most conditions, allows noninvasive and accurate detection of atherosclerotic plaques and stenoses, their effect on intraluminal blood flow, and the presence of venous thrombosis.

Invasive Contrast Arteriography

Angiography is the definitive test of abnormal peripheral artery anatomy but is often inconclusive about the physiologic condition of the tissues. Adverse effects of contrast media and catheter-related complications must be weighed against the benefits of this procedure. Contrast media have a direct toxic effect on vascular endothelium; can produce renal failure, especially in diabetic patients; may cause peripheral vasodilation with hypotension; may result in seizures and stroke in neurologic patients; and can cause severe idiosyncratic and allergic reactions. Catheter-related complications, including embolization, catheter breakage, and vascular disruption, vary with operator skill and anatomic location but average 0.5%. Overall mortality rate from angiography is 0.03%.[13] Emergency angiography is usually required in these circumstances: (1) acute arterial embolus or thrombosis if the clinical diagnosis is uncertain, (2) consideration of emergency vascular bypass grafting, and (3) characterization of vascular abnormality before emergency surgical correction. A decision to proceed with angiography should be made with the vascular surgeon.

Computed Tomography and Magnetic Resonance Imaging

Computed tomography (CT) scan is the most useful diagnostic modality for the evaluation of the abdominal aorta.[14] In the peripheral arteriovascular system, CT scans are useful primarily for atherosclerotic, infected, and false aneurysms. Magnetic resonance imaging (MRI) scan has an undefined role but is a promising technology in the evaluation of vascular disease. The ability to make axial, coronal, and sagittal sections provides accurate visualization of anatomy. MRI scan detects changes in the relaxation variables of tissues before obvious structural changes, uniquely differentiating blood, thrombus, fat, and fibrosis.

MANAGEMENT

The management of acute arterial occlusion depends on the degree and cause of ischemia. Patients with limb-threatening ischemia from embolism receive emergency Fogarty catheter embolectomy. Patients with limb-threatening ischemia caused by in situ thrombosis require direct or Fogarty catheter thrombectomy combined with vascular bypass grafting. Thrombectomy alone often fails as a result of recurrent thrombosis. Patients who have a lesion that cannot be bypassed, who have evidence of irreversible ischemia, or who are too ill to tolerate revascularization are treated with primary amputation.

A patient with non-limb-threatening ischemia from embolism is treated with emergency Fogarty catheter embolectomy. Non-limb-threatening ischemia from in situ thrombosis is best managed nonoperatively with immediate systemic heparinization and possibly with intraarterial thrombolytic therapy (see Figure 82-1).

Elective surgical repair of an asymptomatic atherosclerotic peripheral arterial aneurysm is usually accomplished by excision of the aneurysm with end-to-end anastomosis or graft interposition. Infected true and false peripheral aneurysms require aneurysm resection, debridement of infected tissue, and ligation of the proximal and distal uninfected arteries. Autogenous vein bypass through uninfected tissue planes is attempted. Prosthetic grafts carry a high risk of graft infection. The surgical approach to noninfected false aneurysms is similar to that of peripheral atherosclerotic aneurysms.

Patients with thoracic outlet syndrome who have cervical ribs, arterial involvement, or significant neurologic symptoms require surgical decompression with removal of anomalous fibromuscular bands and resection of the first rib, if present. Subclavian and subclavian-axillary aneurysms may be treated with resection and end-to-end anastomosis, graft reconstruction, or surgical revision. Patients with distal embolic occlusions are treated with Fogarty catheter embolectomy. Axillary and subclavian vein thromboses are best managed with surgical thrombectomy or systemic thrombolytic therapy. Patients with only brachial plexus involvement and minimal signs and symptoms should be followed closely with conservative treatment.

Surgical treatment of peripheral AV fistulas requires interrupting the fistula tract and restoring both arterial and venous continuity with end-to-end anastomosis or graft interposition. If anatomic location precludes surgical intervention, percutaneous transvascular embolization with liquid tissue adhesives (e.g., isobutyl-2-cyanoacrylate) is usually successful.

Noninvasive Therapy

Acute Anticoagulation with Heparin IV heparin remains an important and effective initial therapy for the ED treatment of patients with acute arterial embolism, acute arterial thrombosis, and subclavian vein thrombosis. Heparin should be immediately and empirically administered to these patients in standard IV doses (80 U/kg by IV bolus, followed by a maintenance infusion of 18 U/kg/hr). Heparin quickly reduces thrombin generation and fibrin formation, minimizing clot propagation, which can intensify limb ischemia and jeopardize tissues. Relative contraindications include recent neurosurgery (especially within 2 weeks), major surgery within 48 hours, childbirth within 24 hours, a known bleeding diathesis, thrombocytopenia, a potentially hemorrhagic lesion, or active bleeding.

Thrombolytic Therapy Low-dosage intraarterial thrombolytic therapy is being used with increasing frequency for acute arterial occlusion. Patients with limb-threatening ischemia are not candidates for this therapy because clot lysis generally takes 6 to 72 hours. Patients cannot tolerate several more hours of ischemia without substantial tissue or limb loss, and immediate Fogarty catheter embolectomy is still the treatment of choice in most patients with an acute arterial embolus. Consideration of thrombolytic therapy is generally reserved for patients with in situ thrombosis and non-limb-threatening ischemia.

Intraarterial thrombolytic agents induce clot lysis in the small, distal runoff vessels, decreasing outflow resistance and enabling the native artery to remain open longer. Thrombolysis often uncovers a critical stenosis that, untreated, may lead to another episode of thrombosis. After successful thrombolytic therapy, most patients require secondary bypass grafting or percutaneous transluminal angioplasty. Streptokinase, urokinase, and tissue plasminogen activator (t-plasminogen activator) have all been used successfully. IV administration of a thrombolytic agent to treat arterial occlusion is less effective than direct administration into the clot. Clots more than 30 days old are more organized and less likely to achieve successful lysis.

Invasive Therapy

Fogarty Catheter Thrombectomy The Fogarty catheter is most frequently used for iliac, femoral, and popliteal embolectomy, often with only local anesthesia.[15] Aortic saddle embolus is removed by sequentially passing the Fogarty catheter through bilateral common femoral arteriotomies.

Newly formed in situ thrombosis can often be successfully removed with the Fogarty catheter. An older thrombus adheres more firmly to the damaged vessel wall, requiring direct surgical thrombectomy. The Fogarty catheter is not used in the venous system because of the venous valves.

Peripheral Percutaneous Transluminal Angioplasty The initial success and long-term patency achieved by angioplasty depend on the location of the lesion and the extent of atheromatous disease. Proximal larger-caliber arteries (e.g., iliac, femoropopliteal) have the best initial and long-term results. Discrete stenotic lesions (<5 cm) have better long-term patency rates than those vessels that are diffusely involved or with multiple involved segments. Balloon angioplasty has become the accepted sole treatment for isolated stenotic lesions in the renal, iliac, and superficial femoral vessels.

Transluminal angioplasty with intravascular stent placement is being used in more distal vessels, including the popliteal and tibial circulation, as well as in more complex and diffuse lesions in patients who are prohibitive surgical risks.[16] Its value in these patients remains to be determined.

Recanalization devices include the percutaneous atherectomy catheter, percutaneous angioscope, hot-tip laser, excimer laser, and high-speed rotating wire and drill.[16]

Grafting Vascular grafting is often used by the vascular surgeon and is associated with a variety of complications that can be diagnosed in the ED. Autogenous vein grafts (usually a reversed greater saphenous vein) provide excellent long-term patency for small arteries. Vein grafts respond to arterial pressure with gradual intimal proliferation and medial fibrosis. They may develop atherosclerosis, which can lead to graft stenosis and thrombosis. False aneurysms may form along the suture line.

Polytetrafluoroethylene prosthetic grafts are widely used in medium and large arteries that are impossible to bridge with smaller vein grafts. Prosthetic grafts have a higher rate of thrombosis than venous grafts. Distal emboli may result from poor fixation of luminal fibrin. If the prosthetic graft has not been adequately covered by viable tissue, it can erode into adjacent structures and hollow viscera. Prosthetic graft infection is a devastating complication requiring removal of the entire graft.

Vascular grafts may be used to bypass arterial occlusions and reconstruct a diseased arterial bifurcation, or they may be interposed between sections of resected artery. The two most common complications of both prosthetic and vein grafts are (1) thrombosis and (2) development of a false aneurysm at one or more suture lines. Bypass grafting is most often used as palliative treatment for symptoms of atherosclerotic occlusive disease. Patients with localized unilateral stenosis (<3 to 5 cm in length) may have a comparable rate of success with percutaneous transluminal angioplasty with or without stent placement.[17]

Patients with calf claudication from superficial femoral or popliteal occlusive disease usually do not experience rapid progression of disease if they stop smoking and maintain an active exercise regimen. Patients who have progression of disease, significant rest pain, or tissue loss require surgical revascularization.

Sympathectomy Lumbar sympathectomy is no longer used for treatment of ischemia resulting from arterial occlusion because no evidence shows an increase in blood flow to muscle. The benefit of sympathectomy in symptomatic Raynaud's phenomenon is unclear, but it remains a valuable method to treat Buerger's disease.[18]

Hyperbaric Therapy

Scant objective evidence indicates that hyperbaric therapy alters the long-term course of chronic obliterative vascular disorders. Success has been achieved with healing chronic diabetic ischemic ulcers and salvaging ischemic skin grafts and flaps.[19]

CHRONIC ARTERIAL INSUFFICIENCY

Arteriosclerosis Obliterans

Arteriosclerosis obliterans (atherosclerotic occlusive disease, chronic occlusive arterial disease, obliterative arteriosclerosis) is the peripheral arterial presentation of atherosclerosis, encompassing occlusive disease of the aorta and its branches to the extremities. Most often, atherosclerosis obliterans affects the lower abdominal aorta, the iliac arteries, and the arteries supplying the lower extremities. Upper extremity manifestations are uncommon.

Arteriosclerosis obliterans is responsible for 95% of cases of chronic occlusive arterial disease. It is most common in persons older than 50, but as many as 19% of cases occur in patients between ages 30 and 49. Men are affected more often than women, 5:1 to 10:1. Approximately one third of patients with arteriosclerosis obliterans have coexistent coronary artery disease. The incidence of diabetes mellitus is 20% to 30%.[20]

As in other atherosclerotic disease, risk factors for arteriosclerosis obliterans include cigarette smoking, hyperlipidemia, and hypertension. Of patients with arteriosclerosis obliterans, 70% to 90% are smokers when first examined, 75% have hyperlipidemia, and 30% have hypertension.[20]

Clinical Features and Differential Diagnosis Acute arterial occlusion from embolism, thrombosis, or trauma is ruled out primarily by history. Atheromatous emboli from proximal ulcerated plaques or aneurysms can cause small scattered ischemic lesions in the toes, feet, or legs, which may cause blue toe syndrome (see Figure 82-3). The peripheral pulses are present in the blue toe syndrome. Exercise-induced claudication must be distinguished from the nocturnal muscle cramps that frequently occur during rest in elderly patients. Aortoiliac occlusive disease must be differentiated from osteoarthritis of the hip, in which symptoms tend to be more variable from day to day, are not relieved completely with rest, and are not reliably reproduced by the same amount of exercise. Pseudoclaudication from the cauda equina syndrome is caused by narrowing of the lumbar canal from spondylosis, disease of the intervertebral disks, or spinal cord tumor. Symptoms mimic intermittent claudication but are less closely related to exercise and rest than true claudication.

The cause of lower extremity ulcers should be carefully determined. Approximately 5% of lower extremity ulcerations are caused by *arterial insufficiency.*[21] These are usually located distal to the ankle, typically at the terminal portion of the digits, around the nail beds, or between the toes, caused by friction of one toe on another. Less common locations include the metatarsal heads, heel, and malleoli. Arterial insufficiency ulcers are painful but improve when the extremity is in a dependent position. They are associated with evidence of coexistent chronic arterial insufficiency (absence of hair growth on dorsum of feet, skin atrophy, absent pulses, and nail deformities). Ulcers are initially small, shallow, and dry. The base is gray, yellow, or black, with minimal or no granulation tissue. The rim of the ulcer is sharp and indolent, showing no signs of cellular proliferation or epithelialization.

Approximately 90% of lower extremity ulcers are caused by *chronic venous insufficiency.*[21] These typically occur proximal to or in the region of the ankle, especially in the vicinity of the medial malleolus. Venous stasis ulcers are only mildly painful and improve with elevation of the extremity. Evidence of longstanding chronic venous insufficiency, including edema, prominent superficial veins, and stasis dermatitis, is present. Ulcers are moderate in size with a weeping base and extensive granulation tissue. A rapidly developing ulcer is more suggestive of venous insufficiency.

Most of the remaining lower extremity ulcers are caused by *diabetic neuropathy,* alone or with arterial insufficiency.[21] The location reflects sites of repeated trauma, including the toes, heels, and plantar surface of the feet, especially the metatarsal heads. Neurotrophic ulcers are characteristically painless. Patients may have evidence of coexistent peripheral arterial insufficiency. The ulcers are deep and penetrating, often with suppurative drainage caused by an associated underlying infection or chronic osteomyelitis. Neurotrophic ulcers are usually surrounded by a rim of thick callus.

Hypertensive ulcers are rare and reflect longstanding, uncontrolled hypertension. These ulcers are typically located in the vicinity of the lateral malleolus and start as painful, reddish blue areas of infarcted skin. A hemorrhagic bleb develops, then breaks down into a superficial ulcer. This ischemic area can reach a size of 5 to 10 cm. The appearance is an ischemic ulcer with sharply demarcated borders, little granulation tissue, and minimal drainage. The pain is the most severe of all lower extremity ulcers.

Multiple ischemic ulcerations above and below the ankle should suggest vasculitis or atheromatous embolization. Ulcers with regular edges in unusual locations may be factitial or may result from subcutaneous injection of illicit drugs. Thickened, rolled, and elevated edges with a central depression containing granulation tissue are characteristic of malignant ulcers.

Management The first step in determining treatment is to identify patients whose symptoms are the result solely of arteriosclerosis obliterans without coexistent thromboembolic disease. Treatment is then dictated by the accurate classification of symptomatic patients into two groups: those with functional ischemia and those with limb-threatening ischemia.[22] All patients' initial assessments and treatments should be made in conjunction with appropriate vascular surgery consultation.

Patients with limb-threatening ischemia constitute a surgical emergency. Angiography should be arranged in consultation with a vascular surgeon to determine the presence of sufficiently localized disease to permit emergency bypass grafting.[22] Patients with functional ischemia may require outpatient arrangements for noninvasive vascular testing or elective invasive contrast arteriography to determine treatment options such as bypass grafting. Ischemic ulcers or skin lesions should be cultured in the ED. Systemic antibiotics should be instituted if infection is present. Wet to dry dressings may help debride ulcers containing fibrin, debris, or infection. Radiographs of the underlying bones should be obtained to rule out osteomyelitis. Patients with ischemic rest pain require hospitalization even if they are not surgical candidates. Bed rest, a warm environment, and maintenance of the limb in a dependent position usually relieve pain.

Buerger's Disease (Thromboangiitis Obliterans)

First described by Buerger in 1908, thromboangiitis obliterans is an idiopathic inflammatory occlusive disease primarily involving the medium and small arteries of the hands and feet.[23] Patients are usually men between 20 and 40 years of age who use tobacco, although recent reports indicate an increasing frequency of this disease in women. Buerger's disease affects all races but is more prevalent in the Middle and Far East. The incidence in the United States is 20 in 100,000.[24] The exact pathogenesis of Buerger's disease is unknown, but virtually all patients are smokers.

Thromboangiitis obliterans is characterized by segmental acute and chronic inflammation in the smaller arteries of both upper and lower extremities. The initial arterial inflammatory process progresses to affect the adjacent veins and nerves, often leading to associated venous thrombosis and progressive fibrous encasement of these structures. This is recognized clinically as painful, tender, reddened, or dark nodules over a peripheral artery with either a reduced or an absent pulse (*phlebitis migrans*).

Clinical Features Clinical criteria for the diagnosis of Buerger's disease include (1) a history of smoking, (2) onset before age 50, (3) infrapopliteal arterial occlusive lesions, (4) either upper limb involvement or phlebitis migrans, and (5) absence of atherosclerotic risk factors other than smoking. A characteristic symptom of Buerger's disease is foot or instep claudication caused by infrapopliteal arterial occlusion. Intense rubor of the affected extremity, particularly with dependency, is also characteristic. Foot pulses may be absent in the presence of normal femoral and popliteal pulses. Involvement of the hands is often bilateral and symmetric, leading to the development of hand claudication or fingertip ulcers. Phlebitis migrans occurs early in the disease. Approximately 50% of patients experience Raynaud's-type triphasic color response to cold. In the upper extremities the digital arteries are usually more involved than the radial or ulnar arteries.[24]

Diagnostic Strategies Adherence to diagnostic clinical criteria should be sufficient for ED diagnosis of Buerger's disease. Noninvasive vascular laboratory testing can confirm the diagnosis and determine the extent of involvement. Although rarely required, angiography demonstrates multiple segmental occlusions.

Differential Diagnosis In patients older than 50 who have signs of peripheral ischemia, arteriosclerosis obliterans is a more likely diagnosis. In young women, autoimmune diseases such as scleroderma or systemic lupus erythematosus should be considered.[24]

Management Permanent complete abstinence from tobacco is the only known effective treatment for Buerger's disease. If a patient does not completely stop smoking, alternating periods of quiescence are followed by exacerbations, with severe arterial insufficiency. Patients who permanently abstain from smoking have a benign clinical course. Despite this, many individuals who have Buerger's disease continue to smoke even though severe pain at rest, tissue loss, and eventually amputation occur.

With early symptoms without threat of tissue loss, patient education and follow-up with a vascular surgeon are sufficient. Vascular surgery treatment options are varied for patients with severe symptoms or threatened tissue loss. Intractable pain can be controlled with epidural anesthesia. Intraarterial or IV prostaglandin E_1 and antithrombotic agents, including aspirin and heparin, have been used successfully.[24] Patients with large-vessel arterial occlusion may benefit from arterial reconstruction. Sympathectomy is still a valuable treatment in advanced cases for cutaneous ulceration or vasospastic symptoms.[18] Because patients with Buerger's disease demonstrate good healing, intensive conservative treatment is usually successful in preventing surgical amputation.

ACUTE ARTERIAL OCCLUSION

Arterial Embolism

Despite advances in diagnosis and treatment, acute arterial embolus continues to be associated with substantial morbidity and mortality. As in recent decades, the incidence of arterial embolic disease appears to be increasing. Approximately 50% of acute arterial occlusions are caused by arterial embolism. The other 50% are caused by in situ thrombosis.[3]

Differential Diagnosis The clinical differentiation of arterial embolism and thrombosis is reviewed earlier under Pathophysiology.

Phlegmasia cerulea dolens is a massive iliofemoral deep venous thrombosis. The initial symptom may be acute onset of a swollen and painful leg. As swelling continues, secondary arterial insufficiency may occur. In acute arterial embolus, leg swelling is not usually present, especially not at the onset of pain. In addition, acute embolus produces a sharply demarcated pallor; phlegmasia cerulea dolens causes a cyanotic-appearing leg.

Aortic dissection may involve the arteries of the upper or lower extremity and may mimic acute embolus. A history of progressive severe pain, the presence of aortic insufficiency, and involvement at multiple sites suggest dissection. Acute neurologic syndromes (e.g., transverse myelitis, spinal subarachnoid hemorrhage, ruptured intervertebral disk) may produce sudden onset of unilateral or bilateral lower extremity weakness or sensory loss that mimics an acute aortic saddle occlusion.

Cold, blue extremities may result from low-output states such as hypovolemia, decreased cardiac output, sepsis, dehydration, MI, and pulmonary emboli in patients with longstanding atherosclerotic disease.

Management Acute arterial embolus is a surgical emergency. The likelihood of limb salvage decreases after 4 to 6 hours. On the basis of clinical diagnosis alone, full doses of IV heparin should be administered immediately to minimize clot propagation. Patients whose history and physical examination clearly indicate an acute arterial embolus should have immediate Fogarty catheter embolectomy without prior angiography. In these patients, preoperative US and angiography are rarely useful diagnostically and prolong the limb's ischemic status.

If the differentiation of acute embolus and in situ thrombosis is uncertain, pretreatment angiography is required and usually diagnostic. Patients with acute emboli generally show minimal signs of atherosclerosis, occlusion at the site of an arterial bifurcation, sharply demarcated cutoffs, and lack of flow distal to the occlusion. In patients with in situ thrombosis, arteriography shows diffuse atherosclerosis, occlusion at sites other than arterial bifurcations, a tapered irregular cutoff, and well-developed collateral vessels. In general, emboli tend to lodge at arterial bifurcations, whereas arterial thrombi do not (see Table 82-1).

Intraarterial thrombolytic therapy for acute embolus remains investigational. Immediate limb-threatening ischemia precludes consideration of treatment with thrombolytic therapy in most patients. Potential risks of thrombolytic therapy in arterial embolus patients with non-limb-threatening ischemia include partial clot lysis with further distal embolization or recurrent embolic events from the primary source of the initial embolus.[25]

Atheroembolism (Blue Toe Syndrome)

Atheroemboli are microemboli consisting of cholesterol, calcium, platelet aggregates, and hemorrhagic debris that break off from proximal atherosclerotic plaques or aneurysms and lodge in distal end arteries (Figure 82-2). In the CNS, atheroembolism causes TIAs and strokes. In the peripheral vascular system, atheroemboli characteristically are found in the lower extremities with cool, painful cyanotic toes in the presence of palpable distal pulses (Figure 82-3).

Clinical Features The typical presentation of atheroembolism is the sudden onset of a small painful area on the foot, typically the toe, which is cyanotic and tender.[26] If bilateral involvement is present, the distribution is not symmetric. Posterior tibial and dorsalis pedis pulses are present. The physical examination should be directed toward identification of a proximal source, such as an atherosclerotic aneurysm in the aorta, iliac, femoral, or popliteal arteries.

Differential Diagnosis A variety of conditions may mimic the blue toe syndrome. Acrocyanosis is painless, has a symmetric distribution, and may be located in the hands,

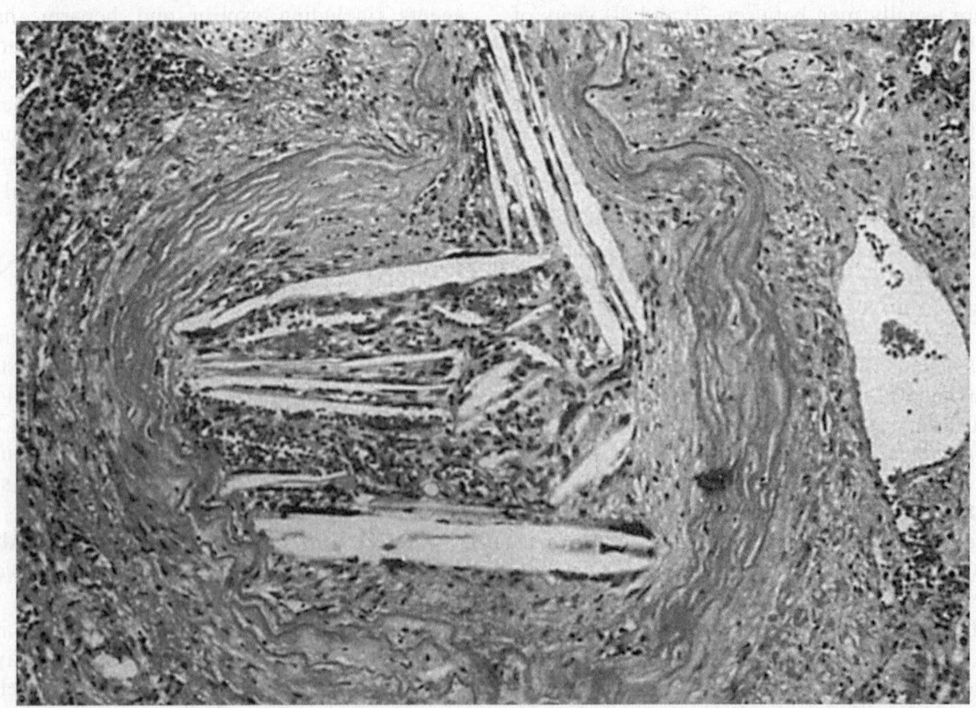

Figure 82-2. **Photomicrograph of cholesterol embolus lodged in peripheral arteriole. *Courtesy Arthur C. Aufderheide, MD.***

nose, and lips. Poor peripheral perfusion as a result of low cardiac output must also be considered. The cutaneous manifestations of vasculitis typically are palpable purpuric lesions and associated with constitutional symptoms of low-grade fever, myalgias, and weight loss. Previous frostbite may leave the extremities sensitive to cold. Local injury to the foot of the diabetic patient is easily differentiated.

Management Treatment is directed toward identifying and removing the proximal source of atheroembolism. Angiography is the most accurate diagnostic method to determine the source of emboli. If the cause is an aortic aneurysm and the patient is a surgical candidate, operative repair should be performed. Stenotic lesions in the iliac or femoral arteries can be treated with local endarterectomy, vascular bypass, or angioplasty.[16] Medical management with aspirin, dipyridamole, crystalline warfarin sodium (Coumadin), or steroids has variable results.

Arterial Thrombosis

Approximately 50% of acute arterial occlusions are caused by in situ thrombosis.[3] Acute arterial thrombosis is almost always superimposed on a complicated atherosclerotic lesion but can be caused by vasculitis or trauma (see Pathophysiology). In patients with limb-threatening ischemia, angiography is required to evaluate the feasibility of emergency bypass grafting. In patients with non-limb-threatening ischemia, angiography may be required if the clinical distinction of acute embolism and thrombosis is difficult (see Table 82-1).

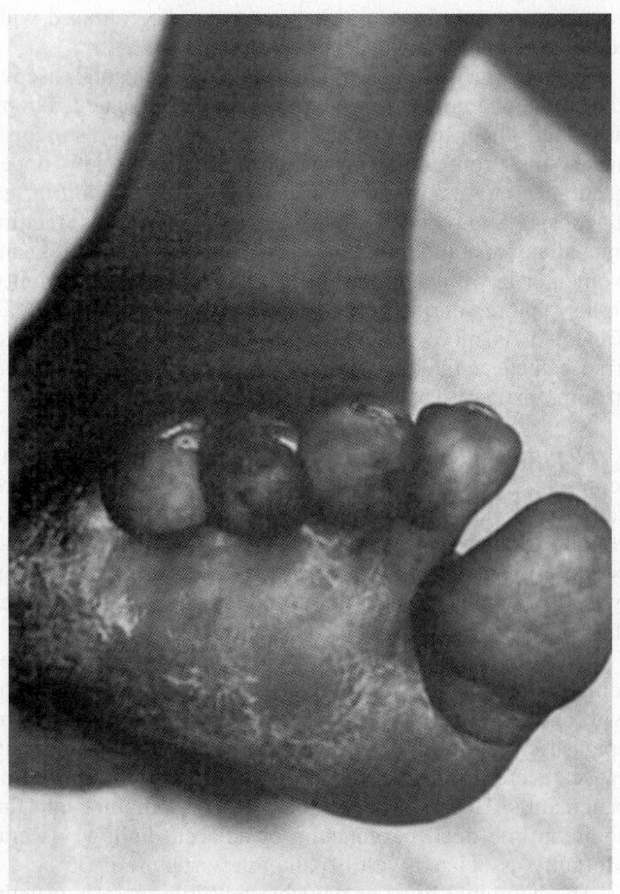

Figure 82-3. **Clinical presentation of atheromatous emboli, or blue toe syndrome.** ***Courtesy Gary R. Seabrook, MD.***

Management Systemic heparinization should be immediately established in the ED. Patients with severe limb-threatening ischemia require emergency direct or Fogarty catheter thrombectomy combined with bypass grafting. Simple thrombectomy alone often fails as a result of rethrombosis. Patients who have atherosclerotic disease not amenable to vascular bypass, who are too ill to tolerate revascularization, or who have irreversible ischemia require primary amputation. Patients with non-limb-threatening ischemia are initially best managed nonoperatively with heparin anticoagulation and consideration of treatment with low-dosage intraarterial thrombolytic therapy.

PERIPHERAL ARTERIAL ANEURYSMS

A true aneurysm is an abnormal localized dilation of the intact wall of any vessel caused by a combination of mural weakness and hemodynamic forces. Aneurysms enlarge at a rate governed by the cause of the lesion. Those caused by atherosclerosis progress slowly over years; those caused by trauma or infection enlarge over days, weeks, or months. The primary risk of central aneurysms (abdominal aorta, iliac arteries, and visceral arteries) is rupture (see Chapter 81). Peripheral arterial aneurysms rarely rupture; instead they are complicated by thrombosis or embolism that jeopardizes distal tissues.[27]

The cause of an aneurysm depends on its anatomic location. Lower extremity aneurysms are most often atherosclerotic in origin. Upper extremity aneurysms are usually caused by localized trauma. Visceral aneurysms result from abnormal hemodynamics, atherosclerosis, or infectious causes.

Lower Extremity

Femoral and popliteal artery aneurysms almost always occur in older men with advanced atherosclerosis. Twenty-five percent of patients have distal atheroembolism or thromboembolism; an additional 15% have total occlusion from in situ thrombosis.[27]

Popliteal Aneurysms Popliteal aneurysms are the most common peripheral aneurysms and occur bilaterally in approximately 60% of patients.[27] An abdominal aortic aneurysm occurs in almost 80% in patients with bilateral popliteal aneurysms. Most patients have claudication, thromboembolic events, atheroembolic events, or gangrene. Aneurysmal dilation can cause venous compression with associated deep venous thrombosis.

Femoral Aneurysms Femoral aneurysms are the second most common peripheral aneurysms and manifest similar to popliteal aneurysms. Femoral aneurysm dilation can also compress the femoral nerve, producing anterior thigh pain or weakness.

Diagnosis of both popliteal and femoral aneurysms is made by palpation of a pulsatile mass. Bilateral plain radiographs may show unilateral or bilateral calcified aneurysms. US and CT scan are diagnostic. Arteriography yields definitive diagnosis and indicates involvement of distal vessels. Patient with a lower extremity aneurysm should be evaluated for the presence of other aneurysms.

Asymptomatic patients often undergo elective surgical excision of the aneurysm and restoration of arterial continuity by end-to-end anastomosis or graft interposition. Simultaneous repair of coexisting abdominal aorta or contralateral extremity aneurysms combined with vascular bypass is typically done. Patients with limb-threatening thromboembolic events are first treated with Fogarty catheter embolectomy.[27]

Upper Extremity

Peripheral arterial aneurysms in the upper extremities are rare. Atherosclerosis generally spares the upper extremities, making localized trauma the most common cause.

Subclavian Artery Aneurysms The causes of proximal subclavian artery aneurysms are thoracic outlet obstruction, trauma, and rarely atherosclerosis. Subclavian aneurysms from atherosclerosis represent severe disease; 30% to 50% of these patients also have aortoiliac or other peripheral aneurysms.[28] Symptoms depend on the aneurysm's anatomic location. Patients may have chest, neck, and shoulder pain from acute expansion. Compression of the right recurrent laryngeal nerve can lead to voice change. Compression of the trachea can lead to stridor or other respiratory complaints. The chest radiograph may reveal a superior mediastinal mass, easily confused with a neoplasm.

Subclavian-Axillary Artery Aneurysms The subclavian artery can be compressed by a complete cervical rib that articulates with the first rib, producing a poststenotic dilation in the proximal subclavian and distal axillary artery. This syndrome occurs more often in women and in the dominant upper extremity. Cervical ribs occur in only 0.6% of the population.[29]

Axillary Artery Aneurysms Axillary artery aneurysms are most often caused by blunt trauma from inappropriate and prolonged use of crutches. Humerus fracture and anterior shoulder dislocation are less common causes.[28]

Subclavian, subclavian-axillary, and axillary artery aneurysms share the common complications of thromboembolism and limb-threatening ischemia, neuromuscular and sensory dysfunction from brachial plexus compression, and CNS ischemia produced by retrograde thromboembolism in the vertebral and right carotid circulation. The physical examination should be directed accordingly. A systolic bruit with a palpable thrill is common.

Arteriography to confirm the diagnosis and determine involvement of distal vessels is the diagnostic procedure of choice. Surgical treatment consists of aneurysm resection, vascular grafting, and reestablishment of arterial continuity.

Ulnar Artery Aneurysms (Hypothenar Hammer Syndrome) The rare syndrome of ulnar artery aneurysm is associated with occupational trauma in which the heel of the palm is used to hammer, push, or twist objects.[30] Patients are often mechanics, carpenters, and machinists.

The ulnar artery normally fits snugly in the bony canal at the hypothenar eminence under the hook of the hamate bone. Long-term repetitive damage to this region results in aneurysm formation.[30] The aneurysm itself may secondarily develop a mural thrombus that repeatedly embolizes to the superficial palmar arch or to a digital artery. Symptoms consist of paresthesias, pain, coolness, and cyanosis, most often in the little and ring fingers and occasionally in the middle and index fingers. The thumb is characteristically spared because of its radial artery blood supply. Diagnosis is easily made by finding a pulsatile or nonpulsatile tender mass in the hypothenar eminence of the dominant hand. Allen's test may demonstrate occlusion of the ulnar artery. Angiography of the distal vessels is diagnostic. Proximal angiography rules out the subclavian and axillary arteries as embolic sources. Treatment requires surgical resection of the aneurysm and reestablishment of ulnar artery continuity. Adjunctive preoperative thrombolytic therapy may be helpful.[30]

Viscera

Splenic Artery Aneurysms Splenic artery aneurysms account for 60% of all visceral arterial aneurysms. They are the only aneurysms that are more common in women, with a female/male ratio of 4:1.[31] The development of aneurysms in the splenic artery has been attributed to systemic arterial fibrodysplasia, portal hypertension, and increased splenic AV shunting that occurs in pregnancy.

Splenic artery aneurysms are most often asymptomatic. Symptomatic patients exhibit vague left upper quadrant or epigastric discomfort and occasional radiation of pain to the left shoulder or subscapular area. Most splenic artery aneurysms are less than 2 cm in diameter; therefore a pulsatile mass is not palpable. Occasionally a systolic bruit may be heard.

Only 2% of splenic artery aneurysms result in life-threatening rupture.[31] More than 95% of ruptures occur in young women during pregnancy and may be confused with ectopic pregnancy or placental abruption.

Splenic artery aneurysms are usually an incidental discovery on the abdominal radiograph as signet ring calcifications in the left upper quadrant. US, CT, and MRI can distinguish aneurysms from other cystic lesions in the left upper quadrant.[31] An angiogram is usually required to confirm the diagnosis. Symptomatic splenic artery aneurysms require immediate operative intervention, particularly in pregnant women or in women of childbearing age. Maternal mortality from rupture during pregnancy is approximately 70%. Treatment is more controversial in asymptomatic patients. Transcatheter embolization has been successfully performed in some patients and is an alternative to surgery.[32]

Hepatic Artery Aneurysms Hepatic artery aneurysms represent 20% of visceral artery aneurysms. The lesions are caused by atherosclerosis, infection (most often as a complication of IV drug abuse), major abdominal trauma, and polyarteritis nodosa. Hepatic artery aneurysms affect men twice as often as women and usually occur in patients older than 60 years of age.

Most aneurysms remain asymptomatic. Unruptured symptomatic aneurysms generally produce symptoms consistent with cholecystitis: vague, persistent, right upper quadrant or epigastric pain radiating to the back. Large aneurysms may cause severe upper abdominal discomfort, similar to that of pancreatitis. Hepatic artery aneurysms may rupture into the common bile duct, peritoneum, or adjacent hollow viscera. Mortality associated with hepatic artery rupture is 35%.

An abdominal bruit or palpable pulsatile mass is usually not present on physical examination. Aneurysmal calcification may be seen on a plain abdominal radiograph, but the diagnosis can be made reliably only by angiography. US and CT can be used to detect asymptomatic hepatic artery aneurysms.[32]

Because of the high mortality rate associated with aneurysmal rupture, an aggressive approach to patient management is warranted. Surgical resection of the aneurysm is performed in operative candidates. Transarterial catheter occlusion can be used in patients who are high surgical risks.[33]

Superior Mesenteric Artery Aneurysms Superior mesenteric artery aneurysms are the third most common visceral aneurysms. Nearly 60% are infected aneurysms caused by nonhemolytic streptococci from left-sided bacterial endocarditis. Atherosclerosis and trauma are much less common causes. Patients are usually less than 50 years of age; men and women are affected equally.

Patients generally have intermittent upper abdominal pain consistent with abdominal angina. Fifty percent have a pulsatile abdominal mass on physical examination. The stigmata of subacute bacterial endocarditis may be present. Plain abdominal films may show a calcified aneurysm. Angiography is necessary to confirm the diagnosis.

Management of superior mesenteric artery aneurysm should address any underlying infectious process. The surgical approach is difficult and varies with the condition of the patient, the shape of the aneurysm (saccular or fusiform), and the intraoperative assessment of bowel viability.

Infected Aneurysms

Mycotic Aneurysms The term *mycotic aneurysm* has been a source of confusion in the medical literature. No direct association exists with fungal disease. Although the term has been used to describe any infected aneurysm regardless of cause, it should be reserved for infected aneurysms resulting from bacterial *endocarditis,* as originally described in 1885 by Osler.[34,35]

Septic emboli from infective endocarditis may implant in one of two ways. First, hematogenous seeding of bacteria can occur in nonaneurysmal arteries whose vessel walls have been damaged by preexisting atherosclerosis. Second, septic emboli may also become lodged in the vasa vasorum of larger vessels, causing vessel wall ischemia and infection. In smaller vessels, septic emboli tend to lodge at arterial bifurcations, AV fistulas, or sites of arterial stenosis. Mycotic aneurysms are most common in the aorta, superior mesenteric artery, and intracranial and femoral arteries.

The infecting organism in mycotic aneurysms reflects the bacteriology of infective endocarditis. *Streptococcus viridans* is the most common organism, although IV drug abusers are most often infected by *Staphylococcus aureus.* Patients who have mycotic aneurysms tend to be 30 to 50 years of age. The mortality rate is reported to be 25% (Table 82-2).[34,35]

Atherosclerotic Arteries The most common current cause of an infected aneurysm is sepsis with hematogenous spread of bacteria to atherosclerotic arteries. Large vessels (especially the aorta) rather than peripheral arteries are the most common site. Organisms associated with these infected aneurysms are *Salmonella, Staphylococcus,* and *Escherichia coli.* Patients tend to be older than 50 and to have well-established atherosclerosis. Perforation often occurs before diagnosis and carries a mortality rate of 75%.[34]

Preexisting Aneurysms The incidence of infection in preexisting atherosclerotic aneurysms is estimated at 3% to 4%. Some patients with ruptured aneurysms have a higher incidence of positive bacterial culture results than those who have elective surgical treatment of an asymptomatic aneurysm. Gram-positive organisms, especially *Staphylococcus,* predominate (60%). Mortality is extremely high (90%) because of aneurysm rupture.[34,35]

Posttraumatic Pseudoaneurysms Posttraumatic infected aneurysms result from invasive hemodynamic monitoring, angiography, and IV drug use. The most common artery affected is the femoral because of its involvement in groin injection. *S. aureus* is isolated in 30% to 70% of cases. Because of the more peripheral location and early identification, mortality is low (5%).[36]

The clinical presentation of an infected aneurysm varies with anatomic location and underlying pathophysiologic process. Patients with infected abdominal aneurysms are often misdiagnosed. Onset is usually insidious; low-grade fever may be present for several months. Common findings are fever (75%), back and abdominal pain (33%), and

Table 82-2. Clinical Characteristics of Infected Aneurysms

	Mycotic aneurysm	Infection of atherosclerotic arteries	Infection of existing aneurysm	Posttraumatic infected false aneurysm
Cause	Endocarditis	Bacteremia	Bacteremia	Drug addiction Trauma
Age (years)	30-50	>50	>50	<30
Incidence	Rare	Most common	Unusual	Very common
Location	Aorta Visceral Intracranial Peripheral	Atherosclerotic Aortoiliac Intimal defects	Infrarenal Aorta	Femoral Carotid
Bacteriology	Gram-positive cocci	*Salmonella* Others	*Staphylococcus* Others	*Staphylococcus aureus* Polymicrobial
Mortality	25%	75%	90%	5%

From Wilson SE, Van Wagenen P, Passaro E Jr: *Curr Probl Surg* 15:1, 1978.

palpable aneurysm (53%). More peripheral aneurysms, especially infected femoral pseudoaneurysms, are characterized by a tender groin mass, some manifestation of sepsis, or bleeding.[37] Almost all are easily palpable on physical examination. Although rare, fungal infections should be considered in patients who are chronically immunosuppressed, have been treated recently for disseminated fungal disease, or have diabetes mellitus.[38]

Laboratory findings are usually not diagnostic. Bacteremia often is continuous, and blood culture findings are positive for bacterial growth in approximately 70% of cases. Positive blood culture results in a patient with a preexisting aneurysm should prompt treatment as an infected aneurysm until disproven; however, negative blood culture results alone do not rule out this diagnosis. Angiography should be performed when an infected aneurysm is suspected.[38] Indium-111-labeled white blood cells are used to confirm or rule out infected aneurysms.[39]

Treatment must include both antibiotics and surgical repair. Antibiotic therapy is usually continued for at least 6 to 8 weeks, although some advocate lifelong treatment after successful surgical repair.[40] The most important intervention is timely repair.[34,35] Without surgery, all patients will have aneurysm rupture with exsanguinating hemorrhage.[35]

Traumatic Aneurysms

Traumatic aneurysm refers to a pseudoaneurysm that follows perforation of the arterial wall, with formation of a perivascular hematoma. Chronic traumatic aneurysms may or may not be associated with an AV fistula. Pseudoaneurysm is a synonym for *false aneurysm*.

The usual presentation is a pulsatile mass found near the course of an extremity artery, with a history of trauma more than 1 month earlier.[41] The expanding aneurysm may compress associated peripheral nerves and produce neuropathy. Distal perfusion is usually well maintained, and thromboembolism is rare. A loud systolic and possibly a separate faint diastolic murmur are characteristic.

The diagnosis can be verified with many methods, including conventional angiography, digital subtraction arteriography, and CT scan. Surgical excision of the aneurysm with end-to-end anastomosis or graft interposition is indicated as soon as possible after diagnosis to decrease the risk of complications, including rupture, thrombosis, or neurologic dysfunction caused by continued expansion.

VASOSPASTIC DISORDERS

Vasospastic disorders are characterized by an abnormal vasomotor response in the distal small arteries. Blood flow in the peripheral circulation is controlled by local, autonomic, and humoral mechanisms.[11] The cause of the heightened vasospastic response is unknown (see Pathophysiology).

Raynaud's disease is the most common vasospastic disorder and occurs five or more times as often in women as in men. By definition, Raynaud's disease has no evidence of an underlying cause. The diagnosis is correct in 95% of cases using these criteria: (1) episodes are precipitated by cold or emotion; (2) symptoms are bilateral; (3) gangrene is absent or is minimal and confined to the skin; (4) no disease or condition that may cause a secondary Raynaud's phenomenon is present; and (5) symptoms have been occurring for at least 2 years.[43]

The classic Raynaud's attack is triphasic: the fingers become white, then blue, and finally red. This is produced initially by complete closure of the palmar and digital arteries (and possibly arterioles), producing cessation of capillary perfusion. When a slight relaxation of arterial spasm occurs, a slight flow of blood returns into the dilated capillary bed, where it rapidly dissipates, producing cyanosis. Arterial spasm usually spontaneously resolves, arterial flow returns to baseline, but reactive hyperemia produces a red extremity. Attacks are often precipitated by cold and emotional stress. Raynaud's disease usually follows a benign course. True histologic changes within the vessel wall are absent. Reassurance, education, and continued primary care follow-up observation are the only treatment necessary for true Raynaud's disease.

Raynaud's phenomenon is Raynaud's disease that has an identifiable underlying disorder. Connective tissue disorders, including scleroderma, rheumatoid arthritis, and systemic lupus erythematosus, have the highest association with Raynaud's phenomenon. Treatment should be directed toward identifying the underlying disorder and minimizing threatened tissue loss if present.[42]

Benign livedo reticularis is caused by spasm of the dermal arterioles and may involve all parts of the upper and lower extremities, and include the trunk. It is most common when skin is exposed to a cool environment. It is never associated with histologic vascular abnormality and quickly resolves when the exposed skin is covered or the environment is warmed. *Secondary livedo reticularis* can occasionally accompany peripheral vascular disease manifestations of other conditions similar to the causes of Raynaud's phenomenon.[42]

Acrocyanosis is the least common of the vasospastic disorders and is characterized by persistent painless symmetric cyanosis of the fingers, the hands, and less often the feet. The disease is benign and not associated with either vascular abnormality or an underlying disorder. Pain, trophic skin changes, and ulceration do not occur. This disorder occurs more often in women, is intensified by exposure to cold, and lessens with warming. The diagnosis is made by the bilateral and persistent nature of the findings, localized to the hands or feet in the presence of normal arterial pulsations. The involved extremities are nearly always cold; excessive perspiration is common. Except for reassurance and protection from cold, treatment is usually unnecessary.[42]

Primary erythromelalgia is a rare syndrome of paroxysmal vasodilation with burning pain, increased skin temperature, and redness of the feet and less often the hands. However, secondary erythromelalgia can occur in patients with underlying disease processes, most often systemic lupus erythematosus, myeloproliferative disorders, hypertension, venous insufficiency, or diabetes mellitus. Erythromelalgia is as common in children as adults, but in children it is less likely to be associated with an underlying systemic illness. Attacks are not triggered by cold and usually occur during modest ambient temperatures. Skin temperature of the involved digits is high compared with the patient's core temperature. Symptoms may remain mild for years or may become so severe that disability results. Tissue loss and trophic skin changes do not occur. Although rest, elevation of the extremities, and cold compresses or immersion in ice may provide temporary relief, no consistently effective treatment has been found for the multiple, often daily episodes of pain that occur with erythromelalgia.[42]

THORACIC OUTLET SYNDROME

Thoracic outlet syndrome involves compression of the brachial plexus, subclavian vein, or subclavian artery at the superior aperture of the thorax. Thoracic outlet syndromes were previously categorized by cause, as scalenus anticus, costoclavicular, hyperabduction, cervical rib, and first thoracic rib syndromes. They are now most easily divided into three types—neurologic, venous, and arterial—depending on the predominant symptoms.

Compression of the brachial plexus causes the *neurologic* type of thoracic outlet syndrome and constitutes approximately 95% of all cases.[43] Onset of symptoms occurs between ages 20 and 50 years, with women predominating about 3 to 1. Compression or thrombosis of the subclavian vein constitutes the *venous* type of thoracic outlet syndrome and is responsible for 4% of all cases. It occurs most often in men 20 to 35 years of age. The *arterial* type of thoracic outlet syndrome is rare, occurring in approximately 1% of all cases, but is potentially the most serious of the three types. Men and women are affected equally in a bimodal age distribution of young adults (from cervical rib compression) and patients over age 50 (from localized atherosclerosis caused by arterial compression). Figure 82-4 demonstrates the relationship between anatomic abnormalities and neurovascular compression.

Principles of Disease

Roos[43] describes four basic concepts of thoracic outlet syndromes: (1) patients who have a thoracic outlet syndrome develop an anatomic abnormality predisposing them to symptoms under certain conditions; (2) brachial plexus compression or irritation constitutes approximately 95% of all thoracic outlet syndrome cases and is rarely caused by compression of the subclavian artery; (3) bedside testing for thoracic outlet syndrome based on positional compression of the subclavian artery is insensitive and unreliable; and (4) in advanced or refractory cases, the causative anatomic abnormalities must be surgically corrected.

The subclavian artery courses over the first rib between the scalenus anticus muscle anteriorly and the scalenus medius posteriorly. From this point it passes under the clavicle to the axilla, where the brachial plexus lies posteriorly and laterally. Four anatomic abnormalities have been associated with thoracic outlet syndrome.

Cervical rib syndrome results from an uncommon abnormality (0.5% to 0.7% of all chest radiographs) and is bilateral in 70% of patients.[43,44] It occurs twice as often in women as men. Most cervical ribs are incomplete, attached to a fibrous band on the scalene tubercle of the first rib. The site of compression is the scalene hiatus, made up of the scalene anterior muscle frontally, the scalene medius posteriorly, and the cervical rib inferiorly.

Scalenus anticus syndrome results when the neurovascular bundle is compressed as it passes through the interscalene triangle. The compression is caused by variations in the insertion of the anterior scalene muscle. In some patients the subclavian artery passes through the body of the muscle.

Costoclavicular syndrome results when the shoulders are moved backward and downward. Causes include hypertrophy of the subclavius muscle, abnormalities of the first rib, and past clavicular fractures.

Hyperabduction syndrome results from the neurovascular

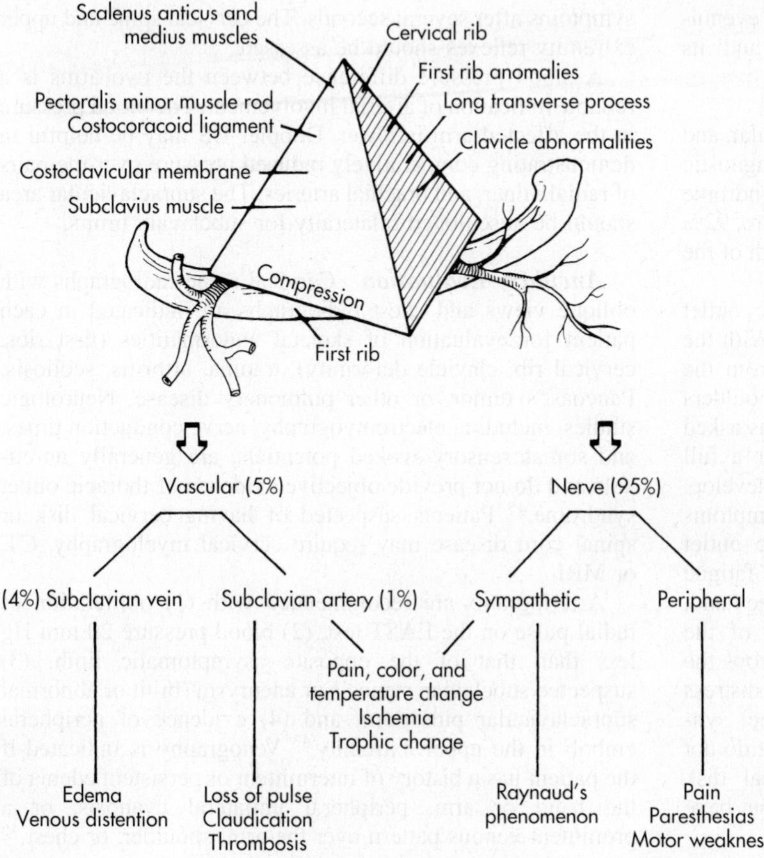

Figure 82-4. **Interrelationships of muscle, ligament, and bone abnormalities in the thoracic outlet that may compress neurovascular structures.** *From Urschel HC Jr, Razzuk MA:* N Engl J Med *286:1140, 1972.*

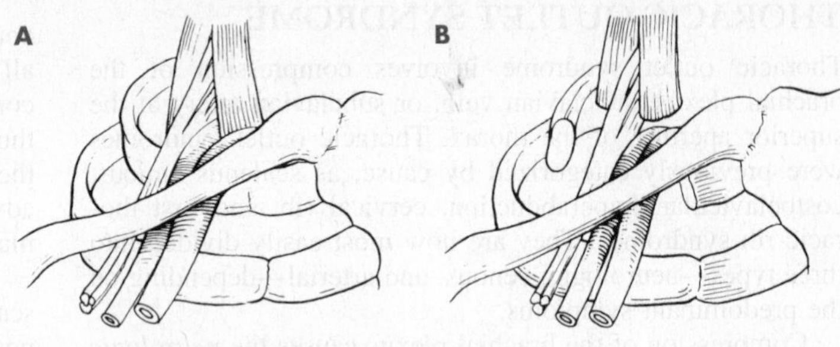

Figure 82-5. **A, Thoracic outlet compression in costoclavicular space. B, Decompression of thoracic outlet by resection of first rib with disarticulation of the costochondral joint.** *From Etheredge S, Wilbur B, Stoney RJ:* Am J Surg *138:175, 1979.*

compression that occurs when the arms are placed in the hyperabducted position. The site of compression is in the retroclavicular space anterior to the first rib or at the point where the neurovascular bundle passes beneath the pectoralis minor muscle.

The neurologic and venous compression type of thoracic outlet syndrome can be associated with any underlying anatomic abnormality. Bony abnormalities (cervical rib, first thoracic rib, or clavicle) are the most common causes of the arterial type of thoracic outlet syndrome (Figure 82-5, *A*).

Clinical Features

Compression or irritation of the brachial plexus most often affects the lower two nerve roots, eighth cervical (C8) and first thoracic (T1), producing pain and paresthesias in the ulnar nerve distribution. The second most common anatomic pattern is involvement of the upper three nerve roots of the brachial plexus (C5, C6, and C7), with symptoms referable to the neck, ear, upper chest, upper back, and outer arm in the radial nerve distribution. Venous compression eventually progresses to intimal damage and subclavian vein thrombosis, with venous engorgement and swelling of the affected extremity. Persistent subclavian artery compression eventually results in poststenotic aneurysm formation and its pathologic sequelae.

Physical Examination The Adson, costoclavicular, and hyperabduction maneuvers are unreliable as diagnostic tests.[45] Only 1% of all patients with thoracic outlet syndrome have involvement of the subclavian artery. Furthermore, 92% of asymptomatic patients have variation in the strength of the radial pulse during positional changes.[43-45]

The most reliable test in screening for thoracic outlet syndrome is the *elevated arm stress test* (EAST).[45] With the patient sitting, the arms are abducted 90 degrees from the thorax and the elbows flexed 90 degrees, with the shoulders braced slightly behind the frontal plane. The patient is asked to open and close the fists slowly but steadily for a full 3 minutes and to describe any symptoms that develop. Normally the patient performs this test without symptoms other than mild fatigue. The patient with thoracic outlet syndrome, however, usually has early heaviness and fatigue of the involved limb, gradual onset of numbness of the hand, and progressive aching through the arm and top of the shoulder. Within the 3 minutes the patient usually drops the hand to the lap for relief of the progressive, crescendo distress that becomes intolerable. Patients with carpal tunnel syndrome may experience dysesthesias in the fingers but do not have shoulder or arm pain. Patients with cervical disk syndromes may have pain in the neck and shoulder but have no arm or hand symptoms.

The EAST evaluates all three types of thoracic outlet syndrome: neurologic, venous, and arterial. Radial pulses may be palpated by the examiner during the test. The presence of a radial pulse and a positive EAST test result are strong indications that the basis of symptoms is neurologic involvement of the brachial plexus.

The hands should be observed for changes in skin color, warmth, moisture, or muscular atrophy. Triceps muscle strength (innervated by C7) should be tested bilaterally. Muscle strength of the interosseous muscles (innervated by C8 and T1) should be tested by asking the patient to spread the fingers apart against resistance. The muscles innervated by the radial nerve are tested by the patient hyperextending the thumb and dorsiflexing the wrist against resistance. The median nerve innervates the thenar muscles, which can be tested by asking the patient to abduct the thumb away from the palm with the thumb pointing straight to the ceiling. *Tinel's sign* ("electric shock" to tips of fingers) is an indication of carpal tunnel compression of the median nerve and is elicited by percussing the volar aspect of the wrist. Gentle pressure with the thumb in the supraclavicular fossa over the brachial plexus may reproduce thoracic outlet symptoms after several seconds. The cervical spine and upper extremity reflexes should be assessed.

A blood pressure difference between the two arms is a reliable indication of arterial involvement. The blood pressure in the affected arm is lower. Doppler US may be helpful in demonstrating comparatively reduced pressure over the pairs of radial, ulnar, and brachial arteries. The supraclavicular area should be auscultated bilaterally for subclavian bruits.

Ancillary Evaluation Cervical spine radiographs with oblique views and chest radiographs are indicated in each patient for evaluation of skeletal abnormalities (first ribs, cervical rib, clavicle deformity), trauma, arthritis, scoliosis, Pancoast's tumor, or other pulmonary disease. Neurologic studies, including electromyography, nerve conduction times, and somatosensory-evoked potentials, are generally unreliable and do not provide objective evidence of thoracic outlet syndrome.[45] Patients suspected of having cervical disk or spinal cord disease may require cervical myelography, CT, or MRI.

Arteriograms are recommended with (1) obliteration of radial pulse on the EAST test, (2) blood pressure 20 mm Hg less than that of the opposite asymptomatic limb, (3) suspected subclavian stenosis or aneurysm (bruit or abnormal supraclavicular pulsation), and (4) evidence of peripheral emboli in the upper extremity.[43] Venography is indicated if the patient has a history of intermittent or persistent edema of the hand or arm, peripheral unilateral cyanosis, or a prominent venous pattern over the arm, shoulder, or chest.[46]

Differential Diagnosis

The differential diagnosis of thoracic outlet syndrome includes herniated cervical disk, cervical spondylitis, spinal cord tumor, ulnar nerve compression at the elbow, carpal tunnel syndrome, orthopedic shoulder problems (sprain, rotator cuff injury, tendinitis), trauma, postural palsy, angina pectoris, and a variety of neuropathies, including multiple sclerosis, alcoholism, and diabetes.

Patients with a herniated cervical disk have more severe persistent pain radiating in a sharply demarcated dermatomal distribution (usually C4-5 or C5-6) and often have localized tenderness of the cervical spine at the affected level. Carpal tunnel syndrome is characterized by nocturnal symptoms of pain and paresthesias and an associated Tinel's sign on physical examination. Brachial plexus compression and irritation can be confused with other vascular conditions, such as Raynaud's disease, vasospastic disorders, vasculitis, or arterial ischemia.[43] Unilateral symptoms should suggest thoracic outlet syndrome, whereas bilateral symptoms suggest a systemic process. Subclavian or axillary venous thrombosis from thoracic outlet syndrome must be differentiated from thrombophlebitis or mediastinal venous obstruction from a benign or malignant process (Pancoast's tumor).

Management

Treatment varies, depending on whether the involvement is neurologic, arterial, or venous. In patients with only brachial plexus involvement and with minimal signs and symptoms, conservative treatment with physiotherapy and shoulder girdle exercises is sufficient. Surgery is reserved for patients with significant neurologic signs and symptoms. This includes intolerable pain or progressive loss of function and strength of the arm or hand. First rib and anomalous muscle or fibrous tissue resection is the surgical treatment of choice and provides consistent relief of symptoms and minimal morbidity (Figure 82-5, *B*).[43]

Patients with arterial complications of thoracic outlet syndrome (thrombosis, thromboembolism, or acute ischemia) require immediate heparinization and angiography; Fogarty catheter embolectomy, if appropriate; and emergency or urgent surgical exploration. Patients with axillary and subclavian vein thromboses require immediate heparinization and venography and are treated with surgical thrombectomy or systemic thrombolytic therapy.[47]

Disposition

The correct diagnosis of thoracic outlet syndrome can be achieved in more than 90% of patients with a careful history, physical examination, and bedside testing alone.[44] Neurologic, orthopedic, or vascular surgery consultation is indicated according to the pathologic condition.

PERIPHERAL ARTERIOVENOUS FISTULAS

Acquired peripheral AV fistulas are most often caused by trauma (gunshot wounds, stab wounds, or surgery). Malignancy, infection, and arterial aneurysms are less common sources. Patients generally seek medical care several months after an invasive surgical procedure or penetrating injury.

Differential Diagnosis

The correct diagnosis of an AV fistula can usually be made with clinical examination alone. A constant systolic and diastolic (to-and-fro) murmur associated with a palpable thrill is characteristic. Sixty percent of AV fistulas are also associated with a coexisting false aneurysm. Patients with peripheral venous disease may have similar cutaneous manifestations (varicose veins and stasis pigmentation) but lack vascular bruits. Infection in the form of bacterial endarteritis may complicate large fistulas.

Management

Acquired peripheral AV fistulas usually increase in size with time if treatment is delayed. Vessel dilation, peripheral ischemia, and cardiac output increase. The fistula usually is repaired best with a direct surgical approach, interrupting the fistula tract and restoring both arterial and venous continuity with end-to-end anastomosis or graft interposition.[48] Transcatheter embolization with detachable balloons and liquid acrylic tissue adhesives (e.g., isobutyl-2-cyanoacrylate) is being used for surgically inaccessible fistulas.[49]

VASCULAR ABNORMALITY CAUSED BY DRUG ABUSE

Principles of Disease

The vascular complications of parenteral drug use have risen significantly in both frequency and severity over the past decade.[50] These IV or intraarterial injuries may result in acute arterial ischemia, infected pseudoaneurysms, lymphatic obstruction, or direct neurologic injury.

Acute arterial ischemia may result from direct drug effects or endogenous catecholamine release after injection. Endothelial wall damage may stimulate platelet aggregation and thrombus formation. Precipitated crystals, talc, or foreign body emboli may cause arterial occlusion. Necrotizing arteritis can produce ischemia and is especially prevalent in patients who abuse IV methamphetamine.

Infected pseudoaneurysms associated with AV fistulas result from a through-and-through puncture of the artery with simultaneous contamination from either skin flora or organisms inoculated by contaminated needles or drug. These fistulas are the most common vascular lesion resulting from IV drug abuse. Secondary infection of the vascular structure may be covered by a surrounding soft tissue infection (cellulitis or abscess). Infected aneurysms at sites distant from the injection can occur.

IV drug abusers may have unilateral hand edema or "puffy hand syndrome" develop because of gradual obliteration of the superficial venous vessels and chronic lymphatic obstruction. Direct injury to adjacent nerves, polyneuritis, and ischemic neuritis may result from IV drug abuse. Coexisting serious or life-threatening infections include cellulitis, septicemia, and bacterial endocarditis.[50]

Clinical Features

Patients may withhold information about the use of IV drugs, so this possibility should be considered in all patients, especially patients with a fever. Objective evidence such as track marks may be present.

Distal ischemia after intraarterial injection most often occurs in the upper extremity after injection of the brachial or radial artery. The immediate onset of a severe, burning pain at the time of injection is a characteristic hallmark.[51] Patients have a painful, edematous upper extremity with patchy blue-purple skin discoloration. Distal pulses are generally present, but the skin temperature of the involved extremity is decreased. Because patients tend to seek attention early, the site of injection may be identifiable over the radial or brachial artery. Evidence of gangrene, pregangrenous changes, or neuromuscular deficits may accompany this syndrome.

Patients with infected pseudoaneurysms have a painful mass develop several days to weeks after injection, with resultant bleeding or "hitting pink." The mass is usually pulsatile, and 50% have an associated bruit.[50] Infected pseudoaneurysm is part of the differential diagnosis of cutaneous abscess or cellulitis in an IV drug user. Infected pseudoaneurysms are most often encountered in the lower extremities (80%). All patients should be carefully evaluated for sepsis, metastatic infection, and bacterial endocarditis. A peripheral vascular examination with careful documentation of pulses should be performed. A radiograph of the affected extremity can rule out a subcutaneous needle or foreign body. Angiography is the diagnostic procedure of choice for patients with suspected pseudoaneurysm or distal ischemia. US is often unable to distinguish an aneurysm from an abscess or cellulitis.

Management

Therapeutic considerations for acute ischemia from intraarterial injection are primarily conservative. Intraarterial vasodilators, heparin, low-molecular-weight dextran, thrombolytic therapy, analgesics, systemic warming to stimulate vasodilation, antibiotics, elevation of the affected limb to promote venous drainage, and physical therapy have not significantly altered the outcome or amputation rate in this patient population. Surgical treatment is reserved for delayed amputation, with the goal of preserving as much tissue as possible. Gradual resolution of symptoms without surgical intervention is the most common outcome.

Patients with infected pseudoaneurysms require aneurysm resection, debridement of infected tissue, and ligation of the proximal and distal uninfected arteries. Autogenous vein bypass through uninfected tissue planes may require an extensive surgical approach.[52]

Methicillin-resistant *S. aureus* and gram-negative rods are increasing in frequency as the causative agents in infections and vascular injury resulting from drug abuse. IV nafcillin is recommended for mild infections, nafcillin and a second- or third-generation cephalosporin for major infections, and vancomycin and a second- or third-generation cephalosporin or an aminoglycoside for patients who are bacteremic or overtly septic.[50]

COMPLICATIONS

Long-Term Central Venous Access

Hickman-Broviac Catheter The Hickman-Broviac double-lumen catheter was introduced in 1979 and is in common use today. The smaller Broviac line is often used for the administration of IV therapy; the larger Hickman line is reserved for additional venous access and blood withdrawal (Figures 82-6, *A,* and 82-8, *B*). This catheter generally is inserted into the cephalic, subclavian, external, or internal jugular vein, with the distal tip advanced to just above the right atrium.[53] The proximal end exits through a subcutaneous tunnel from the lower anterior chest wall. A felt cuff (Dacron) is used to anchor it in place subcutaneously. The Hickman-Broviac catheter is made of polymeric silicone rubber that is of low thrombogenic potential but extremely flexible and soft. Because of the pliability of the material, the catheter must be treated gently. Clearing an obstructed catheter with a guidewire may perforate the catheter. Forcing fluid through the catheter by positive pressure carries the risk of catheter rupture or catheter embolus. For this reason, no syringe larger than 5 ml should be used for irrigation.

Routine Care and Use The smaller Broviac line is most often used for the infusion of total parenteral nutrition (TPN) or fat emulsions. This line should be irrigated with 6 ml of normal saline solution between different infusions to prevent mixing of incompatible solutions, development of precipitation, and resultant catheter occlusion. The larger Hickman line should be used to withdraw blood. This line should be irrigated with 6 ml of *heparinized* saline after blood withdrawal to prevent clot formation in the catheter lumen. When a clamp is used, it should be placed over a piece of tape wrapped around the line. The clamp should have a smooth surface since teeth or prongs may sever or abrade the line.

Routine care and frequency of catheter dressing changes vary with the preference of the treating physician.[53-56] Most patients become skilled in routine catheter maintenance and are a reliable source of information. The need for absolute sterile technique when manipulating the catheter cannot be overemphasized.

Catheter Occlusion Patients with Hickman catheters may exhibit complete or partial obstruction to flow in either

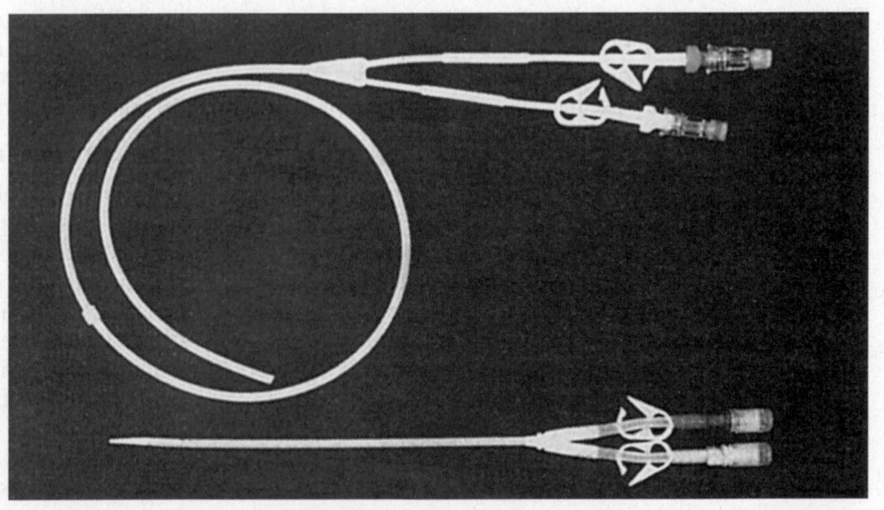

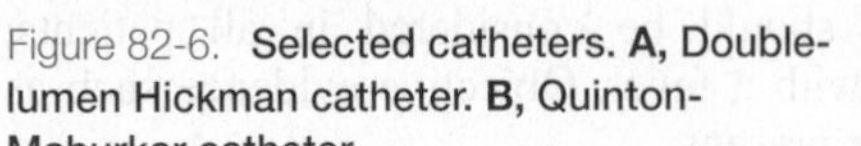
Figure 82-6. **Selected catheters. A, Double-lumen Hickman catheter. B, Quinton-Mahurkar catheter.**

line in the ED. For those with complete obstruction to flow, these differential diagnoses, in decreasing order of frequency, are (1) clots within the catheter lumen, (2) precipitants within the catheter lumen, and (3) mechanical obstruction. In patients with catheters that accept infusions at normal rates but cannot be aspirated, these differential diagnoses, in decreasing order of frequency, are (1) catheter lodged against the wall of the vessel, (2) occluding fibrin sheath around the catheter tip, (3) ball valve or mural thrombus, and (4) central venous thrombosis. Patients who have intermittent complete occlusion and withdrawal occlusion have a type of mechanical obstruction called *pinch-off syndrome,* in which the catheter lumen is compromised from mechanical forces acting on it between the clavicle and the first rib. Clots within the catheter lumen, obstructing fibrin sheaths, and ball valve or mural thrombus often respond to low-dose intracatheter urokinase; central venous thrombosis, precipitants in the catheter lumen, and mechanical obstruction do not respond (Box 82-1).

Precipitants within the catheter lumen most often result from failure to clear the line with saline after TPN, flushing the line with a heparin solution instead. Heparin precipitates with TPN fluid-producing solids. Clots within the catheter lumen usually result from failure to flush the line with a heparinized saline solution after blood aspiration.

A chest radiograph should be obtained in all patients with persistently occluded catheters to confirm catheter position and integrity. The catheter tip should be positioned just above the right atrium.[53] Persistent right atrial placement may cause perforation of this thin-walled heart chamber. Comparison with previous radiographs may be necessary to ensure lack of movement or displacement. In patients with withdrawal occlusion but appropriate catheter position, and without clinical evidence of subclavian vein thrombosis, the catheter may be lodged against the vessel wall. The patient's changing body position, raising the arms above the head, or performing Valsalva's maneuver may relieve withdrawal occlusion. If this is unsuccessful, further treatment can be considered when the presentation and history are consistent with a type of catheter occlusion that responds to low-dose intracatheter urokinase (see Box 82-1). Urokinase (5000 U) should be injected into the catheter and left for 30 minutes before aspiration is again attempted. If this is also unsuccessful, a second dose of urokinase can be injected and the procedure repeated.[57] Contraindications to thrombolytic agents should be considered, although low-dose therapy for occluded catheters appears well tolerated.[57,58]

Mechanical obstruction has a variety of causes, including pinch-off syndrome. The catheter is intermittently obstructed during both administration and withdrawal of fluids. A chest radiograph demonstrates narrowing of the catheter lumen as it passes between the clavicle and the first rib. This condition is typically detected within 3 weeks after catheter placement; the catheter must be removed because of fragmentation or embolization if left in place.[59]

Because engorged collateral circulation or swelling in the affected extremity is not universally present with subclavian vein thrombosis, this diagnosis should be considered in all patients who are unresponsive to declotting attempts. Catheter removal with systemic heparinization or catheter maintenance with high-dose thrombolytic therapy is a therapeutic option for subclavian vein thrombosis.[60,61] Mechanical occlusion is rare and requires catheter replacement with a surgical approach. Because of variations in approach by different consultants, early consultation is recommended in patients who have occluded central venous catheters (Figure 82-7).

Catheter Laceration If an external catheter laceration or fracture occurs, the catheter should be clamped distal to the laceration close to the chest wall. The catheter can be repaired as long as the damage is more than 4 cm from the chest wall. After clamping, as an interim measure, the EP can insert a 14-gauge, 2-inch Angiocath into the catheter; remove the stylus; tape securely; and flush with heparin. The catheter can then be used while a repair kit (e.g., Evermed) is obtained.[62]

Catheter-Related Infections Catheter infections can be categorized as local or systemic. Local infections primarily involve the skin and subcutaneous tissues surrounding the exit site with erythema, tenderness, and no clinical or laboratory evidence of sepsis. Skin organisms are primarily responsible for local infections, especially coagulase-negative staphylococci.[55] Studies show that local infections usually do not require catheter removal and resolve with antibacterial therapy alone.[63]

The source of systemic infection in patients with Hickman-Broviac catheters may be difficult to localize, particularly in immunosuppressed patients. The most common sites of systemic infection in any patient with a central venous catheter, in decreasing order of frequency, are the urinary tract, anorectal area, upper respiratory tract, and the catheter.[55] The most common organisms causing catheter infection are coagulase-negative staphylococci, *S. aureus,* and *Candida albicans.* In immunocompromised patients with Hickman-Broviac catheters, gram-positive organisms now are responsible for more cases of sepsis than gram-negative bacteria. Accordingly, initial empiric therapy should include an antistaphylococcal drug, in addition to the usual gram-negative coverage. All patients who have a suspected vascular access infection should have two blood cultures drawn. Comparison of blood cultures drawn simultaneously through the catheter and from a peripheral blood vessel may assist in determining whether the catheter is the source of infection. Infections that do not extend through the vessel

Box 82-1 Differential Diagnosis of Occluded Chronic Indwelling Catheters

Complete Occlusion

Clot in catheter lumen*
Precipitate in catheter lumen
Mechanical obstruction

Withdrawal Occlusion

Catheter against vessel wall
Fibrin sheath*
Ball valve/mural thrombus*
Subclavian vein thrombosis

Intermittent Complete Occlusion and Withdrawal Occlusion

Pinch-off syndrome

*Usually responds to low-dose intracatheter urokinase.

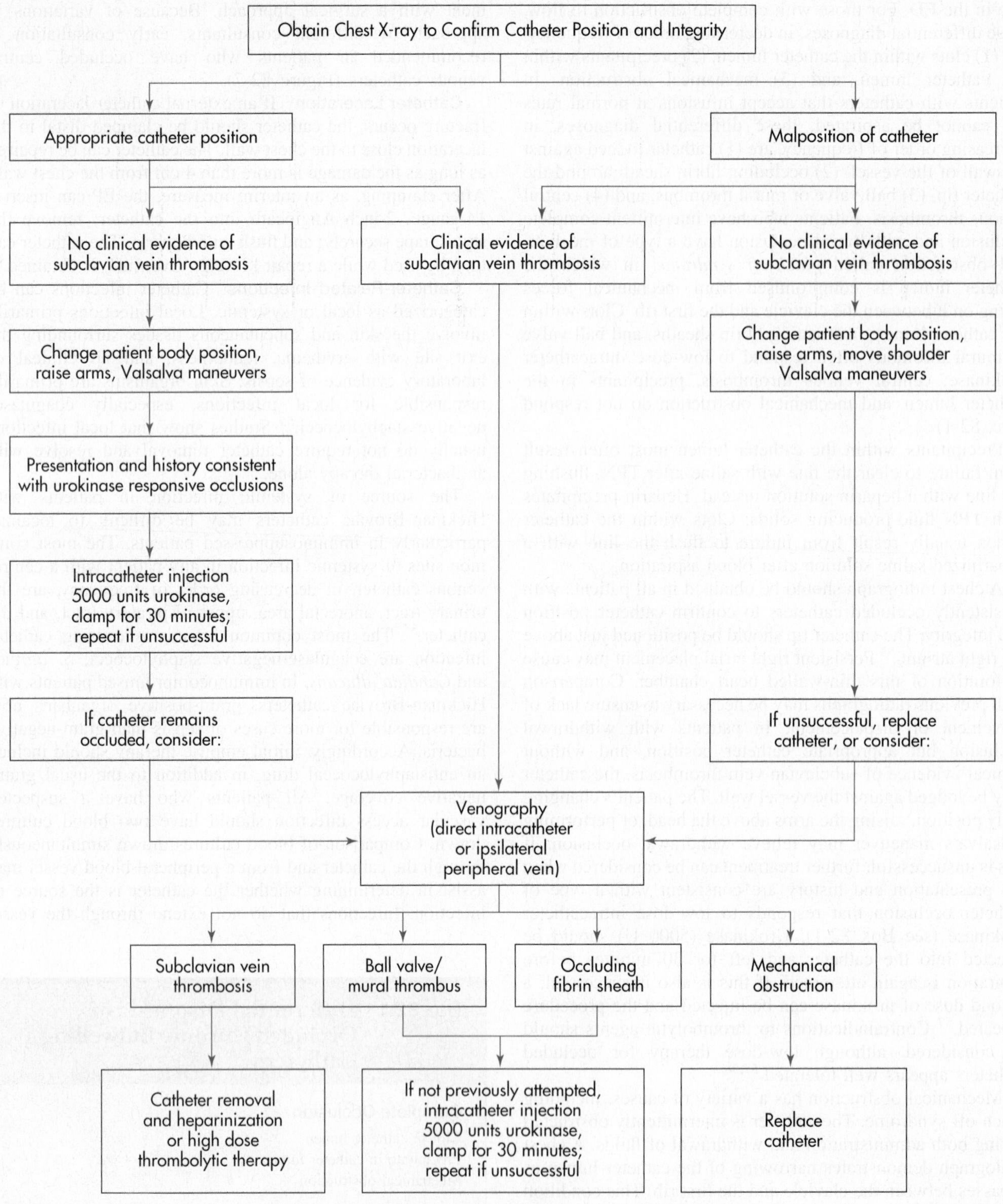

Figure 82-7. **Approach to occluded indwelling venous catheter.**

wall (*pericatheter infections*) can be successfully treated without catheter removal. Catheter removal is mandatory in patients with continued positive blood culture results despite therapy and in those with vascular access infections caused by *Candida* species.[63]

Catheter-related septic central venous thrombosis can progress through and around the vessel wall to cause a *perivascular infection* or abscess. This rare but devastating complication is associated with serious morbidity and a reported mortality as high as 83%. Because of the lack of specific clinical findings, the most prominent diagnostic feature is continued bacteremia after catheter removal. Diagnosis is confirmed by venography or CT scan.[64] Removal of the catheter, IV administration of antibiotics, and anticoagulation constitute appropriate initial therapy. Surgical treatment with thrombectomy and possible abscess drainage is indicated after failure of an adequate course of antibiotics and anticoagulation. Thrombolytic agents have been used as an adjunct for catheter-related septic venous thrombosis, but the risk/benefit ratio has not been established.[65] In patients who require catheter removal, a quantitative culture of the number of organisms on the catheter's surface correlates well with a positive blood culture result for the same organism. This technique involves rolling the catheter on a culture medium. Broth culture of catheter tips may be less reliable in determining whether the catheter is the source of infection.[66]

Groshong Catheter The Groshong catheter is a single, thin-walled silicone rubber catheter designed for prolonged venous cannulation. It differs from the Hickman-Broviac catheter in insertion, design, and maintenance. A decreased outer diameter/inner diameter ratio allows insertion into a smaller vein through a smaller introducer sheath. The catheter can be inserted under local anesthesia without fluoroscopy, using the Seldinger technique and a peel-away catheter introducer sheath. After catheter placement in the subclavian, internal, or external jugular vein, a subcutaneous tunnel is created with a stainless steel tunneling device through which the catheter is threaded. A cuff (Dacron) stabilizes the catheter's placement in subcutaneous tissues and reduces the chance of inadvertent removal or retrograde infection.[67]

The Groshong catheter is constructed with a closed end and a vocal cord–type integral valve at the distal end (Figure 82-8, *A*). This pressure-sensitive two-way valve at the intravascular end minimizes back-bleeding, eliminating the need for heparin flushes or external clamping, but permits blood sampling with gentle negative pressure. Patency of the catheter is maintained with 5 ml of saline flush once a week. A 20-ml saline irrigation is necessary after any blood transfusion or if blood is observed in the catheter lumen. A 30-ml saline irrigation is performed before blood sampling after infusion of hyperalimentation solutions.

Groshong catheters offer the advantage of bedside placement, minimal back-bleeding, elimination of heparin flushes, and elimination of external clamping when changing injection caps or connecting tubing. A lower incidence of complete obstruction to flow from clots or precipitants within the catheter lumen, however, has not been shown.[68] Groshong catheters are otherwise subject to the same complications as described for Hickman-Broviac catheters.

Vascular Access for Hemodialysis

Quinton-Mahurkar Catheter The Quinton-Mahurkar is the preferred catheter for providing immediate and short-term vascular access for hemodialysis. Its advantages include bedside placement and a functional life up to 18 months.[69] This single, flexible polyurethane cannula has two separate D-shaped channels, each connected by a molded Y piece to a color-coded external port (Figure 82-6, *B*). To protect against a disconnected cap, each limb of the Y piece has an attached clamp. The Quinton-Mahurkar catheter is placed by the Seldinger technique, most often in the subclavian vein and less often in the femoral vein.

Mortality from central venous catheter hemodialysis is low (0 to 1.25 per 1000 catheterizations), but morbidity is high, with a reported overall complication rate near 30%.[70]

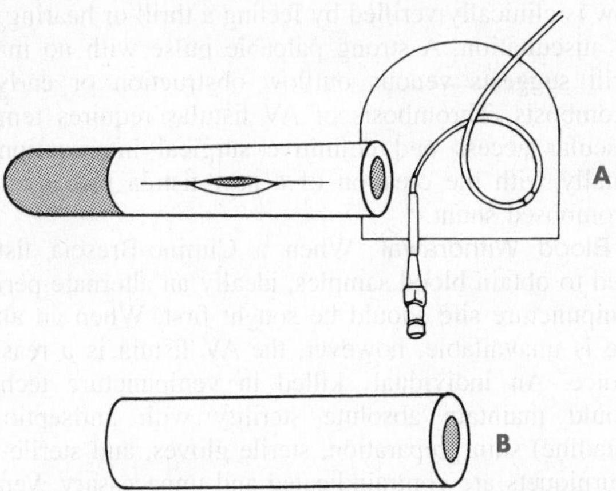

Figure 82-8. **A, Groshong catheter with closed distal end and vocal cord–type valve. B, Hickman catheter with open distal end.** ***From Delmore JE:*** **Gynecol Oncol** ***34:216, 1989.***

The most common complications are catheter-related infections and thrombosis.

A Quinton-Mahurkar catheter can be used to obtain blood samples. After blood withdrawal, the line should be flushed with more than 10 ml of normal saline solution, followed by 5000 U of heparin in 1 ml of saline to prevent intracatheter clot formation. The catheter may also be used for the administration of IV therapy. Routine care and use are otherwise similar to that previously described for chronic indwelling central venous catheters.

Cimino-Brescia Fistula and Prosthetic Bridge Fistula The subcutaneous Cimino-Brescia fistula is the preferred means of vascular access for long-term hemodialysis. The fistula is created through a side-to-side and side-to-end anastomosis using the radial artery and the cephalic forearm vein. The high blood flow and pressure on the venous side of the fistula "arterialize" the veins, which takes 3 to 5 weeks. The Cimino-Brescia fistula is well tolerated by patients, has a low infection rate, and has the longest functional use of any vascular access method. The fistula has a 90% patency rate at 12 months, which gradually decreases to approximately 75% at 4 years.

An alternative to the Cimino-Brescia fistula is the *arteriovenous bridge fistula.* Formed by a prosthetic conduit, this fistula connects a superficial artery (usually the radial or brachial) with a large antecubital vein. The prosthetic material is usually expanded polytetrafluoroethylene. AV bridges may be constructed in the leg between the superficial femoral or femoral artery and the saphenous vein. Lower extremity arterial bridges have a higher blood flow rate and therefore are less likely to thrombose but are also associated with a higher rate of infection produced by their proximity to the bacteria-laden perineum.

Thrombosis Thrombosis is the most common complication of a subcutaneous AV fistula or prosthetic graft. ED personnel must avoid circumferential bandages, tourniquets, or blood pressure cuffs in the fistula-bearing arm because these objects restrict venous outflow and may predispose to thrombosis. A tourniquet should not be used. The opposite arm or the fistula itself can be used to acquire blood or vascular access (without using a tourniquet). Normal graft flow is clinically verified by feeling a thrill or hearing a bruit on auscultation. A strong palpable pulse with no matching thrill suggests venous outflow obstruction or early graft thrombosis. Thrombosis of AV fistulas requires temporary vascular access and definitive surgical intervention later, usually with the creation of a new fistula proximal to the thrombosed shunt.

Blood Withdrawal When a Cimino-Brescia fistula is used to obtain blood samples, ideally an alternate peripheral venipuncture site should be sought first. When an alternate site is unavailable, however, the AV fistula is a reasonable choice. An individual skilled in venipuncture techniques should maintain absolute sterility with antiseptic (e.g., Betadine) skin preparation, sterile gloves, and sterile gauze. Tourniquets are contraindicated and unnecessary. Venipuncture should be performed on the well-developed venous side of the fistula. After blood acquisition, gentle pressure should be maintained for 5 minutes, taking care not to occlude the vessel lumen. The site should then be observed for several minutes to ensure that bleeding does not occur. A prosthetic AV bridge fistula can also be used to obtain blood samples. Venipuncture is achieved by careful perforation of the superficial wall of the prosthetic graft; otherwise, the technique is identical.

Clinically differentiating a Cimino-Brescia fistula from a prosthetic AV bridge fistula may be difficult. The prosthetic portion of an AV bridge fistula connects the arterial to the venous vessels in an H shape and is tunneled for some distance beneath the skin, giving the appearance of a single, large blood vessel. The prosthetic fistula will have a thrill but will not be as pulsatile as a Cimino-Brescia fistula when gently palpated. If asked, most patients are knowledgeable about their fistula.

Peripheral IV access is also best established at an alternate site. When an alternate site is unavailable and the patient requires timely IV access, the Cimino-Brescia fistula or bridge fistula can be used, following the guidelines given for venipuncture. Careful attention to sterile technique, operator skill, and avoidance of tourniquets can provide timely venipuncture or IV therapy while preventing infectious or thrombotic complications. If an IV line is used in a fistula, early removal after alternative IV access is desirable.

Infection Infections of an AV fistula or graft are potentially life threatening and are manifested by signs of septicemia and local inflammation. Once the diagnosis of infected fistula is considered, blood cultures should be obtained and IV antibiotics for gram-positive skin organisms administered. Prosthetic graft infection cannot be eradicated with IV antibiotics alone and requires prosthetic graft removal. Infections are the second leading cause of death of patients receiving long-term dialysis.

Steal Phenomenon Vascular steal from the ulnar artery via the palmar arch occasionally occurs in patients with atherosclerotic disease distal to the shunt, particularly diabetic patients. Patients with this condition may experience fingertip ischemia during periods of increased shunting (hemodialysis or increased activity). The steal phenomenon usually requires graft ligation with construction of a new fistula in the opposite extremity.

Venous Hypertension Acute venous hypertension may occur in the first few weeks after fistula construction. This is a true surgical emergency. The early rise in venous pressure produces marked swelling of the extremity and severe venous stasis disease. Characteristic skin pigmentation, edema, and occasionally venous ulceration are seen. Management of venous hypertension requires hospitalization and urgent ligation of the vein immediately distal to the fistula before a potentially exsanguinating vessel rupture.

Bleeding Patients may also present to the ED with bleeding from their fistula after dialysis. Persistent, gentle pressure, taking care not to occlude blood flow, usually resolves this problem.

KEY CONCEPTS

- Acute arterial occlusion is a limb-threatening emergency requiring immediate heparinization and Fogarty catheter embolectomy. The clinical diagnosis is based on some variant of the "five Ps": pain, pallor, pulselessness, paresthesias, and paralysis. Confirmatory tests are unnecessary and increase the limb's ischemic status.
- Atheroembolism (blue toe syndrome) is associated with cool, painful cyanotic toes in the presence of palpable distal pulses. A proximal source should be localized, most often an atherosclerotic aneurysm in the aorta or the iliac, femoral, or popliteal artery.
- Popliteal aneurysms are bilateral in 60% of patients and often coexist with an abdominal aortic aneurysm.
- The classic Raynaud's attack is triphasic: the fingers become white, blue, then red. Raynaud's disease has no detectable underlying cause and usually a benign course. Raynaud's phenomenon has an underlying disorder, usually connective tissue disease.
- The only reliable clinical test for detection of thoracic outlet syndrome is the elevated arm stress test (EAST).
- Complications of parenteral drug abuse include acute arterial ischemia, infected pseudoaneurysms, lymphatic obstruction, and direct neurologic injury.
- Acute venous hypertension may occur in the first few weeks after construction of an arteriovenous fistula. Hospitalization is required for ligation of the vein before a potentially exsanguinating vessel rupture occurs.

REFERENCES

1. Haimovici H: Landmarks and present trends in vascular surgery. In Haimovici H, editor: *Vascular surgery,* ed 3, East Norwalk, Conn, 1989, Prentice Hall.
2. Rutherford RB: Arterial aneurysms: etiologic considerations. In Rutherford RB, editor: *Vascular surgery,* ed 3, Philadelphia, 1989, Saunders.
3. Brewster DC, Chin AK, Fogarty TJ: Arterial thromboembolism. In Rutherford RB, editor: *Vascular surgery,* ed 3, Philadelphia, 1989, Saunders.
4. Kumagai K et al: Increased intracardiovascular clotting in patients with chronic atrial fibrillation, *J Am Coll Cardiol* 16:377, 1990.
5. Haimovici H: Muscular, renal and metabolic complications of acute arterial occlusions: myonephropathic-metabolic syndrome, *Surgery* 85:461, 1979.
6. Fisher DF et al: Dilemmas in dealing with the blue toe syndrome: aortic versus peripheral source, *Am J Surg* 148:836, 1984.
7. Cotran RS, Kumar V, Robbins SL: *Pathologic basis of disease,* ed 4, Philadelphia, 1989, Saunders.
8. Bandyk DF: Vascular injury. In Condon RE, Nyhus LM, editors: *Manual of surgical therapeutics,* ed 7, Boston, 1988, Little, Brown.
9. Elkin DC, Warren JV: Arteriovenous fistulas: their effect on the circulation, *JAMA* 134:1524, 1947.
10. Perry MO: Acute limb ischemia. In Rutherford RB, editor: *Vascular surgery,* ed 3, Philadelphia, 1989, WB Saunders.

11. Halperin JL, Coffman JD: Pathophysiology of Raynaud's disease, *Arch Intern Med* 139:89, 1979.
12. Plummer D: Principles of emergency ultrasound and echocardiography, *Ann Emerg Med* 18:1291, 1989.
13. Hessel S, Adams D, Abrams H: Complications of angiography, *Radiology* 138:273, 1981.
14. Gomes MN, Choyke PL: Improved identification of renal arteries in patients with aortic aneurysms by means of high-resolution computed tomography, *J Vasc Surg* 6:262, 1987.
15. Fogarty TJ et al: A method of extraction of arterial emboli and thrombi, *Surg Gynecol Obstet* 116:241, 1963.
16. Wholey MH: Advances in balloon technology and reperfusion devices for peripheral circulation, *Am J Cardiol* 61:87G, 1988.
17. Morin JF et al: Factors that determine the long-term results of percutaneous transluminal dilatation for peripheral arterial occlusive disease, *J Vasc Surg* 4:68, 1996.
18. Persson AV, Anderson LA, Padberg FT Jr: Selection of patients for lumbar sympathectomy, *Surg Clin North Am* 65:393, 1985.
19. Myers RAM, Marzella L: Hyperbaric medicine: what is it, how is it used? *MMJ* 37:559, 1988.
20. Juergens JL, Spittell JA Jr, Fairbairn JF: *Peripheral vascular diseases,* ed 5, Philadelphia, 1980, Saunders.
21. Litchfield R et al: Differential diagnosis of leg ulcers, *JAMA* 78:364, 1979.
22. Kempczinski RF: Management of chronic ischemia of the lower extremities. In Rutherford RB, editor: *Vascular surgery,* ed 3, Philadelphia, 1989, Saunders.
23. Buerger L: Thromboangiitis obliterans: a study of vascular lesions leading to presenile spontaneous gangrene, *Am J Med Sci* 136:567, 1908.
24. Lie JT: Thromboangiitis revisited, *Pathol Annu* 23:257, 1988.
25. Sicard GA et al: Thrombolytic therapy for acute arterial occlusion, *J Vasc Surg* 2:65, 1985.
26. Falanga V, Fine MJ, Kapoor WN: The cutaneous manifestations of cholesterol crystal embolization, *Arch Dermatol* 122:1194, 1986.
27. Evans WE, Hayes JP: Popliteal and femoral aneurysms. In Rutherford RB, editor: *Vascular surgery,* ed 3, Philadelphia, 1989, WB Saunders.
28. Ho PK et al: Aneurysms of the upper extremity, *J Hand Surg* 12A:39, 1987.
29. Scher LA et al: Vascular complications of thoracic outlet syndrome, *Vasc Surg* 3:565, 1986.
30. Pineda CJ et al: Hypothenar hammer syndrome: form of reversible Raynaud's phenomenon, *Am J Med* 79:561, 1985.
31. Stanley JC, Zelenock GB: Splanchnic artery aneurysms. In Rutherford RB, editor: *Vascular surgery,* ed 3, Philadelphia, 1989, WB Saunders.
32. Mandel SR et al: Nonoperative management of peripancreatic arterial aneurysms: a 10-year experience, *Ann Surg* 205:126, 1987.
33. Baker JS et al: Splanchnic artery aneurysms and pseudoaneurysms: transcatheter embolization, *Radiology* 163:135, 1987.
34. Wilson SE, Van Wagenen P, Passaro E Jr: Arterial infection, *Curr Probl Surg* 15:9, 1978.
35. Reddy DJ, Ernst CB: Infected aneurysms. In Rutherford RB, editor: *Vascular surgery,* ed 3, Philadelphia, 1989, Saunders.
36. Reddy DJ et al: Infected femoral artery false aneurysms in drug addicts: evolution of selective vascular reconstruction, *J Vasc Surg* 3:718, 1986.
37. Miller BM et al: *Histoplasma* infection of abdominal aortic aneurysms, *Ann Surg* 197:57, 1983.
38. Shetty PC et al: Mycotic aneurysms in intravenous drug abusers: the utility of intravenous digital subtraction angiography, *Radiology* 155:319, 1985.
39. Brunner MC et al: Prosthetic graft infection: limitations of indium white blood cell scanning, *J Vasc Surg* 3:42, 1986.
40. Mehmet OC et al: Review of salmonella mycotic aneurysms of the thoracic aorta, *J Cardiovasc Surg* 30:99, 1989.
41. Feliciano DV et al: Delayed diagnosis of arterial injuries, *Am J Surg* 154:579, 1987.
42. Spittel JA Jr: Vasospastic disorders. In Spittel JA Jr, editor: *Clinical vascular disease,* Philadelphia, 1983, Davis.
43. Roos DB: Thoracic outlet nerve compression. In Rutherford RB, editor: *Vascular surgery,* ed 3, Philadelphia, 1989, Saunders.
44. Roos DB: Congenital anomalies associated with thoracic outlet syndrome, *Am J Surg* 132:771, 1976.
45. Roos DB: New concepts of thoracic outlet syndrome that explain etiology, symptoms, diagnosis and treatment, *Vasc Surg* 13:313, 1979.
46. Lang EK: Arteriography and venography in the assessment of thoracic outlet syndromes, *South Med J* 65:129, 1972.
47. Drury EM et al: Lytic therapy in the treatment of axillary and subclavian vein thrombosis, *J Vasc Surg* 2:821, 1985.
48. Beall AC et al: Surgical management of traumatic arteriovenous aneurysms, *Am J Surg* 106:610, 1963.
49. Berenstein A et al: Percutaneous embolization of arteriovenous fistulas of the external carotid artery, *AJNR Am J Neuroradiol* 7:937, 1986.
50. Benitez PR, Newell MA: Vascular trauma in drug abuse: patterns of injury, *Ann Vasc Surg* 1:175, 1986.
51. Geelhoed GW, Joseph WL: Surgical sequelae of drug abuse, *Surg Gynecol Obstet* 139:749, 1974.
52. Trout HH, Smith CA: Lateral iliopopliteal arterial bypass as an alternative to obturator bypass, *Am Surg* 48:63, 1982.
53. Bjeletich J, Hickman RO: The Hickman indwelling catheter, *Am J Nurs* 62, 1980.
54. Krzywda E: Unpublished data, 1990, Medical College of Wisconsin.
55. Pessa ME, Howard RJ: Complications of Hickman-Broviac catheters, *Surg Gynecol Obstet* 161:257, 1985.
56. Quebbeman EJ: Unpublished data, 1990.
57. Anderson AJ et al: Hickman catheter clots: a common occurrence despite daily heparin flushing, *Cancer Treat Rep* 71:651, 1987.
58. Sharma GVRK et al: Thrombolytic therapy, *N Engl J Med* 306:1268, 1982.
59. Hinke DH et al: Pinch-off syndrome: a complication of implantable central venous access devices, *Radiology* 177:353, 1990.
60. Lokich JJ et al: Complications and management of implanted venous access catheters, *J Clin Oncol* 3:710, 1985.
61. Fraschini G et al: Local infusion of urokinase for the lysis of thrombosis associated with permanent central venous catheters in cancer patients, *J Clin Oncol* 5:672, 1987.
62. Anderson MA, Aker SN, Hickman RO: The double-lumen Hickman catheter, *Am J Nurs* 272, 1982.
63. Hampton AA, Sherertz RJ: Vascular-access infections in hospitalized patients, *Surg Clin North Am* 68:57, 1988.
64. Kaufman J et al: Catheter-related septic central venous thrombosis: current therapeutic options, *West J Med* 145:200, 1986.
65. Schuman ES: Outpatient management of Hickman catheter sepsis, *Infect Surg* 103, 1987.
66. Moyer MA, Edwards LD, Farley L: Comparative culture methods on 101 intravenous catheters: routine, semiquantitative, and blood cultures, *Arch Intern Med* 143:66, 1983.
67. Malviya VK et al: Vascular access in gynecologic cancer using the Groshong right atrial catheter, *Gynecol Oncol* 33:313, 1989.
68. Delmore JE et al: Experience with the Groshong long-term central venous catheter, *Gynecol Oncol* 34:216, 1989.
69. Grabner DA, Dinerstein C: The Quinton-Mahurkar dual lumen subclavian catheter: preliminary clinical information, *Dial Transplant* 12:847, 1983.
70. Vanholder R, Hoenich N, Ringoir S: Morbidity and mortality of central venous catheter hemodialysis: a review of 10 years' experience, *Nephron* 47:274, 1987.

83 Venous Thrombosis and Pulmonary Embolism

Craig F. Feied

PERSPECTIVE

Venous thromboembolism (VTE) is a single disease with manifestations that include deep vein thrombosis (DVT), pulmonary thromboembolism (PTE), superficial vein thrombosis (SVT), and chronic venous insufficiency (CVI). PTE, the most serious complication of venous thrombosis, is the third most common cause of death in the United States, with at least 780,000 clinically apparent cases occurring annually.

As imaging studies improve, it becomes increasingly apparent that virtually every case of DVT embolizes to some extent. The frequency and severity of pulmonary embolism are not related to the presence or absence of DVT symptoms; two thirds of patients with proven PTE have no symptoms of DVT, and half of patients with proven DVT but no symptoms of PTE have undiagnosed pulmonary emboli of significant size.[1] Despite the frequency and the gravity of PTE, the diagnosis is often missed. The patient's history can only suggest the disease, and no physical finding is necessary or sufficient to make the diagnosis. The diagnosis of VTE usually cannot be made or excluded on the basis of clinical judgment; specific diagnostic tests are essential when VTE is suspected. If the diagnosis is missed at the initial presentation, delaying therapeutic anticoagulation for only 24 hours, the risk of recurrent embolism increases from 4% to 23%, with a fivefold increase in the likelihood of death within 1 year.[2,3]

Historical Background

Until the 1930s, PTE was viewed as an almost universally fatal disease, with surgery the only treatment despite an operative mortality of nearly 100%. In the 1930s, heparin came into widespread clinical use as an antithrombotic agent. The beneficial effects of anticoagulation in thromboembolic disease were so immediately and dramatically apparent that anticoagulation rapidly became the mainstay of management, replacing surgical intervention in all but a small subset of critical cases. In the late 1960s and early 1970s, two large-scale clinical trials demonstrated the usefulness of fibrinolytic agents in attaining rapid clot resolution, and a National Institutes of Health (NIH) consensus committee established fibrinolysis as the standard of care for hemodynamically unstable PTE.[4]

Epidemiology

Deep Vein Thrombosis DVT causes more than 600,000 hospitalizations in the United States each year. Many more cases go unrecognized, however, and the true incidence is unknown. Although clinical diagnosis can result in both false-positive and false-negative results, clinical estimates of the incidence of DVT and PTE always underestimate the magnitude of the problem when compared with the findings of prospective studies and with autopsy findings. In orthopedic patients, for example, the rate of DVT found by prospective evaluation is 10 times greater than the rate found by clinical diagnosis and retrospective review.[5] Studies that depend on clinical recognition of disease underestimate the incidence of DVT because nonobstructing thrombus usually causes no symptoms, and the symptoms that occur with obstructing thrombus are often vague and nonspecific.

Pulmonary Embolism More than 400,000 cases of PTE are missed annually in the United States, resulting in the death of more than 100,000 patients who would have survived with the proper diagnosis and treatment. About 10% of deaths from PTE occur within 60 minutes after the initial onset of symptoms. Those who survive an initial event are at increased risk for recurrent PTE and development of pulmonary hypertension, which occurs in up to 70% of patients and carries its own attendant mortality and morbidity.[6]

One of every nine people will develop DVT before age 80, and VTE accounts for one of every 20 deaths after age 50. The incidence of clinically recognized DVT and PTE is 0.2% per year in the general population and 1% per year in those over age 75.[7] Autopsy studies demonstrate that most cases of DVT and PTE go undiagnosed, even when they are the immediate cause of death, so the true incidence in the general population is much higher than the recognized incidence.

Unrecognized fatal PTE is common in the ED as well. Transesophageal echocardiography identifies unsuspected pulmonary embolism in 36% of ED patients who have cardiac arrest with pulseless electrical activity.[8]

Autopsy Evidence

A carefully performed autopsy is the gold standard for assessing the incidence of fatal PTE. Autopsy results consistently demonstrate that up to 60% of patients dying in the hospital will have evidence of PTE and that the diagnosis will be missed antemortem in more than 70% of cases. The incidence of in-hospital DVT is highest (approaching 70%) in patients undergoing surgical repair of a fractured hip without prophylaxis, but the problem is not confined to surgical patients. In the absence of prophylactic measures, acute DVT may be demonstrated in about 15% of all general medical patients placed at bed rest for a week, in about 30% of medical intensive care unit (ICU) patients, and in 20% to 50% of those with pulmonary disease, acute myocardial infarction (MI), or stroke (cerebrovascular accident).[9,10] At least half of these patients can be shown to have had PTE, even though the majority will have had none of the classic symptoms of PTE.[1,11]

These cases of occult VTE are clinically significant. When general medical inpatients are randomized to receive prophylactic subcutaneous heparin or no prophylaxis against VTE, heparin reduces mortality by 30%.[12] VTE is not restricted to postoperative patients and those at bed rest in the hospital. Autopsy studies have found a similar incidence and pattern of PTE for in-hospital and out-of-hospital deaths. Just as the incidence of VTE is generally underestimated, the mortality risk associated with DVT and PTE as a primary or comorbid diagnosis is also generally underestimated. Large-scale studies show that in some populations the 1-week mortality of patients diagnosed with PTE is nearly 40% and the 1-year mortality nearly 60% despite early diagnosis and treatment.[3,13]

PRINCIPLES OF DISEASE

Anatomy and Physiology

Venous The peripheral venous system functions both as a reservoir to hold extra blood and as a conduit to return blood from the periphery to the heart and lungs. Primary collecting veins of the lower extremity are passive, thin-walled reservoirs that are tremendously distensible. Most are suprafascial, surrounded by loosely bound alveolar and fatty tissue that is easily displaced. These suprafascial collecting veins can dilate to accommodate large volumes of blood with little increase in back pressure; the volume of blood sequestered within the venous system at any moment can vary by a factor of two or more without interfering with the normal function of the veins. Blood passes from the superficial veins through perforating veins into the subfascial veins of the deep venous system and then back to the heart and lungs.

Pulmonary The pulmonary arterial tree contains 26 branchings, of which only the first three are visible on a pulmonary arteriogram. Normal pulmonary arteries are highly distensible, making the lungs a primary capacitance circuit for the cardiovascular system. Bronchial arteries anastomose with pulmonary arteries in the distal vascular tree, and bronchial arterial flow often is sufficient to prevent pulmonary parenchymal infarction even when segmental or subsegmental pulmonary arteries are completely blocked by PTE.

Pathophysiology

Under normal conditions, microthrombi (tiny aggregates of red cells, platelets, and fibrin) are continually formed and lysed within the venous circulatory system. Under pathologic conditions, microthrombi may escape the normal fibrinolytic system to grow and propagate. PTE occurs when fragments of thrombus break loose and are carried via the vena cava and the right side of the heart to lodge in the pulmonary arterial tree.

Deep Vein Thrombosis With respect to the risk of death and of long-term sequelae, the *site* of DVT is much less important than was formerly believed. Fatal PTE, chronic cor pulmonale, and significant local morbidity can result from DVT at any site in the body. Calf vein thrombosis eventually propagates above the knee in about 80% of cases, but it often embolizes to cause hemodynamic collapse and death without ever extending above the knee. Upper extremity DVT is no more benign than calf DVT; both spontaneous and catheter-associated upper extremity thrombosis can cause death from massive PTE. Even superficial phlebitis cannot be considered benign, since investigation often reveals occult deep vein extension, and progression to fatal embolism is common.

The body's natural circulating anticoagulant effect depends principally on three plasma proteins: antithrombin III, protein C, and protein S. Together, these plasma proteins prevent minor vessel injury from triggering runaway thrombus propagation and uncontrolled intravascular coagulation.

The fibrinolytic system, when working correctly, ensures that thrombus is lysed wherever it is not needed. Plasmin, the body's principal fibrinolytic enzyme, degrades the fibrin that binds individual blood components into a thrombus. A circulating inactive form of plasmin (plasminogen) is converted into plasmin by plasminogen activators. Urokinase plasminogen activator (u-plasminogen activator, urokinase) is produced in renal cells and excreted in the urine. Tissue plasminogen activator (t-plasminogen activator, TPA) is found in the endothelial cells of vessel walls and acts on thrombus in situ. TPA is released in response to physiologic stimuli, such as segmental venous stasis, vessel wall injury, exercise, and thrombin. Most of the action of TPA is limited to the surface of a thrombus, where plasmin is formed when plasminogen and TPA together bind to fibrin, but naturally circulating TPA does produce a mild systemic lytic state in which circulating fibrinogen is consumed. Disturbances of the fibrinolytic system lead either to increased bleeding or to the inappropriate extension of otherwise appropriately formed thrombus.

Thrombophlebitis Properly treated, superficial thrombophlebitis that does not progress to involve the deep veins can be benign. Deep thrombophlebitis, on the other hand, carries a high morbidity and mortality. Unfortunately, clinical examination cannot distinguish isolated superficial vein phlebitis from thrombophlebitis that also involves deeper veins, and SVT may not remain superficial. The deep and superficial venous systems communicate through hundreds of perforating veins up and down the leg, and thrombus can propagate through a perforating vein at any time. One fifth of patients with apparently superficial thrombophlebitis actually have an associated DVT at presentation, and many more will progress to deep system involvement over time.[14]

Without anticoagulation, approximately 10% of hospitalized patients with superficial thrombophlebitis will develop PTE, and 20% of these patients will die. Superficial and deep thrombophlebitis are best regarded as a single clinical entity, of which the major sequelae are CVI and PTE.[15]

Embolization and Embolism Except in pregnant patients and patients with significant trauma, virtually all lower extremity DVT starts in the *calf veins,* although it has spread proximally in more than 80% of cases before clinical symptoms become apparent and the diagnosis is made.[16] DVT need not spread proximally to cause fatal PTE, however; the largest autopsy series ever to look for the source of fatal PTE found that 25% of lethal pulmonary emboli and 33% of massive pulmonary emboli arise from isolated calf vein thrombi.[17] Up to half of patients with isolated calf vein thrombosis have symptomatic PTE, and emboli from calf veins are large or massive in 40% of cases.[18,19]

Thrombus in the *ileofemoral deep veins* nearly always embolizes. Current techniques can demonstrate PTE in 60% to 80% of patients with DVT in the popliteal or femoral veins, even though about half these patients have no clinical symptoms to suggest PTE. As thrombus progresses proximally from the calf to the thigh, the frequency of clinically recognized embolization increases. Thrombus that has reached the popliteal segment of the femoral vein embolizes in more than 60% of cases, and by the time it has propagated proximally into the thigh, it embolizes in at least 80% of patients.[11,17,20] For thrombus above the popliteal segment of the femoral vein, proximity of venous thrombus is not associated with risk of subsequent embolization.[20]

Significant lung perfusion defects are found in a substantial number of patients with spontaneous or catheter-related upper extremity DVT, and massive PTE is responsible for the death of 10% of patients with a known upper extremity DVT who die in hospital.[21] Pulmonary emboli are found in a third of patients with catheter-associated thrombosis, and a 20% mortality is seen in those with PTE.

The source of embolism is found within the upper venous tree (vena cava, jugular, subclavian, and innominate veins) in 8% of fatal pulmonary emboli.

Nonthrombotic Pulmonary Embolism Other substances besides thrombus are capable of passing through the systemic venous circulation and lodging in the pulmonary vasculature, most often amniotic fluid, fat, and air. Pulmonary embolism has also resulted from such diverse sources as contaminants of intravenous (IV) drug preparations, mercury, barium, broken catheters, parasites, tumor, brain tissue, bullets, cardiac vegetations, marrow, and bile. Each of these types of embolism requires the routine supportive care used in thromboembolism, but none is appropriately managed with anticoagulants or fibrinolytic agents.

Amniotic Fluid Embolism Amniotic fluid embolism may occur in the setting of abortion or in the immediate postpartum period, but it usually occurs near the end of the first stage of labor. Successful management of amniotic fluid embolism must include emptying the uterus. The infusion of fresh frozen plasma, platelets, cryoprecipitate, or whole blood may be required because disseminated intravascular coagulation (DIC) typically occurs and principally accounts for a mortality exceeding 80%.

Fat Embolism Fat emboli have been reported in a variety of unusual clinical settings but most often occur after fractures of the long bones, especially fractures of the tibia and the femur. Contrary to some published reports, fat globules in sputum, urine, or blood are not diagnostic of fat embolism; fat globules may be found in the body fluids of healthy patients. Unlike thromboemboli, fat emboli may pass through the pulmonary circulation and into the systemic arterial circulation, where virtually any end organ may be affected. Petechiae may appear on the chest, axillae, neck, fundi, and conjunctivae. The cerebral circulation is at particular risk, and patients may have central nervous system symptoms ranging from headache or irritability to disorientation, convulsions, and coma. An acute respiratory distress syndrome is often seen, and thrombocytopenia may develop. The only treatment of potential value is high-dose steroid therapy. Heparin is not recommended because it may increase the production of toxic fatty acids in the lungs.

Pulmonary Air Embolism Air embolism is generally iatrogenic in origin but may occur in a variety of other clinical circumstances, from the use of pressurized underwater breathing apparatus to the use of air-powered surgical or dental drills and saws. Vaginal insufflation is a cause of fatal venous air embolism associated with orogenital sex. Most cases occur during pregnancy, when air more easily passes beneath the fetal membranes and into the circulation of the subplacental sinuses, leading to immediate circulatory collapse with a high maternal and fetal mortality. In many cases of vaginal insufflation, the air embolism is both venous (leading to circulatory collapse) and arterial, leading to cerebral circulatory impairment and coma.

The clinical syndrome of venous air embolism includes a loud, churning, machinery-like murmur that is heard over the precordium. Air bubbles may be detected within the heart sonographically. Although it is often taught that the formation of an air lock in the right ventricle or in the pulmonary arterial circulation requires 5 ml/kg body weight of IV air, circulatory collapse has resulted from infusion of the 20-ml priming volume of air contained in an ordinary IV infusion set that had not been flushed with saline.

To prevent air lock formation, the patient should be placed in a left lateral position in an attempt to trap air within the right atrium. Aspiration via a Swan-Ganz or other right-sided heart catheter may be successful. Emergency thoracotomy and direct needle aspiration of intracardiac air are appropriate for a patient with air embolism in full arrest who does not respond quickly to closed-chest cardiopulmonary resuscitation (CPR). Hyperbaric treatment may be used to decrease the size of the air bubbles within the cerebral circulation or the pulmonary arterial tree, permitting the bubbles to travel more distally and reducing the amount of pulmonary or cerebral circulation that is affected.

Other Substances *Bile* emboli have been identified at autopsy after percutaneous transhepatic drainage for a pancreatic cancer obstructing the bile duct. *Tumor* embolism is more common than usually realized, may masquerade as thromboembolism, and is often misdiagnosed antemortem. *Bone marrow* embolism usually is associated with fractures of the long bones, but may also occur with fractures of the sternum and ribs sustained during closed-chest CPR.

Pulmonary Thromboembolism

Hemodynamic Effects When thrombus occludes a portion of the pulmonary vasculature, pulmonary vascular resistance rises, forcing an increase in pulmonary arterial and right ventricular pressures. If the cross-sectional area removed from circulation is small, the hemodynamic effects may be negligible. If 50% or more of the vascular tree is occluded, sustained significant pulmonary hypertension and acute cor pulmonale occur. A murmur of acute tricuspid regurgitation indicates that the pulmonary arterial pressure exceeds 40 mm Hg. If a sufficiently large fraction of the pulmonary vasculature is occluded, right-sided heart failure and hemodynamic collapse will occur. Most deaths from PTE are caused by hemodynamic collapse.

Even slight elevations of pulmonary arterial pressure can cause substantial mortality and morbidity. A minimal pressure increase above a patient's premorbid baseline is an independent predictor for the development of cardiac disease even when the absolute level of the pulmonary arterial pressure, overall pulmonary function, coronary arteries, and systolic cardiac function are within the normal range.[22] Because PTE is most often silent and because it is a disease of recurrences, many patients accumulate multiple small chronic pulmonary emboli and go on to develop chronic cor pulmonale.[6]

Respiratory Effects Some of the mechanisms whereby PTE causes disturbances of oxygen tension (Po_2) and carbon dioxide tension (Pco_2) remain obscure, but much can be understood through the simple application of classic models of respiratory physiology. The initial result of PTE is to reduce or abolish pulmonary blood flow in some areas of the lung, converting normally ventilated lung into physiologic ventilatory dead space. Ventilation going to this portion of the lung is wasted, and the effect is as though the patient had suddenly reduced respirations without a corresponding decrease in metabolic requirements.

Receptors driving the respiratory centers can detect even a slight hypoxemia and hypercarbia. The patient attempts to compensate for this primary drop in effective ventilation by increasing total minute ventilation through increased depth or frequency of respirations. If the hypoperfused area is small, increased oxygen extraction may provide adequate tissue oxygen delivery, and an increase in ventilation may be so subtle as to be clinically unrecognized. A 15% increase in minute ventilation may be accomplished almost without being detectable, either by an increase from 12 to 14 respirations/min or by an increase of only 75 ml in tidal volume. If the size of the newly created alveolar dead space (i.e., the hypoperfused region) is large, the compensatory effort will be more overt, with prominent tachypnea and dyspnea. In massive PTE (angiographically defined as the blockage of flow to an area greater than that served by two lobar arteries) respiratory collapse may ensue. If pulmonary vascular resistance increases to the point where cardiac output cannot be maintained, increased oxygen extraction can result in very low venous Po_2 levels.

Pulmonary pseudoshunt Abnormal blood gas results in patients with PTE are sometimes said to arise from a pseudoshunt because they behave as though a portion of pulmonary blood has been shunted through an unventilated path. The mechanism is straightforward; portions of the pulmonary circulation have been blocked by thrombus, and very little blood can pass through those areas. The rest of the blood must flow through the remaining portions of the pulmonary vascular tree, thus creating areas of low flow but normal ventilation (ventilation/perfusion [$\dot{V}/\dot{Q}$] ratio >1) along with areas of high flow but normal ventilation ($\dot{V}/\dot{Q}$ ratio <1). The small amount of blood that passes through the area of decreased flow has an increased opportunity to equilibrate with alveolar gas. This gives a small volume of blood with a normal or slightly increased Po_2 and a normal or slightly decreased Pco_2. The much larger amount of blood passing through an area of increased flow has a shortened opportunity to equilibrate with alveolar gas and will have a decreased Po_2 and an increased Pco_2.

This may be understood by thinking of the blood flowing past each alveolus as divided into a "normal" volume and an "extra" volume. Equilibration is not strongly time dependent, so even though the velocity of flow increases, the normal volume of blood equilibrates normally with the normal volume of gas in the alveolus. The extra volume of blood that follows afterward is exposed to an alveolus that is already deoxygenated and high in CO_2. This extra volume of blood has no opportunity to become oxygenated or to release CO_2; in a sense, it has been "shunted" through an unventilated portion of lung. Mixed arterial blood reflects the reduced $\dot{V}/\dot{Q}$ ratio of this large volume of poorly equilibrated blood.

In other words, the nonperfused part of the pulmonary system has been converted into physiologic dead space. Removal of perfusion from 25% of alveoli is roughly equivalent to reducing a patient's minute volume by 25% without decreasing metabolic demands.

Other causes of impaired gas exchange The simple model of V/Q mismatch and increased physiologic dead space explains most of the respiratory abnormalities that may be seen in PTE, but other factors also play a role. Immediately after the event, pain and anxiety typically cause relative hyperventilation, which raises the Po_2 and lowers the Pco_2. After 24 hours of decreased blood supply, a dramatic decrease in local surfactant production may produce an area of atelectasis. In many cases this is followed by transudation of fluid, with the development of alveolar infiltrates (indistinguishable from those seen in an infectious pneumonia) and a further impairment of gas exchange. Rales are commonly heard during this phase, and sometimes there is a pulmonary rub. Additional mechanisms proposed for the hypoxemia seen in acute PTE include (1) right-to-left shunting through a patent foramen ovale, (2) true intrapulmonary shunting through pulmonary arteriovenous anastomoses that are forced open in the setting of pulmonary hypertension, and (3) increased oxygen extraction as a result of decreased cardiac output. The release of neurohumoral factors may cause pulmonary vasoconstriction with widespread bronchoconstriction and wheezing, requiring more compensatory effort from the patient. Finally, if the anastomotic circulation from the bronchial arteries is insufficient in the area of the embolism, pulmonary infarction will produce pain and splinting with further associated global or regional hypoventilation.

When all available theoretic, clinical, and experimental evidence is considered, physiologic alterations in massive PTE clearly tend to produce hypoxemia, but compensatory mechanisms permit relative sparing of the PO_2 at the expense of the Pco_2, which may be normal, high, or low. Small pulmonary emboli produce no detectable alteration in arterial Po_2, Pco_2, or pH.

Chronic Cor Pulmonale Massive or recurrent PTE leads to chronic disability in most patients. Chronic PTE is an important cause of chronic cor pulmonale because pulmonary arterial endothelium is relatively incapable of lysing thrombus, and most thromboembolus that lodges in the pulmonary circulation remains permanently within the lungs. Abnormalities seen on the $\dot{V}/\dot{Q}$ scan or the angiogram often resolve, but the resolution occurs through organization, retraction, and recanalization of thrombus. The affected vessels remain lined with stiff, organized thrombus, and gas exchange continues to be significantly impaired in the most distal portions of the pulmonary vascular tree. Most important, the elastic distensibility of recanalized vessels is greatly reduced, and they can no longer perform their usual function as the capacitive portion of the cardiopulmonary circuit.[23] In a distensible circuit, increases in flow velocity produce little or no increase in pressure, but in a nondistensible circuit, resistance and pressure are a function of the flow velocity. After recanalization of thrombus leaves pulmonary arterioles relatively nondistensible, any attempt to increase cardiac output causes an increase in pulmonary vascular resistance. Cardiac output can only increase if pulmonary arterial pressure increases enough to overcome this extra resistance. If the disease is extensive, pulmonary arterial pressures may be as much as five times normal, making any exercise impossible. Disease of this severity is almost invariably fatal within a few years.

Chronic Venous Insufficiency Recanalization of thrombosed deep veins results in a valveless channel, leading to chronically elevated ambulatory venous pressure within the legs and a clinical postphlebitic syndrome. This postphlebitic venous insufficiency syndrome is responsible for chronic pain, edema, hyperpigmentation, and ulceration, as well as many cases of recurrent DVT and PTE.

Even when valvular incompetence is isolated to popliteal venous segments or deep veins of the calf, ambulatory venous pressures can be very high. Up to 60% of patients with isolated failure of valves in the popliteal segment of the femoral vein develop severe signs of CVI, and isolated calf vein thrombophlebitis results in clinical postphlebitic syndrome in 20% to 40% of patients.[24]

Just as thrombotic damage to valves within the deep system produces deep venous insufficiency, damage to perforating valves (valves that lead between the deep and superficial systems) can produce similar symptoms through a syndrome of superficial venous insufficiency. When high-pressure blood enters the superficial system through failed perforating valves, it invariably causes secondary failure of valves all along the superficial veins. This allows venous blood to escape from its normal antegrade flow path and to flow in a retrograde direction down into an already congested leg. Over time, these incompetent superficial veins become visibly dilated and tortuous, at which point they are called *varicose veins*.

Risk Factors

Some patients are at particularly high risk for VTE because of identifiable underlying medical conditions or environmental conditions. All the recognized risk factors, or markers, have their roots in Virchow's triad of venous stasis, hypercoagulability, and endothelial injury. The most common identifiable risk factors for VTE are a history of DVT or PTE, recent surgery or pregnancy, limb immobilization, confinement to bed, and underlying malignancy. Risk markers are helpful in raising the suspicion of disease but are not useful in ruling out DVT or PTE, because many patients who present with VTE have no clinically recognizable risk factors, even after a detailed laboratory investigation (Box 83-1).

Box 83-1 Risk Factors for Venous and Pulmonary Thromboembolism

AIDS (lupus anticoagulant)
AMI
Antithrombin III deficiency
Behçet's disease
Blood type A
Burns
Catheters (indwelling venous infusion catheters)
Chemotherapy
Congestive heart failure
Drug abuse (IV drugs)
Drug-induced lupus anticoagulant
DVT in the past
Estrogen replacements
Fibrinogen abnormality
Fractures
Hemolytic anemias
Heparin-associated thrombocytopenia
Homocysteinuria
Hyperlipidemias
Immobilization
Inflammatory bowel disease
Malignancy
Obesity
Old age
Oral contraceptives
PE in the past
Phenothiazines
Plasminogen abnormality
Plasminogen activator abnormality
Polycythemia
Postoperative
Postpartum period
Pregnancy
Protein C deficiency
Protein S deficiency
Resistance to activated protein C
SLE (lupus)
Superficial phlebitis
Trauma
Varicose veins
Venography
Venous pacemakers
Venous stasis
Warfarin (first few days of therapy)

AIDS, Acquired immunodeficiency syndrome; *SLE*, systemic lupus erythematosus.

History of Deep Vein Thrombosis Persons with a history of prior venous thrombosis are 5 to 30 times more likely to have a new DVT in response to a triggering event than those who have not had prior episodes. VTE recurrence rates are as high as 30% during a 5-year follow-up.[25] Patients with prior VTE include many with other irreversible risk factors, and the sequelae of prior DVT include permanent venous abnormalities, such as endothelial irregularity, chronic venous stasis, and valvular damage, all of which predispose to a recurrence.

Varicose Veins Without prophylaxis, more than half of patients with varicose veins will develop DVT when subjected to a secondary risk factor such as surgery. This is twice the incidence seen in comparable patients without varicose veins.

Hematologic Abnormalities The previous category of "idiopathic venous thrombosis" has been replaced by an ever-increasing number of quantifiable defects in hemostasis. Identifiable hematologic abnormalities are responsible for approximately 50% of clinically detected venous thromboembolic episodes, but these hypercoagulable states usually are not diagnosed until after a patient has already had several clinically recognized episodes of DVT or PTE. Primary or acquired coagulopathy should be sought in all patients with DVT or PTE, even when other risk factors such as surgery, pregnancy, or immobilization are present, because hidden hematologic abnormalities may cause thrombosis only when other risk factors act as coprecipitants.

Primary thrombogenic and hypercoagulable states may be produced by disorders of platelet number or function, defects of intrinsic or extrinsic coagulation, low levels of circulating anticoagulants, high levels of procoagulant factors, resistance to anticoagulant factors, excessive inhibitors of fibrinolysis, or insufficient fibrinolytic activation. They may be congenital or acquired. Congenital syndromes of increased platelet adhesion have been described, and acquired increases in platelet adhesiveness are seen in many clinical settings, including the immediate postoperative period, pregnancy, and the puerperium.

A primary deficiency of protein C or protein S leads to a hypercoagulable state in which patients often have episodes of DVT or PTE before age 35. These patients are also at risk for premature arteriosclerotic syndromes and MI at an early age. Acquired deficiency of these proteins can result from cancer, chemotherapy, vitamin K deficiency, oral anticoagulants, surgery, and DIC.

Among the inherited coagulopathies, antithrombin III deficiency deserves special mention because heparin is ineffective as an anticoagulant in the absence of antithrombin III. In *familial antithrombin III deficiency* the circulating levels may be reduced to half the normal amounts, with a correspondingly high risk for venous thrombosis. More than half of affected persons have PTE before age 50. Patients with severe liver disease may also develop venous thrombosis from an acquired antithrombin III deficiency.

Deficiencies of protein C, protein S, or antithrombin III each account for approximately 5% of the cases of DVT. Resistance to activated protein C, most often due to a point mutation known as *factor V Leiden,* is a more common defect that appears in 7% of the general population and underlies 20% to 50% of the cases of thrombophlebitis in patients who lack another recognized causative factor. Affected persons are asymptomatic until factor V is activated, at which point they are resistant to the inhibitory effects of protein C.

A high plasma level of procoagulant factor VIII is a strong independent factor that increases the risk of DVT recurrence nearly sevenfold. Patients who have persistently elevated levels of factor VIII after an episode of VTE may be candidates for prolonged anticoagulation.

Impaired fibrinolytic activity can occur in many ways. Plasminogen levels may be low, or plasminogen itself may be defective because of structural abnormalities. Fibrinogen and fibrin may have abnormal structures that resist degradation by plasmin. Patients may have high levels of circulating inhibitors of fibrinolysis or low levels of plasminogen activators. Thrombosis related to reduced fibrinolytic activity has been documented in congenital syndromes as well as in postoperative patients, in women taking oral contraceptives (OCs), and during pregnancy and the puerperium.

Polycythemia and Thrombocytosis The risk of thrombosis increases linearly with increasing hematocrit, and 40% of deaths in patients with polycythemia vera are related to arterial or venous thrombosis. It would seem logical that thrombocytosis should also raise the risk of thrombosis, but the opposite is true: platelet counts above 1 million lead to a reduced likelihood of thrombosis and an increased likelihood of bleeding problems.

Surgery Perioperative DVT may occur in response to even minimal venous endothelial injury. Widespread use of anticoagulant prophylaxis has greatly reduced postoperative DVT and PTE in Europe, but prophylaxis remains underutilized in the United States. Without prophylaxis, DVT occurs in up to half of general surgery patients and in up to 80% of patients after some types of orthopedic surgery.

Catheter-Associated Thrombosis Femoral central lines have a high associated morbidity; 25% to 33% of patients develop DVT after femoral vein cannulation, and the incidence of femoral vein thrombosis increases to 50% when concentrated dextrose solutions are infused.[26] The risk is associated with even brief episodes of femoral vein cannulation, and low-intensity prophylactic anticoagulation is not protective.

Subclavian and axillary vein thromboses once were rare and reportable entities, but increases in the prevalence of transvenous pacemakers and long-term central venous catheters have made catheter-associated subclavian vein thrombosis (and resultant pulmonary embolism) a common clinical entity.[27] Subclavian vein thrombosis may be associated with any indwelling catheter but is most common in patients receiving infusions of chemotherapeutic agents or parenteral alimentation. Significant local thrombi can develop around catheters that have been in place for only 24 hours. Removal of a thrombosed central line should not be undertaken lightly, because sudden collapse and death from massive PTE can follow removal of a central venous catheter that is anchoring an otherwise mobile thrombus. Catheter-associated thrombi are a common source of fatal embolism; fatal emboli may arise from any type of intravascular catheter or device, including ventriculovascular shunts and intracardiac defibrillator leads.

Anesthesia General anesthesia is an independent risk factor for the development of DVT after surgery. The incidence of DVT is much lower after epidural anesthesia than after general anesthesia.[28]

Immobility Immobility is one of the most important risk factors for VTE. After 1 week, DVT can be identified in 15% of patients at bed rest in a general medical ward and in twice as many ICU patients. The incidence of VTE at autopsy is 15% in patients dying from any cause after less than 1 week at bed rest, but this increases to 80% in patients who die after more prolonged immobilization without prophylaxis.[29] In hemiparetic stroke patients, DVT occurs in 60% of paralyzed legs but in only 7% of nonparalyzed legs.[30] Pregnant patients placed at bed rest for premature labor or preterm rupture of membranes are at 20 times higher risk of VTE than comparable pregnant patients who are not placed at bed rest.[31]

Autoimmune Disease and Immunodeficiency VTE is common in patients with systemic lupus erythematosus (SLE). The lupus anticoagulant (LA) is associated with a sixfold increase in risk and the anticardiolipin antibody with a twofold increase. LA also causes VTE in patients with acquired immunodeficiency syndrome (AIDS) and in other autoimmune diseases besides SLE. Phenothiazines and other drugs can cause secondary increases in LA.

Cancer Patients who develop spontaneous DVT or PTE and have no recognized risk factors deserve special surveillance for cancer because they may be at high risk for occult malignancy. This recommendation has been controversial, but prospective studies validating the risk estimate are convincing. The relative risk for cancer is 19 times higher for patients under age 50 who have had DVT than for patients without a history of DVT.[32] Cancer is newly diagnosed within 2 years in up to 25% of patients with DVT who have no other identifiable risk factor.[33]

Colon and ovarian cancer are the malignancies most often

associated with VTE, but PTE may be associated with many other types of cancer. The incidence of autopsy-confirmed PTE is approximately 30% in patients who die with ovarian or biliary cancer and about 15% in those who die with stomach cancer. The incidence of PTE is less than 6% in patients with cancers of the esophagus and larynx and in those with leukemia, myelomatosis, and lymphoma. The largest number of pulmonary emboli occurs in patients with palliatively treated cancers of the peritoneal cavity.

Chemotherapy Chemotherapy independently increases the risk of DVT and PTE. Some chemotherapeutic agents decrease circulating anticoagulants, such as antithrombin III, protein C, or protein S. Others cause an increase in circulating procoagulants, such as von Willebrand's factor.

Inflammatory Bowel Disease Ulcerative colitis and Crohn's disease are associated with higher risk of DVT and PTE because of increases in fibrinogen, factor VIII, and platelet activity and decreases in antithrombin III and α_2-macroglobulin levels.

Stroke and Neurotrauma The incidence of recognized DVT is extremely high after stroke; up to half of patients develop acute DVT within a median time of 5 days.[30] Compression hosiery and other prophylactic measures can dramatically reduce the incidence of DVT in this population.

Neurotrauma often is followed by syndromes of defibrination, DIC, and VTE. DVT is a complication in up to 40% of neurosurgical patients.

Coronary Artery Disease MI and congestive heart failure are independent risk factors for DVT and PTE. Patients admitted for acute MI who "rule in" and who do not receive anticoagulation have a 26% to 38% incidence of DVT, whereas control patients admitted for acute MI but who are eventually "ruled out" have a much lower incidence. This may be related to the duration of bed rest traditionally used in patients with confirmed MI. The presence of lipemic serum also increases the speed and extent of thrombus formation in response to vascular injury.

Pregnancy and Puerperium PTE is the most common nontraumatic cause of maternal death during pregnancy and the postpartum period and is responsible for up to half of all obstetric morbidity and mortality. The absolute incidence of recognized pregnancy-associated thromboembolism is 1 to 4 per 1000 births. Three fourths of clinically apparent cases of VTE occur before delivery, and one half occur in the first 15 weeks of pregnancy.[34] Bed rest during pregnancy increases the risk of VTE twentyfold.[31]

Septic *pelvic vein* thrombophlebitis is a serious complication of postpartum endometritis that often results in death from septic pulmonary emboli. The diagnosis is difficult to make in patients with endometritis, and thus anticoagulation has been recommended as part of the routine therapy of significant postpartum endometritis.

Ovarian vein thrombosis is a serious puerperal complication that presents as severe localized adnexal pain, often involving the flank or abdomen. Fever is common. Ovarian vein thrombosis may be diagnosed by computed tomography (CT), magnetic resonance imaging (MRI), or color flow ultrasonography (US), but the diagnosis usually is made laparoscopically.

Exogenous Estrogens Hormone replacement therapy increases the risk of VTE about fourfold in women without any other recognized thrombotic abnormalities.[35] OC use also increases the risk of DVT and PTE by 7 to 18 events per 100,000 women annually, for a relative risk 3 to 12 times higher than that of the general population.[36] There is no significant difference between second-generation and third-generation OCs with respect to the risk of VTE.

Blood Cell Surface Antigens Type A blood is associated with lower levels of antithrombin III and higher levels of factor VIII than type O blood. Patients with non-O blood type have a risk of venous thrombosis two to four times higher than those with type O blood. White blood cell HLA surface antigens Cw4, Cw5, and Cw6 are also associated with a higher incidence of venous thromboembolic disease, although the excess risk has not been quantified.

Advancing Age Although PTE is more common in older patients, neither age nor gender is an independent risk factor.

Childhood and Adolescence The diagnosis of VTE is made in about 1:2000 pediatric hospitalizations, and PTE is the cause of death in about 1:2000 pediatric autopsies. In Canada the incidence of recognized VTE is nearly 1:100,000 children per year, with a mortality of about 2% per episode.[37]

Obesity Obesity, defined as weight greater than 20% above ideal weight, has long been accepted as a risk factor for DVT and PTE, but the evidence supporting this association has been questioned. When associated factors such as history, illness, immobility, and age are taken into account, obesity may not be an independent risk factor.

CLINICAL FEATURES

Venous Thrombosis

The clinical diagnosis of DVT is unreliable even in the presence of classic signs and symptoms. The presence of tenderness, erythema, edema, and a palpable cord on examination of the lower extremities does not prove thrombophlebitis, and their absence does not rule it out.

Pain on passive dorsiflexion of the foot often is misreported as a positive Homans' sign. *Homans' sign* actually is spontaneous maintenance of the relaxed foot in abnormal plantar flexion. Both the real Homans' sign and the pseudo–Homans' sign were repudiated by Homans, however, because neither of them has any positive or negative predictive power for any specific disease state.

DVT may be clinically unrecognized because it is nonobstructing and causes no symptoms, or because the symptoms are too vague and nonspecific to trigger a diagnostic workup given the clinical setting. A patient with a fractured tibia, for example, has an obvious reason to have pain, swelling, and discoloration in the leg. A coronary artery bypass graft (CABG) patient with a saphenous vein graft donor site is likewise expected to have leg swelling and pain, along with chest pain from the median sternotomy.

Unfortunately, even when classic findings are present, only 50% of patients actually have DVT, and at least 50% of patients *with* DVT lack any of these findings. DVT often cannot be diagnosed or excluded on the basis of clinical findings, and diagnostic tests are usually required when the diagnosis of DVT is being considered. Any otherwise unexplained diffuse leg pain or swelling warrants consideration of possible DVT.

Phlegmasia Dolens Incomplete venous obstruction usually produces a cerulean or violaceous congested extremity with intact pulses, but extensive obstruction of both superficial and deep venous systems can masquerade as arterial blockage to produce a limb that is white (alba), painful, edematous, cold, and pulseless. If venous outflow cannot be reestablished quickly, amputation is usually necessary.

Mondor's Disease Thrombophlebitis of a subcutaneous vein leading from the breast to the axilla is known as *Mondor's disease.* This entity is painful and can be disfiguring because spontaneous fibrosis of the vessel often leads to retraction of subcutaneous tissues, with puckering and hardening of one quadrant of the breast. Mondor's disease of the penis has also been described.

Venous Insufficiency

Subjective symptoms of venous insufficiency include burning, swelling, throbbing, cramping, and leg fatigue. About half of patients with superficial venous reflux have subjective symptoms. Objective findings may include edema, calor, rubor, local tenderness, skin discoloration, stasis dermatitis, lipodermatosclerosis, atrophie blanche, or chronic nonhealing leg ulceration. In contrast to the pain of arterial insufficiency or venous obstruction, pain caused by venous insufficiency often is improved by walking. Warmth tends to aggravate the symptoms, and cold tends to relieve them. Leg elevation and compression stockings often ameliorate or prevent the pain of venous insufficiency. CVI affects approximately 5% and chronic leg ulcer approximately 1% of the adult population of developed countries.

Variceal Hemorrhage Bleeding from lower extremity varicosities is common and occasionally is fatal. Oversewing a ruptured vessel is a traditional approach that results in short-term control but leads to delayed healing and early recurrences, because it does nothing to ablate the dilated superficial thin-walled vessel that has ruptured. Follow-up with a venous specialist for consideration of sclerotherapy is advised.

Pulmonary Thromboembolism

PTE is relatively common, but its manifestations are nonspecific, and definitive tests can be invasive or difficult to interpret, leading to misdiagnosis. Three classic presentations of PTE are described in the literature: pulmonary infarction or hemorrhage, submassive embolism without infarction, and massive embolism. In this idealized scheme, patients with pulmonary infarction have pleuritic chest pain and may be difficult to distinguish from patients with pleuritis or with an infectious pneumonitis. Patients with *submassive embolism* (angiographically defined as the blockage of flow to an area less than that served by two lobar arteries) have acute and unexplained dyspnea either on exertion or at rest, and their disease may be confused with infection, congestive heart failure, asthma, or hyperventilation. Patients with *massive embolism* (blockage of flow to an area larger than that served by two lobar arteries) classically have acute cor pulmonale, often with syncope, and typically are thought to have MI or hypovolemic or septic shock. To some extent the modern experience still fits these idealized historical categories. Approximately 12% of patients with the pulmonary infarction syndrome may have neither dyspnea nor tachypnea. Some patients with circulatory collapse do not have dyspnea, tachypnea, or pleuritic pain. A normal arterial P_{O_2} (>80 mm Hg) is more prevalent in patients with the pulmonary infarction syndrome (27%) than in patients with the isolated dyspnea syndrome (11%). The belief that pulmonary infarction implies smaller, more distal emboli is supported by the observation that a high-probability $\dot{V}/\dot{Q}$ lung scan is less prevalent among the pulmonary infarction group (32%) than the isolated dyspnea group (65%).[38]

Unfortunately, most patients with acute PTE will exhibit only a few subtle clinical findings. The classic presentations of acute PTE are rarely seen, and the clinical presentation of PTE may precisely mimic that of innumerable other diseases. The classic triad of signs and symptoms (hemoptysis, dyspnea, and chest pain) occurs in fewer than 20% of patients in whom the diagnosis is made. Retrospective identification of signs and symptoms in an inpatient population with proven PTE shows that even for patients in whom the diagnosis has been successfully made, the clinical manifestations of PTE are nonspecific and protean (Tables 83-1 and 83-2). Even when a patient has classic signs and symptoms of "obvious" PTE, the clinical diagnosis is unreliable.

The diagnosis of PTE is even more difficult when a patient has one of the many common atypical presentations. Patients with PTE often have isolated or primary complaints of abdominal pain, back pain, significant fever, productive cough, new-onset reactive airway disease, hiccoughs, new-onset atrial fibrillation, DIC, or any of a host of other symptoms and signs. The chest pain of PTE, as with that of myocardial ischemia, can present in a variety of typical and atypical ways. Common presentations include sudden onset of sharp respirophasic pain, insidious chest wall tenderness, abdominal or shoulder pain, or even a heavy nonpleuritic substernal chest pressure indistinguishable from angina pectoris. In severe disease, gallop sounds and a murmur of tricuspid regurgitation may be appreciated. In subacute disease, a pleural or pericardial rub may sometimes be heard.

Tenderness on palpation of the chest wall, back, or abdomen is a common finding and may even be an isolated presenting symptom in patients with PTE.[39] Palpation may seem to reproduce the pain of PTE, as well as that of pneumonia and of any other intrathoracic syndrome that affects the intercostal nerves. Pleuritic chest pain should

Table 83-1. Symptoms in Patients with Angiographically Proven PTE

Symptoms	Percent
Dyspnea	84
Chest pain, pleuritic	74
Apprehension	59
Cough	53
Hemoptysis	30
Sweating	27
Chest pain, nonpleuritic	14
Syncope	13

Table 83-2. Signs in Patients with Angiographically Proven PTE

Sign	Percent
Tachypnea >16/min	92
Rales	58
Accentuated second sound	53
Tachycardia >100/min	44
Fever >37.8° C	43
Diaphoresis	36
S_3 or S_4 gallop	34
Thrombophlebitis	32
Lower extremity edema	24
Cardiac murmur	23
Cyanosis	19

prompt consideration of PTE, because PTE may account for up to one fifth of presentations of young, active patients with pleuritic chest pain who lack other classic signs, symptoms, or known risk factors for PTE.[40,41] Just as unexplained leg symptoms should raise the possibility of DVT, unexplained chest symptoms should suggest the possibility of PTE.

The two cardinal symptoms that should prompt consideration of PTE are unexplained chest pain and shortness of breath. Shortness of breath is the most common complaint associated with unexpected death within a few weeks after discharge from an ED, and is a common presenting complaint in patients with PTE.

Paradoxical Embolism Paradoxical embolism is the passage of venous emboli into the systemic circulation via a patent foramen ovale or other intracardiac defect. The foramen ovale remains patent in more than 27% of the adult population. Isolated calf vein DVT is responsible for 63% of the cases of peripheral arterial embolization through a patent foramen ovale and is an important cause of stroke.

DIAGNOSTIC STRATEGIES

The diagnosis of venous thromboembolic disease is made when either DVT or PTE has been detected. In some patients the diagnosis of DVT may be more readily made, whereas in others the diagnosis of PTE is more accessible. Once the diagnosis of VTE has been made, therapeutic decisions depend on the extent and location of thrombosis or embolism. Obstructing iliofemoral DVT is an indication for regional fibrinolysis, so the iliofemoral portion of the deep veins should be examined. Similarly, acute right-sided heart strain from PTE is an indication for systemic or catheter-directed fibrinolysis, so the workup must be sufficient to make this treatment decision.

The diagnosis is made (1) if DVT is demonstrated by duplex US, venography, CT, MRI, or some other technique; (2) if V/Q scanning is convincingly positive; or (3) if pulmonary angiography, spiral CT, or another convincing test is positive. The diagnosis is considered disproved if the patient has a negative pulmonary angiogram or a normal perfusion scan with a relatively low clinical likelihood of disease. A definitive test is important, because the patient with a nondiagnostic $\dot{V}/\dot{Q}$ scan may still have PTE, even after a negative duplex US, venogram, and chest radiograph.

Deep Vein Thrombosis

Contrast venography, B-mode US, magnetic resonance venography, and computed tomographic venography can produce an actual picture of the deep vessels and their contents. These images often reveal small mural thrombi and free-floating thrombi that are functionally silent because they do not obstruct the deep veins. Imaging can also permit identification of extensive thrombus that fully occludes venous collaterals or accessory veins but does not produce a major impediment to venous outflow.

Maximum Venous Outflow The maximum venous outflow (MVO) measurement is a noninvasive test that measures obstruction to venous outflow from the lower leg, physiologic information that cannot be obtained from anatomic imaging studies such as duplex US or venography. The test is sensitive to significant intrinsic or extrinsic venous obstruction from any cause, at almost any level. Unfortunately, the test does not detect nonobstructing or minimally obstructing thrombus. The MVO test has been largely supplanted by imaging technologies that have much higher overall negative predictive values.

B-Mode Ultrasound Imaging Color flow duplex US is B-mode ultrasound in which Doppler sampling is used to color-code regions of the display based on flow direction and velocity or volume. Noninvasive duplex US has replaced venography as the initial maging study of choice for patients with suspected lower extremity DVT, but the test is neither as sensitive nor as specific as contrast venography. Applying pressure to the leg with the imaging transducer causes normal deep veins to collapse easily, but veins containing thrombus are resistant to compression. This difference is exploited to aid in the detection of thrombus. A negative scan requires centimeter-by-centimeter compression testing of the deep venous system, an exacting task.

The B-mode Doppler test is best at detecting obstructing thrombus in the femoral vein and is less sensitive below the popliteal trifurcation (at the knee) and above the saphenofemoral junction (at the groin). Only half of patients with proven symptomatic PTE will have a positive lower extremity venous US scan, so a negative scan is not a diagnostic endpoint. A nondiagnostic $\dot{V}/\dot{Q}$ scan plus a single negative result from lower extremity venous US does not exclude the diagnosis of PTE.[42]

Contrast Venography Although it remains the gold standard, contrast venography is not an entirely satisfactory test for the diagnosis of venous thrombosis. When used for diagnosis of DVT, the finding of a fully occlusive "cutoff" lesion or an outlined filling defect is conclusively positive, but a negative interpretation has less predictive power. Veins filled with thrombus that has partially recanalized may appear normally opacified with contrast even when the patent channel is small and slitlike. Eccentric mural thrombus may be invisible in views taken perpendicular to the vessel wall where the thrombus is attached. Free-floating pedunculated thrombi may be missed if the contrast medium surrounding the thrombus is too highly concentrated.

Venography has fallen gradually into disfavor because it is time-consuming and requires a high degree of technical expertise to obtain acceptable images. Also, up to 10% of patients develop proven DVT after a negative venogram, either because the venogram initially missed seeing the DVT or because IV contrast can trigger DVT by causing endothelial injury.[43] The morbidity and mortality of this invasive technique cannot be ignored; extravasation into the dorsum of the foot may cause sloughing of tissue, and anaphylactoid reactions to contrast material occur in 3% of patients, sometimes resulting in death.

Radionuclide Tests The radiolabeled substances used in scintigraphic lung scanning may be injected into a foot vein in the manner usually used for contrast venography. The leg, thigh, and pelvis may then be scanned as the radionuclide ascends through the venous circulation to the lungs. The resulting images are of low contrast and are difficult to read, but if positive, they can be helpful. A negative nuclear venogram cannot rule out DVT and should not be taken as evidence against the diagnosis.

Radiolabeled fibrinogen scanning is primarily of historical interest because it can require several days to yield results. Also, fibrinogen is a human blood product with an unavoidable risk of infection. A newer thrombus-tagging radiopharmaceutical recently was released for clinical use. Technetium 99m apcitide binds to glycoprotein IIb/IIIa receptors on the surface of activated platelets, making the agent specific for acute thrombi. Radiolabeled monoclonal antibodies to mature and immature thrombus have also shown promise as a more rapid and reliable alternative test for venous thrombosis and PTE.

Laboratory Tests

Many different biochemical changes have been recognized in patients with DVT and PTE. The same changes occur in many other diseases that produce pulmonary air space alterations, however, and they are neither sensitive nor specific for PTE. As yet, no known blood or serum test proves or excludes the diagnosis of PTE.

Clotting Function Tests of clotting function are normal in most patients with PTE. Anticoagulation remains a mainstay of therapy for PTE, although progression of thrombus and recurrent embolism can occur in patients who are fully anticoagulated. In fact, new PTE in the hospital occurs despite therapeutic anticoagulation with heparin in 3% of patients who have nonfloating deep vein thrombus without PTE at presentation, in 13% of those who present with a floating thrombus but no PTE, in 11% of those who already have PTE at presentation but have no floating thrombus, and in 39% of those presenting with PTE who have a floating thrombus visible at venography.[44]

Hemoglobin and Hematocrit PTE does not alter a patient's hemoglobin or hematocrit, but a finding of polycythemia should raise the clinical suspicion simply because it is a known risk factor for thrombosis.

White Blood Cell Count An elevated white blood cell count is neither sensitive nor specific because it may be either normal or elevated (as high as 20,000) in patients with DVT and PTE.[45] Both CVI and DVT can mimic leg cellulitis, and true cellulitis is a common complication of both diseases.

Erythrocyte Sedimentation Rate The erythrocyte sedimentation rate (ESR) usually is normal in patients with PTE, but it may be elevated to any level by an underlying comorbid disease process.

Platelet Count Progressive thrombocytopenia has been associated with new onset of thromboembolism in hospitalized patients, but the platelet count usually is normal in patients with PTE. The onset of thrombocytopenia in a patient who is receiving heparin should raise the suspicion of heparin-induced thrombocytopenia, a syndrome of fulminant thrombosis that is refractory to treatment. Paradoxically, thrombocytosis is more likely to be associated with hemorrhagic complications than with thrombotic effects.

D-Dimer Radioimmunoassay Monoclonal antibody radioimmunoassay has been used to identify and quantify D-dimer, a unique degradation product produced by plasmin-mediated proteolysis of cross-linked fibrin. The gold standard D-dimer test is performed using a quantitative enzyme-linked immunosorbent assay (ELISA) and is considered positive if the assay is greater than 500 ng/ml.

Although offering great promise, the D-dimer test has not been studied sufficiently to define its precise clinical use. The test is nonspecific and thus must not be considered diagnostic of PTE when positive. A negative test must be interpreted in the context of the pretest probability of PTE. Moderate or high pretest suspicion should not be deterred by a negative test, because D-dimer testing will miss about 7% of the cases of VTE. Depending on the patient population and the specific brand of ELISA used, the negative predictive value can be as low as 78%, the sensitivity as low as 80%, and the positive predictive value as low as 30%.[46-50]

An increasing number of qualitative tests for D-dimer are being commercially marketed as substitutes for the gold standard quantitative ELISA. These tests are much less expensive and easier to perform but also much less sensitive and reliable than ELISA.[51] Many patients with proven pulmonary embolism have normal D-dimer test results using these simple commercial assays.[52] Whether quantitative or qualitative, D-dimer testing remains promising but imprecisely defined in VTE.

Hypercoagulable States

Screening tests for protein C, protein S, lupus anticoagulant, antithrombin III deficiency, and factor V Leiden (resistance to activated protein C) are helpful in ruling out these important risk factors. The tests are especially helpful to guide long-term therapy after a confirmed diagnosis of DVT or PTE.

Arterial Blood Oxygen

Arterial blood gases have a zero predictive value in a typical population of patients in whom PTE is suspected. This is because the population being tested includes some patients who have PTE as well as a larger group who do not have PTE but do have some pulmonary pathology that affects pulmonary gas exchange more than PTE does. When arterial oxygen tension (Pao_2) is measured, and any reasonable level of Pao_2 is chosen as a dividing line, the incidence of PTE will be higher in the group with a Pao_2 above the dividing line than in the group below the divider. This seemingly counterintuitive result may be demonstrated mathematically for any test finding with a Gaussian distribution. Clinical evidence that it is true for the Pao_2 in patients with suspected PTE has been available since the early work of Menzoian and Williams[53] (Table 83-3).

Improved diagnostic tests have shown that PTE often does not produce obvious abnormalities of pulmonary gas ex-

Table 83-3. Arterial Oxygen Tension and Incidence of PTE

Po_2 selected	Incidence of PE in patients below the selected Po_2	Incidence of PE in patients above the selected Po_2
80 mm Hg	45/101 (44.6%)	9/19 (47.4%)
70 mm Hg	39/87 (44.8%)	15/33 (45.5%)
65 mm Hg	29/69 (42%)	25/51 (49%)

change; many patients are initially asymptomatic, and most have a normal Pao_2. Even in a population of classically symptomatic patients with large or massive PTE, about 1 in 5 has a normal Po_2, and 1 in 20 has a Pao_2 level above 100 mm Hg on room air.[53-55] Pao_2 levels have no predictive value in the evaluation of patients with suspected PTE.

Alveolar-Arterial Oxygen Gradient

Although routinely used in the past, the alveolar-arterial (A-a) gradient has no discriminatory ability in the diagnosis of PTE. The Pao_2 is very sensitive to the minute ventilatory volume; thus if the patient takes one or two extra breaths per minute, the Pao_2 may be normal even when pulmonary gas exchange is significantly impaired. Compared with Pao_2, the A-a oxygen gradient is a more sensitive measure of impaired gas exchange because if the minute volume rises without an increase in cellular respiration, the Pco_2 will drop proportionately. The A-a gradient is the difference between the measured arterial oxygen and the alveolar oxygen, which is predicted by the formula $Fio_2(P_{atm} - P_{H_2O}) - (1.25 \times Pco_2)$, with Fio_2 the fraction of inspired oxygen. For an intubated patient on 100% oxygen at sea level, this is approximately $(Fio_2 \times 715) - (1.25 \times Pco_2)$. On room air at sea level, this expression simplifies to $150 - (1.25 \times Pco_2)$.

The A-a gradient will never be zero because pulmonary gas exchange is not perfect, but in the absence of impaired pulmonary gas exchange, the A-a gradient should be less than 10 mm Hg in young persons and less than 20 mm Hg in older persons. A useful rule of thumb is that the A-a gradient should be no greater than 10 plus one tenth of the patient's age. The A-a gradient is a better measure of gas exchange than the Po_2 alone, but it remains nonspecific and insensitive for detection of PTE. Small pulmonary emboli do not impair pulmonary gas exchange, and nearly every type of pulmonary pathology can affect the A-a gradient. A large PTE often causes an increased A-a gradient, but a normal arterial blood gas (normal Po_2, Pco_2, pH, and A-a gradient for age) will be seen in up to 23% of patients with symptomatic PTE.[54,55] The A-a gradient is normal in many more patients with small emboli in whom the diagnosis is never made.

Even when the A-a gradient is abnormal, this is not a positive predictor of PTE. Most patients with an abnormal A-a gradient have some pulmonary pathology other than PTE as the cause for their impaired gas exchange.

Pulse Oximetry

Pulse oximetry is of no discriminatory value in the diagnostic evaluation of a patient with suspected PTE. Most patients with PTE will have a normal oxygen saturation, and most patients with an abnormal oxygen saturation will have a cause other than PTE. Pulse oximetry is used in patients with suspected PTE to (1) identify those who require immediate supplemental oxygen and (2) monitor patients whose oxygen saturation might drop.

Chest Radiography

Chest radiographic findings are both nonspecific and insensitive for PTE. Most thromboemboli go undiagnosed, and most chest radiographs in patients with PTE are normal. The most common chest radiographic interpretations in patients with a proven diagnosis of PTE are cardiac enlargement (27%), normal (24%), pleural effusion (23%), elevated hemidiaphragm (20%), pulmonary artery enlargement (19%), atelectasis (18%), and parenchymal pulmonary infiltrates (17%).[56]

Two rare chest radiographic findings have been classically associated with PTE but may occasionally be seen in other clinical entities as well. The first is *Hampton's hump,* a triangular or rounded pleural-based infiltrate with the apex toward the hilum, usually located adjacent to the diaphragm (Figure 83-1). The second is *Westermark's sign,* a dilation of the pulmonary vessels proximal to the embolism along with collapse of distal vessels, sometimes with a sharp cutoff. If present, Westermark's sign is the earliest detectable chest radiograph abnormality (Figure 83-2).

The development of a focal infiltrate within 3 days after the onset of symptoms in a patient with clinically suspected PTE is consistent with a confirmed diagnosis of PTE.

Echocardiography

An echocardiogram should be considered in every patient with pulmonary embolism, because the presence of right-sided heart strain from PTE is a strong predictor of subsequent death. Early fibrinolysis can reduce the mortality by 50% in these patients, thus positive echocardiographic findings should prompt consideration of immediate fibrinolysis.[57]

Acute pulmonary hypertension causes both the right ventricle and the pulmonary arteries to dilate, and the ratio of right-to-left ventricular end-diastolic diameters correlates well with angiographic indices of the severity of the obstruction. These indirect signs are of value in assessing the severity of proven PTE but should not be relied on for the primary diagnosis of PTE, because they also are seen in patients with right ventricular infarction and with other causes of pulmonary hypertension. The diagnosis of PTE cannot reliably be made on the basis of the transthoracic echocardiogram alone, unless thrombus in transit actually is visible in the right side of the heart.[58]

Transesophageal echocardiography (TEE) can reveal thrombus in the central pulmonary arteries, and the specificity of the test is high. Unfortunately, the sensitivity and negative predictive value of TEE are too low to permit its use as a screening tool.

Ventilation/Perfusion Scanning

Nuclear scintigraphic $\dot{V}/\dot{Q}$ scanning of the lung is a relatively noninvasive test that is most often nondiagnostic, but it remains the initial study of choice for most patients with suspected PTE because in many cases it is capable of ruling the diagnosis in or out with acceptable confidence

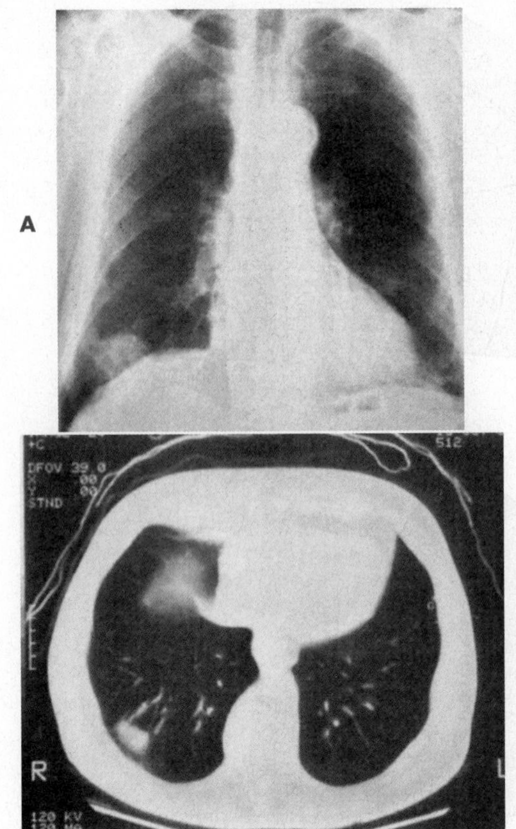

Figure 83-1. **Pulmonary infarction caused by thromboembolism: Hampton's hump as seen on chest radiograph (A) and CT scan (B).**

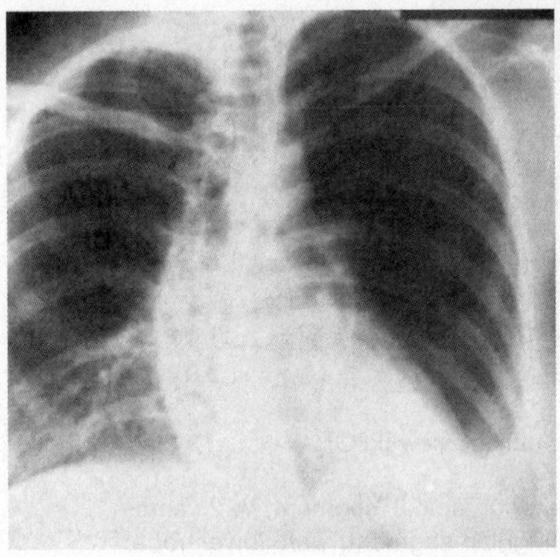

Figure 83-2. **Chest radiograph showing relative paucity of pulmonary vessels on the left (Westerman's sign). A left pleural effusion is also present.**

levels. The $\dot{V}/\dot{Q}$ scan should be obtained as soon as possible once the diagnosis of PTE is considered; the likelihood of a nondiagnostic perfusion pattern increases with time because decreased perfusion leads to loss of surfactant and to secondary air space abnormalities.[59]

Indications A $\dot{V}/\dot{Q}$ scan is indicated for any patient in whom the diagnosis of PTE is suspected and no alternative diagnosis can be established. It is also indicated for patients with DVT without symptoms of PTE. A repeat V/Q scan is indicated before anticoagulation is discontinued in a patient with DVT or PTE caused by irreversible risk factors, because recurrence of symptoms after cessation of anticoagulation is common. If a reference $\dot{V}/\dot{Q}$ scan is available for comparison, the patient may be spared a future angiogram.

Pregnancy Both perfusion and ventilation scans are acceptable diagnostic modalities in the pregnant patient. The fetal radiation exposure from a $\dot{V}/\dot{Q}$ scan is 50 mrem, one tenth of the maximum permissible fetal gestational exposure dose of 500 mrem recommended for radiation workers. No effects have ever been documented at such a small dose. Much of the fetal exposure comes from accumulation of radioisotope in the maternal urinary bladder, and a brisk diuresis may reduce fetal exposure by approximately 50%.

Technique Perfusion scans are performed by IV infusion of radioisotope-labeled microaggregates of albumin that are trapped as they pass through the pulmonary microcirculation and are detected by a gamma camera positioned over the patient's chest. A normal patient in the supine position will have blood flow that is evenly distributed from side to side and from top to bottom; thus if the pulmonary circulation is unimpaired, the scan will demonstrate a uniform distribution of the radioisotope. Reduced blood flow to an area of the lung will result in a relative paucity of emissions emanating from that area. Perfusion defects as small as 3 cm in diameter may be detected by a skilled examiner if a complete eight-view scan is performed. It is important that anterior, posterior, right and left lateral, and all four orthogonal oblique views be obtained. The right and left anterior oblique (RAO and LAO) views provide the best assessment of the anterior contralateral midlung. The lingula is best seen on the RAO, and the right middle lobe is best seen on the LAO view. Right and left posterior oblique (RPO and LPO) views demonstrate defects in the lateral basal segments of the lower lobes that may otherwise be missed on routine lateral views because of overlapping emissions (Figure 83-3).

Perfusion The perfusion scan is neither sensitive nor specific for PTE. An area of infarction the size of a walnut, for example, will not be detected. Small thrombi often cause small, distal, pleural-based infarcts that can produce severe pleuritic chest pain without being detectable scintigraphically. Even large or massive emboli may not be detected if they are incompletely obstructing and do not asymmetrically decrease regional perfusion enough to be detected on a perfusion scan. Many pathologic processes other than PTE can cause perfusion defects on a lung scan, including local parenchymal collapse, consolidation, vasoconstriction, chronic obstructive pulmonary disease, and congestive heart failure.

Ventilation A ventilation scan increases the specificity (but not the sensitivity) of abnormal perfusion scans when segmental or larger perfusion defects are present.[60] Just as a perfusion scan measures the distribution of blood flow through the pulmonary arterial tree, a ventilation scan measures the distribution of radioactive gas or aerosol as it washes through the bronchoalveolar tree. Abnormalities of ventilation may show up as regions of poor or delayed inflow or as areas of retention and delayed washout.

Mismatch Initially, PTE causes an area of blocked perfusion and normal ventilation, shown as a $\dot{V}/\dot{Q}$ scan

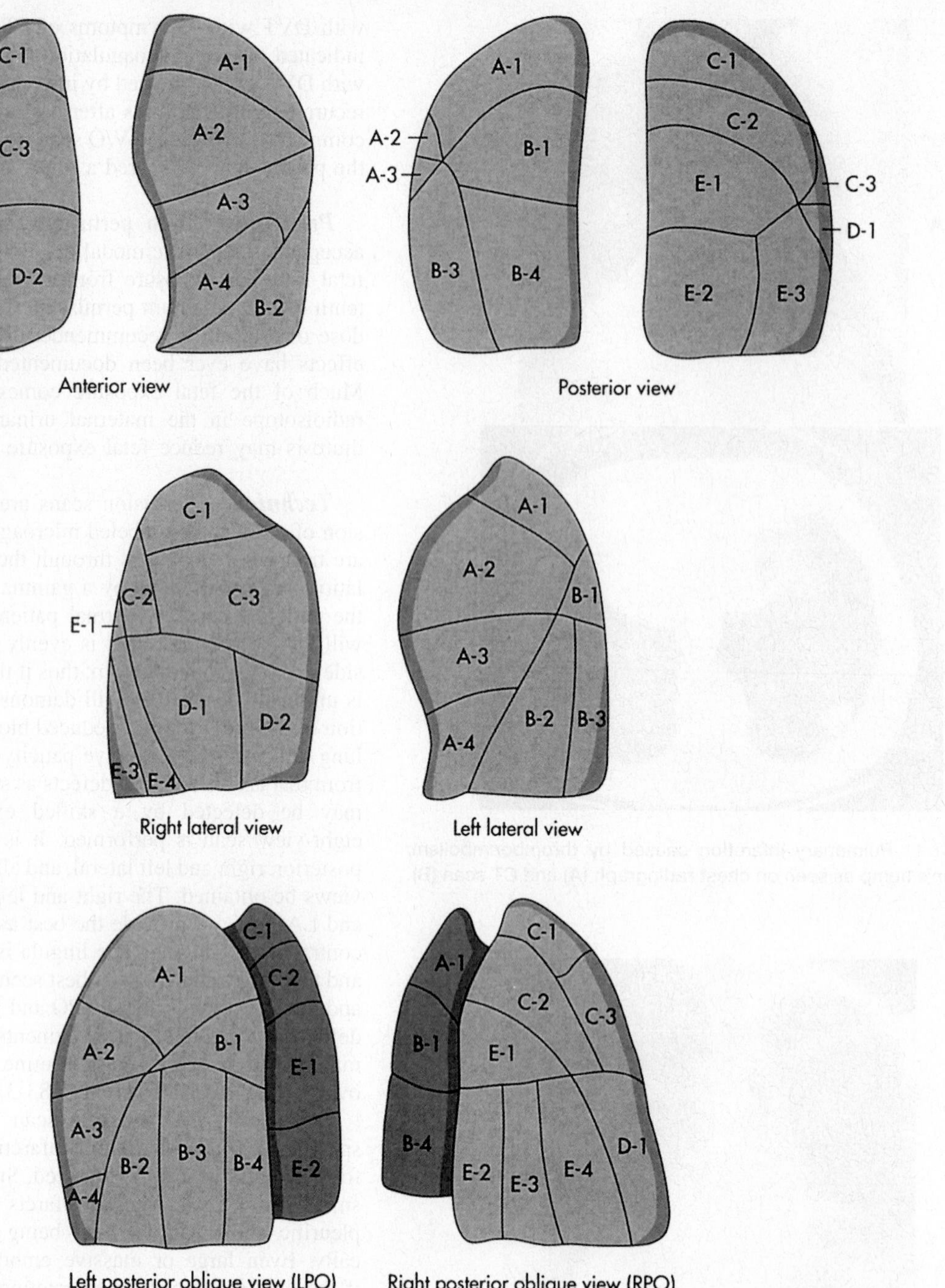

Figure 83-3. **Pulmonary anatomy.** ***Left upper lobe:*** **A-1, posterior apical segment; A-2, anterior segment; A-3, superior lingular segment; A-4, inferior lingular segment.** ***Left lower lobe:*** **B-1, superior segment; B-2, anteromedial segment; B-3, lateral basal segment; B-4, posterior basal segment.** ***Right upper lobe:*** **C-1, apical segment; C-2, posterior segment; C-3, anterior segment.** ***Right middle lobe:*** **D-1, lateral segment; D-2, medial segment.** ***Right lower lobe:*** **E-1, superior segment; E-2, posterior basal segment; E-3, lateral basal segment; E-4, anterior basal segment.**

mismatch. This mismatch often is absent when PTE causes secondary ventilation abnormalities because of splinting, atelectasis, infiltrates, effusions, bronchospasm, and other confounding factors. In practice, a large ventilation defect with a small perfusion defect is more suggestive of primary air space disease than of PTE. A ventilation defect smaller than the perfusion defect is more consistent with PTE than with pulmonary air space disease.

Interpretation Lung scanning is a surprisingly imprecise test for the diagnosis of PTE. Only 41% of patients with PTE found through pulmonary angiography will have a high-probability lung scan. The combination of clinical assessment and $\dot{V}/\dot{Q}$ scan is sufficient to diagnose or to exclude PTE in only a few patients.[60]

$\dot{V}/\dot{Q}$ scan patterns are properly categorized as normal, high probability, or nondiagnostic. Most patients with PTE have nondiagnostic scans. Under currently accepted models of radiographic and clinical assessment, if a perfusion scan is abnormal, it is either high probability or nondiagnostic. Referring to a nondiagnostic scan as "low probability" is inappropriate and misleading, and may encourage the clinician to falsely exclude the diagnosis of PTE.[61] If a radiologist's reading of a scan includes the obsolete low-probability terminology, clarification should be sought. Many such scans show no perfusion defects and should be considered normal, whereas others are nondiagnostic and must be followed up with further investigation.

A *normal* perfusion pattern means that the patient has less than a 5% chance of PTE being identified if angiography is performed. An *abnormal but nondiagnostic* pattern means that the patient has a 15% to 85% likelihood of having PTE. A *high-probability* pattern means that the patient has an 85% or greater likelihood of PTE being found at angiography.

$\dot{V}/\dot{Q}$ scan results should always be interpreted in the context of the clinical presentation, because an individual patient with PTE may have a scan pattern in any one of the $\dot{V}/\dot{Q}$ categories. The categories are simply rank-order groupings based on the empiric probability that patients with a given pattern of perfusion and ventilation defects will go on to have a positive pulmonary angiogram.

Caveats on Classification The modern lung scan classification scheme is not used in its entirety at every institution. At some institutions, $\dot{V}/\dot{Q}$ scans are never reported as normal, no matter what the actual pattern of perfusion. This is unfortunate because normal perfusion is the scan pattern with the highest predictive value.

Some institutions continue to report nondiagnostic $\dot{V}/\dot{Q}$ patterns using obsolete and clinically confusing terminology, such as moderately high, indeterminate, intermediate, low, ultra-low, or near-normal probability. Diagnostic $\dot{V}/\dot{Q}$ patterns classified as high probability or normal may be relied on to guide the clinical management of patients when the prior clinical assessment is concordant with the scan result. Regardless of the language used, however, a nondiagnostic $\dot{V}/\dot{Q}$ pattern is not an acceptable endpoint in the workup for PTE.

Many scans initially are read by residents or by radiologists with limited experience in the interpretation of nuclear scintigraphic scans. The final reading often is different from the preliminary report. An incorrect or incomplete understanding of the published criteria often leads to an incorrect categorization even when the underlying interpretation of the scan is correct. Finally, even when appropriate criteria are correctly applied, the categorization of $\dot{V}/\dot{Q}$ scans according to published criteria represents an oversimplification.

A $\dot{V}/\dot{Q}$ reading should always include accompanying detail explaining what views were imaged and exactly what pattern of defects was seen. In a patient with profound hypoxemia and hypotension, for example, a small, focal, peripheral area of decreased perfusion would be inconsistent with the massive embolism necessary to cause such severe symptoms. In this case the clinician would look for some other cause of shock. In a patient with localized pleuritic chest pain and a high clinical probability of PTE, on the other hand, even a normal $\dot{V}/\dot{Q}$ scan is consistent with a small, pleural-based PTE.

High Probability High-probability $\dot{V}/\dot{Q}$ scans have a sensitivity of 41% and a positive predictive value of 87%. This means that 87% of patients with this pattern will have a positive angiogram, but the test only detects 41% of all the patients with a positive angiogram. When the clinical pretest probability of PTE is moderate to high, a high-probability $\dot{V}/\dot{Q}$ result is an acceptable endpoint to the workup.

Nondiagnostic Nondiagnostic $\dot{V}/\dot{Q}$ patterns have a positive predictive value of 21% for PTE, thus if the scan is assumed positive for PTE, it will be incorrect 79% of the time. Likewise, a nondiagnostic scan is only 43% sensitive and thus cannot be used to exclude the diagnosis. A nondiagnostic $\dot{V}/\dot{Q}$ pattern does not change the prior clinical likelihood that a given patient has had PTE. Regardless of whether the patient has a high or a low prior clinical likelihood of PTE, a nondiagnostic $\dot{V}/\dot{Q}$ result is never an acceptable endpoint in the workup.

Normal Normal $\dot{V}/\dot{Q}$ patterns (no perfusion defects) exclude embolism with a specificity of 96%. If a normal $\dot{V}/\dot{Q}$ pattern is presumed negative, it will be correct 96% of the time but will miss 2% of PTE cases. At least 4% of patients with this normal pattern will be found to have PTE if angiography is performed. In fact, PTE was proved in 9% of the PIOPED study patients who underwent angiography after a normal $\dot{V}/\dot{Q}$ scan.[60] A normal $\dot{V}/\dot{Q}$ pattern is not a guarantee that the patient does not have PTE, but it is an acceptable endpoint for the workup of PTE when the clinical likelihood is also low.

Serial Scans For the small fraction of patients in whom an adequate pulmonary angiogram, spiral CT, or other definitive test cannot be performed, the specificity of $\dot{V}/\dot{Q}$ scanning may be enhanced over a period of days by the use of serial scans. Scintigraphic perfusion abnormalities that change over time (with or without treatment) are characteristic of PTE and are not seen in any other common cause of segmental or subsegmental scintigraphic defects. An otherwise nondiagnostic $\dot{V}/\dot{Q}$ scan is considered positive for PTE if the size or shape of the perfusion defect is improved or worsened on a repeat scan.

In the absence of pharmacologic fibrinolytic therapy, resolution of $\dot{V}/\dot{Q}$ defects occurs over several weeks by means of natural fibrinolytic processes that recanalize occluded pulmonary arteries to produce a circumferential fibrotic plaque with an open central channel. Unfortunately, the timing of this process cannot be predicted because the natural fibrinolytic process is highly idiosyncratic. In many patients, all $\dot{V}/\dot{Q}$ defects have resolved within a few weeks after the initial occlusion, even though the bulk of the clot material remains lining the vascular tree of the lung.[23] In 60% of cases, however, some or all of the $\dot{V}/\dot{Q}$ defects may be permanent.[62]

Clinical Application The $\dot{V}/\dot{Q}$ scan is a relatively insensitive and nonspecific test, and excessive reliance on the scan pattern leads to potential errors in clinical management at two extremes: (1) failing to obtain a confirmatory angiogram for patients with a high-probability scan but only a low clinical probability, and (2) inappropriately withholding further workup and treatment from patients with a nondiagnostic scan or a normal scan with moderate or high clinical probability.

The terminology used to report scan results can adversely influence patient outcome.[61] When nondiagnostic scans are correctly reported as nondiagnostic in patients with normal cardiopulmonary reserves, the mortality from PTE is 0.14%.

When the same scan patterns are incorrectly reported as "low probability" in patients with poor cardiopulmonary reserves, the mortality from PTE is 50 times higher, at 7.8%. The "low-probability" reading leads many clinicians to discount the likelihood of PTE, when at least 15% of these patients will have a positive angiogram.

In the absence of proven DVT, patients with an abnormal but nondiagnostic perfusion scan require a pulmonary angiogram or other definitive test to prove or disprove the diagnosis of PTE.[61]

Pulmonary Angiography

Pulmonary angiography is both the most invasive and the most reliable test for PTE. A positive result is apparent as a dye "cutoff" (blockage of flow) or an intraluminal filling defect. A complete negative study requires the visualization of the entire pulmonary tree bilaterally through selective cannulation of each branch of the pulmonary artery and injection of contrast material with multiple views of each area. With 26 branchings of the pulmonary vessels, even a well-performed angiogram will not detect emboli in vessels smaller than third-order or lobular arteries. Embolic obstruction of these smaller arteries is common at postmortem examination. Small emboli cannot be seen angiographically, which explains the patients with pleuritic chest pain who die from a massive PTE shortly after a negative pulmonary angiogram. This also explains the sudden onset of pleuritic chest pain and delayed development of a small sterile effusion, with negative $\dot{V}/\dot{Q}$ scan and pulmonary angiogram. Continued surveillance will reveal recurrent thromboembolic disease in many such patients.

Predictive Value

Although pulmonary angiography is generally accepted as the gold standard in the diagnosis of PTE, the test is not infallible. Angiography may falsely diagnose PTE in the presence of an intraluminal tumor or an extrinsic mass, and it may be falsely negative when thrombus is small and distal.

When reviewers independently examine the same angiogram, all usually agree that a positive angiogram is positive when the defect is lobar, but they agree only 66% of the time when the embolus is subsegmental.[63] Reviewers agree that a negative angiogram is negative only 81% of the time, which drops to 54% when the angiogram is of poor quality. Individual reviewers are uncertain of the diagnosis in 8% of patients. Technical or patient care factors prevent the completion of 1% of pulmonary angiograms, and 3% are inadequate. In the PIOPED study, negative angiograms were judged to be false negatives in 4 of 675 cases (0.6%); in these four cases, autopsy showed a missed thromboembolism within 6 days of the angiogram.[63]

Pulmonary angiography will remain the "court of last resort" in the diagnosis of PTE for the immediate future because no better test is yet available. When performed carefully, a positive pulmonary angiogram provides virtually 100% certainty that an obstruction to pulmonary arterial blood flow does exist, and a negative pulmonary angiogram provides greater than 90% certainty in the exclusion of PTE.

Timing A stable patient with a nondiagnostic $\dot{V}/\dot{Q}$ scan and adequate cardiac reserves who has been fully anticoagulated can wait a number of hours for angiography. Angiography should not be delayed in patients who are unstable, have evidence of right-sided heart failure, have underlying cardiac disease, or cannot be fully anticoagulated. Angiography is less likely to be diagnostic after a patient receives fibrinolytic therapy because such patients may have complete resolution of angiographic findings (as well as resolution of scintigraphic perfusion defects) within 90 minutes of the initial infusion.

Mortality and Morbidity Angiographic complications historically have included anaphylactoid reactions to contrast material, dysrhythmias, cardiac arrest, and endocardial injury or frank perforation by the catheter. With modern techniques, however, pulmonary angiography is a very safe procedure. The frequency of complications (about 9%) is *not* related to the pulmonary arterial pressure, the amount of contrast material used, or the presence or absence of PTE.[63] The incidence of myocardial perforations and dysrhythmias is very low. Angiographic mortality (maximum estimated rate of 0.5%) is almost exclusively seen in patients who are already moribund at the start of the procedure.[60,63] Pregnant patients are at no special risk when undergoing pulmonary angiography. The mortality risk of undiagnosed PTE is high, and the risks of pulmonary angiography are low enough to justify its continued routine use in the evaluation of patients with suspected PTE.

Computed Tomography

A *spiral (helical) CT scan* offers several advantages over traditional CT scans. The spiral technique permits very rapid scanning over a large area, so the entire lung can be imaged while the patient holds a breath. The entire scan can be performed during the first circulation pass of an injected bolus of venous contrast, and vessels can be tracked from cut to cut at high spatial resolutions. Vessels can be enhanced during image reconstruction using *CT angiography* (CTA). This technique has shown great promise in the detection of PTE by a relatively noninvasive method. Unlike lung scans and pulmonary angiography, the CT scan also often provides evidence for an alternative diagnosis when the patient does not have PTE.

Some groups have already abandoned pulmonary angiography and perfusion lung scanning in favor of spiral CT, citing studies that suggest spiral CT has comparable sensitivity and specificity. Unfortunately, others have shown spiral CT to be less reliable in diagnosing or excluding PTE. Meta-analysis suggests an overall sensitivity of only 68%, with some convincing evidence that even in experienced hands, spiral CT may have only a 53% sensitivity and 82% negative predictive value for PTE compared with standard pulmonary angiography.[64,65] The acquisition of images with new, multidetector CT scanners may lead to significant improvements in diagnostic accuracy. It seems likely that $\dot{V}/\dot{Q}$ scans and invasive pulmonary angiography may be completely replaced by CTA within the next few years.

Magnetic Resonance Imaging

Pulmonary vessels containing blood flowing at normal velocities normally have little or no intraluminal signal on MRI. Increased intraluminal signal intensity may occur as a result of occlusive PTE, nonocclusive thrombus, tumor, atheromatous plaque, or other alterations in flow dynamics. Electrocardiographically gated spin-echo MR images can detect thrombus in the central pulmonary vessels but cannot

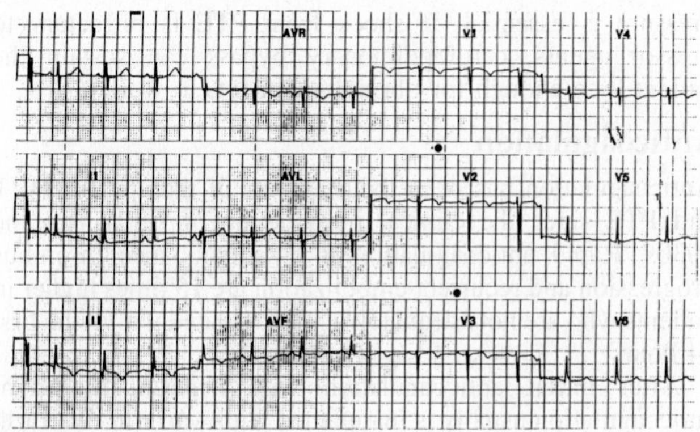

Figure 83-4. **ECG showing S_1-Q_3-T_3 pattern suggestive of pulmonary thromboembolism.**

yet reliably distinguish thrombus from other low-flow states, particularly in small-caliber vessels. With many new approaches under development, the role of *MR angiography* (MRA) for the diagnosis of PTE is likely to increase in the future.

Computed Tomographic and Magnetic Resonance Venography

CT venography (CTV) is a promising modality with as yet unproven clinical value. Veins of the pelvis and extremities can be imaged with the same bolus of contrast used to perform CTA, but the sensitivity and specificity of the approach remain to be determined. *MR venography* (MRV) is somewhat more advanced, is becoming widely available as a clinically useful test for venous pathology, and offers great promise for the near future because it can detect venous obstruction in areas of the body where no other diagnostic test is useful. Spin-echo and gradient-recalled acquisition in steady state (GRASS) MR images can reliably detect thrombus in deep veins of the calf, thigh, and pelvis. Unfortunately, MRV still depends on operator experience, and false-negative results still present a problem.

A significant advantage of CTV and MRV is that they often reveal other causes for leg pain and edema in patients who do not have DVT. Because US and contrast venography are insensitive for the diagnosis of pelvic vein and distal calf vein thrombosis, many have adopted MRI as the new gold standard for these clinical conditions. It is likely that CTV and MRV will replace direct contrast venography as the gold standard for the diagnosis of all venous thromboses.

Electrocardiography

The most common electrocardiographic (ECG) abnormalities in patients with PTE are tachycardia and nonspecific ST-segment–T-wave abnormalities. Aside from these nonspecific patterns, any ECG abnormality is as likely as another. The classic abnormalities are related to right-sided heart strain: tall peaked P wave in lead II (P pulmonale), right axis deviation, right bundle branch block, atrial fibrillation, and S_1-Q_3-T_3 pattern (Figure 83-4). Such ECG abnormalities may suggest PTE, but their absence has no predictive value. Only 20% of patients with proven PTE will have any of the classic findings, and 25% will have ECG results that are unchanged from their baseline state.[66]

Pulmonary Function Tests

Pulmonary function tests are insensitive for PTE because they measure parameters that are altered only when a large fraction of the pulmonary circulation is obstructed. The tests also most often are nonspecific because underlying pulmonary disease and prior PTE cause many false-positive results. The end-tidal–arterial CO_2 gradient, late dead space fraction, and dead space/tidal volume ratio are under investigation as diagnostic tests for PTE.

DIFFERENTIAL CONSIDERATIONS

Pneumonia

Pneumonia and PTE are often confused and may sometimes be indistinguishable except by angiography or autopsy. The two share common signs and symptoms of dyspnea, tachypnea, cough, hemoptysis, hypoxia, tachycardia, pleuritic pain, fever, cyanosis, and hypotension. Shaking chills, purulent sputum, anad positive blood cultures support the diagnosis of infectious pneumonia, whereas no response to antibiotics, bloody sputum that is nonpurulent, and culture-negative effusion support the diagnosis of PTE. Unfortunately, many patients cannot be correctly diagnosed by clinical means. The $\dot{V}/\dot{Q}$ scan may be normal even with a large infectious infiltrate, but it is often nondiagnostic when there is an infiltrate because any process that can cause parenchymal abnormalities on the chest radiograph may also interfere with perfusion and ventilation. The correct diagnosis of PTE is virtually always missed in patients with pneumonia who also develop PTE.

Asthma

Patients with asthma typically present to the ED with dyspnea, shortness of breath, tachycardia, tachypnea, and other findings that would suggest PTE in a nonasthmatic patient. Small, recurrent pulmonary emboli can present as bronchospasm of insidious onset even in young patients. At autopsy, half of patients whose death was clinically attributed to severe asthma may be found to have died from other causes of respiratory collapse, including 10% with unsuspected PTE.[67]

The bronchospasm of PTE responds to most medications used to treat asthma, so the true diagnosis may be elusive. Occult PTE, like congestive heart failure, should always be considered before a diagnosis of primary reactive airway disease is made in an older patient with no history of childhood asthma. Severe asthmatic decompensation that is unusually refractory to treatment should also suggest PTE. Unfortunately, local shunting caused by air space disease renders the $\dot{V}/\dot{Q}$ scan unreliable in asthma, so angiography or spiral CT may be necessary to prove or disprove the diagnosis.

Pleurisy and Pleuritis

Pleurisy implies a primary pleural inflammatory process, often characterized by pleural effusion and pleuritic chest pain. The clinical diagnosis of pleurisy is rarely correct; most patients with chest pain and an effusion have pleural inflammation that is secondary to another primary process. Many patients given this diagnosis actually have pneumonia with infiltrates that are not yet visible on the chest radiograph. Others may have a small pulmonary infarct from distal thromboemboli, a traumatic contusion, a subdiaphragmatic process causing pleural irritation, or neuritis from herpes zoster. Some may have a primary pleural process, such as tuberculous, viral, or autoimmune pleurisy, but no reliable means can prove this during a brief ED visit. Accordingly, unexplained pleuritic chest pain should prompt a careful search for a specific cause, including PTE, before pleurisy, a diagnosis of exclusion, is made.

Angina

Angina pectoris will be the initial diagnosis in a sizable minority of patients with symptomatic acute PTE. In some patients this represents true ischemic cardiac pain induced by the PTE, whereas in others the diagnosis of cardiac angina is simply incorrect.

Myocardial Infarction

In some patients the symptoms of PTE can mimic those of acute MI, and in the absence of prophylactic measures, hospitalized patients with MI are at high risk for secondary VTE. The possibility of confusion between acute MI and PTE is especially high in those with impending arrest. Absence of bradycardia in patients with PTE is the only significant premorbid clinical difference between those who die from acute MI and those with acute MI who die from unrecognized PTE. Pulseless electrical activity is common in patients with PTE, but the arresting rhythm is asystole in most coronary care unit deaths from unsuspected PTE.[8]

Carcinoma

Infarction from PTE can produce an isolated nodule, suggesting a diagnosis of bronchogenic carcinoma. The two conditions may produce an identical defect on the $\dot{V}/\dot{Q}$ scan, and the pulmonary angiogram may be unable to distinguish between clot and a tumor mass obstructing pulmonary blood flow. Chest CT is often helpful, but an open lung biopsy may be required to rule out carcinoma.

MANAGEMENT

General and Supportive Care

In patients with acute VTE the treatment goals are to (1) prevent death from a current embolic event, (2) reduce the likelihood of recurrent embolic events, and (3) minimize the long-term morbidity of the event.

Supportive and symptomatic therapy for the patient should not be forgotten in the rush to diagnose and treat life-threatening VTE. Pain relief often is needed, and oxygen may be helpful as a pulmonary vasodilator even when the patient is not hypoxemic. Shock must be managed with inotropic or pressor agents and with fluid resuscitation (if indicated) while fibrinolytic therapy or surgical intervention is being prepared.

Supportive measures can buy time but should never replace a primary therapeutic intervention. The ability of fluid or pressors to sustain a patient's blood pressure is not predictive of a good outcome. With proven or strongly suspected PTE the need for such measures mandates immediate fibrinolysis or thrombectomy.

Volume expansion usually is not beneficial for a hypotensive patient with massive PTE. Even if volume expansion succeeds in raising systemic blood pressure, the patient with acute pulmonary hypertension already faces an excessive right ventricular afterload, so volume expansion will usually worsen right ventricular function. If a patient has frank shock from PTE, norepinephrine may be the preferred agent because restoration of cardiac output and coronary perfusion pressure is essential. If shock from PTE is refractory to pressor agents, cardiopulmonary bypass can sustain the patient long enough for fibrinolytic agents to work.[68]

Anticoagulation

Anticoagulation has been the mainstay of therapy for DVT and PTE since the clinical introduction of heparin in the 1930s. Rapid anticoagulation is essential, since thrombus progression and recurrent embolization are 15 times higher in patients who are not adequately anticoagulated within the first 24 hours.[2]

After initial anticoagulation with heparin, long-term anticoagulation usually is maintained with warfarin. Warfarin should never be started without prior heparinization, because warfarin will reduce the levels of the anticoagulants protein C and protein S before it reduces the levels of procoagulant proteins, producing a clinically important hypercoagulable state in the first 5 days.

Heparin The most frequently used drug in the treatment of acute VTE is heparin. Some form of heparin is indicated for all patients with VTE except those with antithrombin III deficiency, in whom heparin is ineffective. Heparin anticoagulation does not guarantee a successful outcome; extension of DVT and recurrent PTE may occur despite effective heparin anticoagulation. Nonetheless, prompt intensive anticoagulation with heparin can reduce the mortality of PTE from more than 30% to less than 10% by inhibiting thrombus propagation and thus reducing the size and frequency of recurrent emboli.

Heparin does not dissolve existing thrombus; it interferes with the coagulation cascade to inhibit the action of thrombin and slow the formation of new thrombus. This allows natural fibrinolytic mechanisms to reduce the size and extent of existing thrombus, but these natural mechanisms act slowly and are ineffective against a large clot burden at any site. When VTE is treated with heparin, some recanalization and reduction in clot size eventually occur in 30% to 60% of patients, but natural fibrinolytic mechanisms completely clear large occlusive thrombi from the peripheral circulation in only 3%.[69]

Because heparin works by activating antithrombin III, a deficiency of antithrombin III renders heparin ineffective as an anticoagulant. Alternative anticoagulants (e.g., hirudins) must be used in patients with antithrombin III deficiency.

When VTE is suspected, heparin should be started without delay. In patients with DVT, failure to achieve a therapeutic activated partial thromboplastin time (aPTT) value within the first 24 hours leads to a 23% incidence of new embolism, compared to only 6% for patients with a therapeutic aPTT.[2]

Patients with active DVT or PTE are hypercoagulable and require a higher initial dose of heparin than that used for prophylaxis or arterial thrombosis. When traditional approaches to heparin dosing are used, 60% of patients do not achieve a therapeutic aPTT value within the first 24 hours. To achieve effective anticoagulation in 24 hours, unfractionated heparin in an initial bolus of 100 to 150 U/kg (about 10,000 units for a 70-kg patient) should be given, and maintenance infusions started at 18 U/kg/hr.[70] The aPTT should be monitored 6 hours after each change in therapy, with a target aPTT of at least 1.5 times the control value. Any subtherapeutic aPTT should be addressed immediately with rebolus and increased infusion rate. Even with extremely high aPTT results, the infusion should be interrupted for only 1 hour, with a 10% decrease in heparin dosage.

Subcutaneous Unfractionated Heparin Subcutaneous unfractionated heparin is not effective as primary therapy for VTE or as prophylaxis against recurrence in patients with prior VTE. It contributes little to the prophylaxis or treatment of VTE now that fractionated low-molecular-weight heparins are widely available.

Low-Molecular-Weight Heparin Low-molecular-weight heparin (LMWH) is rapidly replacing unfractionated heparin in many settings because it is more effective for prophylaxis and treatment of DVT and PTE, has a lower incidence of bleeding complications, and is easier to administer.[69,71] Although hepatic transaminases are occasionally elevated with LMWH therapy, they spontaneously return to normal with no adverse outcomes.

It is neither necessary nor useful to monitor the aPTT when giving LMWH. The drug is most active in a tissue phase and is more active against factor Xa than against factor IIa, thus the aPTT usually is not prolonged, even when the patient is fully anticoagulated.

Although enoxaparin is the only LMWH approved by the U.S. Food and Drug Administration (FDA) for treatment of DVT and PTE, dalteparin and ardeparin probably are also safe and effective (at a higher dose than that approved for prophylaxis) for treatment of patients with active DVT or PTE. The drugs are not equivalent, and dosing is highly product specific.

Enoxaparin (Lovenox) is administered by subcutaneous injection. The adult dose for treatment of DVT or PTE is 1 mg/kg every 12 hours, or 1.5 mg/kg as a single injection every 24 hours. The adult dose for routine prophylaxis is 30 mg every 12 hours. In patients undergoing abdominal surgery, the prophylactic dose is 40 mg once daily, with the first dose given 2 hours before surgery. Enoxaparin is available in prefilled syringes designed for self-administration at home. In the event of bleeding complications, 1 mg of protamine sulfate can neutralize 1 mg of enoxaparin.

Dalteparin (Fragmin) is approved for postoperative DVT prophylaxis in abdominal surgery, with once-daily dosing of 2500 units subcutaneously. If necessary, 1 mg of protamine can neutralize 100 units of dalteparin.

Ardeparin (Normiflo) is approved for DVT prophylaxis in patients undergoing hip and knee surgery, at a dose of 50 U/kg every 12 hours. If necessary, 1 mg of protamine can neutralize 100 units of ardeparin.

Pregnancy Subcutaneous LMWH has largely supplanted IV unfractionated heparin for prophylaxis and treatment in pregnancy. Unlike warfarin, heparin is not teratogenic and may be administered throughout pregnancy until onset of active labor. LMWH can more than triple the rate of live birth (from 20% to 75%) in patients with recurrent pregnancy loss due to inherited or acquired thrombophilia.[72] LMWH does not increase the risk of malformations, low birth weight, or stillbirth. It is not known whether a twofold increase in the risk of preterm delivery is caused by the underlying thrombophilia or the heparin itself. Heparins do not cross the placenta and are not secreted in breast milk.

Uterine hemostasis is unaffected by heparin. If anticoagulation is indicated, fractionated or unfractionated heparin should be restarted after delivery as soon as the episiotomy has been repaired and any wound bleeding has resolved.

Warfarin Warfarin interferes with the action of the vitamin K–dependent clotting factors II, VII, IX, and X, as well as the action of the anticoagulant factors protein C and protein S. Warfarin causes a temporary hypercoagulable state during the first 5 days of therapy, because the anticoagulants protein C and protein S have short half-lives compared with the procoagulant vitamin K–dependent proteins. To prevent progression and recurrence of DVT and PTE, concomitant heparin must be given when warfarin is started in patients with VTE. Heparin must be continued for at least 5 days after the initiation of warfarin.

This early hypercoagulability is not a rare or theoretic problem but a real and important clinical issue. The incidence of progressive thrombosis and embolization is 40% when patients are started directly on warfarin, compared to only 8% when full heparin anticoagulation is given before warfarin.[73] Warfarin-induced hypercoagulability also causes the syndrome of *warfarin skin necrosis,* in which areas of skin and portions of the distal extremities become gangrenous and may require amputation. Discontinuation of warfarin therapy results in a second temporary hypercoagulable state,[74] which may contribute to the high rate of recurrent VTE seen shortly after cessation of warfarin.[75]

Warfarin anticoagulation usually is effective against venous thrombosis when the international normalized ratio (INR) is above 2.5. Patients with prior thrombosis from an irreversible hypercoagulable state, however, may require a target INR above 3.0 to prevent recurrent thrombosis.[76]

Warfarin causes significant hemorrhage in a substantial minority of patients. Hemorrhagic complications are controlled by the transfusion of fresh frozen plasma and by parenteral vitamin K (10 mg subcutaneously, intramuscularly, or rarely, intravenously). Parenteral vitamin K will reverse the warfarin effect within a few hours. Vitamin K is thrombogenic in patients with an existing hypercoagulable state and should not be used unless mandated by significant bleeding complications.

Warfarin is teratogenic and cannot be used in pregnancy. It is secreted in breast milk only in minute quantities, however, and may be used safely by nursing mothers.

Duration Most patients with an initial DVT should be anticoagulated for 6 months or longer. A subset of patients who have a reversible or time-limited cause of venous thrombosis and no irreversible risk factors may be candidates for a 3-month course of oral anticoagulation. For patients without a known reversible risk factor, continuing warfarin indefinitely beyond 3 months results in a 95% reduction in the frequency of recurrent VTE with only a slight increase in bleeding risk.[77,78] Long-term anticoagulation is indicated for patients with a second episode of VTE or with a known irreversible risk factor.[78] Regardless of the duration of anticoagulation, DVT and PTE often recur shortly after cessation of therapy.

Complications Heparin-related major bleeding complications occur in 4% of patients treated for VTE.[79] The risk of serious hemorrhage increases when unfractionated heparin prolongs the aPTT to more than three times control values, but the risk of bleeding does not rise incrementally with further prolongation of the aPTT. The risk of hemorrhage is increased by the concomitant use of aspirin or other platelet inhibitors. Fresh frozen plasma and platelet transfusions are ineffective when excessive bleeding is caused by heparin, but the anticoagulant effect of heparin may be reversed by protamine sulfate (15 mg infused over 3 minutes).

In addition to bleeding complications, heparin may cause *heparin-associated thrombocytopenia* (HAT), an immune complex–mediated consumptive thrombocytopenia that often triggers a fulminant thrombotic syndrome with a very high mortality. If HAT occurs, heparin must be discontinued immediately, and fibrinolysis must be considered at the first sign of disseminated thrombosis.

Plasma testing can identify the two thirds of patients with HAT who do not have a cross-reaction to the LMWH enoxaparin, but the drug of choice for patients with HAT is *lepirudin* (Refludan), a nonheparin hirudin anticoagulant that is a highly specific, direct inhibitor of thrombin. All thrombin-dependent assays are affected by hirudins, and the aPTT is prolonged by therapeutic doses of the drug. The dose of lepirudin is 0.4 mg/kg given slowly over 15 to 20 seconds as a bolus, followed by 0.15 mg/kg/hr as a continuous IV infusion. The maximum bolus dose is 44 mg, and the maximal initial infusion dose is 16.5 mg/hr. The dose is adjusted to maintain a therapeutic aPTT prolongation (1.5 to 2.0 times the control value). Lepirudin is renally excreted; thus the maintenance dose must be reduced in patients with a reduced creatine clearance. When given with fibrinolytics, the initial IV bolus of lepirudin is reduced to 0.2 mg/kg and the continuous IV infusion reduced to 0.1 mg/kg/hr.

Chronic Venous Insufficiency Anticoagulation is essential because it can greatly reduce mortality, but anticoagulation alone is far from adequate therapy for most patients with DVT or PTE. Anticoagulation can slow or stop the progression of new thrombus but does nothing to remove existing thrombus. In many cases, deep vein thrombus treated in this way fails to recanalize, leaving a chronic obstruction to outflow that is poorly tolerated by the patient. In other cases the thrombus recanalizes incompletely, leaving a narrowed channel that still produces resistance to outflow. Even when spontaneous recanalization is complete, the leg usually is dysfunctional; if not removed in time, thrombus destroys venous valves and produces a valveless channel that leads to profound venous reflux and venous hypertension.

When patients with DVT are treated with anticoagulants alone, 65% sustain venous valve damage that results in permanently altered patterns of venous return. Depending on the location and size of thrombus and the intensity and duration of anticoagulation, 30% to 80% will develop a lifelong postphlebitic syndrome of venous insufficiency, with recurrent pain, swelling, stasis dermatitis, ulceration, and recurrent DVT and PTE.[80]

The valves of the popliteal segment are particularly important for the preservation of calf muscle pump function and normal venous outflow from the lower leg. More than half of patients with valve damage from thrombosis isolated to the popliteal segment will develop postphlebitic symptoms.

CVI can affect the upper extremities as well. Subclavian vein thrombosis treated with anticoagulation alone often leads to permanent outflow obstruction or CVI, with extension to occlude the superior vena cava in 10% of patients and progression to PTE in 36%.[27]

Fibrinolysis

Deep Vein Thrombosis Fibrinolytic therapy for DVT has intrinsic appeal because removing an abnormal clot seems intuitively preferable to leaving it in place. In addition to restoring a widely patent outflow channel, lysis of thrombus can preserve and restore normal venous valve structure and function if performed early enough in the disease process.[81] This is important because postphlebitic symptoms are directly related to the extent and location of venous valve damage. For catheter-associated venous thrombosis, fibrinolysis is now accepted therapy. Complete lysis of local thrombus is achieved without a significant systemic lytic state in most patients who receive direct intrathrombus infusion.

Evidence also supports the routine use of fibrinolytic therapy for some patients with non-catheter-related DVT. Compared with anticoagulation alone, lytic therapy for DVT produces more rapid clot resolution, more complete clot resolution, a marked reduction in late symptoms, and a reduced likelihood of recurrent DVT and PTE. Compared with heparin, fibrinolysis can double the likelihood of achieving a normal venogram and normal lower extremity physiologic function, can reduce the rate of recurrent DVT by 50%, and can reduce the incidence of a crippling postphlebitic syndrome by up to 70%.[82,83]

Many centers now have a significant experience with a variety of techniques for dissolving thrombus within the deep veins. The greater the reduction in the amount of thrombus and the earlier it can be accomplished, the greater the benefit to the patient. Compared with systemic infusions, transcatheter delivery of fibrinolytic agents directly into the bulk thrombus has a higher success rate with fewer systemic effects.[84]

Pulmonary Thromboembolism Fibrinolytic agents have been used for the treatment of PTE for more than 30 years and are well-established as the treatment of choice for patients with hemodynamic compromise from PTE. Immediate fibrinolytic therapy is recommended for patients with PTE who are hypotensive, have massive PTE, have had syncope with persistent hemodynamic compromise, are significantly hypoxemic, or have other evidence of depleted cardiopulmonary reserves. Immediate fibrinolysis may also be indicated for patients with acute right ventricular strain from PTE, even in the absence of hemodynamic compromise. Further study is required to assess the risk-benefit ratio of fibrinolysis for less severe PTE presentations. Of those who survive a PTE and have recurrences, many will develop chronic pulmonary hypertension if treated with heparin alone, because heparin fails to dissolve the thrombus that accumulates in the lungs. Carbon monoxide diffusion, a primary measure of pulmonary gas exchange, also becomes normal immediately after the administration of lytic agents but remains permanently impaired when patients with PTE are treated only with anticoagulants.[85]

Natural fibrinolytic processes often do recanalize pulmonary vessels and restore flow, but the vessels remain lined with organized fibrous clot. The stiffened vessels have lost their natural elasticity and can no longer perform their normal capacitive volume function. This stiffening and loss of pulmonary vascular volume is reflected in elevated pulmonary vascular resistance and pulmonary artery pressures that are high at rest and become even higher with minimal exercise, even many years after the original PTE. Patients who receive lytic therapy, on the other hand, have normal resistance and normal arterial pressures at rest and at exercise.

PTE is a disease of recurrences, and the progressive accumulation of new microthrombi with each episode is significant in the development of pulmonary hypertension and cor pulmonale. Lytic therapy helps to prevent pulmonary hypertension by (1) removing large-vessel pulmonary arterial thrombus that would otherwise only recanalize, (2) dissolving microemboli from the microcirculation of the lung, and (3) reducing the rate of recurrent embolization.[86]

Mortality Benefit Virtually all the mortality of DVT occurs when fragments of thrombus embolize to the pulmonary circulation. In some populations the 1-week mortality rate of patients with PTE treated with heparin is nearly 40%, and the 1-year mortality rate is nearly 60%.[3] When given immediately and followed by intensive chronic anticoagulation, heparin can reduce the short-term mortality of PTE from more than 30% to 10% or less, but 1 in 10 patients still dies from the disease.

Early fibrinolytic therapy greatly reduces the death rate from PTE. Patients treated with lytic agents have much more rapid and complete resolution of pulmonary vascular obstruction than patients treated with heparin alone, with superior hemodynamic improvement, as measured by right atrial, right ventricular, and pulmonary arterial pressures; Pao_2; and pulmonary vascular resistance. Patients treated with lytic therapy also have 25% to 60% fewer recurrences of PTE than those treated with heparin alone.[57,86]

Unstable patients treated with lytic agents are significantly more likely to survive than those treated only with anticoagulants. Fibrinolysis has been in common use for hemodynamically unstable patients with PTE since the 1980s. The last study attempting to randomize hemodynamically unstable patients was halted before completion in the mid-1990s because all the patients receiving heparin died and all those receiving fibrinolytics survived.[87]

The mortality benefit when patients receive fibrinolysis in addition to anticoagulation is not limited to those who are hemodynamically unstable. Mortality decreases by more than 50%, from 11% to 5% or even less, when hemodynamically stable patients with evidence of right ventricular strain receive fibrinolysis rather than heparin as their primary therapy.[57,86] This mortality benefit extends beyond the immediate period; the early recurrence rate for VTE is 18% after treatment with heparin but only 8% after treatment with lytics. Fibrinolysis is not without risk: intracranial bleeding occurs in about 0.5% of patients treated with heparin and in up to 1.2% of those treated with fibrinolytic agents.[57] This increased risk is far outweighed, however, by the overall mortality benefit of fibrinolytic agents for patients with VTE extensive enough to produce right ventricular strain.

Routine Fibrinolytic Therapy The benefits of fibrinolytic therapy probably outweigh the recognized risks of the therapy for many hemodynamically stable patients with DVT or PTE. Early lysis of clot, whether in the deep veins or in the lungs, can restore normal structure and function to these critical parts of the circulatory system, significantly reducing short-term and long-term morbidity. Additional study will establish whether the benefit exceeds the risk sufficiently to establish fibrinolytic therapy as a potential primary mode of treatment for every patient with DVT and PTE.

In the absence of invasive procedures, about 4% of patients receiving fibrinolytic agents or heparin will experience significant bleeding. If invasive procedures are performed, fibrinolysis causes significantly more local bleeding than heparin. For patients with a high-probability $\dot{V}/\dot{Q}$ scan and a concordant clinical likelihood, the added risk of bleeding after invasive procedures can be avoided if fibrinolysis is initiated without a confirmatory pulmonary angiogram. The rate of significant bleeding with lytic therapy is three times higher in patients who have received an angiogram.

Risk of intracranial bleeding is the main deterrent to the routine use of fibrinolytic therapy for thromboembolic disease. Fibrinolysis may cause intracranial bleeding in up to 1.2% of patients treated for PTE, and the benefits of fibrinolysis must exceed this level of risk to be justified.[57] The mortality benefit for hemodynamically unstable patients is unquestionable, and the twofold mortality benefit for hemodynamically stable patients with right ventricular strain from PTE holds up even when intracranial bleeds are taken into account. The mortality benefit in other clinical settings is less well established.

If serious noncompressible bleeding complications result from lytic therapy, the infusion of lytic agent should be stopped. Fresh frozen plasma and cryoprecipitate may be effective at reversing the lytic state. *Aminocaproic acid* (an inhibitor of plasminogen activators) may be given as a 5-g IV bolus administered over 30 minutes, followed by a maintenance infusion of 1 g/hr until the bleeding has resolved.

The recognition of hemorrhagic risks associated with anticoagulation and fibrinolysis should not prevent the appropriate use of anticoagulants and fibrinolytic agents.[88]

Alteplase and Other Regimens Because most deaths from PTE occur soon after the first symptoms are apparent, the fastest-acting available agent and the fastest-acting safe infusion regimen are recommended. At this time the only FDA-approved fibrinolytic regimens for PTE are alteplase, streptokinase, and urokinase. Urokinase is no longer available because of intrinsic concerns about the manufacturing process. Streptokinase is given as a loading dose of 250,000 units over 30 minutes and an infusion of 100,000 U/hr for 24 hours. Streptokinase is rarely used for treatment of PTE because it is highly antigenic and because the 24-hour infusion is associated with a high incidence of bleeding complications.

The approved alteplase (Activase) regimen for PTE is 100 mg as a 2-hour continuous IV infusion. Many centers believe it is safer and more effective to use the 90-minute front-loaded regimen that was approved for acute MI: 100 mg as a 15-mg IV bolus, followed by 50 mg infused over the next 30 minutes, then 35 mg infused over the next 60 minutes. For patients less than 67 kg, a weight-adjusted regimen is preferred: an initial 15-mg IV bolus, followed by 0.75 mg/kg infused over the next 30 minutes (not to exceed 50 mg), then 0.50 mg/kg infused over the next 60 minutes (not to exceed 35 mg). For critically ill patients unlikely to survive the infusion period, very rapid infusion of 50 or 100 mg of alteplase may be given over 10 or 15 minutes.

Although not labeled by the FDA for this indication, the newer recombinant plasminogen activator *reteplase* works even more quickly than alteplase for patients with PTE. Reteplase (Retavase) is given as two IV doses of 10 units each. Each dose is infused over 2 minutes, with the second dose given 30 minutes after the first. Besides reteplase, other new fibrinolytic agents under investigation for use in PTE include tenecteplase, prourokinase, and recombinant staphylokinase.

When alteplase is used for iliofemoral DVT, pulse-spray catheters have been used to deliver 24-hour or longer regional infusions of 1 mg/hr. Reteplase has also been used for iliofemoral DVT at infusion rates of 0.5 to 1.0 U/hr.

Full anticoagulation with heparin or LMWH is not a contraindication to fibrinolysis. If IV unfractionated heparin is used, the infusion may be paused during the active phase of fibrinolysis and restarted approximately 2 hours after initiation of therapy with alteplase or reteplase. Bleeding complications have not been consistently shown to increase when heparin is continued concurrently with alteplase in patients with PTE.

Contraindications

Heparin and fibrinolytic agents are relatively or absolutely contraindicated in a variety of situations that place the patient at high risk for bleeding complications, but more than half of patients with PTE are eligible for fibrinolytic therapy. Many clinical conditions are relative or minor contraindications to anticoagulation but are absolute or major contraindications to lytic therapy. The list of contraindications has changed as more has been learned about lytic therapy (Table 83-4). Advanced age is not a contraindication to fibrinolysis because the benefits of lytic therapy increase with age more than the risks increase. A history of prior nonhemorrhagic stroke is not a contraindication. Pregnancy is not a contraindication; pregnant patients with hemodynamically significant PTE have been successfully treated with fibrinolytic agents at all stages of pregnancy, including preterm labor.

Embolectomy

In the prefibrinolytic era, immediate pulmonary embolectomy was the only effective therapy for patients with massive PTE and was indicated whenever angiographically demonstrated emboli caused severe right-sided heart failure and systemic hypotension that could not be managed with pressor agents. At present, embolectomy is reserved for the patient with severe pulmonary or cardiac compromise who is not a candidate for fibrinolysis, for whom there is insufficient time to achieve fibrinolysis, or in whom fibrinolytic therapy has failed. The procedure carries an operative mortality of 25% to 40% or more, and regardless of the embolism's size, patients who do not become hypotensive will do better without surgery if further embolization can be prevented.

Transvenous catheter embolectomy is an alternative approach. A suction-tip catheter is placed in contact with the thrombus under fluoroscopic guidance, and the thrombus is held by suction while the catheter is withdrawn.

Cardiopulmonary Bypass

Portable percutaneous (femorofemoral) cardiopulmonary bypass machines are increasingly available within the ED, and patients with profound hypoxemia or shock from massive PTE are excellent candidates for emergency bypass with extracorporeal membrane oxygenation. This temporizing measure can be instituted rapidly and will support a subset of patients long enough for fibrinolysis or surgical embolectomy to correct the underlying problem.[68] The placement of large femoral arterial and venous catheters for bypass is not a contraindication to lytic therapy if the catheters are placed correctly and not removed until after the lytic state has resolved.

Table 83-4. Contraindications to Anticoagulation and Fibrinolysis

Clinical setting	Thrombolysis	Heparin
Active major external bleeding	Absolute	Absolute
Active internal bleeding (even if minor)	Absolute	Absolute
Recent neurosurgery (past 8 weeks)	Absolute	Relative
Recent hepatic or renal biopsy	Absolute	Relative
Recent ocular surgery (past 8 weeks)	Absolute	Relative
Severe heparin-induced thrombocytopenia	Not contraindicated	Absolute
Major trauma	Relative	Relative
Recent surgery (including organ biopsy)	Relative	Not contraindicated
Recent major vessel puncture (current cannula acceptable)	Relative	Not contraindicated
Immediately postpartum	Relative	Relative
Recent past history of GI bleeding	Relative	Relative
HTN uncontrolled at the time of thrombolysis	Relative (strong)	Relative
Longstanding diastolic HTN over 110 torr	Relative	Relative
Recent prolonged CPR	Relative	Relative
Current pregnancy	Relative	Not contraindicated
Diabetic retinopathy with recent hemorrhage	Absolute	Relative
Bacterial endocarditis	Relative	Not contraindicated
Mild heparin-associated thrombocytopenia	Not contraindicated	Relative
CNS cancer	Relative	Relative

Presumptive Fibrinolysis or Thoracotomy

Massive PTE is found in 36% of ED patients in cardiac arrest who have pulseless electrical activity as the initial cardiac rhythm.[8] CPR and Advanced Cardiac Life Support (ACLS) protocols are ineffective when cardiac arrest is caused by obstruction of the pulmonary tree; conventional CPR will not result in any oxygenated blood reaching the cerebral circulation, and the mortality in this setting approaches 100%. Although the evidence is anecdotal, case reports describe satisfactory outcomes after presumptive bolus administration of fibrinolytic agents in patients with cardiac arrest and a strong presumptive diagnosis of PTE. For presumptive therapy in cardiac arrest, reteplase (10-unit IV bolus) and alteplase (50-mg IV bolus) have been used.

Case reports also document resuscitation after bilateral thoracotomy and massage of the pulmonary vessels to dislodge a saddle embolus and restore circulation to at least a portion of the pulmonary vascular tree. Thoracotomy in this setting is of unproven benefit. It should not be attempted unless cardiopulmonary bypass and embolectomy will be immediately available in the operating room if the patient is resuscitated. ED thoracotomy is contraindicated in patients who have received fibrinolytic therapy.

Prevention of Recurrence

Approximately 25% of patients who survive their first PTE will have a clinically recognized recurrence, even if appropriately diagnosed and treated.[25] Prevention is critically important because if a patient survives the first few hours of a symptomatic PTE, most mortality risk and much morbidity are associated with future recurrences.

Heparin Prophylaxis Some form of heparin prophylaxis is recommended for almost all surgical patients and for medical patients whose activity is severely restricted. In these groups, heparin reduces DVT by 68% and PTE by 49%.[89] Prophylactic heparin also reduces mortality by 30% in a general population of unselected medical patients.[12] When a patient with prior thromboembolic disease must undergo surgery or enforced bed rest, full-dose anticoagulation is strongly indicated because without prophylaxis, the incidence of recurrence is virtually 100%.

Gradient Compression Stockings An effective compression garment can significantly reduce the incidence of DVT and PTE. True gradient compression stockings (30 to 40 mm Hg or higher) are highly elastic and provide a gradient of compression that is highest at the toes and gradually decreases to the level of the thigh. Compression stockings of this type have proven effectiveness in the prophylaxis of thromboembolism, reducing the incidence of DVT by nearly 70% in high-risk populations.[90] External compression is also effective as adjunctive therapy in the treatment of patients with active DVT.[91]

The ubiquitous white stockings known as "antiembolic stockings" or "Ted hose" produce a maximum compression of 18 mm Hg (less after washing) but are rarely fitted to provide even this inadequate gradient compression. They are of limited efficacy in prophylaxis against thromboembolism.

Gradient compression stockings are an inexpensive, effective, safe, and non-invasive form of prophylaxis and adjunctive therapy. Whenever possible, gradient compression stockings with 30 to 40 mm Hg of pressure should be placed on patients with superficial phlebitis and on those with suspected or proven DVT before they leave the ED. Jobst, Juzo, Medi, Venosan, and Sigvaris are manufacturers of effective gradient compression hose that may be stocked in the ED.

Intermittent Pneumatic Compression Active pneumatic sequential compression devices for the legs are an effective form of prophylaxis against thromboembolism, offering a reduction in risk comparable to that obtained with gradient compression stockings. Unfortunately, nursing compliance with orders for the devices is poor; external pneumatic compression devices were incorrectly applied or nonfunctioning in 22% of ICU patients and in 52% of patients on a nursing unit.[92]

Combined Prophylaxis Combined therapies are more effective than any single modality of prophylaxis. For high-risk patients, such as those with a prior history of VTE, many clinicians use a synergistic combination of three proven modalities: subcutaneous LMWH, gradient compression stockings (30 to 40 mm Hg), and an active intermittent pneumatic leg or foot compression device.

Vena Cava Filters Transvenous implantation of an "umbrella" filtering device within the vena cava may be necessary in trauma patients, in those who cannot tolerate a period of anticoagulation, and in patients with proven recurrence of DVT or PTE despite intensive anticoagulation. When properly positioned, vena cava filters prevent the largest thrombi from passing upward into the pulmonary arteries and can reduce the mortality of PTE. Filters do not prevent smaller pulmonary emboli from reaching the pulmonary circulation, and large emboli may bypass the filters or may originate above the filter. Vena cava filters are a supplement, not a substitute, for anticoagulation; many patients have died from PTE with a vena cava filter in place. In high-risk patients with proximal DVT, an initial beneficial effect of vena cava filters for the prevention of PTE is counterbalanced by an increase in recurrent DVT, with no net difference in mortality.[93]

DISPOSITION

Ambulation versus Bed Rest

In patients with acute DVT, bed rest almost certainly increases the risk of embolization because immobility encourages the propagation of fresh, friable thrombus. Anticoagulation alone does not protect against this problem; in patients at bed rest, heparin anticoagulation slows but does not prevent the progression of thrombus. The current trend is to recognize the overwhelming contribution of stasis to thrombogenesis and to keep patients ambulatory in compression hose from the first day.[91]

Treatment Approaches

The initial treatment of phlebitis is based on the patient's history and risk factors and the results of a detailed US examination. For patients with superficial or deep vein thrombophlebitis, treatment approaches depend largely on the localization of thrombus using duplex US.

Uncomplicated Superficial Disease A patient with no risk factors and no prior thromboembolic history who develops purely superficial phlebitis that does not involve the greater saphenous vein (GSV) above the knee will usually respond to nonsteroidal antiinflammatory agents, strict use of gradient compression hose, increased ambulation, and early repeat examination. Duplex US is absolutely indicated and bed rest absolutely contraindicated in this setting.

Complicated Superficial Disease Full outpatient anticoagulation with subcutaneous LMWH is the appropriate therapy for a patient with superficial phlebitis who has a history of deep vein thrombophlebitis, any known irreversible risk factors for venous thrombosis, decreased mobility, or involvement of the GSV above the knee. Antibiotics should be used if clinical evidence suggests that phlebitis may be septic and when the GSV is involved in the proximal thigh. Lysis of ascending GSV thrombus or surgical interruption of the saphenofemoral junction with removal of the saphenous vein must be considered if GSV phlebitis approaches the junction.

Limited Disease Although thrombus in the muscular venous sinuses is known to embolize, an outpatient regimen of full-dose subcutaneous LMWH, gradient compression hose, increased ambulation, and early repeat duplex US probably is safe for patients with small isolated thrombi involving only small venous channels in the peroneal and soleal plexus. If outpatient treatment is attempted, these patients should be followed with serial duplex US until the thrombus is seen to regress.

Tibial, Popliteal, or Femoral Disease Deep vein thrombophlebitis involving the tibial veins carries almost the same risk of PTE as does DVT in the popliteal and more proximal thigh veins. Standard therapy for all these patients includes hospitalization and full-dose anticoagulation with IV unfractionated heparin. Strict gradient compression therapy may help to improve outcome. Maintenance of ambulation is required in Europe but is only beginning to be accepted in the United States. Alternative treatment approaches include full-dose subcutaneous fractionated LMWH, fibrinolytic agents, and in some cases the placement of a vena cava filter.

Outpatient treatment remains controversial. Profit-oriented insurers and hospitals can see a financial benefit to outpatient treatment of DVT and PTE, but risks remain for both the clinician and the patient because some of these patients will die from pulmonary embolism.

KEY CONCEPTS

- If an abnormal perfusion lung scan is not high probability, it is nondiagnostic and is never a valid endpoint for the diagnostic workup. Fibrinolysis is indicated for PTE patients with hemodynamic compromise, syncope and persistent hemodynamic instability, or significant hypoxemia. It should also be strongly considered for patients unlikely to survive a further insult and those with evidence of right ventricular strain due to PTE.
- Anticoagulation should be started as soon as the diagnosis of VTE is seriously considered. Delays in treatment are associated with significantly worse outcomes and an increased risk of recurrences that persists for many weeks.
- Venous thrombosis is rarely benign at any location. Calf vein DVT and upper extremity DVT often cause fatal PTE, and seemingly superficial thrombophlebitis often involves the deep veins or progresses to involve them.
- 80% of ventilation/perfusion scans and pulmonary angiograms will be normal because the proper use of these tests is to rule out VTE in a population of at-risk patients with a 21% prevalence of the disease.

REFERENCES

1. Meignan M et al: Systematic lung scans reveal a high frequency of silent pulmonary embolism in patients with proximal deep venous thrombosis, *Arch Intern Med* 160:159, 2000.
2. Hull RD et al: Relation between the time to achieve the lower limit of the APTT therapeutic range and recurrent venous thromboembolism during heparin treatment for deep vein thrombosis, *Arch Intern Med* 157:2562, 1997.
3. Heit JA et al: Predictors of survival after deep vein thrombosis and pulmonary embolism: a population-based, cohort study, *Arch Intern Med* 159:445, 1999.
4. National Institutes of Health consensus development conference statement: Thrombolytic therapy in thrombosis, *Ann Intern Med* 93:141, 1980.
5. Jaureguito JW et al: The incidence of deep venous thrombosis after arthroscopic knee surgery, *Am J Sports Med* 27:707, 1999.
6. Madani MM, Jamieson SW: Chronic thromboembolic pulmonary hypertension, *Curr Treat Options Cardiovasc Med* 2:141, 2000.
7. Oger E: Incidence of venous thromboembolism: a community-based study in Western France, EPI-GETBP Study Group, Groupe d'Etude de la Thrombose de Bretagne Occidentale, *Thromb Haemost* 83:657, 2000.
8. Comess KA et al: The incidence of pulmonary embolism in unexplained sudden cardiac arrest with pulseless electrical activity, *Am J Med* 109:351, 2000.
9. Hirsch DR, Ingenito EP, Goldhaber SZ: Prevalence of deep venous thrombosis among patients in medical intensive care, *JAMA* 274:335, 1995.
10. Ibarra-Perez C et al: Prevalence and prevention of deep venous thrombosis of the lower extremities in high-risk pulmonary patients, *Angiology* 39:505, 1988.
11. Moser KM et al: Frequent asymptomatic pulmonary embolism in patients with deep venous thrombosis, *JAMA* 271:223, 1994.
12. Samama MM et al: A comparison of enoxaparin with placebo for the prevention of venous thromboembolism in acutely ill medical patients, Prophylaxis in Medical Patients with Enoxaparin Study Group, *N Engl J Med* 341:793, 1999.
13. Siddique RM et al: Thirty-day case-fatality rates for pulmonary embolism in the elderly, *Arch Intern Med* 156:2343, 1996.
14. Verlato F et al: An unexpectedly high rate of pulmonary embolism in patients with superficial thrombophlebitis of the thigh, *J Vasc Surg* 30:1113, 1999.
15. Blumenberg RM et al: Occult deep venous thrombosis complicating superficial thrombophlebitis, *J Vasc Surg* 27:338, 1998.
16. Cogo A et al: Distribution of thrombosis in patients with symptomatic deep vein thrombosis: implications for simplifying the diagnostic process with compression ultrasound, *Arch Intern Med* 153:2777, 1993.
17. Havig O: Deep vein thrombosis and pulmonary embolism: an autopsy study with multiple regression analysis of possible risk factors, *Acta Chir Scand Suppl* 478:1, 1977.
18. Meissner MH et al: Early outcome after isolated calf vein thrombosis, *J Vasc Surg* 26:749, 1997.
19. Barnes RW et al: Perioperative asymptomatic venous thrombosis: role of duplex scanning versus venography, *J Vasc Surg* 9:251, 1989.
20. Monreal M et al: Deep venous thrombosis and the risk of pulmonary embolism: a systematic study, *Chest* 102:677, 1992.
21. Monreal M et al: Upper-extremity deep venous thrombosis and pulmonary embolism: a prospective study, *Chest* 99:280, 1991.
22. Cooper R et al: Elevated pulmonary artery pressure: an independent predictor of mortality, *Chest* 99:112, 1991.
23. Sharma GVRK, Folland ED, McIntyre KM: Long-term hemodynamic benefit of thrombolytic therapy in pulmonary embolic disease, *J Am Coll Cardiol* 15:65A, 1990.

24. Lindhagen A et al: Venous function five to eight years after clinically suspected deep venous thrombosis, *Acta Med Scand* 217:389, 1985.
25. Heit JA et al: Predictors of recurrence after deep vein thrombosis and pulmonary embolism: a population-based cohort study, *Arch Intern Med* 160:761, 2000.
26. Dailey RH: Femoral vein cannulation: a review, *J Emerg Med* 2:367, 1985.
27. Prandoni P, Bernardi E: Upper extremity deep vein thrombosis, *Curr Opin Pulm Med* 5:222, 1999.
28. Poikolainen E, Hendolin H: Effects of lumbar epidural anaesthesia and general anaesthesia on flow velocity in the femoral vein and postoperative deep vein thrombosis, *Acta Chir Scand* 149:361, 1983.
29. Gibbs NM: Venous thrombosis of the lower limbs with particular reference to bedrest, *Br J Surg* 45:209, 1957.
30. Warlow C, Ogston D, Douglas AS: Venous thrombosis following strokes, *Lancet* i:1305, 1972.
31. Kovacevich GJ et al: The prevalence of thromboembolic events among women with extended bed rest prescribed as part of the treatment for premature labor or preterm premature rupture of membranes, *Am J Obstet Gynecol* 182:1089, 2000.
32. Goldberg R et al: Occult malignant neoplasm in patients with deep venous thrombosis, *Arch Intern Med* 147:251, 1987.
33. Bastounis EA et al: The incidence of occult cancer in patients with deep venous thrombosis: a prospective study, *J Intern Med* 239:153, 1996.
34. Gherman RB et al: Incidence, clinical characteristics, and timing of objectively diagnosed venous thromboembolism during pregnancy, *Obstet Gynecol* 94:730, 1999.
35. Lowe G et al: Thrombotic variables and risk of idiopathic venous thromboembolism in women aged 45-64 years: relationships to hormone replacement therapy, *Thromb Haemost* 83:530, 2000.
36. Burkman RT: Cardiovascular issues with oral contraceptives: evidenced-based medicine, *Int J Fertil Womens Med* 45:166, 2000.
37. Andrew M et al: Venous thromboembolic complications (VTE) in children: first analyses of the Canadian Registry of VTE, *Blood* 83:1251, 1994.
38. Stein PD, Henry JW: Clinical characteristics of patients with acute pulmonary embolism stratified according to their presenting syndromes, *Chest* 112:974, 1997.
39. Dreyfuss AI, Weiland DS: Chest wall tenderness as a pitfall in the diagnosis of acute pulmonary embolism, *Arch Intern Med* 144:2057, 1984.
40. Branch WTJ, McNeil BJ, Branch WT Jr: Analysis of the differential diagnosis and assessment of pleuritic chest pain in young adults, *Am J Med* 75:671, 1983.
41. Hull RD et al: Pulmonary embolism in outpatients with pleuritic chest pain, *Arch Intern Med* 148:838, 1988.
42. Daniel KR, Jackson RE, Kline JA: Utility of lower extremity venous ultrasound scanning in the diagnosis and exclusion of pulmonary embolism in outpatients, *Ann Emerg Med* 35:547, 2000.
43. Hull RD et al: Clinical validity of a negative venogram in patients with clinically suspected venous thrombosis, *Circulation* 64:622, 1981.
44. Monreal M et al: Recurrent pulmonary embolism: a prospective study, *Chest* 95:976, 1989.
45. Afzal A et al: Leukocytosis in acute pulmonary embolism, *Chest* 115:1329, 1999.
46. Goldhaber SZ et al: Quantitative plasma D-dimer levels among patients undergoing pulmonary angiography for suspected pulmonary embolism, *JAMA* 270:2819, 1993.
47. Scarano L et al: Failure of soluble fibrin polymers in the diagnosis of clinically suspected deep venous thrombosis, *Blood Coagul Fibrinolysis* 10:245, 1999.
48. van der Graaf F et al: Exclusion of deep venous thrombosis with D-dimer testing: comparison of 13 D-dimer methods in 99 outpatients suspected of deep venous thrombosis using venography as reference standard, *Thromb Haemost* 83:191, 2000.
49. Lee AY et al: Clinical utility of a rapid whole-blood D-dimer assay in patients with cancer who present with suspected acute deep venous thrombosis, *Ann Intern Med* 131:417, 1999.
50. Sijens PE et al: Rapid ELISA assay for plasma D-dimer in the diagnosis of segmental and subsegmental pulmonary embolism: a comparison with pulmonary angiography, *Thromb Haemost* 84:156, 2000.
51. Farrell S, Hayes T, Shaw M: A negative SimpliRED D-dimer assay result does not exclude the diagnosis of deep vein thrombosis or pulmonary embolus in emergency department patients, *Ann Emerg Med* 35:121, 2000.
52. Kutinsky I, Blakley S, Roche V: Normal D-dimer levels in patients with pulmonary embolism, *Arch Intern Med* 159:1569, 1999.
53. Menzoian JO, Williams LF: Is pulmonary arteriography essential for the diagnosis of pulmonary embolism? *Am J Surg* 137:543, 1979.
54. Stein PD et al: Arterial blood gas analysis in the assessment of suspected acute pulmonary embolism, *Chest* 109:78, 1996.
55. Prediletto R et al: Diagnostic value of gas exchange tests in patients with clinical suspicion of pulmonary embolism, *Crit Care (Lond)* 3:111, 1999.
56. Elliott CG et al: Chest radiographs in acute pulmonary embolism: results from the International Cooperative Pulmonary Embolism Registry, *Chest* 118:33, 2000.
57. Konstantinides S et al: Association between thrombolytic treatment and the prognosis of hemodynamically stable patients with major pulmonary embolism: results of a multicenter registry, *Circulation* 96:882, 1997.
58. Jackson RE et al: Prospective evaluation of two-dimensional transthoracic echocardiography in emergency department patients with suspected pulmonary embolism, *Acad Emerg Med* 7:994, 2000.
59. Davis RB et al: Indeterminate lung imaging: can the number be reduced? *Clin Nucl Med* 11:577, 1986.
60. PIOPED Investigators: Value of the ventilation/perfusion scan in acute pulmonary embolism: results of the Prospective Investigation of Pulmonary Embolism Diagnosis (PIOPED), *JAMA* 263:2753, 1990.
61. Hull RD et al: The low-probability lung scan: a need for change in nomenclature, Arch Intern Med 155:1845, 1995.
62. Wartski M, Collignon MA: Incomplete recovery of lung perfusion after 3 months in patients with acute pulmonary embolism treated with antithrombotic agents, THESEE Study Group, Tinzaparin ou Heparin Standard: Evaluation dans l'Embolie Pulmonaire Study, *J Nucl Med* 41:1043, 2000.
63. Stein PD et al: Complications and validity of pulmonary angiography in acute pulmonary embolism, *Circulation* 85:462, 1992.
64. Drucker EA et al: Acute pulmonary embolism: assessment of helical CT for diagnosis, *Radiology* 209:235, 1998.
65. Harvey RT et al: Accuracy of CT angiography versus pulmonary angiography in the diagnosis of acute pulmonary embolism: evaluation of the literature with summary ROC curve analysis, *Acad Radiol* 7:786, 2000.
66. Bell WR, Simon TL, DeMets DL: The clinical features of submassive and massive pulmonary embolism, *Am J Med* 62:355, 1977.
67. Illig H: [Death from or in asthma?] *Med Klin* 73:357, 1978.
68. Kawahito K et al: Resuscitation and circulatory support using extracorporeal membrane oxygenation for fulminant pulmonary embolism, *Artif Organs* 24:427, 2000.
69. van Den Belt AG et al: Fixed dose subcutaneous low molecular weight heparins versus adjusted dose unfractionated heparin for venous thromboembolism, *Cochrane Database Syst Rev* (2):CD001100-2000.
70. Wheeler AP, Jaquiss RD, Newman JH: Physician practices in the treatment of pulmonary embolism and deep venous thrombosis, *Arch Intern Med* 148:1321, 1988.
71. Breddin HK: Prophylaxis and treatment of deep-vein thrombosis, *Semin Thromb Hemost* 26(suppl 1):47, 2000.
72. Brenner B et al: Gestational outcome in thrombophilic women with recurrent pregnancy loss treated by enoxaparin, *Thromb Haemost* 83:693, 2000.
73. Brandjes DPM et al: Acenocoumarol and heparin compared with acenocoumarol alone in the initial treatment of proximal-vein thrombosis, *N Engl J Med* 327:1485, 1992.
74. Palareti G et al: Activation of blood coagulation after abrupt or stepwise withdrawal of oral anticoagulants: a prospective study, *Thromb Haemost* 72:222, 1994.
75. Schulman S et al: A comparison of six weeks with six months of oral anticoagulant therapy after a first episode of venous thromboembolism, Duration of Anticoagulation Trial Study Group, *N Engl J Med* 332:1661, 1995.
76. Rosove MH, Brewer PM: Antiphospholipid thrombosis: clinical course after the first thrombotic event in 70 patients, *Ann Intern Med* 117:303, 1992.

77. Kearon C et al: A comparison of three months of anticoagulation with extended anticoagulation for a first episode of idiopathic venous thromboembolism, *N Engl J Med* 340:901, 1999.
78. Schulman S et al: The duration of oral anticoagulant therapy after a second episode of venous thromboembolism, Duration of Anticoagulation Trial Study Group, *N Engl J Med* 336:393, 1997.
79. Zidane M et al: Frequency of major hemorrhage in patients treated with unfractionated intravenous heparin for deep venous thrombosis or pulmonary embolism: a study in routine clinical practice, *Arch Intern Med* 160:2369, 2000.
80. Kahn SR et al: Long-term outcomes after deep vein thrombosis: postphlebitic syndrome and quality of life, *J Gen Intern Med* 15:425, 2000.
81. Hermans H et al: Valvular function and prostacyclin production following clot lysis and balloon thrombectomy in thrombosed canine veins, *Proc Am Venous Forum* 4:35, 1992.
82. Mewissen MW et al: Catheter-directed thrombolysis for lower extremity deep venous thrombosis: report of a national multicenter registry, *Radiology* 211:39, 1999.
83. Turpie AG et al: Tissue plasminogen activator (rt-PA) vs heparin in deep vein thrombosis: results of a randomized trial, *Chest* 97(suppl 4):172S, 1990.
84. Verhaeghe R et al: Catheter-directed lysis of iliofemoral vein thrombosis with use of rt-PA, *Eur Radiol* 7:996, 1997.
85. Sasahara AA, Sharma GVRK: Does thrombolytic therapy alter the prognosis of pulmonary embolism? *Haemostasis* 16(suppl 3), 1986.
86. Goldhaber SZ et al: Alteplase versus heparin in acute pulmonary embolism: randomised trial assessing right-ventricular function and pulmonary perfusion, *Lancet* 341:507, 1993.
87. Jerjes-Sanchez C et al: Streptokinase and heparin versus heparin alone in massive pulmonary embolism: a randomized controlled trial, *J Thromb Thrombolysis* 2:227, 1995.
88. Goldhaber SZ: Thrombolytic therapy in venous thromboembolism: clinical trials and current indications, *Clin Chest Med* 16:307, 1995.
89. National Institutes of Health consensus development conference statement: Prevention of venous thrombosis and pulmonary embolism, *JAMA* 256:744, 1986.
90. Wells PS, Lensing AW, Hirsh J: Graduated compression stockings in the prevention of postoperative venous thromboembolism: a meta-analysis, *Arch Intern Med* 154:67, 1994.
91. Partsch H, Blattler W: Compression and walking versus bed rest in the treatment of proximal deep venous thrombosis with low molecular weight heparin, *J Vasc Surg* 32:861, 2000.
92. Comerota AJ, Katz ML, White JV: Why does prophylaxis with external pneumatic compression for deep vein thrombosis fail? *Am J Surg* 164:265, 1992.
93. Decousus H et al: A clinical trial of vena caval filters in the prevention of pulmonary embolism in patients with proximal deep-vein thrombosis, Prevention du Risque d'Embolie Pulmonaire par Interruption Cave Study Group, *N Engl J Med* 338:409, 1998.

Section V GASTROINTESTINAL SYSTEM

84 Esophagus, Stomach, and Duodenum

Mark Lowell
William G. Barsan

ESOPHAGEAL OBSTRUCTION

Perspective

Although most ingested foreign bodies pass asymptomatically through the gastrointestinal (GI) tract, it is estimated that approximately 1500 people die each year from complications related to their ingestion.[1] Eighty percent of foreign body ingestions occur in the pediatric age group, with coins being the most commonly impacted object. In adults, most impactions are due to pieces of food, particularly meat and bones. Patients with preexisting esophageal abnormalities are at greater risk of foreign body impaction. Denture wearers are also at increased risk because of impaired oral sensation. Prisoners, alcoholics, psychiatric patients, and mentally retarded patients also have increased rates of foreign body ingestion.

Principles of Disease

The adult esophagus is approximately 25 to 30 cm in length. Superiorly, it begins in the hypopharynx as a transverse slit posterior to the larynx and approximately at the level of the cricoid cartilage. On either side of this cephalad slit are the piriform recesses, which are blind pouches that may occasionally harbor a foreign body. Throughout its course, the esophagus has four natural areas of narrowing that may cause impaction of a foreign body: at the cricopharyngeus muscle (the upper esophageal sphincter), the aortic arch, the left mainstem bronchus, and the diaphragmatic hiatus. Most impactions occur in the proximal third of the esophagus and, if large enough, can impinge on the trachea, leading to airway compromise.

The esophagus comprises two main bands of muscle: an inner circular layer and an outer longitudinal layer. The resting tone of these muscles causes the inner epithelium to fold in on itself, effectively obliterating the lumen. Elastic fibers enable the esophageal lumen to expand and allow passage of a food bolus. The upper one third of the esophagus, including the cricopharyngeus muscle, contains striated muscle to allow for the voluntary initiation of swallowing. The middle portion of the esophagus is a mixture of skeletal and smooth muscle, and the distal third comprises only smooth muscle.

Although it is relatively fixed at its origin, the esophagus becomes mobile as it traverses the mediastinum. Thus it can be easily displaced by adjacent structures such as an enlarged left atrium or ventricle, a goiter, or a mediastinal tumor. Displacement of the esophagus may alter its shape enough to impede the passage of a food bolus or foreign body.

Clinical Features

Esophageal obstruction may be partial or complete. The patient with complete obstruction is unable to swallow, is often drooling, and may be violently retching in an attempt to regurgitate the obstructing bolus. The patient may complain of pain from the neck to the substernal and epigastric area, although the perceived level of obstruction may not correlate with the actual site of the obstruction.

Proximal obstructions may present as a "cafe coronary," characterized by sudden cyanosis and collapse caused by food (usually an unchewed piece of meat) lodging in the upper esophagus or oropharynx leading to airway obstruction. Similarly, "steakhouse syndrome" results when a large piece of food, usually improperly chewed, is swallowed and causes esophageal obstruction in the distal esophagus. The obstruction may be transient with spontaneous passage of the bolus or may be complete or partial. Intense discomfort develops shortly after swallowing a large piece of meat, and the patient is usually unable to swallow anything else. Ingestion of alcohol and absence of teeth are predisposing factors. Although it may occur in a patient with a normal esophagus, abnormalities such as carcinoma, peptic stricture, or a Schatzki's ring are identified in almost 90% of patients with an esophageal obstruction.[2] Schatzki's ring is a fibrous, diaphragm-like stricture near the gastroesophageal junction present in up to 15% of the population.

Aside from naturally occurring areas of anatomic narrowing, there are other pathologic causes of esophageal stenosis that may lead to symptoms of obstruction. Intrinsic causes of luminal narrowing include carcinoma and webs. An esophageal web is a thin structure composed of mucosa and submucosa. Although webs can occur in isolation, they are also seen in the Plummer-Vinson syndrome, which is characterized by anterior webs, dysphagia, iron deficiency anemia, cheilosis, spooning of the nails, glossitis, and thin friable mucosa in the mouth, pharynx, and upper esophagus. Women 30 to 50 years of age are usually affected. Patients usually present with dysphagia that is initially intermittent and worse with solids. If untreated, it may progress and become more constant.[3]

Extrinsic compression of the esophagus can occur in a variety of conditions. In the neck, thyroid enlargement from goiter or carcinoma may cause dysphagia. Symptoms may also be seen with a pharyngoesophageal or Zenker's diverticulum, a progressive outpouching of the pharyngeal mucosa as a result of increased pressure generated by failure of proper relaxation of the cricopharyngeus muscle. Noisy deglutition, dysphagia, foul breath, and a palpable compressible mass in the neck may be present. Laryngotracheal aspiration when the patient is supine results from the emptying of contents from the diverticulum.

Congenital anomalies of the aortic arch may cause dysphagia in both children and adults. In children, respiratory symptoms are also usually present and commonly predominate. In adults, an anomalous right subclavian artery is the most common vascular cause for dysphagia, which often will not become manifest until the fourth decade of life. The most common symptoms in adults are dyspnea on exertion and dysphagia. Vascular compression of the esophagus with dysphagia may also occur with aneurysms of the aortic arch and great vessels. Bronchogenic carcinoma can cause dysphagia by direct involvement of the esophagus or by compression with nodes.

Esophageal foreign bodies can present atypically in small children or mentally impaired individuals. They may present with choking, refusing to eat, vomiting, blood-stained secretions, or respiratory distress.[4]

Diagnostic Strategies

Plain radiographs of the neck should be obtained if a foreign body in the throat is suspected. Coins are easily visualized. Disk batteries have a characteristic radiographic "double-density" appearance.[5] Small bones or radiopaque objects may be visualized. However, failure to demonstrate a foreign body on radiographs does not rule out its presence.

If available, endoscopy is the procedure of choice for both diagnosing and treating esophageal foreign bodies. When endoscopy is unavailable, a radiographic contrast study may help in diagnosis. However, because of difficulties in performing endoscopy after contrast administration, it may be advisable to consult with the endoscopist before performing any study in a patient with a suspected esophageal foreign body. If an esophageal perforation is suspected, a water-soluble contrast agent (e.g., Gastrografin) should be used first because barium induces an inflammatory response in tissues. However, failure to visualize a clinically suspected perforation warrants a repeat examination utilizing barium as the contrast agent. Since barium may obscure subsequent endoscopic visualization, a minimal amount of thin barium should be used. The use of a swallowed barium-soaked cotton ball to identify the site of obstruction is not recommended because it adds an additional foreign body to be removed.

Plain radiographs followed by contrast studies have false-negative rates of less than 1% and false-positive rates of less than 20%.[6,7] Computed tomography (CT) scanning of the neck and chest may be helpful in identifying a foreign body, as well as in visualizing changes in the surrounding tissues associated with perforation.[8]

Differential Considerations

Esophageal foreign bodies must be distinguished from foreign bodies in the airway. This can be especially difficult in small children. Radiographically, esophageal foreign bodies lie in the frontal plain and are best visualized in anteroposterior (AP) views. Tracheal foreign bodies tend to lie sagittally.

Patients with esophageal obstruction may present with retrosternal pain that can appear similar to an acute ischemic cardiac syndrome. The presence of odynophagia suggests an underlying mucosal lesion.

Management

Flexible endoscopy by an experienced endoscopist is the procedure of choice for removal of esophageal foreign bodies. Other techniques are available to the emergency physician should a qualified endoscopist not be immediately available.

Upper Esophagus Oropharyngeal foreign bodies can usually be removed with a Kelly clamp or McGill forceps under direct visualization. Smooth upper esophageal foreign bodies can often be removed with a Foley catheter. This procedure requires an experienced technician, a cooperative patient, and fluoroscopic guidance. The patient is placed in a prone position, and the catheter is passed into the esophagus past the point of the foreign body impaction. The balloon is then inflated and the catheter withdrawn, pulling the foreign body with it. Controversy exists regarding the safety of this technique because there is no direct control of the foreign body.[9-11] Prophylactic endotracheal intubation may be warranted to prevent the foreign body from entering the airway.

When these maneuvers fail to dislodge the esophageal foreign body, consultation with a qualified endoscopist is indicated.

Lower Esophagus Lower esophageal obstruction is usually the result of an impacted food bolus and can often be treated effectively in the ED. Administration of 1 mg glucagon intravenously (up to a total of 2 mg) may cause enough relaxation of the esophageal smooth muscle to allow passage of the bolus in approximately 50% of patients.[12,13] Because glucagon affects smooth muscle only, it is only effective for impactions in the lower esophagus. Many emergency physicians will give the patient a trial of glucagon while arranging for endoscopy. Side effects of glucagon include vomiting, nausea, dizziness, and flushing. It should not be used in patients with sharp-edged, potentially damaging foreign bodies or in patients with insulinoma, pheochromocytoma, and Zollinger-Ellison syndrome.[14]

Effervescent agents are sometimes effective in accelerating the passage of an obstructing food bolus. Although the mechanism of action is unclear, it is hypothesized that the carbon dioxide released from bubbles escaping the fluid acts to disrupt the impacted food bolus and to distend the distal esophagus. The administration of carbonated beverages (including soft drinks) results in the passage of the obstructing food bolus in 60% to 80% of patients treated.[15,16] Studies combining the use of glucagon and an effervescent agent show rapid relief of symptoms in 65% to 75% of patients.[17,18] It has been recommended that effervescent agents be avoided in cases of complete obstruction and cases where an obstruction has been present for over 24 hours because of the theoretical potential of inducing perforation of a possibly ischemic distal esophagus.[19] The use of meat tenderizer (papain) to soften a food bolus is not recommended. Although intact mucosa is resistant to papain's effects, an inflamed mucosa becomes much more inflamed when exposed to this proteolytic enzyme and is more likely to perforate.[20]

Patients with sharp-edged, distal foreign bodies, those who have contraindications to use of the aforementioned agents, and those who do not respond to treatment should be evaluated with endoscopy. It is unclear whether contrast radiographic studies, performed to document the presence of obstruction, are of any benefit in symptomatic patients.

Endoscopy should be performed immediately for patients experiencing significant distress and for children with impaction of an alkaline button battery. These batteries contain concentrated sodium or potassium hydroxide in addition to metals such as zinc, lithium, and mercury. Leakage of any of these can lead to systemic toxicity. Larger batteries have greater risk of impaction and leakage. Batteries that pass into the stomach should be followed radiographically and clinically to ensure passage. Assistance with the management of a patient with button battery ingestion can be obtained though the National Button Battery Ingestion Hotline at (202) 525-3333.

Urgent intervention is also indicated for sharp objects, disk batteries, coins in the proximal esophagus, and impactions that impair the handling of secretions.[21] It is unclear whether patients with mild to moderate symptoms of esophageal obstruction from a suspected food bolus require immediate endoscopy. In such cases, some authors believe that emergent intervention is unnecessary if the patient is still able to handle secretions because the bolus will often pass on its own.[22] Others believe that the softened bolus makes endoscopic removal more difficult and predisposes to complications.[23] Any object remaining in the esophagus for over 24 hours carries a higher risk of complications.

Most authors advocate follow-up endoscopic evaluation in all cases after an esophageal obstruction to rule out underlying pathologic conditions.

Stomach Certain foreign bodies that pass into the stomach still require endoscopic retrieval. Objects longer than 5 cm and wider than 2 cm will rarely pass the stomach. All sharp and pointed foreign bodies (e.g., toothpicks, bones) should be removed before they pass the stomach because 15% to 35% may cause intestinal perforation.[24] Smaller objects that pass into the stomach can be followed with stool inspections and with serial radiographs if necessary to ensure passage.

ESOPHAGEAL PERFORATION

Perspective

Esophageal perforation is a potentially life-threatening condition that must be identified and treated early to minimize morbidity and mortality. Although first reported by Boerhaave in the early 1700s as a result of forceful vomiting, it can also result from any Valsalva-like maneuver, including childbirth, cough, or heavy lifting. In modern times, spontaneous perforation accounts for only 15% of cases, with iatrogenic injuries accounting for the remainder. These usually occur as a complication of upper endoscopy, dilation, sclerotherapy, or other GI procedures. It has also been reported as a complication of both nasogastric tube placement and endotracheal intubation, including after the use of the esophagotracheal Combitube.[25,26] Other causes of perforation include foreign body ingestion, caustic substance ingestion, severe esophagitis, carcinoma, and direct injury due to blunt or penetrating trauma.

Principles of Disease

Over 90% of spontaneous esophageal ruptures occur in the distal esophagus. In contrast, rupture resulting from blunt trauma to the neck or thorax usually occurs in the proximal and middle third of the esophagus. Most iatrogenic injuries occur at the pharyngoesophageal junction, since the wall in this area is thin, and there is no serosal layer to reinforce it. Another site of frequent iatrogenic injury is the esophagogastric junction. In this area, the esophagus curves anteriorly and to the left as it enters the abdomen, and an endoscope has a greater likelihood of perforating the posterior wall.

Once a perforation occurs, saliva and gastric contents can enter the mediastinum. Rapid spread of an infectious or inflammatory response to the surrounding tissues and organs occurs because of the thinness of the esophageal wall. Changes in intrathoracic pressure during respiration draw contaminants deeper into the mediastinum. The presence of gastric enzymes and other foreign material in the mediastinum induces an intense inflammatory response that may result in enough fluid buildup to displace adjacent structures.

Clinical Features

The presenting features vary with the site of injury. Patients with an upper esophageal perforation usually present with neck or chest pain, dysphagia, respiratory distress, and fever.

Odynophagia, nausea, vomiting, hoarseness, or aphonia may also result.

Perforation of the lower esophagus may present with abdominal pain, pneumothorax, hydropneumothorax, and pneumomediastinum.[27] The pain often radiates into the back, to the left side of the chest, and to the left or both shoulders.[28,29] Most patients have mediastinal or cervical emphysema, which may be noted by palpation or by a "crunching" sound heard during auscultation (Hamman's sign). Abdominal examination may reveal epigastric or generalized abdominal tenderness, often with guarding and involuntary rigidity. Patients with severe mediastinitis may present in fulminant shock.

Pain or fever following esophageal instrumentation should be considered a perforation until proven otherwise. It should be noted that symptoms due to iatrogenic perforation may not appear until several hours after the procedure.

Diagnostic Strategies

Radiographic studies are used to establish the diagnosis of an esophageal perforation. A chest radiograph and an upright abdominal radiograph are usually obtained first. Radiographic abnormalities may be detected in up to 90% of patients, and include findings such as subcutaneous emphysema, pneumomediastinum, mediastinal widening, pleural effusion, or pulmonary infiltrate.[30] Radiographic changes may not be present in the first few hours following the perforation.

Patients with suspected perforation should have contrast radiographic studies performed. Barium sulfate is superior in identifying small perforations; however, it may incite an inflammatory response in tissues. For this reason, water-soluble agents (e.g., Gastrografin) should be used first. If a clinically suspected perforation is not identified, the examination should be repeated using barium.

CT of the chest may be used if a contrast study does not demonstrate a clinically suspected perforation. Findings such as mediastinal air, extraluminal contrast, or fluid collections or abscesses adjacent to the esophagus confirm a perforation. These can be found after the initial perforation has healed. CT scan also allows evaluation of other adjacent areas that may suggest an alternate diagnosis. Endoscopy may be useful, especially in cases of trauma; however, small perforations may be difficult or impossible to visualize.

Laboratory studies are usually not helpful early after a perforation, although an elevated white blood count may be noted.

Differential Considerations

Misdiagnosis occurs in more than half of patients with esophageal rupture because the differential diagnosis includes the numerous causes of chest and abdominal pain including pulmonary embolism, acute myocardial infarction, aortic dissection, perforated ulcer, pneumothorax, lung abscess, pericarditis, or pancreatitis. It is important that esophageal perforations be diagnosed as soon as possible, since the morbidity and mortality of the disorder increase with time.

Management

Certain patients with esophageal perforation require aggressive management. These include patients with Boerhaave's syndrome, clinically unstable patients, patients with perforations that contaminate the mediastinum or pleura, patients with intraabdominal perforations, or patients with perforations with an associated pneumothorax.[31] Broad-spectrum intravenous antibiotics should be initiated early. The combination of a second-generation cephalosporin and an aminoglycoside usually provides adequate coverage.[32] Patients should be kept NPO, and a nasogastric tube should be considered to eliminate oral and gastric secretions. Early surgical consultation is warranted.

There is growing evidence that some perforations can be managed conservatively with close observation in certain low-risk patients. These patients would include those who are clinically stable (minimal symptoms and fever with no clinical signs of shock), those whose perforation resulted from endoscopic injury following dilation, and those who present a long time after their procedure and have demonstrated no ill effects. The latter patients usually have small perforations of the cervical esophagus.[33-35] Most authors advocate treatment with suction and antibiotics as noted above.

ESOPHAGITIS

Perspective

Esophagitis is defined as inflammation of the esophagus. The most common cause of esophagitis is gastroesophageal reflux disease (GERD), which is discussed in the following section. Other important causes of esophagitis that may be encountered in the ED include infectious esophagitis, pill esophagitis, and injuries from the effects of caustic ingestion, radiation, or sclerotherapy.

Principles of Disease

Infectious Esophagitis Esophageal infections in the immunocompetent host are relatively rare. Iatrogenic alterations in host defenses through the use of immunosuppressive agents, potent chemotherapeutic agents, and broad-spectrum antibiotics have increased the incidence of esophageal infections. The spread of the human immunodeficiency virus (HIV) has also led to an increase in esophageal infection, although the epidemiology has been changing as more effective antiretroviral agents have become available. In addition to iatrogenic immunosuppression, diseases that weaken immunologic defenses in otherwise normal hosts can also predispose the esophagus to infections. These conditions include diabetes mellitus, alcoholism, underlying malignancy, use of corticosteroids, and advanced age. Changes that occur in the mucosal barrier of the esophagus as a result of these conditions result in an increased susceptibility to infection. The *Candida* species (primarily *Candida albicans*) are the most common esophageal pathogens.

The use of inhaled steroids for asthma has led to candidal infection in otherwise healthy patients. As empiric antifungal prophylaxis in immunosuppressive states has become more common, viral esophagitis has become more prominent. Herpes simplex 1 and cytomegalovirus are the most common viral pathogens. Bacteria, mycobacteria, other fungi, and parasitic organisms such as *Trypanosoma cruzi, Cryptosporidium,* and *Pneumocystis* are uncommon causes of infectious esophagitis and are usually diagnosed by culture or biopsy.

Pill Esophagitis Pill esophagitis is estimated to occur in approximately 10,000 people per year in the United States.[36] However, because most cases are unreported, the true incidence is unknown. It results when a pill or capsule fails to pass into the stomach and remains in contact with the esophageal mucosa for a prolonged period. The contents can become exposed, resulting in inflammation and injury. It has been reported in all age groups. Predisposing factors include advanced age, decreased esophageal motility, and extrinsic compression. Large pills are more likely to be retained, as are those coated with gelatin. It should be noted that pills can stick to a normal esophagus, especially when taken without water or while in the supine position. Any area of the esophagus can be affected, although sites of natural compression may be more susceptible. Sustained-release compounds may be more damaging than standard preparations.[36] Injury can range from minor irritation to frank ulceration, hemorrhage, and ultimately stricture formation. Some of the more common offending medications include antibiotics (especially the tetracycline family) and antivirals, aspirin and other nonsteroidal antiinflammatory drugs (NSAIDs), potassium chloride, quinidine, ferrous sulfate, alprenolol, alendronate, and pamidronate.

Other Causes Esophagitis from caustic substance ingestion occurs most commonly in children, although adults may do so in a suicide attempt. Strongly acidic or alkaline substances are the offending agents. The degree of injury depends on the concentration of the substance, the volume ingested, and the time in contact with tissue. Strong acids produce coagulation necrosis, which results in eschar formation that usually limits the damage. In contrast, alkali produces liquefaction necrosis, which continues to injure as long as the substance is in contact with tissue.[37]

Patients undergoing radiation treatment for underlying malignancy may develop esophagitis. The degree of injury is related to the total dosage of radiation received. The mucosa becomes inflamed and friable. Agents used during sclerotherapy can also cause esophagitis.

Clinical Features

Bleeding can result from esophagitis of any type. This can range from localized oozing as a result of inflammation to frank hemorrhage. Ulceration and perforation can also result. Inflammation may also spread to surrounding tissues, resulting in complications such as mediastinitis.

Infectious Esophagitis Most commonly, infectious esophagitis causes severe odynophagia. Dysphagia of both solids and liquids may also be present. Pain may be so severe that the patient refuses to eat or drink. Chest pain may also be present, and may be described as acute in onset, constant, and not affected by standard antacid measures. Heartburn and nausea may also be presenting symptoms. Some immunocompromised patients may have fever or bleeding without dysphagia or odynophagia.

Pill Esophagitis Patients with pill esophagitis present with odynophagia. Most patients have no prior history of esophageal disease and present with sudden onset of pain worsened by swallowing. Dysphagia may be present. Although some patients may present complaining of a pill that has become "stuck," the history of pill ingestion may be difficult to obtain because symptoms may begin hours after the offending pill is taken. Atypical presentations include a burning type pain suggesting GERD as the etiology.

Other Patients with caustic injuries may present with pain in the mouth, chest, or epigastrium. Dysphagia and vomiting may be present. Patients may be drooling. Airway compromise may be present due to direct injury or resulting edema. Later, perforation may occur, and strictures are a common long-term complication. Radiation-induced esophagitis usually causes odynophagia and dysphagia. Strictures may ultimately develop.

Diagnostic Strategies

Endoscopy is the best method of diagnosing both pill-induced and infectious esophagitis. With infectious esophagitis, direct visualization may reveal characteristic signs of infection, such as white plaques of Candida or herpetic vesicles. Definitive diagnosis can be made via brushings and biopsies. Radiographic studies are usually not helpful because the findings are nonspecific. A strong clinical suspicion is necessary to diagnose pill esophagitis. The other causes of esophagitis are usually clinically apparent.

Differential Considerations

Symptoms of esophagitis include dysphagia and odynophagia. Chest pain may also be a component, and therefore an acute coronary syndrome must be considered. Esophageal pain is more likely to be positional and related to swallowing. Other causes of esophageal pain include GERD, esophageal motility disorder, foreign body, and perforation.

Management

Infectious Esophagitis For infectious esophagitis, therapy should be directed at the causative organism. Candidal esophagitis can be treated with some of the newer antifungal agents such as fluconazole (200 mg po daily for 3 to 4 weeks), ketoconazole (300 to 400 mg po daily for 3 to 4 weeks), or itraconazole (100 to 200 mg po daily for 3 to 4 weeks).[38] Initial treatment for herpes simplex esophagitis includes antivirals such as acyclovir (400 mg po 5 times per day for 7 to 14 days or 5 to 10 mg/kg IV q 8 hr for 7 to 14 days), famciclovir (500 mg po tid for 7 to 14 days), or valacyclovir (500 mg po bid for 7 to 14 days).[39] For cytomegalovirus, initial treatment can begin with ganciclovir (5 mg/kg IV q 12 hr for 2 to 3 weeks) or foscarnet (60 mg/kg IV q 8 hr or 90 mg/kg IV q 12 hr for 2 to 3 weeks).[40] It should be noted that optimal treatment regimens have not yet been described.

If the causative organism cannot be adequately identified, or if the patient is severely debilitated, admission to the hospital may be required. For patients discharged from the ED, follow-up should be arranged as appropriate (e.g., gastroenterology, infectious disease). In addition to antibiotic therapy directed at the infecting organism, treatment with antacids, topical anesthetics, or sucralfate may provide symptomatic relief.

Pill Esophagitis If a patient with suspected pill esophagitis has persistent symptoms, endoscopy may be necessary. It will also help determine alternate etiologies. The best treatment for pill esophagitis is prevention. Patients should be instructed to drink at least 4 ounces of liquid with any pill. All medications should be taken in an upright position, and should remain upright for several minutes following medication ingestion. Patients with underlying esophageal abnormalities, or those that are bedridden, should avoid the use of pills whenever practical. No data exist supporting any specific treatment, although intuitively anti-acid medication may prevent further erosion of damaged mucosa.[41]

Other Management of caustic injuries includes rinsing of the mouth and dilution of the substance with water. Airway compromise or involvement may require aggressive management. Emesis or gastric lavage is contraindicated, since it reexposes tissues to the agent. Charcoal is not indicated. Patients usually undergo delayed endoscopy to evaluate the extent of injury. A patient who presents with the history of caustic substance ingestion without obvious clinical findings should be admitted and observed.

Treatment of radiation esophagitis is supportive. Patients who cannot eat or drink should be admitted for intravenous fluid therapy.

GASTROESOPHAGEAL REFLUX DISEASE

Perspective

Asymptomatic reflux of gastric contents from the stomach into the esophagus occurs in most people several times a day as a normal physiologic phenomenon. When reflux becomes symptomatic, or histopathologic alteration in the upper gastrointestinal or respiratory tract results from these episodes, GERD is said to exist. In the United States, symptomatic reflux in the form of heartburn occurs daily in 7% of adults, weekly in 14%, and monthly in 40%.[42]

Principles of Disease

In the normal individual, several mechanisms prevent reflux of gastric contents into the esophagus. The major barrier to gastroesophageal reflux is the lower esophageal sphincter (LES). The anatomic relationship between the cardia of the stomach and the left side of the esophagus (known as the angle of His) contributes to prevention of reflux. When reflux does occur, gravity, peristalsis, normal swallowing of saliva, and secretions from esophageal glands help clear refluxed gastric contents back into the stomach. Factors operate at the mucosal level to minimize the damage caused by refluxate.[43] The presence of a hiatal hernia (a prolapse of a portion of the stomach through the diaphragmatic esophageal hiatus), formerly thought to be synonymous with GERD, plays a variable role in contributing to the symptoms of GERD.[44]

Clinical Features

Symptoms The most common manifestation of GERD is reflux esophagitis, of which the most common symptom is heartburn, defined as a burning sensation that begins in the subxiphoid area and radiates toward the neck. Reflux may also cause a dull discomfort, localized pressure, or severe squeezing pain across the middle of the chest. This type of pain has been postulated to be a result of acid-induced esophageal spasm, but this is believed to be uncommon. The patient may appear comfortable or may have associated diaphoresis, pallor, nausea, and vomiting, leading to the consideration of an ischemic cardiac syndrome. A detailed history is often helpful in differentiating cardiac chest pain from reflux, although the distinction may not be possible in the ED.

Other symptoms of GERD include regurgitation (the spontaneous appearance of acid or bitter material in the mouth or pharynx) or water brash (a vagally mediated hypersalivation response that may produce as much as 10 ml of saliva in 1 minute). Dysphagia and odynophagia may also be a presenting complaint, and may be associated with more serious complications (see below).

Any condition or agent that decreases LES pressure, decreases esophageal motility, or prolongs gastric emptying will predispose patients to reflux (Box 84-1). Positions that place the esophagus in a dependent position to the stomach or increase intraabdominal pressure tend to precipitate reflux. Stooping, bending, leaning forward, Valsalva-type maneuvers, and assuming a supine position are common precipitants.

GERD can manifest itself in extraesophageal locations. Reflux-induced asthma may result from either aspiration of gastric contents into the lung or activation of a vagal reflex arc from the gut to the lung. Although both asthma and GERD have been shown to coexist in many individuals, it is difficult to identify GERD as the etiology of the asthma, and there is no diagnostic test to define which patients have GERD-associated asthma.[45-47] Chronic persistent cough (without wheezing) can also result from reflux.[48]

If the refluxate reaches the proximal esophagus, otolaryngologic manifestations may result, even in the absence of esophageal symptoms. Laryngeal and tracheal stenosis can result from repeated exposure to refluxate; it is postulated that subglottic stenosis in patients intubated for prolonged periods may be due to GERD.[49] GERD may also cause dysphonia, cough, globus sensation, repetitive throat clearing, and frequent sore throat or laryngitis.[50] Refluxate that enters the oropharynx may lead to dental problems, such as erosion of the lingual sides of the teeth as a result of acid exposure.

Complications Repetitive exposure to acid can lead to changes in the esophageal mucosa. Continued reflux can lead to thinning of the normal stratified squamous epithelial layer. With the development of esophagitis, an inflammatory

Box 84-1 Agents and Conditions Related to Gastroesophageal Reflux

Decreased LES Pressure
- Anticholinergic drugs
- Benzodiazepines
- Caffeine
- Calcium channel blockers
- Chocolate
- Ethanol
- Fatty foods
- Nicotine
- Nitrates
- Peppermint
- Progesterone, estrogen, pregnancy

Decreased Esophageal Motility
- Achalasia
- Diabetes mellitus
- Scleroderma

Increased Gastic Emptying Time
- Anticholinergic drugs
- Diabetic gastroparesis
- Gastric outlet obstruction

response occurs within the mucosa and submucosa with infiltration of polymorphonuclear leukocytes. The inflammatory response is the result of chemical irritation of the esophageal mucosa from reflux of gastric acid, pepsin, and bile acids. Both acid and alkaline reflux produce the same pathologic changes. Continued exposure can lead to further endoscopically visible changes of erosion, ulceration, and scarring. Ultimately stricture formation may result. The most severe histologic consequence of GERD is replacement of the normal stratified squamous epithelium with metaplastic columnar epithelium in a condition known as Barrett metaplasia. Histologically, it is characterized by a villous architecture with goblet cells. There is a strong correlation between the development of Barrett metaplasia and adenocarcinoma of the esophagus.

Diagnostic Strategies

GERD is a common problem, and additional diagnostic testing is rarely necessary, assuming other more serious etiologies of the patient's symptoms have been excluded. Patients with dysphagia or odynophagia should be referred for further study.

Differential Considerations

The emergency physician must not fail to consider acute ischemic cardiac syndromes as the cause of the patient's symptoms. Radiation of pain is an inconstant finding in both esophageal and cardiac chest pain. The pain seen with reflux may radiate into the neck, jaws, shoulders, back, arms, and abdomen. Radiation into the back is more often ascribed to the esophagus. Radiation of pain into one arm or into the neck or jaw is not a helpful distinguishing feature. Radiation of pain into the abdomen is present approximately three times more often in reflux than in ischemic heart disease. Radiation into both arms is rarely seen in reflux, whereas it may be present in approximately one quarter of patients with ischemic heart disease. Precipitation of pain by exercise and relief by rest may occur in pain from reflux, as well as in ischemic heart disease. Emotional precipitation of pain occurs in reflux, although it is also seen with coronary artery disease.[51] The occurrence of reflux after meals is another important feature in the history. A feeling of "fullness" after meals occurs commonly and is helpful in differentiating reflux from coronary artery disease.

Relief of chest pain from reflux by antacids is a key point in the history; however, the emergency physician should not place too much weight upon this point as evidence against a cardiac etiology. The relief is often short lived, and pain may recur in a short time. Esophageal pain may be brought on by swallowing. The physical examination in patients with esophageal reflux is not usually helpful in diagnosis. Thus the history is by far the most valuable aid.[52] The emergency physician must maintain an acute awareness of the diverse presentations of ischemic heart disease, however, and should be cautious in attributing chest pain to esophageal causes based solely on historical elements.

Management

Because of the multifactorial causes of GERD, many treatment options exist. Pharmacologic therapy of GERD includes acid-neutralizing agents, agents that decrease acid production, agents that act on the LES or affect motility, and agents that protect the mucosa. Most gastroenterologists recommend a stepwise approach to the treatment of GERD. The first step requires lifestyle modification. Patients should be instructed to avoid sleeping in the fully recumbent position to both decrease the number of reflux episodes and to facilitate clearance of refluxate. The following should also be avoided: eating before retiring at night; wearing tight garments and heavy physical exercise after meals; anticholinergic drugs or consumption of foods or agents that decrease LES tone such as cigarettes and alcohol; and direct irritants to the esophagus such as coffee, citrus fruit, and tomato-based products.[53] Overweight patients may experience relief with weight loss. Avoidance of fatty foods and consumption of smaller meals may also help alleviate symptoms. Many patients will self-medicate with antacids or over-the-counter-strength H_2 receptor antagonists, which have been demonstrated to relieve and prevent symptoms.[54]

Patients may present to the ED when self-directed therapy has failed. The next step adds the use of prescription-strength H_2 blockers, which have become the main method of therapy for GERD. Endoscopic healing has been noted in 70% to 90% of patients with mild esophagitis who are treated with H_2 blockers.[55,56] The success rate is less for severe esophagitis, although symptomatic improvement may occur in the absence of endoscopic improvement. Higher doses than those recommended for gastric disorders are frequently necessary, and bid dosing is recommended. Choices include cimetidine 400 mg po bid, ranitidine 150 mg po bid, famotidine 20 mg po bid, or nizatidine 150 mg po bid. These agents are generally regarded as safe and effective, although some question the long-term effects of acid suppression on stomach bacterial flora.[57]

Previously, some physicians used a prokinetic drug for patients whose symptoms suggest a superimposed motility disturbance (e.g., regurgitation, choking, abdominal distention). In addition to improving propulsive activity of the stomach and small and large intestine, the increased esophageal peristalsis and LES tone would make it effective therapy for reflux by improving the clearance of refluxate.[58] Cisapride (Propulsid) was formerly used for this purpose, but was withdrawn from the marketplace by the manufacturer because of adverse cardiac effects.

Patients whose symptoms fail to respond despite the above treatment are candidates for dual therapy with a proton pump inhibitor (PPI). These drugs have been demonstrated to be more efficacious than H_2 blockers, presumptively due to the greater degree of acid suppression.[59] The long-term use of PPIs has been associated with consequences such as bacterial proliferation, changes in the gastric mucosa, delayed gastric emptying, and hyperplasia of enterochromaffin-like cells, so these patients should be followed closely.

Patients who fail to respond to all of the above measures should be referred to a gastroenterologist for further diagnostic evaluation, such as esophageal manometry or ambulatory pH monitoring. Medically refractory patients may be candidates for antireflux surgery.

Another agent that may be of benefit in refractory cases of symptomatic esophageal reflux is sucralfate, the salt of aluminum hydroxide and sucrose octasulfate. It may have an advantage in that it also absorbs and inactivates bile salts.[60-62] This is not a Food and Drug Administration (FDA)–approved indication for its use.

Although the emergency physician can initiate antireflux therapy, the patient with clinically suspected reflux should be referred to a physician capable of performing further diagnostic tests to confirm the diagnosis and provide follow-up care. Further testing may include esophageal pH monitoring, an upper GI series, esophageal manometry, or esophagoscopy.[63]

GASTRITIS

Perspective

Strictly speaking, gastritis is a histologic diagnosis denoting inflammation of the gastric mucosa. Hence, the diagnosis of gastritis can only be made by endoscopy and biopsy. However, it is common practice for clinicians to use the term *gastritis* to refer to symptoms of dyspepsia. To further confuse the picture, gastroenterologists will frequently use the term to refer to the endoscopic finding of an edematous, friable mucosa. However, without accompanying inflammation, this is more appropriately termed gastropathy rather than gastritis.[64] Controversy exists regarding how to best classify the entities that cause gastritis or gastropathy. This section will consider gastritis and gastropathy together as one entity, since the distinction makes little difference in the ED setting. Regardless of the cause, up to 50% of the population will have endoscopic evidence of gastritis or gastropathy by age 50.

Principles of Disease

The most common cause of gastritis is infection with *Helicobacter pylori.* Although most patients are asymptomatic at the time of initial exposure, acute infection with *H. pylori* can cause severe gastritis and upper gastrointestinal symptoms. Suppurative gastritis (also known as *acute phlegmonous gastritis*) can result from a bacterial infection of the stomach wall, usually from a gram-positive coccus or a gram-negative rod. Patients usually have an underlying mucosal abnormality such as cancer, ulcer, or preexisting gastritis.[65] Rarer infectious causes of gastritis include mycobacterial, viral, parasitic, and fungal organisms.

Gastritis can also result from exposure to drugs. Aspirin or other NSAIDs are the most common offending agents. Inflammation occurs as a result of prostaglandin inhibition both locally and systemically, and is probably a precursor to gastric ulcer formation. Other drugs implicated in causing gastritis are potassium preparations and iron supplements.

Gastritis can result from both short- and long-term exposure to ethanol, although some authors feel that the long-term effects are more likely due to *H. pylori* rather than the ethanol itself.

The presence of corrosive agents in the stomach can induce gastritis. Intrinsic substances such as bile or ingested substances such as acids, alkali, and corrosive agents can induce an inflammatory response and subsequent gastritis.

Any condition that causes hypovolemia and/or hypotension can lead to gastritis. Ulcer formation may ultimately result. This may be a major causative factor in intensive care unit patients who develop gastritis and upper gastrointestinal bleeding.

Other causes of gastritis include radiation, autoimmune reactions, Crohn's disease, and sarcoidosis. These disorders can only be diagnosed by biopsy.

Clinical Features

There are no symptoms that are characteristic of gastritis. Acute gastritis may cause abdominal pain, nausea, and vomiting, although most patients are asymptomatic unless ulcers or other complications develop. By definition, it is not possible to diagnose gastritis or gastropathy based on clinical features alone. However, a good clinical history such as recent NSAID use or alcohol ingestion in the setting of the above symptoms may enable the emergency physician to make a presumptive clinical diagnosis of gastritis.

Acute infection with *H. pylori* may cause epigastric abdominal pain, nausea, and vomiting. Systemic signs such as fever are usually absent. Symptoms may last days to weeks. If the infection goes untreated, chronic gastritis may result. Patients with phlegmonous gastritis usually present with a toxic appearance. Patients with gastritis as a result of decreased mucosal blood flow may present with symptoms of abdominal pain and upper GI bleeding, in addition to those of their underlying disease.

Complications of gastritis include perforation and gastric outlet obstruction.

Diagnostic Strategies

Because the diagnosis of gastritis is usually made empirically in the ED, no specific diagnostic tests are necessary. Ancillary tests should be ordered as clinically indicated to rule out other possible diagnoses or to assess for complications of gastritis such as bleeding, obstruction, or perforation.

Differential Considerations

Before making the diagnosis of gastritis, other diseases that cause nausea, vomiting, and upper abdominal pain must be excluded. These include pancreatitis, biliary tract disease, and small bowel obstruction.

Management

Treatment of presumptive gastritis can be started in the ED. H_2 antagonists have been shown to improve symptoms of dyspepsia in patients taking NSAIDs. Dosages should begin at the low end and be tapered up as necessary. Patients with persistent symptoms should be referred to a gastroenterologist for further diagnostic evaluation.

PEPTIC ULCER DISEASE

Perspective

Gastric and duodenal ulcers are usually grouped together as peptic ulcer disease (PUD) because of the similarity in their pathogenesis and treatment. Approximately 4 million people in the United States are affected by PUD each year.[66] The annual cost to the health care system is estimated to be over 15 billion dollars.[67] Increased understanding of the etiology and pathogenesis of PUD over the past decade has led to the advent of new and effective therapies. PUD is now considered to have two main etiologies: *H. pylori* infection and NSAID use. Approximately 1% of PUD is caused by increased levels of circulating gastrin from gastrin-secreting tumors (Zollinger-Ellison syndrome). These patients have increased parietal cell mass and hypersecretion of acid leading to ulcer formation.

Principles of Disease

Histologically, the stomach comprises different types of cells with varying secretory functions. Mucous cells secrete acidic mucus, parietal cells secrete hydrochloric acid (via the hydrogen-potassium ATPase, the "proton pump") and intrinsic factor, chief cells secrete pepsinogens, and enterochromaffin-like cells release substances such as histamine and gastrin. Acid secreted by the parietal cells can generate a hydrogen ion concentration gradient of greater than one million to one within the lumen of the stomach.

Many mechanisms exist to protect the gastric mucosa from the digestive effects of the hydrochloric acid, proteolytic enzymes, bile, and other injurious substances to which it is exposed. Normally a gastric mucosal barrier to intraluminal gastric acid is present and prevents the back-diffusion of hydrogen ions from the gastric lumen. Sodium ions are barred from moving in the opposite direction. This ionic impermeability protects the gastric mucosa from damage in a hostile environment. Damage to the gastric mucosal barrier from any cause (Box 84-2) will allow hydrogen ions and digestive enzymes to contact the gastric mucosa, leading to inflammation, bleeding, and potential ulceration.

The identification of *H. pylori* has proven to be a landmark discovery that has markedly changed our understanding of peptic ulcer disease. *H. pylori* is an S-shaped, gram-negative rod whose natural habitat is the human stomach between the epithelial cell surface and the overlying mucus. Infection with *H. pylori* is a primary risk factor for development of PUD. It is estimated that 95% of patients with duodenal ulcer and 84% of patients with gastric ulcer are infected with *H. pylori.*[68] *H. pylori* is more prevalent in lower socioeconomic groups and is probably spread via the fecal-oral route, although oral to oral and iatrogenic transmission have been suggested. It is found in all age groups, although it is believed that infection is acquired during childhood. Its presence is believed to cause mucosal inflammation that disrupts the normal defense mechanisms and leads to ulceration. It also increases the risk of gastric carcinoma and, less often, lymphoma. Not all people infected with *H. pylori* develop PUD, and it is unclear what role environmental and host factors such as diet play. It is now accepted that almost all non–NSAID-related ulcers are due to *H. pylori.* Eradication of infection with *H. pylori* results in more rapid healing of ulcers, prevents relapse, and diminishes the rate of ulcer complications. The most effective means of diagnosis and optimal management, including the most effective antibiotic regimens, are still being defined. Currently available tests include a urea breath test, antibody testing, and direct mucosal biopsy during endoscopy. As of yet, none of these are of practical use for the ED patient.

The second most common cause of peptic ulcer formation is the use of NSAIDs. NSAIDs have both a direct and indirect effect on the gastric mucosa. NSAIDs are weak acids that remain in the nonionized form in the acidic milieu of the stomach lumen. This allows free diffusion into the mucosal cells, where ionization occurs. Since ionized forms cannot cross the cell membrane, the NSAID becomes "ion trapped" within the cell. The increased intracellular concentration of NSAID damages the cell, most likely as a result of inhibition of mucosal prostaglandin secretion, reduced mucus production, and diminished cell turnover.[69] Since administration of enteric coated NSAIDs that are not absorbed in the stomach does not diminish the incidence of ulcer formation, a second systemic mechanism of injury also exists. It is believed that the inhibition of cyclooxygenase by NSAIDs leads to a diminished level of protective prostaglandins in the stomach. Additionally, the antiplatelet aggregation effect of NSAIDs may increase the amount of bleeding associated with the development of NSAID-induced ulcers. It should be noted that NSAIDs differ in their ulcerogenic potential, with ibuprofen having one of the lowest risks of GI toxicity.[70]

PUD also occurs in infants and children. Infants with PUD usually present with poor feeding, vomiting, or failure to thrive, but hematemesis may be the first sign. Toddlers and preschool children may have abdominal pain or vomiting and bleeding. Eighty percent of ulcers in this age group are stress ulcers. Older children and adolescents usually have primary PUD, with presentations similar to that of adults.

Box 84-2 Substances and Conditions That Damage the Gastric Mucosal Barrier

Bile
Cigarette smoking
Ethanol
Glucocorticoids
Helicobacter pylori
NSAIDs
Pancreatic secretions
Shock states
Stress

Clinical Features

Presenting Symptoms The most common symptom of PUD is abdominal pain, occurring in 94% of patients with an ulcer.[71] Classically, ulcer pain is described as nonradiating epigastric pain of a burning or gnawing quality, although pain in the chest, back, or other areas of the abdomen may be noted. It usually occurs 2 to 3 hours following a meal or at night. Pain that awakens a patient from sleep between midnight and 3 AM is classic for ulcer disease because gastric acid output is high at about 2 AM in most people. Ulcer pain is usually not present on awakening in the morning because gastric acid output is at its lowest at this time. Colicky pain is rarely gastric or duodenal in origin. Well-defined periods of exacerbation and remission are usually present with duodenal ulcer and aid in the diagnosis. A constant pain for weeks or months at a time is uncommonly caused by ulcer disease. Relief of pain after eating is another feature of gastric or duodenal ulcer. The pain from duodenal ulcer is usually worse immediately preceding a meal, and the complex of pain-eating-relief is typical for duodenal ulcer.

Although some patients with ulcers may vomit, consideration of alternate diagnoses such as gastric volvulus, gastric outlet obstruction, small bowel obstruction, pancreatitis, or biliary tract disease should be considered first. Relief of abdominal pain with antacids is an important aspect of the history. Antacids usually afford relief of pain in both PUD and gastritis. Ninety percent of patients with PUD have pain relief with antacids, and 75% with gastritis have relief. Patients with duodenal ulcer usually experience pain relief within 5 minutes.

Physical findings in patients with PUD are usually minimal. Mild epigastric tenderness may be elicited. A positive stool guaiac may be evidence of a bleeding ulcer, but other causes of occult bleeding must be considered.

Complications The most serious complications of PUD include hemorrhage, perforation, penetration, and gastric outlet obstruction. Hemorrhage is the most common complication, occurring in 15% of patients. Older patients are at greater risk. Approximately 7% of patients will experience perforation, which occurs when an ulcer erodes through the wall and leaks air and digestive contents into the peritoneal cavity. Penetration is pathologically similar to perforation, except that the ulcer erodes into another organ such as the liver (usually from a gastric ulcer) or the pancreas (usually from a duodenal ulcer) instead of into the peritoneal cavity. Gastric outlet obstruction occurs in 2% of ulcer patients, as a result of edema and scarring near the gastroduodenal junction. Symptoms may manifest as gastroesophageal reflux, early satiety, weight loss, abdominal pain, and vomiting.

Pain patterns may be helpful in diagnosing some of the complications of PUD. Pain from a perforated duodenal ulcer is usually appreciated first in the epigastrium but becomes generalized within a short time. Vomiting is present in 50% of patients, and peritoneal findings usually result. Pneumoperitoneum commonly occurs after duodenal ulcer perforation, and the accumulated air under the diaphragm may cause referred pain to the shoulder. One or both shoulders may be involved, depending on the location of the free air.

A history of ulcerlike anterior abdominal pain that begins to radiate into the back suggests penetration of a duodenal ulcer. The pain is usually described as steady, and is perceived at the level of the lower thoracic and upper lumbar vertebrae. Relief of the pain with antacids and food often vanishes, and the pain becomes refractory to treatment. Also, pain radiation may occur to the chest, right upper quadrant, and left upper quadrant in up to 20% of patients. The sudden onset of pain, especially if unrelated to eating, suggests either ulcer perforation or gastric volvulus.

Diagnostic Strategies

The initial diagnosis of PUD is usually made clinically. Ancillary tests may be of benefit in evaluating possible complications of PUD in patients who present in distress. They may also be of benefit in providing indirect evidence of another disease. A complete blood count (CBC) may diagnose anemia, and liver enzymes may help elucidate a hepatic or biliary tree etiology. Electrolytes may provide indirect evidence of disease, and amylase and lipase should be considered to rule out pancreatitis, and may provide indirect evidence of a posterior penetrating ulcer.

Abdominal and chest radiographs should be ordered if perforation or penetration is suspected or if a pulmonary etiology is being considered, although negative films do not definitively rule out these diagnoses. Electrocardiography should be performed in any patient suspected of having a cardiac etiology. Any female patient of childbearing age should have a pregnancy test performed. As noted earlier, several methods exist for diagnosing infection with *H. pylori,* although at this time none is of practical application in the ED.

Differential Considerations

Fifty percent of patients with symptoms of dyspepsia will have no identifiable etiology. These patients are classified as having non-ulcer dyspepsia (NUD). The official criteria for diagnosing NUD are chronic recurrent upper abdominal pain or discomfort for a period of at least 1 month, with symptoms present more than 25% of the time, and an absence of evidence of organic disease.[72]

NUD may be caused by peptic ulcers that are not yet large enough to appear endoscopically. Gastritis due to hypersecretion of gastric acid, *H. pylori* infection, bile reflux, or viral infection may cause NUD, although these should be identifiable endoscopically or pathologically. Maldigestion or malabsorption of carbohydrates can present as NUD in patients with lactase deficiency or in patients who consume large quantities of nonabsorbable sugars such as sorbitol, mannitol, and fructose. Intestinal parasites such as *Giardia lamblia* or *Strongyloides stercoralis* may cause NUD, as can chronic pancreatitis. NUD may also be caused by gastric motility disorders, which have been reported in 25% to 60% of patients with NUD. Abnormalities in the biliary tract such as increased resting pressure of the sphincter of Oddi, or incomplete relaxation of the sphincter upon gallbladder contraction may lead to bile duct distention and pain.[73]

Many other disorders can produce epigastric pain that mimics the pain of an ulcer. It can be difficult to distinguish between gastritis and PUD. The discomfort associated with gastritis is often mild to moderate in severity and described as a hot, burning pain or bloating. In particular, burning pain is twice as common in gastritis as in PUD. Esophageal disorders such as GERD, esophagitis, or esophageal spasm can present with abdominal symptoms. Mesenteric ischemia ("abdominal angina") should be considered, especially in elderly patients and those with underlying vascular disease and/or atrial fibrillation. Aortic dissection must also be considered. Other abdominal sources such as the biliary tract and pancreas should be considered. The emergency physician must not fail to consider an atypical presentation of an acute cardiac syndrome or other intrathoracic process as the cause of the abdominal pain. Finally, abdominal pain may be secondary to a psychiatric disorder. Recent studies have suggested that some patients may have an altered perception of visceral pain, and have increased sensation of pain when the stomach or small intestine is dilated.

Management

Treatment of presumptive PUD may be initiated from the ED. Lifestyle changes may help. Bland diets and frequent small feedings are often used, although no study has proven their effectiveness. Agents that exacerbate gastric or duodenal ulcer disease should be avoided, including aspirin, ethanol, and cigarette smoking. Since PUD is a result of either infection with *H. pylori* or NSAID use, the emergency physician may begin treatment based on the presumed etiology. For NSAID-related ulcers, treatment should begin by discontinuing the offending agent. For documented NSAID-induced ulcers, a PPI is the preferred method of treatment, although H_2 blockers are also effective.[74]

If NSAIDs are not being used by a patient with suspected PUD, it is currently recommended to treat for *H. pylori* infection. Dyspeptic symptoms without proven ulcer may also be an indication for treatment, but that decision may be best left to a gastroenterologist. Antacid therapy may be started with a PPI or H_2 blocker. It should be noted that nonendoscopic testing for *H. pylori* is available (e.g., antibody detection, urea breath test); however, its role in the evaluation of ED patients is not yet defined.

Recommended regimens include: lansoprazole 30 mg po bid × 14 days, clarithromycin 500 po bid × 14 days, and amoxicillin 1 g po bid × 14 days—available commercially as PrevPac; omeprazole 20 mg po bid × 14 days, clarithromycin 500 po bid × 14 days, and amoxicillin 1 g po bid × 14 days; lansoprazole 30 mg po bid × 14 days *or* omeprazole 20 g po bid × 14 days, and clarithromycin 500 mg po bid × 14 days and metronidazole 500 mg po bid × 14 days; or lansoprazole 30 mg po bid × 14 days *or* omeprazole 20 g po bid × 14 days and bismuth subsalicylate (Pepto-Bismol) 525 mg po qid × 14 days and metronidazole 500 mg po tid × 14 days and tetracycline 500 mg po qid × 14 days.[75]

GASTRIC VOLVULUS

Perspective

Gastric volvulus is a rare cause of severe abdominal pain that occurs when the stomach rotates upon itself more than 180 degrees, creating a closed loop obstruction. Only 400 cases have been reported in the literature, although its true incidence is unknown because some types of volvulus are intermittent and resolve spontaneously. The peak age of occurrence is in persons aged 40 to 50 and is usually associated with the presence of a paraesophageal hernia. Approximately 20% of cases occur in infants under 1 year of age and are due to congenital diaphragmatic defects.[76] If an acute volvulus is not identified and corrected early, it may lead to gastric ischemia, perforation, and death. The mortality from acute gastric volvulus is 15% to 20%.

Principles of Disease

The stomach is fixed at only two points, the esophagocardiac junction and the pylorus. The remainder of the organ is relatively distensible and mobile, and can occupy various positions within the abdomen. When a person is supine, the stomach lies entirely above the umbilicus, whereas it descends below the umbilicus in the erect position. Regardless of its position, the stomach maintains its familiar morphology because of ligamentous attachments to the surrounding organs. A primary (or subdiaphragmatic) volvulus occurs when the stabilizing ligaments are too lax or are congenitally abnormal in such a way that the stomach is able to twist upon itself. Approximately one third of cases are of this type.

Secondary (or supradiaphragmatic) volvulus occurs in patients with diaphragmatic defects such as a paraesophageal hiatal hernia, an elevated diaphragm, gastric ulcer or carcinoma, diaphragmatic paralysis, extrinsic pressure on the stomach from other organs, or abdominal adhesions.[77] The combination of one of the above factors and ligamentous laxity makes a volvulus more likely to occur.

Gastric volvulus can be classified based on its axis of rotation. The most common form is organoaxial volvulus, which occurs when the stomach twists on its long axis. Less commonly, the stomach folds on its short axis from the lesser to greater curvature and is classified as a mesenteroaxial volvulus. Approximately one third of gastric volvulus are of this type.

Clinical Features

Presenting Symptoms The presenting features of a gastric volvulus can be variable based on the type. Primary volvulus may present with the sudden onset of severe abdominal pain. The upper abdomen may demonstrate marked distention. Patients with secondary volvulus may have their predominate symptoms in their chest, with pain radiating to the back and shoulders along with accompanying dyspnea. The abdominal examination may be unremarkable. Vomiting is usually present and may be persistent and severe. The combination of severe epigastric pain and distention, vomiting, and inability to pass a nasogastric tube (Borchardt's triad) should make one strongly consider the possibility of a gastric volvulus.[78]

A volvulus may be chronic if the rotation is minimal and there is no vascular compromise. Symptoms usually consist of mild intermittent upper abdominal pain. Early satiety, dyspnea, bloating, eructation, and upper abdominal fullness may be present. It is unknown how often a chronic volvulus can lead to an acute volvulus.

Complications If not recognized, volvulus can lead to bowel ischemia and necrosis of the stomach. Untreated, this may lead to shock and death. Fortunately, the frequency of gastric infarction is low (reported between 5% and 28% for organoaxial volvulus) because of the redundant blood supply of the stomach. Other complications include ulceration, perforation, hemorrhage, pancreatic necrosis, and omental avulsion.

Diagnostic Strategies

A plain abdominal radiograph often demonstrates a large, gas-filled loop of bowel in the abdomen or chest. A barium swallow may help visualize the abnormality. There are no laboratory findings specific for volvulus, although elevations in amylase and alkaline phosphatase have been reported.

Differential Considerations

The differential diagnosis of gastric volvulus includes any disease that can present with sudden upper abdominal pain and vomiting. Perforated peptic ulcer, gastric outlet obstruction, and biliary tract disease should be considered. Symptoms of a secondary volvulus may lead one to consider an acute cardiac syndrome.

Management

Treatment of an acute gastric volvulus is surgical, with the goal of reducing the volvulus and preventing its recurrence by repairing any predisposing defects. Mortality increases with delayed diagnosis due to complications of ischemia. Acutely, one should attempt passage of a nasogastric tube, as this may occasionally reduce the volvulus. There have been reports of reductions of volvulus using endoscopy, but this is probably best reserved for those patients who cannot tolerate an operation or who have no evidence of vascular compromise.[79]

DYSPHAGIA

Perspective

Precise motor control of the act of swallowing is necessary to ensure that material is successfully transferred from the mouth through the esophagus into the stomach. This includes the muscles of the oropharynx, the upper esophageal sphincter (UES), the body of the esophagus, and the LES. Failure at any one of these levels results in a motility disorder, the primary symptom of which is dysphagia, which literally means "difficulty swallowing."

Principles of Disease

Normal Physiology Swallowing is a complex phenomenon requiring both voluntary and involuntary skeletal muscle activity. Control of swallowing is coordinated via the swallowing center in the medulla. Afferent sensory input involves the trigeminal, glossopharyngeal, vagus, and spinal accessory cranial nerves; efferent motor activity travels via the trigeminal, facial, glossopharyngeal, vagus, and hypoglossal cranial nerves. The act of swallowing begins a process of both simultaneous and sequential activity in all three esophageal zones. A rapidly progressive pharyngeal contraction transfers the food bolus through a relaxed UES into the esophagus, where a moving ring-like contraction begins in the upper esophagus and propagates distally, making the transition from striated to smooth muscle, culminating with the propulsion of the bolus through a relaxed LES. Three mechanisms have been described that regulate the peristaltic wave, ensuring a smooth transition from the striated muscle in the upper esophagus to the smooth muscle of the middle and lower esophagus and coordination of UES and LES activity. These mechanisms include sequential firing of vagal afferents that begin in the brainstem, an intramural neural mechanism that responds to local stimuli, and myogenic propagation of the contraction through the myocytes themselves.[80]

Physiologically, swallowing can be divided into oral, pharyngeal, and esophageal phases. The oral phase involves preparation of the food bolus by mastication and lubrication. The tongue then propels the bolus into the pharynx by progressive anteroposterior contractions. In the pharyngeal phase of swallowing, events are initiated by delivery of the food bolus to the oropharynx. Voluntary contraction of the pharyngeal muscles seals the nasopharynx by elevation of the soft palate. The oropharynx is sealed by the upward movement of the tongue against the palate. The larynx and hyoid bone are elevated to seal off the respiratory passage. The cricopharyngeus muscle, or UES, relaxes, and the bolus is swept into the esophagus by sequential peristaltic waves initiated in the upper pharynx. During the esophageal phase, the bolus is propelled toward the stomach by sequential peristaltic waves. Peristalsis can be initiated by swallowing or in response to luminal distention of the gut or changes in the pH or osmotic environment of the mucosa. The lower sphincter normally maintains a degree of tone sufficient to prevent reflux of gastric contents. When the food bolus reaches the lower sphincter, the sphincter relaxes to allow passage of the bolus and then regains its degree of resting tone.

Pathophysiology Disturbances of the interactions between the components of the upper GI tract will lead to a motility disorder. The motor disorders of the body of the esophagus are only now beginning to be better understood. The major primary esophageal motility disorders are achalasia, diffuse esophageal spasm, hypercontractile esophagus ("nutcracker esophagus"), and nonspecific motor disorder. Of these, the only two that are well defined are achalasia and diffuse esophageal spasm. Controversy exists as to whether or not the other entities are true disease states, since symptoms are not always associated with manometric abnormalities, and correction of the abnormalities does not always result in symptom improvement. Motor disorders may be the primary cause of other esophageal abnormalities such as GERD or esophageal diverticula.

Clinical Features

Dysphagia can be produced by a large number of entities. A thorough history will reveal the diagnosis in most patients (Box 84-3).[81-83] One should determine the location where the bolus sticks; the duration of the dysphagia and whether symptoms are intermittent or progressive; whether solids, liquids, or both are involved; whether it is associated with pain; and whether the patient has any previous gastroesophageal history (e.g., esophageal reflux). Any family history of neurologic disease should be obtained.

The examination should include a thorough evaluation of the head and neck and a detailed neurologic examination. The patient should be observed while swallowing. Difficulty in initiating the swallow, misdirection of the bolus with regurgitation or aspiration, and unusual posturing of the patient when swallowing should be noted. Many patients with neuromuscular disorders depend on gravity to swallow, and having the patient swallow in the prone position may be helpful in diagnosis.

Oropharyngeal Dysphagia Oropharyngeal causes of dysphagia inhibit the initiation of swallowing. Neuromuscular diseases cause approximately 80% of oropharyngeal dysphagias, with most remaining etiologies being localized structural lesions. Most neuromuscular causes of dysphagia result in misdirection of the bolus, sticking, and the need for repeated swallowing attempts. Patients may drool and turn the head and neck to the side to facilitate swallowing. Liquids, especially of extreme temperatures, usually cause dysphagia more commonly than solids, and symptoms are more often intermittent. Progressive unremitting dysphagia is usually not caused by neuromuscular disorders of the oropharynx. Cerebrovascular accidents are probably the most common cause for neuromuscular dysphagia, especially those involving the vertebrobasilar system and posteroinferior cerebellar arteries and when some degree of dysarthria is present. The mechanism in such cases is pharyngeal weakness, with failure of the cricopharyngeus muscle to relax. Weakness of the tongue may occur, resulting in poor transfer of the bolus, or weakness of the buccal muscles may produce drooling and difficulty initiating the swallow.[84]

The second most common cause of neuromuscular dysphagia is polymyositis or dermatomyositis. These disorders are characterized by inflammatory and degenerative changes in striated muscle that can produce dysphagia from weakness of the palate, pharynx, and upper esophagus. Dysphagia is seen in approximately 25% of patients with these disorders at the time of treatment.[85]

Other neuromuscular causes of oropharyngeal dysphagia are listed in Box 84-3. One that deserves particular mention is myasthenia gravis. Two thirds of patients with myasthenia gravis can have dysphagia, and occasionally it is the presenting symptom. The dysphagia becomes progressively worse with repeated swallowing attempts and temporarily reversible with edrophonium.

Disorders in the pharyngeal phase of swallowing may lead to misdirection of the bolus, pain, sticking, or multiple swallowing attempts. Tongue weakness can result in oral regurgitation. Inability to seal the nasopharynx because of obstruction or muscular weakness can cause nasal regurgitation. Inefficient laryngeal elevation from muscular weakness or a fixed larynx can result in laryngotracheal aspiration. Delayed aspiration can occur with pharyngeal weakness and

Box 84-3 Causes of Dysphagia

Neuromuscular

Vascular

Cerebrovascular accident

Immunologic

Dermatomyositis
Multiple sclerosis
Myasthenia gravis
Polymyositis
Scleroderma

Infectious

Botulism
Diphtheria
Poliomyelitis
Rabies
Sydenham's chorea
Tetanus

Metabolic

Lead poisoning
Magnesium deficiency

Other

Alzheimer's disease
Amyotrophic lateral sclerosis
Brain tumor
Depression
Diabetic neuropathy
Familial dysautonomia
Muscular dystrophies
Metabolic myopathies (e.g., thyrotoxicosis)
Parkinson's disease

Obstructive

Achalasia
Aortic aneurysm
Esophageal motility disorder
Esophageal rings
Esophageal stricture
Esophageal webs
Foreign bodies
Hypertrophic cervical spurs
Inflammatory lesions (tonsillitis, retropharyngeal abscess)
Left atrial enlargement
Neoplasm
Thyroid enlargement
Vascular anomalies
Zenker's diverticulum

Other

Alcoholism
Decreased saliva production (Sjögren's syndrome, postirradiation)
Diabetes
GERD

with pooling of food in the piriform recesses or in a diverticulum. Inability to contract the pharyngeal muscles is often compounded by failure of the cricopharyngeus to relax. Failure of relaxation of the cricopharyngeus with or without pharyngeal weakness causes misdirection of the bolus or necessitates repeated swallowing attempts. Inflammatory lesions of the tongue or oropharynx can result in odynophagia and even complete inability to swallow because of pain.

Esophageal Dysphagia Dysphagia from upper esophageal lesions is usually perceived 2 to 4 seconds after the initiation of swallowing. Dysphagia that the patient localizes to the substernal or retrosternal area may be anatomically accurate, but localization to the neck may be referred from anywhere in the esophagus.

The motor disorders of the esophagus are only now beginning to be understood. The two best-defined motility disorders are achalasia and diffuse esophageal spasm. Other disorders such as nutcracker esophagus and nonspecific motor disorder have been described, but controversy exists as to whether these entities are true disease states, as symptoms are not always associated with manometric abnormalities, and correction of the abnormalities does not always result in symptom improvement.

Achalasia is a disorder of unknown cause in which there is a marked increase in the resting pressure of the LES and absent peristalsis in the body of the esophagus. Although it can occur at any age, most patients are between 20 and 40 years of age. Dysphagia is the most common presenting symptom and usually begins insidiously with equal frequency for solids and liquids. Patients may report that maneuvers that increase esophageal pressure (raising arms above the head, standing erect with back straight) will help pass the food. Odynophagia from esophageal spasm may also be seen early in the course of achalasia. The symptoms are often worse with rapid eating and during periods of stress. The patient may also report chest pain as a symptom. As dilation occurs above the sphincter, retention of undigested food in the esophagus occurs and the patient may be aware of gurgling while eating. Regurgitation of the undigested material can occur after a meal (prompting consideration of the diagnosis of an eating disorder) or with changes in position or vigorous exercise. The regurgitated food usually has no acid taste, although bacterial contamination may lead to fermentation of the undigested food. Laryngotracheal aspiration may occur, especially at night, and may cause nocturnal coughing. Physical examination is usually unremarkable except for weight loss.[86,87]

Radiographically, a dilated esophagus is seen proximal to a narrowed gastroesophageal junction that has a beak-like appearance.

The second type of intrinsic motor disorder of the esophagus is diffuse esophageal spasm. Manometrically, simultaneous prolonged strong esophageal contractions are noted to be interspersed over normal peristaltic waves. If a barium swallow is obtained during a spasm, findings such as a "corkscrewing" or curling of the esophagus may be noted. Diffuse spasm may be precipitated by swallowing very hot or cold liquids. Symptoms include chest pain, dysphagia, or both.

"Nutcracker esophagus" is the term used to describe prolonged, high-intensity peristaltic waves. Many authors feel that this represents a variant of diffuse esophageal spasm. Nonspecific motor disorder includes repetitive esophageal contractions, nontransmitted esophageal contractions, or low-amplitude esophageal contractions.

Diagnostic Strategies

Given the myriad causes of dysphagia, a careful history and physical examination are essential. If the problem is thought to be in the mouth and upper esophagus, a swallowing study (video-esophagram) should be obtained. If a motor disorder is suspected, a swallowing study may prove helpful as well, but this may not detect intermittent dysfunction. In such cases, referral to a gastroenterologist for manometric examination may be required. At that time, additional provocative studies can be performed.

Differential Considerations

The differential diagnosis of lower esophageal dysphagia includes acute coronary syndromes. Substernal chest pain is the main symptom in 80% to 90% of patients with esophageal motility disorders. The chest pain can be similar to angina, described as crushing or squeezing with similar patterns of radiation to cardiac chest pain. Nitroglycerin may relieve the pain of spasm as well, further confusing the picture.

Symptoms that suggest an esophageal etiology of chest pain are pain that is prolonged and nonexertional, pain that interrupts sleep, pain related to meals, relief with antacids, and presence of other symptoms of esophageal disease such as heartburn, dysphagia, or regurgitation.[88] Because of considerable overlap in symptoms, the emergency physician must exclude a cardiac diagnosis before attributing chest pain to an esophageal cause.

Management

Esophageal motility disorders are generally treated by gastroenterologists, since the diagnosis is usually made manometrically. Achalasia is the only motility disorder for which reasonably good studies support specific treatment. Pharmacologic therapy is directed at decreasing the tone of the LES. Nitrates and calcium channel blockers have been used with some success; however, reflux symptoms may be exacerbated.[89] Other therapies used with some degree of success have included botulinum toxin injection, pneumatic dilation, and surgical intervention.

Although no definitive therapy has been described for any of the other motility disorders, the emergency physician should be familiar with those that may be used in the therapy of these disorders. It should be noted that medical therapy of esophageal motility disorders is rather limited, and clinical results are usually minimal. Anticholinergic drugs such as hyoscyamine sulfate (Levsin) or dicyclomine (Bentyl) have also been used because they decrease the amplitude of esophageal peristalsis and LES pressure.[90] These drugs may also exacerbate reflux symptoms because they cause delayed gastric emptying and decreased esophageal peristalsis.

Calcium channel blockers decrease both LES pressure and the amplitude of esophageal contractions. Nifedipine has been used successfully in some patients.[91] Diltiazem has been shown to be effective in patients with nutcracker esophagus.[92] Verapamil has been shown to decrease LES pressure when administered intravenously to healthy volunteers, but no effects have been noted using an oral dose.[93,94] Psychotropic medications such as alprazolam and trazodone have been used to treat some esophageal motility disorders. Although no study has demonstrated specific beneficial manometric effects, it is believed that the improvement may be secondary to treatment of an underlying functional disorder such as panic attacks or depression.[95]

PHARMACOLOGIC AGENTS FOR UPPER GASTROINTESTINAL DISORDERS

Antacids

By the time most patients present to the ED with upper GI complaints, most have already tried some form of antacid therapy, since these agents are readily available as over-the-counter preparations. Antacids afford pain relief in most patients with PUD. Doses with low neutralizing capacity (as low as 30 mEq) promote ulcer healing. Antacids may also work by binding bile acids or inhibiting pepsin.

The choice of antacid should be individualized. The magnesium-containing antacids can produce diarrhea in up to 25% of patients. Magnesium-containing antacids can also lead to an increase in serum magnesium levels and should be avoided or used with caution in patients with impaired renal function. Aluminum-containing antacids may lead to constipation, and prolonged use may lead to phosphate depletion. Calcium-containing antacids have been marketed as both neutralizing acid and as a means of calcium supplementation, especially for postmenopausal women. Calcium-containing antacids have been traditionally believed to cause the most acid rebound, a paradoxic increase in gastrin secretion and acid production. Calcium antacids can also lead to constipation, and their excess consumption can lead to hypercalcemia, alkalosis, and renal insufficiency (the milk-alkali syndrome).

Antacids can also decrease the absorption of warfarin, digoxin, some anticonvulsants, and some antibiotics. The recommended dose of antacids in the treatment of peptic ulcer disease is 400 mmol/day divided over four doses, usually delivered 1 and 3 hours after meals and at bedtime. Antacids are the least expensive drugs available to treat PUD, but their use is somewhat limited by side effects and inconvenient dosing schedules.

Histamine Blockers

Histamine has been identified as the most important factor in stimulating the parietal cells of the gastric mucosa to secrete acid. Type 2 histamine receptors (H_2) are located on the parietal cells of the stomach. The discovery of the ability of H_2 blockers to inhibit gastric acid production was a major advance in antiulcer therapy because ulcers cannot develop in the absence of acid. These drugs are highly selective competitive inhibitors of histamine for the H_2 receptor on parietal cells and reduce both the volume of gastric juice and its hydrogen ion concentration. All of the currently available H_2 blockers are rapidly absorbed after an oral dose, reaching peak levels within 1 to 2 hours. All have half-lives of approximately 2 to 3 hours, so the effects last for about 6 hours. Most are now available over the counter in lower dosage strength. H_2 blockers are effective in treating duodenal ulcer and, to a lesser extent, gastric ulcer. They are widely prescribed for symptoms of dyspepsia and work well in patients with episodic heartburn. All H_2 blockers are mainly hepatically and renally metabolized with the exception of nizatidine, which is almost exclusively renally metabolized. Dosages of all these agents should be reduced in patients with renal failure.

H_2 blockers are safe and generally well tolerated. Side effects are rare, including central nervous system (CNS) effects such as somnolence, dizziness, and confusion. Transient increases in liver enzymes may be noted. Some patients may exhibit abnormalities in cardiac conduction, as there are H_2 receptors found in the heart. Cimetidine has been shown to cause gynecomastia. Dosing of the various agents is summarized in Table 84-1.

Proton Pump Inhibitors

The H^+/K^+ ATPase ("proton pump") is located on the apical portion of the parietal cell and is responsible for the production of hydrogen ions in gastric acid. The available PPIs irreversibly bind to stimulated proton pumps to block secretion of hydrogen ions. Although they have no effect on the volume of gastric juice produced, production of acid can be reduced by up to 95%. Both basal and stimulated gastric acid secretion are reduced. The antisecretory effects last up to 72 hours. Because, at the cellular level, additional proton pumps are continually recruited to produce more acid in response to stimulation, several doses of a PPI are necessary to achieve maximal anti-acid effect (sometimes up to 4 days). Numerous clinical trials have shown PPIs to be much more effective than H_2 blockers at acid inhibition.[96,97]

All available PPIs are acid-labile prodrugs that are inactivated in gastric juice. Thus all oral preparations are manufactured as enteric-coated granules. As they are hepatically metabolized, dosage should be reduced in patients with hepatic failure. Side effects are usually minimal. Currently, PPIs are indicated for the short-term treatment of active duodenal ulcer and severe erosive esophagitis and in the treatment of symptomatic GERD that has not responded to therapy with H_2 blockers. They are also used at significantly higher dosages in patients with Zollinger-Ellison syndrome.[98] Dosing of the various agents is summarized in Table 84-2.

Prostaglandins

Prostaglandins exert protective effects on the gastric mucosa, although the exact mechanisms are still debated.[99] Inhibition of gastric acid secretion, increased secretion of mucus and bicarbonate, and stimulation of mucosal blood flow have all been demonstrated.[100] Misoprostol (Cytotec) is an analog of prostaglandin E_1 with a longer duration of action and greater potency than endogenous prostaglandins. It should be used only for prevention of NSAID-induced gastric ulcers in high-risk patients. The dose is 200 μg 4 times a day with food, but crampy abdominal pain and diarrhea may require the use of a somewhat less effective dose of 100 μg 4 times a day.[101] Misoprostol is an abortifacient and therefore is contraindicated in any female patient of childbearing age who is not using contraception.

Other Agents

Sucralfate (Carafate) binds to epithelial cells and especially to ulcerated surfaces, providing a protective layer that inhibits further acid damage. Its mechanism of action is not completely understood, although it has been shown to enhance epithelial growth, suppress acid secretion, and inhibit growth of *H. pylori.* The usual dose is 1 g 4 times a day given 30 to 60 minutes before meals.

Bismuth compounds such as bismuth subsalicylate (Pepto-Bismol) decrease pepsin activity, increase mucus secretion, and form a barrier to further acid damage in ulcer craters. They also increase prostaglandin synthesis and retard hydrogen ion diffusion through the mucosal barrier.[102] Bismuth may also help heal ulcers through its bactericidal action on *H. pylori.*

KEY CONCEPTS

- The combined use of glucagon and an effervescent agent can cause rapid relief of acute lower esophageal obstruction in up to 75% of patients.

Table 84-1. Summary of Histamine Receptor Antagonists

	GERD	PUD
Nizatidine	150 mg bid	300 mg qhs or 150 mg bid; 150 mg qhs (maint)
Famotidine	20 or 40 mg bid × 12 weeks	40 mg qhs or 20 mg bid; 20 mg qhs (maint)
Cimetidine	800 mg bid or 400 mg qid × 12 weeks	800 mg qhs × 4-6 weeks; 400 qhs (maint)
Ranitidine	150 mg bid (150 mg qid for erosive esophagitis)	150 mg bid or 300 mg qhs; 150 mg qhs (maint)

Maint, Maintenance dosage.

Table 84-2. Summary of Proton Pump Inhibitors

	GERD	PUD	Zollinger-Ellison syndrome
Omeprazole	20-40 mg qd × 4-12 weeks; followed by 20 mg qd (maint)	20-40 mg daily × 4 weeks (DU); 8 weeks (GU); 10-20 mg qd (maint)	60 mg/day
Rabeprazole	20 mg qd × 4-8 weeks; 20 mg qd (maint)	20 mg qd × 4 weeks	
Lansoprazole	15 mg qd; 30 mg po for erosive esophagitis; 15 mg qd (maint)	15 mg qd × 4 weeks (DU); 30 mg qd × 8 weeks (GU); 15 mg qd (maint)	60 mg/day
Pantoprazole	40 mg qd × 8 weeks for erosive esophagitis	N/I	

DU, duodenal ulcer; *GU,* gastric ulcer; *maint,* maintenance dosage; *N/I,* not an approved indication in the United States.

- Radiographic contrast studies of patients with suspected perforation of the esophagus or stomach should first be performed with water-soluble agents like Gastrografin.
- GERD should receive stepwise treatment with (1) lifestyle modification and over-the-counter antacids or H_2 receptor antagonists, then (2) prescription-strength H_2 antagonists, then (3) dual therapy with the addition of a proton pump inhibitor, and finally (4) antireflux surgery.
- Oropharyngeal dysphagia is most commonly caused by a neuromuscular disorder (e.g., stroke, polymyositis, or myasthenia gravis), whereas esophageal dysphagia is usually caused by an intrinsic motility disorder (e.g., achalasia or esophageal spasm).

REFERENCES

1. Hamilton K, Polter D: Foreign bodies and bezoars. In Feldman M, Sleisenger MH, Scharschmidt BF, editors: *Sleisenger and Fordtran's gastrointestinal and liver disease,* ed 6, Philadelphia, 1998, WB Saunders.
2. Choudhry U, Boyce HW: Treatment of esophageal disorders caused by medications, caustic ingestion, foreign bodies, and trauma. In Wolfe MM, editor: *Therapy of digestive disorders,* Philadelphia, 2000, WB Saunders.
3. Pope CE II: Rings, webs, diverticula. In Sleisenger MH, Fordtran JS, editors: *Gastrointestinal diseases,* ed 5, Philadelphia, 1993, WB Saunders.
4. *Guidelines for the management of ingested foreign bodies.* ASGE Publication 1026, February 1995.
5. Maves MD, Lloyd TV, Carithers JS: Radiographic identification of ingested disc batteries, *Pediatr Radiol* 16:154, 1985.
6. Brady PG: Esophageal foreign bodies, *Gastroenterol Clin North Am* 20:691, 1991.
7. Taylor RB: Esophageal foreign bodies, *Emerg Med Clin North Am* 5:301, 1987.
8. Braverman I et al: The role of CT imaging in the evaluation of cervical esophageal foreign bodies, *J Otolaryngol* 22:311, 1993.
9. Taylor RB: Esophageal foreign bodies, *Emerg Med Clin North Am* 5:301, 1987.
10. Campbell JB, Quattromani FL, Foly LC: Foley catheter removal of blunt esophageal foreign bodies: experience with 100 consecutive children, *Pediatr Radiol* 13:116, 1983.
11. Ginaldi S: Removal of esophageal foreign bodies using a Foley catheter in adults, *Am J Emerg Med* 3:64, 1985.
12. Glauser J et al: Intravenous glucagon in the management of esophageal food obstruction, *J Am Coll Emerg Physicians* 8:228, 1979.
13. Ferrucci JT, Long JA: Radiologic treatment of food impaction using intravenous glucagon, *Radiology* 125:25, 1977.
14. Votey S, Dudley JP: Emergency ear, nose, and throat procedures, *Emerg Med Clin North Am* 7:117, 1989.
15. Mohammed SH et al: Dislodgement of impacted esophageal foreign bodies with carbonated beverages, *Clin Radiol* 37:589, 1986.
16. Rice BT et al: Acute esophageal food impaction treated by gas-forming agents, *Radiology* 146:299, 1983.
17. Kaszar-Siebert DJ et al: Treatment of acute esophageal food impaction with a combination of glucagon, effervescent agent, and water, *Am J Roentgenol* 154:533, 1990.
18. Robbins MI et al: Treatment of acute esophageal food impaction with glucagon, an effervescent agent, and water, *Am J Roentgenol* 162:325, 1994.
19. Choudhry U, Boyce HW: Treatment of esophageal disorders caused by medications, caustic ingestion, foreign bodies, and trauma. In Wolfe MM, editor: *Therapy of digestive disorders,* Philadelphia, 2000, WB Saunders.
20. Webb WA: Management of foreign bodies of the upper gastrointestinal tract, *Gastroenterology* 94:204, 1988.
21. Faigel DO, Fennerty MB: Miscellaneous diseases of the esophagus. In Yamada T et al, editors: *Textbook of gastroenterology,* Philadelphia, 1999, Lippincott Williams and Wilkins.
22. Webb WA: Management of foreign bodies of the upper gastrointestinal tract, *Gastroenterology* 94:204, 1988.
23. Brady PG: Esophageal foreign bodies, *Gastroenterol Clin North Am* 20:691, 1991.
24. Webb WA: Management of foreign bodies of the upper gastrointestinal tract, *Gastroenterology* 94:204, 1988.
25. Ahmed A, Aggarwal M, Watson E: Esophageal perforation: a complication of nasogastric tube placement, *Am J Emerg Med* 16:64-66, 1998.
26. Richards CF: Piriform sinus perforation during esophageal-tracheal Combitube placement, *J Emerg Med* 16:37-39, 1998.
27. Faigel Douglas O et al: Miscellaneous diseases of the esophagus. In Yamada T, editor: *Textbook of gastroenterology,* Philadelphia, 1999, Lippincott Williams and Wilkins.
28. Keighley MRB et al: Spontaneous rupture of the esophagus, *Br J Surg* 59:649, 1972.
29. Datta CK, Brannon JV: Spontaneous rupture of esophagus (Boerhaave syndrome): a review of literature and a case presentation, *W Va Med J* 75:180, 1979.
30. Younes Z, Johnson D: The spectrum of spontaneous and iatrogenic esophageal injury, *J Clin Gastroenterol* 29:306-317, 1999.
31. Baehr PH, McDonald GB: Esophageal disorders caused by infection, systemic illness, medications, radiation, and trauma. In Feldman M, Sleisenger MH, Scharscmidt BF, editors: *Sleisenger and Fordtran's gastrointestinal and liver disease,* ed 6, Philadelphia, 1998, WB Saunders.
32. Orringer MB: Tumors, injuries, and miscellaneous conditions of the esophagus. In Greenfield LJ, editor: *Surgery: scientific principles and practice,* Philadelphia, 1993, JB Lippincott.
33. Baehr PH, McDonald GB: Esophageal disorders caused by infection, systemic illness, medications, radiation, and trauma. In Feldman M, Sleisenger MH, Scharscmidt BF, editors: *Sleisenger and Fordtran's gastrointestinal and liver disease,* ed 6, Philadelphia, 1998, WB Saunders.
34. Niezgoda JA, McMenamin P, Graeber GM: Pharyngoesophageal perforation after blunt neck trauma, *Ann Thorac Surg* 50:615, 1990.
35. Sawyer R, Phillips C, Vakil N: Short- and long-term outcome of esophageal perforation, *Gastrointest Endosc* 41:130, 1995.
36. Kikendall, JW: Pill esophagitis, *J Clin Gastroenterol* 28:298, 1999.
37. Swann LA, Munter DW: Esophageal emergencies, *Emerg Med Clin North Am* 14:557, 1996.
38. Fraimow HS, Klein RS: Treatment of esophageal infections in the immunocompromised host. In Wolfe MM et al, editors: *Therapy of digestive disorders,* Philadelphia, 2000, WB Saunders, p 771.
39. Fraimow HS, Klein RS: Treatment of esophageal infections in the immunocompromised host: In Wolfe MM, editor: *Therapy of digestive disorders,* Philadelphia, 2000, WB Saunders, p 775.
40. Fraimow HS, Klein RS: Treatment of esophageal infections in the immunocompromised host. In Wolfe MM et al, editors: *Therapy of digestive disorders,* Philadelphia, 2000, WB Saunders, p 776.
41. Faigel DO, Fennerty MB: Miscellaneous disease of the esophagus. In Yamada T et al, editors: *Textbook of gastroenterology,* Philadelphia, 1999, Lippincott Williams and Wilkins.
42. Nebel OT, Frones MF, Castell DO: Symptomatic gastroesophageal reflux: incidence and precipitating factors, *Am J Dig Dis* 21:953, 1976.
43. Orlando RC: Reflux esophagitis. In Yamada T, editor: *Textbook of gastroenterology,* Philadelphia, 1999, Lippincott Williams and Wilkins.
44. Mittal RK: Hiatal hernia: myth or reality? Proceedings of a symposium: First Multi-Disciplinary International Symposium on Supraesophageal Complications of Reflux Disease, *Am J Med* 103:33S, 1997.
45. Harding SM et al: Asthma and gastroesophageal reflux: acid suppressive therapy improves asthma outcome, *Am J Med* 100:395, 1996.
46. Larrain A et al: Medical and surgical treatment of nonallergic asthma associated with gastroesophageal reflux, *Chest* 99:1330, 1991.
47. Sontag SJ: Gastroesophageal reflux and asthma. Proceedings of a Symposium: First Multi-Disciplinary International Symposium on Supraesophageal Complications of Reflux Disease, *Am J Med* 103:84S, 1997.
48. Ing AJ: Cough and gastroesophageal reflux. Proceedings of a Symposium: First Multi-Disciplinary International Symposium on Supraesophageal Complications of Reflux Disease, *Am J Med* 103: 91S, 1997.

49. Gaynor EB: Gastroesophageal reflux as an etiologic factor in laryngeal complications of intubation, *Laryngoscope* 98:972, 1998.
50. Kahrilas PJ: Gastroesophageal reflux disease, *JAMA* 276:983, 1996.
51. Davies HA: Anginal pain of esophageal origin: clinical presentation, prevalence, and prognosis, *Am J Med* 92:5S, 1992.
52. Areskog M, Tibbling L, Wranne B: Esophageal dysfunction in non-infarction coronary care unit patients, *Acta Med Scand* 205:279, 1979.
53. Fisher RS: Treatment of gastroesophageal reflux disease. In Wolfe MM, editor: *Therapy of digestive disorders,* Philadelphia, 2000, WB Saunders.
54. Wolfe MM: H_2-receptor antagonists vs OTC medications: how beneficial have they been? *Pract Gastroenterol* 20:10, 1996.
55. Johnson DA: Medical therapy for gastroesophageal reflux disease, *Am J Med* 92:88S, 1992.
56. Pignon JP et al: Critical review of randomized double-blind trials in the medical treatment of gastroesophageal reflux, *Gastroenterol Clin Biol* 11:668, 1987.
57. Driks MR et al: Nosocomial pneumonia in intubated patients given sucralfate as compared with antacids or histamine type 2 blockers: the role of gastric colonization, *N Engl J Med* 317:1376, 1987.
58. Fisher RS: Treatment of gastroesophageal reflux disease. In Wolfe MM et al, editors: *Therapy of digestive disorders,* Philadelphia, 2000, WB Saunders.
59. Brunner G et al: Efficacy and safety of long-term treatment with omeprazole in patients with acid-related diseases resistant to ranitidine, *Can J Gastroenterol* 3:72, 1989.
60. Williams RM et al: Multicenter trial of sucralfate suspension for the treatment of reflux esophagitis, *Am J Med* 83:61, 1987.
61. Richter JE: A critical review of current medical therapy for gastroesophageal reflux disease, *J Clin Gastroenterol* 8:72, 1986.
62. Nagashima R: Mechanisms of action of sucralfate, *J Clin Gastroenterol* 3:117, 1981.
63. Mattox HE, Richter JE: Prolonged ambulatory esophageal pH monitoring in the evaluation of gastroesophageal reflux disease, *Am J Med* 89:345, 1990.
64. Yardley JH, Hendrix TR: Gastritis, gastropathy, duodenitis, and associated ulcerative lesions. In Yamada T, editor: *Textbook of gastroenterology,* ed 3, Philadelphia, 1999, Lippincott Williams and Wilkins.
65. Tytgat GNJ: Gastritis. In Bouchier IAD et al: *Gastroenterology: clinical science and practice,* ed 2, Philadelphia, 1993, WB Saunders.
66. Munnangi S, Sonnenberg A: Time trends of physician visits and treatment patterns of peptic ulcer disease in the United States, *Arch Intern Med* 157:1489, 1997.
67. Del Valle J et al: Acid peptic disorders. In Yamada T, editor: Textbook of gastroenterology, ed 3, Philadelphia, 1999, Lippincott Williams and Wilkins.
68. Kuipers EJ, Thijs JC, Festen HPM: The prevalence of *Helicobacter pylori* in peptic ulcer disease, *Aliment Pharmacol Ther* 9:59, 1995.
69. Del Valle J et al: Acid peptic disorders. In Yamada T, editor: *Textbook of gastroenterology,* Philadelphia, 1999, Lippincott Williams and Wilkins.
70. Henry D et al: Variability in risk of gastrointestinal complications with individual nonsteroidal anti-inflammatory drugs: results of a collaborative meta-analysis, *BMJ* 312:1563, 1996.
71. Del Valle J et al: Acid peptic disorders. In Yamada T, editor: *Textbook of gastroenterology,* Philadelphia, 1999, Lippincott Williams and Wilkins.
72. Talley NJ et al: Functional dyspepsia: a classification with guidelines of diagnosis and management, *Gastroenterol Int* 4:145, 1991.
73. Fisher RS, Parkman HP: Management of nonulcer dyspepsia, *N Engl J Med* 339:1376, 1998.
74. Wolfe MM: Therapy and prevention of NSAID-related gastrointestinal disorders. In Wolfe MM editor: *Therapy of digestive disorders,* Philadelphia, 2000, WB Saunders.
75. American College of Gastroenterology Guidelines, *Am J Gastroenterol* 93:2330, 1998.
76. Miller DL et al: Gastric volvulus in the pediatric population, *Arch Surg* 126:1146, 1991.
77. Godshall D, Mossallam U, Rosenbaum R: Gastric volvulus: case report and review of the literature, *J Emerg Med* 17:5, 837, 1999.
78. Hamilton K, Polter D: Foreign bodies and bezoars. In Feldman M, Sleisenger MH, Scharschmidt BF, editors: *Sleisenger and Fordtran's gastrointestinal and liver disease,* ed 6, Philadelphia, 1998, WB Saunders.
79. Hamilton K, Polter D: Foreign bodies and bezoars. In Feldman M, Sleisenger MH, Scharschmidt BF, editors: *Sleisenger and Fordtran's gastrointestinal and liver disease,* ed 6, Philadelphia, 1998, WB Saunders.
80. Diamant NE: Neuromuscular mechanisms of primary peristalsis. Proceedings of a Symposium: First Multi-Disciplinary International Symposium on Supraesophageal Complications of Reflux Disease, *Am J Med* 103:40S, 1997.
81. Mathog RH, Fleming SM: A clinical approach to dysphagia, *Am J Otolaryngol* 13:133, 1992.
82. Richter JE: Heartburn, dysphagia, odynophagia, and other esophageal symptoms. In Sleisenger MH, Fordtran JS, editors: *Gastrointestinal diseases,* ed 5, Philadelphia, 1993, WB Saunders.
83. Hess GP: An approach to throat complaints: foreign body sensation, difficulty swallowing, and hoarseness, *Emerg Med Clin North Am* 5:313, 1987.
84. Seaman WB: Pharyngeal and upper esophageal dysphagia, *JAMA* 235:2643, 1976.
85. Tandan R, Bradley WG: Dermatomyositis and polymyositis. In Isselbacher KJ et al editors: *Harrison's principles of internal medicine,* New York, 1994, McGraw-Hill.
86. Pitcher JL: Dysphagia in the elderly: causes and diagnosis, *Geriatrics* 28:64, 1973.
87. Clouse RE: Motor disorders. In Sleisenger MH, Fordtran JS, editors: *Gastrointestinal diseases,* ed 5, Philadelphia, 1993, WB Saunders.
88. Alban-Davies H et al: Angina-like esophageal pain: differentiation from cardiac pain by history, *J Clin Gastroenterol* 7:477, 1985.
89. Kikendall JW, Mellow MH: Effect of sublingual nitroglycerin and long-acting nitrate preparations on esophageal motility, *Gastroenterology* 79:703, 1980.
90. Katzka DA, Castell DO: Esophageal motor disorders and chest pain. In Bayless TM, editor: *Current therapy in gastroenterology and liver disease,* ed 4, St Louis, 1994, Mosby.
91. Richter JE et al: Oral nifedipine in the treatment of noncardiac chest pain in patients with the nutcracker esophagus, *Gastroenterology* 93:21, 1987.
92. Cattau EL Jr et al: Diltiazem therapy for symptoms associated with the nutcracker esophagus, *Am J Gastroenterol* 86:272, 1991.
93. Becker BS, Burakoff R: The effect of verapamil on lower esophageal sphincter pressure in normal subjects and in achalasia, *Am J Gastroenterol* 78:773, 1983.
94. Allen M et al: Comparison of calcium channel blocking agents and an anticholinergic agent on esophageal function, *Aliment Pharmacol Therapeut* 1:153, 1987.
95. Katzka DA, Castell DO: Esophageal motor disorders and chest pain. In Bayless TM, editor: *Current therapy in gastroenterology and liver disease,* ed 4, St Louis, 1994, Mosby.
96. Lauritsen K et al: Effect of omeprazole and cimetidine on duodenal ulcer: a double-blind comparative trial, *N Engl J Med* 312:958, 1985.
97. Maton PN: Omeprazole, *N Engl J Med* 324:965, 1991.
98. Shamburek RD, Schubert ML: Control of gastric acid secretion, *Gastrointestinal Pharmacology* 21:527, 1992.
99. Wallace JL: Prostaglandins, NSAIDs, and cytoprotection, *Gastrointestinal Pharmacology* 21:631, 1992.
100. Walt RP: Misoprostol for the treatment of peptic ulcer and antiinflammatory drug-induced gastroduodenal ulceration, *N Engl J Med* 327:1575, 1992.
101. Graham DY, Agrawal NM, Roth SH: Prevention of NSAID-induced gastric ulcer with misoprostol: multicenter, double-blind, placebo-controlled trial, *Lancet* 2:1277, 1988.
102. Hixson LJ et al: Current trends in the pharmacotherapy for gastroesophageal reflux disease, *Arch Intern Med* 152:717, 1992.

85 Liver and Biliary Tract

David A. Guss

HEPATIC DISORDERS

The liver is one of the largest organs in the body, serving a multitude of critical functions. The average weight of the normal adult liver is 1500 g. It receives approximately 30% of the resting cardiac output via the portal vein and the hepatic artery. The liver can be affected by a variety of disorders and, because of its varied synthetic and metabolic functions, may show a broad range of clinical signs and symptoms. Acute and chronic diseases of the liver are common in the general population and represent one of the more common causes for presentation to the ED.

Hepatitis

Perspective *Hepatitis* is a generic term referring to inflammation of the liver. Hepatitis, although most commonly a consequence of viral infection, can be secondary to bacterial, fungal, or parasitic infection; a result of toxic exposure; a side effect of prescribed medication; or a consequence of an immunologic disorder. Hepatitis in its generic context represents the most common variety of liver disease encountered by the emergency physician.

Viral Hepatitis Although many viruses are associated with some degree of measurable liver inflammation, the most significant and potentially severe cases of viral hepatitis are caused by type A (infectious), type B (serum), type C (posttransfusion), and delta viruses. Although a common cause of hepatitis, Epstein-Barr virus, the causative agent of mononucleosis, is more important clinically for its nonhepatic effects.

Epidemiology In 1997 there were 11.7 cases of hepatitis A per 100,000 population in the United States. The incidence for hepatitis B was 3.9 and hepatitis C was 1.4 per 100,000 population.[1] The number of cases of hepatitis A remained stable during the 10 years between 1988 and 1997, but had declined by almost 60% for hepatitis B and increased by almost 50% for hepatitis C.[1] Widespread use of the hepatitis B vaccine, along with changes in sexual practices among homosexual males, is largely responsible for the decline in rates of hepatitis B. It is expected that the relatively recent introduction of an effective hepatitis A vaccine will have a similar effect on the incidence of this infection.

Hepatitis A virus (HAV), the causative agent of type A hepatitis, is a RNA virus in the group of enteroviral picornaviruses.[2] It is spread by the fecal-oral route either directly or through contaminated water or foodstuffs. Transmission via contact with blood is a theoretical possibility but is exceedingly rare. HAV can occur sporadically but is notorious for its association with epidemics. HAV infection is common worldwide; serologic evidence of previous infection exists in almost 100% of the adult population in some regions. In the United States, close to one half of all urban-dwelling adults are seropositive for antibody for HAV.[3] Approximately one third of reported cases occur in children under 15 years of age and the fewest number are in the group over 40.[4] The incidence of hepatitis A infection varies among different ethnic groups. In the United States, the incidence among American Indians and Alaskan natives is 121 per 100,000 population compared to Asians with an incidence of 5 per 100,000 population.[4] High rates of seropositivity in association with the relatively small number of reported episodes supports the notion that many cases are anicteric and may be asymptomatic. Occult disease appears to be more common in the pediatric age group. It is estimated that as many as 70% of cases in children are asymptomatic.[4] The typical incubation period for HAV is 30 days, with a range of 15 to 45 days. Viremia is of relatively short duration and is most prominent before onset of symptoms. Fecal shedding and the period of greatest infectivity occur before the onset of symptomatic disease and have generally waned by the time jaundice appears (Figure 85-1). HAV is not associated with a chronic carrier state.

Hepatitis B virus (HBV) is a DNA virus associated with hepatitis B. It is contained in a 42-nm structure called the *Dane particle.* Within this enveloped virion is the viral DNA, which is both single- and double-stranded; DNA polymerase; hepatitis B surface antigen (HBsAg); and hepatitis B core antigen (HBcAg). Hepatitis B e antigen (HBeAg), detectable in the serum of infected patients, is thought to be a degradation product of HBcAg.[5] Compared with HAV, for which there is only a single antigenic variety, there are eight subtypes of HBV as defined by surface antigen. HBV, which is principally transmitted by parenteral exposure, can be transmitted via intimate contact as well. The highest rates of infection are among intravenous (IV) drug users and homosexual men. Blood transfusion, previously a common source of infection, has been eliminated because of modern blood-bank screening techniques.

HBsAg has been detected in a variety of bodily secretions, including saliva, semen, stool, tears, urine, and vaginal secretions. Although the presence of HBsAg is not synonymous with infectivity, HBV DNA has been identified in several of these fluids and is likely to be infectious.[6] The typical interval between exposure and onset of clinical illness is between 60 and 90 days; however, serologic markers of infection generally appear within 1 to 3 weeks (Figure 85-2).[7] Approximately 10% of adults and 90% of neonates infected with HBV will become chronic carriers of HBsAg.[8] These groups serve as important reservoirs of infection and major sources of exposure risk for the health care worker. The overall prevalence of HBsAg in the United States is low but can be significant in many subpopulations (Table 85-1). Health care workers who come in contact with blood with some regularity have a prevalence of HBsAg of 1% to 2%, and 15% to 30% show serologic evidence of previous infection.[9]

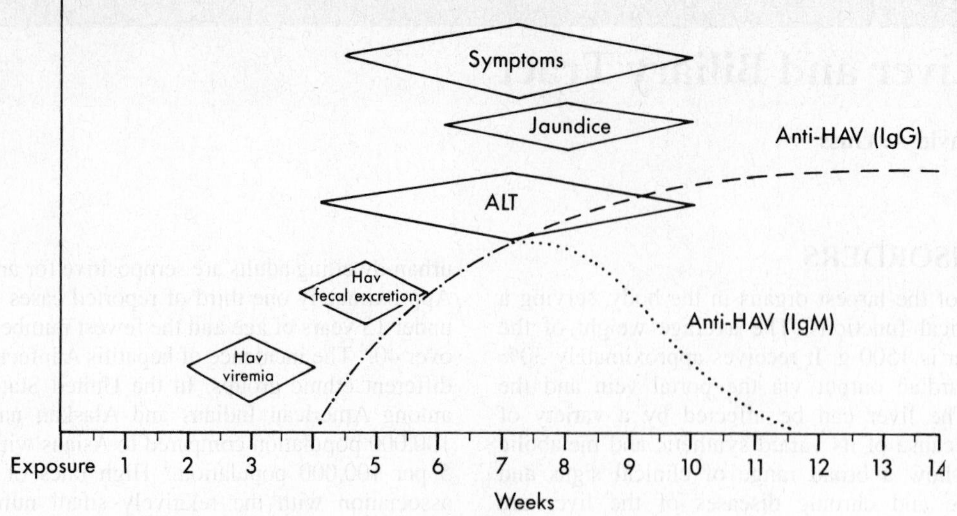

Figure 85-1. **Acute hepatitis A virus infection.**

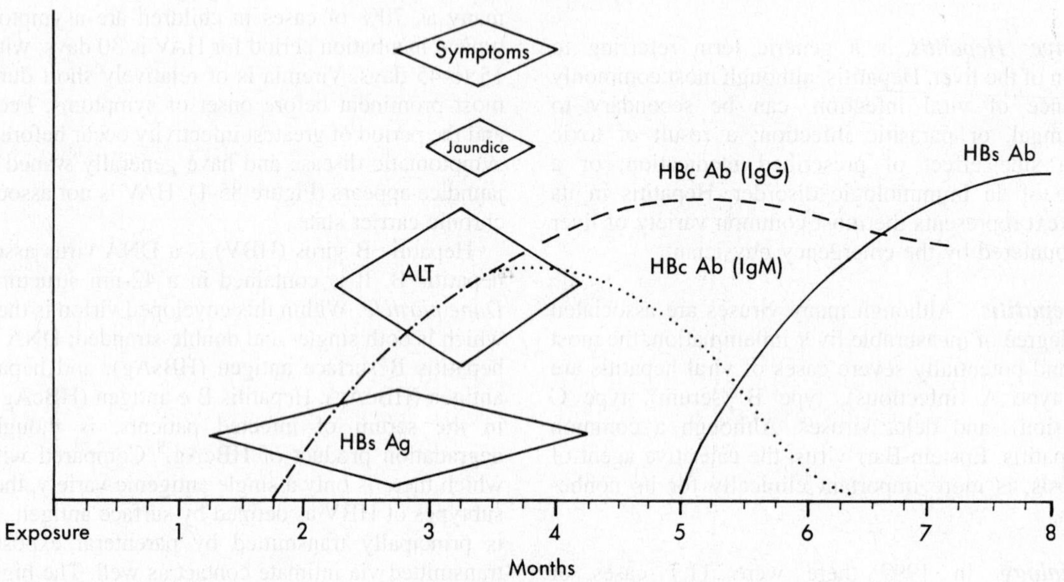

Figure 85-2. **Acute hepatitis B virus infection.**

Table 85-1. Prevalence of Hepatitis B Serologic Markers

Population	HBsAg (%)	All markers
Immigrants from areas with endemic HBV	13	70-85
Intravenous drug users	7	60-80
Homosexual males	6	35-80
Household contacts of HBV carriers	3-6	30-60
Health care workers, frequent blood exposure	1-2	15-30
Health care workers, infrequent blood exposure	0.3	3-10
Prisoners (men)	1-8	10-80
Healthy adults first time blood donors	0.3	3-5

Modified from Centers for Disease Control and Prevention: *MMWR* 39(RR-2), 1990.

What was historically referred to as non-A non-B hepatitis is caused by at least two distinct RNA viruses—hepatitis C and hepatitis E. Hepatitis C, linked to transfusions, is common in the United States. Hepatitis E, which is associated with fecal-oral transmission, is encountered most often in Asia, Africa, and the Soviet Union.[10] The historic risk of hepatitis in patients receiving blood transfusions was about 0.45% per unit transfused. The screening of donor blood for surrogate markers (aminotransferases) and antibody to hepatitis C has decreased this risk to 0.03% per unit.[11] Although hepatitis C has been most prominently associated with transfusions, only 10% of patients with this disease report a previous history of having received blood or blood products.[12] Approximately 4% to 8% of cases are linked to occupational exposure in health care workers, and 23% to 60% are associated with IV drug use.[13] In as many as 40% to 57% of cases of hepatitis C, no identifiable source of infection is present.[12-14] The incubation period of hepatitis C is 30 to 90 days, with a mean of 50 days, whereas hepatitis E has an incubation similar to that of HAV—15 to 60 days.[15] Approximately 50% of patients with hepatitis C go on to develop chronic hepatitis, and cirrhosis develops in 20% of this group within a decade.[16,17] In the United States it is estimated that 2.7 million people are chronically infected with HCV.[18]

Hepatitis delta virus (HDV) was discovered by Rizzetto et al in 1977 while they were working on liver specimens from patients with chronic HBV infection.[19] It is a defective RNA virus that can infect only patients who are actively producing HBsAg, which is required for its viral coating. HDV is worldwide in its distribution. In the United States, the incidence of HDV antibody is between 4% and 30% of patients with chronic HBV infection.[20,21] As a consequence of the routine association with chronic HBV infection, it is likely that many cases of HDV are misdiagnosed as acute or reactivated HBV. HDV is spread in a manner similar to HBV, being most common among IV drug users, promiscuous homosexual men, and hemophiliacs. Infection with HDV can occur either concomitantly with HBV (coinfection) or subsequent to earlier HBV infection (superinfection). In cases of coinfection, the course of the illness is generally dominated by HBV; however, the delta virus seems to carry an increased risk of fulminant disease.[22,23] In cases of superinfection, the presentation may span the gamut from acute self-limited disease to fulminant hepatitis or chronic infection.

Hepatitis G virus, also referred to as hepatitis G/Gbv-C virus, is the most recently identified virus associated with hepatitis. It is a RNA virus in the Flaviviridae family. Transmission of the virus seems to occur through blood transfusion, parenteral exposure to blood or blood products, and possibly during intimate sexual contact. The virus has been identified in patients with acute and chronic hepatitis. However, it is generally felt to be an innocent bystander with disease manifestations attributed to coinfection with another hepatitis virus.[24-26]

Principles of Disease The pathophysiology of viral hepatitis is incompletely understood. In the most common varieties of hepatitis, liver injury appears to be related to the development of the immunologic response to infection rather than to the cytopathologic effect of the virus. HDV appears to be an exception having significant direct cytotoxic potential.

Clinical Features The clinical presentation of viral hepatitis is highly variable. A significant number, possibly a majority, of cases are asymptomatic. The protean nature of symptoms and the common occurrence of anicteric disease can result in misdiagnosis. The most common symptoms are malaise, fever, and anorexia, followed by nausea, vomiting, abdominal discomfort, and diarrhea. The first symptom leading to physician consultation is commonly jaundice. A small number of patients with HBV develop a prodromal illness characterized by arthralgia or arthritis and dermatitis. The joint involvement is generally polyarticular and is most common in the small joints of the hands and the wrists. Joint fluid usually is noninflammatory but can have cell counts as high as 90,000 cells/mm^3. The characteristic dermatitis is urticarial but may be macular, papular, or petechial.

Fulminant hepatitis is characterized by acute onset and progresses to hepatic failure and encephalopathy over a period of days. Although most often encountered with HBV and HDV and least frequently with HCV, fulminant hepatitis can occur in association with all viral etiologies.[27] The overall incidence of fulminant hepatitis is 1% to 2% of all cases. The hallmarks of fulminant disease are altered mentation and spontaneous mucosal bleeding.

Physical findings include elevated temperature, scleral or cutaneous icterus, and abdominal tenderness. If significant vomiting has occurred, tachycardia and supine or orthostatic hypotension may be noted. Hepatomegaly may be detected and, when present, is generally characterized by a smooth, homogeneous, and tender liver surface. Even if liver enlargement is not appreciated, the patient often has tenderness to percussion over the lower right ribs. Scleral icterus is generally noticeable earlier than cutaneous discoloration, particularly in people of pigmented races. Muddy sclera, commonly found among African-American patients, may obscure or confuse this finding. An alternative in this setting is examination of sublingual or subungual surfaces. Scleral icterus usually is not clinically apparent, even to the most astute observers, until serum bilirubin is above 2.5 mg/dl. Spider angiomata and splenomegaly, although more commonly associated with cirrhosis, may be detected with acute presentations. Gray or acholic stools are distinctly uncommon.

Diagnostic Strategies Laboratory tests are critically important in diagnosing hepatitis and determining specific cause. The most useful tests are measurements of the hepatic aminotransferases and bilirubin. The typical case is associated with elevations (tenfold to 100-fold) of serum aspartate aminotransferase (AST) and alanine aminotransferase (ALT), with ALT generally elevated in excess of AST. Bilirubin may be moderately increased (5 to 10 mg/dl) and occasionally is markedly elevated (15 to 25 mg/dl). Hyperbilirubinemia typically emerges several days to a week or more after the onset of clinical symptoms. Both fractions of bilirubin—direct reacting and indirect reacting—are elevated in close-to-equal proportions. Alkaline phosphatase and lactate dehydrogenase may be elevated but are rarely more than two to three times normal. Prothrombin time (PT) is a useful test to assess the degree of hepatic synthetic dysfunction. Elevation of the PT may be the first clue of a complicated course. The white blood count (WBC) generally is not useful because values range from low overall counts with a lymphocytic predominance to marked polymorphonuclear leukocytosis.

Although determination of the precise cause of hepatitis can rarely be achieved during the primary visit to the ED, it is important to initiate this evaluation as soon as possible. Identification of the causative agent has significant impact on prognosis and public health issues. In this regard, it is important to be able to interpret the significance of certain serologic tests (Table 85-2).

Acute HAV is diagnosed by the presence of immunoglobulin M (IgM) HAV antibody, whereas prior infection is determined by the measurement of an immunoglobulin G (IgG) antibody. Acute HBV infection is characterized by the presence of HBsAg and IgM antibody to HBcAg. HBsAg alone should not be relied on to make the diagnosis of acute HBV because it can be either absent late in the course of acute disease or present chronically unrelated to the cause of the current episode. Anti-HBcAg antibody is generally the best indicator of previous HBV infection, whereas anti-HBsAg antibody is the best marker for immunity to HBV.

Currently, the diagnosis of hepatitis C is based on the exposure history and the elimination of other causes. The

Table 85-2. Serologic Markers in Hepatitis

Serologic marker	Abbreviation	Interpretation
Antibody to HAV	Anti-HAV	A combination of IgG and IgM antibody defining infection with HAV, acute or past
IgM antibody to HAV	Anti-HAV IgM	Antibody to HAV, indicating acute infection
Hepatitis B surface antigen	HBsAg	Surface antigen associated with acute or chronic HBV infection
Hepatitis B e antigen	HBeAg	Antigen associated with active infection, acute or chronic, and indicative of high infectivity
Antibody to B surface antigen	HBsAb	Antibody indicative of acute or past infection or immunization
Antibody to B core antigen	HBcAb	A combination of IgG and IgM antibody defining infection with HBV, acute or past
IgM antibody to B core antigen	HBcAb-IgM	Antibody to B core antigen, indicating acute infection with HBV
Antibody to B e antigen	HBeAb	Antibody to e antigen, possibly representing resolving HBV infection and decreased infectivity
Antibody to HDV	Anti-HDV	Antibody defining infection with HDV; HBsAg should be present
Antibody to HCV	Anti-HCV	A new antibody that defines infection with HCV, acute or past

serologic assay for an antibody to this virus facilitates a definitive diagnosis but there can be a delay between the onset of symptoms and the development of assayable antibody.[15,28,29] Furthermore, the HCV test does not distinguish acute from chronic infection.

Diagnosing HDV requires an aggressive search because the disease can easily be mistaken for acute or chronic HBV infection. A serologic test for the antibody to HDV (anti-HDV) is available. The presence of this antibody in conjunction with IgM antibody to HBcAg suggests coinfection of HDV and HBV. Anti-HDV in association with IgG antibody to HBcAg supports the diagnosis of superinfection.

The temporal relationships between infection, clinical symptoms, and serologic responses for the two most common causes of viral hepatitis, HAV and HBV, are delineated in Figures 85-1 and 85-2.

Complications of acute hepatitis are most commonly related to fluid or electrolyte imbalance as a result of inadequate oral intake or refractory emesis. Severe vomiting can result in upper gastrointestinal (GI) bleeding as the result of an esophageal tear. The most severe complication of acute disease is the development of liver failure heralded by the emergence of hepatic encephalopathy. Most patients with viral hepatitis have self-limited disease that goes on to symptomatic and histologic resolution in 2 to 4 weeks. Approximately 10% of patients with hepatitis B and as many as 50% of those with hepatitis C will develop chronic disease. A small but significant number of these patients will go on to develop cirrhosis and eventually die.

Differential Considerations The protean nature of the symptoms and signs associated with viral hepatitis makes the differential diagnosis of this disorder quite broad. Beyond a variety of nonhepatic viral illnesses, one must consider all of the infectious, chemical, and immunologic etiologies of hepatic inflammation in addition to biliary tract disease. A viral cause is often suggested by the exposure and medical history but requires serologic tests for confirmation. Alcoholic hepatitis usually is associated with a history of chronic or excessive alcohol consumption, less marked elevation of hepatic transaminases, and AST levels elevated above those of ALT. Extrahepatic obstruction, cholecystitis, and cholelithiasis are excluded by their lack of association with significant elevation of aminotransferases. On occasion, abdominal ultrasound is required to eliminate these other causes.

Management Treatment of viral hepatitis is primarily symptomatic. The most common requirement is to correct fluid and electrolyte imbalance that may have occurred as a consequence of poor oral intake or excessive diarrhea or vomiting. Antiemetics should be used; they may allow resumption of adequate oral intake, thereby avoiding hospital admission. In the anorectic or nauseous patient, fluid intake should be encouraged, with avoidance of solids until they are palatable. Medications requiring primarily hepatic metabolism generally do not need to be discontinued or the dosage modified unless there is suspicion of significant hepatic dysfunction as evidenced by prolongation of PT. Nonessential drugs with hepatotoxic potential should not be taken. Alcohol consumption should be completely discontinued until signs of liver injury have disappeared. Although a variety of active interventions (e.g., corticosteroid administration) have been suggested, no reliable data suggest that such therapies offer clear benefit; they may even be harmful.

Disposition Hospital admission is rarely required for patients with viral hepatitis and is generally reserved for the individual with significant fluid and electrolyte imbalance or refractory vomiting. Patients with less severe illness may require hospitalization for concomitant medical problems or if suitable living arrangements are not available. Altered sensorium or prolonged PT beyond 5 seconds over control may suggest fulminant disease or an increased likelihood of a complicated course, necessitating admission for observation. The emergence of fulminant disease should lead to consideration of transfer to a facility that can offer liver transplantation.

Anxiety about disease communicability may affect the ease of a disposition. Patients with possible HAV infection should be advised to practice meticulous personal hygiene, not to share toiletries, and to ensure cleaning of utensils and

Table 85-3. Postexposure Hepatitis Prophylaxis

Hepatitis A

Nature of exposure	Recommended treatment
Close personal contact	ISG 0.02 ml/kg IM
Day care center	
Employee	ISG 0.02 ml/kg IM
Attendee	ISG 0.02 ml/kg IM
School contacts	None
Hospital contacts	None
Workplace contacts	None
Food-borne source	
Within 2 weeks of exposure	ISG 0.02 ml/kg IM
After 2 weeks of exposure	None
After common source outbreaks have begun to occur	None

Hepatitis B

Nature of exposure	Source	Exposed individual: Unvaccinated	Exposed individual: Vaccinated
Percutaneous/mucosal	HBsAG$^+$	1. HBIG* 2. HB vaccine†	1. Test HBsAb; if –, then a. HBIG b. HB vaccine
	Known source High-risk HBsAg$^+$	1. HB vaccine 2. Test source; if +, then HBIG	1. Test HBsAb; if – and source HBsAg$^+$ a. HBIG b. HB vaccine
	Low-risk HBsAg$^+$	1. HB vaccine	1. None
	Unknown source	1. HB vaccine	1. None
Intimate sexual	HBsAg$^+$	1. HBIG 2. HB vaccine‡	1. None
Household/workplace	HBsAg$^+$	1. None	1. None
Perinatal	HBsAg$^+$	1. HBIG§ 2. HB vaccine	NA

Hepatitis C

Unknown benefit from prophylaxis; ISG 0.06 ml/kg IM should be considered for parenteral exposures from patients with evidence of viral hepatitis and negative serologies

Hepatitis delta

Same as for Hepatitis B

Modified from Centers for Disease Control and Prevention: *MMWR* 39(RR-2), 1990.
*HBIG, hepatitis B immune globulin, dose 0.6 ml/kg IM.
†HB vaccine, hepatitis B vaccine, dose 20 μg IM deltoid (adequate vaccination requires three injections, so all patients should be referred for follow-up).
‡Vaccine required only if repeated sexual contacts are likely to occur over an extended period of time and the source becomes a chronic carrier.
§Dose of HBIG 0.5 ml/kg.

kitchenware between uses. In those patients with suspected HBV or HDV infection, the relatively low risk of transmission in lieu of intimate personal contact or parenteral exposure should be emphasized.

The emergency physician assumes specific public health responsibilities when managing a patient with viral hepatitis. Viral hepatitis is a reportable disease, and the emergency physician is required to complete appropriate health department notification forms. The emergency physician should provide immunoprophylaxis for the patient's family members and close personal contacts. Although the nature of prophylaxis depends on the specific viral cause, it is wise to offer γ-globulin to household contacts immediately, pending serologic determination. Table 85-3 outlines the guidelines for immunoprophylaxis. Patients with HAV infection who process or handle food must not return to work while potentially infectious. Although infectivity is greatly diminished by the time jaundice emerges, it is best to delay return to work until after jaundice has cleared.

Special Considerations The risks associated with percutaneous or mucosal exposure to blood or blood products have recently been brought into sharp focus as a result of the human immunodeficiency virus (HIV) epidemic. Antedating this epidemic is the long-standing risk associated with HBV. There has been effective preexposure and postexposure prophylaxis for HBV for almost two decades. The risks from HBV are exemplified by the relatively high rates of seropositivity for HBV infection among health care workers compared with the general population (see Table 85-1). Health care workers in an ED are in particular jeopardy because of frequent contact with blood and interaction with patient groups at higher risk of harboring infective virus. Seropositivity among ED nurses is 30%, and among ED physicians it has been reported at between 12% and 15% (see Table 85-1).[22,23,30-32] It is estimated that the 1-year risk of infection among ED physicians is 0.25%, with a 30-year risk approaching 1 in 13. During a 30-year career, the risk of death from HBV is estimated at 1:540.[33] A recent analysis conducted in an inner-city ED identified markers for hepatitis C in 18% of patients. The health risk this might pose to staff is unknown.

As a result of the considerable risk, all ED personnel involved in patient care or custodial work should be vaccinated for HBV before or soon after employment. The vaccine is highly effective and associated with minimal acute or delayed toxicity. A complete three-injection series of vaccine is associated with the development of protective antibody in approximately 95% of individuals.[34] Centers for Disease Control and Prevention (CDC) data suggest that optimal immunologic response results from deltoid injection.[35] HBV immune globulin (HBIG) is recommended for immediate passive immunization in individuals not previously immunized but exposed to potentially infective material. HBIG alone diminishes the risk of HBV infection by 75%.[9] Unvaccinated, exposed people should receive HBIG 0.06 ml/kg intramuscularly (IM) in addition to the HB vaccine. Concerns related to the potential risk of HIV infection from gamma-globulin preparations are unfounded. Figure 85-3 outlines an approach for managing health care workers exposed to blood or other potentially infectious secretions.

A safe and effective vaccine for HAV is available; however, health care workers are not currently on the list of those recommended for routine immunization.[4]

The risk of seroconversion after percutaneous exposure from an HCV-positive source is about 1.8%[14] Despite health care workers' theoretical risk to bloodborne HCV exposure, the prevalence of HCV infection in this group is approximately 1% to 2%, which is no greater than the prevalence in the general population.[14] There is no effective vaccine for HCV and no accepted pre- or postexposure prophylaxis.

Key Concepts

- Viral hepatitis is a common ED disorder that can be caused by an increasingly large number of agents.
- Clinical presentation is highly variable, with many cases, particularly in the pediatric age range, being anicteric or asymptomatic.
- The process of identifying the etiologic agent should be initiated in the ED because it affects both prognosis and public health interventions.
- Many of the etiologic agents of viral hepatitis represent a potential threat to health care workers necessitating proper preexposure and postexposure prophylaxis.

Alcohol-Related Liver Disease

Perspective Alcoholism is a major medical and social problem in the United States; an estimated 10 million people are chronic alcoholics.[36] Alcohol and its metabolites are toxic to most organ systems and are contributory to disease or death from many different causes. The liver is the most common site of injury from chronic ethanol ingestion. Alcoholic liver disease is ranked as the fourth leading cause of death among men aged 25 to 64 years living in urban areas. Cirrhosis, most commonly linked to chronic alcohol consumption, is the ninth most common overall cause of death and years of productive life lost.[37]

Principles of Disease Alcohol is largely eliminated by metabolic degradation in the liver. Approximately 2% to 15% of alcohol is excreted unchanged in the urine or expired air.[38,39] Alcohol is degraded in the liver by three enzyme systems: 1) cytosolic alcohol dehydrogenase and aldehyde dehydrogenase, 2) peroxisomal catalase, and 3) microsomal oxidases. The action of alcohol dehydrogenase on ethanol results in a decreased oxidized nicotinamide adenine dinucleotide/reduced nicotinamide adenine dinucleotide (NAD^+/NADH) ratio that plays a significant role in many of the metabolic effects of ethanol and may contribute to liver injury. The precise pathogenesis of alcoholic liver disease is unknown and probably multifactorial. There is evidence linking coexistent malnutrition, accumulation of toxic metabolites (e.g., acetaldehyde), excessive production of NADH, induction of microsomal enzymes, and alteration of immune function.[38,39]

Regardless of the precise mechanism of injury, there appears to be genetic heterogeneity with respect to susceptibility to liver damage. Women and possibly American Indians appear to have an increased propensity for injury, relative to white men.[40,41] A study of Portuguese adults identifies certain histocompatibility antigens with enhanced risk of ethanol-related hepatic injury.[42] Although susceptibility to alcohol varies, in general there is rough correlation between the amount of ethanol ingested and the risk of developing liver disease. The risk of liver injury increases as daily consumption exceeds 80 g of ethanol daily in men and 20 g in women. For men this is equivalent to a six pack of beer, four to six glasses of wine, or three to four mixed drinks daily.[36]

The most common variety of alcohol-induced liver disease is steatosis. Fatty infiltration of the liver is most likely a consequence of altered fatty acid metabolism resulting from the diminished NAD^+/NADH ratio, which favors triglyceride production.[43] Fatty infiltration appears to be a direct result of the duration and amount of alcohol consumed and, in general, is reversible when the patient ceases ethanol consumption. Beyond enlargement of the liver, which is usually painless, this tends to be a benign disorder.

Clinical Features Alcoholic hepatitis is a potentially severe form of alcohol-induced liver disease and a more common cause for people to present to the ED. Although

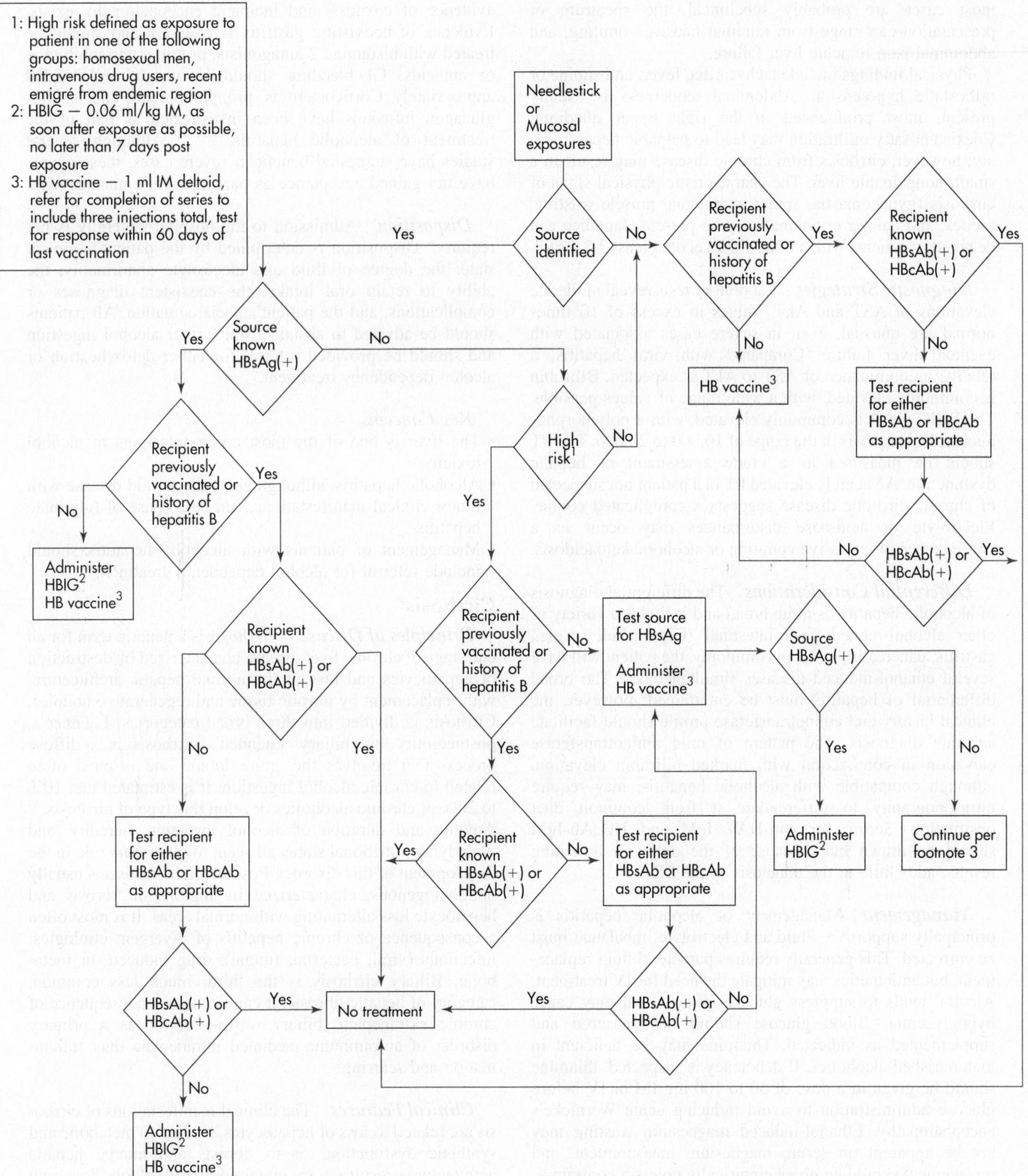

Figure 85-3. **Management of health care workers exposed to blood or other infectious secretions.**

most cases are probably subclinical, the spectrum of presentation can range from minimal nausea, vomiting, and abdominal pain to acute liver failure.

Physical findings include tachycardia, fever, and supine or orthostatic hypotension. Abdominal tenderness is usually present, most pronounced in the right upper quadrant. Coexistent fatty infiltration may lead to palpable hepatomegaly; however, cirrhosis from chronic disease may result in a small, nonpalpable liver. The characteristic physical signs of cirrhosis (gynecomastia, spider angiomata, muscle wasting, ascites, and palmar erythema) may be present. Jaundice can be noted in patients with a bilirubin level of at least 2.5 mg/dl.

Diagnostic Strategies Laboratory tests reveal moderate elevations of AST and ALT. Values in excess of 10 times normal are unusual, even in severe cases associated with eventual liver failure. Compared with viral hepatitis, a relative predominance of AST to ALT is expected. Bilirubin is commonly elevated, with a wide range of values possible. The WBC count is commonly elevated, with a polymorphonuclear leukocytosis in the range of 10,000 to 20,000. The PT should be measured as a crude assessment of hepatic dysfunction. An acutely elevated PT in a patient not suspected of chronic cirrhotic disease suggests a complicated course. Electrolyte or acid-base disturbances may occur as a consequence of excessive vomiting or alcoholic ketoacidosis.

Differential Considerations The differential diagnosis of alcoholic hepatitis is quite broad and includes a variety of other alcohol-related gastrointestinal (GI) maladies (e.g., gastritis, pancreatitis). Not uncommonly, the patient will have several ethanol-induced diseases simultaneously. The broad differential of hepatitis must be entertained; however, the clinical history and aminotransferase profile should facilitate accurate diagnosis. The pattern of mild aminotransferase elevation in conjunction with marked bilirubin elevation, although compatible with alcoholic hepatitis, may require ultrasonography to differentiate it from common duct obstruction. Serum for anti-HAV IgM and HBcAb-IgM should be drawn but, because of the delay in obtaining results, adds little to the diagnosis in the ED.

Management Management of alcoholic hepatitis is principally supportive. Fluid and electrolyte imbalance must be corrected. This generally requires parenteral fluid replacement, but antiemetics may mitigate the need for IV treatment. Alcohol tends to suppress gluconeogenesis and may cause hypoglycemia. Blood glucose should be measured and supplemented as indicated. Thiamine may be deficient in malnourished alcoholics. If deficiency is suspected, thiamine should be given in a dose of 50 to 100 mg IM or IV before glucose administration to avoid inducing acute Wernicke's encephalopathy. Ethanol-induced magnesium wasting may not be apparent on serum magnesium measurement, and replacement should be given empirically unless a contraindication such as renal failure or known hypermagnesemia exists. Magnesium can be given as a sulfate salt in a dose of 1 g IV or IM or as oral replacement in a dosage of 200 to 1,000 mg daily as an oxide, chloride salt, or amino acid conjugate.

The overall nutritional status of the patient should be addressed with the administration of a high-calorie, vitamin-supplemented diet. Protein content may require restriction if evidence of cirrhosis and incipient encephalopathy exists. Evidence of coexisting gastritis is common and should be treated with histamine 2 antagonists, proton pump inhibitors, or antacids. GI bleeding should be sought and treated appropriately. Corticosteroids, propylthiouracil, and insulin-glucagon infusions have been investigated as part of the treatment of alcoholic hepatitis.[36,44-48] Although several studies have suggested benefit in severe cases, these agents have not gained acceptance as part of routine management.

Disposition Admission to the hospital generally is not required. Disposition is determined by the patient's clinical state: the degree of fluid and electrolyte abnormality, the ability to retain oral intake, the coexistent diagnoses or complications, and the patient's social situation. All patients should be advised to abstain from further alcohol ingestion and should be provided referral for either detoxification or alcohol dependency treatment.

Key Concepts

- The liver is one of the most common targets of alcohol toxicity.
- Alcoholic hepatitis, although generally a mild disease with minor clinical manifestations, can be a cause of fulminate hepatitis.
- Management of patients with alcoholic hepatitis should include referral for alcohol dependency treatment.

Cirrhosis

Principles of Disease *Cirrhosis* is a generic term for an end stage of chronic liver disease characterized by destruction of hepatocytes and loss of the normal hepatic architecture, with replacement by fibrotic tissue and regenerative nodules. Cirrhosis is divided into three broad categories: Laënnec's, postnecrotic, and biliary. Laënnec's cirrhosis is a diffuse process that involves the entire lobule and is most often related to chronic alcohol ingestion. It is estimated that 10% to 20% of chronic alcoholics develop this type of cirrhosis.[44] Amount and duration of alcohol ingestion, heredity, and underlying nutritional status all seem to play some role in the development of this disorder. Postnecrotic cirrhosis is usually nonhomogenous, characterized by regions of fibrosis and hepatocyte loss alternating with normal areas. It is most often a consequence of chronic hepatitis of divergent etiologies: infectious (viral, bacterial, fungal), drug induced, or metabolic. Biliary cirrhosis is the third, much less common, category of hepatic fibrosis. It can occur as a consequence of chronic extrahepatic biliary obstruction or as a primary disorder of autoimmune-mediated intrahepatic duct inflammation and scarring.

Clinical Features The clinical manifestations of cirrhosis are related to loss of hepatocytes, leading to metabolic and synthetic dysfunction, or to fibrosis and altered hepatic architecture, resulting in impaired portal blood flow and portal hypertension. Typically, the patient with cirrhosis complains of chronic fatigue and poor appetite. With the exception of those with biliary cirrhosis, many patients with cirrhosis can be asymptomatic until they develop some dramatic complication such as GI bleeding, ascites, or hepatic encephalopathy. Patients with biliary cirrhosis generally complain of pruritus or develop obvious jaundice before end stage cirrhosis or complications develop. Primary biliary cirrhosis may be associated with other immune-mediated disorders; these patients may have signs and symptoms characteristic of scleroderma or CREST—calcinosis cutis, Raynaud phenomenon, esophageal motility disorder, sclerodactyly, and telangiectasia—syndrome.[49]

Physical examination may reveal muscle wasting, thinning of the skin with patchy ecchymosis, spider angiomata, palmar erythema, Dupuytren's contracture, and, in men, gynecomastia or testicular atrophy. Jaundice is generally absent in mild or early cases. The liver may not be palpable if it is extensively scarred, but a large regenerative nodule, tumor, or fatty infiltration can result in hepatomegaly. Ascites is common, particularly in advanced disease, and may be present in association with a characteristic pattern of abdominal wall vein distention known as *caput medusae.*

Diagnostic Strategies Laboratory tests are not specific. Aminotransferase levels are rarely more than minimally elevated. Bilirubin may be increased but usually not until cirrhosis is far advanced. Elevation of alkaline phosphatase out of proportion to other liver enzymes is suggestive of biliary cirrhosis. Coagulation studies are commonly abnormal, and the serum albumin level is low as a result of impaired hepatic synthetic function. Mild-to-moderate anemia and thrombocytopenia are often present in Laënnec's cirrhosis. Elevated blood urea nitrogen (BUN) or creatinine should suggest dehydration or hepatorenal syndrome.

Ancillary tests are rarely of use in the emergency setting. Ultrasonography is highly sensitive for the detection of ascites, but a carefully performed physical examination can generally yield equivalent results.[50] Patients with ascites and fever or abdominal pain should have paracentesis performed to eliminate the possibility of spontaneous bacterial peritonitis. Nuclear or computed tomography (CT) scan imaging may reveal a hepatic or splenic appearance characteristic of cirrhosis and portal hypertension but, in general, these tests should be deferred to an elective setting.

Management Treatment of cirrhosis in the ED is limited. Fluid and electrolyte imbalances should be corrected, and vitamin and nutritional supplements should be provided. Most patients can be discharged with referral to a general internist for further evaluation and treatment. Ascites associated with respiratory compromise or significant discomfort can be treated with paracentesis and removal of up to 1 to 2 L of fluid. Removal of larger quantities can result in fluid and electrolyte abnormalities and should, therefore, result in admission for observation. If spontaneous bacterial peritonitis is a consideration, diagnostic paracentesis should be done.

A low-sodium diet in conjunction with low-dosage diuretics, preferably an aldosterone antagonist, may be of use in the chronic management of ascites and edema. Coagulopathy noted before a planned invasive procedure or in conjunction with active bleeding should be corrected with fresh-frozen plasma. Uncomplicated prolongation of PT can be treated with vitamin K supplement, but this is often ineffective. GI bleeding should be treated aggressively. Early consultation with a gastroenterologist for endoscopy will often permit identification of a bleeding site and initiation of appropriate adjunctive treatment. The presence of a newly elevated creatinine value may herald the onset of hepatorenal syndrome and requires admission for optimal fluid and electrolyte management.

Complications of cirrhosis include GI bleeding, ascites with or without infection, encephalopathy, and hepatorenal syndrome. Although GI bleeding is often related to esophageal or gastric varices, more than one half of cases result from some other source (e.g., gastritis or a duodenal ulcer)[51] (see Chapter 23). Ascites occurs as a consequence of portal hypertension, impaired hepatic lymph flow, hypoalbuminemia, and renal salt retention. Although ascites generally causes little more than unsightly abdominal distention and discomfort, it can become massive and lead to respiratory embarrassment. Spontaneous infection of ascites is an important and often subtle complication and is discussed separately. Encephalopathy occurs as a result of impaired hepatic metabolic function and portal hypertension. The pathophysiology of this complication, its diagnosis, and treatment are presented in the next section. Hepatorenal syndrome is defined as renal failure occurring in the setting of cirrhosis without obvious renal pathology. The mechanism of this almost universally fatal complication is not understood. An unexplained elevation of creatinine or BUN suggests an emerging hepatorenal state.

Key Concepts

- Cirrhosis is an advanced stage of liver disease from a variety of causes.
- The clinical presentation in the ED of patients with cirrhosis is most often a complication of cirrhosis such as ascites, variceal bleeding, or hepatic encephalopathy.
- Impaired hepatic synthetic and metabolic function in patients with cirrhosis may require correction of coagulopathy before invasive procedures and modification of medication dosing.

Hepatic Encephalopathy

Principles of Disease Hepatic encephalopathy is a clinical state of disordered cerebral function occurring because of acute or chronic liver disease. The pathophysiology of hepatic coma is complex and related to the diseased liver's failure to adequately perform its normal metabolic functions, which can occur as a result of hepatocellular dysfunction or portal systemic shunting. Ammonia, formed primarily in the GI tract by the action of bacteria on proteinaceous compounds, is a common marker of this process. Normally, absorbed ammonia is converted to urea in the liver. In the setting of severe hepatic disease, ammonia accumulates and crosses the blood-brain barrier and combines sequentially with α-ketoglutarate and glutamate to form glutamine. Although serum ammonia levels correlate inconsistently with the severity of encephalopathy, there is a close association with cerebrospinal fluid (CSF) glutamine levels.[52] Whether glutamine is itself toxic or simply represents a marker for disordered central nervous system (CNS) metabolism is unknown. Other agents presumed to play a role in the pathophysiology of this disorder include mercaptans, octopamine, γ-aminobutyric acid, and the aromatic amino acids, particularly tryptophan.

Clinical Features The clinical manifestations of hepatic encephalopathy vary depending on the severity of the process. Presenting symptoms run the gamut from mild cognitive dysfunction, irritability, and confusion to profound coma. Table 85-4 summarizes the four stages of hepatic encephalopathy. Asterixis, a low-amplitude, alternating flex-

Table 85-4. Grades of Hepatic Encephalopathy

Grade	Clinical description
I	Disordered sleep, irritability, depression, mild cognitive dysfunction
II	Lethargy, disorientation, confusion, personality changes, asterixis
III	Somnolence or marked disorientation, confused speech, inability to follow commands, possible asterixis
IV	Coma

ion and extension of the wrist when it is held in extension is characteristic of mild to moderate degrees of encephalopathy. A similar finding may be elicited in the dorsiflexed foot or in the head with extension of the neck. Fetor hepaticus, a musty breath odor presumably caused by mercaptans, may be appreciated in severe cases.

Physical examination commonly reveals signs of cirrhosis, including spider angiomata, testicular atrophy, muscle wasting, superficial bruising, gynecomastia, and ascites.

Diagnostic Strategies Laboratory tests may be normal or indicative of fulminant liver failure or chronic cirrhosis. Serum ammonia levels are generally elevated but, as previously mentioned, do not necessarily correlate with the severity of encephalopathy. Laboratory tests reflective of hepatic synthetic function, albumin and protime, are generally abnormal. The electroencephalogram is abnormal in most cases, but the pattern of generalized slowing with high-voltage bursts of triphasic or delta waves is not specific.[52,53]

Differential Considerations The differential considerations in patients with hepatic encephalopathy include the full gamut of causes of altered sensorium. Structural CNS disorder, seizure or postictal state, infection, trauma, endocrine and metabolic abnormalities, toxic ingestion, and hypothermia are all considerations. The diagnosis can be narrowed if there is a history of previous episodes of hepatic encephalopathy or it is recognized the patient has severe underlying liver disease and physical signs are supportive. It may be useful to obtain a full electrolyte panel, glucose, toxicology screen, head CT scan, and CSF examination to eliminate potentially life-threatening conditions.

Management Aggressive management of the patient with hepatic encephalopathy is supported by the high rate of reversibility. As is the case with any comatose patient, attention is first drawn to the airway not only for respiratory support but for prevention of aspiration. These patients are generally hemodynamically stable; however, they do have an increased incidence of GI bleeding. Hypokalemia, alkalosis, and GI bleeding contribute to increased ammonia production or absorption and must be corrected when present. Relatively mild degrees of hyponatremia, hypoglycemia, azotemia, or dehydration will often have a disproportionate effect on cerebral function and require immediate correction. All CNS-depressant drugs must be discontinued, and care should be taken not to prescribe even mild sedatives.

Lactulose and neomycin represent the principal therapeutic agents in the management of this disorder. Lactulose is a poorly absorbed sugar metabolized by colonic bacteria yielding lactic acid. The salutary effects of this agent are related both to the acidification of the fecal stream, resulting in the trapping of ammonia as ammonium in the stool, and to its cathartic action. The usual dosage of lactulose is 15 to 30 ml orally three or four times daily or in a quantity sufficient to result in several loose bowel movements daily. The principal adverse effect is excessive diarrhea, with resultant fluid and electrolyte imbalance. Neomycin is a poorly absorbed aminoglycoside. It is believed to act by reducing colonic bacteria responsible for the production of ammonia. Neomycin is administered orally at a dosage of 0.5 g every 4 to 6 hours. Ototoxicity or renal injury may occur in patients with impaired renal function. In obtunded patients, lactulose and neomycin can be administered via nasogastric tube. An alternate route for neomycin is by rectal enema. Long-term management requires diet modification, with significant protein restriction. Alternative therapies, still undergoing clinical evaluation, include metronidazole, levodopa, branched-chain amino acid infusions, bromocriptine, and more recently the benzodiazepine antagonist, flumazenil.[54-58]

Disposition Although most patients with hepatic encephalopathy will require hospitalization, individuals with grade I or II encephalopathy without complicating factors and a supportive home environment can be managed at home. In addition to a prescription for lactulose, a diet with limited amounts of protein is essential to effective ongoing management.

Key Concepts

- The differential diagnosis of hepatic encephalopathy includes all causes of altered sensorium. Although clinical setting may point to the correct diagnosis a broad evaluation including chemistry studies, toxicology, head CT scan, and CSF examination may be required.
- Management of hepatic encephalopathy includes correction of underlying electrolyte abnormalities and strict protein restriction.

Spontaneous Bacterial Peritonitis

Perspective Spontaneous bacterial peritonitis (SBP) is defined as acute bacterial infection of ascites in patients with liver disease, without an apparent external or intraabdominal focus of infection. Although the syndrome is not new, it was only after the work of Harold Conn in the late 1960s and early 1970s that this potentially fatal disorder was recognized with any regularity. Although the disease remains most common in patients with cirrhosis secondary to alcohol, it can occur in any patient with ascites that results from cirrhosis.[59,60] Retrospective studies have identified SBP in 5% to 27% of patients admitted to the hospital with cirrhosis and ascites.[61,62]

Principles of Disease The pathophysiology of SBP remains speculative but is most likely related to a combination of impaired phagocytic function in the liver in conjunction with portal systemic hypertension, which can cause bowel mucosal edema and transmural migration of enteric organisms. Additional contributing factors may include impaired opsonic and complement activity in ascitic fluid. The bacteriology of SBP reveals a predominance of gram-negative enteric organisms. *Escherichia coli* is most common, isolated in 47% to 55% of cases, followed by *Streptococcus* sp (18% to 26%), *Klebsiella* sp (11%), and *Streptococcus pneumoniae* (8% to 20%).[59,60] Polymicrobial and anaerobic infections have been reported but are not common.

Clinical Features The clinical presentation can be variable, ranging from the acute onset of severe abdominal pain, fever, chills, and hemodynamic instability to the slow, insidious onset of abdominal discomfort, low-grade fever, or hepatic encephalopathy. Although by definition ascites must be present for SBP to occur, free peritoneal fluid may not always be clinically apparent. Similarly, elevated temperature, a common occurrence in SBP, may not be detected in 20% to 50% of cases.[63]

Physical examination may reveal only mild tenderness or abdominal rigidity and guarding with rebound tenderness. The broad spectrum of manifestations and nonspecific physical findings requires consideration of the diagnosis of SBP in any patient with ascites associated with fever, abdominal pain, or unexplained clinical deterioration.

Diagnostic Strategies Although diagnosis is made by culture of the ascitic fluid, treatment decisions should be made in advance of these results. An ascitic fluid granulocyte count more than 500 cells/mm^3 correlates with positive cultures in more than 90% of cases; however, it is recommended the emergency physician initiate treatment for SBP if the neutrophil count is greater than 250 cell/mm^3.[60-64] An ascitic fluid pH of less than 7.34 or a pH gradient between arterial blood and ascitic fluid of more than 0.10 is also a reliable early indicator of SBP but is more cumbersome to obtain and therefore of less clinical utility.[64,65] Other laboratory parameters (e.g., aminotransferase, bilirubin, and peripheral blood count) although commonly abnormal, are nonspecific and more often are a consequence of underlying liver disease than infection. A PT should be obtained in advance of paracentesis, and fresh-frozen plasma should be administered if significant coagulopathy is identified.

Differential Considerations The differential diagnosis of SBP includes all of those entities that may lead to peritonitis and abdominal pain in patients with or without liver disease.

Management Treatment of SBP requires IV antibiotics. The choice of agents should take into account the anticipated bacteriology of the process. A third-generation cephalosporin such as cefotaxime is considered to be a drug of choice with a demonstrated cure rate of 85%.[63] An alternative would be an ampicillin sulbactam combination. Ampicillin and an aminoglycoside is a rational and effective combination but somewhat less desirable due to the risk of renal toxicity.

Disposition Spontaneous bacterial peritonitis is a risk in any patient with ascites. It has been shown that the risk of SBP is markedly increased in patients with ascitic fluid protein levels of less than 1 g/dl.[62,63,66] Other important risk factors include serum bilirubin level greater than 3.2 mg/dl, platelet count less than 98,000/mm^3, and previous history of SBP.[67] Antibiotic prophylaxis of high-risk patients can reduce SBP incidence by 60% to 80% and be cost effective.[62,63,66,68] Recommended regimens include norfloxacin 400 mg daily and ciprofloxacin 750 mg once weekly.[62,63,69] If a high-risk patient with ascites is identified in the ED and contraindications are absent, prophylactic therapy should be initiated. Referral to a primary care physician or gastroenterology specialist is recommended.

Key Concepts

- SBP should be considered in any patient with ascites presenting with abdominal pain, fever, or unexplained clinical deterioration.
- Diagnosis is dependent upon sampling of ascitic fluid and measurement of cell count. An ascitic fluid granulocyte count greater than 250 cells/mm^3 is an indication for antibiotic treatment.
- Identification of high-risk patients with ascites is an indication for initiation of SBP prophylaxis with an orthoquinolone antibiotic.

Drug-Induced Liver Disease

Perspective Injury to the liver can occur as a result of exposure to a variety of chemical agents. Ethanol, the agent most commonly incriminated, has already been discussed. Most of the other agents associated with hepatic toxicity are commonly prescribed medicinals or drugs available over the counter. Although hepatic injury represents a relatively small proportion of all adverse drug reactions, it may account for up to 5% of hospital admissions for jaundice.[70] For reasons not entirely clear, the incidence of liver injury related to drugs appears to increase with age. Notable exceptions to this generalization include valproic acid and aspirin, which more often cause hepatic damage in children.

Principles of Disease The pathogenesis of liver injury as a result of drug exposure is variable. It may occur as a result of a direct cytotoxic effect of the primary agent or, as is more often the case, a major or minor metabolite. Alternatively, toxicity can be related to a hypersensitivity or allergic reaction. Antimetabolites (e.g., azathioprine, comfrey tea) have been associated with hepatic injury caused by venoocclusive disease, whereas oral contraceptives have been implicated in cases of hepatic vein thrombosis.[71-73]

Not all agents commonly associated with hepatic toxicity will cause injury in all patients. This is a consequence of variations in metabolic pathways, simultaneous ingestion of other substances that may facilitate toxicity, amount and duration of drug exposure, or patient idiosyncrasy. Isoniazid is an example of an agent that appears to have differential toxicity depending on both the patient's age and the rate of conversion to a particular toxic metabolite, acetyl hydrazine. Acetaminophen is the classic example of a drug that is relatively nontoxic when taken in the usually recommended amounts but universally toxic and potentially fatal when taken in significant excess (see Chapter 142).

Generally, the pattern of drug-induced liver injury is one of hepatocellular necrosis or cholestasis. Although specific agents tend to cause damage characterized by a particular pattern of injury, there is considerable overlap. Cellular necrosis is commonly associated with anesthetic agents (e.g., halothane, the antimicrobials amphotericin and ketoconazole, or the antidysrhythmic amiodarone). A cholestatic picture is characteristic of chlorpromazine, haloperidol, anabolic or oral contraceptive steroids, and erythromycin estolate.

Clinical Features The clinical presentation for drug-induced liver disease is highly variable. Many patients will be asymptomatic, with injury apparent only by moderate elevations of aminotransferase levels. Alternatively, patients may experience painless jaundice resulting from agents associated with cholestatic pathology or as a result of acute hepatitis indistinguishable from virally induced disease.

Physical examination will vary in accordance with the nature of the underlying pathology. The liver can be enlarged and tender. A rash is frequently seen in halothane-induced hepatitis, consistent with its presumed allergic causation. Aminotransferase levels are commonly elevated, but only mildly so in cholestatic cases. Bilirubin is often elevated, most dramatically in cases associated with cholestasis. Eosinophilia is frequently seen in cases of chlorpromazine and halothane-induced injury.

It can be difficult to differentiate drug-induced liver injury from infectious causes or extrahepatic biliary obstruction. A careful history in conjunction with knowledge of the drugs commonly associated with hepatic toxicity should facilitate diagnosis (Table 85-5). On occasion, particularly in cases with a cholestatic presentation, abdominal ultrasound and liver biopsy may be necessary.

Management Management consists of discontinuing the offending agent(s) and instituting the usual supportive measures recommended in the treatment of acute hepatitis. For patients with cholestasis and significant pruritus, a bile acid sequestering agent such as cholestyramine may provide relief. Although drug-induced liver disease is generally a benign disorder, it can be associated with fulminant hepatic failure or subsequent cirrhosis.

Disposition Mild cases of drug-induced hepatitis can be managed effectively on an outpatient basis. Telephone consultation with a gastroenterology specialist is recommended to aid in the diagnosis and assure reliable follow-up.

Table 85-5. Common Agents Involved in Hepatic Injury

Agent	Injury pattern
Acetaminophen	Cytotoxic
Amiodarone	Cytotoxic
Amphotericin	Cytotoxic
Anabolic steroids	Cholestatic, venoocclusive
Azathioprine	Cytotoxic, cholestatic, venoocclusive
Carbamazepine	Cytotoxic, cholestatic
Chlorpromazine	Cholestatic
Cis-platinum	Cytotoxic
Contraceptive steroids	Cholestatic, hepatic vein thrombotic
Cyclophosphamide	Cytotoxic
Erythromycin estolate	Cholestatic
Gold salts	Cytotoxic, cholestatic
Haloperidol	Cholestatic
Isoniazid	Cytotoxic
Ketoconazole	Cytotoxic
Lovastatin	Cytotoxic
Methoxyflurane	Cytotoxic
Methotrexate	Cytotoxic
Methyldopa	Cytotoxic
Phenobarbital	Cholestatic
Phenytoin	Cytotoxic
Quinidine	Cytotoxic
Tetracycline	Cytotoxic, fatty infiltrative
Salicylate	Cytotoxic
Valproic acid	Cytotoxic
Verapamil	Cholestatic

Hepatic Abscesses

Hepatic abscesses fall into two broad categories, pyogenic and amebic. Although there may be similarities in clinical presentation, the pathophysiology and treatment differ significantly.

Pyogenic Abscess

Principles of Disease Pyogenic hepatic abscess is an uncommon entity, present in only 8 to 16 cases per 100,000 hospital admissions. The disorder increases in frequency with age and is distributed equally between men and women.[74] Liver abscesses are most commonly associated with biliary tract obstruction or cholangitis, but they may be related to diverticulitis, pancreatic abscess, omphalitis, appendicitis, inflammatory bowel disease, or bacteremia of any cause.[75-77] In a significant number of cases no underlying cause for liver abscess is identified.[78]

Solitary and multiple abscesses occur with approximately equal frequency, both occurring most often in the right lobe of the liver. Cases with multiple lesions tend to define a more severely ill group associated with adverse prognosis. Bacteriologic study reveals both anaerobic and aerobic organisms. *E. coli; Klebsiella, Pseudomonas,* and *Enterococcus* sp; anaerobic streptococci; and various *Bacteroides* sp are the microbes most commonly isolated.[79,80]

Clinical Findings Clinical presentation is characterized by the onset of high fever, chills, right upper quadrant pain, nausea, and vomiting. Patients generally present acutely and appear quite ill, particularly if there is underlying cholangitis. A more insidious chronic presentation, although atypical, has been described. Physical findings include elevated temperature, right upper quadrant tenderness, hepatomegaly, and occasionally dullness to percussion and decreased breath sounds over the right lower chest. Jaundice may be apparent, especially if coexistent biliary tract obstruction is present.

Diagnostic Strategies Laboratory findings include leukocytosis in 70% to 80% of cases, elevated alkaline phosphatase in up to 90%, and bilirubin in excess of 2 mg/dl in 50% of patients. Serum aminotransferase levels are commonly elevated to two to four times normal.[74,81] Chest radiographs may reveal a right pleural effusion, a basilar atelectasis, or an elevated right hemidiaphragm.[82]

A variety of imaging techniques are useful in delineating hepatic abscesses, including ultrasonography, nuclear scan with technetium or gallium, CT scan (Figures 85-4 and 85-5), and magnetic resonance imaging (MRI) scan. In the ED, ultrasonography and the CT scan are the most sensitive and expeditious modalities.[83]

Differential Considerations The differential diagnosis of pyogenic hepatic abscess includes amebic liver abscess, hepatitis and cholangitis, and pancreatic and subphrenic abscess. Although clinical evaluation may not allow definitive diagnosis, appropriate use of imaging techniques generally does.

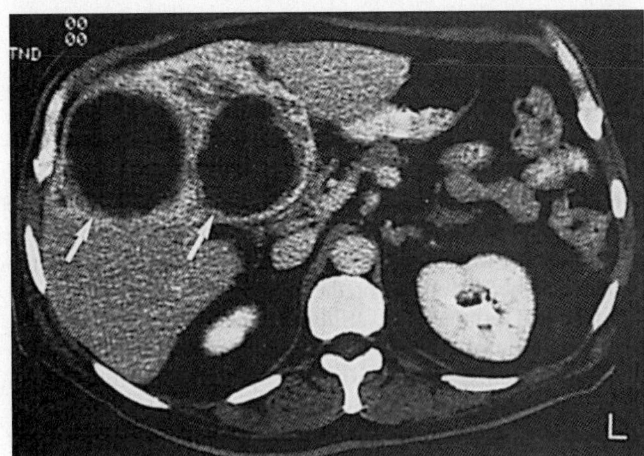

Figure 85-4. **Contrast computed tomography scan of liver showing large cystic masses with irregular, contrast-enhancing borders in a patient with pyogenic liver abscess caused by *Streptococcus milleri*.**

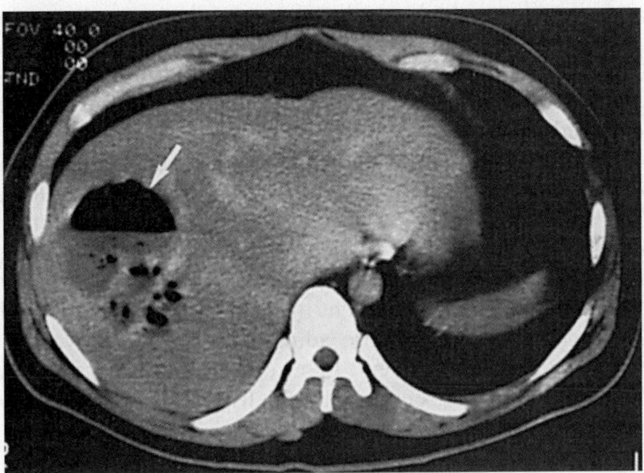

Figure 85-5. **Contrast computed tomography scan of liver showing pyogenic liver abscess. Complex cystic mass with air-fluid level caused by gas-producing *Klebsiella* sp. pneumonia.**

Management The initial treatment of a pyogenic hepatic abscess entails hemodynamic stabilization, IV antibiotics, and pain control. Pending definitive microbial identification, broad-spectrum antibiotic coverage should be provided. Triple antibiotic coverage is warranted and should include an aminoglycoside or third-generation cephalosporin for gram-negative coverage plus metronidazole or clindamycin for anaerobes and ampicillin for streptococcal species. Definitive treatment requires drainage. This is most commonly accomplished percutaneously, with open surgical drainage reserved for complex cases associated with intraperitoneal soiling, intestinal perforation, or biliary obstruction.[84-88]

Complications include rupture of the abscess into the peritoneal cavity or an adjacent anatomic structure (e.g., the thoracic cavity, lung, pericardium).

Disposition Patients with pyogenic hepatic abscess uniformly require admission to the hospital. Consultation with a general surgeon, gastroenterologist, or interventional radiologist will be necessary.

Amebic Abscess

Principles of Disease Amebiasis is one of the most common protozoan infections worldwide. It is estimated that up to 10% of the world's population and approximately 1% to 2% of the U.S. population are infected. Transmission is generally via the fecal-oral route and is usually the consequence of ingesting contaminated water or foodstuffs. The illness is more common in homosexual men, presumably as a result of oral-anal contact during sexual activity. One limited but fatal outbreak of intestinal disease in the Midwest was traced to a contaminated colonic irrigation apparatus.[89] Although intestinal disease is by far the most common manifestation of infection, extraintestinal disease is not rare, with the liver most commonly affected. *Entamoeba histolytica* is the only ameba responsible for invasive disease, and recent evidence suggests that only certain varieties of *E. histolytica* are pathogenic.[90] Pathogenic amebae reach the liver after invasion of the intestinal mucosa and transit via the portal vein. As with a pyogenic abscess, involvement of the right lobe is more common.

Clinical Features Clinical presentation is generally acute, with fever, chills, abdominal pain, nausea, and vomiting. Coexistent diarrhea is common in children but is present in less than one third of adults. Careful questioning of patients without diarrhea often yields a history of intestinal illness several weeks before. Many patients complain of cough, which can serve to misdirect attention from the liver. Chronic illness of several months' duration, although less common than the acute presentation, has been described.[91]

Physical examination reveals an elevated temperature, right upper quadrant tenderness, hepatomegaly, and findings of dullness and decreased breath sounds over the right lower chest.

Diagnostic Strategies Laboratory parameters are not specific. Neutrophilic leukocytosis is common. Alkaline phosphatase is elevated in 75% of cases and aminotransferases in 50%. Hyperbilirubinemia is uncommon and when present is indicative of biliary obstruction.[92] The chest radiographs may reveal a right pleural effusion, a basilar atelectasis, or an elevated right hemidiaphragm. Ultrasound imaging of the liver can be diagnostic, revealing a peripherally based mass with well-circumscribed borders and an inhomogeneous hypoechoic center. Technetium, CT, and MRI scanning are alternative imaging modalities if ultrasonography is inconclusive.

Diagnosis is supported by identifying a pathogenic protozoan in the stool. However, even in cases of invasive intestinal disease, the yield from this site may be low. Serologic testing is generally required to establish a definitive diagnosis. Agar gel diffusion, counterimmune electrophoresis, or rapid enzyme immunoassay are positive in most cases.[93,94] Indirect hemagglutination remains positive for an extended period and is therefore not helpful in establishing the presence of acute infection.

Differential Considerations In a review of 75 cases of amebic liver abscess seen in a single ED over 5 years, the correct diagnosis was made in only 31.5% of patients.[95] The differential diagnosis of an amebic liver abscess includes, most prominently, pyogenic abscess, followed by biliary tract disease, hepatitis, pneumonia, appendicitis, and pancreatitis. Respiratory symptoms and abnormal chest radiographic findings may cause confusion with pulmonary illnesses. Hepatic imaging is helpful in establishing the correct diagnosis; however, differentiation from pyogenic illness may still be difficult.

Management Management of amebic hepatic abscess consists of supportive therapy and initiation of amebicidal therapy. Metronidazole, 750 mg by mouth or IV three times daily for 7 days, is the treatment of choice. Most patients will respond to this regimen. Percutaneous catheter drainage is required only in refractory or complicated cases.

The most serious complication of amebic liver disease is rupture into adjacent anatomic structures. Involvement of the lung occurs in 20% to 35% of cases, often presenting with signs and symptoms of massive pleural effusion or consolidative pneumonia.[92] Rupture into a bronchus can present with cough productive of an anchovy paste–like substance, necrotic debris, or frank hemoptysis. Abdominal pain with peritonitis can result from rupture into the abdominal cavity. Involvement of the pericardium occasionally is seen with lesions in the left lobe of the liver and can be catastrophic, either acutely as a consequence of pericardial tamponade or chronically from constrictive pericarditis.

Disposition Select patients with amebic liver abscess can be managed as outpatients. This approach is best suited for individuals with mild clinical disease, stable living circumstances, and access to medications as well as follow up care. Patients with more severe disease, evidence of complications, or questionable social circumstances should be admitted to a medical service.

Miscellaneous Disorders of the Liver

Chronic Hepatitis Chronic hepatitis is defined as persistent inflammation of the liver for at least 6 months. Chronic disease is generally divided into two broad categories: chronic persistent hepatitis (CPH) and chronic active hepatitis (CAH). CPH is characterized clinically by a lack of symptoms, persistent mild complaints, or intermittent episodes of moderate hepatitis. Despite persistent elevation of aminotransferases, CPH rarely progresses to hepatic failure or cirrhosis. CAH, on the other hand, commonly progresses to cirrhosis. CAH initially may follow a clinical course indistinguishable from that of CPH; however, biopsy of the liver, even early in the sequence of disease, reveals diffuse inflammation, bridging necrosis, and evidence of scarring and macronodular cirrhosis.[96]

The causes of chronic hepatitis include all of the recognized etiologies of acute hepatitis: viral, immunologic, toxic, and metabolic. Although any of the hepatitis viruses can go on to cause chronic disease, it is rare with HAV. It may occur in 5% to 10% of patients with HBV infection, in 50% to 60% of those with HCV, and probably in an even greater percentage of patients with HDV infection.[2,21,97-99] The incidence of chronic disease from other etiologies is closely related to the reversibility of the metabolic or immunologic disorder or to the duration of exposure to the incriminated toxic substance.

Chronic hepatitis, in its precirrhotic stage, is not a common reason for arrival at the ED. It is not unusual, however, for an elevated aminotransferase level to be detected during the course of evaluation of some seemingly unrelated entity. Evaluation is generally limited to obtaining a careful history and ordering appropriate viral serologies (HBsAg, HBeAg, and anti-HCV). The active treatment of CAH is no longer experimental but goes beyond the bounds of the ED. Referral to an internist or gastroenterology specialist is advisable.

Liver Disease in Pregnancy The two primary hepatic disorders associated with pregnancy are benign cholestasis and acute fatty liver. Cholestasis is not rare and appears to have a familial linkage. Onset is in the third trimester and is heralded by the development of progressive pruritus. Bilirubin may be elevated, but not dramatically, so jaundice is commonly absent. Laboratory tests reveal elevated alkaline phosphatase, 5′-nucleotidase, and bilirubin. Although the chief concern to the mother is discomfort from pruritus, the illness can bode poorly for the fetus. There is an increased incidence of prematurity, stillbirth, and fetal distress.[100,101] Malabsorption of vitamin K can result in serious coagulopathy in the fetus, predisposing to spontaneous intracranial hemorrhage.[102] Treatment is supportive and should include subcutaneous vitamin K. The illness resolves without incident after delivery.

Acute fatty liver of pregnancy is a malignant disorder that, if unrecognized, can progress rapidly to maternal and fetal demise. The incidence is about 1 in 7000 live births.[103] The illness occurs in the latter part of the third trimester and is more common in primigravidas and twin pregnancies.[102,104] The initial clinical features include fatigue, anorexia, nausea, and vomiting. Abdominal pain may be present, most prominently in the midepigastrium and right upper quadrant. Physical examination may reveal mild jaundice and abdominal tenderness. The liver may not be palpable because of the enlarged uterus.

Abnormal laboratory findings include moderate elevation of aminotransferases (5 to 10 times normal) and bilirubin, hypoglycemia, and evidence of disseminated intravascular coagulation (prolonged PT and partial thromboplastin time, hypofibrinogenemia, elevated fibrin split products, and thrombocytopenia). Treatment involves aggressive fluid and electrolyte support, glucose administration, and movement toward immediate delivery. Liver disease generally resolves without permanent sequelae after delivery.[103]

Hepatic Cancer

Hepatocellular carcinoma is the most common primary hepatic malignancy. This tumor is much more common in underdeveloped areas of the world, particularly in regions where chronic HBV infection is prevalent. In parts of China and Africa, the incidence of hepatocellular carcinoma approaches 100 in 100,000; in the United States, it is 4 or 5 per 100,000.[105] It has been estimated that HBV is causally related to the development of hepatoma in 75% to 90% of cases worldwide.[106] Associations beyond HBV include infection with *Clonorchis* and schistosomiasis, chronic alcoholic liver disease, primary biliary cirrhosis, hemochromatosis, and several chemical agents (e.g., estrogens, androgens, thorotrast, vinyl chloride).[107]

Metastases to the liver are much more common in the United States than is primary malignancy, occurring as a result of a wide variety of tumors of GI, lung, breast, or other origin.

The clinical presentation of hepatic carcinoma or metastases is nonspecific. Symptoms may include nausea, vomiting, jaundice, or right upper quadrant abdominal pain. Physical examination may reveal signs of recent weight loss or cachexia. The linkage of hepatocellular carcinoma with cirrhosis results in many of these patients manifesting that process. An enlarged liver, particularly in patients with a history of cirrhosis, is strongly suggestive of malignant transformation. Although laboratory tests (e.g., blood count, aminotransferase measurements, bilirubin measurement) are often abnormal, they are nonspecific and generally of little aid in diagnosis. Alpha-fetoprotein is often elevated in patients with a hepatoma but is nonspecific and of limited use in diagnosis. Ultrasound imaging, CT scan, or MRI scan of the liver are all effective means of identifying tumor. Liver biopsy is recommended for definitive diagnosis of hepatoma, whereas biopsy of an alternative site may be preferable in cases of metastatic disease.

Management of these patients in the ED is limited to supportive measures, provision of analgesic agents, and possibly nutritive supplementation. Hepatitis B serologies should be obtained in cases of hepatoma to determine linkage with chronic HBV infection and to assess infection risk to family members.

BILIARY TRACT DISORDERS

Cholelithiasis

Perspective The biliary tract comprises hepatic bile canaliculi, intrahepatic and extrahepatic bile ducts, the common bile duct, and the gallbladder. Bile, required for absorption of fats and fat-soluble nutrients, is produced in the canaliculi. During the fasting state, approximately 50% of the bile produced flows directly into the duodenum; the other half is stored in the gallbladder. The gallbladder serves to acidify and concentrate the bile and can store up to 50 ml of bile for immediate availability at the time of feeding. The presence of food in the stomach—in particular, fat—results in both vagal impulses and the secretion of cholecystokinin-pancreozymin, which serve as potent stimuli for gallbladder contraction. Removal of the gallbladder generally is not associated with measurable changes in intestinal fat absorption or clinical symptomatology.[108]

The principal cause of biliary tract disease is related to the development of gallstones. It is estimated that 20% of women and 8% of men have gallstones, resulting in approximately 500,000 operations annually.[109,110]

Principles of Disease There are two categories of gallstones: cholesterol and pigmented. The cholesterol stones most commonly occur as a consequence of an elevated concentration of cholesterol in bile relative to the other principal constituents of bile, that is, bile acids and phospholipids. Bile acids and lecithin, the primary bile phospholipid, act in concert to solubilize cholesterol. As cholesterol levels rise or bile acids and lecithin levels decline, cholesterol has an increasing tendency to form crystals. These crystals, particularly in an incompletely emptying gallbladder, serve as a nidus for stone formation.[111] Factors associated with an enhanced risk of cholesterol stone formation include increased age, female gender, massive obesity, rapid weight loss, cystic fibrosis, parity, drugs (e.g., clofibrate and oral contraceptive agents), and familial tendency. The hereditary risk of cholelithiasis is most dramatically demonstrated by the high concordance for stone formation in monozygotic twins and the exceedingly high incidence of cholelithiasis in Pima Indians.[112,113]

There are two varieties of pigmented stones: black and brown. Black stones occur exclusively in the gallbladder and contain a high concentration of calcium bilirubinate. They are more commonly encountered in the elderly and have a strong association with disease causing intravascular hemolysis (e.g., sickle cell anemia and hereditary spherocytosis). Brown stones are associated with infection and can form in both the gallbladder and the intrahepatic and extrahepatic bile duct system. Although bacterial infections are most commonly incriminated, parasites (e.g., *Ascaris lumbricoides* and *Clonorchis sinensis*) have also been linked to brown stone formation.[114] Both types of pigmented stones contain calcium bilirubinate and therefore may be visible on plain abdominal radiographs. For a stone to be radiopaque it must contain at least 4% calcium by weight (Figure 85-6).[115]

Clinical Features The most common clinical manifestation of cholelithiasis is biliary colic. The pathophysiology of this process is not entirely clear, but it appears to be related to the passage of small stones from the gallbladder through the cystic duct into the common bile duct. The term *colic* is often misleading; these individuals commonly complain of steady pain rather than intermittent or cramping discomfort. The pain is most often perceived in the right upper quadrant but may be located in a wide region of the upper abdomen. Radiation of pain, if it occurs, is generally to the base of the scapula or shoulder. Associated symptoms include nausea and vomiting, which may be severe enough to lead to fluid and electrolyte imbalance. Patients with biliary colic commonly admit to similar self-limited occurrences in the past and may offer an association between symptom onset and eating. A relationship between fatty food ingestion and symptoms is as likely to occur in patients with gallstones as it is in those without. Physical examination usually reveals mild tenderness without guarding or rebound in the right upper quadrant or epigastric region.

Diagnostic Strategies There are no pathognomonic clinical laboratory findings; most commonly obtained test results are within normal limits. Important tests to obtain include ALT and AST to evaluate for the presence of hepatitis, bilirubin and alkaline phosphatase for evidence of common duct obstruction, and amylase or lipase for the presence of pancreatitis.

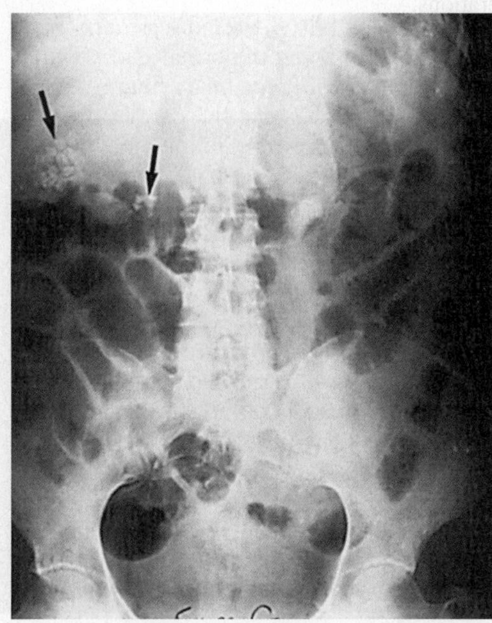

Figure 85-6. **Plain flat plate (kidney, ureter, bladder [KUB]) radiograph of abdomen with calcified gallstones and pancreatic calcifications. This patient also has bilateral staghorn calculi and calcified iliac vessels.**

The diagnosis of biliary colic is made clinically in conjunction with demonstration of stones in the gallbladder. Plain radiographs have little role in the evaluation of cholelithiasis because only 10% of stones have sufficient calcium to allow visualization.[116] Historically, oral cholecystography (OCG) with ipanoic acid was the procedure of choice for imaging the gallbladder and identifying stones. This technique can identify gallstones in 95% of patients with cholelithiasis in whom visualization of the gallbladder can be achieved. However, in large series, as many as 25% of patients' gallbladders will not be visualized after a single dose of ipanoic acid and 8% after a second dose.[117] Nonvisualization may indicate underlying gallbladder disease but, alternatively, can be a result of noncompliance with contrast ingestion or impaired hepatic function.

Ultrasonography is the procedure of choice for investigating the gallbladder. Ultrasound imaging can be performed rapidly, does not require the overnight delay necessary with OCG, is at least as sensitive, and provides the added use of permitting evaluation of surrounding structures (Figure 85-7).[116] Ultrasonography can also be employed by the emergency physician at the bedside, adding further convenience to the patient and reducing turnaround times.[118] OCG remains an option for the patient with clinical suspicion of cholelithiasis in the uncommon circumstance when ultrasound imaging has failed to identify the gallbladder.

Differential Considerations The differential diagnosis of biliary colic includes cholecystitis, acid peptic disease of the stomach or duodenum, pancreatitis, and hepatitis. Patients with cholelithiasis may occasionally present with chest pain and generate concern referable to cardiopulmonary syndromes. The clinical history in conjunction with normal laboratory test values (ALT, AST, and amylase and alkaline phosphatase), gallstones on ultrasound imaging, and minimal or no tenderness in the right upper quadrant favor the diagnosis of cholelithiasis. A chest radiograph and electrocardiogram may be required to help eliminate cardiopulmonary considerations.

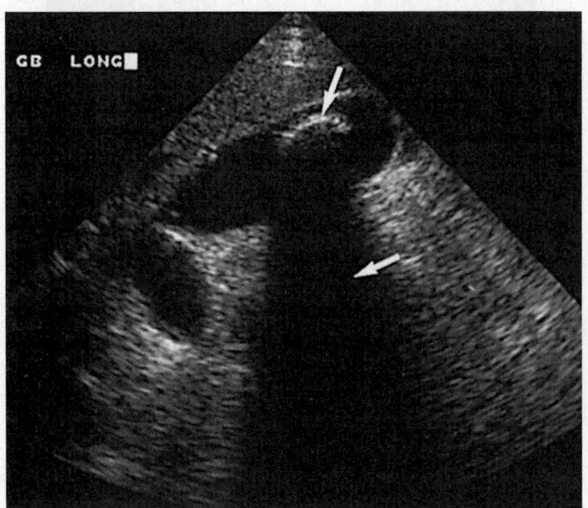

Figure 85-7. **Ultrasound image of gallbladder showing solitary, large gallstone in distended gallbladder. Both stone and typical shadow are well seen.**

Management The initial management of biliary colic is directed at fluid and electrolyte correction and symptom relief. Vomiting is managed with antiemetics and, if necessary, nasogastric suction. Pain can often be controlled with antispasmodics (e.g., glycopyrrolate), the nonsteroidal anti-inflammatory ketorolac, and, if necessary, opiate analgesic agents. Clinical evidence of volume depletion should be treated with IV fluids.

The definitive management of cholelithiasis, traditionally and most commonly, involves surgical removal of the gallbladder; however, other options exist. Oral administration of bile acid (e.g., chenodeoxycholate or ursodeoxycholate) over a period of months to years can result in dissolution of small to medium-size stones, whereas methyltert-butyl ether irrigation of the gallbladder has been shown to dissolve stones over a period of hours or days.[119-122] Most recently, the technique of extracorporeal shock wave lithotripsy has been applied successfully to a select cohort of patients with solitary stones of less than 20 mm diameter.[123,124]

The most common complication of biliary colic is fluid and electrolyte imbalance as a result of vomiting. Other adverse consequences might include Mallory-Weiss tear from uncontrolled emesis and cholangitis from unrecognized and persistent common bile duct obstruction.

Special Considerations Biliary colic is an uncommon disease in children and, when it occurs, is most often associated with an underlying hemolytic disorder (e.g., sickle cell anemia or spherocytosis). ED management need not be modified for the pediatric patient.

Cholelithiasis may be encountered in pregnant women. Diagnosis in this population is made more difficult by the common occurrence of nausea and vomiting, particularly in the first trimester, and the presence of an enlarged uterus in later pregnancy, which interferes with anatomic relationships and abdominal examination. Ultrasound imaging is of considerable diagnostic use in this setting. Treatment in the ED is comparable with that for the nonpregnant patient; however, definitive therapy is generally delayed until after parturition.

Cholecystitis

Perspective Acute cholecystitis is defined as sudden inflammation of the gallbladder. The incidence of the disease is variable; estimates range from 5% to 19% of patients operated on for biliary tract disorders.[125,126] The risk factors for cholecystitis mirror those for cholelithiasis: increasing age, female gender, increasing parity, and obesity.[127] Although gallstones play a prominent role in the pathogenesis of cholecystitis, approximately 2% to 12% of cases are categorized as acalculous.[128]

Principles of Disease Obstruction of the cystic duct appears to be the critical factor in the development of gallbladder inflammation. Gallstones are identified in 95% of patients with cholecystitis and may be located in the common bile duct in many patients with acalculous cholecystitis. Causes of cystic duct obstruction unrelated to stone disease include tumor, lymphadenopathy, fibrosis, parasites, and kinking of the duct. Regardless of cause, obstruction of the cystic duct leads to filling and distention of the gallbladder. The ensuing inflammatory reaction may be related to mucosal ischemia from increased hydrostatic pressure or to the action of cytotoxic products of bile metabolism (e.g., lysophosphatidylcholine).[129] Although bacteria are isolated from the bile of inflamed gallbladders in 50% to 75% of cases, the role of infection in the pathogenesis of cholecystitis is not completely understood.[130] Coliforms (e.g., *E. coli*) represent the most common isolates, but anaerobes have been identified in as many as 40% of cases.[131]

Clinical Features The most common presenting symptom of cholecystitis is pain, usually localized to the right upper quadrant. Although the pain may initially be described as colicky, it will become constant in virtually all cases. A prior history of similar but less severe and self-limited symptoms is a valuable diagnostic clue, as is a prior history of documented gallstones. Radiation of pain is generally to the tip of the scapula on the right. Nausea and vomiting are generally present, and the patient may complain of fever.

Most often physical examination reveals temperature elevation, tachycardia, and tenderness in the right upper quadrant or epigastric region, often with guarding or rebound. Murphy's sign, which is described as tenderness and an inspiratory pause elicited by palpation of the right upper quadrant during a deep breath, is compatible with, but not specific for, gallbladder inflammation. Fever and tachycardia may not always be present, so cholecystitis should remain a diagnostic consideration in the absence of these findings in patients with right upper quadrant pain and tenderness.

Diagnostic Considerations A polymorphonuclear leukocytosis with left shift is common but not invariably present. Serum aminotransferase, bilirubin, and alkaline phosphatase may be mildly elevated but are more often within normal limits. An elevated amylase should suggest the diagnosis of pancreatitis, either instead of or in addition to cholecystitis. Plain abdominal radiographs may reveal calcified stones, gas in the gallbladder, or an upper quadrant sentinel loop. However, these findings are so uncommon and nonspecific that plain film radiographs are not recommended unless other diagnostic considerations are present.

Ultrasound imaging is the most useful test in the ED setting. Visualization of the gallbladder without identification of stones has an extremely high negative predictive value for cholecystitis, whereas the presence of stones, a thickened gallbladder wall, and pericholecystic fluid has a positive predictive value in excess of 90%.[132]

Nuclear scintigraphy with technetium-99m-labeled iminodiacetic acid (IDA) is generally considered the most sensitive and specific imaging test for cholecystitis. IDA administered IV is taken up by hepatocytes and secreted into the bile canaliculi. Failure to outline the gallbladder within 1 hour of administration of IDA in the face of hepatic and common duct visualization proves cystic duct obstruction. In the appropriate clinical setting, this finding is diagnostic of cholecystitis. Conversely, visualization of the gallbladder and common duct within 1 hour of administration has a negative predictive value of 98%.[133,134] Scintigraphy with IDA loses its sensitivity as serum bilirubin rises above 5 mg to 8 mg; however, scintigraphy with diisopropyl IDA (diisopropyl iminodiacetic acid or mebrofenin) allows visualization of the biliary tree in patients with total serum bilirubin in the range of 20 mg to 30 mg.[135]

Differential Considerations Diagnostic considerations in the patient suspected of having cholecystitis include hepatitis, hepatic abscess, pyelonephritis, right lower lobe pneumonia or pleurisy, pancreatitis, acid peptic disease of the duodenum with perforation or penetration, and appendicitis. Up to 20% of patients with acute cholecystitis may be misdiagnosed when only clinical criteria are considered.[136] Accurate diagnosis often requires the use of sonographic or, less commonly, scintigraphic studies.

Management Basic supportive measures provide the foundation for initial management of acute cholecystitis. Volume status should be optimized with IV crystalloid administration. Emesis can be managed with antiemetics and nasogastric suction. This latter technique may have the added benefit of diminishing the stimulus for biliary secretion and excretion, thereby adding to pain relief. Narcotic analgesic agents are useful for pain control. Despite the questionable role of microbial infection in the pathogenesis of cholecystitis, antibiotics are recommended. Unless clinical evidence of sepsis exists, coverage with a single broad-spectrum antibiotic (e.g., a second-generation or third-generation cephalosporin) is adequate.

The most serious complication of cholecystitis is gangrene of the gallbladder, with necrosis and perforation. Localized perforation may lead to pericholecystic abscess or fistula formation, the latter predisposing to gallstone ileus at a later date. Patients with diabetes mellitus are at increased risk for bacterial invasion of the gallbladder wall and the development of emphysematous cholecystitis.

Disposition Admission for antibiotics and pain management is required. Surgery is recommended for patients with cholecystitis; however, the timing of the operation is not universally accepted. Surgery usually is performed after symptoms have subsided but during the acute hospitalization. Immediate cholecystectomy or cholecystotomy is reserved for the complicated case in which the patient has gangrene or perforation.

Special Considerations Cholecystitis is uncommon in the pediatric age group but, when it occurs, should be managed as it is in the adult. When cholecystitis occurs in the pregnant woman, it poses challenging diagnostic and therapeutic issues. Initial therapy is identical to that for the nonpregnant patient, but the issue of surgical intervention requires an individualized consultation between surgeon and obstetrician.

Acalculous cholecystitis occurs in approximately 5% to 14% of cases.[88] It is more common in the elderly and is most often encountered in patients that are recovering from nonbiliary tract surgery. Over the last decade, acalculous disease has been increasingly encountered as a complication of advanced AIDS, usually secondary to infection with cytomegalovirus (CMV) or *Cryptosporidium.*[137] As compared to calculous disease, acalculous cholecystitis tends to have a more acute and malignant course with a mortality rate as high as 41%.[138] The techniques used to diagnose acalculous disease are identical to those for other forms of cholecystitis but are less sensitive and specific. Sonographic findings include thickening of the gallbladder wall, pericholecystic fluid, and lack of response to cholecystokinin.[139] Scintigraphic findings are the same as in calculous disease.

Emphysematous cholecystitis is an uncommon variant of cholecystitis, occurring in approximately 1% of cases. It is characterized by the presence of gas in the gallbladder wall, presumably consequent to the invasion of the mucosa by gas-producing organisms (e.g., *E. coli, Klebsiella* sp, and *Clostridium perfringens*). It is more common in diabetic patients and, as opposed to simple cholecystitis, has a male predominance and is acalculous in up to 50% of cases.[139-141] Clinical presentation and physical findings are similar to cholecystitis. Plain radiographs or CT scans of the abdomen will reveal gas in the gallbladder wall. Because of a high incidence of gangrene and perforation, emergency cholecystectomy is recommended.[130] Antibiotic coverage should include penicillin, an aminoglycoside, and clindamycin or an ampicillin-sulbactam combination agent. Mortality of emphysematous cholecystitis is approximately 15%.[141]

Key Concepts

- The vast majority of patients with cholecystitis will have gallstones; however, approximately 5% will have acalculous disease. This group of patients tends to have more severe disease and is at increased risk for complications.
- Despite an unclear relationship between bacterial infection and pathophysiology, antibiotic therapy is recommended.
- Patients with acalculous and emphysematous cholecystitis are at increased risk for gangrene and perforation and should have emergent cholecystectomy.

Cholangitis

Perspective Acute obstructive cholangitis was first described by Charcot in 1877. In one large series, it was reported to occur in approximately 8% of patients admitted for biliary tract disease.[142] Cholangitis is most often a consequence of common duct blockage by a gallstone but may be associated with malignancy or a benign stricture.

Principles of Disease The key factors in the pathogenesis of cholangitis are obstruction, elevated intraluminal pressure, and bacterial infection. Unexpectedly, incomplete obstruction is more commonly encountered than complete blockage.[142] Bacteria may gain access to the obstructed common duct either in a retrograde manner from the duodenum, via lymphatics, or from portal vein blood.[143] The most commonly encountered organisms are similar to those encountered in other varieties of biliary tract disease: *E. coli* and *Klebsiella, Enterococcus,* and *Bacteroides* sp.

Clinical Features Patients most often experience fever, chills, nausea, vomiting, and abdominal pain. The classic triad of physical findings first described by Charcot are right upper quadrant pain, fever, and jaundice. Although these findings are compatible with cholangitis, they can also be seen with both cholecystitis and hepatitis. Sepsis is a common complication and may be heralded by tachycardia, tachypnea, and frank hypotension. The presence of Charcot's triad along with the clinical signs of sepsis and altered sensorium is referred to as Reynolds' pentad.

Diagnostic Considerations Common laboratory abnormalities include polymorphonuclear leukocytosis, hyperbilirubinemia, elevated alkaline phosphatase, and moderately increased aminotransferases. ABG measurements are useful to assess base deficit as an early sign of sepsis.

Sonography can be helpful if it demonstrates common and intrahepatic ductal dilatation, whereas identification of stones in the gallbladder or common duct suggests the underlying cause of obstruction (Figure 85-8). Although nuclear scintigraphy cannot determine the cause, it appears to be a more sensitive means to diagnose early obstruction. Several studies have demonstrated a high incidence of nonvisualization of the biliary tree with cholescintigraphy in patients with common duct obstruction when sonography failed to identify dilatation.[144,145]

Alternative imaging techniques include CT scan, percutaneous transhepatic cholangiography (THC), and endoscopic retrograde cholangiopancreatography (ERCP). Although these techniques may be more expensive and take longer to accomplish, the latter two have the added benefit of offering potential therapeutic benefit. Endoscopic cholangioscopy can permit culture of bile, direct removal of obstructing stones, or decompression of the biliary tree by sphincterotomy or stent placement.[146]

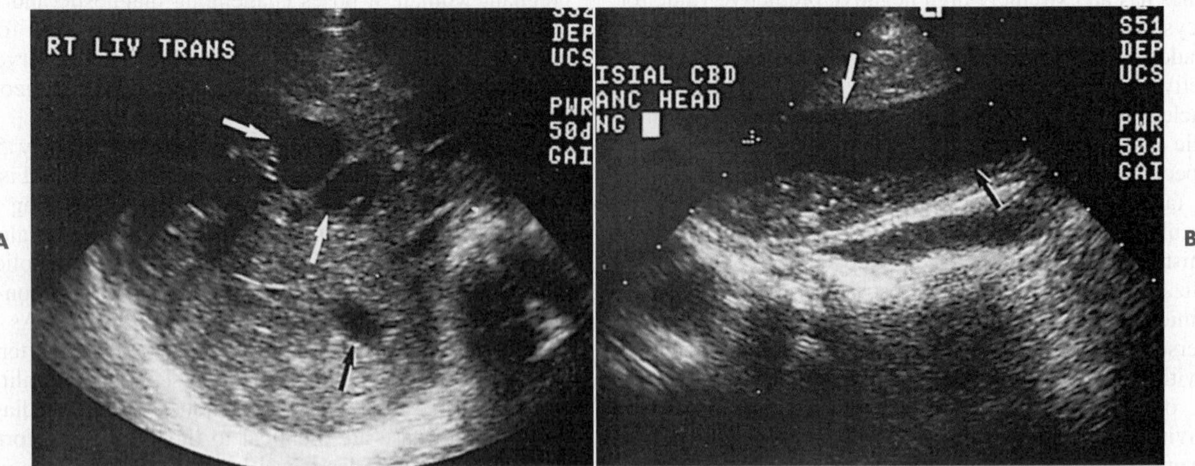

Figure 85-8. Abdominal ultrasounds image. **A,** Multiple dilated intrahepatic ducts in patient with common bile duct obstruction. **B,** Significant dilated common bile duct in same patient. Duct measures 2 cm.

Differential Considerations Although patients with cholangitis, in general, will have a higher fever and appear more ill than those with cholecystitis, there can be considerable variability and overlap. The presence of jaundice is the clinical sign most helpful in differentiating these two disorders. An elevated bilirubin is characteristic of cholangitis and uncommon in cholecystitis. Ultrasonographic evidence of dilated common and intrahepatic ducts is usually required to distinguish cholangitis from cholecystitis.

Management Treatment of cholangitis includes hemodynamic stabilization with crystalloid fluid and, if necessary, vasopressors. Broad-spectrum antibiotic coverage should be initiated immediately after blood cultures are obtained. Ampicillin, an aminoglycoside, and clindamycin or metronidazole are suggested. Mezlocillin, an acyl-ureidopenicillin with activity against gram-positive, gram-negative, and anaerobic organisms, is secreted into the bile and may be a reasonable single-agent alternative to triple-drug therapy.[147] The key to successful treatment is early biliary tract decompression. This can be achieved with THC, ERCP, or surgery.

Disposition Patients with cholangitis will require admission, preferably to a monitored setting. Prompt consultation with a service that can provide for biliary tract decompression (surgery, interventional radiology, or gastroenterology) is necessary.

Key Concepts

- Cholangitis is an emergent condition resulting from extrahepatic bile duct obstruction and bacterial infection.
- Effective management requires prompt administration of broad-spectrum antibiotics and early biliary tract decompression.
- Biliary tract decompression can be achieved surgically, transhepatically, or via ERCP.

Sclerosing Cholangitis

Sclerosing cholangitis is an idiopathic inflammatory disorder affecting the biliary tree. It is characterized by diffuse fibrosis and narrowing of the intrahepatic and extrahepatic bile ducts. It is commonly associated with inflammatory bowel disease, particularly ulcerative colitis; however, in 25% of cases it appears as an isolated disorder.[148]

Patients may arrive at the ED with complaints of weight loss, lethargy, jaundice, and pruritus. Rarely, these patients develop infective cholangitis. Prompt diagnosis may be more difficult in these cases because of the sclerotic nature of the bile ducts and the failure to demonstrate dilation on ultrasound imaging. Surgical exploration or ERCP is often required for diagnosis. The management of noninfected cases is primarily symptomatic. Cholestyramine, a bile acid sequestrant, may diminish pruritus.

AIDS Cholangiopathy

Patients with advanced HIV disease, generally with CD4 counts less than 200/mm^3, may develop any one of a series of disorders that have been collectively referred to as AIDS cholangiopathy. Included in this category are bile duct stricture, papillary stenosis, or sclerosing cholangitis.[137] The precise pathophysiology is not completely understood but is related to infection with either CMV, *Cryptosporidium*, Microsporidia, or *Mycobacterium avium* complex. Clinical presentation may be similar to other causes of cholangitis with fever and right upper quadrant pain. Laboratory values include increased levels of alkaline phosphatase and minor elevation of transaminases. As compared to other etiologies of cholangitis, bilirubin is less commonly elevated. Ultrasonography is generally helpful in identifying bile duct stricture, thickening, or dilation. IDA scans are useful as they are in other causes of cholangitis. Management involves endoscopic sphincterotomy or stent placement in conjunction with treatment of the underlying infective agent.

Porcelain Gallbladder

The porcelain gallbladder is a dramatic radiographic finding caused by either linear or punctate calcifications within the gallbladder wall. Most patients are women, with a mean age in the 50s. Gallstones are commonly present. The gallbladder may be palpable in the right upper quadrant and is usually nontender. Patients with this disorder should be referred for cholecystectomy because of the high incidence of associated carcinoma.

Malignancy

Carcinoma of the biliary tract is uncommon. Gallbladder carcinoma is the most common malignancy, accounting for 5% of all cancers found at autopsy. It occurs predominately in women over the age of 50.[149] Cholelithiasis and porcelain gallbladder appear to be major risk factors. Metastatic disease to regional nodes and the liver is common at the time of initial diagnosis because of the relatively silent nature of early disease. Symptoms include chronic right upper quadrant pain and jaundice. Physical examination may reveal a palpable mass in the right upper quadrant. These tumors will occasionally perforate, and the patient may have symptoms of pericholecystic abscess. Noninvasive imaging techniques may be of some aid in identifying the tumor. Ultrasound imaging is more sensitive than the CT scan, but even the sequential use of both tests fails to identify malignancy in 49% of cases.[150] Radionuclide imaging is nonspecific, revealing no image in most circumstances.

Carcinoma of the extrahepatic bile ducts is less frequent than gallbladder malignancy and, compared with gallbladder cancer, is more common in men. Jaundice is the finding most often encountered. A palpable gallbladder (Courvoisier's sign) may be present on physical examination in one third of cases.[151] Diagnosis is suggested by the presence of dilated intrahepatic and extrahepatic bile ducts on sonography. THC and ERCP may serve to delineate better the location and extent of tumor. Scirrhous carcinomas may have a radiographic appearance similar to that of sclerosing cholangitis and may be effectively differentiated only with surgical biopsy. Both gallbladder and ductal carcinomas have a similarly dismal prognosis, with 5-year survival in the range of 5% to 13%.[152,153]

Carcinoma of Vater's ampulla is more common in the elderly and, like ductal malignancy, displays a male predominance. The critical location of the ampulla results in relatively early symptomatology and thus more prompt diagnosis. Ultrasound imaging is the most useful initial imaging technique, but GI endoscopy and ERCP are generally necessary to provide the definitive diagnosis. Early diagnosis contributes to the more favorable prognosis, with 5-year survival ranging from 32% to 62%.[154]

REFERENCES

1. Centers for Disease Control and Prevention: summary of notifiable diseases, United States, 1997, *MMWR* 46:3, 1998.
2. Balistreri WF: Viral hepatitis, *Pediatr Clin North Am* 35:637, 1988.
3. Szmuness W et al: Distribution of antibody to hepatitis A antigen in urban adult populations, *N Engl J Med* 295:755, 1976.
4. Centers for Disease Control and Prevention: Prevention of hepatitis A through active or passive immunization: recommendations of the advisory committee on immunization practices, *MMWR* 48:1, 1999.
5. Lee HS, Vyas GN: Diagnosis of viral hepatitis, *Clin Lab Med* 7:741, 1987.
6. Sherlock S: The natural history of hepatitis B, *Postgrad Med J* 63(suppl 2):7, 1987.
7. Edwards MS: Hepatitis B serology: help in interpretation, *Pediatr Clin North Am* 35:503, 1988.
8. Thomas HC: Hepatitis B viral infection, *Am J Med* 85(suppl 2A):135, 1988.
9. Centers for Disease Control and Prevention: Recommendations for protection against viral hepatitis, *MMWR* 34:32, 1985.
10. Centers for Disease Control and Prevention: Enterically transmitted non-A, non-hepatitis: Mexico, *MMWR* 36:36, 1987.
11. Donahue JG et al: The declining risk of post-transfusion hepatitis C virus infection, *N Engl J Med* 327:369, 1992.
12. Alter MJ, Sampliner R: Hepatitis C: and miles to go before we sleep, *N Engl J Med* 321:1538, 1989.
13. Centers for Disease Control and Prevention: Non-A, non-B hepatitis: Illinois, *MMWR* 39:31, 1989.
14. Centers for Disease Control and Prevention: Recommendations for prevention and control of hepatitis C virus (HCV) infection and HCV-related chronic disease, *MMWR* 47:1, 1998.
15. Hoofnagle JH: Hepatitis. In Mandell GL, Douglas RG, Bennett JE, editors: *Principles and practice of infectious disease,* New York, 1990, Churchill Livingstone.
16. Seeff LB, Dienstag JL: Transfusion-associated non-A, non-B hepatitis: where do we go from here? *Gastroenterology* 95:530, 1988.
17. Alter MJ et al: The natural history of community acquired hepatitis C in the United States, *N Engl J Med* 327:1899, 1992.
18. Alter M et al: The prevalence of hepatitis C virus infection in the United States, 1988 through 1994, *N Engl J Med* 341:556, 1999.
19. Rizetto M et al: Immunofluorescence detection of a new antigen-antibody system associated to hepatitis B virus in liver and in serum of HBs Ag carriers, *Gut* 18:997, 1977.
20. Chatzinoff M, Friedman LS: Delta agent hepatitis, *Infect Dis Clin North Am* 1:529, 1987.
21. Bonino F, Smedile A, Verme G: Hepatitis delta virus infection, *Adv Intern Med* 32:345, 1987.
22. Smedile A et al: Influence of delta infection on severity of hepatitis B, *Lancet* 2:945, 1982.
23. Govindarajan S et al: Fulminate B viral hepatitis: role of delta agent, *Gastroenterology* 86:1417, 1984.
24. Alter M et al: Acute Non-A-E hepatitis in the United States and the role of hepatitis G virus infection, *N Engl J Med* 336:741, 1997.
25. Alter H et al: The incidence of transfusion-associated hepatitis G virus infection and its relation to liver disease, *N Engl J Med* 336:747, 1997.
26. Hadziyannis S: Fulminant hepatitis and the new G/GBV-C flavivirus, *J Viral Hepatitis* 5:15, 1998.
27. Lee W: Acute liver failure, *N Engl J Med* 329:1862, 1993.
28. Kuo G et al: An assay for circulatory antibodies to a major etiologic virus of human non-A, non-B hepatitis, *Science* 244:362, 1989.
29. Cossart Y: Laboratory investigation of hepatitis C: a review, *Pathology* 31:102, 1999.
30. Trott A: Hepatitis B exposure and the emergency physician: risk assessment and hepatitis vaccine update, *Am J Emerg Med* 5:54, 1987.
31. Iserson KV, Criss EA: Hepatitis B: prevalence in emergency physicians, *Ann Emerg Med* 14:119, 1985.
32. Iserson KV et al: The prevalence of hepatitis B serologic markers in emergency physicians, *Am J Emerg Med* 2:394, 1984.
33. Iserson KV, Criss EA, Wright AL: Hepatitis B and vaccination in emergency physicians, *Am J Emerg Med* 5:227, 1987.
34. Centers for Disease Control and Prevention: Update on hepatitis B prevention, *MMWR* 36:353, 1987.
35. Centers for Disease Control and Prevention: Suboptimal response to hepatitis B vaccine given by injection into the buttock, *MMWR* 34:105, 1985.
36. Diehl AM: Alcoholic liver disease, *Med Clin North Am* 73:815, 1989.
37. Centers for Disease Control and Prevention: Premature mortality in the United States: public health issues in the use of years of potential life lost, *MMWR* 35:15, 1986.
38. Lieber CS: Alcoholic liver disease: new insights in pathogenesis lead to new treatments. *J Hepatol* 32(S1):113, 2000.
39. Lieber CS: Alcohol and the liver: metabolism of alcohol and its role in hepatic and extrahepatic diseases. *Mt Sinai J Med* 67:84, 2000.
40. Morgan MY, Sherlock S: Sex related differences among 100 patients with alcoholic liver disease, *BMJ* 1:939, 1977.
41. Lamarine RJ: Alcohol abuse among Native Americans, *J Commun Health* 13:143, 1988.
42. Monteiro E et al: Histocompatibility antigens: marker for susceptibility to and protection from alcoholic liver disease in a Portuguese population, *Hepatology* 8:455, 1988.
43. Lieber CS: Metabolism and metabolic effects of alcohol, *Med Clin North Am* 68:3, 1984.
44. Pimstone NR, French SW: Alcoholic liver disease, *Med Clin North Am* 68:39, 1984.
45. Bird GL, Williams R: Treatment of advanced alcoholic liver disease. *Alcohol Alcohol* 25:197, 1990.
46. Bird G et al: Insulin and glucagon infusion in acute alcoholic hepatitis: a prospective randomized controlled trial, *Hepatology* 14:1097, 1991.
47. Carithers RL Jr et al: Methylprednisolone therapy in patients with severe alcoholic hepatitis: a randomized multicenter trial, *Ann Intern Med* 110:685, 1989.
48. Black M, Tavill AS: Corticosteroids in severe alcoholic hepatitis, *Ann Intern Med* 110:677, 1989.
49. Heathcote J: The clinical expression of primary biliary cirrhosis, *Semin Liver Dis* 17:23, 1996.
50. Neighbor ML: Ascites, *Emerg Med Clin North Am* 7:683, 1989.
51. Bosch J et al: Portal hypertension, *Med Clin North Am* 73:931, 1989.
52. Fraser C, Arieff AI: Hepatic encephalopathy, *N Engl J Med* 313:865, 1985.
53. Gammal SH, Jones EA: Hepatic encephalopathy, *Med Clin North Am* 73:793, 1989.
54. Morgan MH, Read AE, Speller DCE: Treatment of hepatic encephalopathy with metronidazole, *Gut* 23:1, 1982.
55. Mousseau DD, Butterworth RF: Trace amines in hepatic encephalopathy, *Prog Brain Res* 106:277, 1995.
56. Egberts EH et al: Branched chain amino acids in the treatment of latent portal systemic encephalopathy: a double blind placebo controlled crossover study, *Gastroenterology* 88:887, 1985.
57. Morgan MY: The treatment of chronic hepatic encephalopathy, *Hepatogastroenterol* 38:377, 1991.
58. Scollo-Lavizzori G, Steinmann E: Reversal of hepatic coma by benzodiazepine antagonist (R015-1788), *Lancet* 1:1324, 1985.
59. Conn HO, Fessel JM: Spontaneous bacterial peritonitis in cirrhosis: variations on a theme, *Medicine* 50:161, 1971.
60. Wilcox CM, Dismukes WE: Spontaneous bacterial peritonitis: a review of pathogenesis, diagnosis and treatment, *Medicine* 66:447, 1987.
61. Hallak A: Spontaneous bacterial peritonitis, *Am J Gastroenterol* 84(4):345, 1989.
62. Guarner C, Soriano G: Spontaneous bacterial peritonitis, *Semin Liver Dis* 17:203, 1997.
63. Gilbert J, Kamath P: Spontaneous bacterial peritonitis: an update, *Mayo Clin Proc* 70:365, 1995.
64. Stassen WN et al: Immediate diagnostic criteria for bacterial infection of ascitic fluid: evaluation of ascitic fluid polymorphonuclear leukocyte count, pH, and lactate concentration, alone and in combination, *Gastroenterology* 90:1247, 1986.
65. Attali P et al: pH of ascitic fluid: diagnostic and prognostic value in cirrhotic and noncirrhotic patients, *Gastroenterology* 90:1255, 1986.
66. Andreu M et al: Risk factors for spontaneous bacterial peritonitis in cirrhotic patients with ascites, *Gastroenterology* 104:1133, 1993.
67. Guarner C et al: Risk of a first community-acquired spontaneous bacterial peritonitis in cirrhotics with low ascitic fluid protein levels, *Gastroenterology* 117:414, 1999.
68. Das A: A cost analysis of long term antibiotic prophylaxis for spontaneous bacterial peritonitis in cirrhosis, *Am J Gastroenterol* 93:1895, 1998.

69. Rolachon A: Ciprofloxacin and long-term prevention of spontaneous bacterial peritonitis: results of a prospective controlled trial, *Hepatology* 22:1171, 1995.
70. Lewis JH, Zimmerman HJ: Drug-induced liver disease, *Med Clin North Am* 73:775, 1989.
71. Bach N, Thung SN, Schaffner F: Comfrey herb tea-induced hepatic veno-occlusive disease, *Am J Med* 87:97, 1989.
72. Rollins BJ: Hepatic veno-occlusive disease, *Am J Med* 81:297, 1986.
73. Maddrey WC: Hepatic vein thrombosis (Budd-Chiari syndrome): possible association with the use of oral contraceptives, *Semin Liver Dis* 7:32, 1987.
74. Rustgi AK, Richter JM: Pyogenic and amoebic liver abscess, *Med Clin North Am* 73:847, 1989.
75. Chu KM et al: Pyogenic liver abscess. An audit of experience over the past decade, *Arch Surg* 131:148, 1996.
76. Land MA, Moinuddin M, Bisno AL: Pyogenic liver abscess: changing epidemiology and prognosis, *South Med J* 78:1426, 1985.
77. Greenstein AJ, Sachar DB: Pyogenic and amebic abscesses of the liver, *Semin Liver Dis* 8:210, 1988.
78. Seeto R, Rockey D: Pyogenic liver abscess. Changes in etiology, management, and outcome, *Medicine* 75:99, 1996.
79. Branum GD et al: Hepatic abscess changes in etiology, diagnosis, and management, *Ann Surg* 212:655, 1990.
80. Srivastava ED, Mayberry JF: Pyogenic liver abscess: a review of aetiology, diagnosis and intervention, *Dig Dis* 8:287, 1990.
81. Frey CF et al: Liver abscesses, *Surg Clin North Am* 69:259, 1989.
82. Barnes PF et al: A comparison of amoebic and pyogenic abscesses of the liver, *Medicine* 66:472, 1987.
83. Gyorffy EJ et al: Pyogenic liver abscess: diagnostic and therapeutic strategies, *Ann Surg* 206:699, 1987.
84. Rajak CL et al: Percutaneous treatment of liver abscesses: needle aspiration versus catheter drainage. *AJR* 170:1035, 1998.
85. Ch YS et al: Pyogenic liver abscess: treatment with needle aspiration, *Clin Radiol* 52:912, 1997.
86. Miller FJ et al: Percutaneous management of hepatic abscess: a perspective by interventional radiologists, *J Vasc Interv Radiol 8:241, 1997.*
87. Barakate M et al: Pyogenic liver abscess: a review of 10 years' experience in management, *Aust N Z J Surg* 69:205, 1999.
88. Chou F et al: Single and multiple pyogenic liver abscesses: clinical course, etiology, and results of treatment, *World J Surg* 21:384, 1997.
89. Centers for Disease Control and Prevention: Amebiasis associated with colonic irrigation—Colorado, *MMWR* 30:10, 1981.
90. Sargeunt PG, Williams JE, Grene JD: The differentiation of invasive and non-invasive *Entamoeba histolytica* isoenzyme electrophoresis, *Trans R Soc Trop Med Hyg* 75:519, 1978.
91. Katzenstein D, Rickerson V, Braude A: New concepts of amoebic liver abscess derived from hepatic imaging: serodiagnosis and hepatic enzymes in 67 consecutive cases in San Diego, *Medicine* 61:237, 1982.
92. Reed SL, Braude AI: Extraintestinal disease: clinical syndromes diagnostic profile, and therapy. In Ravdin J, editor: *Amebiasis: human infection by* Entamoeba histolytica, New York, 1988, John Wiley & Sons.
93. Kraoul L et al: Evaluation of a rapid enzyme immunoassay for diagnosis of hepatic amoebiasis, *J Clin Microbiol* 35:1530, 1997.
94. Parija S, Karki B: Detection of circulating antigen in amoebic liver abscess by counter-current immunoelectrophoresis, *J Med Microbiol* 48:99, 1999.
95. Hoffner R et al: Common presentation of amebic liver abscess, *Ann Emerg Med* 34:351, 1999.
96. Boyer JL: Chronic hepatitis—a perspective on classification and determinants of prognosis, *Gastroenterology* 70:1161, 1976.
97. Alter HJ et al: Detection of antibody to hepatitis C virus in prospectively followed transfusion recipients with acute and chronic non-A, non-B hepatitis, *N Engl J Med* 321:1494, 1989.
98. Garcia G, Gentry KR: Chronic viral hepatitis, *Med Clin North Am* 73:971, 1989.
99. Payne JA: Chronic hepatitis: pathogenesis and treatment, *Dis Mon* 34:109, 1988.
100. Yip DM, Baker AL: Liver diseases in pregnancy, *Clin Perinatol* 12:683, 1985.
101. Reyes H: Review: intrahepatic cholestasis. A puzzling disorder of pregnancy, *J Gastroenterol Hepatol* 12:211, 1997.
102. Rustgi VK: Liver disease in pregnancy, *Med Clin North Am* 73:1041, 1989.
103. Castro M et al: Reversible peripartum liver failure: a new perspective on the diagnosis, treatment, and cause of acute fatty liver of pregnancy, based on 28 consecutive cases, *Am J Obstet Gynecol* 181:389, 1999.
104. Riely CA: Acute hepatic failure at term: diagnostic problems posed by broad clinical spectrum, *Postgrad Med* 68:118, 1980.
105. Di Bisceglie AD: Hepatocellular carcinoma: molecular biology of its growth and relationship to hepatitis B virus infection, *Med Clin North Am* 73:985, 1989.
106. Beasley RP: Hepatitis B virus: the major etiology of hepatocellular carcinoma, *Cancer* 61:1942, 1988.
107. Lisker-Melman M, Martin P, Hoofnagle JH: Conditions associated with hepatocellular carcinoma, *Med Clin North Am* 73:999, 1989.
108. Krondyl A, Vavrinkova H, Michalec C: Effect of cholecystectomy on the role of the gallbladder in fat absorption, *Gut* 5:607, 1964.
109. Cooper AD, Young HS: Pathophysiology and treatment of gallstones *Med Clin North Am* 73:753, 1989.
110. Young M: Acute diseases of the pancreas and biliary tract, *Emerg Med Clin North Am* 7:555, 1989.
111. Colcock BP, McManus JE: Experience with 1,356 cases of cholecystitis and cholelithiasis, *J Surg Obstet Gynecol* 101:161, 1955.
112. Comess LJ, Bennett PH, Burch TA: Clinical gallbladder disease in Pima Indians, *N Engl J Med* 277:894, 1967.
113. Schoenfield IJ et al: Gallstones—interdepartmental clinical case conference, UCLA School of Medicine, *West J Med* 124:299, 1976.
114. Maki T: Pathogenesis of calcium bilirubinate gallstones: role of *E. coli*, β-glucuronidase and coagulation by inorganic ions, polyelectrolytes and agitations, *Ann Surg* 164:90, 1966.
115. Trotman BW et al: Evaluation of radiographic lucency or opaqueness of gallstones as a means of identifying cholesterol of pigment stones, *Gastroenterol* 68:1563, 1975.
116. Carroll BA: Preferred imaging techniques for the diagnosis of cholecystitis and cholelithiasis, *Ann Surg* 210:1, 1989.
117. Mujahed Z, Evans JA, Whalen JP: The non-opacified gallbladder of oral cholecystography, *Radiol* 112:1, 1974.
118. Cardenas E: Limited bedside ultrasound imaging by emergency medicine physicians, *West J Med* 168:188, 1998.
119. Ahmed A, Cheung RC, Keeffe EB: Management of gallstones and their complications, *Am Fam Physician* 61:1673, 2000.
120. Tomida S et al: Long-term ursodeoxycholic acid therapy is associated with reduced risk of biliary pain and acute cholecystitis in patients with gallbladder stones: a cohort analysis, *Hepatol* 30:6, 1999.
121. Petroni ML et al: Repeated bile acid therapy for the long-term management of cholesterol gallstones, *J Hepatol* 25:719, 1996.
122. Allen MJ, Barody TJ, Buglios TF: Rapid dissolution of gallstones by MTBE, *N Engl J Med* 312:217, 1985.
123. Sackman M et al: Shock wave lithotripsy for gallbladder stones, *N Engl J Med* 318:393, 1988.
124. Thistle JL, Peterson BT: Biliary lithotripsy: a perspective, *Ann Intern Med* 111:868, 1989.
125. LaMorte WW et al: The role of the gallbladder in the pathogenesis of cholesterol gallstones, *Gastroenterol* 77:580, 1979.
126. Glenn F, Dillon LD: Developing trends in acute cholecystitis and choledocholithiasis, *J Surg Obstet Gynecol* 151:528, 1980.
127. Friedman GD, Kannel WB, Dauber TR: The epidemiology of gallbladder disease: observations in the Framingham study, *J Chron Dis* 19:273, 1966.
128. Kadakia SC: Biliary tract emergencies, *Med Clin North Am* 77:1015, 1993.
129. Jivegard L, Thornell E, Svanik J: Pathophysiology of acute obstructive cholecystitis: implications for nonoperative management, *Br J Surg* 74:1084, 1987.
130. Nahrwold DL: Acute cholecystitis. In Sabiston DC Jr, editor: *Textbook of surgery*, ed 14, Philadelphia, 1991, WB Saunders.
131. Finegold SM: Anaerobes in biliary tract infection, *Arch Intern Med* 139:1338, 1979.
132. Cooperberg PL, Jibney RG: Imaging the gallbladder, *Radiol* 163:605, 1987.
133. Pare P, Shaffner EA, Rosenthall L: Non-visualization of the gallbladder by ^{99}m-TcHiVA cholescintigraphy as evidence of cholecystitis, *Can Med Assoc J* 118:384, 1978.

134. Weissman HS et al: An update in radionuclide imaging in the diagnosis of cholecystitis, *JAMA* 246:1354, 1981.
135. Grossman SJ, Joyce JM: Hepatobiliary imaging, *Emerg Med Clin North Am* 9:853, 1991.
136. Halasz NA: Counterfeit cholecystitis: a common diagnostic dilemma, *Am J Surg* 130:189, 1975.
137. Tanowitz H et al: Gastrointestinal manifestations, *Med Clin North Am* 80:1395, 1996.
138. Kalliafas S et al: Acute acalculous cholecystitis: incidence, risk factors, diagnosis, and outcome, *Am Surg* 64:471, 1998.
139. Sharp KW: The acute abdomen, *Surg Clin North Am* 68:269, 1988.
140. Garcia-Sancho Tellez L et al: Acute emphysematous cholecystitis. Report of twenty cases, *Hepatogastroenterol* 46:2144, 1999.
141. Joshi N: Infections in patients with diabetes mellitus, *N Engl J Med* 341:1906, 1999.
142. Salk RP et al: Spectrum of cholangitis, *Am J Surg* 130:143, 1975.
143. Sievert W, Vakil NB: Emergencies of the biliary tract, *Gastroenterol Clin North Am* 17:245, 1988.
144. Kaplun L et al: The early diagnosis of common duct obstruction using cholescintigraphy, *JAMA* 254:2431, 1985.
145. Miller DR, Egbert RM, Braunstein P: Comparison of ultrasound and hepatobiliary imaging in the early detection of acute total common duct obstruction, *Arch Surg* 119:1933, 1984.
146. Brugge W, Van Dam J: Pancreatic and biliary endoscopy, *N Engl J Med* 341:1808, 1999.
147. Gerecht WB et al: Prospective randomized comparison of mezlocillin therapy along with combined ampicillin and gentamicin therapy for patients with cholangitis, *Arch Intern Med* 149:1279, 1989.
148. Schaffner F: Sclerosing cholangitis. In Berk JE, editor: *Gastroenterology,* ed 4, vol 6, Philadelphia, 1985, WB Saunders.
149. Fromm D: Carcinoma of the gallbladder. In Sabiston DC Jr, editor: *Textbook of surgery,* ed 13, Philadelphia, 1986, WB Saunders.
150. Fultz PJ, Skucas J, Weiss SL: Comparative imaging of gallbladder cancer, *J Clin Gastroenterol* 10:683, 1988.
151. Orloff MJ, Marassi NP: Tumor of the extrahepatic bile ducts. In Berk JE, editor: *Gastroenterology,* ed 4, vol 6, Philadelphia, 1985, WB Saunders.
152. Arnaud JP et al: Primary carcinoma of the gallbladder—review of 143 cases, *Hepatogastroenterol* 42:811, 1995.
153. Wilkinson DS: Carcinoma of the gall-bladder: an experience and review of the literature, *Aust N Z J Surg* 65:724, 1995.
154. Hayes DH et al: Carcinoma of the ampulla of Vater, *Ann Surg* 206:572, 1987.

86 Pancreas

Sally A. Santen
Robin R. Hemphill

The pancreas is a retroperitoneal organ extending across the posterior abdomen in the epigastrium. The head of the pancreas sits in the loop of the first part of the duodenum whereas the tail lies against the hilum of the spleen. The main pancreatic duct goes from the tail through the body, to the head of the pancreas and with the common bile duct enters the second part of the duodenum through the sphincter of Oddi. Accessory ducts and anomalies are not uncommon. Anterior to the pancreas from right to left is the transverse colon, the lesser sac of the omentum, and the stomach. Posteriorly lies the bile duct, portal vein, splenic vein, vena cava, aorta, and superior mesenteric artery. To the left are the psoas muscle, kidney, and adrenal gland. Because of the close proximity, inflammation of the pancreas may not only injure these structures, but can also mimic a variety of diseases.

The pancreas has both essential exocrine and endocrine functions. Exocrine products include amylase, lipase, trypsin, chymotrypsin, elastase, carboxypeptidase, phospholipase, and other enzymes. In addition, bicarbonate is produced in greatest quantity from this organ. The bicarbonate serves to neutralize gastric acids as well as the enzymes that break down proteins, carbohydrates, and fats. Cholecystokinin, pancreozymin, and secretin, as well as other factors, control secretion of these enzymes. The endocrine functions of the pancreas are managed by insulin, glucagon, pancreatic polypeptide, and somatostatin.

Diabetes is the most common disorder of the pancreas, followed by pancreatitis. Acute pancreatitis is an inflammatory process of the pancreas usually associated with abdominal pain, elevated pancreatic enzymes, and variable involvement of other regional tissues or remote organ systems. Severe pancreatitis may result in chronic pancreatitis resulting from permanent alterations in function and morphology. Chronic pancreatitis is an ongoing inflammation of the pancreas. Acute pancreatitis may still develop in this population. Pancreatic abscesses, necrosis, and pseudocysts are complications of pancreatitis. Pancreatic tumors may develop from the endocrine or nonendocrine structures. These tumors may cause acute pancreatitis, but usually present in a more indolent fashion. The most common is adenocarcinoma originating from the pancreatic ducts.

ACUTE PANCREATITIS

Perspective

The first reports of pancreatitis date to the 1700s, whereas the first accurate study and description were completed by Fitz in 1889.[1] He noted that performing surgery in the early stages of this disease was "extremely hazardous." Since then our understanding of pancreatitis has advanced; however, treatment remains largely supportive rather than curative. Advances in care have decreased hospital mortality from 25% to 30% to 6% to 10% over the past 30 years.[2] Most patients with pancreatitis have a mild course; however, 25% of cases are severe, with a 9% mortality. Children are at increased risk for mortality, with rates of 20% to 25%. Severity is also increased in obese patients.[3-5] Disease progression and outcome are difficult to predict at onset.

Pancreatitis can be divided into mild or severe pancreatitis. The severity of pancreatitis is defined by the presence of organ failure or local complications such as necrosis, pseudocysts, or abscess.[6] About 20% to 30% of cases will be severe, although on initial presentation the severity may not be apparent. The morbidity and mortality of severe pancreatitis are significant. Mortality occurs in about 10% of all pancreatitis and in about 30% of severe pancreatitis. Death in the first week is usually from pulmonary failure, multiorgan failure, or cardiovascular collapse.[7] Later deaths are more likely to be from infective complications.[8] About 40% of fatal pancreatitis on autopsy was undiagnosed. Therefore, pancreatitis should be suspected in moribund patients with multiorgan failure. Pancreatitis is more severe in some obese patients, in whom mortality increases from 5% to 36%.

The incidence of pancreatitis is 12/100,000, although this incidence varies with the age, gender, and social characteristics of the population studied.[9] Gallstones are the most common obstructive cause of pancreatitis and occur more commonly in women than men, with peak symptomatic incidence between 50 and 60 years of age. Some anatomic variations of the duct result in increased risk of obstruction.[10] Many gallstones are asymptomatic; however, for people with gallstones between 8 and 20 per 1,000 person years will develop pancreatitis.[9] Alcoholic pancreatitis is more common in men than women. In most (but not all) populations, this is the second leading cause of pancreatitis after obstructive causes. It occurs after 5 to 10 years of heavy drinking.

Principles of Disease

Pathophysiology The pathogenesis of pancreatitis is multifactorial although poorly understood. The initial cause of pancreatitis is thought to include direct cellular toxicity or increased ductal pressure. Many mechanisms are recognized, from obstruction of the pancreatic or bile ducts, direct toxicity of the pancreatic cells from toxins or infections, and idiopathic. Regardless of the etiology, the final common pathway is premature activation of pancreatic enzymes such as trypsinogen and zymogen either in the ducts or in the acinar cells.[3,10,11] This activation causes the release of enzymes that are intended to digest dietary proteins and fats that instead lead to cellular breakdown and pancreatic tissue autodigestion. Initially the injury is localized, creating focal pancreatic injury and edema. With increasing severity, the inflammation causes necrosis of the pancreas and spreads to the surrounding fat and tissues. There may be necrosis of the pancreatic ducts as well as the vascular structures, leading to hemorrhage.[12,13] Necrosis of more than 30% of the pancreas increases both morbidity and mortality.[14]

The enzyme activation, inflammation, and necrosis commonly create a fluid collection in 30% to 50% of patients with severe pancreatitis.[15] Over time a fibrinous or granulation wall may develop around this fluid collection, creating a pseudocyst. Thus, pseudocysts are not present in the initial phases of pancreatitis, but instead develop over 4 to 6 weeks. Fluid collections, necrotic areas, or pseudocysts may become infected in 1% of cases, usually after several weeks.[15]

As stated previously, inflammation of the pancreas can affect surrounding tissues. Irritation of the surrounding bowel is common, creating bowel wall edema, ileus, and third spacing of fluid. Formation of ascites is common, and together with bowel edema can cause significant intravascular fluid loss and hypotension.

Because of the release of inflammatory mediators, the initial localized inflammatory response caused by pancreatitis may become a systemic inflammatory response resulting in multiple organ failure. This is a sepsis-like response and any system can be involved, potentially resulting in myocardial depression, adult respiratory distress syndrome (ARDS), disseminated intravascular coagulation (DIC), or renal failure.[16]

Etiology Eighty percent of pancreatitis is caused by either gallstones (about 45%) or alcoholism (about 35%) (Box 86-1).[3] The exact mechanism of biliary pancreatitis is not clear. Either a stone within the bile duct applies transmural pressure on the pancreatic duct or a stone in the common channel of the pancreatic duct and common bile duct causes obstruction. Obstruction or pressure on the pancreatic duct causes bile reflux or increased pressure of pancreatic secretions. Either mechanism leads to the activation of pancreatic enzymes setting off the cascade of pancreatitis. Many cases that were presumed to be idiopathic are actually due to small stones, sludge, or crystals that are too small to be seen by ultrasound examination but may be noted on endoscopic retrograde cholangiopancreatography (ERCP).[17,18]

Alcohol is the cause of about 35% of pancreatitis cases. The mechanism by which alcohol is toxic to the pancreas is not well understood. Possible mechanisms include toxic effects of the ethanol metabolite acetaldehyde, ethanol-related lipid metabolism, or spasm of the sphincter of Oddi. Patients with alcoholic pancreatitis have usually had 5 to 10 years of chronic alcohol use before the onset of pancreatitis.[3,19] Underlying chronic pancreatitis may precede and follow exacerbations of acute pancreatitis.

In addition to alcohol, there are a number of other medications and toxins that cause pancreatitis, including didanosine, pentamidine, organophosphates, and selected scorpion bites. The list of definite and potential drugs causing pancreatitis is quite extensive (Box 86-2). Another cause of pancreatitis is hypertriglyceridemia, with levels less than 500 mg/dl being implicated, although often the level is above 1,000 mg/dl. In pregnancy, both gallstones and increased triglycerides levels can cause pancreatitis.[3] When this occurs, both maternal and fetal mortality is high (20%).

Both blunt and penetrating abdominal trauma can disrupt the ductal system and the pancreatic cells, setting off the enzyme cascade that will result in acute pancreatitis. Pancreatitis may also develop in 1% to 10% of ERCP procedures, resulting from iatrogenic ductal injury.[20] Likewise, postoperative pancreatitis is well recognized and has a higher mortality than other etiologies.

Although both viral and bacterial etiologies for pancreatitis are known, the two most common viral causes of pancreatitis are mumps and coxsackie B. Pancreatitis is more common in patients with human immunodeficiency virus (HIV) than in the general population.[21] In addition to the common etiologies, this population is at risk for pancreatitis from opportunistic infections, HIV-specific medications, and AIDS-related cancers.[22-24] Ultimately, the cause of acute pancreatitis is idiopathic in about 10% of cases.[12]

The etiology of pancreatitis in adults and children is similar, although incidences are different. Trauma (including child abuse), infection, and idiopathic causes make up 70% of the etiologies in children.[3] Hereditary pancreatitis is an

Box 86-1 Etiology of Pancreatitis

Toxic
Alcohol, methanol
Drugs
Scorpion bites in Trinidad

Metabolic
Hypercalcemia (often from hyperparathyroid)
Hyperlipidemia and hypertriglyceridemia (>1000 mg/dl)

Obstructive
Biliary tract disease
Ampullary tumors
Pancreas divisum with obstruction of the accessory duct
Periampullary duodenal diverticula
ERCP and postpancreatography
Pancreatic neuroendocrine tumors
Pancreatic carcinoma
Sphincter of Oddi fibrosis, stricture, tumor, or hypertension

Infectious
Viral
Adenovirus
Coxsackievirus
CMV
EBV
Echovirus
Hepatitis A, B, C virus
HIV
Varicella
Rubella

Other infections
Aspergillus
Campylobacter
Clonorchiasis
Cryptococcus
Cryptosporidium
Dysentery
Vasculitis
Lupus
Polyarteritis nodosa, malignant hypertension

Other Etiologies
Diabetic mellitus, DKA
Crohn's disease
Cystic fibrosis
Emboli (atherosclerotic)
Hemochromatosis
Hereditary pancreatitis
Hypothermia
MAI
Mumps
Mycobacterium TB
Mycoplasma sp
Legionella sp
Leptospirosis
Salmonella typhimurium
Scarlet fever
Streptococcal food poisoning
Toxoplasma
Tuberculosis
Ascariasis
Ischemia from hypoperfusion
Perforated ulcer
Postoperative
Pregnancy
Reye's syndrome
Trauma
Uremia
Idiopathic

autosomal dominant trait with the onset frequently noted during childhood. Other causes include infections and congenital anomalies.[25]

Clinical Features The clinical spectrum of pancreatitis ranges from mild to life threatening. It should be suspected in all patients with epigastric abdominal pain, regardless of age. After diagnosis, the complications of severe pancreatitis should be sought.

By history, almost all patients have abdominal pain, most commonly in the midepigastric area; however, the pain can also be in the right or left upper quadrant. If there is significant inflammation, the pain may be diffuse and the patient may have difficulty localizing the discomfort. The onset is relatively rapid, increasing in severity over 30 to 60 minutes. The pain is generally described as constant and severe, and may radiate to the mid-back. The degree of pain does not correlate with the severity of disease.[12] Even though gallstones are frequently the cause of pancreatitis, the onset of pain is not usually related to eating. Nausea and vomiting frequently are present along with the pain. Although mild pain may be improved by lying on the side or sitting up, typically there is little relief with position change, moving, eating, vomiting, or bowel movement.[26] Colicky pain or pain that waxes and wanes may suggest another diagnosis. About 50% of patients will have had a history of similar abdominal pain that may represent biliary colic or mild pancreatitis.[26]

On physical examination, vital signs may be stable but are frequently abnormal. Hypotension, tachycardia, and shock indicate severe disease with complications or an alternate diagnosis. Vital signs may also be influenced by pain (tachycardia, tachypnea, hypertension) or alcohol withdrawal (tachycardia, hypertension, fever). A low-grade fever is present in about half of patients with pancreatitis after 1 to 3 days in the absence of infection.[12,14] High fever is uncommon during the acute presentation of pancreatitis because serious infection is a late complication. Pulse oximetry should be measured to determine the presence of hypoxia, which is an indicator of systemic complications and severe disease.

Patients with pancreatitis generally appear restless and in moderate distress. They may be jaundiced if an obstructing stone is present. The cardiopulmonary examination may be significant for rales or diminished breath sounds if the patient is hypoventilating from pain or if a pleural effusion is present. Observation of the abdomen may be normal or notable for distention. Only rarely will there be evidence of blood within the peritoneum or retroperitoneum resulting from severe hemorrhagic pancreatitis. Blood within these areas is classi-

Box 86-2 Drug-Induced Pancreatitis

Definite	Possible
Acetaminophen	Bumetanide
Azathioprine	Carbamazepine
Cimetidine	Chlorthalidone
Cisplatin	Clonidine
Corticosteroids	Colchicine
Didanosine	Cyclosporin
Erythromycin	Cytarabine
Estrogens	Diazoxide
Ethyl alcohol	Enalapril
Furosemide	Ergotamine
l-Asparaginase	Ethacrynic acid
Mercaptopurine	Indomethacin
Metronidazole	Isoniazid
Methyldopa	Isotretinoin
Nitrofurantoin	Mefenamic acid
Octreotide	Opiates
Organophosphates	Phenformin
Pentamidine	Piroxicam
Ranitidine	Procainamide
Tetracycline	Rifampin
Salicylates	Thiazides
Sulfonamides, trimethoprim-sulfamethoxazole, sulfasalazine	
Sulindac	
Valproic acid	

cally described by Cullen's sign (discoloration around the umbilicus) and Grey Turner's sign (discoloration of the flank). Auscultation of the abdomen may reveal normal, decreased, or absent bowel sounds depending on whether the patient has a concomitant ileus. Because the pancreas is a retroperitoneal organ, palpation of the abdomen generally reveals epigastric guarding, with rebound being a less common finding.[12] Murphy's sign may be present if the pancreatitis developed secondary to a biliary source. Very rarely the physician may see evidence of subcutaneous fat necrosis, which appears as red nodules most prominent on the extremities. Other physical findings such as the stigmata of alcoholism or xanthomas of hyperlipidemia may help point to the etiology of the pancreatitis.

Complications Many patients with pancreatitis follow a mild course; however, complications are common and may be severe related to local damage and systemic injury. The multiorgan involvement is multifactorial, arising from the direct release of pancreatic enzymes into the bloodstream and perhaps more importantly, from the initiation of the systemic inflammatory response via mediators. This can affect most of the major organ systems.[4,10,12,14]

Shock may result from multiple sources of volume loss. Fluid sequestration occurs in both the pancreas and the bowel lumen and wall. There may also be hemorrhage into necrotic pancreatic tissue. Release of vasodilator and cardiodepressive substances may occur.

About 18% to 30% of patients may have pulmonary complications. These include (1) degradation of surfactant by pancreatic phospholipases, (2) pleural effusions (more commonly on the left and frequently with elevated amylase), (3) hypoxia from atelectasis, hypoventilation, and intrapulmonary shunting, and (4) ARDS. ARDS, from the loss of surfactant as well as from the inflammatory mediators causing capillary leak, is rare but has a 60% mortality.[4]

Metabolic complications of pancreatitis include both hyperglycemia and hypocalcemia. Hyperglycemia is caused by decreased insulin and increased glucagon. The mechanisms for hypocalcemia are (1) sequestration or saponification of calcium in areas of fat necrosis; (2) hypoalbuminemia, hypomagnesemia, hyperglucagonemia; and (3) inactivation of parathyroid hormone.

Coagulopathy develops from circulating proteases affecting the coagulation cascade. Acute tubular necrosis can cause acute renal failure and results from circulating inflammatory mediators or from hypotension and hypoperfusion.

Late complications occur after the second week of illness and include local structure involvement, abscess formation (1% to 4%), gastric bleeds from stress ulcers, splenic vein thrombosis, rupture of pancreatic pseudoaneurysms, fistula formation, splenic rupture, venous thrombosis, and right hydronephrosis.[3] Pancreatic pseudocysts develop in 1% to 8% of patients after 4 to 6 weeks and are more common in alcoholic pancreatitis.[27] Long-term complications of pancreatitis include recurrent or chronic pancreatitis, diabetes mellitus, and digestive and malabsorption problems.

Diagnostic Strategies

Laboratory Tests The diagnosis of acute pancreatitis and the differentiation from other abdominal disorders depend on careful clinical assessment in conjunction with abnormality of certain laboratory values and supportive radiographic findings. The elevation of amylase has been the cornerstone of the diagnosis of pancreatitis although it is an imperfect assay.

Amylase is an enzyme that cleaves carbohydrates. It is produced primarily in the salivary glands and pancreas although it can also be found in small amounts in the fallopian tubes, ovary, testis, muscle, intestines, and other organs. Pancreatic amylase can be differentiated from other sources by electrophoresis, a test that is not readily available in the ED. Elevations of amylase may be seen in normal individuals as well as in ectopic pregnancy, macroamylasemia, parotitis, renal failure (decreased clearance), mesenteric ischemia, bowel obstruction or infarction, perforated duodenal ulcer, acute peritonitis from other causes, and other diseases.[28] Because of the other nonspecific sources of amylase, elevations of amylase are about 70% specific for the diagnosis of pancreatitis.[12,26] In acute pancreatitis amylase rises within 6 to 24 hours and peaks in 48 hours, normalizing in 5 to 7 days. Sensitivity of amylase decreases after the first 24 to 48 hours.

In addition to the unclear origin of amylase, there are several other limitations to using amylase to diagnose acute pancreatitis. The use of different assays and the lack of an international standard lead to varying measured levels of "normal" amylase across institutions. Different studies have used varied threshold levels in making the diagnosis. Complicating matters is that there is no universal gold standard to diagnose pancreatitis; amylase, autopsy, computed tomography (CT), and laparoscopy have all been used. Thus, amylase is commonly used as an imperfect standard with which to make the diagnosis of pancreatitis because of its low cost and rapid availability. However, it is difficult to determine the precise value of this test to the clinician trying to make the initial diagnosis, particularly in the presence of an unclear clinical presentation. According to the literature, the sensitivity of amylase for the diagnosis of pancreatitis ranges from 79% to 95% depending on the comparative choice of gold standard test.[28] As expected, the sensitivity and specificity of amylase vary dependent upon the cut-off value selected to make the diagnosis of pancreatitis. Amylase is about 40% specific when the upper limit of normal of amylase is chosen, 50% to 60% when two times the upper limit is chosen, and 70% to 100% when five times the upper limit is used.[28] The higher cut-off of amylase gives a related drop in sensitivity. In up to 25% of patients with pancreatitis, especially in alcoholics and patients with hypertriglyceridemia or chronic pancreatitis, the amylase can be normal.[28] Importantly, the emergency physician should be aware that mild amylase elevations in patients presenting with acute abdominal pain of unclear etiology, particularly in the elderly, should raise the suspicion of an acute surgical abdomen. Essentially, amylase levels alone, whether normal, mildly elevated, or extremely elevated, do not diagnose pancreatitis unless accompanied by the appropriate clinical picture.

Lipase is a pancreatic enzyme that hydrolyzes triglycerides and has been used both as an adjunctive test and an alternative test for the diagnosis of pancreatitis. Unfortunately, its use has many of the same pitfalls as amylase. In the presence of pancreatic inflammation it increases within 4 to 8 hours and peaks at 24 hours. The levels will fall over 8 to 14 days.[28] Lipase, like amylase, exists in other tissues. Improved assays have rendered lipase more specific than amylase. Yet, there are still cases of nonpancreatic elevations of lipase such as duodenal ulcers, bowel obstruction, and idiopathic elevations.[28,29] Comparisons between amylase and lipase are limited by the lack of a true gold standard for the diagnosis of pancreatitis as well as the choice of cut-off values used for the diagnosis. Despite these limitations, lipase is at least equally sensitive and probably more specific than amylase (specificity 80% to 99%).[28] At five times the upper limits of normal, lipase is 60% sensitive and 100% specific.[28] The use of two times the upper limit of normal for lipase has been recommended to decrease the possibility of missing the diagnosis of pancreatitis.[28] Using elevation of either amylase or lipase as evidence of disease will increase the sensitivity but decrease the specificity. Requiring both levels to be elevated does the reverse. Several expert authors recommend using lipase over amylase when seeking the diagnosis.[4,12,28,30]

The degree of elevation of amylase or lipase is not a marker of disease severity.[10,31] In a study of patients with pancreatitis, patients with amylase elevation less than three times normal had an equal severity of disease compared to those with higher elevations of amylase. In fact, alcoholics will frequently have lower amylase levels but may develop more severe disease than nonalcoholic patients.[31] In a patient with prolonged abdominal pain or the history of pancreatitis, an elevated amylase for longer than a week may suggest pseudocyst or pancreatic abscess. Contrary to earlier studies, using the amylase to lipase ratio does not indicate a specific etiology of pancreatitis.[10]

There are several new tests still under development and not yet widely available. These include urine and serum assays for trypsinogen, tests for elastase, and others. Urinary trypsinogen-2 shows a sensitivity of 94% and specificity of 95% when either CT findings or three times the normal amylase are used as the gold standard.[32-34] In addition, the following tests under investigation may increase sensitivity for the diagnosis of pancreatitis and improve prognostic capability: phospholipase A2, CRP, IL-6, trypsinogen, trypsin activation peptide, and leukocyst elastase.[10,26]

In evaluating a patient with abdominal pain, amylase, lipase, and other blood tests are necessary to narrow the differential, detect complications, and determine prognosis. Although the levels of amylase and lipase may be very high, they are not reliable prognostic indicators. Ranson developed a two-step list of primarily laboratory parameters, performed at admission and after 48 hours, to determine mortality from pancreatitis (Box 86-3).[35,36] With this in mind, additional testing should consist of a complete blood count (CBC), a lactate dehydrogenase (LDH), and a comprehensive metabolic panel (which will include liver enzymes, calcium, renal function, and glucose). Patients with liver disease should have coagulation studies performed to determine the degree of liver dysfunction. Arterial blood gas tests should be used selectively in patients who are acidotic or hypoxic. This information can be used for treatment decisions and to determine prognosis based upon Ranson's criteria. Magnesium should be checked in alcoholics and in those patients with electrolyte abnormalities. Both hypocalcemia and hyperglycemia are common in pancreatitis. Hyperglycemia results from glucagon and insulin abnormalities. Calcium is best determined using the ionized calcium level. Serum calcium is falsely lowered by low albumin levels that may be present in patients with pancreatitis. The creatinine and blood urea nitrogen (BUN) will note the presence of hypovolemia and renal involvement.

Elevation in liver enzymes may result from biliary-induced pancreatitis or from other diseases of the liver or

Box 86-3 Ranson's Criteria

At Admission	Within 48 Hours of Admission
Age >55 years	Hematocrit fall >10%
WBC >16,000/mm^3	BUN rise >5 mg/dl
Glucose >200 mg/dl	Calcium <8 mg%
LDH >350 IU/L	PO_2 <60 mm Hg
AST >250 SF units	Base deficit >4 mEq/L
	Fluid sequestration >6 L

Substitute if Gallstone Induced Admission	Within 48 Hours of Admission
Age >70 years	Hematocrit fall >10%
WBC >18,000/mm^3	BUN rise >2 mg/dl
Glucose >220 mg/dl	Calcium <8 mg%
LDH >400 IU/L	Base deficit >5 mEq/L
AST >250 SF units	Fluid sequestration >4 L

Add the Total Number of Signs at 48 Hours	Mortality
0-3	1%
3-4	15%
5-6	40%
>7	100%

biliary tract. In addition, liver enzymes may increase from the pressure on the common bile duct that results from the surrounding pancreatic inflammation. Mild elevations of bilirubin are common in all types of pancreatitis as well as many other liver disorders. For the patient diagnosed with pancreatitis, higher elevations of aspartate transaminase (AST) and LDH are related to worse prognosis according to Ranson's criteria.

When elevated, the pattern of liver enzyme elevation may help determine the etiology of the pancreatitis (Table 86-1). Alanine aminotransferase (ALT) is the best single marker for biliary etiology levels greater than three times baseline support the diagnosis of biliary pancreatitis.[3,4,21] The higher the elevation of ALT, the greater the specificity and predictive value for gallstones. ALT levels more than 150 IU/L have 96% specificity, positive predictive value (PPV) of 95%, and 48% sensitivity for gallstone pancreatitis. Significant rises in AST, alkaline phosphatase, and bilirubin are also more likely to be related to biliary pancreatitis but are not as sensitive as ALT.[21]

The CBC may be notable for an elevated white blood cell count and the hematocrit may be either high or low. Early in the course, the hematocrit may be elevated because of third space volume loss. A decrease in hematocrit is a poor prognostic factor because it indicates intraabdominal hemorrhage and severe pancreatitis. An electrocardiogram should also be done early to determine whether the patient's abdominal pain may be cardiac in origin.

There are several scoring systems for judging the prognosis of the patient with acute pancreatitis. The most commonly used is Ranson's criteria, which was developed in 1974 (see Box 86-3). Five criteria on admission note the degree of local inflammation, whereas the six criteria at 48 hours note the development of systemic complications. Ranson noted that the model did not work well for patients with gallstone pancreatitis, so he revised the criteria to reflect the improved mortality. Although Ranson's criteria has 90% negative predictive value, the obvious drawback to the use of this system in the ED is that the scoring cannot be completed until 48 hours after diagnosis.[4,37] Although it is a simple and well-known scoring system, it may result in delayed recognition of illness severity[26]; therefore, the APACHE-II (Acute Physiology and Chronic Health Evaluation) system may also be used to judge severity.[37-40] This score includes 12 physiologic variables, age, and chronic health status to generate a total point score. The score can be performed on admission and throughout the hospital stay. Different studies use different cut-off numbers to determine sensitivity and specificity. In one study, APACHE-II scores greater than 7 at admission indicated severe disease with a sensitivity of 68% and specificity of 67%.[38] A score greater than 13 is associated with high likelihood of death.[3] The difficulty with the APACHE score is that it is time-consuming to calculate because it includes multiple variables. Both the Ranson and APACHE scores are better in predicting patients with disease of low to moderate severity. In severe disease the scoring system becomes less accurate.[10] In patients with AIDS, Ranson's criteria may not be as accurate because of HIV-induced changes in the laboratory values such as calcium and LDH.[22,23]

Because numerous factors contribute to disease severity and prognosis in patients with acute pancreatitis, a symposium of gastroenterologists has created a uniform definition for severe pancreatitis.[15] This definition includes extensive local injury or systemic complications (Box 86-4), a greater than level 2 on Ranson's criteria at 48 hours, or an APACHE score of greater than 7.[15,22]

Radiographic Studies

Abdominal radiographs are frequently ordered for patients with abdominal pain. Although these films will not help diagnose acute pancreatitis, they may help exclude other causes of abdominal pain such as bowel obstruction or perforation. In pancreatitis, abdominal series may show an ileus with a sentinel jejunal loop or spasm of the transverse colon and dilation of the ascending colon. Pancreatic calcifications of chronic pancreatitis or gallstones may also be seen. The chest radiograph included in an abdominal series may show left sided or bilateral pleural effusions, atelectasis, or ARDS. Up to 80% of radiographs in patients with pancreatitis will have some abnormal finding.[26] Unfortunately, many of these findings are nonspecific.

Table 86-1. Sensitivity and Specificity for the Etiology of Pancreatitis of Liver Enzymes[21]

	Sensitivity (%)	Specificity (%)	PPV (%)
ALT >150 mmol/L	48	96	95
AST	44	95	87
Alkaline phosphatase >300 units/L	24	95	87
Bilirubin 2.8 mg/dl	38	93	89

Box 86-4 Severe Pancreatitis

Local Complications of the Pancreas

Pseudocyst
Related ascites
Fistula
Pancreatic necrosis

Systemic Complications

Infection (by culture)
Refractory hypotension
Renal failure (creatinine >2.0 mg/dl if no renal insufficiency or rise >1 mg/dl)
New onset pulmonary insufficiency (O_2 saturation <90% without chronic pulmonary disease)
Symptomatic pulmonary effusion
ARDS
New onset cardiac dysfunction
Acidemia (pH <7.25)
Gastrointestinal bleeding (>500 ml/24 hours)
New onset DIC (platelet ≤100,000 mm³, fibrinogen <1 g/L, FSP elevated)

Since laboratory tests cannot completely exclude gallstones as the etiology of pancreatitis, another diagnostic test is recommended.[3] CT and ultrasound are complementary studies in the evaluation of pancreatitis. Ultrasound images the biliary tract with better accuracy than CT; however, the pancreas and pseudocysts are less well visualized by this modality because of overlying bowel gas present in more than half of cases. It is recommended that an ultrasound be performed within the first 24 hours of admission to determine whether gallstones or dilation of the common bile duct (CBD) are present.[7,30] In one study that compared the results of CT and ultrasound among patients with pancreatitis, ultrasound resulted in a change in treatment in 55% of patients compared with no changes after CT. CT was 39% sensitive for biliary disease whereas ultrasound was 83% sensitive.[41] In another study ultrasound was 94% sensitive for gallstones but only 19% for CBD stones and 38% for CBD dilation.[42] Because of these limitations, when gallstone pancreatitis is highly suspected, an ERCP may be necessary to determine the presence of and to remove CBD stones early in the hospital stay.[43]

There are two reasons to perform CT in pancreatitis. The first is to rule out other causes of abdominal pain; the second is to evaluate for the presence of peripancreatic complications such as hemorrhage, pseudocyst, abscess, or vascular abnormalities.[44] The Atlanta international symposium recommended CT in patients with (1) an uncertain diagnosis; (2) severe clinical pancreatitis, abdominal distention, tenderness, fever higher than 102° C, and leukocytosis; (3) a Ranson score of more than 3 or APACHE score of more than 8; (4) no improvement within 72 hours; and (5) acute deterioration. Patients in whom the diagnosis is clear may wait to have the CT performed as an inpatient. The main indication for obtaining a CT in the ED is to exclude other diagnoses. Patients with a clear diagnosis of pancreatitis and without evidence of obstructive etiology may have an imaging study, CT and/or ultrasound, performed as necessary as an inpatient.

If a CT scan is obtained, a dynamic helical CT with oral and intravenous contrast is recommended. This is to help differentiate unopacified bowel from a pancreatic abscess or pseudocyst. CT may also be used to stage the severity and prognosis of acute pancreatitis.[3,13] Grades A (no abnormality) and B (focal or diffuse pancreatic enlargement) indicate lower levels of inflammation. Grade C shows mild peripancreatic inflammation and is associated with an increased risk of complication. Grade D (enlarged pancreas with fluid in the anterior pararenal space) and Grade E (enlarged pancreas with two or more fluid collections) are associated with significant risk of infection, and have mortality of up to 15%. Pseudocysts on CT are noted as encapsulated collections of fluid that develop after about 4 weeks of pancreatitis.

Differential Considerations

Pancreatitis must be differentiated from other abdominal processes, cardiopulmonary disorders, and systemic diseases (Box 86-5). It is important to note that a number of acute surgical conditions may mimic pancreatitis in presentation and may cause elevated amylase such as bowel perforation, ischemic bowel, and ruptured ectopic pregnancy.

Box 86-5 Differential Diagnosis for Pancreatitis

Abdominal Disorders

Perforated viscus
Peptic ulcer disease
Cholecystitis, gall bladder colic
Cholangitis
Gastroenteritis
Nephrolithiasis or pyelonephritis
Bowel obstruction
Mesenteric ischemia
Abdominal aortic aneurism
Ectopic pregnancy

Cardiopulmonary Disorders

Myocardial infarction
Pericarditis
Pneumonia
ARDS
Pleural effusion

Systemic Diseases

Sickle cell crisis

Management

The management of pancreatitis is primarily supportive, with rehydration and pain control. A group of British gastroenterologists has described three overlapping phases of management: (1) diagnosis and assessment of severity, (2) management and monitoring according to disease severity, and (3) detection and management of complications.[7]

The supportive care given to the patient with acute pancreatitis has multiple objectives. The first is volume replacement. Because of vomiting and fluid sequestration, most patients with pancreatitis are dehydrated. Fluids should be replaced with normal saline, and this may require several liters. Vital signs and urine output should be used to judge the adequacy of volume replacement.

A second objective is pain control. Abdominal pain associated with pancreatitis is severe and will generally require narcotic analgesia. Meperidine historically has been used in pancreatitis and biliary disease. Although morphine may increase the tone of the sphincter of Oddi, there is no evidence to show that it worsens the disease process in pancreatitis. Patient-controlled analgesia may be the most effective method of pain control.[30] Antiemetics are indicated for nausea or vomiting.

A third objective is the removal of inciting factors such as alcohol and food. The patient should have nothing by mouth because oral intake stimulates the release of pancreatic enzymes. In the past, nasogastric suction, although uncomfortable for the patient, was almost routinely employed. Controlled trials have shown that the use of nasogastric suction does not decrease pain or length of hospital stay.[45-47] At this time, nasogastric suction is indicated only in cases of intractable vomiting or ileus.

Objective four is reevaluation for complications of pancreatitis. Hypotension should be corrected with large volumes of normal saline (up to 6 L). Airway control is appropriate for respiratory failure or continued shock. Hyperglycemia should be treated cautiously as it may self correct as the pancreatitis resolves. Hypocalcemia may result in decreased albumin or hypomagnesemia, so ionized calcium and magnesium levels should be checked before initiating replacement therapy. If the magnesium level is low, its replacement will frequently raise the calcium level. If there is true hypocalcemia and the patient is experiencing symptoms, then treatment is appropriate. Calcium gluconate should be used if the calcium must be replenished. However, the serum potassium should be normalized before calcium replacement because calcium will cause intravascular potassium shifts.

In the cases of gallstone pancreatitis, gastroenterology consultation is appropriate to discuss the use of ERCP. Early operative removal of gallstones and the gallbladder has been shown to increase mortality[48]; however, early removal of common bile duct stones by ERCP may reduce morbidity. At this time there are conflicting opinions regarding the optimal timing of ERCP in the presence of gallstone pancreatitis.[49] Early endoscopic sphincterotomy (in 24 to 48 hours) and stone removal are recommended in the setting of cholangitis, sepsis, and evidence of severe obstructive pancreatitis.[3,6,42,50,51] In mild pancreatitis, early ERCP has not consistently been shown to improve morbidity. In addition, there is approximately a 5% rate of pancreatitis with ERCP and papillotomy as well as other complications associated with the procedure (bleeding and perforation). With this information in mind it is appropriate to involve the consultant early in the case so a well-coordinated plan can be determined.

Theoretically the following medications should moderate the pathophysiology of pancreatitis: histamine 2 (H_2) blockers decrease the release of secretin by inhibition of gastric acid, glucagon directly suppresses pancreatic exocrine secretion, and octreotide inhibits pancreatic secretion. However, these therapies have not been shown to be clinically effective.[3,4,6] In addition, atropine, calcitonin, somatostatin, fluorouracil, and inhibitors of inflammatory mediators have not been shown to be effective in small studies.[4,6,12,16,46] Aprotinin, gabexate, and lexifant are still under investigation and may have some utility in pancreatitis.[3,6] Peritoneal lavage to wash out inflammatory mediators has not been shown to be effective.

For patients with severe pancreatitis an H_2 blocker, although not helpful for the acute disease, may decrease stress-induced ulcers. In patients with severe or necrotizing pancreatitis, there is some evidence that antibiotics may be effective in reducing sepsis[3,6,8,52]; therefore, broad-spectrum antibiotics such as imipenem or cefuroxime are indicated in patients with sepsis or severe pancreatitis.

Surgical intervention or percutaneous drainage may be necessary for cases of infected pancreatic necrosis, infected pseudocyst, or unresolved pseudocyst. Surgery is preferred when percutaneous drainage is not effective or not possible (extensive pancreatic necrosis or deteriorating clinical status).[14,30]

Disposition

The course of acute pancreatitis is unpredictable and complications may occur hours or days after the onset of illness; therefore, all patients with acute pancreatitis should be admitted to the hospital. Patients with evidence of severe pancreatitis should be admitted to the intensive care unit, especially if there is evidence of pulmonary insufficiency or cardiovascular problems such as hypotension or poor urine output. This includes patients with a score of more than 2 on Ranson's criteria on admission or other evidence of organ failure or local complications.[3,12]

In smaller hospitals without appropriate intensive care facilities, patients with evidence of severe pancreatitis should be transferred. If one suspects or confirms the cause of pancreatitis to be gallstones, discussion with a specialist (gastroenterologist or surgeon) is necessary. Pediatric patients have increased morbidity and mortality with pancreatitis and should be considered for early transfer to a pediatric facility.

CHRONIC PANCREATITIS

Principles of Disease

Chronic pancreatitis is an ongoing inflammatory process leading to irreversible structural damage and impairment of exocrine and endocrine pancreatic function. Normal pancreatic structure is replaced with fibrotic tissue and the pancreatic ducts become strictured in some areas and dilated in others. It is seen in about 4 per 100,000 population.[10] In 70% to 80% of cases, the etiology is chronic alcohol use, although the exact mechanism by which alcohol causes chronic pancreatitis is unclear. The risk of chronic pancreatitis increases with the duration and amount of alcohol consumption.[53] The ingestion of 150 g a day of alcohol for an average of 5 to 15 years is associated with chronic pancreatitis; 5% to 15% of chronic alcoholics develop this disease.[10,53,54] It is possible that small amounts of alcohol in people sensitive to it may also induce chronic pancreatitis. Three theories exist as to the mechanism by which alcohol causes chronic pancreatitis: (1) direct cellular toxicity, (2) alcohol-induced precipitation of proteinaceous fluid in the ductules that cause obstruction and calcification, and (3) injury caused by recurrent acute pancreatitis leading to irreversible damage and chronic inflammation.[55] Chronic pancreatitis can continue even after the cessation of alcohol use, although it is more commonly associated with alcoholic relapse.

Other causes of chronic pancreatitis include hyperlipidemia, ductal obstruction, trauma, hyperparathyroidism, alpha1-antitrypsin deficiency, hereditary pancreatitis, and tropical pancreatitis (cassava fruit is implicated).[53] Idiopathic chronic pancreatitis occurs in about 10% of patients. There is a bimodal distribution of idiopathic chronic pancreatitis occurring in the second and fifth decades. In the 25% of unknown causes, occult alcohol may be the culprit. In children the most common causes are cystic fibrosis and hereditary pancreatitis.

Chronic pancreatitis has been classified and reclassified several times. One useful system uses both underlying pathology and probable etiology. Chronic calcific pancreatitis, usually seen in alcoholics, is characterized by patchy fibrosis, ductal injury, intraductal protein plugs, and stones. Chronic obstructive pancreatitis results from obstruction of the main pancreatic duct by tumors or strictures. Chronic inflammatory pancreatitis is seen in association with autoimmune diseases and is characterized by diffuse fibrosis and inflammatory changes. The final type is a silent perilobular fibrosis with an unclear etiology.[56]

As in acute pancreatitis, chronic inflammation can cause local injury such as pseudoaneurysms, splenic vein thrombosis, pancreatic ascites, or pancreatic fistulas. Pancreatic pseudocysts occur in up to 25% of chronic pancreatitis cases.[10] Rarely, pseudocysts can erode into vascular structures or can become infected. Narrowing of the bile duct from extrinsic pressure or strictures may lead to elevated liver enzymes and jaundice. Approximately 5% of patients develop duodenal obstruction secondary to inflammation around the head of the pancreas. Thus, the acutely ill patient with chronic pancreatitis may be manifesting the primary disease or a complication of this disease. The most common endocrine complication is the presence of glucose intolerance in many patients with chronic pancreatitis. Over years, insulin-dependent diabetes develops in between 30% and 50% of patients.

Chronic pancreatitis has a high morbidity in terms of pain and complications. In addition, patients with chronic pancreatitis have an excess mortality of about 20%; however, the cause of death is more likely to be related to other consequences of alcoholism rather than directly to pancreatitis.[54]

Clinical Features Chronic pancreatitis may present in several ways. The patient may have chronic pain or have an acute flare of the chronic underlying disease. These flares may be severe, and if the patient is relatively well in between, it may be difficult to distinguish this episode from a recurrent one of acute pancreatitis.[53] When present, the pain is epigastric, usually radiating to the back and associated with nausea and vomiting. Often, the patient can relate the similarity to previous attacks of acute pancreatitis or flares of chronic pancreatitis. Use of alcohol or eating exacerbates the pain. There is no correlation between remaining pancreatic function and the degree of pain.[10] Several studies have shown that the pain diminishes over years of chronic disease.[53]

Over time, about 15% of patients with chronic pancreatic disease may develop symptoms of pancreatic exocrine function insufficiency including maldigestion, malabsorption, diarrhea, steatorrhea, or weight loss. Malabsorption occurs after approximately 90% of the pancreas is nonfunctional. Functional endocrine insufficiency will develop in approximately one to two thirds of patients with chronic disease.[53] This insufficiency may be present in the absence of pain because of the overall loss of functioning pancreatic tissue. The symptoms primarily manifest as hyperglycemia; however, the development of diabetic ketoacidosis is rare. Many patients with chronic pancreatitis have an insufficiency of glucagon as well and are malnourished, so hypoglycemia may also develop.[53]

On physical examination patients may appear in significant discomfort. Their general appearance is frequently one of chronic illness from alcoholism, poor nutrition, and malabsorption. On abdominal examination there is frequently tenderness without peritoneal signs. The abdomen should be carefully palpated for a mass that might represent a pseudocyst or tumor. Stigmata of chronic alcohol abuse may also be present. Jaundice may be noted from pressure on the common bile duct or from alcohol-related liver injury.

Diagnostic Strategies

The diagnosis of chronic pancreatitis is frequently made clinically rather than from laboratory values. The serum levels of amylase and lipase are initially elevated in chronic pancreatitis but as the disease progresses, these levels decrease and become normal. The degree of elevation of amylase and lipase is not prognostic. In the patient with the appropriate clinical picture, normal amylase and lipase are consistent with a diagnosis of chronic pancreatitis.

As in acute pancreatitis, a complete blood count and complete metabolic profile should be checked. The white blood cell count is usually normal. There may be elevations of hepatic enzymes (alkaline phosphatase, bilirubin, or transaminases) either from alcoholic hepatitis or from compression on the biliary duct from pancreatic inflammation or a mass in the head of the pancreas. Elevations in serum glucose may also be seen; hypoglycemia is less common. Sudan stain of the stool may show fat globules. Decreased albumin and calcium are common because of the chronic nature of the disease.

On abdominal radiographs, pancreatic calcifications that are pathognomonic of chronic pancreatitis are seen in 30% to 50% of patients.[10,53] Pancreatic calcifications are more common in alcohol-related chronic pancreatitis. Patients with calcifications have had pancreatitis for an average of several years; therefore, these patients should be evaluated for long-term complications such as diabetes and malabsorption.

Abdominal imaging in the ED with CT scan or ultrasound is not necessary for patients with chronic pancreatitis. Imaging should be reserved for cases where the pain is prolonged, significantly increased, or unresponsive to treatment, or when the diagnosis is in question. Although ultrasound is useful in diagnosing the cause of acute pancreatitis, it is less useful in chronic pancreatitis, with a sensitivity of 60% and specificity of 80% to 90%.[10,53] The primary findings on ultrasound are pancreatic calcifications and some ductal abnormalities. CT is 90% sensitive for chronic pancreatitis and is the preferred modality when imaging is indicated. It diagnoses chronic pancreatitis and complications such as pseudocysts.[53] CT findings consistent with chronic pancreatitis are dilated intrapancreatic ducts or microcalcifications.

Although ERCP is not an ED procedure, it can be helpful in diagnosing pancreatic duct abnormalities and measuring pancreatic function. Some gastroenterologists consider the ductal abnormalities seen on ERCP to be the gold standard for the diagnosis of chronic pancreatitis.[53] In the future, endoscopic ultrasound and magnetic resonance imaging cholangiopancreatography may assume a greater role in the evaluation of chronic pancreatitis.

Differential Considerations

The diagnosis of chronic pancreatitis is usually straightforward in the alcoholic patient with hyperamylasemia who has chronic abdominal pain and a history of similar, previous flares of pancreatitis. However, the emergency physician should not be lulled into complacency and forget that other abdominal processes (both unrelated to the pancreas or complications of pancreatitis) still exist in the differential (see Box 86-5). In addition, other chronic abdominal disease such as peptic ulcers, irritable bowel, gallstones, and endometriosis may present with recurrent abdominal pain. Finally, narcotic-dependent patients in withdrawal may have vomiting and abdominal pain that may be difficult to differentiate from chronic pancreatitis.[54]

Management

The initial management of chronic pancreatitis is supportive. Depending upon the patient's clinical status and electrolyte values, fluids and electrolytes may need to be replaced. An "alcohol cocktail" with thiamine, multivitamins, and folate is often indicated because patients are frequently malnourished. Antiemetics should be used to treat recurrent emesis.

Patients with chronic pancreatitis may have normal laboratory values despite significant pain, and patients with chronic pain syndromes may not exhibit signs of autonomic hyperactivity when experiencing exacerbations of their underlying disease. In patients unknown to the ED, this may lead to a concern that the patient is drug seeking. Although this possibility is ever-present in the ED setting, the emergency physician should be on the side of treatment in all cases except those of obvious abuse. Either morphine or meperidine may be used, and should be titrated. Tramadol (Ultram) was used effectively in one study.[57] The use of narcotics may be needed over extended periods. In the ideal medical system, the primary care physician monitors the narcotic prescription because narcotic dependence may eventually become an issue.[53]

The removal of inciting factors, especially alcohol, is important. Patients with significant pain should have nothing by mouth, although as in acute pancreatitis, a nasogastric tube is not indicated. The use of oral pancreatic replacement enzymes increases the amount of trypsin in the duodenum and may provide a negative feedback to the release of pancreatic secretions.[10] Therefore pancreatic replacement enzymes will not only help treat malabsorption but may also decrease the pain in some patients.[53] In theory, proton pump inhibitors or H_2 receptor blockers may reduce pancreatic stimulation; however, these have not been shown to decrease pain or improve recovery.[10] Octreotide is also under investigation to treat the pain of chronic pancreatitis.

Beyond the ED treatment, endoscopic dilation, ductal stone removal, or stenting of the pancreatic ducts may be a helpful treatment adjunct. Common bile duct stenting may also be necessary because obstruction occurs in about 5% to 10% of cases.[10] For cases of severe pain or for the drainage of pseudocysts, pancreatic resection and a Whipple procedure are sometimes recommended. Celiac plexus blocks have also been used for pain control.[53]

Disposition

In general, patients with chronic pancreatitis are managed as outpatients and present to the ED with exacerbations or complications. Because acute pancreatitis can present in patients with chronic pancreatitis, the same prognostic indicators for severity of acute pancreatitis should be noted. Patients with severe disease should be admitted to the intensive care unit. Patients with dehydration, abdominal pain unresponsive to medications, or questionable diagnosis should be admitted for evaluation and treatment. After a careful ED evaluation, in the absence of dehydration, unstable vital signs, or uncontrolled pain, a patient may be treated as an outpatient with close follow-up.

PANCREATIC CANCER

Perspective

Pancreatic cancer is not commonly an ED diagnosis; however, pancreatic cancer may be found on CT, or a patient with known cancer may present with complications. Pancreatic cancer is a particularly lethal cancer, with death occurring in approximately 99% of patients. It is the fifth most common cause of cancer-related mortality in the United States. The disease is diagnosed in approximately 27,000 Americans a year or 9 to 10 people per 100,000. Less than 10% of patients survive 10 years, and the 5-year survival is only 2% despite aggressive surgery and advances in chemotherapy.[58,59]

Principles of Disease

Little is known about the causes of pancreatic cancer.[60] It has been noted that heavy smoking increases the risk by 2 to 3 times. In one study, chronic pancreatitis increased the risk of pancreatic cancer approximately 4% in patients followed over 20 years. Pancreatic cancer is more common in diabetic patients, although this may be the result of development of diabetes in patients with pancreatic cancer. There is a small familial aggregation of pancreatic cancer.

Ductal adenocarcinomas make up 95% of malignant pancreatic tumors. The pancreatic head is the most common location of origin in about 70% of cases. The tumor extends locally into adjacent structures and can metastasize via hematogenous or lymphatic spread to liver, peritoneum, lungs, bones, and brain. Neuroendocrine tumors, such as gastrinomas, vasoactive intestinal peptide (VIP)-omas, and glucagonomas make up the remaining cases. These types of tumors have a better prognosis.

Clinical Features The presentation of pancreatic cancer is variable because progression of the disease is indolent. The tumor has usually been present for several months before the cancer is diagnosed; therefore, patients may present with pain of long duration or with one of the many complications of this cancer. One of the most common presentations is weight loss that is usually the result of anorexia rather than malabsorption. The abdominal pain is usually a dull, constant pain in the epigastrium that may radiate to the back. The patient may present with jaundice from common bile duct obstruction. Progressive jaundice develops in about 75% of patients. An enlarged and palpable, but painless, gallbladder in the presence of jaundice is most commonly associated with pancreatic cancer (termed Courvoisier's sign). Glucose intolerance may also develop. As the tumor enlarges, patients may develop evidence of bowel obstruction. Pancreatic cancer (as well as other cancers) may render patients hypercoagulable and result in thromboembolic presentations. Varices and gastrointestinal bleeding may be caused by compression of the portal system by the tumor.

Neuroendocrine tumors of the pancreas are rare and present with symptoms that are the result of the hormones that they produce. For example, insulinomas may present with hypoglycemia. Gastrinomas are related to Zollinger-Ellison syndrome and recurrent peptic ulcers. VIP-omas present with extreme watery diarrhea, hypokalemia, and achlorhydria. Glucagonomas present with glucose intolerance and necrolytic migratory erythema.[61] Some tumors produce multiple hormones.[61] Other nonfunctional tumors my also be noted incidentally on CT as small pancreatic masses. Diagnosis is made by abnormal levels of hormones and the appropriate clinical syndrome. Fifty percent of pancreatic neuroendocrine tumors are malignant.[62]

Diagnostic Strategies

The diagnosis of pancreatic cancer may be made by ultrasound, although CT scan provides better imaging of the cancer. Percutaneous ultrasound, CT-guided biopsy, or ERCP-guided biopsy can be used for tissue diagnosis. Histologic samples are needed to differentiate ductal adenocarcinoma from islet cell tumors, other metastatic cancers, and lymphoma. Serologic markers have not proven satisfactory for diagnosis or follow-up although several oncogenes and tumor markers are under study.

Management

Complete resection of the carcinoma is the only effective treatment. Unfortunately, few tumors (5% to 10%) are diagnosed at a stage where this may be possible. In patients with unresectable tumors, the median survival is approximately 6 months. Palliative surgery may be performed to relieve obstruction. Biliary drainage by percutaneously or ERCP-placed stents may also improve jaundice. Chemotherapy and radiation therapy may decrease tumor size to ease pain and prolong survival in some patients.[63] Treatment of neuroendocrine tumors is aimed both at tumor growth by excision and hormone excess.[62-64]

In the ED, patients may present with complications of the cancer such as bowel obstruction, jaundice, or pain control issues. Given the grim prognosis of the disease and significant pain associated, narcotics should not be withheld.

KEY CONCEPTS

- Most cases of acute pancreatitis are caused by gallstones (45%) and alcoholism (35%). Other etiologies include medications, toxins, and trauma.
- The clinical spectrum of acute pancreatitis ranges from mild (epigastric discomfort often associated with vomiting) to life threatening (severe abdominal pain in the presence of an acute abdomen and hemodynamic instability due to systemic complications). The mortality of severe pancreatitis approaches 30%.
- There is no perfect test for diagnosing acute pancreatitis. The most useful tests include serum amylase and lipase. Unfortunately, both tests can be normal in up to 25% of cases, and mild elevations are not specific for acute pancreatitis and can be seen in many other acute surgical disorders causing abdominal pain. Both tests are highly specific for pancreatitis when serum levels are elevated five times above the upper limits of normal.
- Emergent abdominal CT should be performed in patients with clinically suspected pancreatitis who appear acutely ill (to exclude peripancreatic complications such as hemorrhage, pseudocyst, or abscess) and in patients with an uncertain diagnosis (to exclude other surgical causes of acute abdominal pain).
- Since the course of acute pancreatitis is unpredictable, all patients should be hospitalized for pain control, hydration, observation, and the management of complications. Patients with severe pancreatitis (having more than two of Ranson's criteria, an APACHE score over 7, or evidence of systemic complications) should be cared for in an ICU.

REFERENCES

1. Leach SD, Gorelick FS, Modlin IM: Acute pancreatitis at its centenary, *Ann Surg* 212:109, 1990.
2. Neoptolemos JP et al: Acute pancreatitis: the substantial human and financial costs, *Gut* 42:888-891, 1998.
3. Steinberg WM: Diagnosis and management of acute pancreatitis, *Cleve Clin J Med* 64:182, 1997.
4. Steinberg W, Tenner S: Acute pancreatitis, *N Engl J Med* 330:1198, 1994.
5. Martinez J et al: Obesity: a prognostic factor of severity in acute pancreatitis, *Pancreas* 19:15, 1999.
6. Tenner S, Banks PA: Acute pancreatitis: nonsurgical management, *World J Surg* 21:143, 1997.
7. British Society of Gastroenterology: United Kingdom guidelines for the management of acute pancreatitis, *Gut* 42:S1, 1998.
8. Kramer KM, Levy H: Prophylactic antibiotics for severe acute pancreatitis: the beginning of an era, *Pharmacother* 19:592, 1999.
9. Moreau JA et al: Gallstone pancreatitis and the effect of cholecystectomy: a population based cohort study, *Mayo Clin Proc* 63:466, 1988.
10. Banks PA: Acute and chronic pancreatitis. In Feldman M, Scharschmidt BF, Sleisenger MH, editors: *Gastrointestinal and liver disease,* Philadelphia, 1998, WB Saunders.
11. Steer ML: Pathogenesis of acute pancreatitis, *Digestion* 58:46, 1997.
12. Mergener K, Baillic J: Fortnightly review: acute pancreatitis, *Lancet* 316:44, 1998.
13. Balthazar EJ, Freeney PC, van Sonnenberg E: Imaging and intervention in acute pancreatitis, *Radiol* 194:297, 1994.
14. Baron TH, Morgan DE: Acute necrotizing pancreatitis, *N Engl J Med* 340:1412, 1999.
15. Bradley E: A clinically based classification system for acute pancreatitis, *Arch Surg* 128:586, 1993.
16. Horman J: The role of cytokines in the pathogenesis of acute pancreatitis, *Am J Surg* 175:76, 1998.
17. Lee SP, Nicholls JF, Park HZ: Biliary sludge as a cause of acute pancreatitis, *N Engl J Med* 326:589, 1992.
18. Ros E, et al: Occult microlithiasis in "idiopathic" acute pancreatitis, *Gastroenterol* 101:1701, 1991.
19. Ranson JHC: Etiologic and prognostic factors in human acute pancreatitis, *Am J Gastenterol* 77:633, 1982.
20. Freeman ML: Complications of endoscopic biliary sphincterotomy: a review, *Endosc* 29:288, 1997.
21. Tenner S, Dubner H, Steinberg W: Predicting gallstone pancreatitis with laboratory parameters: a meta-analysis, *Am J Gastroenterol* 89:1863, 1994.
22. Manocha AP et al: Prevalence and predictors of severe acute pancreatitis in patients with acquired immune deficiency syndrome (AIDS), *Am J Gastroenterol* 94:784, 1999.
23. Dutta SK, Ting CD, Lai LL: Study of the prevalence, severity and etiologic factors associated with acute pancreatitis in patients infected with human immunodeficiency virus, *Am J Gastroenterol* 92:2044, 1997.
24. Dassopoulos T, Ehrenpreis E: Acute pancreatitis in human immunodeficiency virus-infected patients: a review, *Am J Med* 107:78, 1999.
25. Benkov KJ, Compton CC: Weekly CPC exercises, *N Engl J Med* 340:215, 1999.
26. Ranson JHC: Diagnostic standards for acute pancreatitis, *World J Surg* 21:136, 1997.
27. Maringhini A et al: Pseudocysts in acute nonalcoholic pancreatitis, *Dig Dis Sci* 44:1669, 1999.
28. Vissers RJ, Abu-laban RB, Mchugh DF: Amylase and lipase in the emergency department evaluation of acute pancreatitis, *J Emerg Med* 17:1027, 1999.
29. Frank B, Gottlieb K: Amylase normal, lipase elevated: is it pancreatitis? *Am J Gastroenterol* 94:463-469, 1999.
30. Banks PA: Practice guidelines in acute pancreatitis, *Am J Gastroenterol* 92:377-386, 1997.
31. Lankisch PG, Burchard-Reckert S, Lehnick D: Underestimation of acute pancreatitis: patients with only a small increase in amylase/lipase levels can also have or develop severe acute pancreatitis, *Gut* 44:542-544, 1999.
32. Kemppainen EA et al: Rapid measurement of urinary trypsinogen-2 as a screening test for acute pancreatitis, *N Engl J Med* 336:1788-1793, 1997.
33. Kemppainen EA et al: Advances in the laboratory diagnostics of acute pancreatitis, *Ann Med* 30:169-175, 1998.
34. Kylanpaa-Back ML et al: Reliable screening for acute pancreatitis with rapid urine trypsinogen-2 test strip, *Br J Surg* 87:49-52, 2000.
35. Ranson JHC, Rifkind KM, Turner JW: Prognostic signs and nonoperative peritoneal lavage in acute pancreatitis, *Surg Gynecol Obstet* 143:209-219, 1976.
36. Ranson JHC et al: Prognostic signs and operative management in acute pancreatitis, *Surg Gynecol Obstet* 139:69-81, 1974.
37. Agarwal N, Pitchumoni L: Assessment of severity in acute pancreatitis, *Am J Gastroenterol* 86:1385-1391, 1991.

37a. Demmy TL et al: Comparison of multiple parameter prognostic systems in acute pancreatitis, *Am J Surg* 156:492-496, 1988.

38. Wilson C, Heath DDI, Imrie CW: Prediction of outcome in acute pancreatitis: a comparative study of APACHE II, clinical assessment and multiple factor scoring systems, *Br J Surg* 77:1260-1264, 1990.
39. Demmy TL et al: Comparison of multiple parameter prognostic systems in acute pancreatitis, *Am J Surg* 156:492-496, 1988.
40. Sanctis JT et al: Prognostic indicators in acute pancreatitis: CT vs APACHE, *Clin Radiol* 52:842-848, 1997.
41. Harvey RT, Niller WT: Acute biliary disease: initial CT and follow-up US vs. initial US and follow-up CT, *Radiol* 213:831-836, 1999.

42. Liu CL, Lo CM, Fan ST: Acute biliary pancreatitis: diagnosis and management, *World J Surg* 21:149-154, 1997.
43. Pezzilli R et al: Ultrasonographic evaluation of the common bile duct in biliary acute pancreatitis patients, *J Ultrasound Med* 18:391-394, 1999.
44. Dazell DP et al: Acute pancreatitis: the role of diagnostic imaging, *Crit Rev Diagn Image* 39:339-363, 1998.
45. Naeije R et al: Is nasogastric suction necessary in acute pancreatitis? *BMJ* 2:659-660, 1978.
46. Loiudice TA et al: Treatment of acute alcoholic pancreatitis: the roles of cimetidine and nasogastric suction, *Am J Gastroenterol* 79:553-558, 1984.
47. Levant JA et al: Nasogastric suction in the treatment of alcoholic pancreatitis: a controlled study, *JAMA* 229:51-52, 1974.
48. Kelly TR, Wagner DS: Gallstone pancreatitis: a prospective randomized trial of the timing of surgery, *Surg* 104:600-605, 1988.
49. Folsch UR: The role of ERCP and sphincterotomy in acute biliary pancreatitis, *Endosc* 30:A253-255, 1998.
50. Gupta R, Johnson CD, Toh SKC: Early ERCP is an essential part of the management of all cases of acute pancreatitis, *Ann Roy Coll Surg Engl* 81:46-50, 1999.
51. Fan ST et al: Early treatment of acute biliary pancreatitis by endoscopic papillotomy, *N Engl J Med* 328:228-232, 1993.
52. Pederzoli P et al: A randomized multi-center clinical trial of antibiotic prophylaxis of septic complications in acute necrotizing pancreatitis with imipenem, *Gynecol Obstet* 176:480-483, 1993.
53. Mergener K, Baillie J: Chronic pancreatitis, *Lancet* 350:1379-1385, 1997.
54. Apte MV, Keogh GW, Wilson JS: Chronic pancreatitis: complications and management, *J Clin Gastroenterol* 29:225-240, 1999.
55. Ammann RW, Mauellhaupt B: Progression of alcoholic acute to chronic pancreatitis, *Gut* 35:552-556, 1994.
56. Sarles H: Definition and classification of pancreatitis, *Pancreas* 1991:6, 1991.
57. Wilder-Smith CH et al: Effect of tramadol and morphine on pain and gastrointestinal motor function in patients with chronic pancreatitis, *Dig Dis Sci* 44:1107-1116, 1999.
58. Rosewicz S, Wiedenmann B: Pancreatic carcinoma, *Lancet* 349: 485-489, 1997.
59. Haycox A et al: Current practice and future perspectives in detection and diagnosis of pancreatic cancer, *Aliment Pharm Therap* 12:937-948, 1998.
60. Lowenfels AB, Maisonneuve P: Pancreatic cancer: Development of a unifying concept, *Ann NY Acad* 880:191-200, 1999.
61. Wermers RA, Fatourechi V, Kvols LK: Clinical spectrum of hyperglucagonemia associated with malignant neuroendocrine tumors, *Mayo Clin Proc* 71:1030, 1996.
62. Eriksson G, Oberg K: Neuroendocrine tumors of the pancreas, *Br J Surg* 87:128-131, 2000.
63. Hugier M, Mason NP: Treatment of cancer of the exocrine pancreas, *Am J Surg* 177:257-265, 1999.
64. Pelley RJ, Bukowski RM: Recent advances in systemic therapy for gastrointestinal neuroendocrine tumors, *Curr Opin Oncol* 11:32-37, 1999.

87 Small Intestine

Susan P. Torrey
Philip L. Henneman

SMALL BOWEL OBSTRUCTION

Perspective

The signs and symptoms of intestinal obstruction have been recognized for centuries. This clinical entity has been treated with a variety of interventions, including enemas and insufflation of the rectum, metallic mercury ingestion, therapeutic bleeding, and percutaneous intestinal puncture.[1,2] By the late nineteenth century proximal intestinal decompression was reliably utilized to provide temporary symptomatic relief of intestinal obstruction. Antibiotics and improved surgical techniques have significantly improved the prognosis for patients with small bowel obstruction.

Patients with small bowel obstruction account for 20% of hospital admissions for acute abdominal complaints.[2-4] Approximately 300,000 operations are performed in the United States each year for relief of intestinal obstruction.[5] Aggressive treatment has resulted in a current mortality of less than 5%, a substantial improvement over the expected 60% mortality associated with this disease in 1900.[6] When strangulation complicates small bowel obstruction, however, the mortality rate increases to as much as 30%.[7] Death from small bowel obstruction occurs most often in the elderly or in patients with significant underlying illness.

The term *mechanical obstruction* implies a physical barrier to the flow of intestinal contents. Within this definition, *simple obstruction* refers to the situation where the intestinal lumen is partially or completely occluded at one or more points, thus producing proximal intestinal distention, but without the compromise of the intestinal vascular supply. A *closed-loop obstruction* implies that a segment of bowel is obstructed at two sequential sites, usually by twisting about a constricting adhesive band or hernia opening. This mechanism of obstruction has a high risk of compromising intestinal blood flow with resulting intestinal ischemia, a condition referred to as *strangulation obstruction.* It is important to note that not all closed-loop obstructions have intestinal ischemia, and that other types of obstruction may eventually involve vascular compromise.

In contrast to mechanical obstruction, *neurogenic* or *functional obstruction* occurs when intestinal contents fail to pass through the bowel lumen because of disturbances in gut motility, rather than actual blockage. This entity is also commonly referred to as an *adynamic ileus.* When intestinal peristalsis fails, dilation of the involved intestinal tract will develop. Adynamic ileus is most commonly seen after abdominal surgery, but can be caused by other common medical conditions (Box 87-1). Focal decrease in peristaltic activity may occur because of a localized inflammatory

Box 87-1 Causes of Adynamic Ileus

Abdominal trauma
Infection (retroperitoneal, pelvic, intrathoracic)
Laparotomy
Metabolic disease (hypokalemia)
Renal colic
Skeletal injury (rib fracture, vertebral fracture)
Medications (e.g., narcotics)

Box 87-2 Lesions Causing Small Bowel Obstruction

Intrinsic
Congenital (atresia, stenosis)
Inflammatory (Crohn's, radiation enteritis)
Neoplasms (metastatic or primary)
Intussusception
Traumatic (hematoma)

Extrinsic
Hernias (internal and external)
Adhesions
Volvulus
Compressing masses (tumors, abscesses, hematomas)

Intraluminal
Foreign body
Gallstones
Bezoars
Barium
Ascaris infestation

process (e.g., pancreatitis, cholecystitis, or appendicitis) and result in gas and fluid accumulation in an isolated segment of bowel. This segmental ileus is called a *sentinel loop.*

Pseudoobstruction refers to a poorly understood disorder of intestinal motility associated with a number of medical conditions, including amyloidosis, collagen vascular disease, diabetes, and hypothyroidism, as well as several metabolic disorders (hypokalemia, hypocalcemia, and uremia). The signs and symptoms of intestinal obstruction are present, but there is no evidence of an underlying lesion on diagnostic evaluation. Supportive care is recommended, but the results of treatment are often disappointing.

Principles of Disease

There is a relationship between the progressive physiologic changes that occur in patients with small bowel obstruction and the corresponding clinical manifestations. Mechanical small bowel obstruction initially causes mild proximal intestinal distention that results from the accumulation of normal gastrointestinal secretions and swallowed air above the obstructing lesion. This distention stimulates peristalsis above and below the obstruction, which accounts for the frequent loose bowel movements that may accompany partial and even complete small bowel obstruction in the early stages.[1,2] Early bowel distention stimulates epithelial cell secretory activity, resulting in the addition of more fluid, increasing bowel dilation, and the creation of a self-perpetuating process. This situation is worsened by the inability of the distended bowel to absorb fluid and electrolytes at a normal rate. Further increases in intraluminal pressure result in capillary and lymphatic obstruction, with subsequent edema of the bowel wall. Perforation will occur if this process continues uninterrupted. In addition, vomiting and intraperitoneal fluid sequestration further compound volume losses, leading to extracellular fluid depletion, hypovolemia, and eventually, shock.

The rise in intraluminal pressure is much more abrupt with a closed-loop obstruction because the intestinal contents are also prevented from retrograde flow. Strangulation occurs with the development of venous congestion, small vessel rupture, intramural and mesenteric hemorrhage, and arterial insufficiency.[8] It is also not uncommon for the loop of distended bowel to further twist on itself, resulting in large artery occlusion. Either sequence of events will then progress rapidly from intestinal ischemia to infarction.

Necrosis of the bowel and leakage of contaminated contents cause bacterial peritonitis and sepsis. While the proximal small bowel normally contains few bacteria, this changes quickly during times of intestinal stasis. Simple intestinal obstruction has been shown to be associated with increased bacterial translocation to mesenteric lymph nodes. In one series, 59% of the patients undergoing laparotomy for simple small bowel obstruction had bacteria (most commonly *Escherichia coli*) cultured from mesenteric lymph nodes, compared with only 4% of patients operated on for other reasons.[1,3]

The most common causes of small bowel obstruction are listed in Box 87-2. In developed countries, postoperative adhesions are now responsible for more than 50% of all small bowel obstruction. It is estimated that as many as 15% of abdominal surgeries will eventually result in small bowel obstruction from adhesion.[9] A particularly high incidence of small bowel obstruction is found after gynecologic or intestinal surgeries, as well as in those patients who have previously undergone surgery in the presence of peritonitis or significant abdominal trauma.[10] Other important causes of small bowel obstruction include hernias and neoplasms, each with an incidence of approximately 15%.[1-3] Hernias can be either external or internal. External hernias involve the abdominal wall (e.g., inguinal, femoral, or incisional), whereas internal hernias typically involve mesenteric defects from prior surgery. Although hernias account for a relatively small portion of bowel obstruction, they are extremely important to recognize because this group has a high rate of strangulation (28% with hernias versus 8% with adhesive obstruction[3]). Anatomically this occurs because many obstructions caused by hernias are of the closed-loop type. When neoplasm is associated with small bowel obstruction, the cause is most often colon cancer, followed by pancreatic, gastric, and gynecologic malignancies.

There are several less common causes of small bowel obstruction that are nonetheless interesting and pertinent to the practice of emergency medicine. *Gallstone ileus* is rare in the general population, but accounts for 25% of nonstrangulated small bowel obstructions in those patients over the age of 65.[11] In this entity, a gallstone erodes through an inflamed gallbladder wall into a loop of adjacent small bowel. The stone then passes through the bowel lumen until it meets some narrowing, typically the distal ileum, where it produces mechanical obstruction. Given the elderly patient population in which this problem occurs, it is not surprising to find a 15% to 18% mortality. Another unique cause of small bowel obstruction is an *obturator hernia.* This typically occurs in elderly emaciated women with significant concomitant medical illness but no previous abdominal surgery.[12] It is believed that women with a wider pelvis and more oblique obturator canal are predisposed to the development of obturator hernia in the presence of decreased preperitoneal fat due to emaciation and chronic increased intraabdominal pressure resulting from associated medical disease. This hernia is difficult to detect, and often diagnosed when it presents as small bowel obstruction. Both of these uncommon causes of small bowel obstruction occur in the elderly population, which is becoming an increasing percentage of the emergency department population.

Another uncommon but noteworthy cause of small bowel obstruction is *small bowel volvulus.* This condition results from abnormal twisting of a loop of bowel around the axis of its own mesentery. Although volvulus of the colon (sigmoid and cecum) is common, volvulus of the small bowel is rare. Primary small bowel volvulus occurs in an otherwise normal abdominal cavity, and is seen most often in adult populations in parts of Africa, the Middle East, and the Indian subcontinent. It is rarely seen in Europe and North America. Secondary causes of small bowel volvulus include malformation and malrotation of the intestine, or tethering the loop of bowel at its apex as a result of postoperative adhesions.[13] The need for suspicion and early surgical intervention cannot be overemphasized, since this classic closed-loop obstruction has a high incidence of strangulation, 60% in one series.[3]

Intussusception occurs in all age groups but is primarily a disease of infancy and early childhood, constituting the most common cause of bowel obstruction in early childhood. Only 5% of all intussusceptions occur in adults, and intussusception accounts for only 5% of small bowel obstruction in adults. An intussusception occurs when a segment of bowel telescopes into an adjacent segment, resulting in obstruction and ischemic injury to the intussuscepting segment. In striking contrast to the idiopathic nature of most childhood intussusceptions, a mechanical cause is present in more than 90% of adult cases. Tumors, either benign or malignant, act as the lead point of intussusception in over 65% of adult cases. Recently, there have been several reports of adult intussusception associated with acquired immunodeficiency syndrome (AIDS).[14] In this setting the lesions are most often in the ileum, caused by lymphoma or unusual inflammatory processes, including atypical mycobacterial infection.

Signs and symptoms caused by intussusception in the adult are nonspecific, and may occasionally be chronic or recurrent in nature. Abdominal pain is a prominent complaint, often associated with some symptoms suggestive of obstruction (nausea, vomiting, and abdominal distention). Radiographic features of intussusception are also nonspecific. Plain films may reveal evidence of partial or complete bowel obstruction. Occasionally, a sausage-shaped soft tissue density, outlined by two strips of air, may be seen. It has recently been recommended that ultrasonography may be useful in the diagnosis of adult and pediatric cases. The mainstay of diagnosis, however, remains contrast studies, and while reduction of the intussusception may simultaneously occur, surgery is always recommended for adults because of the high incidence of pathologic lesions.

Clinical Features

History Patients with small bowel obstruction typically complain of regularly recurrent bouts of poorly localized abdominal pain lasting from seconds to minutes. The painful spasms occur every few minutes with proximal intestinal obstruction, and less frequently with more distal obstruction. The pain is described as crampy in nature, and each episode has a characteristic crescendo-decrescendo pattern. A change in the description of the pain from intermittent and colicky to constant and severe may signal the development of complications, such as intestinal ischemia or perforation.

In general, the more proximal the obstruction, the greater the patient's discomfort and the shorter the delay between onset of symptoms and presentation. Several hours of severe colicky pain in association with bilious vomiting and mild abdominal distention is typical of proximal intestinal obstruction, whereas a day or two of progressively worsening pain and more prominent abdominal distention is typical of distal obstruction. When vomiting does occur with distal intestinal obstruction, it is often feculent from bacterial proliferation. Patients with complete intestinal obstruction eventually develop obstipation, while those patients with early or partial obstruction may continue to pass stool or flatus.

Physical Examination The physical examination should begin with a brief but thorough assessment of the patient's degree of distress, vital signs, and general condition. These important parameters will determine the urgency of the evaluation and management of the patient.

Examination of the abdomen should include inspection for distention and a careful search for surgical scars and external hernias. Auscultation may reveal hyperactive bowel sounds, in particular rushes or high-pitched "tinkles" produced by forceful peristaltic efforts. Late in the course of bowel obstruction, the bowel sounds may become hypoactive or absent. Percussion may elicit tympany with distal obstruction and ileus. Palpation may reveal a tender mass, especially with a closed-loop cause of obstruction. A rectal examination should be performed to evaluate the rectal vault and to check for gross or occult blood. A recent prospective study of patients with abdominal pain defined six clinical variables that had high sensitivity and positive predictive value for the diagnosis of bowel obstruction.[15] These included history of previous surgery, history of constipation, age over 50, vomiting, abdominal distention, and increased bowel sounds.

The presence of peritoneal signs usually indicates late obstruction with complications including strangulation. However, aggressive abdominal palpation in the setting of bowel dilation can give the false impression of peritonitis, as quick compression/decompression of dilated bowel may elicit a significant pain response. Determining the presence of pain with cough or gentle shaking of the patient's pelvis, along with percussion tenderness, is often helpful to differentiate peritonitis from pain due to rapid decompression of dilated loops of bowel. Other clues to serious complications include alterations of the vital signs with tachycardia, hypotension, and fever indicating early sepsis. Unfortunately, a number of studies document that even experienced physicians cannot reliably distinguish between strangulation and simple intestinal obstruction on the basis of examination alone.[2-3,8]

Complications Complications associated with small bowel obstruction include hypovolemia, intestinal ischemia and infarction, peritonitis and sepsis, and respiratory compromise from elevation of the diaphragms or aspiration of gastrointestinal material. The incidence of complications is, in part, related to the degree of intestinal dilation, which in most cases is directly related to delays in presentation, diagnosis, and initiation of appropriate treatment. Early diagnosis and management in the ED can prevent or minimize much of the preoperative morbidity associated with this disease.

Complications related to surgical management of small bowel obstruction include recurrence of the obstruction, hemorrhage, wound infection, abscess formation, sepsis, and short bowel syndrome.[3] Much of the eventual postoperative morbidity and mortality is related to the patient's underlying medical condition. Whether treated surgically or conservatively, the long-term recurrence rate of adhesive small bowel obstruction is significant—53% after an initial episode and 83% after second and further episodes.[6]

Diagnostic Strategies

Routine laboratory testing yields nonspecific findings. Leukocytosis is common with both simple and strangulated obstructions and is not a reliable marker for intestinal compromise. Serum markers of intestinal compromise and ischemia, including creatine phosphokinase (CPK), amylase, and lactate, are only elevated late in the course of bowel obstruction. Electrolytes and renal function are appropriate tests if prolonged volume loss is evident.

Conventional and special radiographic examinations of the abdomen are the most useful diagnostic adjuncts for the evaluation of patients with suspected small bowel obstruction. These studies may confirm or exclude the presence of bowel obstruction; identify the site, severity, and cause of the obstruction; and help distinguish simple obstruction from strangulation.[8,16,17] Answers to these pivotal questions determine the need for urgent surgical intervention versus a period of conservative, nonoperative management.

An adequate plain film examination of the abdomen requires at least two films, one with the patient supine and the other with the patient in the upright or decubitus position. An upright chest film may be added to exclude the presence of free subdiaphragmatic gas, an uncommon finding in bowel obstruction. Plain films demonstrate the presence of small bowel obstruction in 50% to 60% of cases and are suggestive of obstruction in another 20% to 30%.[10] The cause of obstruction is only rarely demonstrated on conventional abdominal radiographs. The ability to correctly predict the site of obstruction is often limited by fluid-filled loops or abnormal positioning of small bowel.[17] Despite these potential limitations, plain radiographs are still the appropriate starting point for the diagnostic evaluation of a patient with suspected small bowel obstruction.

Typical plain film findings with small bowel obstruction are distended loops of small bowel proximal to the site of obstruction followed by normal or collapsed bowel distal to the obstruction. The supine view may show dilated loops of bowel that are sharply angulated or arranged in a series of parallel segments reminiscent of a stepladder. Upright or decubitus films may demonstrate multiple intraluminal air-fluid levels (Figure 87-1). In general, the greater the number of dilated loops of bowel, the more distal the site of obstruction. Colonic gas is usually negligible unless the films are done early in the course of the obstruction or in the presence of a partial small bowel obstruction.[1,2]

When the obstructed intestine contains more fluid than gas, the classic findings described above may be absent. In this setting, small pockets of gas may become trapped between the *valvulae conniventes* of the small bowel and may appear as an oblique series of round radiolucencies on the upright film—the so-called "string of pearls" sign, which is very suggestive of small bowel obstruction.

Two subtle plain film findings suggest the presence of a closed-loop obstruction: the coffee-bean sign and the pseudotumor sign.[8] The coffee-bean sign refers to distended, air-filled, and U-shaped bowel loops that are separated by edematous bowel wall. The pseudotumor sign refers to the presence of a fluid-filled loop of bowel that resembles a mass. These are revealing signs as to the type of obstruction, but are seldom seen or properly interpreted.

Patients with adynamic ileus or gastroenteritis may have plain film findings that are similar to those of intestinal obstruction. However, in this setting, the radiologic findings tend to involve the entire gastrointestinal tract, including the colon, and air-fluid levels are not as prominent as with mechanical obstruction. The air-filled loops of bowel are also not dilated in gastroenteritis or other causes of adynamic ileus.

Since the first reports describing the role of computed

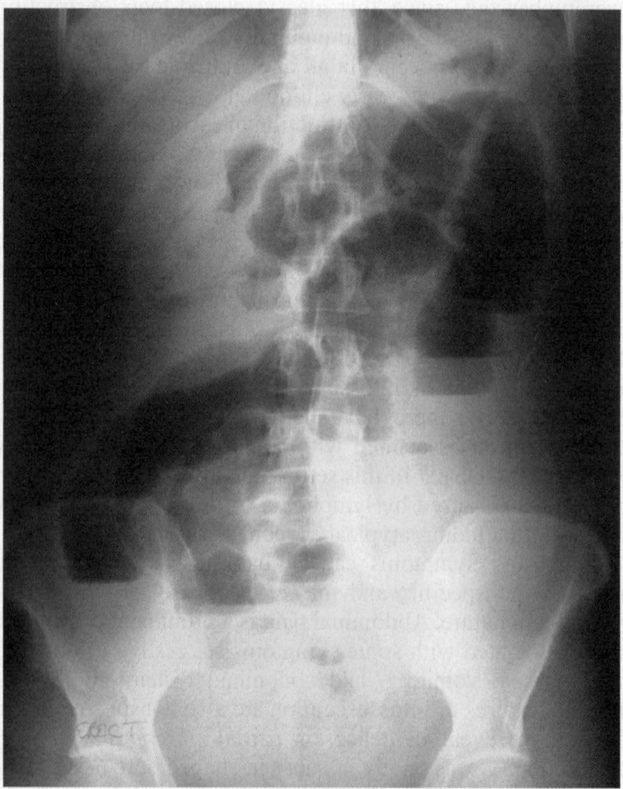

Figure 87-1. **Upright abdominal film revealing multiple air-fluid levels and small bowel dilation, consistent with a diagnosis of small bowel obstruction.**

tomography (CT) in bowel obstruction in the early 1990s, this modality has been increasingly utilized. It is considered complementary to standard radiography in the evaluation of small bowel obstruction. CT has been shown to be an excellent way to demonstrate intussusception, volvulus, and extraluminal lesions like abscesses and tumors.[4,17] This modality is especially helpful and should be used as an early imaging technique in the setting of known abdominal malignancy or inflammatory bowel disease, or when an abdominal mass is discovered on examination. CT scans have high sensitivity, specificity, and accuracy in the diagnosis of small bowel obstruction.[4,17,18] In high-grade obstructions, in particular, these numbers are greater than 90%.[4] CT scan can demonstrate both closed-loop obstruction and findings suggestive of strangulation.[9,19-22] In the vast majority of cases CT scan is not required in the ED to make the diagnosis of bowel obstruction. Its main use is in better defining the site of obstruction and possible cause.[10,23-26]

Differential Considerations

The diagnosis of small bowel obstruction should be considered in any patient with abdominal pain and vomiting, especially if there is a prior history of abdominal surgery. It is often difficult to distinguish between mechanical obstruction, adynamic ileus, and pseudoobstruction on clinical grounds alone.

Other clinical diagnoses that must be considered range from benign to life-threatening, and include gastroenteritis, cholelithiasis and cholecystitis, pancreatitis, peptic ulcer disease, appendicitis, ischemic bowel syndromes, myocardial infarction, and pregnancy. Each of these diagnoses has typical signs, symptoms, and diagnostics that help to differentiate it from small bowel obstruction, but in the early presentation it may be a surprising challenge to accurately exclude each diagnosis from the differential list.

Management

The initial management of small bowel obstruction has remained largely unchanged for several decades and consists of aggressive fluid resuscitation, bowel decompression, and timely surgical consultation.

All patients with small bowel obstruction should be admitted to the hospital. IV hydration should be initiated with an isotonic crystalloid solution administered through large-bore catheters. Enteral decompression via nasogastric suction should take place early in the patient's course to remove accumulated gas and fluid proximal to the obstruction. There is no convincing argument for the use of a long intestinal tube (e.g., Cantor, Miller-Abbott) over a nasogastric tube.[27] Placement of a nasogastric tube is a noxious procedure for patients. Local anesthetics applied to the nose and posterior pharynx may improve the patient's tolerance of the procedure.

There is no convincing research to recommend routine use of antibiotics in the conservatively managed patient. However, the demonstration of bacterial proliferation during intestinal stasis and obstruction suggests that broad-spectrum antibiotics are appropriate when surgery is planned, and when there is any suggestion of vascular compromise or intestinal perforation.[2] Antibiotic use should provide coverage of gram-negative and anaerobic organisms that colonize the intestinal contents (e.g. second-generation cephalosporins).

"Never let the sun set or rise on a bowel obstruction" is an oft-quoted surgical adage that has stood the test of time because of the preoperative difficulty in distinguishing strangulation from simple bowel obstruction.[1-3] Proponents of early surgical intervention cite the similar clinical and radiographic presentations of simple and strangulated obstructions, and argue that any delay in surgical therapy may increase morbidity. Although no debate exists over the need for surgery if there are signs of peritoneal irritation or fever, some surgeons advocate a trial of conservative therapy in the absence of findings suggestive of strangulation. Up to 75% of patients with partial small bowel obstruction, and 35% to 50% of those with complete obstruction, will have resolution of symptoms when treated with IV fluid and bowel decompression alone.[28-31] Patients with early postoperative bowel obstruction, adhesive obstruction, and obstruction secondary to Crohn's disease are more likely to respond to nonoperative management. Surgical intervention should be planned if substantial relief is not attained within a short time after nasogastric tube placement or if symptoms persist after 48 hours of conservative treatment. A practical point is that obstruction occurring in a patient without a previous history of laparotomy is not likely to be caused by peritoneal adhesions. Such de novo obstruction, and the underlying cause, usually will not resolve without surgery.

Neither advanced age nor known abdominal malignancy is a contraindication to operative interventions. The patient with known abdominal cancer who does not have widespread intraabdominal metastases should be treated like any other patient with small bowel obstruction. The patient should receive a trial of bowel decompression, followed by surgery if symptoms do not resolve. From 20% to 40% of patients with abdominal neoplasms and small bowel obstruction have a benign cause for the obstruction.[32,33] In addition, the incidence of strangulation with obstruction due to malignancy is uniformly reported to be low. Therefore a trial of tube decompression is a safe and often successful option.

Laparoscopy may be of benefit in managing some patients with small bowel obstruction.[34-37] Bowel obstruction has traditionally been a relative contraindication for laparoscopy because of the potential for bowel distention and the risk of enteric injury. However, as experience with this surgical approach has increased, surgeons have begun to demonstrate that this is a safe and effective method of diagnosing and treating acute bowel obstruction in selected patients, particularly in the patient with adhesive obstruction.

Key Concepts

- Bowel obstruction should be considered in all patients who present with crampy abdominal pain and vomiting, particularly when there is a history of previous abdominal surgery.
- The diagnosis of small bowel obstruction is usually made on the basis of plain radiographs, with the upright abdominal x-ray revealing air-fluid levels and dilated loops of small bowel in the majority of cases. Abdominal CT scan may be of help in confirming the diagnosis when x-ray findings are nondiagnostic.
- ED management should include volume assessment and resuscitation, bowel decompression, and surgical consultation. A significant percentage of small bowel obstruction caused by adhesions may be managed without surgery.

ACUTE MESENTERIC ISCHEMIA

Perspective

Acute mesenteric ischemia primarily affects patients over the age of 50 years, especially those with significant cardiovascular or systemic disease. The acute form of this disease results in the rapid development of intestinal injury and is much more common than the chronic form of mesenteric ischemia. Chronic mesenteric ischemia results when splanchnic blood flow is inadequate to fully support the functional demands of the intestines, yet not so compromised as to threaten bowel viability. The incidence of acute mesenteric ischemia is difficult to determine, but has been reported at 0.1% of hospital admissions, and several authors report the increasing occurrence in our aging population.[38,39] Acute vascular compromise of the intestine remains an important and life-threatening cause of acute abdominal pain in patients presenting to the ED.

Acute mesenteric ischemia was described in the eighteenth and nineteenth centuries in the sporadic reports of several physicians. An understanding of the exact physiology, however, awaited the classic experimental work of Litten in 1875, who described the results of ligation of mesenteric vessels in animals.[40] In 1895, Elliot described the first patient to recover following resection of infarcted intestine, probably due to mesenteric venous thrombosis. He created two stomas and reanastomosed them 2 weeks later. Thus the diagnosis of gangrenous bowel by laparotomy and its treatment by resection with anastomosis, a sequence of events that is still common today in patients with acute mesenteric ischemia, were first performed more than 100 years ago.

The concept of mesenteric revascularization as the treatment of acute mesenteric ischemia was introduced in the 1950s. Even with the advent of this significant surgical advance, however, morbidity and mortality rates remained high. Today, most physicians use an aggressive approach to the patient with suspected acute mesenteric ischemia as was first proposed in the 1970s. The single most important step in this approach is early diagnosis.

Acute mesenteric ischemia is actually caused by four distinct etiologies, each with a select group of risk factors, signs and symptoms on presentation, and varying nuances in the evaluation and management of the patient. The most common cause of acute mesenteric ischemia is arterial embolus, which accounts for at least 50% of cases. Arterial thrombosis and venous occlusion by thrombosis represent 15% of acute presentations each. The remaining 20% of mesenteric ischemia is caused by nonocclusive vascular disease.[41,42] The importance of early diagnosis and aggressive intervention in patients with suspected acute mesenteric ischemia is underscored by mortality rates that climb to 70% to 90% once intestinal infarction has occurred.[38,43] The mortality of this lethal disease has changed little in the last several decades, and probably will not change until a reliable screening test for the disease is found.

Principles of Disease

The severity of intestinal injury is inversely proportional to mesenteric blood flow and is a function of the state of the systemic circulation, the number and caliber of involved vessels, the status of the collateral circulation in the region, and the duration of the ischemia.[39,41-42,44] The extent of the damage ranges from reversible impairments in mucosal function to transmural infarction and necrosis of part or all of the bowel served by the compromised vasculature.[41]

Blood supply to the abdominal organs derives from three major vessels: the celiac trunk, the superior mesenteric artery (SMA), and the inferior mesenteric artery (IMA). Abdominal organs receive their blood supply based on embryological development. The esophagus, stomach, proximal duodenum, liver, gallbladder, pancreas, and spleen are supplied by the celiac trunk. The SMA supplies the distal duodenum, jejunum, ileum, and colon to the splenic flexure. The descending and sigmoid colon and the rectum are supplied by the IMA. There is an abundant system of collateral vessels and significant territorial overlap of blood flow that can be clinically significant.[46]

Approximately 20% to 25% of the cardiac output is delivered to the small and large intestine, with two thirds going to the SMA distribution and one third to the IMA.[41] Eighty percent of this flow is destined for perfusion of the mucosa because of its high metabolic requirement. Accordingly, the visceral mucosa is very sensitive to decreased perfusion. With the onset of hypoperfusion, a redistribution of intramural blood flow favoring the superficial layers of the mucosa takes place. Below a critical level of blood flow, however, the intestinal villi become ischemic and significant alterations in mucosal function occur.

The countercurrent exchange mechanism in the small intestinal villi initiates and perpetuates ischemic damage to the tissue.[41,47] As epithelial cells become necrotic, there is release of endothelial factors, which leads to the attraction and activation of neutrophils and macrophages into the ischemic tissue. These cells release protease enzymes, tissue necrosis factor, platelet activating factor, arachidonic acid byproducts, and toxic oxygen radicals that cause further endothelial damage, increased vascular permeability, vasoconstriction, inflammation, and further necrosis. This initial ischemic insult is compounded if and when perfusion is reestablished, since restoration of blood flow permits further recruitment of inflammatory cells to the area. Ischemic disruption of the normally impenetrable mucosal barrier allows the release of bacteria, toxins, and vasoactive mediators into the systemic circulation. Cardiac depression, multisystem organ failure, septic shock, and death may occur even before the development of intestinal ischemia. Necrotic changes can be seen as soon as 10 to 12 hours after the onset of symptoms but may develop in more delayed fashion.

Mesenteric Arterial Embolism The median age of patients presenting with mesenteric arterial emboli is 70 years. Approximately two thirds of these patients are women. The vast majority of arterial emboli resulting in acute mesenteric ischemia involve the SMA. The source of SMA emboli is usually the heart, either left atrial or ventricular thrombi that fragment during or after a dysrhythmia, or valvular lesions. Emboli consisting of tumor and cholesterol have also been reported.[48] Emboli typically lodge 4 to 7 cm from the vessel's origin at a point of anatomic narrowing such as the takeoff of a major arterial branch. More than 50% of SMA emboli are found immediately distal to the origin of the middle colic artery. Risk factors for mesenteric arterial emboli include coronary artery disease, valvular heart disease, and dysrhythmias, in particular atrial fibrillation.[41] Risk factors are listed in Box 87-3. These are important to

Box 87-3 Factors Associated with Mesenteric Arterial Embolism

Coronary Artery Disease
Post–myocardial infarction mural thrombi
Congestive heart failure

Valvular Heart Disease
Rheumatic mitral valve disease
Nonbacterial endocarditis

Dysrhythmias
Chronic atrial fibrillation

Aortic Aneurysms or Dissections

Coronary Angiography

recognize in an effort to increase early consideration and diagnosis of this disease.

Mesenteric Arterial Thrombosis The SMA, which originates from the ventral surface of the abdominal aorta at a 45-degree angle, is commonly narrowed by atherosclerosis. This is the most common site for thrombus formation in the mesenteric circulation. In contrast to arterial embolism, the more proximal nature of thrombus formation results in greater visceral damage and a less favorable prognosis. SMA thrombosis usually occurs in patients with chronic, severe, visceral atherosclerosis. Up to 50% of these patients will give a history of "abdominal angina," or abdominal pain after meals. Thus risk factors associated with mesenteric arterial thrombosis include the elderly, diffuse atherosclerosis (coronary, cerebral, or peripheral vascular disease), and hypertension.

Nonocclusive Mesenteric Ischemia Nonocclusive mesenteric ischemia has only been defined in the last 50 years as intraoperative and postmortem examinations have revealed ischemic bowel without obvious vascular obstruction.[49-51] The pathogenesis of nonocclusive mesenteric ischemia is multifactorial, but a common pathway involves mesenteric vasoconstriction, usually in response to low-flow states associated with decreased cardiac output or the administration of vasoactive medications. Factors contributing to the development of nonocclusive mesenteric ischemia include many systemic diseases associated with hypotension, as well as medications that produce splanchnic vasoconstriction (Box 87-4). Nonocclusive mesenteric ischemia is seen in patients of all ages and often develops during hospitalization for other medical or surgical problems.

Mesenteric Venous Thrombosis Mesenteric venous thrombosis is the least common cause of acute mesenteric ischemia. It occurs in a younger patient population, and the mortality rate is lower than other causes, ranging from 20% to 50%.[52] Mesenteric venous thrombosis usually occurs in association with an underlying medical condition, including hypercoagulable states, inflammatory processes within the abdomen, local trauma, and conditions associated with relative venous stasis (Box 87-5). Historically, up to 60% of patients with mesenteric venous thrombosis have a history of peripheral deep venous thrombosis.[41]

Box 87-4 Factors Associated with Mesenteric Venous Thrombosis

Hypercoagulable States
Polycythemia vera
Sickle cell disease
Antithrombin III deficiency
Protein C or S deficiency
Malignancy
Myeloproliferative disorders
Estrogen therapy/OCP
Pregnancy

Inflammatory Conditions
Pancreatitis
Diverticulitis
Appendicitis
Cholangitis

Trauma
Operative venous injury
Postsplenectomy
Blunt or abdominal trauma

Miscellaneous
Congestive heart failure
Renal failure
Decompression sickness
Portal hypertension

Box 87-5 Factors Associated with Nonocclusive Mesenteric Ischemia

Cardiovascular Disease Leading to Low-Flow States
Congestive heart failure
Dysrhythmias
Cardiogenic shock
Postcardiopulmonary bypass

Preceding Hypotensive Episode
Septic shock

Drug-Induced Splanchnic Vasoconstriction
Digoxin
Vasopressors
Ergot alkaloid poisoning
Cocaine abuse

Clinical Features

History Patients over 50 years of age with risk factors for mesenteric ischemia who experience the sudden onset of severe abdominal pain that lasts for more than 2 hours should be suspected of having acute mesenteric ischemia.[38,53] Patients with acute mesenteric ischemia typically complain of severe, poorly localized, colicky abdominal pain. Associated symptoms may include nausea, vomiting, and frequent bowel movements as the bowel attempts to empty itself. The most consistent complaint is pain that is initially out of proportion to the physical findings. This characteristic finding is noted because only visceral structures are initially ischemic, and the parietal peritoneum is spared. Mesenteric ischemia can also be more subacute in its presentation with the insidious onset of less severe and vague abdominal pain, abdominal distention, and occult gastrointestinal bleeding.

Physical Examination Physical findings may be nondiagnostic in the early phases of mesenteric ischemia. As the disease progresses, abdominal distention and diffuse abdominal tenderness without guarding develop. Transmural intestinal injury leads to peritoneal signs (involuntary guarding and rebound tenderness). Late in the ischemic episode, the abdomen is grossly distended, with absent bowel sounds and exquisite tenderness to palpation. Heme-positive stool develops in 25% of patients and often occurs as a relatively late finding.[41] Historical details and physical findings referable to other parts of the body may suggest the etiology of the acute impairment in mesenteric blood flow.

Complications Delays in diagnosis permit progression of the disease process and the development of transmural intestinal ischemia with its correspondingly high morbidity and mortality. Yet even with early diagnosis and aggressive management, a complicated course is to be expected. Secondary reperfusion injury is common, and bowel initially believed to be viable at the time of operation may become ischemic and infarct in the postoperative period. Other postoperative complications include wound infections, intraabdominal abscesses, sepsis, and pneumonia. This patient population is also at risk for many life-threatening complications because of its significant concurrent illness, including myocardial infarction, pulmonary embolism, and renal failure.

Diagnostic Strategies

Routine laboratory and standard radiographic evaluation are usually not helpful in the diagnosis of mesenteric ischemia. An increase in the peripheral white blood cell (WBC) count is a common but nonspecific finding, and although a normal count makes the diagnosis of acute intestinal ischemia less likely, it does not exclude the diagnosis. Hemoconcentration, metabolic acidosis with base deficit, and hyperamylasemia are present in more than one half the cases of acute mesenteric ischemia but are likewise nonspecific findings. A significant emphasis has been placed on the role of serum lactate levels in ischemia, but a consensus regarding its utility has yet to be reached.[39] The sensitivity of this serum marker is high, approaching 100% particularly when bowel infarction is present, but it has a disappointing specificity, ranging from 42% to 87% in varying series.[54,55] A recent retrospective review of mesenteric ischemia noted an elevated serum lactate level at the time of diagnosis to be most useful as a significant predictor of mortality.[56] The seromuscular enzyme CPK rises 3 to 4 hours after vascular occlusion, but has limited specificity and sensitivity. Other seromuscular enzymes (LDH, AST) and mucosal enzymes (alkaline phosphatase) are even less sensitive and specific than CPK.[41]

Plain radiographs should be obtained to rule out other causes of acute abdominal pain, such as bowel obstruction or free air. Plain radiographs are most often normal in the presence of acute mesenteric vascular compromise. By the time any changes characteristic of acute intestinal ischemia are apparent, transmural damage has already taken place. Subtle signs of acute mesenteric ischemia on plain abdominal radiographs include adynamic ileus, distended air-filled loops of bowel, and bowel wall thickening from submucosal edema or hemorrhage. In advanced stages of ischemia, pneumatosis of the bowel wall may be detected as intraluminal gas dissects into the submucosa.[42,57] Another late, and often pre-terminal, sign of necrotic bowel is the presence of gas within the portal venous system.

Further radiographic examinations must be selected judiciously. Barium contrast studies are contraindicated because residual contrast can limit visualization of the mesenteric vasculature during diagnostic angiography.[42] Duplex ultrasonography may be of some benefit in visualizing flow in the SMA and celiac axis. Unfortunately, many patients suspected of mesenteric ischemia often have dilated, air-filled loops of bowel, which make ultrasonography extremely difficult.

In the setting of intestinal ischemia, the abdominal CT scan is capable of demonstrating indirect evidence of bowel ischemia such as edema of the bowel wall and mesentery, abnormal gas patterns, intramural gas, and ascites. Occasionally, direct evidence of mesenteric venous thrombosis is seen. Although some studies find CT scanning to be as sensitive as angiography,[58,59] it should not be considered the first study of choice. Nonetheless, the diagnosis of acute mesenteric ischemia will occasionally be made by CT scan given the prevalence of this test in the evaluation of abdominal pain. Finally, one must keep in mind that similar to plain films, a large percentage of patients may have normal or nonspecific CT findings, and thus the diagnosis of mesenteric ischemia cannot be ruled out on the basis of a normal CT scan.[39]

Angiography remains the "gold standard" in the diagnosis of mesenteric ischemia and is unique among other diagnostic modalities in that it may assist with both diagnosis and therapy. Preoperative angiography is useful in diagnosis of either mesenteric artery embolus or thrombus. It allows for identification of the site and type of occlusion, as well as evaluation of the splanchnic circulation, thus facilitating plans for prompt revascularization. Classically, the angiographic finding with SMA embolus is the "mercury meniscus" sign appearing 3 to 8 cm distal to the origin of the SMA (Figure 87-2). Thrombosis of the SMA typically reveals an occlusion just distal to the origin of the vessel. Additionally, angiography will provide definitive diagnosis of nonocclusive mesenteric ischemia.[38] There are two clinical situations, however, in which angiography is contraindicated in the setting of nonocclusive disease: shock and vasopressor therapy.[39] In these instances diagnosis during laparotomy is preferred, since the underlying mesenteric arterial vasoconstriction may result in either a false-positive or false-negative diagnosis of acute mesenteric ischemia. Broad patient-selection criteria must be used if early diagnosis and effective intervention are to be possible. Therefore a significant number of negative angiograms should be accepted.[38]

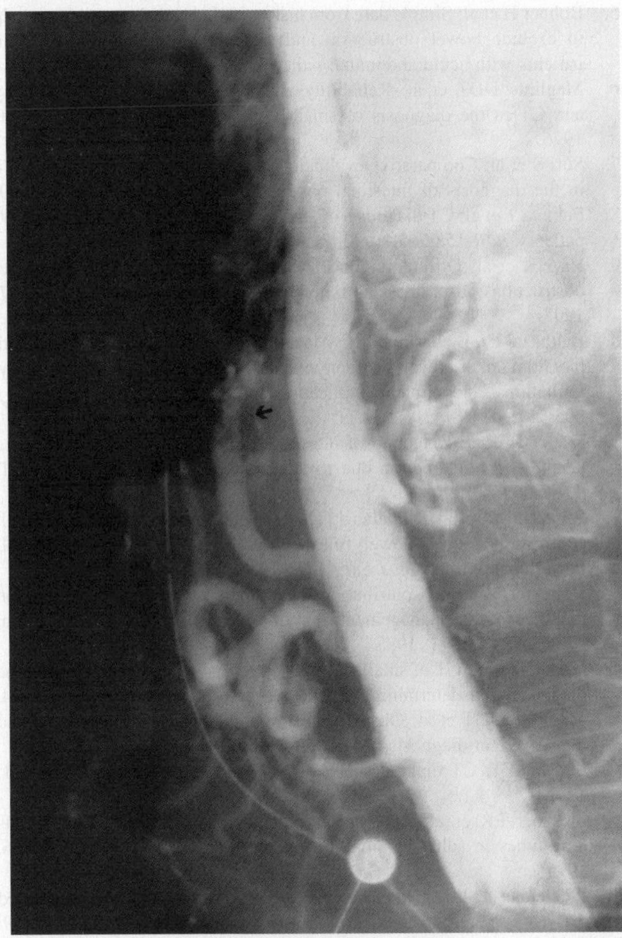

Figure 87-2. **Angiogram demonstrating a superior mesenteric artery embolus (*arrow*).** ***Courtesy of Mark LeQuire, MD, Department of Radiology, Carolinas Medical Center, Charlotte, NC.***

Differential Considerations

Mesenteric ischemia occurs most often in patients over 50 years of age, but the diagnosis should be considered in all patients, regardless of age, who have the sudden onset of severe abdominal pain. The severe and colicky nature of the pain may also suggest cholecystitis, peptic ulcer disease, perforation of bowel, nephrolithiasis, diverticulitis, and bowel obstruction. The significant pain, often out of proportion to the physical findings, may also suggest the possibility of pancreatitis and abdominal aortic aneurysm rupture.

Management

Early diagnosis achieved by aggressive utilization of angiography remains the key to successful patient outcome. Therapeutic intervention must take place as soon as the diagnosis of acute mesenteric ischemia is made if tissue salvage is to be maximized and mortality minimized.

Initial resuscitative efforts should include correction of hypovolemia and hypotension, as well as any accompanying metabolic abnormalities. In the patient population at risk for mesenteric ischemia, successful resuscitation may require invasive hemodynamic monitoring. Control of dysrhythmias, congestive heart failure, and other factors contributing to relative hypoperfusion of the bowel is a priority. If vasopressors must be used to support blood pressure, the lowest possible dose should be infused, and alpha agonists should be avoided, with inotropes being the preferred agent. Enteral decompression via nasogastric tube placement is recommended. Broad-spectrum antibiotic therapy that covers bowel flora should be initiated early, particularly once surgery is anticipated.

Once the patient is stabilized, routine laboratory and plain film examination can be performed to exclude other more common causes of abdominal pain. If an expeditious evaluation does not reveal an alternative diagnosis, angiography should be performed. Even when the decision to operate has been made on clinical grounds, a preoperative angiogram may improve management of the patient at laparotomy.[38] In addition, once the diagnosis of acute mesenteric arterial compromise is confirmed, infusion of papaverine through the angiography catheter directly into the SMA reduces or eliminates mesenteric vasoconstriction. Use of this vasodilator in both nonocclusive and occlusive forms of mesenteric ischemia has improved survival 20% to 50%.[60]

Papaverine is a potent inhibitor of phosphodiesterase, the enzyme necessary for degradation of cyclic adenosine monophosphate (cAMP). Increased cAMP levels cause vascular smooth muscle relaxation and relief of vasoconstriction. Since papaverine is 90% metabolized by the liver on its first pass, few if any systemic effects are noted during its use. The dosing is 60 mg bolus into the SMA, followed by a 30 to 60 mg/h continuous infusion at a concentration of 1 mg/mL.[41]

The surgical management of acute mesenteric ischemia is both challenging and controversial. Treatment principles range from pharmacologic manipulation without operation to revascularization procedures to bowel resection. The underlying cause of intestinal hypoperfusion is often not amenable to surgical correction, as with mesenteric venous occlusion and nonocclusive disease, and the role of operation may be limited to the resection of already infarcted bowel.

If a revascularization procedure is to be undertaken in the presence of arterial occlusive disease, it is completed before any evaluation of bowel viability is performed. The reason behind this therapeutic sequence is that bowel that initially appears irreversibly damaged may exhibit significant recovery on restoration of blood flow. Obviously necrotic bowel is resected, but in the presence of extensive ischemic damage, the surgeon may choose to leave bowel of questionable viability in place and to reevaluate its viability during a subsequent operation.[61,62] This "second-look" operation, typically performed 12-24 hours after the initial procedure, may permit a more limited resection.

Percutaneous transluminal angioplasty (PTA) has been described for both acute and chronic mesenteric ischemia from thrombosis of the SMA. In the acute setting, it appears to have an increased risk of recurrence and potential for extensive bowel loss.[41] With chronic intestinal ischemia, particularly in elderly patients who are poor surgical candidates, mesenteric angioplasty is a good option, with the majority of patients having complete symptomatic improvement and continued relief of symptoms during followup.[63]

Intraarterial infusion into the SMA of thrombolytic agents has been used successfully for stable patients with mesenteric ischemia following acute emboli,[64,65] but only on a case report basis. Close monitoring and frequent clinical reassessment, as well as serial angiograms, are necessary after the infusion of thrombolysis. The main drawbacks to the use of thrombolytic agents are the difficulty in assessing bowel viability without laparotomy, the possible time delay of 12 to 18 hours before clot resolution, and the potential of clot fragmentation and involvement of more distal branches that are less amenable to surgical revascularization.[62]

In the patients surviving the initial episode of acute mesenteric ischemia, recurrent thrombosis is a potential problem requiring long-term anticoagulation. Coumadin is started after mesenteric arterial embolism and mesenteric venous thrombosis. Antiplatelet therapy is begun following mesenteric arterial thrombosis and nonocclusive mesenteric ischemia. The 2-year mortality following mesenteric ischemia is as high as 70%. This grave prognosis, however, was mainly related to cardiovascular comorbidity rather than recurrent mesenteric ischemic events.[66]

Key Concepts

- There are four different acute mesenteric ischemia syndromes, each having a specific set of risk factors or associated medical conditions that are critical in raising the index of suspicion during initial presentation.
- The diagnosis of acute mesenteric ischemia may be suggested by "pain out of proportion" to examination findings, heme-positive stool, elevated serum lactate levels, and classic findings on plain film or CT scan, but none of these provide enough sensitivity to ensure diagnosis before bowel infarction occurs.
- An aggressive approach to diagnosis and management, including early utilization of angiography, has provided some improvement in the dismal prognosis of acute mesenteric ischemia, although mortality from this disease is still greater than 50%.

REFERENCES

1. Holder WD: Intestinal obstruction, *Gastroenterol Clin North Am* 17:317, 1988.
2. Bass KN, Jones B, Bulkley GB: Current management of small-bowel obstruction, *Adv Surg* 31:1, 1998.
3. Mucha P: Small bowel obstruction, *Surg Clin North Am* 67:597, 1987.
4. Maglinte DDT et al: The role of radiography in the diagnosis of small-bowel obstruction, *AJR* 168:1171, 1997.
5. Ray NF et al: Abdominal adhesiolysis: inpatient care and expenditures in the United States in 1994, *J Am Coll Surg* 186:1, 1998.
6. Barkan H, Webster S, Ozeran S: Factors predicting the recurrence of adhesive small-bowel obstruction, *Am J Surg* 170:361, 1995.
7. Ellis H: The clinical significance of adhesions: focus on intestinal obstruction, *Eur J Surg* 163(suppl 577):5, 1997.
8. Balthazar EJ: CT of small-bowel obstruction, *AJR* 162:255, 1994.
9. Beck DE et al: Incidence of small-bowel obstruction and adhesiolysis after open colorectal and general surgery, *Dis Colon Rectum* 42:241, 1999.
10. Cox MR et al: The operative etiologies and types of adhesions causing small bowel obstruction, *Aust NZ J Surg* 63:848, 1993.
11. Reisner RM, Cohen JR: Gallstone ileus: a review of 1001 reported cases, *Am Surg* 60:441, 1994.
12. Lo CY, Lorentz TG, Lau PWK: Obturator hernia presenting as small bowel obstruction, *Am J Surg* 167:396, 1994.
13. Roggo A, Ottinger LW: Acute small bowel volvulus in adults, *Ann Surg* 216:135, 1992.
14. Begos DG et al: The diagnosis and management of adult intussusception, *Am J Surg* 173:88-94, 1997.
15. Bohner H et al: Simple data from history and physical examination help to exclude bowel obstruction and to avoid radiographic studies in patients with acute abdominal pain, *Eur J Surg* 164:777, 1998.
16. Maglinte DDT et al: Reliability and role of plain film radiography and CT in the diagnosis of small-bowel obstruction, *AJR* 167:1451, 1996.
17. Suri S et al: Comparative evaluation of plain films, ultrasound and CT in the diagnosis of intestinal obstruction, *Acta Radiol* 40:422, 1999.
18. Fukuya T et al: CT diagnosis of small-bowel obstruction: efficacy in 60 patients, *AJR* 158:765, 1992.
19. Ha HK et al: Differentiation of simple and strangulated small-bowel obstructions: usefulness of known CT criteria, *Radiology* 204:507, 1997.
20. Balthazar EJ, Liebeskind ME, Macari M: Intestinal ischemia in patients in whom small bowel obstruction is suspected: evaluation of accuracy, limitations, and clinical implications of CT in diagnosis, *Radiology* 205:519, 1997.
21. Frager D et al: Detection of intestinal ischemia in patients with acute small-bowel obstruction due to adhesions or hernia: efficacy of CT, *AJR* 166:67, 1996.
22. Peck JJ, Milleson T, Phelan J: The role of computed tomography with contrast and small-bowel follow-through in management of small bowel obstruction, *Am J Surg* 177:375, 1999.
23. Donckier V et al: Contribution of computed tomography to decision making in the management of adhesive small bowel obstruction, *Br J Surg* 85:1071, 1998.
24. Frager D et al: CT of small-bowel obstruction: value in establishing the diagnosis and determining the degree and cause, *AJR* 162:37, 1994.
25. Maglinte DDT et al: Obstruction of the small intestine: accuracy and role of CT in diagnosis, *Radiology* 188:61, 1993.
26. Stewart ET: CT diagnosis of small-bowel obstruction, *AJR* 158:771, 1992.
27. Fleshner PR et al: A prospective, randomized trial of short versus long tubes in adhesive small-bowel obstruction, *Am J Surg* 170:366, 1995.
28. Pickleman J, Lee RM: The management of patients with suspected early postoperative small bowel obstruction, *Ann Surg* 210:216, 1989.
29. Sosa J, Gardner B: Management of patients diagnosed as acute intestinal obstruction secondary to adhesions, *Am Surg* 59:125, 1993.
30. Seror D et al: How conservatively can postoperative small bowel obstruction be treated? *Am J Surg* 165:121, 1993.
31. Cox MR et al: The safety and duration of non-operative treatment for adhesive small bowel obstruction, *Aust NZ J Surg* 63:367, 1993.
32. Butler JA et al: Small bowel obstruction in patients with a prior history of cancer, *Am J Surg* 162:624, 1991.
33. Tang E, Davis J, Silberman H: Bowel obstruction in cancer patients, *Arch Surg* 130:832, 1995.
34. Freys SM et al: Laparoscopic adhesiolysis, *Surg Endosc* 8:1202, 1994.
35. Francois V et al: Postoperative adhesive peritoneal disease: laparoscopic treatment, *Surg Endosc* 8:781, 1994.
36. Ibrahim IM et al: Laparoscopic management of acute small-bowel obstruction, *Surg Endosc* 10:1012, 1996.
37. Strickland P et al: Is laparoscopy safe and effective for treatment of acute small-bowel obstruction? *Surg Endosc* 13:695, 1999.
38. Kaleya RN, Boley SJ: Acute mesenteric ischemia: an aggressive diagnostic and therapeutic approach, *Can J Surg* 35:613, 1992.
39. Ruotolo RA, Evans SRT: Mesenteric ischemia in the elderly, *Clin Geriat Med* 15:527, 1999.
40. Boley SJ, Brandt LJ, Sammartano RJ: History of mesenteric ischemia: the evolution of a diagnosis and management, *Surg Clin North Am* 77:275, 1997.
41. Castellone JA, Powers RD: Ischemic bowel syndromes: a comprehensive, state-of-the-art approach to emergency diagnosis and management, *Em Med Report* 18:189, 1997.
42. McKinsey JF, Gewertz BL: Acute mesenteric ischemia, *Surg Clin North Am* 77:307, 1997.
43. Mamode N, Pickford I, Lieberman P: Failure to improve outcome in acute mesenteric ischemia: seven-year review, *Eur J Surg* 165:203, 1999.
44. Walker JS, Dire DJ: Vascular abdominal emergencies, *Emerg Med Clin North Am* 14:571, 1996.
45. Reference deleted in pages.

46. Rosenblum JD, Boyle CM, Schwartz LB: The mesenteric circulation: anatomy and physiology, *Surg Clin North Am* 77:289, 1997.
47. Mitsudo S, Brandt LJ: Pathology of intestinal ischemia, *Surg Clin North Am* 72:43, 1992.
48. Krupski WC, Selzman CH, Whitehill TA: Unusual causes of mesenteric ischemia, *Surg Clin North Am* 77:471, 1997.
49. Wilcox MG et al: Current theories of pathogenesis and treatment of nonocclusive mesenteric ischemia, *Dig Dis Sci* 40:709, 1995.
50. Howard TJ et al: Nonocclusive mesenteric ischemia remains a diagnostic dilemma, *Am J Surg* 171:405, 1996.
51. Bassiouny HS: Nonocclusive mesenteric ischemia, *Surg Clin North Am* 77:319, 1997.
52. Rhee RY, Gloviczki P: Mesenteric venous thrombosis, *Surg Clin North Am* 77:327, 1997.
53. Bradbury AW, Brittenden J, Ruckley CV: Mesenteric ischemia: a multidisciplinary approach, *Br J Surg* 82:1446, 1995.
54. Lange H, Jackel R: Usefulness of plasma lactate concentration in the diagnosis of acute abdominal disease, *Eur J Surg* 160:381, 1994.
55. Murray MJ et al: Serum lactate levels as an aid to diagnosing acute intestinal ischemia, *Am J Surg* 167:575, 1994.
56. Newman TS et al: The challenging face of mesenteric infarction, *Am Surg* 64:611, 1998.
57. Wolf EL, Sprayregen S, Bakal CW: Radiology in intestinal ischemia: plain films, contrast, and other imaging studies, *Surg Clin North Am* 72:107, 1992.
58. Klein HM et al: Diagnostic imaging of mesenteric infarction, *Radiology* 197:79, 1995.
59. Taourel PG et al: Acute mesenteric ischemia: diagnosis with contrast-enhanced CT, *Radiology* 199:632, 1996.
60. Levine J, Jacobson E: Intestinal ischemic disorders, *Dig Dis* 13:3, 1995.
61. Levy PJ, Krausz MM, Manny J: Acute mesenteric ischemia: improved results: a retrospective analysis of ninety-two patients, *Surgery* 107:373, 1990.
62. Schneider TA et al: Mesenteric ischemia: acute arterial syndromes, *Dis Colon Rectum* 37:1163, 1994.
63. Allen RC et al: Mesenteric angioplasty in the treatment of chronic intestinal ischemia, *J Vasc Surg* 24:415, 1996.
64. Regan F, Karlstad RR, Magnuson TH: Minimally invasive management of acute superior mesenteric artery occlusion: combined urokinase and laparoscopic therapy, *Am J Gastroenterol* 91:1019, 1996.
65. Turégano-Fuentes P et al: Acute arterial syndromes in mesenteric ischemia, *Dis Colon Rectum* 38:778, 1995.
66. Klempnaueer J et al: Long-term results after surgery for acute mesenteric ischemia, *Surgery* 121:239, 1997.

88 Acute Appendicitis

Jeannette M. Wolfe
Philip L. Henneman

PERSPECTIVE

Epidemiology

Appendicitis is a common condition requiring emergency surgery. About 7% of people will develop appendicitis sometime during their lifetime. Most cases occur in adolescents and young adults, with the incidence in men being slightly higher than in women.[1,2] The incidence of appendicitis in the United States has actually decreased since the early part of the century. This may be due to increased fiber in American diets causing better-formed stools, or improved hygiene resulting in fewer enteric infections.[3]

Historical Perspective

The earliest evidence of appendicitis is suggested by the presence of right lower quadrant adhesions in an Egyptian mummy from the Byzantine era. In 1492 Leonardo da Vinci drew pictures of the colon and the appendix and called the structure an "orecchio," which literally means ear. The first appendix was removed incidentally in 1735 by Claudius Amyand during the repair of a scrotal hernia in an 11-year-old boy. The appendix had perforated and a cutaneous fecal draining fistula had developed.[4] The half-hour operation was done without anesthesia and the boy fully recovered. In 1880 in Europe, Lawson Tait performed the first successful planned appendectomy by removing a gangrenous appendix from a 17-year-old woman. Six years later Reginald Fitz, a pathologist, coined the term "appendicitis" when he read his classic paper at the first meeting of the Association of American Physicians. Fitz correctly described many of the pathophysiologic changes associated with appendicitis and advocated early surgery. Three years later, Charles McBurney described a point "determined by the pressure of one finger" between "one and a half and two inches from the anterior spinous process," which when palpated was associated with the greatest discomfort in patients with acute appendicitis. The general acceptance that appendicitis was a surgical disease didn't occur until several decades later. The popularity of early surgical intervention finally surged in the early 1900s after King Edward VII suffered a perforated appendix and was operated on days before his coronation.[4,5]

PRINCIPLES OF DISEASE

Pathophysiology

The appendix is a hollow, muscular, closed-ended tube arising from the posterior medial surface of the cecum, about 3 cm below the ileocecal valve. Its average length is approximately 10 cm and its normal capacity is 0.1 to 0.3 ml. The role of the appendix in human physiology is unknown, but it may serve some type of immunologic function as suggested by the abundance of lymphoid tissue.[2] Innervation of the appendix is derived from sympathetic and vagus nerves from the superior mesenteric plexus. Afferent fibers that conduct visceral pain from the appendix accompany the sympathetic nerves and enter the spinal cord at the level of the tenth thoracic segment. This causes referred pain to the umbilical area.

The anatomic location of the appendix affects the clinical presentation as well as the subsequent risk of developing appendicitis. In a study of 10,000 autopsies, the appendix was located behind the cecum in the retrocecal fossa in 65% of cases, and down in the pelvis in 31%.[6] Interestingly, this ratio is somewhat reversed in patients who undergo surgery for appendicitis. It is possible that a retrocecal appendix is less likely to become obstructed because of the position of its lumen.[7]

The majority of patients who develop appendicitis do so because of an acute obstruction of the appendiceal lumen. This is usually from an appendicolith, but obstruction can also be caused by calculi, tumor, parasite, or foreign object. Of historical note, in the early nineteenth century one of the more common causes of acute appendicitis related to foreign objects was ingested lead shells buried in quail meat.[8]

After acute obstruction, intraluminal pressure rises because mucosal secretions are unable to drain. The resulting distention stimulates visceral afferent pathways and is perceived as a dull, poorly localized pain. Abdominal cramping may occur because of hyperperistalsis. Next, ulceration and ischemia develop as the intraluminal pressure exceeds the venous pressure and bacteria and polymorphonuclear cells begin to invade the appendiceal wall. The appendix may appear grossly normal at this time, with evidence of pathology apparent only by microscopic examination.[9] With time, the appendix becomes swollen and begins to irritate surrounding structures, including the peritoneal wall. The pain then becomes more localized to the right lower quadrant. Continued swelling and ischemia may lead to necrosis and perforation through the appendiceal serosal layer, resulting in abscess formation or diffuse peritonitis. The time required for the appendix to perforate is highly variable but usually occurs within 24 to 36 hours.[3] Elderly patients are prone to earlier perforation because of anatomic changes associated with aging, such as a narrowed appendiceal lumen, thinner mucosal lining, decreased lymphoid tissue, and atherosclerosis.[10]

In about one third of cases, no direct cause of obstruction is noted. In these cases it is surmised that inflammation is caused by viral, bacterial, or parasitic infection, with subsequent mucosal ulceration or lymphoid hyperplasia.[2,3]

CLINICAL FEATURES

History

Appendicitis is classically described as starting with the vague onset of dull periumbilical pain, and the development of anorexia, nausea, and vomiting. The pain then migrates to the right lower quadrant, and a low-grade fever may develop. In most instances, the patient has not experienced pain similar to this episode in the past.[2] Unfortunately, the presentation may be highly variable. If the appendix is retrocecal or retroiliac, the pain may start in the right lower quadrant without migration and may be blunted by the presence of overlying bowel.[11] If the appendix is elongated, the pain may be referred to the flank, pelvis, or right upper quadrant. Other less typical symptoms seen with appendicitis are increased urinary frequency and the desire to defecate.[2,3]

Physical Examination

The most common finding on physical examination is localized abdominal tenderness, usually in the right lower quadrant. The pain may be noted over McBurney's point, an area 2 cm from the anterosuperior iliac spine. However, because only 35% of patients have the base of their appendix within 5 cm of this point, it is not uncommon for pain to be localized to other areas in the lower abdomen.[12]

Other physical findings that may be present are guarding and rigidity. Both of these findings reflect the tensing of the abdominal wall musculature to protect the underlying bowel. The difference between the two is that guarding is usually voluntary and the patient can often be persuaded to relax. Rigidity is involuntary and implies more significant underlying pathology.[2]

Rovsing's sign is the referred tenderness to the right lower quadrant when the left lower quadrant is palpated. *Psoas sign* is the increase of pain when the psoas muscle is stretched as the patient is asked to extend his or her hip. *Obturator sign* is the elicitation of pain as the hip is flexed and internally rotated.

Rebound tenderness is a late finding in patients with appendicitis and occurs most often after the appendix has ruptured or infarcted. The presence of rebound tenderness can be suspected if the patient reports abdominal pain with coughing or gentle rocking of the pelvis. Classically, rebound tenderness is detected by gradually pressing over the area of tenderness for 5 to 10 seconds and then quickly withdrawing the hand to just above the skin level. A positive response is when the patient reports increased pain as the hand is removed. Because this is a painful procedure for the patient, it should not be repeated unnecessarily.[11]

Isolated rectal tenderness may rarely be the only site of localized pain in patients with a low-lying appendix. In general, however, it has a very low diagnostic value, especially if there is concurrent right lower quadrant pain.[13,14] Although a single rectal examination may provide other important information, such as the discovery of a rectal mass or occult blood, multiple examinations are not justified.

Although any of the above signs may be present in patients with acute appendicitis, a review of 10 studies that examined 13 classic signs and symptoms of appendicitis identifies three findings that are highly predictive of appendicitis: right lower quadrant pain, rigidity, and migration of initial periumbilical pain to the right lower quadrant.[2] Conversely, the presence of pain for more than 48 hours, a history of similar episodes of pain, the lack of migration and right lower quadrant pain, and the lack of worsening pain with movement or cough make appendicitis less likely.[2,13] Vital signs are often normal, particularly early in the course. A low-grade fever (<38° C) is present in about 15% of patients. This increases to about 40% if perforation has occurred.[15]

Special Considerations

Children Young children with acute appendicitis are often misdiagnosed, and in the vast majority the correct diagnosis is made only after perforation has occurred. This may be due to children's inability to accurately communicate discomfort and because many common childhood illnesses are associated with anorexia, nausea, and vomiting.[16] Very young children with perforation may also present with grunting. Children may be more prone to perforation because of the thinness of the appendiceal wall. They also may be more likely to develop diffuse peritonitis because their omentum is immature and may be unable to wall off infection.[17]

Women The diagnosis of acute appendicitis in women of childbearing age is especially problematic. As many as

45% of women with symptoms suggestive of appendicitis will have a normal appendix at surgery, and up to one third of women with true appendicitis are initially misdiagnosed. Gynecologic disease can easily masquerade as appendicitis because of the close proximity of the right ovary, fallopian tube, and uterus to the appendix.[18-20] Approximately 25% of women with signs suggestive of acute appendicitis ultimately have gynecologic disease.[2,21] The clinical and laboratory distinction between these two entities can be very difficult. Findings that may be more suggestive of gynecologic pathology are listed in Box 88-1. Of note, although cervical motion tenderness is more common in patients with pelvic inflammatory disease, it does not differentiate women with and without appendicitis. In one study, almost 25% of women with acute appendicitis were noted to have cervical motion tenderness.[18]

Because recognizing appendicitis in women is probably most difficult during the childbearing years, ancillary testing with ultrasound, computed tomography (CT), or ultimately laparoscopy can be very helpful.

Pregnant Women Pregnant women carry an overall risk of developing appendicitis similar to the general population.[22,23] Of the three trimesters, appendicitis appears to occur slightly more often in the second trimester. The reason for this is unknown. The diagnosis of appendicitis during pregnancy can be difficult because early symptoms of appendicitis, such as nausea and vomiting, occur frequently in a normal pregnancy. Laboratory values are even less helpful because leukocytosis is common during pregnancy. The enlargement of the uterus can also change the location of the appendix and cause atypical right upper quadrant pain. Because the correct diagnosis is often delayed, the rate of perforation is about two to three times higher in pregnant patients compared with the general population. Although maternal death from appendicitis is extremely rare, fetal abortion occurs in about 20% of cases in which the appendix is perforated.[22,23] Because morbidity is high, extra caution should be taken in treating pregnant women who have abdominal pain. The liberal use of ultrasound and early surgical and gynecologic consultation should be strongly considered.

Elderly Patients Elderly patients are three times more likely to have a perforated appendix at surgery compared with the general population. There appear to be multiple causes for this, including the previously noted age-related anatomic changes of the appendix that weaken the appendiceal wall. Elderly persons also commonly delay seeking medical care for multiple reasons, such as early nonspecific symptoms, reluctance and inability to leave their home, and difficulties in accurately communicating worsening symptoms. Diagnosis can be further delayed after physician examination because of atypical presentations and minimally abnormal lab tests.[10,24]

Box 88-1 Abdominal Pain in Women

More Suggestive of Appendicitis

Anorexia
Pain localized to the right lower quadrant

More Suggestive of Pelvic Inflammatory Disease

Several days of symptoms
History of pelvic inflammatory disease
Diffuse lower abdominal pain
Bilateral adnexal pain
Cervical motion tenderness
Vaginal discharge
Illness in first 2 weeks of menstrual cycle

Complications The complication rate after the removal of a normal or an acutely inflamed appendix is about 3% and increases approximately three to four times if perforation occurs.[15] The most common complication is infection. Localized wound infection occurs in about 2% to 7% of cases, and deep intraabdominal abscess occurs in 0.8% to 2%, with the higher percentages representing cases in which perforation has occurred.[25] Other complications include small bowel obstruction, pneumonia, and urinary retention and infection. Although some have suggested that fallopian tube damage from a ruptured appendix may account for significant tubal infertility,[26] this has not been confirmed by more recent studies.[27,28]

Morbidity in cases of uncomplicated appendicitis is less than 0.1%, but it increases to almost 4% with perforation and can climb much higher in elderly patients with perforation.[29]Although reported perforation rates vary, the overall average is about 20% to 30%. This increases greatly at the extremes of age. The elderly have perforation rates of about 30% to 60%, and children less than 3 years can have perforation rates as high as 80% to 90%.[10,17] Perforation of the appendix has been reported as the most common abdominal disorder resulting in malpractice claims and the fifth most expensive cause of claims against emergency physicians.[30,31]

Delay in definitive management of patients with acute appendicitis can lead to increased perforation rates and complications. This delay can be caused by one or more of the following: patient delay in seeking medical care, physician delay in consulting a surgeon, administrative delay caused by patient transfer based on insurance status, surgical delay in the decision to operate, or hospital delay in the availability of the operating room. Several recent studies suggest that the greatest delay in patients with complicated appendicitis is delayed patient presentation for medical care.[11,32] One study shows the average patient delay in seeking medical care for simple appendicitis is 17 hours, versus 32 hours for perforated disease.[1] Uninsured patients and those covered by Medicaid have the highest adjusted risk for ruptured appendix, and this is believed to be related to presentation to the hospital based on fear of financial burden.[33,34]

DIAGNOSTIC STRATEGIES

Ancillary Tests

The diagnosis of appendicitis is, in general, based on the patient's history and the physical examination. Ancillary testing is unnecessary if the diagnosis is clear and may delay definitive management. Routine testing often yields nonspecific results.

Leukocyte Count

About 80% to 90% of patients with acute appendicitis will have a white blood cell (WBC) count above $10{,}000/mm^3$.

This percentage is slightly lower in elderly patients and the very young.[15,35-38] Unfortunately, the leukocyte count is not a very specific test and is often elevated with other causes of abdominal pain. Repeat measurement of the leukocyte count after an observation period is also of limited value because about 25% of patients with acute appendicitis will not have a rise from their initial count.[36]

C-Reactive Protein

The C-reactive protein is an acute-phase reactant that increases over 6 to 12 hours and peaks 2 to 3 days after inflammation or injury. As a result, it may not be elevated in early appendicitis. The reported sensitivity of C-reactive protein for appendicitis varies from 40% to 99%. A recent meta-analysis suggests an overall sensitivity of 62% and a specificity of 66%.[39]

Urinalysis

Urinalysis is helpful in differentiating urinary tract disease from acute appendicitis. Mild, sterile pyuria may be seen with appendicitis, especially if the appendix is irritating the ureter. Significant pyuria, greater than 20 WBCs/hpf, is more suggestive of urinary tract disease.[16] A urine or serum pregnancy test is appropriate for all women of childbearing age to identify obstetric problems.

Special Studies

Diagnostic Scores Diagnostic scoring systems using aspects of the history, physical examination, and routine ancillary tests have been developed in an attempt to decrease the number of normal appendixes and perforated appendixes removed. Although some retrospective studies have shown a benefit in using these systems, they have not performed consistently well when prospectively evaluated.[2,40]

Plain Film Radiographs Plain abdominal radiographs are not useful in diagnosing appendicitis because of their very low sensitivity and specificity.[41] One recent study shows that plain film radiographs are normal in over 50% of patients with acute appendicitis, specific conditions are suggested in only 10% of radiographs, and the radiographic abnormalities identified do not correlate with the final disease in over 50% of cases.[41] Because of their limited value, abdominal radiographs are not recommended in the evaluation of appendicitis unless there is a significant concern of bowel obstruction.

Barium Enemas Barium enemas have a sensitivity of about 80% to 90% for detecting appendicitis.[42,43] Positive findings suggestive of appendicitis include nonvisualization of the entire appendix, pressure defects in the surrounding cecum, and spasms in the cecum or ileum. Obstructive appendicitis is essentially ruled out if the entire appendix fills with contrast dye.[43] Unfortunately, it is not uncommon for a normal appendiceal lumen not to be visualized with this technique, and therefore a barium enema is probably most helpful when other colon pathology is high in the differential diagnosis.[42]

Nuclear Medicine Scans Nuclear studies have been used in the past two decades to evaluate equivocal cases of acute appendicitis. The patient's WBCs are labeled with a nuclear tag, and over a period of several hours a series of gamma camera scans are performed to look for localized areas of inflammation with increased nuclear uptake.[42,44] The sensitivities of these studies vary with the type of nuclear tag. Hexamethyl-propyleneamineoxime (HMPAO), a neutral lipophilic complex, shows the most promise, with sensitivities of 87% to 93% in several small studies.[42,45-47] The disadvantages of nuclear studies include poor interreader reliability, scanning delays of several hours, false positives, and nonspecific findings caused by other inflammatory changes in the pelvis or urinary tract.[42]

Ultrasonography Graded compression ultrasound has been prospectively shown to improve the clinical accuracy of the diagnosis of acute appendicitis.[48,49] It may be particularly helpful in women of childbearing age in which pelvic pathology mimicking appendicitis is of concern. The reported sensitivity and specificity of ultrasound for acute appendicitis is 75% to 90% and 85% to 95%, respectively.[48-53]

Ultrasound is considered positive for appendicitis if the appendix is noncompressible and has a diameter of greater than 6 to 7 mm (Figure 88-1). The advantages of ultrasound are its inexpensive cost, the lack of radiation or dye exposure, and the ability to immediately scan a patient without a time delay for contrast filling. It also allows the ultrasonographer to correlate the patient's pain with the direct visualization of underlying abdominal contents. The major disadvantage of ultrasound is that the visualization of an abnormal appendix is operator dependent and can be especially difficult in patients who are obese, have strictures, or have a retrocecal appendix. It also may be limited in patients who have significant tenderness and cannot tolerate the graded compression. Once the appendix has perforated, it becomes more difficult to identify via ultrasound. The visualization of a normal appendix is even more problematic, with reported rates of only 2% to 45%.[49,54] Therefore, although a positive ultrasound study for appendicitis has a very high positive predictive value (90%), a negative study, especially one in which the appendix is not seen, is not helpful unless alternative pathology is identified.[55]

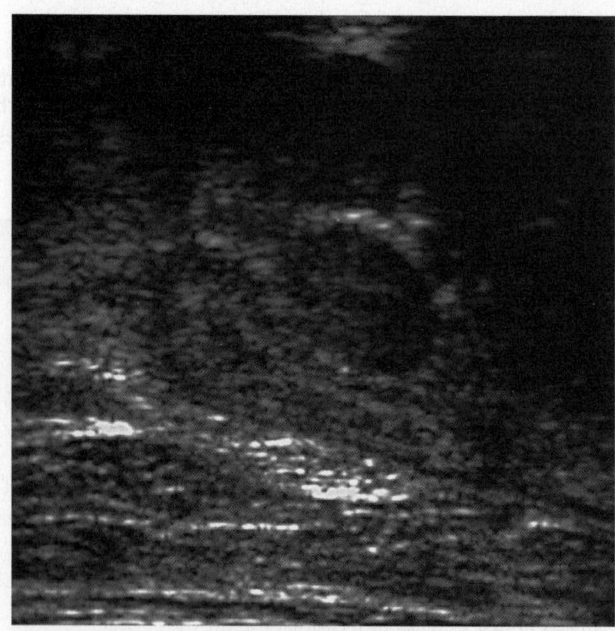

Figure 88-1. **Ultrasound of acute appendicitis.**

Computed Tomography CT has been prospectively studied and has also been shown to improve the clinical accuracy of the diagnosis of appendicitis.[49,56] CT findings suggestive of appendicitis include an enlarged appendix (a diameter measuring greater than 6 mm), pericecal inflammation, and the presence of an appendicolith (Figure 88-2). The sensitivity and specificity vary by study and technique (Table 88-1).[42,49,50,56-61] Of the different modalities, rectal contrast, thin cut, helical CT appears to be the most advantageous. This technique allows the patient to be scanned after a 15-minute prep time, completely avoids oral and intravenous (IV) contrast, and consistently shows opacification and distention of the distal cecum, which helps identify the appendix.[59,60]

The advantage of CT over ultrasound is that the appendix can usually be visualized, the technique itself is standardized and not operator dependent, and alternative pathology for the patient's pain is often found. Because a negative CT examination for appendicitis has a high negative predictive value, treatment decisions (including discharging patients from the ED) can be made more confidently based on CT results.[49] CT is also very helpful in differentiating between appendiceal and pelvic pathology.[62]

The biggest disadvantage of CT is the radiation exposure. This can be decreased by up to 67% by doing a 15-cm scan through the cecum and pelvis. This exposes the patient to approximately 300 mRads (the equivalent of radiation exposure of one abdominal plain film) and decreases the overall cost of the scan.[60,62]

Table 88-1. Sensitivity and Specificity of Appendicitis by CT Scan

Type of scan	Sensitivity (%)	Specificity (%)
Noncontrast conventional CT	87-96	97
Oral and IV contrast conventional CT	96	89-96
Helical CT with oral and rectal contrast	Up to 100	95
Helical CT with rectal contrast	97-98	94-98

Data from references 42, 49, 50, 56-62.

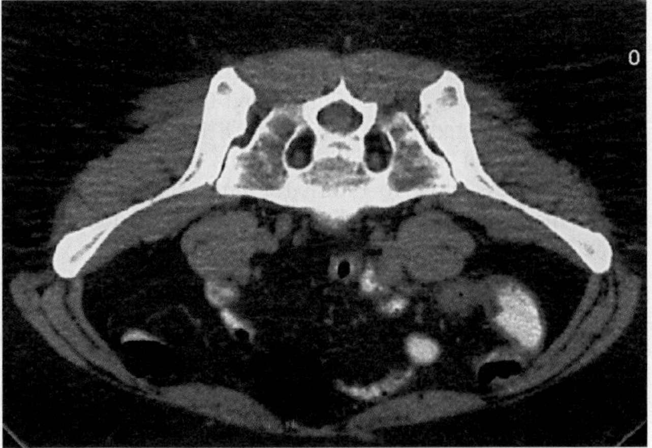

Figure 88-2. **Oral contrast CT of acute appendicitis.**

Magnetic Resonance Imaging Magnetic resonance imaging (MRI) has recently been studied in patients with suspected appendicitis. Although the data at this point are limited, they suggest that MRI, especially T-2 weighted images, may be very sensitive in picking up appendicitis. Changes seen on MRI in patients with acute appendicitis include appendiceal intraluminal fluid seen as a markedly hyperintense center, edema of the appendiceal wall, and periappendiceal signal intensity consistent with fluid and inflammation. The potential benefits of MRI are that it spares the patient ionizing radiation and that the entire appendix is usually visualized.[63,64]

Laparoscopy Laparoscopy can be performed for either diagnosis or definitive treatment (see below). Its greatest advantage is in female patients of childbearing age who may have appendicitis or localized pelvic inflammatory disease. Because laparoscopy is usually performed under general anesthesia, it realistically should be considered only after ultrasound or CT examinations have been performed. Unfortunately, preliminary data on minilaparoscopy, which can be done at the patient's bedside, have not been promising because of the limited ability to adequately visualize the appendix.[65]

Summary

Historically, ancillary tests have been most helpful in patients who do not present with the classical presentation of acute appendicitis. Several studies have recently challenged this view and suggest that even patients with a high clinical suspicion of appendicitis may benefit from preoperative studies (specifically ultrasound or helical CT with rectal contrast).[48,49,66-68] The authors of these studies believe this would decrease the number of normal appendixes removed without increasing the perforation rate, and tests would be cost effective because they would decrease unnecessary surgery and hospital costs (the cost of one negative laparotomy would pay for about 18 to 22 CT scans).[66,67]

At present, ultrasound and CT appear to be the most promising and readily available tests. Which of these tests is chosen to further evaluate equivocal patients should probably be customized to the individual patient and available resources. Patient factors to consider include age, gender, body habitus, and the likelihood of pelvic pathology. Institutional factors include the availability of the test, the expertise of the individual performing and interpreting the test, and the preference of the surgeon. Some institutions are now developing protocols that utilize both tests. One recent study of 108 children with equivocal findings of acute appendicitis followed nondiagnostic ultrasound examinations with rectal contrast, limited, abdominopelvic CT. Ultrasound correctly diagnosed 40% of the children with acute appendicitis, the contrast limited CT scan was 94% sensitive in the remaining children, and the negative laparotomy rate was only 6%.[49]

DIFFERENTIAL DIAGNOSIS

Because an elongated appendix can irritate almost any abdominal structure, the differential diagnosis of appendicitis is quite extensive. The more common diseases that can mimic appendicitis are listed in Box 88-2.

Box 88-2 Differential Diagnosis for Appendicitis

Nonspecific abdominal pain
Gastroenteritis
Ascending diverticulitis
Gallbladder disease
Inflammatory bowel disease
Typhilitis
Renal colic

Women
Ovarian cyst
Ovarian torsion
Pelvic inflammatory disease
Ectopic pregnancy

Children
Henoch-Schönlein purpura
Testicular torsion
Epiploic appendicitis
Mesenteric adenitis/ileocolitis
Meckel's diverticulum

MANAGEMENT

A strategy to evaluate patients with right lower quadrant pain is listed in Figure 88-3. Patients should be instructed not to eat or drink and they should undergo a complete physical examination, including rectal and pelvic examinations. Dehydrated patients should receive bolus intravenous crystalloid fluid; hydrated patients should receive maintenance fluid. Parenteral antiemetics should be given to patients who are nauseated or vomiting.

In general, pain medication is underprescribed in patients with appendicitis. Patients with moderate to severe pain should be given appropriate doses of a short-acting opiate such as morphine or fentanyl. Ideally this should be done in consultation with the surgeon. A recent study shows that physical examination findings in patients going to the operating room with clinical appendicitis are unchanged after opiate administration.[69] Patients who have been evaluated by a surgeon and are undergoing a further diagnostic study should be given longer-acting opiates to keep them comfortable throughout the study. The effect of the opiate can always be temporarily reversed by the surgeon with naloxone if there is a concern that the examination is hindered by the drug.

Once the decision to operate has been made, prophylactic antibiotics should be given to cover gram-negative and anaerobic organisms. Intravenous second-generation cephalosporins, such as cefotetan or cefoxitin, provide good coverage. Preoperative antibiotics have been shown to decrease the incidence of postoperative wound infections.[70,71] If the appendix has already perforated, more complete coverage with ampicillin, gentamicin, clindamycin, or advanced penicillin combinations such as piperacillin and tazobactam may be preferred.

The appendix can be surgically removed either through the traditional open technique or through laparoscopy. The major advantage of laparoscopy is that it allows the surgeon to visualize other areas of abdominal and pelvic pathology if the appendix appears grossly normal. Other reported advantages are a quicker recovery time, reduced postoperative pain, earlier return to work, and decreased hospital costs.[72-74] All of these advantages, however, have been challenged by opponents of laparoscopy.[75] They believe that many of the studies are methodologically flawed and yield inconsistent results. Ultimately, the greatest differences in outcomes and overall costs seem to be based less on operative technique and more on the pathology of the appendix at the time of its removal. Based on 1999 data from the University Health Consortium of 118 academic medical centers, the average length of stay for uncomplicated acute appendicitis was 2.3 days, and cost (not charge) was $4667. This increased to 5.9 hospital days and $8954 if a complication such as perforation occurred.[76]

The gross visualization of the appendix during surgery can sometimes be misleading. Macroscopic signs of appendicitis include serosal vascular congestion, fibrinous or purulent film engulfing the appendix, and visible perforation or pus.[52] About 7% to 32% of appendixes that appear grossly inflamed will not have evidence of disease on pathology report. Conversely, 10% to 24% of appendixes that appear grossly normal may have microscopic evidence, in the form of leukocyte infiltration or wall ulceration, of acute appendicitis.[75,77] Because early signs of appendicitis may be determined only by microscopic investigation, the traditional practice of surgeons has been to remove a normal appendix. This has been challenged with the recent introduction of laparoscopy, and many institutions will now leave in a grossly normal-appearing appendix. Their reasoning is that appendicitis in a grossly normal appendix represents early disease that is probably curable with a short course of antibiotics. Consequently, they recommend a 3-day course of antibiotics if a grossly normal appendix is seen and no other abdominal pathology is identified during laparoscopy.[77,78]

Another approach with patients who have evidence of obvious perforation and abscess formation is to nonoperatively drain the abscess and treat the patient with intravenous antibiotics, with interval removal of the appendix 6 weeks later.[79,80] Recently, it has even been suggested that the appendix may not have to be removed after successful abscess resolution.[80]

DISPOSITION

Patients who have a low suspicion of appendicitis may be sent home after early follow up is arranged with the emergency physician, their primary care doctor, or the surgeon. They should be kept on a liquid diet and informed that they may have "appendicitis" and that it is critical that they be reevaluated in the next 6 to 8 hours. They should understand what signs and symptoms of appendicitis to expect so they know to return for immediate reevaluation should these develop. This discussion should be documented in the ED chart.

To minimize the risk of medical malpractice, the diagnosis of gastroenteritis should be made with caution and only in patients with nausea, vomiting, and diarrhea. Patients who require significant doses of opiates to control their pain should not be discharged without a specific diagnosis that can be safely treated as an outpatient.[81]

If follow up cannot be arranged, if the patient or family members appear unreliable, or if a significant language or

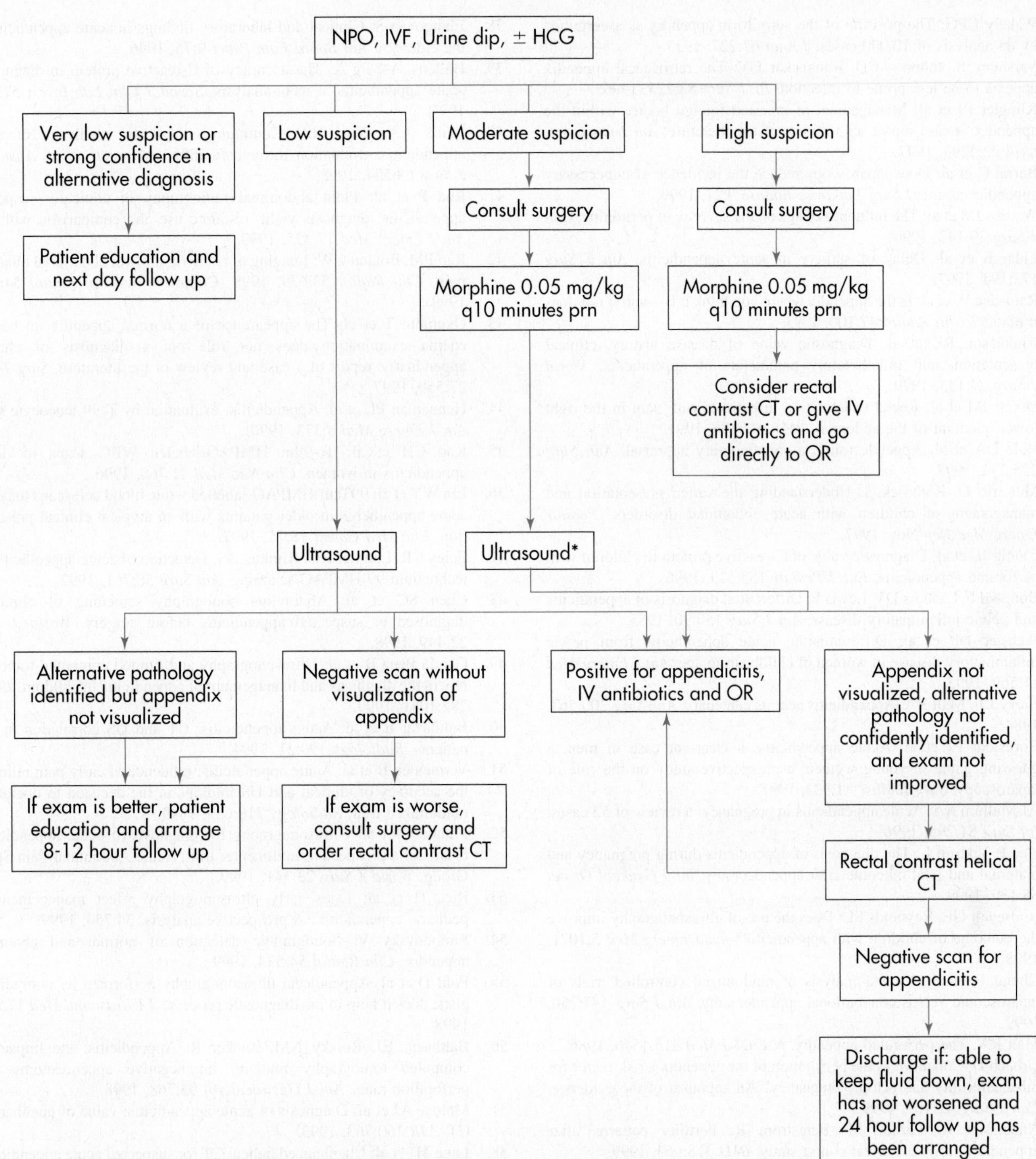

Figure 88-3. **Evaluation of right lower quadrant pain.**

transportation barrier exists, admission for observation should be strongly considered.

KEY CONCEPTS

- Classic appendicitis is a clinical diagnosis.
- Ultrasound and rectal contrast helical CT should be considered in equivocal cases, especially in female patients.
- Patients considered to be at very low risk for appendicitis may be sent home if they appear reliable and close follow up is arranged.

REFERENCES

1. Korner H et al: Incidence of acute nonperforated and perforated appendicitis: age-specific and sex-specific analysis, *World J Surg* 21:313, 1997.
2. Wagner J, Mckinnery P, Carpenter J: Does this patient have appendicitis? *JAMA* 276:1589, 1996.
3. Feldman: *Sleisenger & Fordtran's gastrointesteinal and liver disease,* ed 6, Philadelphia, 1998, WB Saunders.
4. Seal A: Appendicitis: a historical review, *Can J Surg* 24:427, 1981.
5. Smith S: Appendicitis, appendectomy and the surgeon, *Bull Hist Med* 70:414, 1996.

6. Wakely CPG: The position of the vermiform appendix as ascertained by an analysis of 10,000 cases, *J Anat* 67:227, 1933.
7. Varshney S, Johnson CD, Rangnekar GV: The retrocaecal appendix appears to be less prone to infection, *Br J Surg* 83:223, 1996.
8. Klingler PJ et al: Management of ingested foreign bodies within the appendix: a case report with review of the literature, *Am J Gastroenterol* 92:2295, 1997.
9. Barrat C et al: Does laparoscopy reduce the incidence of unnecessary appendicectomies? *Surg Laparosc Endosc* 9:27, 1999.
10. Watters JM et al: The influence of age on the severity of peritonitis, *Can J Surg* 39:142, 1996.
11. Eldar S et al: Delay of surgery in acute appendicitis, *Am J Surg* 173:194, 1997.
12. Ramsden W et al: Is the appendix where you think it is—and if not does it matter? *Clin Radiol* 47:100, 1993.
13. Andersson RE et al: Diagnostic value of disease history, clinical presentation, and inflammatory parameters of appendicitis, *World J Surg* 23:133, 1999.
14. Dixon JM et al: Rectal examination in patients with pain in the right lower quadrant of the abdomen, *BMJ* 302:386, 1991.
15. Hale DA et al: Appendectomy: a contemporary appraisal, *Ann Surg* 225:252, 1997.
16. McLario D, Rothrock S: Understanding the varied presentation and management of children with acute abdominal disorders, *Pediatr Emerg Med Rep* Nov, 1997.
17. Chung JL et al: Diagnostic value of C-reactive protein in children with perforated appendicitis, *Eur J Pediatr* 155:529, 1996.
18. Bongard F, Landers DV, Lewis F: Differential diagnosis of appendicitis and pelvic inflammatory disease, *Am J Surg* 150:90, 1985.
19. Webster DP et al: Differentiating acute appendicitis from pelvic inflammatory disease in women of childbearing age, *Am J Emerg Med* 11:569, 1993.
20. Barry J Jr, Malt RA: Appendicitis near its centenary, *Ann Surg* 200:567, 1984.
21. Borgstein PJ et al: Acute appendicitis: a clear-cut case in men, a guessing game in young women: a prospective study on the role of laparoscopy, *Surg Endosc* 11:923, 1997.
22. Al-Mulhim AA: Acute appendicitis in pregnancy: a review of 52 cases, *Int Surg* 81:295, 1996.
23. Hee P, Viktrup L: The diagnosis of appendicitis during pregnancy and maternal and fetal outcome after appendectomy, *Int J Gynecol Obstet* 65:129, 1999.
24. Roosevelt GE, Reynolds SL: Does the use of ultrasonography improve the outcome of children with appendicitis? *Acad Emerg Med* 5:1071, 1998.
25. Chung R et al: A meta-analysis of randomized controlled trials of laparoscopic versus conventional appendectomy, *Am J Surg* 177:250, 1999.
26. Malt RA: The perforated appendix, *N Engl J Med* 315:1546, 1986.
27. Urbach D, Cohen M: Is the perforation of the appendix a risk factor for tubal infertility and ectopic pregnancy? An appraisal of the evidence, *Can J Surg* 42:101, 1999.
28. Andersson R, Lambe M, Bergstrom R: Fertility patterns after appendicectomy: historical cohort study, *BMJ* 318:963, 1999.
29. Fauci AS et al (editors): *Harrison's principles of internal medicine*, ed 14, New York, 1998, McGraw-Hill.
30. Trautlein JJ, Lambert RL, Miller J: Malpractice in the emergency department: review of 200 cases, *Ann Emerg Med* 13:709, 1984.
31. Reynolds SL, Jaffe DM, Glynn W: Professional liability in a pediatric emergency department, *Pediatrics* 87:131, 1991.
32. Hale DA et al: Appendectomy: improving care through quality improvement, *Arch Surg* 132:153, 1997.
33. Braveman P et al: Insurance-related differences in the risk of ruptured appendix, *N Engl J Med* 331:444, 1994.
34. O'Toole SJ et al: Insurance-related differences in the presentation of pediatric appendicitis, *J Pediatr Surg* 31:1032, 1996.
35. Paajanen H et al: Are serum inflammatory markers age dependent in acute appendicitis? *J Am Coll Surg* 184:303, 1997.
36. Lyons D et al: An evaluation of the clinical value of the leucocyte count and sequential counts in suspected acute appendicitis, *Br J Clin Pract* 41:794, 1987.
37. Lau W et al: Leucocyte count and neutrophil percentage in appendicectomy for suspected appendicitis, *Aust N Z J Surg* 59:359, 1989.
38. Elangovan S: Clinical and laboratory findings in acute appendicitis in the elderly, *J Am Board Fam Pract* 9:75, 1996.
39. Hallens, Asberg A: The accuracy of C-reactive protein in diagnosing acute appendicitis: a meta-analysis, *Scand J Clin Lab Invest* 57:373, 1997.
40. Malik AA, Wani NA: Continuing diagnostic challenge of acute appendicitis: evaluation through modified Alvarado score, *Aust N Z J Surg* 68:504, 1998.
41. Roa P et al: Plain abdominal radiography in clinically suspected appendicitis: diagnosis yield, resource use and comparison with CT, *Am J Emerg Med* 17:325, 1999.
42. Rao PM, Boland GW: Imaging of acute right lower abdominal quadrant pain, *Clin Radiol* 53:639, 1998 (Comment in: *Clin Radiol* 54:271, 1999).
43. Okamoto T et al: The appearance of a normal appendix on barium enema examination does not rule out a diagnosis of chronic appendicitis: report of a case and review of the literature, *Surg Today* 27:550, 1997.
44. Henneman PL et al: Appendicitis: evaluation by Tc99 leucocyte scan, *Am J Emerg Med* 8:373, 1990.
45. Kao CH et al: Tc-99m HMPAO-labeled WBC scans to detect appendicitis in women, *Clin Nuc Med* 21:768, 1996.
46. Lin WY et al: 99Tcm-HMPAO-labelled white blood cell scans to detect acute appendicitis in older patients with an atypical clinical presentation, *Nuc Med Comm* 18:75, 1997.
47. Foley CR, Latimer RG, Rimkus DS: Detection of acute appendicitis by technetium 99 HMPAO scanning, *Am Surg* 58:761, 1992.
48. Chen SC et al: Abdominal sonography screening of clinically diagnosed or suspected appendicitis before surgery, *World J Surg* 22:449, 1998.
49. Garcia Pena B et al: Ultrasonography and limited computed tomography in the diagnosis and management of appendicitis in children, *JAMA* 282:1041, 1999.
50. Balthazar E et al: Acute appendicitis: CT and US correlation in 100 patients, *Radiology* 190:31, 1994.
51. Vermeulen B et al: Acute appendicitis: influence of early pain relief on the accuracy of clinical and US findings in the decision to operate: a randomized trial, *Radiology* 210:639, 1999.
52. Franke C et al: Ultrasonography for diagnosis of acute appendicitis: results of a prospective multicenter trial: Acute Abdominal Pain Study Group, *World J Surg* 23:141, 1999.
53. Rice H et al: Does early ultrasonography affect management of pediatric appendicitis? A prospective analysis, 34:754, 1999.
54. Simonovsky V: Sonographic detection of normal and abnormal appendix, *Clin Radiol* 54:533, 1999.
55. Pohl D et al: Appendiceal ultrasonography performed by nonradiologists: does it help in the diagnostic process? *J Ultrasound Med* 17:217, 1998.
56. Balthazar EJ, Rofsky NM, Zucker R: Appendicitis: the impact of computed tomography imaging on negative appendectomy and perforation rates, *Am J Gastroenterol* 93:768, 1998.
57. Malone AJ et al: Diagnosis of acute appendicitis: value of unenhanced CT, *AJR* 160:763, 1993.
58. Lane MJ et al: Unenhanced helical CT for suspected acute appendicitis, *AJR* 168:405, 1997.
59. Rao PM et al: Helical CT technique for the diagnosis of appendicitis: prospective evaluation of a focused appendix CT examination, *Radiology* 202:139, 1997.
60. Rao PM et al: Helical CT combined with contrast material administered only through the colon for imaging of suspected appendicitis, *AJR* 169:1275, 1997.
61. Lane M et al: Suspected appendicitis: nonenhanced helical CT in 300 consecutive patients, *Radiology* 213:341, 1999.
62. Rao PM, Feltmate CM, Rhea JT: Helical computed tomography in differentiating appendicitis and acute gynecologic conditions, *Obstet Gynecol* 93:417, 1999.
63. Inescur L et al: Acute appendicitis: MR imaging and sonographic correlation, *AJR* 168:669, 1997.
64. Hormann M et al: MR imaging in children with nonperforated acute appendicitis: value of unenhanced MR imaging in sonographically selected cases, *AJR* 171:467, 1998.
65. Mutter D et al: Value of microlaparoscopy in the diagnosis of right iliac fossa pain, *Am J Surg* 176:370, 1998.

66. Rhea JT et al: A focused appendiceal CT technique to reduce the cost of caring for patients with clinically suspected appendicitis, *AJR* 169:113, 1997.
67. Rao PM et al: Effect of computed tomography of the appendix on treatment of patients and use of hospital resources, *N Engl J Med* 338:141, 1998.
68. Rao PM et al: Introduction of appendiceal CT: impact on negative appendectomy and appendiceal perforation rates, *Ann Surg* 229:344, 1999.
69. Wolfe J et al: Does the administration of morphine to patients with acute appendicitis change exam findings or disposition? *Acad Emerg Med* 6:500, 1999 (abstract).
70. Antimicrobial prophylaxis in surgery, *Medical Letter* 37:79, 1995.
71. Bauer T et al: Antibiotic prophylaxis in acute nonperforated appendicitis, *Ann Surg* 209:307, 1989.
72. Garbutt JM et al: Meta-analysis of randomized controlled trials comparing laparoscopic and open appendectomy, *Surg Laparosc Endosc* 9:17, 1999.
73. Steyaert H et al: Laparoscopic appendectomy in children: sense or nonsense, *Act Chir Belg* 98:119, 1998.
74. Chung R et al: A meta-analysis of randomized controlled trials of laparoscopic versus conventional appendectomy, *Am J Surg* 177:250, 1999.
75. Fingerhut A, Millat B, Borrie F: Laparoscopic versus open appendectomy: time to decide, *World J Surg* 23:835, 1999.
76. Personal conversation with Peter Lindenauer, BMC, by permission of Sue Mertens, University Health Consortium 2000.
77. Champault G et al: Recognition of a pathological appendix during laparoscopy: a prospective study of 81 cases, *Br J Surg* 84:671, 1997.
78. Barrat C et al: Does laparoscopy reduce the incidence of unnecessary appendicectomies? *Surg Laparosc Endosc* 9:27, 1999.
79. Yamini D et al: Perforated appendicitis: is it truly a surgical urgency? *Am Surg* 64:970, 1998.
80. Ein SH, Shandling B: Is interval appendectomy necessary after rupture of an appendiceal mass? *J Pediatr Surg* 31:849, 1996.
81. Rusnak R, Borer J, Fastow J: Misdiagnosis of acute appendicitis: common features discovered in cases after litigation, *Am J Emerg Med* 12:397, 1994.

89 Acute Gastroenteritides

Robert A. Bitterman

INVASIVE BACTERIAL ENTERITIS (Table 89-1)

Campylobacter Enteritis

Epidemiology *Campylobacter* is the most common bacterial cause of diarrhea in patients who seek medical attention, and is found in the stools of 5% to 14% of these patients.[1,2] Most cases occur in young children, but all ages are affected. The disease is more common during the summer months. Opportunistic infections with *Campylobacter* species are often found in homosexual men or patients with acquired immunodeficiency syndrome (AIDS), even in the absence of symptoms of diarrhea or proctitis. *Campylobacter* species are a common cause of "backpacker's" diarrhea, along with *Giardia,* which is usually acquired by drinking from wilderness water sources.

Pathophysiology *Campylobacter* organisms are small gram-negative bacteria. *C. jejuni, C. coli,* and *C. fetus* are the most common subspecies isolated. *C. cinaedi* and *C. fennelliae* are isolated almost exclusively from male homosexuals. *Campylobacter* species produce disease primarily by direct invasion of the colonic epithelium, and may induce inflammatory changes endoscopically indistinguishable from inflammatory bowel disease.

Infection is transmitted by the fecal-oral route through contaminated food and water, or by direct contact with fecal material from infected animals or persons. The primary reservoirs for *Campylobacter* species are chickens and common birds such as pigeons, blackbirds, starlings, sparrows, and canaries.[3]

Clinical Presentation The incubation period for *Campylobacter* enteritis is approximately 2 to 5 days. Disease onset is usually rapid, consisting of fever, cramping abdominal pain, and diarrhea. Constitutional symptoms of anorexia, malaise, myalgias, and headache are the rule, and some patients experience backache, arthralgias, and vomiting. The clinical picture can mimic acute appendicitis. The diarrhea often lags 24 to 48 hours after the onset of fever and abdominal pain. Typically, the stools are loose and bile colored but progress to become watery, grossly bloody, or melenic more than 50% of the time. Either gross or occult blood is found in 60% to 90% of patients with *Campylobacter* gastroenteritis. At the height of the illness, patients usually pass more than eight to ten stools per day.[1]

Most patients are well within a week or less; however, diarrhea can persist for weeks. Rare cases have been fatal. Relapses are common, although generally milder than the original episode.

Diagnostic Strategies Diagnosis is made by stool culture. Laboratory findings include a leukocytosis and stool positive for occult or gross blood and fecal leukocytes. Blood cultures will sometimes be positive. Sigmoidoscopy reveals a nonspecific inflammatory colitis, and *Campylobacter* infection must be considered before a new diagnosis of inflammatory bowel disease is made.

Differential Considerations The differential diagnosis of campylobacteriosis includes all organisms that produce typical infectious diarrhea or fecal leukocytes (Box 89-1), but particularly salmonellosis, shigellosis, and *Escherichia coli* 0157:H7.

Table 89-1. Epidemiologic Aspects of Invasive Bacterial Enteritis

Pathogen	Sources	Incubation period (I) and duration (D) untreated	Features
Campylobacter	Contaminated food/water, wilderness waters (backpacker's diarrhea), birds, animals	I: 2-5 days D: 5-14 days	May cause bloody diarrhea May mimic acute appendicitis or inflammatory bowel disease; recurrence common
Salmonella	Grade A shell eggs, poultry, unpasteurized milk, domestic pets	I: 8-24 hr D: 2-5 days	Family and cafeteria-type food poisoning outbreaks common; increased incidence in patients with cancer or immunodeficiency
Shigella	Person-to-person, confined populations, poor hygiene, waterborne	I: 24-48 hr D: 4-7 days	Toxigenic watery diarrhea, followed by invasive picture; may produce severe dysentery
Yersinia	Food/water/milk, person-to-person, dogs, cats, pigs	I: 12-48 hr D: 5-14 days	Appendicitis/terminal ileitis-like syndrome; postinfection polyarthritis; long duration of fecal excretion of the organism
Vibrio parahaemolyticus	Raw or inadequately cooked seafood, especially shrimp	I: 8-24 hr D: 1-2 days	High attack rates, summer months; self-limited
E. coli 0127:H7	Raw ground beef, raw milk, meats, person-to-person, waterborne, travel	I: 3-8 days D: 5-10 days	Bloody diarrhea/hemorrhagic colitis; hemolytic-uremic syndrome or thrombotic thrombocytopenic purpura
Plesiomonas	Uncooked shellfish, travel	I: 1-2 days D: 5-20 days	Severe abdominal cramps and vomiting, with dehydration

Box 89-1 Fecal Leukocytes in Acute Diarrhea

Commonly Present

Campylobacter
Salmonella
Shigella
Yersinia
Vibrio vulnificus
Vibrio parahaemolyticus
E. coli serotype 0157:H7
Plesiomonas shigelloides
Amebic dysentery
Ulcerative colitis
Crohn's disease of the colon
Clostridium difficile (usually)
Stongyloides stercoralis (usually in immunocompromised patients)
Aeromonas hydrophila (occasionally)
Ischemic or radiation colitis

Commonly Absent

Viruses
Enterotoxigenic *E. coli*
Cryptosporidium
Isospora belli
Giardia lamblia
Enteromonas hominis
Aeromonas hydrophila (usually)
Clostridium difficile (occasionally)
All toxin-induced bacterial food poisoning
- *Staphylococcus aureus*
- *Bacillus cereus*
- *Clostridium perfringens*
- Noncholera vibrios
- *Vibrio cholerae*
- Scombroid fish toxins
- Ciguatera fish toxins

Management Treatment with antibiotics is not needed for patients who are clinically much improved when contacted regarding their culture result. Otherwise, treatment with ciprofloxacin or norfloxacin produces a rapid clinical and bacteriologic cure.[4] Relapses occur less often in patients treated with a quinolone compared with those who are untreated. Erythromycin is an acceptable alternative.[5] *Campylobacter* organisms are generally resistant to TMP-SMX. See Table 89-2 for antibiotic regimens. Because *Campylobacter* infection is an invasive enteritis, antimotility agents are not recommended.

Salmonellosis

Epidemiology *Salmonella* organisms are gram-negative bacilli that cause more than 2 million infections in the United States each year, most during the summer months.[6,7] *Salmonella* accounts for 10% to 15% of all cases of acute food poisoning reported to the Centers for Disease Control and Prevention (CDC).[3,8] The organism affects all age groups, but particularly children.

Almost all *Salmonella* infections are acquired by the ingestion of contaminated food or drink.[8-10] Direct person-to-person transmission can occur, but most human infections

Table 89-2. Antibiotic Therapy for Diarrhea in Immunocompetent Adults

Pathogen	Antibiotic*†	Dose
Campylobacter	1. Ciprofloxacin	500 mg PO bid × 7 days
	2. Erythromycin	500 mg PO qid × 7 days
Salmonella	1. Ciprofloxacin	500 mg PO bid × 7 days
	2. TMP/SMX	160 mg/800 mg PO bid × 7 days
Shigella	1. Ciprofloxacin	500 mg PO bid × 7 days
	2. TMP/SMX	160 mg/800 mg PO bid × 7 days
Vibrio parahaemolyticus	1. Tetracycline or doxycycline	500 mg PO qid × 7 days
		100 mg PO qid × 7 days
E. coli 0157:H7	1. None recommended	
Enterotoxigenic *E. coli*	1. Ciprofloxacin	500 mg PO bid × 7 days
	2. TMP/SMX	160 mg/800 mg PO bid × 7 days
Plesiomonas hominis	1. TMP/SMX	160 mg/800 mg PO bid × 7 days
	2. Ciprofloxacin	500 mg PO bid × 7 days
Clostridium difficile		
Diarrhea	1. Metronidazole	250 mg PO qid × 10-14 days
	2. Vancomycin	125 mg PO qid × 10-14 days
Colitis	1. Metronidazole or vancomycin	500 mg PO qid × 10-14 days; 1 g IV q day
Aeromonas	1. TMP/SMX or tetracycline	500 mg PO bid × 7 days
	2. Ciprofloxacin	160 mg/800 mg PO bid × 7-14 days
		500 mg PO qid × 7-14 days
Giardia lamblia	1. Metronidazole	250 mg PO tid × 5 days
	2. Furazolidone	100 mg PO qid × 7-10 days
Entamoeba histolytica	Symptomatic intestinal disease	
	1. Metronidazole followed by iodoquinol	750 mg PO tid × 10 days; 650 mg PO tid × 20 days
	2. Paromomycin	500 mg PO tid × 7 days
Cryptosporidium	1. Paromomycin	500-750 mg PO qid × 14-21 days
	2. Indomethicin	50 mg PO tid
Isospora belli	1. TMP/SMX	160 mg/800 mg PO qid × 10 days then bid for 3 wk
Cyclospora cayetanensis	1. TMP/SMX	160 mg/800 mg PO bid × 7 days
Strongyloides stercoralis	1. Ivermectin	200 μg/kg/PO day × 1-2 days
	2. Thiabendazole	50 mg/kg/day in two doses × 2 days (max 3 g/day)
Enterobius vermicularis	1. Mebendazole or pyrantel pamoate	100 mg PO × 1 dose, repeated after 2 wk
		11 mg/kg PO × 1 dose, (max 1 g) repeated after 2 wk
	2. Albendazole	400 mg PO × 1 dose, repeated after 2 wk

*Another quinolone agent, norfloxacin, can be substituted for ciprofloxacin in the treatment of diarrheas. The equivalent dosage is 400 mg bid.
†1 indicates drug of first choice; 2 indicates alternative drug(s).

are related to the vast reservoir of salmonellosis in lower animals. Poultry products such as turkey, chicken, duck, and eggs constitute the most common source of *Salmonella.*

Unpasteurized milk and domestic pets are other sources. Approximately 10% of household dogs and cats excrete *Salmonella,* and pet reptiles, such as turtles, snakes, and iguanas, have been responsible for outbreaks of salmonellosis.[6,11,13] Rattlesnake meat and medicinal preparations have been associated with *Salmonella arizonae* infections, especially among Hispanic populations in the southwestern United States.

Cooking contaminated foods decreases the possibility of infection but does not eliminate it. *Salmonella* may survive cooking deep inside certain foods where temperatures may not reach the lethal range (e.g., large turkeys and soft-cooked eggs). Very large outbreaks of *Salmonella* infections have been traced to contaminated, unbroken grade A shell eggs.[6] These outbreaks have not resulted from the usual contamination during the cooking or storage processes, but rather from *Salmonella* passed from an infected hen into the egg. The means by which the *Salmonella* contaminates the eggs is unknown. There may be fecal contamination of the eggs before deposition of the shell, or transovarian transmission, or both.[14] Although the organism is present in the uncracked egg, thorough cooking usually eradicates or reduces it to clinically insignificant levels.

Common raw egg–based sources of *Salmonella* infections include hollandaise sauce, homemade eggnog, caesar salad dressing, and French toast mix. *Salmonella enteritidis* is the species universally associated with egg-related infections.[53] Patients convalescing from *Salmonella*-related enterocolitis and persons with asymptomatic infection may continue to excrete *Salmonella* organisms for weeks or months, thus serving as sources of infection.

Pathophysiology Ingested *Salmonella* organisms penetrate the intestinal mucosal cells and lodge in the lamina propria. The subsequent inflammatory reaction produces the gastroenteritis. Different *Salmonella* serotypes show marked variations in invasive potential and are associated with particular presentations: *Salmonella typhi* with enteric fever (typhoid fever), *Salmonella choleraesuis* with septicemia, *Salmonella typhimurium* with acute gastroenteritis, and *S. enteritidis* infections from grade A shell eggs.[6]

Relatively large numbers of *Salmonella* must be ingested to produce illness. However, a carrier state can be induced with ingestion of 10 to 100 times fewer bacteria. In infants and adults with certain underlying diseases, a much smaller inoculum may produce illness. Decreased gastric acidity or an alteration of intestinal flora resulting from the administration of antibiotics can impressively reduce the size of the required inoculum. Approximately one third to one half of patients hospitalized with salmonellosis have some type of major underlying disease, such as leukemia, lymphoma, cancer, or AIDS. The incidence of *Salmonella* enteric fever is markedly increased in immunodeficient patients with cancer or AIDS.[15,16] Patients with sickle cell anemia, other hemolytic anemias, or AIDS are unusually susceptible to *Salmonella* bacteremia.[15] Protracted salmonellosis and higher morbidity and mortality rates occur in patients older than 65 years of age.

Clinical Presentation Family outbreaks and sporadic cases are more common than large epidemics. After an incubation period of 8 to 48 hours, the typical patient with *Salmonella* gastroenteritis presents with fever, colicky abdominal pain, and loose, watery diarrhea, occasionally with mucus and blood. Nausea and vomiting are common, but are rarely severe or protracted. Mild to moderate diffuse abdominal tenderness is present in most patients, but occasionally severe tenderness and even rebound can occur. Symptoms usually abate within 2 to 5 days, and recovery is uneventful.

Diagnostic Strategies Diagnosis is made by stool culture. The peripheral white blood cell (WBC) count is usually normal unless bacteremia is present. Fecal leukocyte tests are positive, and sometimes occult blood is also present in the stool. Blood cultures are occasionally positive and should be drawn in all severely ill patients. The possibility of an underlying disease or immunodeficiency state should be considered in every patient with a severe *Salmonella* infection.

Differential Considerations Family or communal outbreaks may suggest staphylococcal-related food poisoning, but this entity has a shorter incubation period, is not associated with fever, and produces the typical toxigenic, noninvasive, diarrheal picture. Vomiting is also much more prominent in cases of staphylococcal-related food poisoning than in most *Salmonella* infections.

Management Discharged patients whose stool cultures return positive for *Salmonella* should be contacted by telephone to ascertain their condition. Most patients with *Salmonella* gastroenteritis will have clinically improved by the time their culture results are available. These patients do not require antibiotic treatment. Patients who are not improving should be treated to effect cure, and those who represent a public health risk should be treated to eradicate the carrier state and prevent spread of the organism. The antibiotic of choice for outpatient management of *Salmonella* gastroenteritis is either ciprofloxacin or norfloxacin.[5] The quinolones are clinically effective and eradicate the organisms from the stool, thus preventing the carrier state or relapses from occurring. Ciprofloxacin has also been demonstrated to be effective in the treatment of chronic *S. typhi* carriers. Patients requiring inpatient therapy are best treated with intravenous (IV) ceftriaxone until sensitivity studies become available.[17,18]

Follow-up with the patient's personal physician should be arranged. Food handlers or health care personnel should not be allowed to work until the carrier state has abated. Repeated stool cultures and further decisions regarding job or school situations will be required. Personal hygiene should be stressed because untreated patients may continue to shed infective organisms in the stool for weeks or even months. As with other invasive pathogens, the use of antimotility drugs alone is contraindicated. These drugs prolong fever and diarrhea and increase the incidence of bacteremia and the carrier state in patients with *Salmonella* enteritis. However, administration of loperamide is safe when given concomitantly with an appropriate antibiotic.

Prevention of salmonellosis depends on adequate cooking and minimizing the time that foods are allowed to stand at room temperature to reduce the chance of bacterial growth to an infectious inoculum. Careful personal hygiene, including hand washing, is also important.

Shigellosis

Epidemiology Shigellosis, or bacillary dysentery, is worldwide in distribution and particularly common in countries lacking effective sanitation. Approximately 25,000 to 40,000 cases are reported annually in the United States, but many more undoubtedly occur. *Shigella sonnei* is responsible for approximately 75% of the infections occurring in this country; *Shigella flexneri* causes most of the remaining cases, with *Shigella dysenteriae* responsible for a small percentage of cases.[2]

Shigella infections are common in confined populations, such as those in mental or penal institutions, in nursing homes, or on Indian reservations. Spread is by the fecal-oral route, and humans are the only natural hosts. *Shigella* can be found in large numbers around the bases of toilets used by infected persons, and they readily pass through toilet tissue onto the fingers. *Shigella* may be recovered in cultures taken as long as 3 hours after contamination. Shigellosis also has been transmitted by mouth-to-mouth resuscitation of patients and through the use of mannequins in CPR training. In the last few years a number of large outbreaks have been associated with recreational water venues such as swimming pools, water parks, fountains, hot tubs, and spas.[19]

Pathophysiology Unlike *Salmonella,* which requires a very large inoculum to produce disease, as few as 50 to 100 *Shigella* bacilli can cause infection. No other enteric pathogen is so efficient in producing overt disease in humans. Infection is generally superficial, localized to the epithelial lining of the mucosa; therefore bowel perforation or invasion into the bloodstream is extremely rare. Bleeding occurs from superficial ulcerations of the mucosa.

Many patients infected with *Shigella* will not have dysentery develop, but will have only a watery diarrhea of short duration. The watery diarrhea is caused by exotoxin-induced secretion of water and electrolytes by the small bowel, whereas the bloody mucoid dysentery is the result of colonic mucosal invasion by the organisms. Systemic manifestations may also be toxin induced because bacteremia is rarely found.

Clinical Presentation The incubation period is usually 24 to 48 hours, and the clinical manifestations that follow can vary considerably or have a bimodal presentation. Mild, watery diarrhea with few if any constitutional symptoms or asymptomatic infection occurs in a significant proportion of infected individuals. Colicky abdominal pain, followed shortly by high fever and diarrhea, is the more common clinical presentation. The stools are liquid and greenish, contain shreds of mucus and undigested food, and average 7 to 12 daily. Only 20% to 30% of culture-proven cases develop bloody mucoid stools.

When true dysentery develops, it is ordinarily preceded by a recognizable period of watery diarrhea lasting a few hours to a few days. Patients with dysentery have grossly bloody diarrhea, tenesmus, and significant constitutional symptoms, such as fever, nausea, vomiting, headache, and myalgias. Convulsions and other neurologic manifestations are common in children. If symptoms are severe enough, profound dehydration and even circulatory collapse can occur.

Generally, shigellosis is a self-limited disease. Patients become afebrile in 3 to 4 days, and the abdominal cramping and diarrhea resolve within 1 week. A significant number of untreated patients will continue to shed organisms in the stool for 2 or more weeks, and approximately 10% of patients will have a relapse unless treated with antibiotics.

Diagnostic Strategies Most cases of shigellosis remain undiagnosed. Patients seen in the ED with mild, watery diarrhea and few if any constitutional symptoms are sent home with conservative management, and no investigative procedures are performed. However, shigellosis should be considered in every patient with an acute febrile illness associated with diarrhea, especially those patients who appear ill or who have dysenteric stools.

Fecal white blood cells are present in cases of shigellosis, regardless of the gross appearance of the stool, and usually in large numbers.[2] Thus finding leukocytes in watery stools can help identify shigellosis even in the absence of classic dysenteric stools. Occult blood is usually present in the stools of all shigellosis patients. Blood leukocytosis is common, and a significant leftward shift in the differential count is almost always present. Blood cultures for *Shigella* are rarely positive. Sigmoidoscopic examination reveals diffuse mucosal inflammation, often with multiple ulcerations.

A definitive diagnosis of shigellosis is made with stool culture. Stool cultures are positive in more than 90% of cases when stool is obtained during the first 3 days of illness; however, only approximately 75% are positive if samples are obtained more than 1 week after the onset of diarrhea.

Differential Considerations The major differential diagnosis of shigellosis includes salmonellosis, *Campylobacter* enteritis, *E. coli* 0157:H7 infection, amebic dysentery, and ulcerative colitis.

Management Treatment is primarily the correction of fluid and electrolyte abnormalities. Discharged patients whose stool cultures return positive for *Shigella* organisms should be contacted by telephone, and the use of antibiotics considered. If *S. sonnei* or *S. flexneri* is cultured, the decision to administer antibiotics is based on the patient's clinical condition and the feasibility of sanitary control. Asymptomatic patients or ones improving do not need to be treated with antibiotics unless necessary for public health measures. Patients who are not improving should be treated. Antibiotics shorten the clinical course and eradicate the pathogen from the stool, often within 48 hours.[20] Whenever *S. dysenteriae* is isolated, the patient should be treated for public health reasons to prevent outbreaks of dysentery, even if the patient is asymptomatic when the culture result returns.

In the United States, over 50% of *Shigella* organisms are resistant to ampicillin, and 25% to 45% are resistant to TMP-SMX.[2,5] No resistance has been found to the quinolone agents ciprofloxacin or norfloxacin, and one of them should be considered the drug of choice unless sensitivity studies demonstrate that the organism is sensitive to either ampicillin or TMP-SMX.

Antimotility agents may prolong the fever, diarrhea, and excretion of *Shigella* in the stools and are contraindicated in patients with invasive shigellosis. However, they may be safe when used simultaneously with antibiotics. Follow-up stool cultures should be done in patients treated for *S. dysenteriae* to ensure eradication of the organism. Follow-up cultures, however, are not necessary in patients treated for *S. sonnei* or *S. flexneri,* provided that the patient improves clinically.

Yersinia enterocolitica Gastroenteritis

Epidemiology *Yersinia enterocolitica,* a gram-negative, aerobic bacterium, is a member of the family Enterobacteriaceae, along with *Salmonella, Shigella,* and *E. coli. Y. enterocolitica* is increasingly being recognized as a human pathogen all over the world, particularly in Scandinavia, Europe, Canada, and Japan. In some areas, such as Ontario and Quebec, Canada, it is now much more common than *Shigella* and is approaching the incidence of *Salmonella* as a cause for gastroenteritis in children. In the United States it is increasingly found to cause gastroenteritis and other enteric syndromes that can mimic appendicitis. *Yersinia* infections are most common in childhood.[2,3]

Pathophysiology Yersiniosis is an invasive infection of the intestine, particularly the terminal ileum, and the mesenteric lymph nodes. Infection originates from contaminated food or drink. The consumption of contaminated milk or contaminated raw pork has accounted for sporadic cases and several large outbreaks of infection. Fecal-oral transmission to humans from a variety of animals, particularly dogs, cats, and pigs, and direct person-to-person spread probably occur, but communicability appears to be low.[21]

Clinical Presentation The initial clinical picture of *Yersinia* enterocolitis resembles that of infection by other invasive intestinal organisms: fever; colicky abdominal pain; watery, greenish, and sometimes bloody diarrhea; and constitutional symptoms of anorexia, vomiting, and malaise. However, in *Y. enterocolitica* gastroenteritis, the abdominal pain and diarrhea usually persist for 10 to 14 days or longer.

A substantial number of patients with yersiniosis, in particular adolescents and young adults, develop an ileocecitis. In these cases, lower abdominal pain with little or no diarrhea predominates and may perfectly mimic acute appendicitis. Large gastrointestinal outbreaks have been traced to contaminated milk, largely because physicians noticed an extraordinary jump in the number of negative appendectomies.[21]

Postinfection manifestations, such as erythema nodosum or a persistent polyarthritis, may occur in as many as 2% to 5% of patients, mainly adults.[2]

Diagnostic Strategies Leukocytosis sometimes occurs with *Yersinia* enterocolitis, and blood cultures are almost always negative. Fecal stains show leukocytes, as in other invasive diarrheas, and occasionally red blood cells (RBCs) as well. If performed, contrast radiography of the small bowel shows mucosal abnormalities consistent with terminal ileitis. Radiographic studies of the large bowel and sigmoidoscopy usually show normal colonic mucosa.

Ultrasonography can show a typical sonographic picture of bacterial ileocecitis and may differentiate bacterial enteritis from acute appendicitis and save some patients needless surgery.[22]

Culturing the organism from the stool is the only definitive way to diagnose yersiniosis. Stool cultures require special techniques and a long time for growth. Patients with *Yersinia* enterocolitis routinely continue to shed organisms in the stools well into convalescence, long after the diarrhea subsides. The mean duration of fecal shedding is approximately 6 weeks.

Differential Considerations The diagnosis should be suspected when a patient has prolonged abdominal pain and diarrhea after what appears to be a common, usually self-limited gastroenteritis syndrome, or the patient has appendicitis or a mesenteric adenitis-like syndrome. *Y. enterocolitica* infection should also be considered in the differential diagnosis of regional enteritis, which it can very closely mimic.[22]

Management Generally, *Y. enterocolitica* infection is self-limited at the diarrheal stage and resolves without treatment. As with other invasive gastrointestinal pathogens, antiperistaltic drugs are not recommended.

Treatment with antibiotics has not been proven essential or efficacious in the management of uncomplicated *Yersinia* enterocolitis or in the pseudoappendicitis syndrome. However, because *Yersinia* organisms take a long time to grow on culture, in most studies the duration of illness before antibiotics were started was 1 to 2 weeks. *Yersinia* organisms are usually susceptible to TMP-SMX, which is the treatment of choice when antibiotic therapy is indicated.[17] The drug has not been shown to decrease the fecal shedding of the organism. Quinolones are an effective alternative.[5] Treatment should be considered in patients who are still significantly ill at the time a culture returns, particularly if they are immunocompromised or have a significant underlying medical illness, or in cases in which the fecal shedding could represent a public health hazard.

Vibrio parahaemolyticus Gastroenteritis

Epidemiology *Vibrio parahaemolyticus* bacilli are gram-negative, marine vibrios present in the coastal seawaters of the United States, Japan, and other temperate-zone nations. It is by far the most common etiology of bacterial enteritis in Japan, causing up to 70% of cases. It has also been implicated in many outbreaks of acute diarrheal illness in the coastal areas of the United States, often from eating raw oysters.[23-25] Raw fish is the most common infection vehicle in Japan, whereas inadequately cooked seafood, usually shrimp, is the most common source in the United States. Several epidemics of *V. parahaemolyticus* infections have occurred on cruise ships.[26] Food poisoning from vibrios can be partly explained by the fact that vibrios are not detected by standard techniques used to check fishing waters, nor are they eliminated by the usual commercial decontamination procedures for shellfish.[27,28]

The illness appears to be limited to the warmer months of the year when large numbers of vibrios are present in coastal seawaters and the temperature favors bacterial multiplication in unrefrigerated seafood. *V. parahaemolyticus* grows rapidly at room temperature, and within 3 to 4 hours a few organisms can multiply to an infectious inoculum. Attack rates are quite high, but there is no evidence of secondary spread among family members of infected patients.[24]

Pathophysiology Unlike other vibrios, *V. parahaemolyticus* produces disease by an infectious process rather than one mediated through an enterotoxin. It causes an intense, inflammatory response in the intestinal mucosa. Stools contain numerous leukocytes and are occasionally grossly bloody. *V. parahaemolyticus* appears to be pathogenic only for humans; no other known host exists. Vibrios are not found in the feces of asymptomatic persons.

Clinical Presentation Symptoms usually appear 8 to 12 hours after the ingestion of contaminated food, but the incubation period can range from 4 to 48 hours. The most predominant symptom is acute diarrhea, but the volume of fluid lost is generally not great. Moderately severe abdominal cramps usually occur, and many patients also exhibit systemic symptoms of fever, nausea, and headache. Vomiting can occur but generally is not prominent. The illness is almost invariably self-limited and seldom lasts longer than 24 to 48 hours.[24]

V. parahaemolyticus infection should be suspected when a common-source outbreak of acute diarrheal disease occurs in persons exposed to fresh or frozen seafood. It should also be considered when fecal WBCs are present in cases of acute diarrhea linked to food poisoning.

Diagnostic Strategies The diagnosis of *V. parahaemolyticus* infection can be confirmed within 24 hours by culturing the stools on thiosulfate-citrate-bile salt-sucrose (TCBS) agar.

Management Because the disease is self-limited, most patients require no therapy. Antibiotic treatment appears to shorten neither the course nor the duration of pathogen excretion, although tetracycline may benefit patients with particularly severe or extended infections. An occasional patient may require fluid replacement. Antimotility agents are not indicated.

Because *V. parahaemolyticus* is widely present in coastal waters, the only effective preventive measures are through the application of adequate cooking, refrigeration, and hygienic practice in the preparation of seafood for human consumption.

Hemorrhagic *Escherichia coli* Serotype 0157:H7 Gastroenteritis

Epidemiology *E. coli* serotype 0157:H7 is an important and common cause of bloody diarrhea in the United States, Canada, the United Kingdom, and South America. Its incidence is about the same as that of *Shigella* in many parts of the United States, particularly in the Pacific Northwest.[29] Infection is most common in children and the elderly. Patients with a previous gastrectomy are also at risk, probably because of loss of the gastric acidity defense. Large outbreaks of *E. coli* 0157:H7 hemorrhagic colitis have occurred, primarily in nursing homes, with mortality rates as high as 35%.[3,7,30,31]

Inadequately cooked hamburger has caused many large outbreaks.[32] *E. coli* 0157:H7, present in the intestines of healthy cattle, contaminates the meat during slaughter, and the grinding process then transfers the organisms from the surface of the meat to the interior. United States Department of Agriculture (USDA) food safety regulations now require that hamburger be cooked thoroughly, to the point that the juices are no longer pink, to effectively kill *E. coli* organisms. Outbreaks have also occurred from apple cider, raw milk, seed sprouts, contaminated municipal water supplies, and person-to-person spread in daycare centers.[10,33]

Food handlers with *E. coli* 0157:H7–related diarrhea have contaminated meals responsible for institutional outbreaks. Person-to-person spread occurs, and this explains the secondary infections that occur later in workers caring for persons with *E. coli* 0157:H7 colitis.[7,30]

Pathophysiology *E. coli* 0157:H7 is one of more than 30 serotypes of *E. coli* known to produce *Shigella*-like toxins called *vertoxins,* which are cytotoxic to the intestinal vascular endothelial cells and cause hemorrhagic colitis. *E. coli* 0157:H7 does not cause an invasive infection.[29,34]

Clinical Presentation After an incubation period of 4 to 9 days, patients initially produce watery diarrhea that becomes bloody hours to days later. More than 95% of patients will report bloody stools.[29] The amount of blood varies, but stools passed may consist wholly of blood, and the infection may masquerade as gastrointestinal (GI) bleeding from noninfectious causes.

The bloody diarrhea is typically accompanied by severe abdominal cramps, pain, and often vomiting. Fever is not a prominent symptom. Fecal leukocytes are found but in small numbers, which contrasts strikingly with the sheets of white cells seen in *Shigella* dysentery. Endoscopic, histologic, and radiographic studies demonstrate only nonspecific changes consistent with an inflammatory hemorrhagic colitis.[29]

Uncomplicated infection resolves spontaneously over 7 to 10 days. A carrier state may last another 1 to 2 weeks, but it also resolves spontaneously. Chronic diarrhea is rare.[35]

Complications *E. coli* 0157:H7 hemorrhagic colitis produces two serious complications, hemolytic uremic syndrome (HUS) and thrombotic thrombocytopenic purpura (TTP). HUS is especially common in children, occurring in 20% to 25% of cases. Approximately 5% to 10% of elderly patients in nursing home outbreaks acquire HUS, and 50% to 80% of these patients die. TTP is seen in 2% to 3% of cases, most often in immunosuppressed patients. HHS or TTP typically occurs 5 to 20 days after onset of infection, and the diarrhea can be totally resolved and forgotten by the time a diagnosis is established. Death from *E. coli* 0157:H7 hemorrhagic colitis alone or from one of the complications is common and occurs primarily among the elderly.[31,36]

Diagnostic Strategies Diagnosis requires specific stool culture techniques. In addition to the routine battery of media used for stool cultures, specimens should be plated onto sorbitol-MacConkey medium. The 0157:H7 strains of *E. coli* are sorbitol negative at 18 to 24 hours on this media and can be rapidly identified using various serologic tests, such as latex agglutination or fluorescent antibody testing. DNA probes aid in the diagnosis and are used by the CDC to determine the etiology of widespread outbreaks.[37] Clinical laboratories must establish rapid identification systems for this organism.

Differential Considerations Hemorrhagic *E. coli* infections are misdiagnosed as ischemic colitis, inflammatory bowel disease, intussusception, or another infectious colitis. The examining physician should test for *E. coli* 0157:H7 when considering a diagnosis of one of these entities.

Management Limited studies to date have not demonstrated antibiotic therapy to shorten the clinical course or eradicate the organism. Moreover, treatment with antibiotics to which the organism is resistant probably increases the risk of developing HUS by eliminating competing bowel flora.[29,30,36]

Aeromonas hydrophila Gastroenteritis

Epidemiology *Aeromonas* species are gram-negative, facultative, anaerobic, rod-shaped bacteria of the family Vibrionaceae. *Aeromonas* organisms are ubiquitous in fresh and brackish water in the United States and also contaminate the food supply.[2,8] Drinking untreated water, usually from private wells or springs, causes most cases of diarrhea from *Aeromonas* bacteria.[23] *Aeromonas* infection has not been associated with consumption of shellfish. Predisposing factors include age, underlying disease such as colon cancer or inflammatory bowel disease, and recent hospitalization or antibiotic treatment. *Aeromonas* infection causes 10% to 15% of all cases of diarrhea in children.[38] It does occur in normal adults but is most often seen in immunocompromised patients. It is a particularly common cause of diarrhea in patients with AIDS.[15,16]

Pathophysiology The exact mechanism by which *Aeromonas* species produce diarrhea has not yet been explained. Both enterotoxins and cytopathic toxins may be produced, and the organisms may have some invasive characteristics.

Clinical Presentation Typical symptoms are watery diarrhea, abdominal cramps, vomiting, and occasionally fever. Children tend to have a more acute, severe illness than do adults. In untreated patients, diarrhea tends to persist for 2 to 10 weeks, the illness being much more prolonged in adults than in children. Generally, fecal leukocytes and occult blood are absent from the stool; however, patients can have a severe colitis, including fever, fecal leukocytes, and bloody diarrhea, which can mimic Crohn's disease or ulcerative colitis. An association of inflammatory bowel disease exists with acute *Aeromonas*-associated diarrhea. What role, if any, *Aeromonas* species play in the activation of inflammatory bowel disease remains unknown.

Diagnosis is made by stool culture, but *Aeromonas* infection should be strongly suspected in children or the immunocompromised patient, particularly those with a history of drinking from untreated water sources.

Management Antibiotic treatment results in prompt resolution of all symptoms. Treatment also eradicates the organism from the stools. TMP-SMX is the drug of choice, but both the quinolones and tetracyclines effectively treat *Aeromonas*-related diarrhea.[5,17]

Plesiomonas shigelloides Gastroenteritis

Epidemiology *Plesiomonas shigelloides* is a gram-negative, facultative, anaerobic bacterium of the family Vibrionaceae. *Plesiomonas* has been recovered in up to 17% of immunocompetent patients who have acute diarrhea.[15,16] Infection is strongly associated with eating uncooked shellfish, usually raw oysters, in the 48 hours before the onset of illness. A strong association also exists between *Plesiomonas* infection and foreign travel, especially to Mexico. Sporadic diarrheal illness occurs in both normal and immunocompromised hosts. Large outbreaks have occurred, usually resulting from oyster consumption.[8]

Pathophysiology The mechanism of disease production is enteroinvasion by the organisms. *Plesiomonas* does not appear to produce enterotoxins.

Clinical Presentation The incubation period is only 1 to 2 days. Most patients have significant diarrhea and vomiting, severe abdominal cramps, and some degree of dehydration. Stools are generally bloody and contain mucus, with fecal leukocytes present. Symptoms last anywhere from 5 to 40 days and are usually shorter in children and longer in adults.

Diagnosis of *P. shigelloides* infection should be considered in patients with a typical invasive-appearing diarrhea, especially if the stools are bloody or when the onset of illness is shortly after the ingestion of raw shellfish or foreign travel, particularly to Mexico.

Diagnostic Strategies Definitive diagnosis is via stool culture. However, the laboratory must be notified because unless oxidase testing is done, *Plesiomonas* species may be indistinguishable from normal Enterobacteriaceae on nonselective culture media. Patients with *Plesiomonas* infections should be evaluated for possible immunodeficiency.

Management Antibiotic treatment results in rapid clinical and bacteriologic cure. *P. shigelloides* is usually resistant to ampicillin but susceptible to TMP-SMX, the quinolones, cephalothin, gentamicin, and chloramphenicol. Current recommended treatment is TMP-SMX, 160 mg/800 mg PO bid for 7 days or, alternatively, ciprofloxacin, 500 mg PO bid, or norfloxacin, 400 mg PO bid for 7 days.[5,39] Follow-up evaluation is not necessary, unless the patient is immunodeficient or does not respond clinically.

TOXIN-INDUCED BACTERIAL GASTROENTERITIS (Table 89-3)

Staphylococcal Food Poisoning

Epidemiology Staphylococcal-related food poisoning is caused by the multiplication of an enterotoxin-forming strain of *Staphylococcus* organisms in the food before ingestion. Contamination of food with *Staphylococcus* organisms is extremely common because the organism can be grown from the hands of approximately 50% of persons. Most protein-rich foods will support the growth of staphylococci, especially ham, eggs (even hard boiled), custard-filled pastries, mayonnaise, and potato salad.[3,40] Contaminated foods need sit at room temperature for only a few hours for the staphylococci to grow and produce sufficient enterotoxin to elicit disease if ingested. Foods containing sufficient enterotoxin to produce violent illness are usually normal in appearance, odor, and taste. Large outbreaks are common, particularly in institutions.[3,7,8]

Pathophysiology The staphylococcal enterotoxin is a heat-stable toxin, and once it is present in food, reheating or even boiling will not prevent illness. The toxin has no local effect on the digestive tract. It is absorbed, and symptoms are mediated by a direct effect of the absorbed toxin on the central nervous system (CNS). The disease can be reproduced by the parenteral injection of the enterotoxin.[40]

Clinical Presentation The illness has an explosive onset, beginning 1 to 6 hours after ingestion of the contaminated food. Cramping and abdominal pain, with violent and often-repeated retching and vomiting, are the predominant symptoms. Diarrhea is variable; it is usually mild, occasionally absent entirely, and infrequently profuse. Fever is occasionally present. Although often violent, staphylococcal food poisoning is short-lived, usually subsiding in 6 to 8 hours and rarely lasting as long as 24 hours. The patient is often recovering when first seen by a physician. Attack rates are very high, often greater than 75% of the population at risk.[40]

The short incubation period and multiple cases in persons eating the same meal are highly suggestive of this disease. Examination of the stool is noncontributory, and no practical laboratory test is available to confirm the diagnosis. The epidemiologic circumstances, however, usually provide adequate suggestive evidence.

Management Rapid, uncomplicated, spontaneous recovery is the rule. In adults an IV or intramuscular injection of promethazine hydrochloride, 25 mg, prochlorperazine, 10 mg, or droperidol, 2.5 to 5 mg, may control vomiting. IV fluids to correct saline depletion are needed in 10% to 15% of patients, particularly in the young or debilitated. Antibiotics are of no value because staphylococcal food poisoning is caused by preformed enterotoxin and not by viable microorganisms. Strict personal hygiene of food handlers and immediate refrigeration of foods not due for immediate consumption are the most important preventive measures. Ordinary refrigerator temperatures prevent production of the enterotoxin. Food should not be allowed to stand for long periods before being served.

Clostridium perfringens Food Poisoning

Epidemiology *Clostridium perfringens* is probably the most common cause of acute food poisoning in the United States, constituting almost one fourth of all bacteria-associated food-borne illnesses. Most cases of *C. perfringens* food poisoning occur in fairly large outbreaks and are caused by the ingestion of meat or poultry dishes.[3,8,41] Most market meats and poultry are heavily contaminated with *C. perfringens,* type A, heat-resistant spores. The organism is also ubiquitous in the environment and in human and animal feces. Typically, poisoning results from ingesting food that is cooked more than 24 hours before consumption, allowed to cool slowly at room temperature, and then served either cool or rewarmed. During this period of incubation, spores that

Table 89-3. Epidemiologic Aspects of Toxin-Induced Bacterial Enteritis

Pathogen	Sources	Incubation period (I) and duration (D) untreated	Features
Preformed toxins			
Staphylococcus	Food-handler related; potato salad, mayonnaise, confections	I: 1-6 hr D: 6-10 hr	Very high attack rates, large outbreaks
Bacillus cereus emetic toxin	Fried rice	I: 2-4 hr D: 10 hr	High attack rate, almost always fried rice
Bacillus cereus diarrheal toxin	Vegetables, meats, especially gravies	I: 6-14 hr D: 24-36 hr	Food reheated or sitting out for long periods
Scombroid	Mahimahi, tuna, bluefish	I: 5-60 min D: 6 hr	Peppery or bitter taste, histamine intoxication, high attack rates
Ciguatera	Large, predacious, coral reef fish	I: 2-6 hr D: 7-14 days	High attack rates, neurologic symptoms with gastrointestinal symptoms, chronic paresthesias
Toxins produced after colonization			
Clostridium perfringens	Meat, poultry, gravies, "steam table" meats	I: 6-24 hr D: 24 hr	Food reheated or sitting out for long periods
Vibrio	Seafood, especially raw shellfish	I: 24-48 hr D: 6-8 days	Summer months, dehydration common
Escherichia coli	Usually unsanitary drinking water	I: 24-72 hr D: 1-7 days	Travelers, dehydration common in children
Clostridium difficile	Overgrowth of normal flora	I: 5-14 days D: Variable	Antibiotic-associated colitis, cytopathic toxin
Aeromonas	Untreated drinking water	I: 1-5 days D: 2-10 wk	Common and severe in children, chronic watery diarrhea in adults, occasionally mimics inflammatory bowel disease

survived cooking germinate, and clostridia grow to sufficient numbers to constitute an infectious inoculum.

Pathophysiology Ingestion of live organisms is required to produce disease, but illness is not caused by infection; rather, it is from an enterotoxin produced by sporulation of the organism in the GI tract. The enterotoxin is responsible for all the symptoms of *C. perfringens* food poisoning.

Clinical Presentation Symptoms usually appear within 6 to 12 hours but can occur up to 24 hours after ingestion of the contaminated food. Frequent, watery diarrhea and moderately severe abdominal cramping are the major symptoms. Fever, nausea, and vomiting are rare. The illness is self-limited and rarely lasts for more than 24 hours.

C. perfringens food poisoning should be considered in a patient who has an acute onset of abdominal cramps and diarrhea shortly after eating a suspect meat or poultry dish and when others who ate the same meal are similarly ill. Leukocytes and erythrocytes are not present on stool examination.

Complications A rare type of *Clostridium* food poisoning, termed *enteritis necroticans,* occurs after the ingestion of foods heavily contaminated with the type C strain of *C. perfringens.* The illness is characterized by an acute onset of severe abdominal pain, vomiting, diarrhea, prostration, and shock and may be rapidly fatal. Postmortem examination reveals a diffuse, hemorrhagic, necrotizing enteritis of the jejunum, ileum, and colon.

Management Occasionally a patient will need IV fluid replacement. Antibiotics are of no value because of the natural history of the disease. Food poisoning from *C. perfringens* can be prevented by avoiding long periods of warming or cooling of foods that have already been cooked.

Bacillus cereus Food Poisoning

Epidemiology *Bacillus cereus* is an aerobic, spore-forming, gram-positive rod that is a common cause of food-borne illness. The organism is ubiquitous in soil and in raw, dried, and processed food. As with other bacterial pathogens commonly isolated from raw foodstuffs and the environment, the disease is associated with improper food handling.[8]

B. cereus causes two distinct clinical syndromes: an emetic form produced by a heat-stable, staphylococcal-like enterotoxin and a diarrheal form resulting from a heat-labile enterotoxin similar to that of *E. coli.* The emetic form is almost always caused by the ingestion of contaminated fried rice; the diarrheal syndrome is usually associated with meats or vegetables.[3,42]

Pathophysiology *B. cereus* is found in uncooked rice. Its heat-resistant spores survive boiling and then germinate when boiled rice is left unrefrigerated (a common practice in Chinese restaurants to avoid clumping of grain). The vegetative forms then multiply and produce toxin. Flash frying or brief rewarming before serving is often not sufficient to destroy the preformed, heat-stable toxin. Spores also survive cooking, and if the food is left sitting at room temperature, they will germinate. The vegetative forms then grow and produce toxin.

Clinical Presentation The emetic syndrome is clinically indistinguishable from that caused by staphylococcal enterotoxin. After an incubation period of 2 to 3 hours, profound vomiting and abdominal cramping occur in all patients. Diarrhea is present in approximately 25% to 30% of persons affected. The duration is short, usually less than 10 hours, and patients recover uneventfully.

The diarrheal syndrome begins after an incubation time of 6 to 14 hours and is characterized by diarrhea in all patients and by abdominal cramps in approximately 75%. Vomiting occurs in only 20% of cases. The duration of illness ranges from 20 to 36 hours. Symptoms are essentially the same as for food poisoning produced by *C. perfringens,* although vomiting is even less common with *C. perfringens.*

B. cereus food poisoning should be suspected in two clinical scenarios: first, whenever an illness predominantly found in the upper GI tract that is similar to staphylococcal food poisoning develops less than 6 hours after eating fried rice, and second, whenever a predominantly lower intestinal tract illness occurs 6 to 24 hours after a suspect meal, usually of meats or vegetables.

Diagnostic Strategies Isolation of 10^5 or more organisms from incriminated foods confirms the diagnosis. Stool cultures are sometimes positive, but the organisms can also be present in the stools of healthy persons.[42]

Management Both syndromes are generally mild and self-limited. Antibiotics are not indicated because symptoms are mediated by enterotoxins. Parenteral antiemetics effectively comfort patients presenting with violent vomiting. *B. cereus* food poisoning is preventable if boiled rice and other cooked foods are promptly eaten or refrigerated and not left to sit at room temperature.

Cholera and Noncholera Vibrios

Epidemiology Other halophilic marine *Vibrio* species in addition to *V. parahaemolyticus* have shown a dramatic increase as a cause for acute gastroenteritis associated with seafood. Their epidemiology is identical to that of *V. parahaemolyticus:* ubiquitous in coastal seawater, outbreaks associated with the eating of raw or inadequately cooked shellfish, and an incidence markedly limited to the warmer months of the year.[24] Outbreaks of true cholera continue to occur sporadically along the gulf coast of the United States from inadequately cooked crabs or oysters.[24] Cholera outbreaks in South America and India have led to an increasing number of cases of cholera imported into the United States.[43]

Pathophysiology The difference between these species and *V. parahaemolyticus* lies in their mechanism of pathogenesis. *V. parahaemolyticus* produces disease directly by an invasive intestinal infection, whereas these strains produce an enterotoxin in vivo that is responsible for the diarrhea. Therefore symptoms resemble other forms of enterotoxin-induced gastroenteritis, not those caused by invasive pathogens. The enterotoxin of the noncholera vibrio is antigenically similar to *V. cholerae* enterotoxin and produces a similar diarrheal illness, although much less severe.[24]

Clinical Presentation Patients experience copious watery diarrhea, abdominal cramps, and often nausea and vomiting within 24 to 48 hours after ingesting contaminated seafood. Almost half lose enough fluids to require hospitalization. A low-grade fever may occur. The median duration of illness is approximately 7 days, quite unlike the 1- to 2-day course of *V. parahaemolyticus.*[24]

Another *Vibrio* species, *Vibrio vulnificus,* can produce an invasive gastroenteritis. *V. vulnificus* is also associated with eating raw seafood, especially raw oysters. Septicemia is common, and mortality approaches 50% in patients with significant underlying diseases, particularly chronic liver disease.[27,28] Physicians should advise all patients with chronic liver disease, alcoholism, AIDS, other immunodeficiency states, and any significant chronic disease to avoid all raw shellfish.[27,28]

Diagnostic Strategies Because these are noninvasive vibrios, unlike *V. parahaemolyticus,* stained fecal smears will not show leukocytes or erythrocytes. Stool cultures will quickly identify the organisms if plated on appropriate TCBS medium.

Management Most patients will lose enough fluids to require rehydration therapy. The World Health Organization (WHO) oral rehydration formula has been used successfully to treat cholera worldwide.[43] In the ED, use of either oral or IV fluid hydration is dictated by the clinical picture. The role of antibiotics in the treatment of intestinal infections caused by noncholera vibrios is not clearly established. However, appropriate antibiotics, particularly tetracyclines, have been shown to decrease both the severity and the duration of cholera and may have the same effect on the diarrheal disease caused by these marine vibrios.[24] Prevention, as with *V. parahaemolyticus,* depends on proper handling and avoidance of inadequately cooked seafood.

Scombroid Fish Poisoning

Epidemiology Scombroid fish poisoning is a growing problem in the United States. The disease takes its name from the suborder Scombroid (e.g., tuna, mackerel, and related species) and results from the ingestion of a wide variety of dark-meat fish. The fish species most commonly implicated are mahimahi, tuna, and bluefish.[44] Restaurants serve these fish under various names such as mackerel, swordfish, bonito, dolphin, amberjack, or the generic "tuna salad sandwich."

Most cases occur in Hawaii and Florida, followed by California, New York, Washington, and Connecticut. However, scombroid poisoning can occur in any location where "fresh fish" are flown in on a regular basis.[45]

Pathophysiology Scombroid fish poisoning results from the ingestion of heat-stable toxins produced by bacterial action on the dark meat of the fish. The responsible bacteria are normal constituents of the surface marine flora of the fish rather than contaminants. The histidine decarboxylase activity of these organisms produces histamine and histamine-like substances, which cause the symptoms of scombroid fish poisoning. High levels of histamine in the fish correlate directly with the occurrence of the illness. Formation of the scombrotoxins is directly related to improper preservation and refrigeration of the fish from the time they are caught until the time they are cooked. Generally, the problem is caused by improper refrigeration by the supplier, rather than the fault of the restaurant serving the fish.[45]

Clinical Presentation The symptoms of scombroid fish poisoning resemble histamine intoxication. While eating the fish, the patient may note a metallic, bitter, or peppery taste. Symptoms usually develop abruptly within 20 to 30 minutes and consist of facial flushing; diarrhea; severe, throbbing headache; palpitations; and abdominal cramps. Sometimes dizziness, dry mouth, nausea, vomiting, and urticaria also occur. The facial flushing resembles a sunburn and can extend over the entire skin surface. The conjunctivae are usually injected. The duration of the major symptom complex is generally less than 6 hours, and although weakness and fatigue persist longer, the clinical course is usually benign. The attack rate is very high; most persons sharing the same toxic fish will become ill.[45]

Management Parenteral antihistamine therapy, such as diphenhydramine, 50 mg, or cimetidine, 300 mg, intramuscular (IM) or IV, usually promptly relieves all symptoms. Rarely, IV fluids are necessary. The disease is preventable if fish are properly handled, especially if they are refrigerated early and adequately.[46] This is not an allergic reaction, so patients should not be told they are allergic to these fish, nor should they be prohibited from eating them again in the future.

Ciguatera Fish Poisoning

Epidemiology Ciguatera fish poisoning is a common public health problem, with appreciable economic significance. It is endemic in tropical regions—especially the Caribbean and the Indo-Pacific islands—but is found worldwide. It is responsible for more than half of all fish-related food poisonings in the United States.[2,4] Fish caught around Hawaii and Florida cause the most cases, but because the responsible ocean fish are now commonly transported inland, cases may be seen virtually anywhere in the country.[47]

Ciguatoxin is produced by the marine dinoflagellate—a unicellular plankton—*Gambierdiscus toxicus,* which attaches itself to marine algae and is passed up the food chain. The lipid-soluble toxin accumulates in the tissues of the larger predacious coral-reef fish, with the highest concentrations in the viscera and roe. It does not affect the fish in any way. Only humans suffer its ill effects—part of the price we pay for our privileged position at the top of the food chain.

More than 400 fish species that frequent coral reefs have been implicated as ciguatoxin carriers, but fewer than 50 are commercially important species. Red snapper, grouper, amberjack, barracuda, sea bass, sturgeon, jack tuna, king mackerel, and moray eels are the most common carriers.[48,49]

Pathophysiology Ciguatera fish poisoning results from the ingestion of a neurotoxin called *ciguatoxin.* Ciguatoxin is heat and acid stable, odorless, and tasteless. It is not deactivated by cooking or freezing, nor is it eliminated by drying, salting, smoking, marinating, or pickling. No one is able to tell whether a fish contains sufficient amounts of the toxin to produce illness.[48-50] Ciguatoxin has both anticholinesterase and cholinergic properties, but its toxicity is probably due to its inhibition of calcium regulation, through the passive cell membrane sodium channels.[48]

Clinical Presentation Ciguatera fish poisoning is most commonly seen in the spring and summer months. The incubation period is generally short, approximately 2 to 6 hours, but a delay of 12 to 24 hours is not unusual. Attack rates are very high; 80% to 90% of those exposed become ill. Symptoms tend to be related to the amount of toxin ingested and vary considerably in their severity. A person who has recently ingested ciguatoxin is likely to have much more serious symptoms from a second exposure.[48-50]

Classically, patients develop both GI and neurologic symptoms. The GI symptoms (e.g., nausea, vomiting, profuse watery diarrhea, crampy abdominal pain, and diaphoresis) tend to appear earlier. The panoply of neurologic symptoms consists largely of dysesthesias and paresthesias around the throat and the perioral area; "burning feet," which may resemble alcoholic peripheral neuropathy; "loose, painful teeth"; and sometimes CNS changes, such as ataxia, weakness, vertigo, visual hallucinations, and even confusion and coma.[49,51]

One symptom highly suggestive of ciguatera fish poisoning is sensory reversal dysesthesia, in which cold objects are perceived to be warm and vice versa. Patients describe such distortion of temperature perception very vividly. Another classic feature is either a return or a worsening of the symptoms after ingestion of alcohol.[48-50]

Ciguatera poisoning lasts an average of 1 to 2 weeks, but at least half of its victims are still symptomatic at 8 weeks. The neurologic symptoms, particularly the paresthesias and dysesthesias, tend to persist longer than the GI symptoms and have been reported up to years later. It can be a chronic, nagging problem.

Differential Considerations Ciguatera fish poisoning should be strongly considered in patients with a combination of GI and neurologic symptoms, particularly dysesthesias. Sensory reversal dysesthesia and marked worsening of the symptoms with alcohol ingestion are highly suggestive of ciguatera toxicity.

The disease is sometimes misdiagnosed as acute gastroenteritis with "hyperventilation syndrome" because of the combination of GI symptoms and paresthesias, particularly when they occur about the mouth and acral areas. Similarly, ciguatera toxicity has sometimes been ascribed to malingering because the paresthesias are often transient and vague and lack traditional dermatome patterns.

Other disorders that should be considered include paralytic or neurotoxic shellfish poisoning, eosinophilic meningitis, botulism, organophosphate insecticide poisoning, and tetrodotoxin poisoning.[47,48]

Management Treatment of ciguatera fish poisoning is primarily supportive. IV fluids are given to replace volume losses from vomiting and diarrhea, and analgesics are given as needed. In severe cases, the toxin may display some anticholinesterase activity, manifested as bradycardia and hypotension, which can be treated with atropine and dopamine. Patients must be told to abstain from alcohol of any kind until all symptoms even possibly related to the toxicity have completely resolved.

Pruritus may be managed with an H_1 antagonist such as terfenadine at a dosage of 60 mg bid. Amitriptyline, 25 mg bid, can bring about a rather dramatic reduction in both the pruritus and the dysesthesias, two of the most disturbing and protracted symptoms.

Dramatic recovery from ciguatera fish poisoning has been reported after the use of IV mannitol, 1 g/kg of a 20% solution infused over 30 minutes.[49,51] In all the patients, CNS manifestations were markedly reduced within minutes after mannitol infusion. These reports are as yet empirical and uncontrolled, and the mechanism of action is unclear; nevertheless, the use of mannitol should be considered in patients who are seriously ill from ciguatera fish poisoning.[49,51]

Enterotoxigenic *Escherichia coli*

Epidemiology Enterotoxin-producing *E. coli* is recognized as a major cause of acute diarrheal disease throughout most of the world. In some U.S. cities, enterotoxin-producing *E. coli* has been responsible for 60% to 80% of moderate to severe cases of pediatric diarrheal disease. It is also a major cause of diarrhea in adults, particularly in persons traveling to underdeveloped areas, such as Mexico, the Middle East, Asia, and parts of the Mediterranean. The disease has been most intensely studied in North American visitors to Mexico, where it occurs in 40% to 60% of travelers studied, often incapacitating them or forcing a change in their plans (see section on traveler's diarrhea later in this chapter).[52]

Infection is acquired from contaminated food or drink. Unpeeled fruits, leafy vegetables, unsanitary drinking water, and the most deceitful vehicle—ice prepared from impure water—are the most common sources. Most tourists are rather careful about their food and drink, although there seems to be a poor correlation between individual eating habits and the incidence of traveler's diarrhea.[53]

Pathophysiology For an *E. coli* strain to cause diarrhea, it must possess both a surface factor that allows colonization (although not invasion) of the small intestine and the ability to secrete an enterotoxin that causes the outpouring of fluids and electrolytes into the small bowel lumen. The enterotoxin-induced secretion occurs in the absence of any demonstrable histologic damage to intestinal epithelial cells or to the capillary endothelial cells.[2]

E. coli produces both heat-labile and heat-stable toxins. The heat-labile enterotoxin causes the secretion of water and electrolytes into the intestinal lumen by the stimulation of adenyl cyclase, which results in an increase in cyclic adenosine monophosphate (cAMP). The heat-stable toxin probably exerts its effect through the stimulation of guanylate cyclase in mucosal cells and tends to have a more rapid onset of action. Either or both toxins may be produced by any enterotoxic strain of *E. coli.* The intestinal fluid losses are qualitatively identical to those in cholera and other toxigenic diarrheas.[2]

Clinical Presentation After an incubation period of 24 to 72 hours, an abrupt onset of watery diarrhea follows. Severity varies from a fulminant, cholera-like disease to the much more common and milder "turista," in which the symptoms of mild, watery diarrhea and abdominal cramps are more troublesome than life threatening. Fever is unusual. Vomiting occurs in fewer than half of the adults and is seldom responsible for significant fluid losses. Even in severe cases, the diarrhea seldom lasts longer than 48 to 72 hours, and the response to either oral or IV fluids is uniformly good. Milder disease generally subsides more gradually, occasionally persisting for 1 week or longer.

E. coli enterotoxin–induced disease should be suspected when a child or adult has frequent, watery diarrhea and little other symptoms. Most often it is passed off as "mild, nonspecific gastroenteritis," and resolves spontaneously. Anyone who acquires toxigenic diarrhea while visiting a developing nation probably has this disease. *E. coli* is by far the most common cause of traveler's diarrhea.

Diagnostic Strategies No easy, rapid means of laboratory diagnosis of enteropathogenic *E. coli* exists because *E. coli* is part of the normal colonic flora, and its ability to produce enterotoxin is not restricted to any specific serotype. Stool preparations show no erythrocytes or leukocytes.

Clostridium difficile Antibiotic–Associated Enterocolitis

Epidemiology Severe colitis can occur with the oral or parenteral administration of several antimicrobial drugs, particularly clindamycin. Other antibiotics that have been associated with colitis include lincomycin, ampicillin, cephalosporins, tetracycline, penicillin, chloramphenicol, sulfa products, and erythromycin. *Clostridium difficile,* a toxin-producing bacterium, is the cause of antibiotic-induced colitis. It occurs primarily in adults. Patients with constipation and those treated with constipating agents, especially diphenoxylate hydrochloride (Lomotil), or narcotics are particularly prone to developing antibiotic-associated colitis (AAC). These conditions favor multiplication of the clostridia and a buildup of toxin in the colon.[54]

Many if not most cases of *C. difficile* colitis are of nosocomial origin, transmitted among hospitalized patients by the hands of hospital personnel or from patient to patient. Up to 20% of inpatients acquire the organism, although only about a third become symptomatic.[54,55] Some nosocomial infections occur even in the absence of antibiotic therapy.[56]

Pathophysiology The disease is unique in that an organism normally found in the colon causes illness only after the administration of antimicrobial agents. *C. difficile* proliferate when the normal bowel flora is substantially reduced by antibiotic therapy. The organisms must then produce sufficient quantities of a cytopathic toxin for the disease to occur. This cytopathic toxin destroys the colonic mucosa rather than inducing the secretion of fluids and electrolytes as occurs with other types of toxin-induced diarrhea.[55]

The mucosa becomes hyperemic and edematous. Raised, yellowish-white plaques, loosely adherent to the mucosa, occur in patches, primarily in the rectosigmoid area, but can occur in any part of the colon. The disease was named *pseudomembranous enterocolitis* because of these pseudomembrane-like plaques.

Clinical Presentation Symptoms may appear during the course of antimicrobial therapy or sometimes up to 3 or 4 weeks after discontinuation of antibiotics. Because the toxin alters the intestinal mucosa, the illness presents more like an invasive diarrhea than a toxigenic one. Typically, patients have fever, crampy abdominal pain, and watery, sometimes bloody, diarrhea. Fecal leukocytes are generally, but not invariably, present. Children tend to have more severe infections than adults. The disease continues to have a significant mortality.[7,56]

Diagnostic Strategies Stool tissue culture toxin assays are the primary method to diagnose *C. difficile* infection.[54,55,57] Although quite sensitive and specific, they require 48 to 72 hours for completion. Stool cultures can confirm the presence of *C. difficile* in the feces of patients with AAC. However, a positive stool culture is not diagnostic because *C. difficile* is often present in the feces of normal subjects or in persons receiving antibiotics who do not have an enteritis. Cultures are seldom used clinically, but are often part of epidemiologic studies.[54,55] In patients with a typical history and physical findings, a tentative diagnosis can be made by sigmoidoscopy or colonoscopy.

Differential Considerations It is important to differentiate diarrhea with colitis from simple antibiotic-associated diarrhea. Simple antibiotic-induced diarrhea is common. From 3% to 10% of all patients treated with antibiotics, particularly children, develop diarrhea. These patients experience mild, watery diarrhea and no associated constitutional symptoms or evidence of a cytopathic toxin-induced colitis.

Management Many cases of antibiotic-associated colitis are self-limited, provided that the offending agent is discontinued. When stopping the antibiotic does not resolve the diarrhea, or when it is severe, empiric antibiotic treatment should be started promptly to eradicate *C. difficile*. Either oral metronidazole or oral vancomycin may be used to treat *C. difficile* colitis. The dosage of metronidazole is 250 mg PO qid for 10 to 14 days. Metronidazole is also effective when administered intravenously. The dose of vancomycin is 125 to 250 mg PO qid for 10 to 14 days, except in critically ill patients, for whom the recommended dosage is 500 mg PO qid for 10 to 14 days.[5,54,55] Patients significantly ill with colitis should be admitted to the hospital and started on both IV metronidazole and oral vancomycin.[56]

Vancomycin is generally not effective if given intravenously because it does not reach effective intraluminal concentrations. Because vancomycin is much more expensive than metronidazole and both seem to be equally effective, oral vancomycin is reserved for patients who do not respond to metronidazole therapy or for those who are extremely ill at the time of presentation.

Patients generally become afebrile and show clinical improvement within 36 to 72 hours, and the diarrhea resolves over 5 to 7 days, even though toxin assays and stool cultures may remain positive for weeks. From 5% to 55% (average 25%) of patients suffer a relapse regardless of the antibiotic chosen, its dosage, or the duration of treatment. Nearly all of these patients will respond to another course of antibiotic therapy.[5,55]

Adding the yeast *Saccharomyces boulardii,* 500 mg PO bid for 4 weeks, to antibiotic treatment dramatically decreased the number of recurrences of *C. difficile*–associated disease in patients with previous episodes. However, no benefit results when *S. boulardii* is given to patients with an initial episode.[5,58] No serious adverse reactions have occurred with the use of *S. boulardii.*[58]

Although toxicity from parenteral vancomycin is common, no adverse effects have been reported with its *oral* use in the treatment of *C. difficile* colitis. Antimotility or constipating agents are contraindicated in these patients because of the risk of toxic megacolon and the possibility of increasing the level of cytopathic toxin in the colon.

ACUTE VIRAL GASTROENTERITIS

Etiology and Epidemiology

Viral gastroenteritis is the second leading cause of illness in the United States. Parvovirus-like agents such as the Norwalk virus are primarily responsible for disease in adults and older children, whereas human reovirus-like agents, also called *rotaviruses,* cause most diarrheal disease in infants and young children. Rotaviruses also cause epidemics in adults, especially those in contact with sick children, such as parents and hospital personnel.[59,60]

The attack rates for both infections may reach 50%, and the incubation period is short, so explosive outbreaks are common. Transmission of viral gastroenteritis is generally from person to person by the fecal-oral route, but water- or food-borne outbreaks are also common. Large outbreaks of Norwalk virus have occurred from municipal or semipublic water sources, recreational swimming, stored water on cruise ships, cafeteria sandwiches, food handlers, or shellfish.[61] The ingestion of raw oysters has caused many large outbreaks.[61] Nosocomial spread of infection is also common.[62]

Other enteric viruses, such as astrovirus and picornaviruses, are common causes of diarrhea in HIV-infected patients.[60,63]

Pathophysiology

Viruses distort the absorptive cells of the microvilli of the small bowel, decreasing their absorptive surface and causing diarrhea from decreased absorption of fluid and electrolytes. The histologic picture resembles tropical sprue, and, indeed, transient malabsorption of fats and sugars occurs in patients with viral gastroenteritis, which may persist for a week or more after infection.[60]

Virus-induced diarrheal stools contain more sodium, chloride, and bicarbonate than normal stools, but this is not comparable to the almost isotonic fluid loss of bacterial toxin–induced diarrhea. Potassium loss is usually not significant unless symptoms are prolonged.

Clinical Presentation

Viral gastroenteritis occurs primarily in two epidemiologically distinct clinical forms. Outbreaks caused by rotaviruses are usually sporadic, occasionally epidemic, and typically occur in the winter months in infants and children 6 to 24 months of age. The incubation period is 24 to 72 hours, followed by an abrupt onset of vomiting, watery diarrhea, and low-grade fever, but little or no associated abdominal pain. Vomiting is a prominent and constant early manifestation of rotavirus enteritis but rarely persists beyond the first 36 hours. The diarrhea generally lasts for 4 to 7 days and may be followed by steatorrhea in approximately 20% to 40% of patients. A number of children have significant dehydration requiring hospitalization and IV fluid replacement, but the disease is rarely life threatening.

Overt clinical disease may occur among family and adult contacts of ill children, but it is uncommon. Studies show that most adults with rotavirus infections are asymptomatic. When symptoms do occur, they are usually mild, perhaps because these episodes are reinfections as 60% to 90% of older children and adults have antibodies to rotaviruses (see also Chapter 124).[59,60]

The second clinical entity is characteristically epidemic and is responsible for family and community-wide outbreaks of gastroenteritis among school-age children, family contacts, and adults. This form is generally caused by the Norwalk virus. After an incubation period of 20 to 36 hours, diarrhea, nausea, and mild abdominal cramps occur. Vomiting is not prominent. Fever is generally absent. Anorexia, headache, malaise, and myalgias may be present. The illness is self-limited, usually lasting only 24 to 48 hours. Generally, most adults have mild symptoms, and most do not seek medical attention.[59,60]

Diagnostic Strategies

The diagnosis of rotavirus gastroenteritis should be entertained in children with significant vomiting, diarrhea, low-grade fever, moderate dehydration, and a normal WBC count, especially in those 6 to 24 months old who become symptomatic during the winter months. An elevated BUN value and a compensated metabolic acidosis are common findings. Serum electrolyte determinations demonstrate that the dehydration is usually isotonic.

In adults the diagnosis of viral gastroenteritis is usually one of exclusion. The physician diagnoses viral enteritis when a patient has mild intestinal symptoms, does not appear ill, and further history and physical examination uncover no reason to suspect a bacterial pathogen, inflammatory disease, or any other etiology. No investigation beyond the physical examination is done, and the patient is sent home with appropriate instructions. Some of these patients may have mild bacterial infections, but these are also generally self-limited, and treatment is not different.

A laboratory diagnosis can be made by demonstration of the viruses in stools by electron microscopy or various methods used for the detection of viral antigens, such as counterimmunoelectrophoresis or enzyme-linked immunoabsorbent assay. In rotavirus illness, because of the huge numbers of viruses present in the stools, these antigen-detection methods are quite sensitive and specific, in addition to being the most practical for the average hospital laboratory. Rotazyme testing is probably indicated only in more serious cases of diarrhea. Fecal leukocytes and erythrocytes are not found in viral gastroenteritis.[60]

Management

The most important aspect of therapy for acute viral gastroenteritis is fluid replacement. Many children require hospitalization, with IV fluid and electrolyte repletion. After vomiting subsides, this can generally be achieved by the oral route. No specific antiviral therapy is indicated. Antidiarrheal agents are not recommended in children. In adults they are generally not needed but may be comforting. Because spread is primarily by the fecal-oral route, scrupulous hand washing and other hygienic practices are the best preventive measures.

PROTOZOAN GASTROINTESTINAL INFECTION (Table 89-4)

Coccidia: *Cryptosporidium* and *Isospora belli*

Epidemiology *Cryptosporidium* and *Isospora* are intestinal protozoan parasites that commonly cause diarrhea in the young of many animal species such as cattle, lambs, pigs, goats, cats, dogs, chickens, and birds. In humans, cryptosporidiosis is a worldwide problem, most often seen in persons who handle animals, children in daycare centers, healthy male homosexuals, and immunocompromised patients.[64,65] *Cryptosporidium* is the most common cause of chronic

Table 89-4. Epidemiologic Aspects of Protozoan Gastroenteritis

Pathogen	Sources	Incubation period (I)	Features
Entamoeba histolytica	Fecally contaminated food and water sources	3 wk to 4 mo	Infection may be commensal or intermittently symptomatic or produce severe dysentery
Giardia lamblia	Water-borne, fecal-oral, day care centers, travelers, backpackers, AIDS, male homosexuals	1-3 wk	5%-10% of U.S. population, malabsorption syndromes or commensal
Coccidia			
Cryptosporidium and *Isospora*	Fecal-oral, water-borne, animals, day care centers, AIDS	5-10 days	Profuse watery diarrhea, self-limited in the immunocompetent, persistent in the immunocompromised
Cyclospora cayetanensis	Fresh fruit, berries, lettuce, water supply	1 wk	Explosive, protracted, watery diarrhea; fatigue, weight loss
Strongyloides stercoralis	Occupational exposure to soil, travel to endemic areas in United States (Kentucky, Tennessee, Ohio) or overseas	Weeks to months	Eosinophilia, sepsis, and hyperinfection syndrome in AIDS patients
Enteromonas hominis	Fecal-oral, male homosexuals	?	Chronic watery diarrhea, especially in children

diarrhea in persons with AIDS.[15,16] Congenital immunodeficiency and treatment with cancer chemotherapeutics or other immunosuppressive drugs are also predisposing factors. The organism is highly infectious and is easily transmitted from person to person. Nosocomial spread, household contact infections, and large outbreaks in daycare centers or in other facilities where personal hygiene is poor occur commonly.[65] In addition to zoonotic spread and person-to-person spread, indirect transmission occurs by exposure to fecally contaminated environmental surfaces, toys, food, and recreational water venues such as community swimming pools, water parks, decorative fountains, hot tubs, and spas.[19] *Cryptosporidium* oocysts are highly resistant to chlorine and common disinfectants. Large outbreaks of cryptosporidiosis have originated from community swimming pools.[66]

The oocysts are also small (2 to 6 μm) and may not be removed from contaminated water by standard filtration systems used in the treatment of public water supplies.[67] Thirteen thousand cases of cryptosporidiosis caused by contamination of a filtered public water system occurred in one Georgia city, and an estimated 400,000 people became ill in Milwaukee in 1993, also from a municipal water supply, even though the treated water met federal and state standards for drinking water.[67,68] Contamination of rivers and streams by *Cryptosporidium* has been reported in a number of states.[12] In children, cryptosporidiosis is more common in the late summer and early fall and is often associated with intestinal infection from other organisms, particularly *Giardia.*

Isosporiasis is generally an opportunistic infection. It occurs primarily in patients with AIDS, especially Haitians with AIDS, and in homosexual men. In the homosexual community, isosporiasis is a sexually transmitted disease similar to giardiasis and amebiasis.[69,70]

Pathophysiology The pathophysiology is the same for both coccidial organisms. Disease is acquired by ingestion of oocysts. Excystation occurs, and the trophozoites and all other developmental stages are found only at the surface of the intestinal epithelial membranes. Infection is noninvasive; no tissue phase exists. Profuse fluid loss results from a combination of enterotoxin-induced secretions and malabsorption. In cryptosporidiosis, a biliary reservoir may contribute to the chronicity of the infection and the inability to eradicate the organism.[65]

Clinical Presentation The clinical presentations of cryptosporidiosis and isosporiasis are indistinguishable. After an incubation period of approximately 1 week, symptoms may develop insidiously or suddenly. Infection is characterized by profuse watery diarrhea, crampy abdominal pain, anorexia, nausea, malaise, weight loss, and flatulence. The diarrhea and abdominal pain are often exacerbated by eating. Immunocompromised patients can have enormous stool fluid losses: 3 to 4 L/day is common, and losses may reach 10 to 20 L/day. Physical examination usually reveals only signs of dehydration. Minimal diffuse abdominal tenderness may be present, but fever and leukocytosis are uncommon. Eosinophilia does not occur. Stool examinations for blood or fecal leukocytes are almost uniformly negative in adults but occasionally are positive in children.[19,23,65]

The patient's immune status is the primary determinant of whether the infection is self-limited or persistent. Diarrhea in immunocompetent persons usually resolves after 1 to 3 weeks, but it can continue longer or become chronic. In immunodeficient patients, especially those with AIDS, chronic, persistent diarrhea is the rule rather than the exception, causing significant discomfort and morbidity unless the infection is responsive to treatment.[15,16,70]

Asymptomatic infections can occur from either *Cryptosporidium* or *Isospora,* and a carrier state has been demonstrated for *Cryptosporidium.*[70] In one U.S. study of immunocompetent patients who underwent upper endoscopy for a variety of reasons, 13% were found to harbor cryptosporidia in the second portion of the duodenum. None of the patients had diarrhea.[71]

Diagnostic Strategies The diagnosis of either coccidial infection is made by documenting the oocysts in the stool. Acid-fast stains are the current preferred method; they are fast, simple, inexpensive, and reliable. Yeast are morphologically similar to coccidia but are not acid fast. Patients with diarrhea from *Cryptosporidium* generally excrete large numbers of oocysts continually, so the organism can be readily identified in the stools by experienced examiners. *Isospora* oocysts, however, may be shed only intermittently and in much smaller numbers, so multiple stool samples often must be obtained and concentrated to successfully identify this parasite.[69,72]

Management In immunocompetent persons, *Cryptosporidium* infection is generally self-limited; symptomatic therapy and fluid replacement are all that is necessary. No proven effective antibiotic treatment has been found for cryptosporidiosis.[5,65,73]

Immunocompetent patients shed the infective oocysts in the stools when symptomatic and continue shedding oocysts after resolution of their clinical illness for 2 to 3 weeks, sometimes for 4 to 6 weeks, creating obvious infection-control problems.[64]

Treatment of cryptosporidiosis in immunocompromised patients is usually ineffective. The most successful interventions occur when the underlying immunodeficiency can be reversed. Patients taking immunosuppressant agents (e.g., prednisone, cyclophosphamide, or cancer chemotherapeutic drugs) generally recover if the drugs can be discontinued. Patients with AIDS usually continue to have significant watery diarrhea until death. Prostaglandin inhibitors, such as indomethacin, may decrease the secretory diarrhea.[74] Zidovudine (azidothymidine, or AZT) is probably the best treatment for *Cryptosporidium* diarrhea in patients with AIDS because it directly enhances host immunity by suppression of HIV replication.[65] Patients severely infected with *Cryptosporidium* are often incontinent and have large numbers of infectious oocysts in their feces, so strict enteric precautions are necessary to prevent nosocomial spread. Paromomycin (Humatin, 500 to 750 mg PO tid or qid) sometimes ameliorates cryptosporidiosis, particularly in combination with azithromycin, but no good evidence exists that any drug is routinely effective.[5,73,75,76]

Isosporiasis, in marked contrast to cryptosporidiosis, responds promptly to antibiotic therapy. The treatment of choice for isosporiasis is TMP-SMX 160 mg/800 mg PO qid for 10 days, then bid for 3 weeks. In patients with sulfonamide sensitivity, as is common in AIDS patients, pyrimethamine, 50 to 75 mg PO daily, may be effective.[69]

Chronic suppressive therapy with either twice daily doses of TMP-SMX or daily doses of pyrimethamine is often required because *Isospora* infection recurs in more than 50% of patients.[69,70]

Patients seen in the ED whose examination for parasites later reveals *Cryptosporidium* or *Isospora* should be contacted. Recovering patients need only have the diagnosis and its ramifications explained to them. Patients who are not recovering, and those who are known or thought to be immunosuppressed, should have appropriate treatment and follow-up arranged.

Coccidia: *Cyclospora cayetanensis*

Epidemiology *Cyclospora* is a coccidian parasite widely distributed throughout the world that produces disease very similar to *Cryptosporidium* and *Isospora.* It is acquired from contaminated foods, primarily fresh fruit, raspberries and other berries, lettuce, and contaminated water supplies.[77-79] It is occasionally the cause of traveler's diarrhea. It infects all classes of vertebrates, reptiles, and rodents, and the vast majority of cases occur during the spring and summer seasons, often in large outbreaks.[76,79] The average incubation period is 1 week.[80]

Pathophysiology The exact mode of *Cyclospora* transmission and mechanism of disease is not well elucidated. The organism is ingested in the oocyst stage, sporulates in the gut, and produces an explosive watery diarrhea. The histological picture looks similar to tropical sprue, but it is unknown if symptoms are toxin induced or secondary to direct infection of the small bowel.[80]

Clinical Presentation Typically the patient presents with an acute onset of explosive watery diarrhea and abdominal cramps. Constitutional symptoms are relatively mild, and fever is uncommon.

The disease is generally self-limited in immunocompetent hosts, but tends to be prolonged, frequently 2 to 3 weeks in duration, and relapsing diarrhea is common. Sustained fatigue and weight loss are common.[77,79,80]

Diagnostic Strategies The clinical picture may be suggestive, but finding the oocysts in the stools confirms the diagnosis. Fecal leukocytes are absent. The oocysts measure 8 to 10 μm in diameter, and are extraordinarily difficult to distinguish from *Cryptosporidium.* In fact, the CDC will not accept the diagnosis unless confirmation is made by an experienced reference laboratory. In some studies the disease was misdiagnosed in up to 70% of cases, creating "pseudo-outbreaks." Health departments that identify *Cyclospora* infection should contact the CDC's Parasitic Division for confirmation.[77,78]

Differential Considerations The primary confusing organism is *cryptosporidium* because the symptoms of the two entities are often indistinguishable. *Cryptosporidium* tends to be associated with animal contact, day care centers, or immunocompromised patients. *Isospora* and *Aeromonas hydrophila* infections should also be considered in the differential.

Management The disease tends to be self-limited in immunocompetent persons, but treatment with sulfa medications is very effective for cyclosporiasis, unlike treatment for cryptosporidiosis.

The drug of choice is TMP/SMX DS, 1 tablet po bid for 7 days in immunocompetent patients, and 1 tablet po qid for 10 days, then 1 tablet po three times per week in AIDS patients. The children's dose is TMP 5 mg/kg plus SMX 25 mg/kg bid for 7 days. Thorough washing of fresh produce before consumption decreases, but does not eliminate, the risk of transmission. Irradiation may be the future solution.[5,77,78,80]

Giardiasis

Epidemiology *Giardia* is the most common cause of water-borne diarrheal outbreaks in the United States.[23,72,81] Community-wide epidemics have closed down ski resorts in Colorado and affected entire towns. The mode of transmission in such cases is contamination of municipal water supplies with cyst-infested feces from humans or animals, particularly beavers or muskrats, but also dogs, raccoons, and other animals. Campers and backpackers in the mountainous West, especially the Rocky Mountains or northern Cascades, commonly acquire giardiasis, called "backpackers diarrhea," from drinking fecally contaminated water from the "pristine mountain streams."[72] Only rarely is *Giardia* infection communicated by contaminated food.

Giardia may be spread by sexual or other close person-to-person contact in which fecal contamination may occur, particularly among homosexual men, and in day care centers and institutions for the mentally retarded. The prevalence of *Giardia* is 5% to 10% in the general U.S. population, 5% to 25% in homosexual men, and 25% to 30% in children in day care centers.[72]

Many cases of acute symptomatic giardiasis in the United States are found in persons returning home from travel elsewhere. Travelers to any underdeveloped country can acquire giardiasis, but it is especially common in those who visit the republics of the former Soviet Union, the Caribbean states, and Latin America, where the water supplies appear to be heavily contaminated with *Giardia* cysts.[52] Visitors to the former Soviet Union, particularly the city of Leningrad, experience attack rates approaching 60%, the disease ruefully known among its victims as "the Trotskys."[82,83]

Patients with decreased gastric acidity, for any reason, are more susceptible to *Giardia* infection. Giardiasis is also more frequent in patients with various immunoglobulin deficiencies; a relative deficiency of intestinal IgA may be the reason.

Pathophysiology *Giardia* trophozoites infect the duodenum, jejunum, and upper ilium. Encystation occurs in the gut lumen, and cysts passed in the feces maintain viability for long periods. After the cysts are ingested by the next host, excystation to the active trophozoites occurs in the proximal small bowel, completing the life cycle. The trophozoites rapidly multiply by binary fission to enormous numbers. A single diarrheal stool may contain billions of parasites or hundreds of millions of cysts. The trophozoites are capable of superficial invasion of the mucosa, but malabsorption probably causes most symptoms.

Clinical Presentation Most patients harboring *Giardia* are asymptomatic. The most common symptoms of acute infection are abdominal distention, colicky pain with audible borborygmi, flatulence, and frequent stools that are pale, loose, explosive, and often offensive-smelling. The onset is usually sudden and follows an incubation period of 1 to 3 weeks. It can persist or be chronically intermittent and produce a malabsorption-like illness, particularly in patients with an immunoglobulin deficiency.

Diagnostic Strategies Routine tests (e.g., blood counts, electrolytes, or radiographic studies) are generally not helpful. Eosinophilia does not occur. Stool examination is the primary means of diagnosis. In the acute phase of *Giardia* infection, rapid bowel transit allows trophozoites to appear in the stool in addition to the more hardy cystic form of the parasite. Trained observers using standard stool examination techniques will readily identify *Giardia* in more than 95% of acute cases if three or more stool specimens are studied. Finding *Giardia* in subacute, chronic, or asymptomatic infection, however, can be much more difficult. The trophozoites may be passed only intermittently and in much smaller numbers. Concentration techniques should be used to enhance chances of finding the cysts in the stools. Diagnosis may require small-bowel sampling techniques such as duodenal-jejunal aspiration by endoscopy or duodenal-jejunal biopsies. Stool antigen tests may also prove diagnostic.[83]

Differential Considerations *Enteromonas hominis,* a flagellate parasite like *Giardia,* can produce an intestinal infection that mimics giardiasis. *Enteromonas* is also found most commonly in children and male homosexuals.[84] Even when all techniques fail to confirm a clinically suspected case of giardiasis, an empirical diagnosis may be supported by a successful trial of appropriate antibiotics.

Management All patients harboring *Giardia* should be treated, even if they are asymptomatic. Asymptomatic cyst passers, especially children and food handlers, pose a threat of infection to others and are at risk of developing intermittent chronic symptoms at a later date.[83]

The treatment of choice in both asymptomatic and symptomatic patients is metronidazole 250 mg PO tid for 5 days for adults and 5 mg/kg PO tid (maximum 250 mg po tid) for 5 days for children.[5,83]

Common side effects of metronidazole include nausea, headache, dry mouth, and a metallic taste. An Antabuse-like reaction may occur in patients who concomitantly drink alcohol. Furazolidone is the only alternative drug available as a suspension, which may be helpful in treating children. However, its cure rates average only 80%. The recommended dosage is 100 mg PO qid for adults or 1.5 mg/kg PO qid for children, up to the adult dose, for a total of 7 to 10 days. Nausea and vomiting are common side effects, and rarely a hemolytic anemia occurs in patients with G6PD deficiency.[5,83]

Giardiasis must be considered a family infection. To prevent reinfections, other household members and sexual contacts should be examined, and if found to harbor the parasite, treated appropriately.[83]

Acute Intestinal Amebiasis

Epidemiology *Entamoeba histolytica* is a ubiquitous organism. It is estimated that at least 10% of the world's population is infected with *E. histolytica,* and 10% of these infections cause clinical disease. Its prevalence rate in the United States is approximately 4%. High-risk groups include travelers, male homosexuals, patients with AIDS, and institutionalized persons, especially the mentally retarded. Most cases acquired in the United States are asymptomatic; acute amebic dysentery is rare and most often occurs in travelers returning from underdeveloped countries where the disease is endemic.[85]

E. histolytica exists in trophozoite and cystic forms. The trophozoites infect the colon and may produce symptomatic disease. Infectious cysts are passed in the feces and are highly resistant to environmental factors. Transmission is usually from ingestion of cysts present in fecally contaminated food or water. Homosexual men commonly acquire amebic infection from cysts ingested through anal-oral sexual practices. In most male homosexuals, the infection is asymptomatic. *E. histolytica* can be regarded as a harmless commensal in this group. A diligent search for other organisms should be completed before ascribing diarrhea to amebas. Coinfection with other enteric pathogens occurs frequently in male homosexuals.[15,16]

Pathophysiology The factors that determine whether infection with *E. histolytica* will be commensal or invasive are poorly understood. Varying strain virulence and host susceptibility are determinants. In young children, pregnant women, persons with malnutrition or underlying systemic disease, or persons taking corticosteroids, amebiasis is often more fulminating.[86]

Invasive trophozoites characteristically produce colonic ulcerations that have rounded or punched-out margins and are elevated by a submucosal inflammatory reaction from the advancing trophozoites. The bases of the ulcers are covered with whitish or yellowish exudate. Usually no diffuse mucosal inflammation exists between ulcers. However, should diffuse inflammation occur, the picture becomes indistinguishable from that of idiopathic ulcerative colitis or Crohn's disease.

Clinical Presentation In most patients, *E. histolytica* lives commensally without producing symptoms. Acute amebic dysentery follows an incubation period as short as 1 week or as long as 1 year. The onset is abrupt, with fever; severe abdominal cramps; profuse, bloody diarrhea; and tenesmus.

Chronic amebic dysentery is the common symptomatic form. The onset is gradual. Usually, intermittent diarrhea is present with two or four foul-smelling stools daily, often containing blood-streaked mucus. Vague abdominal cramps, flatulence, weight loss, and low-grade fever are present. Symptomatic periods may alternate with asymptomatic periods lasting for months or years. The only physical finding may be slight right lower quadrant tenderness and occasional tender hepatomegaly. The diagnosis is elusive because cysts or trophozoites are difficult to demonstrate.

The stools of patients with symptoms contain mucus and leukocytes, although not in large numbers. Eosinophilia does not occur except in rare cases of ameboma. Liver function tests are generally normal unless the disease is complicated by liver abscess, which is the most common serious complication of amebic colitis.[85]

Diagnostic Strategies Definitive diagnosis of intestinal amebiasis depends on the laboratory identification of the organisms in the stools. The stools must be examined before the administration of antibiotics, antidiarrheal agents, antacids, enemas, or radiographic procedures using barium sulfate. All of these agents destroy trophozoites or distort cysts and thus interfere with the recovery of amebas. A rectal biopsy or mucosal exudate obtained at sigmoidoscopy may reveal the amebas even when multiple previous stool examinations have been negative. To obtain mucosal exudate, it is important to use a glass or metal pipette because amebas adhere to cotton swabs.

Serologic tests are quite sensitive and specific for active amebic infection. Because administration of steroids to patients with amebic colitis is potentially fatal, and identification of the parasite in stools is difficult, a serologic test for amebiasis should be done in all newly diagnosed cases of inflammatory bowel disease before initiation of steroid therapy.[87]

Differential Considerations Amebiasis should always be considered in cases of acute dysenteric-like colitis and in the differential diagnosis of any chronic diarrhea, especially when the feces contain blood-streaked mucus. Amebiasis should also be suspected in male homosexuals with acute colitis. Patients with AIDS, however, rarely develop amebic dysentery. In AIDS patients the infection is almost uniformly commensal and without consequence.[15,88] Patients with nondysenteric amebiasis are often misdiagnosed as having irritable bowel syndrome, diverticulitis, or regional enteritis.

Management Substantial controversy exists over whether asymptomatic cyst passers should be treated. In asymptomatic male homosexuals and patients with AIDS, the infection is almost always commensal and no treatment is indicated. When these patients present with diarrhea, other enteric pathogens are usually causative and should be ruled out before implicating *E. histolytica.* Asymptomatic food handlers and persons intimately involved in the care of others should be treated for public health reasons.[85]

For treatment of benign cyst passers, oral iodoquinol is 80% to 85% effective, relatively nontoxic, and probably the initial drug of choice. For mild to moderate intestinal infection, metronidazole is added (see Table 89-2).[5] Patients with severe infections should be treated in the hospital. Therapy is usually effective, but relapses can occur. Standard precautions to prevent fecal-oral spread are the best preventive measures.

Enterobiasis

Epidemiology *Enterobius vermicularis,* also known as *pinworm* or *seatworm,* is perhaps the most prevalent parasite in the United States. It is estimated that 20% to 30% of all children are infected with pinworms, and a total of 30 to 40 million persons are infected. Adult worms are small, spindle-shaped, white to yellowish round worms that live in the cecum and adjacent portions of the large and small bowel. The female averages 10 mm in length, and the male is 3 mm. The gravid female migrates through the anal canal at night and oviposits her eggs (usually more than 10,000) onto the perineal area. The eggs become infective larvae 4 to 6 hours after deposition, and once ingested, the larvae are released in the small intestine and migrate down to the cecum. Approximately 1 month from the time of ingestion, newly developed, gravid females are again discharging eggs.[72]

The human body is the only natural host of *E. vermicularis.* The most common means of infection, particularly in children, is by the direct transfer of eggs from the anus to the mouth by way of contaminated fingers. Retrograde infection, which happens primarily in adults, may sometimes occur. In this situation, larvae hatch in the perineal region, reenter the anus, and migrate to the cecum. Spread within family and children's groups occurs readily, either by direct transfer of eggs or by airborne transmission. The eggs, which are relatively resistant to desiccation, also contaminate night clothes and bed linens, where they remain viable and infective for 2 to 3 weeks.

Pathophysiology Because *E. vermicularis* does not penetrate the mucosa, there are no anatomic lesions. The movement of the worms or the presence of the eggs on the perineum usually causes local tingling or itching. Scratching causes irritation of the skin, which can lead to excoriations, eczematous dermatitis, and secondary bacterial infections. In women, gravid female worms can migrate through the vagina and uterus into the fallopian tubes, where they may evoke vaginitis, endometritis, or salpingitis. Young girls with pinworms may have a much higher incidence of urinary tract infections than persons not infected.[72]

Clinical Presentation The most common symptom is pruritus ani. This usually occurs at night in relation to the nocturnal migration and oviposition. Scratching may lead to secondary skin changes and bacterial infection. Restlessness, insomnia, and enuresis are probably a result of the pruritus.

Diagnostic Strategies Adult worms may be recognized in the perineal area, and in suspected cases nocturnal examination of this area using a flashlight may confirm infection. Worms can sometimes also be seen on the surface of stool. The most reliable way to diagnose infection is to examine material taken from the perineal area for ova. The cellophane tape test is simple and reliable. The tape is folded, sticky side out, over the end of a tongue blade, pressed firmly against the perineal area, and then spread on a glass slide with toluene and examined under the low power of a microscope. The typical eggs are identified easily.

A single cellophane tape test will detect approximately 50% of infections. If done daily for 3 days, the test will detect 90% of infections; after 5 days it will detect 99%. Examining stool specimens for ova is rarely helpful, but scrapings from under the fingernails may reveal the ova.[72] Eosinophilia is not found because the worm does not have a tissue phase.

Management All infected individuals in a family or communal group should be treated simultaneously. It is the usual accepted practice also to treat empirically all other members of the same group at the same time, even if they are not infected. The drug of choice is either mebendazole (Vermox), a single oral dose of 100 mg chewed well, or pyrantel pamoate (Antiminth), a single oral dose of 11 mg/kg (maximum 1 g). With either drug, a second dose should be administered 2 weeks later because mature worms seem to be more vulnerable than young worms. Treatment is effective in 90% to 95% of infections.[5]

The ease of airborne dissemination of the eggs, their resistance to desiccation, and the poor hygienic practices of children ensure reinfection. Ova are also resistant to ordinary fumigants and disinfectants, making control in schools, institutions, and the home very difficult.

Table 89-5. Causes of Diarrhea in Patients with AIDS

Frequency	Organism
Most common	*Cryptosporidium*
	Cytomegalovirus
Common	*Entamoeba histolytica* (probably commensal, not causative)
	Giardia lamblia
	Mycobacterium avium-intracellulare
	Salmonella species, especially *typhimurium*
	Aeromonas hydrophila
	Microsporidia
	Astrovirus/picornavirus
	Clostridium difficile
	Campylobacter jejuni
Less common	Viruses—herpes simplex, rotavirus, adenovirus, Norwalk agent
	Cyclospora
	Isospora belli
	Enteromonas hominis
	Strongyloides stercoralis
	Blastocystis hominis
	Shigella species
	Yersinia enterocolitica

Miscellaneous Protozoan Infections

Infections with other parasites appear to be increasing in the United States, primarily as a result of widespread international travel and the AIDS epidemic. Substantial increases have been noted with *Strongyloides stercoralis, E. hominis,* and *Blastocystis hominis* (Table 89-5).[15,16,84]

DIARRHEA IN PATIENTS WITH AIDS

Epidemiology

Diarrhea is the most common manifestation of gastrointestinal disease in patients with AIDS and may be either the presenting symptom or a life-threatening complication of the disease. The occurrence rate is greater than 90% in developing countries and 50% to 60% in the United States.[15,16,74,88,89]

Patients who are HIV positive and those with active AIDS are more susceptible to infection both from the usual enteric organisms and from opportunistic organisms. Diarrheal diseases are much more problematic in AIDS patients because of their diminished immunity and underlying poor nutritional status.[15,16]

A vastly different profile of pathogens causes diarrhea in AIDS patients compared with normal immunocompetent individuals. Also, the ramifications of the disease are significantly more serious, requiring a much more aggressive diagnostic evaluation and treatment regimen.

Pathophysiology

Mucosal biopsy specimens in patients with AIDS show crypt epithelial cell degeneration, villous atrophy, chronic inflammation, and often mild fibrosis. These nonspecific changes may be associated with many inflammatory or infectious processes, but because a significant percentage of AIDS patients with diarrhea have no pathogen identified, HIV itself may produce an enteropathy.[70,74,88,89]

In the homosexual population, unprotected receptive anal intercourse and anal-oral contact among multiple partners provide exposure to a diverse spectrum of enteric pathogens. In the heterosexual IV drug–abusing population, infection spreads primarily from water- and food-borne transmissions of the organisms. Patients with AIDS are unable to combat these intestinal pathogens, probably because of a combination of their T-lymphocyte functional deficiency and underlying HIV-induced enteropathy.

Etiology

A known enteric pathogen can be identified in approximately 80% to 85% of AIDS patients with diarrhea. Multiple organisms may be present in as many as 20% to 25% of patients. Male homosexuals with AIDS develop diarrhea more often than other AIDS patients.[15,89]

Table 89-5 lists the causes of diarrhea in patients with AIDS. *Cryptosporidium* and cytomegalovirus (CMV) infections are the two most common causes. The incidence of each is 15% to 40%.[16,88,89] Chronic persistent diarrhea is most often from one of the coccidia, *Cryptosporidium* or *Isospora belli.* CMV and *Mycobacterium avium-intracellulare* also produce a chronic illness, although most patients are dead within 6 months of diagnosis. In underdeveloped countries, the coccidia are by far the most common cause of diarrhea in patients with AIDS; *Cryptosporidium* is the etiologic agent in more than 50% of patients and *Isospora* in approximately 15%.[70]

Salmonella infections, especially *S. typhimurium,* are much more common in the immunocompromised host.[88] One unusual source of *Salmonella* is rattlesnake meat preparations. Hispanic persons in particular use rattlesnake powder or capsules as a treatment for a variety of ailments. *S. arizonae* is the usual species associated with rattlesnake meat.[90]

E. histolytica, although commonly found, is generally considered commensal. It is extremely rare for amebae to cause invasive disease in patients with AIDS.[38,70] For unknown reasons *Campylobacter, Shigella, Yersinia, V. parahaemolyticus,* viruses (non-CMV), *Neisseria gonorrhoeae,* and *Chlamydia trachomatis* are unusual causes of diarrhea in patients with AIDS.

Astrovirus and picornavirus infections commonly cause diarrhea in AIDS.[63] The protozoan parasite *Microsporidia* may account for as much as 50% of the unexplained chronic, watery, nonbloody diarrhea that occurs with HIV infection.

Clinical Presentation

In AIDS patients, diarrhea presents in one of three ways. First, at the time of HIV seroconversion patients usually experience diarrhea, nausea, anorexia, and malaise in association with an acute infectious mononucleosis–like syndrome. Second, diarrhea may be the presenting symptom of full-blown AIDS, with associated fever, malaise, anorexia, and significant weight loss. Third, and the most common presentation, however, is for diarrhea to start well after AIDS has been clinically apparent. These patients typically have a chronic debilitating infection develop that rarely remits spontaneously. It is often accompanied by profound weight loss, major nutritional impact, and a diminished sense of well-being. Many cases are refractory to treatment and persist until death, or may even be the cause of death.[74,88,89]

In AIDS, the presenting signs and symptoms generally do not allow one to consistently classify diarrheas as outlined for the immunocompetent host earlier in this chapter. This is in part because many patients with AIDS have multiple, concomitant enteric pathogens. However, some clinical pictures are typical. Patients with a fulminating clinical course usually have a disseminated infection, such as infection with CMV or *M. avium-intracellulare.* Massive weight loss is also associated with those two organisms and the coccidia, *Cryptosporidium* or *Isospora.* Voluminous, watery diarrhea is usually due to one of the coccidial organisms. Patients with a proctocolitis-like picture most often have herpes simplex virus or CMV infection. Strongyloidiasis should be considered in any immunocompromised patient who deteriorates suddenly and has polymicrobial sepsis, meningitis, or adynamic ileus.[88]

Complications

The most common complications are dehydration and malnutrition resulting from both fluid loss and malabsorption. CMV can produce GI hemorrhage, perforation, or toxic megacolon.[91] *M. avium-intracellulare* often produces severe anemia, weight loss, and a rapid downhill course of persistent weakness, malaise, and malabsorption. Bacteremia can be found in as many as 40% to 45% of AIDS patients with diarrhea, usually caused by *M. avium-intracellulare* or *Salmonella* species.[15,16,74]

Diagnostic Strategies

The diagnostic approach for AIDS patients with diarrhea is entirely different from that in an immunocompetent host. In 80% to 90% of cases, one or more enteric pathogens are found; of the pathogens identified, 55% to 75% are treatable.[15,16,74,89] Known pathogens are detected less frequently in patients being treated with antivirals.[15] Diarrhea in AIDS patients is generally not self-limiting but requires medical intervention to effect resolution. Therefore each patient deserves a diagnostic evaluation, although the approach and intensity of the diagnostic workup remain controversial.[15] Box 89-2 summarizes one logical approach.

AIDS patients with diarrhea should have one or more stool specimens cultured for enteric bacteria and examined by multiple stain preparations for ova, parasites, and mycobacteria. The usual bacterial enteric pathogens are readily identified, but the protozoan infections can be difficult to find. Multiple stool specimens may have to be examined to diagnose *Giardia lamblia* and *Isospora belli,* in part because these oocysts are generally shed only intermittently and in small numbers. In patients with severe diarrhea from *Cryptosporidium,* the first stool examination is usually positive, but in less severe cases additional samples may have to be studied to effect the diagnosis. Specialized techniques are necessary to detect most of the viral agents.

Blood cultures are a valuable diagnostic tool. Bacteremia may be found in up to 40% of patients, and in 20% of cases a positive blood culture may be present when the stool cultures and examinations fail to reveal a pathogen.[88] The most common organisms that produce bacteremia are *M. avium-intracellulare, Salmonella,* and occasionally *Shigella* or *Campylobacter.* Most cases of *M. avium-intracellulare* bacteremia occur in heterosexual IV-drug abusers.[88] A routine complete blood count (CBC) demonstrating eosinophilia suggests parasitic infection with *Strongyloides stercoralis.*[88]

Box 89-2 Diagnostic Protocol for Evaluating Diarrhea in Patients with AIDS

A. Initial evaluation—indicated in all patients
   1. Stool cultures for enteric bacteria—*Salmonella, Shigella, Campylobacter, Yersinia*
   2. Stool examinations by various stains, especially acid-fast stains, for ova, parasites, and mycobacteria; *C. difficile* toxin assay
   3. Blood cultures
   4. Proctosigmoidoscopy in patients with clinically severe colitis or a proctocolitis picture, especially male homosexuals

B. Further evaluation—indicated if initial studies are negative or to look for multiple organisms present if a patient fails to respond to appropriate therapy for an identified pathogen
   1. Repeat stool cultures and examinations, possibly add culture for viruses
   2. Proctosigmoidoscopy or gastroduodenoscopy performed to obtain duodenal fluid and small bowel and colonic biopsies, which are examined for:
      a. Duodenal fluid examination for ova and parasites
      b. Duodenal and colonic biopsies cultured for mycobacteria, cytomegalovirus, and herpes simplex; colonic biopsy tissue is also cultured for bacterial enteric pathogens (add gonorrhea and chlamydia testing in patients with acute proctitis)
      c. Biopsy specimens examined by multiple stains (e.g., acid-fast, hematoxylin-eosin, Giemsa, silver, periodic acid-Schiff) for protozoa, mycobacteria, and cells containing viral inclusion bodies

If the aforementioned tests are negative, endoscopy should be performed to obtain mucosal biopsies from the rectum or colon. Rectal biopsy, which can be performed easily even in seriously ill patients, is an indispensable tool in the diagnosis of CMV infection.[15] Viral inclusion bodies with clear halos typical of CMV can be demonstrated. Stained examinations of the biopsy tissue may also diagnose *M. avium-intracellulare, Cryptosporidium,* or *Giardia* infections that were missed on stool examinations. Herpes simplex virus can be identified microscopically by detecting multinucleated giant cells or through cultures obtained at the time of endoscopy.

Small bowel biopsies and duodenal aspirates are indicated when stool examination, cultures, and sigmoidoscopy fail to lead to a diagnosis. Small bowel studies are most helpful for detecting *Cryptosporidium,* CMV, *M. avium-intracellulare, Giardia,* or *I. belli.*[15,16]

Differential Considerations

Kaposi's sarcoma, even if it involves the bowel, rarely produces diarrhea. Symptomatic oral and esophageal candidiasis is common in patients with AIDS, but diarrhea from *Candida* has not been reported. Diarrhea can be a side effect of drugs used to treat AIDS, such as dideoxyinosine (ddI), and must be differentiated from infectious causes.[16,70,89]

Antibiotic-associated colitis from *C. difficile* should be considered when the diarrhea follows antibacterial therapy. Ulcerative colitis can mimic or be mimicked by CMV colitis.[15] Aphthous ulceration, particularly of the colon, should be considered when cultures and endoscopy biopsy specimens fail to reveal evidence of infection with common infectious pathogens, herpes simplex virus, or CMV. Empiric corticosteroid therapy may cause dramatic improvement in these patients.[92] Acute proctitis should be differentiated from diarrhea or acute colitis, because the investigative evaluation and treatment regimens are distinctly different.

Management

Treatment of diarrhea in patients with AIDS includes diet, antimotility agents, and antimicrobial agents. Diets that are lactose-free and low in fat often diminish the diarrhea caused by malabsorption. Patients should avoid intestinal stimulants such as caffeine, raw or inadequately cooked seafood, rattlesnake preparations, and untreated water. Varying success has been reported with the standard antimotility agents, such as diphenoxylate or loperamide. In patients with cryptosporidiosis, these agents commonly cause a marked increase in crampy abdominal pain. Long-acting morphine sulfate derivatives have afforded much better clinical relief in a consistent fashion.[15,88]

Specific antimicrobial therapy can lead to marked symptomatic improvement in 55% to 75% of patients in whom a pathogen has been identified. Many patients will show substantial improvement after therapy, even when the organism or the diarrhea has not been eliminated. Antimicrobial therapy should be dictated by the results of the diagnostic evaluation. Empiric use of antimicrobials is not indicated; no one antimicrobial agent can possibly provide reasonable coverage of the wide variety of causative organisms found in these patients. This is in distinct contrast to the situation encountered in normal, immunocompetent patients discussed earlier. The possibility of multiple organisms must always be considered, especially when patients do not respond to known effective antimicrobial agents for an identified pathogen.

Table 89-6 summarizes the treatment of pathogens causing diarrhea in patients with AIDS. Ganciclovir is a nucleoside analog similar to acyclovir. It is effective in inducing clinical remission in up to 80% of patients with gastrointestinal CMV.[5,16,88,93,94] Foscarnet is also effective. The dosage of both drugs should be reduced in patients with low creatinine clearance.[5,94]

However, treatment of the other most common cause of diarrhea in patients with AIDS, cryptosporidiosis, has been much less successful.[5,15,70,73] Paromomycin, particularly in combination with azithromycin, may be beneficial.[5,76,80] Infection with *Cryptosporidium's* coccidial cousins, *I. belli* and *C. cayetanensis,* however, can be cured with TMP-SMX.[5,69]

Although *E. histolytica* is one of the most common pathogens found in these patients, most practitioners consider it commensal and withhold treatment except when evidence of amebic dysentery arises.[70,88] *M. avium-intracellulare* has not been very responsive to therapy, and generally death ensues within 6 to 8 months of diagnosis. Virtually all of the other organisms listed in Table 89-5 are susceptible to the usual therapeutic agents, although higher dosages and longer courses of therapy are often required. Recurrences of either the opportunistic organisms or the usual enteric organisms are common. Chronic suppressive antimicrobial therapy may be indicated to prevent relapse or reinfection.[88]

Patients with AIDS enteropathy or infectious enteritis not responsive to antimicrobial therapy may respond to zidovudine (AZT) because it enhances host immunity by suppressing HIV replication.

TRAVELER'S DIARRHEA

Epidemiology

It is said that "travel expands the mind and loosens the bowels." Diarrhea is by far the most common health problem of the 12 million persons who travel from an industrialized nation to a developing country each year. Travel to high-risk areas such as Mexico, Latin America, Africa, the Middle East, or Asia is associated with diarrheal attack rates of 30% to 50%. However, few travelers to industrialized countries develop diarrhea. Among visitors to the United States, the attack rate is less than 4%. Traveler's diarrhea is more common in young adults than in senior citizens.[82,95]

Pathophysiology

The syndrome is caused by an infection acquired by ingesting fecally contaminated food or water. High-risk items include raw leafy vegetables, raw or undercooked meats or seafood, unpeeled fruits, unpasteurized dairy products, and tap water. The most deceitful vehicle of all is ice, which is often made from water contaminated with bacteria that survived freezing.[53]

Once an organism is ingested, rapid and dramatic change occurs in the traveler's intestinal flora. When the ingested inoculum overcomes an individual's defense mechanisms, diarrhea develops. Most often this is from the elaboration of enterotoxins that produce a secretory diarrhea. When organisms are invasive, rather than toxigenic, a typical infectious enteritis develops.

Etiology (Table 89-7)

Enterotoxigenic *E. coli* is responsible for 40% to 50% of all cases of traveler's diarrhea and may be acquired anywhere in the world. The organisms adhere to the wall of the small bowel, where they multiply and produce an enterotoxin that causes fluid secretion and diarrhea. The other infectious bacterial agents, particularly *Shigella, Salmonella,* and *Campylobacter,* account for 20% to 30% of cases. *V. parahaemolyticus* is an increasingly common cause because of its association with raw or inadequately cooked seafood. The organism commonly causes diarrhea in persons traveling to Japan or Asia or those vacationing on cruise ships.[26,52,82,95]

Plesiomonas shigelloides is typically associated with uncooked shellfish, especially oysters. It is also associated with travel to Mexico. *Plesiomonas* produces a typical invasive enteritis. *E. coli* 0157:H7 and enteroinvasive *E. coli* each cause up to 5% of traveler's diarrhea.[3,7] Another type of *E. coli,* enteroadherent *E. coli,* may be the cause of a significant number of the previously undiagnosed cases of traveler's diarrhea.[96]

Norwalk virus and rotavirus may cause up to 10% of traveler's diarrhea in Mexico.[52] *Giardia* is the most common parasite acquired by travelers and accounts for 3% to 5% of all cases. Travelers to the former Soviet Union, particularly Leningrad and Moscow, have a very high risk for acquiring giardiasis. Amebiasis is rare.[82]

Table 89-6. Treatment of Pathogens Causing Diarrhea in Patients With AIDS

Organism/treatment regimen	Comments
Cytomegalovirus	
Foscarnet 90 mg/kg IV q12hr × 14-21 days (diluted in 100 ml D_5W, infused over at least 1 hr)	
Ganciclovir 5 mg/kg q12hr IV × 14 days (diluted in 100 ml D_5W, infused over 1 hr)	Effective, but 75% recurrence rate within 8 to 9 weeks; maintenance therapy may be warranted
Cryptosporidium	
Paromomycin 1 g PO bid × 12 weeks *plus* azithromycin 600 mg QD × 4 wks	Disease generally chronic, despite treatment
Somatostatin analogs?	
Antiviral therapies	
Indomethicin 50 mg PO q8hr	
Cyclospora cayetanensis	
TMP/SMX 160 mg/800 mg qid PO × 10 days, then 1 tab PO 3x/wk	
Entamoeba histolytica	Treatment not recommended unless amebic dysentery develops (see Table 89-2)
Giardia lamblia	
Metronidazole 250-750 mg PO tid × 5 to 10 days	Patient's symptoms may resolve despite continued enteric presence of *Giardia*
Mycobacterium avium-intracellulare	
Clarithromycin 500 mg PO bid *plus* ethambutol PO 15 mg/kg/day	
Antituberculous regimens or ciprofloxacin 500-750 mg PO bid × 10-14 days	Mixed results with antituberculous drugs, more drug resistant than TB strains of mycobacteria; little evidence that treatment prolongs life
Salmonella species	
Ciprofloxacin 500-750 mg PO bid × 10-14 days	Bacteremia common; maintenance therapy often required
Ceftriaxone 1-2 g IV q12hr × 7-10 days	
Herpes simplex virus	
Acyclovir 5 mg/kg PO or IV tid × 7-10 days	Proctitis picture, especially in male homosexuals
Campylobactor jejuni	
Ciprofloxacin 500 mg bid × 7-10 days	40% recurrence rate; erythromycin acceptable alternative
Isospora belli	
Trimethoprim-sulfamethoxazole (TMP-SMX) 160 mg/800 mg PO qid × 10 days, then bid for 3 weeks	50% recurrence rate; chronic suppressive therapy usually recommended
Aeromonas hydrophila	
Ciprofloxacin 500 mg PO bid × 14 days or TMP-SMX 160 mg/800 mg PO bid × 14 days	Associated with drinking untreated water
Enteromonas hominis	
Metronidazole 250-750 mg PO tid × 10 days	Increasingly common in male homosexuals, possibly commensal; treatment indicated when no other pathogens found in the presence of appropriate symptoms
Blastocystis hominis	
Metronidazole 750 mg PO tid × 10 days or furazolidone 100 mg PO qid × 7-10 days	Possibly more common in children
Shigella species	
Ciprofloxacin 500 mg PO bid × 7 days	Most species resistant to ampicillin, and increasingly resistance is found to TMP-SMX
Yersinia	
Ciprofloxacin 500 mg PO bid × 7 days	Appendicitis-like picture; bacteremia possible
Strongyloides stercoralis	
Ivermectin 200 μgm/kg/d × 1-2 days	Migration of the larvae through the bowel wall may be accompanied by gram-negative bacteremia and a hyperinfection syndrome in AIDS patients; in disseminated strongyloidiasis, therapy should be continued for at least 5 days

Table 89-7. Causes of Traveler's Diarrhea

Agent	Estimated incidence (%)*
Bacteria (approximately 80%-85%)	
Enterotoxigenic *E. coli*	45-50
Shigella	8-12
Campylobacter	7-9
Enteroinvasive *E. coli* (hemorrhagic strain 0157:H7)	5-6
Salmonella	3-5
Others, such as *Vibrio, Aeromonas, Plesiomonas,* shigelloides, *Yersinia,* other types of *E. coli*	1-5
Viruses (approximately 5%-10%)	
Rotavirus	5-10
Norwalk agent and others	0-5
Parasites (approximately 5%-6%)	
Giardia lamblia	4-5
Cryptosporidium	3-4
Entamoeba histolytica	0-1
Strongyloides stercoralis	0-1
Unknown	5-10

*Rough estimates, which vary depending on destination.

Clinical Presentation

Traveler's diarrhea typically begins abruptly and results in four or five loose or watery stools per day for 1 to 3 days. Approximately one third of patients will be temporarily confined to bed, and the symptoms may last more than a week in 10% of patients. Onset is usually within the first 3 to 4 days of travel but may occur at any time, including after the patient arrives home. Patients may not associate their diarrhea with recent travel because the incubation time of the infection, particularly if it is parasitic, may have been long enough to allow them to return home before the symptoms began.

Associated symptoms include abdominal cramps, nausea, bloating, urgency, and occasionally vomiting, fever, chills, headache, malaise, tenesmus, and bloody stools. Symptoms depend on whether the cause is "toxigenic" or "infectious," as discussed earlier. Traveler's diarrhea may ruin one's trip, but it is rarely life threatening.

Prevention

Diet Traditionally, instruction regarding food and beverage preparation has been touted to prevent traveler's diarrhea. Most travelers, however, do not follow such advice. Ideally, a tourist should eat foods that are freshly prepared and served piping hot. High-risk foods should be assiduously avoided, and travelers should follow the Peace Corps adage of "boil it, cook it, peel it, or forget it."[97]

Thirsty travelers should be advised to avoid ice and to drink beverages such as tea and coffee that are made with boiled water, canned or bottled carbonated beverages, and wine.[52,53]

Boiling water is by far the most reliable method to make it safe for drinking and brushing teeth. Travelers and outdoor enthusiasts should be advised to bring the water to a vigorous boil and allow it to cool without adding ice. Boiling destroys virtually all bacteria, viruses, and parasitic cysts. A pinch of salt in each quart improves the taste. When boiling is not feasible, water can be chemically disinfected with 2% tincture of iodine drops or tetracycline hydroperiodide tablets, such as Globaline or Potable-Aqua, available from pharmacies and sporting goods stores.[98]

Nonantimicrobial Medications The non-antimicrobial agent most studied in the prevention of traveler's diarrhea is bismuth subsalicylate (Pepto-Bismol). Two tablets, or two ounces, taken four times per day has been shown to decrease the incidence of traveler's diarrhea by 65%. This dosage, however, contains the daily equivalent of eight 5-grain aspirin tablets. Bismuth subsalicylate should not be used in the following situations: patients who are allergic to salicylates, those taking large doses of salicylates for arthritis, and patients taking oral anticoagulants, uricosuric drugs, or methotrexate. Salicylates have antiplatelet effects, inhibit the activity of uricosuric drugs, and increase the toxicity of methotrexate by decreasing its renal clearance. Pepto-Bismol also turns the tongue and stool black and may cause mild tinnitus and interfere with the bioavailability of doxycycline.[99]

Antiperistaltic agents such as diphenoxylate and loperamide are not effective prophylactic agents. Controlled studies have indicated that the use of diphenoxylate actually increases the incidence of traveler's diarrhea; slowing of the gut allows more time for organisms to colonize and elaborate toxin or produce infection.[96]

Antimicrobials A single daily dose of prophylactic antibiotics such as doxycycline (100 mg) double-strength TMP-SMX (160 mg/800 mg), ciprofloxacin (500 mg), or norfloxacin (400 mg) can effectively prevent traveler's diarrhea in up to 90% of persons. The regimen is started the day before travel and continued until 2 days after returning home.

The risks of prophylactic treatment include allergic reactions, skin rashes, photosensitivity reactions, serious hematologic reactions, Stevens-Johnson syndrome, and other infections that may be induced with antibiotic therapy, such as antibiotic-associated colitis or *Candida* vaginitis.[52,98]

The main argument, however, against the widespread use of prophylactic antibiotics in millions of travelers each year has been the risk of emergence of organisms resistant to the antibiotics used. Resistance to doxycycline is now found in many parts of the world. TMP-SMX resistance is common in tropical areas. The quinolones are the most effective agents.[5,52,96,98,100]

Management

Diet In most patients, fluid and electrolyte balances can be maintained by drinking potable fruit juices, bottled beverages, or caffeine-free soft drinks.

Nonantimicrobial Medications Adsorbents such as kaolin or pectin are ineffective in treating traveler's diarrhea. They may give the stools more consistency, but have not been shown to decrease cramps or the frequency of stooling, or to shorten the course of an infectious diarrhea.

Nonantimicrobial agents such as bismuth subsalicylate, paregoric, codeine, diphenoxylate, or loperamide may provide prompt but temporary symptomatic relief. Loperamide (initial dose 4 mg followed by 2 mg after each unformed stool

Box 89-3 Current Recommendations for the Prevention and Treatment of Traveler's Diarrhea

1. Provide instruction regarding sensible dietary practices and drinking-water management.
2. Inform patients about prophylaxis but do not encourage it. The basis of this recommendation is threefold: first, the modest benefit from bismuth subsalicylate as opposed to its aspirin-related complications; second, the ramification of widespread use of prophylactic antibiotics in terms of adverse medication reactions or the emergence of resistant organisms; third, the availability of highly successful treatment strategies.
3. Patients who request prophylaxis should be steered toward the use of bismuth subsalicylate rather than antibiotic. However, the emergency physician may judiciously recommend the use of prophylactic antibiotics for travel in special clinical circumstances, such as in patients with significant underlying medical illnesses, immunocompromised persons, or a short 2- to 3-day trip to a very high-risk area. In these cases one of the quinolones, norfloxacin or ciprofloxacin, is recommended.
4. Institute prompt antimicrobial therapy once traveler's diarrhea occurs.
   a. Toxigenic/nondysentery: loperamide combined with TMP-SMX or one of the quinolones used alone.
   b. Infectious/dysentery: norfloxacin or ciprofloxacin-alone or in combination with loperamide.
   c. The rare traveler with persistent symptoms, particularly fever, chills, or blood or mucus in the stools, unresponsive to antimicrobial therapy within 24 to 48 hours should seek immediate medical attention.

for 2 days; total dosage no more than eight 2 mg capsules/day) has been shown to provide significantly more relief than bismuth subsalicylate (30 ml PO every 30 minutes for 3 to 5 hours on each of 2 days; 240 ml/day).[96] Antimotility agents alone, however, should never be given to patients when an invasive bacterial infection is suspected, and they should be discontinued if symptoms persist longer than 48 hours.

Antimicrobials Antibiotics have a role in the treatment of all clinical presentations of traveler's diarrhea. Antibiotic therapy can provide prompt relief of symptoms, decrease the rate of stooling, and shorten a typically 1- to 3-day illness to a few hours.[82,101,102]

In toxigenic, nondysenteric traveler's diarrhea, 3 days of treatment with the combination of loperamide and TMP-SMX is extremely effective (98% response rate: one half of persons so treated pass their last unformed stool in less than 1 hour).[103] In patients with high fever, bloody stools, or the typical bacterial/invasive picture, the treatment of choice is norfloxacin, 400 mg bid, or ciprofloxacin, 500 mg bid. The duration of treatment is generally 3 to 5 days, although even one double dose may be all that is necessary. Supplementing quinolone therapy with loperamide appears to enhance clinical resolution of symptoms.[100,101]

Quinolone agents are also preferred over TMP-SMX for patients traveling to areas known to have organisms with high resistance to TMP-SMX, or where *Campylobacter* is common. Worldwide there has been a steady, continual increase in resistance to doxycycline and TMP-SMX in the bacterial enteric organisms that cause traveler's diarrhea. In some countries, the incidence of resistance for *Salmonella* and *Shigella* is as high as 50%. Fortunately, little resistance has been reported to the quinolone agents, norfloxacin, or ciprofloxacin.[3,5,82]

In addition, persons with dysentery failing to respond to TMP-SMX should promptly be switched to one of the quinolone antibiotics. The quinolone agents are not recommended for use in children and pregnant women.[96]

A summary of current recommendations for the prevention and treatment of traveler's diarrhea is outlined in Box 89-3. Further detailed information on traveler's diarrhea and the other medical problems of travelers can be found at the Center for Preventive Services section of the CDC's website, *www.cdc.gov/travel.htm.* The website contains a plethora of travel-related information. The CDC's "Yellow Book," *Health Information for International Travel,* can be downloaded for free at *www.cdc.gov/travel/reference.htm,* and the CDC provides up-to-the-minute travel information through its Traveler's hotline phone number of 877-FYI-TRIP.

KEY CONCEPTS

- Treatment should be considered in patients who are still significantly ill at the time a culture returns, particularly if they are immunocompromised or have a significant underlying medical illness, or in cases where the fecal shedding could represent a public health hazard.
- Patients with sickle cell anemia, other hemolytic anemias, or AIDS are unusually susceptible to *Salmonella* bacteremia.
- Most patients with *Salmonella* gastroenteritis will be clinically improved by the time their culture results are available. These patients do not require antibiotic treatment. Patients who are not improving should be treated to effect cure, and those who represent a public health risk should be treated to eradicate the carrier state and prevent spread of the organism.
- Antimotility agents alone are not generally recommended for invasive enteritis. These can prolong fever and diarrhea and increase the incidence of bacteremia and the carrier state.
- *In Y. enterocolitica* gastroenteritis, the abdominal pain and diarrhea usually persist for 10 to 14 days or longer. A substantial number of patients with yersiniosis, in particular adolescents and young adults, develop an ileocecitis. In these cases, lower abdominal pain with little or no diarrhea predominates and may perfectly mimic acute appendicitis.
- The symptoms of scombroid fish poisoning, which resemble histamine intoxication and usually develop abruptly within 20 to 30 minutes of eating the fish, consist of facial flushing; diarrhea; severe, throbbing headache; palpitations; and abdominal cramps, and generally last less than 6 hours. The mainstay of therapy is antihistamine administration.
- Many cases of *C. difficile* antibiotic-associated enterocolitis are self-limited, provided that the offending agent is discontinued. When stopping the antibiotic does not resolve the diarrhea, or when it is severe, empiric antibiotic treatment should be started promptly. Either oral metronidazole or oral vancomycin may be used to eradicate *C. difficile* colitis.

- *Giardia* is the most common cause of water-borne diarrheal outbreaks in the United States. Most patients harboring *Giardia* are asymptomatic. The most common symptoms of acute infection are abdominal distention, colicky pain with audible borborygmi, flatulence, and frequent stools. All patients harboring *Giardia* should be treated, even if they are asymptomatic.
- Diarrhea is the most common manifestation of gastrointestinal disease in patients with AIDS and may be either the presenting symptom or a life-threatening complication of the disease. Diarrhea in the AIDS patient is generally not self-limiting but requires medical intervention to effect resolution. Therefore each patient deserves a diagnostic evaluation.
- Enterotoxigenic *E. coli* is responsible for 40% to 50% of all cases of traveler's diarrhea and may be acquired anywhere in the world. A single daily dose of prophylactic antibiotics can effectively prevent traveler's diarrhea in up to 90% of persons. The regimen is started the day before travel and continued until 2 days after returning home.

REFERENCES

1. Altekruse SF et al: *Campylobacter jejuni:* an emerging food-borne pathogen, *Emerg Infect Dis* 5:1, 1999.
2. Goodman L et al: Infectious diarrhea, *Dis Mon* 45:268, 1999.
3. Tauxe RV: Emerging food-borne diseases: an evolving public health challenge, *Emerg Infect Dis* 3:1, 1997.
4. Wistrom J et al: Empiric treatment of acute diarrheal disease with norfloxacin, *Ann Intern Med* 117:202, 1992.
5. Editorial Board: Drugs for parasitic infections, *Med Let* 3:1, 2000.
6. Angulo FJ, Swerdlo DL: *Salmonella enteritidis* infections in the United States, *J Am Vet Med Assoc* 213:1729, 1998.
7. Mead PS: Food-related illness and death in the United States, *Emerg Infect Dis* 5:607, 1999.
8. Olsen SJ, et al: Surveillance for food borne-disease outbreaks: United States, 1993-1997, *MMWR* 49(SS-1), 2000.
9. VanBeneden CA et al: Multinational outbreak of salmonella infections due to contaminated alfalfa sprouts, *JAMA* 281:158, 1999.
10. Taormina PJ et al: Infections associated with eating seed sprouts: an international concern, *Emerg Infect Dis* 5:626, 1999.
11. Meriman J, Hoar B, Angulo FJ: Iguanas and *Salmonella marina* infection in children: a reflection of the increased incidence of reptile-associated salmonellosis in the US, *Pediatrics* 99:399, 1997.
12. Fayer R et al: *Cryptosporidium parvum* in oysters from commercial harvesting sites in the Chesapeake Bay, *Emerg Infect Dis* 5:1, 1999.
13. Centers for Disease Control and Prevention: Reptile-associated salmonellosis: selected states, 1996, 1998, *MMWR* 48:1009, 1999.
14. Food and Drug Administration: Update on *S. enteritidis* in shelled eggs, *FDA Drug Bull* Feb 6, 1989.
15. Weber R et al: Enteric infections and diarrhea in HIV-infected persons, *Arch Intern Med* 159:1473, 1999.
16. Angulo FJ, Swerdlow DL: Bacterial enteric infections in persons infected with HIV, *Clin Infect Dis* 21(suppl 1):S84, 1995.
17. Editorial Board: Choice of antimicrobial drugs, *Med Lett* 36:53, 1994.
18. Smith ME: Comparison of ofloxacin and ceftriaxone for short-course treatment of enteric fever, *Antimicrob Agents Chemother* 38:1716, 1994.
19. Centers for Disease Control and Prevention: Outbreak of cryptosporidiosis associated with a water sprinkler fountain: Minnesota, *MMWR* 47:856, 1998.
20. Murphy S et al: Ciprofloxacin and loperamide in the treatment of bacillary dysentery, *Ann Intern Med* 118:582, 1993.
21. Oloughlin EV, Gall DJ, Pai CH: *Yersinia enterocolitica:* mechanisms of microbial pathogenesis and pathophysiology of diarrhea, *J Gastroenterol Hepatol* 5:2, 1990.
22. Pylaert JBCM et al: Incidence and sonographic diagnosis of bacterial ileocaecitis masquerading as appendicitis, *Lancet* ii:84, 1989.
23. Centers for Disease Control and Prevention: Surveillance for waterborne disease outbreaks, United States 1997-1998, *MMWR* 49(SS-4):1, 2000.
24. Hlady WG, Klontz, KC: The epidemiology of vibrio infections in Florida, *J Infect Dis* 173:1176, 1996.
25. Centers for Disease Control and Prevention: Outbreak of *Vibrio parahaemolyticus* infections associated with eating raw oysters: Pacific Northwest, 1997, *MMWR* 47:457, 1998.
26. Koo D, Maloney K, Tauxe R: Epidemiology of diarrheal disease outbreaks on cruise ships, 1986 through 1993, *JAMA* 275:545, 1996.
27. Hlady WG, Mullen RC, Hopkins RS: *Vibrio vulnificus* from raw oysters: leading cause of reported deaths from food-borne illness in Florida, *J Fla Med Assoc* 80:536, 1993.
28. Mouzin E et al: Prevention of *Vibrio vulnificus* infections: assessment of regulatory educational strategies, *JAMA* 278:576, 1997.
29. Dundass, Todd WT: *E. coli* 0157:H7 review article, current opinion, *Infect Dis* 11:171, 1998.
30. MacDonald KL, Osterholm MT: The emergence of *Escherichia coli* 0157:H7 infection in the United States: the changing epidemiology of food-borne disease, *JAMA* 269:2264, 1993.
31. Slutsker L et al: *Escherichia coli* 0157:H7 diarrhea in the United States: clinical and epidemiologic features, *Ann Intern Med* 126:505, 1997.
32. Centers for Disease Control and Prevention: *Escherichia coli* O157:H7 infections associated with eating a nationally distributed commercial brand of frozen ground beef patties and burgers: Colorado, 1997, *MMWR* 46:777, 1997.
33. Cody SH et al: An outbreak of *Escherichia coli* 0157:H7 infection from unpasteurized commercial apple juice, *Ann Intern Med* 120:202-209, 1999.
34. Tarr PI et al: *Escherichia coli* 0157:H7 and the hemolytic uremic syndrome: importance of early cultures in establishing the etiology, *J Infect Dis* 162:553, 1990.
35. Belongia EA et al: Transmission of *Escherichia coli* 0157:H7 infection in Minnesota child day-care facilities, *JAMA* 269:883, 1993.
36. Boyce TG, Sverdlow DL, Griffin PM: *Escherichia coli* 0157:H7 & the hemolytic-uremic syndrome, *N Engl J Med* 333:364, 1995.
37. Bender JB et al: Surveillance for *E. coli* O157:H7 infections in Minnesota by molecular subtyping, *N Engl J Med* 337:338, 1997.
38. San Joaquin VH, Pickett DA: *Aeromonas*-associated gastroenteritis in children, *Pediatr Infect Dis* 7:53, 1988.
39. Holmberg SD et al: *Plesiomonas* enteric infections in the United States, *Ann Intern Med* 105:690, 1986.
40. Centers for Disease Control and Prevention: Outbreak of staphylococcal food poisoning associated with pre-cooked ham: Florida, 1997, *MMWR* 46:1189, 1997.
41. Lund BM: Food-borne disease due to *Bacillus* and *Clostridium* species, *Lancet* 336:982, 1990.
42. Centers for Disease Control and Prevention: *Bacillus cereus* food poisoning associated with fried rice at two child daycare centers: Virginia, 1993, *MMWR* 43:177, 1994.
43. Centers for Disease Control and Prevention: Imported cholera associated with a newly-described toxigenic *Vibrio cholera* 0139, 1993, *MMWR* 42:501, 1993.
44. Bishai WR, Sears CL: Food poisoning syndromes, *Gastroenterol Clin North Am* 22:579, 1993.
45. Centers for Disease Control and Prevention: Scombroid fish poisoning: Illinois, South Carolina, *MMWR* 38:1, 1989.
46. Bartholomew BA et al: Scombrotoxic fish poisoning in Britain: features of over 250 suspected incidents from 1976 to 1986, *Epidemiol Infect* 99:775, 1987.
47. Morris PD, Campbell DS, Freeman JI: Ciguatera fish poisoning: an outbreak associated with fish caught from North Carolina coastal waters, *South Med J* 83:380, 1990.
48. Gollop JH, Pon EW: Ciguatera: a review, *Hawaii Med J* 51:91, 1992.
49. Beadle A: Ciguatera fish poisoning, *Military Med* 162:319, 1997.
50. Centers for Disease Control and Prevention: Ciguatera fish poisoning: Texas, 1997, *MMWR* 47:692, 1998.
51. Blythe DG et al: Clinical experience with IV mannitol in the treatment of ciguatera, *Bull Soc Pathol Exot* 85:425, 1992.
52. Editor, Advice for travelers, *Med Let* 40:470, 1998.

53. Sheth NK, Wisniewski TR, Franson TR: Survival of enteric pathogens in common beverages, an in vitro study, *Am J Gastroenterol* 83:658, 1988.
54. Gerding BN et al: *Clostridium difficile*-associated diarrhea and colitis, *Infect Control Hosp Epidemiol* 16:459, 1995.
55. Kelly CP, LaMont JT: *Clostridium difficile* infection, *Ann Rev Med* 49:375, 1998.
56. Frost F et al: Increasing hospitalization and death possibly due to *Clostridium difficile* diarrheal disease, *Emerg Infect Dis* 4:1, 1998.
57. Bartlett JG: How to identify the cause of antibiotic-associated diarrhea, *J Crit Illness* 9:1063, 1994.
58. McFarland LV et al: A randomized placebo-controlled trial of *Saccharomyces boulardii* in combination with standard antibiotics for *Clostridium difficile* disease, *JAMA* 271:1913, 1994.
59. Kapikian AZ: Viral gastroenteritis, *JAMA* 269:627, 1993.
60. Kapikian AZ: Overview of viral gastroenteritis, *Arch Virol Suppl* 12:7, 1996.
61. Daniels NA et al: A food-borne outbreak of gastroenteritis associated with Norwalk-like viruses: first molecular traceback to deli sandwiches contaminated during preparation, *J Infect Dis* 181:1467, 2000.
62. Kohn MA et al: An outbreak of Norwalk virus gastroenteritis associated with eating raw oysters, *JAMA* 273:466, 1995.
63. Grohmann GS et al: Enteric viruses and diarrhea in HIV-infected patients, *N Engl J Med* 329:14, 1993.
64. Cordell RL, Addiss DG: Cryptosporidiosis in child care settings: a review of the literature and recommendations for prevention and control, *Pediatr Infect Dis J* 13:310, 1994.
65. Guerrant RL: Cryptosporidiosis: an emerging, highly infectious threat, *Emerg Infect Dis* 3:1, 1997.
66. Bell A et al: A swimming pool-associated outbreak of cryptosporidiosis in British Columbia, *Can J Public Health* 84:334, 1993.
67. Hayes EB et al: Large community outbreak of cryptosporidiosis due to contamination of a filtered public water supply, *N Engl J Med* 320:1372, 1989.
68. MacKenzie WR et al: A massive outbreak in Milwaukee of *Cryptosporidium* infection transmitted through the public water supply, *N Engl J Med* 331:161, 1994.
69. Ackers JP: Treatment of *Isosporiasis, Semin Gastrointest Dis* 8:33, 1997.
70. Mannheimer SB, Soave R: Protozoal infections in patients with AIDS, *Dis Clin North Am* 8:483, 1994.
71. Robert WG et al: Evidence of cryptosporidiosis in patients undergoing endoscopy: evidence for an asymptomatic carrier state, *Am J Med* 87:537, 1989.
72. Cevallos AM, Farthing MJG: Parasitic infections of the gastrointestinal tract, *Curr Opin Gastroenterol* 6:112, 1990.
73. White AC et al: Paromomycin for cryptosporidiosis in AIDS: a prospective, double-blind trial, *J Infect Dis* 170:419, 1994.
74. Simon D, Brandt LJ: Diarrhea in patients with the acquired immunodeficiency syndrome, *Gastroenterol* 105:1238, 1993.
75. Armitage et al: Paromomycin and zithromycin treatment of cryptosporidiosis, *Arch Intern Med* 152:2497, 1992.
76. Smith NH et al: Combination drug therapy for cryptosporidiosis in AIDS, *J Infect Dis* 178:900, 1998.
77. Centers for Disease Control and Prevention: Outbreaks of cyclosporiasis in the United States and Canada 1997, *MMWR* 46:521, 1997.
78. Colley DG: Widespread food-borne cyclosporiasis outbreaks present major challenges, *Emerg Infect Dis* 2:354, 1996.
79. Herwaldt BL et al: An outbreak in 1996 of cyclosporiasis associated with imported raspberries, *N Engl J Med* 336:1548, 1997.
80. Sterling CR, Ortega YR: Cyclospora: an enigma worth unraveling, *Emerg Infect Dis* 5:20, 1999.
81. Centers for Disease Control and Prevention: Giardiasis surveillance: United States, 1992-1997, *MMWR* 49(SS-7):1, 2000.
82. Chak A, Banwell JG: Traveler's diarrhea, *Gastroenterol Clin North Am* 22:549, 1993.
83. Ortega YR, Adam RD: Giardia: overview and update, *Clin Infect Dis* 25:545, 1997.
84. Spriegel JR, Sagg KG, Tsang TK: Infectious diarrhea secondary to *Enteromonas hominis, Am J Gastroenterol* 84:1313, 1989.
85. Weinket R et al: Prevalence and clinical importance of *Entamoeba histolytica* in two high-risk groups: travelers returning from the tropics and male homosexuals, *J Infect Dis* 161:1029, 1990.
86. Berkelman RL: Emerging infectious diseases in the United States 1993, *J Infect Dis* 170:272, 1994.
87. Farmer RG: Infectious causes of diarrhea in the differential diagnosis of inflammatory bowel disease, *Med Clin North Am* 74:29, 1990.
88. Smith PD et al: NIH Conference: gastrointestinal infections in AIDS, *Ann Intern Med* 116:63, 1993.
89. Sanchez-Mejoradag G, Ponce de Leons S: Clinical patterns of diarrhea in AIDS: etiology and prognosis, *Rev Invest Clin* 46:187, 1994.
90. Babu K et al: Isolation of salmonellae from dried rattlesnake preparations, *J Clin Microbiol* 28:361, 1990.
91. Orloff JJ et al: Toxic megacolon in cytomegalovirus and colitis, *Am J Gastroenterol* 84:794, 1989.
92. Bach MC et al: Aphthous ulceration of the gastrointestinal tract in patients with AIDS, *Ann Intern Med* 112:465, 1990.
93. Buckner FS, Pomeroy C: Ganciclovir treatment of cytomegalovirus gastroenteritis, *Clin Infect Dis* 17:644, 1993.
94. Dietrerich DT et al: Treatment of cytomegalovirus infections in AIDS, *Am J Gastroenterol* 88:542, 1993.
95. Black RE: Epidemiology of traveler's diarrhea and relative importance of various pathogens, *Rev Infect Dis* 12(Suppl 1):S73, 1990.
96. Ericsson CD: Traveler's diarrhea, *Curr Opin Gastroenterol* 6:100, 1990.
97. Kozicki M, Steffen R, Schar M: "Boil it, cook it, peel it, or forget it": does this rule prevent traveler's diarrhea? *Int J Epidemiol* 14:169, 1985.
98. Centers for Disease Control and Prevention: *Health information for international travel.* The most current version can be downloaded for free at the CDC website at *www.cdc.gov/travel/reference.htm.*
99. DuPont HL et al: Prevention of traveler's diarrhea by the tablet formulation of bismuth subsalicylate, *JAMA* 257:1347, 1987.
100. DuPont HL, Ericsson CD: Drug therapy: prevention and treatment of traveler's diarrhea, *N Engl J Med* 328:1821, 1993.
101. Taylor DN et al: Treatment of travelers' diarrhea: ciprofloxacin plus loperamide compared with ciprofloxacin alone, *Ann Intern Med* 114:731, 1991.
102. Petruccelli BP et al: Treatment of traveler's diarrhea with ciprofloxacin and loperamide, *J Infect Dis* 165:557, 1992.
103. Erickson CD et al: Treatment of traveler's diarrhea with sulfamethoxazole and trimethoprim and loperamide, *JAMA* 263:257, 1990.

90 Large Intestine

Robert A. Bitterman
Michael A. Peterson

DISORDERS OF COLONIC MOTILITY

Congenital Megacolon: Hirschsprung's Disease (also see Chapter 165, Gastrointestinal Disorders)

Perspective Hirschsprung's disease (HD) is caused by a congenital absence of the myenteric parasympathetic nerve ganglia of the distal colon. HD occurs in 20 of every 100,000 persons and accounts for approximately 20% of neonatal intestinal obstructions. The disorder is usually evident in early infancy, but some individuals with less severe disease are not diagnosed until adolescence or early adulthood.[1]

Principles of Disease During development, neural crest cells normally migrate in a cephalad to caudad manner along the gastrointestinal (GI) tract. A genetic defect leads to incomplete migration and a distal aganglionic bowel segment of variable length. This aganglionic segment may extend proximally from the anus to involve 4 to 25 cm of distal colon; rarely is more of the colon involved.[2] This aganglionic segment cannot relax to permit passage of stool, thus the more proximal colon becomes greatly dilated.

Clinical Features The majority of patients are diagnosed before 1 year of age, although up to 18% may not be diagnosed until the age of 5. The age of diagnosis seems to depend on the extent of the disease; persons with shorter segment involvement with milder disease are sometimes not diagnosed until later in life.

Symptoms may begin at birth with failure to pass meconium or may appear in the next few weeks. Abdominal distention, anorexia, and failure to pass stool are characteristic. The abdomen is distended and the enlarged colon, filled with impacted fecal material, is palpable. Rectal examination reveals no ampullary dilation and no impacted feces present in the rectal vault. This is in direct contrast to the widely dilated rectum full of impacted feces seen in acquired megacolon. Commonly, after the rectal examination, the patient with HD has an explosive discharge of feces and gas, providing temporary relief of symptoms.

HD should be considered in any infant with symptoms and signs of obstructive bowel disease and in infants or young children with enterocolitis. Of patients with HD, 5% eventually develop life-threatening enterocolitis, possibly because of an impaired ability to combat a challenge by *Clostridium difficile*.[2] Adults may be diagnosed when chronic constipation is unresponsive to medical management.

Diagnostic Strategy When there are significant lengths of aganglionic bowel, plain-film radiographs of the abdomen usually show nonspecific intestinal obstruction. A barium enema will show the narrowed aganglionic segment with a proximally dilated colon (Figure 90-1). If only a very short segment of bowel is affected, the barium enema may not show the very distal aganglionic zone. Definitive diagnosis is made by a rectal biopsy, which demonstrates the absence of myenteric ganglia.[1,3]

Differential Considerations In younger children, other causes of obstruction include volvulus and rectal strictures. In older children and adults, HD may be confused with chronic constipation or acquired megacolon.

Management ED management is supportive. Treatment is similar to other causes of intestinal obstruction (see the section on large bowel obstruction later in this chapter). In cases of suspected enterocolitis characterized by fever, bloody diarrhea, and abdominal distention, aggressive management is warranted and includes fluid resuscitation and antibiotics.

Disposition Patients suspected of having HD should be admitted for an evaluation to include a rectal biopsy. The treatment is surgical removal of the aganglionic segment, which is curative.

Key Concepts

- HD should be suspected in any adult with chronic refractory constipation, especially if there is coexistent megacolon.

Acquired Megacolon

Perspective *Acquired megacolon* refers to a subacute or chronic disorder. Megacolon is defined as a colon measuring 6 cm or more in diameter. A dilated colon with an acute onset of symptoms implies large bowel obstruction and is discussed later in this chapter. The underlying disorder in all cases of acquired megacolon is severe chronic constipation of either organic or psychoneurogenic origin.

The more common organic causes are postoperative anorectal stricture, radiation proctitis, anorectal injury, lymphogranuloma venereum, and endometriosis. Myxedema and infiltrative diseases such as scleroderma and amyloidosis can decrease colonic motility and produce marked colonic distention. Megacolon can also result from metabolic abnormalities, such as hypokalemia. Patients with neurologic disorders such as paraplegia are also prone to megacolon, because control of the voluntary muscles for defecation is lost.

Another cause is infection with *Trypanosoma cruzi,* or Chagas' disease, which is endemic in South and Central America; it results in destruction of the intramural ganglia and leads to chronic megacolon.[4] Over the past 20 years, many persons have immigrated to the United States from the Latin American countries, resulting in an increase of Chagas' disease in this country.[5]

Psychogenic megacolon is seen in young children usually as an extension of problems with toilet training. Institution-

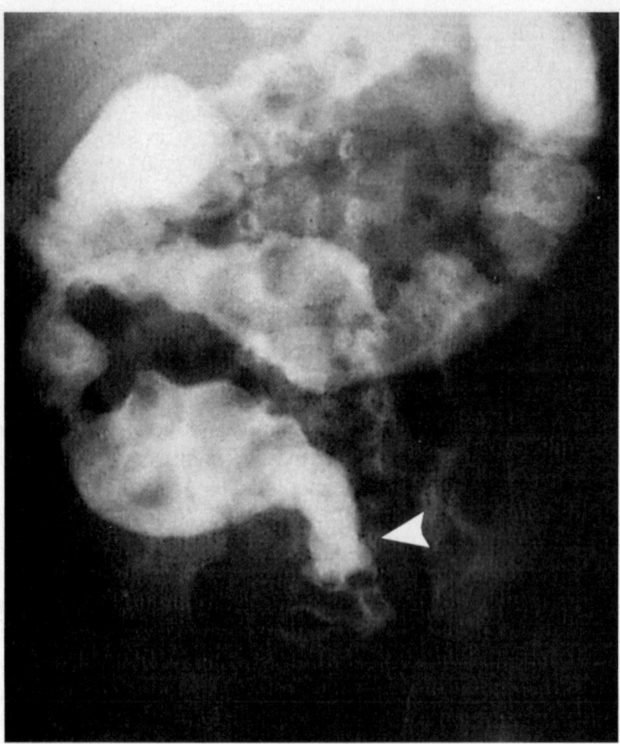

Figure 90-1. **Barium enema in a 2-week-old infant demonstrating narrowed distal colon-rectum of HD.**

alized psychotic patients may also develop megacolon. Severe constipation, perhaps because of inactivity and voluntary inhibition of defecation, is probably the cause.

Principles of Disease Chronic constipation leads to partial mechanical obstruction of the lower colon, rectum, or anus, resulting in a dilated colon with decreased motor tone.

Clinical Features The diagnosis is easy to establish by the history and rectal examination. The history is one of long-term constipation, usually with concomitant laxative abuse. In children with psychogenic megacolon, the onset of symptoms is usually the time when toilet training begins, not early infancy. Rectal examination results are distinctive in acquired megacolon; fecal material fills a cavernous ampulla as opposed to the snug, empty rectal segment of HD. Patients with long-standing megacolon are prone to sigmoid volvulus or fecal impactions.

Diagnostic Strategy Laboratory analysis, including electrolytes and a complete blood count (CBC), is helpful in assessing for potential causes such as hypokalemia and anemia associated with colon carcinoma.

A barium enema can confirm the diagnosis and is sometimes necessary to demonstrate strictures or to rule out cancer or other causes of acquired megacolon.

Differential Considerations Patients with dilated segments of colon may also be manifesting a late presentation of HD. Systemic diseases that cause constipation and may be associated with megacolon include endocrine disorders such as thyroid disease, and neurologic disorders such as Parkinson's disease and multiple sclerosis. Carcinoma of the colon or rectal trauma with subsequent stricture formation may also present as megacolon.

Management Treatment of megacolon depends on its cause. Megacolon with an organic cause is best treated by resolving the underlying problem, such as resecting strictures. Psychogenic megacolon usually requires the long-term use of stool softeners, bulk laxatives, enemas, and, in institutionalized patients, good nursing care. In children, treatment is based on education regarding normal bowel habits, but usually a long course of mineral oil and enemas is required until the child acquires a regular pattern of bowel movements.

Disposition Patients without acute signs or symptoms suggestive of progressive bowel obstruction can be managed on an outpatient basis.

Key Concepts

- Progressive bowel obstruction may be congenital or acquired.
- Management of acquired megacolon must reflect the pathophysiology and the degree of symptomatology.

Irritable Bowel Syndrome

Perspective Irritable bowel syndrome may be defined as an abnormal state of intestinal sensation and motility, which leads to abdominal pain with constipation or diarrhea that is modified by psychosocial factors, and for which no anatomic cause can be found. It is primarily a disease of young to middle-aged adults, with a female predominance of approximately 2:1. Surveys show that as many as 15% of the general population report symptoms consistent with the diagnosis of irritable bowel syndrome.[6] Clearly, not all of those affected seek medical attention. Those who do have a higher incidence of abnormal personality traits, excessive patterns of illness behavior, and higher anxiety levels.[7] Generally, psychologically distressed patients seek medical attention for their bowel problems, whereas other people ignore these symptoms or treat themselves.

Principles of Disease The precipitating cause of irritable bowel syndrome is largely unknown, although there has been a proven association with severe gastroenteritis and periods of psychological stress. The basic pathophysiologic abnormalities are alterations in both intestinal motility and sensation. Resting pressures in the sigmoid colon are increased in patients with constipation and decreased in patients with diarrhea; interestingly these findings are absent during sleep. This may be representative of a general hyperresponsiveness of all smooth muscle in affected patients, some demonstrating increased sensitivity of bladder and pulmonary smooth muscle.[7] Patients also exhibit an exaggerated pain response to intestinal stimulation.

Clinical Features The diagnosis of irritable bowel syndrome is based on a characteristic symptom complex related to physical and emotional stress and the exclusion of organic disease. Although there have been several sets of criteria developed to diagnose irritable bowel syndrome, the most concise and extensively used are the Manning Criteria (Box 90-1).[6,8]

The typical patient describes symptoms occurring intermittently for months or years, usually in strong association with episodes of psychosocial stress. Either diarrhea or

Box 90-1 Manning Criteria for the Diagnosis of Irritable Bowel Syndrome

Abdominal pain plus two or more of the following:
- Pain relieved by defecation
- Pain associated with looser stools
- Pain associated with more frequent stools
- Abdominal distention
- Feeling of incomplete evacuation
- Mucus in stools

Box 90-2 Differential Diagnosis of Irritable Bowel Syndrome

- Intestinal infection
- Inflammatory bowel disease
- Carcinoma
- Aortic aneurysm
- Mesenteric ischemia
- Laxative abuse
- Lactose intolerance
- Intermittent volvulus
- Intussusception

constipation may predominate, or diarrhea may alternate with constipation. However, in any individual patient, the nature and character of the symptoms tend to remain constant.

Diarrhea consists of loose, sometimes watery stools in small amounts that often contain excessive mucus. The frequency of diarrhea and its relation to meals is highly variable. Nocturnal diarrhea is distinctly unusual but occasionally occurs. Constipation is often described as the infrequent passage of small, hard pellets known as *scybala.* There may be "pencil-like" stools, reflecting heightened anal sphincter or rectal tone, or the passage of a large amount of mucus.

Abdominal pain is usually crampy or aching in character and is localized in the lower abdomen, often over the sigmoid colon. The pain is usually relieved with the passage of stools or flatus.

A whole host of extracolonic symptoms is common. Such symptoms include anorexia, nausea, belching, excessive bloating, heartburn, back pain, weakness, faintness, and palpitations. Significant weight loss is unusual.

Findings on physical examination are nonspecific. The patient may appear anxious and usually has mild, vague, diffuse lower abdominal tenderness. Sometimes a feces-filled sigmoid colon is palpable. Rectal examination reveals an ampulla characteristically empty of feces. Sigmoidoscopic examination is usually normal but may show increased spasm, mucus, or mucosal vascular engorgement.

Diagnostic Strategy There are no specific laboratory tests for irritable bowel syndrome. One must always be aware of the lack of specificity that exists when a diagnosis is made by exclusion and keep constantly attuned to clues that may point to an organic cause. Laboratory investigation should be guided by the clinical examination and the need to exclude other potential causes of abdominal pain and diarrhea or constipation. Consider stool examination for occult blood, bacteria, and ova and parasites (especially *Giardia lamblia*). A CBC is helpful to detect anemia that is possibly secondary to a GI malignancy.

An abdominal computed tomography (CT) scan, barium enema, or colonoscopy may be indicated if there is a concern for another etiology of the symptoms.

Differential Considerations See Box 90-2.

Management The goal of therapy is to allow the patient to adjust to a chronic condition. The most important factor is an effective doctor-patient relationship in which the physician can provide compassion, education, and reassurance while excluding organic disease. That irritable bowel syndrome has a significant psychologic component without a specific identifiable lesion does not undermine the legitimacy of the patient's complaints. Any implication that the problem is all emotional will be taken as a rejection by the patient and should be avoided.

Treatment modalities that may be beneficial include a high-fiber, low-fat diet; bulk-forming agents, such as bran or psyllium seed preparations; and avoidance of caffeine, sorbitol (sugarless gum or candy), and foods that tend to bother the patient. Some patients may benefit from behavioral therapies such as biofeedback and stress management. The judicial use of anxiolytic, antispasmodic, antidiarrheal, or antidepressant agents may be beneficial. Drug therapy is best reserved for severe or refractory symptoms.

Disposition Patients with known or suspected irritable bowel syndrome and without significant findings on the abdominal examination may be treated at home. Good follow-up should be established. Irritable bowel syndrome is a diagnosis of exclusion and is usually made in the primary care setting. Most of the tests used to confirm this diagnosis are not available to the emergency physician. The emergency physician may elect to try various medical therapies, but the most successful treatment is through a good relationship with a primary care physician.

Key Concepts

- Nocturnal diarrhea, significant weight loss, or age over 50 at onset of symptoms suggests a diagnosis other than irritable bowel syndrome.
- There should be no significant abdominal tenderness in patients with irritable bowel syndrome.
- In elderly patients, exclude abdominal aortic aneurysm and ischemic colitis.
- Ongoing follow-up is essential for evaluation and management.

Diverticular Disease

Diverticular disease, especially diverticulitis, is a disorder commonly encountered in the ED. All patients in the correct age range with lower abdominal pain or lower GI bleeding should be suspected of having diverticular disease.

Diverticulosis

Perspective *Diverticulosis* refers to the mere presence of diverticula of the colon, without evidence of inflammation. The frequency of diverticulosis is directly related to advancing age: 50% of persons by age 65 years and 65% of persons by age 85 years will have diverticula.[12] Diverticula are strikingly isolated to Western civilizations, suggesting that the highly refined low-fiber Western diet is responsible for an abnormal increase in bowel wall muscle tone.[9] Most persons with diverticulosis of the colon are asymptomatic; only 10% to 20% will at some time develop symptoms such as pain, inflammation, or bleeding.[10]

Principles of Disease Diverticulosis is a disorder of colonic muscle function. An increase in tone of the muscle layers of the bowel wall causes a shortening of the bowel, with muscle thickening, particularly of the taeniae coli (the longitudinal muscles), resulting in saclike protrusions (diverticula) of the colonic mucosa through the muscularis. These saclike protrusions occur at sites of relative weakness in the bowel wall where small colonic arteries penetrate the muscular layers.

Diverticula occur most commonly in the sigmoid colon and are usually confined to the sigmoid area. However, they may be present in more proximal parts of the colon or involve the entire colon. For unknown reasons, persons of Japanese, Chinese, or Hawaiian ancestry are prone to the development of diverticula in the cecum and ascending colon. Uncomplicated asymptomatic diverticula do not require any particular evaluation or treatment.

Painful Diverticular Disease

Principles of Disease Painful diverticular disease can occur with otherwise uncomplicated diverticulosis. Symptoms are similar to those of irritable bowel syndrome, and manometric studies reveal similar muscle motor abnormalities with both disorders. In both irritable bowel syndrome and painful diverticular disease there is a heightened response to food ingestion or emotional stimuli, resulting in a marked increase in the amplitude of muscle contractions. As a consequence, intraluminal pressure is increased, stretching the bowel wall and causing pain. These similarities have prompted suggestions that the irritable bowel syndrome may be a precursor to colonic diverticulosis.[9]

Clinical Features Patients with diverticulosis may experience recurrent, intermittent, but usually nonpersistent left lower quadrant abdominal pain and tenderness. The pain often follows a meal as a result of the gastrocolic reflex and may be relieved with defecation or the passage of flatus. Flatulence is common. An attack may be accompanied by either diarrhea or constipation. On examination, there may be mild tenderness or fullness in the left lower quadrant, but signs of peritoneal inflammation such as rebound tenderness, muscle guarding, fever, and leukocytosis are absent.

Diagnostic Strategy The diagnosis of diverticulosis should be suspected when a patient over 40 years of age complains of lower abdominal pain, constipation or diarrhea or both, and increased flatulence. Although historically the barium enema has been the diagnostic modality of choice, colonoscopy can also establish the diagnosis and has been shown to be both safe and more accurate in detecting carcinoma and colonic polyps, in addition to diverticula.[10]

Differential Considerations See Box 90-3.

Management Treatment of painful diverticular disease is directed toward the relief of painful bowel spasm and toward reducing further formation of diverticula. Muscle spasm may be relaxed by the local application of heat or by the administration of anticholinergics, which reduce sigmoidal contractions. Sedatives may alleviate tension or anxiety, which can increase sigmoid muscle contractions. The patient should be started on a high-fiber diet. Bulk laxatives and stool softeners are used to decrease intraluminal pressure and prevent constipation. Antibiotic use is not necessary in the absence of signs of diverticulitis.

Box 90-3 Differential Considerations in Painful Diverticular Disease

Ovarian cyst with or without torsion
Ureterolithiasis
Irritable bowel syndrome
Ectopic pregnancy
Carcinoma of the bowel
Ischemic bowel

Disposition If there is no evidence of diverticulitis (fever, peritoneal findings, or significant abdominal tenderness), patients can usually be managed on an outpatient basis. Patients should be reevaluated in a few days to ensure improvement in their symptoms.

Key Concepts

- Painful diverticular disease manifests with transient abdominal pain and tenderness and doesn't require emergent imaging studies or antibiotics.

Diverticulitis

Principles of Disease Diverticulitis is present when inflammation of a diverticulum occurs, and is the most common complication of diverticulosis. The frequency increases with age; only 2% to 4% of patients with diverticulitis are under 40 years of age.[11]

Diverticulitis begins when fecal matter is sequestered in the diverticular sac and becomes inspissated and hard, forming a fecalith that abrades the mucosa or compromises the blood supply of the sac. Inflammation develops and leads to microperforation of the thin wall. In uncomplicated diverticulitis, the inflammatory process is confined to the colonic wall by the serosa (termed *peridiverticulitis*). If there is perforation of the serosa, the inflammation may form a localized pericolic abscess or spread to produce frank peritonitis.

Clinical Features The clinical signs and symptoms of acute diverticulitis and their severity depend on the amount of contamination resulting from the perforation and the ability of the host defenses to localize the resulting inflammatory process. The predominant symptom in patients with classical sigmoid diverticulitis is persistent abdominal pain. Initially, the pain may be vague and generalized, but it quickly becomes well localized to the left lower quadrant. Low-grade fever, malaise, and a change in bowel habits, usually constipation, are common. Urinary symptoms are commonly present secondary to inflammation near the bladder or ureter. Occasionally the patient will have anorexia, nausea, and vomiting.

Examination reveals tenderness localized to the left lower quadrant. Distention is common, but bowel sounds are usually normal. Traditionally it has been stated that a mass, or phlegmon, composed of inflamed loops of matted bowel or a frank abscess, is palpable in patients with diverticulitis. However, pain, muscular rigidity, or abdominal guarding may preclude the palpation of a mass even if one is present. In most patients, a mass will not be found clinically. The rectal examination may reveal generalized tenderness. Examination of the stool for occult blood will be positive in more than 50% of cases, but gross bleeding is unusual.[12]

Complications of diverticulitis include abscess or fistula formation, perforation, and obstruction. When the inflammatory process progresses beyond peridiverticulitis to true abscess formation, the pain and tenderness will become much more severe and signs of acute peritonitis will be present. The peritoneal irritation still usually remains localized.

Generalized peritonitis results when the perforation of the diverticulum spills into the free peritoneal space. Patients then have severe abdominal pain, fever, guarding, rigidity, and rebound tenderness. Patients with immunodeficiency diseases, those taking steroids or other immunosuppressive drugs, or the elderly may not demonstrate the expected inflammatory indicators such as elevated temperature, elevated white blood (WBC) count, or clinical signs of peritonitis. The risk of perforation is high in the immunocompromised patient: 43% compared to 14% for the nonimmunocompromised patient.[10] The signs and symptoms of cecal or right-sided diverticulitis are difficult to distinguish from those of acute appendicitis.[13]

Partial colonic obstruction occurs in a significant number of patients with acute diverticulitis, probably because of inflammation, spasm, and edema. Complete obstruction occurs in less than 10% of patients and can be difficult to distinguish from obstruction secondary to carcinoma.[14]

Fistulas may develop after repeated attacks. The most common fistula is a colovesical fistula. Patients with colovesical fistulas have characteristic symptoms of pneumaturia, fecaluria, or symptoms of an ordinary urinary tract infection.

Diagnostic Strategy Mild sigmoid diverticulitis is usually diagnosed on clinical grounds alone. Patients over 40 years of age with persistent abdominal pain and tenderness, especially in the left lower quadrant, should be suspected of having diverticulitis.

Most patients will have an elevated WBC count, with an increase in immature forms. The red blood cell (RBC) analysis is usually normal; if an iron deficiency anemia is present, it should suggest carcinoma rather than diverticulitis.

Abdominal radiographs generally show nonspecific ileus and mild distention. Radiographic studies are done primarily to exclude colonic obstruction or perforation, which may be evidenced by free intraperitoneal air. Contrast radiographic studies and endoscopy are generally avoided in acute diverticulitis for fear of inducing a perforation. However, in select situations, a limited water-soluble contrast study has been found to be safe and useful.[12] After resolution of the acute diverticulitis, barium enema examinations are indicated to exclude other colonic pathology and to look for some of the complications of diverticulitis such as fistula formation. The barium enema also is used to exclude colon carcinoma, because these two diseases can mimic each other. Similarly endoscopy, particularly with the newer pediatric endoscope, has sometimes proven useful in making a diagnosis or in excluding carcinoma, thus avoiding unnecessary surgical procedures.

The examination of choice to discover the extent of acute diverticulitis is an abdominal CT scan.[15] The CT scan has been shown to be as accurate as contrast enema studies in defining the colonic involvement of the diverticulitis. It is accurate in demonstrating the presence of abscesses and the extent of pericolonic inflammation, and may demonstrate or exclude other intraabdominal pathology. One study shows that in 46% of patients admitted with a diagnosis of acute diverticulitis, a CT scan revealed a different diagnosis such as appendicitis or tuboovarian abscess. Thus the CT scan is especially useful when the clinical picture is unclear, as is common in the elderly.[16] The CT scan also has the advantage of not inducing perforation.[17] Ultrasound has not been proven to be an accurate diagnostic modality for diverticulitis.[10]

Before initiating diagnostic studies, such as contrast studies, colonoscopy, or a CT scan, the emergency physician should discuss the diagnostic approach with the physician who will be managing the patient on an ongoing basis.

Differential Considerations The most important differential diagnosis in acute sigmoid diverticulitis is carcinoma of the colon with a localized perforation. Other diseases to consider include ischemic colitis, ulcerative colitis, bacterial colitis, ectopic pregnancy, and pelvic infections such as tuboovarian abscess. Cecal diverticulitis is usually mistakenly diagnosed as acute appendicitis because of the frequency of the latter and the relative rarity of the former.

Chronic diverticulitis may appear initially as a fibrotic colonic stricture, with partial or total colon obstruction. This can be difficult to differentiate from a colon carcinoma.

Management Most episodes of diverticulitis are not severe and resolve with medical management alone. Patients should be treated with bowel rest, parenteral fluids, analgesics, intravenous antibiotics, and frequent reexaminations. When the diagnosis is not in doubt and the disease is mild, a reliable patient can be treated at home with a clear liquid diet, nonopioid analgesics, and oral antibiotics such as either trimethoprim-sulfamethoxazole and metronidazole, or ciprofloxacin and metronidazole. Close follow-up care is mandatory. Failure of outpatient treatment is an indication for admission. Uncertainty about the diagnosis is also a reason for hospitalization.[12]

When patients are to be admitted for acute diverticulitis, analgesia and antibiotic therapy should be initiated in the ED. Treatment is directed against both facultative and obligate, anaerobic, gram-negative bacteria. Well-studied, equally effective regimens are listed in Box 90-4. Alternate regimens include ticarcillin-clavulanic acid or imipenem, with or without an aminoglycoside.[9,17,18]

The treatment of generalized peritonitis, perforation, or evidence of gas in the bowel wall is immediate surgical intervention. Intraabdominal abscess formation secondary to diverticulitis also requires prompt surgical consultation; abscesses less than 5 cm in diameter can be treated with antibiotics alone.[15] Immediate surgery has been avoided in some patients with abscesses by using CT- or ultrasound-guided percutaneous catheter drainage of the abscess cavity.[12] When indicated, traditional surgical intervention has been a multistage procedure, starting with surgical drainage followed by a diverting colostomy. If the catheter drainage procedure plus conservative management and antibiotics are effective, an elective one-stage resection of the involved colonic segment can be performed later.[17,19]

Approximately 10% to 25% of patients managed medically for acute diverticulitis experience recurrent attacks and

Box 90-4 Recommended Inpatient Antibiotic Therapy for Acute Diverticulitis

1. Cefoxitin 2 to 3 g IV q 8 hr
2. Aminoglycoside plus a specific anaerobic agent:
   Gentamicin or tobramycin 5.1 mg/kg IV qd
   plus
   Metronidazole 500 mg IV q 6 hr or clindamycin 300 to 600 mg IV q 6 hr

Box 90-5 Differential Diagnosis of Lower Gastrointestinal Bleeding

Diverticular disease
Colonic angiodysplasia
Colitis, infectious or inflammatory
Neoplastic lesions
Anorectal diseases (hemorrhoids, fistulas, fissures)
Upper GI and small bowel lesions

have an increased risk of complications. It is generally thought that patients who have had two episodes of acute diverticulitis should undergo elective resection of the involved colon.[9] In patients under age 40 years, the recurrence rates are even higher, with as many as 25% readmitted in under 1 year and up to 20% requiring emergency surgery. In these relatively young patients with diverticulitis, consideration should be given to elective sigmoid resection after a single severe attack of diverticulitis, even if the patient has a satisfactory response to medical treatment.[11,17]

Disposition Patients with peritoneal findings, those who have already failed outpatient management, or those who have significant abdominal tenderness with an unclear diagnosis should be admitted. Elderly and immunocompromised patients have unreliable physical examinations and poorer overall outcomes and should also be admitted. Generalized peritonitis mandates the need for urgent surgical consultation.

Key Concepts

- Diverticulitis is uncommon in patients under 40 years of age.
- Symptoms of chronic weight loss or bleeding suggest carcinoma.
- Older patients, especially those over the age of 60, may have ischemic colitis.

Hemorrhage from Diverticula (See also Chapter 23, Gastrointestinal Bleeding.)

Principles of Disease Bleeding may occur from a diverticulum as a result of an entrapped fecalith eroding a branch of a colonic artery on the dome of the diverticulum. Recently, NSAID use has also been implicated as a contributor to diverticular bleeding. Bleeding is a common complication of diverticulosis; though usually mild, it can be massive and life-threatening. Diverticulosis is actually the most common cause of significant lower GI hemorrhage.

Clinical Features Bleeding caused by diverticulosis of the colon is characteristically sudden, unexpected, and often profuse from the onset. Most patients do not have symptoms of inflammation at the time of hemorrhage, although many will have had a previous episode of diverticulitis.

The clinical course is most often surprisingly benign. Blood flows at a steady but moderate rate, and the capacity of the colon to accommodate a large volume of lost blood contributes to the apparent suddenness of rectal bleeding. Thus the volume lost is often very large, but the signs of hypovolemia may be deceptively mild.

Diagnostic Strategy A CBC is helpful in indicating the extent of blood loss, but may underrepresent the amount of acute bleeding in the ED. For bright red bleeding, anoscopy or proctoscopy should be performed to exclude internal hemorrhoids or another rectal lesion as the source. Consider a nasogastric tube if no bleeding source is found, because 10% to 15% of patients with hematochezia have an upper GI source.[10] If the bleeding is occurring at a mild to moderate rate, sigmoidoscopy or colonoscopy is the procedure of choice and is diagnostic in approximately 50% of patients. Bleeding can often be controlled with the colonoscope as well. If colonoscopy fails to determine the site of bleeding and the bleeding continues, angiography or nuclear scintigraphy should be performed. Continued severe bleeding may require surgical intervention.

Management Most patients will lose enough blood to require a transfusion, but in 75% to 95% of patients the bleeding stops spontaneously or with conservative management. Should the bleeding continue, definitive management depends on localizing its source. Selective arterial catheterization may be diagnostic and also therapeutic, by directly infusing a vasopressor to slow or stop the bleeding from diverticula. Early recurrent bleeding occurs in 15% to 20% of patients, but the time saved allows for stabilization and preparation for surgery.[9]

Differential Considerations See Box 90-5.

Disposition Most patients with lower GI bleeding who have either profuse bleeding or an unclear source should be admitted to the hospital for observation and investigation into the cause of the bleeding.

Key Concepts

- A CBC may not accurately reflect the amount of acute blood loss.
- In 10% to 15% of patients with lower GI bleeding, the source is located in the upper GI tract.
- Diverticulosis is the most common cause of significant lower GI bleeding.

STRUCTURAL COLON DISORDERS

Large Bowel Obstruction

Perspective Colonic obstruction is primarily a disease of the elderly because its two most common etiologies, carcinoma and diverticulitis, are age-related diseases. Volvulus, which causes 10% to 13% of large bowel obstructions, also occurs more often in the elderly.[20] Other causes of large bowel obstruction include inflammatory processes, ischemic colitis, Crohn's disease, radiation colitis, and foreign bodies.

Paralytic ileus secondary to injury, illness, or electrolyte abnormalities, and pseudoobstruction, particularly after intraabdominal procedures such as cesarean sections, can cause functional large bowel obstructions. Pseudoobstruction, in which the colon appears obstructed without a definable obstructive lesion, may also be encountered in elderly patients with chronic illnesses such as renal failure, congestive heart failure, or hypothyroidism.[14,21-24]

Large bowel obstruction is much less common than small bowel obstruction. The usual causes of small bowel obstructions—adhesions and hernias—rarely cause obstruction of the colon.

Principles of Disease Once the colon is obstructed distally, intraluminal pressures rise to the point that arterial flow is compromised, leading to colon wall death and perforation. Intestinal secretions, which are normally absorbed in the large intestine, pool there and contribute to dehydration. In a distended, ischemic colon, bacteria invade local nodes, which eventually leads to sepsis.[8]

Clinical Features Symptoms of acute large bowel obstruction are typically insidious, often developing over several days. Diffuse, colicky lower abdominal pain, obstipation, and distention may eventually be followed by nausea and vomiting. Vomiting may be late in appearance or even absent in large bowel obstruction, depending to some extent on the competence of the ileocecal valve. Feculent vomiting rarely occurs and, when it does, is due to proliferation of bacteria in the stagnant intraluminal fluids proximal to the obstruction.[23,25]

Distention is the most constant and prominent physical finding. High-pitched bowel sounds may be audible. Fever, marked abdominal tenderness, or peritonitis suggests the presence of strangulation of the gut, as is seen with volvulus. In such circumstances, the pace of diagnostic and therapeutic interventions must be quickened.

Diagnostic Strategy The hidden fluid losses that occur with large bowel obstruction can be substantial and are further exacerbated by anorexia, vomiting, underlying medical illness, or diuretic therapy. Dehydration may be difficult to ascertain in the elderly patient; the urine specific gravity test, in the absence of underlying renal disease, provides a relatively accurate assessment of the patient's volume status. A blood sample for CBC and a set of electrolytes should also be obtained. A WBC count over 20,000/mm^3, particularly if the patient's pain is out of proportion to clinical findings, suggests the presence of gangrenous bowel. The electrolytes may reveal hypokalemia or other abnormalities that may suggest paralytic ileus or substantial fluid loss with secondary dehydration.[23,25]

The diagnosis of obstruction is confirmed by supine and upright abdominal radiographs (Figure 90-2). Classically the bowel is dilated to a width of 6 cm or greater. A width of 10 cm or greater should prompt concerns of imminent perforation. Free air may be present if perforation has occurred. A water-soluble contrast enema or colonoscopy may be necessary to differentiate mechanical obstruction from either paralytic ileus or pseudoobstruction. It is also beneficial to localize the point of obstruction before operating. A CT scan is less helpful in obstruction unless intussusception or diverticular abscess is suspected.

Differential Considerations Any occurrence of large bowel obstruction should raise suspicion for cancer of the colon and prompt an evaluation for the same. Volvulus, unlike a slowly progressive neoplasm, tends to present with an abrupt onset. Diverticulosis can cause an obstruction when chronic, intermittent diverticulitis is followed by fibrosis and stricture formation, or when an acute episode of diverticulitis is complicated by a pericolic abscess and intestinal compression.

Management Treatment of large bowel obstruction consists of (1) correction of fluid and electrolyte abnormalities, (2) intestinal decompression with nasogastric suction, (3) administration of broad-spectrum antibiotics, and (4) relief of obstruction. Treatment of obstruction secondary to carcinoma is always surgical.

Key Concepts

- High fever, persistent tachycardia, or peritoneal signs suggest perforation of the bowel.
- Immunocompromised patients with perforated bowel typically have unimpressive abdominal examinations.

Volvulus

Volvulus of the colon accounts for approximately 10% to 13% of all large bowel obstructions in the United States, and is exceeded only by carcinoma and diverticulitis as a cause of acute large bowel obstruction. Its incidence is estimated at 3 per 100,000 in the United States.[26] Volvulus results from the rotation of a segment of bowel about its mesenteric axis sufficient to produce obstruction of the lumen and cause vascular occlusion as well. It can occur only if a freely movable segment of bowel has its points of fixation in close approximation. In the colon these areas are the sigmoid colon and the cecum, representing 60% and 40% of cases, respectively. Volvulus of the transverse colon or splenic flexure is rare.[20]

The pathogenic twisting of a mobile piece of bowel is the only feature that volvulus of the sigmoid and the cecum have in common. The epidemiology, clinical manifestations, and treatment are different.

Sigmoid Volvulus

Perspective In the United States, sigmoid volvulus occurs almost exclusively in two groups of persons: patients of all ages who have severe psychiatric or neurologic disease and elderly patients with debilitating diseases who lead lives of inactivity. The usual history is one of severe, chronic constipation. It is distinctly uncommon for volvulus to occur in a person who leads an active life and who has no serious mental or physical illnesses, although it can occur in pregnancy.[27] In parts of South America, such as Brazil, where megacolon secondary to Chagas' disease is common, volvulus also is common.[4]

Principles of Disease The chronic, severe constipation leads to debilitation and lengthening of the chronically distended colon, particularly in the sigmoid region. This produces the redundant sigmoid loop, attached by a narrow mesenteric root, which is the *sine qua non* for sigmoid volvulus. There is evidence that genetic factors may predispose one to development of volvulus, although this is not clear.

Clinical Features Early symptoms of acute sigmoid volvulus are intermittent cramping, lower abdominal pain,

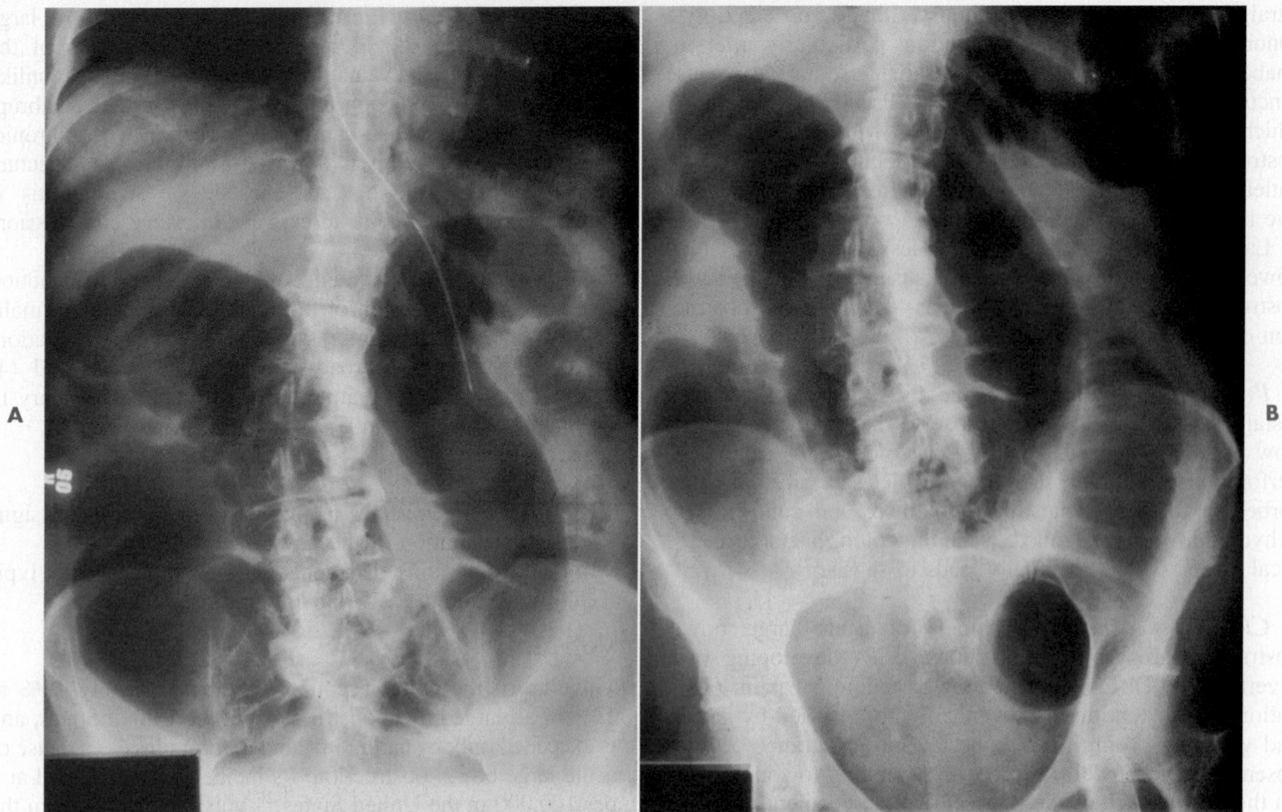

Figure 90-2. **Large bowel obstruction at sigmoid colon caused by "apple core" carcinoma. A, Erect. B, Supine.**

and progressive abdominal distention. Later come nausea, vomiting, dehydration, and obstipation. Most patients relate similar episodes in the past that were terminated spontaneously by the passage of large amounts of flatus and stool, giving instant relief of pain and distention. Patients characteristically are seen late in the course of their illness; they often wait for days before seeking medical attention, which probably reflects the high incidence of sigmoid volvulus in psychiatric and nursing home patients.

The most common physical findings are diffuse abdominal tenderness and marked distention and tympany. Respiratory embarrassment can occur because of distention elevating the diaphragm. Fluid and electrolyte sequestration, dissimilar to small bowel obstruction, is not usually a problem. Fever, marked abdominal tenderness, or peritonitis suggests that strangulation is present. Perforation is unusual because the sigmoid colon in older patients is usually thickened, accounting for its ability to withstand massive distention and high intraluminal pressures.

Diagnostic Strategy The diagnosis should be sought in the case of any institutionalized patient with an acute abdomen. In approximately 80% of cases, the diagnosis can be confirmed by a plain-film radiograph of the abdomen. It shows a tremendously dilated single loop of colon in the left half of the abdomen, with both ends down in the pelvis and the bow positioned superiorly, a "bent innertube" picture (Figure 90-3). If necessary, a barium enema can reveal the pathognomonic twisted "bird's beak" or "ace of spades" deformity (Figure 90-4).[4,26] High WBC counts of 20,000/mm^3 to 25,000/mm^3 and marked polymorphonuclear predominance with many immature forms strongly suggest that strangulation is present. If the diagnosis is in doubt, a CT scan can also be helpful, demonstrating specific findings that can be pathognomonic (such as the mesocolon "whirl sign") and in some cases indicating gangrene.

Management Initial treatment consists of the stabilizing maneuvers previously discussed in the section on large bowel obstruction. Once the diagnosis of sigmoid volvulus is made, a surgeon should be consulted. The therapy of choice for nonstrangulating sigmoid volvulus is decompression and detorsion, using a rectal tube via the sigmoidoscope. Success is achieved in 85% to 95% of patients, with a mortality rate of approximately 2%. Sometimes a barium enema is successful when the rectal tube is not.[20,28]

Failure of tube decompression, or suspected strangulation, demands immediate operative reduction. After nonoperative decompression, the recurrence rate of sigmoid volvulus approaches 90%. Most authors recommend elective resection after the first episode of sigmoid volvulus in all patients except those with a short life expectancy (because of terminal illness or severe underlying medical disease) and risk factors that contraindicate surgery.[8,26]

Disposition All patients should be admitted for continued intestinal decompression and elective resection (in low-risk candidates) to prevent recurrence.

Key Concepts

- High fever, significant leukocytosis (WBC count >20,000/mm^3), or peritoneal signs suggest bowel strangulation or perforation.
- The treatment of choice for a nonstrangulated sigmoid volvulus is manipulation with a sigmoidoscope.

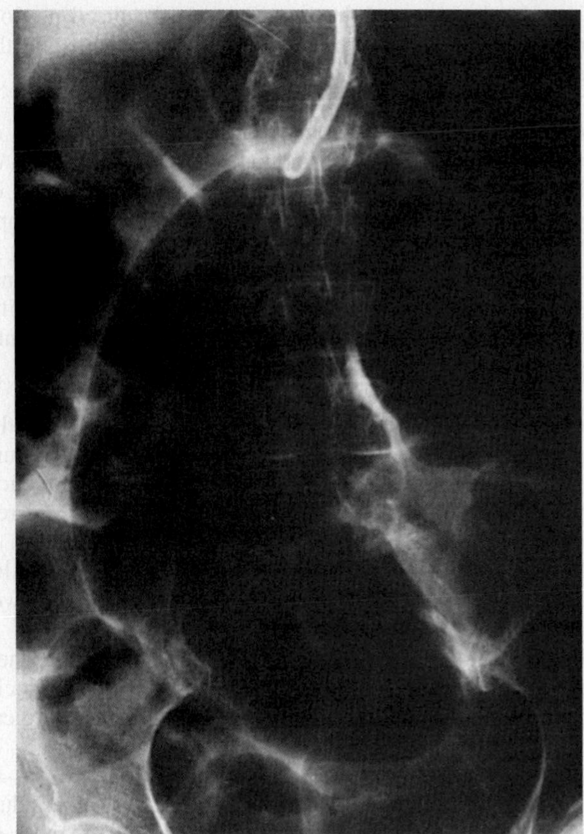

Figure 90-3. **Plain-film radiograph of abdomen demonstrating large, dilated loop characteristic of sigmoid volvulus.**

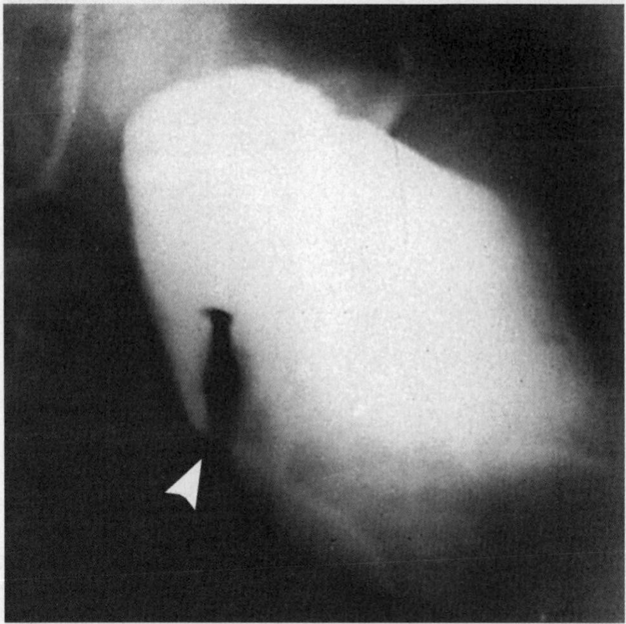

Figure 90-4. **Characteristic "bird's beak" of volvulus shown on barium enema.**

Cecal Volvulus

Perspective Volvulus of the cecum occurs in all ages but is most common in persons 25 to 35 years of age.

Principles of Disease Unlike in sigmoid volvulus, severe, chronic constipation is not an underlying factor, and there is no association with psychiatric or neurologic diseases. Hypofixation (presumably congenital) of the cecum, proximal ascending colon, and terminal ileum to the posterior abdominal wall is a prerequisite for cecal volvulus. Rotation of the hypermobile cecum, usually 360 degrees around the mesenteric pedicle of the ileocecal artery, produces a closed-loop obstruction. This rotation is often precipitated by distal colonic obstruction from neoplasm, inflammation, or other causes.

There is a relatively high incidence of previous abdominal surgery in patients with cecal volvulus, the surgery possibly having disturbed the fixation of the cecum to the posterior wall. Marathon runners may be predisposed to cecal volvulus, possibly because of congenital hypofixation coupled with a thin and flexible mesentery.[2]

Clinical Features The clinical manifestations are essentially those of an acute small bowel obstruction. There is an acute onset of severe, colicky abdominal pain, followed by nausea and vomiting. The abdomen is diffusely tender and greatly distended.[23]

Diagnostic Strategy A plain-film abdominal radiograph is usually diagnostic, but it may be confusing unless one remembers that lack of lateral fixation allows the mobile cecum to be seen anywhere in the abdomen. Usually there is one large, dilated ovoid segment of colon in the midabdomen, with distended small bowel loops and a relatively empty distal large bowel (Figure 90-5), the characteristic "coffee bean" deformity. If the ileocecal valve is incompetent, reflux of gas into the small bowel may give the appearance of a small bowel obstruction. Free air may indicate bowel perforation.

Management Experience suggests that nonoperative decompression is often unsuccessful and unreliable, although successful laparoscopic cecopexy has been reported.[26] Operative treatment is preferred. Mortality is high, 10% to 15% if the bowel is viable, increasing to 30% to 40% if gangrenous bowel is present at the time of operation.[29,30]

Key Concepts

- Cecal volvulus should be suspected in any case of small bowel obstruction, especially in young patients with no other predisposing factors for obstruction.
- Plain-film radiographs usually show a dilated segment of colon.
- Management is usually operative.

Intussusception (See also Chapter 165, Gastrointestinal Disorders)

Perspective Intussusception is the invagination of a proximal piece of bowel into the lumen of an adjacent distal piece that usually occurs in children aged 3 months to 5 years. On rare occasions it can occur in adults, usually from a lesion that serves as a lead point for the invagination. Twenty percent of intussusceptions were colonic in one series.[31]

Principles of Disease In adults, unlike in children, a pathologic lesion is usually involved in the intussusception.[32] A pathologic lesion serves as an object that the normal peristaltic process in the intestine can push along, as it would any intestinal contents. Because the lesion is attached to the intestine, it pulls the intestinal wall along with it, telescoping

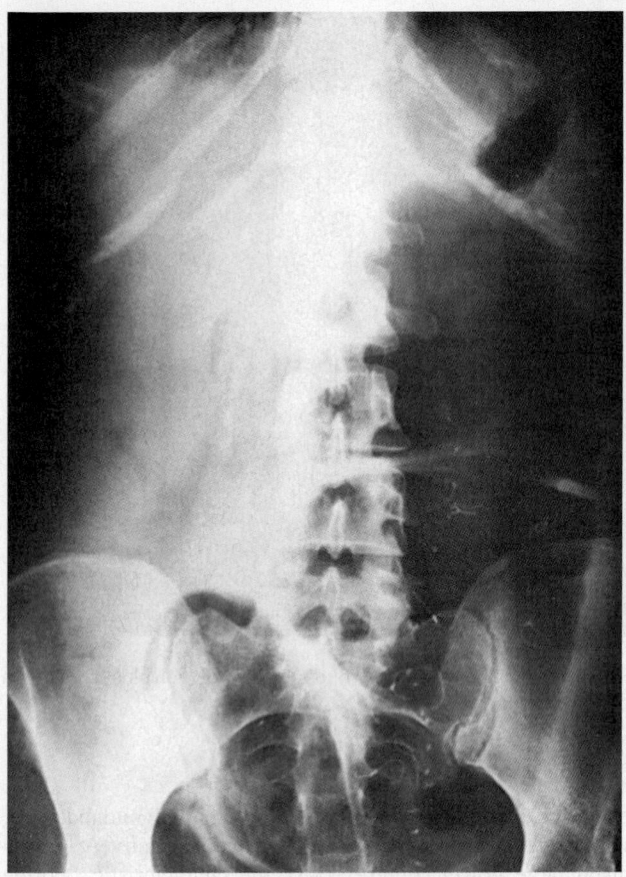

Figure 90-5. **Plain-film radiograph demonstrating distended colon characteristic of cecal volvulus. Note presentation in left lower quadrant and absence of right-sided gas shadows.**

the proximal portion of the intestine into the distal portion. Compression of the mesenteric vessels occurs as the mesentery is invaginated and results in bowel edema.

Clinical Features The clinical picture may be one of either acute intestinal obstruction, with hours or days of abdominal distention, abdominal pain, and constipation, or may be much more indolent, with weeks to months of crampy abdominal pain. Unlike in children, intestinal bleeding is present in adults only 20% of the time, and an abdominal mass is almost never felt.[31] Because of its nonspecific symptoms, adult intussusception is often not diagnosed until surgery is performed.

Diagnostic Strategy CT scan of the abdomen is the diagnostic test of choice for adult intussusception. Barium enemas are also accurate but, unlike in children, the reduction that may accompany barium enema is usually not desired before surgery because of the risk of a seeding from a malignant lead point (Figures 90-6 and 90-7). Plain-film abdominal radiographs usually show nonspecific bowel obstruction.

Enema or insufflation techniques are contraindicated when there is evidence of peritonitis, perforation, sepsis, or shock. Patients with these problems require prompt surgical intervention.

Management There is controversy about whether adult intussusception should be primarily resected or reduced before resection. A reasonable approach is to use the former for large bowel intussusception, in which malignancy rates are high, and the latter in a selective fashion for the small bowel.

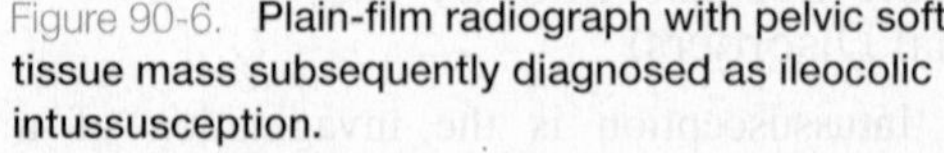

Figure 90-6. **Plain-film radiograph with pelvic soft tissue mass subsequently diagnosed as ileocolic intussusception.**

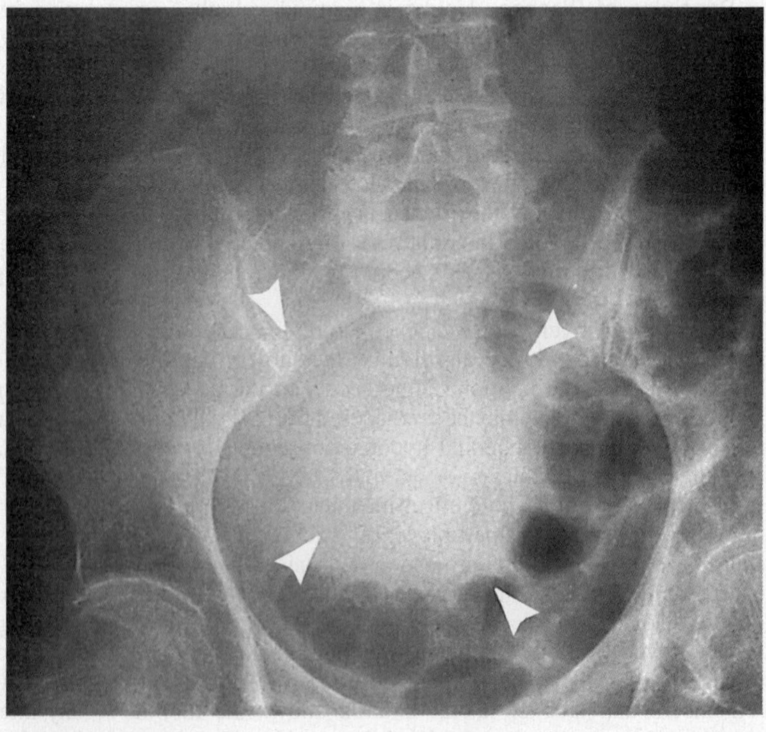

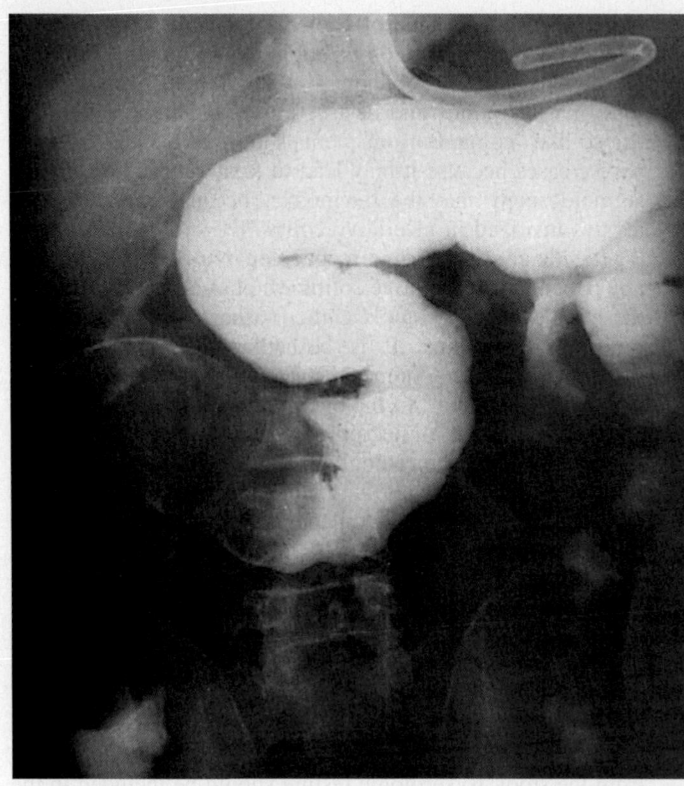

Figure 90-7. **Enterocolic intussusception with thin layer of barium around invaginating intestine.**

Disposition All patients should be admitted for definitive treatment and evaluation of the cause of the intussusception.

Key Concepts
- A number of causes of bowel obstruction must be excluded.
- Lead points for intussusception in adults must be identified in order to exclude malignancy.

INFLAMMATORY BOWEL DISEASE
Ulcerative Colitis

Perspective Ulcerative colitis affects all age groups, with the highest incidence in the third and fourth decades of life. Approximately 60 to 120 out of every 100,000 persons in the United States has ulcerative colitis.[33,34] The disease occurs almost exclusively in industrialized nations, is more common in urban than in rural settings, and involves family history in 10% to 15% of cases. Caucasians are affected four times more often than other races, but there is no gender differential.

Principles of Disease Although the cause of ulcerative colitis remains unknown, there is strong evidence that several different disease processes end up in a final common pathway involving a disordered immune response with inflammation of colonic mucosa. The immune response appears to be genetically and environmentally influenced and to require the presence of antigens from normal bacterial flora.[34,35]

Ulcerative colitis always arises first in the rectum and is confined to the rectum in 10% to 38% of cases. More often, the disease spreads continuously to the upper parts of the colon; pancolitis, involvement of the entire colon, occurs in about 10% of cases. Even with less than total involvement, the disease is strikingly and uniformly continuous. There are no skip areas like those seen in Crohn's disease of the colon.[36]

In severe cases, the typical mucosal appearance consists of a thick inflammatory exudate composed of pus, blood, and mucus covering irregular, shallow ulcers interspersed with islands of swollen mucosa, so-called *pseudopolyps.* Increased mucosal friability is a characteristic finding in ulcerative colitis, as is the microscopic "crypt abscess" formed by the accumulation of WBCs, RBCs, and pus. Blood loss is not great because the inflammation is superficial. As the disease becomes chronic, the colon becomes a rigid, foreshortened tube that lacks its usual haustral markings.[37]

Clinical Features Previously undiagnosed ulcerative colitis manifests with a spectrum of severity. Approximately 10% of the patients will have an acute onset of fever, crampy abdominal pain, tenesmus, urgency, and the frequent painful passage of stools containing blood, mucus, and pus. The rest will give a history of an insidious, often cyclic or recurrent course of fever, abdominal pain, anorexia, weight loss, and mild diarrhea, usually but not always bloody. Between episodes, these patients may be asymptomatic and have normal stools (Box 90-6). Patients with known ulcerative colitis may come to the ED with acute exacerbations.

Recurrences are often associated with emotional stress, infections or other acute illnesses, pregnancy, dietary indiscretions, use of cathartics or antibiotics, or withdrawal of antiinflammatory or corticosteroid medications. Bloody diarrhea is the predominant symptom, but the picture will be similar to the acute onset described above. Extracolonic manifestations may be present in up to 20% of cases; these include anterior uveitis, peripheral arthritis, and skin lesions

Box 90-6 Clinical Presentation of Ulcerative Colitis

Initial Signs and Symptoms

1. Chronic insidious recurrent abdominal pain, anorexia, weight loss, and mild diarrhea
2. Acute onset of bloody diarrhea, abdominal pain, with or without tenesmus, vomiting, and fever

Complications

1. Toxic megacolon
2. Perforation
3. Large bowel obstruction
4. GI hemorrhage
5. Perirectal abscess
6. Anal fistula

such as erythema nodosum.[34] Any of the symptoms and signs of acute colitis can be masked by chronic steroid use and the generally poor nutritional status of the patient. Peritonitis is sometimes missed in patients taking high doses of corticosteroids, even in cases of colonic perforation.

Toxic megacolon occurs in up to 5% of cases and usually occurs during the initial acute episode. The patient will appear septic, apathetic, and lethargic, with high fever, chills, tachycardia, and progressive abdominal pain, tenderness, and distention. The cause of toxic dilation is unknown, but precipitating factors may include use of antidiarrheal agents, vigorous use of cathartics or enemas, or barium enema examinations.[38] Toxic dilation occurs predominantly in the transverse colon, probably because in the supine position air collects in the transverse colon.[38]

Perforation is another serious complication with a mortality rate exceeding 15%. It can occur with or without toxic megacolon. Approximately 25% of patients with toxic megacolon will have perforation.

Other complications of ulcerative colitis include obstruction of the colon caused by benign stricture formation, which occurs in approximately 10% of patients. Massive GI hemorrhage secondary to ulcerative colitis may be seen in up to 3% of patients, and may require surgery. Anorectal complications such as perirectal abscesses or anal fistulas occur in approximately 15% of patients. They tend to occur during the first year of the disease process and correlate somewhat with severity of the disease. Anorectal problems are much more common, severe, and extensive in patients with Crohn's disease than in patients with ulcerative colitis.[39]

There is an increased risk of developing colon carcinoma in patients with long-standing, extensive ulcerative colitis. The risk is clearly related to the severity and the duration of the disease process, especially after it has been present for 10 to 15 years. The risk appears to be approximately 1% per person per year among those with pancolitis.[34] Patients with ulcerative colitis may also develop anemia from intestinal blood loss, or hypoproteinemia from malabsorption.

Diagnostic Strategy The diagnosis of ulcerative colitis should be suspected in anyone with bloody diarrhea. The most useful diagnostic study for acute colitis is fiberoptic endoscopy and intestinal biopsy. A barium enema of the colon is no longer the method of choice for establishing the initial diagnosis of ulcerative colitis, but it may be helpful in chronic cases. The enema may show a rigid, shortened colon, with loss of haustrations and destruction of mucosal pattern, the "hose-like" colon. Barium enema should be avoided in acute, severe cases because it may lead to toxic megacolon. Gentle sigmoidoscopy may be diagnostic, because the rectum is always involved in ulcerative colitis.[40]

The diagnosis of toxic megacolon must be suspected in any patient with ulcerative colitis who has a sharp decrease in the number of daily stools without a corresponding amelioration of symptoms. It is best diagnosed by plain-film radiography of the abdomen. The transverse colon is dilated, usually greater than 8 cm; over 6 cm is abnormal (Figure 90-8). Often islands of necrotic tissue or gas in the bowel wall itself are seen on the radiograph. Films should be examined for the presence of free air, indicative of perforation. The barium enema must be avoided in cases of suspected toxic megacolon because it may precipitate perforation.

Differential Considerations Infectious agents, especially *Campylobacter, Shigella,* enterohemorrhagic *Escherichia coli,* and *C. difficile* (antibiotic-associated colitis), can produce diseases clinically and sigmoidoscopically indistinguishable from ulcerative colitis. Acute amebiasis may also mimic ulcerative colitis. Amebiasis can be difficult to identify from the stool, so serologic testing should be included in the workup. In patients with acquired immunodeficiency syndrome (AIDS), the chronic diarrhea and diffuse colonic involvement of Kaposi's sarcoma may mimic chronic ulcerative colitis. Histoplasmosis and cytomegalovirus can cause similar symptoms. Diseases that must be excluded, particularly in the elderly, include diverticulitis, ischemic colitis, radiation colitis, and carcinoma of the colon.

By far the most important differential diagnosis is Crohn's disease of the colon. Differentiation is accomplished primarily by gross examination via colonoscopy and examination for characteristic histologic changes on biopsy. However, the gross and microscopic changes are not pathognomonic, and in up to 20% of cases it may be impossible to distinguish between the two disease processes.[41] Ulcerative colitis that is limited to the rectum may be confused with syphilis, gonorrhea, and lymphogranuloma venereum.

Management Initial treatment usually consists of sulfasalazine, a 5-acetylsalicylic acid (5-ASA) derivative, 2 to 6 g/day in divided doses with meals, plus the use of oral steroids. Other more expensive 5-ASA derivatives without the toxicity of sulfasalazine may be substituted if needed.[42,43] Both corticosteroid and 5-ASA enemas have also proven helpful. The use of antibiotics is controversial. Close follow-up for these patients with a primary care physician should be arranged.[44,45]

The treatment of choice for significant acute ulcerative colitis, characterized by high fever, significant anemia (hematocrit <30%), tachycardia, and stools more frequent than six to eight per day, is high-dose intravenous steroids. Hydrocortisone 100 mg or methylprednisolone 20 mg IV every 6 to 8 hours may be used. Immunomodulating agents such as azathioprine, mercaptopurine, and cyclosporine may be used in refractory cases. For patients with disease resistant to medical therapy, a colectomy, which is curative, may be considered.

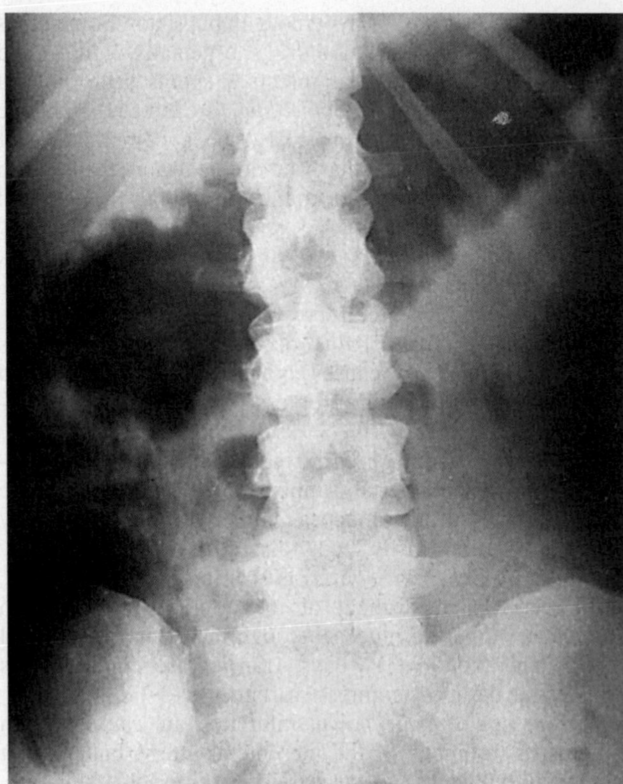

Figure 90-8. **Toxic megacolon secondary to ulcerative colitis. Smooth indentations along margin of colon represent pseudopolyps.**

Disposition Patients with known ulcerative colitis with mild exacerbations, or those with isolated ulcerative proctitis, can be managed as outpatients. Any patient with an acute colitis suspicious for new-onset ulcerative colitis should be admitted for diagnostic investigation and initial control of the disease process if the diagnosis is confirmed.

Patients with known ulcerative colitis with a more severe exacerbation, or with suspected toxic megacolon, should be hospitalized. The disease is explosive and unpredictable and requires the skill of an experienced physician.

Key Concepts

- The diagnosis of toxic megacolon must be suspected in any patient who has a sharp decrease in the number of daily stools without a corresponding amelioration of symptoms.
- Indications for inpatient treatment include high fever, tachycardia, or progressive abdominal pain.

Crohn's Disease

Perspective Crohn's disease affects about 30 to 60 persons per 100,000 in the United States. Approximately 20% of patients with Crohn's disease have colonic disease alone and, of those patients with small bowel disease, 30% will develop coexistent colon involvement. Both sexes are equally affected, and the disease is three to eight times more common in Jewish than in non-Jewish populations. Onset is generally between the ages of 15 and 40 years, although a person of any age may be affected. The incidence of Crohn's disease in the United States has been doubling every 10 years for the past 3 decades.[21,39]

Principles of Disease The cause of Crohn's disease is unknown, although it is believed that the mechanism of disease is similar to that described in the section on ulcerative colitis. Crohn's disease is characterized by chronic inflammation extending through all layers of the bowel wall and involving the mesenteric and regional lymph nodes as well. The important features distinguishing it from ulcerative colitis are as follows: (1) chronic inflammation involves all layers of the bowel, not just the mucosa and submucosa; (2) the disease process is not continuous (rather, segments of normal bowel are interspersed, producing so-called *skip areas*); (3) rectal involvement is not common, but anorectal complications such as fistulas and abscesses are common; and (4) there is characteristic small bowel involvement.

Clinical Features Patients may have one of three patterns of disease: (1) inflammatory disease, (2) strictures, or (3) fistulas. The inflammatory pattern is similar to the chronic type of ulcerative colitis. Patients have chronic diarrhea associated with abdominal cramps, fever, anorexia, and weight loss. Grossly bloody stools, which are the hallmark of ulcerative colitis, are, however, less common in Crohn's disease. In approximately half of patients, perianal disease is the initial complaint. Those with strictures may develop toxic megacolon, while those with fistulas may suffer from abscess formation. Extraintestinal manifestations of Crohn's disease, each occurring in approximately 10% of patients, include aphthous ulcers, erythema nodosum, iritis or episcleritis, and arthritis (either monoarticular arthritis, sacroiliitis, or ankylosing spondylitis). Gallstones are found in 35% to 60% of patients with Crohn's disease. Recurrences are common, and the disease tends to progress despite a patient's apparent clinical well-being.[21,46]

Diagnostic Strategy Crohn's disease should be suspected in any patient whose symptoms show a picture consistent with a chronic inflammatory colitis. Clues to the diagnosis are the presence or history of anorectal problems such as fistulas or abscesses, the absence of bloody diarrhea, sparing of the rectum, and concomitant small bowel involvement. The diagnosis may be confirmed by sigmoidoscopy, a rectal biopsy, or contrast radiography studies. A barium enema will show changes consistent with regional enteritis: skip areas of inflammation and noninvolvement of the rectum. A CT scan of the abdomen with oral and rectal contrast is the diagnostic procedure of choice when abscess formation is suspected.

Differential Considerations In younger patients, the prime differential diagnosis includes ulcerative colitis or invasive infectious enteritis such as with *Campylobacter, Shigella, C. difficile* antibiotic-associated colitis, *herpes simplex virus,* or even *Chlamydia.* Patients with the typical regional enteritis picture of acute terminal ileitis or "pseudoappendicitis" must be evaluated for infection with *Yersinia enterocolitis.*[41] Studies have shown that as many as 50% to 80% of cases of acute terminal ileitis are due to *Yersinia* infections.[41] Yersiniosis also has a high frequency of secondary manifestations such as erythema nodosum or monoarticular arthritis, similar to that in Crohn's disease or ulcerative colitis. However, the perirectal abscesses, fistulas, and colonic skip lesions or stenosis are not seen with *Yersinia* infection. Chemical colitis associated with the popular practice of "cleansing enemas" should also be considered.

The most important consideration in elderly patients suspected of having Crohn's disease of the colon is ischemic colitis. At one time there was thought to be a peak in the incidence of Crohn's disease after age 50 years. It is now known that this later peak was due primarily to patients with colonic ischemia or infectious colitis who were misdiagnosed.[47] Hemorrhagic colitis from enteropathogenic *E. coli* serotype 0157:H7 must also be considered, particularly in nursing home patients who have ingested inadequately cooked ground beef.[48,49]

Management Management is similar to that for ulcerative colitis except for the following: metronidazole (10 to 20 mg/kg/day) has become an important addition to the treatment of Crohn's disease involving the perineum and colon. Success with metronidazole has been reported in patients with refractory chronic perineal manifestations of Crohn's disease. Recurrence rates are high, generally necessitating long-term maintenance therapy at reduced dosages. Metronidazole may also be used for the patient with Crohn's colitis, or ileocolitis of mild to moderate severity, who does not respond to or cannot tolerate sulfasalazine.[21,23]

Methotrexate, which has several significant side effects, is used in patients requiring ongoing steroid treatment, in an attempt to reduce their steroid use. Antibiotics may be used when suppurative complications occur, but with the exception of metronidazole are not used for primary therapy. One recent promising therapy is enteric-coated fish oil, which has been shown to reduce the frequency of relapses.[50] Surgery may be required for complications such as abscesses or strictures. In general, therapy for Crohn's colitis is less effective than that for ulcerative colitis.

Disposition Any patient with undiagnosed, nonspecific mild colitis needs a thorough investigation to determine its cause, but this does not have to be done in the hospital. Reliable patients can be worked up on an outpatient basis, provided they do not appear ill and have a physician who can coordinate their evaluation and treatment. Those with severe symptoms or significant dehydration require hospitalization. Those with evidence of toxic megacolon or abscess formation require surgical consultation in addition to hospitalization.

Key Concepts

- Metronidazole is a key component in the treatment of Crohn's disease.
- Recurrences are more common than in ulcerative colitis.
- Unlike ulcerative colitis, Crohn's disease affects all layers of the bowel, and may afflict the small bowel in addition to the colon.

ISCHEMIC COLITIS

Perspective

Colonic ischemia is a disease of the elderly; 90% of cases occur in patients older than 60 years.[51] Many patients have associated potentially obstructing colonic lesions such as diverticulitis, fecal impaction, or carcinoma distal to the area of colitis. Most younger patients with ischemia of the colon have associated vascular disease, arteriosclerotic heart disease, diabetes mellitus, or hypercoagulable states. Some cases are related to vasoconstrictive drugs, especially digitalis and cocaine.[52] Certain intestinal infective agents such as *Entamoeba histolytica* and *Cytomegalovirus* can cause ischemic colitis. Chronic ischemia may also be a complication of abdominal surgery, particularly abdominal aortic aneurysm repair. Colonic ischemia accounts for about half of all mesenteric ischemia.

Principles of Disease

There are essentially three types of ischemic colitis:[53]

Gangrenous ischemic colitis occurs when a complete loss of arterial flow causes bowel wall infarction and gangrene, which can progress to perforation, peritonitis, and death.

Stricturing ischemic colitis results from a gross impairment of the arterial supply, leading to hemorrhagic infarction of the mucosa, which ulcerates, heals by fibrosis, and finally leads to stenosis.

Transient ischemic colitis is caused by a transient, reversible impairment of the arterial supply, which causes a partial mucosal slough that heals by mucosal regeneration in a few days. Transient ischemic colitis is by far the most common variant.

Some cases of large bowel infarction are caused by an embolus or thrombus of the mesenteric artery, but in most patients ischemia occurs secondary to arteriolar shunting, spasm, or poor perfusion of mucosal vessels. Most cases involve the splenic flexure, which is supplied by end-arteries. The rectum is usually spared, because its blood supply is different from the rest of the colon and less dependent on the inferior mesenteric artery.[47]

Clinical Features

The onset of ischemic colitis is characteristically acute, with generalized lower abdominal pain, usually in the left lower quadrant, followed within 24 hours by bloody diarrhea or rectal bleeding. However, one quarter of patients will have no abdominal pain at all. Vomiting and fever are rare. On examination, the abdomen may be distended with tenderness over the involved intestine. Peritoneal findings are indicative of bowel necrosis. Further symptoms depend on the type of ischemic colitis present. With the gangrenous type, both symptoms and signs progress rapidly, and may resemble an acute bowel obstruction with sepsis. With an impaired but not complete loss of blood supply, the patient's symptoms tend to linger but do not progress. Mild to moderate crampy abdominal pain and rectal bleeding may continue for days or weeks, but then usually resolve spontaneously and rarely recur.

Diagnostic Strategy

There are no specific serum markers proven in the diagnosis of intestinal ischemia. Plain-film abdominal radiographs are often nonspecific but may show the classic finding of "thumbprinting." Thumbprinting represents local areas of swelling within the bowel mucosa caused by submucosal edema and hemorrhage.

Colonoscopy may reveal only blood oozing from above or the generalized response of the colon to injury by inflammation, ischemia, or infection. The segmental distribution and rectal sparing of the disease process are suggestive but are not diagnostic. Colonoscopy is preferred over sigmoidoscopy. A barium enema is contraindicated in cases of gangrenous ischemic colitis, because perforation is common. In patients with suspected transient or stricturing ischemic colitis and who are not manifesting acute abdominal pain, a barium enema may be diagnostic, demonstrating thumbprinting (most common), longitudinal ulcers, and eccentric deformities of the bowel wall. Angiography is rarely diagnostic because of the peripheral vascular nature of the disease.[54] CT scan is normal in early stages of bowel infarction, although it may show nonspecific findings such as bowel wall thickening and pneumatosis. Color flow duplex imaging is highly specific but not sensitive.

Differential Considerations

Ischemic colitis often mimics or is mimicked by infectious colitis, inflammatory bowel disease, or even colon carcinoma.[51,54] Infection is still the most common cause of new-onset colitis in the elderly. Enterohemorrhagic *E. coli* serotype 0157:H7 produces an infectious colitis that closely resembles colonic ischemia. It affects primarily older women and has occurred in nursing home epidemics.[48] The source is usually contaminated meat. Once ingested, the organism produces a cytotoxin that results in the hemorrhagic colitis. Antibiotic-associated colitis caused by *C. difficile* infection may also mimic colonic ischemia.

Many cases of colitis in the elderly once considered to be Crohn's disease or ulcerative colitis in retrospect were really colonic ischemia. The features considered atypical in these elderly patients, such as segmental distribution of the disease, infrequent rectal involvement, high rate of spontaneous recovery, low rate of recurrence, lack of adequate response to usual inflammatory bowel disease therapy, and frequent progression to fibrotic stenosis with delayed obstruction, are now recognized as characteristic of colonic ischemia.[47] Always consider the diagnosis of ischemic colitis whenever contemplating the diagnosis of inflammatory bowel disease in an elderly patient.

Management

When ischemic colitis is suspected, a surgeon should be consulted. Gangrenous ischemic colitis or evidence of perforation requires immediate surgery as soon as the patient is stabilized. Ischemic colitis without evidence of peritonitis or perforation is generally self-limited and requires only conservative management, including bowel rest, parenteral fluids, and antibiotics.[51] Vasopressors should be avoided, if possible. Low blood-flow states (hypotension) should be aggressively reversed.

Disposition

All patients with acute symptoms in whom surgery is not indicated should be admitted to the hospital for supportive therapy and observation. Symptoms generally resolve within 24 to 48 hours.

Key Concepts

- Always consider the diagnosis of ischemic colitis whenever contemplating the diagnosis of inflammatory bowel disease in the elderly.
- Thumbprinting of the colon on plain abdominal radiographs suggests ischemic colitis.
- Surgical consultation is warranted in all cases of suspected ischemic colitis.

RADIATION PROCTOCOLITIS

Perspective

Injury of the colon and rectum can occur from radiation used in the treatment of abdominal and pelvic malignancies, usually carcinoma of the cervix, testis, prostate, or urinary bladder. The effect may be immediate or delayed many years after treatment, so the possibility of radiation-induced enteritis should be considered in anyone with intestinal disturbances who has undergone pelvic irradiation.

Incidence depends on many variables, including the technique and dosages of radiation, diet, the patient's nutritional state, and whether previous operations have fixed the bowel in the pelvis. Approximately 25% to 50% of patients undergoing irradiation for cancer of the cervix will develop symptoms of proctocolitis. In patients irradiated for carcinoma of the bladder, radiation proctitis occurs almost invariably because of the difficulty in shielding the rectum.[22]

Principles of Disease

Early symptoms during or just after radiation therapy are caused by damage of the absorptive mucosal cells. The mucosa shows edema, hyperemia, and inflammation that usually reaches a maximum within a few weeks and then subsides. Later symptoms are the result of induced ischemic bowel disease from endarteritis. Localized strictures are common. The anterior wall of the rectum is the most common site involved because it lies closest to the cervix and bladder.

Clinical Features

Patients actively undergoing radiation treatment that exposes the colon may experience diarrhea, tenesmus, cramps, and abdominal pain. Symptoms often begin in the second week of treatment and resolve by the sixth week. There are some patients whose symptoms do not resolve, exhibiting chronic radiation damage. These patients are prone to such long-term complications as fistulas, strictures, and proctitis. Fistulas may occur with abscess formation, or to the bladder or vagina. Intermittent bleeding is also common in late stages because of the formation of weak-walled telangiectasias in the irradiated area.[22]

Diagnostic Strategy

The diagnosis of acute radiation damage to the colon is made clinically with the appropriate history of recent radiation exposure. In delayed onset of disease, where there is not a clear relationship with a radiation insult, or when symptoms are prolonged well after radiation treatment, other diagnoses such as a stricture from carcinoma must be excluded.

Differential Considerations

Patients who have acute symptoms suggestive of radiation proctocolitis may have inflammatory bowel disease or an infectious enterocolitis; those with more chronic symptoms may have inflammatory bowel disease ischemic colitis.

Management

Treatment is supportive. Diarrhea or fecal incontinence may be improved by bulk-forming agents and the judicious use of antimotility agents. Patients may require chronic iron supplementation or even periodic transfusions if telangiectasias bleed chronically. Strictures are managed initially with enemas, stool softeners, and pain control, and with dilation or surgery as needed.

Disposition

Most cases of radiation-induced proctocolitis can be managed at home with consultation of the radiation oncologist. If the diagnosis is in doubt or symptoms are severe, hospitalization may be necessary.

Key Concepts

- Radiation proctocolitis may occur during or just after radiation exposure, or many years later.
- Delayed development or symptoms that persist long after radiation treatment should prompt an evaluation for other causes, such as carcinoma of the colon.

REFERENCES

1. Harrison MW et al: Diagnosis and management of Hirschsprung disease: a 25-year perspective, *Am J Surg* 152:49, 1986.
2. Doig CM: Hirschsprung's disease in mimicking conditions, *Dig Dis* 12:106, 1994.
3. Klein MD, Philippart AI: Hirschsprung's disease: three decades experience at a single institution, *J Pediatr Surg* 28:1291, 1993.
4. Jones IT, Fazio VW: Colonic volvulus: etiology and management, *Dig Dis* 7:203, 1989.
5. Kirchhoff LV: American trypanosomiasis (Chagas' disease)—a tropical disease now in the United States, *N Engl J Med* 329:639, 1993.
6. Paterson WG et al: Recommendations for the management of irritable bowel syndrome in family practice, *CMAJ* 161:154-160, 1999.
7. Maxwell PR et al: Irritable bowel syndrome, *Lancet* 350:1961-1965, 1997.
8. Manning AP: Towards positive diagnosis of the irritable bowel, *BMJ* 2:653-654, 1978.
9. Rege RV, Nahrfold DL: Diverticular disease, *Curr Probl Surg* 26:133, 1989.
10. Stollman NH, Raskin, JB: Diverticular disease of the colon, *J Clin Gastroenterol* 29:241-252, 1999.
11. Freischla CJ et al: Complications of diverticular disease of the colon in young people, *Dis Rectum* 29:639, 1986.
12. Floch MH: Update on diverticulitis: diagnostic and therapeutic options, *J Crit Illness* 8:43, 1993.
13. Cubbay N: Diverticular disease of the right colon (letter), *J Clin Pathol* 41:1025, 1988.
14. Deans GT et al: Malignant obstruction of the left colon, *Br J Surg* 81:1270, 1994.
15. Ferzoco LB et al: Acute diverticulitis, *N Engl J Med* 338:1521-1526, 1998.
16. Cho KC et al: Sigmoid diverticulitis: diagnostic role of CT-comparison with barium enema studies, *Radiology* 176:111, 1990.
17. Schwartz JT: Acute diverticulitis: choosing therapy wisely, *J Crit Illness* 5:119, 1990.
18. Editorial Board: Choice of antimicrobial drugs, *Med Lett* 36:53, 1994.
19. Morris J et al: The utility of computed tomography in colonic diverticulitis, *Ann Surg* 204:132, 1986.
20. Jones IT, Fazio VW: Colonic volvulus: etiology and management, *Dig Dis* 7:203, 1989.
21. Strong SA, Fassio VW: Crohn's disease of the colon, rectum, and anus, *Surg Clin North Am* 73:933, 1993.
22. Otchy DP, Nelson H: Radiation injuries of the colon and rectum, *Surg Clin North Am* 75:1017, 1993.
23. Richards WO, Williams LF Jr: Obstruction of the large and small intestine, *Surg Clin North Am* 68:355, 1988.
24. Lopez-Kostner F et al: Management and causes of large-bowel obstruction, *Surg Clin North Am* 77:1265-1290, 1997.
25. Buechter KJ et al: Surgical management of the acutely obstructed colon: a review of 127 cases, *Am J Surg* 156(3 pt 1):163, 1988.
26. Frizelle FA, Wolff BG: Colonic volvulus, *Adv Surg* 29:131-139, 1996.
27. Mangiante EC et al: Sigmoid volvulus—a four decade experience, *Am Surg* 55:41, 1989.
28. Friedman JD et al: Experience with colonic volvulus, *Dis Colon Rectum* 32:409, 1989.
29. Tejler G, Jiborn H: Volvulus of the cecum: a report of 26 cases and review of the literature, *Dis Colon Rectum* 31:445, 1988.
30. Rabinovici R et al: Cecal volvulus, *Dis Colon Rectum* 33:765, 1990.
31. Eisen LK et al: Intussusception in adults: institutional review: *J Am Coll Surg* 188:390-395, 1999.
32. Prater JM et al: Adult intussusception, *Am Fam Phys* 47:447, 1993.
33. Papadakis KA, Targan SR: Current theories on the causes of inflammatory bowel disease, *Gastroenterol Clin North Am* 28:283-296, 1999.
34. Andres PG, Friedman LS: Epidemiology and the natural course of inflammatory bowel disease, *Gastroenterol Clin North Am* 28:225-281, 1999.
35. Scholmerich J: Inflammatory bowel disease, *Endoscopy* 31:667-673, 1999.
36. Podolsky DK: A review article: inflammatory bowel disease, *N Engl J Med* 325:928, 1991.
37. Archambault A: Ulcerative colitis: an overview, *Can Fam Physician* 36:343, 1990.
38. Danovitch SH: Fulminant colitis and toxic megacolon, *Gastroenterol Clin North Am* 18:73, 1989.
39. Farray FA, Peppercorn MA: Advances in the management of ulcerative colitis and Crohn's disease, *Consultant* 28:39, 1988.
40. Miner TB, Biddle WL: Modern treatment of ulcerative colitis, *Comprehensive Ther* 15:38, 1989.
41. Farmer RG: Infectious causes of diarrhea in the differential diagnosis of inflammatory bowel disease, *Med Clin North Am* 74:29, 1990.
42. Courtney MG et al: 5-Aminosalicylic acid treatment of ulcerative colitis compared to sulfasalazine, *Lancet* 339:1279, 1992.
43. Singleton JW et al: Mesalamine capsules for the treatment of active Crohn's disease: results of a 16-week trial, *Gastroenterology* 104:1293, 1993.
44. Peppercorn MA: Advances in drug therapy for inflammatory bowel disease, *Ann Intern Med* 112:50, 1990.
45. Brattsand R: Overview of newer glucocorticosteroid preparations for inflammatory bowel disease, *Can J Gastroenterol* 4:407, 1990.
46. Brinberg DE, Berkeley BE: Crohn's disease: a comprehensive approach to management, *Postgrad Med* 86:257, 1989.
47. Bower TC: Ischemic colitis, *Surg Clin North Am* 73:1037, 1993.
48. Cohen MB, Giannella RA: Hemorrhagic colitis associated with *Escherichia coli* 0157:H7, *Adv Intern Med* 37:173, 1992.
49. Berkelman RL: Emerging infectious diseases in the United States 1993, *J Infect Dis* 170:272, 1994.
50. Belluzi A et al: Effect of enteric coated fish-oil preparation on relapses in Crohn's disease, *N Engl J Med* 334:1558-1560, 1996.
51. Greenwald DA, Brandt LJ: Colonic ischemia, *J Clin Gastroenterol* 27:122-128, 1998.
52. Brown DN et al: Ischemic colitis related to cocaine abuse, *Am J Gastroenterol* 89:1558, 1994.
53. Cappell MS: Intestinal (mesenteric) vasculopathy. II. Ischemic colitis and chronic mesenteric ischemia, *Gastroenterol Clin North Am* 27:827-860, 1998.
54. Toursarkissian B, Thompson RW: Ischemic colitis, *Surg Clin North Am* 77:461, 1997.

91 Anorectum

Wendy C. Coates

PRINCIPLES OF DISEASE

The anorectum marks the end of the alimentary canal. From its beginning at the rectosigmoid junction at the level of the third sacral vertebra (S3), the rectum follows the sacral curvature for 12 to 15 cm, then sharply turns posteriorly and inferiorly at the puborectalis muscle (Figure 91-1). Here the anal canal begins its 4-cm course to the anal verge, the orifice where stool exits the body. It is supported by three muscle groups, the levator ani and the internal and external anal sphincters. Anal valves are located 2 cm proximal to the anal verge at the dentate line. Above the valves are the anal crypts that contain mucous glands to lubricate the area during defecation. They are a nidus for abscess and fistula formation if occluded. Proximal to the crypts are the columns of Morgagni, where the epithelium of the anal canal changes from pink columnar (like the rectum) to squamous.[1-4]

The superior, middle, and inferior hemorrhoidal arteries provide the blood supply to the anorectum. They arise from the inferior mesenteric, internal iliac, and internal pudendal arteries, respectively. The superior hemorrhoidal veins drain into the portal system, while the inferior hemorrhoidal veins drain into the caval system. Lymphatic drainage is to the inferior mesenteric nodes above the dentate line and to the inguinal nodes from all areas of the anorectum.[2]

Sympathetic and parasympathetic nervous systems function together to retain the contents of the rectum until evacuation is desired. Continence is maintained when sympathetic fibers from L1 to L3 (upper rectum) and presacral nerves (lower rectum) inhibit contraction of rectal smooth muscle while L5 fibers cause the internal sphincter to contract. Elimination occurs when parasympathetic fibers from the anterior roots of S2 to S4 cause the rectal wall to contract and the internal sphincter to relax. Voluntary external sphincter control is mediated by motor branches of the pudendal nerve (S2, S3) and the perineal branch of S4. The levator ani is supplied by the pudendal nerve and pelvic branches of S3 to S4 fibers. Sensory perception of rectal distention involves extramural receptors to parasympathetic fibers from S2 to S4. The abundant sensory nerve endings of the distal anal epithelium perceive sensations that are transmitted via the pudendal nerve.[2,4]

Defecation begins as the rectum becomes distended, the internal sphincter relaxes, and stool enters the anal canal. At an appropriate time and place, the external sphincter is relaxed to complete the process of elimination. Sometimes voluntary straining is needed to assist in the passage of stool. By performing the Valsalva maneuver, the abdominal muscles contract, the rectal angle straightens, and the pelvic floor descends. To postpone defecation, the external sphincter contracts voluntarily. This relaxes the rectal wall and quells the urge to defecate unless there is an underlying sphincter disorder or an overwhelming volume of stool.[1]

CLINICAL FEATURES

History

A complete history of anorectal and gastrointestinal (GI) symptoms, and the presence of systemic disease, elucidates the diagnosis of most anorectal disorders (Box 91-1 and Figure 91-2). Common complaints include bleeding, swelling, pain, itching, and discharge. The standard questions of time and circumstances of onset, duration, quality, and radiation should be asked. Next, alterations in bowel habits of the individual patient should be noted. These include changes in color, frequency, or consistency of the stool, and the presence of straining, flatus, and incontinence of solid or liquid stool. People with underlying GI disorders (e.g., Crohn's disease, cancer, or polyps) are predisposed to different presentations of anorectal problems. Similarly, those with underlying systemic diseases like acquired immunodeficiency syndrome (AIDS), cancer, diabetes mellitus, and coagulopathies are prone to serious complications of anorectal conditions. Finally, patients should be asked directly about the use of the anus for sexual purposes.[5-7]

Rectal Bleeding The color, amount, and relationship to defecation are important factors in establishing the cause of rectal bleeding. Approximately 10% to 20% of the population experiences rectal bleeding at some time.[8] Pain and bright red blood signify anal fissures or hemorrhoids. Fissure pain is sharp, sudden in onset, and not associated with swelling, whereas pain from a prolapsed or thrombosed hemorrhoid is gnawing, continuous, and of more gradual onset. Painless rectal bleeding occurs in internal hemorrhoids, cancer, or precancerous lesions.

The relationship of bleeding to defecation is important. Visible blood on the toilet paper is usually caused by anal fissures or external hemorrhoids; however, minute quantities can result from any irritating condition. Bright red blood that drips into the toilet bowl or streaks around the stool is caused by internal hemorrhoids. Blood mixed with stool originates proximal to the rectum, whereas melena indicates a very proximal source. Bloody mucus is associated with cancer, inflammatory bowel disease, and proctitis.[1,7,8]

Swelling and Masses Patients who complain of a swelling near the anus or have the sensation of rectal fullness often list hemorrhoids as their chief complaint. Painful swellings that bleed are usually thrombosed hemorrhoids, but other painful lesions such as abscesses, pilonidal disease, and hidradenitis suppurativa must be considered. Painless, itchy swellings may be caused by condylomata acuminata or secondary syphilis. A mass protruding through the anal orifice may signal rectal prolapse.[1,7] Perianal and rectal carcinoma should be considered in older persons and those with long-standing anorectal complaints.[9]

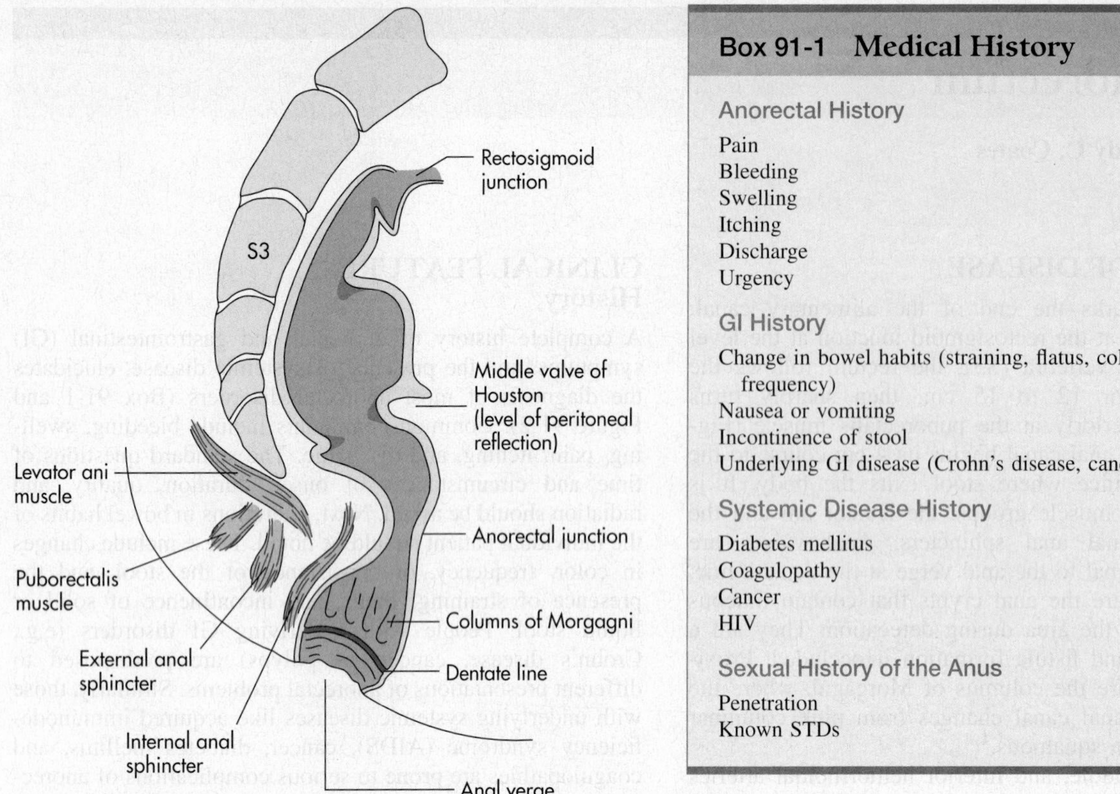

Figure 91-1. **Anorectal anatomy.**

Box 91-1 Medical History

Anorectal History

Pain
Bleeding
Swelling
Itching
Discharge
Urgency

GI History

Change in bowel habits (straining, flatus, color, consistency, frequency)
Nausea or vomiting
Incontinence of stool
Underlying GI disease (Crohn's disease, cancer, polyps)

Systemic Disease History

Diabetes mellitus
Coagulopathy
Cancer
HIV

Sexual History of the Anus

Penetration
Known STDs

- Pain?
  - Yes → Bleeding?
    - Yes → Swelling?
      - Yes → Hemorrhoids
      - No → Anal fissure
    - No → Swelling?
      - Yes → Abscess, Pilonidal cyst, Hidradenitis
      - No
        - Episodic pain? Yes → Proctalgia fugax
        - Urgency? Yes → Incontinence
  - No → Bleeding?
    - Yes → Polyps, Adenoma
    - No → Swelling?
      - Yes → Itch?
        - Yes → Condylomata acuminata
        - No → Procidentia
      - No → Itch? Yes → D/C?
        - Yes → Proctitis
        - No → Pruritus ani

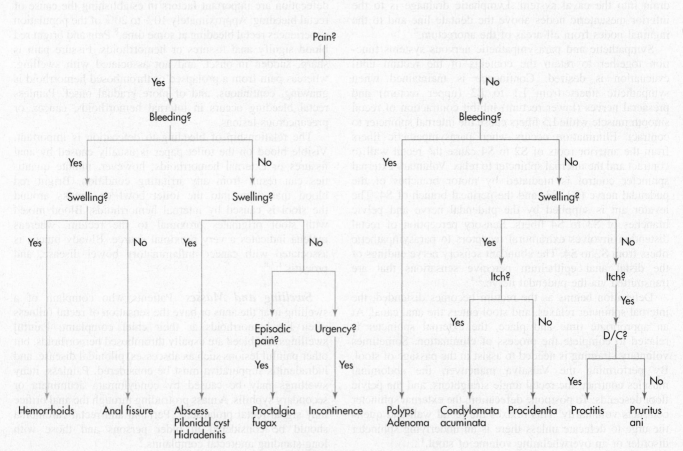

Figure 91-2. **Algorithm for anorectal complaints.**

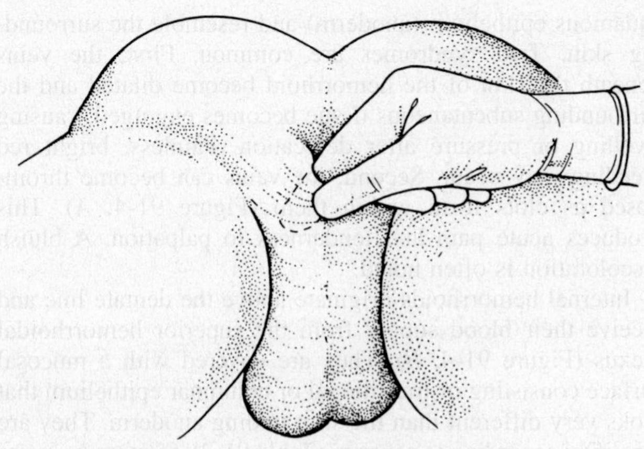

Figure 91-3. **Bidigital rectal examination.**

Pain and Itching Severe, episodic anorectal pain that is not associated with bleeding or swelling is proctalgia fugax. Perianal itching (pruritus ani) is caused by any lesion that makes hygiene difficult to maintain.

Physical Examination

The physical examination should take place in a private location with attention to the patient's modesty. The patient can then relax the external sphincter to facilitate a complete examination. The patient is placed in the left lateral decubitus position and covered with a sheet. The buttocks are inspected for dermatologic manifestations of disease and then gently spread apart to expose the anal orifice. Elements of personal hygiene are noted, in addition to anatomic disruptions such as fissures, skin tags, lesions, hemorrhoids, or abscesses. The patient is asked to strain to assess the integrity of the pelvic floor and note prolapse of hemorrhoids or rectal mucosa. Next, a well-lubricated gloved finger is placed flat against the anal opening, exerting gentle pressure until the external sphincter relaxes and allows the finger to enter the anus. Anal sphincter tone can be assessed by asking the patient to squeeze. By sweeping the finger in a circumferential manner, accessible areas of the anorectum can be examined for masses and areas of tenderness. The cervix or prostate is palpated. A bidigital examination reveals masses and tender areas at the distal portion of the anal canal and perineum (Figure 91-3). Upon withdrawal, the contents on the glove can be assessed for frank or occult blood, mucus, or pus.[1,5]

Direct visualization can be accomplished by anoscopy. With the patient similarly positioned, the lubricated anoscope is inserted into the anus with the obturator in place. The obturator is removed and a circumferential view of the rectal mucosa is possible. Attention is directed at sites of bleeding, hemorrhoids, masses, or abnormal tissue, and finally the dentate line and anal epithelium.

MANAGEMENT OF SPECIFIC ANORECTAL PROBLEMS

Hemorrhoids

Perspective The history of ancient and modern civilization may have been altered by hemorrhoids. When the Philistines defeated the Israelites, the book of I Samuel reports the fate of the avengers: "A deadly panic had seized the whole city, since the hand of God had been very heavy upon it. Those who escaped death were afflicted with hemorrhoids, and the outcry from the city went up to the heavens."[10] In 1815 the battle of Waterloo marked the defeat of Napoleon's army. Speculation purports that the great leader suffered from hemorrhoids at the time of his defeat.[11]

Hemorrhoidal disease continues to afflict modern man with a 4.4% incidence in the U.S. population. Both sexes are affected, and there is an increased frequency among whites, rural dwellers, and those from high socioeconomic status.[12]

Principles of Disease The cause of hemorrhoids is controversial. Hippocrates believed that bile and phlegm heated the blood and caused engorgement of hemorrhoidal vessels. Today, the anal vascular cushion theory is the most widely accepted. Rather than forming a continuous ring around the anal canal, the submucosa forms three distinct cushions of tissue that are richly supplied with small blood vessels and muscle fibers. Blood supply to these cushions is from the superior rectal artery with some contribution from the middle and inferior hemorrhoidal arteries, which explains why hemorrhoidal bleeding is bright red. The muscularis submucosa cushions the anal canal during defecation to prevent injury and to aid in fecal continence.[13]

As the supportive tissue deteriorates, usually starting in the third decade, venous distention, prolapse, bleeding, and thrombosis occur. Some controversy exists whether straining and constipation cause this by producing venous backflow when intraabdominal pressure increases.[1,13] In pregnant women, direct pressure on a hemorrhoidal vein can produce symptomatic hemorrhoids. Some familial predisposition is recognized, but whether this is a result of genetic factors or acquired factors such as diet is unknown. Hemorrhoids are not varicose veins; they are normal structures that manifest symptoms when the muscularis submucosa weakens and the anal cushions are displaced distally.[13] Conditions that increase sphincter tone correlate with a higher prevalence of hemorrhoids.[14] Portal hypertension does not cause hemorrhoids. The incidence of symptomatic hemorrhoids is similar in patients with and without portal hypertension. Rectal bleeding in this population may be caused by rectal varices that are vascular communications between the superior and middle hemorrhoidal veins.[1,15,16] A major exception to this observation occurs in the pediatric population in which children with portal hypertension are prone to hemorrhoidal exacerbations.[17,18]

Clinical Features A careful history is needed to confirm the presence of hemorrhoids, because many patients use this term to refer to any perianal condition. Bleeding with defecation is the most common complaint, and unless the hemorrhoids are thrombosed it is usually painless. Patients report seeing variable amounts of bright red blood on the toilet paper or in the toilet bowl. The few patients with substantial blood loss should be managed appropriately. Many complain of swelling, itching, mucoid discharge, or simply the presence of a moist perianal area. Further history should address recent stool patterns, such as diarrhea or constipation; chronic medical problems, such as portal hypertension or bleeding disorders; and a dietary and family history.

Hemorrhoidal symptoms are exacerbated by frequent bowel movements, prolonged sitting, heavy lifting, and straining while defecating. Although straining is cited as a cause of hemorrhoids, it may also be a result of them when the patient is constipated from the fear of defecating.[1] Physical examination should address the type and degree of hemorrhoids. This can be accomplished by a visual inspection at rest and during straining. Nonprolapsing hemorrhoids can be visualized on anoscopy as a focus of bleeding, or as they bulge when the patient is asked to strain while the anoscope is removed.[1]

Hemorrhoids are classified according to their location and severity (Table 91-1). External hemorrhoids originate below the dentate line and receive their blood supply from the inferior hemorrhoidal plexus. They are covered with modified squamous epithelium (anoderm) and resemble the surrounding skin. Two syndromes are common. First, the veins beneath the skin of the hemorrhoid become dilated and the surrounding subcutaneous tissue becomes engorged, causing swelling or pressure after defecation. Painless, bright red bleeding may occur. Second, the veins can become thrombosed as clots form within them (Figure 91-4, *A*). This produces acute pain and tenderness to palpation. A bluish discoloration is often noted.

Table 91-1. Types of Hemorrhoids

Type	Origin	Epithelium
External	Inferior hemorrhoidal plexus Proximal to dentate line	Modified squamous epithelium (anoderm)
Internal	Superior hemorrhoidal plexus Distal to dentate line	Transitional or columnar epithelium (mucosa)
Mixed	Superior and inferior hemorrhoidal plexus Proximal and/or distal to dentate line	Transitional, columnar, or modified squamous epithelium (mucosa and anoderm)

Internal hemorrhoids originate above the dentate line and receive their blood supply from the superior hemorrhoidal plexus (Figure 91-4, *B*). They are covered with a mucosal surface consisting of transitional or columnar epithelium that looks very different than the surrounding anoderm. They are classified according to severity (Table 91-2). Symptoms range from mild, painless bleeding with defecation to irreducible prolapse with unremitting and debilitating pain. First-degree internal hemorrhoids protrude into the lumen of the anal canal, causing a feeling of fullness. Because there are no sensory nerve endings in the mucosal wall, they do not cause pain. Second-degree internal hemorrhoids temporarily prolapse outside the anal canal during defecation but spontaneously return to their normal position at the end of the bowel movement. Both of these are amenable to medical management. Third-degree internal hemorrhoids prolapse spontaneously or during defecation and remain outside the body until they are manually replaced into the anal canal. A throbbing pressurelike pain may accompany bleeding and improves when the hemorrhoids are reduced. Fourth-degree internal hemorrhoids cannot be reduced and are permanently pro-

Table 91-2. Classification of Internal Hemorrhoids by Severity

Type	Prolapse	Mode of reduction	Treatment
First-degree	None	N/A	Medical management
Second-degree	During defecation	Spontaneous	Medical management
Third-degree	May be spontaneous or during defecation	Manual	Medical management Optional surgical repair
Fourth-degree	Permanently	Irreducible	Surgical repair

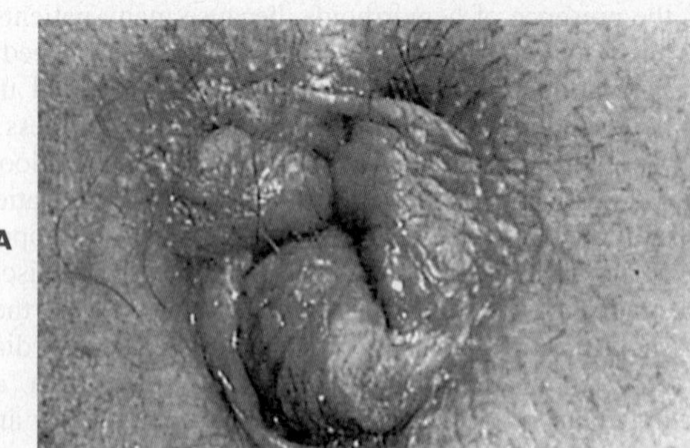

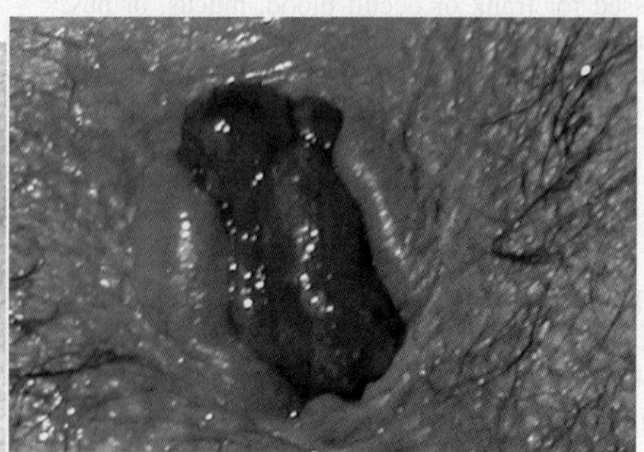

Figure 91-4. **Thrombosed hemorrhoids. A, External. B, Internal. Note the engorged external hemorrhoids that surround the thrombosed internal hemorrhoids. A,** ***Courtesy Michelle Lin, MD, Harbor-UCLA Medical Center;*** **B,** ***Courtesy Gershon Effron, MD, Sinai Hospital of Baltimore. In Seidel HM et al:*** **Mosby's guide to physical examination,** ***ed 4, St Louis, 1999, Mosby.***

lapsed. Continued prolapse leads to the formation of a thrombus with possible progression to gangrene. Definitive treatment for the intense pain and thrombosis is surgical.[1,19]

Management The symptoms of nonthrombosed external and nonprolapsing internal hemorrhoids can be ameliorated by the standard regimen, *WASH,* aimed at overcoming the problems that led to their formation (Box 91-2). Anal canal pressures decrease significantly in *warm water* (40° C).[20] Patients can direct a shower stream at the area for several minutes or take sitz baths. Mild oral *analgesic* agents improve the pain. The use of topical anesthetics, steroid creams, and suppositories is controversial. Prolonged use of topical corticosteroids produces atrophic skin changes and is discouraged.[1] *Stool softeners* can make the passage of stool easier to avoid straining. A *high-fiber diet* (20 to 30 g of dietary fiber per day) produces stool that is passed more easily.

Patients with second- or third-degree internal hemorrhoids also benefit from this regimen; however, permanent resolution of their symptoms may require surgical intervention (Table 91-3). These patients can be discharged from the ED on the WASH regimen and referred to a surgeon for banding, sclerotherapy, or elective hemorrhoidectomy. Patients with acute, gangrenous, fourth-degree internal hemorrhoids should be referred for emergent hemorrhoidectomy.[14,19]

Acutely thrombosed external hemorrhoids can be excised (*not* incised and drained) in the ED to provide prompt relief within the first 48 hours after the onset of symptoms (Figure 91-5). Incision results in incomplete evacuation of the clot, subsequent rebleeding, and swelling because vessels are lacerated. Excision provides long-term relief and prevents the formation of skin tags.[1] This procedure should not be attempted by the emergency physician in pediatric patients, pregnant women, or immunocompromised patients.[14] If not excised, the thrombosed external hemorrhoid and its associated symptoms will resolve spontaneously after several days when the hemorrhoid ulcerates and leaks the dark accumulated blood. Residual skin tags may persist.[1]

Box 91-2 The WASH Regimen

W Warm water
A Analgesic agents
S Stool softeners
H High-fiber diet

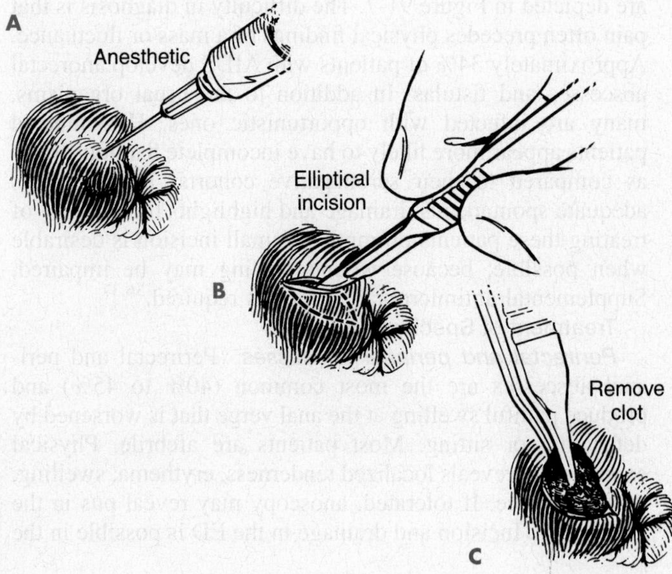

Figure 91-5. **Excision of thrombosed external hemorrhoid. A, Field block with local anesthetic. B, An elliptical incision is made around the hemorrhoid. C, The thrombosed hemorrhoid is removed.** *From Larson S. In Rosen P et al, editors: Atlas of emergency procedures, St Louis, 2001, Mosby.*

Anal Fissures

Principles of Disease The development of an anal fissure is the most common cause of the sudden onset of intensely painful rectal bleeding. A superficial tear in the anoderm results when a hard piece of feces is forced through the anus, usually in patients who are constipated. Although anyone can experience an anal fissure, it is most common in the 30- to 50-year age bracket.[21] It is the most commonly encountered anorectal problem in pediatric patients, especially infants.[22,23] Men and women are affected equally. Approximately 99% of fissures in men and 90% in women

Table 91-3. Surgical Management of Hemorrhoids

Classification	Management
Thrombosed external hemorrhoids	Excision in ED
Second- and third-degree internal hemorrhoids	Elective surgical repair Banding Sclerotherapy Hemorrhoidectomy
Fourth-degree hemorrhoids (nonthrombosed)	Nonemergent hemorrhoidectomy
Thrombosed or gangrenous	Emergent hemorrhoidectomy
Fourth-degree internal hemorrhoids	Thrombosed or gangrenous fourth-degree internal hemorrhoids

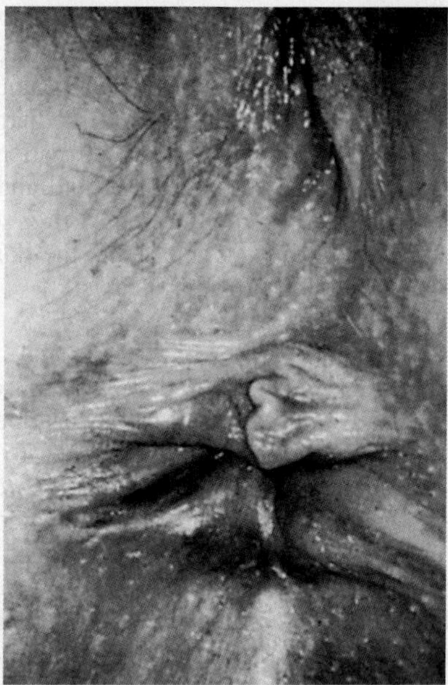

Figure 91-6. **Lateral anal fissure.** *Courtesy Gershon Efron, MD, Sinai Hospital of Baltimore. In Seidel HM et al:* **Mosby's guide to physical examination,** *ed 4, St Louis, 1999, Mosby.*

occur along the posterior midline where the skeletal muscle fibers that encircle the anus are weakest. Anterior midline fissures are more common in women.[1,24,25] Fissures that occur elsewhere should alert the emergency physician to diseases such as leukemia, Crohn's disease, human immunodeficiency virus (HIV) infection, tuberculosis (TB), or syphilis.[26]

Those not treated promptly may become chronic and display a classic "fissure triad" of deep ulcer, sentinel pile, and enlarged anal papillae (Figure 91-6). A sentinel pile forms when the skin at the base of the fissure becomes edematous and hypertrophic.[21,24] A resolving sentinel pile can form a permanent skin tag and may be associated with a fistulous tract.

Clinical Features The patient complains of a sudden, searing pain during defecation that may be accompanied by a small amount of bright red blood on the stool or toilet paper. This is followed by a nagging, burning sensation that lasts for a few hours from internal sphincter spasm. Subsequent bowel movements are excruciating, and the external sphincter can exhibit a reflex spasm. Physical examination must be performed cautiously to avoid further spasm and pain. With the patient in the left lateral decubitus position, the buttocks are separated, and the perianal skin is gently retracted. The depth of the fissure, its orientation to the midline, and the presence of a coexisting sentinel pile or edema are noted. Rectal examination during an acute exacerbation is often impossible because of pain and sphincter spasm.[21]

Management Treatment using the WASH regimen (see Box 91-2) focuses on eliminating constipation with a bulking agent, stool softener, and high-fiber diet. Warm sitz baths and limited use of topical anesthetic creams may be helpful.[21,27] Parental encouragement to pediatric patients helps prevent encopresis that can result from a fear of painful bowel movements. Most uncomplicated fissures will resolve in 2 to 4 weeks. Topical agents aimed at reducing sphincter pressures may be effective adjuncts to therapy. These include nitrates (glyceryl trinitrate ointment) or nifedipine 0.2% gel twice daily.[28] Injection of botulinum toxin has been shown to be effective in relaxing the sphincter tone by inhibiting acetylcholinesterase release, but it caused reversible fecal incontinence in 7% of patients.[29] Long-term treatment of recurrent fissures focuses on reducing resting anal pressures, and may require anal dilation under anesthesia or surgical correction of the internal sphincter to reduce its tone.[21,24,29]

Abscesses and Fistulas

Principles of Disease In the fifth century BC, Hippocrates outlined the cause and treatment of anorectal abscesses and fistulas. King Louis XIV of France was relieved of the condition by surgery. Anorectal abscesses and fistulas are most common in adults who are 30 to 50 years old, and men are afflicted more often than women (2:1 to 7:1).[1,30] There is a peak incidence in infants (85% male) that is associated with congenital abnormalities.[31,32]

A popular explanation of anorectal abscesses is the cryptoglandular theory in which the ducts of the mucus-producing anal glands at the base of the anal crypts become occluded.[30] Other abscesses are caused by inflammatory bowel disease, trauma, cancer, radiation injury, and infection (TB, lymphogranuloma venereum [LGV], actinomycosis).[1,33] Common bacterial causative agents are *Staphylococcus aureus, Escherichia coli, Streptococcus, Proteus,* and *Bacteroides.*

Management

General Approach *Abscesses* are the acute manifestations of a continuum of anorectal infections, whereas *fistulas* are the chronic sequelae.[21] Symptoms vary depending on the site of infection, but incision and drainage is required in all cases (Table 91-4). Delay of medical management might allow extension of the infection and eventual compromise of the sphincter mechanism.[21,34] Adjunctive antimicrobial therapy is indicated in patients who are immunocompromised, diabetic, or have valvular heart disease.[35] Tetanus status should be verified. The sites of anorectal abscess formation are depicted in Figure 91-7. The difficulty in diagnosis is that pain often precedes physical findings of a mass or fluctuance. Approximately 34% of patients with AIDS develop anorectal abscesses and fistulas. In addition to the usual organisms, many are infected with opportunistic ones. HIV-infected patients appear more likely to have incomplete fistulous tracts as compared to their seronegative cohorts. This prevents adequate spontaneous drainage and highlights the urgency of treating these patients promptly. A small incision is desirable when possible, because wound healing may be impaired. Supplemental antimicrobial therapy is required.[36,37]

Treatment of Specific Abscesses

Perirectal and perianal abscesses Perirectal and perianal abscesses are the most common (40% to 45%) and produce painful swelling at the anal verge that is worsened by defecating or sitting. Most patients are afebrile. Physical examination reveals localized tenderness, erythema, swelling, and fluctuance. If tolerated, anoscopy may reveal pus in the anal crypts. Incision and drainage in the ED is possible in the

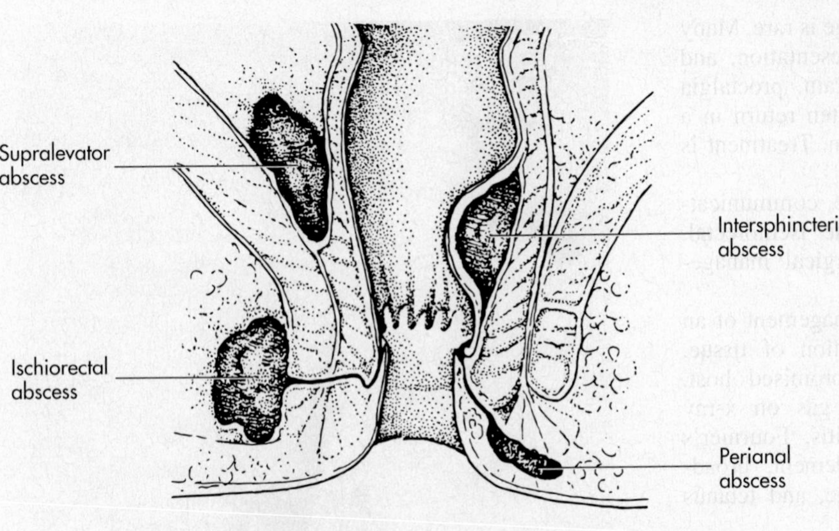

Figure 91-7. **Location of common anorectal abscesses.**

Table 91-4. Types of Abscesses

	Perianal	Ischiorectal	Intersphincteric	Supralevator	Postanal
Incidence	40%-45%	20%-25%	20%-25%	<5%	5%-10%
Location	Outside anal verge	Buttocks	Lower rectum	Above levator ani	Deep to external sphincter
Symptoms	Painful perianal mass	Buttock pain	Rectal fullness	Perianal and buttock pain	Rectal fullness Pain near coccyx
Fever, ↑WBC	–	±	±	+	+
Associated fistula	++	+	+++	+++	–
ED incision and drainage	+	±	–	–	–

absence of complicating factors (e.g., diabetes mellitus, extremes of age, and immunocompromised hosts). Some patients may be unable to tolerate the procedure without general or regional anesthesia. Incision and drainage should not take place in a sterile surgical procedure area. The WASH regimen (see Box 91-2) may alleviate postoperative discomfort. Antibiotics are unnecessary in healthy adults except in cases involving associated cellulitis.[1,6]

Ischiorectal abscess Approximately 20% to 25% of abscesses form outside the sphincter muscles in the buttocks, and patients complain of severe pain. The diagnosis is obvious if an indurated mass on the buttocks is seen, but is more difficult if the abscess is deep. Patients often have fever and leukocytosis.[1] If there is no induration, a needle aspirate can confirm the presence of pus. Although many patients require drainage under general anesthesia, superficial abscesses can be treated in the ED in a fashion similar to that used for the perianal abscess. If the patient is febrile, a short course of antibiotics may be considered, beginning with a parenteral dose prior to drainage followed by 3 to 7 days of an oral agent.[1]

Intersphincteric abscess One fourth of abscesses form in the space deep to the external sphincter and inferior to the levator ani. The infection tracks cephalad to appear as a mass in the rectum that may be confused with a thrombosed internal hemorrhoid. Patients complain of continuous rectal pressure and a throbbing pain exacerbated by defecation or sitting. They may be febrile and have leukocytosis. There may be no external evidence of inflammation, but rectal examination reveals an erythematous, indurated, sometimes draining mass. Associated fistulas and inguinal lymphadenopathy are common.[1,30,35] Drainage in the operating room is required, so that the entire abscess and fistula network can be treated.[35]

Supralevator abscess Accounting for fewer than 5% of abscesses, supralevator abscesses cause perianal and buttock pain associated with fever and leukocytosis. External evidence of this disease is usually absent, which often delays the diagnosis.[35] Approximately 23% of patients are obese or have diabetes mellitus, and others have concurrent disorders such as Crohn's disease, pelvic inflammatory disease, or diverticulitis.[1] A tender mass may be palpated on rectal or pelvic examination. Emergency surgical treatment is indicated.

Postanal abscess Postanal abscesses are uncommon and occur posterior to the rectum, deep to the external sphincter, and inferior to the levator ani. Patients complain of severe rectal discomfort and coccygeal pain. They are usually febrile and have continuous pain that does not change with position.

Rectal examination is painful, but anal drainage is rare. Many of these abscesses are missed on initial presentation, and patients are diagnosed with lumbosacral strain, proctalgia fugax, sciatica, or coccygodynia. Patients often return in a few days with an abscess draining at the skin. Treatment is surgical.[1]

Horseshoe abscess Occasionally a large, communicating, horseshoe-shaped abscess forms in the ischiorectal, intersphincteric, or supralevator spaces. Surgical management is necessary.

Necrotizing infection A delay in the management of an anorectal abscess may lead to the destruction of tissue, especially in the diabetic or immunocompromised host. Widespread cellulitis, necrotic tissue, and gas on x-ray suggest the possibility of necrotizing fasciitis, Fournier's gangrene, or tetanus. Wide surgical debridement, broad-spectrum antibiotics with anaerobic coverage, and tetanus prophylaxis are required.[1]

Treatment of Fistulas A *fistula* is a connection between two epithelium-lined surfaces. Anorectal fistulas develop in 50% to 67% of patients with ischiorectal abscesses.[1,34] Other causes include Crohn's disease, trauma, foreign body reactions, TB, and cancer.[21] Evidence to support these diagnoses should be sought, because the anorectal complaint may represent the presenting symptom of the disease. Patients notice a recurrent or persistent perianal discharge that becomes painful when one of the openings becomes occluded. Bidigital rectal examination may reveal a tract in the perineum or canal.[21] Probing of fistulous tracts is not recommended, because the danger of creating a new tract outweighs the benefit of identifying the path of the existing fistula.[35] Evaluation may include intrarectal ultrasound.[38] Spontaneous resolution of fistula-in-ano is rare. Most fistulas produce recurrent abscesses if untreated, so all patients should be referred for surgical management. A new method of treating fistulas with fibrin glue has been suggested.[39] Fistulotomy generally is not performed at the time of drainage of the abscess.[35]

Pilonidal Disease

Principles of Disease Little nests of hair in the sacrococcygeal area were first described in 1847 by Anderson (Latin *pilus,* hair; *nidus,* nest), who originally believed the lesions to be scrofula.[40] One hundred fifty years later, physicians have yet to agree on the cause and best mode of treatment. Pilonidal abscesses and subsequent sinus tracts afflict young adults with a 4:1 male predominance and are more common in obese and hirsute individuals. The disease is rare in persons over 40 years of age, even among those who were afflicted in their youth. The lesions arise in the midline of the sacrococcygeal area in the natal cleft and should not be confused with anal fistulas, perirectal abscesses, hidradenitis suppurativa, or granulomatous diseases (syphilis, TB).[1] Much of our understanding of pilonidal disease comes from experience in World War II, when the condition was rampant among jeep drivers.[41]

The debate between congenital predisposition and acquired disease seems to favor the latter.[41,42] This theory asserts that bacteria enter the usually sterile hair follicle and produce inflammation and edema that occlude the opening to the skin surface. The contents expand until the hair follicle ruptures, and the material spreads into the subcutaneous fatty tissue where a foreign body reaction leads to abscess formation. The purulent material subsequently tracks cephalad and drains to the skin via a laterally displaced epithelialized tract. Diagnosis is made by establishing the presence of a painful, fluctuant area in the presacral skin (Figure 91-8). In chronic or recurrent disease, visible or palpable tracts of 2- to 5-cm length may be identified with openings approximately 5 cm above the anus. These sinuses usually contain hairs and cellular debris.[41,43]

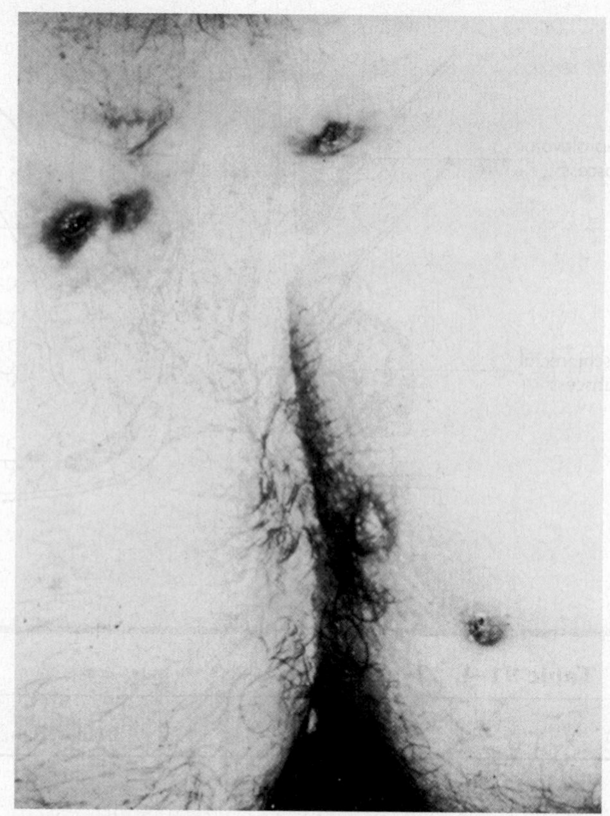

Figure 91-8. **Pilonidal sinus with multiple openings over sacrum and buttocks.** ***Modified from Corman ML:*** **Colon and rectal surgery,** ***ed 3, Philadelphia, 1993, JB Lippincott.***

Management Treatment options vary from conservative therapy to extensive surgical management.[41,44] Antibiotics can supplement surgical drainage in cases accompanied by cellulitis but should never be the primary mode of treatment.[1] ED management of pilonidal disease involves drainage of the acute abscess for relief of symptoms. To prevent reaccumulation of debris, a longitudinal incision *off* the sacral midline should be made (Figure 91-9). To decrease the usual 40% recurrence rate, the patient can be referred for follicle removal and unroofing of sinus tracts after the acute inflammation subsides (usually 1 week). A higher cure rate by shaving the hairs in the natal cleft every 3 weeks has been reported.[41] For patients whose disease is recalcitrant, wide excision and plastic surgery techniques are used.

Hidradenitis Suppurativa

Perianal *hidradenitis suppurativa* is an infection of the apocrine glands first described by Velpeau in 1839 and named

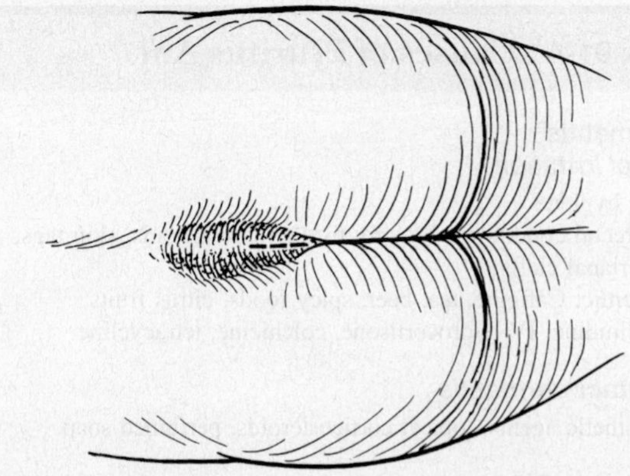

Figure 91-9. **Incision and drainage of pilonidal cyst. The incision is made lateral to the midline.** *From Larson S. In Rosen P et al, editors:* **Atlas of emergency procedures,** *St Louis, 2001, Mosby.*

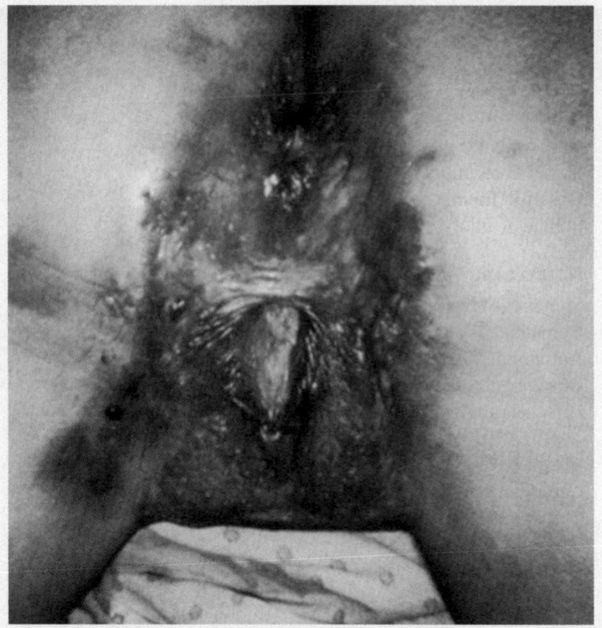

Figure 91-10. **Hidradenitis suppurativa.** *Modified from Corman ML:* **Colon and rectal surgery,** *ed 3, Philadelphia, 1993, JB Lippincott.*

by Verneuil in 1864, based on the Greek words *hidros* (sweat) and *aden* (gland).[45,46] It is most common in young adults and is related to poor skin hygiene, hyperhidrosis, obesity, acne, diabetes mellitus, and smoking. Patients are commonly misdiagnosed with pilonidal disease or fistula-in-ano. The differential diagnosis also includes sebaceous cysts, furuncles, granulomas (TB or syphilis), and Crohn's disease. Occluded apocrine ducts are infected with strains of *Staphylococcus, Streptococcus, E. coli,* or *Proteus.* Extension through the dermis spreads the infection to neighboring ducts, and a network of sinus tracts forms. This cycle leads to extensive scarring.[42,45]

Patients complain of a pustule in the perianal area, which may be associated with fever, leukocytosis, and malaise. One or more tender pustules may drain pus and have surrounding cellulitis (Figure 91-10). Local lymphadenopathy is common. Treatment begins with careful attention to perianal hygiene, warm compresses, and broad-spectrum antibiotics. Drainage of isolated lesions may provide symptomatic relief, but the recurrence rate approaches 40%. Referral to a surgeon for wide excision of advanced chronic disease may be necessary.[1,45]

Proctalgia Fugax

Proctalgia fugax is an intensely painful spasm in the rectal area that begins abruptly and lasts for several minutes. It is attributed to a sudden spasm of the levator muscle complex or the sigmoid colon.[47] People who frequent the toilet (e.g., diarrhea or simply an interest in reading) are at greatest risk, and women are more commonly affected than men.[1,35] A psychogenic predisposition is described by Pilling, who found that professionals, managers, and perfectionists are more likely to be afflicted.[48]

Proctalgia fugax can begin abruptly during sleep, defecation, urination, or intercourse.[1] The character of the pain has been compared to a charley horse. It lasts less than 30 minutes and may radiate to the coccyx or perineum. Symptoms during recurrent episodes are consistent for an individual, but each patient has a unique constellation of symptoms.[1] Treatment is often unrewarding, but recommendations include bowel regimens, upward manual pressure on the anus, diazepam, and topical nitrates.[1,49]

Anal Incontinence

Perspective Fecal incontinence is an embarrassing condition that affects parous women, the elderly, and people with a variety of neurologic or traumatic complaints. The delicate balance among the pelvic floor muscles, sphincters, and anorectal sensation is disrupted. *Complete incontinence* is the inability to control passage of solid feces. *Partial incontinence* occurs when there is a loss of control of the passage of flatus or liquid feces.[1,35,50]

Principles of Disease There are many causes of anal incontinence (Box 91-3).[1,35] Injury to muscles and nerves may result from accidental trauma or surgery for anorectal disorders. Similarly, injury or stretching during childbirth can cause immediate or delayed problems. Spinal cord and cauda equina lesions, and the autonomic neuropathy of diabetes mellitus can cause progressive incontinence. Liquid feces may seep around tumors or foreign bodies of the rectum or anal canal. A common "foreign body" is a large impacted stool that occurs in the elderly or those with underlying megacolon. Explosive diarrhea from laxative abuse, inflammation, or infection can temporarily overwhelm a normal sphincter mechanism. Partial incontinence after surgery to correct imperforate anus is common.[1,35] It occurs in children with congenital neurologic conditions such as meningocele, myelomeningocele, and spina bifida. Young children (4 to 7 years) with emotional stress may develop encopresis.[22,51] In otherwise healthy children, sexual abuse involving the anus must be considered.[1]

Clinical Features The physical examination should address the local and systemic factors described previously. The anorectum should be assessed for masses, hemorrhoids, evidence of previous surgery, and neuromuscular function. The anocutaneous reflex, or "anal wink," is elicited by

Box 91-3 Causes of Anal Incontinence

Traumatic
Nerve injured in surgery
Spinal cord injury
Obstetric trauma
Sphincter injury

Neurologic
Spinal cord lesions
Dementia
Autonomic neuropathy (e.g., diabetes mellitus)
Obstetrics: pudendal nerve stretched during surgery
Hirschsprung's disease

Mass Effect
Carcinoma of anal canal
Carcinoma of rectum
Foreign body
Fecal impaction
Hemorrhoids

Medical
Procidentia
Inflammatory disease
Diarrhea
Laxative abuse

Pediatric
Congenital
- Meningocele
- Myelomeningocele
- Spina bifida

After corrective surgery for imperforate anus
Sexual abuse
Encopresis

Box 91-4 Causes of Pruritus Ani

Dermatitis
Fecal irritation
Poor hygiene
Anorectal conditions: Fissure, fistula, hemorrhoids, skin tags, perianal clefts
Systemic: Caffeine, tea, beer, spicy foods, citrus fruits, quinidine, IV hydrocortisone, colchicine, tetracycline

Contact dermatitis
Anesthetic agents, topical corticosteroids, perfumed soap

Systemic Diseases
Dermatologic
Psoriasis, seborrhea
Lichen simplex or sclerosis

Nondermatologic
Chronic renal failure, myxedema, diabetes mellitus, thyrotoxicosis, polycythemia vera
Vitamins A or D deficiency, iron deficiency
Cancers: Bowen's, Paget's, Hodgkin's diseases

Infectious Agents
STDs
Syphilis
HSV
HPV

Other agents
Scabies
Pinworm
Bacterial infection
Fungal infection

touching the skin near the anus with a pin and observing the resulting constriction.[52] Sphincter function is assessed by asking the patient to squeeze the examiner's finger.

Management The approach to management of anal incontinence depends on the cause. Structural and inflammatory conditions may be diagnosed with anoscopy. If a 100-ml enema cannot be retained, the patient may require surgical evaluation.[35] Determination of the cause of incontinence and prompt referral for treatment of underlying conditions are required. In cases of transient incontinence caused by diarrhea, brief therapy with loperamide has been shown to solidify stool and enhance rectal compliance.[35]

Pruritus Ani

Principles of Disease Patients with pruritus ani complain of an uncontrollable urge to scratch the perianal area. Approximately 1% to 5% of the population seeks medical attention to obtain relief from this condition during their lifetime. Others rely on self-treatment to soothe less severe symptoms. The period of peak incidence is during the fifth and sixth decades of life, and it occurs more often in men.[53] The condition is more common in the summer months and is more noticeable at night. The sensation of itching arises when the richly innervated perianal skin becomes irritated. Patients scratch vigorously in an effort to relieve the itching, which leads to a vicious cycle that results in greater irritation and excoriation. The causes of pruritus ani are summarized in Box 91-4.[53-57]

The most common cause is the presence of feces on the perianal skin. Conditions ranging from poor personal hygiene to anatomic disorders of the anorectum allow feces to accumulate in the area. Patients may not clean the area thoroughly after defecation. Disruptions in the anorectal anatomy can lead to uncontrollable fecal collection on the perianal skin. Obesity, deep perianal clefts, copious hair, hemorrhoids, posthemorrhoidal skin tags, rectal mucosal prolapse, anal fissures, and fistulas make the area difficult to clean effectively. Decreased air circulation from wearing tight pants or synthetic undergarments may exacerbate symptoms.

Foods (e.g., caffeine, spicy or citrus foods, tea, and beer) and drugs (e.g., quinidine, colchicine, tetracycline, intravenous hydrocortisone) augment the irritant quality of the feces by altering its pH. Perfumed soaps and drugs, especially local anesthetic creams and ointments, can produce a contact dermatitis. Other dermatologic conditions include psoriasis, seborrhea, lichen simplex, and lichen sclerosis.

Systemic diseases and local infections can produce perianal itching. Chronic renal failure, diabetes mellitus, thyrotoxicosis, myxedema, polycythemia vera, deficiencies of iron or vitamins A or D, and certain cancers (Bowen's, Paget's, Hodgkin's diseases) are systemic causes. Local conditions include pinworms (*Enterobius vermicularis*), scabies (*Sarcoptes scabiei*), bacterial or fungal infections, and dermatologic manifestations of sexually transmitted diseases (e.g., syphilis, herpes simplex virus [HSV], cytomegalovirus [CMV], human papillomavirus [HPV]). Some cases are psychogenic in origin.[58]

Management A careful history and physical examination can identify the etiology of pruritus ani. Questions related to hygienic care of the anus, coexisting anorectal or systemic conditions, diet, and sexual practices must be asked. Pinworms can be identified by applying transparent tape to the perianal area and attaching it to a glass slide. Visualization of eggs under low power of a microscope confirms the diagnosis. The treatment is mebendazole (Vermox) 1 g orally. An alternative treatment is pyrantel pamoate (Antiminth) 1 g orally (11 mg/kg to a maximum of 1 g for pediatric patients). The dose of either may need to be repeated in 2 weeks. Scabies and pediculosis pubis should be treated with lindane 1% lotion or permethrin 5% cream.[53,57] Dermatitis caused by a fungal infection is characterized by sharply demarcated borders and is treated with clotrimazole or nystatin cream. Definitive treatment of concomitant anorectal conditions (e.g., fissures, fistulas, hemorrhoids, skin tags, rectal prolapse) can prevent recurrence of pruritus ani.

Underlying systemic diseases that have perianal manifestations should be treated. Education on personal hygiene is of the utmost importance. Patients should be instructed to clean the area thoroughly with lukewarm water after each bowel movement and pat (rather than rub) it dry with a tissue or towel that is free of chemical irritants. Loose-fitting underwear and exposure to fresh air may aid in alleviating symptoms. The treatment of acute dermatitis includes a short course of topical corticosteroids, calamine lotion, and systemic antihistamines.[53,57] Prevention of recurrent bouts of pruritus ani requires compliance with impeccable anal hygiene, and minimizing those factors that caused the initial exacerbation.

Sexually Transmitted Diseases and Proctitis

Management

General Approach The incidence of sexually transmitted diseases (STDs) has increased in the past few decades and is of particular concern in the patient with HIV (see Chapter 126). The anorectum is often involved because of its increased role in intercourse.[57,59] Semen has a concentrated viral load, and the damaged epithelium of ulcerated anoderm makes an easy portal for entry of the virus.[60] The constellation of infectious diseases that afflicts the anus, rectum, and colon often is termed the "gay bowel syndrome," although it also affects women who engage in anal intercourse.[61] All patients with anorectal infections should be referred for HIV testing.[59,62] A summary of common infections and treatment guidelines is found in Table 91-5. Surgical repair for benign anorectal conditions in HIV-positive patients should be undertaken early in the course of the disease when potential wound healing and patient wellness are at their best.[60]

Treatment of Specific STDs

Gonorrhea Gonorrhea is caused by the gram-negative diplococcus *Neisseria gonorrhoeae* and is most prevalent in young adults. Routine screening in homosexual men reveals that 55% are infected, although not all manifest symptoms.[60] It is postulated that gonorrhea is a cofactor for transmission of HIV.[63] Proctitis (inflammation of the rectum) results from anal intercourse or autoinoculation from vaginal secretions after a 5- to 7-day incubation period. Symptomatic patients complain of pruritus ani, tenesmus, and bloody or thick purulent yellow drainage. Anoscopy reveals proctitis and mucus in the anal crypts. Recovery of the organism directly from the crypts doubles the likelihood of identifying the organism on Gram's stain. Water should be used to lubricate the anoscope, because many lubricants contain an antibacterial agent. Symptoms of disseminated gonococcal infection such as arthritis, skin lesions, perihepatitis, endocarditis, and meningitis may occur.[64]

Chlamydia and lymphogranuloma venereum *Chlamydia trachomatis,* an intracellular organism that is endemic to the tropics, is the most common STD in the United States.[35,65] It causes proctitis in people who practice anal or oral-anal intercourse. Common symptoms include mucoid or bloody discharge, tenesmus, and burning. Some people are asymptomatic carriers of the organism. LGV is a more serious manifestation caused by specific strains of *C. trachomatis* that starts as a painful anal or perianal ulceration. Prominent unilateral lymph nodes coalesce to form a bubo, which must be distinguished from secondary syphilis. Patients often have systemic complaints of fever and malaise. Anoscopic examination reveals an erythematous, friable mucosa. Rectal cultures are generally unreliable because the organism is intracellular. Diagnosis is best achieved by immunofluorescent antibody testing. In its final stage, rectal strictures and rectovaginal fistulas may form.[60]

Herpes simplex virus The clinical symptoms of herpes were recognized as long ago as 100 AD, and genital herpes was described formally in the mid-1700s.[66] There is a 95% seroprevalence of HSV-2 in the HIV-positive population.[60] Herpes proctitis is caused by both strains of the virus, but HSV-2 is responsible for approximately 90% of cases.[64] It is found in people who practice oral-anal or anal intercourse. Symptoms appear 1 to 3 weeks after exposure. Those with proctitis complain of severe rectal pain, bloody mucoid discharge, tenesmus, constipation, and sometimes sacral paresthesias and urinary difficulties. Systemic complaints of fever, malaise, and myalgias may be present.[1,64,66] Physical examination and anoscopy may be impossible without anesthesia.[64] Single or coalesced vesicles and ulcerations occur in the perianal area and rectum, and anoscopy reveals an erythematous, friable, ulcerated rectal mucosa. Chronic mucocutaneous HSV infection is considered diagnostic for AIDS. Definitive diagnosis with viral or immunofluorescent staining relies on proper collection of fluid and scrapings from the base of the vesicle.[1]

Syphilis The number of reported cases of syphilis is increasing. Up to 75% of homosexual men are infected with *Treponema pallidum,* the motile spirochete responsible for the disease.[64] During anal intercourse, the organism enters the rectal mucosa or anoderm and causes an ulcer (chancre) to form within 2 to 6 weeks. This heralds the primary phase of syphilis and may resemble an anal fissure that is not located in the midline.[1,67] Most patients experience discomfort during defecation, mucoid discharge, tenesmus, and inguinal adenopathy. Primary syphilis can be confused with lymphoma, but the diagnosis can be made by visualizing spirochetes on

Table 91-5. Sexually Transmitted Diseases of the Anorectum

Type	Findings	Treatment
Ulcerative		
LGV	Unilateral inguinal adenopathy Fever, malaise Mucoid or bloody discharge	Doxycycline 100 mg PO bid × 21 days If pregnant or allergic to tetracyclines: erythromycin 500 mg PO qid × 21 days
HSV	Rectal pain, tenesmus, constipation Bloody mucoid discharge Vesicles and ulcerations Fever, malaise, myalgias, paresthesias	First episode: Perianal: acyclovir 400 mg PO tid *or* famciclovir 250 mg PO bid × 7-10 days Proctitis: acyclovir 800 mg PO tid × 7-10 days Recurrent: acyclovir 400 mg PO tid *or* famciclovir 125 mg PO bid × 7-10 days
Early (primary) syphilis	Chancre Tenesmus, pain, mucoid drainage Inguinal lymphadenopathy	Benzathine penicillin G 2.4 MU IM once Alternatives: doxycycline or erythromycin
Chancroid (*H. ducreyi*)	Inflammatory lesion progresses to ulcer Inguinal adenitis-bubo	Azithromycin 1 g PO once *or* Ceftriaxone 250 mg IM once *or* Ciprofloxacin 500 mg PO bid × 3 days *or* Erythromycin 500 mg PO qid × 7 days
CMV	Tenesmus, diarrhea, weight loss	Ganciclovir with appropriate disposition
Idiopathic (usually HIV+)	Eccentric, deep, poor healing, multiple	Symptomatic relief or surgical referral
Nonulcerative		
Condylomata acuminata (HPV)	Keratinized vegetative growths in anus or skin Asymptomatic, or pruritus ani, or bleeding	Podophyllin topically or cryotherapy Consider home therapy with podofilox 0.5% solution or gel for limited involvement
Gonorrhea (*N. gonorrhoeae*)	Pruritus ani Tenesmus Purulent yellow discharge	Cefixime 400 mg PO once *or* Ceftriaxone 250 mg IM once *or* Ofloxacin 400 mg PO once *or* Ciprofloxacin 500 mg PO once For pregnant patients: spectinomycin 2 g IM once *plus* erythromycin 500 mg PO qid × 7 days
Chlamydia (*C. trachomatis*)	Mucoid or bloody discharge Tenesmus	Azithromycin g PO once *or* Doxycycline 100 mg PO × 7 days *or* Ofloxacin 300 mg PO bid × 7 days For pregnant patients: erythromycin 500 mg PO qid × 7 days
Syphilis (secondary)	Maculopapular rash Condyloma latum	Benzathine penicillin G 2.4 MU IM once Alternatives: doxycycline or erythromycin

dark field microscopy from scrapings at the base of the ulcer.[1,66] Serologic testing is useful several weeks after the appearance of the chancre. Treponemal tests such as fluorescent treponemal antibody (FTA) become positive earlier than Venereal Disease Research Laboratory (VDRL) or rapid plasma reagin (RPR) (nontreponemal) tests.[66] Patients infected with HIV may take longer to test positive, and in some cases test results remain negative despite infection.[64] Patients with AIDS have a high incidence of neurosyphilis regardless of the stage of syphilis at the time they seek treatment.[68]

In some patients the chancre goes unnoticed, and they are seen initially with secondary syphilis, marked by the appearance of a maculopapular rash that characteristically involves the palms and soles or condyloma latum. The latter is a spirochete-laden, weeping, verrucous lesion in the perianal area that emits a foul odor (Figure 91-11).[1,64] It is easily distinguishable from condyloma acuminatum, which has a drier, more keratinized appearance.[35] Serologic testing results are usually positive. Tertiary syphilis is rare but may be revealed as a rectal gumma with severe perianal pain and paralysis of the sphincters, which may initially cause it to be mistaken for cancer.[64]

Chancroid Chancroid is caused by the gram-negative bacillus *Haemophilus ducreyi,* and begins as an inflammatory pustule or macule that ruptures to form an irregularly shaped ulcer. In several days painful inguinal adenitis develops. It is often a diagnosis of exclusion. All antimicrobial therapy, especially single-dose ceftriaxone, is less effective in HIV-positive patients.[65]

Condylomata acuminata (genital warts) Condylomata acuminata, the most commonly encountered anorectal STD, are caused by HPV. They are most often found in homosexual men but can be seen in heterosexual men, women, and children. The mode of transmission is primarily through sexual intercourse, but it can occur through close contact with infected persons, as often happens in pediatric cases. Because one half of HIV-positive patients have anal warts, HIV testing is recommended.[60,70] The pink-to-gray warts are a result of hyperplastic epithelial growth and appear as vegetative

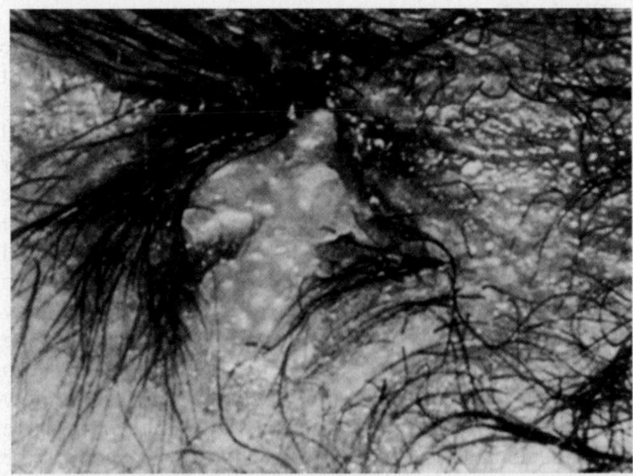

Figure 91-11. **Condyloma latum.** ***Modified from Beck DE, Wexner SD, editors:*** **Fundamentals of anorectal surgery,** ***New York, 1992, McGraw-Hill.***

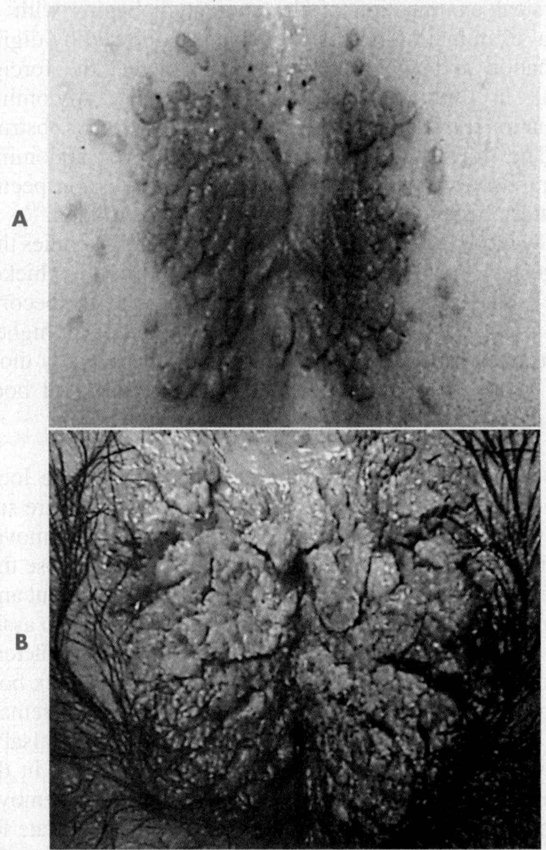

Figure 91-12. **Condylomata acuminata. A, In a child. B, In an adult.** ***Modified from Gordon PH, Nivatvongs S:*** **Principles and practice of surgery for the colon, rectum, and anus,** ***St Louis, 1992, Quality Medical Publishing.***

papilliform growths (Figure 91-12).[1,64] They may coalesce to form a massive patch that obscures the anal verge.[35] Many patients are asymptomatic or complain of pruritus ani, a "hemorrhoid," or bleeding. Evaluation should include anoscopy because the warts often grow within the anal canal.

Box 91-5 Anorectal Lesions in the Patient with HIV

Common Conditions

Anal fissure
Abscess and fistula
Hemorrhoids
Pruritus ani
Pilonidal disease

Common STDs

Gonorrhea
Chlamydia
Herpes
Chancroid
Syphilis
Condyloma acuminata

Atypical Conditions

Infectious: TB, CMV, actinomycosis, cryptococcus
Neoplastic: lymphoma, Kaposi's sarcoma, squamous cell carcinoma
Other: idiopathic anal ulcer

Failure to treat the internal lesions results in recurrence.[1,35,64] The differential diagnosis includes the condyloma latum of secondary syphilis, which has a more flat, moist appearance. Squamous cell carcinoma should be considered if the lesions are indurated. Progression to intraepithelial neoplasia has been reported to be related to the level of immunosuppression.[69]

Outpatient treatment with podofilox 0.5% solution or gel is limited to mild cases of external lesions.[65] Multiple applications of podophyllin resin by the physician may be required. This derivative of the plant *Podophyllum emodi* is a powerful skin irritant, so meticulous application is necessary. Alternate treatments include bichloroacetic acid, immunotherapy, laser, chemotoxic agents, cryotherapy, electrocoagulation, and excision.[35]

Ulcerative lesions in the patient with HIV Anal intercourse has led to a proliferation of anorectal STDs. Most patients who are HIV positive have current or past STD infection, which may be the initial reason for seeking medical attention. One third are anorectal complaints that fall into three categories: (1) routine proctologic conditions seen in the general population, (2) STDs, and (3) opportunistic infections (Box 91-5). The treatment of routine conditions and common STDs is similar except that wound healing may be slower in the patient with HIV.

In immunocompromised patients the differential diagnosis should include opportunistic infections, lymphoma, and Kaposi's sarcoma. Approximately 10% of patients with AIDS develop CMV proctitis with tenesmus, diarrhea, and weight loss. The only clue may be the presence of an anal ulcer that may be indistinguishable from a fissure. Further diagnostic testing and treatment are required.[62] Patients with AIDS often exhibit idiopathic anal ulcerations with pain and bleeding. Before making this diagnosis, other possible causes of the lesions must be considered (see Box 91-5). Symptomatic relief can often be achieved by the WASH regimen (see

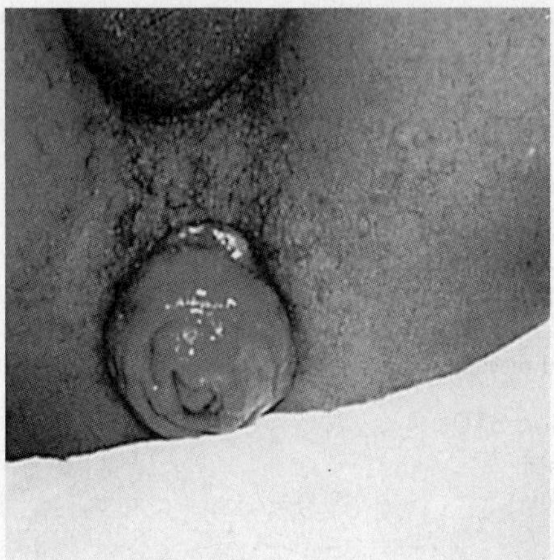

Figure 91-13. **Prolapse of the rectum.** *Courtesy Gershon Efron, MD, Sinai Hospital of Baltimore. In Seidel HM et al:* **Mosby's guide to physical examination,** *ed 4, St Louis, 1999, Mosby.*

Box 91-2), but recalcitrant lesions may require surgical excision.[62,71,72]

Procidentia

Rectal prolapse, or procidentia, is a disease of the extremes of age. It is complete if all bowel layers protrude, or incomplete if only the mucosal layer is involved.[1,35] In adults complete procidentia is most common in older women with a history of excessive straining. The cause is a laxity of attachment structures and it is often accompanied by uterine prolapse or a cystocele. Patients complain of an anal mass during defecation, coughing, or sneezing. It may cause incontinence, bloody or mucoid discharge, and a foul odor.[1,35] Physical examination reveals a red, ulcerated mass protruding from the anus (Figure 91-13). Sphincter tone may be weakened. Reduction should be attempted and, when successful, patients discharged with agents to relieve constipation. Surgical repair is often necessary.[35,50]

In children, procidentia may herald the presence of malnutrition or cystic fibrosis, and occurs during the first 2 years of life. Boys are more commonly affected than girls. Children usually have a mucosal prolapse.[22,73] The parent reports protrusion during defecation with small amounts of mucus or blood. It must be distinguished from a protruding juvenile polyp and intussusception. Reduction of procidentia should be attempted with sedation if necessary.[1] Medical management is successful because the disease is usually self-limited.[73]

Anorectal Foreign Bodies

Perspective The incidence of anorectal foreign bodies is on the rise with the increasing popularity of the anus for sexual gratification. Rectal foreign bodies are also found in children, psychiatric patients, victims of assault, or as a result of iatrogenic injury. Most objects are introduced directly into the anus, but some become lodged there after oral ingestion. It is important to identify and remove foreign bodies to prevent mucosal lacerations, intestinal obstruction, sepsis, and peritonitis. In many cases removal can be done safely in the ED.

Clinical Features

Objects Inserted into the Anus In a few cases, the foreign body is introduced iatrogenically. The two most common are the enema tip and the broken rectal thermometer.[74] However, in most cases the foreign body is placed deliberately by the patient or sexual partner for medicinal or sexual purposes. Objects that are commonly retrieved include fruits and vegetables; household items, especially those whose dimensions resemble the penis; and those purchased specifically with an anal erotic intent (Figure 91-14).[75-85] One can be certain that by the time patients arrive at the ED, they have tried desperately to remove the foreign body at home and have conceived a creative and implausible story to explain the circumstances. This usually focuses on how the object inadvertently found its way into the rectum by the patient accidentally sitting or falling on it. The job of the emergency physician is to ascertain the history in a nonjudgmental manner; to learn the type of foreign body involved; how long it has been there; what attempts have been made to remove it; and whether the patient has fever, abdominal pain, or rectal bleeding.[83] The possibility of assault should always be considered.[83]

Physical examination of the anorectum begins with an external examination for signs of trauma followed by digital examination and anoscopy, which may reveal the foreign body, a lax sphincter, or a mucosal injury. Abdominal examination may demonstrate signs of perforation or obstruction. The foreign body may be visible on abdominal radiographs, or its presence may be inferred by a nonspecific gas pattern, free air, or signs of intestinal obstruction.[80]

Orally Ingested Foreign Bodies Some foreign bodies that are ingested orally, especially toothpicks and fish or chicken bones, pass through the GI tract and subsequently become lodged in the rectum or anal crypts.[74,83,84] Patients at highest risk for ingested foreign bodies are children, especially those in the first 2 years of life; psychiatric patients; and body packers who ingest condoms full of drugs.[71]

Management Optimal treatment depends on the location and type of object found. Generally, objects that are soft and low-lying (<10 cm from anal verge) can be removed safely in the ED.[80] Large, hard, fragile objects, and those that have migrated proximally are difficult to remove without anal dilation under general anesthesia and instrumentation to assist in the passage through the sacral curve and sphincters. Premedication with a benzodiazepine is helpful to relax both the sphincter and the patient, but the patient should remain awake to assist in expulsion by performing the Valsalva maneuver at the appropriate time.[83] With the patient in the lithotomy position, suprapubic pressure can assist in removal (Figure 91-15). Other positions may be more appropriate for a particular foreign body. Several methods are effective for removal. The easiest is to grasp an edge of the foreign body with forceps and apply traction while the patient bears down. Most foreign bodies in the rectum do not have a convenient place to grasp, so other methods are needed. A Foley catheter can be placed beside the foreign body and the balloon inflated proximal to it (Figure 91-16). This breaks the suction of the rectal wall mucosa and provides a way to guide the object out of the rectal vault. Hollow objects may be filled with plaster of Paris, with an inset, inflated Foley catheter to be used as a handle.[83]

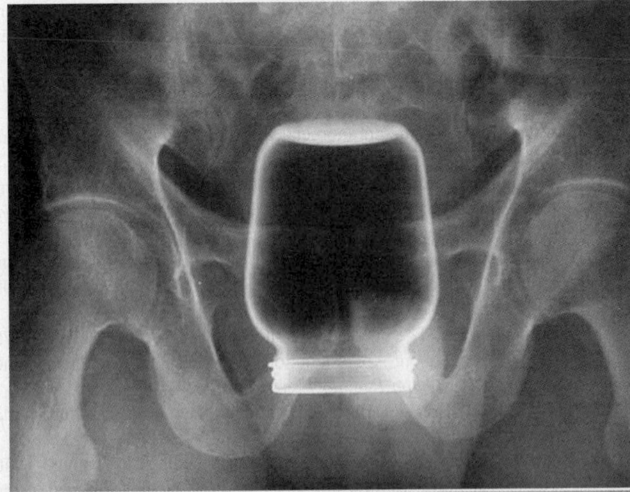

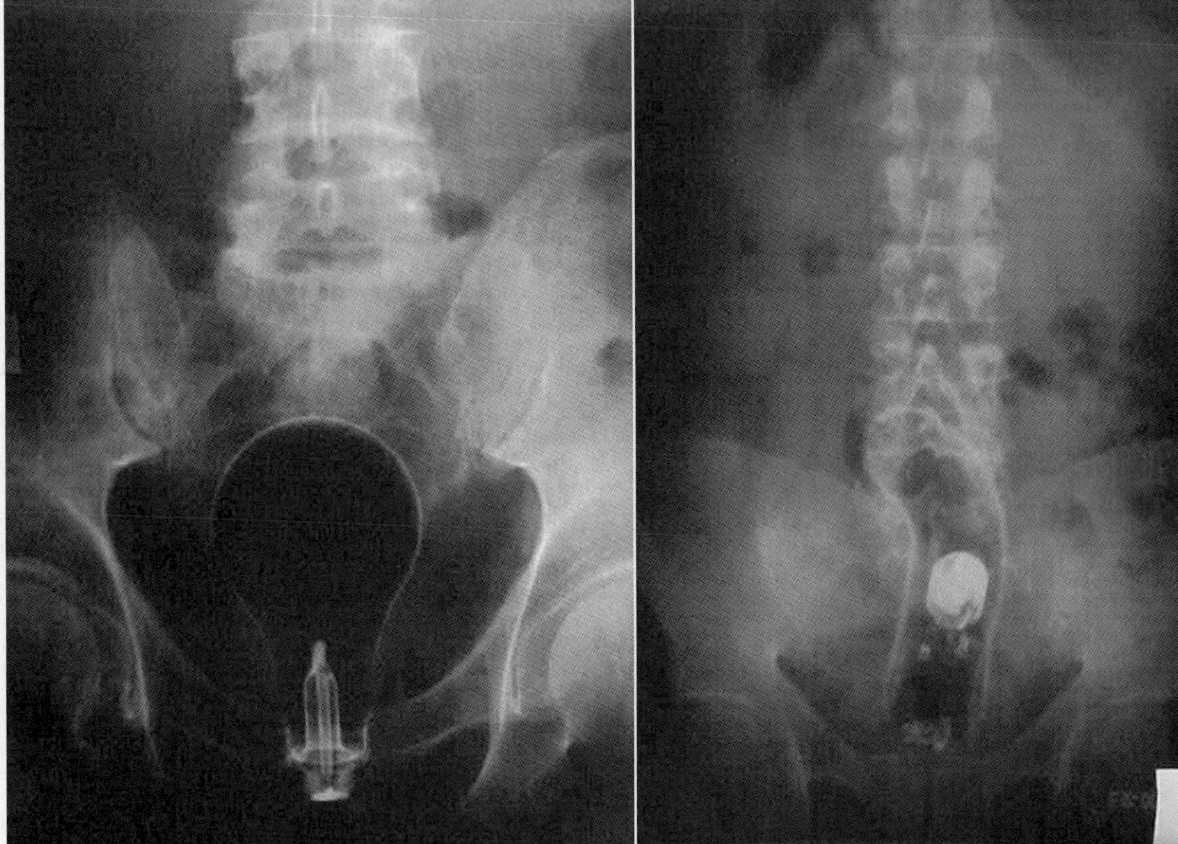

Figure 91-14. **Foreign bodies in rectum. A, Mustard bottle. B, Light bulb. C, Vibrator.**

Other creative ways to remove foreign bodies in the ED have been successful, and an individualized strategy for each patient is essential. After the removal of the foreign body, all patients should undergo sigmoidoscopy to look for mucosal tears and perforations.[76-85] Discharge instructions should warn the patient of signs and symptoms of perforation, peritonitis, and sepsis.

KEY CONCEPTS

- Patients who seek treatment for nonspecific anorectal complaints should be evaluated for the presence of underlying systemic disease (e.g., cancer, diabetes mellitus), because the anus may herald associated conditions.
- Patients with any STD should be evaluated for HIV infection and questioned about the use of the anus for sexual purposes.
- Anorectal conditions can be differentiated according to an algorithm (Figure 91-2) that addresses the presence or absence of pain, bleeding, swelling, and pruritus, in combination with an assessment of the patient's overall health.
- Most anorectal conditions can be symptomatically im-

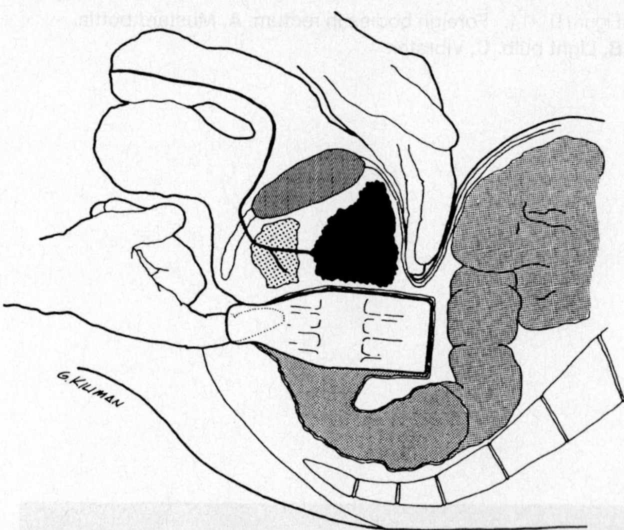

Figure 91-15. **Removal of foreign body from rectum.**

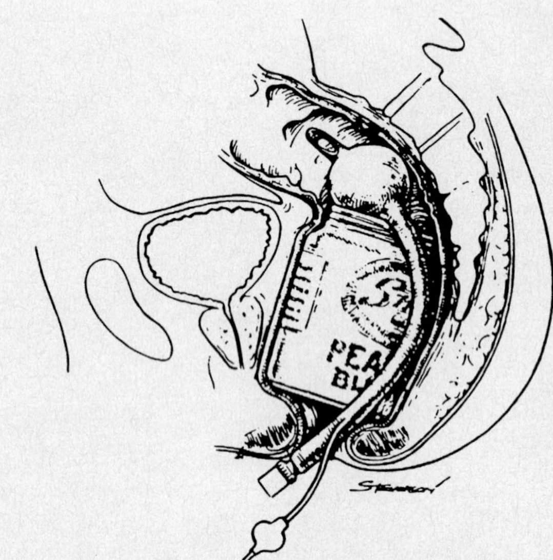

Figure 91-16. **Foley catheter–assisted removal of rectal foreign body.**

proved by adhering to the WASH regimen: *W*arm water, *A*nalgesics, *S*tool softeners, *H*igh-fiber diet.

REFERENCES

1. Corman ML: *Colon and rectal surgery,* ed 4, Philadelphia, 1998, JB Lippincott.
2. Marcio J et al: Anatomy and physiology of the rectum and anus, *Eur J Surg* 163:723, 1997.
3. Moore KL: *Clinically oriented anatomy,* ed 4, Baltimore, 1999, Williams & Wilkins.
4. Pemberton JH: Anatomy and physiology of the anus and rectum. In Beck DE, Wexner SE, editors: *Fundamentals of anorectal surgery,* ed 2, London, 1999, Bailliere Tindall.
5. Jones DJ, Irving MH: ABC of colorectal diseases, *BMJ* 304:974, 1992.
6. Janicke DM, Pundt MR: Anorectal disorders, *Emerg Med Clin North Am* 14:757, 1996.
7. Roberts PL: Patient evaluation. In Beck DE, Wexner SD, editors: *Fundamentals of anorectal surgery,* ed 2, London, 1999, Bailliere Tindall.
8. Jones R, Farthing M: The management of rectal bleeding, *Br J Clin Pract* 47:155, 1993.
9. Levine DS: Colonic and anorectal disorders: diagnosis and treatment, *Geriatrics* 47:22, 1992.
10. *New American bible,* New York, 1970, World Publishing Company.
11. Welling DR et al: Piles of defeat: Napoleon at Waterloo, *Dis Colon Rectum* 31:303, 1988.
12. Johanson JF, Sonnenberg A: The prevalence of hemorrhoids and chronic constipation. An epidemiologic study, *Gastroenterology* 98: 380, 1990.
13. Thomson WHF: The nature of haemorrhoids, *Br J Surg* 62:542, 1975.
14. Delco F, Sonnenberg A: Associations between hemorrhoids and other diagnoses, *Dis Colon Rectum* 41:1534, 1998.
15. Hosking SW et al: Anorectal varices, haemorrhoids, and portal hypertension, *Lancet* 1:349, 1989.
16. Orozco H et al: Colorectal variceal bleeding in patients with extrahepatic portal vein thrombosis and idiopathic portal hypertension, *J Clin Gastroenterol* 14:139, 1992.
17. Heaton ND et al: Symptomatic hemorrhoids and anorectal varices in children with portal hypertension, *J Pediatr Surg* 27:833, 1992.
18. Heaton ND et al: Incidence of haemorrhoids and anorectal varices in children with portal hypertension, *Br J Surg* 80:616, 1993.
19. Orkin BA et al: Hemorrhoids: what the dermatologist should know, *J Am Acad Dermatol* 41:449, 1999.
20. Dodi G et al: Hot or cold in anal pain? a study in the changes in internal sphincter pressure profiles, *Dis Colon Rectum* 29:248, 1986.
21. Hancock BD: Anal fissures and fistulas, *BMJ* 304:904, 1992.
22. Matt JG: Proctologic problems in infants and children: an analysis of 308 cases, *Dis Colon Rectum* 3:511, 1960.
23. Behrman RE, editor: *Nelson textbook of pediatrics,* ed 16, Philadelphia, 1999, WB Saunders.
24. Petros JG et al: Clinical presentation of chronic anal fissures, *Am Surgeon* 59:666, 1993.
25. Goligher J: *Surgery of the anus, rectum, and colon,* London, 1984, Bailliere Tindall.
26. Rosen L et al: Practice parameters for the management of anal fissure, *Dis Colon Rectum* 35:206, 1992.
27. Jensen SL: Treatment of first episodes of acute anal fissure: prospective randomized study of lignocaine ointment versus hydrocortisone ointment or warm sitz bath plus bran, *BMJ* 292:1167, 1986.
28. Antropoli C et al: Nifedipine for local use in conservative treatment of anal fissures, *Dis Colon Rectum* 42:1011, 1999.
29. Jost WH: One hundred cases of anal fissure treated with botulinum toxin: early and long-term results, *Dis Colon Rectum* 40:1029, 1997.
30. Seow-Choen F, Nichols RJ: Anal fistula, *Br J Surg* 79:197, 1992.
31. Endo M et al: Analysis of 1992 patients with anorectal malformations over the last two decades in Japan. Steering committee of Japanese study group of anorectal anomalies, *J Pediatr Surg* 34:435, 1999.
32. Festen C, van Harten H: Perianal abscess and fistula-in-ano in infants, *J Pediatr Surg* 33:711, 1998.
33. Venkatesh KS, Ramanujam P: Fibrin glue application in the treatment of recurrent anorectal fistulas, *Dis Colon Rectum* 42:1136, 1999.
34. Hughes LE: Clinical classification of perianal Crohn's disease, *Dis Colon Rectum* 35:928, 1992.
35. Burnstein M: Managing anorectal emergencies, *Can Fam Physician* 39:1782, 1993.
36. Gordon PH, Nivatvongs S: *Principles and practice of surgery for the colon, rectum, and anus,* ed 2, St Louis, 1998, Quality Medical Publishing.
37. Cataldo PA et al: Intrarectal ultrasound in the evaluation of perirectal abscess, *Dis Colon Rectum* 36:554, 1993.
38. Corfitsen MT et al: Anorectal abscesses in immunocompromised patients, *Eur J Surg* 158:51, 1992.
39. Anderson AW: Hair extracted from an ulcer, *Boston Med Surg J* 37:74, 1847.
40. Armstrong JH, Barcia PJ: Pilonidal sinus disease: the conservative approach, *Arch Surg* 129:914, 1994.

41. Haworth JC, Zachary RB: Congenital dermal sinuses in children—their relation to pilonidal sinus, *Lancet* 2:10, 1955.
42. Billingham RP: Anorectal miscellany: pilonidal disease, anal cancer, Bowen's and Paget's diseases, foreign bodies, and hidradenitis suppurativa, *Prim Care* 26:171, 1999.
43. Manookian C et al: Does HIV status influence the anatomy of anal fistulas? *Dis Colon Rectum* 41:1529, 1998.
44. Khatri VP et al: Management of recurrent pilonidal sinus by simple V-Y fasciocutaneous flap, *Dis Colon Rectum* 37:1232, 1994.
45. Wiltz O et al: Perianal hidradenitis suppurativa: the Lahey Clinic experience, *Dis Colon Rectum* 33:731, 1990.
46. Velpeau A, Verneuil A. Quoted in Paletta C, Jurkiexicz MJ: Hidradenitis suppurativa, *Clin Plast Surg* 14:383, 1987.
47. Harvey RF: Colonic motility in proctalgia fugax, *Lancet* 2:713, 1979.
48. Pilling LF et al: The psychologic aspects of proctalgia fugax, *Dis Colon Rectum* 8:372, 1965.
49. Vincent C: Anorectal pain and irritation: anal fissure, levator syndrome, proctalgia fugax, and pruritus ani, *Prim Care* 26:53, 1999.
50. Hyman NH: Anorectal disease: How to relieve pain and improve other symptoms, *Geriatrics* 52:75, 1997.
51. Weissenberg S: Encopresis. In Corman ML: *Colon and rectal surgery,* ed 3, Philadelphia, 1993, JB Lippincott.
52. Henry MM et al: The anal reflex in idiopathic faecal incontinence: an electrophysiological study, *Br J Surg* 67:781, 1980.
53. Jones DJ: Pruritus ani, *BMJ* 305:575, 1992.
54. Caplan RM: The irritant role of feces in the genesis of perianal itch, *Gastroenterology* 50:19, 1966.
55. Harrington CL et al: Dermatological causes of pruritus ani, *BMJ* 305:955, 1992.
56. Marks MM: The influence of intestinal pH on anal pruritus, *South Med J* 61:1005, 1968.
57. Paré AA, Gottesman L: Anorectal diseases, *Gastroint Clin North Am* 26:367, 1997.
58. Levshin LL: Anorectal symptoms of emotional origin, *Dis Colon Rectum* 4:399, 1961.
59. Bassford TS: Treatment of common anorectal disorders, *Am Fam Physician* 45:1787, 1992.
60. Law CLH et al: Nonspecific proctitis: association with human immunodeficiency virus infection in homosexual men, *J Infect Dis* 165:150, 1992.
61. Jones DJ, Goorney BP: Sexually transmitted diseases and anal papillomas, *BMJ* 305:820, 1992.
62. Kazal HL et al: The gay bowel syndrome: clinicopathologic correlation in 260 cases, *Am Clin Lab Sci* 6:184, 1976.
63. Metcalf AM, Dean T: Risk of dysplasia in anal condyloma, *Surgery* 118:724, 1995.
64. Viamonte M et al: Ulcerative disease of the anorectum in the HIV+ patient, *Dis Col Rectum* 36:801, 1993.
65. Abramowitz M, editor: Drugs for sexually transmitted infections, *Med Lett* 41:85, 1999.
66. Holmes KK et al, editors: *Sexually transmitted diseases,* ed 3, New York, 1999, McGraw-Hill.
67. Craib KJ et al: Rectal gonorrhea as an independent risk factor for HIV infection in a cohort of homosexual men, *Genitourin Med* 71:150, 1995.
68. Bordon J et al: Neurosyphilis in HIV infected patients, *Eur J Clin Microbiol Infect Dis* 14:864, 1995.
69. Bassi O et al: Primary syphilis of the rectum—endoscopic and clinical features, *Dis Colon Rectum* 34:1024, 1991.
70. Orkin BA, Smith LE: Perineal manifestations of HIV infection, *Dis Colon Rectum* 35:310, 1992.
71. Wilcox CM, Schwartz DA: Idiopathic anorectal ulceration in patients with human immunodeficiency virus infection, *Am J Gastroenterol* 89:599, 1993.
72. Miles AJG et al: Persistent ulceration of the anal margin in homosexuals with HIV infection, *J R Soc Med* 84:87, 1991.
73. Corman ML: Rectal prolapse in children, *Dis Colon Rectum* 28:535, 1985.
74. Gordon PH, Nivatvongs S: *Principles and practice of surgery for the colon, rectum, and anus,* ed 2, St Louis, 1998, Quality Medical Publishing.
75. Ahmed A, Cummings SA: Novel endoscopic approach for removal of rectal foreign body, *Gastrointest Endosc* 50:872, 1999.
76. Losanoff JE, Kjossev KT: Rectal "oven mitt": the importance of considering a serious underlying injury, *J Emerg Med* 17:31, 1999.
77. Ooi BS et al: Management of anorectal foreign bodies: a cause for obscure anal pain, *Aust N Z J Surg* 68:852, 1998.
78. Thomson SR et al: Iatrogenic and accidental colon injuries—what to do? *Dis Colon Rectum* 37:496, 1994.
79. Kouralkis G et al: Management of foreign bodies of the rectum: report of 21 cases, *J R Coll Surg Edinb* 42:246, 1997.
80. Cohen JS, Sackier JM: Management of colorectal foreign bodies, *J R Coll Surg Edinb* 41:312, 1996.
81. Campbell JK: Case report: a case of rectal perforation by foreign body presenting as pyrexia of unknown origin, *J R Nav Med Serv* 78:13, 1992.
82. Whatling PJ, Stacey MR: An unusual delivery, *Br J Hosp Med* 51:615, 1994.
83. Fry RD: Anorectal trauma and foreign bodies, *Surg Clin North Am* 74:1491, 1994.
84. Fletcher EC, Varon J: Intestinal obstruction: the marble effect, *Am J Emerg Med* 11:317, 1993.
85. Johnson SO, Hartranft TH: Nonsurgical removal of a rectal foreign body using a vacuum extractor. Report of a case, *Dis Colon Rectum* 39:935, 1996.

92 Renal Failure

Allan B. Wolfson
Richard L. Maenza

ACUTE RENAL FAILURE

RENAL FUNCTION EVALUATION PERSPECTIVE

The kidneys are responsible for the excretion of certain end-products of metabolism (e.g., urea, creatinine, and uric acid) and for control of the concentration of many body fluid constituents (e.g., sodium, potassium, chloride, and hydrogen ions). Plasma is filtered at the glomerulus, creating an ultrafiltrate that is then processed by the proximal and distal tubules and collecting duct. More than 99% of the filtrate is reabsorbed by the tubules; the remainder passes through the ureters, bladder, and urethra and is excreted as urine. The glomerular filtrate contains virtually no red blood cells (RBCs), and its composition is similar to that of interstitial fluid except that it has a protein concentration only 0.02 that of plasma. Water, electrolytes, and small molecules (e.g., glucose and uric acid) are reabsorbed from the glomerular filtrate across the tubular epithelium and are taken up into the plasma of the peritubular capillaries. Other substances are secreted by the tubular epithelium into the urine. The amount of glomerular filtrate formed per minute by both kidneys, termed the glomerular filtration rate (GFR), averages 125 ml/min in adult men and about 100 ml/min in women.

Although renal dysfunction may ultimately result in disturbances in volume regulation, acid-base balance, and electrolyte metabolism, patients often have the cardinal manifestations of hematuria, proteinuria, or azotemia. The last is defined as an increased serum concentration of the end-products of protein metabolism, as reflected principally by urea and creatinine. The evaluation of renal disease in the ED requires the intelligent use of urinalysis, serum and urine chemical determinations, and renal imaging studies to assess the degree of renal dysfunction and to take the first steps in determining its cause.

After discussing these diagnostic studies, this chapter outlines the approach to patients with hematuria, proteinuria, azotemia, or acute renal failure (ARF). Related topics, including urinary tract infection (UTI), urinary tract tumors, nephrolithiasis, renal trauma, acid-base disorders, and treatment of electrolyte abnormalities, are discussed in greater detail in other chapters.

Diagnostic Strategies

Urine Volume Because urine flow does not diminish until the GFR is sharply decreased, urine volume is a poor indicator of renal dysfunction. In fact, urine volume often increases as concentrating ability is lost with advancing renal dysfunction; patients with renal failure typically produce isosthenuric urine. Oliguria, defined as a urine volume of 100 to 400 ml/24 hr, may be seen with prerenal (blood flow–dependent), intrinsic (intrarenal), or postrenal (obstructive) causes of ARF. Alternating oliguria and anuria, although uncommon, is a classic indicator of intermittent obstruction that occurs as urine collects behind an obstructing stone or tumor and then is allowed to flow past as the obstructing material shifts position.

Urinalysis The standard urinalysis consists of dipstick screening for heme pigment, protein, glucose, ketones, pH, leukocyte esterase, nitrite reduction, and microscopic examination of a spun specimen of freshly voided urine.

Heme Heme pigment catalyzes the oxidation of orthotolidine by peroxidase, a reaction that is used to produce a color change on the dipstick reagent strip. The dipstick detects both free hemoglobin (or myoglobin) and hemoglobin contained in RBCs but is more sensitive to the former. Although as few as 3 RBC/hpf (high-power field) can be detected, the dipstick may fail to identify from 10% to 15% of patients with microscopic hematuria, as defined by more than 5 RBC/hpf. The sensitivity of the dipstick can be decreased by substances in the urine that alter the hemoglobin molecule. Vitamin C, for example, can cause a false-negative test result when present in the urine in large quantities. False-negative findings also occur in dilute urine and in urine containing large amounts of protein. False-positive results can be produced by chlorine or other oxidizing agents. A positive dipstick result should prompt microscopic examination of the urine. If red cells are seen, the diagnosis of hematuria is confirmed. If the dipstick result is positive but findings on microscopic examination are negative, pigmenturia (myoglobin or free hemoglobin) should be suspected.

Protein Urine containing large amounts of protein does tend to foam when shaken, but visual inspection alone cannot reliably detect proteinuria. The dipstick test for protein, using the color change of tetrabromophenol blue, can detect protein at concentrations of 10 to 15 mg/dl but does not reliably yield positive results until the concentration is greater than 30 mg/dl. Moreover, the correlation between color intensity and protein concentration is only approximate. The dipstick is three to five times more sensitive to albumin than to globulins and immunoglobulin light chains (e.g., Bence Jones protein), an important limitation. False-positive results are caused by alkaline urine, hematuria, or prolonged immersion of the dipstick in the urine. False-negative results are seen with dilute urine. The sulfosalicylic acid (SSA) test is more sensitive to proteinuria, detecting as little as 5 mg/dl of nonalbumin or albumin protein. Eight drops of 20% SSA are added to 2 ml of urine; turbidity appears if protein is present. False-positive findings may be caused by radiographic contrast agents, penicillin, or sulfonylurea drugs. False-negative results occur in alkaline urine. All specimens that produce a positive dipstick result should be retested using SSA; if the SSA result is significantly more positive than that of the dipstick, a urine electrophoresis should be performed to detect nonalbumin proteins such as the light chains associated with multiple myeloma.[1]

Microscopic Examination After the urine is dipped with the test strip, 10 ml is placed in a conical test tube and spun at 2,000 rpm for 5 minutes (higher speeds may break up casts). The supernatant is discarded. The sediment is resuspended in the residual urine, and a drop is placed on a slide and covered with a cover slip. The periphery of the cover slip, where casts tend to concentrate, is scanned under low power. The slide is then scanned under high power for red cells, white cells, renal tubular epithelial cells, oval fat bodies, bacteria, and crystals. Although some inaccuracy is involved in gauging the degree of hematuria by examining the spun-urine sediment, more reliable quantitative techniques are cumbersome and are rarely available to the clinician. Observations are recorded as the number of cells seen per high-power field. A level of 2 to 3 RBC/hpf in adult men or 2 to 4 RBC/hpf in adult women is commonly accepted as normal; in most studies a finding of 5 RBC/hpf is considered the threshold of abnormality.[2,3]

Casts are formed from urinary Tamm-Horsfall protein, a product of the tubular epithelial cells that gels at low pH and high concentration and when mixed with albumin, red cells, tubular cells, or cellular debris. The composition of a cast thus reflects the contents of the tubule. Casts are described and classified according to their appearance or constituents (e.g., hyaline, red cell, white cell, granular, or fatty casts) (Figure 92-1). Hyaline casts, those that are devoid of contents, are seen with dehydration, after exercise, or in association with glomerular proteinuria. Red-cell casts indicate glomerular hematuria, as seen in glomerulonephritis; the presence of even a few red-cell casts is significant. White-cell casts imply the presence of renal parenchymal inflammation. Granular casts are composed of cellular remnants and debris. Fatty casts, like oval fat bodies, are generally associated with heavy proteinuria and the nephrotic syndrome but have been

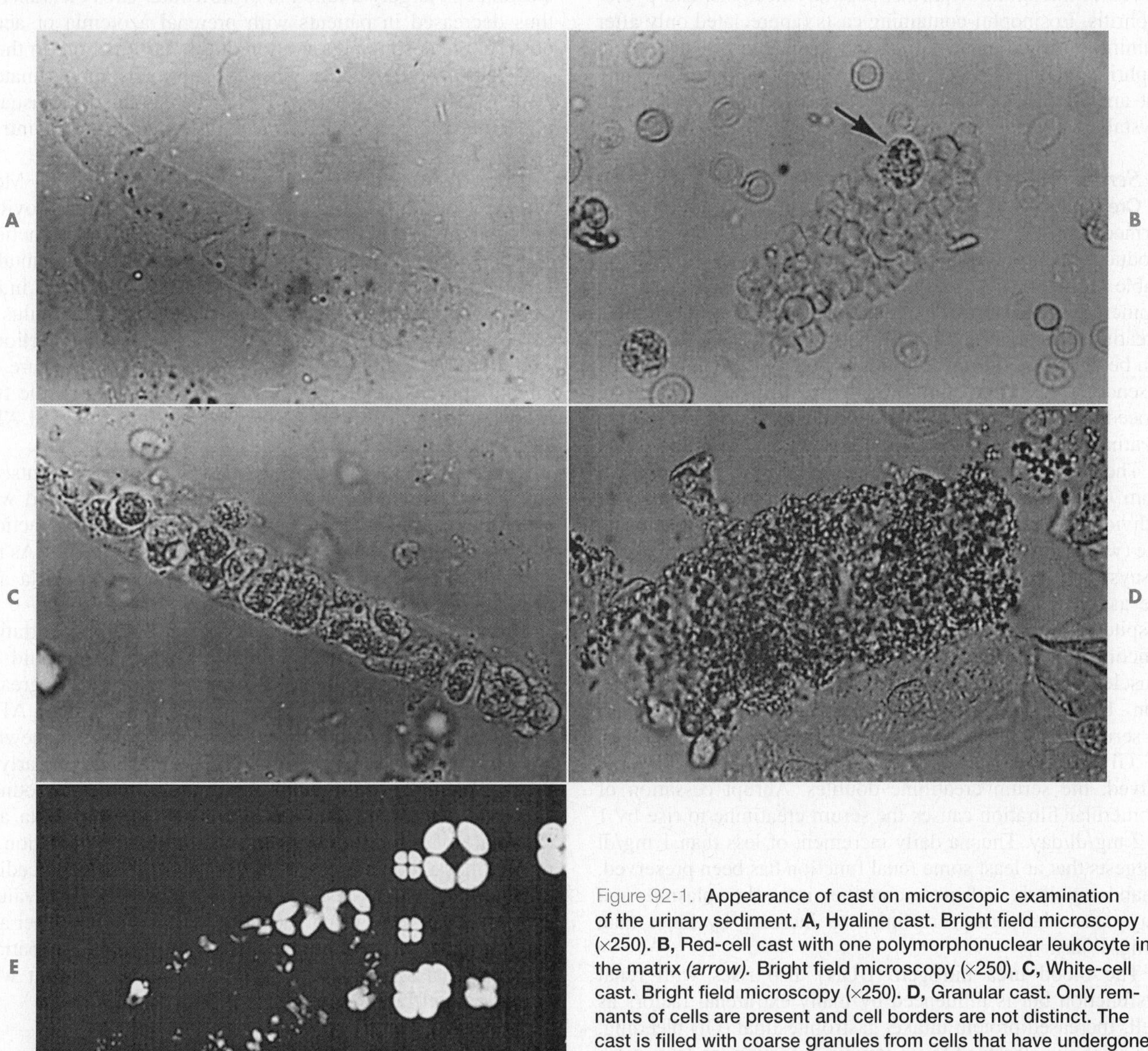

Figure 92-1. **Appearance of cast on microscopic examination of the urinary sediment. A, Hyaline cast. Bright field microscopy (×250). B, Red-cell cast with one polymorphonuclear leukocyte in the matrix *(arrow).* Bright field microscopy (×250). C, White-cell cast. Bright field microscopy (×250). D, Granular cast. Only remnants of cells are present and cell borders are not distinct. The cast is filled with coarse granules from cells that have undergone degeneration. Bright field microscopy (×250). E, Fatty cast. The fat is doubly refractile to polarized light and has a "Maltese cross" pattern. Polarized microscopy (×250).** ***Courtesy the American Society of Clinical Pathologists.***

noted to occur in a substantial proportion of patients with nonglomerular renal disease as well.[4]

Casts may also be classified by size and appearance as hyaline (as described previously), broad, or waxy. In chronic renal disease, casts may be broad (>3 white blood cell [WBC] diameters wide) because of enlargement of those nephrons that are still functioning; they have finely dispersed granules and appear waxy. The term *telescoped sediment* refers to a combination of cellular casts and broad and waxy casts, suggesting ongoing damage of the remaining nephrons.

Microscopic examination of the urinary sediment can be helpful in establishing the cause of ARF. A sediment without formed elements or with only hyaline casts is characteristic of prerenal azotemia or obstruction. Red-cell casts suggest glomerulonephritis or vasculitis. Fatty casts are seen in the nephrotic syndrome and also suggest glomerular disease. In acute tubular necrosis (ATN), the urinary sediment commonly shows granular casts and renal tubular epithelial cells. Large numbers of polymorphonuclear leukocytes are observed in interstitial nephritis, papillary necrosis, and pyelonephritis. Eosinophil-containing casts (appreciated only after staining the sediment) are typical of allergic interstitial nephritis.[5] Uric acid crystals suggest uric acid nephropathy but are extremely nonspecific; oxalic acid or hippuric acid crystals may be seen in ethylene glycol ingestion.

Serum and Urine Chemical Analysis

Creatinine and Blood Urea Nitrogen Creatinine is formed from the breakdown of muscle creatine. The amount produced is proportional to muscle mass and is normally stable from day to day. Creatinine is filtered at the glomerulus, and a small amount is secreted by the tubule. Creatinine clearance, which usually parallels GFR closely, can be determined from a 24-hour urine collection, but in the absence of the information provided by this time-consuming procedure, GFR is commonly estimated from the serum creatinine.

The normal range of the serum creatinine level extends from 0.5 mg/dl in thin persons to 1.5 mg/dl in muscular individuals. Spurious elevations can be caused by acetoacetate (which cross-reacts with creatinine in the commonly used assays) and by certain medications that either cross-react in the assay or reversibly inhibit tubular creatinine secretion despite a normal GFR. Serum creatinine concentration is a function of the amount of creatinine entering the blood from muscle, its volume of distribution, and its rate of excretion. Because the first two are usually constant, changes in serum creatinine concentration generally reflect changes in GFR. Under steady-state conditions, if the GFR is halved, the serum creatinine doubles. Abrupt cessation of glomerular filtration causes the serum creatinine to rise by 1 to 2 mg/dl/day. Thus, a daily increment of less than 1 mg/dl suggests that at least some renal function has been preserved. Rhabdomyolysis releases creatine into the plasma and may cause the serum creatinine to increase by more than 2 mg/dl/day.

The blood urea nitrogen (BUN) also rises with renal dysfunction but is influenced by many extrarenal factors as well. Increased protein intake, gastrointestinal (GI) bleeding, and catabolic effects of fever, trauma, infection, or drugs such as tetracycline and corticosteroids all increase protein turnover and result in increased hepatic urea production and increased BUN. Conversely, BUN tends to be decreased in patients with liver failure or protein malnutrition.

Table 92-1. Typical Urinary Findings in Prerenal Azotemia and ATN

Laboratory test	Prerenal azotemia	ATN
Urinalysis	Normal, or hyaline casts	Brown granular casts, cellular debris
Urine sodium concentration (mEq/L)	<20	>40
Fractional excretion of sodium (%)	<1	>1
Urine/plasma creatinine ratio	>40	<20

Once glomerular filtrate has been formed, renal urea clearance is largely a function of flow rate. Urea clearance is thus decreased in patients with prerenal azotemia or acute obstruction, despite preservation of tubular function. In these individuals the BUN/creatinine ratio, normally approximately 10:1, is usually greater than 10:1, whereas this ratio usually is not markedly increased in cases of uncomplicated intrinsic ARF.

Urine Sodium* and Fractional Excretion of Sodium Measurement of the urine sodium (UNa) concentration provides information on the integrity of tubular reabsorptive function. Normally, UNa concentration parallels sodium (Na) intake. Low UNa concentration thus indicates not only intact reabsorptive function but also the presence of a stimulus to conserve Na. The UNa concentration, as well as the fractional excretion of sodium (FENa),* an additional measure of tubular sodium handling, helps distinguish between the two most common causes of ARF: prerenal azotemia and ATN (Table 92-1).

Urinary indices are most helpful in oliguric patients. In euvolemic individuals who are in sodium balance and who have a moderate sodium intake and normal renal function, UNa is less than 20 mEq/L and FENa is less than 1%.[6] As the stimulus for sodium reabsorption increases, both UNa and FENa decrease.[7,8]

In general, an oliguric patient with a UNa concentration less than 20 mEq/L and FENa less than 1% should be considered to have prerenal azotemia, whereas UNa greater than 40 mEq/L and FENa greater than 1% suggest ATN. Values in patients with prerenal azotemia overlap somewhat with those of patients with nonoliguric ATN, particularly if the renal injury is mild and some capability to retain sodium has been preserved. Thus, intermediate values of UNa and FENa are of little discriminatory use. The administration of mannitol or a loop diuretic within the several hours preceding urine collection may also make interpretation of urine values difficult because the urinary sodium will tend to be higher and the urine less concentrated, causing the results in a patient with prerenal azotemia to resemble those of a patient with intrinsic renal failure (Box 92-1).

*The FENa, a percentage defined as $[(UNa/PNa)/(UCr/PCr)] \times 100$, reflects the fraction of filtered sodium that escapes reabsorption and is excreted in the urine. Note that its calculation requires simultaneous measurement of urine and plasma sodium and creatinine.

Box 92-1 Causes of High or Low FENa and UNa in Patients with Acute Renal Failure

UNa <20 mEq/L, FENa <1%

Prerenal azotemia
Acute glomerulonephritis
Acute obstruction
Contrast-induced ATN (some cases)
Rhabdomyolysis-associated ATN (some cases)
Early sepsis
Nonoliguric ATN (10% of cases)

UNa >40 mEq/L, FENa >1%

ATN (90% of cases)
Chronic obstruction
Diuretic drugs
Osmotic diuresis
Underlying chronic renal failure

From Kelley WN, editor: *Internal medicine,* ed 2, Philadelphia, 1992, JB Lippincott.

In glomerulonephritis, the urinary indices generally reflect intact tubular sodium handling, but the diagnosis is better made by urine microscopy. In obstructive uropathy, the values of the urinary indices depend on the duration of obstruction and cannot be relied on to indicate either the presence or absence of obstruction.

Radiography Renal imaging is often helpful in evaluating the patient with kidney dysfunction, particularly when obstruction is suspected. Intravenous pyelography (IVP) provides an anatomic image of the urinary tract but does not evaluate renal function. The classic findings of obstruction are kidneys that are normal to large in size, nephrograms that become increasingly dense (for up to 24 hours after contrast injection), and delayed opacification of dilated collecting systems. IVP subjects the kidneys of an already azotemic patient to the risk of an additional potential insult from the contrast agent. Patients with a baseline serum creatinine level greater than 2.5 mg/dl are estimated to have approximately a 33% chance that a further significant decrease in renal function will develop, compared with an approximately 2% chance in individuals with a normal baseline creatinine level.

The newer nonionic contrast agents that have been developed appear to have the same potential for nephrotoxicity.[9] In patients with preexisting renal insufficiency, therefore, techniques such as ultrasonography and computed tomography (CT) scanning that do not involve contrast administration are much preferred if available.

Computed Tomography CT scanning may be useful in evaluating some azotemic patients. Hydronephrosis can be recognized without the use of contrast material. Dilated ureters can also often be seen without contrast enhancement and the level of obstruction determined. Moreover, the cause of obstruction (e.g., lymphoma, retroperitoneal hemorrhage, metastatic cancer, or retroperitoneal fibrosis) can often be delineated as well. CT scanning is the technique of choice for visualizing ureteral obstruction at the level of the bony pelvis. Occasionally obstruction severe enough to result in renal failure may not cause detectable proximal dilation of the urinary tract. Bilateral ureteral obstruction produced by malignancy or retroperitoneal fibrosis is the most important cause of this nondilated obstructive uropathy. When noninvasive studies produce negative results, the diagnosis must be made by retrograde pyelography or by antegrade pyelography via a percutaneous nephrostomy.

Ultrasonography Ultrasonography allows accurate measurement of renal dimensions and is a reliable and safe method of excluding obstruction as a cause of ARF. The normal kidney shows an echo-free renal parenchyma surrounding the echogenic central urothelium of the renal pelvis and calices. The sonographic appearance of obstruction is that of an enlarged central sonolucent area that spreads the normal central echodensities. A similar pattern may be produced by renal cysts, but without associated ureteral dilation. Dilation of the collecting system generally is apparent within 24 to 36 hours of the onset of obstruction, but obstruction may be overlooked in patients who are evaluated early in the development of obstructive ARF. Ultrasonography has been reported to be 98% sensitive and 74% specific in demonstrating obstruction (using IVP as the "gold standard") and may also be useful in detecting intrarenal and ureteral calculi.[10,11] However, ultrasonographic resolution is often limited because of the presence of overlying bowel gas.

MANAGEMENT

Approach to Hematuria

Principles of Disease Painless hematuria is estimated to occur in the general population at an incidence of 3% to 4%.[12] Microscopic hematuria is often discovered incidentally on routine urinalysis, but as little as 1 ml of blood in 1 L of urine can cause grossly appreciable hematuria, an occurrence that usually induces the patient to seek medical attention.

Normal individuals pass up to 1 million RBCs into the urine during any 24-hour period. Counts greater than this correspond roughly to the presence of more than 5 RBC/hpf in the spun urine sediment. Although the presence of blood in the urine is not invariably a sign of disease, the finding of hematuria mandates an effort to rule out any treatable underlying disorder. Both gross and microscopic hematuria are caused by similar disorders, but the amount of blood in the urine does not correlate with the severity or the seriousness of the condition causing it.

The causes of hematuria can be divided into hematologic, renal, and postrenal causes; renal causes may be further classified as glomerular or nonglomerular (Box 92-2).[12] Overall, the most common causes of nontraumatic hematuria, in descending order of occurrence, are kidney stones, carcinoma of the kidney or bladder, urethritis, urinary tract infection, benign prostatic hypertrophy (BPH), and glomerulonephritis. The differential diagnosis can be narrowed by taking into account the patient's age and sex (Table 92-2) and by distinguishing between upper and lower urinary tract sources. When gross hematuria is present, cystoscopy can determine whether blood is emerging from one or both ureteral orifices, thereby defining a source in the upper tract. Red-cell casts indicate a renal source, as does associated proteinuria (>500 mg in 24 hours). When differentiating between proteinuria produced by renal parenchymal disease and that simply produced by admixture of urine with extravasated blood, a useful rule of thumb is that 1 ml of whole blood contains approximately 5 billion RBCs and approximately 50 mg of albumin.

The evaluation of the ED patient who has gross or microscopic hematuria should begin with a complete history so that the pattern and character of the hematuria can be defined. Blood noted only on initiation of voiding suggests a urethral source, whereas blood noted only in the last few drops of urine suggests a prostatic or bladder neck source. Total hematuria* (i.e., hematuria present throughout urination) suggests a source in the bladder, ureter, or kidney.* Brown or smoky-colored urine usually has a renal source. Blood clots indicate a nonglomerular renal or lower urinary tract source of bleeding. Hematuria may rarely be cyclic or associated with menses, suggesting endometriosis of the ureter or bladder. Flank pain suggests calculus, neoplasm, renal infarction, obstruction, or infection as cause. Symptoms of frequency, dysuria, or suprapubic pain suggest cystitis or urethritis; in adult men, perineal pain, dysuria, and terminal hematuria suggest prostatitis.

*The same analysis can be applied to microscopic hematuria using a "three glass" collection or urine. Three separate specimens are collected—at the initiation of urination, at midstream, and at termination—and the numbers of red cells are compared.

Box 92-2 Causes of Hematuria

- Hematologic
  - Coagulopathy
  - Sickle hemoglobinopathies
- Renal (glomerular)
  - Primary glomerular disease
  - Multisystem disease (e.g., systemic lupus erythematosus, Henoch-Schönlein purpura, hemolytic uremic syndrome, polyarteritis nodosa, Wegener's granulomatosis, Goodpasture's syndrome)
- Renal (nonglomerular)
  - Renal infarction
  - Tuberculosis
  - Pyelonephritis
  - Polycystic kidney disease
  - Medullary sponge kidney
  - Acute interstitial nephritis
  - Tumor
  - Vascular malformation
  - Trauma
  - Papillary necrosis
- Postrenal
  - Stones
  - Tumor of ureter, bladder, urethra
  - Cystitis
  - Tuberculosis
  - Prostatitis, urethritis
  - Foley catheter placement
  - Exercise
  - Benign prostatic hypertrophy

Other clues as to the cause should be sought by careful questioning. Because glomerulonephritis or interstitial nephritis may be caused by a variety of bacterial, viral, and parasitic infections, any history of recent infection is important. In particular, a recently sore throat suggests the possibility of poststreptococcal glomerulonephritis; a history of foreign travel or residence abroad may suggest schistosomiasis or tuberculosis. Symptoms suggestive of a multisystem disorder (e.g., systemic lupus erythematosus) should also be sought. Because drugs may cause acute interstitial nephritis (AIN), papillary necrosis, or hemorrhagic cystitis, a complete medication history should be elicited. When hematuria is associated with anticoagulant use, underlying disease can be identified in 80% of patients.[13] The family history should be elicited because it may provide a clue to the presence of polycystic or other familial kidney disease, sickle cell disease, or renal calculi. A history of strenuous exercise is important; 15% to 20% of normal individuals exhibit hematuria after strenuous exercise. The mechanism is unclear, but hematuria resolves spontaneously within a few days.[14]

Clinical Features On physical examination, findings of arthritis, skin lesions, hypertension, or edema suggest underlying glomerulonephritis. Because endocarditis or atrial fibrillation may cause renal embolism, the EP should check for a new heart murmur or an irregular rhythm. Costovertebral angle tenderness suggests pyelonephritis or stone disease, and a palpably enlarged kidney suggests polycystic kidney disease or renal malignancy. The prostatic examination may offer clues to the presence of prostatitis, BPH, or cancer. Examination of the external genitalia may reveal a urethral meatal lesion that may be the source of bleeding; in adult women, a pelvic examination should be performed to exclude vulvovaginal sources of blood.

Laboratory Evaluation of hematuria in the ED should include assessment of the blood pressure and measurement of

Table 92-2. Most Common Causes of Hematuria by Age

	<20 yr	20-40 yr	40-60 yr	40-60 yr
Sex	♂ and ♀	♂ and ♀	♂	♀
Causes of hematuria	Glomerulonephritis UTI	UTI Stone Trauma Carcinoma (bladder, kidney)	Carcinoma (bladder) Stone UTI Carcinoma (kidney) BPH if >60	UTI Stone Carcinoma (bladder, kidney)

Adapted from Restropo NC, Carey PO: *Am Fam Physician* 40:149, 1989.
UTI, Urinary tract infection; *BPH,* benign prostatic hyperplasia.

the BUN and serum creatinine levels to gauge the patient's underlying renal function, but urinalysis can be expected to provide more specific information. Red urine that is dipstick-negative and free of red cells on microscopy may be caused by ingestion of beets, red berries, or food coloring; by urate crystals; or by drugs such as phenazopyridine (Pyridium) and rifampin. A finding of red-cell casts, other casts, or lipiduria or significant proteinuria in combination with hematuria suggests intrinsic renal disease and mandates appropriate referral. (The urine should be examined as soon as possible after voiding because structures such as red-cell casts may disintegrate over time.) Microscopic hematuria usually does not produce a positive dipstick test result for protein, but gross hematuria may contribute enough protein to cause a positive result; thus, a finding of proteinuria should be confirmed and the amount quantitated on a 24-hour urine collection. Hematuria in combination with pyuria or bacteriuria suggests UTI; infection should be treated and hematuria reassessed after therapy has been completed. Even if white cells or organisms are not seen on urinalysis, the urine should be cultured to rule out hemorrhagic cystitis, especially when lower tract symptoms are present. Eosinophiluria (appreciable on Wright's stain or Hansel's stain of the urine sediment) suggests AIN.[5,15]

Blood studies should be ordered only as necessary to gauge renal function and to confirm causes suggested by the clinical presentation. In the ED, routine ordering of the full gamut of chemical and serologic studies necessary to rule out all possible causes of hematuria is rarely appropriate. In particular, a platelet count and coagulation studies are extremely unlikely to be helpful in the absence of a suggestive history or other specific clinical clues.

Radiography Ultrasonography The role of urinary tract imaging studies in the immediate evaluation of hematuria is also limited. Visualization of the urinary tract is generally helpful only when the history suggests renal colic or other disorders of the upper urinary tract (e.g., polycystic kidney disease, tumor, or obstruction). Helical CT scanning without contrast has emerged as the imaging modality of choice.[16] Ultrasonography can be used to determine kidney size and shape and to detect renal masses or obstruction. Further imaging studies, if indicated, should be planned after urologic consultation.

If no upper tract lesions are identified on initial imaging studies, cystoscopy is usually the next step in evaluation because it is the most effective means of visualizing the bladder and the male urethra. It is the initial study of choice for patients with active gross hematuria; in fact, some urologists prefer to perform endoscopic procedures promptly during an acute bleeding episode to maximize the chance of localizing the source. In older patients whose urinalysis shows only hematuria and whose history and physical examination are otherwise unhelpful, urinary cytologic examination may also be undertaken.

Patients with hematuria who have no other abnormality revealed by urinalysis; who are otherwise asymptomatic; who are not azotemic, hypertensive, or severely anemic; and who have no evidence of intrinsic renal disease may be monitored as outpatients. (A possible exception may be the patient with a known bleeding disorder.) Others should generally be admitted to the hospital for prompt evaluation. Extensive outpatient evaluation of an isolated episode of hematuria is usually not undertaken in patients less than 40 years of age unless hematuria is persistent, but most patients above the age of 40 should undergo a thorough evaluation after even a single episode of hematuria.

The cause of hematuria can be determined on initial medical and urologic evaluation in 70% to 80% of cases. In others, a diagnosis of small calculi, occult bladder tumor, arteriovenous malformation, or early glomerulonephritis is made only after repeated examination or the development of further signs or symptoms. In 5% to 10% of cases no cause can be determined.

Approach to Proteinuria

Principles of Disease During a 24-hour period, the kidneys normally filter 180 L of plasma containing approximately 12 kg of protein. The 1 to 2 L of urine produced from this filtrate contains only 40 to 80 mg of protein in normal individuals. Abnormal proteinuria is defined as excretion of more than 150 mg/24 hr in adults or more than 140 $mg/m^2/24$ hr in children. Patients with mild to moderate degrees of proteinuria are commonly identified incidentally on routine urinalysis; patients with more severe degrees of proteinuria often seek medical attention because of edema or other effects of hypoproteinemia.

Proteinuria may be classified broadly as glomerular or tubular. *Glomerular proteinuria,* the more common type, results from increased permeability of the glomerular capillaries to plasma proteins. With alteration in the glomerular capillary barrier (e.g., with the nephrotic syndrome and the many varieties of primary and secondary glomerulonephritis), albumin and globulins, which under normal circumstances are restricted from the glomerular ultrafiltrate because of their ionic charge and size, are lost into the urine. Protein losses of 10 g or more per day are not uncommon. *Tubular proteinuria* occurs in patients with normal glomeruli when the smaller proteins that are normally filtered at the glomerulus and then reabsorbed in the tubule appear in the urine because of tubular or interstitial abnormality. This occurs in disorders such as urinary tract obstruction, sickle cell disease, and other causes of acute or chronic interstitial nephritis. In these disorders, daily urinary protein losses rarely exceed 2 g. The term *overflow proteinuria* refers to the urinary loss of small proteins that are present in the blood in excessive concentrations and appear in the glomerular filtrate in amounts exceeding the normal tubular reabsorptive capacity (e.g., the light chains produced in multiple myeloma).

Miscellaneous causes of transient proteinuria include exertion, stress, or fever; excretion of up to 300 mg protein/day can occur during an otherwise normal pregnancy.[2] *Orthostatic proteinuria* is characterized by the occurrence of proteinuria during periods when the patient is upright but not during recumbency; the condition is usually transient and benign. However, persistent proteinuria is a marker for renal disease even in the absence of azotemia or an abnormal urine sediment.

Excretion of more than 2 g of protein in 24 hours is likely to be caused by a glomerular process, whereas excretion of less than 2 g is typical of tubular overflow, or orthostatic proteinuria. In the nephrotic syndrome protein losses exceed the liver's capacity to synthesize albumin and result in hypoalbuminemia. This leads to decreased plasma-oncotic pressure and accumulation of edema fluid in the extravascular interstitial space. Increased aldosterone secretion and further retention of salt and water ensue. Thus, edema is the clinical hallmark of the nephrotic syndrome and is often the initial complaint of patients who have significant proteinuria. Edema ranges in severity from mild dependent peripheral edema or periorbital swelling to frank anasarca with pleural effusions and ascites. Nephrotic-range proteinuria is defined arbitrarily as being greater than 3.5 g/24 hr.

Patients with the nephrotic syndrome are at increased risk for thromboembolic events, including deep venous thrombosis of the lower extremity, renal vein thrombosis, and pulmonary embolism. The reason for this propensity appears to be a hypercoagulable state that may be related in part to urinary loss and decreased plasma levels of antithrombin III, proteins, and fibrinolytic factors.[17] Hyperlipidemia is another typical feature of the nephrotic syndrome; the mechanism is thought to be related indirectly to hypoalbuminemia and decreased oncotic pressure or viscosity. However, the major clinical significance of the nephrotic syndrome is that it indicates the presence of an underlying renal process or systemic disease affecting the glomerulus (Box 92-3).

Clinical Features Evaluation of the patient with proteinuria focuses not only on gauging the severity of proteinuria and the likelihood of complications but on identifying any associated signs of underlying renal disease or systemic illness. One should seek to elicit a history of recent illnesses (including pharyngitis), use of medications or drugs, or a past history of proteinuria, hypertension, edema, or renal disease. In young female patients, the possibility of pregnancy should be kept in mind because pregnancy can exacerbate previously inapparent renal disease; in late pregnancy, proteinuria may be the first sign of preeclampsia. Clues to the presence of systemic diseases that commonly affect the kidneys (e.g., diabetes or collagen vascular disease) should be sought as well. On physical examination the emergency physician should evaluate the blood pressure, note the presence or absence of edema, and assess for signs of systemic disease or renal insufficiency.

Laboratory The laboratory evaluation of the patient with proteinuria should include urinalysis and measurement of the BUN and serum creatinine. Special attention should be given to detecting lipiduria in the form of oval fat bodies (desquamated fat-laden renal epithelial cells), fatty casts, or free fat droplets. The identification of lipiduria is made easier by the characteristic appearance of lipid droplets when viewed under the polarizing microscope ("Maltese crosses") (Figure 92-1, *E*).

Although the finding of isolated proteinuria may or may not be clinically important, proteinuria is almost always significant when it occurs in combination with hematuria. RBCs and red-cell casts suggest glomerulonephritis; proteinuria with pyuria may be seen with acute interstitial nephritis. The combination of proteinuria and glycosuria suggests diabetic nephropathy. A 24-hour urine collection should be ordered to provide an accurate measure of GFR and to quantitate protein excretion.

Abnormal findings on the history, physical examination, or laboratory evaluation greatly increase the probability of the presence of significant renal disease and mandate early referral to an internist or nephrologist. However, in the absence of edema, azotemia, hypertension, active urine sediment, or known systemic illness affecting the kidney, patients with proteinuria may be referred to their primary care provider for follow-up observation. Because transient, mild proteinuria is not uncommon in healthy individuals, patients with mild proteinuria indicated by dipstick (particularly if the urine is concentrated) should always have dipstick testing repeated at follow-up observation before further evaluation is undertaken. Persistent proteinuria may require referral to a nephrologist; in some cases renal biopsy is necessary to establish a diagnosis and guide management.

Box 92-3 Causes of the Nephrotic Syndrome

Primary Renal Disease

Multisystem Disease
- Diabetes mellitus
- Collagen vascular disease
- Systemic lupus erythematosus
- Rheumatoid arthritis
- Henoch-Schönlein purpura
- Polyarteritis nodosa
- Wegener's granulomatosis
- Amyloidosis
- Cryoglobulinemia

Drugs and Toxins
- Heroin
- Captopril
- Heavy metals
- Nonsteroidal antiinflammatory drugs
- Penicillamine
- Others

Allergens

Infection
- Bacterial
- Infective endocarditis
- Poststreptococcal
- Syphilis
- Viral
- Hepatitis B
- Human immunodeficiency virus
- Cytomegalovirus
- Protozoal
- Malaria
- Toxoplasmosis

Malignancy
- Solid tumors
- Multiple myeloma
- Lymphoma
- Leukemia

Miscellaneous
- Hereditary nephritis
- Preeclampsia
- Malignant hypertension
- Reflux nephropathy
- Transplant rejection

ACUTE RENAL FAILURE

Perspective

ARF is a generic term used to describe a precipitous decline in kidney function. Its hallmark is progressive azotemia caused by the accumulation of nitrogenous end-products of metabolism, but this is commonly accompanied by a wide range of other disturbances depending on the severity and duration of renal dysfunction. These include metabolic derangements (e.g., metabolic acidosis and hyperkalemia), disturbances of body fluid balance (particularly volume overload), and a variety of effects on almost every organ system (Box 92-4)

The causes of ARF may be divided into those that decrease renal blood flow (prerenal), produce a renal parenchymal insult (intrarenal), or obstruct urine flow (obstructive or postrenal ARF). Identification of either a prerenal or a postrenal cause of ARF generally makes the prompt initiation of specific corrective therapy possible; if these two broad categories of ARF can be excluded, an intrarenal cause is implicated. The renal parenchymal causes of ARF can be usefully subdivided into those primarily affecting the glomeruli, the intrarenal vasculature, or the renal interstitium.[18] The term *ATN* denotes another broad category of intrinsic renal failure that cannot be attributed to specific glomerular, vascular, or interstitial causes (Figure 92-2).[18]

Box 92-4 Clinical Features of Acute Renal Failure

Cardiovascular
- Pulmonary edema
- Arrhythmia
- Hypertension
- Pericarditis
- Pericardial effusion
- Myocardial infarction
- Pulmonary embolism

Metabolic
- Hyponatremia
- Hyperkalemia
- Acidosis
- Hypocalcemia
- Hyperphosphatemia
- Hypermagnesemia
- Hyperuricemia

Neurologic
- Asterixis
- Neuromuscular irritability
- Mental status changes
- Somnolence
- Coma
- Seizures

Gastrointestinal
- Nausea
- Vomiting
- Gastritis
- Gastroduodenal ulcers
- Gastrointestinal bleeding
- Pancreatitis
- Malnutrition

Hematologic
- Anemia
- Hemorrhagic diathesis

Infectious
- Pneumonia
- Septicemia
- Urinary tract infection
- Wound infection

From Brady HR, Brenner BM, Clarkson MR, Lieberthal W: Acute renal failure. In Brenner BM: *The kidney,* ed 6, Philadelphia, 2000, WB Saunders.

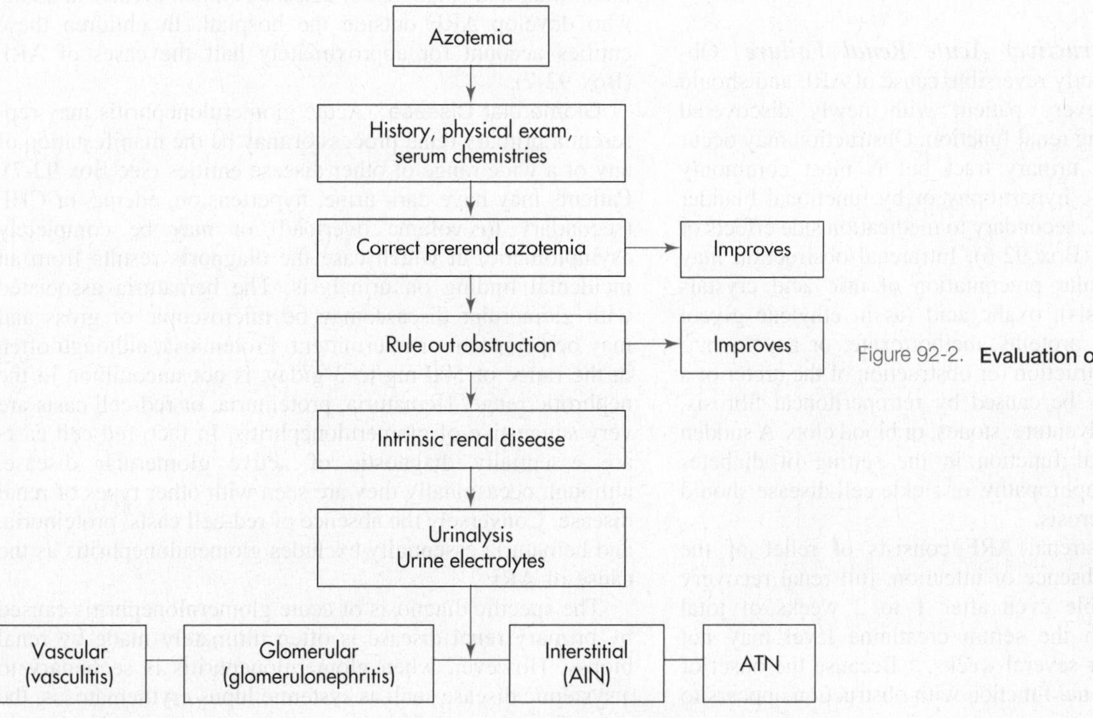

Figure 92-2. **Evaluation of azotemia.**

Principles of Disease

Prerenal Azotemia Decreased renal perfusion that is sufficient to cause a decrease in the GFR results in azotemia. The possible causes can be grouped into entities causing intravascular volume depletion, volume redistribution, or decreased cardiac output (Box 92-5). Individuals who have preexisting renal disease are particularly sensitive to the effects of diminished renal perfusion.

Prerenal azotemia is characterized by increased urine specific gravity, BUN/Cr ratio greater than 10:1, UNa concentration less than 20 mEq/dl, and FENa less than 1%. The condition can generally be corrected readily by expanding extracellular fluid volume, augmenting cardiac output, or discontinuing vasodilating antihypertensive drugs. However, severe prolonged prerenal azotemia can eventuate in ATN.

Patients who have congestive heart failure (CHF) or cirrhosis form an important subset of those with prerenal azotemia. These individuals are often salt-overloaded and water-overloaded, yet their effective intraarterial volume is decreased. Administration of diuretics has the potential to decrease intravascular volume further, resulting in decreased glomerular filtration and prerenal azotemia. For some patients with advanced CHF or hepatic disease, a state of chronic stable prerenal azotemia may be the best achievable compromise between symptomatic volume overload and severe renal hypoperfusion.

Glomerular perfusion may also be decreased in patients with normal intravascular volume and normal renal blood flow who take angiotensin-converting enzyme inhibitors or, more commonly, prostaglandin inhibitors. All nonsteroidal antiinflammatory drugs (NSAIDs), including aspirin, inhibit prostaglandin synthesis. Renal vasodilator prostaglandins are critical in maintaining glomerular perfusion in patients with conditions such as CHF, chronic renal insufficiency, and cirrhosis, in which elevated circulating levels of renin and angiotensin II act to diminish renal blood flow and GFR. In

Box 92-5 Causes of Prerenal Azotemia

Volume Loss
- Gastrointestinal: vomiting, diarrhea, nasogastric drainage
- Renal: diuresis
- Blood loss
- Insensible losses
- Third space sequestration
- Pancreatitis
- Peritonitis
- Trauma
- Burns

Cardiac
- Myocardial infarction
- Valvular disease
- Cardiomyopathy
- Decreased effective arterial volume
- Antihypertensive medication
- Nitrates

Neurogenic
- Sepsis
- Anaphylaxis
- Hypoalbuminemia
- Nephrotic syndrome
- Liver disease

Box 92-6 Causes of Postrenal Acute Renal Failure

Intrarenal and Ureteral
- Kidney stone
- Sloughed papilla
- Malignancy
- Retroperitoneal fibrosis
- Uric acid or oxalic acid, sulfonamide triamterene, or indinavin crystal precipitation
- Methotrexate or acyclovir precipitation[20]

Bladder
- Kidney stone
- Blood clot
- Prostatic hypertrophy
- Bladder carcinoma
- Neurogenic bladder

Urethra
- Phimosis
- Stricture

this setting, decreased production of vasodilator prostaglandins may result in acute intrarenal hemodynamic changes and a reversible decrease in renal function.[19] Other risk factors include advanced age, diuretic use, renovascular disease, and diabetes. This entity is distinct from other renal complications of NSAIDs, including interstitial nephritis and papillary necrosis.

Renal insufficiency secondary to NSAIDs is generally reversible after cessation of the causative agent. For patients who are at increased risk but require treatment with NSAIDs, a short-acting preparation should be prescribed and follow-up monitoring of renal function and serum potassium level should be undertaken in days, rather than weeks. If renal function is unchanged after a short course of treatment, adverse effects from continuing therapy are unlikely, although other potential mechanisms for the production of renal dysfunction (e.g., interstitial nephritis) should be kept in mind.

Postrenal (Obstructive) Acute Renal Failure Obstruction is an eminently reversible cause of ARF and should be considered in every patient with newly discovered azotemia or worsening renal function. Obstruction may occur at any level of the urinary tract but is most commonly produced by prostatic hypertrophy or by functional bladder neck obstruction (e.g., secondary to medication side effects or neurogenic bladder) (Box 92-6). Intrarenal obstruction may result from intratubular precipitation of uric acid crystals (e.g., with tumor lysis), oxalic acid (as in ethylene glycol ingestion), myeloma proteins, methotrexate, or acyclovir.[20] Bilateral ureteral obstruction (or obstruction of the ureter of a solitary kidney) may be caused by retroperitoneal fibrosis, tumor, surgical misadventure, stones, or blood clots. A sudden deterioration of renal function in the setting of diabetes mellitus, analgesic nephropathy, or sickle cell disease should suggest papillary necrosis.

Treatment of postrenal ARF consists of relief of the obstruction. In the absence of infection, full renal recovery is said to be possible even after 1 to 2 weeks of total obstruction, although the serum creatinine level may not return to baseline for several weeks.[21] Because the onset of irreversible loss of renal function with obstruction appears to be gradual, a few days' delay in diagnosis generally is considered acceptable. Still, common sense dictates that obstructions should be detected and relieved as expeditiously as possible.

Intrinsic Acute Renal Failure Of the specific intrarenal disorders that cause ARF, glomerulonephritis, interstitial nephritis, and abnormalities of the intrarenal vasculature are amenable to specific therapy and thus should be carefully considered as possible causes. However, these entities are responsible for only 5% to 10% of cases of ARF in adult inpatients; most are due to ATN. The incidence of glomerular, interstitial, and small vessel disease is much greater in adults who develop ARF outside the hospital. In children these entities account for approximately half the cases of ARF (Box 92-7).

Glomerular Disease Acute glomerulonephritis may represent a primary renal process or may be the manifestation of any of a wide range of other disease entities (see Box 92-7). Patients may have dark urine, hypertension, edema, or CHF (secondary to volume overload) or may be completely asymptomatic, in which case the diagnosis results from an incidental finding on urinalysis. The hematuria associated with glomerular disease may be microscopic or gross and may be persistent or intermittent. Proteinuria, although often in the range of 500 mg to 3 g/day, is not uncommon in the nephrotic range. Hematuria, proteinuria, or red-cell casts are very suggestive of glomerulonephritis. In fact, red-cell casts are essentially diagnostic of active glomerular disease, although occasionally they are seen with other types of renal disease. Conversely the absence of red-cell casts, proteinuria, and hematuria essentially excludes glomerulonephritis as the cause of ARF.

The specific diagnosis of acute glomerulonephritis caused by primary renal disease is often ultimately made by renal biopsy. However, when glomerulonephritis is secondary to a systemic disease such as systemic lupus erythematosus, the

Box 92-7 Intrinsic Renal Diseases that Cause ARF

Vascular
Large vessel
- Renal artery thrombosis or stenosis
- Renal vein thrombosis
- Atheroembolic disease

Small and medium vessel
- Scleroderma
- Malignant hypertension
- Hemolytic uremic syndrome
- Thrombotic thrombocytopenic purpura

Glomerular
Systemic diseases
- Systemic lupus erythematosus
- Infective endocarditis
- Systemic vasculitis (eg, periarteritis nodosum, Wegener's granulomatosis)
- Henoch-Schönlein purpura
- Essential mixed cryoglobulinemia
- Goodpasture's syndrome

Primary renal disease
- Poststreptococcal glomerulonephritis
- Other postinfectious glomerulonephritis
- Rapidly progressive glomerulonephritis

Tubulointerstitial
Drugs (many)
Toxins (eg, heavy metals, ethylene glycol)
Infections
Multiple myeloma

Acute Tubular Necrosis
Ischemia
- Shock
- Sepsis
- Severe prerenal azotemia

Nephrotoxins
- Antibiotics
- Radiographic contrast agents
- Myoglobinuria
- Hemoglobinuria

Other
Severe liver disease[22]
Allergic reactions
NSAIDs[23]

patient's clinical signs and symptoms, in combination with the results of laboratory assessment, aid considerably in narrowing the differential diagnosis. As a rule, extensive laboratory testing to identify the cause of acute glomerulonephritis is not indicated in the ED and is more appropriately performed as part of an inpatient evaluation.

Interstitial Disease AIN is most commonly precipitated by drug exposure or by infection. Drug-induced AIN is poorly understood, but the absence of a clear relationship to the dose and the recurrence of the syndrome on rechallenge with the offending agent suggest that an immunologic mechanism is responsible. The most commonly incriminated drugs are the penicillins, diuretics, anticoagulants, and NSAIDs. AIN has been reported in association with bacterial, fungal, protozoan, and rickettsial infections.

Patients with AIN classically have rash, fever, eosinophilia, and eosinophiluria; but it is common for one or more of these cardinal signs to be absent. Pyuria, gross or microscopic hematuria, and mild proteinuria are observed in some cases. A definite diagnosis sometimes can be made only on renal biopsy. Treatment of AIN is directed at removing the presumed cause; infections should be treated and offending drugs discontinued. Renal function generally returns to baseline over several weeks, although chronic renal failure has been reported to occur.

Intrarenal Vascular Disease Vascular disease of the kidney can be classified according to the size of the vessel that is affected. Disorders such as renal arterial thrombosis or embolism, which affect large blood vessels, must be bilateral (or must affect a single functioning kidney) to produce ARF. Whether to attribute such cases of ARF to prerenal or intrarenal vascular causes is a matter of semantics. The most common cause of thrombosis is probably trauma; thrombosis may also occur after angiography or may be secondary to aortic or renal arterial dissection. Renal atheroembolism is thought to occur commonly—at least on a microscopic level—after arteriography, but is an uncommon cause of ARF. Similarly, patients with chronic atrial fibrillation or infective endocarditis may throw emboli to the kidney; but rarely suffer ARF as a result. Renal arterial embolism can cause acute renal infarction, generally manifested by sudden flank, back, chest, or upper abdominal pain. Urinary findings, including hematuria, are variable. Fever, nausea, and vomiting are not uncommon; in some cases, evidence of embolization to other vessels provides a useful clue. The diagnosis is usually made by renal flow scanning or arteriography. Surgical embolectomy has been reported to restore function when undertaken within several hours of occlusion, but significant return of function has been documented in patients operated on as long as 6 weeks after total occlusion. This is presumably because they develop collateral circulation in association with a preexisting partial occlusion.[24]

An interesting but relatively uncommon type of ARF occurs when an angiotensin-converting enzyme inhibitor is given to a patient with underlying bilateral renal artery stenosis (or unilateral stenosis in a solitary functioning kidney). With inhibition of angiotensin synthesis, efferent arteriolar tone is not maintained and GFR decreases. The condition is reversible with cessation of therapy.

Several diseases that affect the smaller intrarenal vessels can cause ARF (see Box 92-7). Patients whose disease is severe enough to cause ARF are also generally found to have hypertension, microangiopathic hemolytic anemia, and other systemic and organ-specific manifestations.

In recent years, infection with *Escherichia coli* 0157:H7 has emerged as a major cause of hemolytic uremic syndrome, an important cause of ARF in children.[25]

Malignant hypertension, although much less common since the advent of more effective antihypertensive therapy, has by no means disappeared. Patients with scleroderma (systemic sclerosis) may have "scleroderma renal crisis," characterized by malignant hypertension and rapidly progressive renal failure. Whereas vasculitis associated with glomerular capillary inflammation typically causes gross or microscopic hematuria and formation of red-cell casts, vascular involvement of the medium-size vessels, such as that produced by scleroderma, often spares the preglomerular vessels and tends not to produce an active urine sediment. Extrarenal manifestations (rash, fever, arthritis, pulmonary symptoms) are usually evident.

For both malignant hypertension and scleroderma renal crisis, appropriate treatment can produce a gratifying remission of ARF. Patients with malignant hypertension have been reported to recover renal function after aggressive antihypertensive therapy, with temporary maintenance on dialysis if necessary.[26] For individuals who have scleroderma renal crisis, specific therapy with angiotensin-converting enzyme inhibitors has been shown to result in improvement in renal function in a significant proportion of patients.[27]

Acute Tubular Necrosis The term *ATN* refers to a generally reversible deterioration of kidney function associated with a variety of renal insults. Oliguria may or may not be a feature. The diagnosis is made after prerenal and postrenal causes of ARF and disorders of glomeruli, interstitium, and intrarenal vasculature have been excluded. These discrete categories do overlap in a few disorders. For example, ARF associated with multiple myeloma or ethylene glycol toxicity is associated with both intrarenal obstruction and interstitial disease, as well as a probable direct toxic effect on the renal tubule itself.

The most common precipitant of ATN is renal ischemia during surgery or after trauma. The remainder of cases occur in the setting of medical illness, most commonly as a result of the administration of nephrotoxic aminoglycoside antibiotics or radiocontrast agents or in association with rhabdomyolysis. Multiple causes can be identified in some cases; in others a definitive cause is never established.

Several competing theories have been put forward to explain the pathophysiology of ATN.[28] One proposes that casts and cellular debris physically obstruct the tubular lumen, which leads to an increase in intratubular pressure and a consequent decrease in net glomerular filtration pressure. Another theory holds that damage to the renal tubular epithelium allows back-leak of glomerular filtrate into the peritubular capillaries. Other investigators suggest a primarily vascular mechanism for renal failure in which afferent arteriolar vasoconstriction or efferent arteriolar vasodilation is sufficient to decrease glomerular filtration. Yet another view emphasizes the importance of changes in glomerular capillary permeability.

Decreased renal perfusion results in a continuum of renal dysfunction that ranges from transient prerenal azotemia at one extreme to ATN at the other. Early during the period of renal ischemia, renal function can be restored completely by restoring renal blood flow, but at some point, continued hypoperfusion results in renal dysfunction unresponsive to volume repletion and ATN supervenes. ATN may occur in the absence of frank hypotension; even modest renal ischemia may result in ATN in susceptible individuals. Individual susceptibility to ATN may be related to the balance of prostaglandin-mediated vasopressor and vasodilatory influences on the renal vasculature.

Postischemic ATN can occur in the setting of volume loss from the GI tract (upper or lower), skin, or kidneys or can result from severe hemorrhage. In one reported series, 75% of patients with major burns developed ATN.[29] Heatstroke is commonly associated with the development of ATN and is thought to result from a combination of volume loss, hyperpyrexia, and rhabdomyolysis. Another cause of ATN is hyperglycemic hyperosmolar nonketotic coma, which can be associated with loss of as much as 25% of total body water. ATN is also seen in the setting of cardiogenic shock, sepsis, and the "third spacing" of fluids in pancreatitis and peritonitis.

ATN is common in postoperative patients, although not all cases can be attributed to intraoperative hypotension or hemorrhage. Concomitant sepsis, increased age, elevated preoperative BUN and creatinine levels, and longer duration of aortic cross-clamping or cardiopulmonary bypass are associated with a worse prognosis.[30]

Box 92-8 Causes of Pigment-Induced Acute Renal Failure

Rhabdomyolysis and myoglobinuria	Alcoholism
Vigorous exercise	Hypokalemia
Arterial embolization	Hypophosphatemia
Status epilepticus	Hemoglobinuria
Status asthmaticus	Transfusion reactions
Coma-induced and pressure-induced myonecrosis	Snake envenomation
Heat stress	Malaria
Diabetic ketoacidosis	Mechanical destruction of RBCs by prosthetic valves
Myopathy	G6PD deficiency

RBC, Red blood cells.

Nephrotoxins are the other major cause of ATN. Among the most prominent of these are the endogenous pigments myoglobin and hemoglobin. Rhabdomyolysis and ARF resulting from crush injuries first received widespread attention after their description in survivors of the London blitz during World War II, but many other causes of pigment nephropathy have been reported (Box 92-8). Hypotension secondary to fluid loss into damaged muscle is thought to aggravate the effects of myoglobinuria on the renal tubule, as is acidosis. Hemolysis, resulting in the release of hemoglobin into the circulation and hemoglobinuria, can cause ATN but usually only in the presence of coexisting dehydration, acidosis, or other causes of decreased renal perfusion. ATN may be produced by the hemolysis of as little as 100 ml of blood.

ATN associated with rhabdomyolysis is often oliguric; it is characterized by rapid increases in the serum creatinine, potassium, phosphorus, and uric acid levels. Creatine released from muscle is metabolized to creatinine, which may result in serum creatinine increase of more than 2 mg/dl/day, in contrast to the increase of 0.5 to 1.0 mg/dl/day typically seen in other forms of ARF.[31] The BUN/Cr ratio is often less than 10:1. Intracellular potassium released from damaged muscle may raise the serum potassium by 1 to 2 mEq/L in several hours.[30] Likewise, phosphate released from muscle may cause dramatic increases in the serum phosphate level. Uric acid, produced by metabolism of purines released from damaged muscle, may accumulate to levels high enough to suggest acute uric acid nephropathy.

The urine dipstick yields a positive result for heme in only 50% of patients with rhabdomyolysis because myoglobin is rapidly cleared from the serum and therefore may be undetectable in the urine at the time of presentation. Thus, a negative urine dipstick result does not rule out the diagnosis. Serum creatine phosphokinase (CPK) is cleared much more slowly and is therefore a much more sensitive test.

No biochemical parameter can be used to predict which patients who have rhabdomyolysis will develop ARF. In one series of patients in whom alcoholism, muscle compression, and seizures were the most common causes of rhabdomyolysis, ARF developed in only one third. Neither the height of the serum CPK elevation, the presence or absence of myoglobinuria, nor the degree of hyperkalemia correlated well with the development of ARF.[32]

Antibiotics and radiographic contrast agents are other nephrotoxins that are commonly implicated in the development of ATN. The common use of aminoglycosides in the treatment of gram-negative infections has made these antibiotics one of the most common causes of ARF; creatinine elevations are seen in 10% to 20% of patients treated with gentamicin, depending on the population studied and the degree of elevation considered significant. Dose and duration of aminoglycoside therapy are the most important factors associated with nephrotoxicity. Higher doses and longer duration of therapy are associated with higher serum drug levels, leading to greater accumulation of drug in the renal parenchyma. Nephrotoxicity is also correlated with increased age, impaired renal function, dehydration, and exposure to other nephrotoxins. Once-daily administration of a somewhat higher dose is associated with less nephrotoxicity but equal effectiveness.[33,34]

Aminoglycoside-induced ATN typically has a gradual onset. Clinically significant renal dysfunction usually occurs only after several days and often after more than a week of therapy. However, renal failure can develop as long as 10 days after a drug has been discontinued, an observation that appears to be explained by the prolonged tissue half-life characteristic of these agents. Renal function returns to normal after an average of 6 weeks, but it occasionally progresses to permanent renal injury.[35]

Radiographic contrast agents are a common cause of hospital-acquired renal insufficiency. Renal failure produced by these agents may be defined as an increase in serum creatinine level of 50% over baseline with a temporal relation to contrast medium administration and in the absence of other identifiable causes. ATN can occur after any procedure involving contrast, whether by the intravenous or the oral route, but the highest incidence is after arteriography.[36]

Contrast-induced ATN encompasses a spectrum ranging from asymptomatic nonoliguric renal insufficiency to severe renal failure requiring dialysis, but most cases are mild. Typically an increase in the serum creatinine level is noted within 3 days of exposure, with a return to normal within 10 to 14 days.

The most important risk factors for contrast-induced ATN are preexisting renal insufficiency, diabetes mellitus, multiple myeloma, age greater than 60 years, volume depletion, and higher doses of contrast material. Of these, preexisting renal insufficiency is the most important.[37] Significant increases in serum creatinine level are seen in approximately one third of patients who have a baseline serum creatinine level greater than 2.5 mg/dl, but in only 2% of patients who have a normal baseline creatinine level.[38] Similarly, diabetic patients with a serum creatinine level less than 1.5 mg/dl are at low risk for the development of contrast-induced ATN, whereas those whose serum creatinine is greater than 1.5 mg/dl are at significant risk.[39] Multiple myeloma, particularly when dehydration is present, is another reasonably well-documented risk factor. Advanced age also appears to make ATN more likely, possibly because of decreased renal mass and cortical blood flow. The importance of volume depletion as an independent risk factor is controversial; some investigators have shown a protective effect of aggressive volume expansion before contrast exposure.[40] Finally, large doses and repeated doses of contrast are associated with increased risk of ATN, particularly if two studies are performed within 72 hours of one another. In one series, significant changes in the serum creatinine level were twice as likely to develop in patients who received 2 ml/kg or more of contrast material as in patients who received less than 2 ml/kg.[41] The recently introduced low-osmolality contrast media may carry a somewhat lower risk of nephrotoxicity than standard high-osmolality agents.[42]

Clinical Features

Once the presence of azotemia or renal failure has been discovered, the emergency physician should always first consider potentially life-threatening complications (e.g., hyperkalemia and pulmonary edema). Assuming these have been satisfactorily ruled out, the next step is to determine whether the condition represents ARF or is the result of preexisting renal disease. The clinical distinction between ARF and chronic renal failure (CRF) is often difficult; old records and laboratory results are invaluable. The finding of small kidneys on abdominal radiography or of the bony changes of secondary hyperparathyroidism on hand films suggests that renal failure is chronic. Anemia, hypocalcemia, and hyperphosphatemia, on the other hand, should not be relied on to identify patients who have CRF because these abnormalities can develop rapidly in ARF.

In evaluating the patient with azotemia, the history, physical examination, and laboratory studies should seek clues to the cause and identify signs and symptoms of uremia, volume overload, or other complications of renal failure. In attempting to identify the cause of azotemia, the general strategy is to rule out both prerenal and postrenal causes before considering the many intrinsic renal causes. First, potential sources of volume loss and causes of decreased cardiac output should be sought in the history, and the patient should be questioned about light-headedness, bleeding, GI fluid loss, abnormal polyuria, or symptoms of CHF. In men, a history of nocturia, frequency, hesitancy, or decrement of urinary stream suggests prostatic obstruction. A history of lower tract symptoms or of abdominal or pelvic tumor in either sex should likewise be elicited, as should a history of kidney stones or chronic UTI. A documented history of acute anuria (defined as the production of less than 100 ml urine/day) is most often the result of high-grade urinary tract obstruction, although it may also accompany severe volume depletion, severe acute glomerulonephritis, cortical necrosis, or bilateral vascular occlusion. Intermittent anuria, on the other hand, is characteristic of obstructive disease.

The patient should be questioned about medication use and possible exposure to radiographic contrast agents or other exogenous toxins. A history of pharyngitis, hypertension, dark-colored urine, rash, fever, or arthritis suggests intrinsic renal disease or a multisystem disorder. In older patients, symptoms that suggest multiple myeloma should be elicited.

The physical examination should focus on signs of volume depletion such as orthostatic hypotension, tachycardia, and decreased skin turgor; documented short-term changes in body weight offer a valuable clue in assessing volume status, particularly in chronically ill patients. In addition, suspected bleeding should be specifically excluded. Similarly, volume overload should be sought by assessment of jugular venous distention and attention to the presence of rales, an S_3 gallop, or edema. An attempt to percuss the bladder should be made. A distended bladder is percussible when it contains 150 ml of urine, and the dome is palpable abdominally when it contains 500 ml.[2] Prostate examination in adult men or pelvic examination in adult women should not be neglected. Rash, purpura, pallor, or petechiae should be noted, as should arthritis, musculoskeletal tenderness, or findings suggestive of infection or malignancy.

Diagnostic Strategy

Laboratory The laboratory evaluation should begin with a careful dipstick and microscopic urinalysis and measurement of urine output. BUN, serum creatinine, UNa, and FENa levels should be determined to help evaluate renal function and to provide clues as to the cause of ARF. A complete blood count; serum electrolyte calcium, phosphorus, and magnesium levels; electrocardiogram (ECG); and chest roentgenography should be ordered to establish the patient's baseline status and to provide information about possible complications. Other studies may be of value in the ED when the history or physical findings suggest a specific role in immediate diagnosis or management.

Prerenal azotemia should be suspected in the setting of volume loss, volume redistribution, or decreased effective renal perfusion. It is typically associated with a normal urinalysis, high BUN/Cr ratio, increased urine osmolality, UNa concentration less than 20 mEq/L, and FENa less than 1%. A rapid response to volume repletion is also characteristic.

Urethral or bladder neck obstruction is documented by the finding of significant amounts of residual urine in the bladder on catheterization after the patient has voided or attempted to void spontaneously. It should be emphasized that the ability to void does not rule out obstruction. In fact, the urine volume in the presence of obstruction may vary from zero to several liters per day. Flank pain is likewise an insensitive marker for obstruction. Urine indices and the BUN/Cr ratio tend not to be helpful, although an increase in the latter is common in obstruction. The presence of a renal parenchymal disorder can often be diagnosed by its manifestations on microscopic urinalysis or by associated extrarenal manifestations (e.g., with multisystem disease) or the clinical setting (e.g., recent exposure to a new medication). In the absence of these clues, the failure to find evidence for prerenal or postrenal causes in a patient with ARF may also be taken as presumptive evidence of an intrarenal parenchymal process. Among these, the emergency physician should keep in mind the possibility of an acute or ongoing vascular insult because, in this case, timely intervention may be critical in preserving ultimate renal function.

Radiography/Ultrasonography Significant hydronephrosis is usually readily demonstrable by ultrasonography and may indicate either upper or lower tract obstruction. In questionable cases, or if bilateral ureteral obstruction is strongly suspected clinically, the next step is retrograde urography performed by a urologist.[43] IVP is less useful in this setting; in fact, IV contrast material may compound the injury to the kidney.

Management

ED management of ARF is directed to reversing decreases in GFR and urine output (if possible) while minimizing further hemodynamic and toxic insults, maintaining normal fluid and electrolyte balance, and managing other complications of ARF as required. Because renal failure alters the metabolism and action of many drugs, often in ways that are not predictable, the physician must exercise care when prescribing all medications. A compendium of guidelines for drug dosing in renal failure, such as the one by Bennett et al,[44] is of great help for this purpose.

After ensuring that the vital signs are adequate and that the patient is in no immediate danger from volume or metabolic derangements, the next step is to correct prerenal and postrenal factors, if any exist. Intravascular volume should be repleted in hypovolemic patients and maintained in euvolemic patients by matching input to measured and insensible output. Inadequate cardiac output should be augmented when possible. Postrenal or obstructive ARF is treated by restoration of normal urine outflow. Bladder outlet obstruction may be relieved by passage of a Foley catheter, whereas upper tract obstruction may require percutaneous nephrostomy.

When prerenal and postrenal factors have been ruled out, the challenge to the emergency physician is to identify the cause of intrinsic renal ARF, keeping in mind the multitude of known possible causes (see Box 92-7). The clinical setting and physical and laboratory findings often allow the differential diagnosis to be considerably narrowed. The clinical picture is often most consistent with the broad category of ATN.

It has been noted repeatedly that patients who have oliguric ARF have a significantly higher mortality rate and a much greater risk of complications than those who are not oliguric. For example, recovery from oliguric ATN occurs after an average of 15 to 25 days versus 5 to 10 days for nonoliguric ATN. The difference in prognosis may simply reflect a more severe renal insult in patients who are oliguric, and no controlled prospective human studies have been performed to determine whether interventions aimed at converting oliguric to nonoliguric ARF have an effect on renal function or mortality. Nevertheless, because nonoliguric patients are easier to manage, an attempt to increase urine flow is warranted.

Loop diuretics or mannitol are often effective in increasing urine flow once intravascular volume deficits are corrected.[45] The use of furosemide has been shown to decrease dialysis requirements and complications caused by volume overload, although it has not been shown to shorten the clinical course or affect mortality.[46]

Mannitol appears to be most useful when given at the time of or shortly after the renal insult; the recommended dose is 12.5 to 25 g IV. If urine output does not increase, further doses may cause hyperosmolality and clinically significant intravascular volume overload in patients with impaired renal function.[45]

Dopamine (1 to 3 μg/kg/min) has also been used, with and without furosemide, in an effort to increase urine output, but its efficacy has not been validated in prospective studies.[47,48]

Certain specific considerations apply to toxin-induced ATN. Pigment-induced ATN may be prevented by avoidance of hemolysis and muscle injury and by correction of those factors (e.g., dehydration, acidosis) that are known to predispose patients with pigmenturia to the development of renal failure. Once hemolysis or rhabdomyolysis has occurred, treatment is directed at eliminating the cause and preventing the development of renal failure.

Mannitol has been shown to prevent ARF in experimental models of myoglobinuria, presumably by inducing osmotic diuresis and decreasing intratubular deposition of pigment. Furosemide, on the other hand, has not consistently shown a beneficial effect. Other studies have suggested that myoglobin precipitates in an acid urine but not in an alkaline urine. Thus, aggressive volume repletion, alkalinization, and mannitol infusion have been recommended after crush injuries to reduce the likelihood or severity of ARF.[49] This regimen also helps control hyperkalemia.[50] Once ARF has occurred, management is similar to that of other forms of ARF, but early dialysis may be required to control rapidly developing hyperkalemia, hyperphosphatemia, and hyperuricemia.

Patients who have contrast-induced ATN require only supportive therapy but should be hospitalized and seen by a nephrologist. A more significant role for the emergency physician is in preventing the occurrence of contrast-induced ATN, particularly by recognizing risk factors in patients for whom contrast studies are being considered. BUN and serum creatinine levels should be checked before contrast exposure in patients with risk factors. Moreover, before contrast medium is administered to a high-risk patient, it should be established that there is a compelling reason to perform the contrast study and that there is no adequate alternative to using a contrast agent. The patient should be volume replete before the study, the administered dose of contrast should be kept as low as possible, and multiple studies should be avoided as should concomitant use of other nephrotoxins. IV saline, given before and after contrast administration, may be protective.[40]

Volume and Metabolic Complications In addition to these general measures aimed at minimizing decreases in GFR and increasing urine output, a critical component of the management of ARF is the prevention or control of systemic complications. Particularly important are metabolic derangements (e.g., hyperkalemia, hypocalcemia, hyperphosphatemia, and metabolic acidosis) and complications of volume overload (e.g., hypertension and CHF).

Hyperkalemia, the most common metabolic cause of death in patients with ARF, results from an inability to excrete endogenous and exogenous potassium loads. In oliguric patients the serum potassium level typically increases by 0.3 to 0.5 mEq/L/day, but greater increases occur in catabolic, septic, or traumatized patients and in the face of acidosis or exogenous potassium loads from diet or medication.

Hyperkalemia results in serious disturbances in cardiac electrophysiology that may culminate in cardiac arrest. Although some hyperkalemic patients note muscular weakness, most are generally asymptomatic until major manifestations of cardiotoxicity supervene. Thus, hyperkalemia is particularly dangerous and must always be considered and sought out. ECG changes correlate only roughly with the serum potassium level. Mild hyperkalemia (K^+ <6.0 mEq/L) may be cautiously observed without specific treatment while all exogenous sources of potassium are eliminated. If the serum potassium level is greater than 6.5 mEq/L, and particularly if ECG changes are present, urgent intervention is necessary. When cardiotoxicity must be reversed immediately (e.g., when there is hemodynamic compromise), IV calcium (10 ml of 10% calcium gluconate or calcium chloride over 2 minutes) is the treatment of choice. IV insulin (given with glucose to prevent hypoglycemia) and IV bicarbonate temporarily shift potassium to the intracellular space. Bicarbonate should be used with particular caution in patients with renal failure because of its potential to cause volume overload and to provoke hypocalcemic tetany or seizures.[18] Recent reports have documented the safety and efficacy of inhaled albuterol in hyperkalemic patients with *chronic* renal failure; like insulin and bicarbonate, this agent causes potassium to move into cells, thereby controlling hyperkalemia for 2 hours or more.[51] Elimination of potassium from the body is promoted by using a potassium-binding ion exchange resin (sodium polystyrene sulfonate [Kayexalate]), by enhancing urinary potassium excretion, or by dialysis.

Hypocalcemia is a common feature of ARF and can develop rapidly after its onset. Vitamin D–dependent intestinal absorption of calcium is decreased in ARF because of decreased renal synthesis of 1,25-dihydroxyvitamin D. Another factor promoting hypocalcemia is the complexing of calcium with retained phosphate. Rhabdomyolysis-associated ARF in particular is often associated with the deposition of complexed calcium in muscle and other tissues.[52] Asymptomatic hypocalcemia requires no immediate treatment, but incipient or frank tetany should be treated with IV calcium (10 to 20 ml of 10% calcium gluconate over several minutes).

Hyperphosphatemia resulting from decreased renal elimination of phosphate is another common feature of ARF. The serum phosphorus level usually ranges from 6 to 8 mg/dl but may be much higher with rhabdomyolysis or in catabolic states. A calcium-phosphate product greater than 70 may result in metastatic soft tissue calcification. Hyperphosphatemia is often treated with oral calcium-based antacids that bind ingested phosphate in the gut.

Acids produced in normal metabolic processes accumulate in ARF and are buffered in part by serum bicarbonate, resulting in a decrease in the serum bicarbonate level and high-anion-gap metabolic acidosis. Compensatory hyperventilation may be mistakenly attributed to primary cardiac failure or volume overload. The metabolic acidosis associated with ARF is usually mild, and treatment is not generally necessary if the serum bicarbonate level is greater than 10 mEq/L. Overzealous correction may result in hypokalemia, hypocalcemia, or volume overload.

Hypermagnesemia complicates ARF when patients are given magnesium-containing antacids or laxatives.[53] Thus, these products should be avoided (e.g., for treatment of arrhythmia or wheezing) in the setting of ARF.

Hyperuricemia, resulting from decreased renal clearance, is typically in the range of 9 to 12 mg/dl but may be much higher in catabolic patients. For reasons that are unclear, gout rarely complicates ARF. A urinary uric acid/creatinine ratio in excess of 1 suggests that hyperuricemia is the *cause,* rather than the result, of ARF. In this case diuretics, alkalinization of the urine, and dialysis may be necessary.[54]

Disturbances of volume regulation can be expected to occur in most patients with ARF. Some nonoliguric patients excrete salt and water sufficiently well that intravascular volume depletion occurs if adequate fluid replacement is not provided. This prolongs recovery from ARF. Much more commonly, ARF is complicated by volume overload because sodium and water excretion may be inadequate to match even modest intakes. Volume overload is largely responsible for the hypertension often seen in ARF and commonly leads to CHF and pulmonary edema. Iatrogenic volume overload is particularly common and can be prevented only by careful attention to fluid intake and output using prudent estimates of insensible loss. Volume overload can be treated with diuretics or IV nitroglycerin while preparations are being made to initiate dialysis.

Organ System Effects The clinician should be alert to the numerous other important systemic and organ-specific effects of renal failure. Only the more prominent of these can be mentioned here.

Uremia impairs host defenses, particularly leukocyte function. Infection occurs in 30% to 70% of patients with ARF and is a significant cause of morbidity and mortality. Thus, patients with fever require prompt investigation and aggressive treatment.

Pericarditis, which has a prevalence of 12% to 20% in dialyzed patients with end-stage renal disease (ESRD), may also occur in patients with ARF. Chest pain that is worse in a recumbent position is the most common symptom, and most patients have a pericardial friction rub. Fever is common. The ECG may show ST-T wave elevation, low voltage, electrical alternans, or atrial fibrillation. The presence of pericardial effusion is identified most accurately by echocardiography, but tamponade, with typical clinical signs, occurs in some patients. In contrast to the situation in chronic renal failure, pericarditis or pericardial effusion in the setting of ARF is generally an indication for the urgent initiation of dialysis. Patients who have hemodynamically significant tamponade require surgical drainage of the effusion or, occasionally, emergency pericardiocentesis.

Neurologic abnormalities in ARF may be precipitated by electrolyte abnormalities, medications, or uremia. Common symptoms in uremic patients include lethargy, confusion, agitation, asterixis, myoclonus, and seizures.

Anorexia, nausea, vomiting, gastritis, and pancreatitis are also associated with ARF. Gastrointestinal hemorrhage is seen in 10% to 30% of patients; it results from a combination of stress and impaired hemostasis. Gastrointestinal hemorrhage is the second leading cause of death in ARF.

Impaired erythropoiesis, shortened RBC survival, hemolysis, hemodilution, and GI blood loss all play a role in the normocytic normochromic anemia that usually accompanies ARF. Although mild thrombocytopenia may be present, it is the qualitative defect in platelet function associated with ARF that is more significant and that contributes to these patients' bleeding tendencies. In patients with active bleeding or in whom an invasive procedure is being contemplated, the prolonged bleeding time can be corrected pharmacologically. Infusion of 10 U cryoprecipitate normalizes the bleeding time in 1 to 2 hours, with a return to baseline in 24 hours. Administration of 1-deamino-8-D-arginine vasopressin (DDAVP) shortens the bleeding time within 30 minutes.

Disposition

Patients who have new-onset ARF should be admitted to the hospital. If nephrology consultation and dialysis facilities are not available, transfer to another institution is advisable, provided volume and metabolic abnormalities are adequately controlled and the patient is hemodynamically stable.

Decisions regarding dialysis are generally made by the nephrology consultant and take into account many factors, including laboratory test result abnormalities and the presence or absence of symptoms of uremia (e.g., nausea, vomiting, and change in mental status). Many consultants choose to initiate dialysis when the BUN level exceeds 100 mg/dl or the serum creatinine level exceeds 10 mg/dl. Intractable volume overload and life-threatening hyperkalemia are the two most common indications for emergency dialysis.

CHRONIC RENAL FAILURE AND DIALYSIS

CHRONIC RENAL FAILURE

Perspective

The management of patients with chronic renal failure requires the emergency physician to consider different issues from those that are of most concern in patients with acute renal failure. The first and most obvious difference is in the pace of evolution of the patient's illness. An individual with acute renal failure has, by definition, a relatively rapidly evolving clinical course and thus is much more susceptible to the development of clinical manifestations requiring prompt attention. In contrast, a patient with chronic renal disease has most commonly experienced a slowly progressive course of decreasing renal function over months or years and is likely to have either slowly progressive symptoms or acute problems brought on by superimposed illness, trauma, or other physiologic stress. The most common problems requiring emergent intervention are severe hyperkalemia and symptomatic volume overload.

In addition, barring renal transplantation, chronic renal failure is an essentially irreversible condition generally characterized by a relentless decrease in renal function. Thus, whereas preservation of renal function may be a high priority in the patient with known acute renal failure, one does not as a rule need to be as concerned with efforts to reverse the process presumed to have caused chronic renal failure, nor even perhaps with efforts to delineate the exact cause. On occasion however, there may be a reversible component of renal failure that should be addressed. In some cases the underlying pathologic process affecting the kidneys may be arrested or treated; much more commonly, correctable extrarenal factors (e.g., volume depletion or urinary tract obstruction) may be identified.

Finally, in the patient with chronic renal failure who has an acute problem, the focus must be the identification and treatment of intercurrent illness that has caused clinical decompensation, with the goal of returning the patient to a chronically compensated stable status.

Principles of Disease

Pathologically, chronic renal failure is characterized by irreversible nephron loss and scarring. Chronic renal insufficiency denotes a condition in which GFR has been moderately reduced but not to a degree sufficient to cause clinical symptoms; in general, the GFR is reduced by no more than 75%. The term *end-stage renal disease* (ESRD) describes a condition in which renal function has diminished to a very low level and in which serious, life-threatening manifestations can be expected to occur without dialysis or transplantation. At this stage, the kidneys are often shrunken and diffusely scarred to such a degree that it may be impossible to make an etiologic diagnosis, even on pathologic examination.

The causes of chronic renal failure are numerous; their relative frequency primarily depends on the population studied. As with acute renal failure, they can be conveniently classified (Box 92-9) as prerenal (vascular), intrinsic renal (glomerular and tubulointerstitial), and postrenal (obstructive). Glomerular disease accounts for approximately one third to one half the cases of ESRD, of which diabetic nephropathy forms the largest group. Hypertensive nephrosclerosis is another important cause, particularly among African Americans, in whom it may be the cause of 25% or more of cases of ESRD. Among children and adolescents, reflux nephropathy is the most common cause of ESRD. Renal failure related to IV drug use or to human immunodeficiency virus disease is a major consideration in some populations. Clues to other specific causes may be gained from elements of the history, physical examination, or laboratory and imaging studies. Although determining the underlying cause of chronic renal failure can permit the underlying disease to be treated and make possible some improvement in renal function in some cases, this is the exception rather than the rule.

Uremia Regardless of the underlying cause, progressive loss of renal function eventually results in a recognizable syndrome termed uremia. Despite the presence of often impressive laboratory abnormalities, clinical manifestations do not generally appear until GFR has been reduced to perhaps 15% to 20% of normal. Up to that point, the remaining functioning nephrons compensate reasonably well

Box 92-9 Major Causes of Chronic Renal Failure

Vascular

Renal arterial disease
Hypertensive nephrosclerosis

Glomerular

Primary glomerulopathies
Focal sclerosing glomerulonephritis (GN)
Membranoproliferative GN
Membranous GN
Crescentic GN
IgA nephropathy
Secondary glomerulopathies
Diabetic nephropathy
Collagen vascular disease
Amyloidosis
Postinfectious
HIV nephropathy

Tubulointerstitial

Nephrotoxins
Analgesic nephropathy
Hypercalcemia/nephrocalcinosis
Multiple myeloma
Reflux nephropathy
Sickle nephropathy
Chronic pyelonephritis
Tuberculosis

Obstructive

Nephrolithiasis
Ureteral tuberculosis
Retroperitoneal fibrosis
Retroperitoneal tumor
Prostatic obstruction
Congenital

Hereditary

Polycystic kidney disease
Alport's syndrome
Medullary cystic disease

for those that have been injured or destroyed. Beyond that point, the kidney can no longer maintain normal serum levels of certain solutes, and metabolic by-products, collectively termed *uremic toxins,* are retained. These poorly defined substances are thought to be responsible for many of the clinical manifestations of uremia.

Uremia is characterized by derangements in homeostasis and metabolism and by specific effects in multiple organ systems. Homeostatic disturbances generally develop gradually. As the patient becomes unable to promptly excrete an ingested salt or water load, external balance of sodium and water is affected; volume overload or hypernatremia or hyponatremia may result. Inability to concentrate the urine is an early manifestation of renal insufficiency and may be manifested as nocturia. Potassium homeostasis is likewise disrupted, so a relatively small potassium load may lead to dangerous hyperkalemia. Acid-base balance is affected as the kidney fails to clear the daily metabolic acid load because of a decreased ability to excrete ammonium and phosphate; the result is a non–anion-gap acidosis in the earlier stages of chronic renal failure, and a superimposed anion-gap acidosis as GFR decreases further. Calcium and phosphate metabolism is affected early on; retention of phosphate and progressive loss of the kidney's capacity to synthesize 1,25-dihydroxycholecalciferol (1,25-DHCC), the active form of vitamin D, leads to hypocalcemia, secondary hyperparathyroidism, and eventually to the development of renal osteodystrophy.

Uremia causes less dramatic but no less serious derangements in protein, carbohydrate, and lipid metabolism. Nitrogenous by-products of protein catabolism are retained in the blood and are the presumed cause of many of the diverse abnormalities of organ function in renal failure. Most patients with ESRD show decreased glucose tolerance, although it is rarely severe enough to require treatment unless there is a history of overt diabetes. In the latter case, insulin or other hypoglycemic therapy may need to be continued, but generally in a lower dosage than required before renal failure supervened because the normal kidney has a major role in insulin degradation. Incompletely understood alterations in lipid metabolism result in a type IV hyperlipoproteinemia in many ESRD patients.[55]

Clinical Features

Uremia has specific effects on a variety of organ systems. Many of these manifestations are relieved by dialysis, but others are not. A number have been attributed in some degree to retention of nitrogenous wastes and to the previously noted derangements in vitamin D and parathyroid hormone metabolism.

Cardiovascular The cardiovascular system is perhaps the most dramatically affected.[56] Many of the manifestations can be attributed to the effects of chronic volume overload, anemia, hyperlipidemia, alterations in calcium and phosphorus metabolism, and volume- and hormonally mediated hypertension.[57,58] Pericarditis, with or without pericardial fluid accumulation, is also common in ESRD, particularly among the patients who have not been dialyzed.

Pulmonary Similarly, some patients develop uremic pleuritis, with or without associated pleural fluid collections. So-called uremic lung, manifested radiographically by "bat-wing" perihilar infiltrates, represents pulmonary edema and is almost always caused by volume overload or myocardial dysfunction. Noninflammatory pleural effusion caused by volume overload is also fairly common. Of special importance to the emergency physician is the fact that the radiographic appearance of pulmonary edema may at times be misleading, simulating an infectious lobar infiltrate or even assuming a nodular appearance in some cases.[59]

Neurologic Neurologic dysfunction is common in advanced uremia and is usually manifested by lethargy, somnolence, difficulty concentrating, or a frank alteration in mental status. Seizures may also occur, although causes other than uremia per se must be ruled out. Uremic encephalopathy is also commonly manifested by hiccups, asterixis, or myoclonic twitching. The latter should not be confused with tetany caused by hypocalcemia, which is also common in untreated patients with ESRD. Some patients on chronic dialysis therapy develop "dialysis dementia," a syndrome characterized by dementia, altered mental status, and movement disorders that appear to be related at least in part to aluminum overload associated with aluminum-containing medications (e.g., oral phosphate binders) or dialysate.[60,61] In the peripheral nervous system, uremia often causes cramps and a distal sensorimotor neuropathy. A troublesome and very characteristic complaint is the "restless legs syndrome," in which there is persistent neuropathic discomfort in the legs that patients find can be relieved only by movement.

Gastrointestinal Anorexia, nausea, and vomiting are nearly constant features of uremia. These symptoms are thought to be caused by accumulation of nitrogenous wastes because they are often relieved, even in the undialyzed patient, by introduction of a low-protein diet and seem to correlate roughly with the BUN level.

Dermatologic The skin of the patient with chronic renal failure has a characteristic yellowish tinge. "Uremic frost," the result of deposition of urea from evaporated sweat on the skin, is a classic finding that like "uremic fetor," is seen only rarely now with the widespread use of dialysis. Diffuse pruritus is often a major source of discomfort for the ESRD patient; in some cases it may be caused by calcium deposition in the skin secondary to derangements in calcium metabolism.

Musculoskeletal The bones and joints are sites of problems for many patients, particularly those with longstanding renal disease. The complex disturbances of calcium and phosphate metabolism in ESRD result in renal osteodystrophy, a term encompassing several overlapping varieties of bone disease that can cause symptoms of bone pain or frank fractures.[62] Patients with chronic renal disease are generally treated with long-term oral calcium and vitamin D in an effort to prevent both secondary hyperparathyroidism and uremic osteodystrophy. Occasional patients have a poor response to therapy and require parathyroidectomy.

A particular type of arthritis caused by deposition of calcium hydroxyapatite or calcium oxalate crystals in joints is seen in some patients, as are periarticular calcium deposition, spontaneous tendon rupture, myopathy, carpal tunnel syndrome, and a specific ESRD-related amyloid arthropathy.[63-65]

Immunologic Infection remains a leading cause of mortality associated with renal failure.[66] Uremic patients have long been noted to have an increased susceptibility to infection, even when not challenged by the invasive procedures necessitated by dialysis. A variety of immunologic abnormalities have been identified in these individuals.[67-71] Both humoral and cellular immunity have been shown to be affected. Although the relative importance of each in the pathogenesis of infection in renal failure has not yet been clarified, defects in cellular immunity appear to be more significant clinically. Nevertheless, although patients with renal failure should be considered to be immunocompromised, most infections in ESRD patients are caused by common pathogens rather than opportunistic organisms.

Hematologic A rather severe normochromic normocytic anemia, with a hematocrit commonly in the range of 18% to 25%, is nearly universal in untreated ESRD, except among patients with polycystic disease. It is primarily caused by the kidneys' decreased production of erythropoietin, a hormone that stimulates red cell production by the bone marrow. Other contributing factors are increased red cell hemolysis, nutritional deficiencies, and increased bleeding secondary to platelet dysfunction.

Although platelet number is generally normal in uremia, the bleeding time is prolonged because of defective platelet adhesiveness and activation. A common manifestation is the numerous ecchymoses seen in many patients with chronic renal failure.

Diagnostic Strategies

The patient with chronic renal failure, particularly one who is not yet on dialysis, is likely to present to the ED with one of the manifestations previously noted. In cases in which the diagnosis of renal failure has not previously been made, patients most commonly have nonspecific complaints, often of insidious onset, such as generalized weakness, poor appetite, or deterioration of mental functioning. The initial laboratory finding of a reasonably well-tolerated but rather severe anemia may be the first clue to the diagnosis, which is subsequently confirmed by elevated BUN and serum creatinine levels. A prudent next step is to check the ECG for evidence of immediately life-threatening hyperkalemia before proceeding with further laboratory and radiographic investigations.

Once it is established that the patient is in no immediate danger, the emergency physician should attempt to establish that renal failure is indeed chronic, rather than acute. An explicit history to that effect obtained from previous medical records or from the patient or family provides the most straightforward and reliable confirmation, as does the presence of a dialysis access device on physical examination. If such a history is unavailable, the finding of bilaterally small kidneys (readily detected on plain abdominal films or by ultrasonography) is equally good evidence. However, the converse is not necessarily true. A finding of normal-size or large kidneys does not rule out chronic renal failure (Box 92-10); in this case additional diagnostic steps are required to establish the diagnosis. Another good indication of chronicity is the presence of renal osteodystrophy (particularly of the osteitis fibrosa cystica type) on x-ray films of the hands and clavicles because these radiographic changes probably re-

Box 92-10 Causes of Chronic Renal Failure with Normal or Large Kidney Size

Polycystic kidney disease
Amyloidosis
Diabetic nephropathy
Malignant hypertension
Multiple myeloma
Glomerulonephritis (some)
Obstructive uropathy (some)

quire at least a year to develop. Of course, a convincing history of the long-standing presence of the presenting symptoms or of symptoms such as nocturia may be helpful in suggesting chronicity, as may a history of familial kidney disease such as polycystic kidney disease or Alport's syndrome. Laboratory abnormalities such as anemia, acidosis, hyperuricemia, hypocalcemia, and hyperphosphatemia can occur in patients with *acute* renal failure as early as 10 days after onset.[72] Although urinary findings likewise tend not to be helpful, the presence of reliably demonstrated broad waxy casts on microscopic examination is suggestive of chronicity, whereas the finding of an "active" sediment (e.g., red-cell casts) is good evidence for an acute process.

Although, as a rule, chronic renal failure is irreversible and slowly progressive, it is critical that the emergency physician be able to exclude the possibility of potentially reversible factors (in effect, to rule out "acute on chronic" renal failure) and to be sure that treatable causes of chronic renal failure, disorders that if treated might allow for some return of renal function, have not been overlooked. These potentially reversible factors and treatable causes of chronic renal failure are important to keep in mind because they represent the emergency physician's only potential opportunity to reverse the patient's disease rather than simply to manage and ameliorate the results of it (Box 92-11).

Primary among superimposed reversible factors are those that lead to decreased renal perfusion. Of these the most common is volume depletion. Regardless of the initiating cause, the process will be exacerbated by the diseased kidney's impaired ability to conserve sodium and to concentrate the urine appropriately. Decreased renal perfusion caused by cardiac dysfunction of any cause is another extremely common and potentially reversible factor. An uncommonly encountered but important vascular cause of reversible deterioration of renal function is scleroderma renal crisis, a syndrome of accelerated hypertension and severe vasoconstriction in patients with underlying scleroderma that can be reversed by timely treatment with angiotensin-converting enzyme (ACE) inhibitors.[73]

Increased catabolism caused by infection, trauma, surgery, corticosteroids, or GI bleeding is another reversible factor that is often responsible for worsening azotemia and developing uremic symptoms.

Drugs and toxins constitute another important group of reversible factors.[74] Not only may these agents exacerbate renal insufficiency by causing intravascular volume depletion (diuretics), decreased renal perfusion (antihypertensive agents), or increased catabolism (tetracycline), but they can also cause acute tubular necrosis (radiographic contrast

Box 92-11 Reversible Factors and Treatable Causes of Chronic Renal Failure

Reversible Factors

Hypovolemia
Congestive heart failure
Pericardial tamponade
Severe hypertension
Catabolic state/protein loads
Nephrotoxic agents
Obstructive disease
Reflux disease

Treatable Causes

Renal artery stenosis
Malignant hypertension
Acute interstitial nephritis
Hypercalcemic nephropathy
Multiple myeloma
Vasculitis (e.g., systemic lupus erythematosus, Wegener's granulomatosis, polyarteritis nodosa)
Obstructive nephropathy
Reflux nephropathy

material), acute interstitial nephritis (many drugs), or inhibition of renal prostaglandin synthesis (NSAIDs). Particularly noteworthy is the dramatic decrease in renal function produced when an ACE inhibitor is administered to a patient with renal insufficiency caused by bilateral renal artery stenosis (or renal artery stenosis in a solitary kidney).[75]

Postrenal reversible factors are also important because of their frequency, particularly obstructive disease in the older male patient and reflux nephropathy in the child. Papillary necrosis should remain a consideration in the diabetic patient, the patient with sickle cell disease, and the patient with a history of long-term analgesic use. Stone disease, retroperitoneal fibrosis, and even rarer entities such as ureteral tuberculosis should also not be overlooked.

Finally, treatment of the underlying disorder that has caused chronic renal failure can occasionally result in the return of some renal function, most notably in cases of myeloma kidney, some forms of secondary glomerulonephritis, and severe hypertensive disease.[72] Although this consideration must of necessity relate to long-term care and follow-up, it is appropriate that the emergency physician consider this issue to ensure that appropriate evaluation and disposition are arranged.

Management

Individuals with chronic renal failure constitute a group of patients that merit special attention from the emergency physician. These patients are susceptible to infection, bleeding, and the numerous other complications associated with renal failure per se, as well as those that may be associated with the underlying disorder that was the cause of renal failure. Moreover, these patients are more than normally vulnerable to the effects of any intercurrent illness or trauma and the physiologic stresses thereby imposed on a more or less delicately compensated physiologic state. Those who are maintained on chronic hemodialysis or peritoneal dialysis are subject to potential complications entailed by the dialytic therapy itself.

Patients with chronic renal failure are also "special" in that they are uniquely susceptible to iatrogenic illness. First, they are less able to handle fluid and solute loads than are

Box 92-12 Mechanisms of Drug Toxicity in Renal Failure

Excessive drug level
Impaired renal excretion of drug
Impaired renal excretion of active metabolite
Impaired hepatic metabolism
Increased sensitivity to drug
Changes in protein binding
Changes in volume of distribution
Changes in target organ sensitivity
Metabolic loads administered with drug
Misinterpretation of measured serum drug level (i.e., change in therapeutic range)

From Wolfson AB, Singer I: *J Emerg Med* 5:533, 1987.

normal individuals. Just as important, the presence of renal failure significantly alters the metabolism and action of many drugs, often in ways that are not predictable a priori[76] (Box 92-12). Thus, it is imperative that the dose and schedule of every administered agent, even apparently innocuous ones such as antacids and multivitamin preparations, be carefully considered. For this purpose the emergency physician should have access to a compendium such as the one by Bennett et al[77] or be able to consult frequently with the hospital pharmacy.

In light of these considerations, when evaluating the patient with chronic renal failure in the ED, the emergency physician must be prepared not only to make a diagnosis and initiate appropriate treatment, but also to do so while keeping in mind the predictable consequences of chronic renal failure and the necessary modifications of standard treatment they imply. In general, the emergency physician should consult with the patient's nephrologist once the initial evaluation has been completed because management and follow-up monitoring after the patient leaves the ED are often complex.

In the United States, most patients with advancing chronic renal disease are eventually treated with dialysis, but several true emergencies may develop in the patient with ESRD before chronic dialysis has been instituted. Specific diagnostic and therapeutic considerations apply to the management of these conditions regardless of whether they occur in dialyzed or undialyzed patients.

Hyperkalemia Potentially the most rapidly lethal complication of chronic renal failure that the emergency physician must deal with is severe hyperkalemia. As a rule, this condition is clinically silent until it presents with potentially life-threatening manifestations.[78,79] Thus, hyperkalemia must be looked for in every patient with chronic renal disease. These individuals can become severely hyperkalemic when required to handle even modest exogenous and endogenous potassium loads; moreover, even drugs such as β-blockers and ACE inhibitors that have only minimal effects on the serum potassium in normal individuals can cause hyperkalemia in these patients. The inadvertent use of succinylcholine in patients with ESRD can rapidly result in life-threatening hyperkalemia.

An ECG should be obtained whenever hyperkalemia is a possibility, and if signs of hyperkalemia are noted, appropriate therapy should be started immediately, even before laboratory confirmation of a high serum potassium level. ECG changes may be completely absent even when hyperkalemia is severe, however.[80] Thus, a normal ECG does not make laboratory confirmation of a normal serum potassium level unnecessary. A potassium level of 6 mEq/L should be considered potentially dangerous even though many patients with ESRD chronically tolerate levels somewhat above this without ECG changes. A patient with chronic renal failure who is in cardiac arrest should be assumed to be hyperkalemic and treated accordingly while the usual resuscitative measures are taken.

The most rapidly effective treatment for hyperkalemia is IV calcium, which transiently reverses the cardiac manifestations of hyperkalemia without altering the serum potassium level or total-body potassium (Table 92-3). Calcium should be given to buy time in which more definitive measures can take effect. It makes little sense to administer in response to an elevated serum potassium level in the absence of manifestations of hyperkalemia on the ECG.

In treating hyperkalemia, the emergency physician must also keep in mind the ESRD patient's limited ability to tolerate volume and solute loads (see Table 92-3). Thus, repeated doses of IV sodium bicarbonate risk causing volume overload and precipitating pulmonary edema. IV glucose and insulin act less rapidly and also require volume administration. However, if the patient's condition permits, the latter method is preferred because sodium administration can be avoided and hyperkalemia can be controlled for as long as the infusion is continued. Another effective temporizing measure is administration of inhaled albuterol to promote movement of potassium into cells while more definitive maneuvers are being instituted.[81,82]

To remove potassium from the body, sodium polystyrene sulfonate (Kayexalate), a resin that exchanges sodium for potassium ions, can be administered orally or rectally. This drug can continue to control the potassium for hours and, despite the modest sodium load it entails, can be effective as a temporizing measure until dialysis (if necessary) can be instituted. In patients who still retain some renal function, the most effective way to treat hyperkalemia may be to administer an IV diuretic such as furosemide (if the patient is not hypovolemic) and to give volume if necessary. Large doses of diuretic may be necessary to induce a satisfactory diuresis. In light of the potential for ototoxicity with the use of loop-active diuretics, these drugs should be administered by slow infusion rather than by bolus. They should probably be avoided in patients who are also receiving other potentially ototoxic agents.[83] During the course of any of these therapeutic interventions, both the ECG and the serum potassium must be monitored frequently.

Pulmonary Edema Perhaps the most common emergency complaint in the patient with chronic renal failure is pulmonary edema secondary to volume overload. Surprisingly, the diagnosis is not always straightforward. The patient may have a suggestive history of increasing dyspnea on exertion or paroxysmal nocturnal dyspnea, but physical examination may not reveal the expected signs of congestive heart failure and even chest radiography may be deceptive (Figure 92-3).[57] A history of recent weight gain or of the patient being considerably over "dry weight" (typically >5 pounds) is the most reliable clue, and in the absence of

Table 92-3. Treatment of Hyperkalemia

	Dose	Onset/duration of action	Mechanism of action	Comments
Calcium gluconate (10%) or calcium chloride (10%)	10 ml IV (May repeat × 2 prn q5-10min)	1-5 min/~1 hr	Antagonizes membrane effects of K^+	ECG monitoring required Do not mix with HCO_3^- Beware: Hypercalcemia
Sodium bicarbonate	50 mg IV (May repeat × 1 prn)	~10-15 min/1-2 hr	Intracellular movement of K^+	Beware: Volume overload Hypertonicity Alkalosis (Seizures)
Albuterol	10-20 mg (nebulized) by inhalation	30 min/2⁺ hr	Intracellular movement of K^+	Relatively free of significant side effects; tachycardia
Glucose/insulin	10-20 units regular insulin per 100 g glucose	30 min/while infusion continued	Intracellular movement of K^+	Beware: Hyperglycemia Hypoglycemia Infused volume may be decreased by using D10, D20, or D50
Kayexalate	25 gm in 25 ml 70% sorbitol PO q6h ± 50 gm in 50 ml 70% sorbitol by retention enema q6hr	Hours/while continued	Exchange of K^+ for Na^+	Beware: Na^+ overload Enema must be retained × 30-45 min
Dialysis	Hemodialysis Peritoneal dialysis	Minutes/while continued	Removal of K^+ from blood	HD may remove 50 mEq/hr (beware K^+ rebound) PD may remove 15 mEq/hr
IV diuretics (IV fluid if hypovolemic)		Minutes/while diuresis continued (depending on renal function)	Urinary K^+ excretion	Only in patients with residual renal function

From Wolfson AB, Singer I: *J Emerg Med* 6:61, 1988.

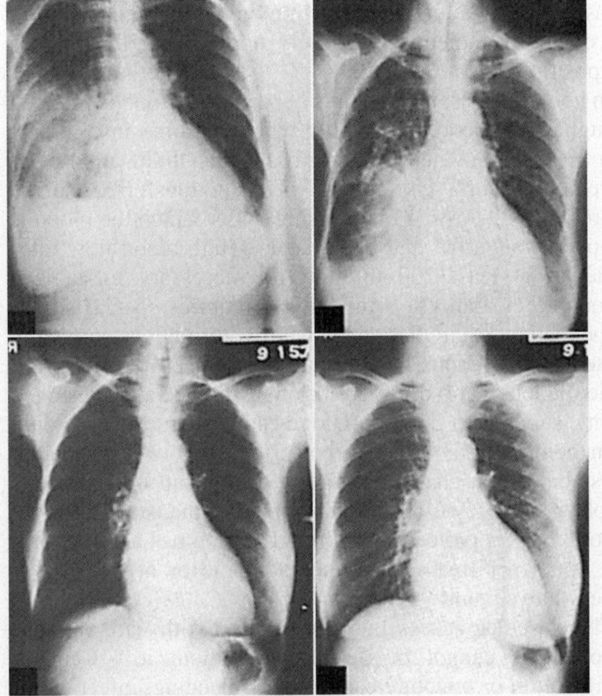

Figure 92-3. **Pulmonary edema simulating right lower lobe pneumonia in dialysis patient. Infiltrate improved drastically, and heart size returned to normal after dialysis and ultrafiltration. A, Chest x-ray film immediately before dialysis showing cardiomegaly and right lower lobe infiltrate interpreted as pneumonia. B, Chest x-ray film 5 hours after initiating dialysis with 2-kg weight reduction. There was marked improvement of infiltrate. C and D, Return of normal lung and cardiac size.** *From Kjellstrand C et al. In Drukker W, Parson FM, Maher JF, editors:* Replacement of renal function by dialysis, *Boston, 1983, Martinus Nijhoff.*

Box 92-13 Treatment of Pulmonary Edema in Renal Failure

Dialysis	Furosemide
Hemodialysis	Bumetanide
Hemofiltration	Nitroglycerin (sublingual, IV, topical)
Peritoneal dialysis	Nitroprusside
Oxygen	Sorbitol
Morphine	
Diuretics	

convincing evidence of another cause for dyspnea, the emergency physician should assume that volume overload is the cause and treat accordingly.

Treatment of pulmonary edema in the patient with chronic renal failure is of necessity somewhat different from that used with other patients (Box 92-13).[84,85] Arrangements for initiation of dialysis should be made as soon as possible because it is the most rapidly effective means to decrease intravascular volume in the absence of renal function. Other immediate measures should be instituted in the meantime. Although such measures may occasionally prove effective enough to avoid dialysis temporarily in patients who possess some residual renal function, the emergency physician should nevertheless anticipate that the extent and rapidity of response to even extremely aggressive medical therapy short of dialysis will be inadequate.

The patient should be placed in the sitting position and high-flow oxygen should be administered by mask. The use of continuous or bilevel positive airway pressure delivered by face mask has been reported to be a useful adjunct in patients with ESRD, as it is in patients without renal failure.[86,87] Sublingual or topical nitroglycerin, or both, can be administered immediately and functions rapidly to reduce both preload and afterload; an IV infusion can be begun promptly and titrated to effect. IV nitroprusside may have an advantage in producing more arteriolar dilation if the patient is hypertensive. IV morphine increases venous capacitance, but as with non–renal failure patients, its routine use as a first-line drug in pulmonary edema has become less common. IV furosemide, although ineffective as a diuretic in patients with advanced renal failure, is a rather potent pulmonary venodilator and may be expected to provide additional relief; patients with residual renal function may respond to large IV doses with some diuresis, although much more slowly than patients without renal compromise.[88] Bumetanide is an appropriate alternative for patients who are allergic to furosemide. The use of ethacrynic acid has been associated with permanent deafness in patients with renal failure.[83] One report notes the efficacy of large doses of oral sorbitol in reducing intravascular volume by causing massive GI fluid loss, but this method has obvious disadvantages.[84]

Infection Because infection is a major cause of morbidity and mortality among patients with ESRD, the possibility of serious infection should be entertained even when the expected classic findings are not all present.[66,68] For example, bacteremia may be manifested by fever alone, just as it is in other patients with impaired immunity. Pneumonia may present with only vague dyspnea or malaise, symptoms that may be attributed to volume overload or uremia. Thus all diagnostic possibilities should be pursued, and empiric broad-spectrum antibiotic coverage is often advisable until infection has been ruled out in the hospital. Bacteremia resulting from vascular access infection is quite common in patients receiving hemodialysis, as is peritonitis in patients undergoing continuous ambulatory peritoneal dialysis.

Urinary tract infection can occur even in patients with minimal urine output or those with long-standing renal failure. Urinary stasis is undoubtedly a predisposing factor. In patients with lower-tract symptoms, infection can usually be diagnosed by urinalysis or culture performed on a few drops of urine; oral antibiotic therapy is usually effective. Upper urinary tract infection presenting with a clinical picture typical of pyelonephritis or renal colic is seen most commonly in patients with polycystic kidney disease and requires parenteral therapy. A clinical diagnosis can be made presumptively in the ED, but invasive measures are sometimes necessary to document infection and guide therapy. For infected cysts, lipid-soluble antibiotics (e.g., clindamycin or trimethoprim-sulfamethoxazole) offer the best antibiotic penetration; surgical intervention for refractory infection sometimes becomes necessary, however.[89,90]

Dialysis Over the past several decades, dialysis techniques have been developed as a substitute for several of the functions of the normal kidney. Dialysis can normalize fluid balance, correct electrolyte and other solute abnormalities, and remove uremic toxins or drugs from the circulation when the patient's kidneys are unable to do so. Dialysis can also, but generally to a lesser degree, reverse some uremic symptoms and permit better long-term control of hypertension, anemia, and renal osteodystrophy.

There are two major dialysis modalities: hemodialysis and peritoneal dialysis. Each is based on technology wherein the patient's blood comes into contact with a semipermeable membrane on the other side of which is a specially constituted balanced physiologic solution. Water and solutes diffuse across the membrane by moving along concentration and osmotic gradients, effectively normalizing the blood's composition.

In hemodialysis, the patient's heparinized blood is pumped through an extracorporeal circuit where it comes into contact with an artificial membrane across which fluid and solute movement occurs. The amount of fluid transferred can be controlled by adjusting the pressure under which the blood is pumped through the dialyzer. Because high blood flow rates (typically at least 200 ml/min) are necessary to achieve reasonable clearances, hemodialysis requires special access to the patient's circulation, generally through a surgically created arteriovenous fistula or an implanted artificial graft. Some patients are dialyzed through a specially designed chronic subclavian catheter (Uldall catheter), most commonly when hemodialysis must be performed before a peripheral access has had a chance to mature or after all of a patient's peripheral sites for access have been exhausted. Chronic hemodialysis is typically performed three times a week for 3 to 5 hours per treatment, either at home or at a specially staffed dialysis unit.

The vascular access must be treated with care because hemodialysis cannot be performed without it.[76] Careless manipulation or puncture can result in bleeding, infection, or thrombosis that may result in loss of the access. The involved arm should never be used for blood pressure determinations, and a tourniquet should never be applied.

In general, blood should be drawn and IV lines established in other locations. In exceptional circumstances, if no other site is available and it is essential to obtain blood samples quickly, the fistula or graft may be used, but with precautions. A tourniquet should not be applied, the area should be cleansed scrupulously before the puncture, and extreme care should be taken not to puncture the back wall of the access. After the puncture, firm but nonocclusive pressure should be applied for at least 10 minutes. The presence of a thrill both before and after the procedure should be documented. Similar precautions are imperative in those exceptional cases in which the fistula or graft must be used for IV access. If this is done, an automated infusion pump is essential to control the infusion rate into these relatively high-pressure blood vessels.

In peritoneal dialysis, the patient's peritoneum functions as the dialysis membrane.[91] Water and solutes diffuse from the peritoneal capillaries across this membrane to equilibrate with sterile dialysate that has been infused into the peritoneal cavity. For acute peritoneal dialysis, dialysate is infused and drained hourly (or even more frequently) for approximately 48 hours through a percutaneously placed stiff temporary catheter. In chronic ambulatory peritoneal dialysis (CAPD), the technique in which patients with ESRD perform dialysis themselves at home, dialysate is infused through a surgically implanted silastic catheter (Tenckhoff catheter) that penetrates the peritoneum and abdominal musculature, passes through a subcutaneous tunnel, and exits through the skin of the lower abdominal wall. Externally the catheter is attached to sterile plastic tubing to which is connected a sterile bag of dialysate. Dialysate is allowed to dwell in the peritoneal cavity for 4 to 8 hours. The patient typically exchanges the fluid four times a day, 7 days a week, discarding the bag of drained fluid and sterilely attaching a bag of fresh fluid, which is then infused. CAPD is truly a continuous form of dialysis and although it is substantially less efficient on an hourly basis than hemodialysis, it achieves a total weekly clearance comparable with that obtained with thrice weekly hemodialysis.[91] A similar technique, continuous cyclic peritoneal dialysis, uses an automatic cycler to perform shorter exchanges while the patient sleeps at night and may offer advantages over CAPD for some patients.[92]

In contrast to hemodialysis, in which a relatively isosmolar dialysate is used and excess intravascular fluid is removed by adjusting the pressure under which the blood is pumped, CAPD uses a hyperosmolar dialysate to remove intravascular fluid by osmotic forces. The typical 1.5% glucose solution generally continues to remove fluid for at least 4 hours before it has substantially equilibrated with the blood. Patients usually use a more concentrated solution (e.g., 4.25% glucose) for fluid removal during the long overnight exchange.

CAPD offers patients with ESRD greater independence than hemodialysis, avoids the dangers of anticoagulation, and achieves smoother control of volume and hypertension without the intermittent rapid shifts of solute typical of hemodialysis. In addition, medications such as insulin and antibiotics can be administered intraperitoneally, allowing smoother absorption and more stable blood levels. The main disadvantage of CAPD is a significant incidence of bacterial peritonitis, which is, however, usually readily treated.

Box 92-14 Indications for Emergency Dialysis

Pulmonary edema
Severe uncontrollable hypertension
Hyperkalemia
Other severe electrolyte or acid-base disturbances
Some overdoses
Pericarditis (possibly)

Indications for Dialysis The decision to initiate chronic dialysis in the patient with ESRD is generally made by the patient's nephrologist in the setting of gradually decreasing GFR and slowly progressive manifestations of renal failure. The absolute value of the BUN or serum creatinine is generally used only as a rough guide as to when chronic dialysis should be instituted. Provision of vascular or peritoneal access will usually have been arranged weeks to months before the anticipated initiation of dialysis to allow the access to mature and to minimize any avoidable mechanical complications of the procedure.

For the patient who comes to the ED with acute renal failure, however, as well as for the patient with chronic renal failure who develops acute problems, it is the emergency physician who must be prepared to make the decision to arrange for dialysis to be provided emergently (Box 92-14). How urgently dialysis must be initiated depends on not only the severity and acuteness of the presenting problem, but also the availability of technical facilities and trained dialysis personnel and the effectiveness of available temporizing measures for the problem at hand.

The most common problem requiring emergent dialysis, particularly in the patient with ESRD, is pulmonary edema secondary to volume overload. Generally, the inciting cause is overingestion of fluid and salt in excess of the patient's greatly diminished renal excretory capacity. Despite the effectiveness of temporizing measures as noted earlier, many of these patients require immediate dialysis—either emergency hemodialysis or, in the case of the CAPD patient, intensification of the usual peritoneal dialysis regimen. Hemodialysis takes time to initiate but, once instituted, can be expected to lead to dramatic improvement in the patient's status within a few minutes. In contrast, the success of peritoneal dialysis in this situation depends on whether the patient can be adequately sustained for the several hours usually required for even hourly peritoneal dialysis exchanges to effect clinically significant changes in intravascular volume status. When hemodialysis is instituted, it is sometimes advisable to begin the procedure using hemofiltration alone ("dry dialysis" using pressure ultrafiltration without dialysate) to avoid the risk of producing circulatory instability or acute neurologic symptoms because of rapid solute shifts.[93] After the patient's volume status has been reduced somewhat, the procedure can proceed using standard hemodialysis.

A related problem that may require emergent, or at least urgent, dialysis is malignant hypertension, particularly when associated with hypertensive encephalopathy or cardiovascular decompensation. Because hypertension in most patients with renal failure is at least in part volume dependent, correction of volume overload, even if clinically inapparent, is a central component of therapy. It must also be kept in mind that hypertensive encephalopathy can occur even at diastolic pressures as low as 100 mm Hg.[94] Temporizing measures such as the administration of IV sodium nitroprusside or nitroglycerin often permit hypertension to be controlled sufficiently so that dialysis can be delayed for several hours, but prolonged administration of sodium nitroprusside carries an increased risk of thiocyanate toxicity in patients with renal failure. In many cases hypertension and associated symptoms are difficult to control until dialysis permits volume overload to be corrected. Because the blood pressure is often dramatically responsive to reduction of circulating volume, it is recommended that other antihypertensive agents that have more prolonged effects be withheld until after dialysis has been able to reduce circulating volume.

Severe hyperkalemia is another common indication for emergent or urgent dialysis, particularly in the patient with acute renal failure who is hypercatabolic. In the patient with chronic renal failure, hyperkalemia is usually caused by excessive potassium intake, but endogenous causes such as hemolysis or rhabdomyolysis must be kept in mind as well.[78,79] A variety of available temporizing measures can be used with varying effectiveness and for various durations to control the serum potassium level, but dialysis remains the most effective means of removing potassium from the body. For rapid control of the serum potassium, hemodialysis, with its high clearance rates, is preferred to peritoneal dialysis. However, because peritoneal dialysis can be continued on a 24-hour basis, it can probably remove at least as great an amount of potassium as daily hemodialysis, and it eliminates the rebound increase in serum potassium often seen after hemodialysis in patients who have been chronically hyperkalemic. Moreover, peritoneal dialysis can often be initiated more easily in a patient who has not previously been dialyzed and is less likely to cause complications related to rapid solute shifts. The rapidity of the fall in the serum potassium with either modality is difficult to predict because 98% of total body potassium resides in the intracellular space and equilibrates rapidly with the blood.

Other severe electrolyte and acid-base disturbances may sometimes require emergent dialysis. Occasional patients with renal failure and severe hypercalcemia uncontrollable by other modalities (e.g., individuals with multiple myeloma causing both renal failure and hypercalcemia) may require dialysis. The occasional patient with renal failure who develops severe hypermagnesemia after inappropriate therapy or magnesium ingestion may require immediate dialysis to reverse life-threatening paralysis or cardiac dysrhythmia.[78] Severe metabolic acidosis in the setting of renal failure is another indication for emergent dialysis, particularly if volume overload precludes the administration of reasonable amounts of bicarbonate. Of note, bicarbonate can also precipitate tetany and convulsions if administered by IV (e.g., to treat acidosis or hyperkalemia) to a patient with hypocalcemia.

A somewhat unusual but related situation is one in which a patient with renal failure has taken an overdose or inadvertently been administered medication that is ordinarily cleared by the kidneys. If the agent is adequately dialyzable and its continued presence in the circulation poses a significant risk to the patient, immediate dialysis can be life saving. An example of such a situation is when a dialysis patient ingests methanol or ethylene glycol. Similarly, ill-advised use of magnesium-containing cathartics or phosphate-containing enemas by patients with ESRD can lead to dangerous hypermagnesemia and hyperphosphatemia, respectively, and may require urgent dialysis.

The serum creatinine and BUN levels themselves should not be considered indications for dialysis. A creatinine of 10 mg/dl or a BUN of 100 mg/dl is often used as a guideline for beginning chronic dialysis in the patient with progressive renal failure. In dialyzed patients, however, the serum creatinine is often considerably greater than 10 mg/dl but is more a reflection of total body muscle mass than the adequacy of dialysis. The BUN is a somewhat better indicator; the level in well-dialyzed individuals is generally in the 50 to 80 mg/dl range and is over 100 mg/dl in less well-dialyzed patients. However, neither blood level correlates more than roughly with uremic symptoms even in undialyzed patients or has any direct bearing on how urgently dialysis should be initiated.

The occurrence of uremic symptoms such as nausea, vomiting, lethargy, or twitching indicates a need for dialysis but does not require dialysis to be initiated immediately. The appearance of pericarditis, even in the absence of cardiac tamponade, has been thought to be an exception. However, it is not uncommon for pericarditis to occur in well-dialyzed ESRD patients as well, and it has not been convincingly demonstrated that pericarditis itself is dangerous or invariably leads rapidly to tamponade.[95-97] In a previously undialyzed patient with progressive renal insufficiency, the appearance of pericarditis indicates that it is time to initiate dialysis, although not necessarily on an emergency basis.

Complications of Dialysis Therapy The emergency physician must be familiar with the particular problems associated with ESRD and dialysis to manage acute problems referred from the dialysis unit or those occurring at home or in the interdialysis period.[76,98-100] Consultation with the nephrologist or dialysis nurse is crucial in arranging a consistent care plan for the dialysis patient with an emergent condition and in ensuring appropriate further acute care or follow-up monitoring.

Hemodialysis

Vascular access–related complications The performance of hemodialysis depends on reliable vascular access, and it is the vascular access device that is responsible for complications of dialysis that most often require evaluation in the ED. It is imperative that these problems be attended to promptly to minimize the risk that the patient's dialysis "lifeline" will be lost.

Bleeding from the dialysis puncture site can occur hours after a hemodialysis treatment, either spontaneously or after inadvertent minor trauma to the site. Patients are usually able to control the bleeding by applying pressure to the area, but they need to be evaluated to exclude significant blood loss. Such bleeding almost always can be stopped by applying firm pressure to the access site; the emergency physician must be careful not to occlude and possibly thrombose the vessel by compressing it too vigorously, and the presence of a thrill immediately after the procedure should be documented on the chart. It may be necessary to keep the patient in the ED for a time to be sure that bleeding does not recur. Recurrent bleeding, especially from an aneurysm or pseudoaneurysm, should be evaluated by a vascular surgeon.

Similarly, if the patient complains that the thrill in the access has been lost, a vascular surgeon should be consulted immediately, because success in reopening a clotted access appears to depend on the time since thrombosis has occurred.[101,102] Although thrombolytic agents such as urokinase or streptokinase are sometimes used, definitive treatment is generally surgical revision. The access device should not be forcefully manipulated or irrigated because rupture of the vessel or venous embolization may result.

Infection of the vascular access is not uncommon and can result in persistent or recurrent bacteremia, as well as loss of the access.[103] Infection appears to be a consequence of contamination at the time of puncture for dialysis; most infections are caused by staphylococci typical of skin flora. Infections are more likely to occur in grafts than in native fistulas.[101,102] The signs and symptoms of an access infection—redness, warmth, and tenderness over the site—are often obvious, but in many cases patients manifest no localizing findings and have only fever or a history of recurrent episodes of fever and documented bacteremia. For this reason, it is common practice to draw blood cultures on all hemodialysis patients who have a fever without an obvious source of infection and to treat them presumptively for an access infection. However, a careful search for other sources of infection should be made before concluding that inapparent access infection is the cause. Infections such as odontogenic abscess, extremity cellulitis (particularly in diabetics), and perirectal abscess can easily be missed.

Although some nephrologists prefer to admit all dialysis patients with fever to the hospital, it is generally possible to manage these individuals on an outpatient basis, provided they otherwise feel well and do not appear to be septic and provided they can care for themselves at home and return promptly if their condition worsens. This course is made more practical by the fact that they can be loaded with IV antibiotics that will dependably maintain adequate blood levels until the time of the next scheduled dialysis treatment, at which time the culture and sensitivity test results can be checked and therapy adjusted accordingly. IV vancomycin is often the drug of choice in this situation because most access infections are staphylococcal, and because this drug is not hemodialyzable and needs to be given only every 5 to 7 days in the chronic dialysis patient. Moreover, its major toxicity is renal. If a gram-negative infection is also thought to be reasonably likely, as in a patient who has had recent episodes of gram-negative bacteremia, a loading dose of a second drug (e.g., aztreonam or an aminoglycoside) can also be administered. The latter agents have a prolonged half-life in ESRD, so patients can be reloaded at the end of the next hemodialysis if cultures prove to be positive.

Nonvascular access–related complications It is not surprising that the hemodialysis procedure itself, which entails invasion of the vasculature, anticoagulation, and often massive shifts of fluid and solutes, is often associated with acute complications such as hypotension, shortness of breath, chest pain, and neurologic abnormalities.

Hypotension that occurs after dialysis is most commonly the result of an acute reduction in circulating intravascular volume and the failure of the patient's homeostatic mechanisms to compensate for it.[104] Because hemodialysis is episodic, each treatment must remove the excess fluid that has accumulated over the period since the last dialysis (generally 2 to 3 days), and patients are often relatively volume-overloaded at the beginning of each treatment. With rapid removal of extracellular fluid, there is inadequate time for transcellular fluid shifts to replace intravascular volume. In addition, hemodialysis may be associated with varying degrees of myocardial and vascular dysfunction caused by acetate that is absorbed from the dialysate or the osmolar shifts associated with dialysis.[105] Autonomic neuropathy may be a contributing factor in many patients with ESRD, as may be the large arteriovenous shunt through the vascular access device. Antihypertensive medications, particularly β-blockers that are required when the patient is in a volume-expanded state, can contribute to the hypotension when intravascular volume is normalized.

Most episodes of hypotension that occur during hemodialysis either resolve spontaneously or are readily managed by either a decrease in blood flow rate or the infusion of small volumes of saline (to effect transient volume expansion) or hypertonic solutions (to transiently reverse acute hypoosmolality). Patients with significant hypotension who do not respond to these maneuvers are often brought to the ED for further evaluation. Dialysis patients should be considered to be at risk for acute myocardial infarction, acute dysrhythmia, and sepsis.[106] These are common causes of hypotension among all emergency patients, and consideration should first be given to these entities (Box 92-15).[76]

Acute hemorrhage is also not uncommon in dialysis patients. Before the widespread availability of human erythropoietin to treat the anemia of ESRD, most patients had a low baseline hemoglobin level, and even relatively modest blood loss had the potential to produce significant symptoms.[107,108] Serum levels of clotting factors are normal in ESRD, but patients are routinely anticoagulated for each hemodialysis treatment. Moreover, transient thrombocytopenia has been reported during the dialysis procedure.[109] However, the qualitative platelet defect characteristic of renal failure represents the most important factor in bleeding that continues beyond the peridialytic period.[110] This abnormality is only partially reversed by dialysis but can be corrected by administration of DDAVP, which causes increased release of factor VIII:VWF polymers from vascular endothelium.

Box 92-15 Differential Diagnosis of Hypotension in Hemodialysis Patients

Hypovolemia
Excessive fluid removal
Hemorrhage
Septicemia
Cardiogenic shock
Dysrhythmia
Pericardial tamponade
Myocardial infarction
Myocardial or valvular dysfunction
Electrolyte disorders
Hyperkalemia or hypokalemia
Hypercalcemia or hypocalcemia
Hypermagnesemia
Vascular instability
Drug related
Dialysate related
Autonomic neuropathy
Excessive access arteriovenous flow
Anaphylactoid reaction
Air embolism

From Wolfson AB, Singer I: *J Emerg Med* 5:533, 1987.

DDAVP has been used successfully to normalize the bleeding time in preparation for surgery in the patient with chronic renal failure.[111] Cryoprecipitate and conjugated estrogen have both been shown to produce similar effects for a longer period.[112,113] Surprisingly, simply correcting the anemia of renal failure by transfusion or treatment with erythropoietin can effectively normalize the bleeding time, apparently by rheologic effect.[114]

GI bleeding, often caused by angiodysplasia or peptic ulcer disease, is common and can be dramatic.[115,116] Occult hemorrhage, however, can challenge the emergency physician's diagnostic skills because symptoms and signs of volume loss tend to be overshadowed by local manifestations of bleeding into a closed space. Thus, spontaneous retroperitoneal or pleural hemorrhage tends to present with flank pain or with chest pain and shortness of breath, respectively.

Occasionally, acute hypotension may be caused by anaphylaxis or an anaphylactoid reaction to some component of the dialyzer or the dialysate; thus, these should be considered if the history is suggestive.[117-119] Acute pulmonary embolism and acute air embolism are two less likely possibilities. The former, although it does occur occasionally in dialysis patients, is unusual. The latter, although reported occasionally in the past, has been all but eliminated by improved dialysis unit monitoring equipment and safety mechanisms.[120]

The emergency physician, however, should not neglect to consider two additional entities in the differential diagnosis of hypotension that are of particular importance in the ESRD patient—acute pericardial tamponade and severe, life-threatening hyperkalemia.

Acute pericardial tamponade may be the result of either sudden pericardial hemorrhage or a compensated pericardial effusion becoming suddenly symptomatic in the face of acute correction of elevated preload. The clinical features of tamponade in the dialysis patient are similar to those in other populations, but the common preexistence of cardiomegaly may make the chest x-ray film difficult to interpret unless it shows the typical "water bottle" shape and a definite increase in heart size from previous examinations.

Similarly, the finding of an elevated central venous pressure is of little use in differentiating tamponade from underlying right-sided heart failure. Even a bedside ultrasonographic examination that shows pericardial fluid, although suggestive, is not proof that tamponade is present because many dialysis patients chronically have appreciable pericardial effusions that do not cause hemodynamic compromise.[94,95] Ultrasonographic demonstration of right ventricular diastolic collapse is more specific, but a definitive diagnosis of tamponade depends on the direct demonstration of equal pressures in the right and left atria on cardiac catheterization.

Emergency pericardiocentesis must occasionally be performed in the ED to relieve acute tamponade, but there is often enough time for the patient to be transported to the catheterization suite or operating room for safer and more definitive therapy in a controlled setting.[76] If immediate pericardiocentesis is believed to be necessary, however, the emergency physician should not hesitate to perform this potentially life-saving procedure, despite the many potential complications and the increased risk of bleeding in patients with ESRD. Similarly, in the case of a dialysis patient who is in cardiac arrest, pericardiocentesis should generally be attempted if initial resuscitative efforts have not been successful.

Severe life-threatening hyperkalemia, although unusual in a dialyzed patient, can occur in the presence of underlying catabolic illness or with a prolonged period of hypotension and low flow. Patients who are hyperkalemic can have profoundly slow heart rates, particularly if they have been treated with β-blockers or calcium channel blockers. If a dialysis patient is in cardiac arrest, it should be assumed that hyperkalemia is present, and separate IV infusions of calcium and bicarbonate should be given immediately.

Shortness of breath in dialysis patients is generally caused by volume overload. In the patient who becomes short of breath while being dialyzed, however, other causes must be sought, primarily sudden cardiac failure, pericardial tamponade, or pleural effusion or hemorrhage. Air embolism and anaphylactoid reactions are unusual causes.[117-120] Often, pneumonia or underlying airways disease is responsible. The hemodialysis procedure itself is associated with transient hypoxemia, but it is generally mild and is usually not associated with significant symptomatology.[121]

Chest pain during dialysis must be taken seriously because almost one half of ESRD patients die of cardiovascular causes, and it is likely that most episodes of chest pain occurring during dialysis are ischemic in origin.[57,66,122,123] Most dialysis patients have risk factors for coronary artery disease, related to either ESRD itself or the underlying condition that led to renal failure, and many have well-documented coronary disease. ESRD is commonly associated with hypertension, hyperlipidemia, and carbohydrate intolerance; in addition, dialysis patients are often anemic, and many are chronically volume overloaded. During hemodialysis these underlying factors may be added to acute physiologic stresses such as transient hypotension and hypoxemia that are often associated with the dialysis procedure, which increases myocardial oxygen demand while decreasing oxygen delivery.

In evaluating the ESRD patient with presumed ischemic chest pain, the EP must keep in mind the potentially reversible factors that may have precipitated the episode. Particularly when a patient whose angina has been stable begins to experience more frequent or more severe anginal episodes, the emergency physician should determine whether increasing anemia, poorly controlled hypertension, or uncorrected volume overload are factors. Coronary artery disease appears to become symptomatic with a lesser degree of obstruction than in other populations. It has been suggested that in patients with ESRD, myocardial oxygen delivery may be significantly impaired with only 50% occlusion of a coronary artery, rather than the 75% occlusion conventionally considered to be significant.[124] Thus, a history of noncritical coronary arterial narrowing should not necessarily rule out ischemia as the cause of chest pain.

Patients who repeatedly experience chest pain while on dialysis should undergo a complete evaluation so that the extent of their coronary disease can be defined and optimal management planned. After repeated, frequent hospital admissions to rule out myocardial infarctions because of chest pain during dialysis, it may be reasonable for the patient's nephrologist and cardiologist to set guidelines for further admissions.

The presence of renal failure and its associated electrolyte and acid-base disturbances does not in general obscure the usual ECG changes of angina or acute myocardial infarction. The pattern of the change of serum cardiac enzymes with acute infarction is also not altered by ESRD, although the "normal" range for these enzymes, which is altered in ESRD, has not been well defined.[125-129] In general, levels of troponin I are the least affected in renal failure compared with CK-MB and troponin T. Treatment of ischemic chest pain is the same as for other populations.

Among nonischemic causes of chest pain, pericarditis should always be a consideration, even in the well-dialyzed patient. The presentation is essentially the same as in nonrenal patients; fever, a friction rub, or atrial dysrhythmias may be associated findings, and signs of pericardial effusion or early tamponade should be sought. Indomethacin is often effective in relieving pain, but some patients eventually require further measures,[130] such as pericardiocentesis with corticosteroid instillation or pericardial stripping.[131] By analogy with the situation in undialyzed uremic individuals, traditional teaching holds that ESRD patients with pericarditis should receive more frequent or intensified dialysis to hasten resolution of the process and to prevent progression to tamponade. The correctness of this view has not, however, been demonstrated in controlled trials.[100]

Neurologic dysfunction during or immediately after hemodialysis is most often caused by disequilibrium syndrome, a constellation of symptoms and signs that is thought to be produced when serum osmolality is lowered rapidly during dialysis, leaving the brain relatively hyperosmolar relative to the extracellular fluid.[67,68] Typically, patients have headache, malaise, nausea, vomiting, and muscle cramps; in more severe cases, there may be altered mental status, seizures, or coma. These symptoms resolve over several hours as fluid and solutes are redistributed across cell membranes. Disequilibrium tends to be worse in patients who require removal of large amounts of fluid; indeed, symptoms are occasionally so severe that the hemodialysis treatment must be terminated prematurely. That the symptoms tend to respond rapidly to infusion of hyperosmolar solutions (e.g., mannitol, hypertonic saline) during dialysis and that the syndrome does not occur in CAPD patients provide additional evidence that rapid changes in osmolarity are the cause of disequilibrium syndrome.

It is dangerous, however, to attribute an altered mental status to disequilibrium syndrome unless other potential causes have been satisfactorily ruled out (Box 92-16), particularly when symptoms persist, fluctuate, or worsen during a reasonable period of observation.[98] Likewise, when seizures occur during dialysis, it is tempting but unwise to attribute them to disequilibrium syndrome without considering other potentially serious causes, even in patients who have had seizures in the past. In particular, the finding of any new focal neurologic abnormality mandates at a minimum an immediate head CT scan to detect intracranial hemorrhage. Similarly, if there is fever or other evidence of infection, meningitis must be a serious consideration. The emergency physician should also consider hyperglycemia and hypoglycemia (especially in the diabetic patient), electrolyte abnormalities, hypoxic states, hypotension of any cause, and other toxic or metabolic causes. The treatment of seizures in patients with ESRD is essentially the same as in other populations.

Complications of peritoneal dialysis As with hemodialysis, most of the complications of peritoneal dialysis are related to the dialysis access device, in this case the peritoneal catheter.[132] In contrast to hemodialysis, however, the dialytic process in CAPD occasions few immediate difficulties. Whatever volume or metabolic problems develop are often a consequence of the fact that the typical CAPD patient is seen by a doctor or nurse only once a month.

Peritonitis is the most common complication of CAPD. Fortunately, it is in general much less severe than other types of peritonitis and can be treated readily on an outpatient basis despite the continued presence of a foreign body—the Tenckhoff catheter—in the peritoneal cavity.[133] Occasionally, when an episode of peritonitis responds poorly to antimicrobial therapy or when a patient has repeated episodes of peritonitis caused by the same organism, the catheter must be removed and the patient sustained on hemodialysis until the infection is completely cleared and a new catheter can be placed.[134] Repeated infections do, however, carry the risk of permanently altering peritoneal permeability or effective surface area and necessitating a permanent switch to hemodialysis.

Peritonitis in CAPD patients is presumably caused by inadvertent bacterial contamination of the dialysate or tubing during an exchange or by extension of an infection of the exit site or the subcutaneous tunnel into the peritoneal cavity. Approximately 70% of cases of peritonitis are caused by *Staphylococcus aureus* or *Staphylococcus epidermidis,* and most of the remainder (approximately 20%) by gram-negative enteric organisms.[133] Fungal infections are uncommon but are generally refractory to medical therapy and are often considered an indication for catheter removal.[135] Polymicrobial infection suggests direct contamination from the GI tract and mandates a search for the site of perforation or fistula, although such a source is identified only in a distinct minority of cases.[136]

The diagnosis of peritonitis is usually made by the patient when a cloudy dialysis effluent is noted, corresponding to the appearance of WBCs in the dialysate. Peritonitis is often, but by no means invariably, accompanied by nonspecific abdominal pain, malaise, or fever. Even in the absence of cloudy fluid, when a patient has fever or abdominal symptoms, it is advisable to consider peritonitis and to check the fluid because early peritonitis may present atypically. In more severe cases, peritonitis is accompanied by nausea, vomiting,

Box 92-16 Differential Diagnosis of Altered Mental Status in Dialysis Patients

Structural

Cerebrovascular accident (particularly hemorrhage)
Subdural hematoma
Intracerebral abscess
Brain tumor

Metabolic

Disequilibrium syndrome
Uremia
Drug effects
Meningitis
Hypertensive encephalopathy
Hypotension
Postictal state
Hypernatremia or hyponatremia
Hypercalcemia
Hypermagnesemia
Hypoglycemia
Severe hyperglycemia
Hypoxemia
Dialysis dementia

severe pain, and hypotension requiring admission to the hospital and mandating consideration of the possibility of acute surgical disease.

In the ED the diagnosis of peritonitis is confirmed by the finding of more than 100 WBC/mm^3 in the peritoneal fluid, with a predominance of neutrophils, or by a positive Gram stain. To obtain a sample of fluid for analysis, the dialysate should be partially drained from the peritoneal cavity. (Draining the peritoneum completely and leaving the peritoneal cavity "dry" is often extremely painful in the presence of peritonitis.) Some of the fluid should be put into an open Vacutainer tube to be sent for cell count and differential. A few drops may be placed on a glass slide for an immediate Gram stain. The remainder of the fluid should be sent to the microbiology laboratory where concentration procedures (e.g., centrifugation) can be performed before Gram stain and cultures are done.

Occasionally, an otherwise asymptomatic patient who has recently begun CAPD notes the appearance of cloudy peritoneal fluid that proves on examination to contain many WBCs with a predominance of eosinophils. This condition, called eosinophilic peritonitis, is thought to represent a transient allergic reaction to some component of the fluid-delivery system.[137] Peritoneal fluid cultures are negative and the condition resolves without antibiotic therapy.

CAPD-associated peritonitis can usually be treated with an initial intraperitoneal loading dose of antibiotic, followed by a 10- to 14-day course of intraperitoneal antibiotics, of which some may be administered by the patient on an outpatient basis. Patients with CAPD are taught how to inject antibiotics into the dialysis bag at the time of an exchange and the proper sterile technique to be used. After making the diagnosis, the emergency physician should contact the patient's nephrologist or dialysis nurse specialist to discuss the choice of antibiotic and to agree on plans for outpatient management and follow-up evaluation or, occasionally if peritonitis is severe or if outpatient management is precluded by psychosocial considerations, for hospitalization.

A common treatment regimen is a loading dose of vancomycin, 30 mg/kg intraperitoneally, and an intraperitoneal or intravenous loading dose of a drug with broad gram-negative coverage (e.g., ceftazidime, aztreonam, or an aminoglycoside) (Table 92-4). Maintenance doses of all of the latter agents may be administered intraperitoneally once daily at the time of an exchange. Vancomycin requires reloading only once every 5 to 7 days.[138] Heparin (1,000 U) may also be added to each 2-L bag for the first few days of treatment to help reduce the formation of fibrin strands that may obstruct the catheter. Patients who usually receive insulin by the intraperitoneal route may have to increase their insulin dosage for a few days until the infection is under control. Patients should be seen by the dialysis nurse in 48 hours to check on the response to therapy and to adjust antibiotic therapy as necessary after reviewing the results of culture and sensitivity testing.

Catheter contamination or leaks from the catheter, tubing, or dialysate bag should be managed in the same fashion as frank peritonitis. The site and cause of leakage should be identified, and damaged elements should be replaced promptly. Occasionally, when there is leakage of peritoneal fluid from around the catheter, surgical correction is necessary.

Individuals who have severe abdominal pain, vomiting, ileus, chills or high fever, or hypotension should be admitted to the hospital. Likewise, patients with severe underlying illness and those who cannot reliably perform exchanges or administer antibiotics at home as necessary require inpatient management. Dialysis exchanges should be continued on the same schedule. The inpatient antibiotic regimen is essentially the same as that used for outpatients.

Table 92-4. Antibiotic Dosages for Treatment of CAPD-Associated Peritonitis

Drug	Loading dose	Maintenance dose
Vancomycin	30 mg/kg IP	30 mg/kg IP q5-7days
Ceftazidine	1 gm IP or IV	1 gm IP in 1 exchange daily
Aztreonam	3 gm IP or IV	1 gm IP in 1 exchange daily
Gentamicin*	2 mg/kg IP or IV	20 mg/L IP in 1 exchange daily

*Caution: ototoxicity.
CAPD, Continuous ambulatory peritoneal dialysis.

Perhaps the most serious potential pitfall in caring for the CAPD patient with abdominal pain or other signs of peritonitis is to overlook other serious intraabdominal conditions whose presentation may mimic that of peritonitis.[139-141] CAPD patients are at increased risk for abdominal or inguinal hernia because of chronically increased intraabdominal pressures; previous abdominal surgery also places them at risk for hernia, as well as for obstruction secondary to adhesions.[142] The manifestations of serious disorders unrelated to dialysis (e.g., acute appendicitis, diverticulitis, cholecystitis, acute pancreatitis, ischemic bowel, or perforated viscus) may also be attributed to ordinary CAPD-associated peritonitis, with the potential for disastrous consequences. The accessibility of the peritoneal fluid for examination may prove helpful in documenting the presence of an inflammatory process, but it also has the potential to mislead the emergency physician as to its cause. Certainly, a finding of brownish or fecal material in the peritoneal drainage should suggest a ruptured viscus until proven otherwise, and immediate surgical consultation should be sought. Detection of localized tenderness, a palpable mass, or an incarcerated hernia on physical examination can be extremely helpful in making the diagnosis. Abdominal radiography may be useful for demonstrating the presence of ileus, but pneumoperitoneum may be caused by the introduction of air during a recent fluid exchange rather than by a perforated viscus.[143] Occasionally, a lateral film demonstrates incarceration of a small portion of bowel protruding through the anterior abdominal wall. Thus, keeping in mind the possibility that disorders other than peritonitis may underlie the patient's symptoms, the emergency physician should maintain a lowered threshold for requesting surgical consultation or admitting the patient to the hospital for observation.

An often alarming but generally harmless occurrence is the appearance of a grossly bloody dialysate in a young female CAPD patient who is otherwise asymptomatic. Unless other findings are present, this is attributable to a small degree of retrograde menstruation that is thought to be common in many women.[144] Scanty, irregular menses are the rule in ESRD; conception can occur but is uncommon, and viable delivery is rare.[145]

Infection of the catheter exit site is another relatively common problem for which the CAPD patient may seek care in the ED.[134] This tends to be caused by typical skin flora and is manifested by the usual local signs of infection. Although not serious in themselves, exit-site infections should be taken seriously because they may lead to infection of the subcutaneous tunnel, which can cause repeated episodes of peritonitis and may ultimately necessitate removal of the catheter. Any visible exudate should be cultured and a Gram stain performed, and an oral antibiotic such as cephalexin should be started, pending the results of culture and sensitivity testing. The patient should be instructed to cleanse the site meticulously several times a day using povidone-iodine or peroxide solution.

Tunnel infections can be difficult to detect on physical examination and may be suspected only after the patient has several bouts of peritonitis caused by the same organism.[146] As with other closed-space infections, they tend to be difficult to eradicate unless the tunnel is partially unroofed and drained.[147]

CAPD patients may also present to the ED with any of several basically mechanical problems, of which the most common is inability to drain the dialysate completely at the time of an exchange.[148] Occasionally this is simply caused by kinking or inadvertent clamping of the external catheter or tubing, but more often it is the result of catheter obstruction by fibrinous debris or kinking or migration of the catheter within the peritoneal cavity. If fluid does not infuse normally, catheter obstruction is most likely. If the fluid infuses easily but fails to drain properly, it may be caused by loculation of the fluid or a check-valve effect of debris or omentum at the catheter tip; rolling the patient from side to side or effecting other changes in position may help. In either case, specific intervention may be guided by a contrast catheterogram.[149] Fibrinolytic agents have been used with success to open occluded catheters, but surgical intervention for catheter replacement is often required.[148]

CAPD patients generally care for themselves completely between routine visits to the nephrologist and dialysis nurse specialist. One consequence of this highly desirable independence, however, is that they may gradually develop volume or metabolic disturbances between visits. Although patients are instructed to weigh themselves daily and to measure their pulse and blood pressure frequently, some become progressively volume overloaded. The result may be only minor worsening of blood pressure control, but occasionally a patient develops acute pulmonary edema and requires immediate attention in the ED. Treatment strategies are the same as for hemodialysis patients, but even with hourly exchanges of 4.25% glucose dialysate solution, improvement may not be rapid, particularly when the presence of 2 L of fluid in the peritoneal cavity restricts lung expansion.

CAPD patients can also become volume depleted, particularly when oral intake is poor or when there has been significant GI fluid loss yet volume continues to be removed by dialysis. Oral or IV rehydration and further instruction on maintaining normal volume status are generally all that is necessary.

Severe metabolic disturbances are much less common among patients with CAPD than hemodialysis patients because with CAPD, dialysis is being performed essentially continuously and the blood remains in near equilibrium with the dialysate. Significant disturbances do occasionally occur, usually in association with hypercatabolic states, major dietary indiscretions, or significant GI fluid loss. One interesting derangement that occurs occasionally in diabetic patients on CAPD is a syndrome of severe hyperglycemia (sometimes even despite continuation of the usual insulin dose) resulting from absorption of glucose from hyperosmolar dialysate, with associated nonspecific symptoms of malaise, weakness, and headache. Although glucose levels may be as high as 1,500 mg/dl in these individuals, they cannot undergo an osmotic diuresis and remain clinically euvolemic.[150] Correction of hyperglycemia must be undertaken carefully to avoid causing rapid osmolar and volume shifts.

MISCELLANEOUS PROBLEMS AMONG PATIENTS WITH END-STAGE RENAL DISEASE

Perspective and Management

A number of vexing symptoms, although not associated with life-threatening illness, often have an important impact on the quality of life and occasionally seriously interfere with everyday functioning.

Nausea and vomiting not caused by medications, underdialysis, or the dialytic procedure itself (e.g., disequilibrium syndrome with hemodialysis or increased intraabdominal pressure with CAPD) occur intermittently and without apparent cause in many ESRD patients. Once anatomic disease of the GI tract has been ruled out (increased gastric rugae are commonly seen on an upper GI radiograph and appear to be without specific import), symptomatic relief can often be obtained with standard antiemetics such as prochlorperazine or trimethobenzamide. Diabetic gastroparesis often responds to metoclopramide, but dystonic reactions may occur unless the dosage is adjusted for renal failure.

Constipation is common among patients who take calcium-containing antacids to bind dietary phosphate. Oral sorbitol is generally effective in relieving constipation and does not have the potential danger of magnesium-containing cathartics. Stool-bulking agents and stool softeners are also helpful. Patients should be instructed not to use phosphate-containing enemas, which carry the risk of exacerbating hyperphosphatemia. Tap-water enemas are usually well tolerated, but water absorption can be considerable with long-term use.

Itching can be extremely distressing to the dialysis patient, and there is no uniformly satisfactory therapy. Most patients achieve some temporary relief with diphenhydramine or hydroxyzine. A variety of oil-based topical remedies for dry skin may be tried; local anesthetics should be avoided because of the risk of inducing an allergic dermatitis and worsening pruritus. Some patients have had success with ultraviolet light therapy, oral activated charcoal, or cholestyramine. When pruritus is clearly associated with severe hyperparathyroidism, parathyroidectomy may be curative.

Muscle cramps, particularly those occurring at night, are thought to be a manifestation of uremic myopathy or neuropathy and are not improved by dialysis. Cramps are usually effectively treated with oral quinine at bedtime or a benzodiazepine. Restless legs syndrome, probably another manifestation of uremic neuropathy, is typically difficult to treat. A variety of agents, including carbamazepine, bromocriptine, and clonazepam, have been recommended for this troublesome complaint.[151] Quinine or benzodiazepines should also be tried, but in some cases, sedatives or even narcotics are necessary.

KEY CONCEPTS

Acute Renal Failure

- The cause of acute renal failure can be classified into prerenal, postrenal, and intrinsic renal causes.
- Management of acute renal failure should be directed first at potentially lethal complications such as hyperkalemia or volume overload, and then at reversal of the underlying cause of renal dysfunction. It is important to avoid any further hemodynamic or toxic insults to the kidneys if at all possible.
- It is critical to consider the patient's impaired renal function when fluid administration regimens and drug dosages are prescribed.

Chronic Renal Failure

- Patients with chronic renal failure have a limited ability to handle fluid and solute loads and altered metabolism of many drugs; therefore fluid administration regimens and drug dosages should be checked carefully.
- The most rapidly lethal complication of chronic renal failure is hyperkalemia. This entity should always be considered a possibility, and appropriate diagnostic and therapeutic interventions should be instituted when indicated.
- Patients with renal failure often present with varying degrees of volume overload. This should be generally the first diagnostic consideration when dyspnea is the presenting complaint.

REFERENCES

1. Dennis VW, Robinson RR: Clinical proteinuria, *Adv Intern Med* 31:243, 1986.
2. Wright WT: Cell counts in urine, *Arch Intern Med* 103:76, 1959.
3. Northway JD: Hematuria in children, *J Pediatr* 78:381, 1971.
4. Braden GL et al: Urinary doubly refractile lipid bodies in nonglomerular renal disease, *Am J Kidney Dis* 11:332, 1988.
5. Nolan CR III, Anger MS, Kelleher SP: Eosinophiluria: a new method of detection and definition of the clinical spectrum, *N Engl J Med* 315:1516, 1986.
6. Steiner RW: Interpreting the fractional excretion of sodium, *Am J Med* 77:699, 1984.
7. Miller TJ et al: Urinary diagnostic indices in acute renal failure: a prospective study, *Ann Intern Med* 89:47, 1978.
8. Espinel CH: The FENa test: use in the differential diagnosis of acute renal failure, *JAMA* 236:579, 1976.
9. Berns AS: Nephrotoxicity of contrast media, *Kidney Int* 36:730, 1989.
10. Ellenbogen PH et al: Sensitivity of grey scale ultrasound in detecting urinary tract obstruction, *Am J Roentgenol* 130:731,1978.
11. Edell S, Zegel H: Ultrasonic evaluation of renal calculi, *Am J Roentgenol* 130:261, 1978.
12. Schoolwerth AC: Hematuria and proteinuria: their causes and consequences, *Hosp Pract* 22:45, 1987.
13. Antolak SJ Jr, Mellinger GT: Urologic evaluation of hematuria occurring during anticoagulant therapy, *J Urol* 101:111, 1969.
14. Siegel AJ et al: Exercise-related hematuria: findings in a group of marathon runners, *JAMA* 241:391, 1979.
15. Corwin HL, Bray RA, Haber MH: The detection and interpretation of urinary eosinophils, *Arch Pathol Lab Med* 113:1256, 1989.
16. Viewig J et al: Unenhanced helical computerized tomography for the evaluation of patients with acute flank pain, *J Urol* 160:1465, 2000.
17. Eberst ME, Berkowitz LR: Hemostasis in renal disease: pathophysiology and management, *Am J Med* 96:168, 1994.
18. Rudnick MR et al: The differential diagnosis of acute renal failure. In Brenner BM, Lazarus JM, editors: *Acute renal failure,* ed 2, Melbourne, 1988, Churchill Livingstone.
19. Clive DM, Stoff JS: Renal syndromes associated with non-steroidal antiinflammatory drugs, *N Engl J Med* 310:563, 1984.
20. Perazella MA: Crystal-induced acute renal failure. *Am J Med* 106:459, 1999.
21. Nadig PW, Yalk WL: Recovery from obstructive disease, *J Urol* 88:470, 1962.
22. Badalamenti S et al: Hepatorenal syndrome, *Arch Intern Med* 153:1957, 1993.
23. Whelton A et al: Effects of celecoxib and naproxen on renal function in the elderly, *Arch Intern Med* 160:1465, 2000.
24. Walter BL, Grunau CFV, Parman SC: Renal artery obstruction, *Ann Emerg Med* 14:607, 1985.
25. Boyce TG, Swerdlow DL, Griffin PM: *Escherichia coli* O157:H7 and the hemolytic-uremic syndrome, *N Engl J Med* 333: 364, 1995.
26. Bakir AA, Bazilinski N, Dunea G: Transient and sustained recovery from renal shutdown in accelerated hypertension, *Am J Med* 80:172,1986.
27. Steen VD et al: Outcome of renal crisis in systemic sclerosis: relation to availability of angiotensin converting enzyme (ACE) inhibitors, *Ann Intern Med* 113:352, 1990.
28. Brady HR et al: Acute renal failure. In Brenner BM, editor: *The kidney,* ed 6, Philadelphia, 2000, WB Saunders.
29. Wilkins RG, Faragher EB: Acute renal failure in an intensive care unit: incidence, prediction and outcome, *Anesthesia* 38:628, 1983.
30. Abel RM et al: Etiology, incidence and prognosis of renal failure following cardiac operations: results of a prospective analysis of 500 consecutive patients, *J Thorac Cardiovasc Surg* 71:323, 1976.
31. Koffler A, Friedler RM, Massry SG: Acute renal failure due to non-traumatic rhabdomyolysis, *Ann Intern Med* 85:23, 1976.
32. Gabow PA, Kaehny WD, Kelleher SP: The spectrum of rhabdomyolysis, *Medicine* 61:141, 1982.
33. Barza M et al: Single or multiple daily doses of aminoglycosides: a meta-analysis, *BMJ* 312:338, 1996.
34. Hatala R, Dinh T, Cook DJ: Once-daily aminoglycoside dosing in immunocompetent adults: a meta-analysis, *Ann Intern Med* 124: 717,1996.
35. Hewitt WL: Gentamicin: toxicity in perspective, *Postgrad Med J* 50(Suppl 7):55, 1974.
36. Berkseth RO, Kjellstrand CM: Radiologic contrast-induced nephropathy, *Med Clin North Am* 68:351, 1984.
37. Lautin EM et al: Radiocontrast-associated renal dysfunction: incidence and risk factors, *Am J Radiol* 157:49, 1991.
38. Byrd L, Sherman RL: Radiocontrast-induced acute renal failure: a clinical and pathophysiological review, *Medicine* 58:270, 1979.
39. Parfrey PS et al: Contrast material-induced renal failure in patients with diabetes mellitus, renal insufficiency, or both, *N Engl J Med* 320:143, 1989.
40. Solomon R et al: Effects of saline, mannitol, and furosemide on acute decreases in renal function induced by radiocontrast agents, *N Engl J Med* 331:1416, 1994.
41. Cochran ST, Wong WS, Roe DJ: Predicting angiography-induced renal function impairment: clinical risk model, *Am J Radiol* 141:1027, 1983.
42. Barrett BJ, Carlisle EJ: Metaanalysis of the relative nephrotoxicity of high- and low-osmolality iodinated contrast media, *Radiology* 188:171, 1993.
43. Lyons K, Matthews P, Evans C: Obstructive uropathy without dilatation: a potential diagnostic pitfall, *BMJ* 296:1517, 1988.
44. Bennett WM et al: *Drug prescribing in renal failure: dosing guidelines for adults,* ed 4, Philadelphia, 1999, American College of Physicians.
45. Solomon R: Managing acute renal failure: do vasodilators and diuretics have a role? *J Crit Illness* 13:709, 1998.
46. Shilliday IR et al: Loop diuretics in the management of acute renal failure: a prospective, double-blind, placebo-controlled, randomized study. *Nephrol Dial Transplant* 12:2592, 1997.

47. Chertow GM et al: Is the administration of dopamine associated with adverse or favorable outcomes in acute renal failure? *Am J Med* 101:49, 1996.
48. Marik PE, Iglesias J: Low-dose dopamine does not prevent acute renal failure in patients with septic shock and oliguria, *Am J Med* 107:387, 1999.
49. Ron D et al: Prevention of acute renal failure in traumatic rhabdomyolysis, *Arch Intern Med* 144:277, 1984.
50. Better OS, Stein JH: Early management of shock and prophylaxis of acute renal failure in traumatic rhabdomyolysis, *N Engl J Med* 322:825, 1990.
51. Allon M, Dunlay R, Copkney C: Nebulized albuterol for acute hyperkalemia in patients on hemodialysis, *Ann Intern Med* 110:426, 1989.
52. Akmal M et al: Hypocalcemia and hypercalcemia in patients with rhabdomyolysis with and without renal failure, *J Clin Endocrinol Metab* 63:137, 1986.
53. Randall RE Jr et al: Hypermagnesemia in renal failure: etiology and toxic manifestations, *Ann Intern Med* 61:73, 1974.
54. Kelton J, Kelly WN, Holmes EW: A rapid method for the diagnosis of acute uric acid nephropathy, *Arch Intern Med* 138:612, 1978.
55. Bagdade JD: Hyperlipidemia and atherosclerosis in chronic dialysis patients. In Drukker W, Parson FM, Maher JF, editors: *Replacement of renal function by dialysis,* ed 2, Boston, 1983, Martinus Nijhoff.
56. Luke RG: Chronic renal failure—a vasculopathic state, *N Engl J Med* 339:841, 1998.
57. Lazarus JM et al: Cardiovascular disease in uremic patients on hemodialysis, *Kidney Int* 7(Suppl 2):S167, 1975.
58. Goodman WG et al: Coronary-artery calcification in young adults with end-stage renal disease who are undergoing dialysis, *N Engl J Med* 342:1478, 2000.
59. Kohen JA, Opsahl JA, Kjellstrand CM: Deceptive patterns of uremic pulmonary edema, *Am J Kidney Dis* 7:456, 1986.
60. Mahoney CA, Arieff AI: Uremic encephalopathies: clinical, biochemical, and experimental features, *Am J Kidney Dis* 2:324, 1982.
61. Fraser CL, Arieff AI: Nervous system complications in uremia, *Ann Intern Med* 109:143, 1988.
62. Llach F, Bover J: Renal osteodystrophies. In Brenner BM, editor: *The kidney,* ed 6, Philadelphia, 2000, WB Saunders.
63. Hoffman GS et al: Calcium oxalate microcrystalline-associated arthritis in end-stage renal disease, *Ann Intern Med* 97:36, 1982.
64. Lotem M, Bernheim J, Conforty B: Spontaneous rupture of tendons: a complication of hemodialyzed patients treated for renal failure, *Nephron* 21:201, 1978.
65. Schwarz A et al: Carpal tunnel syndrome: a major complication in long-term hemodialysis patients, *Clin Nephrol* 22:133, 1984.
66. Port FK: Mortality and causes of death in patients with end-stage renal failure, *Am J Kidney Dis* 15:215, 1990.
67. Goldblum SE, Reed WP: Host defenses and immunologic alterations associated with chronic hemodialysis, *Ann Intern Med* 93:597, 1980.
68. Keane WF, Raij LR: Host defenses and infectious complications in maintenance hemodialysis patients. In Drukker W, Parson FM, Maher JF, editors: *Replacement of renal function by dialysis,* ed 2, Boston, 1983, Martinus Nijhoff.
69. Raskova J et al: B-cell activation and immunoregulation in end-stage renal disease patients receiving hemodialysis, *Arch Intern Med* 147:89, 1987.
70. Ruiz P, Gomez F, Schreiber AD: Impaired function of macrophage Fcχ receptors in end-stage renal disease, *N Engl J Med* 322:770, 1990.
71. Tolkoff-Rubin NE, Rubin RH: Uremia and host defenses, *N Engl J Med* 322:770, 1990.
72. Ziyadeh FN: Approach to the patient with chronic renal failure. In Kelley WN, editor: *Textbook of internal medicine,* ed 3, Philadelphia, 1997, Lippincott-Raven.
73. Thurm LH, Alexander JC: Captopril in the treatment of scleroderma renal crisis, *Arch Intern Med* 144:733, 1984.
74. Abuelo JG: Renal failure caused by chemicals, foods, plants, animal venoms, and misuse of drugs, *Arch Intern Med* 150:505, 1990.
75. Hricik DE et al: Captopril-induced functional renal insufficiency in patients with bilateral renal-artery stenoses or renal-artery stenosis in a solitary kidney, *N Engl J Med* 308:373, 1983.
76. Wolfson AB, Singer I: Hemodialysis-related emergencies: part I, *J Emerg Med* 5:533, 1987.
77. Bennett WM et al: *Drug prescribing in renal failure: dosing guidelines for adults,* ed 4, Philadelphia, 1999, American College of Physicians.
78. Lefkowitz MP, Szerlip HM, Wolfson AB: Electrolyte emergencies. In Wolfson AB, Harwood-Nuss A, editors: *Renal and urologic emergencies,* New York, 1986, Churchill Livingstone.
79. Palevsky PM, Singer I: Disorders of potassium metabolism. In Wolfson AB, editor: *Endocrine and metabolic emergencies,* New York, 1990, Churchill Livingstone.
80. Szerlip HM, Weiss J, Singer I: Profound hyperkalemia without electrocardiographic manifestations, *Am J Kidney Dis* 7:461, 1986.
81. Allon M, Dunlay R, Copkney C: Nebulized albuterol for acute hyperkalemia in patients on hemodialysis, *Ann Intern Med* 110:426, 1, 1989.
82. Montoliu J et al: Treatment of hyperkalemia in renal failure with salbutamol inhalation, *J Intern Med* 228:35, 1990.
83. Pillay VKG et al: Transient and permanent deafness following treatment with ethacrynic acid in renal failure, *Lancet* 1:77, 1969.
84. Anderson CC, Shahvari MBG, Zimmerman JE: The treatment of pulmonary edema in the absence of renal function, *JAMA* 241:1008, 1979.
85. Gehm L, Propp DA: Pulmonary edema in the renal failure patient, *Am J Emerg Med* 7:336, 1989.
86. Huff JS, Whelan TV: CPAP as adjunctive treatment of severe pulmonary edema in patients with ESRD, *Am J Emerg Med* 12:388, 1994.
87. Sacchetti A et al: ED management of acute congestive heart failure in renal dialysis patients, *Am J Emerg Med* 11:644, 1993.
88. Schneider RE et al: Immediate hemodynamic response to furosemide in patients undergoing chronic hemodialysis, *Am J Kidney Dis* 9:55, 1987.
89. Schwab SJ, Weaver ME: Penetration of trimethoprim and sulfamethoxazole into cysts in a patient with autosomal-dominant polycystic kidney disease, *Am J Kidney Dis* 7:434, 1986.
90. Sklar AH et al: Renal infections in autosomal dominant polycystic kidney disease, *Am J Kidney Dis* 10:81, 1987.
91. Levey AS, Harrington JT: Continuous peritoneal dialysis for chronic renal failure, *Medicine* 61:330, 1982.
92. De Fijter CWH et al: Clinical efficacy and morbidity associated with continuous cyclic compared with continuous ambulatory peritoneal dialysis, *Ann Intern Med* 120:264, 1994.
93. Wehle B et al: Hemodynamic changes during sequential ultrafiltration and dialysis, *Kidney Int* 15:411, 1979.
94. Finnerty FA Jr: Hypertensive encephalopathy, *Am J Med* 52:672, 1972.
95. Elkayam U et al: Pericardial involvement in asymptomatic patients undergoing long-term hemodialysis: an echocardiographic study, *Eur J Cardiol* 11:445, 1980.
96. Frommer JP, Young JB, Ayus JC: Asymptomatic pericardial effusion in uremic patients: effect of long-term dialysis, *Nephron* 39:296, 1985.
97. Spector D et al: A controlled study of the effect of indomethacin in uremic pericarditis, *Kidney Int* 24:663, 1983.
98. Wolfson AB, Singer I: Hemodialysis-related emergencies: part II, *J Emerg Med* 6:61, 1988.
99. Wolfson AB: End-stage renal disease: emergencies related to dialysis and transplantation. In Wolfson AB, Harwood-Nuss AH, editors: *Renal and urologic emergencies,* New York, 1986, Churchill Livingstone.
100. Denker BM, Chertow GM, Owers WS Jr: Hemodialysis. In Brenner BM, editor: *The kidney,* ed 6, Philadelphia, 2000, WB Saunders.
101. Butt KMH: Angioaccess. In Drukker W, Parson FM, Maher JF, editors: *Replacement of renal function by dialysis,* ed 2, Boston, 1983, Martinus Nijhoff.
102. Waltzer WC, Rapaport FT, editors: *Angioaccess,* New York, 1984, Grune & Stratton.
103. Francioli P, Masur H: Complications of *Staphylococcus aureus* bacteremia, *Arch Intern Med* 142:1655, 1982.
104. Henderson LW: Symptomatic hypotension during hemodialysis, *Kidney Int* 17:571, 1980.
105. Henrich WL: Hemodynamic instability during hemodialysis, *Kidney Int* 30:605, 1986.

106. Morrison G et al: Mechanism and prevention of cardiac arrhythmias in chronic hemodialysis patients, *Kidney Int* 17:811, 1980.
107. Eschbach JW et al: Correction of the anemia of end-stage renal disease with recombinant human erythropoietin, *N Engl J Med* 316:73, 1987.
108. Eschbach JW et al: Recombinant human erythropoietin in anemic patients with end-stage renal disease, *Ann Intern Med* 111:992, 1989.
109. Hakim RM, Schafer AI: Hemodialysis-associated platelet activation and thrombocytopenia, *Am J Med* 78:575, 1985.
110. Eberst ME, Berkowitz LR: Hemostasis in renal disease: pathophysiology and management, *Am J Med* 96:168, 1994.
111. Mannucci PM et al: Deamino-8-D-arginine vasopressin shortens the bleeding time in uremia, *N Engl J Med* 303:8, 1983.
112. Janson PA et al: Treatment of the bleeding tendency in uremia with cryoprecipitate, *N Engl J Med* 303:1318, 1980.
113. Shemin D et al: Oral estrogens decrease bleeding time and improve clinical bleeding in patients with renal failure, *Am J Med* 89:436, 1990.
114. Vigano G et al: Recombinant human erythropoietin to correct uremic bleeding, *Am J Kidney Dis* 18:4,1991.
115. Zuckerman GR et al: Upper gastrointestinal bleeding in patients with chronic renal failure, *Ann Intern Med* 102:588, 1985.
116. Blackstone MO: Angiodysplasia and gastrointestinal bleeding in chronic renal failure, *Ann Intern Med* 103:805, 1985.
117. Hakim RM et al: Complement activation and hypersensitivity reactions to dialysis membranes, *N Engl J Med* 311:878, 1984.
118. Daugirdas JT et al: Severe anaphylactoid reactions to cuprammonium cellulose hemodialyzers, *Arch Intern Med* 145:489, 1985.
119. Marshall CP et al: Reactions during hemodialysis caused by allergy to ethylene oxide gas sterilization, *J Allergy Clin Immunol* 75:563, 1985.
120. Ward MK et al: Air embolism during haemodialysis, *BMJ* 3:74, 1971.
121. Cardoso M et al: Hypoxemia during hemodialysis: a critical review of the facts, *Am J Kidney Dis* 11:281, 1988.
122. Consensus Development Conference Panel: Morbidity and mortality of renal dialysis: an NIH consensus conference statement, *Ann Intern Med* 121:62, 1994.
123. Bleyer AJ, Russell GB, Satko SG: Sudden and cardiac death rates in hemodialysis patients, *Kidney Int* 55:1553, 1999.
124. Rostand SG, Kirk KA, Rutsky EA: Dialysis-associated ischemic heart disease: insights from coronary angiography, *Kidney Int* 25:653, 1984.
125. Lee TH, Goldman LP: Serum enzyme assays in the diagnosis of acute myocardial infarction, *Ann Intern Med* 105:221, 1986.
126. Martin GS, Becker BN, Schulman G: Cardiac troponin-I accurately predicts myocardial injury in renal failure, *Nephrol Dial Transplant* 13:1709, 1998.
127. Musso P et al: Cardiac troponin elevations in chronic renal failure: prevalence and clinical significance, *Clin Biochem* 2:125, 1999.
128. George SK, Singh AK: Current markers of myocardial ischemia and their validity in end-stage renal disease, *Curr Opin Nephrol Hypertens* 8:719, 1999.
129. Chen P, Tanasijevic M: Use of cardiac troponin-I levels in dialysis patients, *Semin Dial* 13:58, 2000.
130. Minuth ANW et al: Indomethacin treatment of pericarditis in chronic hemodialysis patients, *Arch Intern Med* 135:807, 1975.
131. Buselmeier TJ et al: Uremic pericardial effusion, *Nephron* 16:371, 1976.
132. Gloor HJ et al: Peritoneal access and related complications in continuous ambulatory peritoneal dialysis, *Am J Med* 74:593, 1983.
133. Vas SI: Microbiologic aspects of chronic ambulatory peritoneal dialysis, *Kidney Int* 23:83, 1983.
134. Piraino B, Bernardini J, Sorkin M: The influence of peritoneal catheter exit-site infections on peritonitis, tunnel infections, and catheter loss in patients on continuous ambulatory peritoneal dialysis, *Am J Kidney Dis* 8:436, 1986.
135. Rubin J et al: Fungal peritonitis during continuous ambulatory peritoneal dialysis: a report of 17 cases, *Am J Kidney Dis* 10:361, 1987.
136. Holley JL, Bernardini J, Piraino B: Polymicrobial peritonitis in patients on continuous peritoneal dialysis, *Am J Kidney Dis* 19:162, 1992.
137. Gokal R et al: "Eosinophilic" peritonitis in continuous ambulatory peritoneal dialysis (CAPD), *Clin Nephrol* 15:328, 1981.
138. Boyce NW et al: Intraperitoneal (IP) vancomycin therapy for CAPD peritonitis—a prospective, randomized comparison of intermittent vs. continuous therapy, *Am J Kidney Dis* 12:304, 1988.
139. Steiner RW, Halasz NA: Abdominal catastrophes and other unusual events in continuous ambulatory peritoneal dialysis patients, *Am J Kidney Dis* 15:1, 1990.
140. McDonald RJ et al: Concomitant surgical illness in CAPD patients (abstract), *Perit Dial Int* 8:89, 1988.
141. Royce VL, Jensen DM, Corwin HL: Pancreatic enzymes in chronic renal failure, *Arch Intern Med* 147:537, 1987.
142. Digenis GE et al: Abdominal hernias in patients undergoing continuous ambulatory peritoneal dialysis, *Perit Dial Bull* 2:115, 1982.
143. Kiefer T et al: Incidence and significance of pneumoperitoneum in continuous ambulatory peritoneal dialysis, *Am J Kidney Dis* 22:30, 1993.
144. Blumenkrantz MJ et al: Retrograde menstruation in women undergoing chronic peritoneal dialysis, *Obstet Gynecol* 57:667, 1981.
145. Cattran DC, Benzie RJ: Pregnancy in a continuous ambulatory peritoneal dialysis patient, *Perit Dial Bull* 3:13, 1983.
146. Holley JL et al: Ultrasound as a tool in the diagnosis and management of exit-site infections in patients undergoing continuous ambulatory peritoneal dialysis, *Am J Kidney Dis* 14:211, 1989.
147. Andreoli SP et al: A technique to eradicate tunnel infection without peritoneal dialysis catheter removal, *Perit Dial Bull* 4:156, 1984.
148. Davis R et al: Management of chronic peritoneal catheter malfunction, *Am J Nephrol* 2:85, 1982.
149. Andersen KE, Damgaard M, Torch P: Catheterography in the diagnosis of catheter failure in peritoneal dialysis, *Clin Nephrol* 17:228, 1981.
150. Al-Kudsi RR et al: Extreme hyperglycemia in dialysis patients, *Clin Nephrol* 17:228, 1982.
151. McGee S: Restless legs syndrome, *JAMA* 22:3014, 1991.

93 Genital Infections

Deborah A. Mulligan-Smith

PERSPECTIVE

Patients with genital infections come to the ED with a wide range of signs and symptoms. Some patients complain of vaginal discharge; others have life-threatening peritonitis. It is especially important that the emergency physician accurately diagnose and treat these infections.

Most genital infections are sexually transmitted diseases (STDs), and simultaneous treatment of the patient and sexual contacts prevents further spread in the community. Despite aggressive public education programs, infection with common STDs is on the rise.[1,2] This increase may be due in part to improved surveillance.[2-6] Sexually transmitted diseases have a disproportionate impact on youth, with 3 million adolescents estimated to be infected each year. *Chlamydia trachomatis* infection and gonorrhea are the most common bacterial STDs in the United States.[7] The highest age-specific rates for chlamydia and gonorrhea are found in adolescents and youth in their early twenties.[1,2] Female adolescents and young women are more susceptible to STDs than are older women.[8-10] Early treatment of genital infections in many cases prevents compromise of future reproductive function. There are more than 20 known bacterial, viral, or mycotic causes of sexually transmitted infections. Two or more genital infections may coexist and require appropriate treatment. It is essential that all patients with genital infections receive follow-up care. Finally, the physician may need to consider using alternative drugs to treat genital infections occurring during pregnancy. Table 93-1 lists first-line antibiotic treatment for the entities discussed in this chapter and acceptable alternative therapies.[11]

The economic cost of STDs is staggering, with annual direct and indirect costs estimated to be $10 billion for STDs, much of which is preventable.[1] For chlamydia alone, 75% of the annual $1.5 billion cost is associated with the sequelae of untreated infections that were uncomplicated initially. Screening for chlamydia among females, in particular, has been estimated to be cost-effective, saving as much as $12 for each dollar spent in early detection and treatment.[4,6,7,9,10]

All of the genital infections, including the uncommon ones, discussed in this chapter have been reported in children. STDs are the most common reported infectious diseases among sexually active adolescents.[23] Diagnosis of these infections in children or adolescents requires a particularly aggressive search. Symptoms may be difficult to elicit, and signs may be minimal or absent. Obtaining the information can be difficult because the child's illness is often intertwined with an emotionally charged social situation.[2] Although voluntary sexual contact increases after the age of 10 years, the role of nonsexual physical contact with infected individuals or contaminated objects should not be ignored.[11] The presence of an STD in a prepubertal child is presumptive evidence of sexual abuse and should be investigated.[12]

Often too self-conscious to engage the physician in a health-related dialogue, the adolescent needs a health professional who is innovative, knowledgeable, and caring.[13] Unless otherwise requested, it is advisable to excuse family members and friends from the interview process. The confidential setting allows the patient to freely discuss the sexual health history. The physician should question the sexually active adolescent about the types and frequencies of sexual experiences, birth control methods, and number of partners. By the end of high school, 80% of students are sexually active and 32% report having four or more lifetime sex partners.[1,2] Most states allow treatment of STDs in minors above a statutory age without parental consent.[3,9] The adolescent's potential for poor compliance can be addressed by specific treatment in the ED. The promotion of healthy and responsible sexual decision making is one of the goals of counseling adolescents already engaged in sexual intercourse about contraceptive methods and prevention of STDs.[5]

Table 93-1. First-Line Treatments for Uncomplicated Genital Infections in Nonallergic Patients

Infection	Treatment of nonpregnant patients	Treatment of pregnant patients
Gonorrhea (uncomplicated infection of the cervix, urethra, and rectum)	Cefixime 400 mg po OR ceftriaxone 125 mg IM OR ciprofloxacin 500 mg po OR ofloxacin 400 mg po OR azithromycin 1 g po OR doxycycline 100 mg po bid × 7d	Cefixime 400 mg po OR ceftriaxone 125 mg IM OR spectinomycin 2 g IM
Chlamydia	Azithromycin 1 g po OR doxycycline 100 mg po bid × 7d	Erythromycin base 500 mg po qid × 7 d OR amoxicillin po tid × 7d
Syphilis	Benzathine penicillin G 2.4 million units IM	Same
Chancroid	Azithromycin 1 g po OR ceftriaxone 250 mg IM OR ciprofloxacin 500 mg po bid × 3d OR erythromycin base 500 mg po qid × 7d	Erythromycin base 500 mg po qid × 7d
Lymphogranuloma venereum	Doxycycline 100 mg po bid × 21d	Erythromycin base 500 mg po qid × 21d
Granuloma inguinale	Trimethoprim-sulfamethoxazole DS po bid × 21d OR Doxycycline 100 mg po bid × 21d or until healing occurs	Erythromycin base 500 mg po qid × 21d or until healing occurs
Papillomavirus	Cryotherapy	Same
Herpes simplex virus	Acyclovir 400 mg po tid for 7-10 days OR 200 mg po 5 times a day × 7-10d	Acyclovir for first clinical episode only; not recommended for routine use of recurrent disease
Bacterial vaginosis	Metronidazole 500 mg po bid × 7d OR clindamycin cream 2% (5 g) intravaginally qhs × 7d OR metronidazole gel 0.75% 5 g intravaginally bid × 5d	Metronidazole 250 mg po tid × 7d OR metronidazole gel 0.75% 5 g intravaginally bid × 5d OR clindamycin 300 mg po bid × 7d
Trichomoniasis	Metronidazole 2 g po	Same
Candidiasis	Fluconazole 150 mg po OR intravaginal agents, such as clotrimazole 100 mg vaginal tablet × 7d, miconazole 2% cream, 5 g intravaginally × 7d	Butoconazole 2% cream 5 g intravaginally for 7d OR clotrimazole 1% cream 5 g intravaginally for 7d OR miconazole 2% cream (5 g) intravaginally × 7d

This chapter reviews the management of genital lesions, genital discharge, pelvic inflammatory disease (PID), and toxic shock syndrome.

SPECIFIC DISORDERS

Genital Lesions

Genital lesions vary widely in their morphologic characteristics and treatment. Although not all of these lesions are venereal, it is appropriate to assume so until laboratory testing proves otherwise. This section discusses the management of common genital lesions.

Genital Herpes Simplex The herpes simplex viruses (HSV) encompass two large deoxyribonucleic acid (DNA) strains, HSV-1 and HSV-2, which are structurally and immunologically closely related and are the most common cause of genital ulceration.[14] HSV-1 is usually associated with oral lesions but may cause genital lesions as well. Primary HSV infection generally is responsible for a more significant clinical syndrome than recurrent HSV. Primary HSV illness may last up to 3 weeks. After resolution of the skin lesions, the virus becomes latent by entering spinal nerve root ganglia and is reactivated at irregular intervals by unknown triggers. The recurrent disease is clinically less severe and resolves in 9 to 10 days.[15] With the primary infection, patients report painful, itching, grouped vesicular, or ulcerated lesions. Urethral or cervical involvement results in a mucopurulent discharge. Fever, chills, abdominal pain, myalgias, aseptic meningitis, headache, malaise, lymphadenopathy, and photophobia may be present. The characteristic grouped vesicles on an erythematous base may be obvious if there is penile, vaginal, labial, or prelabial skin involvement. Patients with genital herpes and other ulcerative lesions are at greater risk for human immunodeficiency virus (HIV) infection than the general population.[11]

A nonspecific ulceration or friability may be the only clue to HSV cervicitis. Urethritis often produces a clear, mucoid discharge associated with dysuria. With urethral involvement, dysuria may be sufficiently severe to cause urinary retention. Recurrent HSV infection produces similar, smaller vesicular lesions, but there are usually no systemic manifestations. Many patients report itching, burning or paresthesias a few hours before recurrence of the lesions.[16]

HSV infections are often obvious. If there is doubt or a need to confirm the diagnosis, a simple Tzanck slide preparation reveals the characteristic multinucleated giant cells approximately 50% of the time. Useful stains are Wright's stain and methylene blue. Vesicular contents provide the best material; the liquid is smeared on the slide, stained, and examined microscopically. Direct fluorescent assay and enzyme-linked immunosorbent assay (ELISA) techniques require between 20 minutes and 4 hours and are approximately 80% sensitive compared with tissue culture, the standard for laboratory diagnosis.[17]

Oral acyclovir, 400 mg three times a day for 7 to 10 days or 200 mg five times a day for 7 to 10 days, decreases the duration and severity of the signs and symptoms of genital herpes. The same dosage given for 5 days may be used for symptomatic recurrent infections as intermittent therapy. When treatment is instituted during the prodrome or within 2 days of onset of lesions, some patients with recurrent disease experience limited benefit from therapy. However, because early treatment can seldom be administered, most immunocompetent patients with recurrent disease do not benefit from acyclovir treatment, and it is generally not recommended. IV acyclovir, 10 mg/kg every 8 hours for 10 days, and hospital admission are reserved for patients with severe or systemic symptoms, neurologic complications, or disseminated disease. Acyclovir, 400 mg five times a day for 10 days, is the treatment of choice for first episodes of herpes proctitis.[16] After several untreated recurrences, consider a trial with famciclovir to determine whether there is significant change in duration of symptoms before patient-initiated treatments. Disseminated HSV infection may occur in immunocompromised or pregnant patients with high mortality because of involvement of the central nervous system, lungs, and abdominal viscera. Parenteral therapy is indicated in these cases.

Perhaps the major concern of HSV infections is the possible transmission to the neonate. The virus can infect the intrapartum infant, resulting in chorioamnionitis, abortion, premature delivery, or intrauterine growth retardation. Neonatal problems include encephalitis, disseminated infection, and high mortality.[18] Women with a history of contact with sexual partners with genital HSV should receive screening viral cultures beginning between 32 and 37 weeks of pregnancy. The risk of HSV infection in an infant delivered vaginally to a mother with a first-episode, primary genital infection is between 33% and 50%. The risk of infection to the infant of a mother with recurrent HSV at the time of delivery is 3% to 5%.[19] In general, only the pregnancies of women with clinically suspicious lesions who actually shed the virus near term should be delivered by cesarean section.[19]

Bartholin Cyst and Abscess A Bartholin abscess is a Bartholin gland or duct cyst infected by any number of organisms, including *Neisseria gonorrhoeae, C. trachomatis, Escherichia coli,* and *Proteus mirabilis.* Mixed infections are common.[13,14] The gland normally secretes fluid into the duct that exists at the mucosal surface of the labia. The glands and ducts are neither palpable nor visible unless infected or inflamed. The patient with a Bartholin cyst complains of a relatively painless lump at the lower lateral introitus. On examination, there is a tense, nontender, ovoid mass just lateral and adjacent to the posterior fourchette. Patients with few symptoms can be treated with sitz baths and follow-up monitoring, but large or painful cysts require incision and drainage.

The patient with a Bartholin abscess complains of unilateral swelling and pain at the lower lateral vaginal opening, often making sitting or walking difficult. There are usually no systemic symptoms. Examination reveals an extremely tender, fluctuant, ovoid to spherical mass at the same location as the cyst. There is often surrounding edema and erythema of the labia majora. The Bartholin abscess, like other closed-space infections, requires incision and drainage. The emergency physician should incise the abscess on the mucosal surface of the vestibule just lateral to the hymenal ring. Iodoform gauze, a Penrose drain, or a Word catheter is placed for 24 hours to promote drainage. A Word catheter is a 10 Fr, 5-cm long latex catheter with a 5-ml balloon. After incision, the catheter is placed in the abscess cavity and inflated with water. Sitz baths promote continued drainage. Concurrent vaginal, cervical, or urethral infection requires appropriate antibiotic therapy.[20]

Syphilis Syphilis is a venereal disease caused by the spirochete *Treponema pallidum.* Patients usually go to the ED with one of the three symptom complexes: a genital lesion (chancre), enlarged inguinal lymph nodes (satellite buboes), or the rash of secondary syphilis.[21] Tabes dorsalis, general paresis, and luetic aortitis, manifestations of tertiary syphilis, are rare and occur years after the original infection. A strong correlation between syphilis and HIV infection has been demonstrated in several studies. After appropriate consent and counseling, all patients with confirmed syphilis should receive HIV testing.[22]

Primary Syphilis A small papule develops at the site of inoculation 10 to 90 days after exposure. This papule then becomes a painless, indurated ulcer, the classic chancre, which heals spontaneously in 4 to 5 days. Although serologic tests are often negative at this stage, scrapings obtained from the chancre and examined under dark-field microscopy reveal moving, corkscrew-like treponemes. Approximately 4 weeks after exposure, the infected patient may have firm, rubbery, nontender inguinal adenopathy. Material obtained from the nodes is dark-field positive, and serologic examination usually confirms infection.[23]

Secondary Syphilis The rash of secondary syphilis appears 6 to 20 weeks after exposure. The rash makes diagnosis easy if it is typical, that is, maculopapular, symmetric, and involving the palms and soles. Although this "great masquerader" may mimic virtually any dermatologic condition, a scraping of a syphilitic lesion reveals spirochetes under dark-field examination. Serologic studies are nearly always positive. Condylomata lata (flat warts), patchy alopecia, and loss of the lateral third of the eyebrow are often present. Patients may develop fever, chills, lethargy, generalized lymphadenopathy, and clinical and laboratory evidence of hepatic or renal infection. Many patients, particularly children, may have nonspecific findings such as fever, sore throat, headache, or malaise.[24]

Emergency physicians should initiate treatment for patients with laboratory-proven syphilis (Table 93-2). Patients with persistent signs and symptoms or whose treponemal test titers fail to fall are considered treatment failures. After evaluation for neurosyphilis and HIV infection, patients usually receive the late disease regimen.[25] In general, penicillin-allergic, HIV-infected, and pregnant patients who require treatment for syphilis should receive the appropriate penicillin regimen, after testing and desensitization. Infants should be treated if their mothers had untreated syphilis at delivery, were treated less than 30 days before delivery, or had evidence of relapse or reinfection after treatment. All patients require follow-up evaluation for at least 1 year after treatment or until serologic studies show falling antibody titers.[11]

Lymphogranuloma Venereum Lymphogranuloma venereum (LGV) is an uncommon STD caused by *C. trachomatis.* The initial lesion is a small, shallow, painless, evanescent vesicle, pustule, or ulcer that occurs on the labia, cervix, or penis 7 to 21 days after exposure.[26] The patient usually does not notice the lesion. Two to 12 weeks after exposure, localized inguinal lymph nodes develop that can enlarge, coalesce, and ulcerate impressively.[27] The "groove sign" may appear to be created by the proliferation of inguinal lymphadenopathy superior and inferior to the inguinal ligament. Proctocolitis and perianal fissures may occur in patients with rectal involvement. Fever, headache, myalgias, chills, nausea, vomiting, and hepatomegaly may develop. It is generally acquired as a result of genital contact and may be transmitted by handling objects contaminated by drainage of the ulcerated lesions. Culture is expensive and not commonly available. Serologic testing, either complement fixation or the more specific immunofluorescence, is important to confirm the diagnosis; however, treatment should not be delayed pending these results.[28]

Doxycycline, 100 mg two times a day orally for 21 days, is the treatment of choice. Alternatives include erythromycin, 500 mg four times a day orally, or sulfamethoxazole, 500 mg orally four times a day for 21 days.[11]

Chancroid Chancroid is an increasingly common venereal disease caused by the gram-negative bacillus *Haemophilus ducreyi.* As with syphilis, chancroid is a cofactor in the

Table 93-2. Treatment of Syphilis

Primary, secondary, or early latent	Late latent unknown duration, tertiary (excluding neurosyphilis)	Neurosyphilis
Adults		
Benzathine penicillin G, 2-4 million units in a single dose	Benzathine penicillin G, 2-4 million units IM weekly × 3 weeks	Aqueous crystalline penicillin G 3-4 million units q4h × 10-14d
OR	OR	OR
(In penicillin-allergic, nonpregnant patients)	(In penicillin-allergic, nonpregnant patients)	
Doxycycline 100 mg bid po × 14d	Doxycycline 100 mg po × 30d	Procaine penicillin 2.4 million units IM qd × 10-14d
OR	OR	AND
Tetracycline 500 mg qid po × 14d	Tetracycline 500 mg qid po × 30d	Probenecid 500 mg po qid × 10-14d
Children		
Benzathine penicillin G, 50,000 units/kg IM in a single dose up to 2.4 million units	Benzathine penicillin G, 50,000 units/kg IM weekly up to 2.4 million units/dose × 3 weeks	

transmission of HIV disease. Chancroid manifests 2 to 12 days after exposure as a single small pustule or papule that quickly breaks down into one or more soft, painful chancres. Pain and the puttylike consistency of the ulcers distinguish chancroid from the other causes of genital ulcers.[28] A painful unilateral inguinal bubo develops in 50% of patients. The bubo may rupture and result in considerable tissue destruction.

A Gram's stain prepared from bubo aspirate may reveal short gram-negative bacilli in a linear or parallel ("school of fish") arrangement. The organism is fastidious, so laboratory confirmation is problematic. DNA probes and immunofluorescent testing may be helpful in the future.[15]

Treatment is usually based on clinical presentation. Herpes simplex, LGV, and syphilis may cause similar ulcerative lesions. Because of the high rate of concurrent infections, many experts recommend testing and treatment for syphilis. Azithromycin, 1 g orally in a single dose, is the treatment of choice. Ceftriaxone, 250 mg intramuscularly in a single dose, and erythromycin, 500 mg orally four times a day for 7 days, are also effective.[11]

Granuloma Inguinale Granuloma inguinale is a rare STD caused by the gram-negative pleomorphic bacillus *Calymmatobacterium granulomatis*.[11] The disease begins 1 to 12 weeks after exposure as a painless papule on the genitalia. It slowly and insidiously erodes and enlarges until it forms a beefy-red, velvety ulcer with a rolled border. Subcutaneous granulomas, known as *pseudobuboes,* may develop in the inguinal nodes over the next few months. Extragenital disease involving autoinoculation of the head and neck has been reported in up to 6% of cases. Women with cervical lesions may develop systemic disease, including prolonged spiking fever, anemia, and weight loss. Donovan bodies (monocytes engulfing clusters of organisms that look like microscopic safety pins) confirm the diagnosis; however, few laboratory personnel have experience in identifying this organism. Doxycycline, 100 mg twice a day, or trimethoprim-sulfamethoxazole, 160 and 800 mg twice a day until the lesions heal, are the treatments of choice.[28]

Condylomata Acuminata Condylomata acuminata are sexually transmitted warts caused by the family of human papovaviruses (HPV).[29] HPV is one of the papovavirus family, with over 60 different DNA genotypes. This anogenital expression of HPV infection is the most common viral STD, and the most common STD if subclinical cases are included. The incubation period averages 3 months, but can be up to 12 months. These pedunculated growths occur anywhere in the perineum, vagina, or perianal region and may grow large enough to obstruct the genitourinary tract and thus require extensive surgical procedures.[29] Condyloma in children may be sessile, necrotic growths producing a bloody vaginal discharge.[30] In the ED it is necessary to establish the diagnosis and to screen for other venereal diseases. Over half of the male patients have lesions, which turn white after 3 to 4 minutes of vinegar application. This can demonstrate small or flat lesions not seen with the naked eye. This should be done on all patients requesting evaluation for an STD when HPV infection is suspected. Occasionally it is difficult to distinguish venereal warts from condylomata lata, the flat, wartlike lesions of secondary syphilis, and dark-field microscopy of the aspirate may be required to distinguish these lesions. Cryotherapy is the treatment of choice. In selected patients, podofilox, 0.5% solution twice a day for 3 days, can be applied at home, followed by no treatment for 4 days. This therapy should not be used in pregnancy. Trichloroacetic acid and electrocautery have their proponents.[29] Careful follow-up monitoring is essential because recurrence is common.

Evidence suggests that HPV is carcinogenic. Ninety percent of cervical cancers and half of penile carcinomas contain HPV genomes, usually 16 or 18. Anal intercourse is a risk factor for anal carcinoma.

Vaginal (Genital) Discharge

Patients with vaginitis or cervicitis commonly complain of abnormal vaginal discharge: an increased amount or a change in color or odor, possibly with associated itching, swelling, redness, pelvic pain, or dysuria.[15] A genital discharge rarely is a symptom or sign of life-threatening disease; the problem, however, can be irritating to the patient. Occasionally, a genital discharge does indicate serious gynecologic (PID) or systemic disease (candida vaginitis associated with diabetes mellitus).

The thin, alkalotic vaginal mucosa of the prepubertal girl makes her more vulnerable to infection. In the months preceding first menarche, girls often have a profuse clear or white vaginal discharge. Normal vaginal discharge consisting of desquamated vaginal cells, lactic acid, and secretions from cervical and paralabial glands may be misinterpreted as a vaginal infection. Not uncommonly, the source is a pair of tight-fitting pants, worn often by the patient, interfering with the normal evaporation of the vaginal secretions. This leads to vaginal irritation and trauma.[31]

Many patients with a genital discharge do not have a recognizable disease when they come to the ED, so a wet mount, Gram's stain, and gonorrhea testing may be the only methods to establish the diagnosis. Because many genital discharges are caused by venereal infections, physicians must also screen for other STDs. The eyedropper technique for a single sample or the catheter-within-a-catheter procedure for multiple samples may be used to obtain vaginal samples in a small child. The eyedropper is used to instill a few drops of nonbacteriostatic saline; the material is immediately aspirated and examined. For the catheter-within-a-catheter technique, insert the proximal 4-inch end of an IV butterfly catheter (with the needle removed) into the distal 4 inches of a 12 Fr bladder catheter. Attach a 1- to 3-ml syringe that contains 0.5 to 1.0 ml of sterile saline. Instill the saline and immediately aspirate.[32] Pinworms, which can cause vaginal irritation and pruritus, may be identified by the Scotch tape test.

Gonorrhea Despite heightened awareness and public education on STDs, the incidence of gonorrhea among adolescents remained the same or increased between 1981 and 1991. The prevalence of the disease decreased in older persons for the same interval.[33] *N. gonorrhoeae* is responsible for three patterns of disease in women: asymptomatic carriers (30% to 40%), PID (20% to 40%), and cervicitis (20% to 30%). Patients with cervicitis develop symptoms of increased vaginal discharge, dysuria, and abnormal bleeding 3 to 45 days after infection.[34] The cervix appears friable, erythematous, and congested. A purulent or mucopurulent discharge exudes from the os.[34] The endocervix is the site from which laboratory sampling produces the most positive results. In men, the organism causes dysuria and a purulent discharge 2 to 7 days after exposure. Epididymitis and prostatitis are complications. Although *N. gonorrhoeae* may cause infection of the pharynx, anal canal, or conjunctivae, genital infection remains the most common presentation. Unlike the case in most men, in women, a Gram's stain of the exudate is too insensitive to rule out gonococcus as the causative agent.[11] A culture of the discharge should be plated on Thayer Martin media. This media will curtail the growth of other potentially competing organisms and allow the *N. gonorrhoeae* to flourish. Of special diagnostic significance is the finding that DNA testing is more accurate and reliable in females than are the culture results. The DNA-based tests in women make it possible to detect the presence of a single gonococcal organism in samples of freshly voided urine, tampons, and distal vaginal secretions.[10] For men, a Gram's stain showing the organism is sufficient to make the diagnosis.

Vaginitis is the most common gonococcal infection in children. The thin, friable genital mucosa of the prepubescent girl is susceptible to gonococcal infection, resulting in copious, purulent vaginal discharge. Obtain specimens from the child at the vaginal introitus.[35] Vaginitis, scalp infection, bacteremia, arthritis, meningitis, and endocarditis are manifestations of gonorrhea in the newborn.

Even though resistant strains have developed, many antibiotics are effective against *N. gonorrhoeae*. The treatment for gonorrhea is outlined in Table 93-3.[11,36] Treatment for *C. trachomatis* in addition to therapy directed against gonorrhea is essential because of coinfection in up to 60% of cases. Physicians should prescribe either the ciprofloxacin or the ceftriaxone regimen for pharyngeal infection. Disseminated gonococcal infection from hematogenous spread results in an arthritis-dermatitis syndrome and rarely meningitis and endocarditis. Treatment for the arthritis-dermatitis syndrome or bacteremia should continue for 48 hours after improvement. Meningitis and endocarditis require hospitalization and ceftriaxone, 1 to 2 g intravenously every 12 hours. Ciprofloxacin and all other quinolones are contraindicated in pregnancy and in patients less than 18 years of age. Spectinomycin, 2 g intramuscularly, is indicated in patients who cannot take cephalosporins or quinolones.[11]

***Chlamydia* Cervicitis** *C. trachomatis* is an obligate, intracellular parasite that has the features of both a virus and a bacterium. It is now the most common of all STDs and is one of the principal causes of infertility in women.[3,37] An estimated 1 in 10 adolescent girls and 1 in 20 women of reproductive age are infected. In addition to causing LGV, acute urethral syndrome, and PID, the organism causes mucopurulent cervicitis that is difficult to clinically distinguish from that caused by *N. gonorrhoeae*. Chlamydia causes nongonococcal urethritis and epididymitis in men. Men may also be asymptomatic carriers of the infection. Women with chlamydia cervicitis complain of symptoms similar to those of gonococcal cervicitis. Physical findings include vaginal discharge, cervical edema and erythema, and friability. Yellow (as opposed to white or milky) mucopurulent endocervical discharge obtained on a white cotton-tipped swab and the presence of 10 or more polymorphonuclear leukocytes at 1,000 magnification on Gram's stain is characteristic of chlamydia cervicitis.[15] The absence of intracellular gram-negative diplococci on Gram's stain further supports the diagnosis.

Chlamydial culture using fluorescein-conjugated monoclonal antibody against intracellular inclusions is the diagnostic "gold standard." The test is expensive and requires extreme attention to detail.[38] Several rapid test kits are available.[39-41] MicroTrak uses fluorescent conjugated monoclonal antibodies that react with the organism and appear as small, green fluorescent dots. The technique requires specialized, expert microscopy and trained personnel. Testpack is a visual readout enzyme immunoassay technique that is easy to perform and requires only simple equipment. An antibody-coated solid phase are used to capture chlamydia lipopolysaccharide antigen. The antigen is then detected by a second antibody labeled with enzymes that produce a color reaction. The change in color is read by a spectrophotometer. Both are

Table 93-3. Treatment of Gonorrhea

Uncomplicated infections (urethritis, cervicitis, proctitis)			Disseminated infections (bacteremia and arthritis)*	
Drug of choice		**Concurrent treatment for chlamydia**	**Drug of choice**	**Alternatives**
Cefixime 400 mg po in a single dose OR	A N D	Azithromycin 1 g po OR	Ceftriaxone 1 g IM qd OR	Spectinomycin 2 g IM q12h OR
Ceftriaxone 125 mg IM in a single dose OR		Doxycycline 100 mg po bid × 7d	Ceftizoxime 1 g IV q8h OR	Ciprofloxacin 500 mg IV q12h OR
Ciprofloxacin 500 mg po in a single dose OR			Cefotaxime 1 g IV q8h	Ofloxacin 400 mg IV q12
Ofloxacin 400 mg po in a single dose				

*All regimens should be continued for 1 to 2 days after signs of clinical improvement and then patient can be switched to oral regimen of cefixime 400 mg po bid OR ciprofloxacin 500 mg po bid OR ofloxacin 400 mg po bid to complete 7 days of antibiotic therapy.

highly sensitive and specific.[39,40] Nucleic acid probes use DNA or RNA amplification probes to detect chlamydia in clinical specimens, including urine, tampons, and self-collected distal vaginal secretions.[41] This technique has far better sensitivity and specificity than culture.[4,5,7] A major advantage is that the sample can be split and tested for gonorrhea at the same time.

Azithromycin, 1 g orally in a single dose, is the preferred treatment. Chlamydial infections also respond to doxycycline, 100 mg orally twice a day for 7 days; ofloxacin, 300 mg orally two times a day for 7 days; or an erythromycin base 500 mg orally four times daily for 7 days.[11] The possibility of concurrent infections with *N. gonorrhoeae* and other genital infections should be considered. For the first time, "one-shot" oral therapy (cefixime, 400 mg orally, and azithromycin, 1 g orally) against uncomplicated gonococcal and chlamydial infection is available.[42]

Trichomonas Vaginitis The protozoan *Trichomonas vaginalis* is a common cause of vaginal discharge. Increased number of sexual partners and frequency of sexual activity are associated with higher risk of infection. Trichomonas is seen commonly in the sexually active female adolescent. It can be isolated from the urethra, bladder, and Skene's glands in most infected women. Patients typically complain of a malodorous, itchy, profuse white, or white-tinged discharge. In some, the discharge is grayish, greenish, or frothy. On examination, the vaginal mucosa and the cervix may have a stippled or punctate "strawberry" appearance. The vaginal pH is usually 5.5 or greater. Diagnosis is by wet mount and direct visualization of the motile trichomonads. The organism is pear shaped with three to five flagella at one end and is slightly larger than a leukocyte (Figure 93-1). Treatment is with metronidazole (Flagyl). A single dose of 2 g is the treatment of choice.[42] Provide the medication in the ED. The sexual partner must also receive treatment (see Table 93-1).

Bacterial Vaginosis Bacterial vaginosis is associated with a malodorous discharge that is homogeneous gray or white on examination, a positive amine sniff test, and the finding of clue cells on wet mount. The sniff test is positive if the fishy odor becomes stronger after the addition of a drop of 10% potassium hydroxide to a sample of the discharge. Clue cells are vaginal epithelial cells to which bacteria have become attached (Figure 93-1). Bacterial vaginosis is characterized by an overgrowth of *Gardnerella vaginalis, Mycoplasma hominis,* and *Mobiluncus* species, anaerobes, and other bacteria. There is a relative depletion of lactobacillus species.

Metronidazole, 500 mg two times a day for 7 days, is the treatment of choice. The single-dose therapy that eradicates trichomoniasis is not as effective in treating bacterial vaginosis. Clindamycin, 300 mg twice a day for 7 days, and metronidazole gel 0.75%, 5 g intravaginally twice a day for 5 days, are acceptable alternatives.[11]

Candida Vaginitis *Candida albicans,* a yeastlike organism, is probably the most common cause of vaginitis. Predisposing factors include antibiotic administration, pregnancy, oral contraceptives, steroid administration, restrictive

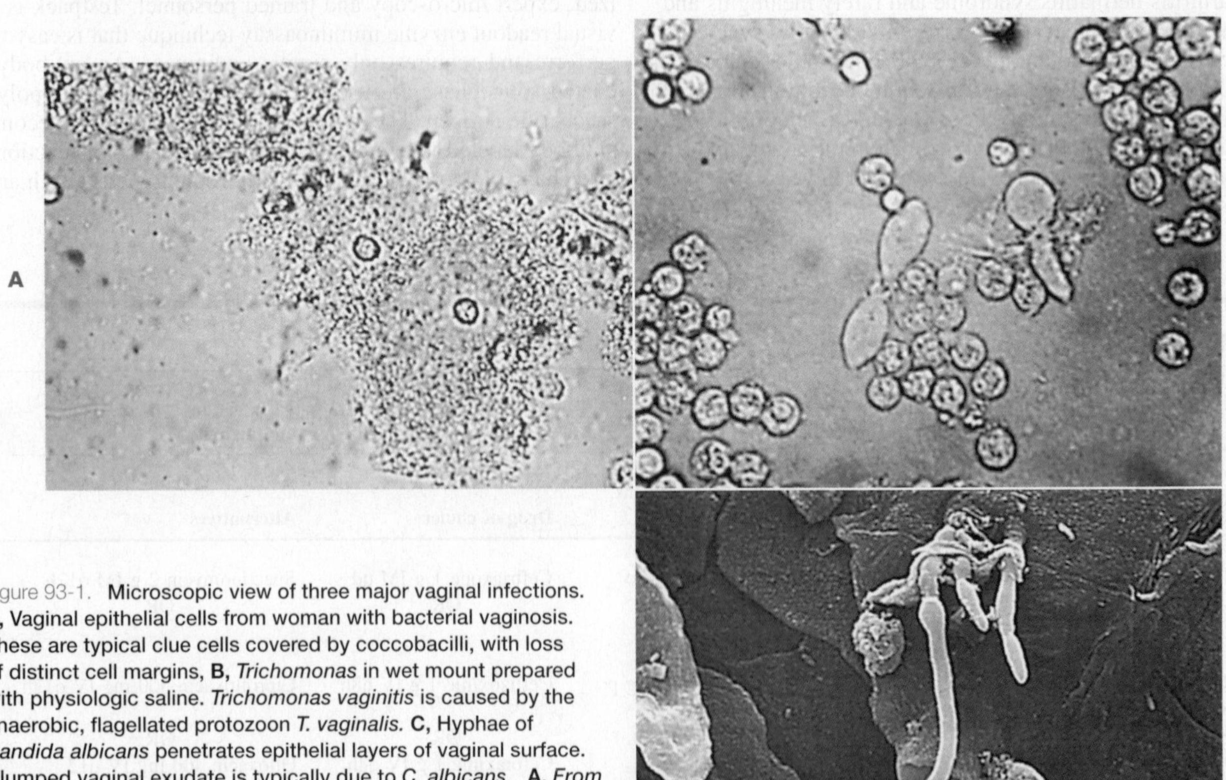

Figure 93-1. Microscopic view of three major vaginal infections. **A,** Vaginal epithelial cells from woman with bacterial vaginosis. These are typical clue cells covered by coccobacilli, with loss of distinct cell margins, **B,** *Trichomonas* in wet mount prepared with physiologic saline. *Trichomonas vaginitis* is caused by the anaerobic, flagellated protozoon *T. vaginalis.* **C,** Hyphae of *Candida albicans* penetrates epithelial layers of vaginal surface. Clumped vaginal exudate is typically due to *C. albicans.* **A,** *From Holmes KK et al, editors:* Sexually transmitted diseases, *New York, 1984, McGraw-Hill;* **B,** *From Gardner HL: Trichomoniasis. In Gardner HL, Kaufman RH, editors:* Benign diseases of the vulva and vagina, *ed 2, St Louis, 1981, Mosby;* **C,** *From Merkus JMWM, Bisschop MPJM, Stolte LAM:* Obstet Gynecol Surv *40:499, 1985.*

clothing, and diabetes. Patients often complain of itching that is severe enough to prevent sleep. Examination reveals a nonodorous, sticky discharge with the texture of cottage cheese. Often the vagina, vulva, and perineal skin exhibit a hyperpigmented, scalded appearance. Confirmation of candidal vaginal infection is made by wet-mount specimen using 10% potassium hydroxide. After 10 minutes, the cellular elements dissolve and the budding spores and pseudohyphae of *C. albicans* ("spaghetti and meatballs") remain (see Figure 93-1). Fluconazole, 150 mg orally in one dose, is the treatment of choice in nonpregnant patients.[43] A number of prescription and over-the-counter antifungal creams, suppositories, and tablets are also effective.[11]

Other Causes of Vaginitis Foreign bodies are an obvious cause of a malodorous discharge. Examination reveals the offending agent, usually a retained hygiene product. Treatment is removal and douche with povidone-iodine (Betadine). Chemical irritant vaginitis commonly occurs after the use of feminine hygiene deodorants, douches, or medications not intended for the vagina. Diagnosis is by history. Stopping the use of the offending agent usually is sufficient treatment.

Atrophic vaginitis results from diminished levels of circulating estrogens and thus is seen only in postmenopausal women. Patients with atrophic vaginitis complain of increased vaginal itching and vulvar discomfort. Topical estrogen creams usually produce relief in 5 to 10 days. Relative lack of estrogen also predisposes the vagina and vulva to infection. Patients with discrete lesions should consult a gynecologist to rule out neoplasm.

Other Causes of Vaginitis in Children

Group A Streptococci Group A streptococci cause 10% of premenarchal vulvovaginitis. The organism is harbored in the nasopharynx. The child self-inoculates by touching the nose and then the vaginal area. The child often has a nonspecific vaginal discharge and an angry red vulvar rash. It is uncommon to note systemic symptoms. Treatment is with a 10-day course of oral penicillin or erythromycin.[31]

Shigella flexneri and *Shigella sonnei* These nonencapsulated gram-negative rods are a common cause of diarrhea. Usually in the young child, direct vaginal contact with infected stool may cause vulvovaginitis. The discharge is painless, pruritic, mucopurulent, or bloody and may occur long after the diarrheal illness. Left untreated, the vaginitis may persist for weeks. Appropriate systemic antibiotics and careful hygiene provide effective control.[31]

Management Purulent, malodorous vaginal discharge in the premenarchal child may be due to a variety of causes other than STDs. Treatment of nonspecific vulvovaginitis in children includes improved toilet hygiene, daily sitz baths in lukewarm clear tap water, daily undergarment changes, discontinuation of chemical irritants (e.g., bubble bath), removal of foreign body, and treatment of specific infection such as pinworms.

Pelvic Inflammatory Disease

Perspective PID is the most serious and most costly infectious disease in postmenarchal women. Approximately 1 million women per year have PID, and nearly one third of them are hospitalized. Chronic pain, infertility, or ectopic pregnancy afflict 25% of diagnosed patients. Half of the cases of ectopic pregnancy in the United States are due to PID. It is estimated that ectopic pregnancy has increased about fivefold over a 20-year period. Among African-American women, ectopic pregnancy is the leading cause of pregnancy-related deaths. The economic cost of PID and its complication are estimated at $4 billion annually.[15]

Principles of Disease PID is an infectious disease with multiple etiologies and presentations. Organisms that cause acute PID may be primary (pathogenic), secondary (opportunistic), or a combination of the two.[44] Predisposing factors to PID include multiple sexual partners, recent menses or abortion, trauma, and the presence of an intrauterine device. The responsible organisms can inflame or infect the cervix, endometrium, myometrium, fallopian tubes, or peritoneum. *N. gonorrhoeae* and *Chlamydia* organisms together account for approximately 80% of all cases of PID.[45] *Mycloplasma hominis* and *Ureaplasma urealyticum* are responsible for a small number of cases.[45] Normal flora in the genitourinary or gastrointestinal tract cause the remaining cases. Patients with altered host response are often infected by multiple organisms. PID, although rarely fatal, is an important cause of ectopic pregnancy, infertility, and chronic pelvic pain.

Clinical Features Patients with PID go to the ED with a constellation of symptoms ranging in severity. The disease falls into three broad syndromes: acute, chronic, and intermediate PID. The definition of these syndromes is somewhat arbitrary, and overlap is common, but the terminology forms a reasonable basis from which to discuss PID. Ascending genital tract infection is rare in premenarchal girls. In this age group, a pelvic infection is more likely a complication of intraabdominal infection. In young, sexually active girls, PID is a major cause of morbidity.

Typically, acute PID is manifested by an increased vaginal discharge, pelvic pain, or symptoms of urethritis, beginning 3 to 5 days after menstruation. A history of antecedent irregular bleeding is elicited in 40% of cases. These symptoms progress over hours to days, and vomiting may also develop. On examination, the hallmark finding is cervical motion tenderness. Bilateral adnexal fullness and tenderness may be present. Peritonitis may develop if the disease is untreated. The white blood cell (WBC) count is often elevated with a left shift, and the erythrocyte sedimentation rate (ESR) is also elevated in most patients. Wet mounts, Gram's stain, and gonococcal cultures are necessary to determine the cause as quickly as possible. Whereas the typical patient with acute PID presents no difficulty in diagnosis, atypical presentations occur commonly. Fewer than 65% of patients with the presumptive diagnosis of acute PID have laparoscopic evidence of the disease. More than 20% of these patients show no demonstrable pelvic pathology.[44] The number and severity of symptoms and signs do not correlate with the severity of disease. The atypical patient may have no fever, vaginal discharge, or adnexal tenderness. The complaint of abdominal pain is absent in 5% of patients.[44]

Like acute PID, the clinical picture of chronic PID is often confusing and vague. Patients complain of constant mild to moderate aching pelvic pain exacerbated by trauma, sexual intercourse, or menstrual periods. Abnormal uterine bleeding is also a common complaint. Exacerbations of acute PID are common. On examination, there is often only nonspecific mild tenderness on palpation. Usually these patients are afebrile without signs of vaginitis, cervicitis, or urethritis. These patients may have lost reproductive capacity because of scarring, tuboovarian abscess, or ovarian dysfunction.

The third group of PID patients (intermediate PID) is the most challenging to diagnose and treat. These patients come to the ED with a clinical picture between that of acute and chronic PID. Intermediate PID is most often caused by *C. trachomatis* or a secondary infection. Symptoms may be those of vaginitis, cervicitis, or more uncommonly urethritis. Pain is steady and aching rather than sharp and increases with intercourse and menstrual periods. On examination, in distinction to chronic PID, unilateral adnexal tenderness, signs of cervicitis, and negative peritoneal signs are the pertinent findings. Generally the WBC and ESR are normal in chronic and intermediate PID. It is important to use laboratory cultures to confirm the diagnosis in these two groups of patients.[15,44]

Differential Considerations The differential diagnosis of PID includes acute appendicitis, endometriosis, corpus luteum bleeding, ectopic pregnancy, and ovarian tumors. Laparoscopy is an increasingly useful and cost-effective tool in diagnosing equivocal or recalcitrant cases.[15]

PID may be complicated by the Fitz-Hugh–Curtis syndrome (gonococcal perihepatitis).[45] The syndrome is an inflammation of the liver capsule that results in bandlike adhesions between the liver and the anterior abdominal wall. Dissemination, usually from *N. gonorrhoeae,* is probably by bacteremia or lymphatic drainage. Typically the patient has a sudden onset of severe, pleuritic, sharp, right upper quadrant pain that occurs days to weeks after symptoms of acute PID. Examination usually reveals profound tenderness over the liver, some lower abdominal tenderness, cervicitis, and culture evidence of PID. Laparoscopy may be required in diagnosis and lysis of adhesions. Failure to consider Fitz-Hugh–Curtis syndrome in the differential diagnosis of right upper quadrant pain may result in unnecessary cholecystectomy and progression of pelvic infection.

Management and Disposition Most patients with chronic and intermediate PID can be managed as outpatients, whereas most with acute PID require hospitalization and intravenous antibiotics. Indications for hospitalization depend somewhat on patient compliance and local practice, but the following are reasonable guidelines:[11]

1. Uncertain diagnosis (e.g., surgical emergencies such as acute appendicitis or an ectopic pregnancy cannot be excluded)
2. Suspected pelvic or tuboovarian abscess
3. Pregnancy
4. Nausea and vomiting precluding oral medications
5. Patient unable to follow outpatient oral regimen
6. Failure to respond to an oral antibiotic regimen
7. Noncompliant patients
8. Patients with HIV infection

Many authors also advocate admission for nulligravidas. Aggressive antibiotic usage and hospitalization are often warranted to avoid the tubal scarring and consequent infertility commonly associated with PID.[15]

Selection of antibiotics for treatment of PID must take into account the polymicrobial etiology of the disease. The most recent treatment recommendations are outlined in Table 93-4.

Sexual assault or abuse and STDs in the adult or child requires special consideration. Recommendations in this chapter are limited to the identification and treatment of STDs. See Chapter 60, Child Abuse, and Chapter 61, Sexual Assault.

The possibility of child sexual abuse should be considered if no obvious risk factor for infection can be identified. Evaluation for determining whether sexual abuse has occurred among children who have infections that can be sexually transmitted should be conducted in compliance with expert recommendations by practitioners who have experience and training in the evaluation of abused or assaulted children.[46] Every state, the District of Columbia, Puerto Rico, Guam, the US Virgin Islands, and American Samoa have laws that require the reporting of child abuse. The exact requirements differ by state, but, generally, if there is reasonable cause to suspect child abuse, it must be reported. The emergency physician should contact their state or local child protection service agency about reporting requirements in their area.

Table 93-4. Initial Treatment of Pelvic Inflammatory Disease

Outpatients	Inpatients
Ceftriaxone, 250 mg IM	Cefoxitin, 2 g IV q6 or cefotetan, 2g q12
OR	AND
Cefoxitin, 2 g IM, + Probenecid 1 g po	Doxycycline, 100 mg IV or po q12h until improvement
AND	THEN
Doxycycline, 100 mg po bid for 10-14 days	Doxycycline, 100 mg po bid to complete 14d
OR	**OR**
Ofloxacin 400 mg po bid for 14 days	Clindamycin, 900 mg IV q8
AND EITHER	AND
Clindamycin 400 mg po qid for 14 days	Gentamicin, 2 mg/kg IV or IM followed by 1.5 mg/kg q8 in patients with normal renal function until improvement (or single daily dosing may be substituted)
OR	THEN
Metronidazole 500 mg po bid for 14 days	Doxycycline, 100 mg po bid to complete 14d

Data from CDC: *MMWR* 47 (No. RR-1): 79-86, 1998.

Toxic Shock Syndrome

Toxic shock syndrome (TSS) was first recognized in 1978 and is associated with tampon usage and menstruation.[47] After an initial increase in incidence, there has been a decrease in frequency in the past several years. Officials for the Centers for Disease Control and Prevention cite a change in tampon composition, a decrease in tampon absorbency, and public awareness as reasons for the decrease.[48]

Criteria for diagnosis of TSS include fever greater than 38.9° C (102° F), an erythematous macular rash, desquamation during the recovery phase, systolic blood pressure of 90 mm Hg or lower for an adult, involvement of at least four organ systems, and absence of other causes for the illness.[49] Most patients report diarrhea, myalgias, vomiting, headache, and sore throat. Elevated serum creatinine, thrombocytopenia, hypocalcemia, azotemia, hyperbilirubinemia, and elevated hepatic enzymes are common laboratory findings. Vaginal cultures of most but not all women with TSS grow *Staphylococcus aureus,* suggesting causation by one or more exotoxins from this bacterium. Blood cultures are negative.

Treatment of TSS is largely supportive, and vigorous fluid resuscitation is important. Multisystem involvement, including adult respiratory distress syndrome, coagulopathy, and myocardial depression, is common. These patients may need invasive monitoring in an intensive care setting. Treatment with antistaphylococcal antibiotics for 7 to 10 days does not alter the course of TSS but may prevent or mollify recurrences.[49]

KEY CONCEPTS

- Most genital infections are sexually transmitted diseases (STDs), and simultaneous treatment of the patient and sexual contacts prevents further spread in the community.
- Despite aggressive public education programs, a well-documented association between infection with common STDs and facilitation of HIV transmission is on the rise.
- Early treatment of genital infections including PID will prevent compromise of future reproductive function.
- Two or more genital infections may coexist and require appropriate treatment.
- Pregnant patients and children are special populations that require specific antibiotic treatment and management.
- It is essential that all patients with genital infections receive follow-up care.

REFERENCES

1. Eng TR, Butler WT, editors: *The hidden epidemic: confronting sexually transmitted diseases,* Institute of Medicine Committee on Prevention and Control of STDs, Washington DC, 1997, National Academy Press.
2. Division of STD Prevention: *Sexually transmitted diseases surveillance, 1997,* US Department of Health and Human Services, PHS, Atlanta, 1998, Centers for Disease Control and Prevention.
3. Fortenberry JD: Health care seeking behaviors related to sexually transmitted diseases among adolescents, *Am J Pub Health* 87:417, 1997.
4. Oh MK et al: Urine based screening of adolescents in detention to guide treatment for gonococcal and chlamydia infections: translating research into intervention, *Arch Pediatr Adolesc Med* 152:52, 1998.
5. American Academy of Pediatrics Committee on Adolescence: Contraception and adolescents, *Pediatrics* 104:1161, 1165, 1999.
6. Position Paper of the Society for Adolescent Medicine: access to health care for adolescents, *J Adolesc Health* 13:162, 1992.
7. Hook EW et al: Diagnosis of genitourinary *Chlamydia trachomatis* infections by using the ligase chain reaction on patient-obtained vaginal swabs, *J Clin Microbiol* 35:2133, 1997.
8. Ziv A, Boulet JR, Slap GB: Emergency department utilization by adolescents in the United States, *Pediatrics* 101:987, 1998.
9. Cohen DA et al: Repeated school-based screening for sexually transmitted diseases: a feasible strategy for reaching adolescents, *Pediatrics* 104:1281, 1999.
10. Shafer MA, Pantell RH, Schacter J: Is the routine pelvic examination needed with the advent of urine-based screening for sexually transmitted diseases? *Arch Pediatr Adolesc Med* 153:119, 1999.
11. Centers for Disease Control and Prevention: 1998 sexually transmitted diseases treatment guidelines, *Morb Mortal Wkly Rep* 47:79, 1998.
12. Dattel BJ et al: Isolation of *Chlamydia trachomatis* and *Neisseria gonorrhoeae* from the genital tract of sexually abused prepubertal females, *Adolesc Pediatr Gynecol* 2:217, 1989.
13. Shafer MA: What teens want in a pediatrician, *Adolesc Health Update* 2:8, 1990.
14. Buntin DM et al: Sexually transmitted diseases: viruses and ectoparasites, *J Am Acad Dermatol* 25:527, 1991.
15. Chambers CV: Sexually transmitted diseases, *Prim Care* 17:833, 1990.
16. Webb DH, Fife KH: Genital herpes simplex infections, *Infect Dis Clin North Am* 1:97, 1987.
17. American Academy of Pediatrics: *2000 Report of the Committee on Infectious Diseases,* Elk Grove, Ill, 2000, the Academy.
18. Brown ZA et al: Effects on infants of a first episode of genital herpes during pregnancy, *N Engl J Med* 317:20, 1987.
19. Soper DE, Mathall CG, Dalton HP: Risk factors for intra-amniotic infection: a prospective epidemiologic study, *Am J Obstet Gynecol* 161:3, 1989.
20. Morton BD, McCarthy LR: Bartholinitis: an unusual etiologic agent, *Obstet Gynecol* 55 (Suppl):975, 1980.
21. Chapel T: The signs and symptoms of secondary syphilis, *Sex Transm Dis* 7:161, 1980.
22. Hook EW III, Marra C: Acquired syphilis in adults, *N Engl J Med* 326:1060, 1992.
23. Kraus SJ: Evaluation and management of acute genital ulcers in sexually active patients, *Urol Clin North Am* 11:155, 1984.
24. Starling S: Syphilis in infants and young children, *Pediatr Ann* 23:334, 1994.
25. Thomas DL, Quinn TC: Serologic testing for sexually transmitted diseases, *Infect Dis Clin North Am* 7:793, 1993.
26. Scieux C et al: Lymphogranuloma venereum: 27 cases in Paris, *J Infect Dis* 160:662, 1989.
27. Thorsteinsson S: Lymphogranuloma venereum: review of clinical manifestations, epidemiology, diagnosis and treatment, *Scand J Infect Dis Suppl* 32:126, 1982.
28. Goens JL, Schwartz RA, de Wolf K: Mucocutaneous manifestations of chancroid, lymphogranuloma venereum, and granuloma inguinale, *Am Fam Physician* 49:415, 1994.
29. Brown DR, Fife KH: Human papillomavirus infections of the genital tract, *Med Clin North Am* 74:1455, 1990.
30. Frasier L: Human papillomavirus infections in children, *Pediatr Ann* 23:354, 1994.
31. Feigin R, Cherry J: *Gynecologic infections in childhood and adolescence: textbook of pediatric infectious diseases,* Philadelphia, 1992, WB Saunders.
32. Pokorny SF, Stormer LVN: Atraumatic removal of secretions from the prepubertal vagina, *Am J Obstet Gynecol* 156:581, 1987.
33. Webster LA, Berman SM, Greenspan JR: Surveillance for gonorrhea and primary and secondary syphilis among adolescents, United States—1981-1991, *MMWR CDC Surveill Summ* 42:1, 1993.
34. McCormack W: Clinical spectrum of infection with *Neisseria gonorrhoeae, Sex Transm Dis* 7:116, 1980.
35. Ingram D: *Neisseria gonorrhoeae* in children, *Pediatr Ann* 23:341, 1994.
36. Portilla I et al: Oral cefixime versus intramuscular ceftriaxone in patients with uncomplicated gonococcal infections, *Sex Transm Dis* 19:94, 1992.
37. Saxer JJ: *Chlamydia trachomatis* genital infections in a community-based family practice clinic, *J Fam Pract* 28:41, 1989.

38. Bauwens JE, Clark AM, Stamm WE: Diagnosis of *Chlamydia trachomatis* endocervical infections by a commercial polymerase chain reaction assay, *J Clin Microbiol* 31:3023, 1993.
39. Reichart CA et al: Evaluation of Abbott Testpack Chlamydia for detection of *Chlamydia trachomatis* in patients attending sexually transmitted diseases clinics, *Sex Transm Dis* 17:147, 1990.
40. Carroll KC et al: Evaluation of the Abbott LCx ligase chain reaction assay for detection of *Chlamydia trachomatis* and *Neisseria gonorrhoeae* in urine and genital swab specimens from a sexually transmitted disease clinic population, *J Clin Microbiol* 25:450, 1998.
41. Gray RH et al: Use of self-collected vaginal swabs for detection of *Chlamydia trachomatis* infection (letter), *Sex Transm Dis* 25:450, 1998.
42. Rein MF: Sexually transmitted diseases, *Compr Ther* 19:136, 1993.
43. Phillips RJM, Watson SA, McKay FF: An open multicentre study of the efficacy and safety of a single dose of fluconazole 150 mg in the treatment of vaginal candidiasis in general practice, *Br J Clin Pract* 44:219, 1990.
44. Bowie WR, Jones H: Acute pelvic inflammatory disease in outpatients: association with *Chlamydia trachomatis* and *Neisseria gonorrhoeae, Ann Intern Med* 95:685, 1981.
45. Reichert JA, Valle RF: Fitz-Hugh-Curtis syndrome: a laparoscopic approach, *JAMA* 236:266, 1976.
46. Groth SJ et al: *Handbook: evaluation and management of the sexually assaulted or sexually abused patient,* Dallas, 1999, American College of Emergency Physicians.
47. Shands KN, Dan BB, Schmid GP: Toxic shock syndrome: the emerging picture, *Ann Intern Med* 94:264, 1981.
48. Reduced incidence of menstrual toxic shock syndrome—United States 1980-1990, *MMWR* 39:421, 1990.
49. Shands KN et al: Toxic-shock syndrome in menstruating women: association with tampon use and *Staphylococcus aureus* and clinical features in 52 cases, *N Engl J Med* 303:1436, 1980.

94 Selected Urologic Problems

Javier I. Escobar II
Edward Rivers Eastman
Ann L. Harwood-Nuss

PERSPECTIVE

Individuals who come to the ED with genitourinary complaints often warrant a rapid but thorough general physical examination. Regions of particular concern include the kidneys, bladder, prostate, and external genitalia.

The Urologic Examination

Kidneys Kidneys are not usually palpable in adults. The right kidney is normally lower than the left. The best method of palpation is illustrated in Figure 94-1. Auscultation over the upper abdominal quadrants and the costovertebral angle should be performed in search of bruits. The presence of a bruit in these areas may signify renal artery stenosis, aneurysm, or an arteriovenous malformation.

Bladder Similarly, the bladder is not palpable in its normal, empty state. When the bladder contains in excess of 150 ml of fluid, it may be palpable or percussible. A bladder that contains 500 ml or more of fluid can often be seen and palpated as a suprapubic mass. Percussion is probably the most reliable method of detecting a distended bladder.

Penis If the patient is uncircumcised, the foreskin should be retracted to inspect for the possibility of infection or tumor. The urethral meatus should be noted both for adequacy of size and proper location. The meatus should be separated with the examiner's thumb and forefinger in search of neoplasm, discharge, or inflammatory lesions.

Scrotum The contents of the scrotum should be palpated. The testes are best examined with the thumb and first finger, palpating gently for consistency, masses, or unusual tenderness. The normal testis is firm and mobile. A hard area within the testis must be considered a neoplasm until proven otherwise, and immediate referral is warranted. The epididymis should be examined. Nodular induration of the epididymis suggests tuberculosis or other chronic inflammation. A mass that is revealed by transillumination may represent a spermatocele. A cystic mass around the testis is likely to be a hydrocele, but note that 10% of testicular neoplasms cause a reactive hydrocele.

Rectum A rectal examination is a mandatory portion of a urologic examination in men and should not be deferred. A 360-degree sweep of the interior of the rectum should be done before careful palpation of the prostate. The surface of the normal adult prostate is approximately the size of a half-dollar, with discrete lateral margins and a firm consistency. The size of the prostate on examination bears little relationship to the degree of urinary obstruction that might be present.

SPECIFIC DISORDERS

Urinary Tract Infections

Perspective

Background Urinary tract infections (UTIs) are second only to respiratory tract infections as a problem encountered by practicing physicians, and they account for approximately 7 million physician visits and 1 million hospitalizations annually.[1,2]

To obtain a better understanding of UTI, it is helpful to review some important terms.

- *Bacteriuria* is the presence of bacteria in the urine.
- *Urinary tract infection* (UTI) describes an inflammatory

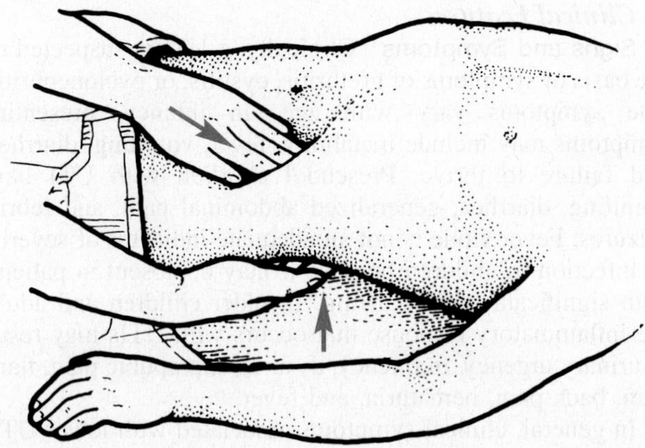

Figure 94-1. **Method of palpation of kidney. Posterior hand lifts kidney upward. Anterior hand feels for kidney. Patient then takes deep breath; this causes kidney to descend. As patient inhales, fingers of anterior hand are plunged inward at costal margin. If kidney is mobile or enlarged, it can be felt between the two hands.** ***Modified from Smith DR:*** **General urology,** ***ed 9, Los Altos, Calif, 1978, Lange Medical Publications.***

response of urothelium to microorganisms in the urinary tract. This term does not distinguish between upper and lower tract infections.

- *Cystitis* refers to inflammation of the bladder resulting in increased urinary frequency, urgency, dysuria, and suprapubic pain. Cystitis can be separated into bacterial and nonbacterial (e.g., radiation).
- *Acute pyelonephritis* is a UTI of the renal parenchyma and collecting system manifested by the clinical syndrome of fever, chills, and flank pain.
- *Uncomplicated urinary tract infection* is an infection that involves a structurally and functionally normal urinary tract. The causative pathogen can generally be eradicated with a short course of standard antibiotics. This type of infection usually occurs in women.
- *Complicated urinary tract infection* is an infection associated with underlying neurologic, structural, or medical problems, all of which may reduce the efficacy of standard antimicrobial therapy. Male patients with UTIs generally fall into this category.
- *Urethritis* refers to inflammation of the urethra.

Epidemiology UTI is a problem that affects all age groups. Routine suprapubic puncture in more than 1000 infants showed a 1% prevalence of bacteriuria. The prevalence of UTI in febrile infants is approximately 5%, regardless of whether UTI is suspected. UTI is more common in boys during the neonatal period but becomes more common in girls during infancy and thereafter.[3-6] When bacteriuria is seen in preschool boys, it is almost always associated with congenital anomalies of the urinary tract. Radiographic abnormalities are found in 45% of female infants and 97% of male infants with UTI.[3] It has been estimated that 0.8% to 1.5% of children have bacteriuria. Infection in either preschool boys or girls is a major problem and accounts for much of the subsequent irreversible renal damage caused by UTIs.[6] One study demonstrated that 1% of school-age females have bacteriuria.[7] The incidence of bacteriuria increases to 4% by young adulthood and 2% per decade thereafter.

Once adulthood is reached, the prevalence of bacteriuria increases in women. It is estimated that 10% to 20% of women will experience a UTI. The prevalence of bacteriuria in young, sexually active women is 2% to 4% and gradually increases to 5% to 10% at age 70 years and to approximately 20% by age 80 years.[8]

Bacteriuria in adult men is uncommon unless cystoscopy or catheterization has occurred. The prevalence is less than 1% from childhood through middle age, but increases to 1% to 3% by age 60 to 65 years, and to 10% by age 80 years. In institutionalized men and women the prevalence of bacteriuria is increased to approximately 25% and 40%, respectively.[8] Nosocomial urinary infections are the most common hospital-acquired infections and account for significant morbidity and mortality.[9]

Principles of Disease

Physiology The urine is sterile along the entire urinary tract from the glomerulus to the external sphincter in men and to the bladder neck in women. The urinary tract maintains its sterility by means of various defenses.[10] A major mechanism is complete emptying. Free, unobstructed flow of urine within the kidney and down the ureter, with complete evacuation of the bladder, is essential. Abnormal anatomy, physiology, or the presence of a foreign body may compromise the host defense mechanisms and predispose to infection.[11-13]

In men the distal urethra is inhabited by staphylococci, streptococci, and diphtheroid organisms. Nevertheless, men generally do not develop infection without predisposing causes.

In women the urethra is short and close to the vulvar and perirectal areas. The organisms that cause UTI in women usually arise from the fecal reservoir, initially colonizing the vaginal introitus and periurethral area. These factors contribute, in part, to the much higher incidence of UTI in women.

Pathophysiology Bacteria most often enter the urinary tract via ascent through the urethra and into the collecting system. Infrequently, bacterial infection of the urinary tract arises from hematogenous or lymphatic sources.

Numerous abnormalities of the urinary tract interfere with its natural resistance to infection. Obstruction from any cause, with resultant stasis of urine, is a major factor. Urinary calculi may cause obstruction and increased susceptibility to the development of a UTI. Any obstruction or impediment to the free flow of urine or complete bladder emptying results in a greatly increased occurrence of UTI. It is crucial that infection in the face of obstruction be diagnosed and relieved promptly.

Vesicoureteral reflux in children plays an important role in UTIs, particularly upper tract infections. Reflux caused by congenital abnormalities or by bladder overdistention (as seen in advanced prostatic hypertrophy) also predisposes to infection. Incomplete bladder emptying may predispose to UTI because of a large residual pool of urine, although this has recently been challenged.[14,15] Various underlying disease states are also associated with an increased frequency of UTI. Diabetic patients have a higher incidence of bacteriuria. Women with sickle cell trait also have a higher incidence of bacteriuria.

As noted earlier, UTIs are more common in women. Marriage, sexual activity, and pregnancy all represent important precipitating factors in the development of UTI in women. There is a 4% to 10% incidence of UTI in pregnant women. Bacteriuria should be sought, confirmed, and promptly treated in this population, as will be discussed.

In young men, bacteriuria is rare and may signify urinary tract disease. UTIs in men generally begin to appear at age 50 years (concomitant with the onset of prostatic hypertrophy) and slowly increase in incidence. The occurrence of UTI in men of any age may warrant referral to a urologist for further evaluation.

The organisms that cause UTIs generally arise from the patient's enteric flora that colonize the perineum and urethra. *Escherichia coli* is the dominant pathogen in more than 80% of first infections in women, men, and children,[8] as well as in 50% of nosocomial UTIs; however, certain patient populations may have unusual organisms. These patients have either a history of frequent hospitalizations or multiple courses of antibiotics given for other diseases. Both of these settings predispose to alterations in the normal gastrointestinal flora. In some disease states the initial episode of infection in the urinary tract may be caused by an unusual pathogen. Typically, this patient group includes those with asthma, chronic obstructive pulmonary disease, or sickle cell disease. A urine culture and sensitivity test should be performed before initiating therapy in this patient population. Patients who fall into this category should be considered to have complicated UTIs and treated accordingly.

Any instrument or catheter passed through the urethra carries bacteria into the bladder. For ambulatory patients the risk is small. A single catheterization in an outpatient setting carries a risk of infection of 1% to 3%.[16] In pregnant or debilitated patients, this risk increases substantially to 10% to 15%.[16]

Bacteriology The majority of UTIs are caused by gram-negative aerobic bacilli, which arise from the gastrointestinal tract. Of these, *E. coli* is the dominant pathogen in more than 80% of cases.[8] *Staphylococcus saprophyticus,* a coagulase-negative gram-positive bacteria, is the second most common cause of UTI, accounting for approximately 11% of cases.[17-20] This species is present in normal skin flora, including the perineal areas, but only in low numbers and it does not appear to be of fecal origin. Sometimes it is falsely identified as *S. albus* or *S. epidermidis.* Other less common organisms may be responsible for infection and include *Proteus, Klebsiella,* and *Enterobacter.*[19] Unusual microorganisms may be found in institutionalized or hospitalized patients and in patients with complicated UTIs. The uropathogens in these patients include more resistant strains of *E. coli, Klebsiella, Proteus,* and *Enterobacter,* as well as *Pseudomonas, Enterococcus, Staphylococcus, Providencia, Serratia, Morganella, Citrobacter, Salmonella, Shigella, Haemophilus influenzae, Mycobacterium tuberculosis,* and fungi.[19,21]

Uropathogenic organisms may elaborate various factors that affect their virulence. These include aerobactin, hemolysins, and fimbriae (pili). Fimbriae, also called *adhesions,* are proteinaceous structures that can attach to specialized receptor sites on host cells. Attachment of bacteria to vaginal and uroepithelial cells ultimately leads to a higher incidence of UTIs.[19,22,23]

The virulence factor of greatest importance is the resistance transfer plasmid. A plasmid is an extrachromosomal piece of deoxyribonucleic acid (DNA) that can be transferred among strains and species of bacteria. Transmission of this genetic material may confer resistance to multiple classes of antibiotics enzymatically. Plasmids may be responsible for 80% to 90% of antimicrobial resistance.[22]

Clinical Features

Signs and Symptoms Clinically, a UTI is suspected on the basis of symptoms of urethritis, cystitis, or pyelonephritis. The symptoms vary with age. In infancy, presenting symptoms may include irritability, fever, vomiting, diarrhea, and failure to thrive. Preschool children with UTI have vomiting, diarrhea, generalized abdominal pain, and febrile seizures. Fever alone is not an adequate indicator of severity of infection in children because it may be absent in patients with significant renal scarring. In older children and adults the inflammatory response that occurs with UTIs may result in urinary urgency, frequency, dysuria, suprapubic pain, flank pain, back pain, hematuria, and fever.

In general, clinical symptoms associated with lower UTIs are localized to the genitourinary system and include urgency, dysuria, frequency, and suprapubic pain. In addition to these symptoms, a patient with an upper UTI may manifest back and flank pain and constitutional symptoms, such as fever, vomiting, and malaise.

Many studies have documented that the correlation between clinical symptoms and the presence and extent of infection is not exact.[16,22,24,25] Stamm et al reported that 30% to 50% of women with symptoms restricted to the lower urinary tract in fact have silent (or subclinical) infection of the kidney.[20]

The importance of differentiating between upper and lower tract infection also entails an understanding of the differences in pathology and pharmacokinetics of antibiotic delivery. Infection of the bladder generally involves only the superficial mucosa, and high urinary concentrations of antibiotics can easily be achieved. The kidney, on the other hand, tends to become infected in the medullary tissue, where it is far more difficult to achieve therapeutic concentrations of antimicrobial agents.

Diagnostic Strategies

Laboratory Tests

Urine collection methods The diagnostic value of microscopic examination depends on the quality of the specimen obtained. In neonates a suprapubic aspirate is a safe procedure for obtaining a urine specimen. Alternatively, in children less than age 6 months, urethral catheterization is more often successful and, like suprapubic aspiration, carries a very low complication rate.

In older children a sterile midstream urine (MSU) sample can be collected from boys. In girls, if the voided specimen is free of cellular elements, it is probably acceptable for analysis. If not, it is appropriate to catheterize the patient. Urine collected with a perineal "bag" is useful only if the culture is negative because of high contamination rates. If a UTI is suspected, the urine should not be collected by perineal bag, but preferably by catheterization or rarely by suprapubic aspiration.

A wide variation in recommendations exists regarding urine collection methods in women. One authority states that it is impossible for an adult woman to cleanse herself properly and collect a midstream voided specimen without perineal contamination. One study has shown that up to 50% of women with sterile bladder urine grew 1000 to 100,000 bacterial colony forming units (CFU) per milliliter from a midstream clean-catch specimen.[26] This finding assumes major significance in the ED evaluation, in which accurate, initial supportive evidence for the diagnosis of UTI is important.

A sterile catheterization is the quickest and most accurate method of obtaining a urine specimen from an adult woman. It is safe, atraumatic, and carries an exceedingly small risk of infection (1% to 3% in most series). This risk increases, however, to 20% if the patient is elderly or debilitated. If the clinician chooses not to catheterize the patient, a clean-catch, MSU specimen should be sought. To assess the possibility of perineal contamination of a urine specimen, it may be helpful to observe the ratio of leukocytes to vaginal epithelial cells. The lower the ratio, the more likely it is that the leukocytes are vaginal contaminants.

In men the time and effort spent instructing adult men in the proper technique of cleansing and collecting a midstream specimen is not efficacious. The specimen is not affected significantly by lack of cleansing or by the timing of specimen collection.[27] It is *not* appropriate to catheterize an adolescent or adult man simply for the purpose of collecting a urine specimen.

Urinalysis Urine cultures constitute the majority of cultures performed by microbiology laboratories, and various screening tests have been developed for the purpose of reducing this burden and its attendant costs. The goal of urine screening tests is to reliably select specimens that will provide negative cultures so that the laboratory can more appropriately focus its attention on higher yield studies.

The most commonly used screening tests measure urinary leukocyte esterase (LE) and nitrite. LE is an enzyme found in neutrophils, and nitrite is produced from urinary nitrate by nitrate reductase, which is present in gram-negative bacteria. Both can be detected by a color change on dipstick testing. The two tests are often combined to improve overall accuracy. Indirect urine dipstick tests for pyuria or bacteriuria are inexpensive and easy to perform and may aid the diagnosis of UTI. However, they should be used with caution because they can be less sensitive than microscopic examination of the urine (urinalysis). Urine dipstick for LE has shown a sensitivity of 75% to 96% for detecting pyuria associated with UTI. However, a recent meta-analysis of screening tests for UTI in children demonstrated that a dipstick test for LE and nitrite may be equal to urinalysis in its ability to detect UTI.[28]

The ability of traditional screening tests to detect UTI in young children appears to be much lower than in older children and adults.[29,30] For this reason, additional screening measures have been proposed, such as Gram's stain and hemocytometry.[31,32] A urine culture should be performed in all infants and children being examined for UTI.[29,30]

The reported sensitivities, specificities, and positive and negative predictive values for any given screening test are varied in the medical literature. Table 94-1 provides average values for a number of these tests. In general, sensitivity diminishes markedly as the threshold accepted for significant bacteriuria decreases (e.g., from 10^5 to 10^2 CFU/ml).[33-35] Perhaps the most effective way to reduce the number of urine cultures ordered by the ED is to limit urine cultures to patients in whom they are truly indicated. In a symptomatic patient, for example, a positive test may support, but does not confirm, the presence of infection; a negative test does not exclude infection.

It has been proposed that symptomatic patients with a

Table 94-1. Characteristics of Several Urine Screening Methods

	Number of specimens	Sensitivity (%)	Specificity (%)	PR+*	PV−†	References
≥100,000 CFU/ml as positive culture						
Slide centrifuge	4161	98	90	65	99	VA‡
Gram's stain (uncentrifuged)	4399	90	82	61	97	9, 10, 14-16
Bioluminescence	7028	91	74	56	97	10-13, 15, 17
Filter-colorimetric	4779	90	62	38	97	11, 15, 16, 18, 19
Leukocyte esterase and nitrate reductase	9324	74	74	51	89	10, 12, 15, 19, 20, VA
Growth photometric	5673	85	85	70	95	10, 11, 14, 21
Disposable filter-colorimetric	1198	91	81	55	97	
Acridine orange	1573	100	68	45	100	17
Particle counting	1058	90	76	31	98	17
≥10,000 CFU/ml as positive culture						
Slide centrifuge	4161	88	95	84	96	VA
Gram's stain (uncentrifuged)	2050	75	86	77	84	9, 14, 16
Bioluminescence	1124	77	83	77	82	11, 13
Filter-colorimetric	3689	77	69	49	87	14, 16, 18, 19
Leukocyte esterase and nitrate reductase	6898	59	83	67	78	19, 20, VA
Growth photometric	4700	68	85	81	80	10, 14, 21

Modified from Olson ML, Shanholter CJ, Willard KE, et al: *Am J Clin Pathol* 96:454, 1991.
*Predictive value of a positive test.
†Predictive value of a negative test.
‡Data presented in this report (combined from initial evaluation and routine clinical laboratory testing).

positive LE test (in the absence of other indications for urine culture) can be treated empirically without a culture. In symptomatic patients, a negative LE test should be followed by urine microscopy. In adults, urine culture should be performed only if the microscopic analysis is also negative or is unavailable, or if the patient is at risk for bacteremia.

Urine microscopy Urine microscopy is another commonly used method of providing clinicians with rapid results and reducing the number of urine cultures performed. Some 96% of infected urine specimens contain 10 white blood cells (WBCs) per mm^3 or greater when counted by a hemocytometer.[36] Various counting chamber methods detect pyuria with an accuracy approaching the hemocytometer.[20,37] Unfortunately, these tests are not widely available; thus direct microscopy is commonly used.

The accuracy of direct microscopy is compromised by a lack of standardization of the technique. Common sources of variability include specimen collection and transport, centrifugation speed and duration, decanting and resuspension techniques, staining, and threshold used for significant numbers of WBCs or bacteria. One method, the slide centrifuge test, avoids many of these sources of error, and high sensitivity and specificity have been reported.[38] Microscopic inspection of uncentrifuged, Gram-stained urine has also given good results.[31,35]

Although no accepted level of pyuria is diagnostic of a UTI, Stamm et al maintain that when pyuria is carefully quantitated using a hemocytometer chamber, pyuria will be found in nearly all cases of acute UTI caused by coliforms. In patients with a low-count coliform infection, those with fewer than eight WBC/mm^3 of urine will have no demonstrable infection. In those with more than eight WBC/mm^3, 85% will have documented infection (coliforms, staphylococci, or *Chlamydia*). (**Note:** The identification of 5 to 10 WBC/hpf in a centrifuged specimen is equivalent to a chamber count of 50 to 100 cells/mm^3.) Despite these controversies and limitations, the most useful test for a presumptive diagnosis of UTI remains the identification of bacteria on a microscopic examination of the urine.

The presence of bacteria on microscopic examination in a symptomatic patient may confirm infection. However, its absence does not exclude it. The limitation imposed by the microscope on the volume of urine may result in a false negative error. The volume of urine seen under a high power field (×570) is approximately 1/30,000 ml. Previous studies have demonstrated that a minimum bacterial count of 30,000/ml must be present for isolation in the urinary sediment.[39] It can be concluded that a negative urinalysis for bacteria does not exclude the presence of bacteria in concentrations less than 30,000/ml. By combining the laboratory findings of pyuria and bacteriuria, in addition to clinical symptoms, the diagnostic yield can be further improved.

Any study of the urine must be done immediately after collection. Urine specimens that are allowed to sit become alkaline, with subsequent dissolution of the cellular elements and a multiplication of bacteria, providing the clinician with markedly unreliable results.

A properly centrifuged specimen should be spun at 2000 rpm for 5 minutes, the supernatant decanted, and the sediment placed on a glass slide with a cover slip. A second slide should be similarly prepared for staining. Gram's stain will aid in differentiating leukocytes, epithelial cells, and bacteria.

In an unstained, uncentrifuged specimen the presence of one organism per oil immersion field indicates a urine culture of greater than 10^4 bacteria/ml. If the urine is Gram's stained, one might detect the presence of more than 10^5 bacteria/ml. If the urine is centrifuged and Gram's stained, one should be able to detect more than 10^4 bacteria/ml.

If the Gram's stain is positive for gram-negative rods, pyuria is also usually present. Coliform infection is the most likely cause. Of these patients, 95% grow in excess of 10^4 coliforms/ml of midstream urine (MSU). Gram's-stained urine is negative in most patients with low-count bacterial infections, and in many cases of infection caused by *S. saprophyticus* and *Chlamydia*. Gram's stain can rule in infection, but it cannot rule it out. Women with no pyuria and negative Gram's stain constitute approximately 25% of patients diagnosed with low-count infection.

Urine culture The definitive diagnosis of UTI is based on the isolation of significant numbers of bacteria on urine culture. Traditionally, growth of 10^5 colony forming units (CFU)/ml has been used as the statistically significant number for the presence of a UTI. However, using an absolute number is fraught with limitations. The presence of 10^5 CFU/ml of bacteria in cultures from a child's urine is associated with a 95% likelihood of infection, where as 10^4 CFU/ml is associated with 50% likelihood for infection.[40]

The symptom complex of dysuria, frequency, urgency, and suprapubic pain may be caused by a wide variety of infectious organisms in numbers far less than the traditional 100,000 CFU/ml. In addition, these same symptoms may represent a significant upper-tract infection or may be caused by urethritis.

Since the benchmark studies by Kass, a quantitative culture of midstream urine revealing 10^5 CFU/ml has been the criterion to diagnose acute bacterial cystitis.[41] His studies, however, were performed in patients with pyelonephritis and asymptomatic bacteriuria. Patients suspected of having a lower UTI were not examined. Subsequently, a distinction was made between acute symptomatic abacteriuria (acute urethral syndrome, pyuria-dysuria syndrome) and acute symptomatic bacteriuria (acute bacterial cystitis). This distinction is made solely on the number of bacteria isolated when cultured. It is postulated that women with a traditionally negative urine culture (10^5 CFU/ml) have infection localized to the urethra, which accounts for the low concentration or absence of bacteria.

A follow-up study by Stamm revealed that 46% of women with dysuria who have a negative urine culture ($<10^5$ CFU/ml) yield bacteriuria with suprapubic aspiration.[26] This suggests that there is probably no difference in urinary tract disease or implications in treatment between the cystitis group and a significant number of those patients thought to have acute urethral syndrome. Of patients with clinical cystitis, 30% to 50% have negative urine cultures according to traditional criteria.[42] Conceptually, patients in both groups should be combined into one: lower UTI. These data suggest that the presence of more than 100 CFU/ml of a known uropathogen (i.e., significant bacteriuria) in a clean voided urine specimen from a symptomatic woman with dysuria is a sensitive and specific indicator of a UTI.

The presence of bacteria on culture in the absence of clinical symptoms does not always indicate infection. Women often carry large numbers of pathogenic bacteria on the perineum, and uncircumcised men may harbor large quanti-

Box 94-1 Groups in Which Urine Culture is Indicated

1. Children
2. Adult men
3. Immunocompromised patients
4. "Treatment failure" (recently completed course of antibiotics with persistent urinary symptoms)
5. Patients with symptoms in excess of 4 to 6 days
6. Elderly patients at risk for developing bacteremia
7. Toxic-appearing patients with signs and symptoms suggestive of pyelonephritis or bacteremia
8. Pregnant women
9. Patients with known chronic or recurrent renal infection
10. Patients with known anatomic urologic abnormalities
11. Patients in whom urinary tract obstruction is suspected (e.g., stones, benign prostatic hypertrophy)
12. Patients with serious medical diseases, to include diabetes mellitus, sickle cell anemia, cancer, or other debilitating diseases
13. Patients with alcoholism, drug dependence
14. Recently hospitalized patients
15. Patients taking antibiotics
16. Patients recently instrumented (e.g., cystoscopy, catheterization)

Box 94-2 High-Risk Groups

Compromised hosts with infected urine warrant a conservative approach. In general, duration of therapy and liberal admission criteria should all be considered carefully. This group is at increased risk for subclinical pyelonephritis, complicated UTI, or antibiotic-resistant pathogens.

Risk Factors (Modified from Stamm):

1. Urban ED
2. Lower socioeconomic status
3. Hospital-acquired infection
4. Indwelling catheter
5. Recent urinary tract instrumentation
6. Known urinary tract abnormality or stone disease
7. Relapse after treatment for UTI
8. UTI before age 12 years
9. Pyelonephritis or more than three UTIs in the past year
10. Symptoms >7 days before treatment
11. Recent antibiotic use
12. Diabetes
13. Immunosuppression (renal failure, chronic illness, drug or alcohol abuse, cancer, elderly)
14. Pregnancy
15. Sickle cell anemia and trait

Modified from Johnson J, Stamm W: *Ann Intern Med* 111:906, 1989.

ties of uropathogenic bacteria on their foreskin. The presence of bacteria in these regions may contaminate otherwise sterile bladder urine during collection.[43]

In this era of cost containment in medicine, it is only natural that this test should be assessed for its relevance in patient care. A number of studies indicate that patients with frequency, dysuria, urgency, and suprapubic pain should be treated on the basis of presentation only; however, a urinalysis and culture are obtained on all women for whom there is uncertainty as to the diagnosis. In general, the list of indications for urine culture (Box 94-1) represents those same high-risk groups reflected in Box 94-2.

The emergency physician customarily orders urine culture and sensitivity without due consideration for the clinical usefulness of both components. In vitro sensitivities seem to contribute little to the general management of most patients with UTIs. There is often poor correlation between the therapeutic response and the in vitro testing. It also represents an additional cost to the patient, with minimal contribution to the therapeutic plan for most outpatients. The exception is the patient who has a complicated UTI.

Imaging The majority of patients with acute cystitis or pyelonephritis do not need emergency imaging of the urinary tract. In certain clinical settings, however, emergency imaging is indicated. Patients with either unusually severe signs and symptoms or an atypical clinical picture may be candidates. For example, a patient with classic signs and symptoms of pyelonephritis but an unremarkable urinalysis may have an obstructive process that has prevented the pyuria and bacteriuria from reaching the bladder. Another example is a patient with a known history of urinary infection under treatment who has persistent fever, chills, and general toxicity. Perhaps one of the most sensitive predictors of a complicated infection (e.g., abscess) is the persistence of fever beyond 72 hours after institution of antimicrobial therapy.[44] Pyelonephritis with obstruction from any cause can rapidly convert the kidney into an abscess, with resultant loss of nephrons and sepsis. Emergency imaging is thus indicated in this circumstance.

First episodes of UTI in selected patients, such as men and girls under age 4 years, generally require evaluation after resolution of their UTI. These patients are at increased risk for having structural anomalies and, if untreated, may develop recurrent UTI or complications such as hydronephrosis, renal scarring, and, ultimately, renal failure. Several imaging studies may be useful in these patients. Intravenous (IV) or excretory urography (pyelography) provides both structural and functional information about the upper urinary tract. However, recent work has focused on gaining this information through safer, less invasive, and less costly methods. Ultrasound has compared favorably with intravenous pyelogram (IVP) in several studies. Radionuclide cystograms compare favorably with voiding cystourethrograms (VCUGs) in the diagnosis of vesicoureteral reflux (VUR) and give less ionizing radiation to the gonads by a factor of 50 to 100. VCUG is the traditional method used for the initial evaluation of the genitourinary tract. Computed tomography (CT) scan is exceptional for diagnosing upper tract complications, such as varying degrees of pyelonephritis, abscesses, pyonephrosis, granulomatous infections, and infected cysts. As with IVP, its disadvantages include cost, radiation exposure time, and contrast-induced reactions.

Ultrasound Many authors recommend ultrasonography as the initial imaging study to exclude obstruction.[45,46] It is a sensitive tool for detecting intrarenal and perinephric abscesses and the presence of hydroureter. It is less accurate in determining the presence of a partially obstructing ureteral stone. Ultrasound can also detect the presence of pyelonephritis and congenital anomalies in pediatric patients.[47] Regardless of the age group, this procedure is relatively inexpensive and avoids the hazards of contrast and radiation exposure.

Intravenous pyelogram IVP has a higher sensitivity and specificity for determining the presence of obstruction as compared with ultrasound. Hydration of the patient is indicated before this study. It is also prudent to obtain renal function studies (BUN, creatinine) to rule out existing renal dysfunction, because patients with preexisting renal disease, diabetes, and multiple myeloma show an increased risk of adverse reactions to contrast media. IVP is not sensitive for detecting the presence of pyelonephritis.

Radionuclide scans Radionuclide scans are also gaining popularity in the early evaluation of UTI. Dimercaptosuccinic acid (DMSA) scans are the most sensitive method of identifying pyelonephritis and are the imaging study of choice in young infant girls with UTI and fever.

Computed tomography scan of the abdomen A contrast-enhanced CT scan of the abdomen is perhaps the best test for assessing kidneys. It has the highest sensitivity for detecting abscess, obstruction, or acute inflammation.[48] As with IVP, its disadvantages include cost, radiation exposure, time, and contrast-induced reactions. As is true for all invasive diagnostic or therapeutic maneuvers, the risk-to-benefit ratio must be determined because significant complications, although rare, do occur after the injection of contrast media.

Urinary Tract Infection in High-Risk Populations

Pregnancy UTI during pregnancy represents a special situation. The incidence of infection in pregnancy is approximately 10%. Untreated bacteriuria is associated with a higher incidence of prematurity and fetal morbidity.[49] Maternal complications include a 20% to 40% incidence of acute pyelonephritis and an increased incidence of postpartum chronic pyelonephritis. The physiologic changes that occur within the urinary tract of pregnant women include ureteral and renal pelvis dilatation and reduced peristalsis throughout the collecting system. During the last trimester, minimal ureteral contractions occur in many patients.

The prevalence of bacteriuria in women does not change with pregnancy.[50] However, in contrast to bacteriuria in nonpregnant females, bacteriuria in pregnant women, even if they are asymptomatic, must be treated. Complications that may result from untreated bacteriuria in pregnancy include premature labor, perinatal mortality, and maternal anemia.[43]

Reasonable antibiotic choices include amoxicillin, cephalexin, and nitrofurantoin. Some authors recommend trimethoprim-sulfamethoxazole if used before the third trimester. Others believe that it should be avoided. Single-dose therapy is not recommended. Admission should be considered in patients who are in their last trimester and who appear ill or have evidence of pyelonephritis and would benefit from treatment with systemic antibiotics. Although pregnant patients with UTI are being treated as outpatients more often than in the past, conservative treatment and close follow-up are warranted.

Diabetes and Sickle Cell Disease Diabetic patients with bacteriuria also have an increased risk for the development of pyelonephritis. Papillary necrosis and perinephric abscess represent two grave complications for this group.

Patients with sickle cell anemia also have shown a predilection for developing papillary necrosis and generalized renal microvascular compromise.

Indwelling Catheters Treatment of asymptomatic bacteriuria in patients with indwelling catheters is not indicated. Antibiotic treatment results in the development of resistant microorganisms. Removal of the catheter results in the spontaneous elimination of bacteria in many patients. Treatment of patients with symptomatic bacteriuria who cannot have the catheter removed includes antibiotic therapy, replacement of the catheter, and strong consideration for hospital admission because this group of patients is at risk for the development of unusual pathogens and bacteremia.

Liberal admission criteria should apply to the patients just discussed and to any compromised patient. In general the emergency physician should be very cautious in outpatient disposition for the entire group of patients listed in Box 94-2. They represent a serious, at-risk group who tend to have abnormal bacteriologic, anatomic, or generalized immune compromises and who fare far less well in the outpatient setting.

Differential Considerations

Bacterial UTI is the most common cause of dysuria, with low-count infections (10^2 to 10^4 organisms/ml) comprising one subgroup.[42] It is important, however, to consider acute urethritis and acute vaginitis in these patients, as well as mechanical trauma or irritation (Tables 94-2 to 94-4 and Figure 94-2). Urethritis caused by *Chlamydia* may be seen in patients with acute dysuria; in fact, *Chlamydia* may be present in up to 20% of women with dysuria.[26] In general, if historical information reveals the presence of multiple sexual partners, a recent change in sexual partners, or a sexual partner with dysuria or discharge, *Chlamydia* should be strongly considered. A pelvic examination should be performed, with appropriate cultures, and a Gram's stain performed in search of either *Chlamydia* or *Neisseria gonorrhoeae*. Other causes of acute dysuria include gonorrhea, trichomonas, and herpes simplex virus.

The dysuria of vaginitis is most often described as "external," the sensation being caused by the passage of urine over inflamed introital tissue. Elderly women may complain of dysuria secondary to atrophic vaginitis. In either case a pelvic examination may be required. Urinary frequency and urgency are seldom if ever associated with a vaginal cause for dysuria.

Acute bacterial cystitis afflicts 6% to 10% of the adult female population each year. The symptoms of dysuria, frequency, urgency, and suprapubic discomfort are associated with significant bacteriuria.

Bacterial infections of the bladder are the most likely cause of dysuria in the female patient (60% to 70%). Most demonstrate positive urine culture with growth exceeding 10^5 CFU/ml of bacteria. However, as described earlier, this number is not absolute, as 30% to 50% of patients have low-count bacterial infections as a cause of their symptoms. It has been suggested that low bacterial counts may represent an early phase of UTI. Finding over 100 CFU/ml in a voided urine specimen of a symptomatic woman is a clear indicator of a true coliform infection.[51]

Table 94-2. Differential Diagnosis of Dysuria Syndromes: Laboratory Findings

	Pyuria	Microscopic hematuria or bacteriuria	Urine culture ($>10^2$ CFU/ml)	Abnormal vaginal fluid or cervical smear	Culture of genital lesions, cervix, or urethra positive for herpes simplex virus, gonorrhea, *Chlamydia trachomatis*
Acute pyelonephritis	+	+	+	−	−
Acute cystitis	+	±	+	−	−
Urethritis caused by sexually transmitted disease:					
Herpes simplex virus	+	−	−	±	+
Neisseria gonorrhoeae	+	−	−	+	+
Chlamydia trachomatis	+	−	−	+	+
Vulvovaginitis (bacterial vaginosis, trichomoniasis, yeast, genital herpes, simplex)	−	−	−	+	±
Noninflammatory dysuria (trauma, irritant, allergy)	−	−	−	−	−

From Stamm WE: *Urology* 32:6, 1988.

Table 94-3. Differential Diagnosis of Dysuria Syndromes: Physical Examination

	Vaginal or cervical discharge, vulvar lesions	Suprapubic tenderness	Flank tenderness, fever
Acute pyelonephritis	−	±	−
Acute cystitis	−	±	−
Urethritis caused by sexually transmitted disease:			
Herpes simplex virus	+	−	−
Neisseria gonorrhoeae	+	−	−
Chlamydia trachomatis	+	−	−
Vulvovaginitis (bacterial vaginosis, trichomoniasis, yeast, genital herpes, simplex)	+	−	−
Noninflammatory dysuria (trauma, irritant, allergy)	−	−	−

From Stamm W: *Urology* 32:6, 1988.

Table 94-4. Clinical Differentiation of Major Causes of Dysuria

Cause	Clinical features
Urinary tract infection	Internal dysuria Frequency, urgency, voiding small volumes Abrupt onset Suprapubic pain Often associated with diaphragm use Presence of pyuria Presence of hematuria (50% of patients)
Sexually transmitted disease	Internal dysuria Occasional history of frequency, urgency, voiding small volumes Gradual onset History of new or multiple sexual partners Vaginal discharge
Vaginitis	External dysuria Gradual onset Vaginal discharge Vaginal odor Pruritus

From Stamm W: *Urology* 32:6, 1988.

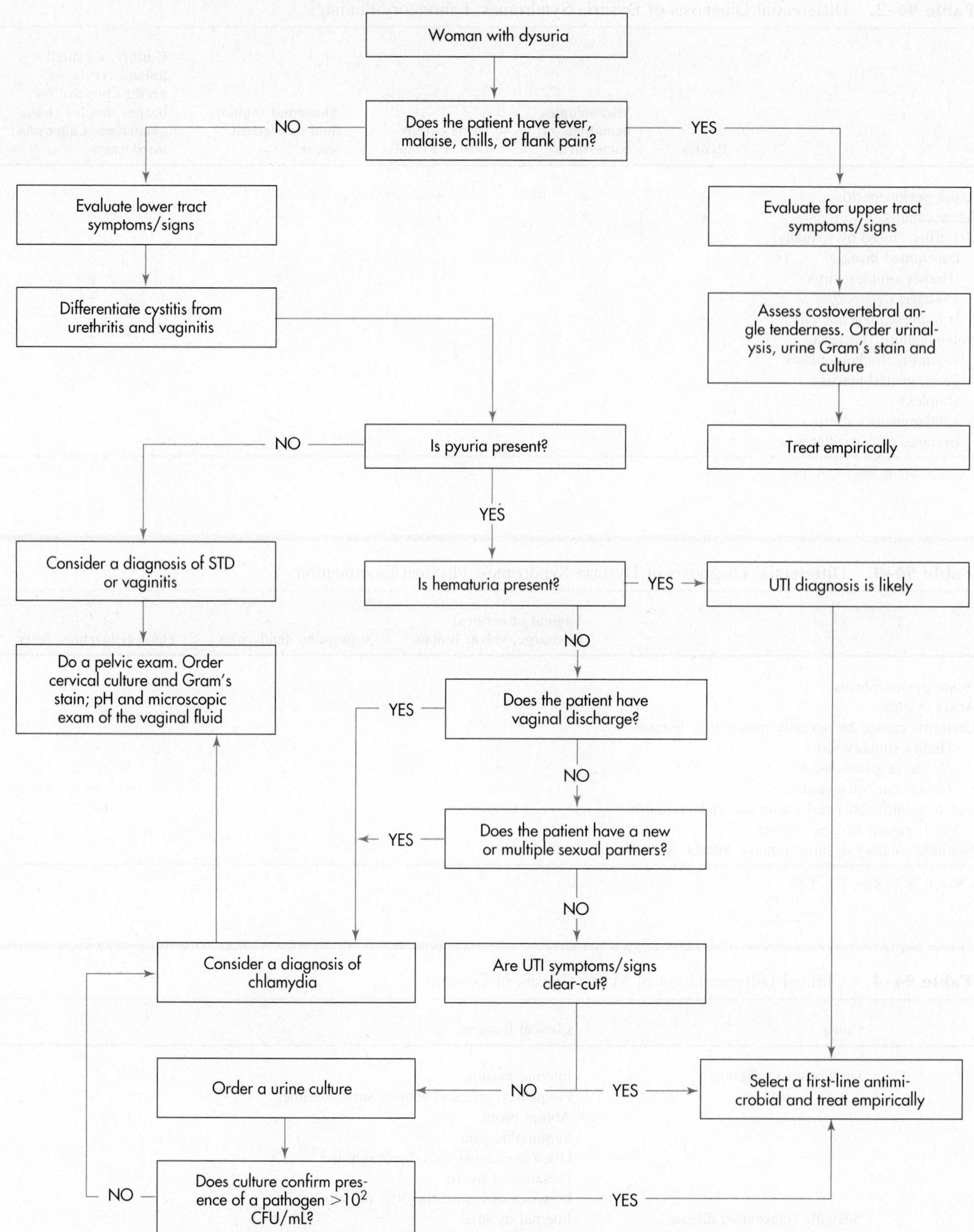

Figure 94-2. **Diagnostic protocol for women with dysuria.** ***From Stamm W:*** **Urology 32:6, 1988.**

Management

Lower UTI Options for treating uncomplicated lower UTI include single-dose therapy, short-course therapy (3 to 5 days), and the more traditional 7- to 10-day course of therapy (Table 94-5).

E. coli remains the most common urinary pathogen and is susceptible to many antibiotic regimens. However, resistance to some commonly used antimicrobials appears to be increasing. A recent study found that over the past decade, resistance to ampicillin increased from 30% to 45%, resistance to carbenicillin increased from 29% to 42%, resistance to tetracycline increased 29% to 40%, and resistance to

Table 94-5. Treatment Regimens for Bacterial Urinary Tract Infections

Condition	Characteristic pathogens	Mitigating circumstances	Recommended empirical treatment*
Acute uncomplicated cystitis in women	*E. coli, S. saprophyticus, P. mirabilis, Klebsiella pneumoniae*	None	3-day regimens: Oral trimethoprim-sulfamethoxazole, trimethoprim, norfloxacin, ciprofloxacin, ofloxacin, lomefloxacin, or enoxacin†
		Diabetes, symptoms for >7 days, recent UTI, use of diaphragm, age >65 yr	Consider 7-day regimen: Oral trimethoprim-sulfamethoxazole, trimethoprim, norfloxacin, ciprofloxacin, ofloxacin, lomefloxacin or enoxacin†
		Pregnancy	Consider 7-day regimen: Amoxicillin, macrycrystalline nitrofurantoin, cefpodoxime proxetil, or trimethoprim-sulfamethoxazole†
Acute uncomplicated pyelonephritis in women	*E. coli, P. mirabilis, K. pneumoniae, S. saprophyticus*	Mild to moderate illness, no nausea or vomiting—outpatient therapy	Oral‡ trimethoprim-sulfamethoxazole, norfloxacin, ciprofloxacin, ofloxacin, lomefloxacin, or enoxacin for 10-14 days
		Severe illness or possible urosepsis—hospitalization required	Parenteral§ trimethoprim-sulfamethoxazole, ceftriaxone, ciprofloxacin, ofloxacin, or gentamicin (with or without ampicillin) until fever gone; then oral‡ trimethoprim-sulfamethoxazole, norfloxacin, ciprofloxacin, ofloxacin, lomefloxacin, or enoxacin for 14 days
		Pregnancy—hospitalization recommended	Parenteral§ ceftriaxone, gentamicin (with or without ampicillin), aztreonam or trimethoprim-sulfamethoxazole until fever gone; then oral‡ amoxicillin, a cephalosporin, or trimethoprim-sulfamethoxazole for 14 days
Complicated UTI	*E. coli, Proteus* species, *Klebsiella* species, *Pseudomonas* species, *Serratia* species, enterococci, staphylococci	Mild to moderate illness, no nausea or vomiting—outpatient therapy	Oral‡ norfloxacin, ciprofloxacin, ofloxacin, lomefloxacin, or enoxacin for 10-14 days
		Severe illness or possible urosepsis—hospitalization required	Parenteral§ ampicillin and gentamicin, ciprofloxacin, ofloxacin, ceftriaxone, aztreonam, ticarcillin-clavulanate, or imipenem-cilastatin until fever gone; then oral‡ trimethoprim-sulfamethoxazole, norfloxacin, ciprofloxacin, ofloxacin, lomefloxacin, or enoxacin for 14-21 days

Modified from Stamm W, Hooton TM: *N Engl J Med* 329:1328, 1993.

*Treatments listed are those to be prescribed before the etiologic agent is known (Gram's staining can be helpful); they can be modified once the agent has been identified. The recommendations are the authors' and are limited to drugs currently approved by the FDA, although not all the regimens listed are approved for these indications. Fluoroquinolones should not be used in pregnancy. Trimethoprim-sulfamethoxazole, although not approved for use in pregnancy, has been widely used. Gentamicin should be used with caution in pregnancy because of its possible toxicity to eighth-nerve development in the fetus.

†Multiday oral regimens for cystitis are as follows: Trimethoprim-sulfamethoxazole, 160-800 mg every 12 hours; trimethoprim, 100 mg every 12 hours; norfloxacin, 400 mg every 12 hours; ciprofloxacin, 250 mg every 12 hours; ofloxacin 200 mg every 12 hours; lomefloxacin, 400 mg every day; enoxacin, 400 mg every 12 hours; macrocrystalline nitrofurantoin, 100 mg four times a day; amoxicillin, 250 mg every 8 hours; and cefpodoxime proxetil, 100 mg every 12 hours.

‡Oral regimens for pyelonephritis and complicated UTI are as follows: trimethoprim-sulfamethoxazole, 160-800 mg every 12 hours; norfloxacin, 400 mg every 12 hours; ciprofloxacin, 500 mg every 12 hours; ofloxacin, 200-300 mg every 12 hours; lomefloxacin, 400 mg every day; enoxacin, 400 mg every 12 hours; amoxicillin, 500 mg every 8 hours; and cefpodoxime proxetil, 200 mg every 12 hours.

§Parenteral regimens are as follows: Trimethoprim-sulfamethoxazole, 160-800 mg every 12 hours; ciprofloxacin, 200-400 mg every 12 hours; ofloxacin 200-400 mg every 12 hours; gentamicin, 1 mg/kg of body weight every 8 hours; ceftriaxone, 1 to 2 g every day; ampicillin, 1 g every 6 hours; imipenem-cilastatin, 250-500 mg every 6-8 hours; ticarcillin-clavulanate, 3.2 g every 8 hours; and aztreonam, 1 g every 8 to 12 hours.

trimethoprim-sulfamethoxazole (TMP-SMX) increased from 15% to 32%.[52]

Proponents of single-dose therapy cite improved compliance, reduced cost, and a lower incidence of adverse effects as advantages. Cure rates of almost 90% have been reported for trimethoprim combined with a sulfonamide. Cure rates are much less satisfactory for the β-lactam antibiotics.[19,53] Controlled trials in large population groups have demonstrated that single-dose therapy is not as effective as other regimens.

Three days of therapy is more effective than single-dose therapy. It shares the advantages of improved compliance, low cost, and reduced side effects and is currently the recommended duration of therapy for uncomplicated lower UTI. Hooton et al found TMP-SMX to be the most cost-effective 3-day regimen when compared with other commonly used antibacterials.[54] Studies indicate that 3-day therapy is effective in pregnancy; it is generally a recommended option, although it is unclear whether this regimen can be used for all lower UTIs or only for asymptomatic bacteriuria.

Interestingly, an indirect comparison shows ofloxacin to be similarly cost-effective; however, it is not considered a first-line agent, nor are the other oral fluoroquinolones.[20,54] Many trials demonstrate the efficacy of the fluoroquinolones and the oral second- and third-generation cephalosporins. Because of increased cost and concerns about the emergence of resistant strains, these agents are generally reserved for complicated, resistant, or recurrent infections.[20,54]

For most uncomplicated UTIs the fluoroquinolones are not significantly more effective than other less expensive antimicrobial agents. Cost must be weighed against advantages, including improved efficacy in the treatment of complicated UTI because of host factors, resistant organisms, and difficult-to-treat pathogens such as *Pseudomonas.* Fluoroquinolones damage developing cartilage in animal studies and should not be used in children.

Seven-day therapy generally offers no benefit over shorter courses. However, it remains an option in pregnancy and with other high-risk conditions (e.g., diabetes) that may result in lower cure rates.

Patients with risk factors for subclinical upper tract infection (see Box 94-2) require traditional treatment with 7 to 10 days of antimicrobial therapy. In addition, these patients require close follow-up to determine response to therapy.

For the lower UTI, numerous antimicrobial agents are highly effective. Nitrofurantoin and trimethoprim are excellent drugs for acute bacterial cystitis. Nitrofurantoin is inexpensive and maintains low serum and high urine levels, with a bacterial resistance pattern that remains unchanged. Adverse reactions are primarily secondary to gastrointestinal disturbance, but may be alleviated by using the macrocrystalline form (Macrodantin).

Folate antagonists, such as trimethoprim, have a broader spectrum of activity than nitrofurantoin. In patients with acute uncomplicated UTIs, antimicrobial susceptibility patterns may be as high as 99%.[55] The addition of sulfamethoxazole further broadens the spectrum to include *Proteus* and *Klebsiella.* Folate antagonists have a higher incidence of adverse effects than nitrofurantoin. These are manifested predominately by gastrointestinal upset, yeast vaginitis, and rash. Addition of the sulfa component further increases the likelihood of side effects.[55]

Except in pregnancy, ampicillin and amoxicillin should not be used empirically as first-line drugs for the treatment of acute UTI. There is a high recurrence rate with ampicillin-resistant strains and an inability to effectively eradicate the vaginal reservoir of pathogenic bacteria.

Controversy exists over whether the time-honored dictum to "force fluids" is beneficial for patients with lower tract infection. It may result in enhanced bacterial washout from the bladder, or it may decrease the concentration of antibiotics. A sounder recommendation is to emphasize regular and frequent bladder emptying. Avoidance of prolonged deferral of voluntary voiding applies to all patients. Individuals who appear symptomatic after intercourse should be encouraged to void before the sexual act. Avorn demonstrated that the ingestion of 300 ml of cranberry juice per day decreases bacteriuria with pyuria in elderly women.[56]

Upper UTI Subclinical pyelonephritis must be considered in the differential diagnosis of any woman with acute dysuria. It occurs most commonly in indigent populations. In several studies, up to 80% of women seen in this setting have upper tract infection or at least tissue invasion. Approximately 30% of patients with symptoms of lower UTI actually have subclinical upper UTI. There also appears to be a relationship between the level of infection and the duration of symptoms. Patients who demonstrate upper tract involvement have symptoms exceeding 5.9 days.[57] Kunin asserts that the most useful guide to upper tract infection is clinical.[19] However, subclinical pyelonephritis should be considered when certain "red flags" are present (see Box 94-2). If a patient has one or more of the listed risk factors, a urinalysis and culture should be performed. If pyuria or white cell casts are present, it is strongly recommended that treatment consist of a conventional full course of antibiotics. Follow-up of these patients is important and should be emphasized.

Mild to moderate pyelonephritis not meeting admission criteria can be safely treated on an outpatient basis with TMP-SMX or a fluoroquinolone for 10 to 14 days. Severe upper UTI requiring admission should be treated with parenteral antibiotics, switching to oral therapy once the patient has been afebrile for 24 to 48 hours. Oral therapy should be continued for 2 weeks. Twenty percent of cultures are resistant to ampicillin, cephalothin, and sulfonamides.[57] Therefore most authors recommend initiating therapy with TMP-SMX, a third-generation cephalosporin such as ceftriaxone, an aminoglycoside, or a fluoroquinolone. Follow-up of these patients is important and should be emphasized. Hospitalization is required in the presence of (1) clinical toxicity, (2) inability to take oral medications, (3) an immunocompromised state, (4) pregnancy, or (5) urologic abnormalities.

UTI in Children

Perspective UTI is a major bacterial disease of childhood. There is a 3% risk for girls and a 1% risk for boys of developing a UTI before age 11 years.[58] An estimated 0.8% to 1.5% of children have bacteriuria. The incidence of UTI in the neonatal period is higher in boys, but becomes higher in girls during infancy and thereafter. In children ages 1 to 3 months UTI is associated with a high incidence of sepsis (30%).[6] After age 3 months, there is a decrease in the incidence of sepsis associated with UTI (5%).[6] Vesicoureteral reflux is a common risk factor for UTI and renal scarring in children.[29,59] Data suggest that the incidence of scar formation after acute pyelonephritis may be as high as 37%.[59]

Principles of Disease As in adults, *E. coli* is the predominant pathogen. There are age-related differences worth noting, however. In older boys, the *Proteus* species is often isolated during UTI, whereas in newborn children, *Klebsiella* is the causative agent.

The route of infection is age related. In the newborn period, it is thought that the bacteria are blood-borne (and often associated with generalized sepsis). In the older age group, as in adults, the ascending urethral route is primarily responsible for generating infection of the urinary tract. Interestingly, in 13% of children an upper respiratory tract infection precedes development of the UTI.[57]

Clinical Features Pyelonephritis may be present *without* overt symptoms. UTI is often overlooked in children because of inappropriate emphasis placed on classic signs and symptoms with little regard to age variables. Nonspecific findings should be considered the rule and not the exception (Table 94-6). Generally, a febrile patient with a UTI indicates pyelonephritis. An elevated BUN level or hypertension in a child older than age 2 months strongly suggests bilateral hydronephrosis or advanced renal parenchymal disease.

Neonates Neonatal UTIs are manifestations of generalized septicemia. Classically, in this age group, feeding difficulties, irritability, and sluggishness are seen. Bacteremia is present in nearly 50% of cases.[58]

Age 1 month to 3 years This age group manifests the most deceptive presentation of UTI. Nonspecific findings are typical. Fever, irritability, abdominal pain, vomiting, and failure to thrive are often seen. Occasionally, gross hematuria may be present.

Age 3 to 11 years In girls, abdominal pain, newly developed enuresis, and irritative voiding symptoms should alert the emergency physician to the possible existence of UTI. In boys, fever is present in association with UTI in more than 50% of cases. Varying degrees of hematuria and irritative symptoms (urgency, dysuria) are present. *Proteus* is a common pathogen in this particular group.

Most cases are simple, uncomplicated infections responsive to commonly used antimicrobial agents. However, certain features, if present, should alert the emergency physician to the possibility of serious underlying disease of the urinary tract. The most significant factors include raised or palpable bladder, hypertension, abnormalities of electrolytes, acidosis, elevated BUN level, evidence of dribbling, poor urinary stream, or straining to void. If any of these are noted, a prompt urologic referral should be considered. In addition, if one is concerned about an obstructive process with an acute febrile UTI, it is appropriate to perform emergency imaging.

Diagnostic Strategies Laboratory studies useful for diagnosing an infection of the urinary tract as discussed in the previous section apply to children as well. However, presumptive treatment may be indicated in high-risk patients based on clinical predictors and screening tests,[60] as shown in Figure 94-3. Additional studies are dictated by the clinical setting and include renal function studies, CBC, serum electrolytes, IVP, voiding cystourethrogram, and ultrasonography. Renal cortical scintigraphy has recently proven to be the most sensitive method of detecting pyelonephritis.[61-63]

Urine collection often poses a challenge in the child with a suspected UTI. The following techniques represent acceptable methods of urine collection:

- Urethral catheterization is acceptable in all infants and is more often successful than suprapubic aspiration. Aseptic technique ensures a low risk of introducing bacteria.
- Suprapubic aspiration is a superb, reliable method if urine is able to be withdrawn, and it carries a very small risk. For patients age 12 months or younger, it is a useful method.
- A plastic bag collection is a reasonably reliable method, but the perineum (in girls) and the glans (in boys) should be properly cleansed before application of the bag. This method can be used to rule out infection, but a positive culture should be confirmed by urethral catheterization.
- A clean-catch urine specimen is preferred for cooperative and continent male patients.

The approach used must reflect the importance of the specimen and its analysis once collected, as well as the ability to repeat the collection before antibiotics are instituted.

Management and Disposition As in adults, there are many options for therapy in children with UTI. Sulfonamides, nitrofurantoin, TMP-SMX, cephalosporins, and aminopenicillins are all effective.[30] Newborns and young infants should be treated with ampicillin and gentamicin as inpatients, and sulfonamides should be avoided. Traditionally, inpatient treatment with parenteral antibiotics has been the rule for young children with suspected pyelonephritis. Recent evidence, however, suggests that oral therapy is acceptable in children with uncomplicated infections.[64] However, the clinician should manage these patients conservatively, and admission is advised for children who are dehydrated, severely ill, not tolerating oral fluids, or have underlying

Table 94-6. Signs and Symptoms of Urinary Tract Infection

Newborn	Infant	Preschooler	School-age child
Poor feeding	Poor feeding	Abdominal pain	Fever
Vomiting	Vomiting	Vomiting	Enuresis
Jaundice	Diarrhea	Strong-smelling urine	Increased frequency of urination
Hypothermia	Fever	Fever	Dysuria
Fever	Strong-smelling urine	Enuresis	Urgency
Failure to thrive		Increased frequency of urination	Costovertebral angle tenderness (flank pain)
Sepsis		Dysuria	
		Urgency	

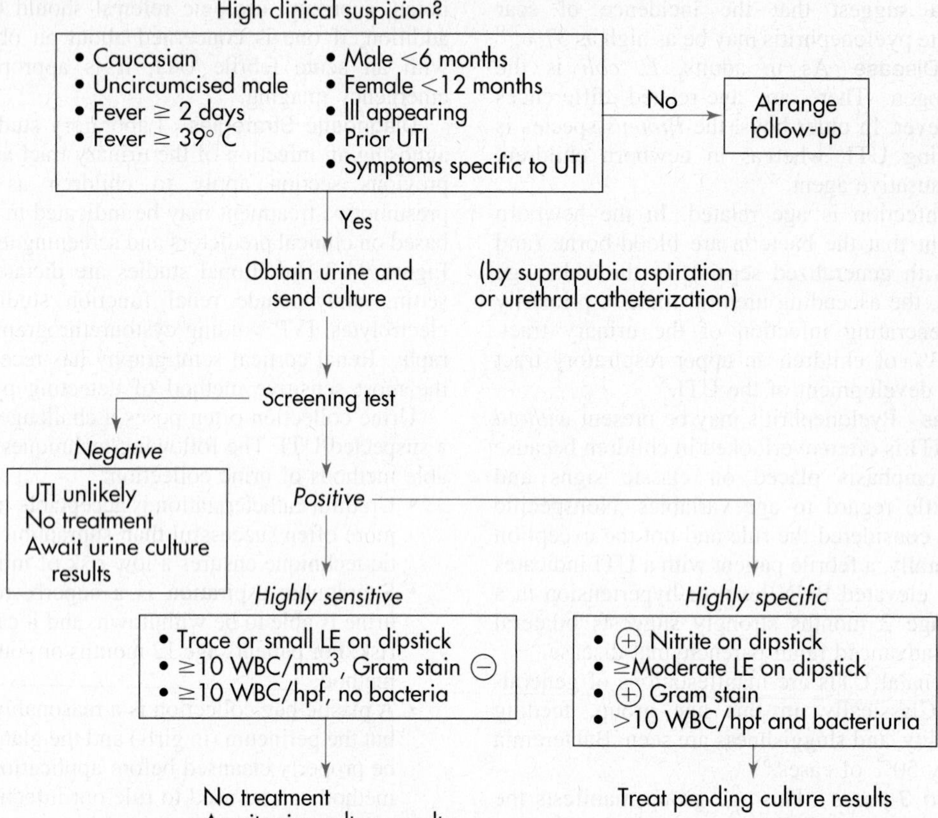

Figure 94-3. **Screening for urinary tract infection (UTI) in febrile children (age 2 to 23 months) in the ED.** ***WBC,*** **White blood count.** ***From Shaw KN, Gorelick MH:*** **Pediatr Clin North Am 46:1111, 1999.**

structural abnormalities of the genitourinary system. In addition, family dynamics, which could affect compliance with medication, should be taken into account when deciding on the disposition of a child with a UTI.

The appropriate duration of therapy is currently a subject of debate. Some authors believe that in children with uncomplicated lower UTI, short-course therapy can be used instead of the traditional 10-day therapy[30,65] Short-course (3-day) therapy is more widely accepted in adolescent girls. Once the decision to discharge a child has been made, the parents should be advised of signs of toxicity and the importance of compliance with medications. Parents should be encouraged to return the child for subsequent evaluation if signs of toxicity occur. The child should be seen in follow-up 2 to 3 days after the ED visit and again 2 to 3 weeks later (or 7 to 10 days after completing the antibiotic course).

UTI in Men

Perspective The incidence of UTIs in men is estimated to be 10 times lower than in women.[58] The route of infection in men is generally ascending, from the urethra to the prostate, bladder, and kidney. Pathogenic organisms responsible for UTI in men are similar in type, regardless of the site of infection in the genitourinary tract. *E. coli* causes 80% of infections in men. It is unusual for either cystitis or pyelonephritis to occur in a normal host. The emergency physician should actively seek predisposing factors, as discussed later.

Specific Disorders

Cystitis Cystitis, in the absence of trauma or instrumentation, is rare. Chronic prostatitis, prostatic hyperplasia with obstruction, and prior instrumentation are the most common predisposing causes. Lack of circumcision and homosexuality are other recognized risk factors.[20,66] Commonly, men with cystitis have symptoms of urinary urgency, frequency, dysuria, nocturia, suprapubic pain, and often low back pain. Gross hematuria occasionally occurs, but fever and chills and flank pain are generally absent. On physical examination, there may be suprapubic tenderness. Pneumaturia may be present and indicative of an infection with gas-forming bacteria. It may also more commonly represent the presence of a vesicoenteric fistula. This is most often caused by diverticulitis, although rectosigmoid carcinoma and regional enteritis are also associated diseases. If fever and chills are present in association with irritative symptoms *and* difficulty in voiding, acute bacterial prostatitis should be strongly considered. The most common pathogens found in men with cystitis are *E. coli, Proteus,* and *Providencia.*

A voided urine specimen should reveal heavy pyuria, bacteriuria, and varying degrees of hematuria. A urine culture is mandatory.

If there are no signs of toxicity, the patient can generally be treated as an outpatient with any of the urinary antibacterial agents (TMP-SMZ, nitrofurantoins, sulfonamides, or fluoroquinolones). However, three qualifying factors must be always addressed when dealing with UTIs in men:

1. It is imperative to eliminate urinary obstruction as a pathogenic mechanism. Infection and obstruction together are catastrophic and may lead to sepsis. Obstruction at the level of the prostate in older men is common and should be considered. Catheterization may be indicated to rule out retention. Obstruction of the upper tracts by urinary calculi should be suggested by the history, in which case an emergency pyelogram or ultrasound is indicated.
2. UTIs in men are often secondary to underlying, serious disease of the genitourinary tract. Therefore all of these patients should be referred to a urologist for diagnostic studies if indicated. Urologic evaluation may not be warranted for those who promptly respond to therapy.[20,67]
3. Urethral catheterization should not be used to collect a urine specimen in a man unless he is in painful urinary retention. If he is unable to produce a specimen in the presence of infectious symptoms, that should represent a major clue as to the cause of the infection. If retention is suspected, however, catheterization for residual urine is indicated. Referral and probable admission are also prudent.

Pyelonephritis Classically, the clinical features in men with acute pyelonephritis are those of flank and costovertebral angle pain, chills and fever, urinary frequency, urgency, and dysuria. The only characteristically helpful sign is costovertebral angle tenderness over the affected kidney. Generalized malaise, nausea, and vomiting are often seen as signs of systemic toxicity. Gross hematuria occasionally occurs. Male patients with this constellation of symptoms should be evaluated carefully for impending gram-negative sepsis.

A voided urine specimen usually reveals leukocytes, occasional leukocyte casts, varying numbers of RBCs, and bacteria. A urine culture is mandatory. Blood cultures should be done if the clinical picture suggests sepsis. CBC, renal function studies, and electrolyte studies are recommended. Uncomplicated pyelonephritis should *not* produce detectable alterations in the BUN level.

For an *adult* male with pyelonephritis, hospitalization may be required. An ultrasound or emergency IVP is indicated if there is a question of obstruction, which is often caused by calculi, stricture, or prostatic hypertrophy. Catheterization for residual urine may be indicated if urinary retention is suspected.

Antibiotic therapy should be instituted in the ED *only* after urine cultures and blood cultures are taken. Appropriate oral therapy includes TMP-SMX, trimethoprim, or an oral fluoroquinolone. IV therapies include TMP-SMX, gentamicin, a fluoroquinolone, or a third-generation cephalosporin.

Urethritis Urethritis is classically divided into gonococcal (GU) and nongonococcal (NGU) origins. Gonococcal urethritis is caused by the gram-negative diplococci *N. gonorrhoeae*. Current evidence exists to support *Chlamydia trachomatis* as the major single cause of nongonococcal urethritis in heterosexual men. It is also now believed to be the most common sexually transmitted infection. *C. trachomatis* is an obligate intracellular bacterium requiring special cell cultures to isolate. The spectrum of diseases for which *C. trachomatis* is responsible is impressive and includes urethritis, epididymitis, cervicitis, salpingitis, conjunctivitis, and neonatal pneumonia.

It has been clearly shown in multiple studies that the two pathogens coexist in men with urethritis up to 30% to 50% of the time. Both *N. gonorrhoeae* and *C. trachomatis* can produce asymptomatic urethral infections. However, nearly all men with gonococcal urethritis have a urethral discharge and symptoms. Furthermore, Gram's stain provides a rapid and sensitive diagnostic test for gonococcal urethritis. Conversely, 25% of patients with *Chlamydia* urethral infection have *no* signs or symptoms. Age, sexual preferences, and race are all determinants of high-risk individuals in whom one should suspect *Chlamydia* infection. The prevalence of *Chlamydia* infection in heterosexual men is 14% in contrast to only 5% in homosexual men. Furthermore, *Chlamydia* urethral infection is more common in men age 20 years old or younger and in African-Americans.[68]

Urethritis in men is caused by a number of entities that may stimulate a man to seek emergency care. Physical examination should be meticulous in search of other sources of urethral irritation. The urethra should be palpated along its penile course and inspected for possible foreign body or periurethral abscess. The meatus should be spread and inspected for ulcerations, neoplasm, or condyloma accuminatum. Herpes virus should be considered. A rectal examination should be performed to assess the prostate.

A diagnosis of urethritis should be suspected if the patient has a history of dysuria or urethral discharge. Urethritis can be tentatively confirmed by examining the discharge, the first-glass urine, or a direct smear of urethral secretions. If an exudate is not present, either through spontaneous discharge or by penile stripping, a urethral secretion can be obtained with a thin cotton swab passed gently up the urethra 1 to 2 cm. The smear should be examined for leukocytes and gonococci after Gram's staining. If there are fewer than five leukocytes per oil immersion field, first-glass and midstream specimens should be examined for leukocytes. The presence of approximately 15 or more leukocytes/hpf in a first-glass specimen and fewer leukocytes in the MSU strongly suggests urethritis. Conversely, the presence of an equal number of leukocytes in the midstream and first-glass urine specimens or the presence of many bacterial rods suggests infection of the bladder, kidney, or prostate.

A careful examination of the Gram's stain may reveal the presence of typical gram-negative intracellular diplococci. The sensitivity and specificity of this finding as diagnostic for gonorrhea approaches 100%. Conversely, one study demonstrates that 33% of patients with proven *Chlamydia* have no leukocytes on a Gram's stain of the urethral smear.[68] Recent research has focused on diagnosing *Chlamydia* or gonorrhea on first-void urine samples, thus avoiding urethral swabs. The LE test has been suggested as an effective screen for asymptomatic urethritis, although this has been refuted.[69,70] In addition, culture for *N. gonorrhoeae* on first-void urine proved 100% sensitive in one study.[71] Polymerase chain reaction and enzyme immunoassay techniques have performed favorably when used on first-void urine for the detection of *Chlamydia.*

With the systematic evaluation outlined, it should be possible to clearly determine the presence of urethritis. However, the decision to treat should be based principally on a history of dysuria and urethral discharge. The coexistence of *N. gonorrhoeae* and *Chlamydia* warrants the treatment regimen detailed in Table 94-7. On occasion, *Trichomonas*

Table 94-7. Treatment of Urethritis

Drug of choice	Dosage/route	Alternatives
Ceftriaxone	125-250 mg 1 M	Cefixime 400 mg PO Ciprofloxacin 500 mg PO Ofloxacin 400 mg PO*
	AND	
Doxycycline	100 mg PO bid × 7 days	Erythromycin 500 mg PO qid × 7 days† Azithromycin 1 g PO‡

*Cannot be used in pregnancy or persons <17 years old.
†Recommended regimen for pregnant patients.
‡Safety in pregnancy and in persons <15 years old not established.

vaginalis is responsible for urethritis. This may be effectively treated with metronidazole (Flagyl).

If a patient has persistent urethritis despite appropriate therapy, one must consider the presence of *Ureaplasma urealyticum,* herpes virus, *Trichomonas,* or *Candida.* One must also consider noncompliance and recurrent infection. Sexual partners should be promptly examined and treated as well because the incidence of complications increases with a delay in treatment.

Postgonococcal urethritis is another entity that may be seen by emergency physicians. This tends to occur in men treated for gonococcal urethritis with a penicillin only, thus allowing the untreated and coexistent *Chlamydia* to produce the recurrent symptoms. This problem should decrease in incidence as appropriate treatment protocols become more widely known and applied.

Prostatitis Prostatitis is seldom clearly established by objective evidence. Indirect parameters often lead physicians to the diagnosis. The history and physical examination provide clues; irritative voiding symptoms and the finding of a tender or "boggy" prostate are suggestive.

Bacterial prostatitis is an infection of the prostate caused primarily by gram-negative organisms. More than 80% of cases are caused by strains of *E. coli;* 20% are caused by *Klebsiella, Enterobacter, Proteus,* and *Pseudomonas* species. Mixed bacterial infections are uncommon. Tuberculous prostatitis may be found in patients with renal tuberculosis. The question of how bacteria infect the prostate gland remains unanswered. Although various routes have been postulated, none have been firmly substantiated.

Acute bacterial prostatitis Acute bacterial prostatitis is an acute febrile illness characterized by chills, low back pain, and perineal pain. Irritative symptoms of voiding are present, including frequency, urgency, dysuria, and varying degrees of bladder outlet obstruction and retention. Patients often also display constitutional symptoms of arthralgia, myalgias, and generalized malaise.

A prostate examination reveals a tender, swollen gland that is firm and warm to touch. If the patient has a spontaneous urethral exudate, it may reveal leukocytes and bacteria. It should be emphasized that the acutely inflamed prostate gland should *not* be massaged because of the possibility of precipitating bacteremia. Fortunately for the clinician, cystitis usually accompanies acute bacterial prostatitis. Thus a culture of voided bladder urine generally reveals the responsible pathogen.

Acute bacterial prostatitis is responsive to therapy with antibacterial agents that, under the circumstances of inflammation, concentrate well in the prostate. The following list represents an appropriate selection of drugs:

1. Oral: Trimethoprim with sulfamethoxazole, one double-strength tablet by mouth bid for 30 days; ciprofloxacin, 500 mg orally bid; norfloxacin, 400 mg orally bid; enoxacin, 400 mg orally bid; or ofloxacin, 400 mg by mouth bid for 30 days.
2. Parenteral: Gentamicin, 3 to 5 mg/kg/day or tobramycin 3 mg/kg/day, plus ampicillin 2 g IV every 6 hours.

If the patient is in a toxic condition with fever, chills, or urinary retention, hospitalization and parenteral antibiotics are warranted. If the patient is having painful urinary retention, urethral catheterization should be avoided. Suprapubic needle aspiration is much safer and more comfortable than a catheter for initial management. A urologist should be consulted in this situation.

General support measures for outpatients should include bed rest, analgesics, antipyretics, hydration, and stool softeners. Nonsteroidal agents may be useful.

Chronic prostatitis Emergency physicians most often deal with chronic prostatitis when an acute exacerbation of the disease occurs. Clinical manifestations vary widely, but most patients complain of some degree of irritated voiding symptoms (frequency, urgency, dysuria), low back and perineal pain, and occasionally myalgias. Fever and chills are uncommon except during an acute exacerbation of the chronic infection. A history of prior episodes of acute prostatitis is often absent.

The physical examination is often unremarkable, including examination of the prostate. The hallmark of chronic bacterial prostatitis is relapsing UTI caused by the same organism. Chronic bacterial prostatitis is the most common cause of recurrent UTI in men.

Except for the macrolides (erythromycin) and the antibiotic bases (lincomycin and clindamycin), most antibacterial agents diffuse poorly from plasma to the prostatic fluid.[72] Unfortunately, these drugs are not effective against most of the pathogens responsible for bacterial prostatitis. Since the introduction of trimethoprim with sulfamethoxazole (Bactrim or Septra), men afflicted with chronic bacterial prostatitis have experienced fairly good cure rates. It is an extremely effective drug against a wide range of gram-positive and gram-negative organisms. Studies have shown that TMP-SMZ not only diffuses into but is actually concentrated in the prostatic fluid. The dosage is one double-strength tablet twice daily, but the optimal duration of therapy is unclear and may range from 4 to 16 weeks. The fluoroquinolones have excellent efficacy and are the drugs of choice for the treatment of chronic bacterial prostatitis. The recommended dosages are as follows: ciprofloxacin, 500 mg bid for 30 days; norfloxacin, 400 mg bid for 30 days; enoxacin, 400 mg bid for 30 days; or ofloxacin, 300 mg bid for 6 weeks.

Renal Calculi

Perspective

Background Renal calculi are common. In this country the prevalence of renal calculi is 7% in men and 3% in women.[73] Renal calculi are primarily seen in middle age, with nearly 70% of all ureteral calculi occurring between the ages of 20 and 50 years. Recurrence of renal calculi is common, with rates approaching 50%.[74] It is believed that most ureteral calculi originate in the kidney and then pass into the collecting system.

Epidemiology Certain clinical features are associated with an increased likelihood of stone formation and should be sought in the initial evaluation of the patients.

Risk factors include age, male gender, and family history. Many conditions are associated with an increased risk of calculi formation. These include primary hyperparathyroidism, milk-alkali syndrome, sarcoidosis, Crohn's disease, laxative abuse, recurrent UTI, and renal tubular acidosis (type I).

Renal calculi form primarily as a result of metabolic abnormalities. Renal colic is more prevalent in hot, arid climates as opposed to wet climates.[75] In the United States the area of highest incidence of stone disease is the Southeast.

Patient occupation is also a risk factor. Kidney stones are most prevalent in white professional men with sedentary lifestyles.

Recurrence of renal calculi is common. In a study of patients having a first stone, recurrence rates of 37% and 50% were demonstrated for 1 and 5 years, respectively.[76] The incidence of recurrence is biphasic, peaking at 1, 2, and 8 years.

Principles of Disease Multiple pathogenic factors interact to cause formation of renal calculi. Renal calculi can be stratified into the following types: calcium, struvite, uric acid, and cystine.

Most stones (75%) are composed of calcium oxalate alone or in combination with calcium phosphate. Hyperexcretion of calcium is a major contributor to stone formation and occurs in various clinical settings. The major dietary sources of calcium are cheese and milk, and hypercalciuria may occur in adults who ingest more than 1 quart of milk daily. Many conditions predispose to hypercalciurea and the development of calculi. Perhaps the most common of these is hyperparathyroidism, in which 67% of patients develop calculi.[58] Peptic ulcer disease may also predispose to calculi formation. These patients tend to ingest large amounts of calcium with food, in addition to absorbed alkali (sodium bicarbonate) and antacids.

The other major component of calcium stones, oxalate, is also influenced by diet. Hyperoxaluria occurs in the presence of small bowel disease—Crohn's disease, ulcerative colitis, and radiation enteritis. With jejunoileal bypass surgery performed for morbid obesity, there is a reported incidence of stone disease of 12%.

Magnesium-ammonium-phosphate (struvite) stones represent approximately 15% of all renal calculi. Struvite stones occur almost exclusively in patients with urinary tract infections and are often referred to as "infection stones." They form as a result of urea-splitting organisms such as *Proteus, Providencia, Klebsiella, Pseudomonas,* and *Staphylococcus.* A distinctive feature of these calculi is the common occurrence of staghorns and coffin-lid crystals, often in the presence of alkali urine.

Uric acid stones comprise 10% of all stones in the United States. The basic causative factor is excessive excretion of uric acid in the urine. Approximately 25% of patients with symptomatic gout have uric acid calculi, and the incidence of uric acid stones increases with the use of uricosuric agents. A distinctive feature of uric acid stones is their radiolucency. These calculi infrequently cause staghorns.

Cystine stones are rare and account for only 1% of stones. They are caused by an inborn error of metabolism, which results in an increased secretion of cystine. Cystine forms staghorns.

Pathophysiology Impaction along the genitourinary tract is a serious complication of renal calculi and can cause several physiologic changes. Once obstruction occurs, there is a rapid redistribution of renal blood flow, resulting in a decrease in the glomerular filtration rate. As both glomerular and tubular function decrease, renal excretion shifts to the unaffected kidney. Obstruction causes a rapid decrease in ureteral peristaltic activity. In the presence of infection, both renal and ureteral function may be impaired. Complete obstruction of the ureters may lead to loss of renal function, with an increased occurrence of irreversible damage after 1 to 2 weeks. Partial obstruction is associated with a lower likelihood of renal injury, but may still result in irreversible damage.

Calculus size and location are important determinants for the resultant degree of disease; however, the major cause of progressive renal damage is the presence of infection. Because the stone behaves as a foreign body, creating stasis and obstruction, decreases in host resistance increase the incidence of infection.

The most important factor that relates to passage of a calculus though the genitourinary tract is its size. The critical size for spontaneous passage is 5 mm. Approximately 90% of stones that are less than 5 mm and located in the lower ureter pass spontaneously within 4 weeks. This number decreases to 15% for stones between 5 and 8 mm. In contrast, 95% of stones larger than 8 mm become impacted along the genitourinary tract, generally requiring lithotripsy or surgical removal. Intervention can in most cases be performed in the outpatient setting.

Ureteral stones originate in the kidney, with gravity and peristalsis contributing to their passage along the ureter. Renal calculi seldom cause complete obstruction. There are five sites along the ureter where calculi are likely to become impacted (Figure 94-4). First, a stone may lodge in the calyx of the kidney or pass into the renal pelvis and become lodged at the ureteropelvic junction. The relatively large renal pelvis (1 cm) narrows abruptly at its distal portion, equaling the diameter of its adjoining ureter (2 to 3 mm). The third region is near the pelvic brim where the ureter arches over the iliac vessels posteriorly into the true pelvis. The most constricted area along the ureter, and a common location for impaction, is at the ureterovesicular junction. This is the site where the ureter enters the muscular coat of the bladder (intramural ureter). At the time of diagnosis, up to 75% of stones are located in the distal third of the ureter. Finally, a calculus may become lodged in the vesical orifice.

Clinical Features

Signs and Symptoms A classic presentation of renal colic typically occurs during the night or early morning. It is usually abrupt in onset with a crescendo of extreme pain that begins in the flank, extends laterally around the abdomen, and radiates into the groin. Pain may radiate into the testicle in men and to the labia majora in women. A constant underlying dull ache in the flank is common between episodes of colic. The cause of colicky, severe flank pain is hyperperi-

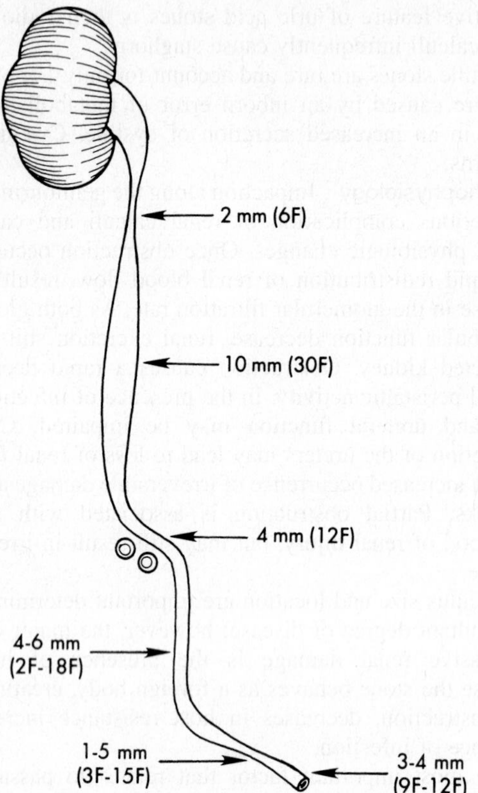

Figure 94-4. **The ureter, showing its variations of caliber.** *After Eisendrath and Rolnick; from Lich R Jr et al: Childhood disorders and diseases. In Harrison JH et al, editors:* Campbell's urology, *ed 4, vol I, Philadelphia, 1978, WB Saunders.*

stalsis of the smooth muscle of the calyces, pelvis, and ureter, whereas the cause of a dull ache can be attributed to acute obstruction and renal capsular tension.

Autonomic nerve fibers that serve both the kidney and testicle (or ovary) are involved in the transmission of pain with renal calculi, and the location of the stone may be suggested by the pattern of pain. A stone located high in the ureter may cause pain that radiates into the testicle (or ovary). As the stone approaches the bladder, the pain may shift to the scrotum or vulva. Symptoms of urinary urgency and frequency often develop as the stone nears the bladder.

Gastrointestinal symptoms of nausea and vomiting are common in patients with renal colic. One third of patients experience gross hematuria, with or without blood clots in the urine. A history of fever and chills strongly suggests superimposed infection and should be regarded as a true emergency.

Physical Examination The patient with renal colic often presents in severe pain, is pacing, and cannot find a comfortable position. The skin is usually pale, cool, and clammy. Pulse rate and blood pressure are often elevated secondary to the extreme pain. Fever is not generally noted and, if present, strongly suggests infection. The abdominal examination may reveal signs of an early ileus with hypoactive bowel sounds. A decrease in peristalsis often accompanies renal colic, but abdominal tenderness is usually absent. It is imperative to auscultate the abdomen in search of bruits over the abdominal aorta and iliac vessels, as the clinical manifestations of aortic abdominal aneurysms may mimic those of renal colic.

Diagnostic Strategies

Laboratory Tests

Urinalysis Considerable information can be obtained from a meticulous urinalysis, and this test should always be performed when renal calculi are suspected.

Urinary pH The mean urinary pH is 5.85. A urinary pH greater than 7.6 should raise suspicion for the presence of urea-splitting organisms because the kidney will not, under normal conditions, produce urine in this alkaline range. Renal tubular acidosis and ingestion of absorbable alkali must also be considered. A pH less than 5 is often associated with the formation of uric acid calculi.

Proteinuria Traces of albumin may be detected and are associated with red blood cells in the urine.

Crystalluria Examination of the crystals present may provide a clue to the stone type.

Sediment Red blood cells are generally found in the urine of patients with urolithiasis. However, the absence of red blood cells in the urine does not exclude the diagnosis. Twenty percent of patients with urolithiasis documented by IVP have no microscopic hematuria. Furthermore, there is no correlation between the degree of obstruction and the absence of hematuria.[77] Pyuria can occur in the absence of infection as a result of ureteral inflammation. However, bacteriuria should be sought especially if other clinical signs of infection, such as fever and chills, are present. Culture should always be done when infection is suspected.

Other laboratory tests Serum uric acid levels are elevated in 50% of all uric acid stone formers. (Salicylates and fasting elevate serum uric acid.) BUN and serum creatinine levels should be measured if indicated.

A CBC may reveal a slightly elevated WBC count in patients with renal calculi. However, a count over 15,000 WBC/mm^3 suggests active infection. Serum calcium and phosphorus levels should be assessed to screen for hyperparathyroidism, sarcoidosis, and other disorders of calcium metabolism, but this metabolic workup may be performed in the outpatient setting.

Imaging Imaging should be performed in patients with a first episode of renal colic. Other indications include patients in whom the diagnosis is unclear and those in whom a proximal UTI, in addition to a calculus, is suspected.

A KUB is the standard, initial radiograph done before injecting contrast media during IVP. A KUB is not a reliable study to diagnose urolithiasis, providing only presumptive evidence for a calculus (<70% specificity), and therefore should be followed by a more definitive study.[78] Radiographic densities may be noted on the KUB. Phleboliths in the pelvic veins are commonly seen. Phleboliths are spherical with a hollow (lucent) center, whereas calculi are usually irregularly shaped. Calcified mesenteric lymph nodes may also add confusion; however, these densities change in position on subsequent films.

Most calculi (90%) are radiopaque. These include calculi composed of calcium oxalate, cystine, calcium phosphate, or magnesium-ammonium-phosphate (Figures 94-5 and 94-6). Uric acid stones, blood clots, and sloughed papillae are seen as "negative" shadow on radiographs. The most commonly

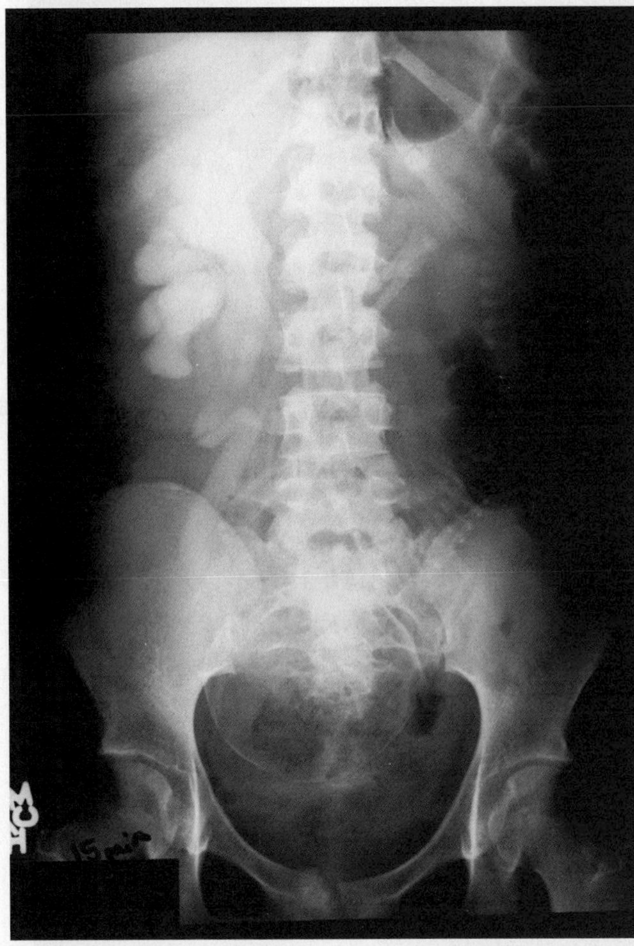
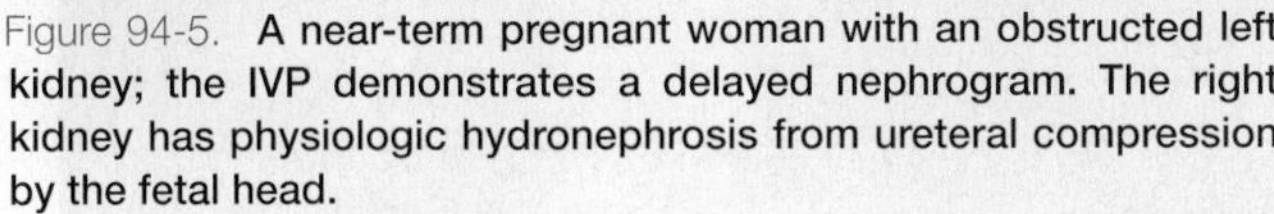

Figure 94-5. **A near-term pregnant woman with an obstructed left kidney; the IVP demonstrates a delayed nephrogram. The right kidney has physiologic hydronephrosis from ureteral compression by the fetal head.**

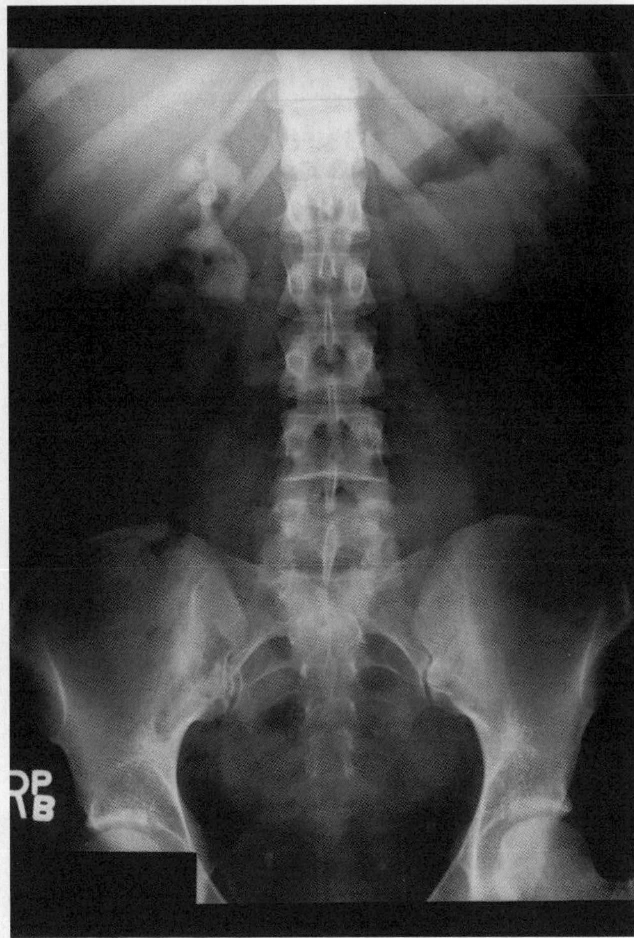

Figure 94-6. **KUB demonstrating a staghorn calculus in the right kidney.**

overlooked calculi lie in the region over the sacrum, where small stones are often obscured by this bony density.

Intravenous pyelogram IVP has traditionally been the cornerstone in ED evaluation of a patient with renal colic. It is very accurate, establishing the diagnosis of calculous disease in 96% of cases and quantifying the presence and severity of obstruction. There are few contraindications to the use of urographic contrast medium, including renal insufficiency and prior reaction to contrast material. The incidence of serious contrast media reactions is extremely low.

After injection of a standard urographic media, a radiograph is taken at 5 minutes. The most reliable and earliest indicator of a calculus is the delay in appearance of contrast media in the 5-minute film. If only a nephrogram is seen at 5 minutes on the affected side, the patient should return to the ED until 60 to 120 minutes have passed (Figure 94-7). This serves two purposes: (1) patient comfort (the radiology examination table is considerably less comfortable than most ED stretchers) and (2) avoidance of unnecessary, repetitive radiographs that do not contribute greatly to localizing the obstruction in the 1- to 2-hour interval. If contrast medium is excreted on the affected side, the degree of hydronephrosis and intensity of obstruction of the kidney can be assessed by the rate of elimination of the dye. The degree of dilation of the ureter above the calculus should be noted. Often the findings may be subtle—there may be only mild dilation of the ureter and calyces.

A helpful finding is columnization. In general, in the absence of a pathologic condition, the ureter should not be seen in its entirety on a single film. The ureter is a dynamic structure, not a passive conduit. Normally it is in various phases of peristalsis. With the onset of obstruction, peristalsis does not cease, but the increase in volume within the ureter results in the columnization of urine and is manifest as such during an excretory urogram.

The pyelogram should not be terminated before dye is allowed to reach the level of the obstructing stone. A column of dye ending at the calculus must be demonstrated for true confirmation to be made.

Occasionally, the patient may become pain-free during the radiographic procedure. This may be caused by two phenomena: (1) the hyperosmolar load of contrast medium often "assists" the passage of the stone or (2) the cessation of pain may signify the onset of complete obstruction.

Ultrasound An alternative to IVP is ultrasound. Ultrasound is less reliable at detecting small ureteral and midureteral stones. However, although only 64% sensitive in detecting calculi, ultrasound shows hydronephrosis with a

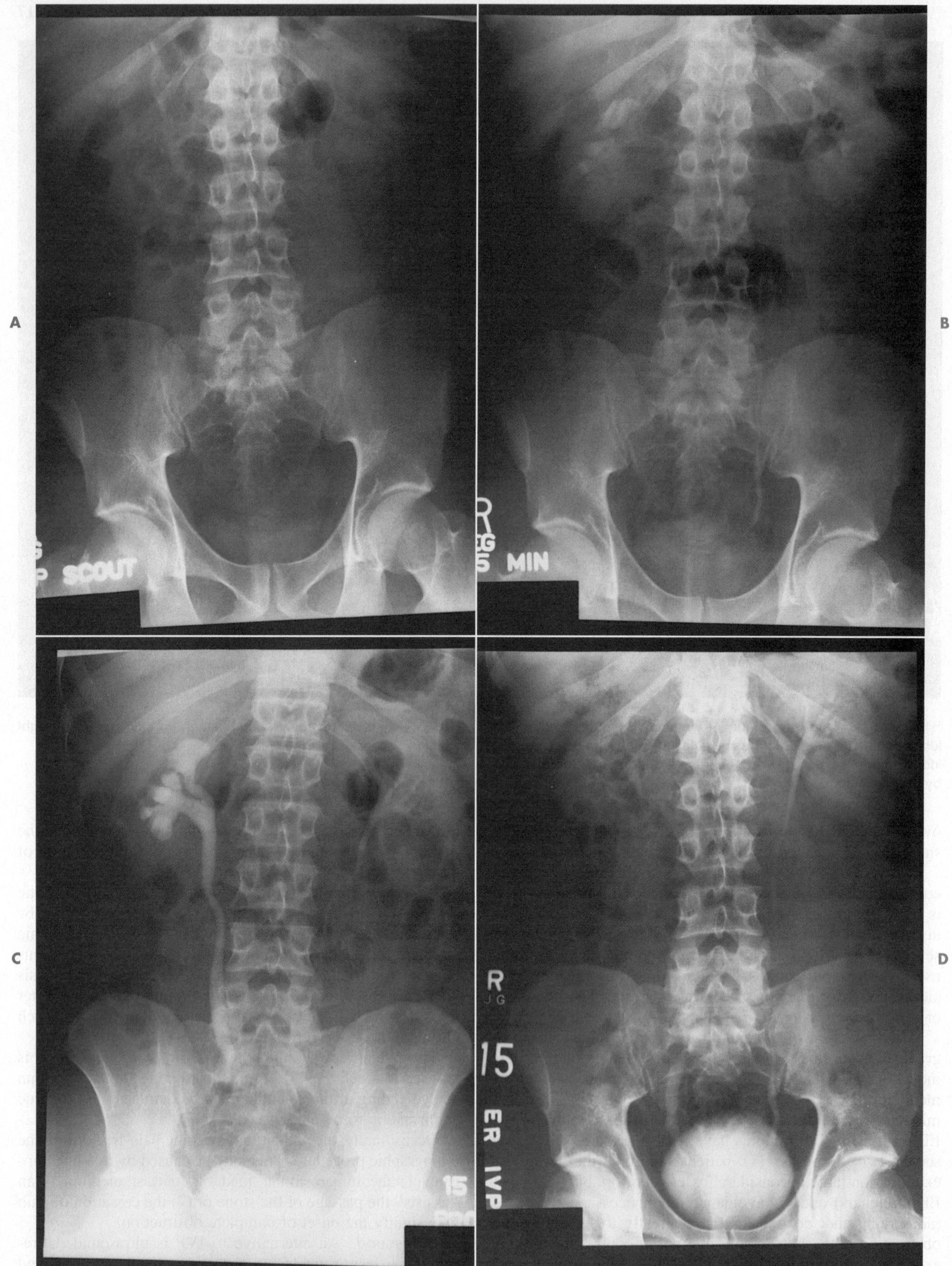

Figure 94-7. **A,** KUB (scout) film in a patient with right renal colic shows a suspicious calcification overlying the second sacral neural foramina. **B,** IVP at 5 minutes shows dilated calyces in the right kidney. **C,** IVP at 15 minutes shows a column of contrast in a dilated ureter. The stone is located in the pelvic ureter and hydronephrosis is demonstrated by the dilated calyces. **D,** An IVP 2 months later at 15 minutes has a delayed right nephrogram consistent with obstruction.

sensitivity of 85% to 94% and a specificity of 100% (Figure 94-8).[79] In a patient with a history of calculi and whose symptoms suggest new renal colic, ultrasound may be the study of choice.

Helical (spiral) computed tomography Helical CT with or without contrast has recently been employed in evaluating renal calculi. Advantages include its ability to detect calculi as small as 1 mm in diameter and direct visualization of complications, such as hydroureter, hydronephrosis, and ureteral edema.[80] Helical CT has advantages over IVP because it can be performed rapidly and does not require intravenous contrast media. Furthermore, other nonurologic causes of symptoms, such as abdominal aortic aneurysms, can be identified. A recent study of nonenhanced helical CT in the evaluation of renal colic found a sensitivity of 97%, a specificity of 96%, and an accuracy of 97%.[80]

Differential Considerations A number of significant clinical entities can produce flank pain (Box 94-3) and should be considered in patients with symptoms suggestive of renal colic. These include acute abdominal aneurysm, pyelonephritis, carcinoma, renal tuberculosis, papillary necrosis, and vascular compromise.

Acute pyelonephritis can cause severe renal pain. Urinalysis should aid in the differential diagnosis by the findings of pyuria and bacteriuria; however, infection occasionally occurs in the presence of an obstructive stone and is a urologic emergency. It is imperative to do an IVP or an ultrasound study in these cases.

Renal carcinoma may also produce flank pain, especially if there has been hemorrhage within the tumor. An abdominal flat plate radiograph (KUB) may demonstrate calcifications overlying the renal shadow that are often seen in renal neoplasms. The IVP may suggest the diagnosis, but a CT scan is the preferred diagnostic study.

Calculous disease complicates renal tuberculosis in 10% of all cases. The finding of sterile pyuria strongly suggests renal tuberculosis; confirmation is made by identifying acid-fast bacilli in the urine.

Papillary necrosis may cause renal colic as a result of the passage of sloughed papillae down the ureter. This is most often seen in diabetics and in patients with a history of acute or chronic UTI. The IVP may be diagnostic; however, a lucent filling defect may simulate a stone, but may instead represent sloughed papilla.

Renal pain, either colicky or noncolicky, is also produced by acute vascular compromise of a kidney. The pain of renal infarction is severe and occasionally associated with microscopic or gross hematuria. The acute vascular changes may be secondary to renal artery embolus, renal vein thrombosis, dissection of the renal artery, rupture of a renal artery aneurysm, aortic dissection, or abdominal aortic aneurysm. If a vascular etiology is suspected, a contrast CT scan or an angiogram should be done. The most common of these relatively rare processes is renal artery embolism, which is most often of cardiac origin (atrial fibrillation, subacute bacterial endocarditis, mural thrombus). An IVP should demonstrate decreased or absent excretion of contrast material. An immediate angiogram is indicated because early diagnosis allows possible salvage of the ischemic kidney. Most renal artery aneurysms are small and seldom manifest themselves. Approximately 60% of renal artery aneurysms are calcified.[81] The dissection or rupture of a renal artery aneurysm is rare and causes shock and flank pain. Renal vein thrombosis often demonstrates microscopic hematuria and proteinuria. The KUB may show an increased renal shadow and, in the early stages, the IVP reveals decreased function of the affected kidney. Predisposing factors for renal vein thrombosis include the nephrotic syndrome, malignancies, and pregnancy.

Renal or perinephric abscess may cause flank pain, fever, and a palpable mass. An IVP with nephrotomograms, ultrasound, or a CT scan should be done. A chest film may demonstrate a pleural effusion or elevation of the diaphragm. Both of these entities are emergencies and demand hospitalization for adequate management and determination of the underlying causes.

Management Patients with ureteral stones are generally in agonizing pain. Often the history, physical examination, and finding of hematuria allow a presumptive diagnosis to be made. Nonsteroidal antiinflammatory drugs (NSAIDs) are an excellent alternative to narcotics or may be used in conjunction with narcotics. Intravenous ketorolac is often administered as a first-line agent for pain caused by renal colic. In addition to their analgesic effects, NSAIDs decrease the pain of renal colic by decreasing ureterospasm and renal capsular pressure secondary to diminishing glomerular filtration rate in the obstructed kidney.

It is entirely appropriate to administer narcotics (morphine sulfate or meperidine in age- and weight-related dosages). There is little evidence in the literature to support the use of anticholinergics for the treatment of acute colic. Reports in the literature describe individuals with factitious hematuria and renal colic. Patients with Munchausen syndrome and those with an analgesic habit often visit the ED in search of drugs. The emergency physician must be aware of this phenomenon because renal colic is a complaint commonly used by individuals seeking narcotics (Box 94-4).[76]

Outpatient Management Most patients with ureteral calculi may be discharged with appropriate referral and careful instructions from the emergency physician. The patient should be instructed to drink a moderate amount of fluids, to take analgesics as needed for pain, and to engage in activity as tolerated. (Caution patients who have occupations that might be hazardous under the influence of either analgesics or the sudden onset of pain.) In addition, patients should strain all urine. This is an important procedure. There are commercially available strainers, or the patient may simply void into a glass jar. The calculus is visible at the bottom. The stone should be saved and submitted to the urologist for analysis. Patients should be told to return immediately if intractable, severe pain recurs, persistent nausea and vomiting develop, or fever and chills occur. Finally, an outpatient urologic evaluation should be scheduled (within 2 weeks).

Indications for Admission (Box 94-5) Admission should be sought for patients who are severely dehydrated, have unrelenting pain or vomiting, or have an underlying infection with hydronephrosis. Sepsis and renal damage are risks in the presence of obstruction and infection. Immediate operative intervention may be indicated to provide drainage and relieve the obstruction.

A patient who returns to the ED with colic may not need a repeat imaging study if the stone was identified previously.

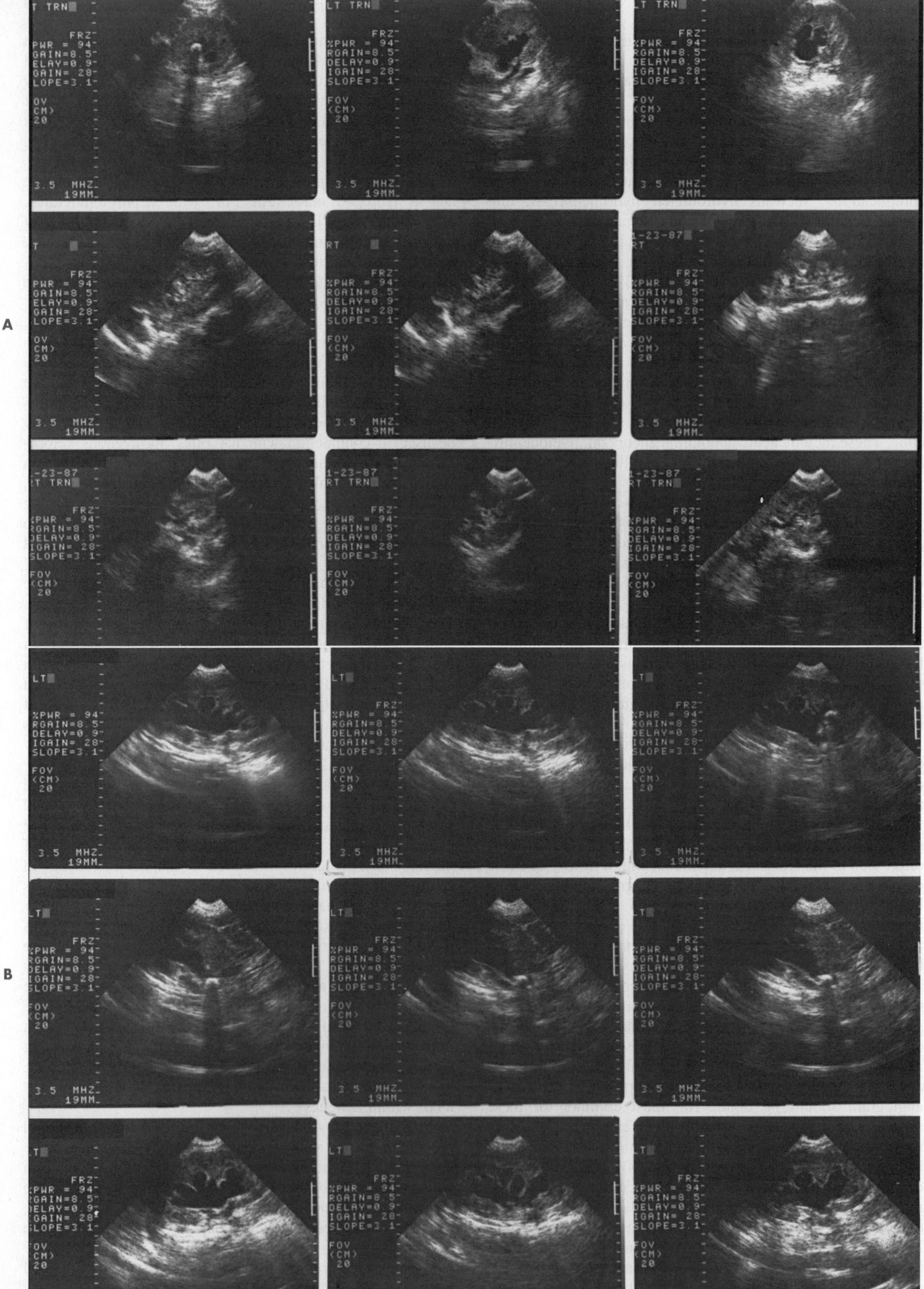

Figure 94-8. **Ultrasound of a patient with renal colic. A, Long 1-1 axis view demonstrates hydronephrosis. B, Transverse cut shows a calcification with an acoustic shadow in the renal calyx.**

Box 94-3 Differential Diagnosis of Urolithiasis

Urologic Disease

Upper urinary tract

Renal infarct
Renal parenchymal tumors
Urothelial tumors
Papillary necrosis
Pyelonephritis
Hemorrhage (blood clot)

Ureter

Urothelial tumors
Hemorrhage (blood clot)
Prior surgery (e.g., stricture)
Metastatic tumors

Lower urinary tract

Urothelial tumors
Urinary retention

Nonurologic Disease

Intraabdominal

Peritonitis (especially appendicitis)
Biliary colic
Intestinal obstruction

Vascular

Abdominal aortic aneurysm
Superior mesenteric artery occlusion

Retroperitoneal

Retroperitonal lymphadenopathy
Retroperitoneal fibrosis
Tumor

Gynecologic

Cervical cancer
Endometriosis
Ovarian vein syndrome

Musculoskeletal

From Lingeman J: Calculous disease of the kidney and bladder. In Harwood-Nuss A, editor: *The clinical practice of emergency medicine,* ed 2, Philadelphia, 1996, JB Lippincott.

In this case a KUB may localize the stone. Urologic consultation is recommended.

Treatment Options Several treatment options are available to the urologist in the management of stones that do not pass spontaneously. Optimal therapy depends on the size, location, and composition of the stone. Extracorporeal shock wave lithotripsy (ECSWL) has proven very effective for stones located in the kidney, with a greater than 85% clearance rate. Upper ureteral stones may also be cleared with a high success rate when ECSWL is done after ureteroscopic manipulation of the stone to a more proximal position. Percutaneous nephrolithotomy, which establishes a tract from the skin to the collecting system, is used on stones too large or hard for ECSWL. Stones unresponsive or unlikely to respond to other techniques may require surgical removal.

Box 94-4 Munchausen-Like Syndrome/ Narcotics-Seeking Patients

History of multiple narcotic allergies
History of uric acid lithiasis
History of contrast allergy
Multiple prior stone events
Itinerant
Factitious hematuria
Noncooperative

From Lingeman J: Calculous disease of the kidney and bladder. In Harwood-Nuss A, editor: *The clinical practice of emergency medicine,* ed 2, Philadelphia, 1996, JB Lippincott.

Box 94-5 Indications for Admission

Obstruction with infection*
Persistent pain
Persistent nausea and vomiting
Urinary extravasation
Hypercalcemic crisis

Relative Indications for Admission

High-grade obstruction
Solitary kidney
Intrinsic renal disease
Size of obstructing stone
Duration of symptoms
Social situation

From Lingeman J: Calculous disease of the kidney and bladder. In Harwood-Nuss A, editor: *The clinical practice of emergency medicine,* ed 2, Philadelphia, 1996, JB Lippincott.

*Potential urologic emergency.

Vesical Calculus

Although calculi generally form in the kidneys, they may also originate in the bladder. There is evidence for assuming that bladder stones constitute a different entity from renal stones. In the United States, bladder stones occur almost exclusively in elderly men, most often as a complication of other urologic disease. The most common cause is infection of the residual bladder urine with urea-splitting organisms *(Proteus).* The other common cause of vesical stones is an indwelling catheter. Predisposing causes to the formation of bladder stones include bladder neck obstruction (usually secondary to prostatic hyperplasia), neurogenic bladder, vesical diverticula, irradiation, and schistosomiasis.

The symptoms are most often pain on voiding and hematuria. The patient may complain of a sudden interruption of the urinary stream. This strongly suggests a vesical stone that intermittently obstructs the bladder outlet. Frequency, urgency, and dysuria are seen in up to 50% of patients and UTI is common.

A physical examination is rarely rewarding because signs may be minimal. Rectal examination may reveal enlarged prostate or a prostatic malignancy. Poor sphincter tone may suggest a neurogenic bladder. Urinalysis generally reveals pyuria and bacteriuria; hematuria is commonly seen as well. Plain radiographs of the pelvis reveal a bladder stone in 50% of cases. IVP may demonstrate obstructive changes in the upper tracts or bladder diverticula.

Acute Scrotal Mass

Perspective The onset of acute scrotal pain and swelling can present a major challenge to the emergency physician. It should be considered a major medical emergency and approached rapidly. Patients with acute scrotal mass may have widely variable signs and symptoms, including a painless mass, severe sharp pain, dull pain, or pain that radiates to the abdomen or thighs. The emergency physician must act quickly to identify emergency conditions in these patients.

Principles of Disease

Anatomy Knowledge of testicular landmarks is essential for examination of the patient with an acute scrotal mass. Figure 94-9 demonstrates the normal anatomy of the scrotum and testis. The normal scrotum is relatively symmetrical, and both testicles are of equal mass and volume. The normal testis is found in the vertical axis with a slight forward tilt, and the epididymis is above the superior pole in the posterolateral position.

Physical Examination The testis should be examined grasping it between the first and second fingers and the thumb. Particular attention should be paid to any tenderness to palpation, discrepancies in size, loss of testicular landmarks, or discoloration. In addition, the epididymis should be nontender, soft, and have a noticeable smooth ridge posterolateral to the testis. Testing of the cremasteric reflex is an essential part of the scrotal examination. The cremasteric reflex is elicited by stroking or pinching the inner thigh and observing an elevation of more than 0.5 cm of the ipsilateral testicle.

Differential Considerations The challenge to the emergency physician in evaluating for acute scrotal mass is the substantial differential diagnosis. Although the differential category is broad, the emergency physician must have a high index of suspicion and rapidly identify testicular torsion. The most common causes of acute scrotal mass are testicular torsion, epididymitis, torsion of appendages, testicular tumor, orchitis, and hernia/hydrocele.

Specific Disorders

Testicular Torsion

Perspective Testicular torsion is estimated to occur in three to four patients per year in a large general hospital (or 1:4000).[82] The average salvageability rate remains low in most series, approximately 50% testicular loss either from atrophy or orchiectomy.[82] There are two peak periods in which torsion is likely to occur: the first year of life and at puberty. One series reports an age range of 5 months to 41 years with the average age of 16.2 years. Clearly, torsion is not limited to the pubertal period. Testicular torsion is 10 times more likely in an undescended testis. It should be high in the differential diagnosis when a patient has a painful inguinal mass and an empty scrotum.

Principles of disease Most torsions are caused by an underlying bilateral anatomic abnormality. There exists a

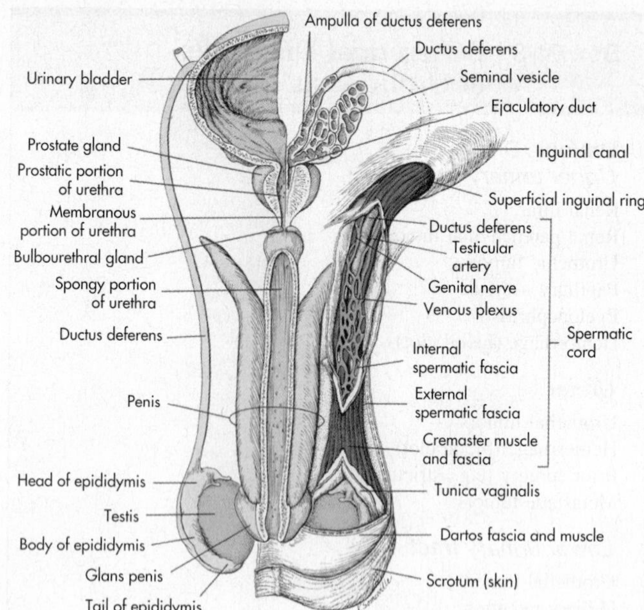

Figure 94-9. **Testes, epididymis, ductus deferens, and glands of the male reproductive system.** ***From Seeley RR et al, editors:*** **Anatomy and physiology, *ed 1, New York, 1989, McGraw-Hill.***

capacious tunica vaginalis with a high insertion about the spermatic cord. The result is a redundant cord. The testis then "dangles" in the scrotum and is mobile. This phenomenon has been likened to the clapper of a bell, hence the term *bell-clapper deformity* of the testicle.

The initial effect of testicular torsion is obstruction of the venous return. As twisting of the cord persists, thrombosis of the vein is followed by arterial thrombosis. The degree of obstruction is a function of the degree of rotation. If the rotation is incomplete, edema and congestion occur. Necrosis develops in the testicle with complete obstruction, and infarction promptly develops when arterial thrombosis occurs. Clinically, there is rapid swelling and edema of the testis and scrotum, with erythema of the scrotal skin following soon after.

The amount of damage is related to the duration and extent of vascular obstruction. A salvage rate of 80% to 100% is possible if the pain lasts less than 6 hours.[82] Continuous pain for 24 hours is usually associated with testicular infarction. Contralateral testicular damage from torsion remains under investigation. It probably does not contribute to male infertility.

Clinical features A well-recognized phenomenon may provide an early clue—nearly 41% of patients report a history of *similar* pain that resolved spontaneously. The pain of torsion usually begins suddenly in the scrotum, but its location may be inguinal or lower abdominal. It is often associated with nausea and vomiting, which are thought to be secondary to the sudden occlusion of the testicular vascular supply. Torsion commonly occurs either after exertion or during sleep. There is a notable absence of urinary symptoms in most patients.

The diagnosis of testicular torsion is often made more difficult by extreme pain, which permits only a superficial examination of the affected hemiscrotum. Generally, the hemiscrotum is swollen, tender, and firm. A reactive hydrocele may be present. The classic signs of a high-riding testis with a transverse lie are not always detectable. Loss of the cremasteric reflex is strongly associated with torsion. The presence of the cremasteric reflex virtually excludes the diagnosis, although rare cases have been reported.[83] In infants and children, many of the signs are often absent.

Examination of the opposite testis is mandatory and should be done with the patient standing. The basic anatomic abnormality that predisposes to testicular torsion is the bell-clapper deformity. Hence the contralateral testicle may be noted to lie in the horizontal axis.

Prehn's sign has been described and used in the past to distinguish torsion from epididymitis. It was believed that relief of scrotal pain by elevating the testis indicated epididymitis; it is not a reliable sign and should not be used to distinguish these two processes. The size of the scrotal mass is also unreliable in determining the underlying process. It in no way indicates the type of pathologic condition present.

Diagnostic strategies A urinalysis should be performed, but it may be unremarkable in testicular torsion. Similarly, a CBC often reveals an absence of leukocytosis. Color Doppler ultrasound has become the test of choice at most hospitals to diagnose testicular torsion if the clinical diagnosis is uncertain. Color Doppler ultrasound has similar sensitivity (86% to 100%) and specificity (100%) to radioisotope scans (80% to 100%, 89% to 100%). In addition to being more specific, color Doppler ultrasound is more rapid and often more practical than radioisotope scans.

Management Manual detorsion should be attempted in most cases while steps are being taken for definitive surgical exploration. Manual detorsion should not be considered curative, but rather a temporizing technique only. Torsion of a testicle may occur in either direction but usually the anterior portion twists medially. After appropriate parenteral analgesics the patient should be placed in the supine position. The anterior portion of the testicle should be twisted laterally unless it appears to shorten the cord or worsen the torsion, in which case detorsion in the reverse direction should be attempted. Cord blocks should be attempted only by the consulting urologist.

No procedure should delay surgical intervention. If the diagnosis is thought to be torsion, the place to prove or disprove it is the operating room. In patients over age 18 years who have a history and physical examination compatible with torsion, no urethral discharge, no cremaster reflex, and no recent urinary tract infection, the diagnosis of torsion should also be strongly entertained with similar expedient referral for exploration. Immediate evaluation and referral to a urologist should be accomplished in the ED and surgery done on an emergency basis.

Disposition Rapid diagnosis in testicular torsion is essential. Once the diagnosis has been established, emergency surgical scrotal exploration and bilateral orchidopexy are performed.

Epididymitis

Perspective Epididymitis is the most common intrascrotal inflammatory disease. It is also the most common misdiagnosis for testicular torsion. It is generally a disease of adult men. The average age for epididymitis is 25 years. Epididymitis rarely affects the prepubertal child in the absence of underlying urinary tract disease. It accounts for more than 600,000 visits to physicians each year in the United States and is responsible for more days lost from military service than any other disease.[72]

Principles of disease Bacterial epididymitis is usually the result of a retrograde ascent of urethral and bladder pathogens. In rare instances, epididymitis may result from hematogenous spread. In the initial stages of epididymitis, there is cellular inflammation that begins in the vas deferens and descends to the lower pole of the epididymis. This descent explains the initial common symptoms of flank and groin pain (secondary to vasitis). The inflammatory process in the lower pole progresses, eventually involving the remaining epididymis and the testis.

In the acute phase the epididymis is swollen and indurated with involvement of both upper and lower poles. The spermatic cord is thickened. The testis may become edematous secondary to passive congestion or to the inflammatory process (orchitis). Resolution of the process may be complete and without sequelae, but peritubular fibrosis often develops, occluding the ductules. If the process is bilateral, it may result in sterility.

Pathophysiology Studies clearly implicate *C. trachomatis* as a major etiologic agent. Through the use of epididymal aspirates during acute epididymitis, it has been demonstrated that in men age 35 years and older, *E. coli* is the predominant pathogen, whereas in men under age 35 years, *Chlamydia* and *N. gonorrhoeae* are the major pathogens.[84] Moreover, nearly two thirds of all cases of acute epididymitis in the younger group are caused by *C. trachomatis.* In addition to the usual pathogens (*Chlamydia, Neisseria,* coliform bacteria), many other organisms are known to cause acute epididymitis, most often in association with systemic infections (e.g., blastomycosis, meningococcus).[58]

The most common cause of nonsexually transmitted bacterial epididymitis in men over age 35 years is infection with coliform organisms or *Pseudomonas* species. Gram-positive cocci are also important pathogens. This age group distinction is important not only from the standpoint of therapy but because bacterial epididymitis in men over age 35 years is commonly associated with underlying urologic pathology.

The older patient (over age 35 years) with epididymitis may give a history of recent genitourinary tract manipulation. Acute or chronic bacterial prostatitis is also an important predisposing condition for the development of epididymitis. In the obtunded, febrile patient with a catheter, it is wise to examine the genitalia to rule out epididymitis as a cause.

The two most common causes of sexually transmitted bacterial epididymitis in young men are *C. trachomatis* and *N. gonorrhoeae,* with *C. trachomatis* clearly the dominant one (nearly two thirds of all cases in the younger age group). Most patients infected with *Chlamydia* do not complain of urethral discharge but have a demonstrable discharge characteristic of nongonococcal urethritis. A sexual history should be obtained, although there is evidence that patients may carry *C. trachomatis* for long periods before clinical epididymitis develops. Of patients with gonococcal epididymitis, 21% to 30% have no history of urethral discharge and no demonstrable discharge 50% of the time. A sexual history is important, but the patient may be reluctant to give a history of recent exposure. Underlying urologic pathology is rare in this age group.

Syphilitic epididymitis probably occurs more often than is generally believed. It may occur early in the secondary stage or 8 to 9 years after the onset of the disease. Diffuse thickening of the superior aspect of the epididymis and rubbery nodules may be palpable.[58] The diagnosis is usually presumptive, having been made on the basis of evidence of syphilis elsewhere. Tuberculous epididymitis is often (41%) the earliest indication of renal tuberculosis, but usually follows a subacute or chronic course, rather than acute. Typically, one might expect to find beading or thickening of the vas deferens. The most common lesion is a "cold abscess" located in the tail of the epididymis, although the disease may cause the more classic, painful inflammation seen with the more usual pathogens. The diagnosis is further suspected by the urine sediment, which typically reveals abacterial pyuria. The diagnosis is confirmed by isolating *Mycobacterium tuberculosis* in the urine. Amiodarone has also been implicated as a cause of noninfectious epididymitis.

Clincial features The pain of epididymitis is usually more gradual in onset, reaching a peak over days, not hours. In 95% of cases of epididymitis, there is a febrile state with an average temperature of 38° C (100.4° F). However, as mentioned earlier, nearly 20% of patients with torsion are also mildly febrile. Urinary tract symptoms may precede the pain.

Examination of the affected scrotum is often difficult. The extreme sensitivity and diffuse changes often mask distinguishing landmarks. In general, edema and erythema of the scrotum are *not* noted in the *early* stage of acute epididymitis. The cremasteric reflex is usually present.

Pain most often begins gradually in the scrotum or groin, radiating along the spermatic cord, and often intensifies over the next few hours. The degree of epididymal swelling varies, but the epididymis often reaches twice normal size over 3 to 4 hours. Fever and generalized toxicity may be seen. A urethral discharge or associated irritative voiding symptoms may accompany the swelling and pain.

There may be tenderness over the groin, lower abdomen, and scrotum. The scrotal skin is usually erythematous and warm. After the initial 3 to 4 hours, the epididymis may be indistinguishable from the testis because of passive congestion. The spermatic cord may be edematous as well. Prostate examination should be performed with proper caution, bearing in mind that the primary infection may be exacerbated by a vigorous massage.

Diagnostic strategies Urinalysis may or may not reveal evidence of bacterial infection. *Chlamydia* are not identified in a routine examination of the sediment, whereas *E. coli* are. If a urethral discharge is present, it must be examined for gram-negative intracellular diplococci and other bacteria.

The presence of more than one gram-negative rod per oil immersion field in the Gram's-stained smear of 1 drop of uncentrifuged urine correlates with the presence of more than 10^3 bacteria/ml of urine. The presence of intracellular gram-negative diplococci on the Gram's stain of the urethral smear correlates nearly 100% of the time with cultures for *N. gonorrhoeae*.

There is often a leukocytosis in the range of 10,000 to 30,000/mm^3. Leukocytosis suggests epididymitis, as does the presence of pyuria in the urine sediment. However, only overwhelming evidence of infection should prevent the strong consideration of torsion as the diagnosis because only 50% of patients with epididymitis have pyuria or bacteria. A urethral Gram's stain and culture are indicated, especially for patients less than age 35 years.

The presence of pyuria, bacteriuria, dysuria, or fever does not exclude a diagnosis of torsion. Any patient with an equivocal examination requires perfusion imaging by color Doppler ultrasonography or nuclear scintigraphy. The diagnosis of epididymitis is confirmed by normal to increased testicular blood flow.

Differential considerations For both age groups, it is recommended that a careful examination of the genitalia be done to rule out other diseases. Three intrascrotal processes commonly confused with epididymitis are torsion, torsion of the testicular appendage, and tumor of the testicle. These are addressed in their respective sections.

Management The treatment for sexually transmitted epididymitis in adults is listed in Table 94-8. Treatment of epididymitis secondary to coliform infection should be guided by the results of the urine analysis and culture. Treatment may be accomplished with various effective antimicrobials, including sulfonamides, TMP-SMZ, ampicillin, cephalosporins, and fluoroquinolones. The emergency physician should not forget the importance of treating the sexual partners of patients with sexually transmitted bacterial epididymitis.

In addition to appropriate antibiotics, general supportive measures are recommended, including bed rest, scrotal support, analgesics, sitz baths, or ice packs. The patient should be referred to a urologist for follow-up. In general, the acute inflammatory process subsides within 2 weeks, although it may be a month or more before the epididymis returns to its normal size.

Complications of the disease include infertility (most often seen in sexually transmitted epididymitis), abscess formation (seen in gonococcal epididymitis), and chronic epididymitis. Ultrasound is indicated for patients not responsive to medical therapy.

Table 94-8. Treatment of Epididymitis

Drug of choice	Dose/route	Alternative
Presumed sexually acquired		
Ceftriaxone	250 mg IM	Ciprofloxacin 500 mg PO
		Ofloxacin 400 mg PO
	followed by	
Doxycycline	100 mg PO bid × 10 days	
	OR	
Tetracycline	500 mg qid × 10 days	
Presumed nonsexually acquired*		
TMP-SMX	One double-strength PO bid × 14 days	Ciprofloxacin 500 mg PO bid × 14 days
		Ofloxacin 400 mg PO bid × 14 days

*Adjust antibacterial therapy with results of urine culture.

Disposition Patients in the older age group should be approached conservatively from the standpoint of admission, recalling that many have urologic pathology as an underlying factor. Patients of any age with systemic signs of toxicity (fever, chills, nausea, vomiting) or complications of acute epididymitis should be hospitalized and treated with parenteral antibiotics. Scrotal abscesses should be sought because emergency surgical debridement and drainage are necessary.

Torsion of Appendages

Perspective In a normal scrotum, several vestigial appendages exist that may undergo torsion and cause an acute, painful scrotal mass. The testicular and epididymal appendages are two vestigial remnants that commonly are involved. Torsion of the appendages is most frequently seen in preadolescent males between ages 3 and 13 years. Torsion of the appendix testis is most common, followed by torsion of the epididymal appendix.

Principles of disease The appendix testis is a müllerian duct remnant, which is attached to the superior pole of the testis between the testis and the epididymis. The appendix epididymis is a wolffian duct remnant attached solely to the epididymis.

The cause of torsion of the appendage is unclear. However, the effects of estrogen before puberty have been thought to cause enlargement and subsequent strangulation of the involved appendage.[85] Similar to testicular torsion, twisting causes obstruction, secondary edema, and sharp pain as the tissue becomes necrotic.

Clinical features The twisted appendage typically presents as an acute scrotal pain and a discrete, painful testicular mass. However, the symptoms are usually less severe than in testicular torsion. Unlike testicular torsion, a history of previous episodes is uncommon, as are complaints of nausea, vomiting, fevers, dysuria, or penile discharge. If the lesion is seen early, it might be rewarding to transilluminate the scrotum. The appendage may appear as a blue-black dot. With the progressive edema it is not uncommon for a reactive hydrocele to develop and mask the small, tender mass of a twisted appendage.

Diagnostic strategies A midstream urinalysis should be performed. The urinalysis generally does not demonstrate pyuria or bacteriuria. Color Doppler ultrasound and nuclear scintigraphy are the diagnostic procedures of choice. An imaging study that demonstrates normal to increased blood flow helps establish the diagnosis.

Differential considerations The emergency physician must consider other diagnoses such as testicular torsion, epididymitis, and testicular tumor.

Management and disposition If testicular torsion can be ruled out with certainty, generally conservative measures remain the standard of care. These include scrotal support, pelvic rest, and analgesia. Resolution of symptoms can be expected within 7 to 10 days. Surgical excision is reserved for severe or refractory cases.

Testicular Tumors

Perspective A tumor of the testis is the most common malignancy to afflict young men, occurring at an average age of 32 years. Testicular cancer comprises 1% of all cancer in men. The differential diagnosis between tumor, torsion, and epididymitis can be extremely difficult. In fact, epididymitis is the most common *incorrect* diagnosis made in cases of testicular tumor (6% to 16% incidence).[82] There is increased prevalence in patients with cryptorchidism in both the nondescended and descended testis.

The vast majority of testicular cancers are seminomas, followed by embryonal cell cancer and teratomas. The cancer spreads by the lymphatic system.

Clinical features Clinically the emergency physician might be confronted with diffuse swelling of the scrotum and its contents, with neither the classically severe pain of torsion or epididymitis nor the palpably hard, painless growth of testicular carcinoma. Although tumors are generally painless ("heaviness" is commonly reported), the patient may have sudden testicular pain because of acute hemorrhage within the tumor. This acute hemorrhage causes an expanding mass effect on the nonpliable tunica albuginea.

Diagnostic strategies Urinalysis should be normal in the presence of tumor. The key to diagnosis is the identification of a distinct *intratesticular* mass. Color Doppler ultrasonography is the initial diagnostic imaging study. A chest radiograph or chest CT may be considered if metastatic spread is suspected. An abdominal CT may be indicated for staging purposes.

Management Suspicion of a testicular tumor is an indication for immediate referral and hospitalization. A radical orchiectomy with high ligation of the spermatic cord is the preferred surgical procedure. The radiosensitive nature of seminomas make the combined treatment of orchiectomy and radiation therapy beneficial for early-stage seminomas. The highly effective chemotherapy agent cisplatin has also improved survival rates.

Orchitis

Perspective Orchitis is an acute infection involving the testis. Because the testis possesses a relatively high threshold of resistance to infection, orchitis is rare without an initial epididymitis. Additionally, orchitis occurs significantly less often than does prostatitis or epididymitis. As in epididymitis, the testis may become infected with a wide variety of organisms.

The two major distinguishing etiologies of orchitis are blood-borne bacterial infection and viral infection. Pyogenic bacterial orchitis is usually secondary to bacterial involvement of the epididymis, with testicular spread occurring secondarily. The most common bacterial pathogens are *E. coli, Klebsiella,* and *Pseudomonas.* Viral orchitis is most commonly caused by mumps. This is rarely seen in prepubertal boys but occurs in 20% to 30% of postpubertal boys with mumps.[82] Granulomatous orchitis occurs in association with syphilis and mycobacterial and fungal diseases, most often in an immunocompromised host.

Clinical features A patient with pyogenic orchitis is usually acutely ill with fever, marked discomfort, and swelling of the testicle. It is common to see a reactive hydrocele, and the testis is swollen and exquisitely tender. The most common picture is that of a coexistent epididymoorchitis. In general, the presumptive signs of infection are present, such as pyuria, leukocytosis, and fever.

A patient with viral orchitis has testicular pain and swelling that commonly begins 4 to 6 days after the onset of parotitis but may occur without parotid involvement. The disease is unilateral in 70% of patients. The clinical course varies, but usually resolution occurs in 4 to 5 days. More than 50% of testes involved with mumps orchitis suffer from atrophy; however, this seldom results in infertility.

Diagnostic strategies A urinalysis, urine culture, and blood cultures should be obtained. If granulomatous orchitis is suspected, its diagnosis depends on specific cultures and often on histologic stains. The diagnosis of testicular torsion should be excluded. If epididymoorchitis is present, it is a difficult entity to distinguish from torsion. Therefore, if the diagnosis is uncertain, color Doppler ultrasonography should be performed.

Management Treatment of pyogenic bacterial orchitis includes antibiotics targeting *E. coli, Klebsiella pneumoniae, Pseudomonas aeruginosa,* staphylococci, or streptococci. Local scrotal measures as outlined in the section on epididymitis are helpful. Admission to the hospital is generally required for patients with systemic signs and symptoms.

Treatment of viral orchitis is supportive only. Admission is guided by the clinical picture, which may range from mild swelling and discomfort to marked pain, high fever, and constitutional symptoms.

Inguinal Hernia and Acute Hydrocele Both inguinal hernia and acute hydrocele are reasonable considerations in the differential diagnosis of an acute scrotal mass. However, both should be readily distinguished by a careful physical examination.

Acute Urinary Retention

Perspective Acute urinary retention (AUR) can be defined as the sudden inability to pass urine. Although there are numerous causes (Box 94-6), the patient with AUR is most often an elderly male with prostatic hypertrophy.

AUR is a common problem in men with advancing age. It is estimated that 10% and 33% of men in their 70s and 80s, respectively, will develop at least one episode of AUR.[86] In women a common cause of urinary retention is an atonic, decompensated bladder that has resulted from years of infrequent voiding. In young patients, urinary retention may be an early manifestation of neurologic disease (e.g., multiple sclerosis, tabes dorsalis, diabetes, syringomyelia). Less common causes of urinary retention include phimosis, paraphimosis, and meatal stenosis.

Psychogenic urinary retention is rare and should be a diagnosis of exclusion, only after appropriate studies on bladder function have been performed by a specialist.

The acute retention of urine may be drug induced, especially in patients who are susceptible (e.g., an elderly man with mild bladder neck obstruction). Drug categories that may directly cause retention include antihistamines, anticholinergics, antispasmodics, and tricyclic antidepressants. Medications that induce bladder neck hypertonicity, resulting in AUR, include ephedrine compounds, amphetamines, and certain "cold" tablets (Box 94-7).

The most common cause of urinary retention in men over age 50 years is prostatic hyperplasia with bladder neck obstruction. Other, less common causes of obstruction in men include carcinoma of the prostate, bladder carcinoma, urethral stricture (secondary to infection or injury), and an atonic or neurogenic bladder.

Clinical Features In elderly men, symptoms and signs may include progressive decrease in the force and caliber of the urinary stream, nocturia, dribbling, prior history of retention, or urologic procedures such as catheterization, dilatation for strictures, and prostatectomy (Box 94-8). Constitutional symptoms such as bone pain and weight loss (suggesting carcinoma of the prostate) should be sought in these patients.

If infection is also present, symptoms such as dysuria, frequency, and urgency may be reported.

Physical examination in men may reveal an enlarged prostate gland, but a normal-size gland does not eliminate it as a source of obstruction. A nodular, firm mass may also be palpated, suggesting carcinoma of the prostate.

A bladder containing 150 ml or more of urine should be palpable and percussible.

Box 94-6 Causes of Acute Urinary Retention in Adults

Penis
- Phimosis
- Paraphimosis
- Meatal stenosis
- Foreign body constriction

Urethra
- Tumor
- Foreign body
- Calculus
- Urethritis (severe)
- Stricture
- Meatal stenosis (female)
- Hematoma

Prostate Gland
- Benign prostatic hypertrophy
- Carcinoma
- Prostatitis (severe)
- Bladder neck contracture
- Prostatic infarction

Neurologic Causes
- Motor paralytic
  - Spinal shock
  - Spinal cord syndromes
- Sensory paralytic
  - Tabes dorsalis
  - Diabetes
  - Multiple sclerosis
- Syringomyelia
- Spinal cord syndromes
- Herpes zoster

Miscellaneous
- Drugs
  - Antihistamines
  - Anticholinergic agents
  - Antispasmodic agents
  - Tricyclic antidepressants
  - α-Adrenergic stimulators
    - "Cold" tablets
    - Ephedrine derivatives
    - Amphetamines

Psychogenic Problems

From Sacknoff EJ, Dretler SP: Urologic emergencies. In Wilkins E, editor: *MCH textbook of emergency medicine,* Baltimore, 1978, Williams & Wilkins.

Box 94-7 Pharmacologic Agents That May Contribute to Acute Urinary Retention

β-Agonists

Isoproterenol
Terbutaline

Narcotics

Morphine
Meperidine
Dilaudid

Anticholinergics

Atropine
Belladonna
Cogentin
Cyclic antidepressants
Antihistamines
Phenothiazines
Propantheline (Probanthine)
Methantheline
Ipratropium bromide
Monoamine oxidase

Musculotropic Relaxants (of Detrusor)

Flavoxate (Urispas)
Nifedipine
Dicyclomine (Bentyl)
Oxybutynin (Ditropan)
Hyoscyamine (Cytospaz)
Estrogen
Diazepam
Indomethacin (NSAIDs)

Box 94-8 Symptoms of Urinary Retention

Obstructive Symptoms

Urinary hesitancy
Straining to void
Decrease in size and force of the urinary stream
Interruption of urinary stream
Sensation of incomplete emptying
Previous episode of urinary retention

Irritative Symptoms

Urinary frequency
Urinary urgency
Dysuria (usually secondary to infection)
Nocturia or nocturnal incontinence

Modified from Lapides J: *Fundamentals of urology,* Philadelphia, 1976, WB Saunders.

Diagnostic Strategies Laboratory studies should be obtained to assess renal function. With both postrenal and prerenal obstruction, the BUN-to-creatinine ratio is elevated. In lower urinary tract obstruction the BUN may be increased because of significant reabsorption. Urinalysis should always be performed to ascertain the presence of coexisting infection. Hematuria suggests the presence of infection, tumor, or calculi.

Imaging studies (IVP, ultrasound, CT scan) are rarely indicated in the ED and are generally reserved for patients with evidence of infection or signs of systemic toxicity.

Management Initial efforts to relieve painful urinary retention are best approached with a standard urethral catheter. A No. 16 or 18 French urethral catheter with a 5 ml balloon may be used. Lidocaine jelly should be inserted into the urethra first, not only to anesthetize the urethra but also to lubricate and distend it.

If a standard urethral catheter cannot be passed, the next step is to attempt to pass a coudé catheter. This type of catheter has an upward deflection in its distal 3 cm, which allows it to pass over an enlarged median lobe of the prostate. It also allows the tip of the catheter to be directed toward the roof of the urethra. The floor of the urethra is more lax, whereas the roof is relatively fixed. A coudé catheter can avoid impinging on the urethral fold.

If a No. 18 French or coudé catheter will not pass into the bladder, further efforts at instrumentation should be stopped. The use of filiforms and followers as well as metal sounds may result in serious tissue damage and should be performed by a specialist.

If there is no consultant available, or if immediate bladder decompression is needed, a percutaneous bladder aspiration may be performed. It is important to ensure that the bladder is palpable and distended to minimize complications. If doubt exists, a 22-gauge needle on a syringe should be passed through the skin to see if urine can be aspirated. This should be done one to two fingerbreadths above the symphysis pubis and directed toward the anus. Alternatively, ultrasound-directed cystostomy may be done. Depending on availability, a number of devices may be used. These include the Cystocath, the Bonana, or the Argyle-Ingram catheter. If these are not available, a central venous set may be used, inserting the 12- to 18-inch tubing into the bladder before the needle is withdrawn[87] (Figure 94-10).

Traditionally, gradual decompression has been recommended to prevent complications such as hematuria, hypotension, and postobstructive diuresis.

The risk of hematuria with release of AUR is 2% to 16%. However, there have been no reported cases of severe hematuria requiring invasive treatment.[88]

Hypotension has been reported after decompression in patients with AUR. AUR results in an increase in systemic blood pressure (SBP) as a result of stimulation of the vesicovascular reflex. Reduction in blood pressure after decompression may be simply normalization of the SBP. Patients at risk for hypotension after decompression include those with advancing age or hypovolemia, in whom the ability to compensate appropriately to sudden changes in SBP is altered.

Postobstructive diuresis is thought to result from a combination of factors, including osmotic diuresis, involvement of natriuretic and diuretic factors, disordered nephron function, altered tubular permeability, and disturbance of sodium-regulating hormones.[88] Patients with comorbidity (renal disease, fluid overload) appear to be at greatest risk for developing postobstructive diuresis.

Nyman reports that gradual emptying of the bladder,

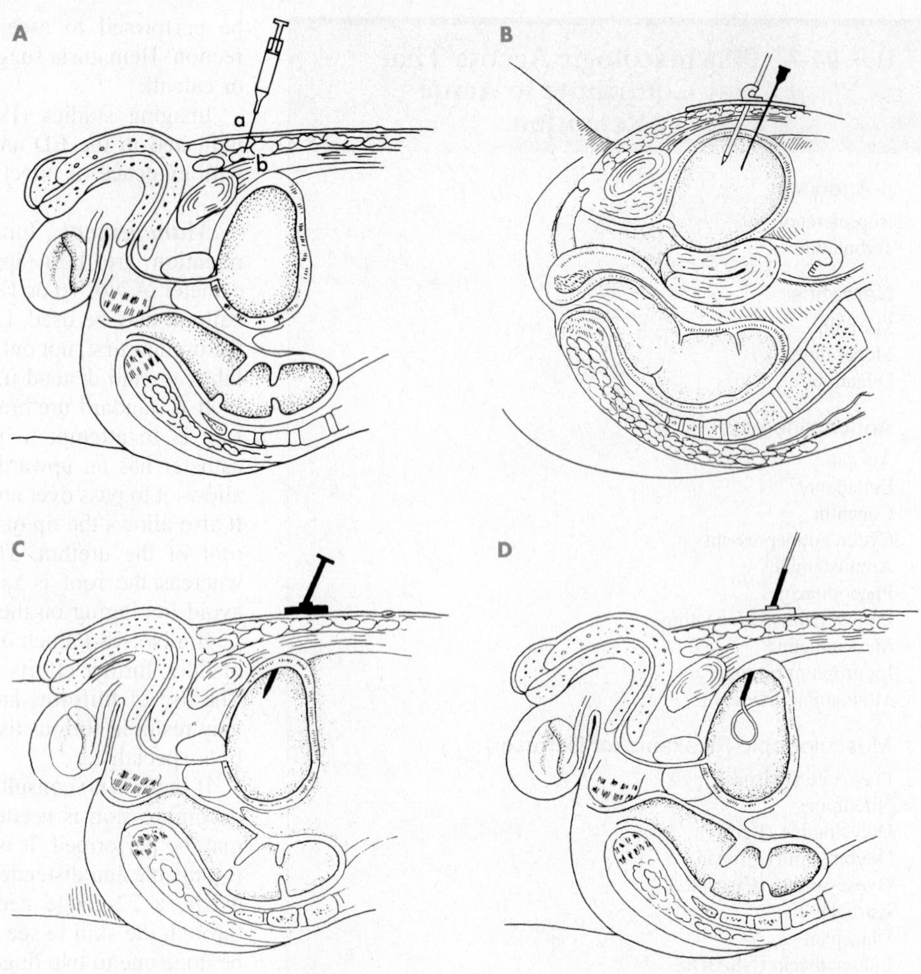

Figure 94-10. **Cystostomy tube placement. A, Anesthetizing trocar track. After skin wheal *(a)* is raised, suprapubic track for trocar is anesthetized, including rectus fascia *(b)*. Anesthetizing until bladder is penetrated will ensure total comfort for patient during trocar insertion. B, Needle localization of bladder. Spinal needle may be used even during trocar insertion to locate bladder. C, Trocar position. Advance trocar until its sheath, as well as point, is fully in bladder. D, Tubing position. Insert enough tubing so that it will not pull out of bladder when bladder empties. *From Robert JR, Hedges JR:* Clinical procedures in emergency medicine, *Philadelphia, 1985, WB Saunders.***

although traditionally recommended, has unproven efficacy.[88] No controlled studies demonstrate that gradual emptying of the bladder reduces the risk of complications. In addition, to avoid large alterations in vesicular pressure, urine would need to be removed in fractions of 50 ml or less, a practice that is impractical in the ED. Surveys of well-intentioned nurses who practice gradual emptying showed that the majority release more than 750 ml initially before clamping the catheter. Although common practice, this technique's physiologic effects are similar to those of complete bladder emptying.

Based on extensive literature review, Nyman recommends quick, complete emptying of the obstructed urinary bladder in all instances.[88]

Disposition Consultation and/or immediate referral is the rule in patients with AUR. After bladder drainage and consultation, patients may be discharged with an indwelling catheter. Patients with signs of serious infection, decreased renal function, volume overload, or inability to care for themselves without reliable home care should be hospitalized.

Removal of the catheter is not prudent, as reaccumulation of urine and recurrence of AUR are inevitable.

Hematuria

Perspective Hematuria is a clinical condition commonly seen by emergency physicians. The prevalence of asymptomatic microscopic hematuria in adult men and postmenopausal women has been reported to range from 10% to as high as 20%.[89] The emergency physician's understanding of the evaluation, workup, and appropriate disposition is essential. Gross or microscopic hematuria should be considered a harbinger of serious urologic disease. In fact, *patients with gross hematuria have approximately five times the yield of life-threatening conditions when compared to those with microhematuria.*[90]

Principles of Disease Bleeding from the lower and middle urinary tract causes approximately 60% of all cases of hematuria. A considerable number are caused by bladder neoplasms. Urologic malignancies have been reported to occur in 2.2% to 12.5% of patients with microscopic hematuria and up to 20% of patients over age 50 years with gross hematuria. A large prospective study of patients with gross hematuria or more than 3 red blood cells/hpf on two of three urinalyses found a potentially life-threatening lesion in 9.1% of these patients.[91,92]

Other sources of bleeding from the bladder commonly include infection of the bladder (hemorrhagic cystitis), varices of the bladder, diverticula, bladder stones, and postradiation changes. Anticoagulation at currently recommended levels does not predispose patients to hematuria. Identifiable genitourinary tract disease is present in most anticoagulated patients with microscopic or gross hematuria.[92] Hemorrhage from the prostate is most often caused by a benign lesion. In fact, bleeding from benign prostatic hyperplasia is the most common cause of gross hematuria

Box 94-9 Most Frequent Causes of Hematuria by Age and Gender

Age 0-20 Years
Acute glomerulonephritis
Acute UTI
Congenital urinary tract anomalies with obstruction

Age 20-40 Years
Acute UTI
Bladder cancer
Urolithiasis

Age 40-60 Years (Women)
Acute UTI
Bladder cancer
Urolithiasis

Age 40-60 Years (Men)
Acute UTI
Bladder cancer
Urolithiasis

Age 60 Years and Older (Women)
Acute UTI
Bladder cancer

Age 60 Years and Older (Men)
Acute UTI
Benign prostatic hyperplasia
Bladder cancer

From Restrop N, Carey P: *Am Fam Phys* 40:149, 1989. Modified from Gillenwater JY, editor: *Adult and pediatric urology,* St Louis, 1987, Mosby.

Box 94-10 Common Causes of Hematuria

Prerenal
Coagulopathy (e.g., hemophilia, idiopathic thrombocytopenic purpura)
Anticoagulation (e.g., use of warfarin sodium [Coumadin, Panwarfin, Sofarin], heparin sodium)
Collagen vascular disease (e.g., systemic lupus erythematosus, scleroderma)
Sickle cell disease, sickle cell trait

Renal
Glomerular
Glomerulonephritis
Lupus nephritis
Benign familial hematuria
Alport's syndrome
Vascular abnormalities (vasculitis, arteriovenous malformation, infarct)

Nonglomerular
Pyelonephritis
Polycystic kidney disease
Granulomatous disease (tuberculosis, cryptococcosis)
Xanthogranulomatous pyelonephritis
Interstitial nephritis
Papillium necrosis, secondary to phenacetin use
Malignant neoplasm (renal cell carcinoma)

Postrenal
Calculus
Ureteritis
Cystitis
Prostatitis
Benign prostatic hyperplasia
Epididymitis
Urethritis
Malignant neoplasm (transitional cell carcinoma)

False
Vaginal bleeding
Recent circumcision
Factitious (automanipulation)
Pigmenturia
- Myoglobinuria
- Hemoglobinuria
- Porphyria
- Intake of certain foods (beets, blackberries, rhubarb)
- Intake of certain drugs (quinine sulfate [Quine, Quinamm], phenazopyridine HCl [Baridium, Pyridium], rifampin [Rifadin, Rimactane], cascara sagrada)

in men age 60 years and older (Boxes 94-9 and 94-10, and Table 94-9).

An attack of renal colic associated with gross hematuria is likely caused by a bleeding site in the kidney or ureter. If a "wormlike" clot is passed, a neoplasm of the kidney or renal pelvis should be suspected.

Hematuria can be divided into glomerular and nonglomerular categories. Hematuria of glomerular origin is frequently associated with dysmorphic erythrocytes, RBC casts, and significant proteinuria in the 2+ to 3+ range on dipstick. IgA nephropathy, Berger's disease, is the most common cause of glomerular hematuria. In contrast, nonglomerular hematuria results in uniformly round erythrocytes and absence of erythrocyte casts and proteinuria.

Clinical Features An appropriate medical history may assist in the evaluation as described in Box 94-11. Certain distinguishing historical features aid the clinician in narrowing the differential diagnosis.

In the presence of glomerular disease, children, typically young males, have hematuria, erythematous skin rash, and fevers suggesting immunoglobulin nephropathy, or Berger's disease. A family history of deafness, renal disease, and hematuria is linked to Alport nephritis. A rash, arthritis, and hematuria are seen with systemic lupus erythematosus. Hematuria, hemoptysis, and microscopic anemia are common presentations of Goodpasture's syndrome. A preceding upper respiratory infection, pharyngitis, skin infection, or rash with associated hematuria suggests poststreptococcal glomerulonephritis.

In the presence of nonglomerular disease, a family history of bleeding disorders or renal cystic disease suggest hemophilia and polycystic kidney disease, respectively. Papillary necrosis should be suspected in diabetics, sickle cell patients, and analgesic abusers. The classic features of urolithiasis, sudden flank pain and hematuria, are common historical complaints. Another common presenting historical complaint is hematuria, dysuria, and frequency consistent with urinary tract infections.

Table 94-9. Results of Hematuria Evaluation in 1000 Adults

Condition	Total No.	Insignificant	Significant		
			Requiring observation	Requiring treatment	Life threatening
Glomerulonephritis	12	0	10	0	2
Renal adenocarcinoma	10	0	0	0	10
Pyelonephritis	7	0	6	1	0
Simple renal cyst	6	0	6	0	0
Renal tubular ectasia	3	0	3	0	0
Papillary necrosis	3	0	3	0	0
Atrophic kidney	1	0	1	0	0
Diffuse intervascular coagulation from stomach cancer	1	0	0	0	1
Pelvic kidney	1	0	1	0	0
Renal arteriovenous fistula	1	0	1	0	0
Renal contusion	1	0	1	0	0
Familial hematuria	1	0	1	0	0
Total renal (%)	47 (4.7)	0	33	1	13
Renal calculus	34	2	22	10	0
Renal pelvic transitional cell cancer	5	0	0	0	5
Ureteropelvic junction obstruction	1	0	1	0	0
Total renal pelvic (%)	40 (4.0)	2	23	10	5
Ureteral calculus	6	0	4	0	2
Ureteral transitional cell cancer	3	0	0	0	3
Total ureteral (%)	9 (0.9)	0	4	0	5
Bladder transitional cell cancer	65	0	0	0	65
Cystitis	43	10	4	29	0
Bladder neck varicosities	33	30	3	0	0
Cystitis cystica	30	29	1	0	0
Bladder neck contracture	8	0	8	0	0
Bladder calculus	6	0	6	0	0
Radiation cystitis	3	0	3	0	0
Interstitial cystitis	2	0	0	2	0
Bladder adenocarcinoma	1	0	0	0	1
Bladder diverticulum	1	0	1	0	0
Positive cytology	1	0	1	0	0
Sigmoid metastases	1	0	0	0	1
Total bladder (%)	194 (19.7)	69	27	31	67
Urethritis/trigonitis	377	355	20	2	0
Benign prostatic hyperplasia	143	107	27	9	0
Recurrent benign prostatic hyperplasia	22	6	8	8	0
Meatal stenosis	20	6	0	14	0
Urethral carbuncle	19	18	0	1	0
Urethral stricture	10	1	3	6	0
Prostate adenocarcinoma	1	0	0	0	1
Urethral prolapse					
Total urethral (%)	593 (59.2)	493	59	40	1
Total diagnostic (%)	883 (88.3)	564 (56.4)	146 (14.6)	(82) 8.2	91 (9.1)

From Mariani A et al: *J Urol* 141:350, 1989.

Diagnostic Strategies

Laboratory Studies Identification of microscopic hematuria can be made by two methods: a dipstick and a microscopic examination of urinary sediment. The dipstick is positive only if there has been lysis of RBCs or with myoglobinuria. The dipstick detects hemoglobin in a concentration greater than 0.003 mg/L. This concentration corresponds to 10,000 red blood cells/mm^3 or 1 to 2 RBCs/hpf of spun urine. Most urine specimens containing red blood cells test positive on the dipstick, but the presence of only a few red blood cells may be missed during a microscopic examination. The urine should be centrifuged for 3 to 5 minutes and examined carefully to distinguish hematuria from hemoglobinuria and myoglobinuria. The presence of erythrocytes establishes the diagnosis of hematuria. Red blood cell casts indicate that the source of bleeding is from the kidney at the glomerular level. Red and white blood cell casts degenerate quickly (as do most cellular elements), so the urine must be examined within 1 hour. Warmth and alkalinity cause rapid lysis and can lead to false-negative

Box 94-11 Medical History of Patients With Hematuria

Exclude pseudohematuria—drugs, vegetable dyes, pigments
Factitious—Munchausen syndrome, narcotic-seeking behavior
Bleeding diathesis
Clots—indicate nonglomerular bleeding; large, thick clots (bladder); small, stringy clots (upper tract)
Gross hematuria—relation to exercise, infection
Relation of gross hematuria to urinary stream—initial (urethra distal to urogenital diaphragm), total (bladder proper or upper urinary tract), terminal (bladder neck or prostatic urethra)
Painful hematuria—urinary tract infection or calculus, papillary necrosis, passage of clots, obstruction, loin-pain hematuria syndrome, glomerulonephritis
Genitourinary history—flank trauma or pain frequency, nocturia, dysuria, prior stones, tissue passage, or infections; vaginal or penile discharge, sexual activity, presence of urinary catheter
Relation to menstruation—endometriosis
Sickle cell disease or trait
Medications
Systemic symptoms—fever, rash, joint pain, weight loss
Infectious etiology—night sweats, sore throat, impetigo, tooth extraction or other invasive procedures, diarrhea, travel to areas endemic for *Schistosoma haematobium*
Risk factors for urologic cancer—age >40 years, tobacco use, analgesic abuse, pelvic irradiation, cyclophosphamide, *S. haematobium,* occupational exposure to dyestuffs and rubber compounds
Family history—hematuria, renal disease, sickle cell disease, deafness, bleeding diathesis
Prior testing—blood pressure, urinalysis serum chemistries, intravenous pyelogram
Pregnancies—proteinuria, hypertension (and month of onset)

results. To visualize erythrocytes optimally, phase contrast microscopy is recommended, although conventional light microscopy is acceptable.

Imaging Emergency imaging studies done in the ED to evaluate nonglomerular hematuria include limited renal ultrasonography, tailored excretory urogram with CT, MRI, and spiral CT without contrast. Because preexisting renal insufficiency is the most important risk factor for renal failure after contrast administration, a serum creatinine determination is recommended before any contrast study.[93]

Differential Considerations

Exercise-Induced Hematuria Strenuous exercise can cause transient hematuria both through direct glomerular excretion of erythrocytes in the urine and through repetitive minor trauma to the bladder (runner's hematuria). In either case, symptoms should resolve spontaneously within 48 hours.[93] Exercise-induced hematuria that does not resolve after 48 hours commonly results from punctate hemorrhagic lesions, suggesting bladder cancer, and can be diagnosed by cystoscopy.

Pseudohematuria Red urine may result from urinary pigments that give a pink-red color to the urine. A microscopic examination of the sediment reveals no red blood cells. The major causes include anthocyanins in beets and berries, phenolphthalein in alkaline urine, depyridium (Pyridium), heavy concentrations of urates, porphyria, and vegetable dyes for food coloring.

Disposition The emergency physician must be cognizant of the acute evaluation and treatment of hematuria, and the appropriate and timely disposition of patients with hematuria. Specifically, a complete urologic evaluation is necessary for the evaluation of tumors. The likelihood of tumors developing within 2 to 5 years after a complete and negative hematuria evaluation is 0% to 3%.[94] Current recommendations include urinalysis and cytology for 3 consecutive years for patients with resolution of hematuria or persistent asymptomatic microhematuria. Patients with gross hematuria should be reevaluated in all instances.[93]

KEY CONCEPTS

- UTI in young children should be treated conservatively and always requires follow-up studies for anatomic evaluation.
- Aortic abdominal aneurysm is most commonly misdiagnosed as nephrolithiasis.
- Testicular torsion is most commonly misdiagnosed as epididymitis.
- Genitourinary neoplasm should always considered in patients presenting with nontraumatic hematuria.

REFERENCES

1. Patton JP, Nash DB, Abruttn E: Urinary tract infections: economic considerations, *Med Clin North Am* 75:495, 1991.
2. Haley RW et al: The nation-wide nosocomial infection rate: a new need for vital statistics, *Am J Epidemiol* 121:159, 1985.
3. Ginsburg CM, McCracken GH: Urinary tract infections in young infants, *Pediatrics* 694:409, 1982.
4. Wettergreen B et al: Epidemiology of bacteriuria during the first year of life, *Acta Paediatr Scand* 74:925, 1985.
5. Hoberman A et al: Prevalence of urinary tract infection in febrile infants, *J Pediatr* 123:17, 1993.
6. Durbin W, Peter G: Management of urinary tract infections in infants and children, *Pediatr Infect Dis J* 3:564, 1984.
7. Kunin CM et al: Urinary tract infection in school children. I. Prevalence of bacteria and associated urologic findings, *N Engl J Med* 266:1287, 1962.
8. Nicolle LE: Urinary tract infection in the elderly, *J Antimicrob Chemother* 33:99, 1994.
9. Morrison AM, Wenzel RP: Nosocomial urinary tract infections due to *Enterococcus, Arch Intern Med* 146:1549, 1983.
10. Childs S: Management of UTIs, *Am J Med* 85:15, 1988.
11. Nielsen KT, Christensen MM, Madsen PO: Risk factors for urinary tract infections, *Infect Urol* 1989.
12. Brettman LR: Pathogenesis of urinary tract infections: host susceptibility and bacterial virulence factors, *Urology* 32:9, 1988.
13. Boscia JA et al: Epidemiology of bacteriuria in an elderly ambulatory population, *Am J Med* 80:208, 1986.
14. Hampson SJ et al: Does residual urine predispose to urinary tract infection? *Br J Urol* 70:506, 1992.
15. Richmann M et al: Risk factors for bacteriuria in men, *Urology* 43:617, 1994.
16. Mariani P, Terndrup TE: Urinary tract infection in women. In Harwood-Nuss A, editor: *The clinical practice of emergency medicine,* ed 2, Philadelphia, 1996, JB Lippincott.
17. Latham RH, Running K, Stamm W: Urinary tract infections in young adult women caused by *Staphylococcus saprophyticus, JAMA* 250: 3063, 1983.
18. Hovelius B, Mardh P: *Staphylococcus saprophyticus* as a common cause of urinary tract infections, *Rev Infect Dis* 6, 1984.
19. Kunin CM: Urinary tract infections in females, *Clin Infect Dis* 18:1, 1994.

20. Stamm WE, Hooton TM: Management of urinary tract infections in adults, *N Engl J Med* 329:1328, 1993.
21. Cox C: Comparison of intravenous fleroxacin with ceftazidine for treatment of complicated urinary tract infections, *Am J Med* 94:1185, 1993.
22. Brettman LR: Pathogenesis of urinary tract infections: host susceptibility and bacterial virulence factors, *Urology* 32:9, 1988.
23. Andriole VT: Urinary tract infections in the '90s: pathogenesis management, *Infect* 20(suppl):S251, 1992.
24. Sheldon CA, Gonzalez R: Differentiation of upper and lower urinary tract infections, *Med Clin North Am* 68:321, 1984.
25. Busch R, Huland H: Correlation of symptoms and results of direct bacterial localization in patients with urinary tract infections, *J Urol* 132:282, 1984.
26. Stamm WE et al: Causes of the acute urethral syndrome in women, *N Engl J Med* 303:409, 1980.
27. Lipsky BA et al: Diagnosis of bacteriuria in men: specimen collection and culture interpretation, *J Infect Dis* 15:847, 1987.
28. Gorelick MH, Shaw KN: Screening tests for UTI in children: a meta-analysis, *Pediatrics* 104:54, 1999.
29. Shaw KN et al: Clinical evaluation of a rapid screening test for urinary tract infections in children, *J Pediatr* 118:733, 1991.
30. Schlager TA, Lohr JA: Urinary tract infection in outpatient febrile infants and children younger than 5 years of age, *Pediatr Ann* 22:505, 1993.
31. Lockhart GR et al: Use of urinary Gram's stain for detection of urinary tract infection in infants, *Ann Emerg Med* 25:31, 1995.
32. Hoberman A et al: Enhanced urinalysis as a screening test for urinary tract infection, *Pediatrics* 91:1196, 1993.
33. Morgan MG, McKenzie H: Controversies in the laboratory diagnosis of community-acquired urinary tract infection, *Eur J Clin Microbiol Infect Dis* 12:491, 1993.
34. Carroll KC et al: Laboratory evaluation of urinary tract infections in an ambulatory clinic, *Clin Microbiol Infect Dis* 101:100, 1992.
35. Weinberg AG et al: Urine screen for bacteriuria in symptomatic pediatric outpatients, *Pediatr Infect Dis J* 10:651, 1991.
36. Stamm WE: Measurement of pyuria and its relation to bacteriuria, *Am J Med* 75:53, 1983.
37. Saito A, Kawada Y: Reliability of pyuria detection method, *Infection* 22:S36, 1994.
38. Goswitz JJ et al: Utility of slide centrifuge Gram's stain versus quantitative culture for diagnosis of urinary tract infection, *Clin Pathol* 99:132, 1993.
39. Kunin CM: The quantitative significance of bacteriuria visualized in the unstained urinary sediment, *N Engl J Med* 265:589, 1961.
40. Carvajal HF, Travis LB: Infections of the urinary tract. In Rudolph AM, Hoffman J, editors: *Pediatrics,* ed 18, Norwalk, Conn, 1987, Appleton & Lange.
41. Kass EH: Bacteriuria and the diagnosis of infections of the urinary tract with observation on the use of methionine as a urinary antiseptic, *Arch Intern Med* 100:179, 1957.
42. Kunin CM, White LV, Hua TH: A reassessment of the importance of "low-count" bacteriuria in young women with acute urinary symptoms, *Ann Intern Med* 119:454, 1993.
43. Schaeffer AJ: Infections of the urinary tract. In Walsh et al, editors: *Campbell's urology,* Philadelphia, 1998, WB Saunders.
44. Kanel KT et al: The intravenous pyelogram in acute pyelonephritis, *Arch Intern Med* 148:2144, 1988.
45. McNicholas MMJ, Griffin JF, Cantwell DF: Ultrasound of the pelvis and renal tract combined with a plain film of abdomen in young women with urinary tract infection: can it replace intravenous urography? *Br J Radiol* 64:221, 1991.
46. MacKenzie JR et al: The value of ultrasound in the child with an acute urinary tract infection, *Br J Urol* 74:240, 1994.
47. Dinkel E et al: Renal sonography in the differentiation of upper from lower urinary tract infection, *Am J Roentgenol* 146:775, 1986.
48. Goldman SM, Fishman EK: Upper urinary tract infection: the current role of CT, ultrasound, and MRI, *Semin Ultrasound CT MR* 12:335, 1991.
49. Bint AJ, Hill D: Bacteriuria of pregnancy: an update on significance, diagnosis, and management, *J Antimicrob Chemother* 33:93, 1994.
50. Stamey TA: *Pathogenesis and treatment of UTI,* Baltimore, 1980, Wilkins & Wilkins.
51. Stamm WE et al: Diagnosis of coliform infection in acutely dysuric women, *N Engl J Med* 307:463, 1982.
52. Dyer IE, Sankery TM, Dawson JA: Antibiotic resistance in bacterial UTI, 1991-97, *West J Med* 169:265a, 1988.
53. Norrby SR: Short-term treatment of uncomplicated lower urinary tract infections in women, *Rev Infect Dis* 12:458, 1990.
54. Hooton TM et al: Randomized comparative trial and cost analysis of 3-day antimicrobial regimens for treatment of acute cystitis in women, *JAMA* 273:41, 1995.
55. Greenberg RN et al: Randomized study of single dose, three-day, and seven-day treatment of cystitis, *J Infect Dis* 153:277, 1986.
56. Avorn J et al: Reduction of bacteriuria and pyuria after ingestion of cranberry juice, *JAMA* 271:751, 1994.
57. Fang L: *Pharmacotherapy* 2:91, 1982.
58. Harrison JH et al, editors: *Campbell's urology,* vol 1, Philadelphia, 1978, WB Saunders.
59. Jakobsson B, Berg U, Svensson L: Renal scarring after acute pyelonephritis, *Arch Dis Child* 70:111, 1994.
60. Shaw KN, Gorelick MH: UTI in the pediatric patient, *Pediatr Clin North Am* 46:1111, 1999.
61. Benador D et al: *Cortical scintigraphy in the evaluation of renal parenchymal changes in children with pyelonephritis,* St Louis, Mosby.
62. Kim SB et al: Clinical value of DMSA planar and single photon emission computed tomography as an initial diagnostic tool in adult women with recurrent acute pyelonephritis, *Nephron* 67:274, 1994.
63. Gleeson FV et al: Imaging in urinary tract infection, *Arch Dis Child* 66:1282, 1991.
64. Hoberman A et al: Oral vs. IV therapy for UTI in young febrile children, *Pediatrics* 104:79, 1999.
65. Petersen KE: Short-term treatment of acute urinary tract infection in girls, *Scand J Infect Dis* 23:213, 1991.
66. Lipsky BA: Urinary tract infections in men, *Ann Intern Med* 110:138, 1989.
67. Krieger JN, Ross SO, Simonsen JM: Urinary tract infections in healthy university men, *J Urol* 149:1046, 1993.
68. Stamm WE et al: *Chlamydia trachomatis* urethral infections in men, *Ann Intern Med* 100:47, 1984.
69. McNagny SE et al: Urinary leukocyte esterase test: a screening method for the detection of asymptomatic chlamydial and gonococcal infections in men, *J Infect Dis* 165:573, 1992.
70. Patrick DM, Rekart ML, Knowles L: Unsatisfactory performance of the leukocyte esterase test of first-voided urine for rapid diagnosis of urethritis, *Genitourin Med* 70:187, 1994.
71. Woods ER et al: First catch urine sediment for *Chlamydia trachomatis* and *Neisseria gonorrhoeae* culture in adolescent males with pyuria, *J Adolesc Health* 12:329, 1991.
72. Ireton RC, Berger RE: Prostatitis and epididymitis, *Urol Clin North Am* 11:83, 1984.
73. Saklayem MG: Medical management of nephrolithiasis, *Med Clin North Am* 81:785, 1997.
74. Ahlstrand C, Tiselius HG: Recurrences during a 10-year follow up after final renal stone episode, *Urol Res* 18:397, 1990.
75. Borghi L et al: Hot occupation and nephrolithiasis, *J Urol* 150:1757, 1993.
76. Seftel A, Resnick MI: Metabolic evaluation of urolithiasis, *Urol Clin North Am* 17:159, 1990.
77. Stewart DP et al: Microscopic hematuria and calculus-related ureteral obstruction, *J Emerg Med* 8:693, 1990.
78. Mutgi A et al: Renal colic: utility of the plain abdominal radiograph, *Arch Intern Med* 151:1589, 1991.
79. Sinclair D et al: The evaluation of suspected renal colic: ultrasound scan versus excretory urography, *Ann Emerg Med* 18:556, 1989.
80. Sheley RC et al: Helical CT in the evaluation of renal colic, *Am J Emerg Med* 17:279, 1999.
81. Zangerle KF, Iserson KV, Bjelland JC: Usefulness of abdominal flat plate radiographs in patients with suspected ureteral calculi, *Ann Emerg Med* 14:316, 1985.
82. Swartz D: The acute scrotal mass. In Harwood-Nuss A, editor: *The clinical practice of emergency medicine,* ed 2, Philadelphia, 1996, JB Lippincott.
83. Rabinowitz R: The importance of the cremasteric reflex in acute scrotal swelling in children, *J Urol* 132:89, 1984.

84. Berger RE et al: The clinical use of epididymal aspiration cultures in the management of selected patients with acute epididymitis, *J Urol* 124:60, 1980.
85. Skoglund RW et al: Torsion of testicular appendage: presentation of 43 cases, *J Urol* 104:604, 1970.
86. Emberton M, Anion K: Acute urinary retention in men: an age old problem, *BMJ* 318:921, 1999.
87. Stewart C: Urinary tract infections in men. In Harwood-Nuss A, editor: *The clinical practice of emergency medicine,* Philadelphia, 1991, JB Lippincott.
88. Nyman MA et al: Management of acute urinary retention: rapid vs gradual decompensation and risk of complications, *Mayo Clin Proc* 72:951, 1997.
89. Thaller TR, Wang LP: Evaluation of asymptomatic microscopic hematuria in adults, *Am Fam Physician* 60:1143, 1999.
90. Mariani AJ et al: The significance of adult hematuria: 1000 hematuria evaluations including a risk benefit and cost effectiveness analysis, *J Urol* 141:350, 1989.
91. Stewart DP et al: Microscopic hematuria and calculus-related ureteral obstruction, *J Emerg Med* 8:693, 1990.
92. Sinclair D et al: The evaluation of suspected renal colic: ultrasound scan versus excretory urography, *Ann Emerg Med* 18:556, 1989.
93. Mariani AJ: The evaluation of adult hematuria: a clinical update
94. Rasmussen OO et al: Recurrent unexplained hematuria and the risk of urologic cancer: a follow up study, *Scand J Urol Nephrol* 22:335, 1989.

Section VII NEUROLOGY

95 Stroke

Rashmi Kothari
William G. Barsan

PERSPECTIVE

Background

Stroke is the third leading cause of death in the United States and the leading cause of adult disability.[1] It afflicts over 700,000 patients per year, with an in-hospital mortality of almost 15% and a 30-day mortality of 20% to 25%.[2-4] Even among survivors, over half are left with a permanent disability and one third need assistance in the activities of daily living.[5] The current cost of stroke is estimated to be over $30 billion per year. In terms of emergency care, almost 2% of all 911 calls and 4% of hospital admissions from the ED involve patients with potential strokes.[6-7]

Stroke can be defined as any vascular injury that reduces cerebral blood flow (CBF) to a specific region of the brain, causing neurologic impairment. The onset of symptoms may be sudden or stuttering and may result in transient or permanent loss of neurologic function. Approximately 80% of all strokes are ischemic, caused by an occlusion of the cerebral vessel.[3-4] The rest are hemorrhagic strokes caused by rupture of the blood vessel into the parenchyma of the brain (intracerebral hemorrhage [ICH]) or into the subarachnoid space (subarachnoid hemorrhage [SAH]). Only ischemic stroke and ICH are discussed in this chapter.

In the past, treatment for stroke consisted of observation, stabilization, and rehabilitation. However, in recent years, with a better understanding of the pathophysiology of neuronal injury and the introduction of new therapies, there has been a shift to early evaluation and treatment. Current interventional treatment regimens include control of hypertension, anticoagulation, thrombolytic therapy, catheter-based interventions, and surgery. The key to success is early identification and treatment of stroke patients before neurologic deficits become irreversible. Emergency physicians play an integral role in the decision-making process involved in the care of these critically ill patients.[8]

PRINCIPLES OF DISEASE

Pathophysiology

The cerebral vasculature supplies the brain with a rich flow of blood that contains the critical supply of oxygen and glucose necessary for normal brain function. When a stroke occurs, there are immediate alterations in CBF and extensive changes in cellular homeostasis. A complete interruption of CBF, which is rare, results in loss of consciousness within approximately 10 seconds and death of vulnerable pyramidal cells of the hippocampus within minutes. In stroke, collateral circulation helps maintain some blood flow to the ischemic region. The normal CBF is 40 to 60 ml/100 g of brain/minute. When CBF drops below 15 to 18 ml/100 g of brain/minute, several physiologic changes occur. The brain loses electrical activity and becomes electrically "silent," although neuronal membrane integrity and function remain intact. Clinically, the areas of the brain maintaining electrical silence manifest a neurologic deficit, even though the brain cells are viable. When CBF is below 10 ml/100 g of brain/minute, membrane failure occurs with a subsequent increase in extracellular potassium and intracellular calcium levels. There is also a rapid depletion in adenosine triphosphate (ATP) coupled with a profound intracellular acidosis.

The areas of the brain in which small amounts of flow are preserved by the collateral circulation in the area surrounding the primary injury are called the *ischemic penumbra.* This border zone of neuronal tissue is of greatest interest to investigators for possible salvage in both ischemic and hemorrhagic stroke.[9] As defined by CBF, the ischemic penumbra constitutes brain tissue with blood flow of 10 to 18 ml/100 g of brain/minute in which electric silence is present but irreversible damage has not yet occurred. In ischemic stroke the duration of occlusion plays a critical role in neuronal survival. Increasing the duration of occlusion increases both the irreversibility of deficits and the amount of cerebral infarction. In experimental animals, occlusion of cerebral vessels usually results in a reversible neurologic deficit if the occlusion lasts less than 2 hours. After 6 hours of occlusion, neurologic deficits in most animal studies are irreversible. In ischemic stroke trials, fibrinolytic or antiplatelet agents have been used to recanalize occluded arteries and reperfuse ischemic areas of the brain within the 2- to 6-hour therapeutic window.[10-14]

In patients with ICH, physical compression and edema caused by the hematoma are thought to play an important role in secondary injury.[15,16] Similar to ischemic stroke trials, investigators have begun looking at the feasibility of ultra-early hematoma evacuation within this 2- to 6-hour window in patients with ICH.[17] Clinical investigators evaluating neuroprotective agents have primarily focused on a longer window of up to 24 hours in patients with both ischemic and hemorrhagic stroke.[18-22] Recent studies using magnetic resonance imaging (MRI) and positron emission tomographic (PET) scanning in humans support this longer time window in some patients.[9,23]

Anatomy and Physiology

Blood is supplied to the brain by the anterior and posterior circulation. The anterior circulation originates from the carotid system and perfuses four fifths of the brain, including the optic nerve, retina, and frontoparietal and anterotemporal lobes. The first branch off the internal carotid artery is the ophthalmic artery, which supplies the optic nerve and retina. As a result, the sudden onset of painless monocular blindness (amaurosis fugax) identifies the stroke as involving the anterior circulation (specifically the carotid artery) at or below the level of the ophthalmic artery. The internal carotid arteries terminate by branching into the anterior and middle cerebral arteries at the circle of Willis.

The anterior cerebral artery supplies the basal and medial aspects of the cerebral hemispheres and extends to the anterior two thirds of the parietal lobe. Perforating branches supply the anterior caudate nucleus, part of the anterior limb of the internal capsule, the anterior third of the putamen, and the anterior hypothalamus. The middle cerebral artery supplies the lenticulostriate branches that supply the putamen, part of the anterior limb of the internal capsule, the lentiform nucleus, and the external capsule. Main cortical branches of the middle cerebral artery supply the lateral surfaces of the cerebral cortex from the anterior portion of the frontal lobe to the posterolateral occipital lobe.

Although the posterior circulation is smaller and supplies only one fifth of the brain, it supplies the brainstem, which is critical for normal consciousness, movement, and sensation. The posterior circulation is derived from the two vertebral arteries that ascend through the transverse processes of the cervical vertebrae. The vertebral arteries enter the cranium through the foramen magnum and supply the cerebellum via the posterior inferior cerebellar arteries. They join to form the basilar artery, which branches to form the posterior cerebral arteries. The posterior circulation supplies the brainstem, cerebellum, thalamus, auditory and vestibular centers of the ear, medial temporal lobe, and visual occipital cortex.

The extent of injury in either an anterior or posterior stroke depends on both the vessel involved and the presence of collateral blood flow distal to the vessel occlusion. A patient with excellent collateral blood flow from the contralateral hemisphere may have minimal clinical deficits despite a complete carotid occlusion. In contrast, a patient with poor collateral flow may have hemiplegia with the same lesion.

Table 95-1. Estimated Number of First-Ever Strokes/TIAs in the United States

Stroke subtype	Estimated number
Large vessel	69,000 (16%)
Small vessel/lacunae	76,000 (17.5%)
Cardioembolic	113,000 (26%)
Stroke of uncommon mechanisms	15,000 (3.5%)
Infarcts of unknown etiology	157,000 (36.5%)
Total stroke/TIAs	430,000 (100%)

Data from Woo D et al: *Stroke* 30:2517, 1999; Petty GW et al: *Stroke* 30:2513, 1999.

Epidemiology

Ischemic Stroke An estimated 430,000 first-ever ischemic strokes occur each year in the United States, of which 10% to 15% are transient ischemic attacks (TIAs). These may occur either from in situ thrombosis or embolic obstruction from a more proximal source, usually the heart. In more than one third of these first-ever strokes, no cause is found (Table 95-1).[24,25]

Approximately one third of all ischemic strokes are thrombotic. These can result from either large- or small-vessel occlusions.[24,25] There is a higher incidence of large-vessel occlusions among men than women and among whites than African Americans.[24,25] Common areas for large-vessel occlusions are cerebral vessel branch points, especially in the distribution of the internal carotid artery. Thrombosis is usually the result of clot formation that develops in the area of an ulcerated atherosclerotic plaque that occurs where there is turbulent blood flow. There is a marked reduction of flow when the stenosis occludes more than 90% of the blood vessel diameter. As further ulceration and thrombosis occur, platelets adhere to the region. A clot then either embolizes or occludes the artery.

Lacunae or small-vessel strokes involve small terminal sections of the vasculature and more commonly occur in African Americans and patients with diabetes and hypertension.[24] A history of hypertension is present in 80% to 90% of patients who have lacunae strokes. The subcortical areas of the cerebrum and brainstem are often involved. The infarctions range in size from a few millimeters to 2 cm and occur most commonly in the basal ganglia, thalamus, pons, and internal capsule. They may be caused by small emboli or by a process termed "lipohyalinosis," which occurs in patients with hypertensive cerebral vasculopathy. Although nearly 20 lacunae syndromes have been described, the most common of these are pure motor strokes, pure sensory strokes, or ataxic hemiparesis. Because they are subcortical and well localized, lacunae strokes do not cause cognitive defects, aphasia, simultaneous sensorimotor findings, and loss of consciousness or memory impairment.

A quarter of all ischemic strokes are cardioembolic.[24,25] Embolization of a mural thrombus in patients with atrial fibrillation is the most common source of these emboli, and patients who have atrial fibrillation are 5 to 17 times more likely to develop a stroke than those who do not have atrial fibrillation.[26] Almost 20% of stroke patients have atrial fibrillation on their admission electrocardiogram (ECG).[26,27] Strokes resulting from atrial fibrillation are more likely to involve large cerebral vessels, be more severe, and have a higher mortality than nonatrial fibrillation-associated strokes.[26,27] Mural thrombi are also commonly found at autopsy in patients with either idiopathic or alcoholic cardiomyopathy or in patients with congestive heart failure. Noncardiac sources of emboli may arise from diseased portions of extracranial arteries and result in an artery-to-artery embolus. One common example is amaurosis fugax, in which emboli from a proximal carotid plaque embolizes to the ophthalmic artery, causing transient monocular blindness. The frequency of arterial embolism and the specific arterial lesions that produce such emboli are not fully known.

Approximately 1% to 2% of patients who have acute myocardial infarctions (MIs) have a subsequent stroke within the first month after their cardiac event.[28,29] Half of these occur within the first 5 days of the MI.[29] Independent predictors of who will develop a stroke after an acute MI are a history of atrial fibrillation (new-onset or chronic), prior stroke, and ST elevation.[29] The use of aspirin reduces the incidence of post-MI stroke by 42%.[30] Ischemic stroke is also associated with alterations in the autonomic function of the heart that may lead to sudden death in 6% to 11% of patients.[31,32] These alterations in autonomic function are thought to be associated with infarcts involving the insular cortex and medullary brainstem.[32,33]

Approximately 3% to 4% of all strokes occur in patients between ages 15 and 45 years. Although atherosclerosis is the most common cause in older patients, younger patients have causes that are often uncommon and reversible. Pregnancy, the use of oral contraceptives, antiphospholipid antibodies (such as lupus anticoagulant and anticardiolipin antibodies), protein S and C deficiencies, and polycythemia all predispose patients to sludging or thrombosis and increase their risk of stroke. Fibromuscular dysplasia of the cerebral vasculature may also lead to stroke, and, in rare instances, prolonged vasoconstriction from a migraine syndrome causes stroke. Recreational drugs such as cocaine, phenylpropanolamine, and amphetamines are potent vasoconstrictors associated with both ischemic and hemorrhagic stroke. Vascular dissections are often associated with severe trauma but can occur from such mild events as turning the head sharply.

A TIA is defined as a neurologic deficit that has complete clinical resolution within 24 hours. TIAs are an important warning sign for the future development of cerebral infarction. Approximately 5% to 20% of the patients who experience a TIA will develop a stroke within 1 month of the event, and up to 50% will experience a stroke within 5 years. The majority of TIAs last less then 30 minutes, but the course can vary.[34] Three or more TIAs occurring within 72 hours are termed *crescendo TIAs.* Although there is a strong relationship between "carotid territory" TIAs and extracranial carotid artery disease, at least 50% of patients with carotid territory TIAs do not have angiographically demonstrable arterial disease. The cause of TIAs in these patients without arterial lesions is unknown. Although clinical deficits resolve within 24 hours, studies indicate that up to 64% have computed tomography (CT) and 81% have MRI evidence of an infarction.[35,36] Almost half of all patients age 65 years and older with "first-ever TIAs" have MRI evidence of a previous, clinically silent, cerebral infarction.[36] These silent infarcts are usually deep, less than 1 cm, and often in the nondominant right hemisphere.

Box 95-1 Location of Hypertensive Hemorrhages

Putamen	44%
Thalamus	13%
Cerebellum	9%
Pons	9%
Other cortical areas	25%

Hemorrhagic Stroke Spontaneous ICH causes 8% to 11% of all acute strokes and is twice as common as SAH. It has a 30-day mortality of up to 50%, with half of these patients dying in the first 2 days. Among survivors, only one in five are living independently at 1 year.[37] There is a higher incidence of ICH among men than women, in Asians than in whites, and it occurs more commonly in young and middle-age African Americans than whites of similar age.[2]

ICH may occur in association with long-standing hypertension (hypertensive hemorrhage), in the elderly with amyloid angiopathy, or in patients with arteriovenous malformations (AVMs). Hypertensive hemorrhage occurs predominantly in older patients and results from degenerative changes in the small penetrating arteries and arterioles, leading to the formation of microaneurysms, most commonly in penetrating vessels of the middle cerebral artery. Two thirds of cases occur within the region of the basal ganglia. The most common sites for hypertensive hemorrhage are listed in Box 95-1. The hematoma that forms usually enlarges, causing local tissue injury and a subsequent increase in intracranial pressure (ICP).

ICH caused by amyloid angiopathy tends to be lobar, occur more commonly in the elderly, and occur with a higher incidence among whites than among African Americans. Sudden increases in blood pressure that occur with such drugs as phenylpropanolamine and cocaine can cause ICH. Other causes include the use of anticoagulants, tumors, and AVMs (especially in the young).

Bleeding from an AVM may be subarachnoid, intraparenchymal, or both. In AVMs the hemorrhage into the subarachnoid space is generally confined to the area of the AVM, and the major clinical presentation results from the intraparenchymal involvement with focal neurologic deficits. AVMs are more likely to bleed into the ventricles and subarachnoid space than are hypertensive ICHs and usually have a less disruptive impact on cerebral function. An AVM produces hemorrhage in younger patients than does hypertensive ICH. These patients may have no history of hypertension.

CLINICAL FEATURES

Ischemic Stroke

The signs and symptoms of an ischemic stroke may occur suddenly and without warning or may have a stuttering, insidious onset. Disruption of the flow to one of the major vascular limbs of the cerebral circulation from stroke results in physiologic disruption to the anatomic area of the brain supplied by that blood vessel. Ischemic strokes can be classified as *anterior* or *posterior* circulation strokes, depending on the vasculature involved. The presence of neurologic deficits is highly dependent on collateral flow. In addition to the vascular supply involved, ischemic strokes can be further described by the temporal presentation of their neurologic deficits. A "stroke in evolution" is one in which focal neurologic deficits worsen over the course of minutes or hours. Approximately 20% of the anterior circulation strokes and 40% of the posterior circulation strokes show evidence of progression. Anterior circulation strokes may progress within the first 24 hours, whereas posterior strokes may progress for up to 3 days. Propagation of a thrombus is postulated as a likely mechanism for progression. A "completed stroke" is one in which a neurologic deficit persists longer than 3 weeks, even if some improvement has occurred.

Anterior circulation strokes (involving primarily the carotid, anterior, and/or middle cerebral arteries) rarely present with complete loss of consciousness unless they occur in the previously unaffected hemisphere of a patient who has experienced multiple previous strokes. Occlusions in the anterior cerebral artery mainly affect frontal lobe function. The patient has altered mentation coupled with impaired judgment and insight, as well as the presence of primitive grasp and suck reflexes. Bowel and bladder incontinence can occur. Paralysis and hypesthesia of the lower limb opposite the side of the lesion are characteristic. Leg weakness is greater than arm weakness in anterior cerebral distribution stroke. Apraxia or clumsiness occurs in the patient's gait.

Marked motor and sensory disturbances are the hallmarks of occlusion of the middle cerebral artery. They occur on the side of the body contralateral to the side of the lesion and are usually worse in the arm and face than the leg. Involvement may occur in only part of an extremity or in the face but is almost always accompanied by numbness in the same region as the motor loss. Hemianopsia, or blindness in half of the visual field, occurs ipsilateral to the lesion. Agnosia, or the inability to recognize previously known subjects, is common, and aphasia may be present if the lesion occurs in the dominant hemisphere. Patients often have a gaze preference toward the affected hemisphere because of disruption of the cortical lateral gaze centers. The clinical aphorism is that a patient looks *at* a destructive lesion (stroke) but *away from* an irritative lesion (seizure focus).

Aphasia, a disorder of language in which the patient articulates clearly but uses language inappropriately or understands it poorly, is also common in dominant-hemisphere stroke. Aphasia may be expressive, receptive, or a combination of both. *Wernicke's aphasia* occurs when the patient cannot process sensory input such as speech and thus fails to understand verbal communication (receptive aphasia). *Broca's aphasia* refers to the inability to communicate verbally in an effective way, even though understanding may be intact (expressive aphasia). Aphasia should be distinguished from dysarthria, which is a motor deficit of the mouth and speech muscles; the dysarthric patient articulates poorly but understands words and word choices. Aphasia is important to recognize because it usually localizes a lesion to the dominant (usually left) cerebral cortex in the middle cerebral artery distribution. *Aphasia* and *dysphasia* are terms that are used interchangeably but must be distinguished from *dysphagia,* which is difficulty in swallowing.

Pathology in the vertebrobasilar system (i.e., posterior circulation strokes) can cause the widest variety of symptoms and as a result may be the most difficult to diagnose. The symptoms reflect cranial nerve deficits, cerebellar involvement, and involvement of neurosensory tracts. The brainstem also contains the reticular activating system, which is responsible for mediating consciousness, and the emesis centers. Unlike anterior circulation strokes, patients with posterior circulation stroke can present with loss of consciousness, and they frequently have nausea and vomiting. The posterior cerebral artery supplies portions of the parietal and occipital lobes, and therefore vision and thought processing are impaired. Visual agnosia, the inability to recognize seen objects, may occur, as well as alexia, the inability to understand the written word. A third nerve palsy may occur, and the patient may experience homonymous hemianopsia. One of the more curious facets of this syndrome is that the patient may be unaware of any visual problem (visual neglect). Vertigo, diplopia, visual field defects, weakness, paralysis, dysarthria, dysphagia, syncope, spasticity, ataxia, or nystagmus may occur with vertebrobasilar artery insufficiency. One of the key features is that the sensory findings such as deficits in pain and temperature perception occur on one side of the face and on the opposite side of the body. Posterior circulation strokes also demonstrate crossed deficits. In contrast, anterior circulation strokes always have findings limited to one side of the body.

A focused neurologic examination should assess level of consciousness, speech, cranial nerve function, motor and sensory function, and cerebellar function. The patient's level of consciousness and fluency of speech can rapidly be assessed in a dialogue with the patient to determine the presence of dysarthria or aphasia. The patient's head should be evaluated for signs of trauma. Pupillary size, reactivity, and extraocular movements provide important information about brainstem function, particularly for cranial nerves (CNs) III through VI; an abnormal third nerve function may be the first sign of tentorial herniation. Gaze preference suggests brainstem or cortical involvement. Central facial nerve weakness from a stroke should be distinguished from the peripheral causes of CN VII weakness (e.g., a Bell's palsy). With a peripheral lesion the patient is unable to wrinkle the forehead. Determination of facial sensation, eyebrow elevation and squinting, smiling symmetry, gross auditory acuity, gag reflex, shoulder elevation, sternocleidomastoid strength, and tongue protrusion complete the cranial nerve evaluation.

Motor and sensory testing is performed next. Moving a relaxed limb assesses muscle tone. Proximal and distal muscle group strength should be assessed against resistance. Truncal ataxia and pronator drift of the arm, which is a sensitive sign of motor weakness, can be tested simultaneously by having the patient sit with eyes closed, arms outstretched, and palms toward the ceiling. Asymmetric sensation to pain and light touch may be subtle and difficult to detect. Double simultaneous extinction is easily tested by the simultaneous light touch of right and left limbs. The patient may feel both the right and left sides being touched individually but may not discern the affected side being touched when both are touched simultaneously. Similarly, the ability to discern a number gently scratched on a forearm (graphesthesia) is another easily tested cortical parietal lobe function. These tests can help differentiate the pure motor deficit of a lacunar stroke from a sensorimotor middle cerebral artery deficit.

Cerebellar testing and the assessment of reflexes and gait complete the examination. Finger-to-nose and heel-to-shin evaluations are important tests of cerebellar functions. Asymmetry of the deep tendon reflexes or a unilateral Babinski sign may be an early finding of corticospinal tract dysfunction. Gait testing is commonly omitted, yet it is one of the most informative parts of the neurologic examination. Observing routine ambulation and heel-to-toe walking can assess subtle ataxia, weakness, or focal cerebellar lesions.

The National Institutes of Health Stroke Scale (NIHSS) is a useful and rapid tool for quantifying neurologic deficit in patients with stroke and can be used in determining treatment options.[38] It has been shown to be reproducible and valid and correlates well with the amount of infarcted tissue on CT scan.[39,40] The baseline NIHSS can determine patients appropriate for fibrinolytic therapy and those at increased risk of hemorrhage. In addition, this test has been used as a prognostic tool to predict outcome and is currently being used to by some stroke centers to stratify patients into treatment trials.[38,41]

Hemorrhagic Stroke

The classic presentation of ICH is the sudden onset of headache, vomiting, severely elevated blood pressure, and focal neurologic deficits that progress over minutes. Similar to ischemic stroke, the patient often has a motor and sensory deficit contralateral to the brain lesion. The patient may present with agitation and lethargy, but may quickly progress to stupor or coma. One third have significant growth in hemorrhage volume within the first few hours.[42] Although headache, vomiting, and coma are common, significant proportions of patients do not have these findings and may present similar to patients with ischemic stroke (Table 95-2). In addition, patients with ICH are likely to have precipitating events such as sexual intercourse, Valsalva maneuver, or labor.

Airway and mental status are of paramount importance in patients with ICH because they can deteriorate precipitously. The respiratory pattern may also be affected in hemorrhagic stroke. Cheyne-Stokes respirations may occur with a large ICH. Putamenal hemorrhages may cause deep, irregular respirations, whereas patients with cerebellar hemorrhage may have a normal respiratory pattern.

The pupillary examination can be extremely helpful in determining the location and extent of the insult. Pontine hemorrhage classically presents with pinpoint pupils because of the interruption of the descending sympathetic tracts and unopposed parasympathetic stimulation. Dilated pupils may result from bleeding into the putamen, whereas blood in the thalamus may present with anisocoria, miosis, or a sluggish pupillary response.

Similar to ischemic stroke, a careful neurologic examination is important in localizing the region and extent of injury. A baseline NIHSS and Glasgow Coma Score (GCS) can be used to assess stroke severity, although the GCS may be more feasible to follow for neurologic deterioration. Cerebellar hemorrhages often present with cranial nerve abnormalities. The parasympathetic fibers course along the outside of cranial nerve III. As a result, compression of the nerve results in loss of pupillary reactivity before anisocoria. As noted previously, the physical examination may be indistinguishable between an ischemic stroke and an ICH, requiring radiographic confirmation.

Table 95-2. Clinical Findings Associated With Ischemic Strokes, ICH, and SAH From the Stroke Data Bank, Harvard and Lausanne and Stroke Registries

Symptom	Ischemic stroke	ICH	SAH
Headache	11%-17%	33%-41%	78%-87%
Vomiting	8%-11%	29%-46%	45%-48%
Decreased level of consciousness	13%-15%	39%-57%	48%-68%
Seizure	0.3%-3%	6%-7%	7%

Data from Bogousslausky J, Van Melle G, Regli F: *Stroke* 19:1083, 1988; Foulkes MA et al: *Stroke* 19:547, 1988; Mohr JP et al: *Neurology* 28:754, 1978.

Table 95-3. Hunt and Hess Scale for Subarachnoid Hemorrhage

Grade	Neurologic status	Predicted 2-month survival (%)*
1	Asymptomatic	70
2	Severe headache or nuchal rigidity; no neurologic deficit	60
3	Drowsy; minimal neurologic deficit	50
4	Stuporous; moderate to severe hemiparesis	40
5	Deep coma; decerebrate posturing	10

*Data from Alvord E et al: Subarachnoid hemorrhage due to ruptured aneurysms, *Arch Neurol* 27:273-284, 1972.

Poor prognostic indicators for patients with ICH include a decreased level of consciousness on arrival, intraventricular hemorrhage, and an ICH volume over 40 ml, all of which can be assessed in the ED (Table 95-3). The ABC/2 technique is a quick and accurate method of measuring ICH volume at the bedside (Figure 95-1).[43]

DIFFERENTIAL DIAGNOSIS

Ischemic Stroke

Extraaxial collections of blood secondary to trauma can mimic stroke. An epidural or subdural hematoma can cause an altered mental status, focal neurologic signs, and rapid progression to coma. Elderly patients who are the age group at highest risk for stroke can be victims of recurrent falls that lead to chronic subdural hematomas. Carotid dissection may occur after neck trauma or sudden hyperextension and may occur with focal neurologic findings, as with an aortic dissection that extends into the carotid arteries. The diagnosis is supported by a compatible history, angiography, or magnetic resonance angiography (MRA).

Other structural lesions that may cause focal neurologic signs include brain tumor and abscesses. Air embolism should be suspected if there are marked atmospheric pressure

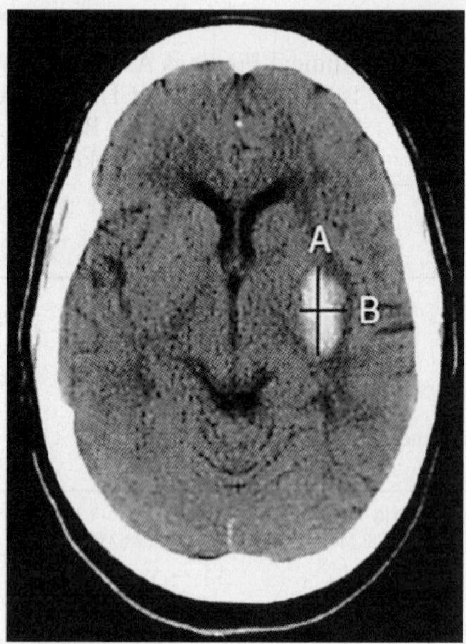

Figure 95-1. **The CT slice with the largest area of hemorrhage is identified. The largest diameter of the hemorrhage on this slice is measured in centimeters (A). The largest diameter 90° to A on the same slice is measured (B). C is the approximate number of 10 mm slices on which the ICH was seen. The volume of the hemorrhage is then A multiplied by B, multiplied by C, divided by 2 (ABC/2).**

changes, such as during scuba diving, or during medical procedures or injuries that may allow air into the vascular system. Seizures, altered mental status, and focal neurologic findings may also occur with air embolism.

Like stroke, giant cell arteritis is a disease of the elderly. It may cause severe headache, visual disturbances, and, rarely, aphasia and hemiparesis. Other symptoms include intermittent fever, malaise, jaw claudication, morning stiffness, and myalgias. The diagnosis is confirmed by temporal artery biopsy. Collagen vascular diseases such as polyarteritis nodosa, lupus, and other types of vasculitis may cause stroke syndromes.

Metabolic abnormalities can also mimic stroke syndromes. Hypoglycemia is often responsible for an altered mental status and is a well-known cause of sustained focal neurologic findings that persist for several days.[43] Wernicke's encephalopathy causes ophthalmoplegia, ataxia, and confusion that can be mistaken for signs of cerebellar infarction.

Migraine is another entity that may present with focal neurologic findings, with or without headache. A seizure followed by Todd's postictal paralysis may mimic stroke, as may Bell's palsy, labyrinthitis, peripheral nerve palsy, and demyelinating diseases. Meniere's disease may be difficult to distinguish from a posterior circulation stroke or TIA. Dizziness, vertigo, hearing loss, and tinnitus in Meniere's disease are common, whereas difficulties with vision, speech, or other focal symptoms are uncommon.

Hemorrhagic Stroke

The differential diagnosis for ICH is similar to that for ischemic stroke and includes migraine, seizure, tumor, abscess, hypertensive encephalopathy, and trauma. Hypertensive encephalopathy and migraine can also present with headache, nausea, and vomiting. Although focal neurologic signs are uncommon, they may occur with these entities. With hypertensive encephalopathy, patients usually have marked elevation in blood pressure and other evidence of end-organ injury, including proteinuria, cardiomegaly, papilledema, and malignant hypertensive retinopathy. These patients usually improve significantly with treatment of their hypertension. Migraines are often associated with an aura, and the patient often has a history of similar headaches. Similar to vertebrobasilar insufficiency, the differentiation between ICH and labyrinthitis can be especially difficult in the elderly. The abrupt onset of vertigo, vomiting, and nystagmus can represent a peripheral process such as labyrinthitis or a central process such as cerebellar or brainstem infarct or hemorrhage. Age greater than 40 years and a history of hypertension or other risk factors for ICH increase the possibility of a cerebellar hemorrhage. Findings specifically referable to the brainstem must be sought. These include hiccups, diplopia, facial numbness, dysphagia, or ataxia. Vertiginous patients often have a strong desire to remain immobile with their eyes closed, but this must not preclude a thorough cranial nerve and cerebellar examination, including assessment of gait. Gross ataxia should be present with cerebellar stroke and absent with labyrinthine disease. A head CT should be strongly considered in patients over age 40 years to assist in differentiating labyrinthitis and cerebellar hemorrhage.

DIAGNOSTIC STRATEGIES

Ischemic Stroke

Although clinical data can help establish the diagnosis, cause, and location of the stroke, confirmatory diagnostic tests are often required to establish the final etiology or to eliminate other causes of the deficits. The immediate ED evaluation should include a blood glucose measurement, cranial CT scan, and an ECG.

An emergency noncontrast cranial CT is the standard imaging technique for evaluating a patient with a potential stroke in the ED.[44] It can quickly differentiate an ischemic stroke from ICH and other mass lesions. This information is crucial for subsequent therapeutic decisions. A CT scan can identify almost all parenchymal hemorrhages greater than 1 cm and up to 95% of all SAH. The majority of ischemic strokes do not have gross signs of infarction on routine CT scan for at least 6 to 12 hours, depending on the infarct's size. However, subtle, ultra-early changes have been noted in up to one third of stroke patients evaluated by CT within 3 hours of symptom onset. These ultra-early changes include the hyperdense artery sign (acute thrombus in a vessel), sulcal effacement, loss of the insular ribbon, loss of gray-white interface, mass effect, and acute hypodensity (Figure 95-2).

The clinical importance of these findings with regard to fibrinolytic therapy administered less than 3 hours after symptom onset is questionable because the ability of treating physicians to identify these findings is poor and their significance is questionable.[45,46] Only acute hypodensity and mass effect have been shown to be associated with an increased risk of ICH after fibrinolysis (compared with treated patients without these findings). However, these findings do not exclude appropriate patients from fibrinolytic therapy because the patients' chance for excellent neurologic outcome at 3 months with these findings was better than placebo-treated patients, and their risk of symptomatic ICH, severe disability, or death at 3 months was no different.[45] The

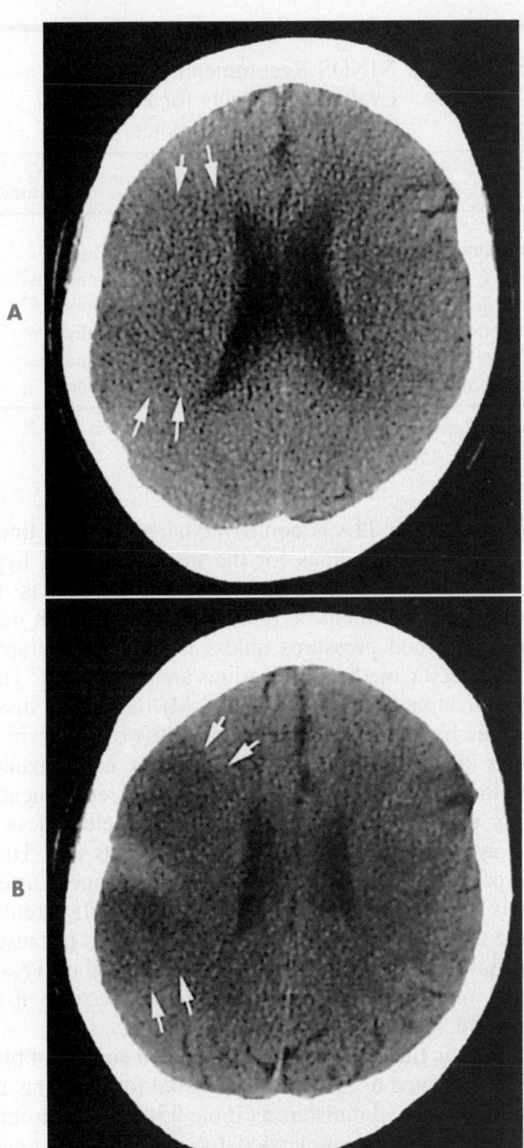

Figure 95-2. **A, CT taken 2 hours and 50 minutes after large right middle cerebral artery occlusion. There are subtle ultra-early ischemic changes, including loss of the gray-white interface *(arrows)*, as well a subtle evidence of sulcal effacement. B, CT of same patient approximately 8 hours after symptom onset showing acute hypodensity *(arrows)* and more prominent sulcal effacement.**

hyperdense artery sign and acute hypodensity of greater than one third of the middle cerebral artery distribution have been associated with poorer outcomes, both in study patients treated with tPA up to 6 hours after symptom onset and in those who were not treated with a fibrinolytic agent.[47-49] A cranial CT scan with contrast is rarely indicated on an emergency basis if the noncontrast cranial CT scan is normal.

An ECG should be obtained because atrial fibrillation and acute MI are associated with up to 60% of all cardioembolic strokes. The hematologic evaluation should include a complete blood count (CBC) with platelet count and coagulation studies. Toxicologic screen and cardiac isoenzyme tests should be considered if appropriate. Elevated blood viscosity even when hematocrit levels are not frankly polycythemic can affect blood flow and prognosis. A platelet count can identify thrombocytosis or thrombocytopenia that may precipitate a thrombosis or hemorrhage. Coagulation studies are especially helpful for patients in whom anticoagulation is being considered or patients with a hemorrhagic stroke. Cocaine or amphetamine ingestion should be considered in patients less than age 40 years who present with either an ischemic or a hemorrhagic stroke. Other ancillary diagnostic tests to consider include an echocardiogram, carotid duplex scan, angiogram, and MRI scan or MRA. Some centers are performing these studies as part of an observation unit protocol in the ED. An echocardiogram can identify a mural thrombus, tumor, patent foramen ovale, or valvular vegetation in patients in whom a cardioembolic stroke is suspected. Echocardiogram should also be considered in patients less than age 65 years with no obvious etiology for their stroke. Carotid duplex scanning may be helpful in patients with known or suspected high-grade carotid stenosis that have worsening neurologic deficit or crescendo TIAs.[50,51] These patients may be candidates for heparinization or emergency carotid endarterectomy. Carotid duplex studies can accurately identify carotid stenosis of greater than 60%, but an angiogram is required to distinguish 95% stenosis from a complete occlusion.

Angiography is the definitive test to demonstrate stenosis or occlusion of both large and small blood vessels of the head and neck. It can detect subtle abnormalities, such as dissection, which may not be demonstrated with other imaging techniques.

The role of MRI in the ED evaluation of stroke continues to evolve. MRI can visualize ischemic infarcts earlier and identify acute posterior circulation strokes more accurately than CT. However, availability, difficulty in accessing critically ill patients, and scan time limit its general use. In addition, although MRI can identify acute ICH, it is considered less accurate at differentiating ischemia from hemorrhage.[52,53] Advances in MRA technology have allowed a noninvasive method of demonstrating large-vessel occlusions of the anterior and posterior circulation, although small intracranial vascular occlusions may not be readily apparent. With the improvement in MRA speed and resolution, MRA is quickly replacing conventional angiography as the diagnostic gold standard for identifying occlusion or stenosis in select patients. Diffusion-weighted imaging (DWI) and perfusion-weighted imaging (PWI) are newer MRI techniques that take minutes to perform and may allow differentiation between reversible and irreversible neuronal injury.[9,54]

Hemorrhagic Stroke

The hematologic evaluation should be performed in the same manner as in the ischemic stroke patient. Particular attention should be directed to the presence of a coagulopathy. A drug screen should be obtained to evaluate for use of sympathomimetics if substance abuse is suspected. Increased sympathetic outflow caused by the hemorrhage may lead to an increase in dysrhythmias. Dysrhythmias may also signal impending brainstem compression from an expanding hemorrhage.

As in ischemic stroke, the cranial CT scan is the diagnostic test of choice to evaluate for an ICH.[37] The CT scan reliably diagnoses up to 95% of ICHs, although very small lesions may not be visible. Hemorrhages of several days' age may appear as isodense regions. Recent advances in MRI technology allow the identification of ICH by MRI even within 1 to 2 hours of hemorrhage onset. However, its use in identifying small hemorrhages is unclear. MRI may be helpful in differentiating ICHs caused by structural abnormalities such as AVMs, aneurysms, and tumors from other causes.[37]

STROKE MANAGEMENT

Ischemic Stroke

With the recent focus on rapid recognition, evaluation, and treatment of stroke, EDs have attempted to streamline the care of these patients to meet recommended time goals (Table 95-4). This has lead to the development of various stroke protocols, critical pathways, and acute interventional stroke teams that are often initiated in the prehospital arena before the patient even arrives at the ED.

In the prehospital setting the focus should be on the ABCs, rapid identification, early hospital notification, and rapid transport.[55] Although it is unusual for patients with ischemic stroke to be unresponsive on presentation, an altered ability to communicate, secondary to dysphasia, may be present. The ischemic stroke patient can usually maintain an airway unless the brainstem is affected or there is significant cerebral edema compressing the opposite hemisphere. Patients with intact protective airway reflexes should be given oxygen if hypoxic (oxygen saturation less than 95%),[56] with the head of the bed slightly elevated[57] and a monitor and intravenous (IV) line established.

Overhydration should be avoided to prevent cerebral edema. However, shock or significant dehydration in the patient with an ischemic stroke should be treated promptly because it may contribute to decreased CBF in the ischemic region. Dextrose-containing solutions should be avoided in normoglycemic patients suspected of having a stroke because elevated blood glucose levels may worsen an ischemic deficit.[58-63] Prehospital personnel should attempt to rapidly ascertain the patient's blood sugar level. If this is not possible, glucose should only be given to diabetic patients in whom hypoglycemia is strongly suspected. ECG monitoring is necessary because of the frequency of cardiac causes of ischemic stroke.[26,28,29]

The circumstances surrounding the stroke and concomitant medical conditions should be ascertained. The initial prehospital responders should document the exact time of stroke onset and the level of neurologic functioning; reversible defects may completely resolve by the time the patient has arrived at the hospital. The level of consciousness, gross focal motor deficits, difficulty with speech, clumsiness, facial asymmetry, and any other focal deficits should be noted. Prehospital stroke scales have been developed to assist in differentiating stroke from nonstroke patients and to identify potential fibrinolytic candidates.[64-67] Early recognition, notification, and transport by prehospital personnel have been valuable in enabling early treatment.[55]

In the ED the ABCs should be reassessed on an ongoing basis because patients may deteriorate rapidly. Even patients with subacute stroke may deteriorate precipitously. They may be found 1 to 2 days after the event has occurred and may have concomitant illnesses, including aspiration pneumonia, dehydration, hypothermia, rhabdomyolysis, or myocardial ischemia. Fever should be thoroughly evaluated by identifying the source of infection and treating promptly. There is strong evidence that even minor degrees of hyperthermia produce worsening of the neurologic injury.[68]

Blood Pressure Management of Ischemic Stroke The management of blood pressure in patients with acute ischemic stroke and TIA is controversial because of limited data. The current guidelines for the management of hypertension in patients with acute ischemic stroke is that antihypertensive treatment be reserved for those with markedly elevated blood pressures unless fibrinolytic therapy is planned or specific medical indications are present.[55,69] These medical indications include (1) acute MI, (2) aortic dissection, (3) true hypertensive encephalopathy, or (4) severe left ventricular failure. A similar approach to the acute management of blood pressure in patients with TIA is recommended.

Table 95-4. NINDS Recommended Stroke Evaluation Targets for Potential Thrombolytic Candidates

	Target time frames
Door to doctor	10 minutes
Door to CT completion	25 minutes
Door to CT reading	45 minutes
Door to treatment	60 minutes
Access to neurologic expertise*	15 minutes
Access to neurosurgical expertise*	2 hours

*By phone or in person.

Oral or parenteral agents should be withheld unless the patient's systolic pressure is greater than 220 mm Hg or diastolic pressure is greater than 120 mm Hg or mean arterial pressure is greater than 130 mm Hg (Table 95-5). If parenteral agents are used, labetalol or enalapril are favored because of ease of titration and limited effect on cerebral blood vessels. Sublingual nifedipine is not recommended because it can produce a precipitous drop in blood pressure.

If fibrinolytic therapy is planned, stringent control of blood pressure is indicated to reduce the potential for bleeding after the thrombolytic is administered (Table 95-5).[70,71] Thrombolytic therapy is not recommended for patients who consistently have a systolic pressure greater than 185 mm Hg or diastolic pressure of 110 mm Hg at the time of treatment. Simple measures can be used to try lowering blood pressure below this level. Recommended approaches include the use of nitroglycerin paste and/or one or two doses of 10 to 20 mg labetalol IV. If more aggressive measures are required to reduce blood pressure below 185/110 mm Hg, the use of tissue plasminogen activator (tPA) is not recommended. Once thrombolytic therapy has been initiated, blood pressure must be monitored closely and hypertension treated aggressively.

Acute Drug Therapy

Two major strategies for acute stroke treatment have been evaluated: recanalization and neuroprotection. To date, only the use of intravenous tPA has been approved by the Food and Drug Administration (FDA) for treatment of patients with acute ischemic stroke. These recommendations were initially based on the results of the National Institutes of Neurological Disorders and Stroke (NINDS) trial, although subsequent long-term follow-up and meta-analysis have supported its use.[72,73]

The current recommendations for the administration of tPA are that it be administered IV at a dose of 0.9 mg/kg to a maximum of 90 mg (10% of the dose given as a bolus

Table 95-5. Emergency Antihypertensive Therapy for Acute Ischemic Stroke

Blood pressure*	Treatment
Nonthrombolytic candidates	
1. DBP >140 mm Hg	Sodium nitroprusside (0.5 μg/kg/min). Aim for 10% to 20% reduction in DBP.
2. SBP >220, DBP >120, or MAP† >130 mm Hg	10 to 20 mg labetalol‡ IV push over 1 to 2 min. May repeat or double labetalol every 20 min to a maximum dose of 150 mg.
3. SBP <220, DBP <120, or MAP† <130 mm Hg	Emergency antihypertensive therapy is deferred in the absence of aortic dissection, acute MI, severe congestive heart failure, or hypertensive encephalopathy.
Thrombolytic candidates	
Pretreatment	
1. SBP >185 or DBP >110 mm Hg	1 to 2 inches of nitropaste or one to two doses of 10 to 20 mg labetalol‡ IV push. If BP is not reduced and maintained to <185/110 mm Hg, the patient should not be treated with tPA.
During and after treatment	
1. Monitor BP	BP is monitored every 15 min for 2 hours, then every 30 min for 6 hours, and then every 1 hour for 16 hours.
2. DBP >140 mm Hg	Sodium nitroprusside (0.5 μg/kg/min).
3. SBP >230 or DBP 121 to 140 mm Hg	(1) 10 mg labetalol‡ IVP over 1 to 2 min. May repeat or double labetalol every 10 min to a maximum dose of 150 mg or give the initial labetalol bolus and then start a labetalol drip at 2 to 8 mg/min. (2) If BP not controlled by labetalol, consider sodium nitroprusside.
4. SBP 180 to 230 or DBP 105 to 120 mm Hg	10 mg labetalol‡ IVP. May repeat or double labetalol every 10 to 20 min to a maximum dose of 150 mg or give initial labetalol bolus and then start a labetalol drip at 2 to 8 mg/min.

BP, Blood pressure; *DBP,* diastolic blood pressure; *MAP,* mean arterial pressure; *SBP,* systolic blood pressure; *tPA,* tissue plasminogen activator.
*All initial blood pressures should be verified before treatment by repeating reading in 5 min.
†As estimated by one third the sum of systolic and double diastolic pressure.
‡Labetalol should be avoided in patients with asthma, cardiac failure, or severe abnormalities in cardiac conduction. For refractory hypertension, alternative therapy may be considered with sodium nitroprusside or enalapril.

followed by an infusion lasting 60 minutes). Treatment must be initiated within 3 hours of the onset of ischemic symptoms in patients who meet strict inclusion and exclusion criteria (Box 95-2). IV tPA is not recommended when the time of stroke onset cannot be ascertained reliably, including strokes recognized on awakening. In addition, caution should be used in treating patients with extensive strokes (NIHSS ≥ 20) or early CT changes of a recent major infarction (e.g., acute hypodensity or mass effect) because they are at increased risk of symptomatic hemorrhage.[74] The use of intravenous tPA beyond the 3-hour window has not been demonstrated, although a meta-analysis of these studies suggests there may be benefit in a specific subset of patients.[11-13,72] Streptokinase is not recommended for use in patients with acute ischemic strokes. Other intravenous fibrinolytic agents are currently being investigated. Preliminary results from a randomized trial of ancrod (a fibrinogen-depleting agent derived from snake venom) shows promise, although it is not FDA-approved at this time.

Recent advances in catheter-based fibrinolysis have been promising and suggest the possibility of extending the therapeutic window beyond the current 3-hour limit.[38,75,76] In the recently published PROACT II study, patients with middle cerebral artery occlusions were 58% more likely to have little or no neurologic disability at 90 days compared with those receiving placebo when treated with prourokinase up to 6 hours after stroke onset. The symptomatic hemorrhage rate (10%) was similar to that seen with intravenous tPA. A combination of low-dose IV tPA followed by intraarterial therapy is currently being evaluated for patients with extensive strokes.[38]

Recent studies have focused on the use of antiplatelet agents in acute ischemic stroke. Data from two large trials involving almost 40,000 patients indicate that the early use of aspirin in patients with acute ischemic stroke who were not treated with a fibrinolytic agent was associated with a small, but significant reduction in stroke recurrence and mortality.[77,78] These studies in combination would suggest that for every 1000 stroke patients treated with aspirin, about nine deaths or nonfatal recurrences would be prevented in the first few weeks, and approximately 13 fewer patients would be dead or dependent at 6 months. The need for acute administration of aspirin in the ED is unclear because patients were given aspirin up to 48 hours after stroke onset. Aspirin should not be given for the first 24 hours in patients receiving a fibrinolytic agent because this has been associated with an increased risk of ICH and death.[79]

Heparin is frequently prescribed for patients with acute ischemic stroke or TIAs, but its value is unproved. No data have established the efficacy of anticoagulants in acute stroke. Heparin may be helpful in preventing recurrent embolism or propagation of a thrombus, but it may increase the risk of bleeding complications, including brain hemorrhage. There is no unanimity about when heparin should be

Box 95-2 Fibrinolytic Therapy for Acute Ischemic Stroke: Inclusion and Exclusion Criteria

Inclusion Criteria

1. Age 18 years or older
2. Clinical diagnosis of ischemic stroke causing a measurable neurologic deficit
3. Time of symptom onset well established to be less than 180 minutes before treatment would begin

Exclusion Criteria

1. Evidence of intracranial hemorrhage on noncontrast head CT
2. Only minor or rapidly improving stroke symptoms
3. High clinical suspicion of SAH even with normal CT
4. Active internal bleeding (e.g., gastrointestinal or urinary bleeding within last 21 days)
5. Known bleeding diathesis, including but not limited to the following:
   a. Platelet count <100,000/mm³
   b. Patient has received heparin within 48 hours and had an elevated activated partial thromboplastin time (greater than upper limit of normal for laboratory)
   c. Recent use of anticoagulant (e.g., warfarin sodium) and elevated prothrombin time >15 seconds
6. Within 3 months of intracranial surgery, serious head trauma, or previous stroke
7. Within 14 days of major surgery or serious trauma
8. Recent arterial puncture at noncompressible site
9. Lumbar puncture within 7 days
10. History of ICH, AVM, or aneurysm
11. Witnessed seizure at stroke onset
12. Recent acute MI
13. On repeated measurements, systolic pressure >185 mm Hg or diastolic pressure >110 mm Hg at time of treatment, requiring aggressive treatment to reduce blood pressure to within these limits

started, the desired level of anticoagulation, or whether a loading dose should be given.[55] Heparin is usually considered in patients at high risk of stroke progression. This includes patients with crescendo TIAs, TIA caused by a cardioembolic source, patients with a high-grade carotid stenosis, those with posterior circulation TIA, and patients with evolving strokes. Heparin should not be initiated in patients with suspected endocarditis or in any patient until a CT scan has ruled out intracranial bleeding. Because of the lack of consensus regarding the use of heparin after stroke, the most prudent course for an emergency physician is to determine the need for heparin therapy in conjunction with the patient's neurologist or the admitting physician.

Low-molecular-weight heparins have more selective antithrombotic actions than heparin and may offer some advantages in stroke management. An early study from Hong Kong reported that treatment with low-molecular-weight heparin (nadroparin) within 48 hours of onset of stroke was associated with a statistically significant improvement in survival and decreased eventual rate of dependency compared with placebo.[80] Unfortunately, subsequent larger, multicenter trials with similar designs were unable to corroborate these findings.[81]

Numerous neuroprotective agents aimed at preventing the cascade of physiologic steps that occur after ischemia and lead to cell death have been studied. These have included antioxidants, calcium channel blockers, N-methyl-D-aspartate (NMDA) inhibitors, glycine, and glutamate receptor antagonist. Although promising in animal and small human trials, none have been demonstrated to be effective in larger, phase III trials.[82-84]

Intracerebral Hemorrhage Management

The patient with a potential ICH requires rapid assessment and transport to a facility that has CT scanning capability and intensive care management. The prehospital management is similar to that for ischemic stroke. The circumstances surrounding the event and other concomitant medical conditions should also be ascertained. An evaluation of the initial level of consciousness, GCS, any gross focal deficits, difficulty with speech, clumsiness, gait disturbance, or facial asymmetry should be noted.

Supportive care involving attention to airway management and perfusion is of the highest priority. Patients with hemorrhagic stroke are more likely to have an altered level of consciousness that may rapidly progress to unresponsiveness requiring emergency endotracheal intubation. Because of increased ICP and intracranial bleeding, manipulation of the airway should be performed as atraumatically as possible. IV access and cardiac monitoring should be initiated. Evaluation of blood glucose level and appropriate dextrose and naloxone administration should be considered in any patient with altered mental status.

There is considerable disagreement regarding the optimal blood pressure management in the patient with ICH. Hypertension may cause deterioration by increasing the ICP and potentiating further bleeding from small arteries or arterioles. On the other hand, hypotension may decrease CBF, thus worsening brain injury. In general, recommendations for the treatment of hypertension in patients with ICH are more aggressive than those for patients with ischemic stroke. The current consensus for ICH is to recommend antihypertensive treatment with parenteral agents for systolic pressure higher than 160 to 180 mm Hg or diastolic pressures higher than 105 mm Hg. Treatment for lower pressures remains controversial.[37,55] Nitroprusside is the agent most commonly recommended because one can obtain a rapid and consistent lowering of the blood pressure to the desired level and adjustments can be made rapidly. Nitroprusside provides a rapid onset, is titratable, and has no effect on mental status. Disadvantages include the need for careful monitoring (ideally with an indwelling arterial catheter) and the theoretical risk of worsening the hemorrhage because of the vasodilatory effects of nitroprusside on cerebral vessels. Labetalol is another therapeutic option.

Hyperventilation and diuretics such as furosemide and mannitol are useful when ICH is complicated by signs of progressively increasing ICP, clinical deterioration associated with mass effect, or impending uncal herniation.[37] These interventions should not be used prophylactically. Diuretics and mannitol move fluid from the intracranial compartment, thereby reducing cerebral edema. Although this effect may be temporarily helpful in the acute setting, the brain tissue re-equilibrates and rebound swelling can occur and worsen the patient's clinical status. These agents can also cause dehydration and lead to hypotension. The use of steroids in cerebral hemorrhage, once a common practice, appears harmful and is not recommended. Other experimental modalities include barbiturate coma and hypothermia.

Seizure activity can cause neuronal injury, elevations in ICH, and destabilization of an already critically ill patient. In addition, nonconvulsive seizure may contribute to coma in up to 10% of patients in a neurologic intensive care unit (ICU).[37] Seizure prophylaxis (phenytoin 18 mg/kg or fosphenytoin 15 to 20 mg PE/kg) should be considered for patients with ICH, especially those with lobar hemorrhage.

Surgery is not beneficial in most cases of ICH. Selected patients with sizable lobar hemorrhage and progressive neurologic deterioration may benefit from surgical drainage. Surgery is more efficacious in patients with cerebellar hemorrhage. The clinical course in cerebellar hemorrhage is notoriously unpredictable. Patients with minimal findings may deteriorate suddenly to coma and death with little warning. For this reason, most neurosurgeons will consider emergency surgery for patients with cerebellar hemorrhage within 48 hours of onset.

DISPOSITION

Ischemic Stroke and Transient Ischemic Attack

Definitions of "stroke centers" remain vague and controversial. However, there is a consensus that emergency medical services (EMS) personnel should transport patients with symptoms consistent with an acute stroke to emergency facilities capable of initiating fibrinolytic therapy within 1 hour of hospital arrival. At a minimum, this requires emergency CT capabilities, a written "acute stroke protocol," and a physician versed in the use of thrombolytic therapy. Intensive care monitoring and neurosurgery capabilities should be available within 2 hours of drug initiation, either at the treating hospital or by helicopter or ground transport to an appropriate health care facility (see Table 95-4).[85]

In most cases, once the diagnosis of an acute stroke or stroke syndrome is established and the patient's condition is stabilized, the patient should be hospitalized for further evaluation and treatment. Patients may deteriorate over the first 24 hours and require close in-hospital monitoring. In addition, patients often require prolonged rehabilitation, including physical therapy and assistance to regain the ability to perform the activities required for daily living. Most patients can be managed on a general medical or telemetry unit. Patients with large acute hemispheric strokes (at risk for herniation), with significant posterior circulation findings, or those treated with a fibrinolytic agent should be monitored in a step-down unit or ICU for at least 24 hours. In some cases, patients with multiple previous strokes who have been thoroughly evaluated, who experience mild new episodes, or who have a completed stroke days to weeks after the event may be treated at home when it is deemed appropriate by the patient's physicians and family.

Patients with new-onset TIAs warrant hospital admission for evaluation and workup. The exception is a patient with only minimal anterior circulation symptoms who can have an extensive ED evaluation. In these patients, the ED evaluation should include a CT scan, a carotid Doppler scan or MRA of their anterior circulation, and an echocardiogram (if indicated). A medically or surgically treatable cause for TIAs (e.g., high-grade carotid stenosis or a mural thrombus) would require in-hospital treatment such as anticoagulation, antiplatelet agents, or carotid endarterectomy. If the patient's symptoms have completely resolved, the workup is negative, and close neurologic follow-up is arranged, the patient can be considered for outpatient therapy. The decision to start the patient on an antiplatelet agent should be made in conjunction with the neurologist.

Hemorrhagic Stroke

All patients with an acute hemorrhagic stroke in whom surgical intervention is a consideration should be admitted to an ICU under the care of a neurologist or neurosurgeon. If this is unavailable at the evaluating institution, the patient should be transported to an appropriate institution.

SUMMARY

Stroke is a major cause of death and disability that challenges the emergency physician to provide stabilization and accurate diagnosis. Recent advances in imaging technology allow this process to occur quickly and accurately. Current research is focused on therapy that may salvage vital brain tissue that is compromised during the ischemic or hemorrhagic event. The ED is the focal point where these patients are identified, stabilized, and the decision for treatment is made. As in other life-threatening diseases, the emergency physician must interact with various disciplines and be intimately involved in the care and decision-making process for these patients.

KEY CONCEPTS

- Patients with the signs and symptoms of an acute ischemic stroke within 3 hours of symptom onset should be evaluated for thrombolytic therapy within the following recommended time frames:

Target time frames	
Door to doctor	10 minutes
Door to CT completion	25 minutes
Door to CT reading	45 minutes
Door to drug treatment	60 minutes

- Carotid Doppler studies are recommended before discharging a patient with TIA.
- Avoid overly aggressive blood pressure management in patients with acute ischemic stroke.
- Accurate time of symptom onset should be documented for all patients with stroke.

REFERENCES

1. American Heart Association: *Heart and stroke facts: statistical supplement,* Dallas, 1994, American Heart Association.
2. Broderick J et al: The Greater Cincinnati/Northern Kentucky Stroke Study: preliminary first-ever and total incidence rates of stroke among blacks, *Stroke* 29:415, 1998.
3. Williams GR et al: Incidence and occurrence of total (first-ever and recurrent) stroke, *Stroke* 30:2523, 1999.
4. Kolominksky-Rabas PL et al: A prospective community-based study of stroke in Germany—The Erlangen Stroke Project (ESPro), *Stroke* 29:2501, 1998.
5. Greshmam GE et al: Epidemiologist profile of long-term stroke disability: the Framingham study, *Arch Phys Med Rehabil* 61:355, 1980.
6. Kothari RU et al: Emergency physicians: accuracy in the diagnosis of stroke, *Stroke* 26:2238, 1995.
7. Kothari RU et al: Frequency and accuracy of prehospital diagnosis of acute stroke, *Stroke* 26:937, 1995.

8. Smith RW et al: Emergency physician treatment of acute stroke with recombinant tissue plasminogen activator: a retrospective analysis, *Acad Emerg Med* 6:618, 1999.
9. Baird AE et al: Enlargement of human cerebral ischemic lesion volumes measured by diffusion-weighted magnetic resonance imaging, *Ann Neurol* 41:581, 1997.
10. The NINDS rt-PA Stroke Study Group: Tissue plasminogen activator for acute ischemic stroke, *N Engl J Med* 333:1581, 1995.
11. Clark W et al for the ATLANTIS Stroke Study Investigators: Recombinant tissue-type plasminogen activator (Alteplase) for ischemic stroke 3 to 5 hours after symptom onset. The ALANTIS study: a randomized controlled trial, *JAMA* 282:2019, 1999.
12. Hacke W et al: Intravenous thrombolysis with recombinant tissue plasminogen activator for acute hemispheric stroke: the European Cooperative Acute Stroke Study, *JAMA* 274:1, 1995.
13. Hacke W et al for the Second European-Australian Acute Stroke Study Investigators: Randomized double-blind placebo-controlled trial of thrombolytic therapy with intravenous alteplase in acute ischaemic stroke (ECASS II), *Lancet* 352:1245, 1998.
14. The Abciximab in Ischemic Stroke Investigators: A randomized, double-blinded, placebo-controlled, dose-escalation study, *Stroke* 31: 601, 2000.
15. Wagner KR et al: Lobar intracerebral hemorrhage model in pigs: rapid edema development in perihematomal white matter, *Stroke* 27:490, 1996.
16. Xi G et al: Role of blood clot formation on early edema development after experimental intracerebral hemorrhage, *Stroke* 29:2580, 1998.
17. Zuccarello M et al: Early surgical treatment for supratentorial intracerebral hemorrhage: a randomized feasibility study, *Stroke* 30:1833, 1999.
18. Clark WM et al for the Citicholine Stroke Study Group: A randomized efficacy trial of citicholine in patients with acute ischemic stroke, *Stroke* 31:2592, 1999.
19. Grotta J: The US and Canadian Lubeluzole Ischemic Stroke Study Group: Lubeluzole treatment of acute ischemic stroke, *Stroke* 28:2338, 1997.
20. Gammans RE et al: ECCO 2000 Study of Citicholine for treatment of acute ischemic stroke: Presented at the 25th International Stroke Conference, New Orleans, Louisiana, February 10-12, 2000.
21. Diener HC: European and Australian Lubeluzole Ischaemic Stroke Study Group: multinational randomized controlled trial of Lubeluzole in acute ischaemic stroke, *Cerebrovasc Dis* 8:172, 1998.
22. RANTTAS Investigators: A randomized trial of tirilazad mesylate in patients with acute stroke (RANTTAS), *Stroke* 27:1453, 1996.
23. Marchal G et al: Prolonged persistence of substantial volumes of potentially viable brain tissue after stroke: a correlative PET-CT study with voxel-based data analysis, *Stroke* 27:599, 1996.
24. Woo D et al: Incidence rates of first-ever ischemic stroke subtypes among blacks: a population-based study, *Stroke* 30:2517, 1999.
25. Petty GW et al: Ischemic stroke subtypes: a population-based study of incidence and risk factors, *Stroke* 30:2513, 1999.
26. Jorgensen HS et al: Acute stroke with atrial fibrillation: the Copenhagen Stroke study, *Stroke* 10:1765, 1996.
27. Lin HJ et al: Stroke severity in atrial fibrillation: the Framingham study, *Stroke* 27:1760, 1996.
28. Maggioni AP et al: Cerebrovascular events after myocardial infarction: analysis of the GISSI trial, *BMJ* 302:1428, 1991.
29. Mooe T, Eriksson P, Stegmayr B: Ischemic stroke after acute myocardial infarction: a population based study, *Stroke* 28:762, 1997.
30. ISIS-2 (Second International Study of Infarct Survival) Collaborative Group: Randomized trial of intravenous streptokinase, oral aspirin, both, or neither among 17,187 cases of suspected acute myocardial infarction: ISIS-2, *Lancet* 2:349, 1988.
31. Silver FL et al: Early mortality following stroke: a prospective review, *Stroke* 45:492, 1984.
32. Tokgozoglu SL et al: Effects of stroke localization on cardiac autonomic balance and sudden death, *Stroke* 30:1307, 1999.
33. Korpelainen JT et al: Dynamic behavior of heart rate in ischemic stroke, *Stroke* 30:1008, 1999.
34. Levy D: How transient are transient ischemic attacks? *Neurology* 38:674, 1988.
35. Fazekas F et al: Magnetic resonance imaging correlates of transient cerebral ischemic attacks, *Stroke* 27:607, 1996.
36. Bhadelia RA et al for the CHS Collaborative Research Group: Prevalence and associations of MRI-demonstrated brain infarcts in elderly subjects with a history of transient ischemic attack: the Cardiovascular Health Study, *Stroke* 30:383, 1999.
37. Broderick JP et al: Guidelines for the management of spontaneous intracerebral hemorrhage: a statement for healthcare professionals from a special writing group of the Stroke Council, American Heart Association, *Stroke* 30:905, 1999.
38. Lewandowski CA and the EMS Bridging Trial Investigators: Combined intravenous and intra-arterial r-TPA versus intra-arterial therapy of acute ischemic stroke: Emergency Management of Stroke (EMS) Bridging Trial, *Stroke* 30:2598, 1999.
39. Brott T: Utility of the NIH Stroke Scale, *Cerebrovasc Dis* 2:241, 1992.
40. Lyden P et al and The National Institute for Neurological Disorders and Stroke rt-PA Study Group: A proposed revision of the NINDS Stroke Scale: results of a factor analysis, *Stroke* 30:2347, 1999.
41. DeGraba TJ et al: Progression in acute stroke-value of the initial NIH Stroke Scale score on patient stratification in future trials, *Stroke* 30:1208, 1999.
42. Brott T et al: Early hemorrhage growth in patients with intracerebral hemorrhage, *Stroke* 28:1, 1997.
43. Kothari RU et al: The ABCs of measuring intracerebral hemorrhage volumes, *Stroke* 27:1304, 1996.
44. Gilman S: Imaging the brain, *N Engl J Med* 338:812, 1998.
45. The NINDS t-PA Stroke Study Group: Intracerebral hemorrhage after intravenous t-PA therapy for ischemic stroke, *Stroke* 2109, 1997.
46. Grotta J et al for the NINDS rtPA Stroke Study Group: Agreement and variability interpreting early CT changes in stroke patients qualifying for intravenous r-tPA therapy, *Stroke* 30:1528, 1999.
47. Manelfe C et al: Association of hyperdense middle cerebral artery sign with clinical outcome in patients treated with tissue plasminogen activator, *Stroke* 30:769, 1999.
48. Marks MP et al: Evaluation of early computed tomographic findings in acute ischemic stroke, *Stroke* 30:389, 1999.
49. Von Kummer R et al: Acute stroke—usefulness of early CT findings before thrombolysis therapy, *Radiology* 205:327, 1997.
50. Executive Committee for the Asymptomatic Carotid Atherosclerosis Study: Endarterectomy for asymptomatic carotid artery stenosis, *JAMA* 273:1421, 1995.
51. Barnett HJ et al: Benefit of carotid endarterectomy in patients with symptomatic moderate or severe stenosis: North American Symptomatic Carotid Endarterectomy Trial Collaborators, *N Engl J Med* 339:1415, 1998.
52. Schellinger PD et al: A standardized MRI stroke protocol-comparison with CT in hyperacute intracerebral hemorrhage, *Stroke* 30:765, 1999.
53. Linfante I et al: MRI features of intracerebral hemorrhage within 2 hours from symptom onset, *Stroke* 30:2263, 1999.
54. Tong DC et al: Correlation of perfusion and diffusion weighted MRI with NIHSS score in acute (<6.5 hour) ischemic stroke, *Neurology* 50:864, 1998.
55. Emergency Stroke Care Task Force: Acute stroke. In Cummins RO, editor: *Advanced cardiac life support*, Chicago, 1997, AHA.
56. Ronning OM, Guldvog B: Should stroke victims routinely receive supplemental oxygen? A quasi-randomized controlled trial, *Stroke* 30:2033, 1999.
57. Elizabeth J et al: Arterial oxygen saturation and posture in acute stroke, *Age Ageing* 22:269, 1993.
58. Weir CJ et al: Is hyperglycemia an independent predictor of poor outcome after acute stroke? Results of a long-term follow-up study, *BMJ* 314:1303, 1997.
59. Broderick JP et al: Hyperglycemia and hemorrhagic transformation of cerebral infarcts, *Stroke* 26:4848, 1995.
60. Yip PK et al: Effect of plasma glucose on infarct size in focal cerebral ischemia reperfusion, *Neurology* 41:899, 1991.
61. Yip PK et al: Effect of plasma glucose on infarct size in focal cerebral ischemia reperfusion, *Neurology* 41:899, 1993.
62. Chew W et al: Hyperglycemia augments ischemic brain injury: in vivo MR imaging spectroscopic study with nicardipine in cats with occluded middle cerebral arteries, *Am J Neuroradiol* 12:603, 1991.
63. Vazquez-Cruz J et al: Progressing cerebral infarction in relation to plasma glucose in gerbils, *Stroke* 21:1621, 1990.
64. Kothari R et al: Early stroke recognition: developing an out-of-hospital NIH Stroke Scale, *Acad Emerg Med* 4:986, 1997.

65. Kothari RU et al: Cincinnati Prehospital Stroke Scale: reproducibility & validity, *Ann Emerg Med* 33:373, 1999.
66. Kidwell CS et al: Design and retrospective analysis of the Los Angeles Prehospital Stroke Screen (LAPSS), *Prehosp Emerg Care* 2:27, 1998.
67. Kidwell CS et al: Identifying stroke in the field: prospective validation of the Los Angeles Prehospital Stroke Screen (LAPSS), *Stroke* 31:71, 2000.
68. Ginsberg MD, Busto R: Combating hyperthermia in acute stroke: a significant clinical concern, *Stroke* 29:529, 1998.
69. Adams JHP et al: Guidelines for the management of patients with acute ischemic stroke, *Stroke* 25:1901, 1994.
70. Brott T et al and The National Institute for Neurological Disorders and Stroke rt-PA Study Group: Hypertension and its treatment in the NINDS rt-PA Stroke Trial, *Stroke* 29:1504, 1998.
71. A Special Writing Group of the Stroke Council: American Heart Association guidelines for thrombolytic therapy for acute stroke: a supplement to the guidelines for the management of patients with acute ischemic stroke, *Circulation* 94:1167, 1996.
72. Wardlaw JM, del Zoppo G, Yamaguchi T: Thrombolysis for acute ischaemic stroke (Cochrane Review). In The Cochrane Library, Issue 4, 1999, Oxford, Update Software.
73. Kwiatkowski TG et al for the NINDS r-tPA Stroke Study Group: Effects of tissue plasminogen activator for acute ischemic stroke at one year, *N Engl J Med* 340:1781, 1999.
74. The National Institute of Neurological Disorders t-PA Stroke Study Group: Generalized efficacy of t-PA for acute stroke: subgroup analysis of the NINDS t-PA Stroke Trial, *Stroke* 28:2119, 1997.
75. Del Zoppo GT, Higashida HT, Furlan AJ for the PROACT Investigators: PROACT: a phase II randomized trial of recombinant pro-urokinase by direct arterial delivery in acute middle cerebral artery stroke, *Stroke* 29:4, 1998.
76. Furlan A et al for the PROACT Investigators: Intra-arterial pro-urokinase for acute ischemic stroke: the PROACT II study: a randomized controlled trial, *JAMA* 282:2003, 1999.
77. International Stroke Trial Collaborative Group: The International Stroke Trial (IST): a randomized trial of aspirin, subcutaneous heparin, both, or neither among 19,435 patients with acute ischaemic stroke, *Lancet* 349:1569, 1997.
78. Chinese Acute Stroke Trial Collaborative Group: CAST: Randomized placebo-controlled trial of early aspirin use in 20,000 patients with acute ischaemic stroke, *Lancet* 349:1641, 1997.
79. Multicentre Acute Stroke Trial—Italy (MAST-I) Group: Randomized controlled trial of streptokinase, aspirin, and combination of both in treatment of acute ischaemic stroke, *Lancet* 346:1509, 1995.
80. Kay R et al: Low-molecular-weight heparin for the treatment of acute ischemic stroke, *N Engl J Med* 333:1588, 1995.
81. Publications Committee for the Trial of ORG 10172 in Acute Stroke Treatment (TOAST) Investigators: Low-molecular-weight heparinoid, ORG 10172 (danaparoid), and outcome after acute ischemic stroke: a randomized controlled trial, *JAMA* 279:1265, 1998.
82. Clark WM et al for the Citicholine Stroke Study Group: A randomized efficacy trial of citicholine in patients with acute ischemic stroke, *Stroke* 31:2592, 1999.
83. Grotta J: The US and Canadian Lubeluzole Ischemic Stroke Study Group: Lubeluzole treatment of acute ischemic stroke, *Stroke* 28:2338, 1997.
84. Gammans RE et al: ECCO 2000 Study of Citicholine for treatment of acute ischemic stroke: presented at the 25th International Stroke Conference, New Orleans, February 10-12, 2000.
85. Barsan WG: Recommendations: emergency department panel. In Marler JR, Jones PW, Emr M, editors: *Proceedings of a national symposium on rapid identification and treatment of acute stroke,* Bethesda, Md, 1997, National Institute of Neurological Disorders and Stroke, NIH Pub No. 97-4239, Washington DC, NIH.

96 Seizures

Charles V. Pollack, Jr.
Emily S. Pollack

PERSPECTIVE

A *seizure* is the clinical manifestation of excessive, abnormal cortical neuron activity. The physical manifestation depends on the area of brain cortex involved and, to a lesser extent, on the specific underlying abnormality. Patients who have recurring seizures without consistent provocation have *epilepsy,* although this term encompasses many disparate clinical syndromes. Seizures may also occur as a predictable response to certain toxic, pathophysiologic, or environmental stresses; these are *reactive* or *secondary seizures,* and patients who have them do not have epilepsy. In the United States, 10% of the population will have at least one seizure in their lifetime; the incidence of epilepsy is less than 1%.[1]

In addition to the distinction between primary (epileptic) and secondary (reactive) seizures, there are many other classifications of ictal events.[2-6] Seizures are termed *generalized* or *focal (partial)* depending on their clinical manifestations. The former type of seizure results from the abnormal electrical event that simultaneously involves both cerebral hemispheres and is accompanied by loss of consciousness; in the latter, abnormal activity is limited to part of one cerebral hemisphere only. Generalized seizures are usually characterized by rhythmic, tonic-clonic muscle contractions, or *convulsions,* although there are *nonconvulsive generalized seizures* as well. Partial seizures can be differentiated further into those during which consciousness is maintained *(simple partial)* and those during which consciousness is impaired *(complex partial).* Finally, partial seizures may become generalized *(partial with secondary generalization).*

Inexperienced witnesses may provide histories insufficient to categorize such seizures. A rule of thumb remains, however, when an accurate history is available: secondary seizures typically are generalized, not partial, in nature. The definitive differentiation among these classifications may require electroencephalographic recording *during* the seizure, sometimes in association with simultaneous video recording.

Seizures in children, as in adults, are classified as primary (idiopathic) and secondary (symptomatic or reactive). The term *cryptogenic* is sometimes used when seizures are thought to be secondary but no cause has been identified. The history is the most important diagnostic tool in evaluating seizures in children. The actual seizure activity is usually not observed, and the emergency physician must rely on a detailed and accurate history for diagnosis.

Some other important terms to describe ictal events include *status epilepticus,* in which seizures occur serially without an intervening return to a normal neurologic condition; *spasm,* which is a specific, debilitating seizure syndrome that occurs in infants; and *myoclonus,* which refers to rhythmic, shocklike muscle contractions also typical for specific seizure syndromes. The *postictal period* is a variable time interval after a seizure, usually characterized by impaired consciousness, but sometimes also marked by self-limited focal paralysis or neurogenic pulmonary edema.

PRINCIPLES OF DISEASE

The pathophysiology of seizures at the neuronal level is incompletely understood, with most of what is known coming from animal studies in which either electrical or pharmacologic stimulation is applied directly to brain cortex. To produce generalized ictus, stimulus must be applied to both hemispheres simultaneously. Some studies demonstrate the concept of recruitment, which occurs when the initiating neurons' abnormal, increased electrical activity activates adjacent neurons and propagates until the thalamus and other subcortical structures are recruited. The clinical seizure activity typically, but not always, reflects the focus of initiation.[1,7,8]

What prompts such initiation is unclear. Proposed mechanisms include disruption of normal structure—whether congenital, maturational, or acquired (as with scar tissue)—and disruption of local metabolic or biochemical function. The latter mechanism is better elucidated because the roles of two neurotransmitters—acetylcholine, which is excitatory to cortical neurons, and gamma-aminobutyric acid (GABA), which is inhibitory—are better recognized. In sensitive neurons, such as those at an ictogenic focus, subtle changes in the local concentrations of these neurotransmitters can produce sustained membrane depolarization, ultimately followed by local hyperpolarization and then recruitment. Recruitment may follow contiguous paths or extend along diverse integrated circuits that are both deep and across the midline.[1,7,8]

When the ictal discharge extends below the cortex to deeper structures, the reticular activating system in the brainstem may be affected, altering consciousness. In generalized seizures, the focus is often subcortical and midline, which explains the prompt loss of consciousness and bilateral involvement.[8,9] Seizures are typically self-limited; at some point, the hyperpolarization subsides and the electrical discharges from the focus terminate. This may be related to reflex inhibition, loss of synchrony, neuronal exhaustion, or alteration of the local balance of acetylcholine and GABA in favor of inhibition.[8,9]

The systemic manifestations of convulsive ictal activity include hypertension, tachycardia, tachypnea, and hyperglycemia from sympathetic stimulation. With more prolonged convulsions, skeletal muscle damage, lactic acidosis, and, rarely, frank rhabdomyolysis may ensue.[1,8,10,11] Autonomic discharge and bulbar muscle involvement may result in urinary or fecal incontinence, vomiting (with significant aspiration risk), tongue biting, and airway impairment.

CLINICAL FEATURES

Primary Seizures

Primary ictal events in adults include those of genetic and of idiopathic origin. Onset is typically during childhood or adolescence, but occasionally idiopathic seizures may begin *de novo* in the adult years. Because this is sufficiently rare, the emergency physician should thoroughly evaluate a first-time seizure in an adult.

Focal seizures in adults, as previously defined, may be classified as simple partial or complex partial. Simple partial seizures are limited in electrical focus to one cerebral hemisphere and do not cause loss of consciousness. Although the specific function of the initiating neurons determines the clinical manifestation of the ictal event (i.e., motor, somatosensory, special sensory, autonomic, or psychic), such clinical manifestations are not sufficiently specific for anatomic localization without performing an electroencephalogram (EEG). Typical features of simple partial seizure include, respectively, focal clonic movements; paresthesias; visual, auditory, olfactory, or gustatory experiences; sweating and flushing; dysphasia; a sense of déjà vu; or unwarranted fear.[7] Motor signs, which by definition remain ipsilateral in simple partial seizures, may spread contiguously in a stepwise fashion ("Jacksonian march") because neuron recruitment occurs in the motor cortex. There is generally no postictal state after a simple partial seizure.

Complex partial seizures are ictal events that involve impairment but not loss of consciousness, either at onset or evolving from focal activity. Amnesia for the ictal event is a consistent finding in a complex partial seizure, although during the episodes the patient may remain responsive to the surroundings. Complex partial seizures typically involve automatisms that are specific to the individual—such as lip smacking, repeated swallowing or verbal phrases, or picking at one's clothing. Complex partial seizures are generally associated with an aura such as a specific smell, taste, visual hallucination, or intense emotional feeling. Unlike generalized seizures, patients maintain higher cortical function during complex partial seizures; for example, patients may drive automobiles, ride bicycles, or play musical instruments. *Psychomotor epilepsy* and *temporal lobe seizures* are other terms applied to such complex partial seizures. However, this terminology is considered outdated because seizures that originate in the temporal lobe may be generalized, simple, or complex partial seizures. Partial seizures may rapidly progress to generalized seizures. A postictal state is common after complex partial seizures and may persist for hours.[1,7,8]

Generalized seizures in adults may be convulsive or nonconvulsive. By definition, patients lose consciousness in a generalized seizure, and no aura is present. Some patients may experience a brief, vague prodrome or dysphoric state just before the ictal event. Convulsive generalized seizures are typified by the grand mal seizure in which the patient loses consciousness; stiffens with generalized muscular hypertonus; and then rhythmically, violently contracts multiple, bilateral, and usually symmetric muscle groups. The muscular force may be sufficiently vigorous to result in posterior shoulder dislocation or fractures of thoracic spine vertebral bodies; significant tongue and buccal injuries may also occur from repeated biting. Dysautonomia, including transient apnea, is a potential manifestation of convulsive generalized seizures; urinary incontinence occurs more often than does fecal incontinence. A generalized convulsive seizure is followed by a postictal state, headache, and drowsiness that may persist for hours. This state must be differentiated in the ED from altered consciousness attributable to other causes. Ictal and interictal EEG findings are abnormal.[1,7,8]

Nonconvulsive generalized seizures include absence, or petit mal, seizures; myoclonic seizures; tonic seizures; and atonic seizures. Absence seizures in adults are further subclassified as *typical* or *atypical.* Typical absence ictus is characterized by the sudden cessation of normal, conscious activity followed by a nonconvulsive, dissociative state that persists for a few seconds to several minutes before suddenly terminating. Eye movements, blinking, or automatisms may be present. There is no postictal state. Absence seizures typically begin in childhood but occasionally develop in older adults, in whom brief 3-Hz spike and wave discharges occur on the EEG. Atypical absence seizures are marked by more complicated motor signs, coexistence with other forms of generalized seizures, inconsistent postictal confusion, and irregular EEG abnormalities.[1,7,8]

Myoclonic and *tonic seizures* are manifested by sudden, brief muscle group contractions without a loss of consciousness. When the entire body is involved, the patient will fall ("drop attack"). Atonic seizures also result in drop attacks, which are so unexpected that significant injury may result. Because there is typically no postictal state associated with these episodes, an altered level of consciousness should prompt the emergency physician to investigate for head trauma or a toxic or metabolic abnormality.

Status epilepticus is defined as serial seizure activity without interictal recovery or the prolonged, continuous seizure activity that lasts longer than 30 minutes and may occur with any type of seizure.[12] The clinical significance can range from life threatening in convulsive generalized status to negligible in typical absence. The most common cause of status epilepticus is discontinuation of anticonvulsant medication. This may be compounded by barbiturate withdrawal when phenobarbital therapy is abruptly withdrawn. Patients may present for the first time with a primary seizure disorder in status. There are many other causes of status epilepticus (Box 96-1).[13,14]

Complex partial status, although not life threatening, should also be treated vigorously to avoid prolonged antegrade amnesia.[7] Clonic simple partial status, also termed *epilepsia partialis continua,* may occur in adults as a result of hyperosmolar conditions such as nonketotic hyperglycemia or uremia and should prompt a thorough metabolic evaluation in the ED.[14]

All classes of primary seizures may recur sporadically, randomly, or predictably. Cyclical recurrence has been reported with awakening, sleep deprivation, and menses, among other factors. Seizures may also be triggered by photic stimulation (particularly strobe lights), specific musical compositions, and tactile stimulation.[1,8,9] The most common cause of recurrent primary seizures is medication noncompliance.[7]

Reactive Seizures

Reactive or secondary seizures do not result from genetic or idiopathic causes. The conditions that cause reactive seizures may be static (e.g., anatomic scarring), progressive (e.g., degenerative cortical disorders), or transient (e.g., acute electrolyte derangements).

Box 96-1 Status Epilepticus: Common Etiologies

Metabolic Encephalopathies

Hyponatremia
Hypocalcemia
Hypoglycemia
Hepatic or renal failure

Infectious Encephalopathies

Central nervous system (CNS) abscess
Meningitis
Encephalitis

CNS Lesions

Neoplasm
Arteriovenous malformations
Acute hydrocephalus
Intracerebral hematomas
Cerebrovascular accident

Intoxications

Cyclic antidepressants
Lead
Strychnine
Camphor

Seizures Caused by Metabolic Derangements Hypoglycemia is a common metabolic cause of reactive seizures. Ictal activity can occur when the plasma glucose level is lower than 45 mg/dl, although some patients may manifest neurologic disturbances at higher levels.[15] A rapid bedside glucose test should be an integral part of seizure evaluation in the ED patient without known epilepsy. Convulsive and nonconvulsive, generalized and partial seizures may all occur during hypoglycemia.[15] Patients at both the extremes of age are particularly susceptible to glucose stress during acute illness. Hypoglycemic seizures respond to glucose therapy; anticonvulsants are unnecessary.

A special cause of hypoglycemia-induced seizures in children is ketotic hypoglycemia. This is the most common cause of childhood hypoglycemia. The first manifestation of the syndrome is classically that of new-onset seizures, which are most likely to be seen initially in the ED. Ketotic hypoglycemia typically affects small-for-age children and is characterized by episodes of symptomatic hypoglycemia associated with periods of caloric deprivation. Prolonged fasting must be avoided and the child's propensity for hypoglycemia anticipated in times of intercurrent illness, such as gastroenteritis, when oral intake may be decreased.[16]

The usual age of onset of ketotic hypoglycemia is between 6 and 18 months, and it may be related to decreased bottle feedings at night and longer periods between meals. The signs and symptoms usually appear in the morning or after a period of fasting. Seizures are often preceded by vomiting and lethargy. Children's blood glucose levels are normal between attacks but are abnormal during periods of relative starvation or under provocation by a ketogenic diet.[16] A presumptive diagnosis can be made in the ED when the typical symptoms are concurrent with hypoglycemia and ketonuria. Symptomatic hypoglycemia in response to provocation with a ketogenic diet confirms the diagnosis. Dietary management alone results in an excellent outcome, and anticonvulsants are unnecessary.[17] Cataracts, probably secondary to recurrent osmotic swelling of the lens, are a common complication, and all patients with ketotic hypoglycemia should be referred for ophthalmologic examination.[18]

Another cause of hypoglycemic seizures unique to children is the so-called *morning-after seizure,* caused by drinking alcohol left unsupervised after a party in the household. This may be an important, although often overlooked, historical inquiry. In adults, hypoglycemia may also result from insulin reaction, a deliberate insulin or hypoglycemic agent overdose, or poor nutrition.

Cation derangements are another common metabolic cause of ictal activity.[19,20] Both hyposmolar and hyperosmolar states can precipitate seizures. Disorders of sodium—the primary cation in the extracellular fluid compartment and thus the primary determinant of serum osmolarity—are most common. Hyponatremia is the most commonly identified electrolyte disorder in hospitalized patients, and sodium levels below 120 mEq/L are often complicated by seizures.[21] The rate at which the sodium level drops, and not the absolute magnitude of the decrease, determines the risk of neurologic manifestations.[20] As a result, correcting hyponatremia should be undertaken slowly in the ED unless seizures are persistent, in which case administration of hypertonic (3%) saline may be indicated. Dilutional hyponatremia is also a potential cause of seizures in young children and may result from overdiluted formula or excessive water swallowing during swimming lessons.[22]

Hypernatremia, which typically occurs as a result of a dehydrating illness or lack of access to free water in the very young and the very old, is also associated with seizures, particularly when serum sodium levels exceed 160 mEq/L. Hypernatremia should also be corrected slowly.[20]

Hypercalcemia reduces neuronal excitability and rarely causes seizures; significant hypocalcemia (7.5 mEq/L), however, is associated with ictal activity. Hypocalcemia may result from hypoparathyroidism, renal failure, or acute pancreatitis, and is typically associated with hypomagnesemia, which can also precipitate seizures, particularly at serum levels lower than 1 mEq/L. Hypomagnesemia is most often seen as a result of poor nutrition, especially in alcoholics. Patients with significant hypomagnesemia or hypocalcemia should be treated for both disorders empirically.[20]

Nonketotic hyperosmolar hyperglycemia is also associated with seizure activity. Partial seizures, including partial status, predominate and do not respond to anticonvulsants, but rather to gradual correction of fluid deficits and glucose excess.[15,23]

Seizures may complicate the course and treatment of renal failure.[24] Ictal activity occasionally complicates uremic encephalopathy, is more common in conjunction with acute fluid and electrolyte shifts during dialysis ("dialysis disequilibrium syndrome"), and can occur as a complication of immunosuppressive therapy after a renal transplant.

Thyroid disease may be associated with generalized seizures. Seizures are the presenting sign of hypothyroidism in up to 20% of patients but are a less common feature of thyrotoxicosis.[25,26] Seizures also occur with hypoparathyroidism as a direct result of the secondary hypocalcemia.[26] Seizures occur in up to one third of patients with hepatic encephalopathy; phenytoin is considered a first-line treatment because benzodiazepines induce coma in these patients.[15,27]

High anion gap acidosis is the most likely acid-base disorder to be associated with seizures.[28] Benzodiazepines should be given for these seizures in the ED because specific treatment is initiated for the underlying metabolic derangement. Seizures may also be a feature of cerebral hypoxia that results from suffocation, respiratory failure, circulatory collapse, or carbon monoxide poisoning.

Hypertensive encephalopathy can also cause seizures. The underlying problem must be addressed while seizure control is attempted with benzodiazepines.[29] Acute intermittent porphyria is an uncommon illness often associated with seizures. Treatment includes glucose and hematin.[27]

Seizures Caused by Infectious Diseases Infectious diseases can cause seizures independent of a purely febrile mechanism. These generally result from primary central nervous system (CNS) infections but occasionally arise from other septic sources. The most important ictogenic infections are meningitis, encephalitis, cerebral abscess, cerebral parasitosis, and the protean CNS manifestations of human immunodeficiency virus (HIV) disease and its associated opportunistic infections.

Seizures can occur as a result of the acute inflammatory response, or as sequelae, to bacterial or viral meningitis. Between 15% and 40% of those patients with meningitis will have at least one seizure during the acute course of their illness; this is more common at both the extremes of age.[30] Partial seizures predominate in most cases, although generalized seizures also occur.[31] After meningitic seizures are terminated with benzodiazepines, phenytoin or phenobarbital therapy should be initiated temporarily.[32]

All viral meningoencephalitides are associated with seizures. These seizures are typically partial motor events, and postictal paralysis is common, particularly with herpetic infections.[15,33] Seizures are the presenting sign in one third of cerebral abscess cases. Although ictal activity is usually generalized, any focal manifestations help establish the location of the lesion.[34]

The parasitic CNS infection neurocysticercosis is relatively common in those areas of the United States with immigrants from Latin America. Seizures complicate 50% to 90% of neurocysticercosis cases.[35] Latent syphilis may also be a cause of adult-onset seizures, and primary HIV disease of the CNS and its attendant infectious and mass lesion complications, such as from toxoplasmosis and lymphoma, are a significant cause of generalized and partial seizures.[15]

Seizures Caused by Drugs and Toxins The list of substances reported to cause seizures either as an idiosyncratic side effect of therapeutic use or as a manifestation of toxic overdose is enormous.[36] The recognition of this etiologic category is of great importance in the ED. Seizure activity should be viewed as a dire sign of toxicity and may herald the onset of life-threatening instability.

Seizures may occur after therapeutic doses of antimicrobials, cardiovascular agents, neuroleptics, and sympathomimetics.[37] Seizures may also result from exposure to plant toxins, insecticides and rodenticides, and hydrocarbons.[56] However, the most common drug- and toxin-associated seizures occur in conjunction with illicit drugs such as cocaine, amphetamines, and phencyclidine; with overdoses of anticholinergic agents such as cyclic antidepressants and antihistamines; as a manifestation of withdrawal from ethyl alcohol and sedative-hypnotics; and with toxic levels and deliberate overdoses of diverse medications such as aspirin, theophylline, isoniazid, lithium, and the anticonvulsants phenytoin and carbamazepine.[38] Standard ED therapeutic measures are usually effective in toxic seizures. In some cases, specific antidotal therapy is available, such as alkalinization for cyclic antidepressant and salicylate overdoses, pyridoxine for isoniazid overdose, and hemodialysis for salicylate and lithium toxicity.

Because of its prevalence in urban ED patient populations, cocaine toxicity deserves special mention.[36] Seizures may occur after isolated recreational or chronic abuse, after overdose, and in "body packers" and "body stuffers."[39,40] Cocaine-related seizures may be a manifestation of direct CNS toxicity or the indirect result of hypoxemia from cardiac toxicity. Cocaine seizures are usually generalized but occasionally are partial.[41] Seizures in cocaine-intoxicated patients must be managed as part of the overall toxic reaction that often includes high fever, rhabdomyolysis, and cardiac arrhythmias (see Chapter 148). Benzodiazepines are the appropriate initial drug therapy.

Ethyl alcohol is another common toxic cause of seizures. Of 472 adult hospital admissions for new-onset seizures, 41% were related to alcohol abuse.[42] Ictal events may occur with acute inebriation but are more common during withdrawal from alcohol.[43-45] Withdrawal seizures are typically generalized, recurrent, and may begin within 6 hours of cessation or decrease of alcohol consumption. Via a phenomenon termed *kindling,* the risk and severity of seizures increase with each episode of withdrawal. Kindling implies that with each episode of alcohol withdrawal, the seizure threshold is lower. Alcoholic patients with seizures must be evaluated for other related, concomitant ictogenic problems (e.g., hypoglycemia, electrolyte derangements, head trauma, coingestion of other toxins, and pregnancy). The preferred treatment for alcohol-associated seizures is benzodiazepines; these drugs substitute for the GABA-enhancing effect of ethanol in the CNS (see Chapter 179).

Of special concern in the consideration of drug- and toxin-induced seizures is ictal activity related to childhood immunizations. Some investigators had thought that pertussis immunization might cause infantile spasm. It now appears that the association between pertussis immunization and the onset of infantile spasm is not causative but rather an unmasking in otherwise predisposed children.[46]

Seizures Caused by Trauma Posttraumatic seizures (PTS) can occur as an acute result of blunt or penetrating head trauma and as posttraumatic sequelae. Immediate posttraumatic seizures occur within 24 hours of injury. Epidural, subdural, and intracerebral hematomas and traumatic subarachnoid hemorrhages can all be acutely ictogenic, particularly as the intracranial pressure rises. Immediate PTS are more common in children than in adults.[47] More often, however, the onset of seizure activity is delayed for at least several hours. Early PTS are those that occur within 1 week of injury, whereas late PTS occur after 1 week. Within the first year after significant head trauma, the incidence of seizures is at least 12 times that of the general population.[48]

The severity of head injury correlates with the likelihood of PTS. The incidence of seizures after injury with neurologic deficit without dural violation is 7% to 39%; when the dura is disrupted, the incidence is 20% to 57%.[49] In head-injured children, the factors predictive of PTS include age less than 1 year, depressed skull fracture, and Glasgow Coma Score between 3 and 8 at ED presentation.[50,51] Of survivors of significant head injury, 10% to 15% will develop posttraumatic epilepsy.[52] Imaging studies should be performed urgently because the likelihood of identifying significant cerebral edema, cerebral contusions, hematomas, and depressed skull fractures is relatively high.

Seizures Associated with Malignancy or Vasculitis Seizures are a common manifestation of primary and metastatic CNS neoplasms. They may also complicate cancer treatment because of postsurgical scarring or chemotherapy-related electrolyte derangements, hematologic abnormalities, or immunosuppression. Although any CNS tumor can be ictogenic, low-grade and slow-growing primary neoplasms (e.g., well-differentiated gliomas and oligodendrogliomas) are implicated most commonly.[53] In these cases, seizures that are most often partial with secondary generalization may be the initial manifestation of the mass.[54] A new-onset seizure in a patient with a non-CNS primary malignancy such as melanoma and tumors of the lung, breast, colon, germ, or renal cells should prompt consideration of CNS metastasis and warrants neuroimaging.

Seizure may also be the presenting manifestation of CNS vasculitis seen in patients with systemic lupus erythematosus and polyarteritis nodosa. These are commonly complex partial seizures that give a general indication of the acute inflammatory focus. Sometimes secondary generalization follows.[55,56]

Seizures Caused by Strokes, Arteriovenous Malformations, and Migraines Infarctive or hemorrhagic stroke is the cause of new-onset seizures in 54% of elderly patients.[57] The overall incidence of seizures with stroke ranges from 4% to 15%; more than half occur within the first week after stroke.[58] The incidence of epilepsy after stroke is 4% to 9%.[58] Seizures that occur acutely with stroke are thought to result from local metabolic alterations in the CNS; these events are transient and the seizures are often focal and self-limited. Seizures that develop later are more likely to be generalized.[58]

Focal seizures also occur in conjunction with unruptured cerebrovascular aneurysms and arteriovenous malformations (AVMs).[15] Arteriography may be required to confirm the diagnosis; unruptured AVMs are easier to detect on an enhanced cranial computed tomography (CT) scan than are the smaller unruptured aneurysms.

Seizures may also coexist with vascular headaches, either coincidentally, via migrainous activation of an epileptic focus, or after vascular headache has induced cerebral infarction that becomes an epileptic focus.[59]

Seizures Caused by Degenerative Disease of the Central Nervous System Approximately 5% of patients with multiple sclerosis develop focal or generalized seizures during their illness. These must be differentiated from tonic spasms that occur in multiple sclerosis. Patients with demyelinating disease should also be evaluated for the other types of reactive seizures.[15]

CNS degeneration associated with aging increases the risk of reactive seizures and epilepsy.[60] Alzheimer's dementia appears to be a significant risk factor for developing new-onset seizures.[61] The elderly are also more likely to have other ictogenic problems (e.g., stroke, brain neoplasm, toxic and metabolic disturbances, and blunt head trauma from falls). Maintenance treatment of elderly patients with epilepsy is often complicated by drug-drug interactions, and breakthrough seizures may result even when patients are compliant.[60] ED management of such patients must include a thorough evaluation for causes of reactive seizures, even though the incidence of primary seizures increases after age 60 years.[1]

Degenerative CNS disease may also cause seizures in younger patients. The neurocutaneous disorders (phakomatoses) include a group of diseases in which neurologic signs and symptoms are associated with characteristic skin lesions. Neurofibromatosis (von Recklinghausen's disease) is characterized by five or more café-au-lait lesions of 0.5 cm diameter or greater, axillary freckling, and subcutaneous nodules. Neurologic symptoms are the result of neurofibromas growing on peripheral and cranial nerves. Seizures and mental retardation are common findings. Optic gliomas and CNS tumors also occur in children with the dominantly inherited syndrome.[62]

Amelanotic nevi or "ash-leaf" spots, shagreen patches, and adenoma sebaceum are the characteristic lesions of tuberous sclerosis. The neurologic symptoms are more severe in children with tuberous sclerosis than in those with neurofibromatosis. A mixed seizure disorder, including infantile spasms and severe mental retardation, is usual. Characteristically, calcified intracranial tumors of varying size line the ventricles and are called *brain stones.*

Sturge-Weber syndrome is a phakomatosis characterized by facial port-wine nevus, hemiplegia, and seizures. The nevus is found in the trigeminal nerve distribution. Progressive hemiplegia and seizures are the result of angiomatous malformations that most typically involve the occipital and parietal cerebral cortex. These lesions may become calcified in a classic "tram track" appearance on a skull film.

Gestational Seizures Seizures associated with pregnancy are divided into two categories: *gestational epilepsy,* in which hormonal and metabolic changes exacerbate underlying epilepsy or adversely influence serum levels of anticonvulsants; and *eclampsia* or *toxemia,* which is a gestational hypertensive encephalopathy manifested by seizures, hypertension, coma, proteinuria, and edema. For the former, antiepileptic therapy should be tailored by the patient's neurologist and obstetrician to maximize seizure control and minimize the risk of teratogenic effects.[63] Convulsive generalized status epilepticus in pregnancy jeopardizes both mother and fetus. Emergency physicians should develop a standing protocol for managing pregnancy-related seizures in conjunction with their consulting obstetricians because of the controversy in this area (see Chapter 172).[63-65]

Psychogenic Seizures

Psychogenic seizures, or pseudoseizures, are functional events that may be associated with alterations in consciousness, abnormal movements and behaviors, and autonomic changes. They are not the result of abnormal CNS electrical activity. Pseudoseizures may be primarily motor and mimic convulsive generalized seizures that are usually readily recognizable; or they may be primarily behavioral and analogous to complex partial seizures, in which case even experienced observers have difficulty differentiating them from true ictus.

Although simultaneous video and EEG recordings may be required to confirm the diagnosis, several typical characteristics of pseudoseizures may aid in differentiating them (Box 96-2).[66,67] In general, patients with pseudoseizures tend to be of lower intelligence or have an underlying anxiety or hysterical personality disorder.[66] Children may also have pseudoseizures. The ED evaluation of these patients is difficult because seizures and pseudoseizures can coexist. All but obviously functional abnormalities should be treated as true ictus pending formal neurologic evaluation. Many patients with pseudoseizures are not deliberately attempting to mislead the examining physician. The longer-term treatment of patients with confirmed pseudoseizures may include direct confrontation, intensive psychotherapy, and a placebo.

Box 96-2 Typical Characteristics of Pseudoseizures[66,67]

- Multiple patterns of seizures with varying initial focal manifestations and precipitants
- Recall of the ictal event
- Asynchronous, thrashing movement of the extremities
- Conversant during the episode
- Abnormal activity stops on command
- Normal pupillary light reaction
- No postictal period (although "postictal" states have been documented after pseudoseizures)
- No response to anticonvulsants
- Prolonged seizure activity
- Absence of the acidemia and elevated serum prolactin levels that accompany true ictus

POSTICTAL STATES

The postictal state that follows most generalized seizures is typically characterized by a decreased level of arousal and responsiveness, disorientation, amnesia, and headache. These conditions may persist for only a few minutes or for many hours and may not be consistent from seizure to seizure. The most important consideration for the emergency physician managing the postictal state is to monitor and investigate the altered mental status after a seizure[68]; otherwise, dangerous underlying metabolic or toxic abnormalities may be overlooked. At the minimum, airway positioning maneuvers, pulse oximetry, rapid glucose determination, and cardiac rhythm monitoring are necessary.

There are two unusual postictal manifestations: postictal paralysis and neurogenic pulmonary edema. Postictal paralysis (or Todd's paralysis) may follow generalized or complex partial seizures and is a focal motor deficit that may persist for as long as 24 hours. Weakness of one extremity or a complete hemiparesis may occur; in the latter case, the patient must be safely restrained to avoid falls caused by a combination of weakness and diminished responsiveness resulting from the postictal state. Todd's paralysis indicates a high likelihood of an underlying structural cause for the seizure.

Neurogenic pulmonary edema (NPE) is a relatively common, although often subclinical, complication of any structural CNS insult, including a seizure, trauma, or hemorrhage. NPE is probably caused by centrally mediated sympathetic discharge and generalized vasoconstriction, coupled with increased pulmonary capillary membrane permeability. After a seizure, NPE can be clinically and radiographically confused with aspiration pneumonia. NPE is managed with ventilatory support, including positive end expiratory pressure and other aggressive measures to reduce intracranial pressure. Hypoxia or other clinical evidence of pulmonary congestion after a seizure should prompt consideration of NPE.[69]

DIAGNOSTIC STRATEGIES

First-Time Seizures

The essential components of the ED seizure evaluation are discussed in Chapter 16. An accurate and thorough history of the ictal event, any known or potential precipitants or exposures, and the patient's medical problems must be obtained. A thorough physical examination, including a complete neurologic examination, is essential. Any identified focal neurologic deficits must be followed for progression or resolution. Appropriate ancillary studies may be comprehensive, but if precipitants (e.g., hypoglycemia or intoxication) are known, may be comparatively limited. There is more debate regarding the role of neuroimaging for seizures in the ED.

Clearly, a cranial CT scan is indicated in any age group when there is suspicion of head trauma, elevated intracranial pressure, intracranial mass, persistently abnormal mental status or focal neurologic abnormality, or HIV disease. An expert panel[70] has made the following recommendations: for patients with first-time seizure, a CT scan should be performed immediately when the provider suspects a serious structural lesion. This suspicion may be based on the presence of a new focal deficit, persistent altered mental status, fever, recent trauma, persistent headache, history of cancer, anticoagulant use, suspicion or known history of AIDS, age greater than 40, and partial onset seizure. Scans may reasonably be obtained on an outpatient, follow-up basis for patients who have completely recovered from the ictal event and for whom no apparent cause has been elucidated; if follow up is unlikely or even questionable, the CT scan should be obtained in the ED to ensure its completion. In patients with known epilepsy and recurrent seizures, the same considerations as above apply, but, in addition, epilepsy patients with a change in seizure pattern, prolonged postictal state, or persistent abnormal mental status should be scanned in the ED.

Initiating anticonvulsant therapy after a single seizure is an issue of considerable controversy. The prompt treatment of any underlying ictal cause discovered in the ED, however, is always appropriate. Disposition plans must be individualized. In one study, Henneman et al note that 46% of adults with new-onset seizures require admission, most for abnormal CT scans or persistent focal abnormalities; 95% of those who retrospectively required admission were correctly identified by using an ED evaluation consistent with that recommended above.[71]

Recurrent Seizures

The initial stabilization of the patient with a known seizure disorder does not differ from that for the new-onset patient; this includes a rapid blood glucose determination. Because the most common cause of seizures in the known seizure patient is noncompliance with medications, the levels of prescribed anticonvulsants should be measured.[7] Supratherapeutic and toxic levels of some anticonvulsants such as phenytoin and carbamazepine, whether attained chronically or after acute overdose, can *cause* seizures. The emergency physician must be cautious about giving a full loading dose of anticonvulsants to patients on chronic therapy before checking a serum level.

Meanwhile, a thorough history and physical examination should focus on intercurrent illness or trauma, drug or alcohol use, potential adverse drug-drug interactions with anticonvulsants, a recent change in anticonvulsant dosing regimens, or a change in ictal pattern or characteristics. Clinical indications should tailor the selection of other laboratory or radiographic tests.[68]

DIFFERENTIAL CONSIDERATIONS

Even when witnessed in the ED, other abnormal movements and states of consciousness can be confused with ictal activity. The disorders in the differential diagnosis include syncope, hyperventilation and breath-holding, certain toxic and metabolic states, transient ischemic attacks, narcolepsy, some movement disorders, and other psychogenic maladies.[7,8,72] Syncope—whether vasodepressive (e.g., "vagal" or micturition syncope), orthostatic, or arrhythmogenic (e.g., paroxysmal ventricular tachycardia or fibrillation, long QT syndrome)—may be confused with ictal events; differentiating among these may be particularly difficult when episodes are recurrent.[13,73]

A sudden loss of consciousness followed by abnormal movements can be ictal or syncopal in origin, hence the consideration "fit versus faint." One series reports that of 946 such patients with episodic attacks of unconsciousness, epilepsy was diagnosed in 40%, and syncope was confirmed in 44%.[74] Generally, ictal tonic-clonic movements are much more forceful and are more prolonged than the "twitches" sometimes associated with fainting. In addition, most seizures are characterized by a postictal state—with the important exception of atonic drop attack ictus—that syncope patients do not manifest.

The cause of an unwitnessed, unprovoked loss of consciousness with a fall, after which the patient presents to the ED, may be difficult to classify. Suggestions of an ictal diagnosis include retrograde amnesia, loss of continence, and evidence of tongue-biting.

Hyperventilation syndrome can be associated with mood disturbances, paresthesias, and posturing movements of the distal extremities.[75] Prolonged breath-holding spells in children can be accompanied by tonic-clonic movements and urinary incontinence.[72] Toxic and metabolic disorders that may mimic ictus include delirium tremens and alcoholic blackouts, the alteration in consciousness associated with hypoglycemia and acute intermittent porphyria, the buccolingual spasms of phencyclidine intoxication; and tonic spasms caused by tetanus, strychnine, and camphor.[7,72] Extrapyramidal reactions may also resemble seizure activity, particularly in children.

Nonictal CNS events, such as transient ischemic attacks, transient global amnesia, and atypical migraines, may present similarly to absence seizures and postictal states such as Todd's paralysis.[72] Carotid sinus hypersensitivity, which can even result from a too-tight necktie, may cause drop attacks.[74] Narcolepsy (recurrent irresistible daytime sleepiness), especially when it occurs with cataplexy (sudden falls), may be associated with hallucinations and abnormal movements. It can be differentiated from seizure activity by the history and response to stimulation. Movement disorders such as hemiballismus and tics are usually associated with other neurologic problems. Finally, dissociative states such as fugue and panic attacks can be confused with seizures. An EEG is an appropriate diagnostic option in unclear cases.

MANAGEMENT

Immediate Management

ED management of the seizing patient begins with active, anticipatory airway management. In generalized ictus, the gag reflex is suppressed and vomiting is often complicated by aspiration of gastric contents. The patient should be placed in a left lateral decubitus position and his or her dentures removed. A bite block should be placed to protect the tongue and allow access for suctioning.

If the patient is persistently apneic or if there is an unavoidable airway threat, the patient should be endotracheally intubated for definitive protection. A benzodiazepine should be used as an induction agent in the hope that its action might terminate the seizure or even obviate the need for tracheal intubation. Trismus may necessitate neuromuscular blockade in selected patients.

Simultaneous to securing the airway and ensuring adequate oxygenation is establishing intravenous (IV) access. In general, the first-line pharmacologic treatment of any active seizure activity is a parenteral benzodiazepine. The IV route is preferred, but diazepam may also be given rectally, endotracheally, or intraosseously.[76-78] Because benzodiazepines directly enhance GABA-mediated neuronal inhibition, they affect both clinical and electrical manifestations of seizures. Benzodiazepines are effective in terminating ictal activity in 75% to 90% of patients.[79]

Benzodiazepines available to the emergency physician include diazepam (Valium), lorazepam (Ativan), and midazolam (Versed). In comparison studies, no one drug is clearly superior.[79] All three may be used in patients regardless of age, and all share the following characteristics: relatively short duration of anticonvulsant action, sedation, and the potential for hypotension and respiratory depression.[80] Pertinent differences among benzodiazepines are the efficacy of diazepam when administered rectally, endotracheally, or intraosseously; a relatively longer duration of seizure suppression with lorazepam; and efficacy of the rectal and intramuscular routes of administration for midazolam. Lorazepam is generally recommended for alcohol withdrawal seizures.[44] The ED dosing of benzodiazepines for seizures is summarized in Table 96-1.

Second-line abortive ED anticonvulsant therapy consists of phenytoin (Dilantin) and phenobarbital. Phenytoin suppresses neuronal recruitment but does not suppress electrical activity at the ictogenic focus.[14] Phenytoin neither sedates patients nor causes respiratory depression, but rapid IV administration of phenytoin in its propylene glycol diluent may cause hypotension and cardiac dysrhythmias. Phenytoin's onset of action is 10 to 30 minutes and IV administration typically requires at least 20 minutes.[80] The duration of action is approximately 24 hours. Continued benzodiazepine dosing is appropriate while phenytoin achieves adequate brain levels.

If levels of phenytoin or phenobarbital are subtherapeutic in a patient already being treated for seizures, ED loading doses can be given intravenously or, alternatively, an adjusted oral dosing schedule can be prescribed to boost the serum level over 24 to 48 hours. This is the only feasible method for anticonvulsants such as carbamazepine and valproate, which cannot be given in large loading doses.

The phenytoin prodrug fosphenytoin is water soluble and can be administered quickly without significant toxicity.[81] Fosphenytoin achieves a free phenytoin level of 2 μg/ml in

Table 96-1. Drugs Used in the Abortive Treatment of Seizures and Status Epilepticus in the ED

Drug	Adult dose	Pediatric dose	Comments
Diazepam	0.2 mg/kg IV at 2 mg/min up to 20 mg	0.2-0.5 mg/kg IV/IO/ET up to 20 mg 0.5-1.0 mg/kg PR up to 20 mg	
Lorazepam	0.1 mg/kg IV at 1-2 mg/min up to 10 mg	0.05-0.1 mg/kg IV	
Midazolam	2.5-15 mg IV 0.2 mg/kg IM	0.15 mg/kg IV then 2-10 μg/kg/min	For pediatric dose, see references 138-140
Phenytoin	20 mg/kg IV at ≤50 mg/min	20 mg/kg IV at 1 mg/kg/min	Use continuous cardiac and blood pressure monitoring during infusion
Fosphenytoin	15-20 PE/kg at 100-150 mg PE/min; may be given IM	—	Safety in pediatric patients has not been established
Phenobarbital	20 mg/kg IV at 60-100 mg/min		May be given as IM loading dose
Valproate	20 mg/kg PR		Dilute 1:1 with water; slow onset
Pentobarbital	5 mg/kg IV at 25 mg/min, then titrate to EEG		Intubation, ventilation, and pressor support are required
Isoflurane	Via general endotracheal anesthesia		Monitor with EEG

ET, Endotracheal; *IM*, intramuscular; *IO*, intraosseous; *PE*, phenytoin sodium equivalents; *PR*, per rectum.

15 minutes, as opposed to 25 minutes with phenytoin itself.[82] Cost analyses of phenytoin versus fosphenytoin use have shown conflicting results. Clinically, fosphenytoin has several advantages: it is better tolerated, more safe, and more stable than phenytoin and it can be given more rapidly IV and it can be given intramuscularly. Using fosphenytoin, however, carries the potential for therapeutic drug monitoring errors and a delayed hypotensive response.[83] Fosphenytoin's use should be considered when convulsive status is refractory to benzodiazepines.

Anticonvulsant experience with phenobarbital is derived primarily from studies of pediatric populations. Phenobarbital is a CNS depressant that decreases both ictal and physiologic cortical electrical activity. Sedation and depression of respiratory drive and blood pressure must be anticipated, and some physicians prefer the nonsedating phenytoin for this reason.[84] The onset of action of phenobarbital is 15 to 30 minutes, and the duration of action is 48 hours.[85] Appropriate ED dosing regimens for phenytoin and phenobarbital are listed in Table 96-1.

Although such agents are being given to abort ongoing seizure activity, the emergency physician must search for other underlying reversible causes. This might prompt administration of dextrose for hypoglycemia, pyridoxine for isoniazid overdose, or magnesium for eclampsia.

As previously discussed, abortive treatment for eclamptic seizures is a subject of much debate. Magnesium is *not* an anticonvulsant, and its efficacy in some eclamptic seizures is largely unexplained; its clinical effect may be a manifestation of local neuromuscular blockade that masks continuing ictal activity.[8,65] Benzodiazepines are often effective in the short term, and phenytoin may also be efficacious in eclampsia. Emergency physicians, in consultation with their obstetric colleagues, should develop a protocol by which eclamptic seizures are managed. The typical dose of magnesium sulfate is 4 to 6 g via IV bolus followed by a 1- to 2-g/hr infusion along with hydralazine. Because hypermagnesemia may cause respiratory arrest, it is essential to monitor patients for the hyporeflexia that precedes respiratory compromise.

Nonpregnant patients who continue to seize in the ED despite management with benzodiazepines, phenytoin, or phenobarbital are likely to meet the clinical criteria for status epilepticus. Additional therapeutic measures include using valproate, barbiturate coma, and general inhalational anesthesia. Valproate, which increases GABA concentration, is not available parenterally but may be given rectally in status (see Table 96-1).[80,84] It is slowly absorbed but may be of use in polydrug-resistant seizures or before prolonged transport when trying to avoid barbiturate coma or general anesthesia.

Barbiturate coma is very effective in terminating seizures by facilitating GABA, although it also suppresses all brainstem function. Previous neurologic consultation is advisable because barbiturate coma may induce respiratory arrest, myocardial depression, and hypotension, while decreasing intracranial pressure and increasing cerebral perfusion.[80]

The preferred agent for barbiturate coma is pentobarbital. Patients require intubation and ventilatory support, continuous cardiac monitoring, and invasive hemodynamic monitoring. Pressors may be required to support the blood pressure. A dosing regimen is provided in Table 96-1.

Isoflurane anesthesia is one final alternative in the management of refractory ictus. Halothane is associated with more hemodynamic and hepatotoxic complications. Isoflurane suppresses electrical seizure foci and is easily titratable. Patients treated with barbiturate coma or inhalational anesthesia will require intubation and mechanical ventilation. Intubation of the seizing patient is best facilitated by using a benzodiazepine as an induction agent and lidocaine (1 mg/kg) as a pretreatment medication. Lidocaine reduces the increase in intracranial pressure that reflexively results from laryngoscopy and intubation.

The visual manifestations of convulsive ictus are extinguished by neuromuscular blockade. When a seizing patient is paralyzed and intubated, the ED cannot assume that pharmacologic therapy has terminated the seizure. Anticonvulsants should be administered and electroencephalographic monitoring of the patient should be arranged.

Long-Term Management

Identifying a new-onset seizure disorder in the ED should prompt consideration for further management in each of three areas: pharmacologic, psychosocial, and legal. The primary dilemma concerns whether to initiate prophylactic anticonvulsant therapy after one seizure. The decision to treat should be based on (1) the risk of seizure recurrence; (2) any underlying, predisposing disease; and (3) the risk of anticonvulsant therapy.

The risk of seizure recurrence is difficult to estimate in the ED. The presence of EEG abnormalities is suggestive of greater risk, but this information is usually unavailable in the ED. Other factors associated with an increased risk of recurrence are partial (versus generalized) ictus, status epilepticus, a history of intracranial surgery or trauma, or the presence of a persistent neurologic abnormality such as Todd's paralysis.[8,86] In adults, the overall risk of seizure recurrence after a single, unprovoked seizure in a prospective study of patients without correctable predisposing factors is 14% at 1 year, 29% at 3 years, and 34% at 5 years.[87] For children, comparable incidences are 26% at 1 year, 40% at 2 years, and 42% at 4 years.[88] By way of comparison, up to 23% of patients can have adverse effects from anticonvulsants significant enough to cause a change in therapy.[89]

The presence of specific underlying conditions may affect the decision to institute long-term therapy. Many authorities recommend treatment after an initial seizure in HIV-positive patients. Alcohol-related seizures are notoriously unresponsive to anticonvulsants. Prophylaxis against PTS beyond the first week after injury is probably unnecessary,[90] but the occurrence of early PTS should prompt at least short-term initiation of therapy.[51]

The side effects of anticonvulsants can be debilitating for the patient. This must be considered before initiating therapy, particularly in women of reproductive age, because anticonvulsants are teratogenic and may precipitate failure of oral contraceptives.[86,91] Some other adverse effects and potential drug-drug interactions of anticonvulsants are listed in Table 96-2.

In the absence of specific underlying conditions that increase risk of recurrence, most authorities do not recommend initiation of anticonvulsant therapy after a single unprovoked seizure in adults or children from the ED.[7,86,92] If the seizure was provoked, the decision should be based on whether the provoking factor can be corrected; if it cannot, anticonvulsant therapy should be instituted.[86] Anticonvulsant

Table 96-2. Important Adverse Effects and Drug-Drug Interactions of Anticonvulsants

Drug	Important adverse effects	Significant drug-drug interactions
Carbamazepine	Dizziness, drowsiness, aplastic anemia, agranulocytosis, rash, hepatotoxicity, teratogenicity	Warfarin, digitalis, calcium channel blockers, tetracycline, erythromycin, oral contraceptives, theophylline
Phenytoin	Gingival hyperplasia, elevated transaminases, nystagmus, rash, myopathy, drug-induced lupus, teratogenicity, "dilantin hypersensitivity syndrome"	Corticosteroids, quinidine, theophylline, cimetidine, digoxin, ciprofloxacin, oral contraceptives, isoniazid, warfarin, disulfiram, cotrimoxazole
Fosphenytoin	Nystagmus, dizziness, pruritus, paresthesia	
Phenobarbital	Drowsiness, hepatitis, teratogenicity, decreased IQ with chronic use in children	Corticosteroids, warfarin, tetracycline, propranolol, quinidine, theophylline, oral contraceptives
Ethosuximide	Drowsiness, ataxia, dizziness, nausea	Isoniazid
Clonazepam	Drowsiness, ataxia	Other CNS depressants
Valproate	Thrombocytopenia, tremor, nausea, hepatotoxicity	Aspirin, erythromycin, isoniazid
Felbamate	Gastrointestinal irritability, headache, dizziness, ataxia	Phenytoin, valproate
Gabapentin	Somnolence, fatigue, ataxia, dizziness, gastrointestinal upset, dyspnea	None significant
Lamotrigine	Rash, dizziness, ataxia, blurred vision, nausea	Carbamazepine, phenobarbital, phenytoin and fosphenytoin, primidone, valproic acid
Felbamate	Anorexia, vomiting, insomnia, somnolence, aplastic anemia, hepatotoxicity	Carbamazepine, phenobarbital, phenytoin and fosphenytoin, primidone, valproic acid
Topiramate	Dizziness, somnolence, ataxia, confusion, fatigue, paresthesias, speech difficulties, diplopia, impaired concentration, nausea	Other anticonvulsants, carbonic anhydrase inhibitors

Table 96-3. Drugs Used for Chronic Anticonvulsant Therapy in Adults

Drug	Indications	Dose mg/kg/day	Therapeutic range μg/mL	Daily doses
Carbamazepine	Partial, GCS	15-25	8-12	3-4
Phenytoin	Partial, GCS	3-8	10-25	1-3
Phenobarbital	Partial, GCS	2-4	15-40	1
Primidone*	Partial, GCS	10-20	5-15	4
Ethosuximide	Absence	10-30	40-100	2
Clonazepam	Absence	0.03-0.3	0.01-0.05	2
Valproate	All	15-60	50-100	4
Felbamate	Partial, GCS, atonic	3600 mg/day	N/A	3

GCS, Generalized convulsive seizure.
*Primidone is a congener of phenobarbital.

dosing regimens in known epileptic patients should only be modified in consultation with the patient's physician.

Drug monotherapy is always preferable in anticonvulsant regimens. As summarized in Table 96-3, the preferred drugs for convulsive generalized seizures are phenytoin, carbamazepine, valproate, phenobarbital, and felbamate. The preferred drugs for nonconvulsive generalized seizures are ethosuximide and valproate. Drugs recommended for the treatment of partial seizures are carbamazepine, phenytoin, phenobarbital, valproate, and felbamate. Dosing should be initiated in the ED, although there is no clear consensus regarding whether a full loading dose of phenytoin or phenobarbital should be given.

The psychological and social implications of the new diagnosis of a seizure disorder should not be underestimated. Fear of seizures and stigmatization are common; employability and insurability may be adversely affected. Although the emergency physician is not usually in a suitable position to arrange for counseling, a referral to local epilepsy support groups may be helpful.

Finally, there are legal implications of diagnosing a new-onset seizure disorder. Each state has regulations regarding driving privileges in patients with seizures, and some states require reporting by the physician. The emergency physician should obey these regulations and inform patients accordingly. Patients should also be advised to refrain from hazardous or isolated activities until cleared to do so by their physician. The need for a MedicAlert bracelet or other medical condition identifier should be stressed.

KEY CONCEPTS

- The possibility of reactive seizures should be considered in all seizure patients who present to the ED, including patients with a history of epilepsy.

- The most common cause of recurrent primary seizures is medication noncompliance; the most common cause of reactive seizures is hypoglycemia.
- Nonconvulsive seizures may be confused with nonictal states, including psychiatric disorders.
- Neuroimaging is recommended for seizure patients when there is suspicion of head trauma, elevated intracranial pressure, intracranial mass, persistently abnormal mental status or focal neurologic abnormality, or HIV disease.
- Primary abortive therapy for seizures in the ED is a benzodiazepine; second-line therapy includes phenytoin or phenobarbital.

REFERENCES

1. Hauser WA, Hesdorffer DC: *Epilepsy: frequency, causes and consequences,* New York, 1990, Demos.
2. Dreifuss FE, Ogunyemi AO: Classification of epileptic seizures and the epilepsies: an overview, *Epilepsy Res* 6(suppl):3, 1992.
3. Gram L: Epileptic seizures and syndromes, *Lancet* 336:161, 1990.
4. Commission on Classification and Terminology of the International League Against Epilepsy: Proposal for revised clinical and electroencephalographic classification of epileptic seizures, *Epilepsia* 30:389, 1989.
5. Commission on Classification and Terminology of the International League Against Epilepsy: Proposal for revised clinical and electroencephalographic classification of epileptic seizures, *Epilepsia* 22:489, 1981.
6. Dreifuss FE: Classification of epileptic syndromes and the epilepsies, *Pediatr Clin North Am* 36:265, 1989.
7. Engel J, Starkman S: Overview of seizures, *Emerg Med Clin North Am* 12:895, 1994.
8. Engel J: *Seizures and epilepsy,* Philadelphia, 1989, FA Davis.
9. Laidlaw J, Richens A, editors: *A textbook of epilepsy,* ed 3, London, 1988, Churchill Livingstone.
10. Orringer CE et al: Natural history of lactic acidosis after grand mal seizures, *N Engl J Med* 297:796, 1977.
11. Meldrum BS, Horton RW: Physiology of status epilepticus in primates, *Arch Neurol* 28:1, 1973.
12. Aicardi J, Chevrie JJ: Convulsive status epilepticus in infants and children: a study of 239 cases, *Epilepsia* 11:187, 1970.
13. Aminoff MJ, Simon RP: Status epilepticus: causes, clinical features, and consequences in 98 patients, *Am J Med* 69:657, 1980.
14. Bancaud J: Kojewnikow's syndrome (epilepsia partialis continua) in children. In Roger J et al, editors: *Epileptic syndromes in infancy, childhood, and adolescence,* London, 1985, John Libbey.
15. Weiner WJ, editor: *Emergent and urgent neurology,* Philadelphia, 1992, JB Lippincott.
16. Pollack ES, Pollack CV: Ketotic hypoglycemia: a case report, *J Emerg Med* 11:531, 1993.
17. Haymond MW, Pagliara AS: Ketotic hypoglycemia, *Clin Endocrinol Metab* 12:447, 1983.
18. Wets B et al: Cataracts and ketotic hypoglycemia, *Ophthalmology* 89:999, 1982.
19. Pollack CV: Medical etiologies of altered mental status, *Top Emerg Med* 13:54, 1991.
20. Riggs JE: Neurologic manifestations of fluid and electrolyte disturbances, *Neurol Clin* 7:509, 1989.
21. Arieff AI: Central nervous system manifestations of disordered sodium metabolism, *Clin Endocrinol Metab* 13:269, 1984.
22. Keating JP, Schears GJ, Dodge PR: Oral water intoxication in infants: an American epidemic, *Am J Dis Child* 145:985, 1991.
23. Khardoi R, Soler NG: Hyperosmolar hyperglycemic nonketotic syndrome, *Am J Med* 77:899, 1984.
24. Lockwood AH: Neurologic complications of renal disease, *Neurol Clin* 7:617, 1989.
25. Tonner DR, Schlechte JA: Neurologic complications of thyroid and parathyroid disease, *Med Clin North Am* 77:251, 1993.
26. Kaminski HJ, Ruff RL: Neurologic complications of endocrine diseases, *Neurol Clin* 7:489, 1989.
27. Rothstein JD, Herlong HF: Neurologic manifestations of hepatic disease, *Neurol Clin* 7:563, 1989.
28. Riley LJ, Ilson BE, Narins RG: Acute metabolic acid-base disorders, *Crit Care Clin* 5:699, 1987.
29. Calhoun DA, Oparil S: Treatment of hypertensive crisis, *N Engl J Med* 323:1177, 1990.
30. Handrick W, Wässer S: Seizures during bacterial meningitis, *Antibiot Chemother* 45:239, 1992.
31. Rosman NP et al: Seizures in bacterial meningitis, *Pediatr Neurol* 1:278, 1985.
32. Shelton MM, Marks WA: Bacterial meningitis: an update, *Neurol Clin* 8:605, 1990.
33. Bale JF: Viral encephalitis, *Med Clin North Am* 77:25, 1993.
34. Chun CH et al: Brain abscess: a study of 45 consecutive cases, *Medicine* 65:415, 1986.
35. Loo L, Braude A: Cerebral cysticercosis in San Diego: a report of 23 cases and a review of the literature, *Medicine* 61:341, 1982.
36. Kunisaki TA, Augenstein WL: Drug- and toxin-induced seizures, *Emerg Med Clin North Am* 12:1027, 1994.
37. Zaccara G, Muscas GC, Messori A: Clinical features, pathogenesis and management of drug-induced seizures, *Drug Safety* 5:109, 1990.
38. Olson KR et al: Seizures associated with poisoning and drug overdose, *Am J Emerg Med* 12:392, 1994.
39. Spivey WH, Euerle B: Neurologic complications of cocaine abuse, *Ann Emerg Med* 19:1422, 1990.
40. Pollack CV et al: Case conference: two crack cocaine body stuffers, *Ann Emerg Med* 21:1370, 1992.
41. Ogunyemi AO et al: Complex partial status epilepticus provoked by "crack" cocaine, *Ann Neurol* 26:785, 1989.
42. Earnest M, Yarnell P: Seizure admissions to a city hospital: the role of alcohol, *Epilepsia* 17:387, 1976.
43. Freedland ES, McMicken DB: Alcohol-related seizures, part I: pathophysiology, differential diagnosis, and evaluation, *J Emerg Med* 11:463, 1993.
44. Freedland ES, McMicken DB: Alcohol-related seizures, part II: clinical presentation and management, *J Emerg Med* 11:605, 1993.
45. McMicken DB, Freedland ES: Alcohol-related seizures, *Emerg Med Clin North Am* 12:1057, 1994.
46. Wentz KR, Marcuse EK: Diphtheria-tetanus-pertussis vaccine and serious neurologic illness: an updated review of the epidemiological evidence, *Pediatrics* 87:287, 1991.
47. Yablon SA: Posttraumatic seizures, *Arch Phys Med Rehabil* 74:983, 1993.
48. Hauser WA: Prevention of post-traumatic epilepsy, *N Engl J Med* 323:540, 1990.
49. Caveness WF: Epilepsy, a product of trauma in our time, *Epilepsia* 17:207, 1976.
50. Lewis RJ, Yee L, Inkelis SH: Clinical predictors of post-traumatic seizures in children with head trauma, *Ann Emerg Med* 22:1114, 1993.
51. Willmore LJ: Post-traumatic seizures, *Neurol Clin* 11:823, 1993.
52. Dugan EM, Howell JM: Posttraumatic seizures, *Emerg Med Clin North Am* 12:1081, 1994.
53. Cascino GD: Epilepsy and brain tumors: implication for treatment, *Epilepsia* 31(suppl 3):S37, 1990.
54. Stein DA, Chamberlain MC: Evaluation and management of seizures in the patient with cancer, *Oncology* 5:33, 1991.
55. Kissel JT: Neurologic manifestations of vasculitis, *Neurol Clin* 7:655, 1989.
56. Adelman DC, Saltiel E, Klinenberg JR: The neuropsychiatric manifestations of systemic lupus erythematosus, *Semin Arthritis Rheum* 15:185, 1986.
57. Ettinger AB, Shinnar S: New-onset seizures in an elderly hospitalized population, *Neurology* 43:489, 1993.
58. Asconapé JJ, Penry JK: Poststroke seizures in the elderly, *Clin Geriatr Med* 7:483, 1991.
59. Bazil CW: Migraine and epilepsy, *Neurol Clin* 12:115, 1994.
60. Scheuer ML, Cohen J: Seizures and epilepsy in the elderly, *Neurol Clin* 11:787, 1993.
61. Romanelli MF et al: Advanced Alzheimer's disease is a risk factor for late-onset seizures, *Arch Neurol* 47:847, 1990.
62. Ricardi VM: Von Recklinghausen's neurofibromatosis, *N Engl J Med* 305:617, 1981.

63. Shuster EA: Seizures in pregnancy, *Emerg Med Clin North Am* 12:1013, 1994.
64. Jagoda A, Riggio S: Emergency department approach to managing seizures in pregnancy, *Ann Emerg Med* 20:80, 1991.
65. Kaplan PW et al: A continuing controversy: magnesium sulfate in the treatment of eclamptic seizures, *Arch Neurol* 47:1031, 1990.
66. Boon PA, Williamson PD: The diagnosis of pseudoseizure, *Clin Neurol Neurosurg* 95:1, 1993.
67. Riggio S: Psychogenic seizures, *Emerg Med Clin North Am* 12:1001, 1994.
68. American College of Emergency Physicians: Clinical policy for the initial approach to patients with a chief complaint of seizure, who are not in status epilepticus, *Ann Emerg Med* 22:875, 1993.
69. Pender ES, Pollack CV: Neurogenic pulmonary edema: case reports and review, *J Emerg Med* 10:45, 1992.
70. Greenberg MK, Barsan WG, Starkman S: Neuroimaging in the emergency department patient presenting with seizure, *Neurology* 47:26, 1996.
71. Henneman PL, DeRoos F, Lewis RJ: Determining the need for admission in patients with new-onset seizures, *Ann Emerg Med* 24:1108, 1994.
72. Morrell MJ: Differential diagnosis of seizures, *Neurol Clin* 11:737, 1993.
73. Moss AJ et al: The long Q-T syndrome: prospective longitudinal study of 328 females, *Circulation* 84:1136, 1991.
74. Huang SKS et al: Carotid sinus hypersensitivity in patients with unexplained syncope: clinical, electrophysiologic, and long-term follow-up observations, *Am Heart J* 116:989, 1988.
75. Perkins GD, Joseph R: Neurologic manifestations of the hyperventilation syndrome, *J Soc Med* 79:48, 1986.
76. Seigler RS: The administration of rectal diazepam for the acute management of seizures, *J Emerg Med* 8:155, 1990.
77. Rusli M et al: Endotracheal diazepam: absorption and pulmonary pathologic effects, *Ann Emerg Med* 16:314, 1987.
78. Lathers CM, Jim KF, Spivey WH: A comparison of intraosseous and intravenous routes of administration for antiseizure agents, *Epilepsia* 30:472, 1989.
79. Leppik IE et al: Double-blind study of lorazepam and diazepam in status epilepticus, *JAMA* 249:1452, 1983.
80. Shepherd SM: Management of status epilepticus, *Emerg Med Clin North Am* 12:941, 1994.
81. Runge J et al: Intravenous phenytoin loading for emergent seizure control, *Ann Emerg Med* 25:139, 1995.
82. Bleck TP: Management approaches to prolonged seizures and status epilepticus, *Epilepsia* 40:S59, 1999.
83. Luer MS: Fosphenytoin, *Neurol Res* 20:178, 1998.
84. Working Group on Status Epilepticus: Treatment of convulsive status epilepticus, *JAMA* 270:854, 1993.
85. Brown T: The pharmacokinetics of agents used to treat status epilepticus, *Neurology* 40:28, 1990.
86. So EL: Update on epilepsy, *Med Clin North Am* 77:203, 1993.
87. Hauser WA et al: Seizure recurrence after a first unprovoked seizure: an extended follow-up, *Neurology* 40:1163, 1990.
88. Shinnar S et al: Risk of seizure recurrence following a first unprovoked seizure in childhood: a prospective study, *Pediatrics* 85:1076, 1990.
89. Ramsay RE et al: A double-blind study comparing carbamazepine with phenytoin as initial seizure therapy in adults, *Neurology* 33:904, 1983.
90. Temkin NR et al: A randomized, double-blind study of phenytoin for the prevention of post-traumatic seizures, *N Engl J Med* 323:497, 1990.
91. Mattson RH et al: Use of oral contraceptives by women with epilepsy, *JAMA* 256:238, 1986.
92. American Academy of Pediatrics Committee on Drugs: Behavioral and cognitive effects of anticonvulsant therapy, *Pediatrics* 76:644, 1985.

97 Headache

Tom Kwiatkowski
Kuman Alagappan

Headache is a common complaint, more frequent than the common cold, and accounts for approximately 2 million visits to the ED per year in the United States.[1] In addition, many more patients will present with headache as part of a constitutional illness, making the symptom of headache one of the most frequent complaints seen in ED practice.

Headache is divided into *primary* and *secondary* disorders. The primary headache disorders include migraine, cluster, and tension-type headaches, which represent greater than 90% of headaches seen in clinical practice.[2] Secondary headache disorders include a variety of organic illnesses, in which head pain is a symptom of an identifiable, distinct pathologic process. To facilitate a standardized approach to headache, the International Headache Society published the *Classification and Diagnostic Criteria for Headache Disorders, Cranial Neuralgias and Facial Pain* in 1988.[3] This comprehensive and widely accepted system includes 13 categories of headache disorders and uses specific operational diagnostic criteria to define each headache type (Box 97-1).

From the perspective of the emergency physician, the vast majority of patients presenting with headache will have a benign primary headache disorder, requiring symptomatic treatment and referral. The real challenge is to identify the very small subset of patients who have headache as a symptom of a serious or potentially life-threatening disease.

PRIMARY HEADACHE DISORDERS

Migraine Headache

Principles of Disease Migraine headaches account for approximately 1 million visits to the ED per year.[4] They typically begin in the second decade of life and are more prevalent among women (18%) than men (6%).[5,6] During childhood, however, there is no gender difference in the prevalence of migraine.[2] After menarche there is a relationship between migraine headache and menses in about 15% of female migraineurs, possibly related to fluctuating estrogen and progesterone levels. After menopause, women also tend to experience fewer migraine headaches.

Historically, migraine headaches have been considered to be vascular in origin. According to this hypothesis, an initial phase of cerebral vasoconstriction resulting in neurologic symptoms (migraine with aura) was followed by a vasodilatory phase, manifested by the typical pounding headache of migraine. Appropriate changes in blood flow have been

Box 97-1 International Headache Society Classification of Headache

1. Migraine
2. Tension-type headache
3. Cluster headache and chronic paroxysmal hemicrania
4. Miscellaneous headaches unassociated with structural lesion
5. Headache associated with head trauma
6. Headache associated with vascular disorders
7. Headache associated with nonvascular intracranial disorder
8. Headache associated with substances or their withdrawal
9. Headache associated with noncephalic infection
10. Headache associated with metabolic disorder
11. Headache or facial pain associated with disorder of cranium, neck, eyes, ears, nose, sinuses, teeth, mouth, or other facial or cranial structures
12. Cranial neuralgias, nerve trunk pain, and deafferentation pain
13. Headache not classifiable

demonstrated for the classic migraine attack, and pain relief provided by vasoconstriction further supported this hypothesis.[7] However, this mechanism does not fully explain the entire spectrum of migraine attacks, and other theories have been proposed regarding its etiology. It is now believed that the pathophysiologic cause of migraine may actually originate in the brainstem within its descending and ascending circuitry, including the ascending pain-modulating projections from the midbrain raphe nuclei.[8] Recent evidence suggests a perturbation of neural activity within this serotonergic system as an important precursor to migraine.[9] Changes in serotonergic activity can alter the cranial circulation, triggering a "vascular phase." In addition to constriction and dilatation of intracranial and extracranial arteries, this neurovascular reaction activates the nociceptive trigeminal vascular system.[10,11] Neural connections between cerebral blood vessels and the trigeminal nerve release neuropeptides that can induce a painful neurogenic or sterile inflammation.[12]

Agonists of the $5\text{-}HT_1$ receptor, such as sumatriptan or dihydroergotamine (DHE), will block the inflammatory process. Effective prophylactic agents are believed to act as antagonists of the $5HT_2$ receptor site.[13]

Migraine is further divided into two major categories. Migraine without aura, or "common migraine," is the most frequent form of migraine and accounts for about 80% of all cases (Box 97-2). "Classic migraine," or migraine with aura, has specific reversible neurologic symptoms that precede the actual headache (Box 97-3) and is seen less frequently.

Clinical Features Migraine headaches tend to be chronic and recurrent. The headache is often unilateral, pulsating in quality, moderate to severe in intensity, and aggravated by routine activities. The side of the headache can vary with individual attacks and may be bilateral in 40% of patients. The onset is usually gradual and the attacks typically last from 4 to 72 hours. Headache frequency is quite variable, and some patients will experience several episodes per month. Associated symptoms include nausea, vomiting, anorexia, photophobia, phonophobia, osmophobia (aversion to odors), blurred vision, light-headedness, and nasal congestion. Some patients will have cognitive impairments producing forgetfulness, irritability, and depression, whereas others may be manic, with outbursts of anger that can be very disruptive in the ED setting. Many patients will have dramatic light and sound sensitivity and will seek a cool, dark, and quiet room.

The aura of classic migraine consists of focal neurologic symptoms that precede and herald the migraine attack. By definition, the aura is fully reversible and typically lasts 10 to 20 minutes, although it may continue for as long as 1 hour. The most common aura is visual and may include scintillating scotomas (bright rim around an area of visual loss), teichopsias (subjective visual image perceived with eyes open or closed), fortification spectrums (zigzagged wall of fortress slowly drifting across visual field), photopsias (poorly formed brief flashes or sparks of light), or blurred vision. Less

Box 97-2 Migraine Without Aura (Common Migraine)

International Headache Society Criteria

A. At least five attacks fulfilling criteria in B, C, D, and E.
B. Attack lasts 4 to 72 hours with or without treatment.
C. Headache has at least two of the following characteristics:
   1. Unilateral location
   2. Pulsating quality
   3. Moderate to severe intensity
   4. Aggravated by walking up stairs or similar routine physical activity
D. During headache, at least one of the following:
   1. Nausea or vomiting (or both)
   2. Photophobia and phonophobia
E. History, physical, and neurologic examination and, if appropriate, diagnostic tests to exclude related organic disease.

Box 97-3 Migraine With Aura (Classic Migraine)

International Headache Society Criteria

A. At least two attacks that fulfill criterion B.
B. At least three of the four characteristics must be present before the diagnosis of classic migraine can be made.
   1. One or more fully reversible aura symptoms indicating focal cerebral cortical or brainstem dysfunction (or both).
   2. At least one aura symptom develops gradually over more than 4 minutes or two or more symptoms occur in succession.
   3. No single aura symptom lasts longer than 60 minutes.
   4. Headache begins during aura or follows with a symptom-free interval of less than 60 minutes (headache may begin before aura).
C. An appropriate history, physical, and neurologic examination with appropriate diagnostic tests must be performed to exclude related organic diseases.

common auras include somatosensory phenomena such as tingling or numbness, motor disturbances, and cognitive or language disorders.[14]

Ophthalmoplegic migraine is a rare syndrome associated with paresis of one or more ocular nerves, most commonly the third cranial nerve. Patients typically present with ipsilateral headache associated with extraocular muscle paresis and occasionally pupillary changes. The ophthalmoplegia or pupillary changes may last for days to weeks and, rarely, may become permanent.[15] Because of the neurologic findings, secondary causes including intracranial aneurysm and mass lesion must be ruled out.

Hemiplegic migraine is characterized by episodic hemiparesis or hemiplegia as an aura to the migraine attack. The progression of the motor deficit is slow or marching in quality and in most cases is accompanied by a sensory disturbance as well. The neurologic symptoms last 30 to 60 minutes followed by a severe pulsating headache. Rarely the motor deficit is persistent, resulting from a true migraine-induced stroke.

Basilar artery migraine presents with an aura referable to the brainstem and is associated with multiple neurologic findings, including visual symptoms (often total blindness), dysarthria, tinnitus, vertigo, bilateral paresthesias, paresis, and altered level of conciousness.[16] The symptoms are stereotyped and resolve spontaneously.

Status migrainosus is a severe migraine headache that persists longer than 72 hours. Associated symptoms are debilitating, and patients often require hospitalization for pain management and supportive care.

Many factors can trigger migraine headaches in predisposed individuals. Common precipitants include sleep deprivation, stress, hunger, hormonal changes, and the use of certain drugs, including oral contraceptives and nitroglycerin.[4] In addition some patients will report specific food sensitivities including chocolate, caffeine, and foods rich in tyramine.[17,18] Alcohol, specifically red or port wine, has also been implicated. In others, certain sensory stimuli such as a strong glare or strong odors can trigger an attack.

Differential Diagnosis Because of their complex symptomatology, migraine headaches may be difficult to distinguish from other secondary causes of headache. Other diagnoses that mimic migraine include ruptured berry aneurysm, arteriovenous malformation, intracranial mass lesions, giant cell arteritis, and cerebrovascular disease.

Diagnostic Evaluation Routine neuroimaging is not necessary for patients with typical recurrent migraine headaches. However, neuroimaging must be considered for patients with new-onset headaches, headaches with a progressive course or change in pattern, headaches that never alternate sides, and headaches associated with any neurologic findings or seizures. Such patients will have a substantially higher likelihood of a secondary cause such as tumor, arteriovenous malformation, or structural lesion.[19] In addition, patients who present with a severe or "worst headache of their life" will require a lumbar puncture to rule out subarachnoid hemorrhage if the computed tomography (CT) scan is negative.

Treatment The pharmacologic treatment of migraine is divided into abortive therapies, which attempt to limit the intensity and duration of a given episode, and prophylactic therapies, which are intended to decrease the frequency and intensity of attacks.[20]

Patients who are unable to control their headaches at home will often present to the ED for better pain control or supportive therapy. There are several approaches to treating the acute headache episode based on the severity of the attack (Table 97-1). In addition, patients with a history of migraine may relate specific interventions that have been successful. The choice of agents will depend on several factors, including the patient's prior response to therapy as previously noted, the existence of comorbid conditions, and the presence or absence of nausea or vomiting. Gastric stasis is common during acute migraine attacks and may limit the effectiveness of oral agents.

For mild to moderate attacks, the International Headache Society (IHS) recommends simple analgesics such as acetaminophen or nonsteroidal anti-inflammatory drugs (NSAIDs). In the presence of nausea or vomiting, adding an agent such as metoclopramide will enhance the absorption and effectiveness of these medications. Appropriate doses and possible side effects are listed in Box 97-1. Of note, indomethacin is available as a rectal suppository.

For moderate to severe attacks, several classes of medications are available to treat the pain in addition to the nausea and vomiting that frequently accompany the headache. Specific agents available for treating severe migraine include DHE and sumatriptan. DHE should be given intravenously (IV) at 1.0 mg slowly over 2 minutes and can be repeated in 1 hour if pain control has not been achieved. Because DHE can cause nausea and vomiting, patients should be pretreated with an antiemetic such as metoclopramide 10 mg IV or prochlorperazine 5 mg IV. Repeated administration of the IV form of DHE has been shown to be very effective in patients with intractable migraine and status migrainosus. Contraindications to using DHE include pregnancy, breast feeding, poorly controlled hypertension, coronary artery disease, and peripheral vascular disease. DHE should not be used if the patient has already taken sumatriptan.

Sumatriptan, the first approved medication of the triptan class, is a selective $5HT_1$ receptor agonist. Other triptans that are available include zolmitriptan, naratriptan, and rizatriptan, but only sumatriptan is available for subcutaneous (SQ) administration and is the most common preparation used in the ED. The initial dose is 6 mg SQ, which may be repeated once in 1 hour if the patient has a partial response to the first dose. Common side effects include tingling, flushing, warm or hot sensations, and heaviness in the chest. Sumatriptan has similar contraindications to DHE including pregnancy, poorly controlled hypertension, and coronary artery disease. Sumatriptan should not be used within 24 hours of administration of an ergotamine-containing medication or DHE.[21]

Neuroleptics have also been shown to be effective in treating acute migraine attacks. Chlorpromazine or prochlorperazine can be administered as a slow 10-mg IV bolus, which can be repeated once in 30 to 60 minutes.[11,22] Because of the incidence of orthostatic hypotension with chlorpromazine, patients should receive a 500-mg bolus of normal saline before its administration. The most common side effects after parenteral administration of these agents include sedation, postural hypotension, and extrapyramidal symptoms including acute dystonic reactions.

Narcotic analgesics such as meperidine should be reserved

Table 97-1. Selected Medications for Acute Migraine Attacks

Medication	Dose and route administered	Comments
Mild to moderate		
Acetaminophen	500 mg to 1000 mg PO	
Aspirin	650 mg to 1000 mg PO	Gastrointestinal upset
Ibuprofen	600 mg to 800 mg PO	Gastrointestinal upset
Naproxen sodium	275 mg to 550 mg PO	Gastrointestinal upset
Indomethacin	25 mg to 50 mg PO 50 mg rectal suppository	Gastrointestinal upset
Moderate to severe		
Dihydroergotamine	1 mg IV or IM; may be repeated in 1 hr	Gastrointestinal upset (pretreat with antiemetic) Cannot be used if sumatriptan already taken Contraindicated with hypertension, coronary artery disease, peripheral vascular disease, and pregnancy
Sumatriptan	6 mg SQ; may be repeated once in 1 hr if partial response	Chest pain, throat tightness, flushing Contraindicated with hypertension, coronary artery disease, peripheral vascular disease, and pregnancy Cannot be used within 24 hours of ergot usage
Prochlorperazine	10 mg IV or IM; may be repeated in 30 to 60 min	Sedation and dystonic reaction
Chlorpromazine	10 mg IV or IM; may be repeated in 30 to 60 min	Significant orthostatic hypotension; therefore saline bolus should be administrated before use of this medication Sedation and dystonic reaction
Metoclopramide	10 mg IV	Dystonic reaction
Ketorolac	30 mg IV or 30 to 60 mg IM	Gastrointestinal upset; avoid medication in elderly and in patients with renal insufficiency
Meperidine	50-100 mg IM or IV	Opioids less efficacious than other treatment modalities
Refractory attack, status migrainosus		
Dihydroergotamine	1 mg IV q8h	Use in conjunction with antiemetic (e.g., metoclopramide, prochlorperazine)
Steroids	Various regimens	Gastrointestinal bleeding, infection, cataracts, aseptic necrosis, memory disturbances

for patients who do not respond or have contraindications to standard migraine therapies. Though frequently used, narcotics have been shown to be less efficacious than other treatments and have the risk of addiction; however, some patients will obtain relief with this class of medications.

The use of steroids for the treatment of migraine remains controversial. Anecdotal evidence suggests they may be effective for prolonged migraine attacks that are refractory to standard therapies and for treating status migrainosus (a migraine attack lasting more than 72 hours).[8,23]

Occasionally, patients will not respond to initial therapy in the ED and will require hospitalization for continued pain control and supportive therapy.

Prophylactic Therapy Prophylactic therapy is indicated for patients who have frequent attacks (more than two to three episodes per month), prolonged attacks lasting more than 48 hours, or attacks that are severe and debilitating. Of note, prophylactic medications are seldom more than 55% to 65% effective.[24]

Several classes of medications are used for the prophylaxis of migraine. Many of these medications have significant side effects, especially among women of childbearing age; therefore, after headaches have decreased, attempts should be made to taper and discontinue treatment when possible.

Beta-adrenergic blocking agents reduce both the frequency and severity of migraine headache and are the most widely used drugs for recurrent migraine.[4] Propranolol has been the most extensively studied medication. However, patients who do not respond to propranolol may respond to another drug in this class including atenolol, metoprolol, timolol, or nadolol.[25] Contraindications to beta-blockers include pregnancy, asthma, heart failure, Raynaud's phenomenon, and diabetes mellitus.[8]

Methysergide, a semisynthetic ergot preparation, has also been widely used for prophylaxis. It is a potent peripheral serotonin antagonist, with a presumed mechanism similar to other ergot drugs. It is contraindicated in patients with coronary artery or peripheral vascular disease, and prolonged use has been associated with retroperitoneal, pulmonary, and endocardial fibrosis.[26]

Other medications used for migraine prophylaxis include calcium channel blockers, tricyclic antidepressants, NSAIDs, anticonvulsants, and monoamine oxidase inhibitors.[8,25]

Cluster Headache

Perspective Cluster headache is the only headache syndrome that is more common in men than in women. It typically occurs in young to middle-aged adults, with a peak incidence in the late twenties. The headaches tend to occur repeatedly over a defined time interval, hence the term "cluster." Several attacks can occur in one day, and a typical cluster period may last 6 to 8 weeks. Several precipitating factors have been implicated, most notably the ingestion of alcohol. Stress and climatic changes may also play a role in susceptible individuals.

Clinical Features Cluster headaches occur suddenly with little warning, and several episodes can occur within a 24-hour period. Each headache lasts from a few minutes up to 2 hours. The patient will typically complain of a unilateral, sharp, stabbing pain in the eye, which may awaken him or her from sleep. The attacks tend to occur exclusively in the territory of the trigeminal nerve.[27] Unlike migraine, the cluster headache patient will present in a predictable fashion (i.e., holding his or her eye, rocking, rubbing the head, and pacing). The attack subsides rapidly, often leaving the patient exhausted.

Up to 30% of patients will have a partial Horner's syndrome with ptosis and miosis.[28] The eye is often injected and tearing and many patients will have unilateral nasal congestion.[7]

Differential Diagnosis Other headache disorders that mimic cluster include migraine, trigeminal neuralgia, and chronic paroxysmal hemicrania (CPH). With migraine, the clinical presentation, gender, and age distribution are usually different. With trigeminal neuralgia, the pain peaks within seconds, lasts only a couple of minutes, and can be provoked by specific trigger points on the face or oral mucosa. CPH is a brief unilateral headache that recurs at least 15 times a day, often induced by rotation or turning of the head or by pressure on the cervical spine.[29]

Treatment Because cluster headaches are abrupt in onset, treatment must be initiated rapidly to be effective. At present, sumatriptan 6 mg SQ is the preferred abortive therapy for the majority of patients if given very early after the onset of the attack[30]; however, by the time a patient presents to the ED, the headache has usually progressed and symptomatic treatment is indicated. High-flow oxygen at a rate 7 to 10 L/min has been shown to abort the headache within several minutes.[31] DHE 1.0 mg IV or IM also has been shown to be effective, but it is less practical than oxygen administration and has more side effects. For patients who do not respond to the above measures, intranasal application of cocaine[24] or lidocaine to produce anesthesia of the sphenopalatine region has been advocated by some but has not gained widespread acceptance.[32]

In addition to acute therapies, several medications have been shown to be effective for the prophylactic treatment of cluster headaches. A short course of oral prednisone may effectively abort a cluster attack in some patients. A recommended regimen is 60 mg of prednisone daily for 10 days, followed by a 1-week taper.[32] To prevent breakthrough headaches after the steroid taper, patients may require the concurrent administration of another prophylactic agent (e.g., verapamil, lithium carbonate, or methysergide).

Tension Headache

Perspective Tension headache is the most common recurrent pain syndrome, affecting more than 75% of the population.[33] Women are affected more frequently than men, and most patients are middle aged. The headaches do not cause significant disability, and patients are able to continue with their normal daily activities.[34] The median frequency of headaches is six per month, and stress and lack of sleep are implicated as triggering factors.[35,36] The average duration of the headache is 4 to 13 hours, with a maximum of 72 hours.[36]

Even though tension headache is the most common headache syndrome, very little is known about its pathophysiology.[33] There is no clear evidence that increased muscle activity is present, and tender areas of the scalp and neck can be found with both tension and migraine headaches. Recent evidence suggests that tension and migraine headaches may be part of a continuum with similar pathophysiology.

Clinical Features Patients will typically complain of a tight, band-like discomfort around their head that is nonpulsating and dull. They also may experience tightening of their neck muscles. The majority will not seek medical assistance because the headache is usually mild in intensity and of relatively short duration. Occasionally, the discomfort can build up slowly and fluctuate in severity over several days. Unlike migraine, symptoms do not worsen with physical activity, and accompanying symptoms such as nausea, vomiting, phonophobia, or photophobia are unusual. Anxiety and depression may coexist with chronic tension headaches.

Differential Diagnosis Tension headache is the least distinct of all the primary headache disorders and its diagnosis is based mainly on the absence of features that would suggest another diagnosis (e.g., migraine). The lack of specificity will often result in the clinician hesitating to make the diagnosis without other diagnostic investigations to exclude organic disease.[37] The most common disorders mimicking tension headache include idiopathic intracranial hypertension, oromandibular dysfunction, cervical spondylosis, sinus or eye disease, and intracranial masses.

Treatment For the majority of individuals, simple analgesics such as aspirin, acetaminophen, or NSAIDs are adequate for pain control. Patients with chronic symptoms may exhibit signs of depression or anxiety, and these patients often respond to medications and nonpharmacologic regimens that treat these conditions. Some nonpharmacologic regimens include meditation, massage, and biofeedback. For long-term management, psychotherapy may be of value in teaching patients to deal with tension effectively.

SECONDARY HEADACHE DISORDERS

Subarachnoid Hemorrhage

Principles of Disease Subarachnoid hemorrhage (SAH) refers to extravasated blood in the subarachnoid space. The blood activates meningeal nociceptors, leading to diffuse occipital pain along with signs of meningismus. SAH accounts for up to 10% of all strokes and is the most common cause of sudden death from a stroke.[38]

Approximately 80% of patients with nontraumatic SAH have ruptured saccular aneurysms.[39] Other causes include arteriovenous malformations, cavernous angiomas, mycotic aneurysms, neoplasms, and blood dyscrasias. SAH may be caused secondarily by an intraparenchymal hematoma that dissects its way into the subarachnoid space.

The risk for aneurysmal SAH increases with age, with most cases occurring between 40 and 60 years of age.[40] In children and adolescents, aneurysms are uncommon, and when SAH occurs it is usually secondary to an arteriovenous malformation.[41] It is estimated that 5% of the general population harbors a berry aneurysm and the risk of rupture may increase with aneurysmal size. Other risk factors associated with SAH include hypertension, smoking, excessive alcohol consumption, and sympathomimetic drugs.[42] There is a familial association of cerebral aneurysms with several diseases, including autosomal dominant polycystic kidney disease, coarctation of the aorta, Marfan's syndrome, and Ehlers-Danlos syndrome type IV.

Of all patients presenting to the ED with headache, 1% to 4% will have SAH. Many patients with SAH die before reaching the hospital, with prehospital mortality ranging from 3% to 26%.[39] Because of the significant morbidity and mortality (50%) associated with this condition and the high likelihood of clinical deterioration in patients who are initially misdiagnosed, emergency physicians must have a very high index of suspicion for SAH and be familiar with its presentation as described in the following sections.[39]

Table 97-2. Hunt and Hess Clinical Grading Scale for Cerebral Aneurysms and Subarachnoid Hemorrhage

Grade	Condition
0	Unruptured aneurysm
1	Asymptomatic or minimal headache and slight nuchal rigidity
2	Moderate or severe headache, nuchal rigidity; no neurologic deficit other than cranial nerve palsy
3	Drowsiness, confusion, or mild focal deficit
4	Stupor, moderate to severe hemiparesis
5	Deep coma, decerebrate posturing, moribund appearance

Clinical Features The majority of patients will present with a sudden, cataclysmic "thunderclap" headache, which is often described as the worst headache of their life. The onset of headache may be associated with exertional activities such as exercise, the Valsalva maneuver, or sexual intercourse in up to 20% of patients.[38] Associated symptoms include nausea and vomiting in about 75% of patients, neck stiffness in 25%, and seizures in 17%.[40] Some patients will experience a headache within the previous 6 to 8 weeks, indicating a warning leak or sentinel hemorrhage. Physical findings depend on the extent of the SAH. Meningismus is present in more than 50% of patients,[41] and up to 20% will have focal findings.[42] Funduscopic examination may reveal retinal or subhyaloid hemorrhages, and patients may also have an isolated third or sixth nerve palsy. Oculomotor (third) nerve compression secondary to an expanding aneurysm will lead to pupillary dilation. About 50% of patients with a ruptured aneurysm will be restless or have an altered level of consciousness. Although the majority will not have focal neurologic signs, when present, they may indicate the site of the aneurysm.[43]

The patient's prognosis is often related to neurologic status at admission. The Hunt and Hess scale stratifies patients according to their clinical signs and symptoms at the time of presentation and is predictive of outcome (Table 97-2).[38,44] Patients who present with a grade I or II hemorrhage tend to have a good prognosis, and patients in grades IV or V tend to do poorly. These patients will have an altered mental status, ranging from stupor to deep coma, together with focal neurologic findings. Patients with grade III hemorrhage present with drowsiness or confusion and are at risk for rapid clinical deterioration.

Diagnostic Studies When the diagnosis of SAH is considered, a CT scan should be ordered emergently. For acute hemorrhage less than 24 hours old, the sensitivity of CT in identifying hemorrhage is greater than 90%; however, it decreases to approximately 50% by the end of the first week.[39] When the CT scan is negative, a lumbar puncture should be performed. Lumbar puncture as a first strategy, postulated to be cost-effective in carefully selected patients who have completely normal physical examinations, may be safe but has not been studied clinically.[45] To differentiate a traumatic lumbar puncture from SAH, the patient's cerebrospinal fluid (CSF) should be spun and the supernatant observed for xanthochromia. The yellowish pigmentation is secondary to the metabolism of hemoglobin to pigmented molecules of oxyhemoglobin and bilirubin, a process that takes approximately 12 hours to occur.[46,47] The method of comparing the red blood cell (RBC) count in the first and last tubes of CSF has been shown to be unreliable.[39] CSF xanthochromia in association with a negative CT scan is diagnostic of SAH. After the diagnosis is established, angiography should be performed to study the vascular anatomy and identify the source of hemorrhage in patients who are candidates for surgical intervention.

Most authorities agree that the presence of xanthochromia as measured by spectrophotometry, which is much more sensitive than visual inspection,[39] is the primary criterion for a diagnosis of SAH. However, because xanthochromia may require up to 12 hours to be present after the initial bleed, patients with persistently bloody CSF without xanthochromia should undergo vascular imaging when the level of clinical suspicion of SAH is high.[39]

Up to 90% of patients with SAH will have cardiac arrhythmias or electrocardiogram (ECG) findings suggestive of acute cardiac ischemia, which may lead to an erroneous primary cardiac diagnosis.[39] Typical ECG findings include ST-T wave changes, U waves, and QT prolongation.[48]

Treatment The management of SAH is complex and includes initial resuscitation, stabilization, and emergent neurosurgical consultation. The goals of management are to treat the acute medical and neurologic complications, prevent recurrent hemorrhage, and forestall the ischemic complications of vasospasm.[49] Because of an altered level of consciousness, patients with SAH of grade III or higher are at risk for respiratory depression and hypercapnia, which can lead to further increases in intracranial pressure (ICP); therefore, these patients may require early endotracheal intubation. Blood pressure must also be closely monitored because of the risk of continued bleeding or recurrent hemorrhage. Nimodipine, a calcium channel blocker, should be started soon after a diagnosis of aneurysmal SAH is made, to lessen the likelihood of ischemic stroke. Because it may cause transient hypotension in some patients, hemodynamic monitoring is required during its administration. The recommended dose is 60 mg by mouth or nasogastric tube every 4 hours.

Analgesics, including opiates, should be used for persistent headache. In patients who are nauseated or at risk for vomiting, antiemetics must also be administered. Agitated patients will require sedation, and all patients should be placed at absolute bed rest in a quiet and dark environment. Clinically evident seizures should be treated with anticonvulsants, but the prophylactic use of these drugs is controversial.[48] The majority of these patients will require hemodynamic and ICP monitoring in an intensive care setting.

Brain Tumor

Principles of Disease Headache is the most common presenting complaint with brain tumor and occurs in about 50% of patients.[50] The majority of patients are elderly and have a cerebral metastasis as a cause of their headache.[51] The most common causes are lung and breast carcinoma followed by malignant melanoma and carcinomas of the kidney and gastrointestinal tract.[43] Primary brain tumors are much less common and typically occur in young adults less than 50 years of age.

The headache can be caused by several mechanisms, including direct involvement or traction on pain-sensitive structures such as meninges or larger cerebral vessels, or as a symptom of increased ICP. The pain patterns produced are highly variable, depending on the location of the mass and the structures involved.[43] Headaches are often but not always on the same side as the tumor. With increased ICP, the pain is often bifrontal or bioccipital and may be accompanied by vomiting. Brain tumors may also disrupt sleep, awakening the patient during the night. This may be related to increases in cerebral pressure that occur with recumbency and sleep-related carbon dioxide retention.[7]

Clinical Presentation The typical patient will present with complaints of a worsening headache that has been present for weeks to months. The headache may have been present initially only on awakening, gradually becoming continuous. The classic triad of brain tumor headache—sleep disturbances, severe pain, and nausea and vomiting—is seen in only one third of patients.[52] Vomiting, when present, may be projectile and not preceded by nausea. If increased ICP is present, the headache is often bilateral and worsened by coughing, sneezing, bending, defecation, and sexual intercourse.[53] Though patients may not complain of focal neurologic deficits, abnormal findings are often found with neurologic testing.[54] Other presentations include seizures, personality changes, and cognitive difficulties.

Diagnostic Evaluation The diagnosis of brain tumor is often suspected from the history and neurologic examination. Neuroimaging with CT or magnetic resonance imaging (MRI) is the most efficient way to confirm the diagnosis. Contrast enhancement on CT will often improve the identification of the underlying mass lesion and help differentiate it from other causes, including abscess, hematoma, or vascular malformation.[55]

Treatment Management consists of urgent referral to neurosurgery and treatment of any acute complications, including increased ICP and seizures. For patients who present with symptoms suggestive of increased ICP (e.g., headache, nausea, vomiting, confusion, weakness), treatment with steroids has been shown to be beneficial. Dexamethasone is the high-potency steroid used most often to treat edema associated with brain tumors. It has several advantages over other glucocorticoids, including a longer half-life, reduced mineralocorticoid effect, and a lower incidence of cognitive and behavioral complications.[54] The exact dose of steroids necessary for each patient varies, depending on the histology, size, and location of the tumor, and the amount of edema present. In general, most patients will require between 8 mg and 16 mg of dexamethasone per day. An appropriate starting dose in the ED is 10 mg IV followed by 4 mg every 6 hours.

Any patient with a seizure (generalized or partial) should be placed on anticonvulsant therapy. Appropriate first-line agents include phenytoin, carbamazepine, and valproic acid. Empiric or prophylactic treatment does not appear to delay or prevent the onset of seizure activity and may expose the patient to unnecessary complications and toxicity.[54]

Giant Cell Arteritis

Principles of Disease Giant cell arteritis, or temporal arteritis, is a systemic inflammatory process of the small and medium-sized arteries. Extracranial branches of the aortic arch and the ophthalmic vessels are most commonly involved, but the process may affect any artery in the body.[55] The mean age of onset is 71 years and it is rare before age 50. Females are more commonly affected than males.

Clinical Presentation Headache is the most common initial manifestation of giant cell arteritis and occurs in 80% to 90% of patients.[56] The headache can be continuous or intermittent and is often worse at night or on exposure to cold. The pain may be described as sharp, throbbing, boring, or aching and is usually localized to the temporal region but may occur anywhere in the head. There may be tenderness over the scalp in the area of the temporal artery, with pain exacerbated when wearing a hat or resting the head on a pillow. Patients may also experience jaw claudication secondary to vascular insufficiency of the masseter and temporalis muscles. Systemic symptoms including fever, anorexia, and weight loss will often be present. About 40% of patients will complain of pain in their large proximal joints, with symptoms referable to the neck, torso, and lower back. This condition, known as *polymyalgia rheumatica,* can occur in the absence of giant cell arteritis.

The most serious complication of giant cell arteritis is permanent visual loss, which eventually occurs in 36% of untreated cases.[57] Amaurosis fugax can also occur before permanent visual loss. Other complications include peripheral neuropathies, transient ischemic attacks, and stroke.

Diagnostic Evaluation The physical examination may reveal tender and indurated superficial scalp arteries that may be pulseless. Visual acuity and visual field testing and a thorough funduscopic examination should also be performed.

The majority of patients will have a significant elevation of the erythrocyte sedimentation rate (ESR), although a normal value does not rule out the diagnosis. Other laboratory abnormalities include mild to moderate anemia, elevated C-reactive protein, and liver function abnormalities.[43] The diagnosis is confirmed by temporal artery biopsy. Because this is a patchy disease, multiple biopsies of a long segment of the artery may need to be examined.

Treatment Because of the risk of visual loss, giant cell arteritis is a medical emergency and treatment should be initiated promptly when the diagnosis is suspected. Steroids are the mainstay of therapy; the recommended initial dose of prednisone ranges from 60 mg/day to 120 mg/day. Symptomatic response usually occurs rapidly over days, although therapy must be continued for months, with close ESR monitoring.

Carotid and Vertebral Dissection

Principles of Disease Carotid and vertebral dissections are more common than previously realized and account for 6% to 10% of strokes in young adults between the ages of 30 and 50.[58] They can be either spontaneous or secondary to trauma, with up to 40% of patients recalling a history of minor trauma preceding the event.[58] Reported mechanisms include neck torsion, chiropractic manipulation, coughing, minor falls, and motor vehicle accidents. Early symptoms and signs are often subtle, and in the absence of neurologic findings delays in diagnosis are common.

The pathologic lesion is intramural hemorrhage within the media of the arterial wall. The hematoma can be localized or extend circumferentially along the length of the vessel, resulting in partial or complete occlusion. Platelet aggregation and thrombus formation also occur, further compromising vessel patency or causing distal embolization. The timing of these events is variable and a patient may experience symptoms of cerebral ischemia days to years after dissection.[59,60]

Clinical Presentation The typical presentation of the patient with carotid or vertebral dissection is the abrupt onset of pain in the neck or face. Neurologic findings may be present on initial evaluation but are often delayed hours to days after the onset of the first symptoms.[58]

Carotid Dissection The classic triad of symptoms for carotid dissection includes unilateral headache, ipsilateral partial Horner's syndrome, and contralateral hemispheric findings that may include aphasia, neglect, visual disturbances, or hemiparesis. The headache is often severe and throbbing but may be subacute and similar to previous headaches. Acute severe retroorbital pain in a previously healthy person with no history of cluster headaches is particularly suggestive of carotid dissection.[7] Most patients will eventually develop signs of cerebral ischemia. Warning symptoms include transient ischemic attacks, amaurosis fugax, episodic lightheadedness, and syncope. Spontaneous dissection of the carotid artery has a favorable prognosis and recurrence is uncommon.[60] Factors associated with a worse prognosis include older age, occlusive disease on angiography, or stroke as the initial presenting symptom.[61]

Vertebral Dissection Vertebral artery dissections are less common than carotid dissections. The classic presentation is a relatively young person who presents with severe unilateral posterior headache and neurologic findings.[62] The majority of patients will develop a rapidly progressive neurologic deficit with symptoms of brainstem and cerebellar ischemia. Common findings include vertigo, severe vomiting, ataxia, diplopia, hemiparesis, unilateral facial weakness, and tinnitus.[63] Spontaneous vertebral artery dissection appears to be relatively rare. Approximately 10% of patients who develop a vertebral dissection will die during the acute phase, secondary to massive stroke. For patients who survive, the prognosis is usually good.[58]

Diagnosis/Treatment The diagnosis of dissection may prove to be difficult. A CT scan should be obtained first but will often be normal in the uncomplicated dissection. Further imaging studies including duplex scanning, magnetic resonance angiography, or catheter angiography will be required to confirm the diagnosis. Treatment is aimed at stroke prevention and usually includes early anticoagulation followed by antiplatelet therapy.

Identifying patients with dissection is challenging. More than 50% of patients see their physician for symptoms before admission. The emergency physician must consider this diagnosis in any young patient who presents with head or neck pain with focal neurologic findings.

Idiopathic Intracranial Hypertension

Principles of Disease Idiopathic intracranial hypertension (IIH) is also known as *pseudotumor cerebri* or benign intracranial hypertension. The term *idiopathic intracranial hypertension*, however, is preferred because this is not always a benign disorder and may have significant neurologic sequelae in affected individuals.

IIH is a relatively common neurologic disease seen primarily in young obese women of childbearing age. Several predisposing factors have been identified, including the use of oral contraceptives, anabolic steroids, tetracyclines, and vitamin A.[64]

Pathophysiology/Clinical Features The pathophysiology of this disease remains controversial, with increased brain water content and decreased CSF outflow considered the two major causative factors.[65] The most prominent symptom is generalized headache, which is often gradual in onset and of moderate intensity. There is no specific localizing pattern, though in some patients, it is worsened by eye movement. It may awaken patients from sleep and is exacerbated by bending forward or the Valsalva maneuver, which impede cerebral venous return.

Visual complaints are common and patients may experience transient visual obscuration several times a day secondary to ischemia of the visual pathways. These episodes can be followed by prolonged periods of visual loss, which can become permanent in up to 10% of patients.[66] On physical examination, patients will have papilledema and visual field defects, including an enlarged blind spot initially followed by loss of peripheral vision. Occasionally, a sixth nerve palsy will be noted.

Diagnosis The diagnosis of IIH should not be made without neuroimaging and measurement of ICP. The diagnostic criteria are as follows:

- Increased ICP (>200 mm H_2O) measured by opening pressure from a lumbar puncture
- Signs and symptoms of increased ICP, with absence of localizing signs
- No mass lesions or ventricular enlargement on neuroimaging

- Normal or low CSF protein and normal cell count
- No clinical or neuroimaging suspicion of venous sinus thrombosis[65]

Treatment Symptomatic treatment often includes lowering ICP and managing the headache. Acetazolamide (a carbonic anhydrase inhibitor) can be used to decrease CSF production alone or with a loop diuretic such as furosemide. Steroids also have been used, although their mechanism of action is unclear. Prolonged therapy is problematic, and rebound IIH often occurs when doses are tapered. Repeated lumbar punctures can be attempted but most patients find this approach objectionable. In patients with impending visual loss or incapacitating symptoms, a ventricular shunt or optic nerve sheath fenestration may be indicated.

Posttraumatic Headache

Headache is the most common symptom following mild or minor head injury. It is part of a complex syndrome that can include dizziness, fatigue, insomnia, irritability, and difficulty with concentration. The prevalence of headache with posttraumatic syndrome is not known because most patients are not admitted for this condition. There are approximately 2 million closed head injuries per year, and it is estimated that 30% to 50% of these patients develop posttraumatic headache (PTHA).[67] Acute PTHA develops hours to days after the injury and resolves within 8 weeks. Chronic PTHA may last from several months to years and may mimic other forms of headache, including tension and migraine headaches.

Patients developing PTHA after minor head injuries have normal neurologic examinations and normal neuroimaging studies. The pathophysiology of their symptoms is unclear and may include both anatomic and functional components. Most patients are more concerned about the cause of the headache rather than the headache itself.

Treatment is symptomatic. For acute PTHA, analgesics such as acetaminophen or NSAIDs are adequate for pain control. For chronic PTHA, treatment must be individualized depending on the type of headache the patient is experiencing. Novel therapies such as antidepressants and beta-blockers may be effective in selected patients.

Acute Glaucoma

Patients with acute angle closure glaucoma present with the sudden onset of severe pain localized to the affected eye that may radiate to the ear, sinuses, teeth, or forehead.[53] Visual symptoms, including blurriness, halos around lights, and scotomas, are typically present, and many patients will also experience nausea and vomiting. The underlying pathophysiology is congenital narrowing of the anterior chamber angle that, under certain conditions, will close, resulting in a significant rise in intraocular pressure (IOP). Episodes can be precipitated by entering a low-light environment such as a movie theater, with resultant pupillary dilatation, or with the use of medications such as mydriatics (e.g., dilated ocular examination), sympathomimetics (e.g., pseudoephedrine), or agents with anticholinergic properties (e.g., antiemetics, antihistamines, antipsychotics, and antidepressants).[64,68]

Physical examination reveals a red eye with a fixed, mid-dilated pupil, corneal clouding, and shallow anterior chamber. The diagnosis is confirmed by demonstrating markedly elevated IOP in the range of 60 to 90 mm Hg (normal <21 mm Hg).

Treatment includes topical miotics, topical beta-blockers, oral carbonic anhydrase inhibitors (e.g., acetazolamide 250 mg four times daily), IV osmotic agents (e.g., mannitol), and prompt referral to an ophthalmologist. The potential for diagnostic confusion between acute glaucoma, iritis, and cluster headache must be recognized. Although cluster headache may present with pain, nausea, and a red eye, vision is not affected and the pupil generally is small and ptotic (from an oculosympathetic paresis).[69] Acute iritis also presents with a painful red eye but only acute angle closure glaucoma will have markedly elevated IOP.

Postdural Puncture Headache

Headache is the most common complication of lumbar puncture, occurring in up to 40% of patients.[70] The incidence is highest in the 18- to 30-year age group and uncommon in young children and adults older than 60. Though the onset is often immediate, patients may not report symptoms for several days. In the majority of affected individuals, the duration of headache is less than 5 days.[70,71]

Pathophysiology The cause of postdural puncture headache (PDPH) is not entirely clear. The most likely explanation is a persistent CSF leak that exceeds CSF production, resulting in CSF hypotension. If sufficient CSF is lost, the brain will descend in the cranial vault when the patient assumes the upright position, leading to increased traction on the pain fibers.[72] Thus the headache is characteristically positional and increases with the upright position and decreases with recumbency. The amount of time a patient remains recumbent after lumbar puncture does not appear to affect the incidence of headache.[7]

Certain factors have been implicated as causes of PDPH, including the size or diameter of the spinal needle, the orientation of the bevel during the procedure, and the amount of fluid withdrawn. Smaller-diameter needles will cause less leakage, and it is postulated that inserting the needle with the bevel up (i.e., bevel pointing up when the patient is in the lateral position) will minimize damage to the dural fibers. Using atraumatic needles or pencil-point needles (e.g., Whitaker[73] or Sprotte[74]) has also been shown to significantly reduce the incidence of PDPH.

Clinical Features The PDPH is typically bilateral, throbbing, and exacerbated by the upright position. Associated symptoms include neck stiffness; nausea; vomiting; auditory disturbances, including tinnitus and hearing loss (hypoacusis); and ocular symptoms, including blurred vision and diplopia.[72]

Treatment Most PDPH headaches resolve spontaneously within a few days with bed rest and mild analgesics. For persistent headaches, oral caffeine 300 mg every 4 to 6 hours or caffeine sodium benzoate (500 mg in 1 L of fluid) may be effective.[70] For severe headaches lasting more than 24 hours, an epidural blood patch (autologous blood clot) will relieve the headache in the majority of patients.[71]

Intracranial Infection

Headache is commonly seen in patients with intracranial infections, including meningitis, brain abscess, encephalitis, and AIDS. The severity and type of headache will vary depending on the specific infection.

With acute bacterial meningitis, the patient will often have a severe bursting headache that rapidly increases in severity over a short period.[75] These patients will typically have significant meningismus, with positive Kernig's and Brudzinski's signs. With viral meningitis patients may also complain of severe headache and nuchal rigidity, but the course is more indolent than with bacterial meningitis.

The severity of headache associated with encephalitis will depend on the type of virus involved. For example, the headache is usually mild with mumps encephalitis. However, with herpes simplex infection, the headache is abrupt and severe and frequently associated with confusion, fever, altered level of consciousness, seizures, and focal neurologic signs.

Patients with brain abscess will often have headache as their presenting complaint.[76] As the infection progresses, vomiting, focal neurologic signs, and depressed level of consciousness typically develop.

Headache is a frequent complaint in patients with human immunodeficiency virus (HIV) infection, and can be caused by a number of conditions, including aseptic meningitis, toxoplasmosis, cryptococcal or tuberculous meningitis, or cytomegalovirus encephalitis.

In the majority of cerebral infections, the mechanism of head pain includes meningeal irritation and increased ICP. In addition, headache may be a general reaction to fever or the toxic products of the infecting agent.[77]

Hypertensive Headache

Contrary to common belief, hypertension is not an important cause of headache, and the occurrence of headache and hypertension in the same patient often is coincidental.[78] Whether some patients with mild to moderate hypertension suffer from headache caused by elevated blood pressure is uncertain. The rate of blood pressure increase is more important as a cause of headache than the absolute blood pressure value. Diastolic pressures lower than 130 mm Hg are rarely the cause of headache.[56]

Nonetheless, the association of headache with severe hypertension is well documented. Acute, severe headache is a prominent symptom of hypertensive encephalopathy and most patients will have a blood pressure in the range of 250/150 mm Hg. Other conditions include headache secondary to toxic agents (e.g., drug-induced hypertension), pheochromocytoma, and eclampsia.

The headache of severe hypertension is typically diffuse, worse when the patient awakes in the morning and gradually subsiding over the course of the day.[78] Treatment is directed at lowering the blood pressure; in most cases, the headache will be relieved within 24 hours. In patients with hypertensive encephalopathy, the headache may persist for days until brain edema has resolved.

Cervicogenic Headache

Cervicogenic headache refers to headaches that originate from disorders of the neck. Diagnosis is based on the presence of the following three distinct sets of symptoms:[79]

1. Unilateral headache triggered by movements of the head or neck or certain head positions.
2. Unilateral headache triggered by pressure on the neck
3. Unilateral headache spreading to the neck or possibly the ipsilateral shoulder or arm

Many of these headaches are reported after a whiplash injury. Even though neck structures play a primary role in the pathophysiology of some headaches, clinical patterns indicating a neck-headache relationship have not been adequately defined.

Medication-Induced Headache

Medication use, abuse, or withdrawal can be a cause of headache and the term *medication-induced headache (MIH)* is used to describe these conditions. MIH is underdiagnosed and often difficult to manage. Though not well understood, it tends to occur in patients with a primary headache disorder (e.g., migraine, tension-type) who use immediate relief medications, often in excessive quantities.[80] Medications that have been implicated include NSAIDs, aspirin or acetylsalicylic acid (ASA), acetaminophen, barbiturate-analgesic combinations plus caffeine with or without codeine, opioids, caffeine, and ergotamine. Women are affected more commonly than men, and the most frequently affected age group is between 30 and 40 years of age.[81] The headache itself is variable and may be accompanied by asthenia, nausea, anxiety, depression, and difficulty with concentration.

The symptomatic medication that leads to the development of this disorder initially provides some pain relief to the patient, but over time tolerance develops, and larger doses are required to obtain symptomatic improvement.[81]

Treatment typically requires complete withdrawal of the medication being overused to achieve long-term results. In addition, these patients will require a comprehensive education and follow-up program involving pharmacologic, dietary, and behavioral components.[81]

Trigeminal Neuralgia

Trigeminal neuralgia is a painful unilateral affliction of the face, characterized by brief electric shock–like (lancinating) pains limited to the distribution of one or more divisions of the trigeminal nerve. Pain is commonly evoked by trivial stimuli (e.g., washing, shaving, smoking, talking, and brushing teeth), but also may occur spontaneously.[82] Individual attacks are brief, lasting a few seconds to less than 2 minutes, and are stereotyped in the individual patient. The lightning-like pains and unilateral grimaces so characteristic of trigeminal neuralgia led to the designation of the term *tic douloureux*.[82] The diagnosis is straightforward in most patients based on clinical criteria. Because these symptoms can be caused by an underlying mass lesion, CT or MRI is imperative in all cases, especially with sensory loss or motor dysfunction.

Several drugs have been effective in treating trigeminal neuralgia, including carbamazepine, phenytoin, and baclofen; however, about 30% of patients fail to respond to medical therapy.[83] In these patients, surgical management, including alcohol or glycerol injection or microvascular decompression, may be indicated.[84]

Cough and Exertional Headache

In some patients, severe headache can be provoked by coughing, sneezing, laughing, heavy lifting or exertion, and the Valsalva maneuver. The pain starts within a few seconds of the precipitant and is typically very brief when associated with cough but can last as long as 24 hours when associated with exertion. The headache is bilateral and throbbing in nature and in the majority of patients resolves spontaneously without persistent neurologic symptoms (e.g., neck stiffness or photophobia). In some patients, the headache may be secondary to structural lesions, especially in the posterior fossa[84]; therefore all patients require CT, or preferably MRI, to rule out intracranial disease including SAH. For patients with benign headache, treatment includes avoiding the underlying triggering mechanism and using analgesics as necessary. For patients with exertional headache, NSAIDs including indomethacin have been effective.

Coital Headache

Coital cephalgia is a recurrent, benign headache associated with sexual activity, and is more common in men than in women. It can occur just before, during, or immediately after orgasm. The headaches are usually dull and throbbing and last from minutes to hours. Occasionally, some patients will experience a sudden, explosive headache that occurs during orgasm. In these patients, SAH must be ruled out.[84,85]

High-Altitude Headache

Headache is one of the cardinal manifestations of acute mountain sickness and can occur at altitudes higher than 5000 feet above sea level in unacclimatized individuals. The headache is throbbing in nature, located in the temporal or occipital areas, and is probably caused by a mild increase in ICP. It is worse at night or in the early morning and exacerbated by the Valsalva maneuver or bending forward.[86] Other findings associated with high-altitude illness include fatigue, nausea, vomiting, dizziness, insomnia, and an altered mental status. Pulmonary edema and cerebral edema occur with severe cases. The treatment for these conditions includes supplemental oxygen and descent to a lower altitude.

KEY CONCEPTS

- Headache is a common presenting complaint in the ED. The emergency physician must distinguish between benign primary headache disorders and the more serious and potentially life-threatening secondary causes of headache.
- The majority of patients will not have abnormal neurologic findings; therefore the key to a successful diagnosis is a thorough and systematic history.
- Patients with the following headache presentations are at risk for serious underlying disease: sudden explosive headache, new-onset headache after age 50, headache associated with papilledema or focal neurologic symptoms, headache after head trauma, subacute headache with increasing frequency or severity, and headache associated with fever, cancer, or immunosuppression.
- The need for diagnostic studies will be dictated by the suspected secondary cause of headache.

REFERENCES

1. Centers for Disease Control and Prevention: *Vital and Health Statistics of the Centers for Disease Control and Prevention/National Center of Health Statistics, National Hospital Ambulatory Medical Survey: Emergency Department Survey,* 1995.
2. Saper JR: Headache disorders, *Med Clin North Am* 83:663, 1999.
3. Daroff RB: Classification and diagnostic criteria for headache disorders, cranial neuralgias and facial pain, Headache Classification Committee of the International Headache Society, *Cephalalgia* 8:1, 1988.
4. Diamond S, Diamond ML: Emergency treatment of migraine: insights into current options, *Postgrad Med* 101:169, 1997.
5. Silberstein S, Merriam G: Sex hormones and headache, 1999 (menstrual migraine), *Neurol* 53:S3, 1999.
6. Boyle CA: Management of menstrual migraine, *Neurol* 53:S14, 1999.
7. Kanner RM: Headache and facial pain. In Portenoy RK, Kanner RM, editors: *Pain management: theory and practice,* Philadelphia, 1996, FA Davis.
8. Capobianco DJ, Cheshire WP, Campbell JK: An overview of the diagnosis and pharmacologic treatment of migraine, *Mayo Clin Proc* 71:1055, 1996.
9. Raskin NH: On the origin of head pain, *Headache* 28:254, 1988.
10. Barre F: Cocaine as an abortive agent in cluster headache, *Headache* 22:69, 1982.
11. Bell R et al: A comparative trial of three agents in the treatment of acute migraine headache, *Ann Emerg Med* 19:1079, 1990.
12. Moskowitz MA: The neurobiology of vascular head pain, *Ann Neurol* 16:157, 1984.
13. Silberstein SD: Serotonin (5-HT) and migraine, *Headache* 34:408, 1994.
14. Campbell JK: Manifestations of migraine, *Neurol Clin* 8:841, 1990.
15. Troost BT: Ophthalmoplegic migraine, *Biomed Pharmacother* 50:49, 1996.
16. Bickerstaff ER: Basilar artery migraine, *Lancet* 1:15, 1961.
17. Moffert AM, Sash M, Scott DF: Effect of chocolate in migraine: a double-blind study, *J Neurol Neurosurg Psychiatry* 37:445, 1974.
18. Monro J, Carini C, Brostoff J: Migraine is a food-allergic disease, *Lancet* 2:719, 1984.
19. Frishberg BM: Neuroimaging in presumed primary headache disorders, *Semin Neurol* 17:373, 1997.
20. Baumel B: Migraine: a pharmacologic review with newer options and delivery modalities, *Neurol* 44:S13, 1994.
21. Edmeads J: Advances in migraine therapy: focus on oral sumatriptan, *Neurol* 45:S3, 1995.
22. Lane PL, McLellan BA, Baggoley CJ: Comparative efficacy of chlorpromazine and meperidine with dimenhydrinate in migraine headache, *Ann Emerg Med* 18:360, 1989.
23. Edmeads J: Emergency management of headache, *Headache* 28:675, 1988.
24. Diener HC, Limmroth V: The treatment of migraine, *Rev Contemp Pharmacother* 5:271, 1994.
25. Tfelt-Hansen P: Prophylactic pharmacotherapy of migraine: some practical guidelines, *Neurol Clin* 15:153, 1997.
26. Graham JR et al: Fibrotic disorders associated with methysergide therapy for headache, *N Engl J Med* 274:359, 1966.
27. Mathew NT: Cluster headache, *Semin Neurol* 17:313, 1997.
28. Sturm JW, Donnan GA: Diagnosis and investigation of headache, *Aust Fam Physician* 27:587, 1998.
29. Nappi G, Russell D: Symptomatology of cluster headache. In Olesen J, Tfelt-Hansen P, Welch KMA, editors: *The headaches,* ed 2, Philadelphia, 2000, Lippincott Williams & Wilkins.
30. Ekbom K: Sumatriptan in the management of cluster headache, *Rev Contemp Pharmacother* 5:311, 1994.
31. Fogan L: Treatment of cluster headache: a double-blind comparison of oxygen *v.* air inhalation, *Arch Neurol* 42:362, 1985.
32. Ekbom K, Solomon S: Management of cluster headache. In Olesen J, Tfelt-Hansen P, Welch KMA, editors: *The headaches,* ed 2, Philadelphia, 2000, Lippincott Williams & Wilkins.
33. Jensen R: Pathophysiological mechanisms of tension-type headache: a review of epidemiological and experimental studies, *Cephalalgia* 19:602, 1999.
34. Spira PJ: Tension headache, *Aust Fam Physician* 27:597, 1998.
35. Jensen R, Paiva T: Symptomatology of episodic tension-type headache. In Olesen J, Tfelt-Hansen P, Welch KMA, editors: *The headaches,* ed 2, Philadelphia, 2000, Lippincott Williams & Wilkins.
36. Iversen HK et al: Clinical characteristics of migraine and episodic tension-type headache in relation to old and new diagnostic criteria, *Headache* 30:514, 1990.
37. Schoenen J, Jensen R: Differential diagnosis and prognosis of tension-type headache. In Olesen J, Tfelt-Hansen P, Welch KMA, editors: *The headaches,* ed 2, Philadelphia, 2000, Lippincott Williams & Wilkins.
38. Becker KJ: Epidemiology and clinical presentation of aneurysmal subarachnoid hemorrhage, *Neurosurg Clin North Am* 9:435, 1998.
39. Edlow JA, Caplan LR: Avoiding pitfalls in the diagnosis of subarachnoid hemorrhage, *N Engl J Med* 342:29, 2000.

40. Locksley HB: Report on the cooperative study of intracranial aneurysms and subarachnoid hemorrhage, Sect. V, Part I: natural history of subarachnoid hemorrhage, intracranial aneurysms and arteriovenous malformations: based on 6368 cases in the Cooperative Study, *J Neurosurg* 25:219, 1966.
41. Linn F et al: Prospective study of sentinel headache in aneurysmal subarachnoid hemorrhage, *Lancet* 344:590, 1994.
42. Levine S et al: Cerebrovascular complications of the use of the "crack" form of alkaloidal cocaine, *N Engl J Med* 323:699, 1990.
43. Newman LC, Lipton RB: Emergency department evaluation of headache, *Neurol Clin* 16:285, 1998.
44. Hunt WE, Hess RM: Surgical risk as related to time intervention in the repair of intracranial aneurysm, *J Neurosurg* 28:14, 1968.
45. Schull MJ: Lumbar puncture first: an alternative model for the investigation of lone acute sudden headache, *Acad Emerg Med* 6:131, 1999.
46. Fishman RA: *Cerebrospinal fluid in diseases of the nervous system,* Philadelphia, 1992, WB Saunders.
47. Roost KT et al: The formation of cerebrospinal fluid xanthochromia after subarachnoid hemorrhage: enzymatic conversion of hemoglobin to bilirubin by the arachnoid and choroid plexus, *Neurol* 22:973, 1972.
48. Sawin PD, Loftus CM: Diagnosis of spontaneous subarachnoid hemorrhage, *Am Fam Physician* 55:145, 1997.
49. Adams HP, del Zoppo GJ, von Kummer R: Management of stroke: a practical guide for the prevention, evaluation and treatment of acute stroke, Caddo, Okla, 1998, Professional Communications.
50. Forsyth PA, Posner JB: Headaches in patients with brain tumors: a study of 111 patients, *Neurol* 43:1678, 1993.
51. Zimm S et al: Intracerebral metastases in solid-tumor patients: natural history and results of treatment, *Cancer* 48:384, 1981.
52. Patchell RA, Posner JB: Neurologic complications of systemic cancer, *Neurol Clin* 3:729, 1985.
53. Welch KMA et al: Headache in the emergency room. In Olesen J, Tfelt-Hansen P, Welch KMA, editors: *The headaches,* ed 2, Philadelphia, 2000, Lippincott Williams & Wilkins.
54. Newton HB et al: Clinical presentation, diagnosis, and pharmacotherapy of patients with primary brain tumors, *Ann Pharmacother* 33:816, 1999.
55. Moltyaner Y, Tenenbaum J: Temporal arteritis: a review and case history, *J Fam Pract* 43:294, 1996.
56. Badran RH, Weir RJ, McGuinness JB: Hypertension and headache, *Scott Med J* 15:48, 1970.
57. Keltner JL: Giant-cell arteritis: signs and symptoms, *Ophthalmol* 89:1101, 1982.
58. Stahmer SA, Raps EC, Mines DI: Carotid and vertebral artery dissections, *Emerg Med Clin North Am* 15:677, 1997.
59. Bogousslavsky J: Dissections of the cerebral arteries: clinical effects, *Curr Opin Neurol* 1:63, 1988.
60. Hart RG, Easton JD: Dissections of cervical and cerebral arteries, *Neurol Clin* 1:155, 1983.
61. Pozzati E et al: Long-term follow-up of occlusive cervical carotid dissection, *Stroke* 21:528, 1990.
62. Caplan LR, Tettenborn B: Vertebrobasilar occlusive disease: review of selected aspects, *Cerebrovasc Dis* 2:256, 1992.
63. Mokri B: Traumatic and spontaneous extracranial internal carotid artery dissections, *J Neurol* 237:356, 1990.
64. Sztajnkrycer M, Jauch EC: Unusual headaches, *Emerg Med Clin North Am* 16:741, 1998.
65. Sorensen PS, Corbett JJ: High cerebrospinal fluid pressure. In Olesen J, Tfelt-Hansen P, Welch KMA, editors: *The headaches,* ed 2, Philadelphia, 2000, Lippincott Williams & Wilkins.
66. Corbett JJ et al: Visual loss in pseudotumor cerebri: follow-up of 57 patients from five to 41 years and a profile of 14 patients with permanent severe visual loss, *Arch Neurol* 39:461, 1982.
67. Packard RC: Epidemiology and pathogenesis of posttraumatic headache, *J Head Trauma Rehabil* 14:9, 1999.
68. Gobel H, Martin T: Ocular disorders. In Olesen J, Tfelt-Hansen P, Welch KMA editors: *The headaches,* ed 2, Philadelphia, 2000, Lippincott Williams & Wilkins.
69. Hedges TR: An ophthalmologist's view of headache, *Headache* 19:151, 1979.
70. Evans RW: Complications of lumbar puncture, *Neurol Clin* 16:83, 1998.
71. Tarkkila PJ, Miralles JA, Palomaki EA: The subjective complications and efficiency of the epidural blood patch in the treatment of postdural puncture headache, *Reg Anesth* 14:247, 1989.
72. Duffy PJ, Crosby ET: The epidural blood patch: resolving the controversies, *Can J Anaesth* 46:878, 1999.
73. Dittmann M et al: Spinal anaesthesia with 29-gauge Quincke point needles and post dural puncture headache in 2378 patients, *Acta Anaesthesiol Scand* 38:691, 1994.
74. Sathi S, Stieg PE: "Acquired" Chiari I malformation after multiple lumbar punctures: case report, *Neurosurg* 32:306, 1993.
75. Drexler ED: Severe headaches: when to worry, what to do, *Postgrad Med* 87:164-170, 173-180, 1990.
76. Weinke T et al: Cryptococcus in AIDS patients: observations concerning CNS involvement, *J Neurol* 236:38, 1989.
77. Marinis M, Welch M: Headache associated with intracranial infection. In Olesen J, Tfelt-Hansen P, Welch KMA, editors: *The headaches,* ed 2, Philadelphia, 2000, Lippincott Williams & Wilkins.
78. Strandgaard S, Henry P: Arterial hypertension. In Olesen J, Tfelt-Hansen P, Welch KMA, editors: *The headaches,* ed 2, Philadelphia, 2000, Lippincott Williams & Wilkins.
79. Sjaastad O, Fredriksen TA, Pfaffenrath V: Cervicogenic headache: diagnostic criteria, *Headache* 30:725, 1990.
80. Mathew NT: Transformed migraine, analgesic rebound, and other chronic daily headaches, *Neurol Clin* 15:167, 1997.
81. Zed PJ, Loewen PS, Robinson G: Medication-induced headache: overview and systematic review of therapeutic approaches, *Ann Pharmacother* 33:61, 1999.
82. Terrence C, Jensen T: Trigeminal neuralgia and other facial neuralgias. In Olesen J, Tfelt-Hansen P, Welch KMA, editors: *The headaches,* ed 2, Philadelphia, 2000, Lippincott Williams & Wilkins.
83. Newton HB et al: Clinical presentation, diagnosis, and pharmacotherapy of patients with primary brain tumors, *Ann Pharmacother* 33:816, 1999.
84. Pascual J et al: Cough, exertional and sexual headaches: an analysis of 72 benign and symptomatic cases, *Neurol* 46:1520, 1996.
85. Banerjee A: Coital emergencies, *Postgrad Med J* 72:653, 1996.
86. Harris MD et al: High-altitude medicine, *Am Fam Physician* 57:1907, 1998.

98 Organic Brain Syndrome

Jeffrey Smith
Jennifer Seirafi

PERSPECTIVE

Physicians in the ED are often confronted with patients who present with signs and symptoms of a confusional state. These patients can pose a diagnostic challenge. Simply determining if such a state is acute, subacute, or chronic can be difficult. The confusional state can be a harbinger of serious medical conditions or psychiatric disorders. The physician in the ED has a unique opportunity to accurately diagnose and manage these patients. He or she must decide who needs prompt intervention, who needs diagnostic evaluation (i.e., laboratory studies, lumbar puncture, a computed tomography [CT] scan of the head) in the ED, who needs hospitalization, and who can be safely discharged. This chapter is divided into the topics of delirium and dementia. The focus will be on the key pathophysiologic and clinical features of delirium and dementia and the management of these patients.

Organic brain syndrome is a nebulous term that encompasses a host of abnormal cognitive states in which the unifying and defining feature is confusion (i.e., the inability to think with normal speed and clarity). The *Diagnostic and Statistical Manual of Mental Disorders (DSM-IV)* no longer classifies delirium and dementia as "organic" mental disorders because of the inaccurate implication that "nonorganic" mental disorders are without a biologic basis.[1] Organic brain syndrome loosely defines a group of cognitive disorders that are secondary to central nervous system (CNS) disease, systemic disorders, or substance-related disorders. In general, acute organic brain syndrome is synonymous with delirium, and chronic organic brain syndrome is synonymous with dementia. The essential finding present in both of these conditions is a confusional state manifesting as global cognitive impairment. Global impairment involves all aspects of higher cortical function; patients may manifest disordered behavior, emotions, judgment, language, abstract thinking, and psychomotor activity. These disorders encompass a wide spectrum of behavioral abnormalities; a patient may be quiet and withdrawn or emotionally labile, agitated, and hallucinating. Although certain aspects of the global impairment are more pronounced in certain individuals, minor deficiencies in other areas of cognitive functioning are usually present.

Several key features best distinguish the disorders of delirium and dementia. These are the time course of disease evolution; the presence of autonomic system involvement; the level of disturbance of consciousness, orientation, and perception; and the acuity of the underlying disease process. In delirium, the widespread cerebral dysfunction typically lasts hours to days, although resolution can take weeks. Delirium is characterized by a disturbance in level of consciousness. The patient usually has some autonomic system abnormalities, as seen in the prototypical condition of delirium tremens, with fever, tachycardia, hypertension, and diaphoresis. Delirium is a direct consequence of an acute systemic or CNS disturbance or insult; milder degrees of disturbance are often not associated with these cognitive impairments. Dementia, which is also characterized by confusion, tends to follow a more gradual course, with the evolution occurring over months to years. There is usually no disturbance in consciousness and perception. There are minimal or no manifestations of autonomic nervous system abnormalities. Most cases of dementia originate in the CNS, and many are irreversible.

When evaluating patients with a confusional state, the physician must keep in mind some basic guidelines. First, he or she must decide whether this state represents delirium or dementia. The diagnosis may seem obvious. However, early symptoms and signs may go unrecognized by the physician unless an adequate history is obtained from the patient and family members and a careful examination, including a brief mental status examination, is performed. Second, supportive care must be provided. This may vary from aggressive airway and cardiovascular support to pharmacologic or physical restraint to simply placing the patient in a quiet room. Third, a diligent search must be initiated for the underlying disease process causing the global cognitive impairment. Always keep in mind that the terms *delirium* and *dementia* are purely descriptive terms that define a group of signs and symptoms but do not define the cause of the altered cognitive state. Finally, and most important, the underlying illness that has been identified must be treated when possible. This is especially crucial with the delirious patient, because immediate initiation of therapy can prevent permanent disability.

Physicians are commonly asked to distinguish a psychiatric or "functional" condition from an acute or chronic organic brain syndrome. Although the distinction may seem intuitively obvious to some physicians, it is not always readily apparent in the emergency setting. In a busy ED the physician must resist the temptation to distinguish psychiatric from organic illnesses prematurely on the basis of a single item in a patient's history or a previous psychiatric illness. To "clear" a patient medically for admission to a psychiatric or detoxification unit, a careful history and examination should be conducted to exclude a medical condition masquerading as a psychiatric disorder. In some patients it is not always possible to exclude a medical problem compounding an apparent psychiatric illness during a brief ED stay, and the medical evaluation should continue after these patients are hospitalized.

DELIRIUM

Perspective

Delirium can be defined as acute cognitive dysfunction secondary to some underlying medical condition. Terms that have been used interchangeably with delirium include *acute organic brain syndrome, acute confusional state, reversible cerebral dysfunction, metabolic encephalopathy, toxic en-*

cephalopathy, and *febrile delirium.* The word *delirium* is derived from the Latin *delirare,* which literally means "to go out of the furrow" (*lira,* Latin "furrow"), but is used figuratively to mean crazy or deranged.[2] The true incidence of delirium in patients in the ED is unknown. However, delirium is present at the time of hospital admission in up to 20% of medical patients.[3] Of hospitalized patients, the prevalence of delirium has been noted to be approximately 10% on a general medical service (16% of patients over 70 years of age), 40% on the neurologic service, 8% to 12% on the psychiatric service, and 35% to 80% on the geriatric service.[4] Geriatric patients are at particularly high risk for developing delirium; however, the incidence is also higher in women, Caucasians, and young children.

Several predisposing factors for the development of delirium have been identified. These factors include age above 60, addiction to drugs or alcohol, and any history of brain damage secondary to trauma or vascular insult.[5] Baseline dementia is also an important risk factor for the development of delirium. The use of physical restraints, malnutrition, any iatrogenic intervention, or the use of more than three medications may precipitate delirium in the elderly hospitalized patient.[6] Predictive factors for the development of postoperative delirium after elective noncardiac surgery include age above 70, alcohol abuse, poor functional or cognitive status, and a markedly abnormal preoperative serum sodium, potassium, or glucose level.[7] Severe psychologic stress and sleep deprivation may facilitate the development of delirium. Once delirium has developed, the patient's basic personality, coping style, intelligence, and level of education can modify manifestations of the acute disability.

Several key features are necessary to make a diagnosis of delirium (Box 98-1). Patients with delirium have disturbances in consciousness, cognition, and perception. These disturbances tend to occur over a short period of time (hours to days). The disturbance in consciousness may present as an inability to focus attention. Deficiencies in cognition may manifest as disorientation and memory deficits. Perceptual disturbances include hallucinations or delusions. The delirious patient may be somnolent or agitated, and the thought process may be mildly disturbed or grossly disorganized. The clinical presentation may be subdued or explosive, and the course can fluctuate over minutes to hours. The patient's sleep-wake cycle may be altered or reversed; agitation is often present during the night. The patient's behavior is unpredictable. Historically, delirium referred to the hyperactive, agitated, emotionally labile patient (i.e., the individual with acute phencyclidine intoxication or delirium tremens). There have been attempts to distinguish between hyperactive and hypoactive delirium.[8] It is important to recognize that the spectrum of delirium is broad and can encompass hyperactive, depressed, and mixed states of consciousness.

Box 98-1 Diagnostic Criteria for Delirium

Clouding of consciousness with reduced ability to focus, sustain, or shift attention. A cognitive change (e.g., memory deficit, disorientation, language disturbance) or perceptual disturbance that is not better accounted for by a preexisting, established, or evolving dementia.

The disturbance develops over hours to days and tends to fluctuate during the course of the day.

Evidence from the history, physical examination, or laboratory findings that the disturbance is caused by a general medical condition, medication or other substance exposure, substance withdrawal, or multiple etiologies.

Modified from American Psychiatric Association: *Diagnostic and statistical manual of mental disorders,* ed 4, text revision, Washington, DC, 2000, American Psychiatric Association.

Principles of Disease

Pathophysiology At a cellular level, delirium is the result of widespread alteration in cerebral metabolic activity, with secondary dysregulation of neurotransmitter synthesis and metabolism. The elderly are particularly susceptible to any change in cerebral biochemical activity. Both the cerebral cortex and the subcortical structures are affected, producing changes in arousal, alertness, attention, information processing, and normal sleep-wake cycle.

Although the exact pathophysiology is not well understood, multiple neurotransmitters have been implicated in causing delirium. Acetylcholine transmission may be one of the important factors in the development of delirium; in addition to anticholinergic medicines causing delirium, serum anticholinergic activity is increased in older patients with delirium.[9] Increased serotonin levels have been found in hepatic encephalopathy, serotonin syndrome, sepsis, and psychedelic drug ingestion.[10] Some of the disturbances that occur in delirium are deficiencies of substrates for oxidative metabolism (e.g., glucose, oxygen); disturbances of ionic passage through excitable membranes; an increase in cytokines; an imbalance of normal noradrenergic, serotonergic, and cholinergic homeostasis; and in select cases, synthesis of false neurotransmitters.[11] Drugs and exogenous toxins can produce delirium by direct effects on the CNS. Although the limbic system appears particularly vulnerable to the effects of these drugs, the cerebral hemispheres and the brainstem can also be profoundly affected.

Tricyclic antidepressants can cause delirium by causing cholinergic inhibition and increasing the concentration of norepinephrine and serotonin at receptor sites.[12] Sedative hypnotics such as the benzodiazepines depress activity in the CNS, especially in the limbic system, thalamus, and hypothalamus. Phenothiazines and other major tranquilizers accumulate in the brain at four times the plasma concentration and have similar depressant effects on the CNS. Barbiturates suppress axon impulse transmission. Narcotics affect CNS activity primarily by interacting with various opioid receptor sites. Depending on the receptor type, the physiologic response may be analgesia, euphoria, sedation, dysphoria, delusions, or hallucinations. Psychedelic drugs probably act as agonists at serotonin receptor sites and increase activity in the cerebral cortex and limbic forebrain. Phencyclidine (PCP) inhibits reuptake of dopamine, norepinephrine, serotonin, and gamma-aminobutyric acid (GABA) and may also act as a false neurotransmitter.

Hyperthermia and hypothermia can cause delirium, probably as a result of changes in the cerebral metabolic rate. In hypothermia, cerebral metabolism decreases 6% to 7% for each 1° C decrease in temperature from 35° to 25° C. Temperature-dependent enzyme systems in the brain are unable to function at low temperatures. In hyperthermia, cellular damage with uncoupling of oxidative phosphorylation begins to occur at temperatures greater than 42° C. Patients suffering from heat stroke may have cerebral edema, degenerative neuronal changes (especially involving Purkinje cells of the cerebellum), and petechiae in the walls of the third and fourth ventricles. Delirium occurring at temperatures below 40° C is multifactorial in origin and not solely caused by increased core temperature.

Delirium caused by metabolic abnormalities such as hyponatremia, hypernatremia, hyperosmolarity, and hypercapnia is associated with a variety of metabolic disturbances at the neuronal and astrocyte level, including impaired energy supplies, changes in resting membrane potentials, and changes in cellular morphology. The high brain ammonia concentration that occurs in hepatic encephalopathy may interfere with cerebral energy metabolism and the sodium-potassium-adenosine triphosphatase (Na-K-ATPase) pump. False neurotransmitters are present in patients with hepatic encephalopathy, and structurally there are increases in the number and size of astrocytes. Acute encephalopathy in renal failure is caused at least partially by increased permeability of the blood-brain barrier to toxic substances such as organic acids. Changes in brain water volume probably play a role in the cognitive impairment that occurs in diabetic ketoacidosis, the nonketotic hyperosmolar state, and hyponatremia.

Most patients who have delirium have reduced cerebral metabolic activity. This reduction in cerebral metabolism is reflected by a decrease in the frequency of electroencephalograph (EEG) background activity. Exceptions are hyperthermia, sedative-hypnotic withdrawal, delirium tremens, and certain drug-induced states in which the cerebral metabolism is either normal or increased.

Etiology Delirium has many causes (Table 98-1). Recreational and prescribed drug use are responsible for most cases of acute delirium.[13] Among the elderly, medications are the most common cause of delirium, accounting for 22% to 39% of cases.[14,15] Acute cognitive dysfunction may be secondary to drug overdose, withdrawal, or adverse or idiosyncratic reactions. Delirium that begins while patients are taking a drug usually disappears after the drug use is stopped. Other agents, including ethanol, cause acute delirium when discontinued abruptly.

The list of commonly prescribed drugs causing delirium is quite extensive and includes antibiotics (antifungal, antimalarial, and antiviral agents; quinolones; and clarithromycin), anticholinergic drugs (antihistamines, antispasmodics, tricyclic antidepressants), anticonvulsants, antiinflammatory agents (corticosteroids, salicylates, nonsteroidal antiinflammatory drugs [NSAIDs]), various cardiovascular medications (β-blockers, antidysrhythmics, antihypertensives, cardiac glycosides), sympathomimetics (phenylpropanolamine), sedative hypnotics, narcotics (transdermal fentanyl [Duragesic], morphine, Dilaudid), miscellaneous drugs (aminophylline, cimetidine, lithium, chlorpropamide), and over-the-counter medications (Compoz, Sominex) that have anticholinergic properties.[16-20] Delirium has also been reported in healthy young adults who consume caffeine-containing stimulants and large quantities of cola.[21-22]

Many "street" drugs with significant abuse potential such as hallucinogens, amphetamines, PCP, cocaine, and MDMA (ecstasy) can cause delirium.[23] Intoxication with any of the alcohols (ethanol, methanol, and ethylene glycol) can cause acute delirium. Ethanol withdrawal causes a full spectrum of symptoms ranging from mild anxiety to florid delirium tremens with agitation and autonomic hyperactivity. Delirium can also occur as part of the withdrawal syndrome associated with barbiturates, sedative hypnotics, opiates, and sympathomimetics.

Table 98-1. Causes of Delirium ("I Watch Death")

Cause	Form
Infectious	Sepsis, encephalitis, meningitis, syphilis, CNS abscess
Withdrawal	Alcohol, barbiturates, sedative hypnotics
Acute metabolic	Acidosis, electrolyte disturbance, hepatic and renal failure, other metabolic disturbances (glucose, Mg^{++}, Ca^{++})
Trauma	Head trauma, burns
CNS disease	Hemorrhage, cerebrovascular accident, vasculitis, seizures, tumor
Hypoxia	Acute hypoxia, chronic lung disease, hypotension
Deficiencies	B_{12}, hypovitaminosis, niacin, thiamine
Environmental	Hypothermia, hyperthermia, endocrinopathies: diabetes, adrenal, thyroid
Acute vascular	Hypertensive emergency, subarachnoid hemorrhage, sagittal vein thrombosis
Toxins/drugs	Medications, street drugs, alcohols, pesticides, industrial poisons: carbon monoxide, cyanide, solvents, etc.
Heavy metals	Lead, mercury

Modified from Wise MG: Delirium: differential diagnosis for delirium: critical items (I WATCH DEATH). In Yudofsky SC, Hales RE, editors: *The American Psychiatric Press textbook of neuropsychiatry,* ed 2, Washington, DC, 1992, American Psychiatric Publishing.

Exposure to industrial chemicals (e.g., carbon disulfide, heavy metals, insecticides, cyanide, and carbon monoxide) can cause a wide range of symptoms that include acute delirium. Delirium has also been reported after the inhalation of typewriter correction fluid and is attributed to the active ingredients trichloroethane and trichloroethylene.[24] In addition, ingestion of certain plants (e.g., nutmeg, foxglove, jimsonweed, and psilocybin-containing mushrooms) can cause delirium.

An acute confusional state can be one of the protean manifestations of a metabolic or nutritional abnormality. The most common metabolic disorder causing acute organic brain syndrome is diabetes mellitus. Hypoglycemia is the most common and readily reversible cause of acute confusion in the diabetic patient. Other causes of acute cognitive impairment in the diabetic patient are hyperglycemia, hyperosmolarity, and acid-base abnormalities. Fluid and electrolyte disorders can be a common cause of altered sensorium, particularly in the child and elderly adult. Dehydration, hypernatremia, hyponatremia, hypercalcemia, hypomagnesemia, hypermagnesemia, hypophosphatemia, or hyperphosphatemia can cause delirium. Other metabolic causes include hypoxemia, hepatic insufficiency, renal insufficiency, and dysfunction of various endocrine glands, including hyperthyroidism, hypothyroidism, Cushing's syndrome, and hyperparathyroidism. Deficiency of niacin, pyridoxine, folic acid, and vitamin B_{12} may be associated with acute confusional states.

Delirium can be a prominent feature of any systemic infection, particularly in very young, elderly, or immunocompromised patients. Infectious and host factors together determine the degree of cognitive impairment. Extracranial infections that are associated with delirium include sepsis (particularly gram-negative sepsis), subacute bacterial endocarditis, Legionnaires' disease, Rocky Mountain spotted fever, malaria, typhoid fever, toxic shock syndrome, and several viral infections, including influenza. Patients with CNS infections, including meningitis, encephalitis, and intracerebral abscess, may have acute cognitive dysfunction.

Acute delirium occasionally can be the first manifestation of an intracranial space-occupying lesion such as a subdural hematoma, tumor (especially frontal lobe), or hydrocephalus. The size and location of the lesion determine whether focal neurologic findings are present.

Other less common causes of delirium include infarction in the distribution of the nondominant middle cerebral artery and the posterior cerebral artery. Patients who have collagen vascular disease with CNS vasculitis may have prominent neuropsychiatric manifestations, including acute delirium. Remote effects of visceral neoplasms unrelated to the presence of metastases can cause paraneoplastic encephalopathy, with symptoms of confusion, catatonia, and dementia.

Patients who are immunocompromised may have multiple and unusual causes of acute delirium. Patients with immunosuppression secondary to malignancy, drugs, or human immunodeficiency virus type 1 (HIV-1) infection may have acute brain dysfunction secondary to infection, complications of drug therapy, or the underlying disease itself. Patients with HIV-1 infection may experience delirium caused by various CNS infections (toxoplasmosis, cryptococcus, cytomegalovirus, herpes simplex, retroviral, or bacterial) or CNS malignancy (lymphoma) with minimal focal neurologic findings. In addition, patients with HIV-1 infection may have delirium secondary to various approved or investigational drugs.

Acute confusional states have been reported to be a more common herald of the onset of physical illness in the elderly than fever, pain, and tachycardia.[25] In addition, the elderly are very susceptible to the toxicities of many commonly prescribed drugs, especially those medications with anticholinergic properties.[26-28] Some of the most commonly prescribed drugs for the elderly, including cimetidine, ranitidine (Zantac), codeine, warfarin, isosorbide, theophylline, nifedipine (Procardia), and digoxin, have been shown to cause significant impairments in tests of recent memory and attention in normal elderly patients. Factors that predispose older adults to delirium include the aging brain, reduced capacity for homeostatic regulation, impaired vision and hearing, and age-related changes in the pharmacokinetics and pharmacodynamics of drugs. The most common cause of delirium in the elderly is multifactorial.[14] Other common causes of delirium in the elderly are infections (especially pneumonia and urinary tract), congestive heart failure, pain (myocardial infarction, ischemic bowel), hypovolemia, sodium depletion, dehydration, malnutrition, and organ failure. Alcoholism and alcohol withdrawal symptoms are also common in the elderly.

Clinical Findings

The clinical manifestations of delirium are as variable as the causes. The clinical presentation can be subtle and unrecognized or dramatic and disruptive in the ED. Patients with an evolving delirium may be in either a hyperactive or a withdrawn state.

Nonspecific prodromal symptoms such as anxiety, restlessness, and insomnia typically progress over hours to days. The most consistent features of delirium are global cognitive impairment, relatively rapid onset of symptoms, and a clinical course that fluctuates over a period of hours to days. The fluctuation in symptoms over hours can be striking. Patients may be agitated and confused at home, yet appear subdued and behave more appropriately during the ED evaluation.

Key aspects of cognitive impairment should be evident to the emergency physician during a careful history and examination of the delirious patient. Disturbance in attention is central to the diagnosis of delirium. The patient is easily distractible and has difficulty remaining focused on a particular topic or interacting with a single individual. Disorientation often accompanies the deficit in attention; however, this finding is not always present. The patient usually is disoriented to time and occasionally is disoriented to place; in extreme cases, there may be disorientation to person. Acute organic brain syndrome, however, may be present in a patient who is completely oriented to person, place, and time. A "mental status examination" that consists solely of questions that assess orientation will not detect delirium in these instances.

The patient with delirium always has some degree of memory impairment. One of the hallmarks of delirium is impairment in short-term memory, with inability to learn and assimilate new information. Remote memory, or memory of past events, is usually preserved. Thought processes and speech may be disorganized. Disturbance in the sleep-wake cycle often occurs early in the course of delirium. A history of insomnia, restlessness, daytime sleepiness, and disturbances in sleep continuity often can be elicited from the patient, family, or friends. Characteristically, the sleep-wake cycle is reversed because patients sleep during the day and are awake throughout the night.

Perceptual disturbances, including misperception of the environment, poorly formed delusions, and hallucinations, are common in patients with acute organic brain syndrome. The delirious patient may experience visual, auditory, tactile, gustatory, or olfactory hallucinations, in contrast to patients with acute functional psychosis, who typically experience only auditory hallucinations. In addition, the delirious patient has a reduced capacity to modulate fine emotional expression and may demonstrate emotional lability. The patient typically manifests undue readiness to laugh, cry, or become angry and may shift rapidly from one form of emotional expression to another.

The evaluation of the cognitively impaired patient must include investigation of a number of key historical points. Because of impairment in cognitive function, the history the emergency physician can obtain from the patient is often incomplete and inaccurate. Family, friends, and prehospital care providers should also be used as sources of information about the patient. The emergency physician should inquire about the patient's medical history and current medical problems, including diabetes, hypertension, kidney or liver disease, and any neurologic or psychiatric problems. It is important to determine whether the patient is immunosuppressed or has risk factors that may predispose to an immunosuppressed state (former transfusions, sexual promiscuity, homosexuality, intravenous [IV] drug use, immunosuppressive therapy, or underlying malignancy). A detailed medication history, including the use of prescribed and over-the-counter medications, alcohol or substance abuse, and use of other medications in the home, is essential. It is important to identify when the symptoms began and whether any prior episodes of similar problems have occurred. Prehospital personnel should be able to provide information about the home environment, medication bottles belonging to the patient or found near the patient, and the possibility of trauma.

The physical examination should begin with a careful assessment of vital signs, noting the presence of fever or hypothermia, hypertension, tachycardia, or abnormal respiratory rate. The delirious patient often has some abnormality in vital signs. The examination should include assessment of the head for signs of trauma and the pupils for symmetry of light reflex; funduscopic examination for hemorrhage or papilledema; examination of the ears for hemotympanum; evaluation of the neck for nuchal rigidity, bruits, and thyroid enlargement; evaluation of the heart and lungs; evaluation of the abdomen for organomegaly and ascites; and examination of the extremities for cyanosis. The skin should be carefully examined for rashes, petechiae, ecchymosis, splinter hemorrhages, and needle tracks. The neurologic examination should include assessment of the cranial nerves, motor strength, sensation, and presence of abnormal movements (e.g., tremor, asterixis, and myoclonus). The reflexes should be assessed for symmetry and presence of hyperreflexia or hyporeflexia. Overlap exists between findings that typically suggest a metabolic or structural neurologic problem. Asterixis is a hallmark of metabolic encephalopathy but can be seen in focal brain disease as either a unilateral or a bilateral finding and can also result from the presence of blood in the subarachnoid space.[28] Focal neurologic signs that typically are associated with structural CNS lesions can also be present in metabolic encephalopathy as a result of hypoglycemia or hyperglycemia, hepatic encephalopathy, uremia, and hypercalcemia.

The emergency physician must be comfortable performing a brief mental status examination on all patients suspected of having acute brain dysfunction. Although the concept is rather obvious, few physicians proceed beyond questions about the patient's orientation to person, place, and time when assessing mental status.[29,30] A physician's inability to diagnose subtle forms of delirium is directly related to failure to perform mental status testing, which all too often is perceived by physicians as time-consuming, awkward to administer, and difficult to interpret.

Mental status testing should include assessment of orientation, memory, attention, concentration, constructional tasks, spatial discrimination, arithmetic ability, and writing. These aspects of cognitive functioning can be assessed in approximately 5 minutes. Typically, disorientation to the environment begins with inability to recall the date, followed by disorientation to day of the week, time, month, year, then eventually place; only in the most severe cases is the person unable to identify self. Memory assessment requires testing the patient's ability to repeat short series of words or numbers (immediate recall), to learn new information (short-term memory), and to retrieve previously stored information (long-term memory). Constructional apraxia is the inability to perform constructional tasks, such as drawing geometric figures, clock faces, or connecting dots. Dysnomia (inability to name objects correctly) and dysgraphia (impaired writing ability) are two of the most sensitive indicators of delirium. Almost all acutely confused patients have writing impairments, including spatial disorganization, misspelling, and tremor.[31]

No single bedside cognitive test that can be administered quickly is ideal. Most of the studies evaluating the ability of the various tests to detect organic cognitive impairment have been based on hospitalized patients. The Mini-Mental Status Examination developed by Folstein and McHugh has been validated more than any other test.[30] For hospitalized patients, this test has a sensitivity of 87% and a specificity of 82% for detecting organic brain syndrome.[32] Some investigators report slightly better results when the test is modified and age is added as a variable in the analysis.[33,34]

The Mini-Mental Status Examination is one of the easiest and most reliable bedside tests that can be administered in the ED. It consists of a short series of questions that test orientation, registration (memory), attention, calculation, recall, and language (Figure 98-1). The registration section tests both immediate and short-term memory; the recall section also assesses short-term memory. The ability to recall two out of three objects has an 81% sensitivity and a 74% specificity for excluding organic brain syndrome. Asking the patient to subtract serial 7s backward from 100 tests attention, concentration, and arithmetic ability. This test is specific but not sensitive for absence of an organic brain syndrome; 40% to 50% of nondelirious, nondemented people fail to perform this test correctly. The Mini-Mental Status Examination can be performed in less than 5 minutes. A total score of 23 or below is considered abnormal and suggests an organic brain syndrome.

The Confusional Assessment Method (CAM) is another useful diagnostic tool and has a sensitivity of 93% to 100% and specificity of 90% to 95%.[35] This simple tool has four key features used for screening for delirium. These features are acute onset and fluctuating course, inattention, disorganized thinking, and altered level of consciousness. To make the diagnosis of delirium, the first two features and one of the last two must be present.

Any bedside cognitive test has limitations. Very mild degrees of cognitive impairment can be missed with bedside screening tests. The patient's level of education and general intelligence can substantially affect the outcome. Furthermore, a single bedside test is ahistorical: it reflects a patient's cognitive functioning at only one point in time. To establish a diagnosis of delirium (or dementia), the physician must show that there has been a decline from the patient's baseline cognitive functioning.

Once the emergency physician establishes that a patient is in a delirious state, it is often difficult to determine the cause of delirium immediately. Delirium is a nonspecific CNS manifestation of a multitude of structural or metabolic insults. The history and physical examination rarely establish the specific cause of the acute brain dysfunction. Further evaluation in the ED is usually necessary to arrive at the cause of the delirium.

All medications or drugs that the patient is taking should be reviewed. It is usually the history and not the physical examination that leads the emergency physician to suspect a specific overdose or adverse reaction to medication as the cause of the patient's delirium. The physical examination is not often helpful in determining the specific drug or class of drugs causing acute cognitive impairment. The one exception

Maximum Score	
	Orientation
5	What is the (year)(season)(date)(day)(month)?
5	Where are we (city)(state)(country)(hospital)(floor)?
	Registration
3	Name three objects: one second to say each. Ask the patient for all three after you have said them. Give one point for each correct answer. Repeat them until all three are learned. Count trials and record number.
	Attention and calculation
5	Serial sevens backward from 100 (stop after five answers). Alternatively, spell WORLD backward.
	Recall
3	Ask for the three objects repeated above. Give one point for each correct answer.
	Language and praxis
2	Show a pencil and watch, and ask subject to name them.
1	Ask the patient to repeat the following: "no ifs, ands, or buts."
3	(Three-stage command): "Take this paper in your right hand, fold it in half, and put it on the floor."
1	Read and obey the following: "Close your eyes." (Written on a piece of paper)
1	Write a sentence. (Must contain a noun, verb, and be sensible. Ignore grammar and punctuation.)
1	Copy this design (interlocking pentagons). Must contain all angles and two must intersect.

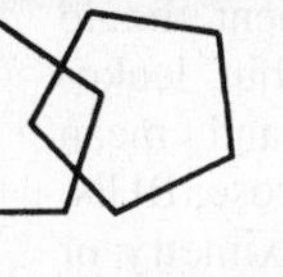

Figure 98-1. **Mini-Mental Status Examination.** *From Folstein MF et al:* J Psychiat Res *12:189, 1975.*

to this rule is toxidromes, which are constellations of signs and symptoms characteristic of intoxication with certain drugs or classes of drugs. Toxidromes can result from anticholinergic poisoning (fever, flushing, dry mucous membranes, tachycardia, and delirium), narcotic overdose (bradypnea, miosis, lethargy), and other drugs such as PCP (vertical nystagmus, bizarre behavior, agitation). Reversal of the symptoms with an antidote can confirm the diagnosis; however, when the history is not helpful, specific toxicology screens based on the physician's clinical suspicion may be useful.

Patients with metabolic or nutritional abnormalities causing delirium may have suggestive, albeit nondiagnostic, findings on examination. The diabetic patient with ketoacidosis may have a fruity breath odor; the patient with hepatic encephalopathy may have ascites and asterixis. Dehydration, hypernatremia, hypercalcemia, and uremia can often be suggested by clinical evaluation; however, laboratory evaluation is necessary to confirm the diagnosis and exclude coexistent conditions. As noted earlier, various systemic and CNS infections can cause delirium, especially in the very young and the elderly. The presence of fever, headache, nuchal rigidity, and photophobia suggests a CNS infection; these findings may not be present in debilitated or immunocompromised patients.

Patients who chronically abuse alcohol may have delirium caused by metabolic abnormalities, infection, nutritional deficiencies, CNS mass lesions (e.g., subdural hematoma), ethanol or other alcohol intoxication, pathologic intoxication, or alcohol withdrawal. Wernicke's encephalopathy produced by thiamine deficiency typically causes abrupt onset of oculomotor disturbances, ataxia, and mental confusion. The oculomotor disturbances range from nystagmus to complete gaze palsy; the ataxia is truncal. Both the oculomotor disturbances and the ataxia may precede the mental confusion by days. Global impairment with disorientation, inattention, and slowed response may proceed to frank stupor and coma if not treated promptly. Alcohol withdrawal syndrome, which occurs after a relative period of abstinence, consists of several clinical manifestations. The earliest and most common manifestation is tremulousness (i.e., "the shakes"), which, in general, presents with a clear but somewhat irritable sensorium. The next most common symptom of alcohol withdrawal syndrome is hallucinosis and disturbed perceptions. These tend to occur with the tremors. Withdrawal seizures occur most commonly within 12 to 24 hours after cessation of drinking. Delirium tremens is the fourth manifestation of alcohol withdrawal and is relatively rare. A precipitating event (e.g., major physical illness, including infection, trauma, liver disease, or metabolic disorder) often leads to the decrease in alcohol intake. The symptoms of delirium tremens usually develop 3 to 5 days after a reduction in alcohol consumption. The patient has delusions, vivid hallucinations, agitation, insomnia, mild fever, and marked autonomic arousal. The hallucinations are primarily visual and may be kinesthetic. Because the patient with delirium tremens has an acute confusional state with fever, meningitis is included in the differential diagnosis until ruled out by cerebrospinal fluid (CSF) analysis. Most cases of delirium tremens subside after 3 days of full-blown symptoms, although it can last weeks. Untreated, the mortality rate for delirium tremens is approximately 5% to 10%. With treatment, the mortality rate is substantially reduced.

Diagnostic Evaluation and Ancillary Studies

Delirium represents a true medical emergency because certain causes of delirium, when untreated, result in increased morbidity or death. It is imperative that the emergency physician proceed in a timely manner with the diagnostic evaluation of the patient. Although some of the causes of delirium require diagnostic testing beyond the scope of what is obtainable or appropriate in the ED, many readily reversible causes can be diagnosed by a series of basic tests available in all EDs.

The laboratory evaluation of the delirious patient should include a complete blood count (CBC) (hemoglobin, leukocyte count with differential, platelet count, and mean corpuscle volume); evaluation of electrolytes, glucose, BUN, and calcium; tests of liver function; and pulse oximetry or arterial blood gas (ABG) evaluation. The CBC will suggest unusual but potentially treatable abnormalities, such as thrombotic thrombocytopenic purpura, megaloblastic anemia, hyperviscosity from myelogenous leukemia, and unsuspected infection. The anion gap should be determined in all patients with altered mental status; an elevated anion gap (>15 mEq/L) may indicate the presence of unmeasured anions, such as sulfate in renal failure, ketoacids in diabetic or alcoholic ketoacidosis, lactate in postictal or hypotensive patients, and exogenous toxins such as ethylene glycol, methanol, or salicylates. A pulse oximeter measurement will detect hypoxemia. Febrile patients and those with suspected occult infection should have urinalysis and a chest radiograph. In the elderly, an electrocardiogram (ECG) should be obtained to exclude a silent myocardial infarction (MI) as a cause of the delirium. Results of this initial screen may be normal, necessitating further evaluation. Despite these diagnostic evaluations, no cause will be found for delirium in up to 16% of patients.[14]

Toxicology screens, although commonly overused and misused as diagnostic tests, have utility in the evaluation of certain patients with delirium. A toxicology evaluation is appropriate when no obvious cause of the alteration in sensorium can be identified. Laboratory techniques for toxicology screens consist of gas-liquid chromatography, high-performance liquid chromatography, and enzymatic analysis. Because various drugs have similar chromatogram patterns, the more information the clinician can provide to the laboratory, the better the yield of the toxicology screen. The mass spectroscope is more sensitive than the chromatogram and permits rapid and accurate determination of virtually any toxin; however, this sophisticated system is expensive and availability is limited.

Additional laboratory studies that may be appropriate when the cause of delirium remains unknown include tests of thyroid function; determinations of levels of B_{12}, folic acid, serum antinuclear antibodies, and urinary porphobilinogen; and screens for heavy metals. Although the results of such tests will not aid in the emergency physician's diagnosis, it may be reasonable to order these studies.

A spinal tap and CSF analysis are essential parts of the ED evaluation in many patients with delirium. Any patient with fever and cognitive dysfunction, even without meningismus, should have a lumbar puncture performed in the ED to rule out meningitis. This is true particularly for any patient who is immunocompromised and unlikely to show all the classic signs of meningitis. Patients with underlying malignancies, hepatic or renal failure, or acquired immunodeficiency syndrome (AIDS); elderly patients; alcoholics; and patients on chronic immunosuppressive therapy such as antimetabolites and steroids may not have the typical symptoms and signs of headache, fever, and stiff neck. Patients with focal neurologic findings, immunocompromised states, or findings of increased intracranial pressure should have a head CT before the spinal tap. They should receive antibiotics in the ED before the CT scan. Patients with subacute presentations suggestive of a CNS infection (i.e., symptoms that develop over days to weeks) who are not toxic-appearing can have antibiotic therapy delayed until after the head CT scan and lumbar puncture. Chronic tuberculous or cryptococcal meningitis does not require initiation of treatment while the patient is in the ED.

The spinal fluid should be sent for routine studies, including cell count, protein, glucose, Gram's stain, acid-fast smear, India ink stain, Venereal Disease Research Laboratories (VDRL) test, and culture. Cryptococcal antigen should be obtained in select patients. Patients with AIDS who have cryptococcal meningitis may have normal or nondiagnostic CSF cell counts, protein, and glucose levels; the diagnostic sensitivity is increased to 95% with an India ink stain and CSF cryptococcal antigen.

Most patients with delirium have a normal or nondiagnostic head CT scan. Patients with a history of trauma, prior neurosurgical procedures, immunodeficiency, or focal neurologic findings should have a head CT scan to detect structural lesions causing delirium. A noncontrast head CT scan is excellent for detecting acute and subacute subdural hematomas, subarachnoid hemorrhage, and most cerebral contusions. Contrast-enhanced CT scans are superior in detecting isodense subdural hematomas, some CNS mass lesions, and enhancing lesions such as toxoplasmosis in the immunocompromised host.

A normal CT scan result does not completely exclude a primary CNS cause of delirium. Early hemispheric infarction, small brainstem lesions, meningitis or encephalitis, closed head trauma, sagittal vein thrombosis, and small isodense subdural hematomas may be missed on CT scan.[36] In addition, approximately 2% to 10% of subarachnoid hemorrhages are not detected by head CT scan and require lumbar puncture for diagnosis. The role of magnetic resonance imaging (MRI) in the evaluation of the delirious patient has not been fully or clearly established. The MRI scan is superior to the CT scan in detecting small intercerebral and brainstem lesions, small brain contusions, and abnormalities of white matter (i.e., leukoencephalopathy). Another imaging technique that is potentially useful beyond the ED evaluation is positive emission tomography (PET) scanning, which provides information regarding cerebral metabolic activity.

Although rarely practical in the emergency setting, the EEG can be a valuable diagnostic tool in determining the presence of delirium. A normal EEG result is incompatible with severe delirium; bilateral diffuse symmetric abnormalities are a relatively consistent feature. In most cases the EEG abnormality consists of relative generalized slowing with or without superimposed fast activity. Such slowing correlates well with the clinical evidence of reduced alertness and wakefulness on the one hand and with diminished cerebral blood flow, oxygen consumption, and metabolic rate on the other. The EEG shows nonfocal slow activity in the 5 to 7 cycles/sec range, a state that rapidly returns to normal as the delirium clears. The sensitivity of the EEG can be increased if a quantitative EEG is obtained. Low-voltage fast predominance on the EEG is noted less commonly in delirium and nearly always in patients with withdrawal from sedative drugs such as alcohol. In delirium tremens, low-voltage fast activity tends to predominate and cerebral blood flow is normal rather than reduced.[37,38]

In mild cases of delirium, the EEG lacks sensitivity. Normal EEG activity is between 8 and 12 cycles/sec. An individual's EEG can be slowed from its normal baseline with mild metabolic encephalopathy, but if that baseline is within upper normal limits and the slowing is not substantial, the EEG result is interpreted as normal. Serial EEG studies would reveal the abnormality because recovery of the patient from delirium would be accompanied by acceleration of the EEG rhythm. Furthermore, clinical changes often precede EEG changes, and normalization of the EEG often trails the return to baseline cognitive status.

Differential Diagnosis

The differential diagnosis of the patient who has apparent delirium includes functional psychiatric disorders and dementia. Depression, mania, paranoia, and schizophrenia may resemble delirium. Several clinical features are helpful in distinguishing between organic and functional syndromes (Table 98-2). Acute organic brain syndrome represents a global cognitive process with clouding of the sensorium, multiple cognitive deficits, and abnormal vital signs. Functional psychiatric syndromes typically have an onset early in life, the patient is oriented, sensorium usually is clear, and cognition is normal. Patients with psychiatric disorders are occasionally unable or unwilling to cooperate with a complete mental status evaluation. In these instances, inconsistent responses to cognitive questions of similar difficulty, poor psychiatric history, normal vital signs, nonfocal neurologic examination, normal laboratory test results, and a normal EEG result support the diagnosis of a psychiatric disorder.

Dementia, like delirium, is characterized by global cognitive impairment. Unlike delirium, dementia tends to be an insidious process that develops over months to years with little fluctuation over hours or days. Typically the patient's vital signs are normal. Dementia primarily occurs in the elderly. However, it is important to remember that patients with dementia are at risk for developing delirium.

Management

Delirium is a medical emergency. The outcome depends on the cause of the delirium, the patient's overall health status, and the timeliness of treatment. The presence of hyperactive or hypoactive delirium has some prognostic significance. The hypoactive form of delirium tends to be more common in the elderly and has a worse overall prognosis, perhaps because it often goes unrecognized.[4] Some patients with delirium have a self-limiting course, whereas others ultimately progress to chronic organic brain syndrome, coma, or death. The initial approach to the delirious patient should focus on diagnosing

Table 98-2. Comparison of Delirium and Acute Psychosis

Characteristic	Delirium	Acute psychosis
Onset	Acute	Acute
Vital signs	Typically abnormal (fever, tachycardia)	Normal
Prior psychiatric history	Uncommon	Common
Course	Rapid fluctuating	Stable
Psychomotor activity	Variable	Variable
Involuntary activity	Possible asterixis, tremor	Absent
Cognition function		
Orientation	Usually impaired	Occasionally impaired
Attention	Globally impaired	May be disorganized
Concentration	Globally impaired	Impaired
Hallucinations	Visual, visual and auditory	Primarily auditory
Delusions	Transient, poorly organized	Systematized
Speech	Pressured, slow, possibly incoherent	Usually coherent
Course	Typically resolves	Responds to therapy, recurrence common

and treating those conditions that can cause increased morbidity if ignored, while providing supporting measures for patients who have a self-limited course.

Prehospital care for the delirious patient should first address the standard ABCs of emergency treatment (airway, breathing, and circulation). If it is impossible to determine whether the patient has a normal oxygen saturation by pulse oximetry during transport, the patient should be placed on supplemental oxygen to treat potential hypoxemia. If the possibility of trauma exists, the cervical spine should be properly immobilized. An IV line should be established to provide normal saline or Ringer's lactate solution, and the serum glucose level should be determined by a bedside method. If the patient is hypoglycemic or if the serum glucose level cannot be assessed, the patient should receive 50 ml of 50% IV dextrose solution or 1 mg of intramuscular (IM) glucagon. For the patient who is neurologically depressed, naloxone hydrochloride should be administered by IV or IM injection. All patients should be placed on a cardiac monitor. Combative patients should be restrained to protect both the patient and the prehospital personnel. Prehospital care providers should attempt to obtain a history of the patient's recent health, current medical problems, and medications from family members or friends at the scene. Whenever possible, a family member or friend should be encouraged to go to the hospital to provide additional information.

After tending to the usual priorities, the emergency physician should focus on the readily treatable causes of acute organic brain syndrome. All patients who have acute delirium can be screened quickly for readily reversible causes such as hypoglycemia, hypoxia, and narcotic overdose.

Acute intoxication from a number of drugs or chemical agents, including tricyclic antidepressants, ethylene glycol, pesticides containing cholinesterase inhibitors, anticholinergic agents, carbon monoxide, and cyanide, requires prompt attention in the ED. Although supportive measures are the mainstay of treatment in most poisonings and intoxications, most of these toxins have specific antidotes. Carbon monoxide poisoning requires immediate treatment with 100% oxygen. Hyperbaric oxygen therapy is recommended in carbon monoxide poisoning if the patient has lost consciousness or has ECG changes consistent with ischemia, severe acidosis, confusion, abnormal neuropsychiatric testing, carbon monoxide levels greater than 25% to 30%, or persistence of symptoms despite 100% oxygen treatment.[39] Pesticide poisoning may require pralidoxime chloride (2-PAM) and large doses of atropine. Suspected anticholinergic overdose causing delirium can be confirmed and reversed with IV physostigmine, although the use of physostigmine is controversial.

Other conditions requiring immediate medical intervention include infections such as acute meningitis, encephalitis, or overwhelming sepsis. Patients who have signs of acute meningitis or overwhelming sepsis should optimally receive antibiotics within the first 30 minutes after arrival to the ED. Other emergency conditions that may present as delirium and require immediate intervention include severe hypothermia, hyperthermia, and CNS vascular conditions, including hypertensive encephalopathy, acute epidural or subdural hematoma, and subarachnoid hemorrhage. Patients with Wernicke's encephalopathy require immediate treatment with 100 mg of IV thiamine, with titration of additional doses until the ophthalmoplegia resolves. Resistance to thiamine may result from hypomagnesemia because magnesium is a cofactor for thiamine transketolase. Glucose administration in patients with severe thiamine deficiency may precipitate Wernicke's encephalopathy. The specific treatment of delirium tremens (and other alcohol withdrawal syndromes) involves the substitution of a long-acting drug that is cross-tolerant for the alcohol. Benzodiazepines are the agents of choice for inducing sedation. Fluids, electrolytes, and thiamine should be given parenterally while carefully searching for precipitating events such as infection.

Other causes of delirium are treated by supportive care in the ED while the identified abnormality is gradually corrected. Delirium secondary to dehydration, hyponatremia, hypernatremia, hypercalcemia, and hepatic or renal disease gradually resolves over hours to days with appropriate treatment. Acute organic brain syndrome secondary to substance abuse usually resolves over several hours as the patient detoxifies.

Supportive care for all patients with delirium includes providing an appropriate environment with adequate lighting, minimizing sensory overload, placing the patient in an area that can easily be observed by staff, and addressing the patient by name. Utilization of sitters may be necessary. Whenever possible, attempt to minimize sensory impairments by replacing glasses and hearing aids.[40] Delirious patients should never remain unobserved, and stretcher side rails should be up at all times. It is important to protect the patient from self-harm or from injuring other patients or staff. Restraints should be a last resort because they can increase agitation and the risk of patient injury.[6] In cases of hyperactive delirium, the patient may need to be restrained physically to protect both the patient and staff. Physical restraints in agitated patients have been associated with significant patient injuries and even death by asphyxiation and should never be used as a substitute for pharmacologic control.[41,42]

Pharmacologic restraint has become the cornerstone in behavioral management. Classes of drugs that have been used for delirium include the antipsychotics and benzodiazepines. The ideal sedating drug should have the following characteristics: low toxicity, ease of administration, short half-life, minimal effects on the cardiovascular and respiratory systems, and no effect on the seizure threshold. Antipsychotic medications that have been used to treat delirium include phenothiazines, butyrophenones, and risperidone. Although no one drug is ideal, the butyrophenones, specifically haloperidol (Haldol), have become the drugs of choice for control of agitation in acute delirium.[31] Phenothiazines and droperidol can cause orthostatic hypotension, lower the seizure threshold, and have anticholinergic effects, making them unacceptable in the treatment of delirium. The opioids, morphine and Demerol, are capable of inducing dysphoria and can exacerbate acute brain failure. They should never be used for behavior control in the agitated delirious patient. Diazepam (Valium) should be avoided as a treatment for agitated behavior in most delirious patients because of its long half-life, respiratory depression, and risk of drug accumulation with repeat dosing. The benzodiazepines, however, are the drugs of choice for delirium caused by withdrawal from alcohol or sedative hypnotics in which a long duration of action is desirable.

Haloperidol is a potent dopamine-blocking medication with virtually no anticholinergic or hypotensive effects. The drug can be easily titrated with IV administration. Although extrapyramidal side effects are common when it is administered on a regular basis for psychosis, the incidence of these side effects in patients receiving IV haloperidol for delirium is strikingly low.[43] One well-known side effect of haloperidol is prolongation of the QT interval, which may lead to ventricular arrhythmias, including torsades de pointes. The incidence varies and can occur with even low-dose IV haloperidol.[44] Dosing should vary with the patient's level of agitation, age, and response to treatment. It is reasonable to start with 1 to 2 mg, increasing the dose as needed. For elderly patients, a lower initial dose of 0.25 to 0.50 mg has been recommended.[45] Hourly doses of 10 to 20 mg may be necessary for delirious medically ill patients in whom agitation is a prominent sign. Patients in intensive care units have received daily doses exceeding 600 mg without serious side effects.[46,47] Droperidol, a butyrophenone pharmacologically similar to haloperidol, has similar sedating properties plus a potent antiemetic effect. Droperidol has been reported to have a faster onset of action than haloperidol,[48] but it has a slightly higher incidence of side effects, including dystonia, hypotension, sedation, and tachycardia. Risperidone has also been reported to be successful in controlling agitation in delirious patients, with a starting dose of 0.5 mg.[49,50] The combination of IV haloperidol and IV lorazepam can achieve more rapid control of agitated behavior than haloperidol alone; in addition, the combination of a benzodiazepine with haloperidol may further reduce the already low incidence of extrapyramidal neuromuscular symptoms, such as acute dystonia, parkinsonism symptoms (e.g., rigidity and akinesia), and akathisia that may occur with IV haloperidol alone.[51] Lorazepam (Ativan) seems to be particularly effective as an adjunct to haloperidol and poses minimal risk to the patient. Both drugs have short half-lives and do not have clinically important major active metabolites. In severe or refractory agitation, 600 mg haloperidol and 240 mg lorazepam have been safely administered daily for more than 2 weeks without untoward effects.[52]

A few comments should be made regarding the legal aspects of treating the patient with delirium. Because the delirious patient is suffering from attention deficits, memory impairment, and disorientation, it is impossible to obtain informed consent regarding proposed diagnostic and therapeutic interventions. Implied consent is appropriate when a true emergency exists because common law recognizes that a reasonable person would want to receive treatment in a true emergency even if impaired awareness at the time of treatment precludes giving informed consent. The physician may render treatment without informed consent to an incompetent patient in a life-threatening emergency situation. A delirious patient who needs urgent but not emergent medical treatment is in a legally ambiguous situation, and the treating physician has several options.[54] Whenever time allows, the physician should involve family members in the evaluation and treatment process. This may be particularly appropriate if there are several equally effective treatment alternatives and if moderate risks are associated with the evaluation and treatment. The physician may also obtain a second clinical opinion before proceeding. Ultimately the course the emergency physician takes when caring for the delirious patient depends on the time available for obtaining consent or appointing an alternative decision-making authority; the risk-to-benefit ratio of diagnostic or therapeutic measures; the availability, sympathy, and decisiveness of family members; and knowledge of the patient's preferences. In addition, the emergency physician must remember to document these proceedings.

Disposition

Patients with delirium secondary to acute drug intoxication may be discharged provided the process readily reverses itself in the ED and the drug has no potentially serious delayed toxicity. Acute intoxication with ethanol, cocaine, heroin, MDMA, or PCP typically clears while the patient is in the ED. For most patients delirious from metabolic, infectious, or CNS processes, admission to the hospital is necessary for further diagnostic evaluation and treatment. The only readily reversible metabolic problem associated with delirium that can be completely managed in the ED is hypoglycemia.

For most patients who have delirium, the outcome is full recovery. After an episode of acute delirium, younger patients may experience mild cognitive dysfunction that lasts weeks to months. Elderly patients, on the other hand, often experience persistent decline in their baseline level of functioning, with a loss of at least one activity of daily living (ADL) following acute delirium.[55,56] Elderly hospitalized patients with delirium have longer hospital stays and higher mortality rates and rates of institutional care after hospitalization.[57] For the elderly, an episode of delirium, especially for those with baseline cognitive impairment, can have significant long-term consequences.

DEMENTIA

Perspective

Dementia is a gradually progressive deterioration of cognitive function. Dementia is not a single disease entity but refers to a highly variable clinical syndrome. Like delirium, there are many different causes, and prognosis depends on the underlying cause. A particular dementia can be classified as either potentially reversible or irreversible. Although most patients with dementia have an irreversible disease process, approximately 10% of dementias are reversible.[58] It is essential that the emergency physician recognize the signs and symptoms of potentially reversible forms of dementia, promptly identify the manifestations of acute illness in the demented patient, and be aware of the normal progression of irreversible dementias.

In 1907 Alzheimer described the clinical history and postmortem findings of a 50-year-old female patient with progressive dementia.[59] For decades, Alzheimer's disease was considered to be an uncommon dementia of younger patients known as "presenile" dementia. The more common dementia of elderly patients was believed to be secondary to atherosclerotic cerebrovascular disease and was referred to as "senile" dementia. Over the past 30 years, research has shown that the neuropathologic changes between the two are identical. Today these two categories of primary degenerative dementias are collectively referred to as *Alzheimer's disease.* Alzheimer's dementia accounts for more than half of all dementias; the remaining cases are attributable to more than 50 known causes.

In 1997 the prevalence of Alzheimer's disease was 2.32 million; this number is expected to quadruple in the next 50 years.[60] At age 60 the prevalence is about 1%, but this doubles every 5 years until it reaches 30% to 50% by 85 years of age.[61] The cost of this disease exceeds $60 billion per year and will increase dramatically as the number of people greater than 80 years old doubles by 2010.[62] The true incidence of dementia is unknown, and the disease is commonly underdiagnosed in lower socioeconomic groups and rural areas. Two million individuals live in nursing homes in the United States; almost 60% of these individuals have some degree of cognitive impairment.

The American Psychiatric Association has defined essential criteria necessary for the diagnosis of dementia (Box 98-2). Several clinical features deserve emphasis. Intellectual impairment must involve both short-term and long-term memory. The cognitive impairment commonly involves abstract thinking, judgment, and other higher cortical functions. Although mild decline in intellectual functioning can be part of the normal aging process, gross intellectual impairment and confusion should never be considered part of normal aging. Another important feature in the diagnosis of dementia is that the cognitive disturbance must significantly interfere with interpersonal relationships, work, and social activities of the individual.

Dementia can be classified according to the degree of cognitive impairment. Mild dementia implies some impairment of work and social activities; however, the capacity for independent adequate personal hygiene and independent living remains intact. With moderate dementia, independent living is hazardous and some degree of supervision is necessary. In severe dementia, continual supervision and often custodial care are needed.

Demented patients often have longer hospitalizations for the same acute medical illness than those without dementia, and the life expectancy of demented patients is 6 to 8 years less than that for nondemented age-matched controls.[63]

Box 98-2 Diagnostic Criteria for Dementia

A. The development of multiple cognitive deficits manifested by both of the following:
   1. Memory impairment (impaired ability to learn new information or to recall previously learned information)
   2. One (or more) of the following cognitive disturbances:
      a. aphasia (language disturbance)
      b. apraxia (impaired ability to carry out motor activities despite intact motor function)
      c. agnosia (failure to recognize or identify objects)
      d. disturbance in executive functioning (i.e., planning, organization, sequencing, abstracting)

B. The cognitive deficits cause significant impairment in social or occupational functioning and represent a significant decline from a previous level of functioning.

C. The deficits do not occur exclusively during the course of a delirium.

Modified from American Psychiatric Association: *Diagnostic and statistical manual of mental disorders,* ed 4, text revision, Washington, DC, 2000, American Psychiatric Association.

Etiology

Dementia may be caused by more than 50 different disease states (Box 98-3). Broadly, dementia may be classified as either primary degenerative dementia or secondary dementia; the latter category includes all the potentially reversible dementias. Primary degenerative dementias include Alzheimer's disease, vascular dementia, the subcortical dementias involving the basal ganglia and thalamus (e.g., progressive supranuclear palsy, Huntington's chorea, Parkinson's disease), and Pick's disease, also known as *dementia of the frontal lobe type.* Most dementia is Alzheimer's type. The second most common cause of dementia is vascular dementia and it accounts for approximately 10% to 20% of all dementias. A smaller percentage are attributable to causes such as anoxic encephalopathy, hepatolenticular degeneration, tumors, and slow virus infections.

Adverse drug reactions and metabolic abnormalities in patients can cause either an acute delirium or a gradual progressive dementia. Drug-induced dementia occurs primarily in the elderly and can be caused by various psychotropic drugs (e.g., sedative-hypnotics, minor or major tranquilizers, lithium, antidepressants), antihypertensive medications, anticonvulsants, anticholinergics, and miscellaneous medications such as L-dopa. Dementia may also be caused by heavy metals and other exogenous agents, such as carbon monoxide, carbon disulfide, and trichloroethylene.

Endocrinopathies that can cause secondary dementia include hypothyroidism, hyperthyroidism, parathyroid disease, Addison's disease, Cushing's disease, and panhypopituitarism. Nutritional deficiencies that cause dementia include thiamine deficiency (Wernicke's syndrome), niacin deficiency (pellagra), B_{12} deficiency, and folate deficiency. Dementia can be caused by intracranial space-occupying lesions and hydrocephalus. Repetitive intracranial trauma, such as boxers

Box 98-3 Classification of Dementias

Primary Cortical Dementias
Alzheimer's disease
Pick's disease

Primary Subcortical Dementias
Huntington's chorea
Parkinson's disease
Progressive supranuclear palsy
Secondary dementia
Drug/toxin-induced
Metabolic or electrolyte disturbance
Intracerebral disorders
Trauma
Mass effect (tumor, hematoma, abscess)
Hydrocephalus
Cerebrovascular disease (multiinfarct dementia)
Endocrinopathies
Infectious (intracranial) chronic meningitis, encephalitis, abscess, HIV-1, slow virus, neurosyphilis
Nutritional
Psychiatric (pseudodementia)
Other (e.g., collagen vascular disease, paraneoplastic)

sustain, can produce a chronic organic brain syndrome without evidence of hematoma or significant contusion (dementia pugilistica).[64] Intracranial processes that may eventually lead to a chronic organic brain syndrome include infections with slow viruses, HIV-1, chronic meningitis (tubercular or fungal), brain abscess, and neurosyphilis. Any patient with dementia who has an HIV-1 infection should be aggressively evaluated for the cause of the dementia and should not be assumed to have cognitive impairment solely resulting from direct HIV-1 infection. Toxoplasmosis, cryptococcal meningitis, herpes virus, cytomegalovirus, varicella-zoster, papovavirus (progressive multifocal leukoencephalopathy), and malignancy can cause progressive cognitive impairment in this compromised group of patients and must be excluded.[65]

Depression in the elderly may closely mimic dementia. Diagnosing pseudodementia, or depression masquerading as dementia, can be difficult and may require therapeutic interventions to confirm the clinical diagnosis of depression.

Principles of Disease

Pathophysiology Dementia is characterized by many different pathophysiologic findings. Alzheimer's disease is the best-understood dementia and has several characteristic anatomic, pathologic, and neurochemical changes. On a broad scale there is cortical atrophy most prominent in the temporal and hippocampal regions, caused by progressive synaptic and neuronal loss in the cerebral grey matter.[66] This is generally followed by loss of white matter (subcortical atrophy). Atrophy secondary to neuronal death is an important manifestation of Alzheimer's disease. Cell loss does occur with the normal aging process, but not to the extent seen in senile dementia. The brain of the patient with Alzheimer's disease typically has diffuse atrophy, with widening of the sulci and some dilatation of the cerebral ventricles, but these characteristics can be found in some normal elderly individuals. Also, not all patients with dementia have gross cerebral atrophy. There is no ischemic component to this disease.

Histologic findings characteristic of Alzheimer's disease are neurofibrillary tangles and senile plaques. The neurofibrillary tangles are intraneuronal paired helical filaments composed of the abnormally phosphorylated protein tau, the structural protein involved in the regeneration of neurites.[62] In demented patients these tangles occur in great numbers throughout the cerebral cortex; only limited numbers can be seen in nondemented elderly patients (primarily in the hippocampus region) and in a variety of other diseases. The density of neocortical tangles correlates with the severity of dementia.[67] Senile plaques are extracellular lesions composed of degenerating neuronal processes and abnormal beta-amyloid protein. These plaques are extensively spread through the cerebral cortex. The plaques can be extremely numerous when the dementia is clinically very mild.[68] Other consistent neurohistopathologic changes in Alzheimer's disease include granulovascular degeneration, Hirano bodies, beta-amyloid deposition in the small cortical blood vessels, and neuronal loss in the limbic area.[69]

Many biochemical abnormalities have been described in patients with Alzheimer's disease. The neurons using acetylcholine as a neurotransmitter in the hippocampus, parietal, and temporal areas are susceptible to these pathological changes.[66] There is a decrease in the neurotransmitter acetylcholine in patients with dementia. The enzyme choline acetyl-transferase (ChAT) synthesizes acetylcholine in the brain. Levels of this enzyme decrease with aging; however, in patients with Alzheimer's disease, the levels may decline to 20% of those of age-matched controlled subjects.

Alzheimer's disease has several risk factors: age, family history, female gender, low education level, and history of head trauma. In recent years new research has led to the discovery of new risk factors and possible mechanisms causing Alzheimer's disease.[70] Apolipoprotein E (ApoE) on chromosome 19 has been associated with both familial and sporadic late-onset Alzheimer's disease.[71] Apo E is responsible for transporting the cholesterol and phospholipids necessary for dendritic and synaptic repair. There are several allelic variants, but those homozygous or heterozygous for the E-4 variant have an increased risk for the development and expression of the disease.[72] Abnormalities on chromosomes 1, 14, and 19 have been associated with Alzheimer's disease. Free radicals have been postulated to cause cross-linking of beta-amyloid, and antioxidants have been shown to reduce formation of beta-amyloid.[62] Also, there may be an inflammatory response associated with Alzheimer's disease; this is supported by the data that indicate antiinflammatory therapy has an inverse association with Alzheimer's disease.[73,74] The use of estrogen replacement therapy in postmenopausal women has been reported to decrease the rate of development of Alzheimer's disease.[75]

Pick's disease is much rarer than Alzheimer's disease and is categorized by a frontal and temporal atrophy caused by cell death. There is a reactive gliosis (proliferation of glial cells) that occurs in these areas. The neurohistopathologic changes associated with this disease include tau-positive inclusions in neurons and glial cells.

In the so-called *subcortical dementias,* the neuropathologic changes involve primarily the basal ganglia. Degenerative changes in this structure can be seen in Huntington's disease, Parkinson's disease, Wilson's disease, and progressive supranuclear palsy.

Approximately 10% to 20% of dementias are secondary to multiple vascular insults to the CNS (multiinfarct dementia [MID]). The multiple infarcts typically involve the cerebral hemispheres and basal ganglia. MID often has an earlier age of onset than Alzheimer's disease and occurs more often in adult men and patients who have risk factors for atherosclerosis. Uncontrolled hypertension, diabetes, atrial fibrillation, tobacco use, hypercholesterolemia, and hypercoagulable states may greatly increase the risk of vascular insult to the CNS. Usually the patient has a history of cerebrovascular infarcts; however, a small number of patients with MID do not have a history of prior strokes. Approximately 10% of dementias are a mixed variety and contain components of both ischemic cerebrovascular disease and senile dementia.

Slow virus infections of the CNS can cause a progressive dementia that is irreversible. In slow virus infections, months to years pass between infection with the virus and appearance of clinical illness. Once the diagnosis has been established, progression may occur over several months or years.

Slow virus infections of the CNS are caused by both conventional viruses and unconventional viral-like agents, known as *prions.* The conventional viruses tend to provoke a mild inflammatory response before the onset of clinical symptoms, whereas the unconventional viruses are insidious, residing within the cells for long periods without causing detectable cytopathic changes. There is a variable presence of elevated levels of circulating antibodies or no detectable immune response.

The CNS inflammatory conditions caused by conventional viruses include subacute sclerosing panencephalitis (SSPE) from the measles virus, progressive multifocal leukoencephalopathy (PML) from the JC virus (a papovavirus), progressive rubella encephalitis, and infection from HIV. The unconventional viral infections include kuru and Creutzfeldt-Jakob disease (CJD). These latter diseases cause a fine vacuolation of the nervous tissue; hence they are referred to as *subacute spongiform viral encephalopathies.*

PML occurs in patients who have immunodeficiency (e.g., AIDS), are taking immunosuppressive medication, or have an underlying malignancy. This disease is consistently associated with disorders of cell-mediated immunity. It is usually caused by a reactivation of the latent JC virus, which resides in either the brain or lymphatic system. The oligodendrocytes are infected by the virus, causing widespread demyelination.

One of the most prevalent slow virus infections causing progressive dementia is HIV-1. HIV may produce a primary neurotrophic disorder in addition to providing the immunologic compromise that permits other viruses to replicate and damage nervous tissue. The most prevalent dementia caused by HIV is HIV dementia or AIDS dementia complex (ADC), which occurs in about a third of patients with AIDS. This is believed to be caused directly by the HIV-1 virus. Pathologic CNS changes occur in 60% of patients with AIDS, and these include atrophy, ventricular widening, meningeal fibrosis, and sulci widening. There are extensive periventricular and central white matter changes. On a cellular level there are multinucleated giant cells present in the perivascular areas. Typical neuropathologic findings include gliosis, focal necrosis of neurons, perivascular inflammation, formation of microglial nodules, multinucleated giant cells, and demyelination.[76-79] Very strong evidence exists that the virus is the direct cause of these changes.

Several of the potentially reversible causes of dementia are also associated with neuropathologic or neurochemical abnormalities. Recent evidence suggests that neurochemical abnormalities may contribute to the depression in pseudodementia. Normal pressure hydrocephalus (NPH) generally affects a younger age group; 50% of patients are less than age 60. Most of the conditions that cause hydrocephalus involve a defect with the arachnoid villi in the uptake of CSF, which results in gradual ventricular dilatation. Primary hydrocephalus is not associated with any predisposing neurologic disease. Secondary hydrocephalus results from some antecedent disorder, such as subarachnoid hemorrhage, head injury, or meningitis.

Several drugs may cause subacute or chronic cognitive dysfunction, particularly in the elderly. Because the elderly patient has a decreased CNS cholinergic reserve, medications with anticholinergic properties such as tricyclic antidepressants often can tip the scales to cognitive impairment. Drug-induced dementia may be dose-related or idiosyncratic. Discontinuation of the suspected drug is frequently the only way to exclude a medication as the cause of cognitive dysfunction.

Ethanol, a commonly abused substance, can cause more than one type of chronic organic brain syndrome. The neurotoxicity of ethanol appears to be independent of thiamine deficiency. Alcoholism can cause cerebral cortical atrophy, but no single alcohol-related dementia syndrome exists. It is estimated that approximately 20% of chronically demented patients have a history of alcoholism. One rare progressive dementia attributable to alcoholism is Marchiafava-Bignami disease, which clinically is similar to frontal lobe dementias and pathologically involves destruction of the central regions of the corpus callosum.[80] Korsakoff's psychosis, which results from thiamine deficiency, is primarily a memory disorder; intellectual functioning is not impaired to the degree of the primary degenerative dementias.

Clinical Features

The symptoms, signs, and progression of chronic cognitive impairment are rarely so diagnostic as to permit identification of the specific cause of the dementia. Typically, gradual progression of symptoms occurs independent of the specific causes. Because Alzheimer's disease is the most common cause of dementia, a more detailed discussion of the progression of this entity will be presented.

Senile dementia begins insidiously. Signs and symptoms of cognitive dysfunction may be present for months to years before the diagnosis is made. The earliest symptoms and signs of Alzheimer's disease are often vague and nonspecific because the patient manifests anxiety, depression, insomnia, frustration, and somatic complaints that are often more prominent than the memory loss. Patients often deny any cognitive deficits and will change the subject of conversations frequently rather than admit their increased forgetfulness. The subtle signs of dementia are often overlooked by physicians in this phase of the disease.[81] Depression is often the initial sign of Alzheimer's disease and is present in up to 40% of cases.[82] Early in the illness, short-term memory is affected, with forgetfulness of recent events such as appointments and names of new acquaintances. Patients often repeat questions. The memory impairment may cause them to withdraw from social situations and recreational pursuits. Complex tasks may cause anxiety and confusion. The patient often has difficulty with interpersonal relationships. The patient's affect may be shallow and labile, and minor events may trigger inappropriate laughter or tears. Compensation for early deficits includes excessive orderliness and avoidance of situations in which the defects may be observed. Patients in this early phase who are treated with antidepressants with strong anticholinergic properties may have their symptoms worsen. Sedative-hypnotics prescribed for anxiety may also increase cognitive dysfunction.

As the dementia progresses, cognitive deficits are more obvious and should be readily apparent on a mental status examination. Recent memory is clearly impaired, and there may be some impairment of remote memory. Most of these patients will demonstrate language deficits and difficulty with spontaneous speech.[83] They will have difficulty naming objects (anomia). They may demonstrate circumstantiality and tangentiality in their thought processes. They make errors in judgment and become lost or confused. Receptive dysphasia, dyslexia, dysgraphia, and dyspraxia may be apparent in more than 50% of these patients. As many as 50% of patients will have delusions, usually of the paranoid type.[82] Atypical presentations of Alzheimer's disease include aphasia, visual agnosia, right parietal lobe syndrome, focal neurological findings, extrapyramidal signs, gait disturbances, and pure memory loss. In the final stage of dementia, patients have marked cognitive impairment, with profound memory disturbances and significant personality changes. These patients will suffer from apraxia, the loss of fine motor skills. They are often bedridden and unable to perform any of the routine activities of daily living.

Family or friends usually bring the patient to the ED because of a sudden worsening in mental status, a change in the patient's activities (e.g., refusal to eat), or a change in the ability of the caregiver to manage the patient. As many as 40% of patients over the age of 55 with dementia have a superimposed delirium on admission to the hospital.[84] Acute confusion superimposed on a baseline dementia may be a more common herald of the onset of physical illness in demented elderly patients than fever, pain, or tachycardia.

Precipitating events causing a deterioration in mental status include stroke, silent MI, pain (i.e., ischemic bowel, dissecting aneurysm), dehydration, and infection. Systemic illnesses more commonly cause acute cognitive decline than primary cerebral events. The most common sites of infection are the urinary tract and lungs. Because Pick's disease dementia affects the frontal and temporal lobes, patients often have frontal lobe release signs, including dramatic behavioral changes of disinhibition and social inappropriateness. This is in contrast to patients with Alzheimer's disease, who initially have memory problems with preservation of social skills until later in the disease process.

Several basal ganglia degenerative disorders have dementia as a prominent finding. These include Huntington's, Parkinson's, and Wilson's diseases, and supranuclear palsy. Several features distinguish cortical and subcortical dementias (Table 98-3). The most striking feature of these dementias is the movement disorder that tends to occur early in the illness. Other features of these dementias include slowness of speech, hypotonia, and dysarthria, which occur early and progress to mutism.

Patients with MID have a stepwise deterioration in mental status with each cerebrovascular insult. The clinical presentation may follow one of two scenarios. In the more common scenario, the patient has suffered several strokes that involve large volumes of cortical and subcortical structures in both hemispheres. The patient exhibits dementia along with other neurologic disabilities (e.g., focal weakness, hyperreflexia, extensor plantar response). The other group of patients have a more subtle presentation. These individuals are characteristically hypertensive and suffer multiple tiny infarcts (lacunae) that involve deep subcortical structures. There may be no focal neurologic residua except progressive dementia with psychomotor retardation.

The clinical manifestations of slow virus CNS infections are protean. After an insidious onset of mental deterioration in subacute sclerosing panencephalitis there is a rapid progression that is associated with myoclonic jerks, incoordination, and ataxia. In PML, neurologic signs and symptoms reflect diffuse asymmetric involvement of both cerebral hemispheres. CJD was initially thought to affect older individuals; however, there have been reported cases in those under 45 years of age.[85] These patients have rapidly evolving dementia with myoclonus. The hallmarks of the disorder are mental deterioration, multisystem neurologic signs, myoclonus, and typical EEG changes that evolve over months. Most patients die within the first 6 months after the onset of clinical symptoms.

AIDS dementia is a subacute dementia with an insidious onset and gradual progression that is often accompanied by motor system abnormalities. The early cognitive impairment includes poor recall, impaired concentration, and difficulty in performing complex sequential tasks. Initially, the symptoms may appear to be manifestations of a depressive illness. Slowing of verbal and motor responses and reduced spontaneity are typically present. A normal level of consciousness may be maintained into the late stages of the illness. The AIDS dementia complex may be more acute after surgery, use of psychoactive drugs, infections, and other stresses. The AIDS dementia complex is primarily of a subcortical nature with a predilection for involvement of frontal white matter. Aphasia and apraxia are uncommon; however, verbal and motor slowing occurs.

Table 98-3. Characteristics of Cortical Versus Subcortical Dementia

	Cortical	Subcortical
Appearance	Unremarkable	Disheveled
Activity	Normal	Slow
Gait	Normal	Posturing, ataxic
Movements	Normal	Tremor, chorea, slow
Speech	Normal	Slow, dysarthric
Language	Anomia, paraphasia	Normal
Cognition	Impaired	Impaired
Memory	Disordered learning	Forgetful
Visual-spatial	Constructional deficit	Sloppy

The most common treatable dementia is pseudodementia or depression. The clinical distinction between depression and dementia is difficult, and the coexistence of depression and dementia is common in mildly demented individuals. A number of distinguishing features may suggest that the problem is depression rather than dementia (Table 98-4). The onset of cognitive changes in pseudodementia can often be pinpointed, and symptoms are usually of short duration before medical help is sought. The progression of symptoms is rapid and the family is usually aware of the severity of the dysfunction. The patient commonly has a history of psychiatric illness. Patients with pseudodementia usually complain of cognitive dysfunction and emphasize their failures and disabilities. The affective change is often pervasive and the patient makes little effort to perform simple tasks. Loss of social skills usually occurs early in the illness, and patients communicate a strong sense of distress and inability to function. Intellectual functioning in pseudodementia is often difficult to assess because of lack of patient cooperation or inconsistent findings on neuropsychometric testing. Attention and concentration are often intact, but patients commonly give answers such as "I don't know" on tests of orientation, concentration, and memory. Memory loss for recent and remote events is usually equally severe, and there may be marked variability in the performance of tasks that have similar degrees of difficulty. Tasks of high capacity (e.g., testing delayed memory with distraction) may be helpful in identifying the depressed patient.[86]

The classic triad of progressive dementia, ataxia, and urinary incontinence occurs in patients with NPH, which affects younger patients than does primary degenerative

Table 98-4. Comparison of Dementia and Pseudodementia

Characteristic	Dementia	Pseudodementia (depression)
Onset	Insidious	More precise, rapid
Prior psychiatric history	Absent	Present
Demeanor	Unconcerned	Distressed
	Conceals deficits	Emphasizes deficits
	Struggles at tasks	Limits effort
	Loss of social skills	Social skills intact
Affect	Shallow, labile	Depressive, pervasive
Cognitive function	Attention impaired	Attention preserved
	Cooperative	Poor effort, despair
	Recent memory more impaired than remote memory	Impaired recent and remote memory
	Consistent testing performance	Variable performance of similar tasks
Course	Chronic, progressive	Response to therapy

dementia. More than half of the reported cases involve individuals less than 60 years of age. Hydrocephalus secondary to prior head trauma or infection has a more favorable prognosis than primary hydrocephalus.

Approximately 20% of reversible dementia is secondary to an intracranial mass. Patients may exhibit focal or nonfocal neurologic findings. A nonfocal neurologic examination can be caused by a tumor in the frontal, subfrontal (i.e., large prolactinoma), or temporal lobe region and occasionally by an extracerebral mass such as a subdural hematoma or meningioma.[87]

Of reversible dementias, 10% to 15% are secondary to medications or chemical intoxications. Elderly patients may have increased susceptibility to the toxicities of commonly prescribed drugs. Age-related changes in metabolism can prolong the half-lives of many medications. Polypharmacy is a common problem in the elderly, which increases the likelihood of adverse drug interactions. A temporal relationship does not always exist between initiation of a medication and onset of cognitive impairment. Furthermore, alcoholism is common in the elderly and may contribute to chronic cognitive impairment. The clinical presentation of a patient with a drug-related or toxin-related dementia may be indistinguishable from that of a patient with a primary degenerative process.

Differential Diagnosis

Subacute or chronic cognitive decline may be secondary to a dementing illness or a manifestation of senescent forgetfulness, delirium, or depression.

Senescent forgetfulness is an inevitable reality of aging. Mild impairment of both short-term and long-term memory usually is present. Unlike dementia, the cognitive disturbance in senescent forgetfulness does not interfere with work or customary social activity.

In most cases, the clinical distinction between delirium and dementia is obvious. In both delirium and dementia, global cognitive processes are impaired. Dementia has an insidious onset, whereas delirium typically is abrupt in presentation. Dementia is a slowly progressive condition; delirium has a fluctuating course varying over the span of hours. The level of consciousness is usually normal in dementia and reduced or agitated in delirium. Hallucinations and fluctuations in psychomotor activity typically are present in delirium and absent from dementia. The dexamethasone suppression test, EEG, CT scan, neuropsychologic testing, and amobarbital interview are not completely reliable in diagnosing pseudodementia.

Diagnostic Strategies

The ED evaluation of the patient with possible dementia should include a medical and psychiatric history plus a collateral history from family and friends. Physical examination should include a detailed neurologic examination with mental status evaluation. Dementia is often unrecognized in the patient who is alert, pleasant, and cooperative. A systematic mental status examination can play a key role in the early identification of dementia in patients who have maintained social and conversational ability.

All patients who have a dementing illness require a basic laboratory and radiologic evaluation to detect treatable dementia (Box 98-4). A thorough examination is not adequate in detecting treatable dementias because of the considerable clinical overlap with irreversible dementias. The basic laboratory evaluation should include CBC, determination of electrolytes and glucose levels, tests of liver and renal function, thyroid function tests, serologic tests for syphilis, and antibody tests for HIV infection. It is important that a serum fluorescent treponemal antibody-absorption test (FTA-ABS) be performed in addition to a VDRL test because the serum VDRL may yield negative results in patients who have tertiary syphilis. The radiologic evaluation should include noncontrast and contrast-enhanced head CT scans.

Certain patients require additional laboratory evaluation, which may include serum B_{12} and folate levels, erythrocyte sedimentation rate (ESR), FANA, urine corticosteroid levels, and urine screens for drugs and heavy metals. Select patients should undergo a lumbar puncture with CSF analysis, MRI scanning, PET scan, EEG (in CJD, characteristic slowing and periodic complexes may be present), neuropsychologic testing, visual evoked potentials, brainstem auditory evoked potentials, and somatosensory evoked potentials.

The laboratory evaluation is frequently unrewarding. In Alzheimer's disease, a cranial CT scan may be normal or show cerebral atrophy, especially in the gyri of the association areas of the cerebral cortex. Cerebral atrophy is a function of age and can occur in both normal and demented patients. The basic usefulness of the CT scan in the evaluation

Box 98-4 Diagnostic Evaluation for Dementia

History (patient, family, friends)
Review of medications
Physical examination, including neurologic evaluation
Mental status examination

Laboratory Evaluation

CBC
Electrolyte, glucose levels
Liver, renal function studies
Urinalysis
Thyroid function studies
VDRL, FTA

Radiographic Evaluation

Chest radiograph
Head CT scan

Additional Evaluation

Blood and urine screens for drugs, heavy metals
Erythrocyte sedimentation rate
HIV screen
Antinuclear antibody
Oxygen saturation, ABG
Serum B_{12} and folate
Lumbar puncture
MRI head scan
EEG
Neuropsychometric testing
Evoked potentials (visual, brainstem auditory, somatosensory)

of dementia is to exclude the presence of hydrocephalus and space-occupying lesions. The EEG is rarely helpful in establishing the diagnosis of senile dementia.

No test allows the clinician to readily distinguish between dementia and pseudodementia. The dexamethasone suppression test (DST) may be used clinically to detect endogenous depression. In the normal individual, administration of IV dexamethasone suppresses release of adrenocorticotropic hormone (ACTH) by the pituitary and produces decreased cortisol production. The DST result is abnormal in 50% of patients with depressive illness (cortisol production is not suppressed by dexamethasone) and only 4% of normal subjects. Some have found this test helpful in detecting pseudodementia; however, it lacks specificity. The evaluation needed to diagnose pseudodementia or concomitant dementia and depression is beyond the scope of ED care. A carefully monitored trial of antidepressants is occasionally necessary to confirm the presence of depression.

Treatment and Disposition

Several questions arise when treating a patient with apparent subacute or chronic cognitive impairment. Why was the patient taken to the ED? What precipitating events have caused a worsening in the baseline mental status? Is there a reversible component to the apparent dementia? Is there a superimposed delirium? Reversible dementias and conditions causing worsening of baseline dementia require early diagnosis and treatment of the underlying disorder if prior cognitive function is to be restored.

Determining reversible causes of dementia during the ED evaluation is occasionally possible on the basis of the history, physical examination, and the head CT scan. Most treatable dementias are secondary to depression, NPH, intracranial mass lesions, and medications. These conditions should be apparent with a careful bedside evaluation and a CT scan. Few reversible causes of dementia can be readily treated in the ED; most patients require hospitalization. Occasionally, individuals who have a gradual decline in cognitive function without an underlying acute medical condition can receive further evaluation as outpatients. Close medical follow-up and strong family support are essential elements when deciding on the feasibility of an outpatient evaluation.

Pharmacotherapy for dementia includes two drugs that have recently been approved by the FDA for the treatment of mild to moderate Alzheimer's disease. These agents are tacrine (Cognex) and donepezil (Aricept). They work by reducing the metabolism of acetylcholine. These drugs do not halt the underlying disease process. They are also associated with peripheral side effects and elevation of liver enzymes. Yet these therapies represent short-term hope for patients with Alzheimer's disease. Several promising agents for treatment include antioxidants, antiinflammatories, and estrogen, but their role has not been clearly defined. The key to altering the course of the disease will require halting synaptic loss. Several new agents, such as nerve growth factor, are currently being investigated to slow the progression of the deficits in dementia.[88]

The main goal in the management of patients with dementia is supportive care. Patients should be in an environment that ensures their personal safety. Employment of home health aides or custodians and occasionally institutionalization may be necessary. Patients should receive adequate supervision to ensure proper nutrition, hydration, and skin care.

Occasionally, medications are needed for symptomatic treatment of agitation, sleep disturbance, and depression. These patients typically do not improve with anxiolytics. Agitation can be controlled with a small dose of the butyrophenone haloperidol (Haldol). The cardiovascular toxicity of this drug is minimal, and it is well tolerated in elderly patients. Temazepam (Restoril) is the drug of choice for sleep disturbance. The half-life of temazepam is 8 to 10 hours at all ages, and the drug bypasses the oxidative hepatic enzyme system. The shorter-acting sedative triazolam (Halcion) should be avoided because it will not maintain sleep throughout the night and may exacerbate mental confusion.

The goal in the management of MID is to prevent further vascular insult by controlling precipitating factors such as hypertension. The prognosis will ultimately depend on the underlying cerebrovascular status. The only slow virus infection that may respond to treatment with some reversal of the cognitive dysfunction is HIV infection.

Occasionally, patients are taken to the ED because of family stress from continuous care of the patient. An honest discussion with family members regarding the home situation often reveals the reason for the present difficulty in managing the patient. A brief nursing home stay or other institutional stay (respite program) may give the family time to mobilize resources to resume care of the patient. Coordinating evaluation, treatment, and ongoing supportive care can be time consuming. A social worker can play a vital role in attempting to deliver comprehensive care to the demented patient.

KEY CONCEPTS

- Delirium is a medical emergency. The delirious patient requires prompt evaluation and treatment. A thorough investigation of possible causes of the delirium must be undertaken in the ED. This may require laboratory and radiographic examinations.
- Dementia has many causes, some of which may be reversible with accurate diagnosis. Resist the temptation to classify dementia as a "futile" disease and search for underlying medical conditions that may be worsening a dementing illness.
- Always be wary of diagnosing patients with behavioral disturbances as having psychiatric illness; many serious medical conditions will be missed. Any abnormal vital signs must be appropriately evaluated.

REFERENCES

1. American Psychiatric Association, *Diagnostic and statistical manual of mental disorders: DSM-IV,* Chicago, 1994, The Association.
2. Hunter R, Macalpine I: *Three hundred years of psychiatry,* London, 1963, Oxford University Press.
3. Francis J, Kappor WN: Delirium in hospitalized elderly, *J Gen Int Med* 128:111, 1990.
4. Inouye SK: Delirium in hospitalized older patients, *Clinics in Geriatric Medicine* 14:745, 1998.
5. Lipowski ZJ: *Delirium: acute confusional states,* New York, 1990, Oxford University Press.
6. Inouye SK, Charpentier PA: Precipitating factors for delirium in hospitalized elderly persons: predictive model and interrelationship with baseline vulnerability, *JAMA* 275:852, 1996.
7. Marcantonio ER et al: A clinical prediction rule for delirium after elective noncardiac surgery, *JAMA* 271:134, 1994.
8. Lipowki AJ: *Delirium: acute confusional states,* Oxford, 1990, Oxford University.
9. Mach JR et al: Serum anticholinergic activity in hospitalized elderly with delirium: a preliminary study, *J Am Geriatr Soc* 43:491, 1995.
10. Chan D, Brennan NJ: Delirium: making the diagnosis, improving the prognosis, *Geriatrics* 54:28, 1999.
11. Adams RD, Victor M, Ropper AH: *Principles of neurology,* ed 6, New York, 1997, McGraw-Hill.
12. Burks J et al: Tricyclic antidepressant poisoning, *JAMA* 230:1405, 1974.
13. Mori E, Yamadoei A: Acute confusional state and acute agitated delirium, *Arch Neurol* 44:1139, 1987.
14. Rudberg M et al: The natural history of delirium in older hospitalized patients: a syndrome of heterogeneity, *Aging* 26:169, 1997.
15. Inouye SK: The dilemma of delirium: clinical and research controversies regarding diagnosis and evaluation of delirium in hospitalized elderly medical patients, *Am J Med* 97:278, 1994.
16. Drugs that cause psychiatric symptoms, *Med Lett* 31:113, 1989.
17. Chen WH et al: Low dose propranolol-induced delirium: 3 cases reported and a review of the literature, *Kaohsiung J Med Sci* 10:40, 1994.
18. Leinonen E et al: Delirium during fluoxetine treatment: a case report, *Ann Clin Psychiatry* 5:255, 1993.
19. Lemesh RA: Accidental chronic salicylate intoxication in an elderly patient: major morbidity despite early recognition, *Vet Hum Toxicol* 35:34, 1993.
20. Steinberg RB et al: Acute toxic delirium in a patient using transdermal fentanyl, *Anesth Analg* 75:1014, 1992.
21. Furlong FW: Possible psychiatric significance of excessive coffee consumption, *Can Psychiatr Assoc J* 20:557, 1975.
22. Shen WW: Cola-induced psychotic organic brain syndrome: a case report, *Rocky Mt Med J* 76:312, 1979.
23. Alciati A et al: Three cases of delirium after "ecstasy" ingestion, *J Psychoactive Drugs* 31:167, 1999.
24. Levy AB: Delirium induced by inhalation of typewriter correction fluid, *Psychosomatics* 27:665, 1986.
25. Hodkinson HM: *Common symptoms of disease in the elderly,* Oxford, 1976, Blackwell.
26. Stewart RB, Hale WE: Acute confusional states in older adults and the role of polypharmacy, *Ann Rev Public Health* 13:415, 1992.
27. Tune L et al: Anticholinergic effects of drugs commonly prescribed for the elderly: potential means for assessing risk of delirium, *Am J Psychiatry* 149:1393, 1992.
28. Levkoff SE et al: Identification of factors associated with the diagnosis of delirium in elderly hospitalized patients, *J Am Geriatr Soc* 36:1099, 1988.
29. Zisook S, Braff DL: Delirium: recognition and management in the older patient, *Geriatrics* 41:67, 1986.
30. Folstein MF, Folstein SE, McHugh PR: The "mini-mental state": a practical method for grading the cognitive state of patients for the clinician, *J Psychiatry Res* 12:189, 1975.
31. American Psychiatric Association Practice Guidelines: Practice guidelines for the treatment of patients with delirium, *Am J Psychiatry* 156(Suppl), 1999.
32. Nelson A, Fogel B, Faust D: Bedside cognitive screening instruments: a critical assessment, *J Nerv Ment Dis* 175:73, 1986.
33. Roca RP: Bedside cognitive examination, *Psychosomatics* 28:71, 1987.
34. Feher EP et al: Establishing the limits of the mini-mental state, *Arch Neurol* 49:87, 1992.
35. Inouye SK et al: Clarifying confusion: the confusion assessment method: a new method for detection of delirium, *Ann Intern Med* 113:941, 1990.
36. Strothen CM: Intracranial disease. In Juhl JH, Grummy AB (editors): *Essentials of radiologic imaging,* Philadelphia, 1987, JB Lippincott.
37. Jacobson SA et al: Conventional and quantitative EEG in the diagnosis of delirium among elderly patients, *J Neurol Neurosurg Psychiatry* 56:153, 1993.
38. Brenner RP: The electroencephalogram in altered states of consciousness, *Neurol Clin* 3:615, 1985.
39. Hyperbaric oxygen therapy: a committee report, *Undersea Hyperb Med Soc,* 20, 1993.
40. Inouye SK, Charpentier PA: A predictive model for delirium in hospitalized elderly medical patients based on admission characteristics, *Ann Intern Med* 119:474, 1993.
41. Pollanen MS et al: Unexpected death related to restraint from excited delirium: a retrospective study of deaths in police custody and in the community, *CMAJ* 158:1603, 1998.
42. O'Halloran RL, Lewman LV: Restraint asphyxiation in excited delirium, *Am J Forensic Med Pathol* 14:289, 1993.
43. Menza MA et al: Decreased extrapyramidal symptoms with intravenous haloperidol, *J Clin Psychiatry* 48:278, 1987.
44. Sharma ND et al: Torsades de pointes associated with intravenous haloperidol in critically ill patients, *Am J Cardiol* 81:238, 1998.
45. Liptzin B: Delirium. In Sadavoy J et al, editors: *Comprehensive review of geriatric psychiatry,* ed 2, Washington, DC, American Psychiatric Press, 1996.
46. Fernandez F et al: Treatment of severe, refractory agitation with a haloperidol drip, *J Clin Psychiatry* 49:239, 1988.
47. Santos AB et al: Managing agitation in the critical care setting, *S Carolina Med Assoc* 88:386, 1992.
48. Thomas H, Schwartz E, Petrilli R: Droperidol versus haloperidol for chemical restraint of agitated and combative patients, *Ann Emerg Med* 21:407, 1992.
49. Sipahimalani A, Massand PS: Use of risperidone in delirium: case reports, *Ann Clin Pyschiatry* 9:105, 1997.
50. Ravona-Springer R et al: Delirium in elderly patients treated with risperidone: a report of three cases, *J Clin Psychopharmacol* 18:171, 1998.
51. Menza MA, Murray GB, Holmes VF: Controlled study of extrapyramidal reactions in the management of delirious medically ill patients: intravenous haloperidol versus intravenous haloperidol plus benzodiazepines, *Heart Lung* 17:238, 1988.
52. Tesar GE, Murray GB, Cassen NH: Use of high-dose intravenous haloperidol in the treatment of agitated cardiac patients, *J Clin Psychopharmacol* 5:344, 1985.

53. Deleted in pages.
54. Fogel BS, Mills MJ, Landen JE: Legal aspects of the treatment of delirium, *Hosp Community Psychiatry* 37:154, 1986.
55. Inouye SK et al: Does delirium contribute to poor hospital outcomes? A three site epidemiologic study, *J Gen Int Med* 13:234, 1998.
56. O'Keefe S, Lavan J: The prognostic significance of delirium in older hospitalized patients, *J Am Geriatr Soc* 45:174, 1997.
57. Cole MG, Primeau FJ: Prognosis of delirium in elderly hospital patients, *Canad Med Assoc J* 149:41, 1993.
58. Weytingh MD, Bossuyt PMM, van Crevel H: Reversible dementia: more than 10% or less than 1%? A quantitative review, *J Neurol* 242:446, 1995.
59. Alzheimer A: Uber eine eigenartige Erkrankuzg de Himrinde, *Allerg Z Psychiatr* 64:146, 1907.
60. Brookmeyer R, Gray S, Kawas C: Projections of Alzheimer's disease in the United States and the public health impact of delaying disease onset, *Am J Public Health* 88:1337, 1998.
61. Geldmacher DS, Whitehouse PJ: Evaluation of dementia, *N Engl J Med* 335:330, 1996.
62. Carr DB et al: Current concepts in the pathogenesis of Alzheimer's disease, *Am J Med* 103(Suppl), 1997.
63. Antonelli IR et al: Unrecognized dementia: sociodemographic correlates, *Aging* 4:327, 1992.
64. Roberts GW, Allsop D, Bruton C: The occult aftermath of boxing, *J Neurol Neurosurg Psych* 53:373, 1990.
65. Levy RM et al: Central nervous system disorders in AIDS. In *AIDS pathogenesis and treatment,* New York, 1988, Marcel Dekker.
66. Gauthier S et al: Alzheimer's disease: current knowledge, management and research, *Can Med Assoc J* 157:1047, 1997.
67. Morris JC et al: Very mild Alzheimer's disease: informant-based clinical, psychometric, and pathologic distinction from normal aging, *Neurology* 41:469, 1991.
68. Morris JC et al: Cerebral amyloid deposition and diffuse plaques in "normal" aging: evidence for presymptomatic and very mild Alzheimer's disease, *Neurology* 46:707, 1996.
69. Morris JC: Relationship of plaques and tangles to Alzheimer's disease phenotype. In: Goate AM, Ashall F, editors: *The pathobiology of Alzheimer's disease,* San Diego, 1995, Academic Press.
70. de Silva HA et al: Abnormal function of potassium channels in platelets of patients with Alzheimer's disease, *Lancet* 352:1590, 1998.
71. Strittmatter WJ et al: Apolipoprotein E: high avidity binding to beta-amyloid and increased frequency of type 4 allele in late onset Alzheimer's disease, *Proc Natl Acad Sci USA* 90:1977, 1993.
72. Roses AD: Apolipoprotein E affects the rate of Alzheimer disease expression: beta-amyloid burden is secondary consequence dependent on APOE genotype and duration of disease, *J Neuropathol Exp Neurol* 53:429, 1994.
73. Selkoe DJ: Alzheimer's disease: genotypes, phenotypes, and treatments, *Science* 275:630, 1997.
74. Breitner JCS et al: Inverse association of anti-inflammatory treatments and Alzheimer's disease: initial results of a co-twin control study, *Neurology* 44:227, 1994.
75. Dubin WR, Weiss KJ, Zeccandi JA: Organic brain syndrome, *JAMA* 249:60, 1983.
76. Navia BA et al: The AIDS dementia complex. II. Neuropathology, *Ann Neurol* 19:525, 1986.
77. Rostad SW et al: Human immunodeficiency virus (HIV) infection in brains with AIDS-related leukoencephalopathy, *AIDS Res Hum Retroviruses* 3:363, 1987.
78. Sharen LR, Cho ES, Epstein LG: Multinucleated giant cells and HTLV-III in AIDS encephalopathy, *Hum Pathol* 17:271, 1986.
79. Kato T et al: Neuropathology of acquired immune deficiency syndrome (AIDS) in 53 autopsy cases with particular emphasis on microglial nodules and multinucleated giant cells, *Acta Neuropathol (Berl)* 73:287, 1987.
80. Weiner WJ, Goetz CG: *Neurology for the non-neurologist,* Philadelphia, 1999, Lippincott Williams and Wilkins.
81. Solari A et al: Agreement in the clinical diagnosis of dementia: evaluation of a case series with mild cognitive impairment, *Neuroepidemiology* 13:89, 1994.
82. Mendez MF et al: Psychiatric symptoms associated with Alzheimer's disease, *J Neuropsychiatry Clin Neurosci* 2:28, 1990.
83. Cummings JL et al: Aphasia in dementia of the Alzheimer type, *Neurology* 35:394, 1985.
84. Erkinjantti T et al: Dementia among medical inpatients: evaluation of 2000 consecutive admissions, *Arch Intern Med* 146:1923, 1986.
85. Will RG et al: A new variant of Creutzfeldt-Jakob disease in the UK, *Lancet* 347:921, 1996.
86. Lachner G, Engel RR: Differentiation of dementia and depression by memory tests: a meta-analysis, *J Nerv Ment Dis* 182:34, 1994.
87. Brisman MH et al: Reversible dementia due to macroprolactinoma: case report, *J Neurosurg* 79:135, 1993.
88. Marx J: NGF and Alzheimer's: hopes and fears, *Science* 247:408, 1990.

99 Brain and Cranial Nerve Disorders

Art Pancioli

Neurologic pathology can be difficult to diagnose in the ED. Clinical entities that can be particularly vexing include cranial nerve pathology, cerebral venous thrombosis (CVT), and multiple sclerosis (MS). This chapter covers some of the neurologic pathology that may provide significant diagnostic and therapeutic challenges to the emergency physician (Table 99-1).

TRIGEMINAL NEURALGIA

Perspective

Trigeminal neuralgia, or *tic douloureux,* is a syndrome featuring painful paroxysms in one or more distributions of the trigeminal nerve. Trigeminal neuralgia is relatively uncommon, with an annual occurrence of 4 individuals per 100,000. Trigeminal neuralgia is more common in women than in men, with a female to male ratio of 1.7:1. Individuals affected are most commonly between 50 and 69 years of age, and symptoms occur more commonly on the right side of the face.[1]

Pathophysiology

Trigeminal neuralgia is an idiopathic disorder. One longstanding theory is based on compression of the trigeminal nerve root. This compression may be caused by a tortuous blood vessel in the posterior fossa, an arteriovenous malformation, or a tumor. Notably, however, structural lesions such as these are not found in all patients with trigeminal neuralgia.[2]

Table 99-1. The Cranial Nerves: Normal Function and Pathologic Considerations

Cranial nerve	Clinical function relevant to emergency medicine	Pathologic features	Possible causes
Cranial nerve I: olfactory nerve	Sense of smell	Unilateral anosmia	*Trauma:* Skull fracture or shear injury interrupting olfactory fibers traversing the cribriform plate *Tumor:* Frontal lobe masses compressing the nerve
Cranial nerve II: optic nerve	Vision	Unilateral vision loss	*Trauma:* Traumatic optic neuropathy *Tumor:* Orbital compressive lesion *Inflammatory:* Optic neuritis (MS) *Ischemic:* Ischemic optic neuropathy
Cranial nerve III: oculomotor nerve	Extraoculomotor function via motor fibers to levator palpebrae, superior rectus, medial rectus, inferior rectus, inferior oblique muscles Pupillary constriction via parasympathetic fibers to constrictor pupillae and ciliary muscles	Ptosis caused by loss of levator palpebrae function Eye deviated laterally and down Diplopia Dilated, nonreactive pupil Loss of accommodation	*Trauma:* Herniation of the temporal lobe through the tentorial opening causing compression and stretch injury to the nerve *Ischemic:* Especially in diabetes, microvascular ischemic injury to nerve causes extraocular muscle paralysis, but usually is papillary sparing (often painful) *Vascular:* Intracranial aneurysms may press on the nerve leading to dysfunction Myasthenia gravis can lead to atraumatic ocular muscle palsy
Cranial nerve IV: trochlear nerve	Motor supply to the superior oblique muscle	Inability to move eye in inward rotation, downward, and laterally Diplopia Patients will tilt head toward unaffected eye to overcome outward rotation of affected eye	Trauma is the most common cause of nerve dysfunction
Cranial nerve V: trigeminal nerve	Motor supply to muscles of mastication and to tensor tympani Sensory to face, scalp, oral cavity (including tongue and teeth)	Partial facial anesthesia Episodic, lancinating facial pain associated with benign triggers such as chewing, brushing teeth, light touch	*Trauma:* Facial bone fracture may injure one section leading to area of facial anesthesia Tic douloureux
Cranial nerve VI: abducens nerve	Motor supply to the lateral rectus muscle	Inability to move affected eye laterally Diplopia upon attempting lateral gaze	*Tumor:* Lesions in the cerebellopontine angle Any lesion, vascular or otherwise, in the cavernous sinus may compress nerve *Elevated intracranial pressure (ICP):* Because of its position and long intracranial length, increased ICP from any cause may lead to injury and dysfunction of the nerve

Cranial nerve VII: facial nerve	Motor supply to muscles of facial expression Parasympathetic stimulation of the lacrimal, submandibular, and sublingual glands Sensation to the ear canal and tympanic membrane	*Hemifacial paresis:* Lower motor neuron lesion with entire side of face paralyzed Upper motor neuron lesion leaves forehead musculature functioning Abnormal taste Sensory deficit around ear Intolerance to sudden loud noises	*Lower motor neuron:* *Infection (viral):* The likely cause of Bell's palsy *Lyme disease:* The most common cause of bilateral cranial nerve VII palsy in areas where Lyme disease is endemic Bacterial infection extending from otitis media *Upper motor neuron:* Stroke, tumor
Cranial nerve VIII: vestibulocochlear nerve	Hearing and balance	Unilateral hearing loss Tinnitus Vertigo, unsteadiness	*Tumors:* Acoustic neuroma Mimics Ménière's disease, perilymphatic fistula
Cranial nerve IX: glossopharyngeal nerve	General sensation to posterior third of tongue Taste for posterior third of tongue Motor supply to the stylopharyngeus	Clinical pathology referable to the nerve in isolation is very rare Occasionally painful paroxysms beginning in the throat and radiating down the side of the neck in front of the ear but behind the mandible	Brainstem lesions Glossopharyngeal neuralgia
Cranial nerve X: vagus nerve	Motor to striated and muscles of the pharynx, larynx and tensor (veli) palatini Motor to smooth muscles and glands of the pharynx, larynx, thoracic and abdominal viscera Sensory from larynx, trachea, esophagus, thoracic and abdominal viscera	*Unilateral loss of palatal elevation:* Patients complain that on drinking liquids the fluid refluxes through the nose *Unilateral vocal cord paralysis:* Hoarse voice	Brainstem lesion Injury to the recurrent laryngeal nerve during surgery
Cranial nerve XI: spinal accessory nerve	Motor supply to the sternocleidomastoid and trapezius muscles	Downward and lateral rotation of the scapula and shoulder drop	Trauma to the nerve
Cranial nerve XII: hypoglossal nerve	Motor supply to the intrinsic and extrinsic muscles of the tongue	*Tongue deviations:* Upper motor neuron lesion causes the tongue to deviate toward the opposite side Lower motor neuron lesion causes the tongue to deviate toward the side of the lesion, and the affected side atrophies over time	Stroke or tumor can cause upper motor neuron lesion Amyotrophic lateral sclerosis (ALS) can cause bilateral lower motor neuron lesion with atrophy Metastatic disease to the skull base may involve the nerve

Clinical Features

Trigeminal neuralgia is a disorder of unilateral facial pain, typically characterized by lancinating paroxysms of pain in the lips, teeth, gums, or chin. The pain of trigeminal neuralgia is commonly associated with physical triggers such as chewing, brushing teeth, shaving, washing or touching the affected area of the face, swallowing, or exposure to hot or cold temperature in the affected area. Trigeminal neuralgia is most commonly found in the maxillary and mandibular divisions of the trigeminal nerve. Rarely, trigeminal neuralgia occurs in the ophthalmic division alone. Patients tend to have clusters of the pain that last a few seconds to several minutes. The attacks can occur during the day or night, but rarely occur during sleep.[2,3]

Diagnostic Strategies

The history and physical examination are the primary diagnostic modalities in the ED. A careful physical examination must be performed to rule out other painful syndromes including odontogenic infections, sinus disease, otitis media, acute glaucoma, temporomandibular joint disease, and herpes zoster. Patients with no local findings to explain the painful syndrome require a very careful neurologic examination. Any evidence of a neurologic deficit should prompt suspicion of a structural lesion, including aneurysm, tumor, or other intracranial lesion such as MS. Notably, 2% to 4% of patients with trigeminal neuralgia also have MS.[4] Patients with normal head and neck examinations and no neurologic deficits who have episodic, unilateral facial pain associated with nonpainful triggers are likely to have trigeminal neuralgia.

Management

Since the 1960s the treatment of choice for trigeminal neuralgia has been the anticonvulsant carbamazepine. This treatment is, however, based on uncontrolled studies, and the mechanism of action of anticonvulsant therapy for trigeminal neuralgia is unclear. The true efficacy of medical therapy is difficult to assess due to a very high rate of spontaneous remission. Nonetheless, carbamazepine appears to be an effective and well-tolerated treatment. The initial dosage of carbamazepine is 100 mg twice daily, then increased to three times daily. The dose may be increased by 100 mg per day, up to a maximum of 1200 mg per day. Due to potential side effects of carbamazepine, complete blood count and liver function studies should be performed periodically on these patients. Additional therapies that have been used for trigeminal neuralgia include phenytoin, baclofen, valproate sodium, lamotrigine, and gabapentin. No medical therapies, however, have been shown to be more effective than carbamazepine.[3]

Surgical management has been an option for patients since the 1950s. Surgical procedures to ablate the painful crises of trigeminal neuralgia include both peripheral approaches and central procedures. Peripheral strategies include medication injection or cryotherapy designed to temporarily block, or permanently ablate, branches of the peripheral trigeminal nerve. Although these are relatively effective initially, recurrence is common. Repeated nerve blocks are not recommended due to a high risk of permanent facial anesthesia.

Central procedures can be divided into percutaneous approaches or open approaches. Percutaneous destruction of the trigeminal ganglion can be done via radio frequency ablation, thermal ablation, glycerol injection, or balloon microcompression. These procedures have the risk of corneal anesthesia, oculomotor paresis, or masticatory weakness.[5]

Open surgical management is the surgical option of choice in most centers. Open surgical treatments include microvascular decompression of the nerve with or without partial ablation. Although the open microvascular decompression procedure has proven very effective, the surgery can have significant side effects. These can include hearing loss, facial anesthesia, cerebrospinal fluid leak, brainstem or cerebellar injury, headaches, meningitis, and death.[6] Recently, gamma knife radiosurgery, which is a minimally invasive, highly directed stereotactic radiosurgery, has been associated with good outcomes in trigeminal neuralgia. This highly specialized technique requires extremely sophisticated stereotactic radio frequency equipment, and is only available in specialized centers.[7]

Disposition

Patients with suspected trigeminal neuralgia should be referred for specialty evaluation. Patients with any physical findings during the head and neck examination should not be considered to have trigeminal neuralgia, and patients with any neurologic deficit require urgent imaging studies to rule out a mass or vascular abnormality.

Key Concepts

- Patients commonly visit multiple physicians in multiple settings before a definitive diagnosis of trigeminal neuralgia is established. A high index of suspicion may provide the patient with more rapid and appropriate specialty consultation and therapy.

FACIAL NERVE PARALYSIS

Perspective

Facial nerve paralysis is an emotionally devastating disorder for the patient and presents a diagnostic challenge to the emergency physician. The acute onset of facial nerve paralysis will often prompt an ED visit, where early diagnosis and early appropriate therapy can improve a patient's chance for recovery of function of the facial nerve. The acute onset of facial nerve paralysis affects approximately 20 to 25 individuals per 100,000 per year without geographic, gender, or race predilections.[8,9]

Principles of Disease

The facial nerve innervates the muscles of facial expression and the muscles of the scalp and external ear, in addition to the buccinator, platysma, stapedius, stylohyoid, and posterior belly of the digastric muscles. The sensory portion of the nerve supplies the anterior two thirds of the tongue with taste, and portions of the external auditory meatus, soft palate, and adjacent pharynx with general sensation. The parasympathetic portion supplies secretomotor fibers for the submandibular, sublingual, lacrimal, nasal, and palatine glands.[10]

The nerve originates from the pontomedullary junction of the brainstem. The nerve enters the internal auditory meatus with cranial nerve VIII. Within the temporal bone the facial nerve has four major branches: the greater and lesser superficial petrosal nerves, the nerve to the stapedius muscle, and the chorda tympani. The facial nerve exits the temporal bone at the stylomastoid foramen. The nerve then enters the parotid gland where it divides to supply the muscles of facial expression.[10,11]

Pathophysiology

Although the complete differential diagnosis for facial nerve paralysis is lengthy, the causes pertinent to emergency medicine can be grouped into several categories: infectious, traumatic, and neoplastic.

Infection

Bell's Palsy Bell's palsy, also commonly called *idiopathic facial paralysis,* has long been postulated to have a viral cause. This disease entity is characterized by an abrupt onset of a lower motor neuron paresis that can progress over 1 to 7 days to complete paralysis. A prodromal illness is described by 60% of patients. Symptoms frequently associated with the facial paresis include ear pain, a perception of sensory change on the involved side of the face, decreased tearing, an overflow of tears upon the cheek (epiphora), abnormally acute hearing (hyperacusis), and an impairment or perversion of taste (dysgeusia).[12]

Treatment approaches can be medical or surgical. The primary medical therapies for Bell's palsy center on reducing inflammatory changes to the nerve with corticosteroids, and treating the presumed viral cause. If these therapies are unsuccessful then surgical decompression may be considered.

The use of corticosteroids for Bell's palsy has been controversial. Their use is based on the belief that edema of the nerve, confined within the facial canal, is causing or contributing to the nerve injury. Based on this theory, most experts currently recommend a course of prednisone with an initial dose of 1 mg/kg/day for 7-10 days with or without a short taper.[8,11,13,14] Although the absolute time frame for steroid initiation remains unclear, experts indicate that therapy should be started as soon as possible. Ideally, steroid therapy would be initiated within the first 24 hours but should be considered for patients without contraindications who seek treatment within 1 week of symptom onset.[13]

A number of publications have advanced the belief that Bell's palsy may be caused by herpes virus infection. One study demonstrated herpes simplex virus type 1 DNA in the endoneural tissue of 11 of 14 patients with Bell's palsy, but not in controls.[15] In one paper, patients treated with prednisone and acyclovir are described as having a more favorable recovery than patients treated with prednisone alone.[16] Recommended antiviral regimens include acyclovir 400-800 mg orally five times daily for 10 days. The newer oral antiviral agents such as valacyclovir and famciclovir have better oral absorption, are better tolerated, and have been recommended as alternatives to acyclovir.[11,13,14] As with steroid therapy, although earlier treatment is preferred, treatment should be considered for patients within 1 week of symptom onset.

Ramsey Hunt Syndrome (Herpes Zoster Oticus) Ramsey Hunt syndrome is characterized by unilateral facial paralysis, a herpetiform vesicular eruption, and vestibulocochlear dysfunction. The vesicular eruption may occur on the pinna, external auditory canal, tympanic membrane, soft palate, oral cavity, face, and neck as far down as the shoulder. There is considerably more pain than is associated with Bell's palsy, and the pain is frequently out of proportion to physical findings. In addition, outcomes are worse than with Bell's palsy, with a lower incidence of complete facial recovery and the possibility of sensorineural hearing loss. Therapy is similar to that for Bell's palsy. Both prednisone and antiviral therapy for 7 to 10 days have been advocated.[11,17]

Lyme Disease Lyme disease is the most frequent vector-borne infection in the United States. It is caused by the spirochete *Borrelia burgdorferi* and is spread by the bite of *Ixodes* genus ticks. Neurologic manifestations can occur in any phase of the disease, and the incidence of facial palsy in patients with neurologic involvement is 35% to 51%. In regions where Lyme disease is endemic, it has been shown to be the leading cause of facial paralysis in children, causing one half of all cases of facial nerve paralysis.[18,19]

Bilateral facial nerve paralysis is rare but can occur with systemic infections. The two diseases most commonly associated with bilateral simultaneous onset of facial paralysis are Lyme disease and infectious mononucleosis. The emergency physician should consider bilateral facial paralysis to be a manifestation of Lyme disease until further testing can confirm or refute this diagnosis.[14,18-20]

Bacterial Facial paralysis can occur from acute bacterial infections of the middle ear, mastoid, or external auditory canal. In the preantibiotic era, facial paralysis was associated with acute otitis media in approximately 2% of cases. Now, however, facial paralysis occurs in only 0.16% of cases of otitis media.[11] Treatment involves intravenous antibiotics and myringotomy for decompression. Malignant otitis externa is another bacterial infection that can be associated with facial paralysis. This disease entity is most commonly seen among immunocompromised patients and is usually caused by a pseudomonal infection. Treatment involves prolonged intravenous antipseudomonal antibiotic therapy and may require surgical debridement.[14,21]

Trauma

Among patients with head trauma, the facial nerve is the most commonly injured cranial nerve. The cause is generally a temporal bone fracture with nerve transection. Surgical exploration is warranted if there is firm evidence after head trauma that the nerve has been transected, indicated by a sudden onset of complete unilateral facial paralysis, loss of electrical activity, and evidence of a displaced fracture involving the facial canal.

Neoplasm

Tumors of the facial nerve itself, or tumors anywhere along the course of the facial nerve that invade or compress the nerve, may lead to facial paralysis. Typically the course is progressive over at least 3 weeks. A sudden onset of paralysis, however, does not rule out an underlying tumor, since facial paralysis secondary to a neoplasm has a sudden onset in approximately 25% of cases.[11] In patients who suffer from recurrent ipsilateral facial paralysis, significant pain, prolonged symptoms, or any other cranial nerve abnormality the suspicion of a tumor must be high.

Clinical Features

The history and physical examination are the primary components of ED evaluation of facial paralysis. The history should focus on symptom onset, concentrating on timing and rapidity of onset and looking for any associated symptoms. A rapid onset of facial paralysis with dysgeusia and hyperacusis preceded by a viral prodrome will lead the clinician toward a diagnosis of Bell's palsy. A history of recurrent ipsilateral paralysis or slow progression of symptoms should alert the physician to the possibility of a tumor. Associated cranial nerve abnormalities, although occasionally seen with Bell's palsy, should also alert the physician to the possibility of a tumor. The Ramsey Hunt syndrome causes significant pain and a vesicular rash, although the rash may follow the facial paresis by a few days. Significant anatomic abnormalities on visual or otoscopic inspection of the ipsilateral ear will be found with bacterial otitis media and otitis externa. Finally, systemic symptoms or bilateral facial paresis, especially in endemic areas, should raise the possibility of Lyme disease.

Diagnostic Strategies

The diagnostic workup of a facial nerve paresis is based on the clinician's index of suspicion that the patient has a disease process other than Bell's palsy. If the clinical history is classic for Bell's palsy, then no imaging or laboratory studies are required. Notably, any history of possible exposure merits serologic evaluation for Lyme disease. Although outpatient testing including electroneurography may ultimately be performed, this is not a part of the ED evaluation.

The physical examination finding of a "central" seventh nerve paralysis (upper-face sparing) should prompt an imaging workup with computed axial tomography (CT) or magnetic resonance imaging (MRI), and consideration should be given to the possibility of an acute stroke or other hemispheric lesion. Any history or physical examination findings suggestive of a possible tumor require imaging with an MRI to rule out a neoplasm. The study of choice will depend on the institution and the consultant.

Disposition

The vast majority of patients who have a seventh nerve paralysis will have clinical Bell's palsy and may be discharged with short-term follow-up. Patients with a possible hemispheric process such as stroke or tumor should be admitted for further evaluation. Patients who might have Lyme disease need antibiotic initiation and referral if they appear nontoxic, and admission if systemically ill.

Patients with a peripheral facial nerve paralysis should have the ipsilateral eye patched and consideration should be given to ophthalmologic follow-up. This is because of the high rate of corneal abrasions and corneal dryness associated with the inability to properly blink or completely close the eye.

Key Concepts

- Recent literature highlights significant potential benefit for patients with clinical Bell's palsy when they are treated early in the course with a combination of corticosteroids and antiviral medication.
- Slowly progressive facial paralysis is suggestive of a neoplasm.
- Recurrent unilateral paralysis may occur with Bell's palsy but is frequently (30%) seen in tumor patients.
- Simultaneous bilateral facial paralysis excludes Bell's palsy as a diagnosis and is suggestive of Lyme disease.
- Patients who have facial muscle paresis with intact forehead movement should be considered to have an upper motor neuron lesion until proven otherwise.
- Lyme disease must be considered a possible cause, especially in endemic regions.

ACOUSTIC NEUROMA

Perspective

Acoustic neuroma is a rare but important cause of sensorineural hearing loss. Patients with asymmetric hearing loss or unilateral tinnitus should be evaluated to rule out acoustic neuroma and thereby prevent further neurologic damage. An acoustic neuroma, also referred to as a vestibular schwannoma, arises from the Schwann cells covering the vestibular branch of the eighth cranial nerve as it passes through the internal auditory canal. The annual incidence of acoustic neuroma is one case per 100,000. The female to male ratio is 1.5:1. Acoustic neuroma is very rarely bilateral, occurring in approximately 5% of cases and generally occurring with Type II neurofibromatosis. Acoustic neuromas, although histologically benign, can cause neurologic damage via direct compression on the eighth cranial nerve and the other structures in the cerebellopontine angle.[23]

Principles of Disease

An acoustic neuroma arises from the Schwann cells covering the vestibular branch of the eighth cranial nerve as it passes through the internal auditory canal. The tumor may compress the cochlear (acoustic) branch of the eighth cranial nerve, causing hearing loss, tinnitus, and dysequilibrium. Continued growth of the tumor may result in compression of structures in the cerebellopontine angle, where the facial and trigeminal nerves may be compressed and damaged. Larger tumors may further encroach upon the brainstem, and if large enough may compress the fourth ventricle, ultimately resulting in signs of increased intracranial pressure (ICP).[24]

Clinical Features

Asymmetric sensorineural hearing loss is the hallmark of acoustic neuroma. Up to 15% of patients with acoustic neuroma, however, will have normal results on an audiogram. These patients typically have symptoms such as unilateral tinnitus, imbalance, headache, fullness in the ear, otalgia, or facial nerve weakness. Thus, patients with asymmetric symptoms should be further evaluated for acoustic neuroma even with the occurrence of a normal audiogram.[25]

Acoustic neuromas are extremely slow-growing tumors. Therefore, symptom onset is generally quite gradual. In one series of 126 cases, the average time from symptom onset to discovery of an acoustic neuroma was approximately 4 years.[26]

Diagnostic Strategies

Any abnormality found during the history or physical examination that might indicate acoustic neuroma should be immediately evaluated with an audiogram. If this test is normal and symptoms remain unexplained, a gadolinium-enhanced MRI may be warranted. This imaging technique is extremely sensitive and has led to earlier diagnosis and a decrease in the mean size at detection of acoustic neuromas. The smaller the tumor at the time of diagnosis, the more options there are for therapy and the better is the potential prognosis.[23]

Differential Considerations

The majority of disease entities in the differential considerations for acoustic neuroma cause symmetric sensorineural hearing loss. Asymmetric sensorineural hearing loss has few causes other than acoustic neuroma. Ménière's disease may present a diagnostic dilemma because it can be asymmetrical. Ménière's disease may be differentiated from acoustic neuroma in that the tinnitus of Ménière's disease is usually intermittent, while the tinnitus of acoustic neuroma is typically continuous. In addition, patients with Ménière's disease typically describe true vertigo, whereas patients with an acoustic neuroma are more likely to describe imbalance or dysequilibrium.

Acoustic neuromas account for 80% of all cerebellopontine angle tumors. Among all other lesions, meningioma is the most common. Meningiomas more frequently cause symptoms of facial palsy or trigeminal nerve abnormality. There may be, however, considerable similarity between the clinical picture of a meningioma and that of an acoustic neuroma in the cerebellopontine angle.[27]

Management

Acoustic neuroma may be removed surgically or with stereotactic radiation. Injuries to the trigeminal, facial, and acoustic nerves, and to the cerebellum, are all possible complications of these procedures.

Disposition

Patients with suspected acoustic neuroma should be referred for an audiogram and evaluation by specialists in either otolaryngology or neurosurgery.

Key Concepts

- The onset of unilateral auditory symptoms requires evaluation and referral.
- Neurologic symptoms of lower cranial nerve dysfunction, ataxia, or raised ICP may be caused by a benign tumor of the cerebellopontine angle.
- The smaller the tumor at diagnosis, the lower the risk of definitive treatment.

DIABETIC CRANIAL MONONEUROPATHY

Perspective

Cranial mononeuropathies are uncommon, but when they occur they will commonly lead to an ED visit. Cranial mononeuropathies attributed to diabetic complications most often affect the extraocular muscles. The oculomotor nerve is the most commonly affected cranial nerve, followed in order by the trochlear and abducens nerves. In one large series in Japan, the incidence of cranial nerve palsies was 1.0% among diabetics and 0.1% among nondiabetics.[28,29]

The incidence of palsy in the third, sixth, and seventh cranial nerves was studied in diabetic patients.[28] The incidence of cranial nerve palsies in diabetic patients was significantly higher than in nondiabetic patients. In this study, the incidence of diabetic complications was compared between those patients with facial palsy and those with ophthalmoplegia. Only one out of nine patients with facial palsy (11%) had diabetic complications, whereas 7 out of 10 patients with ophthalmoplegia (70%) demonstrated diabetic complications. This difference was statistically significant. The authors concluded that ophthalmoplegia appears to be closely related to diabetes, and facial palsy is less strongly correlated with it.[28]

Principles of Disease

The pathologic basis of diabetic mononeuropathy appears to be ischemia of the affected cranial nerve. The ischemic injury to the affected nerve appears to be based on an occlusion of an intraneural nutrient artery serving the nerve. This occlusion will lead to injury primarily to the center of the nerve, because the core fibers are more dependent upon the supply from such nutrient arteries. The peripheral fibers are less affected because they have some supply from collateral vessels. In the oculomotor nerve, the preservation of the circumferentially located parasympathetic fibers explains the pupillary sparing that is usually found in this syndrome. In two studies, the microvascular changes of the intraneural arteries that lead to occlusion were noted in diabetics but absent in nondiabetics.[30,31]

Clinical Features

Patients typically complain of an acute onset of unilateral, retroocular and supraorbital pain, diplopia, and ptosis.[29] Physical findings of a third cranial nerve palsy include the inability to move the eye superiorly and medially. It is also accompanied by ptosis. The pupillary light reflex is usually present. Although less common, the fourth and sixth cranial nerves may be affected. The physical finding associated with a fourth cranial nerve palsy is the inability to move the eye inferolaterally, and with the sixth cranial nerve palsy the patient is unable to move the eye laterally. Because of the long intracranial course of the sixth nerve, a patient with an isolated sixth nerve palsy should be evaluated for an intracranial lesion or increased ICP.[32]

Differential Considerations

Cranial nerve dysfunction demands a thorough history, physical examination, neurologic examination, and cranial imaging such as MRI. Diabetic mononeuropathy must be considered a diagnosis of exclusion, and the differential diagnosis must include trauma, tumor, vertebrobasilar ischemia, and hemorrhage into the brainstem.[33]

Management

Analgesics, patching the affected eye, and antiplatelet therapy constitute the required therapy. The prognosis is good. If the neuropathy does not improve within 3 to 6 months, or if more than one nerve is affected, another cause should be sought. Complete resolution is expected within the first year.

Key Concepts

- Diabetic neuropathy is a diagnosis of exclusion since no definitive diagnostic testing is available.
- Both ischemic and hemorrhagic brainstem lesions must be ruled out in the case of an acute ophthalmoplegia.
- An extraocular mononeuropathy is sufficiently common in patients with diabetes mellitus that the occurrence in isolation should lead the physician to evaluate the patient for previously undiagnosed diabetes.

CEREBRAL VENOUS THROMBOSIS

Perspective

There are no precise studies of the epidemiology of CVT. In a case series, the mean patient age was approximately 38 years, with a female to male ratio of 1.5:1.[34]

Principles of Disease

Cerebral blood is drained by several major veins, which lead into the dural sinuses. The major dural sinuses are the superior sagittal sinus, the inferior sagittal sinus, the straight sinus, the lateral sinuses, and the sigmoid sinuses. Similar to venous thrombosis in other locations, there are multiple causes and predisposing factors that may ultimately lead to CVT. Underlying causes are often divided into infectious or noninfectious categories. Infectious causes include local infections, such as sinusitis, otitis media, cellulitis on the face, and systemic infections. Noninfectious causes include direct injury to the cerebral venous system via trauma, surgery, tumor, dehydration, or any other condition that may predispose a patient to a hypercoagulable state.[34]

Clinical Features

The symptoms associated with CVT are quite varied. This variability stems from differences in thrombus location and acuity of thrombus formation. Headache is the primary feature of CVT in 74% to 90% of affected patients.[34,35] Papilledema is noted in 45% of cases.[35] Lethargy, decreased level of consciousness, or mental status changes may be seen. Seizures are seen in 50% of patients in the acute phase.[34] In addition to the location and acuity of thrombosis formation, a patient's symptom onset will vary based on the extent of collateral vessel growth in the venous territory. Early thrombotic changes may be well compensated for by the collateral venous drainage. Symptoms will appear only when the compensation for venous thrombosis is no longer sufficient. Variability in collateralization between patients also adds to the variability and time course of symptomatology. One study of 102 patients with CVT documents a mean delay of 14 days between the onset of first symptoms and the hospital arrival.[36] The referenced incidence of focal neurologic findings on clinical examination varies between series, ranging from 25% to 71%, and includes seizures.[34,35] Based on the broad spectrum of clinical features, the clinician must have a high degree of clinical suspicion of CVT in the presence of unexplained headache, especially when combined with focal neurologic deficit, papilledema, or seizures.

Diagnostic Strategies

The gold standard for the diagnosis of CVT has long been cerebral angiography. The advent of MRI and magnetic resonance venography (MRV) has significantly improved diagnostic accuracy. CT scanning is also useful in the initial workup of the patient with possible CVT, but CT is not sensitive or specific enough to reliably confirm or exclude it. Findings on CT that are consistent with CVT include hyperdensity of a thrombosed sinus, brain edema, or hemorrhage from swelling secondary to venous congestion. In addition, patients with ventricles that appear smaller than expected for the patient's age may have a CVT.

Similar to CT scanning, MRI can demonstrate local changes secondary to venous congestion, such as brain edema or hemorrhage. In addition, MRI can demonstrate the possibility of CVT based on the lack of what is known as a "flow void." On a normal MRI, a flow void would indicate the presence of blood flow within the sinus. The absence of a flow void indicates a possible thrombus. Diagnostic accuracy, however, is greatly improved through use of MRV. This technique takes advantage of the MRI signal characteristics of flowing blood to create images of venous structures. Combining these imaging techniques further enhances diagnostic accuracy. The presence of a given sinus on conventional MRI and a lack of flow on the MRV are diagnostic of a sinus thrombosis. This combined approach has diagnostic sensitivity similar to that of angiography.[34,37]

Differential Consideration

CVT is difficult to diagnose, and only a high level of suspicion will permit the clinician to detect it. There are numerous causes of nonspecific headache in the differential for CVT. Unexplained headache with either CT findings suggestive of possible CVT or clinical history suggestive of hypercoagulability may lead the clinician to pursue advanced imaging to evaluate a patient for possible CVT.

Management

CVT is a relatively rare disease, and there is a lack of controlled studies evaluating therapy for this condition. Current therapeutic consensus rests on the use of standard heparin to prevent further clot formation and to promote recanalization.[34,35,38,39] Until recently, intravenous heparin was the only option for therapy for patients with CVT. In one placebo-controlled randomized trial of 20 patients, anticoagulation with heparin to a target PTT of 80 to 100 seconds demonstrated benefit, even in patients in which intracranial hemorrhage was seen on CT prior to anticoagulation.[40] In another study of 60 patients randomized to placebo versus low-molecular-weight heparin, no statistical benefit was shown for treatment.[41]

Catheter-based intervention with thrombolysis has been attempted in multiple case series using either urokinase or tissue plasminogen activator. Thrombolysis was shown to be relatively safe and relatively successful in very small case series.[39] In one study of 12 patients, flow was restored completely in six patients, partially in three patients, and could not be restored in the three others. In the three patients in whom flow could not be restored, two had evolution of preexisting intracranial hemorrhage (ICH).[39] Although this new therapy is promising, it should be considered only for cases with symptoms of decreased level of consciousness, elevated ICP, or a rapidly deteriorating neurologic examination.

Disposition

All patients with suspected CVT should be admitted to a unit capable of giving a high level of care with neurologic consultation. Heparinization or catheter-based thrombolysis should be considered.

Key Concepts

- CVT is a relatively rare entity and only a high index of suspicion will lead to the correct diagnosis.
- The onset may be insidious with a considerable delay between onset and arrival in the treatment setting.
- CT scanning is not adequate to rule out CVT. An MRI with MRV is recommended.

MULTIPLE SCLEROSIS

Perspective

MS is an inflammatory disease that affects the central nervous system (CNS). Although the exact etiology remains uncertain, the pathologic manifestation of this inflammatory disease is a demyelination of discrete regions (plaques) within the CNS with a relative sparing of axons. The clinical picture is highly variable, but is classically characterized by episodes of neurologic dysfunction that evolve over days and resolve over weeks.

MS has an overall prevalence in the United States of 0.1%. The peak age at onset is 25 to 30 years, with women being slightly younger at onset than men. The incidence in women exceeds that of men by a ratio of 1.8 to 1. The worldwide prevalence is greatest in the United Kingdom (UK), Scandinavia, and North America. Epidemiologic studies indicate that both genetic and environmental factors are associated with the disease incidence. Data indicating that genetics influence the disease process include a 30% concordance rate among monozygotic twins. In addition, 20% of patients with MS have at least one affected relative. Indicators of environmental influences include the observation that MS is more common in temperate climates. It is rare between 23 degrees north and south latitudes but has a rising incidence above and below 50 degrees north and south latitudes, respectively. Although no exact environmental factor has been identified, if a person emigrates from an area of high prevalence to an area of low prevalence before the age of 20, the risk is diminished. MS is rare in Africans and Asians, but African Americans have a higher incidence than their relatives who remain in Africa.[42] In addition, reports of clusters or miniepidemics support the environmental factors. Thus, an environmental cause superimposed on genetic susceptibility appears likely.[43,44]

Principles of Disease

MS is considered to be an organ-specific autoimmune disease. One theory proposes that genetic factors interact with an environmental trigger or infection to establish pathologically autoreactive T cells in the CNS. After a long and variable latency period (typically 10 to 20 years), a systemic trigger, such as a viral infection or superantigen, activates these T cells. The activated T cells, upon reexposure to the autoantigen, initiate the inflammatory response. This initiates a complex immunologic cascade that leads to the demyelination characteristic of MS. This releases CNS antigens that are hypothesized to initiate further episodes of autoimmune-induced inflammation. The mechanisms underlying this autoimmunity in MS are unknown.[45]

Clinical Features

The clinical picture of MS displays marked heterogenicity. The classic clinical syndrome consists of recurring episodes of neurologic symptoms that rapidly manifest over days and slowly resolve. Variability occurs in age of onset, location of CNS lesions, frequency and severity of relapses, and the degree and time course of progression.

The clinical features of MS can be divided in a manner similar to the divisions of a neurologic examination. They can be divided into aspects of cognitive impairment, cranial nerve dysfunction, impairment of motor pathways, impairment of sensory pathways, impairment of cerebellar pathways, and impairment of bowel, bladder, and sexual functions.[42]

Patients with MS have frequent complaints of poor memory, distractibility, and a decreased capacity for sustained mental effort. Formal neuropsychological testing suggests that cognitive involvement is common and underreported. Specifically, neuropsychological testing has shown that 43% to 65% of patients with MS have cognitive impairment.[46] Notably, there is a correlation between the MRI-based total lesion load and cognitive impairment.[47]

Cranial nerve dysfunction is common in MS. The most common associated cranial nerve abnormality is optic neuritis, a unilateral syndrome characterized by pain in the eye and a variable degree of visual loss affecting primarily central vision. Within 2 years of an attack of optic neuritis, the risk of MS is approximately 20%, and within 15 years it is approximately 45% to 80%.[48,49] Optic neuritis is often the first symptom of MS.[50,51]

Due to lesions in the vestibuloocular connections, the oculomotor pathways may also be affected. This may manifest as diplopia or nystagmus. The nystagmus may be severe enough that the patient may complain of oscillopsia (a subjective oscillation of objects in the visual field). Cranial nerve impairment may also include impairment of facial sensation, which is relatively common. Unilateral facial paresis may also occur. In addition, the occurrence of trigeminal neuralgia in a young person may be an early sign of MS.

Motor pathways are also commonly involved. Specifically, corticospinal tract dysfunction is common in patients with MS. Paraparesis or paraplegia is all too common, and occurs with greater frequency than upper extremity lesions due to the common occurrence of lesions in the motor tracts of the spinal cord. In patients with significant motor weakness, spasms of the legs and trunk may occur when the patient attempts to stand from a seated position. This is manifested on physical examination as spasticity that is typically worse in the legs than the arms. The deep tendon reflexes are markedly exaggerated, and sustained clonus may be demonstrated. Although these symptoms are frequently bilateral, they are generally asymmetrical.[42]

Sensory manifestations are a frequent initial feature of MS and will be present in nearly all patients at some point during the course of the disease. Sensory symptoms are commonly described as numbness, tingling, "pins and needles" paresthesias, coldness, or swelling of the limbs or trunk.[42]

Impairment of the cerebellar pathway results in significant gait imbalance, difficulty with coordinated actions, and dysarthria. Physical examination reveals the typical features of cerebellar dysfunction including dysmetria, dysdiadochokinesis (an impairment of rapid alternating movements), a breakdown in the ability to perform complex movements, an intention tremor in the limbs and head, truncal ataxia, and dysarthria.[42]

Impairment of the bowel, bladder, and sexual functions is also common. The extent of sphincter and sexual dysfunction usually parallels the motor impairment in the lower extremities. Urinary frequency may progress to urinary incontinence with progression of the disease. An atonic bladder may develop, which empties by simple overflow and is often associated with the loss of perception of bladder fullness, and anal and genital hypoesthesia. Constipation becomes common over time, and almost all patients with paraplegia require special measures to maintain bowel habits. Sexual dysfunction, while frequently overlooked, is very common in MS. Approximately 50% of patients become completely sexually inactive secondary to this disease.[42]

Diagnostic Strategies

Although there are no laboratory tests diagnostic for MS, one clinical feature remains relatively unique to this disease. Uhthoff's phenomenon is the eponym for the syndrome in which small increases in the patient's body temperature can temporarily worsen current or preexisting signs or symptoms of MS. Activities such as exercise, a hot bath, exposure to a warm environment, or fever can bring about Uhthoff's phenomenon. This phenomenon reflects subclinical demyelination or preexisting injury to nerves without obvious significant clinical involvement prior to heat exposure or temperature elevation.[42]

The clinical diagnosis rests on the patient having at least two clinical episodes with different neurologic symptoms that occur at different times. Thus MS has commonly been described as having lesions that differ in time and space. It has also been described as a relapsing-remitting disorder with symptoms that fluctuate over time.

Cerebrospinal fluid (CSF) analysis is abnormal in 90% of cases. Fifty percent of patients will have pleocytosis with greater than five lymphocytes per high power field in the CSF. Approximately 70% of patients will have an elevated γ-globulin with immunoglobulin G (IgG) ranging from 10% to 30% of the CSF total protein. Electrophoresis of the CSF demonstrates oligoclonal bands of IgG in 85% to 95% of patients who carry a diagnosis of MS. Note, however, that oligoclonal bands of IgG also will occur in neurosyphilis, fungal meningitis, and other CNS infections. Lumbar puncture (LP) should be considered for all patients with suspected MS, but mass lesions and elevated ICP should be considered and ruled out prior to LP.[52]

MRI is a sensitive test for lesions consistent with MS and is also useful as a marker of disease severity.[53] In patients with an initial neurologic event consistent with CNS demyelination and an MRI with multiple white matter lesions, the 5-year risk of developing MS is 60%. Patients with similar clinical syndromes and a normal MRI have less than a 5% 5-year risk.[54]

Differential Considerations

Other diseases that affect the CNS white matter may appear clinically and radiographically similar to MS. Considerable care must be taken to exclude these disease processes prior to making a diagnosis. These include CNS tumors (especially lymphomas and gliomas), spinal cord compression, vasculitides, Behçet's disease, neurosarcoidosis, postinfectious and postvaccinal encephalomyelitis, human immunodeficiency virus (HIV) encephalopathy, Lyme disease, and vitamin B_{12} deficiency.

Management

Therapy for MS has essentially three arms. The first arm consists of therapies aimed at halting the progression of the disease. The second arm is designed to treat acute exacerbations, and the third arm consists of therapies designed to modify complications.

Therapies aimed at halting disease progress are primarily based on the use of b-interferon or glatiramer acetate. There are two forms of β-interferon; β-1b and β-1a. The interferons are a group of natural compounds that have antiviral and immunomodulatory actions. The side effects include flulike symptoms, depression, anxiety, and confusion. In one study, 560 patients with MS were randomly assigned to receive subcutaneous recombinant interferon β-1a 22 micrograms (n = 189), or 44 micrograms (n = 184), or placebo (n = 187) three times a week for 2 years. The relapse rate was significantly lower at 1 and 2 years with both doses of interferon β-1a than with placebo. Time to first relapse was prolonged by 3 and 5 months in the 22 micrograms and 44 micrograms groups, respectively. The accumulation of burden of disease and number of active lesions on MRI was lower in both treatment groups than in the placebo group. The authors concluded that subcutaneous interferon β-1a is an effective treatment for relapsing-remitting MS in terms of relapse rate, defined disability, and all MRI outcome measures in a dose-related manner, and it is well tolerated.[55]

Another agent is glatiramer acetate. This is a mixture of synthetic polypeptides designed to mimic myelin basic protein. The mechanism of action by which glatiramer acetate exerts its effect is unknown. However, it is thought to act by modifying the immune processes responsible for the pathogenesis of MS. In one study, 251 relapsing-remitting patients with MS were randomized to receive daily subcutaneous injections of glatiramer acetate (previously called *copolymer 1*) or placebo for 24 months. Patients receiving glatiramer acetate had significantly fewer relapses and were more likely to be neurologically improved, whereas those receiving placebo were more likely to worsen. This drug is generally quite well tolerated.[56]

Current recommendations for relapsing-remitting MS are to initiate treatment with b-interferon or glatiramer acetate. These therapies have been demonstrated to decrease the volume of plaques seen on MRI and to diminish relapses.[45]

Acute exacerbations should also be targets for therapy. Although most exacerbations will resolve without therapy, steroids have been demonstrated to diminish the duration of acute exacerbations. More than 85% of patients with relapsing and remitting MS show improvement with intravenous methylprednisolone. Steroids have been shown in controlled trials to speed the recovery of the visual loss of optic neuritis when compared to placebo. In addition, when patients with acute optic neuritis are treated with high-dose steroids, the 2-year rate of development of MS is reduced.[49,57]

The current standard therapy for an acute exacerbation in MS is intravenous methylprednisolone. A typical dose administered intravenously is 250 to 500 mg q12h for 3 to 7 days. It remains controversial whether this should be followed by an oral prednisolone taper. Complications of methylprednisolone therapy include fluid retention, gastrointestinal hemorrhage, anxiety, psychosis, infection, and osteoporosis.

There are several therapies directed toward the complications of MS. The associated spasticity is generally treated with baclofen. This is a highly effective therapy aimed at reducing the painful flexor and extensor spasms. A major side effect is drowsiness that generally diminishes with continued use. Higher dose therapy can cause confusion, especially in the setting of baseline cognitive impairment. For patients with intractable spasticity, baclofen has now become available in intrathecal administration by either bolus therapy or continuous implanted pump therapy. Additional therapies for spasticity include tizanidine, diazepam, and dantrolene.

The tremor and ataxia associated with MS are occasionally treated with propranolol, diazepam, or clonazepam. The results of these therapies, however, are generally unsatisfactory. Pain is often associated with MS and affects the shoulders, pelvic girdle, and face. The facial pain may be indistinguishable from trigeminal neuralgia. Treatment options include carbamazepine, baclofen, or tricyclic antidepressants. Fatigue, which is common, may be treated with amantadine. Both drugs produce partial relief for a minority of patients. In controlled studies the effect of these medications is only slightly better than placebo.[45]

Disposition

Patients with a history of MS who seek treatment in the ED for significant symptoms must first be evaluated to rule out other, non–MS-related pathology. Also, systemic illness, especially infections, can cause an exacerbation and must be ruled out. If the problem is thought to be an exacerbation of MS, most patients will require admission for intravenous steroid therapy. An alternative to admission may be to initiate intravenous steroids in the ED, and arrange for next day follow-up with the primary care physician or neurologist if outpatient intravenous steroid administration is an option. Most important is the index of suspicion that must be maintained by the emergency physician in order to identify early symptoms of MS or a recurrence so that appropriate therapy may be instituted.

Key Concepts

- Any patient with a long-term illness must be evaluated to rule out pathology not related to that illness, before an exacerbation of that illness is assumed to be the cause of the patient's complaint.
- Therapy for patients with MS will require consultation with the patient's primary care provider or neurologist to provide consistent disease management.
- Intravenous methylprednisolone effectively promotes earlier resolution of recurrences.
- Intravenous methylprednisolone has been shown to speed the recovery of vision loss from optic neuritis.

REFERENCES

1. Katusic S et al: Incidence and clinical features of trigeminal neuralgia, Rochester, Minnesota 1945-1984, *Ann Neurol* 27:89, 1990.
2. Tenser RB: Trigeminal neuralgia: mechanisms of treatment, *Neurology* 51:17, 1998.
3. Delzell JE, Grelle AR: Trigeminal neuralgia: new treatment options for a well known cause of facial pain, *Arch Fam Med* 8:264, 1999.
4. Jensen TS et al: Association of trigeminal neuralgia with multiple sclerosis: clinical and pathological features, *Acta Neurol Scand* 65:182, 1982.
5. Taha JM, Tew JM Jr: Comparison of surgical treatments for trigeminal neuralgia: reevaluation of radiofrequency of rhizotomy, *Neurosurgery* 38:865, 1996.
6. McLaughlin M et al: Microvascular decompression of cranial nerves: lessons learned after 4400 operations, *J Neurosurg* 90:1, 1999.
7. Kondziolka D et al: Gamma knife radiosurgery for trigeminal neuralgia, *Arch Neurol* 55:1524, 1998.
8. Adour KK et al: The true nature of Bell's palsy: analysis of 1000 consecutive patients, *Laryngoscope* 88:787, 1978.
9. Hauser W et al: Incidence and prognosis of Bell's palsy in the population of Rochester, Minnesota, *Mayo Clin Proc* 46:258, 1971.
10. The peripheral nervous system. In Clemente CD, editor: *Gray's anatomy,* Philadelphia, 1985, Lea & Febiger.
11. Jackson CG, von Doersten PG: The facial nerve: current trends in diagnosis, treatment, and rehabilitation, *Med Clin North Am* 83:179, 1999.
12. Marenda SA, Olsson JE: The evaluation of facial paralysis, *Otolaryngol Clin North Am* 30:669, 1997.
13. Knox GW: Treatment controversies in Bell's palsy, *Arch Otolaryngol Head Neck Surg* 124:821, 1998.
14. Ruckenstein M: Evaluating facial paralysis: expensive diagnostic tests are often unnecessary, *Postgrad Med* 103:187, 1998.
15. Murakami S et al: Bell's palsy and herpes simplex virus: identification of viral DNA in endoneurial fluid and muscle, *Ann Intern Med* 124:27, 1996.
16. Adour KK: Combination treatment with acyclovir and prednisone for Bell palsy, *Arch Otolaryngol Head Neck Surg* 124:824, 1998.
17. Dickins Jr et al: Herpes zoster oticus: treatment with intravenous acyclovir, *Laryngoscope* 98:776, 1998.
18. Dotevall L, Hagberg LL: Successful oral doxycycline treatment of Lyme disease-associated facial palsy and meningitis, *Clin Infect Dis* 28:569, 1999.
19. Cook SP et al: Lyme disease and seventh nerve paralysis in children, *Am J Otolaryngol* 18:320, 1997.
20. Smith V, Traquina DN: Pediatric bilateral facial paralysis, *Laryngoscope* 108:519, 1998.
21. Joseph EM, Sperling NM: Facial nerve paralysis in acute otitis media: cause and management revisited, *Otolaryngol Head Neck Surg* 118:694, 1998.
22. Jackson CG et al: Facial paralysis of neoplastic origin: diagnosis and management, *Laryngoscope* 90:1581, 1980.
23. The Consensus Development Panel: National Institutes of Health Consensus Development Conference statement on acoustic neuroma, *Arch Neurol* 51:201, 1994.
24. Selesnick SH, Jackler RK: Clinical manifestations and audiologic diagnosis of acoustic neuromas, *Otolaryngol Clin North Am* 25:521, 1992.
25. Wright A, Bradford R: Management of acoustic neuroma, *BMJ* 311:1141, 1995.
26. Selesnick SH et al: The changing clinical presentation of acoustic tumors in the MRI era, *Laryngoscope* 103:431, 1993.
27. Harvey SA, Haberkamp TJ: Pitfalls in the diagnosis of CPA tumors, *Ear Nose Throat J* 70:290, 2000.
28. Watanabe K et al: Characteristics of cranial nerve palsies in diabetic patients, *Diabetes Res Clin Pract* 10:19, 1990.
29. Thomas PK: Clinical features and investigation of diabetic somatic peripheral neuropathy, *Neuroscience* 4:341, 1997.
30. Asbury AK et al: Oculomotor palsy in diabetes mellitus: a clinicopathological study, *Brain* 93:555, 1970.
31. Brown MJ, Asbury AK: Diabetic neuropathy, *Ann Neurol* 15:2, 1984.
32. Clements RS, Bell DSH: Diabetic neuropathy peripheral and autonomic syndromes, *Postgrad Med* 71:50, 1982.
33. Fujioka T et al: Ischemic and hemorrhagic brain stem lesions mimicking diabetic ophthalmoplegia, *Clin Neurol Neurosurg* 97:167, 1995.
34. Villringer A, Einhaüpl KM: Dural sinus and cerebral venous thrombosis, *New Horiz* 5:332, 1997.
35. Wasson J, Redenbaugh J: Transverse sinus thrombosis: an unusual cause of headache, *Headache* 37:457, 1997.
36. Villringer A et al: Pathophysiological aspects of cerebral sinus venous thrombosis (SVT), *J Neuroradiol* 21:72, 1994.
37. Provenzale JM et al: Dural sinus thrombosis: findings on CT and MRI and diagnostic pitfalls, *Am J Roentgenol* 170:777, 1998.
38. Preter M et al: Long-term prognosis in cerebral venous thrombosis: follow-up of 77 patients, *Stroke* 27:243, 1996.
39. Frey JL et al: Cerebral venous thrombosis: combined intrathrombus rTPA and intravenous heparin, *Stroke* 30:489, 1999.
40. Einhaüpl KM et al: Heparin treatment in sinus venous thrombosis, *Lancet* 338:597, 1991.
41. de Bruijn SF, Stam J: Randomized, placebo-controlled trial of anticoagulant treatment with low-molecular-weight heparin for cerebral sinus thrombosis, *Stroke* 30:484, 1999.
42. Francis GS et al: Inflammatory demyelinating diseases of the central nervous system. In Bradley WG et al, editors: *Neurology in clinical practice,* Boston, 1996, Butterworth-Heinemann.

43. Kurtzke JF et al: Multiple sclerosis in the Faroe Islands: transmission across four epidemics, *Acta Neurol Scand* 91:321, 1995.
44. Hogenkamp WE et al: The epidemiology of multiple sclerosis, *Mayo Clin Proc* 72:871, 1997.
45. Giovannoni G, Miller D: Multiple sclerosis and its treatment, *J R Coll Physicians Lond* 33:315, 1999.
46. Rao SM et al: Cognitive dysfunction in multiple sclerosis. I. Frequency, patterns, and prediction, *Neurology* 41:685, 1991.
47. Swirsky-Sacchetti T et al: Neuropsychological and structural brain lesions in multiple sclerosis: a regional analysis, *Neurology* 42:1291, 1992.
48. Wray S: Optic neuritis: guidelines, *Curr Opin Neurol* 8:72, 1995.
49. Beck RW et al: The effect of corticosteroids for acute optic neuritis on the subsequent development of multiple sclerosis, *N Engl J Med* 329:1764, 1993.
50. Ebers GC: Optic neuritis and multiple sclerosis, *Arch Neurol* 42:702, 1985.
51. Kidd D: Presentations of multiple sclerosis, *Practitioner* 243:24, 1999.
52. Mehta PD: Diagnostic usefulness of cerebrospinal fluid in multiple sclerosis, *Crit Rev Clin Lab Sci* 28:233, 1991.
53. Lee KH et al: Magnetic resonance imaging of the head in the diagnosis of multiple sclerosis: a prospective 2-year follow-up with comparison of clinical evaluation, evoked potentials, oligoclonal banding, and CT, *Neurology* 41:657, 1991.
54. Morrissey SP et al: The significance of brain magnetic resonance imaging abnormalities at presentation with clinically isolated syndromes suggestive of multiple sclerosis: a 5-year follow-up study, *Brain* 116:135, 1993.
55. Anonymous: Randomised double-blind placebo-controlled study of interferon β-1a in relapsing/remitting multiple sclerosis. PRISMS (Prevention of Relapses and Disability by Interferon β-1a Subcutaneously in Multiple Sclerosis) Study Group, *Lancet* 352:1498, 1998.
56. Johnson KP et al: Extended use of glatiramer acetate (Copaxone) is well tolerated and maintains its clinical effect on multiple sclerosis relapse rate and degree of disability, *Neurology* 50:701, 1998.
57. Beck RW et al: A randomized, controlled trial of corticosteroids in the treatment of acute optic neuritis, *N Engl J Med* 326:581, 1992.

100 Spinal Cord Disorders

Andrew D. Perron
J. Stephen Huff

PERSPECTIVE

Spinal cord disorders encompass a wide range of pathologic entities and may affect all age groups. Some spinal cord disorders may have catastrophic outcomes if not recognized early in the clinical course. The ultimate neurologic outcome of many of these disorders may depend on an expeditious diagnosis by the emergency physician with appropriate initial therapy, neuroimaging, or consultation for definitive therapy. As with so many other disease processes affecting the nervous system, knowledge of the anatomic organization of the spinal cord and skill in performing a neurologic examination are required for the practitioner to make a correct diagnosis and manage these patients appropriately. This chapter generally concerns processes affecting the spinal cord, its vasculature, and processes compressing the spinal cord. Direct trauma and instability of the spinal column are discussed in Chapter 36.

PRINCIPLES OF DISEASE

Anatomy

In adults, the spinal cord is approximately 40 cm long and extends from the foramen magnum, where it is continuous with the medulla oblongata, to the body of the first or second lumbar vertebra. Like the brain, the spinal cord is covered by three meningeal layers, the inner pial layer, the arachnoid, and the outer dural layer. At its lower end the spinal cord tapers into the conus medullaris where several segmental levels are represented in a small area. The lumbar and sacral nerve roots form the cauda equina as they descend caudally in the thecal sac prior to exit of the spinal canal at the respective foramina. The non–neural filum terminale runs from the tip of the conus and inserts into the dura at the level of the second sacral vertebra.

There are two symmetric enlargements of the spinal cord that contain the segments that innervate the limbs. The cervical enlargement (cord level C5-T1) gives rise to the brachial plexus and subsequently to the peripheral nerves of the upper extremity. The lumbar enlargement (L2-S3) gives rise to the lumbosacral plexus and peripheral nerves of the lower extremity. The space surrounding the spinal cord within the spinal canal is reduced in the area of the enlargements, potentially leaving the cord more vulnerable to compression in these regions. At each segmental level, anterior (ventral) and posterior (dorsal) roots arise from rootlets along the anterolateral and posterolateral surfaces of the cord, respectively. At each level, the anterior root conveys the outflow of the motor neurons in the anterior horn of the spinal cord, and the posterior root contains sensory neurons and fibers that convey sensory inflow.

The arterial supply of the spinal cord is derived primarily from two sources. The single anterior spinal artery arises from the paired vertebral arteries. This anterior spinal artery runs the entire length of the cord in the midline anterior median sulcus and supplies roughly the anterior two thirds of the spinal cord. Blood supply to the posterior third of the spinal cord derives from the smaller paired posterior spinal arteries. Both the anterior and posterior spinal arteries receive segmental contributions from radicular arteries, the largest being the radicular artery of Adamkiewicz, which typically originates from the aorta between T8 and L4. The venous drainage of the cord largely parallels the arterial supply.

The internal anatomy of the spinal cord is divided into

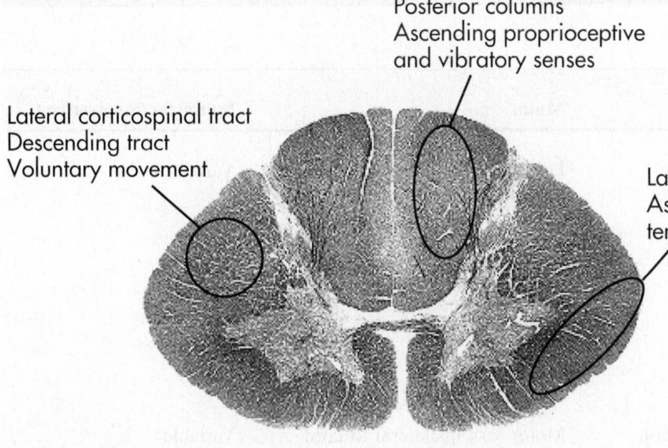

Figure 100-1. **Simplified spinal cord anatomy showing clinically essential motor and sensory tracts.** ***Photomicrograph courtesy of John Sundsten, Digital Anatomist Project, University of Washington.***

central gray matter, which contains cell bodies and their processes, and surrounding white matter, where the ascending and descending myelinated fiber tracts are located. These fiber tracts are organized into discrete bundles, with the ascending tracts carrying sensory information, and the descending tracts conveying the efferent motor impulses and visceral innervation.

For clinical purposes, neuroanatomy of the spinal cord may be greatly simplified (Figure 100-1). Major ascending sensory tracts are represented on the right side of Figure 100-1, with motor tracts on the left side. The posterior columns carry afferent ascending proprioceptive and vibratory information on the ipsilateral side of the cord to the area stimulated; decussation of these fibers occurs in the medulla so that contralateral cortical representation ultimately occurs. In a portion of the lateral column of white matter, the lateral spinothalamic tract conveys afferent information about pain and temperature. (Recall that tracts are named with their point of origin first so that the spinothalamic tract arises in the spinal cord and travels to the thalamus.) The tract is laminated so that sacral fibers are represented most laterally. Crossing of fibers from this tract occurs near the level of entry of the spinal nerve; hence a cord lesion affecting one lateral spinothalamic tract results in decreased or absent pain and temperature perception below the level of injury on the contralateral side of the body.

For clinical purposes the major descending motor tract is represented in the lateral corticospinal tract (which, as the name implies, originates in the cortex and flows toward the spinal cord). This tract also is anatomically organized, with efferent motor axons to the cervical area located medially and the sacral efferent axons located laterally. Decussation of this descending tract occurs in the medulla. The cell bodies of the lower motor neurons (anterior horn cells) are in the ventral portion of the gray matter of the spinal cord.

Classification of Spinal Cord Syndromes

The anatomic organization of the spinal cord lends itself to anatomic pathophysiologic classification of cord dysfunction. The different anatomic syndromes may be the final clinical picture of a variety of clinical processes either extrinsic or intrinsic to the spinal cord. Frequently the syndromes exist in partial or incomplete forms.

Complete (Transverse) Spinal Cord Syndrome Complete spinal cord lesions may occur as either acute or subacute pathologic processes. A complete spinal cord lesion is defined as a total loss of sensory, autonomic, and voluntary motor innervation distal to the spinal cord level of injury. Reflex responses mediated at the spinal level such as muscle stretch ("deep tendon") reflexes may persist, although they may also be absent or abnormal. Autonomic dysfunction may be manifest with hypotension (neurogenic shock) or priapism. The most common cause of the complete transverse cord syndrome is trauma, although this anatomic syndrome is nonspecific as to etiology.[1,2] Other causes of acute complete cord syndrome include infarction, hemorrhages, and entities causing extrinsic compression. Significantly, of patients who develop complete transverse syndromes that persist for more than 24 hours, 99% will not have a functional recovery.[3,4] An important point to consider prior to diagnosing a complete cord lesion is that any evidence of cord function below to the level of injury denotes a partial rather than a complete lesion. For example, signs such as persistent perianal sensation ("sacral sparing"), rectal sphincter tone or voluntary rectal sphincter contraction, or voluntary toe movement suggest a partial cord lesion, which has a better prognosis than a complete lesion.[1]

Spinal shock refers to the loss of muscle tone and reflexes with complete cord syndrome during the acute phase of injury. The intensity of the spinal shock increases with the height of the level in the spinal cord.[5] Spinal shock typically lasts less than 24 hours but has been reported occasionally to last days to weeks.[5,6] A marker of spinal shock is loss of the bulbocavernosus reflex, which is a normal cord-mediated reflex that may be preserved in complete cord lesions. The bulbocavernosus reflex involves involuntary reflex contraction of the anal sphincter in response to a squeeze of the glans penis or a tug on the Foley catheter. The termination of the spinal shock phase of injury is heralded by the return of the bulbocavernosus reflex; increased muscle tone and hyperreflexia follow later.[5,6]

Incomplete Spinal Cord Lesions Incomplete spinal lesions are characterized by preservation of function of various portions of the spinal cord. Of all incomplete spinal lesions, the vast majority can be classified into one of three clinical syndromes: the central cord syndrome, the Brown-Séquard syndrome, or the anterior cord syndrome (Table 100-1).

The Central Cord Syndrome The central cord syndrome, first described by Schneider and colleagues in 1954, is the

Table 100-1. Spinal Cord Syndromes

	Sensory	Motor	Sphincter involvement
Central cord	Variable	Upper extremity weakness, distal > proximal	Variable
Brown-Séquard syndrome	Ipsilateral position and vibration loss Contralateral pain and temperature loss	Motor loss ipsilateral to cord lesion	Variable
Anterior cord syndrome	Loss of pin and touch Vibration, position preserved	Motor loss or weakness below level	Variable
Transverse cord syndrome—complete	Loss of sensation below level of cord injury	Loss of voluntary motor function below cord level	Sphincter control lost
Conus medullaris syndrome	Saddle anesthesia may be present or sensory loss may range from patchy to complete transverse pattern	Weakness may be of upper motor neuron type	Sphincter control impaired
Cauda equina syndrome	Saddle anesthesia may be present or sensory loss may range from patchy to complete transverse pattern	Weakness may be of lower motor neuron type	Sphincter control impaired

most prevalent of the partial cord syndromes.[7,8] It is characterized by bilateral motor paresis, with upper extremities affected to a greater degree than lower extremities, and distal muscle groups affected to a greater degree than proximal muscle groups. Sensory impairment and bladder dysfunction are variable. At times burning dysesthesias in the upper extremities may be the dominant feature.[9] Central cord injury affects the central gray matter and the central portions of the corticospinal and spinothalamic tracts. It is most often caused by a hyperextension injury, with the postulated mechanism being squeezing or pinching of the spinal cord both anteriorly and posteriorly by inward bulging of the ligamentum flavum. The result is contusion to the spinal cord, with the central portion being most affected. This injury classically occurs in the elderly with degenerative arthritis and spinal stenosis in the cervical area but may affect any patient with cervical canal narrowing of any etiology (e.g., congenital narrow canal as seen in achondroplasia or canal narrowing from disk protrusion or tumor). A fall is the most common mechanism of this injury, followed by motor vehicle crashes.[10] The prognosis for patients with central cord syndrome is quite variable, depending on the degree of injury at presentation and patient age.[10,11] In patients less than 50 years old, more than 80% will regain bladder continence and approximately 90% will return to ambulatory status. In those greater than 50 years of age, only 30% regain bladder function, with approximately 50% regaining ambulation.[11]

Brown-Séquard Syndrome Brown-Séquard syndrome, first described in 1846 by the physician it is named for,[12] may be an anatomic or functional hemisection of the spinal cord. Usually the result of penetrating injuries,[13] it may also be the result of compressive or intrinsic lesions. The syndrome has been reported in association with spinal cord tumors, spinal epidural hematoma, vascular malformations, cervical spondylosis, and radiation injury; as a complication of spinal instrumentation; and as resulting from degenerative disk disease.[13] The syndrome in its pure form is characterized by ipsilateral loss of motor function and proprioception/vibration with contralateral loss of pain and temperature sensation below the spinal cord level of injury. Because fibers associated with the lateral spinothalamic tract ascend or descend one to two cord segments before crossing to the contralateral side, ipsilateral anesthesia (pain and temperature modalities) may be noted one or two segments above the lesion, although this observation is variable. The majority of patients with Brown-Séquard syndrome have only partial syndromes of sensory and motor impairment and the classic pattern is not seen.[11,13,14] Brown-Séquard syndrome has the best prognosis of any of the incomplete spinal cord syndromes. Eighty to ninety percent of patients with Brown-Séquard syndrome regain bowel and bladder function, 75% regain ambulatory status, and 70% become independent in their activities of daily living.[11]

The Anterior Cord Syndrome The anterior cord syndrome is characterized by loss of motor function, pinprick, and light touch below the level of the lesion, with preservation of posterior column function including some touch, position, and vibratory sensation. Although most reports of anterior spinal syndrome are after aortic surgery,[15] the syndrome has been reported following severe hypotension, infection, myocardial infarction, vasospasm from drug reaction, and aortic angiography[16] (see the section on spinal cord infarction later this chapter). This lesion may result from a cervical hyperflexion injury resulting in a cord contusion or by protrusion of bony fragments or herniated cervical disk material into the spinal canal. Rarely it is produced by laceration or thrombosis of the anterior spinal artery or a major radicular feeding vessel.[11] Patients present with the characteristic neurologic findings noted above. Functional recovery is variable, with most improvement made in the first 24 hours but little improvement thereafter.[4] Although anterior cord lesions from ischemia are usually incomplete, patients without motor function at 30 days have little or no likelihood of regaining any motor function by one year.[17] Overall only 10% to 20% of patients with this entity regain some muscle function, and even in this group there is little power or coordination.[11]

Conus Medullaris Syndrome/Cauda Equina Syndromes The separation of conus medullaris and cauda equina lesions in clinical practice is difficult because the clinical features of the disorders overlap. Additionally, a combined lesion may occur that masks clear clinical symptoms or signs of either an upper or lower motor neuron type of injury. The conus medullaris is the terminal end of the spinal cord located at approximately L1 in adults. The conus medullaris syndrome may involve disturbances of urination (usually manifested as a denervated, autonomic bladder), as well as sphincter involvement or sexual dysfunction. Sensory involvement may affect the sacral and coccygeal segments, resulting in saddle anesthesia. Pure lesions of the conus medullaris are rare.[18] Upper motor neuron signs such as increased motor tone and abnormal reflexes may be present but their absence does not exclude the syndrome. The conus medullaris syndrome can be caused by central disk herniation, neoplasm, trauma, or vascular insufficiency. Since the conus is such a small structure, with lumbar and sacral segments represented in a small area, a lesion usually causes bilateral symptomatology. This may help distinguish lesions of the conus from those of the cauda equina, which are often unilateral.[18]

The cauda equina ("horse's tail") is the name given to the lumbar and sacral nerve roots that continue on within the dural sac caudal to the conus medullaris. The etiology of the cauda equina syndrome is usually a ruptured, midline intervertebral disk, most commonly occurring at the L4-L5 level. Tumors and other compressive masses may cause the syndrome as well. Like the conus medullaris syndrome, patients generally present with progressive symptoms of fecal or urinary incontinence, impotence, distal motor weakness, and sensory loss in a saddle distribution. Muscle stretch reflexes may also be reduced. The presence of urinary retention is the single most consistent finding, with a sensitivity of 90%.[19] Low back pain may or may not be present.

CLINICAL FEATURES

History

Weakness, sensory abnormalities, and autonomic dysfunction are the cardinal symptoms of spinal cord dysfunction. The tempo and degree of impairment often reflect the tempo of the disease process. A history of cancer should suggest the possibility of metastatic disease. Recent trauma raises the possibility of fracture or disk protrusion. Past medical history is vital, since coagulopathy or other systemic processes may be elicited.

Physical Examination

The physical examination pertinent to spinal cord dysfunction involves testing in three areas: (1) motor function, (2) sensory function, and (3) reflexes. Each component is best tested with the anatomic layout of the spinal cord in mind to help determine the location of the spinal cord dysfunction.

Motor Function Testing of motor function encompasses examination of muscle bulk, tone, and strength. Muscle bulk is easily examined in large motor groups such as the thigh or calf muscles, the biceps, or the triceps. Inspection of the intrinsic hand muscles may also be helpful for determining muscle bulk; wasting may be evident as hollowed or recessed regions of the hand. Decreased mass, asymmetry, or fasciculations should be noted. Tone is tested with repeated passive knee, elbow, or wrist flexion, with the examiner feeling for abnormally increased or decreased resistance. Rapid pronation and supination of the forearm is another useful method to assess tone. Increased tone may be indicative of spasticity or an upper motor neuron lesion, whereas decreased tone corresponds with lower motor neuron, motor end-plate, or muscular problems. Finally, motor strength is graded in both the upper and lower extremities. A rectal examination is performed to assess voluntary sphincter contraction, resting tone, and, as described previously, the bulbocavernosus reflex.

Sensory Function Sensory testing requires a cooperative patient and an attentive examiner. The spinal cord–related modalities that may be clinically useful for emergency physicians include pinprick, light touch (contralateral lateral spinothalamic tract), and proprioception (ipsilateral posterior column). Testing of the patient's response to pinprick, light touch, and proprioception in all four extremities is necessary if a neurologic injury is suspected. Testing of sacral dermatomes may be an important part of the examination in some patients. As previously noted, sacral sparing is an important finding that indicates that spinal cord dysfunction may be incomplete. Recall that the sensory fibers from sacral dermatomes are more peripherally located in the ascending fiber bundles; central or partial cord lesions may ablate sensation in the extremities yet allow some perception of sensation in the sacral area.

Reflexes Muscle stretch ("deep tendon") reflexes may be rapidly tested at the bedside. Responses are graded on a 0 to 4+ scale, with 2 being normal. Hyperactive reflexes suggest upper motor neuron disease (affecting the neurons or their outflow from the brain or spinal cord) as does sustained clonus. Reflexes may be diminished or absent when sensation is lost or when lower motor neuron disease is present. Diseases of muscles or neuromuscular junctions may also decrease reflexes. In acute cord injury, reflexes may be diminished in the acute phase. Again, the bulbocavernosus reflex may be helpful in this assessment as discussed previously.

DIAGNOSTIC STRATEGIES

Historical or physical examination findings that suggest spinal cord dysfunction will prompt further investigations. The basic strategy is to detect or exclude extrinsic compressive lesions or other potentially treatable entities. Magnetic resonance imaging (MRI) has changed the diagnostic approach to the patient with suspected spinal cord dysfunction. Plain radiography and computed tomography (CT) scans may demonstrate bony and some soft tissue abnormalities. Conventional radiography and CT scans will be required in patients with trauma or suspected bony involvement by tumor or degenerative processes, but MRI will show many of these abnormalities and also define the spinal cord. Tissue damage patterns within the cord, such as hemorrhage and edema, may also be detected with MRI. CT myelography may be requested by some consultants. Institutions will vary in procedures that are available.

After imaging studies exclude compressive lesions or other masses affecting the spinal cord, the possibility of inflammatory or demyelinating etiologies remains and lumbar puncture may be useful in diagnosis.

DIFFERENTIAL CONSIDERATIONS

The prime principle in management of spinal cord dysfunction is to consider and exclude potentially treatable lesions. The clinical assessment of spinal cord dysfunction is limited to detecting weakness, sensory alterations, sphincter dysfunction, and perhaps reflex abnormalities. Pain in the back may be present depending on the pathologic process. Since potential functional loss and impact on quality of life are great, the detection of a process where some intervention is possible assumes great importance. For example, a likely diagnosis of spinal cord infarction may be entertained but the pursuit of a treatable process such as spinal cord compression from an epidural hematoma should be seriously considered.[20] This discovery process may involve specialty consultation or obtaining studies not readily available in many emergency settings such as MRI. As a general rule, liberal consultation and imaging are suggested when the possibility of spinal cord dysfunction is considered. The history may suggest an etiology and will guide the tempo of investigation.

The picture of a complete transverse spinal cord syndrome with paraplegia, sensory loss at a clear anatomic level, and sphincter dysfunction cannot be fully simulated by other anatomic lesions. However, incomplete or evolving spinal cord syndromes may be imitated by other processes. It is always prudent to consider an anatomic differential diagnosis—the classic "where is the lesion"—during the diagnostic process. For example, progressive lower extremity weakness and sensory alteration may represent cord dysfunction but could reflect an intracranial vertex mass with bilateral cortical dysfunction. Another example is that of a patient with a rapidly progressive paralysis with areflexia and quadriplegia; ascending paralysis (Landry-Guillain-Barré syndrome [LGBS]) may at times mimic an acute cord lesion. Ataxia has been rarely reported as an isolated finding with spinal cord compression.[21]

Generally speaking, pathologic processes involving the spinal cord may be divided into those affecting the cord or its blood supply primarily, such as demyelination, infection, or infarction, and those that compress the cord, most often originating outside the dura (Box 100-1). Myelitis is a

Box 100-1 Nontraumatic Etiologies of Spinal Cord Dysfunction

Processes Affecting the Spinal Cord or Blood Supply Directly

Demyelination

Multiple sclerosis
Transverse myelitis

Spinal arteriovenous malformation/subarachnoid hemorrhage

Syringomyelia
Traumatic
Tumor

Idiopathic spastic paraparesis

HIV myelopathy
Other myelopathies
Spinal cord infarction

Compressive Lesions Affecting the Spinal Cord

Spinal epidural hematoma

Spinal epidural abscess
Diskitis
Neoplasm
Metastatic
Primary CNS

comprehensive term for spinal cord inflammation with dysfunction, and the etiologies are legion. Although a variety of entities may cause cord compression, the clinical presentation is often similar. The tempo of the process may yield a different clinical picture. For example, in chronic compression, muscle wasting and abnormal reflexes may be present, whereas both of these may be lacking in acute compression.

MANAGEMENT

Just as the clinical manifestations of spinal cord dysfunction are nonspecific as to etiology, the treatment for many of the disease entities is often nonspecific. Steroids are accepted therapy in spinal cord trauma; they are also employed with many causes of cord compression, although rigorous clinical studies are lacking. Radiation treatment is recommended for cord compression by tumor. Surgical consultation for decompression may be considered, although the indications for surgery and timing of surgery are controversial. Involvement of consultants and discussion of what may be understudied therapies are suggested.

The specific diagnosis is needed for treatment and will guide therapy. A discussion of specific disease processes follows.

SPECIFIC DISEASE PROCESSES

As noted earlier, spinal cord disorders may be grouped into those resulting from processes intrinsic to the cord and vasculature and those causing extrinsic compression. The order of this discussion roughly follows the organization of Box 100-1.

Intrinsic Cord Lesions

Multiple Sclerosis

Principles of Disease Demyelination denotes a disease process with the prominent feature of partial or complete loss of the myelin sheath surrounding the axons of the central nervous system (CNS). Multiple sclerosis (MS) is the most common example of such a process; spinal cord involvement may dominate the clinical picture.

Clinical Features The hallmark of MS is CNS lesions that are "scattered in time and space." The demyelinated segments do not transmit action potentials normally, resulting in a wide variety of spinal cord findings, depending on the location and extent of the demyelination. In addition to patchy motor and sensory findings, patients with MS may complain of bladder dysfunction, tremor, or evidence of a transverse partial or complete cord syndrome mimicking a compressive spinal lesion.[22,23] There may be a history of optic neuritis or transient visual problems. Spinal cord lesions in MS primarily involve the lateral corticospinal tracts, the posterior columns, and the lateral spinothalamic tracts. Motor system dysfunction is the most frequent manifestation of MS involvement of the spinal cord, usually as a result of lesions in the lateral corticospinal tracts.

The examination of these patients is often characterized by paresis, increased muscle tone, hyperreflexia, clonus, and a Babinski response. Spinal cord involvement may also result in dysautonomias. Signs of other CNS involvement, such as pallor of the optic discs, may be present.

Diagnostic Strategies Spinal MRI is the imaging test of choice for the diagnosis, since it can exclude motor symptoms and show lesions suggestive of MS.[23-25] Cranial MRI may be helpful in demonstrating other CNS lesions. Cerebrospinal fluid (CSF) testing for myelin basic protein and oligoclonal bands is also a diagnostic option, but no CSF abnormalities are entirely specific for MS.[26,27] Oligoclonal bands in the CSF may aid in the diagnosis but they are significant only if not present in the serum as well.[26]

Differential Considerations The differential diagnosis includes systemic lupus erythematosus (SLE), Lyme disease, neurosyphilis, human immunodeficiency virus (HIV) myelopathy, and others.

Management MS exacerbations may be treated with high-dose methylprednisolone followed by a tapering dose of prednisone. Corticosteroids have been shown to be useful in shortening the amount of time required for recovery from an exacerbation of MS.[23] Consultation and referral are indicated. Immunosuppressive therapy in patients with the chronic progressive form of the disease has met with variable success.[22,23] Since numerous disorders can mimic MS, the definitive diagnosis of the disease is not usually made in the ED.[28]

Transverse Myelitis

Principles of Disease Acute transverse myelitis (ATM) is acute or subacute spinal cord dysfunction characterized by paraplegia, a transverse level of sensory impairment, and sphincter disturbance. It is relatively rare, with a reported annual incidence of 1 per 1.3 million population. Its presentation may be mimicked by compressive lesions, trauma, infection, or malignant infiltration. The exact pathogenesis remains unknown, although it is noted to follow viral infection in approximately 30% of patients and commonly is termed postinfectious myelitis.[29] Other postulated etiologies include infectious, autoimmune, and idiopathic.[30,31] No apparent cause for acute transverse myelitis is found in 30% of patients.[32] Progression of symptoms is usually rapid, with 66% reaching maximal deficit by 24 hours.[32] Symptoms may, however, progress over a period of days to weeks. The thoracic cord region is most often affected by this process (60% to 70%)[32] and the cervical spinal cord is rarely affected.[33]

Clinical Features In addition to motor, sensory, and urinary disturbances, patients with this disease may complain of back pain and may have low-grade fever, raising concern for spinal epidural abscess.

As with MS, the examination of patients can be characterized by weakness progressing to paresis, hypertonia, hyperreflexia, clonus, and a Babinski response. Spinal cord involvement can also result in dysautonomias.

Diagnostic Strategies Evaluation for ATM is primarily done with emergent MRI scanning to exclude compressive lesions. CSF studies are normal in 40% and demonstrate only mildly elevated protein or pleocytosis in the remaining 60%.[34] The most essential aspect of the treatment of ATM is to eliminate a potentially treatable cause such as spinal epidural abscess, neoplasm, or hematoma.

Differential Considerations The differential diagnosis for transverse myelitis includes MS, spinal epidural abscess, spinal neoplasm, and hematoma.

Management Treatment with steroids is of unknown benefit. Anecdotal reports of improvement following steroid administration exist,[32,35] but other investigators have found no benefit to their use.[34] Consultation is suggested, and admission is usually required.

The clinical course of ATM is highly variable, ranging

from complete recovery to death from progressive neurologic compromise.[31] Maximal improvement usually occurs within 3 to 6 months.[36] At the 5-year follow-up of patients with this disease, 30% had a good recovery, 25% had a fair recovery, 30% had a poor recovery, and 15% died due to complications of their disease.[37]

Spinal Subarachnoid Hemorrhage

Principles of Disease Intraspinal hemorrhage is rare and occurs in the same anatomic locations as do intracranial hemorrhages: epidural, subdural, subarachnoid, and intramedullary.[38] Spinal subarachnoid hemorrhage is usually caused by an arteriovenous malformation (AVM).[38,39] Other etiologies include hemorrhage from tumors and cavernous angiomas or spontaneous hemorrhage due to anticoagulation therapy.[40,41] Bleeding may occur exclusively in the subarachnoid space or within the substance of the spinal cord itself.

Clinical Features Patients present with the paroxysmal onset of excruciating back pain at the level of the hemorrhage. This pain may also be in a radicular distribution or into the flank. Patients may complain of headache and exhibit cervical rigidity if the blood migrates into the intracranial subarachnoid space simulating an intracranial subarachnoid hemorrhage.

The patient will present with variable neurologic deficits depending on the magnitude and anatomic location of the hemorrhage. Typically, these deficits include extremity numbness, weakness, or sphincter dysfunction.[42] Nuchal rigidity or signs of meningeal irritation may be present.

Diagnostic Strategies The diagnostic study of choice is the MRI. Lumbar puncture also confirms the diagnosis of blood in the CSF.

Differential Considerations The differential diagnosis includes epidural abscess, tumor, transverse myelitis, ischemia from an aortic catastrophe such as dissection, or an anterior spinal artery thrombosis.

Management Treatment depends on the etiology of the hemorrhage. Neurosurgical referral is obtained for further evaluation and for clot evacuation if compression is present. Angiography may be recommended if AVM is suspected. Spinal epidural and subdural hematomas are discussed later in this section.

Syringomyelia

Principles of Disease Syringomyelia is a cavitary lesion within the substance of the spinal cord. Syrinx is usually a chronic progressive lesion and its location within the cord determines the neurologic findings on examination.

Clinical Features Headache and neck pain are the most common complaints, followed by sensory disturbance, gait disorder, and lower cranial nerve dysfunction.[43]

The classic pattern of sensory deficit is a loss of pain and temperature sensation in the upper extremities, with preservation of proprioception and light touch. This phenomenon is described as a "disassociative anesthesia" because of the discrepant loss of sensory modalities. The sensory deficit is often described as being in a "cape-like" distribution over the shoulders and arms. The anatomic basis for the neurologic findings of syrinx is due to its central location near the central canal. Here it may compress the crossing fibers of the lateral spinothalamic tract that carry pain and temperature fibers. Crude touch, position, and vibratory sensation are typically unaffected. Sensory fibers from the lower limbs are similarly spared.

The symptoms of syringomyelia develop and progress based on the intracavitary pressure and location of the syrinx. The most common features on physical examination are lower limb hyperreflexia, weakness and wasting in the hands and arms, dissociated sensory loss, and gait disorder. Symptoms may be exacerbated by sneeze, cough, or Valsalva maneuver.[44] Ninety percent of patients who develop this process have Arnold-Chiari I malformation (cerebellar tonsils and medulla project into the spinal canal).[45] Syrinx may also result from spinal cord trauma (often months to years later) or compressive tumors or as a sequela of meningitis.[46]

Diagnostic Strategies Syrinx is best seen on MRI. No other study currently in widespread use can equal its diagnostic ability.

Differential Considerations The differential diagnosis for syrinx includes intrinsic spinal tumor and demyelination.

Management If the diagnosis is considered, it is not necessary to perform emergent imaging if follow-up can be arranged, since this is usually a slowly progressive process. In those patients for whom an MRI is obtained and the diagnosis is made, referral to a neurologic surgeon should be made, since symptoms will progress in about two thirds of patients.[47]

Idiopathic Spastic Paraparesis Idiopathic spastic paraparesis is a progressive disorder characterized by progressive weakness and signs of spasticity of the lower extremities. This is at times also referred to as primary lateral sclerosis, which describes the demyelination pattern in the lateral column of the spinal cord. Typically this occurs in older men. Sometimes a heritable form may be discovered. It is a diagnosis of exclusion.[48-50]

HIV Myelopathy HIV myelopathy typically occurs in patients with advanced disease. Weakness, gait disturbance, sphincter dysfunction, sensory abnormalities, and signs of spasticity are present in this progressive process. This is again a diagnosis of exclusion since etiologies such as toxoplasmosis, lymphoma, varicella zoster, and cytomegalovirus (CMV) may simulate this clinical picture in immunocompromised patients. Pathologically, vacuolization of myelin sheaths in the cord may be found. Treatment is directed at the retroviral infection, although there is no proven treatment.[51,52]

Spinal Cord Infarction Spinal cord infarction is another diagnosis of exclusion. Aortic dissection and surgery, as well as global ischemia, are the more common causes, although this may occur as a complication of SLE or be cryptogenic. An anterior spinal cord syndrome is the most common clinical picture. Some recovery may occur, although generally less than in cerebral stroke. The site of clinical dysfunction may be distant from the site of vascular occlusion.[53]

Extrinsic Cord Lesions

Spinal Epidural Hematoma

Principles of Disease Spinal epidural hematoma is a relatively rare condition from a variety of etiologies. Its incidence is placed at 0.1 per 100,000 patients per year.[54,55] Traumatic etiologies include post lumbar puncture (LP) or epidural anesthesia, as well as a complication of spinal surgery. It is more likely to occur in anticoagulated or thrombocytopenic patients, or in those with liver disease or alcoholism.[56,57] Spontaneous bleeding is rare but may be seen from spinal AVM or vertebral hemangioma. Approximately one quarter to one third of all cases are associated with anticoagulation therapy including low-molecular-weight heparin.[2,58,59]

Clinical Features The patient usually presents with sudden, severe, constant back pain with a radicular component. It may be noted to follow a straining episode. The pain is enhanced by percussion over the spine, as well as maneuvers that increase intraspinal pressure such as coughing, sneezing, or straining.[60] Notably, the pain often causes the patient to seek care prior to the development of neurologic signs, possibly leading to delays in diagnosis.[38] Neurologic deficits follow and may progress over hours to days.[55] Again, anticoagulant use or coagulation abnormality may be present.

The patient will be in significant distress. Motor and sensory findings will depend entirely on the level and size of the hematoma, but can include weakness, paresis, loss of bowel or bladder function, and virtually any sensory deficit.

Diagnostic Strategies MRI, as with virtually all suspected intrinsic spinal disorders, is the diagnostic study of choice.[60]

Differential Considerations The differential diagnosis includes abscess, epidural neoplasm, acute disk herniation, and spinal subarachnoid hemorrhage (SAH).

Management Recovery without surgery is rare, and surgical consultation for consideration of emergent decompressive laminectomy must be obtained. Overall mortality is 8%.[55] Functional recovery is related primarily to the length of time the symptoms are present and recovery after 72 hours of symptoms is rare[61] but has been reported.[62]

Spinal Epidural Abscess

Principles of Disease Spinal epidural abscess is an infectious process usually confined to the adipose tissue of the dorsal epidural space where there is a rich venous plexus. It is an uncommon disease entity with an overall frequency of 0.2 to 1.2 per 10,000 hospital admissions.[63,64] Major risk factors include diabetes, intravenous drug abuse, chronic renal failure, alcoholism, and immunosuppression.[65,66] Although the disease may present in subacute or chronic forms, the acute presentation is most frequently seen by the emergency physician. Thoracic and lumbar sites of infection predominate, with cervical epidural abscess being much less common.[67,68] Infection typically extends over 4 to 5 spinal vertebral segments.[69] The dura mater limits the spread of an epidural infection, making subdural or intraspinal spread uncommon. Hematogenous spread of infection to the epidural space is the most common source (26% to 50% of cases),[38,69] either to the epidural space or to the vertebra with extension to the epidural space. Skin and soft tissue infection is the most frequently reported identified source (15%),[65,69] with *Staphylococcus aureus* being the most prevalent organism cultured in more than 50% of cases.[65,69,70] Other frequently identified pathogens include aerobic and anaerobic streptococcus, *Escherichia coli,* and *Pseudomonas aeruginosa.* Multiple organisms are identified in approximately 10% of cases, while in 40% no organism is identified.[70]

Clinical Features The classic clinical presentation of spinal epidural abscess begins with a backache that progresses to localized back pain often associated with tenderness to percussion. Fever, sweats, and rigors are common, reported in 30% to 75% of patients.[38,69,70] The classic triad of back pain, fever, and progressive neurologic deficits, however, is present in a minority of patients and delayed clinical diagnosis is common.[63] Radicular symptoms may not be present initially, but usually develop as the disease progresses.

If untreated, patients develop myelopathic signs, usually beginning with bowel and bladder disturbance. Weakness ensues, followed by paraplegia or quadriplegia. Of note, approximately 10% of patients with spinal epidural abscess present with encephalopathy.[63,69]

Diagnostic Strategies MRI is the imaging modality of choice and needs to be obtained emergently if the diagnosis is entertained. Other diagnostic testing may include a complete blood count (CBC), since leukocytosis is commonly present with an average white blood cell count (WBC) of 13,000 to 16,000/mm^3.[69] The sedimentation rate, while not specific for epidural abscess, is virtually always elevated with this condition.[63,64,69] Plain films are usually normal unless there is osteomyelitis of an adjacent vertebral body. Lumbar puncture is relatively contraindicated, but is often performed as part of evaluation for meningitis. CSF findings are consistent with a parameningeal infection showing elevation of protein and some cellular response.

Differential Considerations Spinal epidural abscess can be mimicked by any compressive spinal lesion including tumor or blood.

Management Urgent surgical consultation for decompression is required. Antibiotics effective against the most common organisms (particularly *S. aureus*) should be started empirically. One such regimen that covers both gram-positive and gram-negative organisms is a third-generation cephalosporin plus vancomycin, both given intravenously, plus rifampin given orally.

Outcome is related to the speed of diagnosis prior to the development of myelopathic signs. The disease is fatal in 18% to 23%, and patients with neurologic deficit rarely improve if surgical intervention is delayed greater than 12 to 36 hours after onset of paralysis.[63,69] Patients operated on before development of neurologic symptoms almost universally have a good outcome.[64]

Diskitis

Principles of Disease Diskitis is an uncommon primary infection of the nucleus pulposus, with secondary involvement of the cartilaginous end-plate and vertebral body. It may occur after surgical procedures or spontaneously, the latter being more common in the pediatric patient population.[71,72] There is an increased incidence of diskitis in immunocompromised patients and in patients with systemic infections. Both an acute and chronic disease course have been described, with the acute course being more common.[71]

Clinical Features Patients present with moderate to severe pain, localized to the level of involvement and exacerbated by almost any movement of the spine. Radicular symptoms are present in 50% to 90% of cases.[73] The lumbar spine is the most common site of disease.

Elevated temperature is noted in more than 90% of

patients.[71] Patients will demonstrate pain with range of motion. Neurologic deficits are the exception with diskitis.

Diagnostic Strategies Plain radiographs are usually not helpful for early diagnosis, but destruction of the disk space is highly suggestive if present. Plain films become positive after 2 to 4 weeks of disease. In addition to disk space narrowing, plain films may show irregular destruction of the vertebral body end-plates. Often there is a latent period (2 to 8 weeks) between the onset of back pain and the development of other clinical symptoms or physical examination findings. MRI is the radiographic study of choice, since it not only can diagnose diskitis, but it can rule out paravertebral or epidural abscess. Laboratory studies often demonstrate an elevated erythrocyte sedimentation rate (ESR), but the WBC is usually normal.[71,72] *S. aureus* is the most common organism, but gram-negative, fungal, and tuberculous infections have all been recognized.

Differential Considerations The differential diagnosis includes spinal epidural abscess, neoplasm, and hematoma.

Management With timely diagnosis and treatment, outcome is generally good, and medical treatment with intravenous antibiotics is usually curative. Surgery is often not necessary.[71-72]

Neoplasm

Principles of Disease Spinal cord tumors are classified according to their relationship to the dura and spinal cord (extradural, intradural/extramedullary, and intradural/intramedullary). Spinal cord tumors produce neurologic symptoms by compression, invasion, or destruction of myelinated tracts. The resulting neurologic symptoms are directly related to both the growth rate and location of the tumor. Spinal cord tumors account for 4% to 10% of CNS tumors, but only 1% of all cancers. Primary tumors occur with an incidence of 1 per 1 million population.[74] Most tumors of the spinal cord, however, are metastatic in origin. Approximately 10% of patients with known cancer will be diagnosed with a spinal metastasis at some point in the course of their disease, and 5% to 10% of patients ultimately diagnosed with cancer first present with a spinal metastasis.[2] Lung cancer, breast cancer, and lymphoma represent greater than 50% of the primary malignancies that subsequently develop spinal metastasis, spreading by both the hematogenous route and direct extension. Most metastases occur in the thoracic spine, and nearly 20% will have disease at multiple levels.[2,75,76]

Clinical Features In 95% of patients with spinal neoplasm, the initial complaint is pain, either in the back at the level of the tumor or in a radicular distribution. Pain is often characterized as dull, constant, and aching, and is said to often worsen with recumbency (unlike the pain of herniated disk).[38] Nighttime pain that is severe is characteristic of spinal neoplasm.[77] Any action that increases intraspinal pressure (Valsalva maneuver, sneeze, cough) may be associated with increased pain.

Neurologic deficits are variable, depending on the location of the lesion. Besides a thorough neurologic examination, a search for possible primary sites should be done on the physical examination.

Diagnostic Strategies Plain-film radiographs are the initial diagnostic test, and 70% to 85% of patients with spinal column involvement will demonstrate some abnormality on these films.[74,77] Patients with neurologic findings and suspicious findings on plain films are candidates for emergent MRI or CT myelogram.

Differential Considerations The differential diagnosis includes any of the compressive lesions (blood, infection). Tumor can also mimic intrinsic lesions such as transverse myelopathy and cord infarction.

Management Acute compressive myelopathy from neoplasm is an oncologic emergency. Immediate treatment is required to preserve function and prevent deterioration. Once paraplegia and incontinence occur, less than 5% of patients will regain ambulatory status.[1,78] Of those patients ambulatory at the time of diagnosis, 60% remain ambulatory.[38] High-dose steroids, radiotherapy, and surgery may all be necessary acute interventions, and consultation with neurosurgeons, neurologists, oncologists, and therapeutic radiologists may be necessary.

KEY CONCEPTS

- Patients with rapid onset and progression of spinal cord symptoms should receive specialized imaging and consultation in the ED.
- MRI is frequently required to make a definitive diagnosis for spinal syndromes.
- With compressive lesions of the spinal cord, duration of neurologic dysfunction is directly related to ultimate neurologic outcome. The diagnosis must be made expeditiously and definitive therapy begun as soon as possible.

REFERENCES

1. Wagner R, Jagoda A: Spinal cord syndromes. In Woolsey RM, Young RR, editors: *Emerg Med Clin North Am* 15:699, 1997.
2. Johnston RA: The management of acute spinal cord compression, *J Neurol Neurosurg Psychiatry* 56:1046, 1993.
3. Guthkelch AN, Fleischer AS: Patterns of cervical spine injury and their associated lesions, *West J Med* 147:428, 1987.
4. Bohlman HH, Freehafer AF, Dejak J: The results of treatment of acute injuries of the upper thoracic spine with paralysis, *J Bone Joint Surg* 67:360, 1985.
5. Shewman DA: Spinal shock and "brain death": somatic pathophysiological equivalence and implications for the integrative unity rationale, *Spinal Cord* 37:313, 1999.
6. Atkinson PP, Atkinson J: Spinal shock, *Mayo Clin Proc* 71:384, 1996.
7. Merriam WF et al: A reappraisal of acute traumatic central cord syndrome, *J Bone Joint Surg* 688:708, 1986.
8. Schneider RC, Cherry G, Pantek H: The syndrome of acute central spinal cord injury, with special reference to the mechanics involved in hyperextension injury of the cervical spinal, *J Neurosurg* 11:546, 1954.
9. Maroon JC: "Burning hands" in football spinal cord injuries, *JAMA* 238:2049, 1977.
10. Tow AM, Kong KH: Central cord syndrome: functional outcome after rehabilitation, *Spinal Cord* 36:156, 1998.
11. Kirschblum SC, O'Connor KC: Predicting neurologic recovery in traumatic cervical spinal cord injury, *Arch Phys Med Rehabil* 79:1456, 1998.
12. Brown-Séquard CE: Lectures on the physiology and pathology of the central nervous system and the treatment of organic nervous affections, *Lancet* 2:593, 659, 755, 821, 1868.
13. Rumana CS, Baskin DS: Brown-Séquard syndrome produced by cervical disc herniation: case report and literature review, *Surg Neurol* 45:359, 1996.
14. Koehler PJ, Endtz LJ: The Brown-Séquard syndrome: true or false? *Arch Neurol* 43:921, 1986.
15. Gharagozloo F et al: Spinal cord protection during surgical procedures on descending thoracic and thoracoabdominal aorta: review of current techniques, *Chest* 109:799, 1996.

16. Rogers FB et al: Isolated stab wound to the artery of Adamkiewicz: case report and review of the literature, *J Trauma-Injury Inf Crit Care* 43:549, 1997.
17. Waters RL et al: Recovery following ischemic myelopathy, *J Trauma* 35:837, 1993.
18. Kim SW: The syndrome of acute anterior lumbar spinal cord injury, *Clin Neurol Neurosurg* 92:249, 1990.
19. Kostiuk JP et al: Cauda equina syndrome and lumbar disc herniation, *J Bone Joint Surg* 68A:386, 1986.
20. Huff JS: Spinal epidural hematoma associated with cocaine abuse, *Am J Emerg Med* 12:350, 1994.
21. Hainline B, Tuszynski MH, Posner JB: Ataxia in epidural spinal cord compression, *Neurology* 42:2193, 1992.
22. Rodriguez M: Multiple sclerosis: basic concepts and hypothesis, *Mayo Clin Proc* 64:570, 1989.
23. Ransohoff RM: Multiple sclerosis: new concepts of pathogenesis, diagnosis, and treatment, *Comp Therapy* 15:39, 1989.
24. Miller DH et al: Magnetic resonance imaging in isolated noncompressive spinal cord syndromes, *Ann Neurol* 22:714, 1987.
25. Gebarski S: The initial diagnosis of multiple sclerosis: clinical impact of magnetic resonance imaging, *Ann Neurol* 17:469, 1985.
26. Swanson JW: Multiple sclerosis: update in diagnosis and review of prognostic factors, *Mayo Clin Proc* 64:577, 1989.
27. Warren KG, Catz I: The relationship between levels of cerebrospinal fluid myelin basic protein and IgG measurements in patients with multiple sclerosis, *Ann Neurol* 17:475, 1985.
28. Herndon RM, Brooks B: Misdiagnosis of multiple sclerosis, *Semin Neurol* 5:94, 1985.
29. Dawson DM, Potts F: Acute nontraumatic myelopathies, *Neurol Clin* 9:585, 1991.
30. Jeffrey DR, Mandler RN, Davis LE: Transverse myelitis: retrospective analysis of 33 cases, with differentiation of cases associated with multiple sclerosis and parainfectious events, *Arch Neurol* 50:532, 1993.
31. Kalita J, Misra UK, Mandal SK: Prognostic predictors of acute transverse myelitis, *Acta Neurolog Scand* 98:60, 1998.
32. Kelley CE, Matthews J, Noskin GA: Acute transverse myelitis in the emergency department: a case report and review of the literature, *J Emerg Med* 9:417, 1991.
33. Misra UK, Kalita J: Transverse myelitis: neurophysiological and MRI correlation, *Paraplegia* 32:593, 1994.
34. Dunne K, Hopkins IJ, Shield JK: Acute transverse myelopathy in childhood, *Dev Med Child Neurol* 28:198, 1986.
35. Dowling PC, Bosch VV, Cook SD: Possible beneficial effect of high-dose intravenous steroid therapy in acute demyelinating disease and transverse myelitis, *Neurology* 30:33, 1980.
36. Sureda B et al: Severe acute transverse myelitis: prognostic factors, *Arch Neurobiol (Madr)* 51:13, 1988.
37. Lipton HL, Teasdale RD: Acute transverse myelopathy in adults: a follow-up study, *Arch Neurol* 28:252, 1973.
38. Schmidt RD, Markovchik V: Nontraumatic spinal cord compression, *J Emerg Med* 2:189, 1992.
39. Aminoff MJ, Barnard RO, Logue V: The pathophysiology of spinal vascular malformations, *J Neurol Sci* 23:255, 1988.
40. Marconi F et al: Spinal cavernous angioma producing subarachnoid hemorrhage: case report, *J Neurosurg Sci* 39:75, 1995.
41. Cordan T et al: Spinal subarachnoid hemorrhage attributable to schwannoma of the cauda equina, *Surg Neurol* 51:373, 1999.
42. Morgan MK, Marsh WR: Management of spinal dural arteriovenous malformations, *J Neurosurg* 70:832, 1989.
43. Rossier AB et al: Posttraumatic cervical syringomyelia, *Brain* 108:439, 1985.
44. Elghazawi AK: Clinical syndromes and differential diagnosis of spinal disorders, *Radiol Clin North Am* 29:651, 1991.
45. Davis CH, Symon L: Mechanisms and treatment in post-traumatic syringomyelia, *Br J Neurosurg* 3:669, 1989.
46. Caplan LR, Norohna AB, Amico LL: Syringomyelia and arachnoiditis, *J Neurol Neurosurg Psychiatry* 53:106, 1990.
47. Dworkin GE, Staas WE: Posttraumatic syringomyelia, *Arch Phys Med Rehabil* 66:329, 1985.
48. Bird TD: Idiopathic progressive spastic paraparesis, *JAMA* 274:1191, 1995.
49. Younger DS, et al: Primary lateral sclerosis: a clinical diagnosis reemerges, *Arch Neurol* 45:1304, 1988.
50. Pringle CE et al: Primary lateral sclerosis, *Brain* 115:495, 1992.
51. Simson DM, Berger JR: Management of the HIV-infected patient, *Med Clin North Am* 80:1363, 1996.
52. de Silva SM et al: Zoster myelitis: improvement with antiviral therapy in two cases, *Neurology* 47:923, 1996.
53. Cheshire WP et al: Spinal cord infarction: etiology and outcome, *Neurology* 47:321, 1996.
54. Tekkok IH et al: Extradural hematoma after continuous extradural anaesthesia, *Br J Anaesth* 67:112, 1991.
55. Hejazi N, Thaper PY, Hassler W: Nine cases of nontraumatic spinal epidural hematoma, *Neurol Med Chir* 38:718, 1998.
56. Dickman CA et al: Spinal epidural hematoma associated with epidural anaesthesia: complications of systemic heparinization in patients receiving peripheral vascular thrombolytic therapy, *Anesthesiology* 72:947, 1990.
57. Mattle H et al: Nontraumatic spinal epidural and subdural hematomas, *Neurology* 37:1351, 1987.
58. Lederle FA et al: Spinal epidural hematoma associated with warfarin therapy, *Am J Med* 100:237, 1996.
59. Wysowski DK et al: Spinal and epidural hematoma and low-molecular-weight heparin, *N Engl J Med* 338:1774, 1998.
60. Boukobza M et al: Spinal epidural hematoma: report of 11 cases and review of the literature, *Neuroradiology* 36:456, 1994.
61. Groen RT, Van Alphen HA: Operative treatment of spontaneous spinal epidural hematomas: a study of the factors determining postoperative outcome, *Neurosurgery* 39:494, 1996.
62. Enomato T et al: Spontaneous spinal epidural hematoma: report of a case, *Neurol Surg* 8:875, 1980.
63. Sampath P, Rigamonti D: Spinal epidural abscess: a review of epidemiology, diagnosis, and treatment, *J Spinal Disord* 12:89, 1999.
64. Rigamonti D, Liem L, Sampath P: Spinal epidural abscess: contemporary trends in etiology, evaluation, and treatment, *Surg Neurol* 52:189, 1999.
65. Curling OD, Gower DJ, McWhorter JM: Changing concepts in spinal epidural abscess: a report of 29 cases, *Neurosurgery* 27:185, 1990.
66. Koppell BS, Tuchman AJ, Mangiardi JR: Epidural spinal infection in intravenous drug abusers, *Arch Neurol* 12:1331, 1988.
67. Nussbaum et al: Spinal epidural abscess: a review of 40 cases and review, *Surg Neurol* 38:225, 1992.
68. Corboy JR, Price RW: Myelitis and toxic, inflammatory and infectious disorders, *Curr Opin Neurol Neurosurg* 6:564, 1993.
69. Hlavin ML et al: Spinal epidural abscess: a ten-year perspective, *Neurosurgery* 27:177, 1990.
70. Danner RL, Hartman BJ: Update of epidural abscess: 35 cases and a review of the literature, *Rev Infect Dis* 9:265, 1987.
71. Maiuri F et al: Spondylodiscitis: clinical and magnetic resonance diagnosis, *Spine* 22:1741, 1997.
72. Honan M, White GW, Eisenberg GM: Spontaneous infectious discitis in adults, *Am J Med* 100:85, 1996.
73. Malik GM, McCormick P: Management of spine and intervertebral disc space infection, *Contemp Neurosurg* 10:1, 1988.
74. Constantini S, Epstein FJ: Primary spinal cord tumors. In Levin VA editor: *Cancer in the nervous system,* New York, 1996, Churchill Livingstone.
75. Schiff D, O'Neill BP, Suman VJ: Spinal epidural metastasis as the initial manifestation of malignancy: clinical features and diagnostic approach, *Neurology* 49:452, 1997.
76. Schiff D, O'Neill BP: Intramedullary spinal cord metastases: clinical features and treatment outcome, *Neurology* 47:906, 1996.
77. Abdu WA, Provencher M: Primary bone and metastatic tumors of the cervical spine, *Spine* 23:2767, 1998.
78. Wong D, Fornasier V, MacNab I: Spinal metastasis: the obvious, the occult, and the imposters, *Spine* 15:1, 1990.

101 Peripheral Nerve Disorders

E. John Gallagher

PERSPECTIVE

Background

The nervous system is traditionally divided into central (CNS) and peripheral (PNS) components. The PNS can be further subdivided into 12 cranial and 31 spinal nerves. This chapter is confined to diseases of the latter. Disorders of the cranial nerves, whether central or peripheral in origin, are discussed in Chapter 99. Because diseases of the neuromuscular junction and the myopathies are located distal to the neuron itself, they are also considered separately in Chapter 102. Radiculopathies, which are disorders of the roots of the PNS, are so commonly associated with musculoskeletal neck and back pain that they are mentioned only briefly here and are discussed in detail in Chapter 47.

The simplest approach to diseases of the PNS parallels the CNS model of separating focal from nonfocal disease. In the PNS, the focal group can be further divided into those with evidence of single versus multiple lesions of peripheral nerves, known respectively as *simple mononeuropathies* versus *multiple mononeuropathies* (or *mononeuropathy multiplex*). The second broad category (i.e., the nonfocal group of peripheral neuropathies) represents the polyneuropathies. These tend to produce bilaterally symmetric symptoms and signs, reflecting the widespread nature of the underlying pathologic process.

A somewhat more complex approach to the PNS, which is more applicable to emergency practice, is proposed in Figure 101-1.

The template in Figure 101-1 is derived from a goal-directed history and physical examination targeted at answering the following three questions, each of which corresponds to a stratum in the algorithm:

1. Are the sensorimotor signs and symptoms symmetric or asymmetric?
2. Are the sensorimotor signs and symptoms distal or both proximal and distal?
3. Is the modality involved exclusively motor, sensory, or mixed (sensorimotor)?

By systematically combining responses to these questions, one can identify seven discrete categories of peripheral neuropathy, each of which contains a finite set of possible diagnoses. Because pure motor or sensory findings tend to occur mainly in an asymmetric, distal distribution, this is the only category in Figure 101-1 subdivided into pure motor and pure sensory abnormalities.

Epidemiology

Although Guillain-Barré syndrome (GBS) is the most commonly encountered emergent peripheral neuropathy in developed countries, its annual incidence is only about 1.2 cases per 100,000.[1] In contrast to the low incidence of acute peripheral neuropathies, several of which are associated with short-term mortality, the vast majority of peripheral neuropathies presenting to the ED are subacute or chronic and are associated with long-term morbidity.

The Neuropathy Association estimates that over 20 million people in the United States suffer from peripheral neuropathy, virtually all of whom belong to the subacute or chronic group. The American Diabetes Association estimates that about 16 million Americans have diabetes mellitus, and that roughly half of these individuals have objective evidence of peripheral neuropathy, although many are asymptomatic.[2] Furthermore, about half of all nontraumatic lower limb amputations occur in diabetics, virtually all of whom have antecedent distal sensorimotor neuropathy.[3]

PRINCIPLES OF DISEASE

Anatomy

The spinal component of the PNS is shown schematically in Figure 101-2. As noted earlier, this does not include the cranial nerves, which are discussed in Chapter 99. The anterior (ventral) and posterior (dorsal) nerve roots exit the spinal cord at each segmental level. Just distal to the dorsal root ganglion they converge to form a mixed (motor and sensory) spinal nerve, of which there are 31 pairs: 8 cervical, 12 thoracic, 5 lumbar, 5 sacral, and 1 coccygeal. The spinal nerves immediately bifurcate into anterior (ventral) and posterior (dorsal) rami. The posterior ramus travels to the back. The anterior ramus innervates the anterolateral portion of the body and supplies all peripheral nerves for the upper and lower extremities via the brachial and lumbosacral plexus, respectively. Interweaving of fibers occurs within a plexus, producing a mixed sensorimotor innervation of peripheral nerves exiting a plexus.

In addition to the motor and sensory modalities of the PNS, the autonomic nervous system also has a peripheral component that innervates cardiac muscle, smooth muscle, and glands. Anatomically and functionally, the autonomic nervous system is divided into two parts: a sympathetic (thoracolumbar) component, and a parasympathetic (craniosacral) component. Autonomic dysfunction may cause systemic abnormalities such as orthostasis, or local problems such as atrophic, dry skin.

Pathophysiology

The PNS has only three basic responses to a wide array of pathologic stimuli. As shown in Figure 101-2, these include (1) the myelinopathies (primary site of involvement is limited to the myelin sheath surrounding the axon), (2) the axonopathies (primary site of involvement is the axon, with or without secondary demyelination), and (3) the neuronopathies (cell body of the neuron itself is primary site of involvement, ultimately affecting the entire nerve). Although overlap occurs, each of these prototypes has a distinctive clinical presentation, electrophysiologic profile, and microscopic appearance.

Electrophysiologic testing—nerve conduction studies

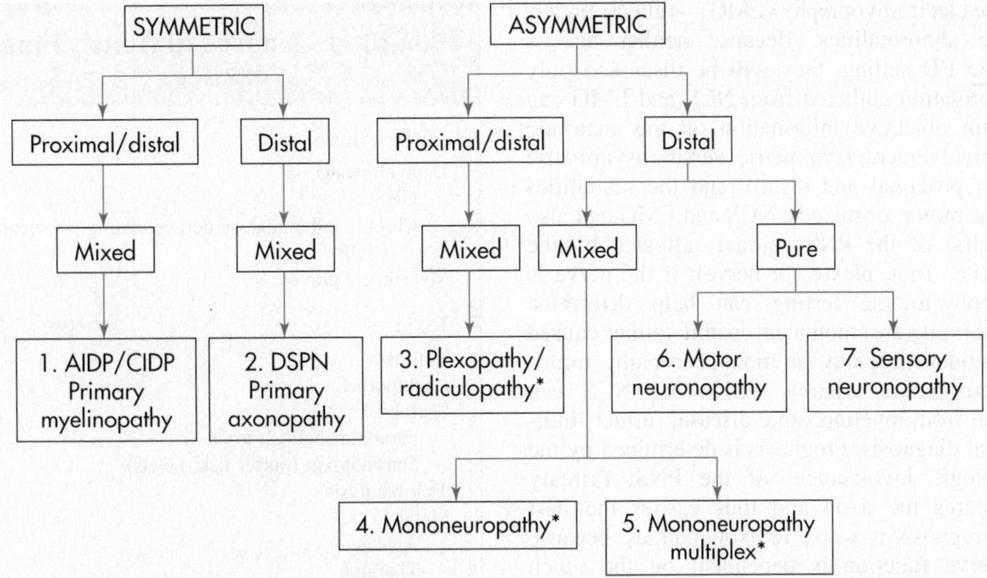

Figure 101-1. **An approach to peripheral neuropathy in the ED.** ***AIDP,*** **Acute inflammatory demyelinating polyneuropathy (Guillain-Barré);** ***CIDP,*** **chronic inflammatory demyelinating polyneuropathy;** ***DSPN,*** **distal symmetric polyneuropathy.**
***A proximal distribution of sensorimotor findings may dominate the clinical picture in patterns 3, 4, and 5, depending on the location of the lesion(s).**

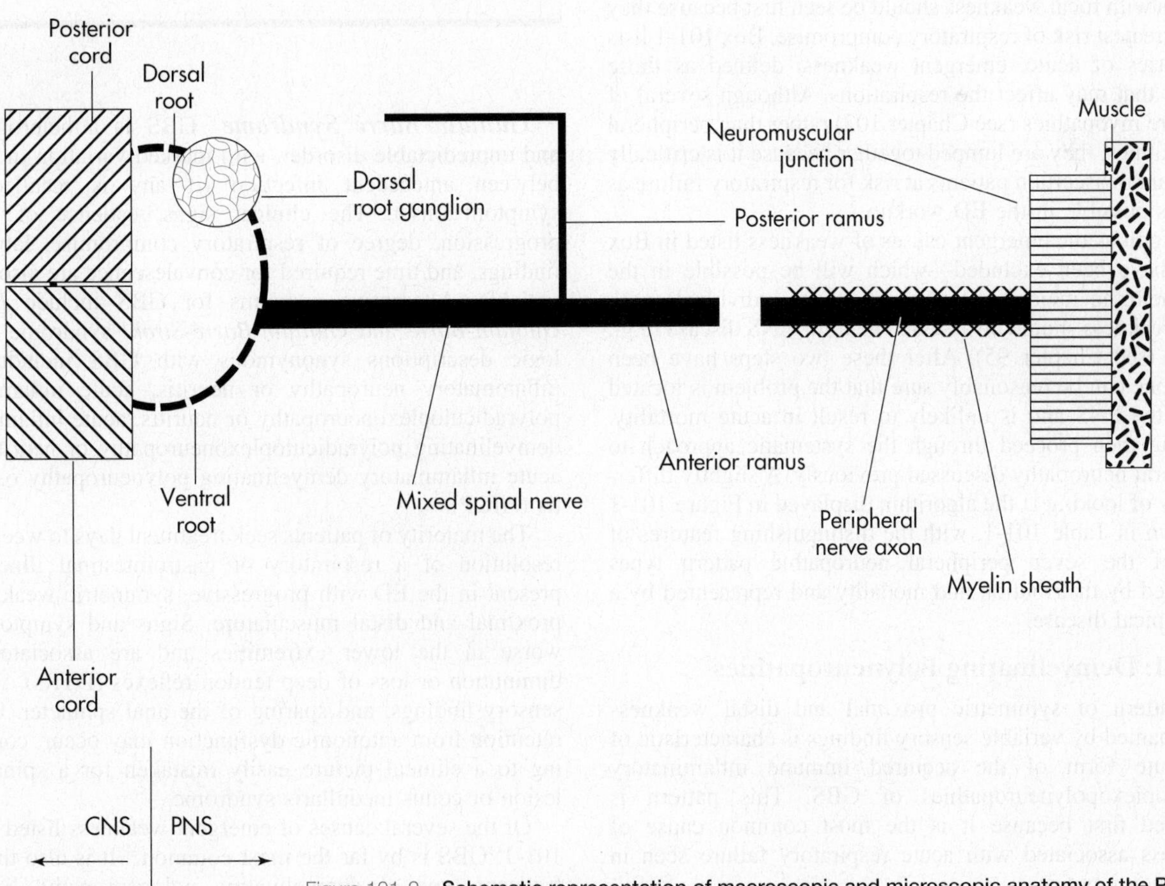

Figure 101-2. **Schematic representation of macroscopic and microscopic anatomy of the PNS and its interface with the CNS. See text for explanation.**

(NCS) and needle electromyography (EMG)—reflects underlying pathologic abnormalities. Because neither test is appropriate to the ED setting, they will be discussed only briefly here. Information gathered from NCS and EMG can be used to obtain objective information on the anatomic distribution of involvement (symmetric versus asymmetric and distal versus proximal and distal), and the modalities involved (sensory, motor, or mixed). NCS and EMG can also identify the level(s) of the PNS neuraxis affected by the disease process (i.e., root, plexus, or nerve); if the nerve is affected, electrophysiologic testing can help determine whether the lesion(s) is (are) mononeuropathic (either caused by an isolated mononeuropathy or mononeuropathy multiplex) or polyneuropathic. Finally, EMG and NCS can distinguish axonal from myelinopathic disease, further limiting the differential diagnosis. Prognosis is determined by the nature of pathologic involvement of the PNS. Primary demyelination spares the axon and thus carries the best prognosis. The prognosis is worse in axonopathies, because reestablishing nerve function is dependent on the much slower process of axonal regeneration. Neuronopathies, which begin with primary destruction of the nerve cell body, produce pure motor or pure sensory syndromes, respectively. Eventually the entire nerve is affected, resulting in the worst prognosis of the three.

CLINICAL FEATURES

The differential diagnosis of any patient coming to the ED with sensory, motor, or sensorimotor historic complaints or physical findings, particularly if localized to the extremities, should include a peripheral neuropathy. Within this group, patients with focal weakness should be seen first because they are at greatest risk of respiratory compromise. Box 101-1 lists the causes of acute, emergent weakness, defined as those entities that may affect the respirations. Although several of these are myopathies (see Chapter 102) rather than peripheral neuropathies, they are lumped together because it is critically important to ascertain patients at risk for respiratory failure as early as possible in the ED workup.

As soon as the emergent causes of weakness listed in Box 101-1 have been excluded—which will be possible in the overwhelming majority of patients—those individuals with focal weakness should be assessed next for CNS disease (e.g., stroke) (see Chapter 95). After these two steps have been taken, one can be reasonably sure that the problem is located within the PNS and is unlikely to result in acute mortality. One can then proceed through the systematic approach to peripheral neuropathy discussed previously. A slightly different way of looking at the algorithm displayed in Figure 101-1 is shown in Table 101-1, with the distinguishing features of each of the seven peripheral neuropathic pattern types described by distribution and modality and represented by a prototypical disease.

Type 1: Demyelinating Polyneuropathies

The pattern of symmetric proximal and distal weakness accompanied by variable sensory findings is characteristic of the acute form of the acquired immune inflammatory radiculoplexopolyneuropathies of GBS. This pattern is discussed first because it is the most common cause of weakness associated with acute respiratory failure seen in emergency practice.

Box 101-1 Causes of Acute, Emergent Weakness

Autoimmune

Demyelinating
- GBS
- Chronic inflammatory demyelinating polyneuropathy (CIDP)

Myasthenia gravis

Toxic

Botulism
Buckthorn
Seafood
- Paralytic shellfish toxin
- Tetrodotoxin (puffer fish, newts)

Tick paralysis
Metals
- Arsenic
- Thallium

Metabolic

Dyskalemic syndromes
- Acquired (especially with thyrotoxicosis)
- Familial

Hypophosphatemia
Hypermagnesemia
Porphyria

Infectious

Poliomyelitis
Diphtheria

Guillain-Barré Syndrome GBS is a heterogeneous and unpredictable disorder, with marked variation in latency between antecedent infection (if any is recalled) and symptom onset. The clinical signs, cadence of disease progression, degree of respiratory compromise, laboratory findings, and time required for convalescence are also highly variable. Alternative eponyms for GBS include *Landry-Guillain-Barré* and *Guillain-Barré-Strohl* syndrome. Pathologic descriptions synonymous with GBS include acute inflammatory neuropathy or neuritis, acute inflammatory polyradiculoplexoneuropathy or neuritis, acute inflammatory demyelinating polyradiculoplexoneuropathy or neuritis, and acute inflammatory demyelinating polyneuropathy or neuritis (AIDP).

The majority of patients seek treatment days to weeks after resolution of a respiratory or gastrointestinal illness and present in the ED with progressive, symmetric weakness of proximal and distal musculature. Signs and symptoms are worse in the lower extremities and are associated with diminution or loss of deep tendon reflexes (DTRs), variable sensory findings, and sparing of the anal sphincter. Urinary retention from autonomic dysfunction may occur, contributing to a clinical picture easily mistaken for a spinal cord lesion or conus medullaris syndrome.

Of the several causes of emergent weakness listed in Box 101-1, GBS is by far the most common.[4] It is also the most frequent type of demyelinating polyneuropathy listed in

Table 101-1. Patterns and Prototypes of Peripheral Neuropathies

Type	Pattern	Prototypical disease	Distribution		Modalities
I	Proximal and distal, symmetric, sensorimotor polyneuropathy	GBS	P/D	S	M > S
II	Distal, symmetric, sensorimotor polyneuropathy	Diabetic DSPN	D	S	S > M
III	Proximal and distal, asymmetric, sensorimotor neuropathy	Brachial plexopathy	P/D	A	S, M
IV	Distal, asymmetric, sensorimotor mononeuropathy (single nerve involved)	CTS (median mononeuropathy)	D	A	S, M
V	Distal, asymmetric, sensorimotor mononeuropathy multiplex (multiple nerves involved)	Vasculitic mononeuropathy multiplex	D	A	S, M
VI	Distal, asymmetric, pure motor neuronopathy	ALS	D	A	M
VII	Distal, asymmetric, pure sensory neuronopathy	Pyridoxine toxicity	D	A	S

A, Asymmetric distribution; *ALS*, amyotrophic lateral sclerosis; *CTS*, carpal tunnel syndrome; *D*, distally located; *DSPN*, distal symmetric polyneuropathy; *GBS*, Guillain-Barré syndrome; *M*, motor findings present; *S*, sensory modalities affected; *P/D*, both proximally and distally located; *S*, symmetric (right and left) distribution.

Box 101-2 Demyelinating Polyneuropathies

GBS
- Fisher variant of GBS (ophthalmoplegia and ataxia)
- Axonal GBS
- Sensory GBS
- Autonomic GBS

Chronic inflammatory demyelinating polyradiculoplexo-neuropathy (CIDP)
Malignancy
HIV
Hepatitis B
Buckthorn
Diphtheria

Box 101-2. In practice, patients with proximal and distal symmetric weakness of relatively acute onset, decreased or absent DTRs, and variable degrees of sensory loss should be managed as if they have GBS or one of its variants, which would place them at risk of respiratory compromise. Conversely, patients with predominantly sensory signs and symptoms are unlikely to develop acute respiratory distress.

About half of patients with GBS have autonomic dysfunction (causing marked fluctuations in pulse and blood pressure), experience a peak of disease severity within a week of onset, have some form of cranial nerve involvement (usually VII), and suffer long-term symptomatic residual of their illness. Nearly one third require ventilatory support. Both the mortality and recurrence rate are about 3%.

In addition to electrophysiologic testing, there are three ancillary tests that may be helpful in the diagnosis of GBS. Cerebrospinal fluid (CSF) analysis is useful when it demonstrates the characteristic picture of elevated protein with a normal or near normal white cell (lymphocyte) count. In the clinical setting of suspected GBS, this finding is highly specific. Early in the disease, however, patients may have normal CSF values. Selective enhancement of the anterior spinal nerve roots on magnetic resonance imaging (MRI) is suggestive, but not diagnostic, of GBS.[5] In more serious cases, axonal degeneration occurs, particularly in association with antecedent *Campylobacter jejuni* infection.[6] Although many investigators regard the inflammation of GBS as a lymphocytic cell-mediated form of delayed hypersensitivity, there is some evidence that circulating anti–myelin sheath autoantibodies also play a role in the disease.[7,8]

Management Individuals with suspected GBS must have their respiratory function followed with FEV_1 or peak flow rate. Any patients unable to perform these tests, and those with values less than 100% predicted, should have an arterial blood gas obtained. Evidence of alveolar hypoventilation (elevated PCO_2) in a patient with an unsecured airway requires a level of intensive monitoring that is impractical in many EDs. Therefore patients with weakness, CO_2 retention, or other evidence of early ventilatory failure should be considered for prophylactic intubation.

In patients with possible GBS who have normal pulmonary function, extensor neck strength can be monitored to predict impending ventilatory failure. All patients with probable GBS should receive neurologic consultation and be admitted to the hospital. Depending on institutional custom, plasma exchange or intravenous immune globulin should be administered. There is sound evidence that both are superior to placebo, and that combination therapy confers no therapeutic advantage over either intervention alone.[9] The role of corticosteroids remains undefined, although the best evidence to date suggests that they are ineffective.[10] Although marked elevations in blood pressure commonly occur, these should not be treated because the autonomic component of this disease can cause blood pressure to drop as precipitously and unpredictably as it rose.

Type 2: Distal Symmetric Polyneuropathies

Most polyneuropathies are characterized by a pattern of distal, symmetric sensorimotor findings, worse in the lower than upper extremities, with a stocking-glove distribution of sensory abnormalities that gradually diminishes as one moves proximally. The motor findings and loss of DTRs, which lag behind the sensory features in most instances, follow a similar pattern of progression from distal to proximal. The diffuse, distal, symmetric nature of this pattern is most consistent with a toxic-metabolic disease process, as yet unidentified, that causes a length-dependent axonopathy. Only the most common causes of distal symmetric polyneuropathies (DSPN) will be discussed, with a more complete listing of other causes shown in Box 101-3.

Diabetic DSPN DSPN is the most common type of peripheral neuropathy seen in emergency practice, with the preponderance of cases occurring in diabetics. Initial symptoms are distal and usually "positive" sensory complaints (e.g., dysesthesias such as tingling or burning) beginning on the plantar surfaces of both feet. At the early stages of a typical DSPN there may be some asymmetry, without evidence of "negative" sensory findings (e.g., numbness), weakness, or reflex loss. At this juncture, it may be impossible to distinguish a focal neuropathic process such as a mononeuropathy from a polyneuropathy, although prior probability strongly favors the latter in this anatomic location. As the process advances, the plantar surfaces of both feet will become dysesthetic before the dorsum of either foot is involved. Weakness of dorsiflexion of the big toe is usually the first motor sign, followed by weakness of foot dorsiflexion, foot drop, loss of ankle jerks, and later a "steppage gait."

Sensory loss continues to move proximally, and before it reaches the knees, the finger tips are usually involved. DTRs are progressively lost, as is proprioception. If the latter becomes severe, patients may develop sensory ataxia. As the neuropathy continues to progress, sensory abnormalities ultimately involve all modalities and extend to a diamond-shaped periumbilical area. Far-advanced disease may affect sensation over the skull vertex and facial midline structures. Atrophy occurs, weakness worsens, and areflexia supervenes. Severely impaired patients may be unable to ambulate or grasp objects.

Management As is the case with most peripheral neuropathies, referral is indicated for management of diabetic DSPNs. However, if discomfort is severe, the etiology of the neuropathy seems likely to be diabetic, and referral will be delayed, it may be necessary to provide symptomatic relief for neuropathic symptoms.

There is good evidence to support use of tricyclic antidepressants as first-line agents, starting with 25 mg of amitriptyline at bedtime (10 mg in the elderly).[11] Carbamazepine 200 to 400 mg q8h or qid should be considered a second-line drug,[11] to be used only if the patient cannot tolerate the side effects of amitriptyline, imipramine, nortriptyline, or desipramine. Among the selective serotonin reuptake inhibitors (SSRIs), paroxetine appears to be effective.[11] Trazodone, phenytoin, and topical capsaicin[12] are equivalent to placebo. No medications have been shown to relieve negative sensory symptoms. Because of the unpredictable and often chronic course of peripheral neuropathies, opioids should generally be avoided. Improving glycemic control can prevent, diminish, or abolish many diabetic DSPNs.

Box 101-3 Distal Sensorimotor Polyneuropathies

- Diabetes mellitus
- Alcoholism
- Neoplastic or paraneoplastic
- Hereditary motor and sensory neuropathies (Charcot-Marie-Tooth)
- Cryptogenic sensorimotor polyneuropathies (CSPN)
- HIV
- Toxins
  - Organic or industrial agents
    - Acrylamide
    - Allyl chloride
    - Carbon disulfide
    - Ethylene oxide
    - Hexacarbons
    - Methyl bromide
    - Organophosphate-induced delayed polyneuropathy (OPIDP)
    - Polychlorinated biphenyls (PCBs)
    - Trichloroethylene
    - Vacor (PNU)
  - Metals
    - Arsenic
    - Gold
    - Mercury (inorganic)
    - Thallium
  - Therapeutic agents
    - Amiodarone
    - Antiretrovirals
    - Dapsone
    - Disulfiram
    - Isoniazid
    - Metronidazole
    - Nitrofurantoin
    - Paclitaxel (Taxol)
    - Phenytoin
    - Simvastatin (and other HMG-CoA reductase inhibitors)
    - Vinca alkaloids (vincristine)
- Nutritional
  - Beriberi (thiamine or vitamin B_1)
  - Pellagra (niacin, B vitamins)
  - Pernicious anemia (vitamin B_{12})
  - Pyridoxine deficiency (vitamin B_6)
- End-organ dysfunction
  - Acromegaly
  - Chronic pulmonary disease
  - Hypothyroidism
  - Renal failure (uremic neuropathy)
- Paraproteinemias
  - Amyloidosis
  - Monoclonal gammopathy of unknown significance (MGUS)
  - Multiple myeloma
  - Waldenström's macroglobulinemia
- Porphyria

Alcoholic DSPN Although the association between alcoholism and peripheral neuropathy has been well-established for centuries, demonstration of a direct neurotoxic effect of alcohol remains elusive. The preponderance of evidence, from both observational studies in humans and experimental data in animal models, suggests that the association between alcohol and peripheral neuropathy may be confounded by nutritional status (i.e., deficiency states might be the true underlying cause of alcoholic peripheral neuropathy).

The clinical and pathologic picture of alcoholic neuropathy is similar to the distal, symmetric, sensorimotor peripheral neuropathy of diabetes. However, in alcoholism the presence of ataxia is more likely to have a contributory cerebellar component. Autonomic skin changes, with atrophy and hair loss, accompany the sensorimotor abnormalities. Often other systemic effects of alcoholism are so severe that the patient may not notice them at all. All patients with suspected alcoholic DSPN should receive dietary supplements and referral for outpatient management.

Toxic and Metabolic Neuropathies Many toxic agents and metabolic derangements produce a neuropathy conforming to the typical picture of an axonopathy causing a DSPN. Box 101-3 lists some of the most common toxic and metabolic causes of peripheral neuropathy.

Type 3: Asymmetric Proximal and Distal Peripheral Neuropathies (Radiculopathies and Plexopathies)

Radiculopathies that conform to this pattern are discussed in detail in Chapter 47. Plexopathies, which are summarized in Box 101-4, are discussed very briefly in this chapter because they are uncommon and often traumatic. Generally, a plexopathy, whether brachial or lumbosacral, is identified by a process of elimination (i.e., a pattern of sensorimotor and reflex abnormalities that fit neither a radicular nor individual peripheral nerve distribution). Although this approach will not exclude a mononeuropathy multiplex on physical examination alone, a careful history should determine whether the patient is at risk for developing a mononeuropathy on the basis of underlying disease.

Radiation (actinic) plexopathy occurs after a variable period of latency following treatment, which may extend to 20 years or more. Almost all series are comprised of women who received radiation treatment for breast cancer.

Among neoplastic causes, most originate from lung or breast. Patients with probable neoplastic brachial plexopathy need imaging studies and may require immediate radiation therapy. Pain control is the focus of management.

Neurogenic thoracic outlet syndrome remains a controversial disorder.[13] Although the pendulum has swung over the past 40 years from a postulated vascular cause of thoracic outlet syndrome to a postulated neurogenic cause, current evidence supporting the high prevalence of compression of the brachial plexus as a cause for thoracic outlet syndrome is in fact only slightly better[14] than was earlier evidence favoring a vascular cause.[15] Cardiothoracic surgeons argue that the syndrome is common, although objective data other than reported postoperative improvement are lacking.[16] On the other hand, neurologists maintain that the paucity of electrophysiologic evidence supports its rarity.

Because of its complexity, there is no reason to expect that one can or should do more in the ED than identify a possible brachial plexopathy. Depending on severity and suspected etiology, one should either admit or refer the patient to a neurologist or neurosurgeon with experience in PNS disease.

Type 4: Isolated Mononeuropathies

The pattern of asymmetric, sensorimotor, usually distal peripheral neuropathy is characteristic of a mononeuropathy. Mononeuropathies are of two main types: isolated and multiple. Multiple mononeuropathies, which are less prevalent in emergency practice than isolated mononeuropathies, are commonly known by the term *mononeuropathy multiplex.* They are discussed in the next section, under Type 5. The isolated mononeuropathies are discussed here.

Box 101-4 Asymmetric Proximal/Distal Peripheral Neuropathies

Brachial Plexopathy

- Open
  - Direct plexus injury (knife or gunshot wound)
  - Neurovascular (plexus ischemia)
  - Iatrogenic (central line insertion)
- Closed
  - Traction injuries
    - "Stingers"
    - Traction neurapraxia
    - Partial or complete nerve root avulsion
  - Radiation
  - Neoplastic
  - Idiopathic brachial plexitis
  - Thoracic outlet

Lumbosacral Plexopathies

- Open
- Closed
  - Traction injuries
    - Pelvic double vertical shearing fracture
    - Posterior hip dislocation
    - Retroperitoneal hemorrhage
  - Vasospastic (deep buttock injection)
  - Neoplastic
  - Radiation
  - Idiopathic lumbosacral plexitis
  - Infectious
    - Herpesvirus (sacrococcygeal)
      - Herpes simplex II
      - Herpes zoster
    - Cytomegalovirus (CMV) polyradiculopathy (HIV)

Isolated mononeuropathies are usually caused by trauma, either blunt or penetrating. If the trauma is blunt, the injury may be secondary to compression from an internal or external source. Entrapment neuropathies are a subset of compression neuropathies occurring at anatomic locations where nerves traverse potentially constricting compartments or tunnels.[17] Isolated mononeuropathies may be acute, intermittent, or continuous. Antecedent peripheral neuropathy may be a risk factor for development of compression neuropathy (so-called "double-crush syndrome"), particularly in diabetics.[18] The isolated mononeuropathies are listed in Box 101-5 and discussed below.

Radial Mononeuropathy The radial nerve arises from C5-T1 roots. As shown in Figure 101-3, after exiting the brachial plexus, it passes behind the proximal humerus in the spiral groove, taking a lateral (radial) course down the upper arm.

At about the level of the antecubital fossa, it bifurcates into the posterior interosseous (pure motor) and superficial radial (pure sensory) nerves. The radial nerve controls extension of the fingers, thumb, wrist, and elbow (triceps). In contrast to the median and ulnar nerves, the radial nerve provides only extrinsic motor innervation to the hand (i.e., it does not supply motor fibers to any muscles that both originate and insert within the hand). In further contrast to the median and

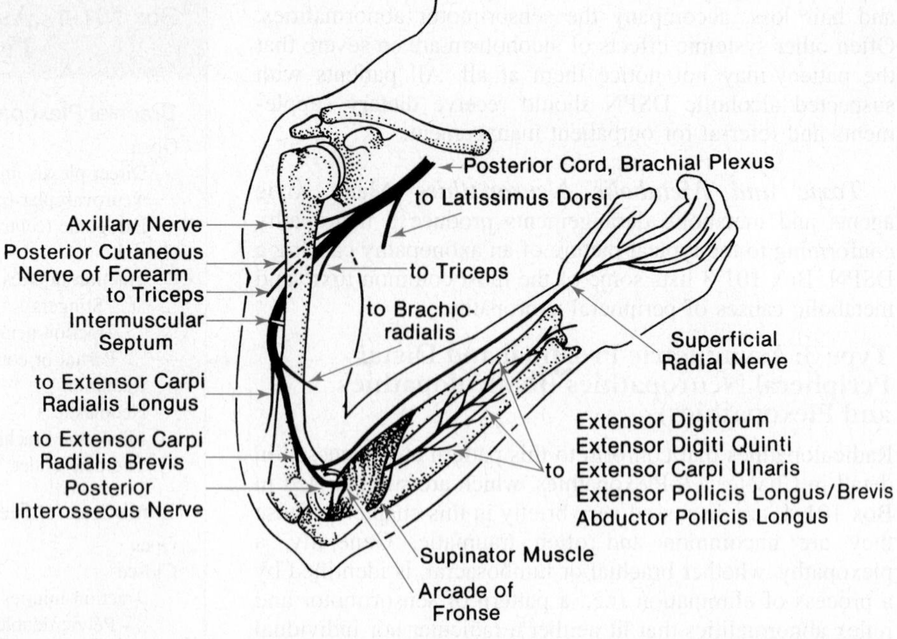

Figure 101-3. **Radial nerve, major branches, right arm, lateral view.** ***From Stewart JD:** Focal peripheral neuropathies, **ed 3, Philadelphia, 2000, Lippincott Williams & Wilkins.***

Box 101-5 Isolated Mononeuropathies

Upper Extremity

- Radial nerve
  - Axilla
  - Humerus
  - Elbow (posterior interosseous neuropathy)
  - Wrist (superficial cutaneous radial neuropathy)
- Ulnar nerve
  - Axilla
  - Humerus
  - Elbow
    - Condylar groove
    - Cubital tunnel
  - Wrist (Guyon's canal)
  - Hand
    - Superficial terminal ulnar neuropathy
    - Deep terminal ulnar neuropathy
      - Proximal hypothenar
      - Distal hypothenar
- Median nerve
  - Axilla
  - Humerus (musculocutaneous mononeuropathy)
  - Forearm
    - Anterior interosseus
    - Pronator syndrome (?)
  - Wrist (carpal tunnel)
  - Hand (recurrent motor branch)
- Suprascapular mononeuropathy
  - Axillary mononeuropathy

Lower Extremity

- Sciatic nerve
- Femoral nerve
  - Iliacus compartment (proximal)
  - Saphenous mononeuropathy (distal)
- Lateral femoral cutaneous (meralgia paresthetica)
- Peroneal nerve
  - Common peroneal mononeuropathy (fibular head, popliteal fossa)
  - Deep peroneal mononeuropathy (anterior compartment)
- Tibial nerve
  - Popliteal fossa (proximal)
  - Tarsal tunnel (distal)
- Sural nerve
  - Popliteal fossa, calf (proximal)
  - Fifth metatarsal base (distal)
- Plantar nerve
  - Distal to tarsal tunnel
  - Interdigital neuropathies (Morton's neuroma)
- Obturator mononeuropathy

ulnar nerves, which supply most of the sensation to the hand, the radial nerve makes a contribution to a cutaneous dorsal area overlying the first dorsal interosseus muscle, sometimes extending part of the way up the dorsum of the thumb, index, and long fingers.

Radial mononeuropathy caused by involvement at the level of the axilla is uncommon. When it occurs, it is usually associated with other upper extremity mononeuropathies or a brachial plexopathy. Although improper use of crutches may cause this syndrome, it usually occurs after an extended period of unconsciousness during which the arm is positioned in such a way that prolonged, deep compression is applied to the axilla. Axillary radial mononeuropathy is distinguished from the more common humeral form by the finding of triceps involvement in addition to typical wrist and finger drop. This occurs because the innervation to the triceps is proximal to the point where the nerve is most vulnerable as it winds around the humeral shaft (see Figure 101-3).

Most radial mononeuropathies are due to so-called "Saturday night palsies." The euphemism is apparently derived from the association of radial mononeuropathy with improper positioning of the arm during deep, commonly inebriated sleep. Consequently, the radial nerve is trapped for a prolonged period between the humeral shaft and some firm surface, causing an external compression mononeuropathy. "Bridegroom's palsy" is another eponym for radial mononeuropathy, so named because the radial nerve may be compressed by the bride's head resting on the bridegroom's arm during sleep.

Because innervation of the wrist and finger extensors occurs distal to this area of the humeral shaft, findings are characterized by wrist and finger drop, and mild numbness over the skin of the first dorsal interosseus muscle. Depending on the level, degree, and duration of compression, some fascicles of the nerve may remain functional, resulting in a partial radial mononeuropathy. Thus the superficial radial nerve may remain intact, resulting in no loss of sensation, or loss of wrist and finger extension may be incomplete.

Because the finger drop of radial mononeuropathy places the hand at a mechanical disadvantage, examination of ulnar function by testing interossei may produce false positive findings of weakness. To adjust for this, the examiner should ask the patient to place the palm on a horizontal supporting surface such as a stretcher. With the fingers extended and no longer "dropped" at the metacarpophalangeal (MCP) joints, interosseous strength can now be fairly tested. Failure to perform this maneuver may cause one to misdiagnose a simple radial mononeuropathy as a brachial plexopathy in an effort to explain what appears to be radial and "partial ulnar" nerve involvement.

Ulnar Mononeuropathy The ulnar nerve includes C7-T1 roots and passes through the brachial plexus to descend medially, without branching, to the ulnar (medial) condylar groove at the elbow. It then enters the cubital canal where it gives off branches to the ulnar wrist flexor and the deep flexors of the fourth and fifth digits.

Just proximal to the wrist, two important sensory branches leave the main trunk to supply cutaneous sensation to part of the hand (Figure 101-4). These are the palmar and dorsal cutaneous branches, which do *not* pass through Guyon's canal. The palmar branch supplies sensation to the hypothenar eminence, and the dorsal branch innervates the ulnar side of the dorsum of the hand, extending out nearly to the tips of the fifth and ulnar half of the fourth digits.

At the wrist, the nerve enters Guyon's canal (Figure 101-5) between the pisiform and hook of the hamate and bifurcates into the superficial terminal sensory branch and the deep motor branch.

The superficial sensory nerve supplies ulnar sensation to the palmar side of the fifth and half of the fourth digit (see Figure 101-5). The deep motor nerve supplies the hypothenar muscles, then crosses to the radial side of the palm to innervate the ulnar intrinsics (all interossei and the ulnar lumbricals of the fourth and fifth digits), terminating in the first dorsal interosseus. The interossei abduct and adduct the fingers, and are all innervated by the ulnar nerve. The lumbrical muscles flex the MCP joints and are evenly divided between the ulnar (fourth and fifth) and median (second and third) digits. The ulnar nerve can be thought of as the complement to the median nerve in the hand, because it supplies all of the muscles and all palmar sensation not innervated by the median.

The ulnar nerve may be injured at two locations near the elbow: in the ulnar condylar groove and distally in the cubital canal. Because the condylar groove is shallow, the ulnar nerve is very superficial in this location and is vulnerable to injury, usually from external pressure or from a fracture or dislocation. A relatively unique feature of the ulnar nerve is its propensity to develop a "tardy ulnar palsy," occurring years after a traumatic event. Many of these delayed ulnar mononeuropathies can be localized to the elbow on electrophysiologic testing.

Some ulnar mononeuropathies occur secondary to compression just proximal to entry into the cubital canal, or are entrapped within the canal itself. Transient symptoms may occur during prolonged flexion or with repeated flexion and extension at the elbow.

Although distinguishing a condylar from a cubital ulnar mononeuropathy is difficult, it is usually possible to localize the problem to the region of the elbow or the wrist. In addition to prior probability heavily favoring the elbow, the presence of sensory abnormalities in an ulnar distribution in the hand and fingers (i.e., usually including the fifth digit and "splitting" the fourth digit) strongly suggests that the lesion is at the level of the elbow rather than the wrist. This is because the ulnar cutaneous innervation to the hand branches off from the main trunk proximal to the nerve entering Guyon's canal (see Figures 101-4 and 101-5). Thus a lesion at the wrist should not produce sensory abnormalities, while one at the elbow would be expected to do so.

Compression of the ulnar nerve within Guyon's canal is rare. When this does occur, it will affect all of the ulnar intrinsics (i.e., the two ulnar [fourth and fifth digits] lumbricals) and all the interossei. However, the ulnar extrinsics (i.e., the deep flexors of the fourth and fifth digits) will not be affected, nor will the ulnar flexor of the wrist. The only sensory abnormalities will be those in the distribution of the superficial terminal sensory branch, sparing other areas of ulnar innervation (see Figure 101-5).

There are three ulnar mononeuropathies that occur distal to Guyon's canal in the hand. The two most common involve the deep terminal branch, either proximal or distal to the separation of the hypothenar branches (see Figure 101-5). If the lesion is proximal, it will produce weakness of all the ulnar innervated muscles of the hand, without sensory loss. If it is distal, the hypothenar ulnar intrinsics will be spared, but the picture will be otherwise similar. Usually this occurs secondary to a laceration or repeated compression in the hand from use of certain tools, a cane, or the handle of a crutch.

Involvement of the superficial terminal branch (see Figure 101-5) presents as pure sensory loss of the palmar surface of the fifth digit and ulnar half of the fourth digit caused by direct compression of this branch occurring just distal to Guyon's canal. The dorsal surface of these two digits should have normal sensation except for the distal tips. This configuration of findings is due to the intact innervation provided by the dorsal and palmar cutaneous branches that

Figure 101-4. **Ulnar nerve, major branches, right arm, anterior view.** *From Stewart JD:* **Focal peripheral neuropathies,** *ed 3, Philadelphia, 2000, Lippincott Williams & Wilkins.*

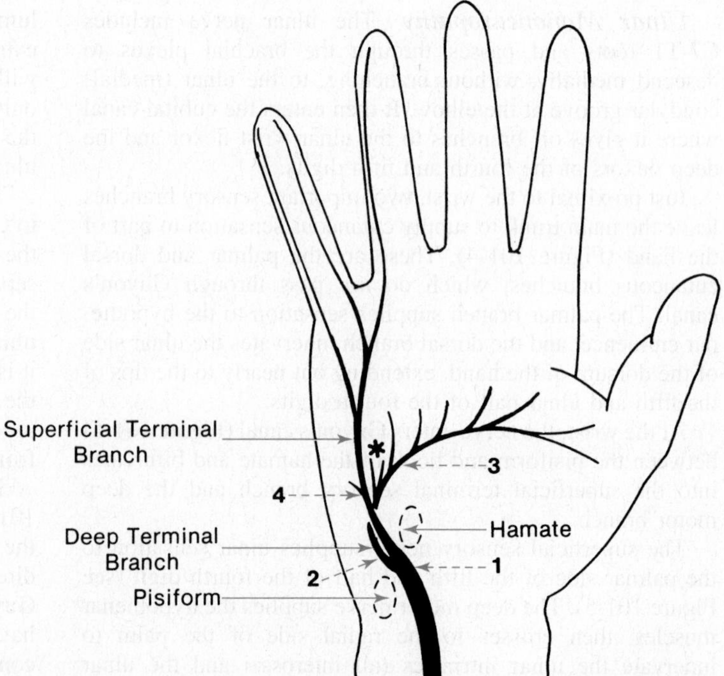

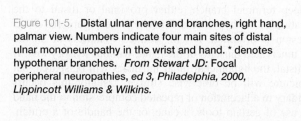

Figure 101-5. **Distal ulnar nerve and branches, right hand, palmar view. Numbers indicate four main sites of distal ulnar mononeuropathy in the wrist and hand. * denotes hypothenar branches.** *From Stewart JD:* **Focal peripheral neuropathies,** *ed 3, Philadelphia, 2000, Lippincott Williams & Wilkins.*

enter the hand without passing through Guyon's canal (see Figure 101-4).

Median Mononeuropathy The median nerve arises from C5-T1 spinal nerve roots and exits the brachial plexus via the lower trunk (Figure 101-6).

Median mononeuropathy is usually diagnosed as carpal tunnel syndrome (CTS), which is the most common of all entrapment neuropathies. Although the patient may complain of bilateral symptoms, a careful history will usually reveal that nocturnal dysesthesia in one hand preceded symptoms in the other. Awakening at night and shaking the hand(s) is a common symptom of CTS. Symptoms are often worsened by activity, and for unclear reasons the pain may spread as high as the arm or shoulder, although the paresthesias are generally confined to the fingers. Many patients on initial questioning will state that their entire hand is involved, although this will not be supported by careful sensory examination. Complaints that the hands are clumsy or weak, especially when holding a glass or opening the lid on a container, are frequent. The skin of the fingers innervated by the median nerve may be drier and rougher to the touch than the corresponding ulnar skin, depending on the duration of entrapment.[19]

Because the nerve has already given off motor branches to the median extrinsic muscles to the hand, when there is motor involvement in CTS it is confined to the median intrinsics, which innervate the **L**umbricals (flexion of the MCP joints), and subserve thumb **O**pposition, **A**bduction, and **F**lexion, therefore known as the LOAF muscles. However, the hallmark of CTS is sensory involvement, with motor abnormalities occurring later. The typical pattern of sensory innervation of the hand by the median, ulnar, and radial nerves shows marked individual variation. The most specific finding for CTS is "splitting" the fourth digit (i.e., normal sensation of the ring finger on the ulnar palmar side with abnormal sensation on the median [lateral] palmar side of the same finger). The most sensitive finding is abnormal sensation of the distal palmar tip of the index finger. If sensory findings are absent in the presence of motor findings consistent with median nerve involvement, it is highly unlikely that the patient has CTS, and an alternative diagnosis should be sought. If there are neither sensory nor motor symptoms evident, none of the provocative tests originally reported to reproduce the sensory symptoms of CTS—of which the most common are Tinel's sign (percussion of the median nerve at the wrist) and Phalen's sign (maximal palmar flexion at the wrist)—has shown adequate sensitivity or specificity to guide the emergency physician in determining which patients should be referred for electrodiagnostic studies.[20-22] As suggested earlier, the best way to examine patients for sensory findings is to touch the distal palmar tips very lightly, asking the patient if the sensation feels "abnormal."

CTS has been associated with many diseases. Those with a reasonably sound evidence base are listed in Box 101-6. Of these, the two most common are diabetes mellitus and pregnancy. CTS associated with systemic illness is commonly bilateral.

Except for pregnant patients, in whom CTS is self-limiting and can usually be treated with nocturnal splinting, all others should be referred for NCS. Because of the dissociation between clinical and electrodiagnostic indicators of CTS, particularly early in the disease, patients with normal electrodiagnostic findings in the face of symptoms suggestive of CTS (with or without signs) should have an MRI.[23] If both of these studies are negative, they should be repeated within a few months if symptoms do not resolve. Thus a patient who arrives in the ED with symptoms and signs consistent with CTS, and a history of normal NCS and MRI in the past, may have undiagnosed CTS that has now progressed to the point that diagnostic studies will be positive. These patients should be referred for repeat testing.[19]

Because of the possibility of development of a disabling "median hand" after inadvertent direct injection of the

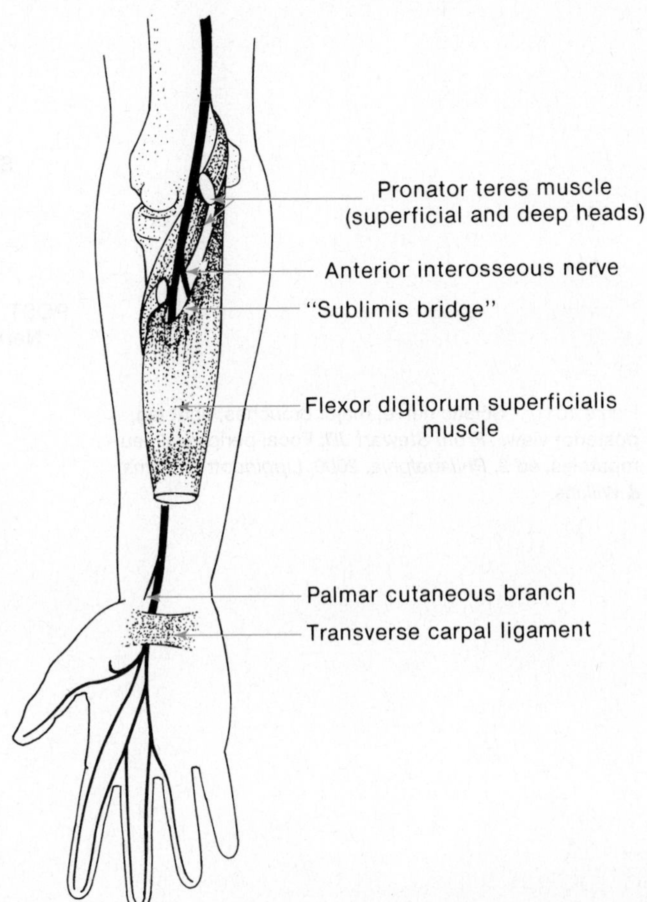

Figure 101-6. **Median nerve, major branches, right arm, anterior view.** *From Stewart JD:* Focal peripheral neuropathies, *ed 3, Philadelphia, 2000, Lippincott Williams & Wilkins.*

Box 101-6 Conditions Associated with Carpal Tunnel Syndrome

Acromegaly
Amyloid
Diabetes mellitus
Hypothyroidism
Pregnancy
Renal failure

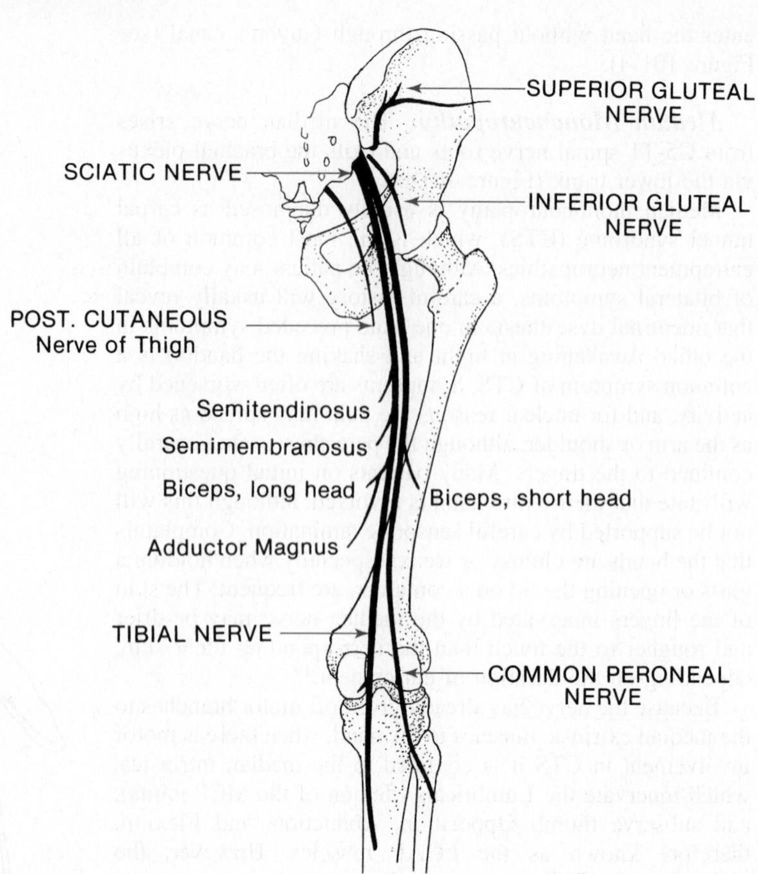

Figure 101-7. **Sciatic nerve, major branches, right leg, posterior view.** *From Stewart JD:* **Focal peripheral neuropathies,** *ed 3, Philadelphia, 2000, Lippincott Williams* **&** *Wilkins.*

median nerve, one should forego injection of the carpal tunnel with steroids in the ED. The physician to whom the patient is referred can decide after NCS whether to recommend splinting, injection, or surgical division of the transverse carpal ligament. Whether this procedure should be performed in the traditional open fashion or through the endoscope is not yet established.[24]

Sciatic Mononeuropathy The sciatic nerve includes L4-S3 spinal nerve roots that pass through the lumbosacral plexus and divide into two terminal branches: the common peroneal and tibial nerves. As shown in Figure 101-7, the nerve exits the pelvis via the sciatic notch, passes behind the hip, and remains deep in the thigh until its terminal bifurcation in the proximal popliteal fossa.

Lesions of the sciatic nerve occur with posterior hip dislocation or with virtually any form of penetrating or blunt trauma that causes formation of a buttock hematoma. Other causes include deep gluteal injection and prolonged supine immobilization on a firm surface. Because the sciatic nerve innervates the hamstrings and provides all sensorimotor function distal to the knee, a complete sciatic mononeuropathy is a devastating injury. Ambulation is extremely difficult because of inability to flex the knee and a flail foot (i.e., neither flexion nor extension is possible at the ankle). Fortunately, many sciatic mononeuropathies are incomplete. For unknown reasons, a partial lesion typically involves only the trunk of the sciatic nerve, which subsequently becomes the common peroneal nerve, sometimes making the two difficult to distinguish from one another clinically. On electrophysiologic studies, evidence of involvement of gluteal muscles or of any muscles innervated by the tibial nerve will readily distinguish a partial sciatic mononeuropathy from a lesion of the common peroneal nerve. Treatment of foot drop requires a posterior splint to maintain the ankle at 90 degrees until a brace can be obtained.

Lateral Femoral Cutaneous Mononeuropathy Lateral femoral cutaneous mononeuropathy (meralgia paresthetica) is a common syndrome believed to be caused by injury to this pure sensory nerve as it passes through or over the inguinal ligament, where it may become entrapped or kinked. Along with facial nerve neuropathy, meralgia paresthetica is one of the most commonly reported mononeuropathies associated with human immunodeficiency virus (HIV).[25] External pressure and obesity may also contribute to nerve injury, causing numbness, dysesthesia, and hyperpathia over the skin of the upper lateral thigh. Regression usually occurs spontaneously, but recurrence is common and may require a release procedure of the inguinal ligament.

Common Peroneal Mononeuropathy The common peroneal nerve is a continuation of one trunk of the sciatic nerve. It is most vulnerable to injury where it winds around the fibular neck (Figure 101-8). It then passes through the fibular canal and bifurcates into its terminal branches, the superficial and deep peroneal nerves. The superficial peroneal nerve innervates the peroneal muscles (foot everters) and supplies sensation to the lateral, distal lower leg and dorsum of the foot. The deep peroneal nerve traverses the anterior compartment and supplies innervation to the dorsiflexors of

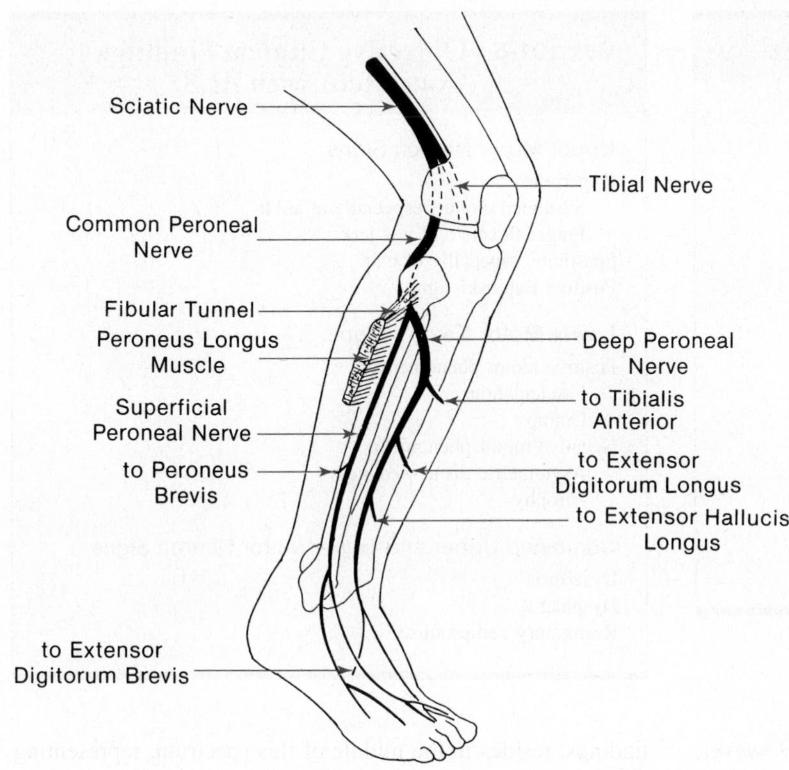

Figure 101-8. **Common peroneal nerve, major branches, right leg, anterolateral view.** *From Stewart JD: Focal peripheral neuropathies, ed 3, Philadelphia, 2000, Lippincott Williams & Wilkins.*

the foot and toes, plus cutaneous sensation between the first and second toes.

Most common peroneal mononeuropathies are idiopathic and are thought to be related to compression where the nerve is superficially located lateral to the fibular neck. Because this common neuropathy is often noted on awakening, it is thought to be secondary to position during sleep. Leg-crossing may also be a risk factor for development of this mononeuropathy. The most striking feature of a complete common peroneal mononeuropathy is foot drop caused by weakness of foot dorsiflexion. At testing, the everters of the foot are also weak, but the inverters, which are innervated by the tibial nerve, remain strong. This may be the single most reliable feature distinguishing sciatic from common peroneal mononeuropathy. Analogous to radial mononeuropathy in the upper extremity, sensory abnormalities in the leg and foot are inconstant and easily overlooked in peroneal mononeuropathy. Most patients with peroneal palsy will recover. Those who do not should be studied electrophysiologically to ensure that the point of compression is not proximal to the fibular neck (i.e., in the popliteal fossa). If the point of peroneal injury appears to be in the region of, or distal to, the fibular neck on EMG, patients whose foot drop does not resolve should be considered candidates for exploration to determine whether the nerve is compressed within the fibular canal.

Treatment of common peroneal palsy may require a posterior splint to maintain the ankle at 90 degrees until the nerve regenerates. This will prevent the foot from falling into sustained equinus (plantar flexion), which in turn allows the intermalleolar distance to narrow, effectively locking the talus out of the ankle mortice.

The treatment of isolated mononeuropathies depends on their etiology, location, and natural history of spontaneous recovery. All penetrating neuropathies should have surgical exploration and repair performed. Blunt trauma may cause a mononeuropathy indirectly by entrapment of a nerve within a fracture, hematoma, or compartment, requiring surgical intervention. Alternatively, nerves may be injured at a point where they are superficial, either by a single direct blow or by sustained pressure caused by immobility (pressure palsies). Most of these will resolve spontaneously over time, depending on the severity of injury and length of the nerve. If entrapment can be confirmed by imaging or electrophysiologic studies, a release procedure is indicated. Many mononeuropathies, ranging from sciatic to CTS, can be identified by MRI. In many instances, when there is disagreement between clinical and EMG findings, MRI may be helpful in selecting patients for exploration by visualizing entrapment or traction.[23,26] Characteristic sonographic findings have also been recently reported in several mononeuropathies.[27]

Of the mononeuropathies that do not require timely surgical exploration, virtually all of the remainder should be referred for electrophysiologic studies and MRI to confirm the location of the neuropathic lesion causing the symptoms.

Type 5: Mononeuropathy Multiplex

Mononeuropathy multiplex (Box 101-7) is characterized by an asymmetric, sensorimotor, usually distal pattern of peripheral neuropathy. Similar to isolated mononeuropathies, sensory abnormalities tend to be located in the same general anatomic region as the accompanying motor findings. Whether DTRs are affected depends on which nerves are involved in the mononeuropathy multiplex. For example, if the process includes the femoral nerve, the knee jerk is likely to be diminished or absent.

Vasculitis Mononeuropathy multiplex is most strongly associated with vasculitis, which is the most common

Box 101-7 Mononeuropathy Multiplex

- Vasculitis
  - Systemic vasculitis
    - Polyarteritis nodosa
    - Rheumatoid arthritis
    - Systemic lupus erythematosus
    - Sjögren's syndrome (keratoconjunctivitis sicca)
  - Nonsystemic vasculitis
- Diabetes mellitus
- Neoplastic
  - Paraneoplastic
  - Direct infiltration
- Infectious
  - Lyme disease
  - HIV
- Sarcoid
- Toxic (lead)
- Transient (polycythemia vera)
- Cryoglobulinemia (hepatitis C)

Box 101-8 Objective Clinical Findings Consistent with ALS

Upper Motor Neuron Signs

- Hyperreflexia
  - Sustained clonus, especially at ankle
  - Finger flexors and jaw jerk
- Spasticity, especially of gait
- Positive Babinski sign

Lower Motor Neuron Signs

- Positive motor phenomena
  - Fasciculations
  - Cramps
- Negative motor phenomena
  - Asymmetric distal weakness
  - Atrophy

Combined Upper and Lower Motor Neuron Signs

- Dysarthria
- Dysphagia
- Respiratory compromise

indication for sural nerve biopsy in most series. However, because diabetes mellitus is far more prevalent than is vasculitis, the most common cause of mononeuropathy multiplex among ED patients is likely to be diabetes.

Diabetes Mellitus Although the role of ischemia in diabetic neuropathies is controversial, evidence for a vascular cause is stronger in the asymmetric diabetic multiple mononeuropathies than in the more common distal, symmetric, predominantly sensory diabetic polyneuropathy (DSPN) seen in a Type 2 peripheral neuropathy. In the treatment of proximal diabetic neuropathy, small uncontrolled trials using immunoglobulin and immunosuppressive therapy have shown improvement in pain, weakness, and gait.[28]

Lyme Disease Peripheral neuropathy occurs in both the early and late stages of Lyme disease. Early in the course of the infection, symptoms usually begin with a radiculitis, extending distally in some patients to produce sensorimotor findings consistent with a mononeuritis multiplex. Inflammation is maximal around spinal and cranial nerve roots, with axonopathic changes predominating over demyelination. Cranial mononeuropathies and a CSF pleocytosis are common at this stage, and the role of antibiotics is unclear. Spontaneous resolution occurs slowly, over weeks to months.[29] In late Lyme disease, the peripheral neuropathy may conform to a distal sensorimotor distribution, radiculopathy, or less commonly, to a mononeuropathy multiplex.

Type 6: Amyotrophic Lateral Sclerosis

Although amyotrophic lateral sclerosis (ALS) and motor neuron disease (MND) are often used synonymously, the latter represents a spectrum of diseases ranging from primary lateral sclerosis (PLS), in which degeneration is confined to upper motor neurons, to progressive muscle atrophy (PMA), in which only lower motor neurons are involved. ALS, which requires the presence of both upper and lower motor neuron findings, resides in the middle of this spectrum, representing the most common form of MND.

In ALS, the primary pathologic process in the PNS component of the disease is a neuronopathy of the anterior horn cell. Because this structure is located proximal to the point where motor and sensory fibers merge to form mixed spinal nerve roots, the signs and symptoms of MND are purely motor (see Figure 101-2). In the CNS, there is loss of Betz cells from the motor cortex with secondary degeneration of the corticospinal tracts. Box 101-8 lists some representative upper, lower, and mixed motor signs. Patients typically demonstrate asymmetric distal weakness without sensory findings. Positive motor phenomena in the form of fasciculations are found in almost all patients at diagnosis, but are rarely an initial complaint. Although there is electrophysiologic evidence of autonomic involvement in ALS, this is generally subclinical.

Most patients with an asymmetric, distal, pure motor neuropathy will have ALS, for which only supportive treatment is available. All patients coming to the ED in whom this diagnosis is suspected should be referred for electrophysiologic confirmation against standardized criteria.[30] This is particularly important because multifocal motor neuropathy, a rare disease that masquerades as ALS, responds dramatically to cyclophosphamide and immunoglobulin administration.[31]

Type 7: Sensory Neuronopathy (Ganglionopathy)

This category of peripheral neuropathy is characterized by a selective or predominant involvement of the dorsal root ganglion, producing a relatively pure sensory syndrome analogous to the pure motor syndrome of ALS discussed above. Although all sensory modalities are affected, proprioception is profoundly altered, leading to sensory ataxia and loss of DTRs without weakness. The distribution is typically asymmetric and distal at the outset, but depending on severity and extent of progression, it may become functionally

Box 101-9 Sensory Neuronopathies (Ganglionopathies)

Herpes
- Herpes simplex I and II
- Varicella zoster (shingles)

Inflammatory sensory polyganglionopathy (ISP)
Paraneoplastic
Primary biliary cirrhosis
Sjögren's syndrome (keratoconjunctivitis sicca)
Toxin induced
- Pyridoxine (vitamin B_6) overdose
- Metals
  - Platinum (cisplatin)
  - Methyl mercury

Vitamin E deficiency

symmetric. Sensory ganglionopathies can now be confirmed by MRI of the spinal cord and surrounding areas, showing degeneration of central sensory projections and localizing the disease process to the dorsal root ganglion.[32]

Some of the more common causes of this type of peripheral neuropathy are listed in Box 101-9.

ANCILLARY DIAGNOSTIC TESTING

Relatively few blood tests contribute to the diagnosis of peripheral neuropathy, and only a small number of these are available in the ED. Ancillary tests that may be indicated in patients referred for evaluation are listed in Box 101-10, along with others that may be ordered selectively, depending on the clinical picture. Expensive batteries of tests purporting to measure a wide variety of antibodies to components of peripheral neuropathies are commercially available, but have not been shown to be useful as screening tests.[33]

Box 101-10 Ancillary Diagnostic Testing in Suspected Peripheral Neuropathy

Obtained in Most Patients

Complete blood count (CBC) with MCV and red cell diameter width (RDW)
Erythrocyte sedimentation rate (ESR)
Glucose
Creatine kinase (CK)
Creatinine

Obtained Only if Indicated

Human chorionic gonadotropin (HCG)
Magnesium
Phosphate
Vitamin B_{12}
Hemoglobin A_{1c}
Serum protein electrophoresis (SPEP) with immune fixation electrophoresis (IFE)
VDRL or RPR screen with fluorescent treponemal antibody-absorption (FTA-ABS) test, as appropriate
Thyroid function
HIV
Rheumatoid factor and antinuclear antibody
Blood, urine, hair, or nails for metal, depending on suspected chronicity of exposure
Specific serum antibodies to components of PNS
CSF for cells, protein
Electrodiagnostic testing
- Nerve conduction studies
- Electromyography

Neurodiagnostic imaging
- MRI
- CT
- Sonography

Quantitative sensory testing
Nerve biopsy (usually sural nerve)

KEY CONCEPTS

- Although peripheral neuropathies only rarely cause respiratory compromise, GBS is by far the most common peripheral neuropathic cause of respiratory arrest.
- Any patient with symmetric weakness, distributed both proximally and distally, with loss or diminution of DTRs and variable sensory abnormalities, should be managed as GBS.
- Once GBS and the other causes of weakness listed in Box 101-1 have been excluded, diseases that place respiratory function at risk have been removed from the differential diagnosis. This effectively eliminates the short-term mortality from peripheral neuropathy.
- In the ED, it will not usually be possible to arrive at the diagnosis of a specific peripheral neuropathy because of the need for confirmatory ancillary testing that is beyond the scope of emergency practice. Rather, the focus should be on identifying one of seven categorical pattern types of peripheral neuropathy shown in Figure 101-1 and listed in Table 101-1.
- One of these seven pattern types can usually be identified by combining three clinical features that are readily obtainable from a goal-directed history and physical: (1) the symmetry or asymmetry of the distribution of findings, (2) their proximal-distal location, and (3) the sensorimotor modalities affected. This approach is summarized as an algorithm in Figure 101-1.
- Identification of one of the seven types of peripheral neuropathy will determine the need for ancillary diagnostic testing, therapeutic intervention, disposition, and the timing of neurologic referral.

REFERENCES

1. Pascuzzi RM, Fleck JD: Acute peripheral neuropathy in adults: Guillain-Barré syndrome and related disorders, *Neurol Clin* 15:529, 1997.
2. Latov N et al: Diabetic neuropathy, *Interdisciplinary Medicine* 4:1, 1999.
3. Centers for Disease Control and Prevention: Lower extremity amputations among persons with diabetes mellitus—Washington, 1988, *MMWR* 40:737, 1991.
4. Barohn RJ, Saperstein DS: Guillain-Barré syndrome and chronic inflammatory demyelinating polyneuropathy, *Semin Neurol* 18:49, 1998.
5. Byun WM et al: Guillain-Barré syndrome: MR imaging findings of the spine in eight patients, *Radiology* 208:137, 1998.
6. Rees JH, Hughes RAC: *Campylobacter jejuni* and Guillain-Barré syndrome, *Ann Neurol* 35:248, 1994.

7. Hartung HP et al: Immunopathogenesis and treatment of the Guillain-Barré syndrome, Part I, *Muscle Nerve* 18:137, 1995.
8. Hartung HP et al: Immunopathogenesis and treatment of the Guillain-Barré syndrome, Part II, *Muscle Nerve* 18:154, 1995.
9. Plasma Exchange/Sandoglobulin Guillain Barré Syndrome Trial Group: Randomized trial of plasma exchange, intravenous immunoglobulin, and combined treatments in Guillain Barré syndrome, *Lancet* 349:225, 1997.
10. Guillain-Barré Syndrome Steroid Trial Group: Double-blind trial of intravenous methylprednisolone in Guillain-Barré syndrome, *Lancet* 341:586, 1993.
11. Barohn RJ: Approach to peripheral neuropathy and neuronopathy, *Semin Neurol* 18:7, 1998.
12. Low PA et al: Double-blind, placebo-controlled study of the application of capsaicin cream in chronic distal painful polyneuropathy, *Pain* 62:163, 1995.
13. Donaghy M et al: Surgery for suspected neurogenic thoracic outlet syndromes: a follow up study, *J Neurol Neurosurg Psychiatry* 67:602, 1999.
14. Lee GW et al: Documentation of brachial plexus compression in the thoracic inlet with quantitative sensory testing, *J Reconstr Microsurg* 16:15, 2000.
15. Roos DB: Historical perspectives and anatomic considerations: thoracic outlet syndrome, *Semin Thorac Cardiovasc Surg* 8:183, 1996.
16. Cheng SW et al: Neurogenic thoracic outlet decompression: rationale for sparing the first rib, *Cardiovasc Surg* 3:617, 1995.
17. England JD: Entrapment neuropathies, *Curr Opin Neurol* 12:597, 1999.
18. Vinik AI: Diabetic neuropathy: pathogenesis and therapy, *Am J Med* 107:17S, 1999.
19. Padua L et al: Multiperspective assessment of carpal tunnel syndrome: a multicenter study. Italian CTS Study Group, *Neurology* 53:1654, 1999.
20. Szabo RM et al: The value of diagnostic testing in carpal tunnel syndrome, *J Hand Surg [Am]* 24:704, 1999.
21. Kuhlman KA, Hennessey WJ: Sensitivity and specificity of carpal tunnel syndrome signs, *Am J Phys Med Rehabil* 76:451, 1997.
22. De Smet L et al: Value of clinical provocative tests in carpal tunnel syndrome, *Acta Orthop Belg* 61:177, 1995.
23. Andre V et al: Clinical, electrophysiological and MRI correlations in carpal tunnel syndrome, *J Radiol* 80:721, 1999.
24. Vasen AP et al: Open versus endoscopic carpal tunnel release: a decision analysis, *J Hand Surg [Am]* 24:1109, 1999.
25. Fuller GN et al: Nature and incidence of peripheral nerve syndromes in HIV infection, *J Neurol Neurosurg Psychiatry* 56:372, 1993.
26. Sawaya RA: Idiopathic sciatic mononeuropathy, *Clin Neurol Neurosurg* 101:256, 1999.
27. Hide IG et al: Sonographic findings in the anterior interosseus nerve syndrome, *J Clin Ultrasound* 27:459, 1999.
28. Younger DS et al: Diabetic peripheral neuropathy: A clinicopathologic and immunohistochemical analysis of sural nerve biopsies, *Muscle Nerve* 19:722, 1996.
29. Duray PH, Steere AC: Clinical pathologic correlation of Lyme disease by stage, *Ann N Y Acad Sci* 539:65, 1988.
30. Subcommittee on Motor Neuron Diseases/Amyotrophic Lateral Sclerosis of the World Federation of Neurology Research Group on Neuromuscular Diseases and the El Escorial "Clinical Limits of Amyotrophic Lateral Sclerosis" workshop contributors: El Escorial World Federation of Neurology criteria for the diagnosis of amyotrophic lateral sclerosis, *J Neurol Sci* 124(Suppl):96, 1994.
31. Chaudhry V: Multifocal motor neuropathy, *Semin Neurol* 18:73, 1998.
32. Lauria G et al: Clinical and magnetic resonance imaging findings in chronic sensory ganglionopathies, *Ann Neurol* 47:104, 2000.
33. Chalk CH: Acquired peripheral neuropathy, *Neurol Clin* 15:501, 1997.

102 Neuromuscular Disorders

Peter Shearer
Andy Jagoda

PERSPECTIVE

Disorders of the neuromuscular unit can cause dramatic clinical pictures, including acute respiratory failure, although they more often have subtle symptoms. Morbidity and mortality are often related to failure of the muscles that maintain airway integrity and drive respiration. In most cases, the pathophysiology of these disorders is well understood and permits for an organization and understanding that is based on the level of the nervous system affected. This facilitates an approach that is based on signs and symptoms, the findings of which direct the urgency of diagnostic testing and treatment.

Processes involving the brainstem and brain can usually be differentiated from those in the spinal cord and in the peripheral nervous system (PNS) based on historical and physical findings. In general, lesions at the level of the brainstem or above produce unilateral weakness; bilateral weakness caused by lesions above the spinal cord is generally associated with a change in mental status or cranial nerve involvement. Lesions of the central nervous system (CNS) result in upper motor neuron signs that include spasticity, hyperreflexia, and extensor plantar reflexes. As a corollary, when bilateral upper motor neuron signs are found in conjunction with normal mental status, diagnostic testing including neuroimaging should focus on looking for a lesion in the spinal cord.

PRINCIPLES OF DISEASE

The neuromuscular unit is divided into four components: the anterior horn cells of the spinal cord, the peripheral nerve, the neuromuscular junction, and the muscle being innervated. The level of the pathology determines associated signs and symptoms (Table 102-1). *Myelopathies* are processes involving the spinal cord. *Radiculopathies* are processes involving the nerve roots as they leave the spinal cord. *Neuropathies* involve the peripheral nerves, and *myopathies* are processes involving the muscles.

Neuropathies involve the axon itself or the myelin sheath (or the Schwann cells that make the myelin sheath) of the nerve. Nerve conduction studies can differentiate the locations of involvement. As the conduction along the axon is disrupted, the subsequent delay in transmission will first cause symptoms in those muscles controlled by longer nerve

Table 102-1. Clinical Characteristics of Neuromuscular Diseases

	History	Strength	DTR	Sensation	Wasting
Myelopathy	Trauma, infection, cancer	Normal to decreased	Increased	Normal to decreased	No
Motor neuron disease (ALS)	Progressive difficulty swallowing, speaking, walking	Decreased	Increased	Normal	Yes
Neuropathy	Recent infection Ascending weakness	Normal or decreased Distal > proximal	Decreased	Decreased	Yes
Neuromuscular junction disease	Food (canned goods) Tick exposure Easy fatigability	Normal to fatigue	Normal	Normal	No
Myopathy	Thyroid disease Previous similar episodes	Decreased Proximal > distal	Normal	Normal	Yes

axons, resulting in a history of weakness beginning in the distal extremities. As the myelin destruction or axonal degeneration progresses, patients will usually note a slowly progressive course of symptoms.

The motor nerve branches into multiple terminals as it approaches the muscle. The neuromuscular junction is composed of the presynaptic membrane, the postsynaptic membrane, and the synaptic cleft. The neurotransmitter is acetylcholine (ACh). The motor synapse is a nicotinic receptor, whereas muscarinic synapses link the CNS with the autonomic nervous system. Disorders of the postsynaptic nicotinic receptors produce weakness. Postsynaptic ACh receptors are continually turned over at a rate that is related to the amount of stimulation. A disorder of transmission often leads to increased production of ACh receptors. Myasthenia gravis (MG) is the prototype of neuromuscular junction diseases.

CLINICAL FINDINGS

History

The history in patients with complaints of weakness initially focuses on establishing the acuity of onset and the potential for airway compromise. Any complaint of difficulty breathing or swallowing raises suspicion for bulbar involvement and concern for life-threatening deterioration. The history must elicit whether the weakness is muscular or nonspecific generalized fatigue. Weakness implies the inability to exert normal force, whereas fatigue implies a decrease in force with repetitive use. When muscular weakness exists, the clinician should determine whether it is focal or generalized, proximal or distal. The history of the present illness must include the duration of symptoms, exacerbating and mitigating factors, and presence of associated symptoms such as fever, weight loss, and bowel or bladder changes.

The patient should be asked about the presence of a preexisting neuromuscular disorder; an acute exacerbation or end-stage degeneration of some genetic muscular dystrophies and MG may be the cause of the current difficulty. Prior episodes or a family history of weakness suggest the familial thyrotoxic forms of the periodic paralyses. A history of a recent illness (often respiratory or diarrheal) supports a diagnosis of the autoimmune causes of weakness such as transverse myelitis. Past history or risk factors for cancer may indicate a metastatic tumor as the cause of a compressive myelopathy. Questions about recent travel can help exclude tick or snake bites, or dietary history may elicit shellfish toxin ingestion or the ingestion of canned goods suggesting botulism.

Box 102-1 Grading Score for Motor Strength

5 = Normal strength
4 = Weak but able to resist examiner
3 = Moves against gravity but unable to resist examiner
2 = Moves but unable to resist gravity
1 = Flicker but no movement
0 = No movement

Physical Examination

The physical examination should first assess the patient's airway and ventilation, and then proceed to localize the level of the lesion. The presence of swallowing and a strong cough suggest that the patient has sufficient protective and ventilatory reserve. More formal bedside spirometric testing is used to establish the ventilatory baseline and provides objective data that can be followed over time. A forced vital capacity of less than 15 ml/kg or a maximal negative inspiratory force of less than 15 mm Hg suggests the need for endotracheal intubation.

The assessment of the vital signs is important because some causes of weakness may result in dysregulation of the autonomic system. A systematic neurologic examination should assess the patient's mental status, cranial nerves, motor function, sensory function, deep tendon reflexes (DTRs), and coordination, including cerebellar function. The motor examination begins by determining whether the weakness is unilateral or bilateral, and which muscle groups are involved. Key components of the examination include motor strength, muscle bulk, and presence of fasciculations. Box 102-1 provides the grading system used in motor strength assessment. Table 102-2 provides the findings used to distinguish upper motor neuron from lower motor neuron processes.

Table 102-2. Distinguishing Upper Motor Neuron (UMN) from Lower Motor Neuron (LMN) Involvement

	DTR*	Muscle tone	Atrophy	Fasciculations	Babinski
UMN	Increased	Increased	No†	No	Present
LMN	Decreased	Decreased	Yes	Yes	Absent

*Deep tendon reflex.
†Not significant, but can occur.

Differential Considerations

Myelopathies A myelopathy will show signs of upper motor neuron dysfunction. Without upper motor neuron function, dominant spinal reflexes produce muscle weakness with increased reflexes, including an extensor plantar reflex (Babinski response). The same reflex arcs will eventually create spasticity in the affected muscles. The weakness will be ascending in nature, and there is often bladder and bowel involvement. When sensory findings are present they often define the distinct level of the lesion.

Motor Neuron Disease Amyotrophic lateral sclerosis (ALS) is the prototypical disease process resulting from a degeneration of the motor neuron without sensory involvement. These patients may complain of dysarthria or dysphagia; however, the characteristic findings are those of combined upper and lower motor neuron dysfunction. Consequently, findings include hyperreflexia, muscle wasting, and fasciculation. Pain is not a component of the clinical picture.

Poliomyelitis affects the anterior horn cells and results in lower motor neuron disease without sensory involvement. The weakness can be symmetric or more often asymmetric. Patients will initially have a clinical picture similar to viral meningitis, with fever and neck stiffness. Currently, most cases follow exposure of an immunocompromised host to the oral polio vaccine, so this should be sought in the history. The cerebrospinal fluid (CSF) analysis resembles that of viral meningitis.

Neuropathies Weakness from a neuropathy will most often be noted in distal muscles first. Depending on the duration of the symptoms, muscle tone and bulk may or may not be affected. As all neurologic outflow from the spinal cord is affected, DTRs are diminished or absent and patients exhibit varying degrees of decreased sensation, muscle wasting, and fasciculation.

Diseases of the Neuromuscular Junction Disorders of the neuromuscular junction cause progressive motor fatigability. The initial depolarization of the muscle causes stimulation of a maximum number of receptors, producing a normal, or nearly normal, strength response. Repeated stimulation leads to diminishing motor strength. This is caused by blockage of the receptors (as in MG) or by a decrease in the amount of ACh released (as in botulism). A decrease in the release of ACh may produce a combination of nicotinic and muscarinic effects leading to anticholinergic findings such as decreased visual acuity, confusion, or urinary retention. In the case of Lambert-Eaton myasthenic syndrome, weakness will be more pronounced at the beginning of muscle use and will improve with repeated use as more ACh builds up in the synaptic cleft with each stimulation. Anticholinergic signs may be present with tachycardia and low-grade fever; dry, flushed skin; and urinary retention.

Myopathies These disorders will usually produce generalized, symmetric weakness. Reflexes are present but markedly decreased, whereas sensation is preserved. Myopathies caused by inflammatory processes may cause muscle tenderness and, over time, some wasting may occur as a result of disuse.

DIAGNOSTIC STRATEGIES

Laboratory Studies

Serum potassium, calcium, and phosphorus should be assessed in patients with acute weakness. Thyroid function tests are recommended in cases of suspected myopathies. A creatine kinase (CK) level will assess for muscular inflammation or rhabdomyolysis. A urinalysis should be performed for the presence of myoglobinuria (positive urine dipstick for blood with no red blood cells seen on microscopy).

Special Studies

Magnetic resonance imaging (MRI) is the preferred test for suspected cases of acute myelopathy. Computed tomography (CT) of the spinal cord with myelography can help to differentiate compressive (herniation, abscess, tumor) from noncompressive causes when an MRI is not available. CSF analysis has limited use in the evaluation of weakness. It is indicated when Guillain-Barré syndrome (GBS) or transverse myelitis is suspected.

SPECIFIC DISORDERS

Disorders of the Neuromuscular Junction

Myasthenia Gravis

Perspective It is rare for the emergency physician to diagnose a new case of MG; more commonly, patients with established disease come to the ED with an exacerbation. In addition, the emergency physician must be cognizant of medication interactions in patients with MG.

Principles of Disease MG has a prevalence of 50 to 125 per million.[1] Age of onset is bimodal, with the first peak in the 20s and 30s, when it affects women more often than men, and a second peak in the sixth and seventh decades, when it affects men more often than women.

MG results from autoantibodies directed against the nicotinic acetylcholine receptor (AChR) at the neuromuscular junction. This leads to complement-mediated destruction of AChRs with a decrease in the total number of available receptors. The autoantibodies further compete with ACh for binding at remaining receptors. Thus with repeated stimulation of the same muscle, fewer and fewer sites are available and fatigue develops.

Muscular weakness and fatigability are the hallmarks of MG. The initial clinical picture often consists of a mononeuropathy involving the ocular or bulbar muscles. Considering the slow clinical progression of MG and the very low likelihood of complications from its progression, the importance of suspecting the diagnosis is to facilitate proper referral for further evaluation.

Clinical Features Ocular symptoms are often the first manifestation of MG. The typical symptoms are ptosis, diplopia, or blurred vision. Ocular muscle weakness may be the first sign in up to 40% of patients, although 85% of patients with MG will eventually have ocular involvement. When present, ptosis is often worse toward the end of the day. Respiratory failure is rarely the initial symptom of MG. Even so, up to 17% of patients may have weakness of the muscles of respiration.[2] Bulbar muscles may be involved, producing dysarthria or dysphagia.

The Lambert-Eaton myasthenic syndrome is a rare disorder often associated with small-cell carcinoma of the lung. Autoantibodies cause an inadequate release of ACh from nerve terminals, affecting both nicotinic and muscarinic receptors. With repeated stimulation the amount of ACh in the synaptic cleft increases, leading to an increase in strength, the opposite of that seen with MG. The classic syndrome includes weakness that increases with use of muscles, hyporeflexia, and autonomic dysregulation. Management primarily focuses on treating the underlying neoplastic disorder, although plasmapheresis and immunoglobulin G (IgG) have been reported to be useful.[3]

Diagnostic Strategies

New-onset MG The diagnosis of MG is based on clinical findings and a combination of serologic testing, the edrophonium test, and electromyographic testing. The first two tests are not usually done in the ED, although serum can be sent for ACh-receptor antibody testing. Results are positive in 80% to 90% of patients with MG. Many patients who are seronegative will still respond to traditional therapy aimed at lowering levels of circulating antibodies, suggesting that antibodies are present but not detected.[1]

The edrophonium (Tensilon) test is a simple, pharmacologic test that can be performed safely at the patient's bedside. It should be noted that the sensitivity and specificity of the test have not been well documented, and there are reports of false positives in cases of botulism and in cases of MG occurring concurrently with other disorders. The test is performed by measuring the distance from the upper to the lower eyelid in the most severely affected eye before and after the intravenous administration of the short-acting AChE blocking agent edrophonium. Because some patients have a severe reaction to edrophonium, an intravenous test dose of 1 to 2 mg is given first. If no adverse reaction is found, and the patient does not dramatically improve in 30 to 90 seconds, a second dose of 3 mg is given. If there is still no response, a final dose of 5 mg is given for a total maximum dosage of 10 mg.[4]

Because of potential bradycardia from edrophonium, atropine should be available at the bedside. Also, because of the potential cholinergic effect of increased airway secretions, this test should be used with caution in asthmatics and patients with COPD.

Another bedside test that can be performed is the ice test.

Box 102-2 Drugs that May Exacerbate MG

Cardiovascular

β-Blockers
Calcium channel blockers
Quinidine
Lidocaine
Procainamide

Antibiotics

Aminoglycosides
Tetracyclines
Clindamycin
Lincomycin
Polymyxin B
Colistin

Other

Phenytoin
Neuromuscular blockers
Corticosteroids
Thyroid replacement

This is based on the observation that cooling decreases symptoms in MG[5] and heat exacerbates symptoms.[6] In a patient with ptosis who is suspected of having MG, the distance between the upper and lower lids is measured (similar to the edrophonium test). An ice pack is then applied to the affected eye for approximately 2 minutes, and then the distance between lids is measured again. A prospective evaluation of this approach that compared patients with MG to patients without MG found the test to be positive (an improvement in distance of at least 2 mm) in 80% of patients with MG and in no patients without MG.[7]

Acute myasthenic crisis An acute myasthenic crisis is defined as respiratory failure leading to mechanical ventilation.[8] It occurs in 15% to 20% of patients with MG,[9,10] usually within the first 2 years of disease onset. Although potentially life-threatening, the mortality from this complication of MG has declined from 40% to 5% since the 1960s with the use of better and more aggressive intensive care unit (ICU) techniques.

Underlying infection, aspiration, and changes in medications most often set off crisis, but the precipitant may not be found in up to 30% of cases.[11] Some patients experience a severe increase in weakness on starting steroids for chronic therapy. Other precipitants can be medications, surgery, and pregnancy (Box 102-2).[8]

The initial step in managing the patient in crisis is stabilization of the airway. In less severe cases in which intubation is not imminent, it is imperative to monitor ventilatory status in the ED pending ICU admission. Airway compromise can be detected by various mechanisms. Arterial blood gas is not necessarily helpful, because functional reserve can be severely diminished by the time a patient develops either hypercarbia or hypoxia. A patient who is not yet intubated but is complaining of shortness of breath or difficulty breathing should have frequent vital capacity measurements. Normally these values range from 60 to

70 ml/kg. When the FVC reaches 15 ml/kg, intubation is necessary. An easy bedside assessment used to follow ventilatory status is to have the patient count from 1 to 25 with one breath.[8] With sequential performance of this, a decline in respiratory function will be detected as the patient fails to count as high as before.

It is important to look for signs of myasthenic crisis in any patient with MG who presents to the ED, even with no complaint of weakness. As previously mentioned, many commonly used drugs can adversely affect the treatment of a patient with MG (see Box 102-2). A patient with stable MG who has an acute medical or surgical condition requires a full neurologic exam. The decision to admit or discharge a patient from the ED should take into account the potential for neurologic deterioration in patients with MG.

Management

Cholinesterase inhibitors Pyridostigmine (15 to 60 mg every 4 to 6 hours) and neostigmine (7.5 to 15 mg every 4 to 6 hours) are the backbone of chronic outpatient therapy and provide symptomatic improvement, although they are not directed at the underlying immunologic basis of the disease. This class of drugs inhibits the hydrolysis of ACh, leading to increased circulating ACh to stimulate the decreased number of receptors and to compete with the antibodies for binding sites. The most common side effects are those of excessive cholinergic stimulation, such as increased airway secretions and increased bowel motility. At extremes there may be bradycardia or even worsening of weakness, simulating a myasthenic crisis. These drugs are often used as adjunctive therapy to control symptoms while other therapy is being instituted, after which they are often discontinued.[12]

The use of intravenous pyridostigmine in the setting of acute exacerbation is controversial. In a review of various therapies for myasthenic crisis, pyridostigmine alone or in combination with prednisolone or plasma exchange appeared comparable to plasma exchange alone. The study reported that 11 of the 63 patients treated for MG crisis suffered cardiac arrest, and that 7 of the 10 patients who developed asystole had received pyridostigmine, although there is no evidence that the pyridostigmine was the cause.[12] In addition, some authors report that most patients with crisis have failed AChE inhibition and may benefit from a rest period from AChE inhibitors.[13]

Thus cholinergic drug therapy should be discontinued during crisis once the patient is intubated. In addition, pyridostigmine may complicate mechanical ventilation by increasing the production of pulmonary secretions.

It has been proposed that acute decompensation and excessive muscarinic stimulation can be caused by overmedication with AChE inhibitors. The prevalence and importance of this cholinergic crisis are debated in the literature. Regardless, the physical examination should distinguish a cholinergic crisis from an exacerbation of the disease. The weakness comes from the excessive stimulation of AChRs by the additional ACh, preventing repolarization, and thus no further muscle contractions can be stimulated. Muscarinic effects of AChE inhibition may include excessive sweating, salivation, lacrimation, miosis, tachycardia, or gastrointestinal hyperactivity.

Immunosuppressant drugs Immunosuppressant drugs are often used for the chronic control of MG. Although they have no role in the acute management of a myasthenic crisis, they may be started before extubation of a patient recovering from crisis. Corticosteroids, azathioprine, and cyclosporine have all been used. Of note, the initiation of corticosteroids in patients with moderate to severe weakness may actually precipitate a worsening of weakness.

Thymectomy Although the association between thymoma and MG is still not fully elaborated, it is well known that thymectomy for patients with thymoma can lead to remission of MG or enable a reduction in other medications. More recently, thymectomy in patients with MG but without thymoma has been shown to have similar benefits and is recommended for patients under 60 years old. Thymectomy in patients between adolescence and 60 years of age leads to remission or improvement in up to 50% of cases.[13] The onset of improvement after thymectomy is often delayed for 2 to 5 years.

Immunomodulatory therapy Plasma exchange (plasmapheresis) and intravenous immune globulin (IV Ig) are forms of short-term immunomodulatory therapy. They are used for patients with severe exacerbations or preoperatively in patients with stable MG.

Plasma exchange removes whole blood from the patient, separates the plasma, and replaces it with donor plasma. Most regimens recommend removal of 2 to 3 liters of plasma three times a week until there is a satisfactory improvement in the weakness. Plasma exchange removes the AChR antibodies and other immune complexes from the blood, and the fall in AChR levels is associated with improvement in symptoms of MG. There is a risk of complications from hypotension or anticoagulation. Because of safety concerns, clinical trials in children have not been done. Although there are no randomized controlled studies of the efficacy of plasma exchange, it is an accepted therapy and is recommended by the American Academy of Neurology for acute exacerbations and for preoperative prophylaxis.[14]

Small uncontrolled studies and case reports of IV Ig for patients not responsive to other therapies began to appear in the 1970s. It is difficult to compare these studies because different protocols and preparations have been used. From 50% to 90% of patients treated with IV Ig have some improvement after infusion. Current consensus suggests a dose of 0.4 g/kg/day for 5 days in cases of uncontrolled acute exacerbations.

There are no blind, controlled comparisons of plasma exchange versus IV Ig. One study concludes that IV Ig is as effective as plasma exchange.[15] Another retrospective study comparing the two techniques found that plasma exchange leads to improved ventilatory status at 2 weeks compared to IV Ig, but it has a higher complication rate.[16] The decision to institute either therapy will be based on the input of the consulting neurologist and the resources available at the admitting hospital.

Botulism

Principles of Disease Botulism is a toxin-mediated illness that can cause acute weakness leading to respiratory insufficiency. In 1998 the Centers for Disease Control and Prevention (CDC) reported 116 cases of botulism in the United States, 65 of which were categorized as infantile botulism.[17] *Clostridium botulinum* is an anaerobic, spore-forming bacterium. Three of eight known toxins produced by *Clostridium botulinum* cause human disease. These are toxin types A, B, and E. Although most cases are isolated events associated with improperly preserved canned foods,[18] there has recently been an increase in the incidence of botulism from wound infections. In 1995 and 1996, 42 cases of wound botulism were reported in heroin users who injected subcutaneously.[19]

Toxin type E is associated with preserved or fermented fish and marine mammals. These are the most important sources of botulism in Alaska, Japan, Russia, and Scandinavia.[20] The botulinum toxin works by binding irreversibly to the presynaptic membrane of peripheral and cranial nerves, inhibiting the release of ACh at the peripheral nerve synapse. As new receptors are generated the patient improves.

Clinical Features The toxin blocks both voluntary motor and autonomic functions. Because the disorder is at the neuromuscular junction, there is no sensory deficit and no sense of pain. The onset of symptoms is 6 to 48 hours after the ingestion of tainted food. There may or may not be accompanying signs and symptoms of gastroenteritis, with nausea, vomiting, abdominal cramps, diarrhea, or constipation. The classic feature of botulism is a descending, symmetric paralysis. The muscles often affected first are the cranial nerves and bulbar muscles, and the patient presents with diplopia, dysarthria, and dysphagia, followed later by generalized weakness. There may be associated blurring of the vision. Because the toxin decreases cholinergic output, anticholinergic signs may be seen in the form of constipation, urinary retention, dry skin and eyes, and increased temperature. Pupils are often dilated and not reactive to light. This can be a point of differentiation from MG. DTRs are normal or diminished.

Infantile botulism occurs from the ingestion of *Clostridium botulinum* spores that are able to germinate and produce toxin in the high pH of the gastrointestinal tract of infants. The same spores are not active in the gut of adults because of the lower pH. It occurs in infants between the age of 1 week and 11 months and has been implicated as a cause of sudden infant death syndrome (SIDS). Because spores can survive in honey, it is recommended that it not be fed to infants. The clinical presentation includes constipation, poor feeding, lethargy, and weak cry; consequently, this diagnosis must be in the differential of the floppy infant.[21]

Diagnostic Strategies The diagnosis is made by both clinical findings and exclusion of other processes. The toxin can be identified in serum and stool, but the assay is not commonly available in most hospitals and requires a prolonged turnaround time. If the suspected food source is available, it should also be tested for the toxin.

Management The treatment is initially focused on stabilizing the airway and supportive measures. There is an antitoxin available that can shorten the disease course, although it is not clear that the antitoxin will decrease ventilator dependence. Nevertheless, the antitoxin should be administered as soon as possible. It is made from horse serum, so allergy testing should be performed before administration.

Tick Paralysis

Principles of Disease The pathogenesis of tick paralysis, also known as *tick toxicosis,* is not fully understood. It is known that a toxin is injected while the tick feeds, and it is referred to as an *ixovotoxin.* The toxin appears to diminish the release of ACh at the neuromuscular junction and also reduces nerve conduction velocity. It may also have effects at autonomic ganglia, leading to pupillary signs.

Clinical Features Tick paralysis is an acute, ascending, flaccid motor paralysis that can be confused with GBS, botulism, and MG. It typically begins with the development of an unsteady gait, followed by ascending, symmetric, flaccid paralysis. Although symptoms usually begin 1 to 2 days after the female tick has attached and begun to feed, delays of up to 6 days have been reported.[22] There may be associated ocular signs, such as fixed and dilated pupils, that can help distinguish it from GBS.

Management A tick can be removed using forceps to grasp it as closely as possible to the point of attachment. Care must be taken not to leave mouth parts in the patient's tissue. Although symptoms may resolve rapidly after removal of the tick, supportive measures such as intubation should not be withheld pending expectation of resolution of symptoms. It has been noted that the toxin of the *Ixodes holocyclus* tick in Australia elaborates a toxin that is very similar to botulinum toxin, and that after removal of this tick symptoms may worsen during the succeeding 24 to 48 hours.[23] Recovery in these patients may also be prolonged.

Disorders of the Muscles

Perspective Newly acquired weakness originating at the muscular level can be divided into two types: inflammatory or toxic-metabolic. Inflammatory disorders usually produce pain and tenderness, but metabolic disorders do not.

Inflammatory Disorders

Principles of Disease The most common inflammatory myopathies are polymyositis (PM) and dermatomyositis (DM). PM may be idiopathic in nature, occur secondary to infections (viral or bacterial), or be seen in conjunction with other disorders such as sarcoidosis or hypereosinophilic syndromes. Inflammatory myopathies cause weakness, pain, and tenderness of the muscles involved. This must be distinguished from simple myalgias related to a fever or cramping that may suggest a myotonia (inability to relax the muscle).

Clinical Features DM and PM can occur at any adult age, although DM may also affect children. There is a slightly increased incidence in women. An associated increased risk of malignancy, especially breast, ovary, lung, gastrointestinal, and lymphoproliferative disorders, after the diagnosis of DM or PM has been shown, although the reported rate of malignancy varies widely. Proximal muscle weakness predominates and leads to complaints of difficulty rising from a seated position or climbing stairs, and weakness in lifting the arms over the head. There is often pain and tenderness in these proximal muscles as well. There is a decrease in reflexes as the weakened muscles fail to contract. Thus the decrease in reflexes is in proportion to the decrease in strength. Fasciculations are not seen, and atrophy is a very late finding.

DM is similar to PM, but it also is associated with classic skin findings. These are more prominent in childhood but are also found in adults. They include a periorbital heliotrope, and erythema and swelling of the extensor surfaces of joints. The facial rash is usually photosensitive and may also involve the exposed areas of the chest and neck.

Diagnostic Strategies Electrolyte abnormalities (see below) must be ruled out and a serum CK checked. If available, the skeletal muscle isoform (MM) should be distinguished from the cardiac muscle isoform (MB). The CK must be interpreted along with the entire clinical picture. The presence of an elevated CK does not establish the cause of weakness as a myopathy because some neuropathies can also produce an elevated CK. Similarly a normal CK does not rule out a myopathy as the cause of weakness. Electromyography and muscle biopsy are used to confirm the diagnosis.[24]

Management PM and DM are usually managed with oral prednisone in a dose of 1 to 2 mg/kg day. When steroids prove ineffective, and during acute exacerbations, cytotoxic drugs such as azathioprine or methotrexate are added. Fortunately, the degree of rhabdomyolysis seen with the inflammatory myopathies is not sufficient to cause renal impairment.

Metabolic Disorders

Perspective Acute, generalized muscle weakness can be seen with severe electrolyte abnormalities from any cause: hypokalemia, hyperkalemia, hypocalcemia, hypercalcemia, hypomagnesemia, and hypophosphatemia. Acute painless myopathies can also be seen with endocrine disorders involving the thyroid, parathyroid, or adrenal glands.

Of particular interest are several disorders referred to collectively as the *periodic paralyses.* This group of entities includes familial periodic paralysis (FPP) of the hyperkalemic and hypokalemic forms, and thyrotoxic periodic paralysis (TPP) that is similar to hypokalemic FPP, except that it is associated with hyperthyroidism.

Familial Periodic Paralysis

Principles of disease Patients with FPP experience intermittent attacks of extremity weakness associated with either hyperkalemia or hypokalemia, although the latter is more common. It is most often associated with an inherited genetic mutation.[25] Patients will usually report a personal and family history of similar episodes.

Clinical features and diagnostic strategies Patients may suffer either isolated or recurrent episodes of flaccid paralysis. The lower limbs are involved more often than the upper, although both can be affected. Bulbar, ocular, and respiratory muscles are usually not involved.[26] The onset is very rapid and uncommonly preceded by a prodrome of myalgias and muscle cramps. Both mental status and sensory function are preserved, but reports of sensory nerve involvement have been documented.[27] Males are more often affected than females. There is a much higher incidence in Asians, particularly Japanese, although it occurs in other ethnic groups.

Attacks may be induced by the injection of insulin, epinephrine, or glucose. The onset of symptoms often follows a high carbohydrate intake and often occurs after a period of rest.[28] A typical complaint is the acute onset of weakness noted on waking in the morning after a large meal the preceding evening. An ECG, which should be done immediately in all patients suffering from acute paralysis, will demonstrate signs of hyperkalemia or hypokalemia. A stat potassium level should be ordered; in the hypokalemic form, the potassium level during an attack falls to values below 3.0 mEq/L.

Management Many cases will resolve spontaneously with supportive care alone. The mainstay of management is the treatment of the underlying hyperkalemic or hypokalemic state. In the hypokalemic state the total body potassium is not depleted, but has shifted intracellularly.[29,30] Thus in the repletion of potassium, caution is necessary to prevent overtreatment. For this reason, intravenous potassium should be used sparingly; one or two 10 mEq doses of potassium chloride (KCl), each administered over 1 hour, should be the maximum given intravenously. This can be done in parallel with oral potassium repletion of 40 mEq and frequent testing of serum potassium levels. Intravenous hydration helps to redistribute the body's potassium stores.

Thyrotoxic Periodic Paralysis The clinical picture of TPP is almost identical to that of hypokalemic FPP, and indeed a small number of patients with hypokalemic FPP have hyperthyroidism. In TPP there are often symptoms related to hyperthyroidism present at the same time the patient comes to the ED complaining of weakness. If present, treatment of the hyperthyroid symptoms, such as tachycardia, may help the treatment of the paralysis as well. There is one case report of TPP in which the patient's weakness did not respond to potassium replacement until propranolol was given to treat the tachycardia.[31] There is probably a genetic feature underlying this disorder, because there is a higher incidence of repeated attacks of hypokalemic periodic paralysis among Japanese and Chinese patients with hyperthyroidism.[32] It is important that all patients have thyroid function testing done after a first episode of hypokalemic paralysis.

KEY CONCEPTS

- In patients with bilateral upper motor neuron signs and a normal mental status, neuroimaging of the spinal cord should be strongly considered.
- A forced vital capacity <15 ml/kg or a maximal negative inspiratory force <15 mm Hg is a potential indications for mechanical ventilation.
- Botulism is a painless descending paralysis with no sensory deficits and no significant alteration of consciousness.
- Any complaint of difficulty in breathing or swallowing should heighten suspicion of bulbar involvement with possible airway compromise.

REFERENCES

1. Drachman DB: Myasthenia gravis, *N Engl J Med* 330:1797, 1994.
2. Massey JM: Acquired myasthenia gravis, *Neurol Clin* 15(3):577, 1997.
3. Penn AS: Lambert-Eaton myasthenic syndrome. In Rowland LP, editor: *Merritt's textbook of neurology,* ed 9, Philadelphia, 1995, Williams and Wilkins.
4. Seybold ME: Office tensilon test for ocular myasthenia gravis, *Arch Neurol* 43:842, 1986.
5. Borenstein S, Desmedt JE: Local cooling in myasthenia: improvement of neuromuscular failure, *Arch Neurol* 32:152, 1975.
6. Gutmann L: Heat-induced myasthenic crisis, *Arch Neurol* 37:271, 1980.
7. Golnik KC et al: An ice test for the diagnosis of myasthenia gravis, *Ophthalmology* 106:1282, 1999.
8. Thomas CE: Clinical features, mortality, complications and risk factors for prolonged intubation, *Neurol* 48:1253, 1997.
9. Fink ME: Treatment of the critically ill patient with myasthenia gravis. In Ropper AH, editor: *Neurological and neurosurgical intensive care,* ed 3, New York, 1993, Raven Press.
10. Cohen MS, Younger D: Aspects of the natural history of myasthenia gravis: crisis and death, *Ann N Y Acad Sci* 377:670, 1981.
11. Mayer SA: Intensive care of the myasthenic patient, *Neurology* 48(Suppl 5):S70, 1997.
12. Berrouschot J et al: Therapy of myasthenic crisis, *Crit Care Med* 25:1228, 1997.
13. Mayer SA: Therapy of myasthenic crisis (letter), *Crit Care Med* 26:1136, 1998.

14. Assessment of plasmapheresis. Report of the Therapeutics and Technology Assessment Subcommittee of the American Academy of Neurology, *Neurology* 47:840, 1996.
15. Gajdos PH et al: Clinical trial of plasma exchange and high-dose intravenous immunoglobulin in myasthenia gravis, *Ann Neurol* 41:789, 1997.
16. Quershi AI et al: Plasma exchange versus intravenous immunoglobulin treatment in myasthenic crisis, *Neurology* 52:629, 1999.
17. Summary of Notifiable Diseases, United States, 1998, *MMWR* 47:1, 1999.
18. Shapiro RL et al: Botulism in the United States: a clinical and epidemiologic review, *Ann Int Med* 129:221, 1998.
19. Passaro D et al: Wound botulism associated with black tar heroin among injecting drug users, *JAMA* 279:859, 1998.
20. Mines D et al: Poisonings: food, fish, shellfish, *Emerg Med Clin North Am* 15:58, 1997.
21. Jagoda A, Renner G: Infant botulism: case report and clinical update, *Am J Emerg Med* 8:318, 1990.
22. Tick paralysis—Washington, 1995, *MMWR* 45:325, 1996.
23. Felz MW et al: A six-year-old girl with tick paralysis, *N Engl J Med* 342:90, 2000.
24. Bartt R: Autoimmune and inflammatory disorders. In Goetz CG, editor: *Goetz textbook of clinical neurology,* Philadelphia, 1999, WB Saunders.
25. Rowland LP: Familial periodic paralyses. In Rowland LP, editor: *Merritt's textbook of neurology,* ed 9, Philadelphia, 1995, Williams and Wilkins.
26. Ober KP: Thyrotoxic periodic paralysis in the United States: report of 7 cases and review of the literature, *Medicine* 71:109, 1992.
27. Inshasi J: Dysfunction of sensory nerves during attacks of hypokalemic periodic paralysis, *Neuromuscul Disord* 9:227, 1999.
28. Miller D et al: Severe hypokalemia in thyrotoxic periodic paralysis, *Am J Emerg Med* 7:584, 1989.
29. Cannon L et al: Hypokalemic periodic paralysis, *J Emerg Med* 4:287, 1986.
30. Miller JD et al: Nonfamilial hypokalemic periodic paralysis and thyrotoxicosis in a 16-year-old male, *Pediatrics* 100:413, 1997.
31. Shayne P, Hart A: Thyrotoxic periodic paralysis terminated with intravenous propranolol, *Ann Emerg Med* 24:734, 1994.
32. Rowland LP: Familial periodic paralysis. In Rowland LP, editor: *Merritt's textbook of neurology,* ed 9, Philadelphia, 1995, Williams and Wilkins.

103 Central Nervous System Infections

Frank W. Lavoie
John R. Saucier

PERSPECTIVE

Background

Central nervous system (CNS) infections have always been among the most perplexing and devastating illnesses. "Epidemic cerebrospinal fever," classically described by Viesseux in 1805, was associated with almost universal mortality.[1] Since that time, epidemiologic changes have occurred in concert with advances in understanding of disease processes and evolution of effective treatment strategies.

The etiologic spectrum of CNS infection has changed considerably as a result of the development and aggressive use of antibiotics and the epidemic emergence of immunocompromising disorders such as infection with the human immunodeficiency virus (HIV). Some of the research on CNS infections has markedly increased in sophistication, which provides insights into pathogenesis, including the role of host mechanisms such as cytokines and other immune components. The pathophysiologic alterations are increasingly understood at the cellular and molecular levels.

Likewise, diagnostic tools have been developed that allow precise pathogen identification, most recently using molecular technologies such as polymerase chain reaction (PCR) tests for viral nucleic acids in cerebrospinal fluid (CSF). The initial treatment methodologies began by demonstrating the efficacy of antiserum treatment by Flexner in 1913 and of antibiotics by Colebrook in 1936.[2,3] The mortality rates were decreased further with the use of high-dose penicillin by Dowling in the 1940s.[4] Unfortunately, despite historical advances, the morbidity and mortality of these disorders remain considerable.

Definitions

CNS infections comprise a broad spectrum of disease entities. Meningitis is defined as "inflammation of the membranes of the brain or spinal cord," and is also called *arachnoiditis* or *leptomeningitis.*[5] *Encephalitis* denotes inflammation of the brain itself, whereas *myelitis* refers to inflammation of the spinal cord. The terms *meningoencephalitis* and *encephalomyelitis* describe more diffusely localized inflammatory processes. Collections of infective and purulent materials may form within the CNS as abscesses. Abscesses may be intraparenchymal, in epidural or subdural intracranial locations, or may be found in intramedullary or epidural spinal locations.

This chapter focuses on the more common acute and subacute CNS infections. Infections of the nervous system with HIV or human T lymphotrophic virus; rabies virus; polio or hepatitis viruses; *Borrelia burgdorferi* (Lyme disease); *Treponema* organisms (syphilis); parasites; rickettsia; and the chronic and slow infections of the CNS (subacute sclerosing panencephalitis, progressive multifocal leukoencephalopathy, and the prion-mediated spongiform encephalopathies, such as Creutzfeldt-Jakob disease and kuru) are not addressed.

Epidemiology

Bacterial meningitis is a common disease worldwide. Meningococcal meningitis is endemic in parts of Africa, and epidemics commonly occur in other countries, including the United States. A variety of other pathogens also are causative.[6-16] The overall incidence of bacterial meningitis in the United States is 5 to 10 cases per 100,000 people per year.[17,18] Men are affected more often than women.[17] The incidence of bacterial meningitis increases in late winter and early spring, but the disease may occur at any time of the year.

Because most cases are unreported, the actual incidence of viral meningitis is unknown. It is estimated to affect between 11 and 27 individuals per 100,000 people.[19,20] A prominent increase of cases is seen in summer months, which is concurrent with seasonal predominance of the enterovirus group of the picornaviruses.

The same organisms responsible for viral meningitis may also be associated with encephalitis. Encephalitis is, however, far less common, and the ratio of cases of meningitis to encephalitis varies according to the specific pathogen. Arbovirus infection is transmitted via an insect vector, although clinical disease develops in only a small percentage of the people bitten. Approximately 11,000 cases (or 5 cases per 100,000 people) of all forms of encephalitis are reported in the United States annually.[21,22]

Although CNS abscesses may occur at any age and any time of year, they are more commonly seen in men than women.[23-26] CNS abscesses are associated with local contiguous and remote systemic infections, intravenous (IV) drug use, neurologic surgery, and cranial trauma. Brain abscess secondary to otitis media most often presents in pediatric or older adult populations. When associated with sinusitis, it most often presents among young adults.[27] Increasingly, CNS abscesses are seen among the immunocompromised population, particularly those with HIV infection.

PRINCIPLES OF DISEASE

Etiology

Meningitis Meningeal inflammation may be caused by a variety of disease processes, but the infectious etiologies predominate. Some of the more common and important infectious etiologic agents in CNS infection, with emphasis on the United States, are listed in Boxes 103-1 and 103-2.[6-11,28] Among the bacterial etiologies, *Streptococcus pneumoniae* remains the predominant pathogen in adult patients, followed by *Neisseria meningitidis* and *Listeria monocytogenes.*[29] *N. meningitidis* is the predominant organism in adults younger than 45 years of age. Five major serogroups cause most meningococcal disease worldwide (A, B, C, Y, and W-135). The serogroup distribution for invasive disease has changed markedly in the United States, with B, C, and Y now most commonly responsible.[30-34] *Listeria* organisms account for up to 25% of the cases of meningitis in the over-60 age group.[35] These pathogens account for the bulk of cases in nontraumatic meningitis, although virtually any organism can be encountered, particularly among patients who are elderly, alcoholic, or immunosuppressed, and those who have cancer.

Meningeal infection may also occur in association with a dural leak secondary to neurosurgery or neurotrauma. *S. pneumoniae, Staphylococcus aureus, Pseudomonas aeruginosa,* and coliform bacteria are seen most commonly in this population.

Viral meningitis may likewise be caused by a variety of etiologic agents.[28] Enteroviruses are statistically encountered most commonly. Unfortunately, precise definition of the etiologic agent is often impossible. Fungal and parasitic meningitides are additional concerns, particularly among immunocompromised patients.[9-11]

Box 103-1 Bacterial, Fungal, and Parasitic Pathogens in CNS Infection

Bacterial

Bacillus sp.
Bacteroides
Borrelia burgdorferi (Lyme disease)
Other *Enterobacteriaceae*
Escherichia coli
Haemophilus influenzae
Listeria monocytogenes
Mycobacterium tuberculosis
Mycoplasma
Neisseria meningitidis
Proteus
Pseudomonas aeruginosa
Staphylococcus aureus
Streptococci
Streptococcus pneumoniae
Treponema (syphilis)
Others

Fungi

Blastomyces
Candida
Cladosporium
Coccidioides
Cryptococcus
Histoplasma
Paracoccidioides
Others

Parasites

Amoebae
Taenia solium (cysticercosis)
Toxoplasma gondii
Others

Rickettsia

Rickettsia rickettsii (Rocky Mountain spotted fever)
Others

Noninfectious meningitides include drug-induced meningitis, carcinomatous meningitis, CNS involvement in serum sickness, vasculitis, systemic lupus erythematosus, Behçet's disease, sarcoidosis, and others (Box 103-3). The differentiation of noninfectious from infectious etiologies can occasionally be perplexing.[36]

Encephalitis Arboviruses and herpes simplex virus (HSV) are the most common causes of endemic and sporadic cases of encephalitis, respectively. Children are the most vulnerable to infection with these viruses, although adults are also commonly affected. Epidemics of viral encephalitis have been attributed to a wide variety of viral agents. Postinfectious encephalomyelitis is also induced by a variety of viral pathogens, most commonly by the measles virus.[37] However, *Mycoplasma pneumoniae* and idiopathic causes are becoming more common in developed countries.[38]

Central Nervous System Abscess The etiologies of CNS abscess are multiple and reflect the primary infective

Box 103-2 Viral Etiologies in CNS Infection

Arboviruses
- Bunyaviruses
  - California encephalitis virus
- Alphaviruses
  - Eastern equine encephalitis virus
  - Western equine encephalitis virus
  - Venezuelan equine encephalitis virus
- Flaviviruses
  - Japanese B encephalitis virus
  - Colorado tick fever virus
  - St. Louis encephalitis virus
- Others

Herpes viruses
- Herpes simplex viruses (HSV)
- Epstein-Barr virus
- Cytomegalovirus
- Varicella-zoster virus

Enteroviruses
- Coxsackieviruses
- Echoviruses
- Poliovirus

Lymphocytic choriomeningitis virus (LCMV)

Retroviruses
- Human immunodeficiency virus (HIV)
- Human T lymphotrophic virus (HTLV)

Paramyxoviruses
- Measles virus
- Mumps virus

Rabies virus

Others

Box 103-3 Noninfectious Meningitides

Drug-induced meningitis
- Nonsteroidal antiinflammatory drugs (NSAIDs)
- Trimethoprim
- Isoniazid
- Others

Carcinomatous meningitis

Serum sickness

Vasculitis

Systemic lupus erythematosus

Behçet's disease

Sarcoidosis

Others

process and the immune state of the human host. A variety of mixed pathogens may be responsible for intracranial abscesses. Streptococci, particularly the *S. milleri* group, have been identified in nearly 50% of brain abscesses.[39] Anaerobic bacteria, predominantly *Bacteroides* species, are commonly seen when the primary infectious process is chronic otitis media or pulmonary disease. *S. aureus* is also often identified, particularly after cranial penetration from surgery or trauma.[40] The Enterobacteriaceae are an additional common isolate. Opportunistic fungal and parasitic etiologies are often seen in the immunosuppressed.[39]

Culture of epidural and subdural abscesses more often yields a single organism, with streptococci most commonly seen when associated with contiguous spread, and *S. aureus* and gram-negative rods most commonly encountered after neurologic trauma.[11] Etiologic agents in spinal abscess are similarly varied. *S. aureus* is most commonly encountered.

Pathophysiology

Bacterial Meningitis The pathogenetic sequence in bacterial meningitis has been well characterized.[9-11,41,42] The first step is nasopharyngeal colonization and mucosal invasion. Although colonization rates vary, virulent microbes use secretion of immunoglobulin A proteases and induce ciliostasis of mucosal cells. After penetration occurs by a variety of mechanisms, bacterial intravascular survival occurs because of the evasion of the complement pathway. The varying capsular properties for each organism protect the bacteria. The third step occurs when the bacteria cross the blood-brain barrier to enter the CSF. The dural venous sinuses, cribriform plate area, and choroid plexus have all been implicated as potential sites of invasion. Although the mechanism of invasion is not completely understood, host defense mechanisms within the CSF are often ineffective; there are low levels of complement, immunoglobulin, and opsonic activity. Bacterial proliferation then occurs, which stimulates a convergence of leukocytes into the CSF.

Meningeal and subarachnoid space inflammation are also associated with the release of cytokines into the CSF, most notably tumor necrosis factor and interleukin 1 and 6.[41,43,44] This results in increased permeability of the blood-brain barrier, cerebral vasculitis, edema, and increased intracranial pressure. A subsequent decrease in cerebral blood flow leads to cerebral hypoxia. Glucose transport into the CSF is decreased coincidentally with an increased use by brain, bacteria, and leukocytes, which depresses CSF glucose concentrations.[45] The increased permeability leads to increased CSF proteins.[46]

Viral Meningitis and Encephalitis Viruses enter the human host through the skin, as in arbovirus injection from a mosquito vector, or via the respiratory, gastrointestinal, or urogenital tracts.[47] Viral replication subsequently occurs outside the CNS and that is most often followed by hematogenous spread to the CNS.[48-50] Additional routes into the CNS include retrograde transmission along neuronal axons and direct invasion of the subarachnoid space after infection of the olfactory submucosa.[51,52]

Fortunately, most systemic viral infections do not result in meningitis or encephalitis. The development and subsequent magnitude of viral infection depend on the virulence of the specific virus, the viral inoculum level, and the state of immunity of the human host.[53,54] The tropism of the virus for specific CNS cell types also influences the focality of disease and its manifestations.[51] Particular viruses may preferentially attack cortical, limbic, or spinal neurons, oligodendria, or ependymal cells. An example is the tropism of HSV for the temporal lobes and the development of temporal lobe seizures and behavioral changes in afflicted patients.

Fungal Meningitis Fungal meningitis probably develops in much the same way as bacterial meningitis, although this has been incompletely studied. Pulmonary exposure followed by hematogenous spread is the primary pathogenetic mechanism in most cases. Immune system defects or immunosuppression compromise host defense mechanisms, with ensuing development of CNS infection.

Central Nervous System Abscess Intraparenchymal brain abscesses, subdural empyema, or intracranial or spinal epidural abscesses form by inoculation of the CNS from contiguous spread of organisms from a sinus, middle ear, or dental infection, or metastatic seeding from a distant site, usually from pulmonary infection, endocarditis, or osteomyelitis.[23-25,40] The primary infection can be identified in 75% to 85% of cases.[23] These conditions may also follow surgery or penetrating cranial trauma, particularly when bone fragments are retained in brain tissue.[55] Otogenic abscesses occur most commonly in the temporal lobe in adults and cerebellum in children, whereas sinogenic abscesses typically occur in frontal areas.[39] Multiple brain abscesses suggest hematogenous spread of organisms, although solitary lesions may also occur. The pulmonary system is the most common source of hematogenous spread.[11]

CLINICAL FEATURES

Symptoms and Signs

Numerous host factors have been implicated in the acquisition of meningitis (Box 103-4).[56,57] Although these factors alone and in combination increase the risk of meningitis, the disease often occurs in patients with none of these factors.

Many patients with meningitis will present with advanced disease; in these patients, the diagnosis of acute meningitis is strongly suspected. The constellation of symptoms that may classically occur in an acute CNS infection consists of fever, headache, photophobia, nuchal rigidity, lethargy, malaise, altered sensorium, seizures, vomiting, and chills.[7,56,58]

Unfortunately, more subtle presentations are also common. Immunosuppressed and geriatric patients present a diagnostic challenge because the classic signs and symptoms of meningitis may not be present. Although some degree of fever is present in most patients, as is a headache and neck stiffness, it is essential that meningitis be carefully considered in any immunosuppressed patient with symptoms or signs of infectious disease. Often, the only presenting sign of meningitis in the elderly patient is an alteration of mental status.

The presentation of fungal meningitis can be obscure even in the healthy adult population. Headache, low-grade fever, lassitude, and weight loss may be present, but often to such a mild degree that the correct diagnosis is not initially considered.[8] This is also true of tuberculous meningitis, which often has a protracted course and a vague nonspecific presentation consisting of fever, weight loss, night sweats, and malaise, with or without headache and meningismus.[7]

The physical findings in meningitis vary, depending on the host, causative organism, and severity of the illness. Nuchal rigidity or discomfort on flexion of the neck is common. Kernig's and Brudzinski's signs are present in approximately 50% of adults.[11] Kernig's sign is present in the patient if the examiner is unable, because of resistance and hamstring pain, to straighten the patient's leg passively to a position of full knee extension when the patient is lying supine with the hip flexed to a right angle.[5] Brudzinski described two signs.[5] The contralateral sign is present if an attempt to passively flex the hip on one side is accompanied by a similar movement of the other leg. The neck sign is present if attempts to passively flex the neck are accompanied by flexion of the hips. Deep tendon reflexes may be increased, and ophthalmoplegia may be present—especially of the lateral rectus muscles.[58]

Box 103-4 Host Factors Predisposing to Meningitis

Age <5 yr
Age >60 yr
Male gender
Low socioeconomic status
Crowding (e.g., military recruits)
Splenectomy
Sickle cell disease
African-American race
Alcoholism and cirrhosis
Diabetes
Immunologic defects
Recent colonization
Dural defect (e.g., traumatic, surgical, congenital)
Continuous infection (e.g., sinusitis)
Household contact with meningitis patient
Thalassemia major
IV drug abuse
Bacterial endocarditis
Ventriculoperitoneal shunt
Malignancy

Some of the systemic findings may include an obvious source of infection such as sinusitis, otitis media, mastoiditis, pneumonia, or urinary tract infection. Various manifestations of endocarditis may be present. Arthritis may be seen with *N. meningitidis* and occasionally with other bacteria.[56] Petechiae and cutaneous hemorrhages are widely reported with meningococcemia but also occur with *Haemophilus influenzae,* pneumococcal organisms, *L. monocytogenes,* and echovirus infections, in addition to staphylococcal endocarditis.[56] Endotoxic shock with vascular collapse often develops in severe meningococcal disease, but shock may be present in the advanced stages of any bacterial meningitis. Any determination of a serious systemic infection should encourage rather than dissuade the clinician from considering the possibility of a concomitant CNS infection.

Patients with encephalitis may also have symptoms of meningeal irritation. An alteration of consciousness occurs in virtually all patients. Fever, headache, and a change of personality are also usually present.[59] Hallucinations and bizarre behavior may precede motor, reflex, and other neurologic manifestations by several days, occasionally prompting an initial diagnosis of a psychiatric disorder.[60] Because focal neurologic deficits and seizures occur much more commonly with encephalitis than meningitis, there may also be diagnostic confusion with a brain abscess.[23,24,61] Distinguishing the etiologic agent in encephalitis is clinically difficult, although HSV encephalitis results in a higher incidence of dysphasia and seizures.[62]

Patients with intracranial abscess may be indistinguishable from those with meningitis or encephalitis. Most patients with intraparenchymal abscess will have a subacute course of illness, with symptoms progressing during the course of 2 or more weeks.[61] However, nuchal rigidity and fever are present in fewer than 50% of cases. Focal neurologic deficits are present in most of these patients. A large number of patients exhibit papilledema, which is a rare finding in meningitis. An abrupt neurologic deterioration that results from uncal herniation or rupture into the ventricular system may occur.

Patients with a subdural or epidural abscess most often have headache, fever, and focal signs, although more subtle presentations are common. Most of the patients with spinal abscess typically present with spinal pain and other symptoms and signs of cord compression, but not necessarily with fever.[63]

Complications

Bacterial Meningitis Some of the immediate complications of bacterial meningitis include coma (with loss of protective airway reflexes), seizures, cerebral edema, vasomotor collapse, disseminated intravascular coagulation, respiratory arrest, dehydration, syndrome of inappropriate secretion of antidiuretic hormone, pericardial effusion, and death (Box 103-5).[6,57,58,64] Various delayed complications include multiple seizures, focal paralysis, subdural effusions, hydrocephalus, intellectual deficits, sensorineural hearing loss, ataxia, blindness, bilateral adrenal hemorrhage (Waterhouse-Friderichsen syndrome), peripheral gangrene, and death.[10,56,58]

Box 103-5 Complications of Bacterial Meningitis

Immediate

Coma
Loss of airway reflexes
Seizures
Cerebral edema
Vasomotor collapse
Disseminated intravascular coagulation (DIC)
Respiratory arrest
Dehydration
Pericardial effusion
Death
Others

Delayed

Seizure disorder
Focal paralysis
Subdural effusion
Hydrocephalus
Intellectual deficits
Sensorineural hearing loss
Ataxia
Blindness
Bilateral adrenal hemorrhage
Death
Others

The case fatality rate for pneumococcal meningitis averages 20% to 25%, with higher fatality rates occurring in patients with serious underlying or concomitant disease or advanced age.[65,66] The prognosis is related to the degree of neurologic impairment on presentation. Overall, 20% to 30% of the survivors of pneumococcal meningitis will have some residual neurologic deficit.[56]

With the advent of antibiotic therapy, the mortality from meningococcal meningitis has markedly decreased to less than 20%, but it remains substantially higher in elderly patients or in those who also have meningococcemia.[66] Although most of the complications and sequelae are less common than with pneumococcal disease, the incidence of Waterhouse-Friderichsen syndrome is dramatically higher when meningococcemia is present.[56] The overall mortality rate in community-acquired gram-negative meningitis is less than 20% since the introduction of the third-generation cephalosporins.[9]

Viral Meningitis With rare exceptions, the overall prognosis for complete recovery from viral meningitis is excellent. Various complications related to the systemic effects of the particular virus include orchitis, parotitis, pancreatitis, and various dermatoses. Usually all of these complications resolve without sequelae.[28]

Viral Encephalitis With the exceptions of HSV meningoencephalitis and varicella-zoster encephalitis, the viral encephalitides are not treatable. The outcome depends on the infecting agent. Encephalitis caused by Japanese encephalitis virus, Eastern equine virus, and St. Louis encephalitis virus is severe, with high mortality rates and virtually universal neurologic sequelae among survivors.[67] Western equine virus and California encephalitis virus cause milder infections, and death is rare. The incidence of neurologic sequelae is highly variable and appears to depend on both the host and the infecting agent.[61,67]

The mortality from HSV encephalitis before the use of acyclovir was 60% to 70%. Acyclovir treatment has reduced the mortality to approximately 30%.[37] Common sequelae observed among survivors include seizure disorders, motor deficits, and changes in mentation.

Tuberculous Meningitis Death from tuberculous meningitis in the adult age group ranges from 10% to 50% of cases, with the incidence directly proportional to the patient's age and the duration of symptoms before presentation. Focal ischemic stroke may result from the associated cerebral vasculitis. In advanced disease up to 25% of patients may require some neurosurgical procedure for obstruction (ventriculoperitoneal shunt or drainage).[68] In most patients some neurologic deficit will develop, but severe long-term sequelae among survivors are unusual.[7,68]

Fungal Meningitis Common CNS complications with fungal meningitis include abscesses, papilledema, neurologic deficits, seizures, bony invasion, and fluid collections. Direct invasion of the optic nerve results in ocular abnormalities in up to 40% of patients with cryptococcal meningitis.[8] The mortality rate is high but variable and is related to the timeliness of diagnosis, underlying illness, and therapeutic regimens.

Central Nervous System Abscess With the early diagnosis afforded by the use of the cranial computed tomography (CT) scan; appropriate antimicrobial therapy; and combined management approaches with surgery, aspiration, and medical therapy, the mortality of brain abscess has declined dramatically from approximately 50% to less than 20%.[23-25] A seizure disorder is the most common sequela of intracranial abscess, occurring in 80% of patients.[9] Other neurologic sequelae of intracranial abscesses, including focal motor or sensory deficits or changes in mentation, are common.[23,24] Complications of spinal abscess primarily result from cord compression, including paralysis, motor and sensory deficits, and bowel and bladder dysfunction. Generalized spread of CNS infection and death may also occur.[63]

DIAGNOSTIC STRATEGIES

Lumbar Puncture

General Considerations Because the consequences of missing a CNS infection are devastating, CNS infection must be presumed to be present until excluded. The mere possibility of the diagnosis of meningitis mandates lumbar puncture unless the procedure is contraindicated by the presence of infection in the skin or soft tissues at the puncture site, or the likelihood of brain herniation.[37] Adherence to this principle prevents a delay in diagnosis, which substantially increases the morbidity and mortality of the disease. Some patients have clinically obvious bacterial meningitis, and CSF examination serves primarily to help identify the organism, thereby facilitating the appropriate treatment. Most patients, however, present more of a diagnostic problem, and analysis of the CSF fluid constitutes the critical step in the elucidation of the presence of CNS infection.

Increased Intracranial Pressure In most patients with bacterial meningitis, lumbar puncture (LP) may be safely performed without antecedent neuroimaging studies. In many circumstances, however, it is advisable to obtain a CT scan of the head before performing a lumbar puncture (Box 103-6). These indications must be carefully weighed against the patient's condition, the probability of meningitis, and the availability of the CT or magnetic resonance imaging (MRI) scan.[9,69-71]

It has been conventionally asserted that an LP in the presence of increased intracranial pressure may be harmful or fatal to the patient. Although data to address this concern are absent, the presence of focal neurologic signs does appear to be associated with a dramatic increase in complications from LP. These patients may deteriorate precipitously during or after the procedure.[72]

Patients with a markedly depressed sensorium that precludes careful neurologic examination, or those with a focal neurologic deficit, papilledema, seizures, or evidence of head trauma must be considered to be at risk for a herniation syndrome that may be exacerbated by an LP. If the presentation is an acute, fulminating, febrile illness and bacterial meningitis is the concerning diagnosis, early initiation of antimicrobial therapy is mandatory because of the association of prognosis and time to treatment.[73] The algorithmic alternatives are therefore (1) immediate LP, followed by initiation of antibiotic treatment before obtaining the results or (2) initiation of antibiotic treatment, followed by a cranial CT scan and then an LP. This latter choice of empiric treatment with antibiotics is now the routine in many institutions. This reflects the efficacy of current methodologies of identification of causative organisms by means other than bacteriologic cultures.

Box 103-6 Indications for CT Scan Before Lumbar Puncture in Suspected Bacterial Meningitis

Profoundly depressed mental status
Papilledema
Focal neurologic deficit
Minimal or absent fever
History or evidence of head trauma (recent or remote)
Recent onset seizure

Cerebrospinal Fluid Analysis

Opening Pressure The normal CSF pressure in an adult varies from 50 to 200 mm water. This value applies only to patients in the lateral recumbent position and may increase severalfold when the patient is in the sitting position. The pressure is often elevated in bacterial, tuberculous, and fungal meningitides, and a variety of noninfectious processes.[37] Pressure may be falsely elevated when the patient is tense or obese or has marked muscle contraction.

Collection of Fluid At least three sterile tubes each containing at least 1 to 1.5 ml of CSF should be obtained and numbered in sequence. A fourth tube may be desirable should later studies such as viral cultures or a Venereal Disease Research Laboratories (VDRL) test for syphilis become necessary. The fluid should be sent to the laboratory for immediate analysis of turbidity, xanthochromia, glucose, protein, cell count and differential, Gram's stain, bacterial culture, and antigen testing (Table 103-1). In certain cases an India ink stain, a bacteriologic stain for acid-fast bacilli, or a VDRL test should be obtained. When only a small amount of fluid can be obtained, the most important studies are the cell count with differential, the Gram's stain, and bacterial cultures. Ideally, the cell count should be performed on both the first and third or fourth tubes to help differentiate true CSF pleocytosis from contamination of the specimen by a traumatic LP.[74]

Turbidity The CSF should be assessed immediately for turbidity or cloudiness by the person performing the LP. Because normal CSF is completely clear and colorless and should be indistinguishable from water, any degree of turbidity is pathologic. Leukocytosis is the most common cause of CSF turbidity; counts greater than 200 cells/mm^3 usually cause clinically detectable changes in CSF clarity.[75]

Cell Count and Differential Normal adult CSF contains no more than 5 leukocytes/mm^3 with at most one granulocyte (PMN)[56,75,76]; therefore, the presence of more than one PMN or a total cell count of more than 5 cells/mm^3 should be considered evidence of CNS infection. In addition, the presence of any eosinophil in the CSF is abnormal, although occasionally basophils may be seen in the absence of disease.[75] Pretreatment with a few doses of antibiotics, although possibly diminishing the yield of Gram's staining and cultures, should not affect the CSF cell counts in meningitis.[9,29,77,78]

Table 103-1. Analysis of Cerebrospinal Fluid

Test	Normal value	Significance of abnormality
Cell count	<5 WBC/mm^3 <1 PMN/mm^3 <1 eosinophil/mm^3	Increased WBC counts are seen in all types of meningitis and encephalitis; increased PMN count suggests bacterial pathogen
Gram's stain	No organism	Offending organism identified 80% of time in bacterial meningitis, 60% if patient pretreated
Turbidity	Clear	Increased turbidity with leukocytosis, blood, or high concentration of microorganisms
Xanthochromia	None	Presence of RBCs in spinal fluid for 4 hr before lumbar puncture; occasionally caused by traumatic tap (if protein >150 mg/dl) or hypercarotenemia
CSF-to-serum glucose ratio	0.6:1	Depressed in pyogenic meningitis or hyperglycemia; lag time if glucose given IV
Protein	15-45 mg/dl	Elevated with acute bacterial or fungal meningitis; also elevated with vasculitis, syphilis, encephalitis, neoplasms, and demyelination syndromes
India ink stain	Negative	Positive in one third of cases of cryptococcal meningitis
Cryptococcal antigen	Negative	90% accuracy for cryptococcal disease
Lactic acid	<35 mg/dl	Elevated in bacterial and tubercular meningitis
Bacterial antigen tests	Negative	>95% specific for organism tested; up to 50% false-negative rate
Acid-fast stain	Negative	Positive in 80% of cases of tuberculous meningitis if >10 ml of fluid

CSF, Cerebrospinal fluid; *PMN,* polymorphonuclear; *WBC,* white blood cell.

The cell counts in bacterial meningitis are usually markedly elevated, sometimes exceeding 10,000 cells/mm^3, and demonstrate a dramatic granulocytic shift.[56] In general, counts exceed 500 cells/mm^3, with a preponderance of polymorphonuclear (PMN) leukocytes. The initial CSF analysis, however, in 6% to 13% of all cases of bacterial meningitis exhibits lymphocytosis (lymphocyte differential count higher than 50%). When only those patients with bacterial meningitis with fewer than 1,000 cells/mm^3 are considered, 24% to 32% have a predominance of lymphocytes.[79,80] In addition, this same population of patients often has only a mild disturbance of CSF glucose and protein levels. In well-established viral meningitis and encephalitis, counts are usually less than 500 cells/mm^3, with nearly 100% of the cells being mononuclear. Early (less than 48 hours) presentations may reveal significant PMN pleocytosis and hence be indistinguishable from early bacterial meningitis.[58]

Similarly, normal cell counts and differentials, although reassuring, do not absolutely exclude bacterial meningitis.[76] Any patient thought to have a clinical syndrome compatible with meningitis requires hospital admission with frequent reevaluation, repeated LP, and antimicrobial therapy. In some patients who have symptoms or signs of meningitis and have a normal initial CSF analysis, CSF pleocytosis may develop within 24 hours; the causative organism may be cultured from the original "normal" CSF.

Brain abscess and parameningeal infections, such as subdural empyema or epidural abscess, usually display CSF cell counts and differentials similar to those of viral meningitis and encephalitis, although the CSF may also be normal.[61]

A traumatic LP is suggested by the presence of a clot in one of the tubes or the clearing of the CSF and a decreasing red blood count (RBC) count from tubes one to three. In the presence of a traumatic lumbar puncture, one may estimate the true degree of CSF white blood count (WBC) pleocytosis with the following formula[75]

$$\text{True CSF WBC} = \text{Measured CSF WBC}$$
$$[(\text{CSF RBC} \times \text{blood WBC})/\text{blood RBC}]$$

Alternatively, when peripheral cell counts are normal, the CSF from a traumatic lumbar puncture should contain around 1 WBC per 700 RBCs.

Gram's Stain A properly performed Gram's stain of a centrifuged specimen of CSF identifies the causative organism approximately 80% of the time in cases of bacterial meningitis.[77] Gram's stain characteristics of the most commonly encountered organisms are described in Table 103-2.[81] The yield from this procedure is diminished by 20% to 30% when there has been prior treatment with antibiotics.[9,10] Misidentification of gram-positive organisms as gram-negative is also known to occur more commonly among pretreated patients because organisms with damaged walls stain unpredictably.[81]

Xanthochromia *Xanthochromia* refers to the yellowish discoloration of the supernatant of a centrifuged CSF specimen. Xanthochromia is abnormal and results from the lysis of RBCs and release of the breakdown pigments oxyhemoglobin, bilirubin, and methemoglobin into the CSF. This process normally begins within 2 hours, and pigments may persist up to 30 days[82]; therefore early analysis of the LP specimen is essential. If a traumatic tap has introduced enough plasma to raise the CSF protein level to 150 mg/dl or more, blood pigments may cause xanthochromia. If the CSF protein level is less than 150 mg/dl, however, and systemic hypercarotenemia does not exist, then xanthochromia of a centrifuged CSF specimen should suggest that subarachnoid hemorrhage has occurred.[75,82,83]

Table 103-2. Gram's Stain Characteristics of Selected Meningeal Pathogens

Pathogen	Typical characteristics
Staphylococci	Gram-positive cocci: singles, doubles, tetrads, clusters
Streptococcus pneumoniae	Gram-positive cocci: paired diplococci
Other streptococci	Gram-positive cocci: pairs and chains
Listeria monocytogenes	Gram-positive rods: single or chains
Neisseria meningitidis	Gram-negative cocci: negative paired diplococci; kidney or coffee bean appearance
Haemophilus influenzae	Gram-negative coccobacilli: "pleomorphic" bacilli
Enterobacteriaceae (including *Escherichia coli*)	Gram-negative rods
Pseudomonas aeruginosa	Gram-negative rods

Glucose When the serum glucose is normal, the CSF glucose is usually between 50 and 80 mg/dl. The CSF glucose is normally in a ratio of 0.6:1 to the serum glucose, except with marked systemic hyperglycemia, when the ratio is closer to 0.4:1. Therefore a CSF-to-serum glucose ratio of less than 0.5 in normoglycemic subjects or 0.3 in hyperglycemic subjects is abnormal and may represent the impaired glucose transport mechanisms and increased CNS glucose use associated with pyogenic meningitis.[56,75,84] Mild decreases in the CSF glucose level may occur with certain viral and parameningeal processes. However, bacterial or fungal meningitis should be presumed to be the cause of low CSF glucose, termed hypoglycorrhachia, until each is clearly excluded.[85] If the serum glucose level has increased rapidly—for example, after IV administration of 50% dextrose in water—equilibration in the CSF may take up to 4 hours, and therefore the interpretation of CSF-to-serum glucose ratios may be unreliable.

Protein The normal CSF protein level in adults ranges from 15 to 45 mg/dl.[74] An elevated CSF protein, usually higher than 150 mg/dl, commonly occurs with acute bacterial meningitis.[56] When a traumatic LP has occurred, the CSF protein can be corrected for the presence of blood by subtracting 1 mg/dl of protein for each 1,000 RBCs.[75,83] Elevated CSF protein concentrations can result from any cause of meningitis, subarachnoid hemorrhage, CNS vasculitis, syphilis, viral encephalitis, neoplasms, and demyelination syndromes.[58,75,86] A greatly elevated CSF protein level (>1,000 mg/dl) in the presence of a relatively benign clinical presentation should suggest fungal disease.[8]

India Ink Preparation India ink staining of the CSF should be performed whenever a diagnosis of cryptococcal meningitis is being considered. The demonstration of budding organisms (Figure 103-1) is virtually diagnostic for cryptococcal disease but occurs in only one third of the cases.[8] A more definitive diagnostic test is the cryptococcal antigen.

Lactic Acid Although nonspecific, elevations in CSF lactic acid concentrations (>35 mg/dl) are potentially indicative of bacterial meningitis.[87] Normal lactate levels (<35 mg/dl) are seen in patients with viral meningitides.[10]

Antigen Detection Counterimmunoelectrophoresis (CIE), latex agglutination, and coagglutination are methods of detecting specific antigens. These tests are particularly useful in patients receiving antibiotic treatment before CSF sampling because the tests depend on the presence of only an antigen and not viable organisms.

The CIE techniques that are performed for the most common bacterial pathogens demonstrate high sensitivity and specificity for bacterial antigens, particularly when performed on CSF, blood, and urine simultaneously.[88] Latex agglutination techniques are, however, more rapid and sensitive and are replacing the use of CIE in many facilities.[89] Although reported results vary, the sensitivities of antigen tests are 50% to 90% for Neisseria organisms, 50% to 100% for *S. pneumoniae,* and approximately 80% for *H. influenzae.*[86] A specific agglutination test for cryptococcal antigen is also highly sensitive (90%) and specific.[90] Cultures are always indicated because a negative antigen test does not exclude the possibility of any particular bacterial or fungal etiology.

Antigen and antibody testing is also being used to identify viral and atypical pathogens.[91-97] These have particular utility in HSV encephalitis. Enzyme-linked immunosorbent assays can detect HSV antibody production.[98] Unfortunately the appearance of antibody in CSF occurs too late to aid in any therapeutic decision analysis. PCR amplification and the identification of HSV DNA have demonstrated a sensitivity of 95% to 100% and a specificity of 100% early in the disease, and have markedly decreased the need for diagnostic brain biopsy in this disorder.[99-102] PCR has also improved diagnosis of tuberculous meningitis, with a sensitivity of 80% to 85% and a specificity of 97% to 100%,[103-106] and is proving to be of value in identifying bacteria, enteroviruses, and other viral etiologies in both immunocompromised and immunocompetent patients.[107-109]

Bacteriologic Cultures Although results are not available for emergency management, bacteriologic cultures of CSF should always be performed. Bacterial culture yields are significantly decreased in patients pretreated with antibiotics. Viral cultures may also be indicated.

Other Tests A variety of additional, nonspecific tests of CSF have been advocated. These include measuring CSF lactate dehydrogenase (LDH), C-reactive protein, and the limulus lysate test; however, none of these have demonstrated a high degree of clinical usefulness. Likewise, the evaluation of CSF chloride as a diagnostic aid for tuberculous meningitis is no longer clinically relevant.

Neuroimaging Techniques

A cranial CT scan or MRI scan is indicated in the evaluation of any patient with presumed CNS infection in whom there is the possibility of an intracranial abscess, intracranial hemorrhage, or mass lesion. In the diagnostic evaluation of acute meningitis, however, a CT scan should not unnecessarily delay LP or antimicrobial therapy. The CT scan may also show hypodense lesions in the temporal lobes in patients with HSV encephalitis, although an MRI scan will reveal this

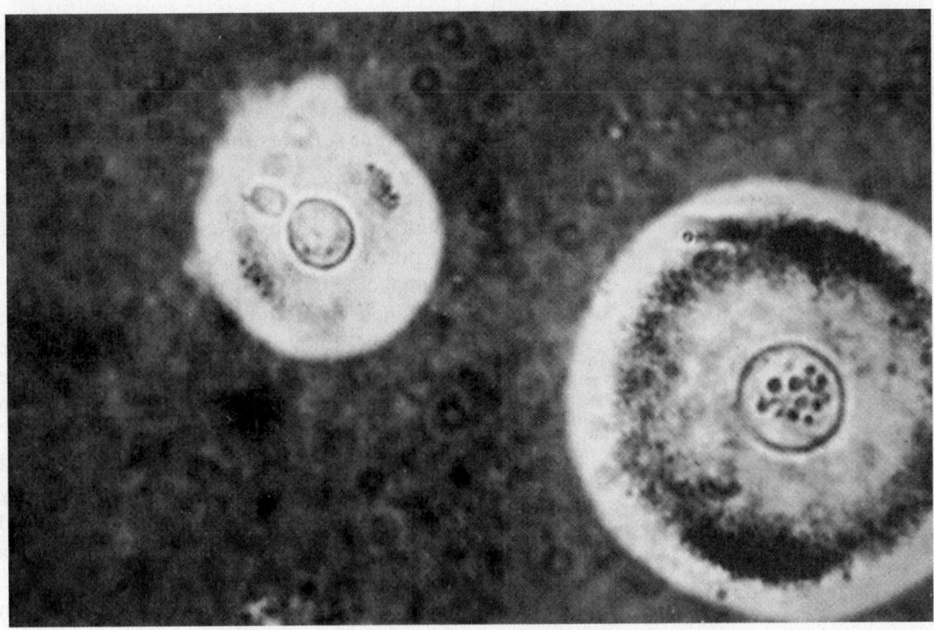

Figure 103-1. **India ink staining of the cerebrospinal fluid.**

abnormality much earlier in the disease process.[10] The contrast-enhanced cranial CT scan or MRI scan is invaluable in the diagnosis of a CNS abscess.[23-25] MRI scanning is also helpful in the evaluation of other infectious and noninfectious encephalitides.

Additional Investigations

As with other infectious diseases, the complete blood count with differential is a nonspecific adjunct in the diagnostic evaluation of a patient suspected to have a CNS infection. The peripheral cell counts are often normal in the presence of significant disease and may even be depressed, particularly in the elderly or the immunosuppressed. A "normal" leukocyte count and differential should never dissuade the EP from performing a diagnostic LP, obtaining a CT scan, or otherwise pursuing the diagnosis of a CNS infection.

Even when antimicrobial therapy has already been administered, two or three blood cultures should be obtained from all patients who are being evaluated for a CNS infection. The blood cultures can identify the causative organisms more often when the meningitis is caused by pneumococcus than meningococcus.[110] Although blood cultures are not immediately useful in the acute diagnosis of meningitis in the ED, they may be of considerable clinical importance later in the management of the disease. The cultures are helpful in identifying a causative organism in only a small minority of cases of brain abscess.[23]

As many as 50% of patients with pneumococcal meningitis also have evidence of pneumonia on an initial chest x-ray study. This association occurs in fewer than 10% of the cases of meningitis caused by *H. influenzae* type B and *N. meningitidis* and in approximately 20% of cases of meningitis caused by other organisms.[111] The identification of a pulmonary infection on chest radiography may assist in identification of causative organisms and appropriate antimicrobial therapy in approximately 10% of cases of brain abscess.[23-25]

Other ancillary investigations such as echocardiography, cultures of other body fluids, and bone scans may be undertaken as necessary to evaluate coexistent or complicated disease. Serum electrolytes, glucose, urea nitrogen, and creatinine levels should be measured to facilitate the interpretation of the CSF glucose level and to establish the level of renal function and the state of electrolyte balance. Although organism-specific abnormalities are uncommon, hyponatremia has been associated with tuberculous meningitis.

A number of characteristic but not pathognomonic electroencephalographic (EEG) abnormalities have been associated with HSV type 1 encephalitis. The presence of focal or lateralized EEG abnormalities in the presence of an encephalitis syndrome should be considered strong evidence supporting a diagnosis of HSV encephalitis.[112]

DIFFERENTIAL CONSIDERATIONS

Patients with meningitis may have symptoms and signs ranging from mild headache with fever to frank coma and shock. To facilitate the discussion of diagnosis and treatment, meningitis may be divided into three clinical syndromes: acute meningitis, subacute meningitis, and chronic meningitis.

Acute meningitis encompasses those patients with obvious signs and symptoms of meningitis who are evaluated in less than 24 hours after the onset of their symptoms and who rapidly deteriorate. In many of these patients the diagnosis of meningitis is not in doubt, and the crucial step is to initiate antimicrobial therapy immediately. The most likely pathogens in this syndrome are *S. pneumoniae* and *N. meningitidis.* Although *H. influenzae* has been reported in this context, it is not commonly implicated in the adult population.[6,29]

In the syndrome of subacute meningitis the symptoms and signs causing the patient to seek care have developed during a period of 1 to 7 days. This includes virtually all cases of viral meningitis, along with most of the bacterial and some of the fungal etiologies.[9-11] The differential diagnosis depends

Box 103-7 Differential Considerations in Chronic Meningitis

Tuberculous meningitis
Fungal CNS infections
Tertiary syphilis
CNS neoplasm
Lupus cerebritis
Sarcoidosis
Rheumatoid arthritis
Granulomatous angiitis
Various encephalitides
Toxic encephalopathies
Metabolic encephalopathies
Multiple sclerosis
Chronic subdural hematoma
Others

on the symptoms and signs at presentation. Among the elderly and immunosuppressed, a change in the patient's mental status may be the only presenting sign in meningitis. Even when a fever is present, the patient's change in mental status may be misattributed to another disease outside the CNS, such as pneumonia or urinary tract infection; neck stiffness may be misattributed to degenerative joint disease. The elderly patient is at high risk for meningitis and, rather than constituting a diagnostic endpoint, the identification of an infection outside the CNS in such a patient is a clear indication for LP because of the risk of bacteremic seeding by the involved organisms.

The differential diagnosis of encephalitis and brain abscess will occur in the context of the subacute meningitis syndrome. Brain abscess should be considered, especially if the fever is minimal or absent or if there are focal neurologic findings.[61] The presence of fever, altered sensorium, headache, seizures, and personality change is consistent with encephalitis. In addition, diagnoses such as subdural empyema, brain tumor, subarachnoid hemorrhage, subdural hematoma, and traumatic intracranial hemorrhage should be considered. In these circumstances a cranial CT scan should be obtained before performing a lumbar puncture.

The spectrum of chronic meningitis includes some of the viral meningitides as well as meningitis caused by tubercle bacilli, syphilis, and fungi. Many of the patients in this group have had symptoms for at least 1 week before presentation and generally have a prolonged indolent course marked by difficult and changing diagnoses and multiple therapies.[7,8] In addition to tuberculous, fungal, and syphilitic meningitides, the differential diagnosis of the chronic meningitis syndrome is extensive (Box 103-7).[11]

MANAGEMENT

Prehospital Care

The field stabilization and transport of the patient with a suspected CNS infection is dictated by the patient's condition. In those cases when the patient is stable and alert with normal vital signs, application of oxygen and rapid transport will suffice, with or without establishing an IV line. If an altered mental status is present, protection or establishment of an adequate airway may be necessary. Shock, if present, may require IV crystalloid infusion. Seizures may usually be managed supportively through protection of the patient's airway and prevention of injury, although prolonged or recurrent seizures may require IV anticonvulsants.

Assessment and Stabilization

Septic shock, hypoxemia, seizures, cerebral edema, and hypotension resulting from dehydration require aggressive management. When possible, a thorough history should be obtained from the patient, family members, or ambulance personnel with particular emphasis on preexisting conditions that may complicate the patient's disease. Some examples include recent neurosurgery, trauma, a history of leukopenia, immunocompromise, or diabetes mellitus.

Hypotension or shock should be treated as indicated with isotonic crystalloid infusion, high-flow oxygen, and pressors. Intravenous dextrose may be required for hypoglycemia secondary to depletion of glycogen stores. Alcoholic or nutritionally compromised patients should also receive 50 to 100 mg of thiamine IV. In those cases of moderate to severe hypotension, central venous pressure monitoring should be initiated and used as a guide for additional IV fluids or vasopressors.

Active airway management with endotracheal intubation may be required, particularly in cases of coma, recurrent seizures, or severe accompanying pulmonary infection. Cardiac monitoring may also be necessary, particularly in elderly patients, those with known coronary disease, and those with an altered mental status. Seizures are a particularly prominent component of the clinical presentation in patients with a brain abscess but may also occur with any CNS infection, especially when an underlying seizure disorder is present.

If acute cerebral edema or an elevated intracranial pressure is present, it should be managed by immediate intubation and adequate ventilation. Osmotic agents such as mannitol or diuretics such as furosemide may be used, but caution should be exercised if shock or uncontrolled hypotension is present. If diuretics or osmotic agents are administered, the emergency physician must ensure that the patient does not become volume depleted and hypotensive.

Definitive Therapy

Bacterial Meningitis Therapy for bacterial meningitis requires antibiotics that penetrate the blood-brain barrier and achieve adequate CSF concentrations, are bactericidal against the offending organism in vivo, and maintain adequate tissue levels to effectively treat the infection.

Until the pathogenetic organism is identified, broad-spectrum coverage of the most common pathogens is necessary (Table 103-3). Many authorities recommend cefotaxime or ceftriaxone, plus vancomycin and rifampin to cover potentially resistant organisms.[113-114] Rifampin is added to vancomycin because vancomycin crosses the blood-brain barrier poorly. High-dose ampicillin is also added if concern exists for *Listeria*.[113,114] In patients allergic to penicillin and cephalosporins, meropenem or chloramphenicol plus vancomycin and rifampin may be effective while awaiting the outcome of desensitization techniques.[29,114]

After the pathogen is identified, more targeted therapy can be instituted. It is prudent to refer to a current antimicrobial reference to guide therapy in all instances, given rapid

Table 103-3. Antimicrobial Therapy for Bacterial Meningitis*

Organism	Treatment of choice	Alternate treatment
N. meningitidis	Penicillin G, 3-4 million IU IV q4hr, or ampicillin, 2 g IV q4hr	Cefotaxime† 2 g IV q4hr, or chloramphenicol, 25 mg/kg IV q6hr
S. pneumoniae	Penicillin G, 3-4 million IU IV q4hr, or ampicillin, 2 g IV q4hr	Cefotaxime† 2 g IV q4hr, or chloramphenicol, 25 mg/kg IV q6hr
H. influenzae	Cefotaxime† 2 g IV q4hr	Chloramphenicol‡ 25 mg/kg IV q6hr, plus ampicillin, 2 g IV q4hr
S. aureus	Nafcillin, 2 g IV q4hr	Vancomycin, 20 mg/kg up to 1 g IV q12hr
E. coli and other gram-negative enterics except *P. aeruginosa*	Cefotaxime† 2 g IV q4hr	Ciprofloxacin, 400 mg IV q12hr
P. aeruginosa	Ceftazidime, 4 g IV q8hr, plus gentamicin, 2.0 mg/kg IV at once then 1.7 mg/kg IV q8hr (adjusted according to renal function), plus 4 mg intrathecally q12hr if required	Ciprofloxacin, 400 mg IV q12hr
L. monocytogenes	Ampicillin, 2 g IV q4hr, plus gentamicin (as for *Pseudomonas*)	Trimethoprim-sulfamethoxazole, 240 mg/1,200 mg IV q6hr

*All doses assume normal metabolic function.
†Or equivalent third-generation cephalosporin (e.g., ceftriaxone, 2 to 3 g IV every 12 hr, or ceftizoxime, 3 g IV every 8 hr).
‡Initial therapy: may be discontinued when in vitro sensitivity to ampicillin has been demonstrated.

changes in etiologic spectrum, drug resistance, and available agents.

The role of corticosteroids in treating acute bacterial meningitis has been controversial. Animal studies demonstrate the salutary effects of the administration of corticosteroids in experimental pneumococcal meningitis, including reduced brain edema, CSF pressure, and CSF lactate levels.[115] An earlier resolution of the clinical and CSF stigmata of meningitis and a decrease in long-term hearing loss are observed in infants and children given dexamethasone with cefuroxime or ceftriaxone compared with those receiving the antibiotic alone, particularly when *H. influenzae* is the offending agent.[116-120] There are few data providing for a proven benefit of corticosteroid therapy in adult human meningitis; however, some authorities recommend it routinely[113,114] and others restrict it to patients with cerebral edema or severely impaired mental status.[42,119]

Viral Meningitis No specific agents are available for treating most types of viral meningitis. Investigational agents in development may reduce symptomatology in enterovirus meningitis[121,122]; however, with the exception of HSV meningitis, the viral meningitides contracted in the United States are generally characterized by a short, benign, self-limited course followed by a complete recovery. The primary therapeutic consideration in cases of viral meningitis is therefore the validity of the diagnosis. Early cases of viral meningitis may be indistinguishable from bacterial meningitis, and this confusion may not be resolved by CSF analysis; therefore when any doubt exists as to the veracity of the diagnosis, appropriate cultures should be drawn and the patient admitted to the hospital. Antimicrobial therapy for presumed bacterial meningitis may be initiated on the basis of the clinical presentation or may be withheld pending the outcome of close clinical observation and repeated LP in 8 to 12 hours.[10]

Viral Encephalitis Specific therapy for meningoencephalitis from human herpes viruses is available. Acyclovir remains the current choice and is capable of substantially improving the patient's outcome. When the diagnosis of herpes meningoencephalitis is suspected or established, IV acyclovir should be administered in a dose of 10 mg/kg every 8 hours.[113,114,123]

Tuberculous Meningitis Early chemotherapeutic intervention in acute tuberculous meningitis improves the patient's prognosis. A strong clinical suggestion of this disease is an adequate indication to begin antituberculous therapy. A standard treatment regimen consists of isoniazid, rifampin, pyrazinamide, and ethambutol or streptomycin.[113,114] Corticosteroids have also been shown to decrease secondary complications.[114,124]

Fungal Meningitis The treatment of fungal meningitis is complex.[8] Four agents are commonly used: amphotericin B, flucytosine, miconazole, and fluconazole. Of these, amphotericin B, either alone or in combination with flucytosine, is the most commonly recommended initial therapeutic regimen.[113,114] These diseases are rarely acutely life-threatening, but rather are slowly progressive. Prolonged therapy, often with multiple agents, is necessary. The initiation of antifungal therapy is rarely indicated in the ED.

Central Nervous System Abscess The treatment of cerebral abscess is complex, and neurosurgical consultation is indicated. The location, size, and number of abscesses influence the choice of medical management, surgical excision, aspiration, or a combination of these modalities.[23,24,39] In general, small multiple abscesses are more appropriately treated medically, whereas large, surgically accessible lesions should be excised. Empiric antimicrobial therapy before identification of specific organisms by aspiration or surgical excision should be guided by the principles of CSF penetration and the coverage of likely pathogens.

Otogenic and sinogenic abscesses are often treated with cefotaxime or ceftriaxone plus metronidazole.[113,114,125] Abscesses with traumatic or neurosurgical causes should have antimicrobial coverage for *S. aureus* or methicillin-resistant *S. aureus*.[113,114] Patients at high risk for tuberculous, fungal, or parasitic abscess should also receive coverage for the suspected etiologic agent. Corticosteroids should be reserved specifically for managing any attendant cerebral edema; in other circumstances, steroid use is associated with increased mortality.[24]

Chemoprophylaxis

Among household contacts the incidence of transmission of meningococcus is approximately 5%; therefore it is recommended that household contacts of bacteriologically confirmed cases receive rifampin (adults, 600 mg; children older than 1 year, 10 mg/kg; children younger than 1 year, 5 mg/kg) orally every 12 hours for a total of four doses.[114] In addition, these contacts should be advised to watch for fever, sore throat, rash, or any symptoms of meningitis. They should be hospitalized with appropriate IV antimicrobial therapy if there are signs that active meningococcal disease is developing because rifampin is ineffective against invasive meningococcal disease. Intimate, nonhousehold contacts who have had mucosal exposure to the patient's oral secretions should also receive rifampin prophylaxis. Health care workers are not at any increased risk for the disease and do not require prophylaxis unless they have had direct mucosal contact with the patient's secretions, as might occur during mouth-to-mouth resuscitation, endotracheal intubation, or nasotracheal suctioning. Azithromycin 500 mg by mouth (PO) or ciprofloxacin 500 mg PO (adults only), or ceftriaxone 250 mg intramuscularly (125 mg intramuscularly for children younger than 15 years), provide single-dose alternatives.[113,114]

There is no indication for chemoprophylaxis in pneumococcal meningitis. Rifampin prophylaxis for the contacts of patients with *H. influenzae* type B meningitis is recommended for nonpregnant household contacts when there are children younger than 4 years of age in the household[113,114] (adults: 600 mg PO; children: 20 mg/kg PO daily for 4 days).

Immunoprophylaxis

A quadrivalent vaccine based on the polysaccharide capsule and conferring protection against groups A, C, Y, and W-135 meningococci has been in routine use by the U.S. military since the 1980s[126,127]; however, the vaccine is relatively ineffective in those under 2 years of age. No licensed vaccine is currently available against the serogroup B meningococcus.[34] The serogroup B capsular polysaccharide has proved to be poorly immunogenic in humans. Efforts are under way to establish an effective group B vaccine by focusing on outer membrane proteins.[128] Additionally, efforts are under way to enhance the immunogenicity and protective efficacy of the group C vaccines by using conjugate methods that link polysaccharides and carrier proteins. Current recommendations for the quadrivalent vaccine are evolving. The vaccine is recommended in established meningococcal epidemics and for travelers to countries where meningococcal disease is currently epidemic. Recently, the Advisory Committee on Immunization Practices has recommended elective vaccination of college freshmen.[34]

The development of effective pneumococcal vaccines has been hampered by the large number of serotypes of the organism. A small number of serotypes, however, are responsible for most clinical pneumococcal disease, and a polyvalent vaccine effective against many of these principal serotypes has been developed.[129] The recommendations for polyvalent pneumococcal vaccine are targeted primarily at prevention of pneumonia, despite a potential beneficial effect for meningitis. A single dose of the vaccine should be considered for elderly or debilitated patients, especially those with pulmonary disease, and for patients with impaired splenic function, splenectomy, or sickle cell anemia. A conjugate vaccine effective against *H. influenzae* type B has been developed for use in the pediatric, but not adult, population.[130] It appears to be approximately 90% protective and has a very low incidence of adverse reactions.[131-135]

Vaccination is also available to confer immune protection against Japanese encephalitis virus, and it is recommended for people performing extensive outdoor activities or spending more than 30 days in endemic areas during transmission seasons.[136] The reported protective efficacy of the vaccine is approximately 90%.[137]

DISPOSITION

With the exception of viral meningitis, all but the most chronic CNS infections require initial inpatient evaluation and treatment. Bed rest, analgesics, and the institution of appropriate IV antimicrobials are indicated.

Some patients with suspected viral meningitides merit hospitalization. These include patients with more severe disease, immunocompromise, suspicion of HSV meningitis, or potential nonviral causes. Some authorities manage patients with classic presentations of viral meningitis as outpatients and ensure close follow-up within 24 hours.[57] Others admit all patients until the more serious causes, such as early bacterial meningitis or encephalitis, can be excluded with absolute certainty.

KEY CONCEPTS

- CNS infection should be considered in all patients with headache, neck stiffness, fever, altered sensorium, or diffuse or focal neurologic findings.
- Lumbar puncture with sampling of cerebrospinal fluid is the only reliable method of assessing the presence or absence of meningitis. In the absence of contraindications, any suspicion of meningitis mandates performance of lumbar puncture.
- Early initiation of antimicrobial therapy is mandatory in any case of suspected acute CNS infection. Antibiotic administration must not be delayed for CSF analysis or performance of neuroimaging studies.
- Antibiotic chemoprophylaxis should be assured for close contacts of patients with meningitis resulting from *Neisseria meningitidis* or *Haemophilus influenzae*. Single-dose and multiple-dose regimens are available.
- Vaccination against *N. meningitidis* is recommended for certain at-risk populations, but does not afford protection against serogroup B infection.
- Concomitant CNS infection should be strongly considered in any patient with another severe systemic infection, such as urinary tract infection or pneumonia.

REFERENCES

1. Viesseux M: Memoire sur le maladie qui a regré à Genève au printemps de 1805, *J Med Chir Pharm* 11:163, 1805.
2. Flexner S: The results of serum treatment in 1300 cases of epidemic meningitis, *J Exp Med* 17:553, 1913.
3. Colebrook L, Kenny M: Treatment of human puerperal, infections and experimental infections in mice with prontosil, *Lancet* 1:1279, 1936.
4. Dowling HF et al: The treatment of pneumococcal meningitis with massive doses of systemic penicillin, *Am J Med Sci* 217:149, 1949.
5. *Stedman's medical dictionary,* Baltimore, 1995, Williams & Wilkins.
6. Durand ML et al: Acute bacterial meningitis in adults: a review of 493 episodes, *N Engl J Med* 328:21, 1993.
7. Alvavez S, McCabe WR: Extrapulmonary tuberculosis revisited: a review of experience at Boston City and other hospitals, *Medicine* 63:25, 1984.
8. Salaki JS et al: Fungal and yeast infections of the central nervous system, *Medicine* 63:108, 1984.
9. Lambert HP, editor: *Infections of the central nervous system,* Philadelphia, 1991, BC Decker.
10. Schlossberg D, editor: *Infections of the nervous system,* New York, 1990, Springer-Verlag.
11. Tyler KL, Martin JB, editors: *Infectious diseases of the central nervous system,* Philadelphia, 1993, FA Davis.
12. Schuchat A et al: Bacterial meningitis in the United States in 1995, *N Engl J Med* 337:970, 1997.
13. Weiss K et al: *Corynebacterium striatum* meningitis: case report and review of an increasing important *Corynebacterium* species, *Clin Inf Dis* 23:1246, 1996.
14. Pruitt AA: Infections of the nervous system, *Neurol Clin* 16:419, 1998.
15. Sigurdardottir B: Acute bacterial meningitis in adults, *Arch Intern Med* 157:425, 1997.
16. Segreti J et al: Acute bacterial meningitis, *Infect Dis Clin North Am* 10:797, 1996.
17. Fraser DW et al: Bacterial meningitis in Bernadillo County, New Mexico, *Am J Epidemiol* 1000:29, 1974.
18. Fraser DN et al: Changing patterns of bacterial meningitis in Olmsted County, Minnesota, *J Infect Dis* 128:300, 1973.
19. Beghi E et al: Encephalitis and aseptic meningitis, Olmsted County, Minnesota, 1950-81: I. Epidemiology, *Ann Neurol* 16:283, 1984.
20. Ponka A, Pettersson T: The incidence and aetiology of central nervous system infections in Helsinki in 1980, *Acta Neurol Scand* 66:529, 1982.
21. Centers for Disease Control: Summary of notifiable diseases, United States, 1987, *MMWR* 36:1, 1988.
22. Johnson RT: Acute encephalitis, *Clin Inf Dis* 23:219, 1996.
23. Schliamser SE et al: Intracranial abscesses in adults: an analysis of 54 consecutive cases, *Scand J Infect* Dis 20:1, 1988.
24. Mampalam TJ et al: Trends in the management of bacterial brain abscesses: a review of 102 cases over 17 years, *Neurosurgery* 23:451, 1988.
25. Yand SY: Brain abscess: a review of 400 cases, *J Neurosurg* 55:794, 1981.
26. Mathiesen GE et al: Brain abscess, *Clin Inf Dis* 25:763, 1997.
27. DeLouvis J et al: Bacteriology of abscesses of the central nervous system: a multicentre prospective study, *BMJ* 2:981, 1977.
28. Specter S et al, editors: *Neuropathogenic viruses and immunity,* New York, 1992, Plenum.
29. Luby JP: Infections of the central nervous system, *Am J Med Sci* 304:379, 1992.
30. Centers for Disease Control and Prevention: Serogroup Y meningococcal disease: Illinois, Connecticut, and selected areas, United States, 1989-1996, *MMWR* 45:1011, 1996.
31. Centers for Disease Control and Prevention: Summary of notifiable diseases, United States, 1997, *MMWR* 46:10, 1997.
32. Diermayer M et al: Epidemic serogroup B meningococcal disease in Oregon: the evolving epidemiology of the ET-5 strain, *JAMA* 281:1493, 1999.
33. Jackson LA et al: Serogroup C meningococcal outbreaks in the United States: an emerging threat, *JAMA* 273:383, 1995.
34. Postgraduate Institute for Medicine: *The changing epidemiology of meningococcal disease in the United States with an emphasis on college health issues,* Englewood, Colo, 1999, Postgraduate Institute for Medicine.
35. Miller LG et al: Meningitis in older patients: how to diagnose and treat a deadly infection, *Geriatrics* 52:43, 1997.
36. Mandell G et al, editors: *Principles and practice of infectious diseases,* ed 4, New York, 1995, Churchill Livingstone.
37. Rowland LP, editor: *Merritt's textbook of neurology,* ed 9, Baltimore, 1995, Williams and Wilkins.
38. Nishimura M et al: Post-infectious encephalitis with anti-galactocerebroside antibody subsequent to *Mycoplasma pneumoniae, J Neurol Sci* 140:91, 1996.
39. Wispelway B, Scheld W: Brain abscess, *Semin Neurol* 12:273, 1992.
40. Small M et al: Intracranial suppuration 1968-1982: a 15-year review, *Clin Otolaryngol* 9:315, 1984.
41. Qualiarello V, Scheld W: Bacterial meningitis: pathogenesis, pathophysiology, and progress, *N Engl J Med* 327:864, 1992.
42. Tunkel MD et al: Bacterial meningitis: recent advances in pathophysiology and treatment, *Ann Intern Med* 112:610, 1990.
43. Saukkonen K et al: The role of cytokines in the generation of inflammation and tissue damage in experimental gram-positive meningitis, *J Exp Med* 171:439, 1990.
44. Ravi V et al: Correlation of tumor necrosis factor levels in the serum and cerebrospinal fluid with clinical outcome in Japanese encephalitis patients, *J Med Virol* 51:132, 1997.
45. Menkes JH: The causes for low spinal fluid sugar in bacterial meningitis: another look, *Pediatrics* 44:1, 1969.
46. Quagliarello VJ et al: Morphologic alterations of the blood-brain barrier with experimental meningitis in the rat: temporal sequence and role of encapsulation, *J Clin Invest* 77:1084, 1986.
47. Root RK, Sande MA, editors: *Viral infections: diagnosis, treatment, and prevention,* New York, 1993, Churchill Livingstone.
48. Monath TP et al: Mode of entry of a neurotropic arbovirus into the central nervous system, *Lab Invest* 48:399, 1983.
49. Bulychev LE et al: Course of infection in guinea pigs, infected aerogenically by Venezuelan equine encephalomyelitis virus (Russian), *Vopr Virusol* 40:122, 1995.
50. Bulychev LE et al: Course of infection in white rats, infected with Venezuelan equine encephalomyelitis virus by a respiratory route (Russian), *Vopr Virusol* 40:79, 1995.
51. Johnson RT: The pathogenesis of acute viral encephalitis and postinfectious encephalomyelitis, *J Infect Dis* 155:359, 1987.
52. Whitley RJ: Viral encephalitis, *N Engl J Med* 323:242, 1990.
53. Kinter RL, Brandt CR: The effect of viral inoculum level and host age on disease incidence, disease severity, and mortality in a murine model of ocular HSV-1 infection, *Curr Eye Res* 14:145, 1995.
54. Oliver KR et al: Susceptibility to a neurotropic virus and its changing distribution in the developing brain is a function of CNS maturity, *J Neurovirol* 3:38, 1997.
55. Tenney JH: Bacterial infection of the central nervous system in neurosurgery, *Neurol Clin* 4:91, 1986.
56. Geiseler PJ et al: Community-acquired purulent meningitis: a review of 1316 cases during the antibiotic era, 1954-1976, *Rev Infect Dis* 2:725, 1980.
57. Scheld WM: Bacterial meningitis and brain abscess. In Isselbacher KJ et al, editors: *Harrison's principles of internal medicine,* New York, 1994, McGraw-Hill.
58. Hoeprich PD, editor: *Infectious diseases: a treatise of infectious processes,* Philadelphia, 1994, JB Lippincott.
59. Whitley RJ et al: Herpes simplex encephalitis: clinical assessment, *JAMA* 247:317, 1982.
60. Fisher CM: Hypomanic symptoms caused by herpes simplex encephalitis, *Neurology* 47:1374, 1996.
61. Benson CA, Harris AA: Acute neurologic infections, *Med Clin North Am* 70:987, 1986.
62. Studahl M et al: Acute viral encephalitis in adults—a prospective study, *Scand J Infect Dis* 30:215, 1998.
63. Maslen DR et al: Spinal epidural abscess, *Arch Internal Med* 153:1713, 1993.
64. Patwari AK et al: Inappropriate secretion of antidiuretic hormone in acute bacterial meningitis, *Ann Trop Paediatr* 15:179, 1995.
65. Sangster G et al: Bacterial meningitis 1940-79, *J Infect* 5:245, 1982.

66. Wenger JD et al: Bacterial meningitis in the United States, 1986B: report of a multistate surveillance study, *J Infect Dis* 162:1316, 1990.
67. Anderson JR: Viral encephalitis and its pathology, *Curr Top Pathol* 76:23, 1988.
68. Kennedy DH, Fallon RJ: Tuberculous meningitis, *JAMA* 241:264, 1979.
69. Weisberg LA: The role of CT in the evaluation of patients with intracranial CNS infectious B inflammatory disorders, *Comput Radiol* 8:29, 1984.
70. Horowitz ST et al: Cerebral herniation in bacterial meningitis in childhood, *Arch Neurol* 7:524, 1980.
71. Klein JO et al: Report of the task force on the diagnosis and management of meningitis, *Pediatrics* 78:959, 1986.
72. Duffy GP: Lumbar puncture in the presence of raised intracranial pressure, *BMJ* 1:407, 1969.
73. Radetsky M: Duration of symptoms and outcome in bacterial meningitis: an analysis of causation and the implications of a delay in diagnosis, *Pediatr Infect Dis J* 11:694, 1992.
74. Sacher RA et al, editors: *Widman's clinical interpretation of laboratory tests,* Philadelphia, 1991, FA Davis.
75. Conly JM, Ronald AR: Cerebrospinal fluid as a diagnostic body fluid, *Am J Med* 75, 1B:102, 1983.
76. Onorato IM et al: A "normal" CSF in bacterial meningitis, *JAMA* 244:1469, 1980.
77. Pickens S et al: The effects of pre-admission antibiotics on the bacteriological diagnosis of pyogenic meningitis, *Scand J Infect Dis* 10:183, 1978.
78. Jarvis CW, Saxena KM: Does prior antibiotic treatment hamper the diagnosis of acute bacterial meningitis? *Clin Pediatr* 11:201, 1972.
79. Powers WJ: Cerebrospinal fluid lymphocytosis in acute bacterial meningitis, *Am J Med* 79:216, 1985.
80. Arevalo CE et al: Cerebrospinal fluid cell counts and chemistries in bacterial meningitis, *South Med J* 82:1123, 1989.
81. Murray PR, editor: *Manual of clinical microbiology,* ed 6, Washington DC, 1995, ASM Press.
82. Kooiker JC: Spinal puncture and cerebrospinal fluid examination. In Roberts JR, Hedges JR, editors: *Clinical procedures in emergency medicine,* ed 2, Philadelphia, 1991, WB Saunders.
83. Fishman RA: *Cerebrospinal fluid in disease of the nervous system,* Philadelphia, 1992, WB Saunders.
84. Powers WJ: Cerebrospinal fluid to serum glucose ratios in diabetes mellitus and bacterial meningitis, *Am J Med* 71:217, 1981.
85. Leonard JM: Cerebrospinal fluid formula in patients with central nervous system infection, *Neurol Clin* 4:3, 1986.
86. Johnson RT et al: Measles encephalitis B-clinical and immunologic studies, *N Engl J Med* 310:137, 1984.
87. Lindquist L et al: Value of cerebrospinal fluid analysis in the differential diagnosis of meningitis: a study in 710 patients with suspected central nervous system infection, *Eur J Clin Microbiol Infect Dis* 7:374, 1988.
88. Feigin RD et al: Countercurrent immunoelectrophoresis of urine as well as of CSF and blood for diagnosis of bacterial meningitis, *J Pediatr* 89:773, 1976.
89. Kaplan S: Antigen detection in cerebrospinal fluid B: pros and cons, *Am J Med* 75:109, 1983.
90. Bouza E et al: Coccidioidal meningitis: an analysis of 31 cases and review of the literature, *Medicine* 60:139, 1981.
91. Glimaker M et al: Detection of enteroviral RNA by polymerase chain reaction in faecal samples from patients with aseptic meningitis, *J Med Virol* 38:54, 1992.
92. Samuelson A et al: Diagnosis of enteroviral meningitis with enzyme immunosorbent assays (EIA) using heat-treated virions and synthetic peptides as antigens, *J Med Virol* 40:271, 1993.
93. Landgren M et al: Diagnosis of Epstein-Barr virus-induced central nervous system infections by DNA amplification from cerebrospinal fluid, *Ann Neurol* 35:631, 1994.
94. Pedneault L et al: Detection of Epstein-Barr virus in the brain by the polymerase chain reaction, *Ann Neurol* 32:184, 1992.
95. Mertens G et al: Detection of herpes simplex virus in the cerebrospinal fluid of patients with encephalitis using polymerase chain reaction, *J Neurol Sci* 118:213, 1993.
96. Kamei S et al: New non-invasive rapid diagnosis of herpes simplex virus encephalitis by quantitative detection of intrathecal antigen with a chemiluminescence assay, *J Neurol Neurosurg Psychiatry* 57:1112, 1994.
97. Musiana M et al: Rapid diagnosis of cytomegalovirus encephalitis in patients with AIDS using in-situ hybridisation, *J Clin Pathol* 47:886, 1994.
98. Aurelius E: Herpes simplex encephalitis B: early diagnosis and immune activation in the acute stage and during long-term follow-up, *Scand J Infect Dis* 89:3, 1993.
99. Gufford T et al: Significance and clinical relevance of the detection of herpes simplex virus DNA by the polymerase chain reaction in cerebrospinal fluid from patients with presumed encephalitis, *Clin Infect Dis* 18:744, 1994.
100. Aslanzadeh J, Skiest DJ: Polymerase chain reaction for detection of *herpes simplex* virus encephalitis, *J Clin Pathol* 47:554, 1994.
101. Aslanzadeh J et al: A prospective study of the polymerase chain reaction for detection of herpes simplex virus in cerebrospinal fluid submitted to the clinical virology laboratory, *Mol Cell Probes* 6:367, 1992.
102. Cinque P et al: The role of laboratory investigation in the diagnosis and management of patients with suspected herpes simplex encephalitis: a consensus report. The EU concerted action on virus meningitis and encephalitis, *J Neurol Neurosurg Psychiatry* 61:339, 1996.
103. Kearns AM et al: A rapid polymerase chain reaction technique for detecting *M tuberculosis* in a variety of clinical specimens, *J Clin Pathol* 51:922, 1998.
104. Bonington A et al: Use of Roche AMPLICOR *Mycobacterium tuberculosis* PCR in early diagnosis of tuberculosis meningitis, *J Clin Microbiol* 36:1251, 1998.
105. Fresquet-Wolf C et al: Value of polymerase chain reaction (PCR) for diagnosis of tuberculoid meningitis (German), *Nervenarzt* 69:502, 1998.
106. Seth P et al: Evaluation of polymerase chain reaction of rapid diagnosis of clinically suspected tuberculous meningitis, *Tuber Lung Dis* 77:353, 1996.
107. Roos KL: Pearls and pitfalls in the diagnosis and management of central nervous system infectious diseases, *Semin Neurol* 18:185, 1998.
108. Read SJ, Kurtz JB: Laboratory diagnosis of common viral infections of the central nervous system by using a single multiplex PCR screening assay, *J Clin Microbiol* 37:1352, 1999.
109. Casas I et al: Viral diagnosis of neurological infection by RT multiplex PCR: a search for entero- and herpesviruses in a prospective study, *J Med Virol* 57:145, 1999.
110. Davey PG et al: Bacterial meningitis B: 10 years experience, *J Hygiene* 88:383, 1982.
111. Carpenter RR, Petersdorf RG: The clinical spectrum of bacterial meningitis, *Am J Med* 33:262, 1962.
112. Lai CW, Gragasin ME: Electroencephalography in *herpes simplex* encephalitis, *J Clin Neurophysiol* 5:87, 1988.
113. Bartlett JG: *1999 Pocket book of infectious disease therapy,* Baltimore, 1999, William & Wilkins.
114. Gilbert DN et al: *Guide to antimicrobial therapy 1999,* Hyde Park, Vt., 1999, Antimicrobial Therapy.
115. Tauber MG et al: Effects of ampicillin and corticosteroids on brain water content, cerebrospinal fluid pressure, and cerebrospinal fluid lactate levels in experimental pneumococcal meningitis, *J Infect Dis* 151:528, 1985.
116. Lebel MH, Freij BJ: Dexamethasone therapy for bacterial meningitis: results of two double-blind, placebo-controlled trials, *N Engl J Med* 319:964, 1988.
117. Kennedy WA, Hoyt MJ, McCracken GH Jr: The role of corticosteroid therapy in children with pneumococcal meningitis, *Am J Dis Child* 145:1374, 1991.
118. Jafari HS, McCracken GH Jr: Dexamethasone therapy in bacterial meningitis, *Pediatr Ann* 23:82, 1994.
119. Trunkel AR, Scheld WM: Acute bacterial meningitis, *Lancet* 346:1675, 1995.
120. McIntyre PB et al: Dexamethasone as adjunctive therapy in bacterial meningitis, *JAMA* 278:925, 1997.

121. Schumm M et al: Chronic enteroviral meningo-encephalitis in X-linked agammaglobulinemia: favorable response to anti-enteroviral treatment, *Eur J Pediatr* 158:1010, 1999.
122. Rotbart HA et al: Treatment of human enterovirus infections, *Antiviral Res* 38:1, 1998.
123. Whitley RJ et al: Vidarabine versus acyclovir in herpes simplex encephalitis, *N Engl J Med* 314:144, 1986.
124. Kumarvelu S et al: Randomized controlled trial of dexamethasone in tuberculous meningitis, *Tuber Lung Dis* 75:203, 1994.
125. Sjolin J et al: Treatment of brain abscess with cefotaxime and metronidazole: prospective study on 15 consecutive patients, *Clin Infect Dis* 17:857, 1993.
126. Hart CA et al: Management of bacterial meningitis, *J Antimicrob Chem* 32:49, 1993.
127. Zangwill KM et al: Duration of antibody response after meningococcal polysaccharide vaccination in U.S. Air Force personnel, *J Infect Dis* 169:847, 1994.
128. Nokleby H, Feiring B: The Norwegian meningococcal group B outer membrane vesicle vaccine: side effects in phase II trials, *NIPH Ann* 14:94, 1991.
129. Butler JC et al: Pneumococcal polysaccharide vaccine efficacy B-an evaluation of current recommendations, *JAMA* 270:1826, 1993.
130. Willis J, editor: *HIB vaccine recommendations,* FDA Drug Bill 15:18, 1985.
131. Peltola H et al: Prevention of *Haemophilus influenzae* type B bacteremic infections with capsular polysaccharide vaccine, *N Engl J Med* 310:1561, 1984.
132. Vadheim CM et al: Eradication of *Haemophilus influenzae* type B disease in southern California: Kaiser-UCLA vaccine study group, *Arch Pediatr Adolesc Med* 148:51, 1994.
133. Harrison LH et al: Postlicensure effectiveness of the *Haemophilus influenzae* type B polysaccharide-*Neisseria meningitidis* outer-membrane protein complex conjugate vaccine among Navajo children, *J Pediatr* 125:571, 1994.
134. Buchanan GA, Darville T: Impact of immunization against *Haemophilus influenzae* type B (HIB) on the incidence of HIB meningitis treated at Arkansas Children's Hospital, *South Med J* 87:38, 1994.
135. Madore DV: Impact of immunization of *Haemophilus influenzae* type B disease, *Infect Agents Dis* 5:8, 1996.
136. Centers for Disease Control and Prevention: Inactivated Japanese encephalitis virus vaccine: recommendations of the Advisory Committee on Immunization Practices, *MMWR* 42:1, 1993.
137. Hoke CH et al: Protection against Japanese encephalitis by inactivated vaccines, *N Engl J Med* 319:608, 1988.

Section VIII PSYCHIATRIC AND BEHAVIORAL DISORDERS

104 Thought Disorders

Robert S. Hockberger
John Richards

PERSPECTIVE

Although written accounts of people exhibiting unusual or bizarre behavior date back more than 3000 years, no detailed descriptions of behavior resembling modern-day schizophrenia can be found before 1800. In the 1800s, Morel introduced the term *dementia praecox* to describe a progressive deterioration of mental functioning and behavior with onset in adolescence to early adult life.[1] In 1911 Bleuler further detailed the specifics of this disorder, which he termed *schizophrenia,* or "split-mindedness."[2] Early authorities differed in their views regarding the pathophysiology of the disorder. Kraepelin viewed schizophrenia as a progressive, degenerative psychologic condition with a uniformly poor prognosis; Meyer believed that the disorder resulted from a combination of biologic, social, and psychologic factors that were potentially treatable. Early treatments for schizophrenia included ice water immersion, the use of barbiturates or insulin to induce prolonged narcosis or coma, seizure induction with pentylenetetrazol (Metrazol), electroconvulsive therapy, and frontal leukotomy.[3] The effectiveness of these treatments was marginal at best, and until recent times most schizophrenic patients were relegated to lifelong institutionalization.

Modern-era pharmacotherapy of schizophrenia, principally with chlorpromazine and haloperidol, began in the early 1950s. This treatment proved so successful that, by the 1960s most psychiatrists believed that individuals with schizophrenia could be successfully managed in the outpatient setting. In 1965 the U.S. Federal Government passed the Community Mental Health Centers Act, initiating the release of medicated schizophrenic patients into the community.[4] Unfortunately, inadequate family support, the unavailability of jobs and low-cost housing, and the lack of funding for social services and outpatient psychiatric care left these individuals isolated without the tools they needed for resocialization. This situation has improved little during the past 30 years, and currently 20% to 40% of homeless people in the United States have major mental illness.[5] The ED serves as the primary entry point into the mental health care system for many of these individuals and is often the only source of treatment for many chronically ill mental patients.[6]

PRINCIPLES OF DISEASE

Schizophrenia is currently viewed as a heterogenous disorder that results from the interaction of biologic and environmental factors. Studies involving adopted twins whose biologic parents have schizophrenia demonstrate a strong genetic basis for the disorder.[7] Although the overall incidence of schizophrenia in the general population is approximately 1%, it increases to almost 10% in first-degree biologic relatives of individuals with the disorder.[8] Research on drugs that mimic schizophrenic-like psychoses, as well as drugs that alleviate the disorder, implicate involvement of the dopaminergic, serotonergic, cholinergic, and glutamatergic systems in the pathophysiology of schizophrenia.[9-12]

Evidence increasingly supports the belief that schizophrenia is a neurodevelopmental disorder resulting from the influence of environmental factors on genetically predisposed individuals. Disruptions in fetal brain development, caused by perinatal hypoxia, poor nutrition, influenza infection, and other insults, may set the stage for development of schizophrenia decades later.[1] New imaging techniques have documented the presence of structural abnormalities, most of which appear to be developmental rather than degenerative, in the brains of many patients with schizophrenia.[9] Recent reviews cite experimental evidence to support the existence of a progressive continuum of psychotic illness.[1,13,14] The continuum begins with unipolar depression, progressing to bipolar illness, then to schizoaffective psychoses, and finally to schizophrenia, depending on the extent of the developmental defect.

CLINICAL FEATURES

Overt signs of schizophrenia usually become manifest during adolescence or early adult life. If questioned carefully, however, many patients will describe a childhood marked by few interpersonal relationships and a sense, on the part of themselves and others, that they were withdrawn and somewhat eccentric.

Phases of Schizophrenia

The development of schizophrenia almost invariably passes through three phases.[15] The *premorbid phase* is characterized by the development of "negative" symptoms that cause deterioration from a previous level of personal, social, and intellectual functioning. Typically, patients progressively withdraw from social interactions and neglect personal appearance and hygiene. It becomes increasingly difficult for them to function at work and school and, ultimately, in their home environment.

The *active phase* is usually precipitated by a stressful event that results in the development of "positive" symptoms such as active delusions, hallucinations, and bizarre behavior. Patients may become agitated or exhibit a hypervigilant withdrawal state characterized by rocking or staring. It is during this phase that they are most likely to be brought to the ED by family, friends, coworkers, or the police.

The *residual phase* resembles the premorbid phase in that patients are left with impaired social and cognitive ability, marked by bizarre ideation or vague delusions and accompanied by peculiar behavior, poor personal hygiene and grooming, and social isolation. Most schizophrenic patients require a sheltered environment to function adequately. Although the disorder has a wide spectrum of severity, the general course for most patients is one of gradual deterioration with periodic episodes of psychotic decompensation, often precipitating another visit to the ED.

Criteria for Schizophrenia

The clinical criteria for the diagnosis of schizophrenia are outlined in the fourth edition of the *Diagnostic and Statistical Manual of Mental Disorders (DSM-IV-TR)* (Box 104-1).[15] First, the patient must exhibit two or more of the following symptoms: delusions, hallucinations, disorganized speech, grossly disorganized or catatonic behavior, and negative symptoms such as flattening of affect, poverty of speech, or an inability to perform goal-directed activities. Second, there must be a sharp deterioration from the patient's prior level of functioning (work, school, self-care, or interpersonal relations), and there must be continuous signs of disturbance (including prodromal symptoms) for at least 6 months. Third, the diagnoses of schizoaffective disorder and mood disorder with psychotic features must be excluded. Fourth, and most important for emergency physicians, the presence of medical conditions that can mimic or cause psychotic symptoms must be excluded. Such conditions include substance abuse, the side effects of some medications, and certain medical disorders (Boxes 104-2 and 104-3).

Box 104-1 Summary of *DSM-IV* Criteria for Schizophrenia

A. Presence of two (or more) characteristic symptoms for 1 month (or more) unless treated
   1. Delusions
   2. Hallucinations
   3. Disorganized speech (derailment or incoherence)
   4. Grossly disorganized or catatonic behavior
   5. Negative symptoms: affect flattening, alogia (poverty of speech), avolition (unable to perform goal-directed activities)

   Note: only one symptom above is required if delusions are bizarre or hallucinations consist of a running commentary.
B. Sharp deterioration from prior level of functioning (i.e., work, self-care, interpersonal relations)
C. Continuous signs of disturbance for 6 months (or more)
D. Schizoaffective disorder and mood disorder when psychotic features have been ruled out
E. Not caused by substance abuse, medication, or a general medical condition

Modified from *Diagnostic and statistical manual of mental disorders*, ed 4-TR, Washington, DC, 2000, American Psychiatric Association.

Delusions

The *DSM-IV* defines delusions as "erroneous beliefs that usually involve a misinterpretation of perceptions or experiences."[15] The delusions seen with schizophrenia are most often persecutory, religious, or somatic. They most often involve a sense of loss of control over the mind or body, such as having one's thoughts stolen, feeling that one is being manipulated by some outside force, or the belief that one's internal organs are rotting away.

Hallucinations

A hallucination is a sensory experience that does not exist, except in the mind of the person experiencing it. Although the hallucinations seen with schizophrenia can involve any sensory modality (auditory, visual, olfactory, gustatory, or tactile), auditory hallucinations (hearing voices) that are pejorative or threatening are especially common.

Disorganized Speech

Patients with schizophrenia experience loosening of associations; that is, their thoughts shift randomly from one topic to another without a logical connection. Their speech often shows lack of content, or not saying much when talking. *Neologisms* (nonsense words invented by the patient) and *perseverations* (frequently repeated words or phrases) are common. Occasionally the person's speech may be so

Box 104-2 Pharmacologic Agents that May Cause Acute Psychosis

Antianxiety Agents
Alprazolam
Chlordiazepoxide
Clonazepam
Clorazepate
Diazepam
Ethchlorvynol

Antibiotics
Isoniazid
Rifampin

Anticonvulsants
Ethosuximide
Phenobarbital
Phenytoin
Primidone

Antidepressants
Amitriptyline
Doxepin
Imipramine
Protriptyline
Trimipramine

Cardiovascular Drugs
Captopril
Digitalis
Disopyramide
Methyldopa
Procainamide
Propranolol
Reserpine

Miscellaneous Drugs
Antihistamines
Antineoplastics
Bromides
Cimetidine
Corticosteroids
Disulfiram
Heavy metals

Drugs of Abuse
Alcohol
Amphetamines
Cannabis
Cocaine
Hallucinogens
Opioids
Phencyclidine
Sedative-hypnotics

severely disorganized that it is totally incoherent, termed *word salad.*

Grossly Disorganized or Catatonic Behavior

As a result of their delusions, hallucinations, and disorganized thinking, schizophrenic patients have great difficulty formulating and producing goal-directed behavior. They are often found wandering about, disheveled, malnourished, apparently talking to themselves, and exhibiting unpredictable and untriggered agitation, such as shouting or swearing. It is this behavior that usually prompts family members, friends, or the police to bring them to the ED. Patients exhibiting catatonia appear to be completely unaware of their environment, maintain a rigid posture, and resist efforts to be moved.

Negative Symptoms

Three negative symptoms—flattening of affect, alogia, and avolition—account for a significant degree of the morbidity associated with schizophrenia. Patients with a *flattened affect* exhibit little facial expressiveness, eye contact, or body language. *Alogia,* or poverty of speech, is manifested by brief, laconic, empty replies to questioning. *Avolition* is characterized by an inability to initiate and persist in goal-directed activities. The emergency physician must be cautious in using the presence of negative symptoms to support a diagnosis of schizophrenia because similar symptoms can be produced by severe depression, chronic environmental understimulation, and treatment with neuroleptic medications.

Box 104-3 Medical Disorders that May Cause Acute Psychosis

Metabolic Disorders
Hypercalcemia
Hypercarbia
Hypoglycemia
Hyponatremia
Hypoxia

Inflammatory Disorders
Sarcoidosis
Systemic lupus erythematosus
Temporal (giant cell) arteritis

Organ Failure
Hepatic encephalopathy
Uremia

Neurologic Disorders
Alzheimer's disease
Cerebrovascular disease
Encephalitis (including HIV)
Encephalopathies
Epilepsy
Huntington's disease
Multiple sclerosis
Neoplasms
Normal-pressure hydrocephalus
Parkinson's disease
Pick's disease
Wilson's disease

Endocrine Disorders
Addison's disease
Cushing's disease
Panhypopituitarism
Parathyroid disease
Postpartum psychosis
Recurrent menstrual psychosis
Sydenham's chorea
Thyroid disease

Deficiency States
Niacin
Thiamine
Vitamin B_{12} and folate

DIAGNOSTIC STRATEGIES

Patients with Known Psychiatric Disorders

Patients with known psychiatric disorders who present with a mild to moderate exacerbation of their symptoms secondary to noncompliance with neuroleptic medication do not require extensive laboratory evaluation.[16] Because some of these patients may have coexisting substance abuse or undiagnosed medical disorders, however, a complete history and physical examination, along with urine toxicology studies, are indicated for most patients.[17-19] Patients exhibiting severe exacerbation of symptoms accompanied by marked agitation, violent behavior, or significantly abnormal vital signs should receive more extensive evaluation.

Patients Without Known Psychiatric Disorders

Schizophrenia is a clinical diagnosis (see Box 104-1). Unfortunately, many toxicologic and medical disorders can mimic schizophrenia. Patients apparently with new onset of psychosis and those with known psychiatric disorders who experience a severe exacerbation of symptoms or exhibit signs or symptoms of organic disease should receive a comprehensive medical evaluation to exclude toxicologic and medical disorders.[20-23]

DIFFERENTIAL CONSIDERATIONS

Medical Disorders

Certain medications and medical disorders may affect thought processes, causing persons to exhibit abnormal behavior (see Boxes 104-2 and 104-3). This behavior may range from mild personality changes to apparent acute psychosis, even in the absence of an underlying psychiatric disorder.[1] Factors that should alert the emergency physician to a medical disorder include (1) history of substance abuse or a medical disorder requiring medication, (2) patient age greater than 35 years without previous evidence of psychiatric disease, (3) recent fluctuation in behavioral symptoms, (4) hallucinations that are primarily visual in nature, (5) presence of lethargy, (6) abnormal vital signs, and (7) poor performance on cognitive function testing, particularly orientation to time, place, and person.[24] These and other factors may be helpful in differentiating functional (psychiatric) from organic (medical) causes of abnormal behavior and can be organized for easy recall into the mnemonic MADFOCS (Table 104-1).[25]

Although the classic textbook differentiation between functional and organic causes of abnormal behavior is straightforward, the evaluation of individual patients may be difficult.[21] A patient with underlying psychiatric disease may develop a medical disorder, which may worsen the patient's behavioral symptoms and further cloud the distinction between functional and organic disease. This evaluation is particularly difficult in the ED when previous medical or psychiatric history is not available, the patient is uncooperative, and the time frame to make a disposition is brief. When the clinical differentiation between functional and organic disease is unclear based on available information, a patient should receive further evaluation to exclude the presence of a toxicologic or medical disorder.

Psychiatric Disorders

A previously undiagnosed patient who presents with an acute functional psychosis may ultimately be given one of several psychiatric diagnoses. A *brief psychotic disorder* involves the sudden onset of psychotic symptoms during the immediate postpartum period or in response to any major stress, such as the loss of a loved one or the psychologic trauma of combat, and lasts from several days to 1 month. Patients with *schizophreniform disorder* have similar symptoms that last longer than 1 month but less than 6 months. Approximately one third of individuals initially given the diagnosis of schizophreniform disorder will recover within 6 months; the other two thirds will retain their symptoms and ultimately be diagnosed as having schizophrenia. Patients with mood disorders may develop psychotic symptoms. If these symptoms are present only during periods of mood disturbance, the diagnosis of *mood disorder with psychotic features* is applied; if they persist for longer than 2 weeks in the absence of prominent mood symptoms, the diagnosis of *schizoaffective disorder* is made. Patients with *personality disorders* may occasionally develop brief psychotic episodes when under stress.

Ganser syndrome is a symptom complex, considered to be emotional in origin, in which the patient may appear to have amnesia, hallucinations, or alterations in consciousness, usually in association with physical complaints. An individual with Ganser syndrome may have psychotic symptoms for no apparent gain except to assume the role of the psychiatric patient.

Table 104-1. Factors in Differentiating Organic and Functional Psychosis: "MADFOCS"

	Organic	Functional
Memory deficits	Recent impairment	Remote impairment
Activity	Psychomotor retardation	Repetitive activity
	Tremor	Posturing
	Ataxia	Rocking
Distortions	Visual hallucinations	Auditory hallucinations
Feelings	Emotional lability	Flat affect
Orientation	Disoriented	Oriented
Cognition	Islands of lucidity	Continuous scattered thoughts
	Perceives occasionally	Unfiltered perceptions
	Attends occasionally	Unable to attend
	Focuses	
Some other findings	Age >40	Age <40
	Sudden onset	Gradual onset
	Physical examination often abnormal	Physical examination normal
	Vital signs may be abnormal	Vital signs usually normal
	Social immodesty	Social modesty
	Aphasia	Intelligible speech
	Consciousness impaired	Awake and alert

Modified from Frame DS, Kercher EE: *Emerg Med Clin North Am* 9:123, 1991.

Persons with a *delusional disorder* experience nonbizarre delusions that may dominate their lives. They may believe that famous people are in love with them (erotomanic type), that they have extraordinary powers with a special relationship to a deity or a famous person (grandiose type), that their sexual partner is unfaithful (jealous type), that they are being malevolently treated in some way (persecutory type), or that they have some physical defect or general medical condition (somatic type). Although patients with somatic delusions may experience tactile or olfactory hallucinations related to the delusional theme (e.g., the sensation of being infested with insects), the other features associated with schizophrenia are not present.

MANAGEMENT

General Approach

Patients with thought disorders may be agitated and hyperactive, may be withdrawn but hypervigilant, or may complain of somatic delusions. In addition, they may have paranoid ideation, may be angry that they have been brought to the ED against their will, or may be frightened because they have been confronted by the police, restrained, and isolated. The presence of such patients in the ED may be disconcerting to staff because these patients are known to be potentially irrational, erratic, and unpredictable in their behavior. Although emergency personnel must remain calm, empathetic, and reassuring in their interactions with patients exhibiting a thought disorder, they also must take steps to ensure staff safety whenever dealing with patients at risk for sudden violence. Such patients include those who have manifested violent behavior before coming to the ED, those who physically or verbally threaten staff, and those who demonstrate an escalating level of agitation despite verbal attempts to calm them.

Each patient should have a complete history and physical examination performed, including a detailed mental status evaluation, to rule out the existence of an organic brain syndrome. Valuable information can be obtained from family members, friends, co-workers, neighbors, paramedical personnel, police, or previous medical records (see Table 104-1).[25]

The most important step in evaluating a patient with a suspected thought disorder is the assessment of the patient's thought processes through a psychiatric interview. This interview attempts to establish a positive physician-patient relationship, to make a correct diagnosis, and to gather the information necessary to render an optimal disposition. The interview should be conducted in a quiet, comfortable room with adequate privacy. The examiner should be sitting, and if possible the interview should proceed to completion without interruption. If the patient is believed to be potentially dangerous but is not in need of immediate restraint, the interview should take place in an open area with security personnel nearby.

The emergency physician should begin with an introduction and should express the desire to be "of help" to the patient. The interview should begin with open-ended questions designed to assess the patient's complaint and understanding of the current circumstances. Good opening questions include "Do you understand why you have been brought here today?"; "You seem to be upset. Can you tell me why?"; and "Do you have any idea why you might be having these symptoms?" The patient's appearance, body language, affect, and speech should be observed during the responses to these questions.

The second portion of the psychiatric interview consists of a formal mental status examination, which may be initiated in a nonthreatening manner by stating, "I am now going to ask you a few questions to see how well you are concentrating."[26] The patient should first be asked questions regarding orientation to time, place, and person because this is the most sensitive test for differentiating organic from functional disease. Patients who are disoriented should receive a detailed medical evaluation to exclude the presence of an organic brain syndrome. Patients who are oriented should be assessed for attention, memory, intellectual functioning, and judgment in an attempt to determine their specific diagnosis, their potential for danger to themselves or others, and their degree of dysfunction and ability to care for themselves in the outpatient setting.

Rapid Tranquilization

When psychotic patients exhibit behavior that is violent or so disorganized and uncooperative that clinical evaluation becomes impossible, the temporary use of physical restraints is indicated while rapid tranquilization is initiated (see Chapter 184). The technique of rapid tranquilization uses serial doses of a high-potency antipsychotic agent until target symptoms, such as agitation and excessive psychomotor activity, are improved. The goal is to facilitate cooperation of the patient without causing unnecessary sedation, which would inhibit further medical and psychiatric assessment. Oral, intramuscular (IM), or intravenous (IV) doses can be given every 30 to 60 minutes until the patient becomes calmer and more cooperative. If the patient is willing, an oral concentrate is preferred because it implies consent and can take effect almost as quickly as IM administration.

Haloperidol (Haldol) is the agent most widely used for rapid tranquilization in the United States.[27-31] The initial dose is 5 to 10 mg for young to middle-age patients and 0.5 to 2.0 mg for elderly patients. Although rapid tranquilization with haloperidol will quickly reduce tension, anxiety, and hyperactivity, delusions and hallucinations may not resolve for several weeks. *Droperidol* (Inapsine), 2.5 to 5 mg IV, is also used.[32,33] Compared with haloperidol, droperidol has a faster onset and shorter duration of action and causes slightly more sedation. It has been found to be effective in sedating uncooperative patients for diagnostic procedures and in treating patients with sympathomimetic drug–induced psychosis. Droperidol does not have antipsychotic activity, however, and should not be considered for maintenance therapy of schizophrenia. Neuroleptics should not be used for pregnant or lactating females, phencyclidine overdose, or anticholinergic drug–induced psychosis. In addition, they should not be used as the sole agent to manage agitation in patients with drug or alcohol withdrawal.

Benzodiazepines are effective in managing agitation in patients who experience withdrawal from alcohol or sedative-hypnotic drugs, who have cocaine intoxication, or who have a contraindication to neuroleptic use. Benzodiazepines are helpful adjuncts to neuroleptic medication in providing rapid tranquilization, particularly in patients exhibiting combativeness or severe agitation, when a greater degree of sedation is desired.[34,35] *Lorazepam* (Ativan), 1 to 2 mg, is frequently mixed with haloperidol, 5 mg, in the same syringe and administered IM or IV for this purpose.

Outpatient Management

The outpatient treatment of schizophrenia involves maintenance therapy using neuroleptic agents, family counseling, and social rehabilitation. Although emergency physicians rarely prescribe outpatient neuroleptic medications, they should be familiar with the complications associated with the long-term use of these agents.

Box 104-4 lists the most common neuroleptic medications currently used in the United States.[36-45] The mechanism of action of these agents appears to be related to their ability to block dopamine receptors in the central nervous system (CNS), particularly dopamine D_2 receptors in the basal ganglia and limbic portions of the forebrain. The earlier, less potent drugs, of which chlorpromazine is the prototype, cause more pronounced sedation, orthostatic hypotension, and cardiovascular toxicity. This is the result of a combination of anticholinergic, antihistaminic, and anti–α-adrenergic effects. The newer, more potent agents (e.g., haloperidol) are safer, especially in older patients, because of their relative lack of these adverse affects. However, these more potent drugs are associated with a higher incidence of extrapyramidal symptoms, such as dystonias, akathisia, akinesia, and rigidity.

The high frequency of severe adverse reactions, poor patient compliance, and the large number of patients with symptoms that are refractory to traditional antipsychotic agents have stimulated attempts to develop alternative agents. These "atypical" neuroleptic agents act by blocking serotonin to a greater extent than dopamine, resulting in a low incidence of extrapyramidal side effects. *Clozapine* has been found to be particularly effective in patients who have failed multiple trials with other antipsychotic drugs and is superior to other neuroleptic agents in reducing negative symptoms.[40] However, clozapine is expensive, has a side effect profile similar to the low-potency antipsychotic agents, and causes agranulocytosis in approximately 1% of patients.[37,39] As a result, it is currently recommended only for the treatment of patients with refractory psychosis. *Risperidone,* another newer neuroleptic agent with improved effects on negative symptoms, has been found to be superior to haloperidol in several short-term trials.[41-46] Because it is expensive, however, risperidone is also currently recommended for use only after conventional antipsychotics have failed.

Because of the high incidence of extrapyramidal symptoms in patients treated with high-potency neuroleptics, it is common practice to administer antiparkinsonian drugs (e.g., benztropine, procyclidine, trihexyphenidyl) at the same time, either to treat the adverse effects or to prevent them. Prophylactic treatment is most useful in patients with a history of extrapyramidal symptoms, those receiving high doses of high-potency antipsychotic agents, and those in whom the occurrence of these symptoms is likely to increase the risk of noncompliance.[47]

Noncompliance with antipsychotic medication remains a leading cause of psychiatric hospitalization. Patients with recurrent psychotic relapses caused by noncompliance are candidates for treatment with long-acting injectable antipsychotic drugs, usually given every 2 weeks. Two such agents available in the United States are fluphenazine decanoate and haloperidol decanoate.[48]

Box 104-4 Common Neuroleptic Agents

Low Potency
- Chlorpromazine (Thorazine)
- Chlorprothixene (Taractan)

Intermediate Potency
- Acetophenazine (Tindal)
- Loxapine (Loxitane)
- Mesoridazine (Serentil)
- Molindone (Moban)
- Perphenazine (Trilafon)
- Thioridazine (Mellaril)
- Triflupromazine (Vesprin)

High Potency
- Droperidol (Inapsine)
- Fluphenazine (Prolixin)
- Haloperidol (Haldol)
- Thiothixene (Navane)
- Trifluoperazine (Stelazine)

Atypical
- Clozapine (Clozaril)
- Olanzapine (Zyprexa)
- Quetiapine (Seroquel)
- Risperidone (Risperdal)

Complications of Neuroleptic Drug Therapy

Dystonia Acute dystonia, the most common adverse effect seen with neuroleptic agents, occurs in 1% to 5% of patients. This reaction is thought to be caused by a disruption of the dopaminergic-cholinergic balance in the nigrostriatal pathways of the basal ganglia, resulting in cholinergic dominance.[47] Dystonic reactions, which can occur at any point during long-term therapy and up to 48 hours after administration of neuroleptics in the ED, involve the sudden onset of involuntary contraction of the muscles of the face, neck, or back. The patient may have protrusion of the tongue (buccolingual crisis), deviation of the head to one side (acute torticollis), sustained upward deviation of the eyes (oculogyric crisis), extreme arching of the back (opisthotonos), or rarely laryngospasm. These symptoms tend to fluctuate, decreasing with voluntary activity and increasing under emotional stress, which occasionally misleads emergency physicians to believe they may be hysterical in nature.

Dystonic reactions should be treated with IM or IV benztropine (Cogentin), 1 to 2 mg, or diphenhydramine (Benadryl), 25 to 50 mg. IV administration usually results in an almost immediate reversal of symptoms. Patients should receive oral therapy with the same medication for 48 to 72 hours to prevent recurrent symptoms.[47]

Akathisia Akathisia is a state of motor restlessness characterized by a physical need to be moving constantly. It occurs most often in middle-age patients during the first few months after the initiation of therapy.[49] Patients are usually observed pacing the room and expressing a sense of inner tension that is not relieved by activity. If asked, they will state that they do not want to be constantly moving but feel physically compelled to do so. This reaction can easily be mistaken for a decompensating psychosis, leading to a vicious cycle in which more medication is given to treat a side effect caused by the same drug. This misdiagnosis can be avoided by carefully evaluating the patient for the exacerbation of positive psychotic symptoms, which are not increased by akathisia. Akathisia is treated with β-blockers (e.g., propranolol, 30 to 60 mg/day) or anticholinergic drugs (e.g., benztropine, 1 mg twice to four times daily). A new potential agent for the treatment of akathisia is glycine, a nonessential amino acid that stimulates glutamatergic neurotransmission.[50] In addition, if possible, the dosage of the antipsychotic agent should be lowered.

Pseudoparkinsonism and Akinesia A clinical picture that may be indistinguishable from Parkinson's disease can occur, particularly in elderly patients during the first month of therapy. Treatment with anticholinergic agents (e.g., benztropine) or antiparkinsonian drugs is usually effective. Akinesia, which is characterized by immobility, withdrawal, and lack of motivation, may be mistaken for a postpsychotic depression. It is responsive to antiparkinsonian drugs, but symptoms usually resolve gradually over time.

Tardive Dyskinesia The most feared neurologic complication of chronic neuroleptic drug treatment is tardive dyskinesia. This syndrome usually appears after several years of treatment and is characterized by involuntary movements, especially of the face and tongue, that are described as writhing, grimacing, and choreoathetoid in nature. The earliest manifestation is often a curling or twisting movement of the tongue. The onset of these symptoms can be falsely attributed to psychologic factors because they intensify under emotional stress, fatigue, and voluntary activity and disappear with sleep.

The reported prevalence of tardive dyskinesia is extremely variable, ranging from 0.4% to 56%, with a mean value of 20%.[36] The incidence of the disorder appears to be directly related to the duration of treatment, total cumulative dosage, evidence of preexisting brain damage, and age of the patient. It is more common in elderly women and patients with associated mood disorders. Once the syndrome has developed, there is no known effective treatment. Discontinuing or lowering the dosage of antipsychotic agents may result in a reversal of symptoms in some patients. Prescribing newer neuroleptics (e.g., clozapine) and co-treatment with benzodiazepines has also been successful in ameliorating symptoms.[51,52]

Orthostatic Hypotension All the antipsychotic agents are capable of causing orthostatic hypotension, an effect related to α-adrenergic blockade. This complication is seen much less with the more potent agents (e.g., haloperidol). Typically, episodes are mild in severity and brief in duration. Symptomatic patients should be treated with oxygen, Trendelenburg's position, and IV crystalloid fluid administration. Pressor agents (e.g., dopamine) should only be used for severe, symptomatic episodes that fail to respond to the previous measures; agents with β-agonist activity (e.g., epinephrine, isoproterenol) are contraindicated in these patients.

Neuroleptic Malignant Syndrome Neuroleptic malignant syndrome (NMS) is a life-threatening complication of neuroleptic drug treatment that affects 0.5% to 1% of patients.[53] It usually occurs in the first few weeks after initiation of treatment, but it can also be seen after a recent increase in drug dosage or after treatment with high doses of neuroleptic agents in the ED. NMS is characterized by high fever, severe muscle rigidity, altered consciousness, autonomic instability, and elevated serum creatine kinase levels. Additional complications can include respiratory failure, gastrointestinal hemorrhage, hepatic and renal failure, coagulopathy, and cardiovascular collapse.

The pathophysiology of NMS is not well understood but is thought to be related to dopamine depletion in the CNS, which leads to defective thermoregulation in the hypothalamus. Predisposing factors include exhaustion, dehydration, and the use of long-acting depot neuroleptics. Treatment consists of early recognition and discontinuation of the neuroleptic agent, fever reduction, rehydration with IV fluids, and general supportive measures. *Dantrolene,* a direct-acting muscle relaxant, should be used in severe cases. It can be administered by continuous rapid IV push at a minimum initial dose of 1 mg/kg, repeated until symptoms subside or up to a maximum cumulative dose of 10 mg/kg.[53] For severe symptoms, dopamine agonists such as bromocriptine, levodopa, and amantadine have shown encouraging results.[53] Because of earlier recognition and treatment, mortality rates with NMS have decreased from 30% to less than 10%.

DISPOSITION

The ultimate disposition of the acutely psychotic patient depends on the underlying cause of the psychosis, whether the patient is a danger to self or others, and the presence of social support in the community.[54-56] Hospitalization is indicated for patients experiencing their first psychotic episode, for patients deemed to be a danger to themselves (suicidal) or others (homicidal), for patients who are grossly debilitated, for patients who are moderately debilitated but have no social support system within the community, and for patients with either functional or organic psychosis that does not clear with a brief period of treatment and observation in the ED. The decision to hospitalize psychotic patients is complex and imprecise and often must be made in a short period with limited information.

A psychiatric short-procedure unit offers a cost-effective alternative to hospitalization.[57] After stabilization, patients are taken from the ED to a separate treatment area, where they are treated for a period of 12 to 24 hours by a small staff of consultants. This unit is used for rapid tranquilization, individual and family crisis intervention, amobarbital interviews, electroconvulsive therapy, and evaluation of patients for underlying medical problems.

KEY CONCEPTS

- In patients exhibiting abnormal behavior, an organic etiology is suggested by (1) new onset of symptoms in a patient over 35 years old, (2) rapid onset of symptoms in a previously normal person, (3) visual hallucinations, (4) abnormal vital signs, and (5) lethargy or disorientation.
- Physical restraints should be considered for patients who have exhibited violent behavior, verbally threaten staff, or demonstrate escalating agitation despite verbal attempts to calm them.
- Rapid tranquilization is best accomplished with the use of high-potency neuroleptics (e.g., haloperidol, droperidol). Benzodiazepines (e.g., lorazepam) are a helpful adjunct for patients with severe agitation.

REFERENCES

1. Jones P, Cannon M: The new epidemiology of schizophrenia, *Psychiatr Clin North Am* 21:1, 1998.
2. Tomlinson WK: Schizophrenia: history of an illness, *Psychiatry Med* 8:1, 1990.
3. Tueth MJ: Schizophrenia: Emil Kraepelin, Adolph Meyer, and beyond, *J Emerg Med* 13:805, 1995.
4. Lewis G et al: Schizophrenia and city life, *Lancet* 340:137, 1992.
5. Opler LA et al: Symptom profiles and homelessness in schizophrenia, *J Nerv Ment Dis* 182:174, 1994.
6. Passuk EL: The impact of deinstitutionalization on the general hospital psychiatric emergency ward, *Hosp Community Psychiatry* 31:623, 1980.
7. Genetics, epidemiology, and the search for causes of schizophrenia, *Am J Psychiatry* 151:3, 1994 (editorial).
8. Schwab SG et al: Support for a chromosome 18p locus conferring susceptibility to functional psychoses in families with schizophrenia, by association and linkage analysis, *Am J Hum Genet* 63:1139, 1998.
9. Michels R, Morzuk PM: Progress in psychiatry, *N Engl J Med* 329:552, 1993.
10. Lieberman JA et al: Serotonergic basis of antipsychotic drug effects in schizophrenia, *Biol Psychiatry* 44:1099, 1998.
11. Tandon R: Cholinergic aspects of schizophrenia, *Br J Psychiatry* S37:7, 1999.
12. Tamminga CA: Schizophrenia and glutamatergic transmission, *Crit Rev Neurobiol* 12:21, 1998.
13. Harrison PJ: The neuropathology of schizophrenia: a critical review of the data and their interpretation, *Brain* 122:593, 1999.
14. Crow TJ, Harrington CA: Etiopathogenesis and treatment of psychosis, *Annu Rev Med* 45:219, 1994.
15. *Diagnostic and statistical manual of mental disorders,* ed 4-TR, Washington, DC, 2000, American Psychiatric Association.
16. Olshaker JS et al: Medical clearance and screening of psychiatric patients in the emergency department, *Acad Emerg Med* 4:124, 1997.
17. Breslow RE, Klinger BI, Erickson BJ: Acute intoxication and substance abuse among patients presenting to a psychiatric emergency service, *Gen Hosp Psychiatry* 18:183, 1996.
18. Elangovan N et al: Substance abuse among patients presenting at an inner-city psychiatric emergency room, *Hosp Community Psychiatry* 44:782, 1993.
19. Dhossche D, Rubinstein J: Drug detection in a suburban psychiatric emergency room, *Ann Clin Psychiatry* 8:59, 1996.
20. Tintinalli JE, Peacock FW IV, Wright MA: Emergency medical evaluation of psychiatric patients, *Ann Emerg Med* 23:859, 1994.
21. Henneman PL, Mendoza R, Lewis RJ: Prospective evaluation of emergency department medical clearance, *Ann Emerg Med* 24:672, 1994.
22. Smith ML: Atypical psychosis, *Psychiatr Clin North Am* 4:895, 1998.
23. Hutto B: Subtle psychiatric presentations of endocrine diseases, *Psychiatr Clin North Am* 21:905, 1998.
24. Anderson WH, Kuehanle JC: Diagnosis and early management of acute psychosis, *N Engl J Med* 305:1128, 1989.
25. Frame DS, Kercher EE: Acute psychosis: functional vs. organic, *Emerg Med Clin North Am* 9:123, 1991.
26. Rund DA, Hutzler JC: *Emergency psychiatry,* St Louis, 1983, Mosby.
27. Smith TE, Docherty JP: Standards of care and clinical algorithms for treating schizophrenia, *Psychiatr Clin North Am* 21:203, 1998.
28. Hillard JR: Emergency treatment of acute psychosis, *J Clin Psychiatry* 59:57, 1998.
29. Battaglia J et al: Haloperidol, lorazepam, or both for psychotic agitation? A multicenter, prospective, double-blind, emergency department study, *Am J Emerg Med* 15:335, 1997.
30. Dubin WR: Rapid tranquilization of the violent patient, *Am J Emerg Med* 7:113, 1989.
31. Clinton JE et al: Haloperidol for sedation of disruptive emergency patients, *Ann Emerg Med* 16:19, 1987.
32. Thomas IT: Droperidol vs haloperidol for chemical restraint of agitated and combative patients, *Ann Emerg Med* 21:407, 1992.
33. Richards JR, Derlet RW, Duncan DR: Chemical restraint for the agitated patient in the emergency department: lorazepam versus droperidol, *J Emerg Med* 16:567, 1998.
34. Garza-Trevino R: Efficacy of the combination of intramuscular antipsychotics and sedatives-hypnotics for control of psychotic agitation, *Am J Psychiatry* 146:1598, 1989.
35. Salzman C et al: Benzodiazepines combined with neuroleptics for management of severe disruptive behavior, *Psychosomatics* 27:17, 1986.
36. Cain JM: Schizophrenia, *N Engl J Med* 334:34, 1996.
37. Alvir JM et al: Clozapine-induced agranulocytosis: incidence and risk factors in the United States, *N Engl J Med* 329:162, 1993.
38. Pickar D et al: Clinical and biologic response to clozapine in patients with schizophrenia, *Arch Gen Psychiatry* 49:345, 1992.
39. Meltzer HY et al: Cost-effectiveness of clozapine in neuroleptic-resistant schizophrenia, *Am J Psychiatry* 150:1630, 1993.
40. Breier A et al: Effects of clozapine on positive and negative symptoms in outpatients with schizophrenia, *Am J Psychiatry* 151:20, 1994.
41. Marder SR, Meibach RC: Risperidone in the treatment of schizophrenia, *Am J Psychiatry* 151:825, 1994.
42. Schooler NR: Negative symptoms in schizophrenia: assessment of the effect of risperidone, *J Clin Psychiatry* 55:22, 1994.
43. McEvoy JP: Efficacy of risperidone on positive features of schizophrenia, *J Clin Psychiatry* 55:18, 1994.
44. Tran PV et al: Double-blind comparison of olanzapine versus risperidone in the treatment of schizophrenia and other psychotic disorders, *J Clin Psychopharmacol* 17:407, 1997.
45. Breier AF et al: Clozapine and risperidone in chronic schizophrenia: effects on symptoms, parkinsonian side effects, and neuroendocrine response, *Am J Psychiatry* 156:294, 1999.
46. Leucht S et al: Efficacy and extrapyramidal side-effects of the new antipsychotics olanzapine, quetiapine, risperidone, and sertindole compared to conventional antipsychotics and placebo: a meta-analysis of randomized controlled trials, *Schizophr Res* 35:51, 1999.
47. Corre KA, Niemann JT, Bessen HA: Extended therapy for acute dystonic reactions, *Ann Emerg Med* 13:194, 1984.
48. Davis JM et al: Depot antipsychotic drugs: their place in therapy, *Drugs* 47:741, 1994.
49. Adler LA: Neuroleptic-induced akathisia: a review, *Psychopharmacology* 97:1, 1989.
50. Heresco-Levy U et al: Efficacy of high-dose glycine in the treatment of enduring negative symptoms of schizophrenia, *Arch Gen Psychiatry* 56:29, 1999.
51. Shapleske J, Mickay AP, Mckenna PJ: Successful treatment of tardive dystonia with clozapine and clonazepam, *Br J Psychiatry* 168:516, 1996.
52. Carpenter WR et al: Diazepam treatment of early signs of exacerbation in schizophrenia, *Am J Psychiatry* 156:299, 1999.
53. Gratz SS, Levinson DF, Simpson GM: Neuroleptic malignant syndrome. In Cain JM, Liberman JA, editors: *Adverse effects of psychotropic drugs,* New York, 1992, Guilford.
54. Hoehn-Saric R, Hatcher ME, Weiskopf C: Disposition of psychiatric emergencies: patient characteristics associated with hospitalization, *Ann Emerg Med* 9:605, 1980.
55. Marson DC, McGovern MP, Pomp HC: Psychiatric decision making in the emergency room: a research overview, *Am J Psychiatry* 145:918, 1988.
56. Hillard JR, Slomowitz M, Deddens J: Determination of emergency psychiatric admission for adolescents and adults, *Am J Psychiatry* 145:1416, 1988.
57. Dubin WR, Fink PJ: The psychiatric short-procedure unit: a cost-saving innovation, *Hosp Community Psychiatry* 37:227, 1986.

105 Mood Disorders

Douglas A. Rund
Marshall G. Vary

PERSPECTIVE

Happiness and sorrow are common emotions but usually cause no impairment in functioning or threat to life. Mood disorder, by contrast, can significantly impair physical, social, and family functioning and can cause psychologic pain, physical pain, and a negative perception of physical health. The term *mood disorders* has replaced "affective disorders" in the fourth edition of the *Diagnostic and Statistical Manual of Mental Disorders* (*DSM-IV-TR*).[1] *Mood* refers to an "enduring emotional orientation that colors the person's psychology," whereas *affect* normally refers to "the outward and changeable manifestation of a person's emotional tone."[2] *Dysphoria* means depressed mood or feeling. The *DSM-IV-TR* assigns psychiatric diagnoses to patients by assessing specific observable and measurable symptoms and signs, facilitating appropriate psychiatric evaluation and communication with psychiatric consultants. Research regarding the neurobiology of mood disorders and genetics may ultimately permit classification of mood disorders by specific, genetically predisposed pathophysiologic derangements.

Epidemiology

In the 1994 National Comorbidity Survey of Psychiatric Disorders the most common psychiatric disorders were major depression and alcohol dependence.[3] Overall, 17.1% of respondents (21.3% of women and 12.7% of men) reported a major depressive episode during their life. In ED patients the overall prevalence of mood disorders is at least 23%.[4] Patients with chronic illness have a much higher prevalence of undiagnosed depression than the general population.[5,6] The lifetime suicide risk for persons with major untreated depressive illness is 15%.[7] Mood disorders are becoming more common, occur at earlier ages, and have increased in every generation born after 1910.[8]

The prevalence of bipolar disorders (manic-depressive disorders) is substantially lower than that of major depression. In the National Comorbidity Study the overall lifetime prevalence of a manic episode was 1.6% (1.7% for women and 1.6% for men). Mood disorders often coexist with other psychiatric disorders, such as anxiety, substance abuse, and attention deficit.

PRINCIPLES OF DISEASE

Current neurobiologic concepts provide the basis for various pharmacologic treatments. The psychosocial theories of depression consider the complex interaction of genetics, environment, and experience, providing the basis for understanding the various psychotherapeutic approaches to treatment.

Neurotransmitters

In the fourth century BC, Hippocrates believed that the body contained four essential humors: blood, phlegm, yellow bile, and black bile. Harmony in the brain required a harmony of humors. "Disharmony" produced mental illness. In the second century AD, Galen believed that "melancholia" resulted from an excess of black bile acting on the brain. Such excesses were caused by noxious stomach vapors, grief, anxiety, excessive wine, and advancing age. Proposed treatments included bloodletting, surgery, special diets, and exercise.[9]

Neurons interact at synapses, where neurotransmitters released at presynaptic sites interact with receptors at postsynaptic sites. Neurotransmitters identified thus far include the biogenic amines (norepinephrine, epinephrine, serotonin, dopamine, glutamine, histamine, acetylcholine, gamma-aminobutyric acid, glycerin), certain neuropeptides, and neurotropic factors.

Theories regarding mood disorders and monoamine neurotransmitters (e.g., norepinephrine) were developed more than 30 years ago.[10,11] *Reserpine,* an antihypertensive medication, depleted cerebral concentrations of norepinephrine and caused clinical depression in a large proportion of patients. *Imipramine,* by increasing cerebral concentrations of norepinephrine at various synaptic sites, alleviated symptoms of depression.

Complex processes in the nervous system cause depression or mania. If the concentrations of neurotransmitters at synaptic sites were the only factors responsible for alleviation of depression, the therapeutic effect of an antidepressant agent would be almost immediate. However, clinical improvement with these agents takes several weeks. Emphasis has now shifted to the study of neurobehavioral systems, intricate regulatory mechanisms, development of preferred neural circuits, and gene transcriptors.[12]

Cerebral Anatomy

Certain areas of the brain are involved in processes that become abnormal during depressive episodes and mania.[13] Stress activates neurons in the *locus ceruleus,* resulting in increased alertness, decreased appetite, increased heart rate, increased cortisol production, and other features of a stress response. The response can be dampened by neurons in the cerebral cortex. Prolonged stress, from which escape appears hopeless, seems to decrease the activity of neurons in the locus ceruleus. Another noradrenergic system, the *medial forebrain bundle,* elicits reward-seeking behavior when stimulated. Prolonged stress decreases levels of norepinephrine in this region and may explain the lack of energy and interest that accompany depression.[14,15]

Serotonergic neurons are located in the brainstem dorsal raphe and project diffusely throughout the brain. The serotonergic system seems to enhance sleep, appetite, libido, and circadian rhythms. Activation decreases aggressive behavior in animal models.[16,17]

Dopaminergic pathways include the tuberoinfundibular

system, originating in the hypothalamus (prolactin secretion); the nigrostriatal system, originating in the substantia nigra (involuntary motor activity); the mesolimbic pathway, in the ventral tegmentum; and the mesocortical pathway, originating in the ventral tegmentum.[18] These pathways regulate emotion, pleasure, learning, and reinforcement. The mesocortical pathway extends to frontal cortical regions that regulate complex cognition concentration and motivation.[19]

Endocrine System

The cortical-hypothalamic-pituitary-adrenocortical system is affected in many patients with depression, causing increased levels of plasma cortisol, apparently from an impaired biofeedback loop regulating cortisol. The thyroid axis malfunctions in 5% to 10% of depressed patients. Thyroid-stimulating hormone levels are elevated, and thyroid replacement therapy facilitates treatment in certain patients.[20]

Genetics

Family studies have repeatedly demonstrated a relationship between genetic inheritance and mood disorders.[21] Monozygotic and dizygotic twins have a high concordance rate, 70% and 35%, respectively, for mood disorder.[22] The mechanisms of genetic transmission are still undetermined but may relate to the synthesis, transport, and action of serotonin.[23,24] The inherited susceptibility to depression may manifest only during severe stress or serious illness.[25]

Psychosocial Theories

The complex neural mechanism that regulates mood responds to and is modified by each person's experience, including events in early childhood, reward and punishment during growth and development, interpersonal relationships, and various kinds of loss. Psychosocial theories of mood disorder form the basis for psychotherapy. Freud noted that personal loss included grief and sadness, but that depression also involved guilt and lowered self-esteem.[26] Freud theorized that suicide in depressed patients is a manifestation of aggression that has been turned against the self in a person otherwise unable to express anger toward loved ones.

The interpersonal theory of depression emphasizes guilt, disputes between partners and family members, role transitions in families and relationships, and problems with social skills necessary to sustain a fulfilling relationship. Cognitive theories have also been applied to depressed individuals, especially when the content of a depressed person's thought involves self-blame, hopelessness, and helplessness. The concept of "learned helplessness" first developed when animals were blocked from escape and subjected to repeated noxious stimuli such as electric shock. They eventually stopped trying to escape and became apathetic, even when escape became available.[27] The concept was later applied to humans and adapted to construct a behavioral mode of therapy for depression.

CLINICAL FEATURES

Major Depressive Disorder

Major depressive disorder is characterized by one or more major depressive episodes, as defined by *DSM-IV-TR* criteria (Boxes 105-1 and 105-2). A major depressive episode is characterized by disturbances in four major areas: mood, psychomotor activity, cognition, and vegetative function.[28]

Box 105-1 Summary of *DSM-IV* Criteria for Major Depressive Episode

A. Five or more of the following symptoms present almost every day during the same 2-week period and representing a change from previous functioning; at least one of the symptoms is either (1) depressed mood or (2) loss of interest or pleasure. **NOTE:** Do not include symptoms caused by a general medical condition, and do not include mood-incongruent delusions or hallucinations.
   1. Depressed mood (can be irritable mood in children and adolescents)
   2. Loss of interest or pleasure in activities
   3. Significant weight loss when not dieting or weight gain or decrease or increase in appetite
   4. Insomnia or hypersomnia
   5. Psychomotor agitation or retardation
   6. Fatigue or loss of energy
   7. Feelings of worthlessness or excessive or inappropriate guilt
   8. Diminished ability to think or concentrate, or indecisiveness
   9. Recurrent thoughts of death (not just fear of dying), recurrent suicidal ideation, or a suicide plan or attempt

B. Symptoms do not meet criteria for a "mixed episode."

C. Symptoms cause clinically significant distress or impairment in social, occupational, or other functioning.

D. Symptoms are not caused by direct physiologic effects of a substance (e.g., drug of abuse, medication) or a general medical condition (e.g., hypothyroidism).

E. Symptoms are not better accounted for by bereavement; after the loss of a loved one, the symptoms persist for longer than 2 months or are characterized by marked functional impairment, morbid preoccupation with worthlessness, suicidal ideation, psychotic symptoms, or psychomotor retardation.

Modified from the *Diagnostic and statistical manual of mental disorders,* ed 4-TR, Washington, DC, 2000, American Psychiatric Association.

Box 105-2 Factors in Evaluating Depression: "In SAD CAGES"

Interest
Sleep
Appetite
Depressed mood
Concentration
Activity
Guilt
Energy
Suicide

The patient must exhibit or experience at least five symptoms for a minimum of 2 weeks.

Mood Disturbances Depressed mood is painful and referred to as being anguished, sad, gloomy, dejected, unhappy, discouraged, or in low spirits. The mood may also involve feelings of anxiety and irritability. The patient's feelings can be so intensely painful that suicide may be seen as the only way to terminate the agony.

Anhedonia refers to the inability to experience pleasure or interest in formerly pleasurable or satisfying activities. The patient must have actually stopped doing the formerly pleasurable activities, for example, the formerly avid tennis or golf player gives up playing entirely. Questions can help to elicit loss of interest or pleasure: "When were you last feeling well?"; "When you were feeling well, what kinds of things did you do for enjoyment?"; "Are you doing those things now?"; and "Are you enjoying them?"[29]

Change in Psychomotor Activity Psychomotor disturbances may take the form of retardation or agitation. *Psychomotor retardation* includes significant slowing of thought processes and physical activity. The patient is slow to answer questions and moves slowly or not at all. Questioning such patients in the ED may be frustrating when the answers come slowly, in short words or phrases, and are low in volume and lack inflection. The "body language" of depression includes sitting slumped over, arms folded, mouth turned down, and eyes closed or downcast. Such slowing clearly affects the patient's work, school, or family functioning. Symptoms may be erroneously attributed to worsening dementia in elderly persons. An alternative presentation is *psychomotor agitation,* in which the patient fidgets, paces, rubs the skin, and is unable to sit still. Other common, almost stereotypical manifestations include hand wringing and tugging at the hair.

Vegetative symptoms include disturbances in three major areas: sleep, appetite, and sexual function. Depressed patients typically report some form of sleep disorder, such as difficulty falling asleep, middle insomnia, or the classic symptoms of early-morning wakening and inability to fall back asleep. Some depressed patients may report sleeping 12 to 14 hours a day and inability to arise in the morning. This may be a more common symptom in depressed teenagers. The depressed patient may lose appetite and weight or may gain weight in a short time. Loss of interest in sexual activity and impotence can be considered vegetative symptoms; they may accompany depression or may be part of the anhedonia associated with depressed mood.

Cognitive Dysfunction Depressed patients are unable to concentrate or think properly, which can cause significant dysfunction in a job or profession. Thought content is negative, such as recurrent thoughts of guilt, failure, worthlessness, and self-criticism. Suicide may preoccupy the patient's thinking and may reinforce feelings of helplessness, perpetuating self-reproach. The patient may formulate a definite plan for ending life. Depressed patients must be questioned about suicidal thoughts and plans, which allows them to describe their pain and may provide them with some relief (see Chapter 109).

Psychosis Psychosis may accompany severe depression. Hallucinations and delusions are classified as mood congruent or mood incongruent. *Mood-congruent* delusions reflect the depressed mood. The patient may report, for example, being "already dead" or feeling like "my insides have rotted away." Hallucinations typically consist of voices saying extremely unpleasant things or punishing the patient for previous wrongs. *Mood-incongruent* delusions do not reflect the depressed mood as clearly and include the paranoid delusions of being followed and having one's thoughts controlled by external forces.

Masked Depression Mood disorders may not be clear at presentation. The depressed patient may have only vague physical symptoms, such as weakness, fatigue, headache, or complaints of pain. Patients may not be aware of their depression and may appear to be frank hypochondriacs. Such symptoms may be the presenting features of a masked, or *hidden,* depression. Clues suggesting mood disturbance include the recent onset of a set of unusual behaviors, trouble at work or job loss, marital difficulties, or self-destructive behavior (e.g., substance abuse, sexual promiscuity).

Children and Adolescents A common and overt presentation of depression in an older child or teenager is a suicide attempt. Such patients should be considered depressed and unstable until subsequent assessment differentiates depression from other conditions in these age groups, including transient psychoses, anxiety disorders, high levels of life stress, and substance abuse.

Symptoms of depression in children and adolescents generally follow the same criteria as for adults. Some children are misdiagnosed as having attention deficit disorder, especially if symptoms involve poor concentration, listlessness, agitation, and withdrawal from daily activities. Depression in these age groups can be misunderstood, masked in its presentation, or simply overlooked by friends, parents, teachers, and physicians. Adequate treatment maximizes the child's potential and minimizes the serious negative impact depression can have on multiple spheres of development. An overdose that "clears" is only the tip of a major issue for each child or adolescent patient and the family.

Elderly Persons Depression is common in elderly persons; losses and grief, serious health issues, and loss of autonomy create a setting conducive to depression. The classic symptoms of moderate to severe depression, with or without psychosis, are typically seen. Depressed patients can present with symptoms involving memory loss, inattention, withdrawal from daily activities, confusion, and lapses in personal and social hygiene that suggest dementia rather than depression. When such symptoms result from depression, the condition is called *pseudodementia.* Serious depression in elderly patients is a highly treatable, reversible condition. Distinguishing it from dementia is essential for further diagnostic and therapeutic follow-up.

Other Depressive Disorders

Seasonal Affective Disorder Seasonal affective disorder is a subclassification of major depressive disorder that is diagnosed when major depression occurs during seasons with less daylight (fall and winter), then either resolves or changes to manic episodes in seasons with more daylight, for at least 2 consecutive years. Phototherapy is an effective and safe treatment for this "winter depression,"[30] which appears to be mediated by ultraviolet radiation through the retina.

Postpartum Depression Symptoms of depression are common in the postnatal period. Up to 65% of mothers report some depressed mood after childbirth, often called "baby blues." Almost one quarter of mothers feel "moderately depressed" or "very depressed" in the postpartum period. Forty-four percent of these women report symptoms lasting a few days; 16% have symptoms a few months; and 3.9% are still depressed 1 year after the birth; 1.5% report thoughts of suicide.[31]

Postpartum depression seems to be more prevalent in those who have mood disorder, are unemployed, or have no assistance with infant care. Severe postpartum depression may negatively influence development in the child.[32]

Dysthymic Disorder Dysthymic disorder is a long-standing, fluctuating, low-grade depression. Some features of a major depressive episode may be present, but marked changes in appetite or psychomotor disturbance are not typically observed. Depressed mood typically begins early in life, and the individual may report having always been depressed. Affected individuals typically are able to carry out their work assignments diligently, but they gain little pleasure from the leisure activities others find enjoyable, such as recreation, time with family, or sexual activity.

Bipolar Disorders

Bipolar disorder is lifelong, with episodic exacerbation of symptoms and deterioration of function characterized by extreme mood swings. Patients with bipolar disorder thus require different forms and intensities of treatment at different times. *Bipolar I disorder* includes at least one *manic* episode, and patients have typically had one or more major depressive episodes. *Bipolar II disorder* involves a *hypomanic* episode and at least one major depressive episode. A hypomanic episode includes the features of a manic episode without psychosis, marked impairment of function, or the need for hospitalization.

Manic Episode As defined by *DSM-IV-TR* criteria (Box 105-3), to be considered manic the disturbance must be severe enough to cause psychosis, the need for hospitalization, or marked impairment in functioning. Bipolar disorders are much less common than major depressive disorder. The overall prevalence of a manic episode is 1.6% in both women and men.[33]

Patients who are experiencing a manic episode may be gregarious, humorous, and engaging. An alternative presentation is one of belligerence and irritability. Initial clues to mania include a history of the patient's behavior immediately before the evaluation and any prior history of bipolar disorder or a history of taking medications almost exclusively prescribed for bipolar disorder, such as lithium. In most cases the manic patient will be brought to the ED by someone else (e.g., family, police, emergency medical services). They often try to leave as soon as possible, display impaired judgment and impulsivity, and may need to be restrained.

Pressured speech is one of the first clinical signs of mania. The patient keeps talking, with no interruption between thoughts or sentences. The speech may be loud and rapid, with creative, amusing, or trivial and irrelevant content. The patient may tell jokes, use puns, or play other word association games. A hallmark of mania is *grandiosity,* which involves feelings of inflated self-esteem and great personal importance. The patient may describe a massive undertaking such as "uniting the world's churches" or "solving world poverty."

Box 105-3 Summary of *DSM-IV* Criteria for Manic Episode

A. Distinct period of abnormally and persistently elevated, expansive, or irritable mood, lasting at least 2 weeks (or any duration if hospitalization is necessary).
B. During the period of mood disturbance, three or more of the following symptoms have persisted (four if the mood is only irritable) and have been present to a significant degree:
   1. Inflated self-esteem or grandiosity
   2. Decreased need for sleep (e.g., feels rested after only 3 hours of sleep)
   3. More talkative than usual or pressure to keep talking
   4. Flight of ideas or subjective experience that thoughts are racing
   5. Distractibility (i.e., attention too easily drawn to unimportant or irrelevant external stimuli)
   6. Increase in goal-directed activity (either socially, at work or school, or sexually) or psychomotor agitation
   7. Excessive involvement in pleasurable activities that have a high potential for painful consequences (e.g., buying sprees, sexual indiscretions, foolish investments)
C. Symptoms do not meet criteria for a "mixed episode."
D. Mood disturbance is sufficiently severe to cause marked impairment in occupational functioning or social activities or to necessitate hospitalization to prevent harm to self or others, or psychotic features are present.
E. Symptoms are not caused by direct physiologic effects of a substance (e.g., drug of abuse, medication) or a general medical condition (e.g., hyperthyroidism).

Modified from the *Diagnostic and statistical manual of mental disorders,* ed 4-TR, Washington, DC, 2000, American Psychiatric Association.

Manic patients have decreased or no need for sleep and typically report being awake for days during a manic episode. They may be involved in a massive project (e.g., writing a novel), may completely disregard consequences of actions, may have difficulty with spending (e.g., credit cards revoked), and may engage in risky behavior (e.g., sexual liaisons with strangers, risky driving) An accurate history must be obtained from family or others who know the patient's behavior.

Manic patients may present to the ED as trauma patients, injured by an action reflecting the patient's grandiosity (e.g., attempting to fly), impulsivity, or belligerence (e.g., fighting, resisting arrest). A manic episode may be punctuated by abrupt periods of tearfulness and profound depression, including suicidal ideation. When depressive and manic features occur concurrently in such a manner, the disorder is termed *mixed* or *bipolar, mixed phase.*

Cyclothymic Disorder Cyclothymic disorder is characterized by a life of mood swings of insufficient severity to meet criteria for a bipolar disorder. Persons with this disorder may have a chaotic life, characterized by frequent mood swings, unstable relationships, and uneven school or work performance.

Box 105-4 Medical Illnesses Associated with Onset of Depression

Neurologic

Parkinson's disease
Stroke
Multiple sclerosis
Head trauma
Sleep apnea

Neoplastic

Pancreatic carcinoma
Brain tumor
Disseminated carcinomatosis

Endocrine

Hypothyroidism
Hyperthyroidism
Cushing's disease
Addison's disease
Diabetes mellitus

Infectious

Human immunodeficiency virus (HIV)

Cardiac

Coronary artery disease
Myocardial infarction

Renal

End-stage renal disease
Renal dialysis

Connective Tissue

Lupus erythematosus
Rheumatoid arthritis

Substance Abuse

Alcohol
Drugs of abuse

Mood Disorders Caused by General Medical Condition

Certain medical illnesses have a well-known association with mood disorder (Box 105-4). In Parkinson's disease, electrical stimulation to a certain area of the substantia nigra alleviates symptoms of depression. Stimulation of an area only 2 mm away can cause acute reversible symptoms of depression, such as crying, not wanting to live, and hopelessness.[34] Parkinson's disease has a well-known association with depression, with up to 40% of parkinsonian patients demonstrating major depression.[35] Further elucidation of neurologic disease will add to the understanding of mood disorders.

Certain malignancies have a well-known association with the onset of depression, including pancreatic carcinoma, brain neoplasm, and disseminated malignancy (e.g., lymphoma).[36] Coronary artery disease,[37] myocardial infarction (MI), end-stage renal disease, acquired immunodeficiency syndrome (AIDS), several endocrine diseases, and connective tissue disease are also associated with major depressive disorder.[38]

Two issues arise in the assessment of patients with depression and serious medical illness (e.g., malignancy, AIDS). First, depression must be distinguished from the symptoms and signs (e.g., weight loss, loss of energy, slowing of activity, sleep disturbance, loss of ability to concentrate) associated with serious medical illness. Alternative criteria for depression can be substituted for *DSM-IV-TR* criteria in patients with serious medical illness: *depressed appearance* for loss of appetite, *social withdrawal* for sleep disturbance, *pessimism* or *self-pity* for energy loss, and *nonreactive mood* for difficulty concentrating.[39] Second, it is important to determine whether the depression associated with terminal, rapidly progressive, or painful illness is understandable or appropriate. Although patients with such diseases may understandably be sad, most do not have major depression. The treatment of major depression in such patients can greatly improve their quality of life.

Mood Disorders Caused by Medications or Other Substances

Certain medications are associated with symptoms of mood disorders (Box 105-5). A medication-induced mood disorder should be considered if the patient has no history of depression before taking the medication.

Intoxication or chronic heavy use of depressants, such as alcohol, sedatives, hypnotics, anxiolytics, and narcotics, can cause symptoms of a major depressive episode; stimulants such as cocaine, phencyclidine (PCP), hallucinogens, and amphetamines can cause symptoms of a manic episode. Mood disorder symptoms can also develop during withdrawal. The symptoms must not occur exclusively during delirium and must cause significant distress or impairment of functioning to qualify for this diagnosis.

When the mood disorder predates the period of substance abuse or lasts longer than 1 month after the period of abuse, the diagnosis may be an underlying mood disorder, such as a major depressive disorder or bipolar disorder, with a comorbid substance abuse or dependence diagnosis.

Substance abuse is typically seen in patients who self-treat underlying depressive symptoms, especially adolescents.

DIAGNOSTIC STRATEGIES

The initial history and physical examination should focus on the presenting complaints and evaluate the possibility that drug abuse, medications, or a general medical condition may be responsible for the patient's condition. The diagnosis of a mood disorder is based on history and observation of the patient's ability and style in relating to family and medical staff. The patient's body language may be helpful. Precipitating events (e.g., loss of job or relationship), accompanying symptoms (e.g., hallucinations, delusions, anxiety disorder, mania), and suicidal intent should be investigated. The patient's history should be confirmed through interviews with family, friends or eyewitnesses to the events that precipitated the ED visit. A tentative diagnosis can be established using *DSM-IV-TR* criteria. Laboratory tests to investigate medical conditions may be necessary (see Box 105-4), but no tests can confirm or exclude mood disorders.

DIFFERENTIAL CONSIDERATIONS

Medical disorders, medications, and substance abuse or withdrawal not only can cause but also can mimic mood disorders. The patient who presents with agitation, for example, might have hypoxia, cocaine intoxication, or

Box 105-5 Medications That Can Cause Depressive or Manic Symptoms

Depressive Symptoms

Antihypertensives

β-Blockers
Captopril
Clonidine
Diltiazem
Enalapril
Nifedipine
Prazosin
Thiazide diuretics

Anticonvulsants

Phenytoin
Valproic acid

Hormones

Anabolic steroids
Contraceptives
Corticosteroids
Thyroid hormone

Sedative-Hypnotics

Barbiturates
Benzodiazepines

Manic Symptoms

Psychiatric agents

Antidepressants
Bupropion
Loxapine
Monoamine oxidase inhibitors (MAOIs)

Antibiotics

Acyclovir
Chloroquine
Interferon
Isoniazid
Norfloxacin
Ofloxacin
Sulfonamides

Other agents

Amantadine
Bromocriptine
Cyclobenzaprine
Cycloserine
Digitalis
Disopyramide
Levodopa
Metoclopramide
Nonsteroidal antiinflammatory drugs
Phenylpropanolamine
Theophylline
Thyroid hormone

alcohol-sedative withdrawal. The patient with symptoms and signs of depression may have an unrecognized malignancy or sedative intoxication.

Antidepressant medications are used to treat a variety of psychiatric and medical disorders, such as anxiety, obsessive-compulsive disorder, posttraumatic stress disorder, smoking cessation, and vasodepressor syncope. As a result, the EP should not automatically assume that a patient taking antidepressant medication is being treated for depression.

Grief and bereavement are normal human reactions to the acute loss of another person, health, social position, or job. The period of mourning is characterized by sadness, diminished sense of well-being (somatic complaints), sleeplessness, and sadness triggered by thoughts of the loss. Normal grief, however, does not include guilt, loss of self-esteem, feelings of worthlessness, suicidal intent, psychomotor retardation, or occupational dysfunction.

Adjustment disorders are behavioral or emotional disorders that occur in response to an identifiable stress or stressors. The emotional component can involve sadness, low self-esteem, suicidal behavior, hopelessness, helplessness, or other self-threatening behavior. Acute adjustment disorder occurs within 3 months of the stressor and does not last longer than 6 months. The stressors are typically not as severe as those precipitating bereavement reaction, and the responses are often more maladaptive. The teenager who ends a romantic relationship, for instance, may attempt drug overdose in response to the stress. In such cases, adjustment disorder is a more likely diagnosis than major depressive episode. The pattern of recurrent maladaptive behavioral responses to stress may be lifelong, but the acute episode should resolve within 6 months.

Borderline personality disorder is characterized by unstable personal relationships, unstable self-image, and inappropriate behaviors. The disorder may include chronic feelings of emptiness, which may be misdiagnosed as depression, or lability of mood, which may be mistaken for mania or hypomania.

Dementia may be confused with depression. Dementia is characterized by abnormal mental status, including abnormalities in tests of memory, calculation, and judgment. Delirium with waxing and waning sensorium, hallucinations, and delusions may involve agitation and restlessness, which might first be considered features of mania or depression.

Differential considerations for manic symptoms include the manic phase of bipolar disorder, stimulant abuse (e.g., cocaine, amphetamines), hallucinogen abuse, alcohol or sedative withdrawal, delirium, hyperthyroidism, other medical conditions causing agitation, brief reactive psychosis, schizoaffective disorder, and schizophrenia.

MANAGEMENT

Emergency Department Stabilization

The creation of a safe and stable environment must be a first priority in management. The patient with an acute manic episode may be disruptive, refuse medical evaluation, and make repeated attempts to leave the ED. Hospital security personnel should be summoned early and, depending on the patient's behavior, can remain to show that disruptive behavior will not be tolerated. When necessary, security personnel can apply physical restraints and search the patient for weapons.

Initiation of treatment for mood disorders is not typically done in the ED. An exception is the acute manic episode with behavior so extreme that the patient or others are threatened. Haloperidol and droperidol are effective agents (see Chapter 104).[40] A typical treatment regimen begins with an intramuscular injection of 5 mg of haloperidol (Haldol). The patient is

Box 105-6 Criteria for Hospitalization of ED Patient with Acute Psychiatric Episode

- Patient demonstrates risk for suicide or homicide or for significant harm to self or others.
- Patient lacks the capacity to cooperate with treatment.
- Patient has inadequate psychosocial support for safe outpatient treatment and compliance.
- Patient has a comorbid condition or complication that makes outpatient treatment unsafe (e.g., acute psychosis, bizarre behavior, need for detoxification).

then monitored for improvement in hallucinations, delusions, agitation, or violent behavior, and another 5-mg dose is administered after 30 to 60 minutes as needed. Most patients respond after a few doses. Benztropine (Cogentin), 1 to 2 mg, is often given initially to prevent extrapyramidal symptoms. Immediate psychiatric consultation should begin during the initiation of rapid tranquilization, since patients undergoing rapid tranquilization will generally require hospitalization (Box 105-6).

Long-Term Treatment

Depression Long-term treatment modalities for depression can be grouped into three broad categories: antidepressant medication, psychotherapy, and electroconvulsive therapy (ECT).

Antidepressant Therapy Many equally effective antidepressants are available for first-episode uncomplicated major depression. After 4 to 6 weeks of therapy the response rate is usually 60% or greater for all agents. However, 10% to 15% of patients quit medication trials,[41] and many patients in general medical practice are inadequately treated.[42]

Coexistent medical illness, psychotic or bipolar symptoms, substance use, and recurrent or refractory depressive symptoms must be considered in the choice of a medication for treatment of depression. Sensitivity to the side effects of the tricyclic antidepressants and the significant risks of serious side effects with monoamine oxidase inhibitors (MAOIs), along with strict dietary limitations, have led to a significant rise in the use of selective serotonin-reuptake inhibitors (SSRIs) as first-line treatment for depression. Side effects of SSRIs include dizziness, sedation, peripheral anticholinergic symptoms, weight gain, sexual dysfunction, neurologic symptoms, cardiovascular symptoms, insomnia, and anxiety. Another antidepressant, ECT, thyroid hormone, or other psychoactive medication may be added in patients with treatment-resistant depression.[43]

Psychotherapy Brief psychotherapy based on the cognitive-behavioral approach is often initially employed in patients with major depression. Interpersonal psychotherapy, psychodynamic psychotherapy, and group or marital/family therapy are also used with some patients.[44] Psychosocial therapeutic support typically includes community-based support groups that focus on specific individual, occupational, or family/marital issues that arise in depression and are amenable to group and supportive intervention.[45-47]

Depressed patients benefit most from a combination of somatic therapy (medication and/or ECT) and psychotherapy. All patients with incomplete therapeutic response, recurrent depression, or comorbid conditions (e.g., anxiety/panic, substance abuse) should receive multimodal treatment.[48]

Electroconvulsive Therapy ECT has a high therapeutic success rate and an excellent safety profile but is not a first-line treatment for uncomplicated major depression. In part, this is a result of an undeserved reputation among laypersons that ECT causes "permanent brain damage." Indications for ECT include severe depression with malnutrition, severe psychosis with agitation, continuing significant suicide risk with ongoing suicidal behaviors, and prolonged catatonia. ECT is used as first-line treatment for patients with recurrent depression who previously had a positive response to ECT. ECT is more often used as a second-line treatment for patients with moderate to severe depression who have not responded to trials of medication or who cannot tolerate the medication because of side effects or concurrent medical conditions.[49]

Bipolar Disorders The primary treatment of bipolar disorder are the mood stabilizers, including lithium, valproate, and carbamazepine. Almost all bipolar patients require a mood stabilizer during exacerbation of depression or mania, and most patients benefit from a mood stabilizer for ongoing supportive maintenance treatment as well. *Lithium* was the first highly effective mood-stabilizing agent used in the treatment of bipolar patients.[50] *Valproate* is a very effective mood stabilizer with dose-related side effects, most of which clear after an initial period of treatment or with reduced dosage.[51] Valproate may be instituted rapidly in acutely manic bipolar patients.[52] Both lithium and valproate serum levels are routinely monitored during therapy. The therapeutic window is much wider for valproate than for lithium. Carbamazepine also produces dose-related side effects but has potentially lethal reactions as well, including blood dyscrasias, exfoliative dermatitis, pancreatitis, and hepatic failure. These conditions are rare and are not reliably predicted by laboratory monitoring.

Mood-stabilizing medications usually take 3 or more weeks to become effective.[53] Some bipolar patients require antipsychotic medications and benzodiazepines in the interim to control symptoms. Some patients with bipolar disorder have persistent psychotic symptoms requiring continuing use of a major neuroleptic, such as haloperidol, olanzapine (Zyprexa), or quetiapine (Seroquel).[54] After 3 weeks a second mood-stabilizing medication or ECT is often added for patients who have a partial response to an initial mood-stabilizing course of treatment.[55] For bipolar patients with a depressive episode, the addition of an antidepressant medication is often helpful.

Bipolar patients are sensitive to psychosocial stressors, changes in medication dosage, and medical illness. This sensitivity can lead to a marked worsening in a patient's level of adaptation and functioning. It is helpful to understand these precipitating stressors when developing a therapeutic support plan for patients. Psychosocial therapeutic support, including individual psychotherapy, supportive community groups, family/marital treatment, and occupational support, can be important in both the acute phase and the maintenance phase of treatment for bipolar patients.

KEY CONCEPTS

- Patients with apparent mood disorders should be evaluated for a medical disorder, medication effect, or drug use that can mimic both depression and mania.
- Mood disorders should be suspected in patients with multiple, vague, nonspecific complaints.
- The differentiation of depression and dementia in elderly patients can be difficult but is important, since depression often responds dramatically to treatment, whereas dementia does not respond.
- Patients with mood disorders should be assessed for their potential for violence or self-harm before discharge from the ED.

REFERENCES

1. *Diagnostic and statistical manual of medical disorders,* ed 4-TR, Washington, DC, 2000, American Psychiatric Association.
2. Dubovsky SL, Buron R: Mood disorders. In *Textbook of psychiatry,* ed 3, Washington, DC, 1999, American Psychiatric Press.
3. Kessler RC et al: Lifetime and 12-month prevalence of DSM-III-R psychiatric disorders in the United States: results from the National Comorbidity Survey, *Arch Gen Psychiatry* 51:8, 1994.
4. Summers WK et al: Psychiatric illness in a general urban emergency room: daytime vs. nighttime population, *J Clin Psychiatry* 341:19, 1979.
5. Cassem EH: Depressive disorders in the medically ill: an overview, *Psychosomatics* 36:S2, 1995.
6. Katon W et al: Distressed high utilizers of medical care, *Gen Hosp Psychiatry* 12:355, 1990.
7. Mueller TI, Deon AC: Recovery, chronicity and levels of psychopathology in major depression, *Psychiatr Clin North Am* 19:85, 1996.
8. Cross-National Collaborative Group: The changing rate of major depression: cross-national comparisons, *JAMA* 268:3098, 1992.
9. Colp R Jr: Psychiatry: past and future. In Sadock BJ, Sadock VA, editors: *Comprehensive textbook of psychiatry,* Philadelphia, 1999, Lippincott, Williams & Wilkins.
10. Schildkraut JJ: The catecholamine hypothesis of affective disorders: a review of supporting evidence, *Am J Psychiatry* 122:509, 1965.
11. Coppen A: The biochemistry of affective disorders, *Br J Psychiatry* 113:1237, 1967.
12. Thase ME: Mood disorders: neurobiology. In Sadock BJ, Sadock VA, editors: *Comprehensive textbook of psychiatry,* Philadelphia, 1999, Lippincott, Williams & Wilkins.
13. Thase ME, Howland RH: Biological processes in depression: an updated review and integration. In Beckhamee EE, Leber WR, editors: *Handbook of depression,* ed 2, New York, 1995, Guilford.
14. Petty F et al: Learned helplessness sensitizes hippocampal norepinephrine to mild restlessness, *Biol Psychiatry* 35:901, 1994.
15. Weiss JM: Stress induced depression: critical neurochemical and electrophysiological change. In Madden J IV, editor: *Neurobiology of learning emotion and affect,* New York, 1991, Raven.
16. Higley TD et al: Cerebrospinal fluid monoamine and adrenal correlates of aggression in free ranging rhesus monkeys, *Arch Gen Psychiatry* 49:436, 1992.
17. Brown GL, Linnoila MI: CSF serotonin metabolite (5-H1AA) studies in depression impulsivity and violence, *J Clin Psychiatry* 51(suppl 4):31, 1990.
18. Kandel ER et al: *Principles of neural science,* ed 3, New York, 1991, Elsevier.
19. Spoont MR: Modulatory role of serotonin in neural information processing: implications for human psychopathology, *Psychol Bull* 112:330, 1992.
20. Joffe RT et al: A placebo-controlled comparison of lithium and triiodothyronine augmentation of tricyclic antidepressants in unipolar refractory depression, *Arch Gen Psychiatry* 50:387, 1993.
21. Tsuang MT, Farone SV: The inheritance of mood disorders. In Hall LL, editor: *Genetics and mental illness: evolving issues for research and society,* New York, 1996, Plenum.
22. Kendler KS, Prescott CA: A twin study of major depression, *Arch Gen Psychiatry* 56:39, 1999.
23. Mann J et al: Possible association of a polymorphism of the tryptophan hydroxylase gene with suicidal behavior in depressed patients, *Am J Psychiatry* 154:1451, 1997.
24. Zhang H et al: Serotonin receptor gene polymorphism in mood disorders, *Biol Psychiatry* 41:768, 1997.
25. Roy A: Genetics of suicide in depression, *J Clin Psychiatry* 60(suppl 2):12, 1999.
26. Freud S: Mourning and melancholia. In *Complete psychological works of Sigmund Freud,* vol 4, London, 1975, Hogwarth.
27. Suomi SJ: Early stress and emotional reactivity in rhesus monkeys. In Ciba Foundation Symposium: *Childhood environment and adult disease,* Chichester, England, 1991, Wiley.
28. Akiskal MS: Mood disorders: clinical features. In Sadock BJ, Sadock VA: *Comprehensive textbook of psychiatry,* Philadelphia, 1999, Lippincott, Williams & Wilkins.
29. Goldberg RJ: *Practical guide to the care of the psychiatric patient,* ed 2, St Louis, 1998, Mosby.
30. Lam RW et al: Effects of light therapy on suicidal ideation in patients with winter depression, *J Clin Psychiatry* 61:30, 2000.
31. Najman JM et al: Postnatal depression—myth and reality: maternal depression before and after the birth of a child, *Soc Psychiatry Psychiatr Epidemiol* 35:19, 2000.
32. Whiffen VE, Gotlib IM: Infants of postpartum depressed mothers: temperament and cognitive status, *J Abnorm Psychol* 98:274, 1989.
33. Hendrick V et al: Gender and bipolar illness, *J Clin Psychiatry* 61:393, 2000.
34. Bejjani B-P et al: Transient acute depression induced by high frequency deep brain stimulation, *N Engl J Med* 340:1476, 1999.
35. Cummings JL: Depression and Parkinson's disease: a review, *Am J Psychiatry* 149:443, 1992.
36. McDaniel JS et al: Depression in patients with cancer: diagnosis, biology, and treatment, *Arch Gen Psychiatry* 52:89, 1995.
37. Gonzalez MB et al: Depression in patients with coronary artery disease, *Depression* 4:57, 1996.
38. Evans DL et al: Depression in the medical setting: biopsychological interactions and treatment considerations, *J Clin Psychiatry* 60:40, 1999.
39. Endicott J: Measurement of depression in patients with cancer, *Cancer* 53(May suppl):2243, 1984.
40. Thomas HT: Droperidol v. haloperidol for chemical restraint of agitated and combative patients, *Ann Emerg Med* 21:407, 1992.
41. McIntyre JS et al: *Practice guideline for major depressive disorder in adults,* Washington, DC, 1996, American Psychiatric Association.
42. Ormel J et al: Outcome of depression and anxiety in primary care, *Arch Gen Psychiatry* 50:759, 1993.
43. Roose SP, Glasssman AH, editors: *Treatment strategies for refractory depression,* Washington, DC, 1990, American Psychiatric Press.
44. Yager J: Patients with mood disorders and marital/family problems, *Annu Rev Psychiatry* 11, 1992.
45. Keller MD et al: A comparison of nefazodone, *N Engl J Med* 342:1462, 2000.
46. Karasu TB: Developmentalist metatheory of depression and psychotherapy, *Am J Psychother* 46:37, 1992.
47. Shea MT et al: Course of depressive symptoms over follow-up: findings from the National Institute of Mental Health Treatment of Depression Collaborative Research Program, *Arch Gen Psychiatry* 42:782, 1992.
48. Scott J: Treatment of chronic depression, *N Engl J Med* 342:1518, 2000.
49. Task Force on Electroconvulsive Therapy: *The practice of electroconvulsive therapy,* Washington, DC, 1990, American Psychiatric Association.
50. Schou M: *Lithium treatment of manic-depressive illness: a practice guide,* ed 5, New York, 1993, Karger.
51. McElroy SL et al: Valproate in the treatment of bipolar disorder: literature review and clinical guidelines, *J Clin Psychopharmacol* 12:42S, 1992.
52. Hirschfeld RMA et al: Safety and tolerability of oral loading divalproex sodium in acutely manic bipolar patients, *J Clin Psychiatry* 60:815, 1999.
53. Compton MT, Nemeroff CB: The treatment of bipolar depression, *J Clin Psychiatry* 61:57, 2000.
54. Sernyak MJ, Woods SW: Chronic neuroleptic use in manic-depressive illness, *Psychopharmacol Bull* 29:375, 1993.
55. Mukherjee S, Sackeim HA, Schnurr DB: Electroconvulsive therapy of acute manic episodes: a review, *Am J Psychiatry* 151:169, 1994.

106 Anxiety Disorders

Eugene E. Kercher

If one strays from the moment, one becomes more anxious. Anxiety is the gap between now and later.

Fritz Pearls[1]

Anxiety and apprehension are common in ED patients. Many medical entities mimic anxiety disorders, and as many as 42% of patients thought to have anxiety disorders are later found to have organic disease. Emergency physicians must thoroughly assess the anxious patient to recognize and appropriately treat anxiety disorder.[2]

PERSPECTIVE

Vigilance is a positive consequence of anxiety, helping people to recognize threats quickly, which produces more learning and more intelligence. The capacity to experience anxiety and the capacity to plan are therefore related, and anxiety accompanies intellectual activity as its "shadow."[3]

The German word *angst* forms the basis for the role of anxiety in psychopathology. In freudian terms, angst means trepidation without an identifiable object, or a vague apprehension about the future. When anxiety has an object, freudians prefer the word *fear.*[4] Lewis[5] translates angst to be agony, dread, fright, terror, consternation, alarm, or apprehension. *Anxiety* is defined as a specific unpleasurable state of tension that forewarns the presence of danger. This uneasiness stems from the anticipation of some imminent danger, the source of which is largely unknown and unrecognized. The discomfort of anxiety is painful and persistently stressful.[1]

Anxiety facilitates performance up to a point of "moderate" anxiety. Beyond this point, further increases in anxiety lead to deterioration of performance. One important function of anxiety is the massive alarm reaction experienced in response to an imminent threat of danger, which prepares an individual to either "fight or flee."[4]

In addition to the well-described adrenergic responses to stress that contribute to survival, some nonadaptive responses may be a source of distress for the patient. The threshold for pain decreases, and the person becomes more aware of bodily discomfort. Respiratory, cardiovascular, gastrointestinal, genitourinary, and neuromuscular complaints are prominent.

Pathologic anxiety (anxiety disorders) occurs when anxiety surpasses a normal response to the "threat" at hand and interferes with normal functioning. Some patients may be unaware that their symptoms are caused by underlying anxiety, whereas others may be consciously anxious.[4]

The emergency physician should not assume anxiety is purely functional because physical discomfort often triggers an anxiety attack. The sudden experience of being sick may induce unacceptable fears of separation, death, or bodily injury. The anxiety state also makes significant metabolic demands, which may actually cause a marginally compensated organ system to fail.

Epidemiology

Millions of individuals each year seek help for what is broadly construed as anxiety or nervousness. Anxiety disorders are among the most prevalent psychiatric disorders, with approximately 25% of the U.S. population experiencing pathologic anxiety during their lifetime.[6] Anxiety is the most common psychiatric problem seen by primary care physicians, with up to 20% of these patients receiving benzodiazepines for 6 months.[7] Most people who frequently use primary care services have significant mood and anxiety difficulties, including panic disorder, generalized anxiety disorder, or depression. Patients with chronic illness and those who make frequent medical visits have higher rates of anxiety and depression.[8] Anxiety is a prominent complaint in 10% to 15% of medical outpatients and 10% of medical inpatients. The prevalence of anxiety disorders surpasses that of any other mental health disorder, including substance abuse. Even the more limited category of *phobia* alone is the most common mental health disorder in women and the second most common in men after substance abuse.[9] In view of the close relationship between alcohol abuse and anxiety disorders, substance abusers may be trying to self-medicate an underlying anxiety disorder.[10]

Anxiety disorders are associated with marked impairment of physical and psychosocial function as well as quality of life. Most patients improve if treated, but only 25% of the patients with panic disorder receive treatment. This low treatment rate results from failure to diagnose, a high degree of patient denial, and physician discomfort with diagnosis and therapy.[11,12]

PRINCIPLES OF DISEASE

No accepted model for emotion has yet emerged.[13] Family studies suggest genetic factors are implicated in anxiety, but the precise nature of the inherited vulnerability is unknown.[14,15] Noradrenergic, serotonergic, and other neurotransmitter systems may be biologic substrates of panic. Studies report that anxious subjects are in a state of "overpreparedness," as indicated by physiologic measures. Heightened arousal has been demonstrated in normal subjects made anxious in the laboratory by a variety of adrenergic-stimulating procedures. Catecholamines increase in normal people as a response to stress, and any change in stimulation seems to increase catecholamine excretion. Anxiety reactions may originate as central nervous system (CNS) arousal states that secondarily provoke peripheral events. The CNS arousal center may be the *locus ceruleus,* which contains at least 50% of all neurons in the CNS, uses norepinephrine as the neurotransmitter, and sends afferent projections to wide areas of the brain by a number of pathways. Other authorities implicate heightened serotonin activity as the basis for panic.[16]

The "benzodiazepine model" has come largely from the

effects of the anxiolytic drugs, specifically the benzodiazepines, on various paradigms for provoking "anxiety" in animals.[4] The neurotransmitter gamma-aminobutyric acid (GABA) is the principal inhibitory neurotransmitter in the CNS.[16] It decreases anxiety by hyperpolarizing other neurons, resulting in less neuronal discharge. Levels of most neurotransmitters in the brain, including GABA, decrease with aging, which may predispose the older person to anxiety.[4]

Other investigators have found anxiety reactions associated with aberrant metabolic changes induced by lactate infusion and hypersensitivity of the brainstem to carbon dioxide receptors.[15]

Psychologic factors, as outlined in psychodynamic, behavioral, and cognitive theories, also may play a causative role in the generation of anxiety in biologically predisposed individuals.

CLINICAL FEATURES

The physical symptoms of autonomic arousal (e.g., tachypnea, tachycardia, diaphoresis, lightheadedness) may be the only manifestation of anxiety (Box 106-1). When present, affective symptoms range from mild edginess to terror and panic. Behavior is characterized by avoidance, including noncompliance with medical procedures, or by compulsions. Cognitive activities include worry, apprehension, obsession, and thoughts about emotional or bodily damage.[17]

Box 106-1 Somatic Symptoms of Anxiety

Respiratory

Hyperventilation
Sense of dyspnea

Cardiovascular

Palpitations
Chest discomfort
Awareness of missed beats

Gastrointestinal

Dry mouth
Difficulty in swallowing
Epigastric discomfort
Excessive flatulence
Frequent or loose stools

Genitourinary

Frequent or urgent micturition
Failure of erection
Amenorrhea
Menstrual discomfort

Neuromuscular

Tremor
Aching muscles
Prickling sensations
Headache
Dizziness, tinnitus

DIFFERENTIAL CONSIDERATIONS

Medical Illness Presenting as Anxiety

Anxiety disorders may present as apparent physical disease, and many physical diseases may be accompanied by symptoms of anxiety. Differentiating between these two scenarios can be a daunting task for the emergency physician. Moreover, many anxious patients also experience significant depression, which should also be evaluated and treated.[18] Several factors help distinguish an organic anxiety syndrome from a primary anxiety disorder[19] (Box 106-2).

Anxiety may be classified as endogenous or exogenous. *Endogenous anxiety,* which arises spontaneously, is not a response to an identifiable external stress of symbolic conflict, although patients may develop conflicts and additional fears to explain their anxiety. *Exogenous anxiety* is an understandable but exaggerated response to an external stress or a psychologic conflict (Box 106-3). In anxiety disorders the somatic symptoms can be so prominent that they occupy all the patient's attention (Box 106-4).

Anxious patients are frequently convinced that their problem is purely physical. The emergency physician must realize that the patient with an anxiety disorder is not in control of the symptoms, is not faking, and cannot immediately identify the correct precipitant. Because the patient may be uncomfortable, uncooperative, impatient, and unreason-

Box 106-2 Predictors of Organic Anxiety Syndrome

1. Onset of anxiety symptoms after age 35.
2. Lack of personal or family history of an anxiety disorder.
3. Lack of childhood history of significant anxiety, phobias, or separation anxiety.
4. Absence of significant life events generating or exacerbating the anxiety symptoms.
5. Lack of avoidance behavior.
6. Poor response to antipanic agents.

Box 106-3 Types of Exogenous Anxiety

- *Traumatic anxiety* is an overwhelming state of panic occurring in the face of great stress, such as rape or a severe physical or medical illness.
- *Separation anxiety* occurs in the face of separation or the threat of separation from a significant person or position.
- *Castration anxiety* is a morbid fear of bodily injury.
- *Instinctual anxiety* is a fear of "something inside welling up" and causing loss of control.
- *Conscience anxiety* is a fear of being "found out" for not acting up to one's standards.
- *Reactionary anxiety* is a response to normal life events, such as birth, marriage, death, loss of position, poverty, and deterioration of physical and mental well-being.

Modified from Dubovsky SJ, Weissberg MP: Anxiety. In *Clinical psychiatry in primary care,* ed 3, Baltimore, 1986, Williams & Wilkins.

able, triage medical personnel must recognize that the patient believes an illness truly exists and is not being consciously manipulative. Moreover, when a patient presents to the ED with anxiety of panic proportions, the possibility of acute medical illness, as well as drug intoxication and withdrawal states, should always be considered.[20]

Anxiety caused by physical illness is usually suggested by the patient's physical findings. The patient should be evaluated for exacerbation of known preexisting disease as well as for symptoms that suggest onset of new illness.[20]

Box 106-4 Definitions of Anxiety Disorders

- *Panic attack* is a discrete period in which there is a sudden onset of intense apprehension, fearfulness, or terror, often associated with feelings of impending doom.
- *Agoraphobia* is an anxiety about, or avoidance of, places or situations from which escape might be difficult.
- *Panic disorder without agoraphobia* is characterized by recurrent and unexpected panic attacks about which there is a persistent concern.
- *Panic disorder with agoraphobia* is characterized by both recurrent unexpected panic attacks and agoraphobia.
- *Agoraphobia without a history of panic disorder* is characterized by the presence of agoraphobia and panic-like symptoms without a history of unexpected panic attacks.
- *Specific phobia* is characterized by clinically significant anxiety provoked by exposure to a specific feared object or situation, often leading to avoidance behavior.
- *Social phobia* is characterized by clinically significant anxiety provoked by exposure to certain types of social or performance situations, often leading to avoidance behavior. Blushing is the cardinal characteristic symptom.
- *Obsessive-compulsive disorder* is characterized by obsessions that cause marked anxiety or distress and by compulsions that serve to neutralize anxiety.
- *Posttraumatic stress disorder* is characterized by reexperiencing of an extremely traumatic event, accompanied by symptoms of increased arousal and by avoidance of stimuli associated with trauma.
- *Acute stress disorder* is characterized by symptoms similar to those of posttraumatic stress disorder that occur immediately in the aftermath of an extremely traumatic event.
- *Generalized anxiety disorder* is characterized by at least 6 months of persistent and excessive anxiety and worry, motor tension, and hypervigilance.
- *Anxiety disorder caused by a general medical condition* is characterized by prominent symptoms of anxiety that are judged to be a direct physiological consequence of a general medical condition.
- *Substance-induced anxiety disorder* is characterized by prominent symptoms of anxiety that are judged to be a direct physiologic consequence of a drug of abuse or medication or toxin exposure.
- *Anxiety disorder not otherwise specified* is included for coding (1) disorders with prominent anxiety or phobic avoidance that do not meet criteria for specific anxiety disorders and (2) anxiety symptoms with inadequate or contradictory information.

Modified from the *Diagnostic and statistical manual of mental disorders,* ed 4-TR, Washington, DC, 2000, American Psychiatric Association.

Cardiac Diseases The symptoms of *myocardial infarction* (MI) and *angina pectoris* are crushing chest pain, shortness of breath, choking or smothering sensations, palpitations, heavy perspiration, and a feeling of impending death. These are also the primary symptoms of acute anxiety, but the pain is rarely the worst symptom, and patients are generally younger.[21] When the differentiation between MI and acute anxiety is unclear, patients should be approached as though they have a cardiac cause. *Cardiac dysrhythmias* can cause palpitations, discomfort, dizziness, respiratory distress, fainting, and anxiety. Patients with panic disorder may have similar symptoms in association with tachycardia and other dysrhythmias, including premature ventricular contractions.[22] Fortunately, most dysrhythmias can be documented and characterized by an electrocardiogram (ECG). *Mitral valve prolapse* (MVP) syndrome can be associated with panic attacks indistinguishable from panic disorder. Most cases of MVP are asymptomatic, however, and possibly not clinically important.[23,24]

Endocrine Diseases Anxiety is the predominant symptom in 20% of patients with *hypoparathyroidism.* Other symptoms include paresthesias, muscle cramps, muscle spasm, and tetany. Most cases result from past surgical removal of the parathyroid glands during thyroidectomy. Diagnosis is suggested by low serum calcium and high phosphate levels and confirmed by parahormone assay.[11] Many patients with anxiety, somatoform, or characterologic disorders are convinced that they have *reactive hypoglycemia.* A normal blood glucose level drawn during an attack can exclude this diagnosis.[22] One half of patients with *pheochromocytoma* have acute attacks of anxiety, headache, sweating, flushing, hypertension, and diarrhea. Pheochromocytoma attacks, like panic attacks, can be precipitated by emotional stress. Pheochromocytoma attacks are more likely to cause crushing back pain, vomiting, and sweating of the whole body; the sweating in panic attacks is more likely to be confined to the hands, feet, and forehead. Pheochromocytoma can be diagnosed by measuring urinary or plasma catecholamines and metabolites.[25] As with panic disorder, *hyperthyroidism* is associated with chronic and acute episodic anxiety. *Thyrotoxicosis* causes anxiety, palpitations, perspiration, hot skin, rapid pulse, active reflexes, diarrhea, weight loss, heat intolerance, proptosis, and lid lag.[26]

Respiratory Diseases Although patients with panic may hyperventilate between attacks, their respiratory distress is episodic.[27] As a result, diseases such as chronic obstructive pulmonary disease (COPD) and congestive heart failure are seldom mistaken for panic disorder.[28] As in panic disorders, *asthma* is characterized by episodic attacks of dyspnea and anxiety. Anxiety also can precipitate and prolong asthma attacks.[29] Asthma is easily differentiated from panic by the good air movement with normal lung sounds that occur during a panic attack. *Pulmonary embolism* causes shortness of breath, hyperventilation, and often acute anxiety. As with anxiety attacks, pulmonary emboli can be recurrent, particularly in individuals with predisposing conditions such as thrombophlebitis, recent surgery, prolonged immobilization, severe heart failure, pregnancy, or malignancy.[22]

Neurologic Diseases *Transient ischemic attacks* (TIAs) include reversible motor and sensory symptoms, and no signs may be evident at evaluation. Anxiety often accompanies these episodes and may be the major symptom on presentation if the TIA has resolved by the time the patient reaches the ED.[22] *Seizure disorders* can cause any psychiatric symptom, including anxiety. Some temporal lobe seizures do not progress to generalized convulsions but present as episodes of anxiety, anger, or other changes in affect. Fearfulness has been found to be the predominant emotion in 61% of patients with partial complex seizures. In a minority of cases, before choreiform movements and flaccid paralysis begin, the prodromal phase of *Huntington's chorea* is dominated by chronic anxiety with episodes of panic anxiety. *Combined systemic disease* (*posterolateral sclerosis*) is a vitamin B_{12} deficiency syndrome that can present as panic. Other symptoms include anxiety, paresthesias, weakness, hyperreflexia, and numerous "soft" symptoms easily misdiagnosed as anxious or hypochondriasis. Patients with severe pernicious anemia may hyperventilate and have other anxiety symptoms, but mental symptoms can occur without anemia.[22] Documentation of pernicious anemia or low serum B_{12} level with impaired absorption establishes the diagnosis.

Drug Intoxication and Withdrawal States Amphetamines, cocaine, and sympathomimetic drugs are used to become euphoric, energetic, and confident. However, patients also become agitated, anxious, or panicky, particularly with large doses or prolonged use. *Caffeine* is a common stimulant and can provoke anxiety symptoms.[30] Lower doses of caffeine can be pleasantly stimulating, but higher doses cause hyperalertness, hypervigilance, motor tension, tremors, gastrointestinal distress, and anxiety. The acute symptoms of caffeine intoxication and generalized anxiety disorder are almost identical. Caffeine, theophylline, theobromine, and related methylxanthines are found in coffee, tea, cola, and many other carbonated drinks.[22] *Yohimbine* is most often used as a stimulant or aphrodisiac but can also produce extreme anxiety. It produces panic anxiety so reliably that it has been useful in experimental anxiety research.[31]

Regular *marijuana* users believe that the drug reduces their anxiety. No perceived rebound of this anxiety occurs when cannabis use is curtailed. Some patients experience the depersonalization associated with marijuana as unpleasant, provoking anxiety, fearfulness, and agoraphobic symptoms.[32] *Khat* is a botanical stimulant that results in symptoms that are stronger than caffeine but weaker than amphetamine. *Amyl nitrite* is used medically as a short-acting vasodilator. It is abused primarily as a sexual stimulant, for prolonging and intensifying arousal, erection, and orgasm. It can cause brief panic anxiety.[22] *LSD* can produce "bad trips," which are often associated with severe generalized anxiety. The effects of LSD are typically abolished within an hour by 50 mg of chlorpromazine or 5 mg of haloperidol.[33]

Sedative-hypnotic drugs (e.g., benzodiazepines, barbiturates, meprobamate, methaqualone, chloral hydrate, paraldehyde, ethchlorvynol, glutethimide) are taken to relieve anxiety or sleeplessness, but their discontinuation can cause *sedative withdrawal* and rebound anxiety. The severity of the withdrawal syndrome depends on the drug, dosage, duration of use, and speed of elimination. In general the intermediate-acting sedative-hypnotics (4 to 6 hours) cause the worst withdrawal. Symptoms include hyperalertness, motor tension, muscle aches, agitation, anxiety, insomnia, hyperactive reflexes and startle response, postural hypotension, tremulousness, nausea, vomiting, convulsions, delirium, and death.

Benzodiazepine withdrawal is rarely fatal but can be very unpleasant. In anxious patients, severe rebound anxiety can occur after only a few weeks' use of recommended therapeutic doses. Lorazepam and alprazolam are short-acting agents, and their abrupt discontinuation is particularly likely to cause panic attacks. Normal people may experience this rebound as stimulating.[22] Although antidepressants are rarely abused, their abrupt withdrawal can cause an abstinence syndrome of insomnia, vivid nightmares, and extreme anxiety.[34]

Alcohol withdrawal in alcohol-dependent individuals presents with severe anxiety symptoms in the context of acute or protracted abstinence syndromes, but it is unclear whether this anxiety is an independent psychiatric disorder or a temporary syndrome related solely to withdrawal.[35]

Panic Attacks in Mental Disorders

Even in the domain of mental illnesses, panic disorder is a diagnosis of exclusion. Several other mental illnesses cause panic attacks as secondary manifestations. The presence of panic attacks often influences the treatment and outcome of the primary illness. Panic attacks can occur as part of *bipolar (manic-depressive) disorder,* in either the manic or the depressed phase. In manic and hypomanic disorders the patient's predominant affect is usually cheerful and euphoric but may be dysphoric, with irritability, extreme anxiety, or panic attacks.[22,36]

Panic attacks are often seen with *schizophrenia,* especially early in its course. Fearfulness, tension, agitation or immobility, disorganized thinking, dilated pupils, extreme insecurity, suspiciousness, and delusions of reference and persecution may characterize schizophrenic panic attacks. Hallucinations often have derogatory accusative content.[22]

Patients with *somatoform disorders* report a variety of somatic symptoms, including panic attacks, and claim to have most of the physical symptoms they are asked about. However, even patients with "pure" anxiety disorders tend to be hypochondriacal. Patients with somatization are more likely to improve transiently on active medication or placebo but rarely respond so well that they stop seeking unnecessary medical attention. Patients with panic disorders, however, seek at least as much psychiatric attention as those with somatoform disorders.[36]

Approximately 50% of patients with a primary panic disorder develop *major depression* (a secondary depression), and almost all are bothered by some degree of depressed mood.[36] Twenty percent of patients with depression have panic attacks; the remainder have considerable anxiety. Depression with panic attacks responds less well to treatment. *Agitated depression with anxiety and psychosis,* sometimes called "involutional melancholia," responds well to electroconvulsive therapy. Depression with anxiety and hostility responds well to antidepressants, but benzodiazepines can exacerbate symptoms.[18]

Posttraumatic stress disorder (PTSD) is an anxiety disorder presumed to be caused by previous terrible experiences. The symptoms are closely related to and worsened by reminders of the trauma. The "flashbacks," in which patients reexperience the original trauma, can have the same symptoms as panic attacks. These patients may avoid crowds or social situations.[37]

Mimicry abounds in nature, where it is often an advantage to disguise the true self. A panic disorder is one of the easier psychiatric diseases to feign because most of the symptoms can be duplicated by intentional hyperventilation. When in doubt, formal psychiatric evaluation is indicated, particularly before prescribing a potentially dangerous or addictive drug therapy. *Social phobias* are narrowly defined as fear of a single, specific social situation, such as public speaking, performing, visiting, using public showers or rest rooms, or eating in public places. *Phobic disorders* (irrational fears) are common psychiatric disorders but are considered normal in children. The objects of fear tend to be things that would have been dangerous to children (e.g. spiders, snakes, bats, cats, enclosed places, the dark, open spaces). Simple phobic disorders probably represent persistence into adult life of instincts that were once useful to survival. Phobia becomes a disorder when it interferes with an individual's life.[36]

When the organic disorders have been excluded, patients regularly troubled by panic attacks are diagnosed as having *panic disorder*[22] (see Box 106-4). *Agoraphobia* is a fear of leaving home, particularly alone. Approximately one half of agoraphobic patients do not have panic attacks. Those with panic attacks are more likely to seek treatment, whereas those with uncomplicated agoraphobia tend to stay at home. Agoraphobia without panic attacks may not differ fundamentally from simple phobias. Most panic disorder patients have multiple phobias, including agoraphobia. The latter is believed to result from the panic patient's increasing attempts to avoid places or situations in which the panic attacks would be particularly inconvenient or difficult to control. Agoraphobic patients particularly avoid places from which escape would be difficult (e.g., bridges, crowded theaters). When they attend theaters, they favor seats on the aisle and near the door. Panic attacks in agoraphobic patients are more likely to include fear of losing control, whereas those not associated with agoraphobia are more likely to include dyspnea and dizziness.

Obsessive-compulsive disorder (OCD) is characterized by recurrent, obtrusive, unwanted thoughts (obsessions), such as fears of contamination, and compulsive behaviors or rituals (compulsions), such as handwashing or checking. OCD is classified as an anxiety disorder because (1) anxiety or tension is often associated with obsessions and resistance to compulsions, (2) anxiety or tension is often immediately relieved by yielding to compulsions, and (3) OCD often occurs in association with anxiety disorders.[17]

Reactive anxiety or *situational anxiety* occurs in reaction to stressful situations (e.g., onset of serious medical illness). The criteria for an adjustment disorder with anxiety include the development of nervousness or anxiety in response to an identifiable stressor.[17]

MANAGEMENT

Initial Evaluation

The patient should first be placed in a quiet area for evaluation. Some patients calm down when removed from the ED environment.[4] If the emergency physician encounters difficulty in calming the patient, supportive family members may help. Often a known and trusted face helps anxious patients make order out of their inner turmoil. Prior discussion and clarification with the family are essential to elicit their support.

Once the patient is calmed, a more formal evaluation can begin. The patient should be allowed to relate the history, and the emergency physician should observe carefully. Direct questions should be avoided, at least initially. Questions regarding drug or alcohol use should be delayed until rapport has been established with the patient. Reassurance should not be premature, because this important treatment modality is more effective when it is delayed until the patient's specific concerns are clarified.

The extent of medical evaluation indicated for the patient with significant anxiety will vary depending on the age and health status of the patient, the nature of the anxiety, and the range and severity of associated symptoms. The emergency physician should consider the anxiogenic effects of medications, including β-adrenergic agonists, theophylline, corticosteroids, thyroid hormones, and sympathomimetics. Potential contributory medical illness (e.g., thyroid dysfunction, hypoglycemic episodes in diabetes, hyperparathyroidism, dysrhythmias, COPD, seizure disorders) and substance use (e.g., caffeine, amphetamines, cocaine) or withdrawal (e.g., alcohol, sedative-hypnotics) must be considered.

If a somatic concern is the major component of the acute anxiety attack, a physical examination with particular attention to the area of complaint is appropriate, even when there is overwhelming evidence of the functional nature of the patient's attack. Anxiety attacks are stressful experiences in themselves and can cause difficulty in marginally compensated organ systems.[22] Careful evaluation reassures the patient and avoids the problem of a premature "medical clearance." Abnormal vital signs and low pulse oximetry readings should alert the emergency physician to organic causes for the anxiety symptoms.[17]

Because of the physical nature of these symptoms, patients often seek treatment in the ED rather than the psychiatric setting. A calm manner and willingness to listen usually relieve some of the patient's initial anxiety. An anxiety or panic reaction may be precipitated by the loss of a significant relationship, a job, a living situation, or self-esteem, as well as by physical illness or injury. Once the patient describes a trigger event, the emergency physician should restate it as if experiencing a similar situation. This gives the patient authoritative approval for expressing embarrassing feelings. A patient who has frequent anxiety reactions is usually suggestible and will respond to reassurance. Conversely, an anxious or unsympathetic physician may only compound the problem.

Even an apparently calm patient may communicate anxiety through worried looks, nervousness, pressured speech, or covert assaults on the emergency physician's confidence. The emergency physician, without being aware of it, may respond empathetically to the patient's overt or hidden anxiety by also becoming anxious. This is a strong clue that the patient is anxious. Without this self-awareness, emergency physicians may focus so much on a patient's physical symptoms that they avoid the uncomfortable feelings associated with not knowing how to address irrational anxiety. Throughout medical training, physicians learn to protect themselves through emotional isolation from the patient. When a patient is very anxious, this protective mechanism may function so well that all awareness of the physician's emotional response toward the patient is ignored.

Careful medical evaluation is important. However, excessive focus on unlikely illness suggests a reason to worry, avoids recognition of crucial psychologic factors, and may increase the patient's anxiety and the severity of symptoms.

After organic illness, medications, and obvious psychiatric causes of the acute anxiety state have been ruled out, the emergency physician should determine whether the anxiety is endogenous or exogenous (see Box 106-3). If the anxiety is paroxysmal, unpredictable, and accompanied by agoraphobia, an endogenous component is likely to be present. Such patients should be referred to a psychiatrist for evaluation. If the anxiety appears to be related to an identifiable external event or circumstance, patients should be encouraged to discuss their feelings. Talking about fears allows the anxious patient some sense of mastery and control over events. These patients often require ongoing advice, support, and assistance in mobilizing necessary resources from family members, friends, and social agencies to achieve realistic expectations.

Anxiety is common in elderly patients, with prevalence rates conservatively estimated at 10% to 15%. Anxiety disorders may be the most common psychiatric ailments experienced by older adults and the least studied in that age group. Older patients with anxiety often have somatic complaints. These patients require an especially careful investigation for underlying medical illness, other psychiatric conditions, and the use of over-the-counter and prescription drugs.[37]

Pharmacologic Treatment

Use of intravenous medication is rare but may be necessary when an anxiety state renders a patient so helpless and out of control that there is a significant threat to the safety of the patient or to persons in the immediate vicinity. It may also be appropriate for the anxious patient undergoing a significant medical illness. Morphine, 1 to 2 mg, is effective in controlling the anxiety associated with congestive heart failure, acute MI, and acute pulmonary embolism. Lorazepam (Ativan), 0.5-mg increments every 20 minutes, can be helpful in alleviating the anxiety associated with substance withdrawal states. Midazolam (Versed), 1 to 4 mg over 2 to 3 minutes, is frequently given to reduce anxiety and increase amnesia for ED procedures.

In the past few years, emergency physicians and the public have become increasingly concerned about the growing use of antianxiety drugs in the United States; 1 million Americans are physically dependent on tranquilizers. When tranquilizers are given in place of understanding, support, and intrapersonal therapies, patients are taught to rely on the external support of a pill rather than on inner resources.

Patients with endogenous anxiety (panic attacks with or without agoraphobia) should be referred to a psychiatrist to establish a good therapeutic relationship before using anxiolytic medication. Benzodiazepines, tricyclics, SSRIs, and MAOIs are safe and effective in endogenously anxious patients who are under psychiatric care (Table 106-1). Recurrence rates of panic attacks are high when drug therapy is discontinued.[15]

Benzodiazepines can be prescribed for motivated patients with acute exogenous anxiety to a time-limited stress. Patients who are cooperative, employed, educated, married, and aware of their problems on a psychologic basis are most likely to respond. Benzodiazepines can be given in one or two daily doses to make use of their short half-lives; alternatively, a bedtime dose may minimize daytime sedation and still manifest a daytime anxiolytic effect. Benzodiazepines should not be prescribed for more than a week. Patients who do not improve within a week are unlikely to benefit from the drug. Patients with a history of alcoholism or drug abuse, who are excessively and emotionally dependent, or who become anxious in response to normal stress are at greater risk of drug dependency. Dependence and abstinence syndromes have been reported to occur with low doses of tranquilizing drugs, especially if they are taken for more than 8 months. Short-acting benzodiazepines (e.g., lorazepam, oxazepam) should be prescribed at low dosages for patients with liver disease or organic brain syndrome and those taking medications that inhibit benzodiazepine metabolism and clearance (e.g., nicotine, cimetidine). Withdrawal rebound symptoms are more common with discontinuation of benzodiazepines than with other antianxiety treatments, and short-acting benzodiazepines produce a more severe abstinence syndrome when they are stopped abruptly. *Clonidine*, in gradually decreasing doses, may ameliorate benzodiazepine withdrawal. All benzodiazepines are effective for generalized anxiety disorder and insomnia; however high-potency benzodiazepines (e.g., alprazolam, clonazepam) are preferred for panic disorder. For some patients, switching from a shorter-acting agent (e.g., alprazolam) to a longer-acting agent (e.g., clonazepam) can be helpful before initiating taper.

Buspirone (BuSpar) is a newer nonbenzodiazepine tranquilizer that does not appear to cause dependency. Buspirone

Table 106-1. Pharmacotherapy for Anxiety Disorders

	SSRIs	TCAs	MAOIs	BZDs	Buspirone	CBT
Panic disorder	+	+	+	+	–	+
GAD	+	+	+	+	+	+
Social phobia	+	–	+	+	–	+
Specific phobia	–	–	–	+/–	–	+
PTSD	+	+/–	+	+/–	–	+
OCD	+	–*	+	+/–†	+/–†	+

BZDs, Benzodiazepines; *CBT,* cognitive-behavioral therapy; *GAD,* generalized anxiety disorder; *MAOIs,* monoamine oxidase inhibitors; *OCD,* obsessive-compulsive disorder; *PTSD,* posttraumatic stress disorder; *SSRIs,* selective serotonin-reuptake inhibitors; *TCAs,* tricyclic antidepressants.

*Clomipramine is effective.

†Used adjunctively with serotonergic antidepressant.

is effective with generalized anxiety disorders. Because of a therapeutic lag in efficacy of several weeks and the need for dose titration, buspirone has had variable and sometimes disappointing results in clinical practice, particularly when used in patients with prior exposure to benzodiazepines.[38]

Many psychiatrists use β-*blockers* to treat anxiety associated with tremor, tachycardia, and stage fright. Because of the risk of extrapyramidal side effects, neuroleptic drugs should be reserved for episodes of psychotic anxiety.[38]

Monoamine oxidase inhibitors (MAOIs) demonstrate high effectiveness for social phobia, panic, generalized anxiety disorders, OCD, and comorbid conditions (e.g., atypical depression). MAOIs, including phenylzine and tranylcypromine, may be difficult to tolerate and may require dietary restrictions.

Tricyclic antidepressants (TCAs) are effective for panic disorder and generalized anxiety disorder, but less so for social phobia, and except for clomipramine (Anafranil) are largely ineffective for OCD. TCAs are also effective for depressive and anxiety symptoms associated with PTSD. TCAs include imipramine (Tofranil), nortriptyline (Pamelor), desipramine (Norpramin), amitriptyline (Elavil), and doxepin (Sinequan). The TCAs have largely been supplanted by the SSRIs as first-line interventions for the treatment of anxiety and depressive disorders.[38]

Selective serotonin-reuptake inhibitors (SSRIs) have become first-line treatment for most anxiety disorders because of their broad spectrum of efficacy for anxiety and depressive conditions. SSRIs are tolerated better and are safer than previous classes of antidepressants, with a lower potential for physical dependence than the benzodiazepines. SSRIs include fluoxetine (Prozac), sertraline (Zoloft), paroxetine (Paxil), fluvoxamine (Luvox), venlafaxine (Effexor), nefazodone (Serzone), and mirtazapine (Remeron).[38]

Long-term use of antidepressants and benzodiazepines for anxious patients is often required to maintain ongoing benefit and prevent relapse.

Nonpharmacologic Therapy

Psychotherapies may be helpful for individuals whose psychologic makeup, coping style, interpersonal dynamics, and situational stressors contribute to the pathologic anxiety. Supportive, insight-oriented, family, and other types of therapy may be helpful when these factors appear prominently in the patient's presentation.[15]

Cognitive-behavioral therapy (CBT) is predicated on the theory that the distress and impairment associated with anxiety and panic are mediated by maladaptive cognitive responses that promote anxiety and avoidance. The core components of CBT for panic disorder include correction of cognitive misperceptions and overreactions to anxiety symptoms, breathing retraining, and muscle relaxation, as well as exposure and desensitization to phobic situations.[15,17]

Meditation (e.g., zen, yoga, transcendental) has been proposed by many authorities, but little clinical data support its efficacy in anxiety disorders.[15] *Biofeedback* appears promising for the treatment of generalized anxiety disorder.[39] *Hypnotic suggestion* may be effective because anxious patients tend to be cognitively scattered, unable to focus their attention, and highly suggestible. A hypnotic state can often be induced by certain stimuli.

These nonpharmacologic techniques take anxious patients out of the future, about which they are frightened, and place them into the present. These techniques should be reinforced by the development of a physically and psychologically healthy lifestyle. A high level of ongoing social support not only protects against vulnerability to illness but also is highly anxiolytic. Regular exercise (e.g., dancing, swimming, bicycling, walking, jogging) also promotes tranquility. Encouraging activity that focuses on hand-eye-ear coordination (e.g., painting, playing keyboard, needlework) helps anxious patients regain and maintain control by bringing them into the present.[40]

DISPOSITION

Many patients with anxiety disorders can be effectively treated in the ED. The emergency physician can proceed with the following general measures:

1. Rule out organic illnesses and medications associated with anxiety.
2. Determine whether anxiety is endogenous or exogenous.
3. Rule out depression.
4. Evaluate the patient's capacity for self-awareness.
5. Assess techniques that have worked in the past.
6. Support coping skills.
7. Give the patient as much control over the care plan as feasible.
8. Offer ongoing support when the patient's strengths are limited.
9. Clarify what is currently frightening the patient.
10. Apply adjunctive techniques as appropriate for the patient's personality and the physician's preference (e.g., neurolinguistics, hypnotic suggestion, breathing exercises).

Patients with panic disorder associated with suicidal or homicidal ideation or with severe depression require urgent psychiatric attention and most likely admission to the hospital. Other patients with suspected endogenous or severe exogenous anxiety disorders should be referred for psychiatric evaluation. The Anxiety Disorders Association of America can be contacted (301-231-9350) for national registry of clinicians and treatment programs specializing in anxiety disorders.

KEY CONCEPTS

- Anxiety may accompany the onset of serious disease, may have significant metabolic demands, and may cause a marginally compensated organ system to fail. As many as 42% of patients thought to have anxiety disorders are later found to have organic disease.
- Anxiety caused by physical illness is usually suggested by the patient's physical findings but may require adjunctive testing.
- Anxiety affects at least 10% to 15% of elderly patients.
- Intravenous medication may be necessary for patients who are a significant threat to themselves or others and for anxious patients with significant medical illness.
- Limited benzodiazepine therapy may be helpful for select patients with exogenous anxiety.

REFERENCES

1. Kercher EE: Anxiety, *Emerg Med Clin North Am* 9:161, 1991.
2. Benjamin GC: Anxiety disorders. In Rosen P et al: *Emergency medicine: concepts and clinical practice,* ed 3, St Louis, 1992, Mosby.
3. Liddell HS: The role of vigilance in the development of animal neurosis. In Hoch P, Zubin J, editors: *Anxiety,* New York, 1949, Grune & Stratton.

4. Barlow DH: *Anxiety & its disorders,* New York, 1988, Guilford.
5. Lewis AJ: Problems presented by the ambiguous word "anxiety" as used in psychopathology. In Burrows GD, Davies B, editors: *Handbook of studies on anxiety,* Amsterdam, 1980, Elsevier/North-Holland.
6. Kessler RC et al: Lifetime and twelve-month prevalence of DSM III-R psychiatric disorders in the United States: results from the National Comorbidity Survey, *Arch Gen Psychiatry* 51:8, 1994.
7. Wells KB et al: Quality of care for psychotropic drug use in internal medicine group practices, *West J Med* 145:710, 1986.
8. Leon AC et al: Prevalence of mental disorders in primary care: implications for screening, *Arch Fam Med* 4:857, 1995.
9. Mathew RJ et al: Psychiatric disorders in adult children of alcoholics: data from the Epidemiologic Catchment Area Project, *Am J Psychiatry* 150:793, 1993.
10. Kushner MG, Sher KJ, Erickson MA: Prospective analysis of the relation between DSM-III anxiety disorders and alcohol use disorders, *Am J Psychiatry* 156:723, 1999.
11. Denko JD, Kaelbling R: The psychiatric aspects of hypoparathyroidism, *Acta Psychiatr Scand* 38(suppl 164):1, 1962.
12. Pollack HM, Smoller JW: The longitudinal course and outcome of panic disorder, *Psychiatr Clin North Am* 18:789, 1995.
13. American Psychiatric Association: *Diagnostic and statistical manual of mental disorders,* ed 4, Washington, DC, 1994, the Association.
14. Pollard CA, Lewis LM: Managing panic attacks in emergency patients, *J Emerg Med* 7:547, 1989.
15. Hollander E, Simeon D, Gorman JM: Anxiety disorders. In Hales RE et al, editors: *Textbook of psychiatry,* Washington, DC, 1999, American Psychiatric Press.
16. Johnson MR, Lydiard RB: The neurobiology of anxiety disorders, *Psychiatr Clin North Am* 18:681, 1995.
17. Stern TA, Herman JB, Slavin PL, editors: *Guide to psychiatry in primary care,* New York, 1998, McGraw-Hill.
18. Gorman JM, Coplan JD: Comorbidity of depression and panic disorder, *J Clin Psychiatry* 57(suppl 10):34, 1996.
19. Rosenbaum JF et al: Anxiety. In Cassem NH, Stern TA, Rosenbaum JF, Jellinek MS, editors: *Massachusetts General Hospital handbook of general hospital psychiatry,* ed 4, St Louis, 1998, Mosby.
20. Coryell W, Noyes R, Clancy J: Excess mortality in panic disorder, *Arch Gen Psychiatry* 39:701, 1982.
21. Katon W et al: Chest pain: the relationship of psychiatric illness to coronary arteriography results, *Am J Med* 84:1, 1988.
22. Dubovsky SJ, Weissberg MP: Anxiety. In *Clinical psychiatry in primary care,* ed 3, Baltimore, 1986, Williams & Wilkins.
23. Muskin PR: Panics, prolapse, and PVCs, *Gen Hosp Psychiatry* 7:219, 1985.
24. Devereaux RB, Kramer-Fox R, Kligfield P: Mitral valve prolapse: causes, clinical manifestations, and management, *Ann Intern Med* 111:305, 1989.
25. Bravo EL, Gifford KW: Pheochromocytoma: diagnosis, localization and management, *N Engl J Med* 311:1298, 1984.
26. Pringuet G, DePerson J: Death anxiety in thyrotoxicosis, *Ann Med Psychol (Paris)* 140:753, 1982.
27. Salkovskis PM, Jones DR, Clark DM: Respiratory control in the treatment of panic attacks: replication and extension with concurrent measurement of behavior and pCO_2, *Br J Psychiatry* 148:526, 1986.
28. Zandbergen J et al: Higher lifetime prevalence of respiratory diseases in panic disorder? *Am J Psychiatry* 148:1583, 1991.
29. Thompson WL, Thompson TL Jr: Psychiatric aspects of asthma in adults, *Adv Psychosom Med* 14:33, 1985.
30. Charney DS, Heninger GR, Jatlow PI: Increased anxiogenic effects of caffeine in panic disorders, *Arch Gen Psychiatry* 42:233, 1985.
31. Mattila M, Seppala T, Mattila MJ: Anxiogenic effect of yohimbine in healthy subjects: comparison with caffeine and antagonism by clonidine and diazepam, *Int Clin Psychopharmacol* 3:215, 1988.
32. Moran C: Depersonalization and agoraphobia associated with marijuana use, *Br J Med Psychol* 59:187, 1985.
33. Leikin JB et al: Clinical features and management of intoxication due to hallucinogenic drugs, *Med Toxicol Adverse Drug Exp* 4:324, 1989.
34. Gawin FH, Markoff RA: Panic anxiety after abrupt discontinuation of amitriptyline, *Am J Psychiatry* 138:117, 1981.
35. Schmekit MA, Hessebrock V: Alcohol dependence and anxiety disorders: what is the relationship? *Am J Psychiatry* 151:1723, 1994.
36. Boyd JH et al: Phobia: prevalence and risk factors, *Soc Psychiatry Psychiatr Epidemiol* 25:314, 1990.
37. Sheikh JI: Anxiety and panic disorders. In Busse EW et al, editors: *Textbook of geriatric psychiatry,* Washington, DC, 1996, American Psychiatric Press.
38. Shatzberg AF, Nemeroff CB: *Textbook of psychopharmacology,* ed 2, Washington, DC, 1998, American Psychiatric Press.
39. Rice KM, Blanchard GB, Purcell M: Biofeedback treatments of generalized anxiety disorder: preliminary results, *Biofeedback Self Regul* 18:93, 1993.
40. Raj A, Sheehan DV: Medical evaluation of panic attacks, *J Clin Psychiatry* 48:309, 1987.

107 Somatoform Disorders

Thomas B. Purcell

PERSPECTIVE

Many patients have functional (nonorganic) complaints, but nonpsychiatrists often fail to recognize subtle presentations of psychiatric disease.[1] In the ED this lack of recognition is probably the result of limited time and the emergency physician's focus on action rather than toward passive listening. Also, many patients with psychiatric disturbances come to the ED at a time when psychiatric consultation is not readily available.[2] Even when psychiatric pathology has been identified or is strongly suspected, emergency physicians are reluctant to attribute somatic complaints to functional etiologies.[3,4] Nevertheless, proper diagnosis and treatment of patients with functional complaints are essential. Misidentification and mismanagement unnecessarily prolong patient distress and add to the overall burden on the health care delivery system.

From 25% to 72% of patient visits to primary care physicians have been attributed to psychosocial distress presenting as somatic complaints.[1,5,6] The prevalence of somatization has risen over the last 30 to 40 years, possibly because of a general decline of patient tolerance for mild and self-limited ailments.[7,8]

CLINICAL FEATURES

Most physicians have experienced somatization; up to 80% of all medical students become convinced they have a disease.[9] *Somatization* refers to a tendency to experience and communicate psychologic distress in the "body language" of physical symptoms in the absence of organic pathology.[10] Patients seek medical attention because they are convinced that their symptoms reflect real physical disease.[11-15]

The term *somatoform disorders* embraces all disorders that have somatization as a common factor. In some cases a demonstrable physical disorder does exist (often iatrogenic), but the patient's complaints will be out of proportion to the physical findings.[12] The symptoms are not feigned or under the voluntary control of the patient.[16,17] Almost any complaint involving any body system may occur, with patients often complaining of fashionable diseases recently popularized by the media.[15] The *environmental somatization syndrome* refers to individuals convinced that their symptoms are caused by exposure to chemical or physical components of the external environment, such as poisonous substances, electromagnetic fields, or ergonomic stress attributed to repetitive movements.[18] In general, it is the *multiplicity* of symptoms, rather than the specific symptom, that is more indicative of somatization.[19,20] In women with more than five and in men with more than three unexplained somatic complaints, the likelihood of a diagnosable psychiatric disorder doubles.[19,21,22]

In general, patients with somatoform disorders tend to be women between ages 20 and 60 who have fewer than 12 years of education, are widowed or divorced, and exhibit low self-esteem. They tend to be self-conscious, vulnerable to stress, anxious, hostile, and depressed.[10,12] Certain patient categories, such as women with chronic pelvic pain, have a high rate of sexual or physical abuse in childhood.[23] Somatizers have difficulty describing their feelings in words, a phenomenon termed *alexithymia* ("without words for mood"), resulting in alternate (somatic) forms of expression.[24] They will steadfastly insist that their symptoms are caused by serious physical disorders, even in the face of conclusive evidence to the contrary.[12] Somatization may be unconsciously motivated by a desire to assume the "sick role" and seek those privileges afforded to a sick person by society, such as release from normal obligations and absolution from blame for their condition.[24,25]

Individual somatic complaints are common in children and adolescents in the general population and generally are not associated with significant social or emotional impairment. Pronounced polysymptomatic somatization, although uncommon in this age group, may occur, and these patients are at increased risk for the later development of major depression, panic attacks, and drug and alcohol abuse.[26]

Somatoform disorders may be subdivided into four specific disorders, each with a somewhat different clinical picture and management approach: somatization disorder, conversion disorder, pain disorder, and hypochondriasis.

Somatization Disorder

Historically referred to as *hysteria* and *neurasthenia,* somatization disorder was given the eponym of "Briquet's syndrome" by Guze in 1975 to avoid the pejorative implications that had come to be associated with the traditional terms.[27] The malady is chronic or repetitive, dating from young adulthood, with numerous physical symptoms and complaints involving a variety of organ systems, but few or no physical findings to explain those symptoms.[28-31]

> **Box 107-1 Summary of *DSM-IV* Criteria for Somatization Disorder**
>
> All the following criteria must be met:
> 1. History of medically unexplained physical symptoms beginning before age 30
> 2. History of all the following:
>   a. Pain related to at least four different sites (e.g., head, abdomen, back, joints, chest) or functions (e.g., during menstruation, during urination)
>   b. At least two gastrointestinal symptoms other than pain
>   c. At least one sexual or reproductive symptom other than pain (e.g., sexual indifference, irregular menses)
>   d. At least one symptom or deficit suggesting a neurologic condition not limited to pain (e.g., paralysis, lump in the throat, blindness)
> 3. Symptoms must not be explainable by any known medical condition, or when there is a related general medical condition, the complaints or impairment must be out of proportion to what might be reasonably expected.
> 4. Symptoms must not be intentionally produced or feigned.
>
> Modified from the *Diagnostic and statistical manual of mental disorders,* ed 4-TR, Washington, DC, 2000, American Psychiatric Association.

The diagnosis of somatization disorder requires several criteria (Box 107-1).[16] This diagnosis is rarely made in the ED, even though it may be suspected, because the proper investigation of this disorder involves time-consuming interviews and may require four to six visits before the establishment of a definitive diagnosis.[4] A short list of symptoms provides a rapid screen for this disorder.[32] The seven symptoms that may best discriminate between patients with and without somatization disorder are (1) dysmenorrhea, (2) the sensation of a "lump" in the throat, (3) vomiting, (4) shortness of breath, (5) burning in the sex organs, (6) painful extremities, and (7) amnesia lasting hours to days. Tested prospectively among patients displaying at least two of these seven symptoms, the diagnosis of somatization disorder is correctly predicted with a sensitivity of 93% and a specificity of 59%. When four or more of these seven symptoms are present, the specificity rises to 100%. Although this screening test may identify patients at high risk for somatization disorder, such patients should still be evaluated more thoroughly to confirm the diagnosis.

True somatization disorder is relatively uncommon, having a prevalence of 0.06% to 2% among the general population and up to 9% among hospitalized patients.[11,16,22,32,33] It tends to run in families and is rarely diagnosed in men,[13,14,16,34,35] although in some cultures the male/female ratio may be equal.[22] The typical patient is a woman in her forties who has a 25- to 30-year history of multiple vague complaints, usually headache, dizziness, nausea and vomiting, syncope, abdominal pain and bowel trouble, fatigue, palpitations, dyspareunia, and dysmenorrhea.[23,31,35-38] Symptoms usually date back to the patient's teens and twenties, with menstrual complaints being common in these age groups.[11,16,31]

Only 33% of patients recover during 10- to 20-year

follow-up,[39] and new symptoms requiring medical attention tend to surface at least every year.[11] Despite a "lifetime of suffering," the life span of these patients is normal.[40]

Somatization disorder is associated with lower socioeconomic groups, alcoholism and other addictions,[17,35,41] and poor education; fewer than 25% graduate from high school.[22,35] Many have occupational, interpersonal, and marital problems.[11,35]

The health care utilization and functional impairment of these patients are astounding. Expenditures for physician services are 14 times greater and overall health care expenditures nine times greater than for unaffected patients. The typical patient spends 7 days in the hospital each year and 7 days sick in bed each month (compared with less than a half day for a control population). More than 82% will stop work because of their health.[35] Once the diagnosis is recognized, however, medical resource use among these patients tends to normalize.[42]

Patients with somatization disorder describe their symptoms in dramatic exaggerated fashion using colorful language, with great detail about how their lives have been disrupted. They usually admit to being sickly throughout life. Although extensive, their narrative suggests no clear diagnostic constellation. Patients offer detailed accounts of multiple prior medical encounters, termed "doctor shopping," and often display multiple abdominal scars because they undergo two to three times the number of surgeries of other patients.[4,35] Their medical records have numerous and exotic test results, and they faithfully consume an impressive array of medications acquired from multiple primary care physicians and specialists. They report allergies to a comprehensive list of antibiotics and analgesics.

These patients are often emotional and vain, exhibit limited interpersonal skills, and have few close personal relationships.[31] They are typically dependent (especially on the physician), and often seductive (yet sexually unresponsive), and highly manipulative.

Of these patients, 68% fulfill the criteria for *histrionic personality disorder.*[43] Somatization disorder may be closely related to some anxiety and affective disorders; more than 80% of patients with somatization disorder report a lifetime history of major depression, and 68% a history of anxiety.[35,36,44,45] These individuals may threaten or attempt suicide. Completed suicide is usually associated with psychoactive substance abuse.[11] Women with this disorder tend to marry men with antisocial personalities. The husband often is overly solicitous, demanding that his wife receive many clinical studies and quick, decisive action. Predictably, he usually shows some degree of dissatisfaction with physicians in general.[31]

Patients who do not meet the full criteria of somatization disorder but have suggestive symptoms for 6 months or longer may be classified as having *undifferentiated somatoform disorder,* which is treated similar to somatization disorder.[16]

Conversion Disorder

Also known as *hysterical neurosis, conversion type,* the rare conversion disorder is characterized by the sudden onset and dramatic presentation of a single symptom, typically simulating some nonpainful neurologic disorder for which there is no pathophysiologic or anatomic explanation.[11] The symptoms, generally conforming to the patient's own idiosyncratic ideas about illness, are not under the patient's voluntary control. Some symptoms provide gratification for unconscious dependency needs; other symptoms provide escape from painful external emotional stimuli (e.g., hysterical paralysis in battle).[41,42,46] Although the symptoms may have a symbolic relationship to the precipitating factors, this is often not the case.[30,46] The most common conversion symptoms are voluntary motor or sensory functions and are therefore called *pseudoneurologic* (Box 107-2).[16] The most common presentations to the ED include pseudoseizures, syncope or coma, and paralysis or other movement disorders.[47]

Box 107-2 Presentations of Conversion Disorder

1. Motor disturbances
   a. Tremors (that worsen when attention is called to the movements)
   b. Seizures (wild, thrashing, writhing, often mimicking copulation)
   c. Paralysis or paresis (often a monoplegia, "stocking glove" weakness, with normal reflexes and limb circumferences)
   d. Aphonia (patient can whisper and cough normally, and vocal cords move normally with respiration)
   e. Coordination disturbances
2. Sensory disturbances
   a. Anesthesia (patient may not find this symptom disturbing)
   b. Blindness and tunnel vision
3. Occasionally, other nonneurologic symptoms, such as vomiting or pseudocyesis

Most patients are women, except for military service and industrial accidents.[16,42,46] Conversion disorder appears in adolescence and early adulthood (but may have later onset) and is more common among lower socioeconomic groups. Symptoms tend to be of sudden onset, waxing and waning in response to environmental stresses.[11,13,14,30,41] The history may show similar symptoms in the past, as well as anxiety, depression, phobias, and sexual disturbances.[30] Up to 29% of patients have a history of past psychiatric illness.[47] Patients may describe their conversion symptoms with a lack of appropriate concern about their profound bodily dysfunction (*la belle indifférence*). Although this time-honored feature has been classically associated with conversion disorder, it may be absent in more than 50% of patients and is also seen in organic disease.[48]

Pain Disorder

Also termed *somatoform pain disorder,*[11] this condition is similar to the conversion disorder in that stressful events are translated into somatic symptoms. The primary and often exclusive symptom is distressful pain that (1) is not intentionally feigned, (2) is persistent in nature, (3) limits daily function, (4) involves one or more organ systems, and (5) cannot be pathophysiologically explained.[16,17,30] The pain most frequently occurs in the face, low back, neck, or pelvic area and causes significant functional impairment, ultimately becoming a major focus in the patient's life.[8,13,14,16,23] One half of all patients have some precipitating traumatic event at the outset (e.g., motor vehicle accident, industrial injury).[11] Chronic pain behavior patterns are typically fixed within 3 months after the onset of symptoms, and patients who do not resume normal activities within 2 weeks deserve reevaluation and a careful psychosocial review.[8] Associated features include frequent visits to physicians despite medical reassurance (doctor shopping), excessive use of analgesics, requests for surgery, and eventually the role of permanent invalid after the pain has forced the patient to discontinue gainful employment.[8,11]

Onset occurs most often in the 30- to 50-year-old age group but can occur at any age. Symptoms such as headaches or musculoskeletal pain are more likely in women.[11,13,16] The pain often approximates real pain from physical disease that the patient has experienced in the past (e.g., the patient with a history of pancreatitis may develop recurrent epigastric pain when stressed). Frequent surgical intervention may produce multiple and genuine iatrogenic pain symptoms.[23]

Hypochondriasis

The term hypochondriasis comes from *regio hypochondriaca,* a Latin term referring to the upper lateral regions of the abdomen inferior to the costal cartilages, especially the area of the spleen, which early physicians presumed to be the seat of this disorder. Hypochondriasis has four characteristics: (1) physical symptoms disproportionate to demonstrable organic disease; (2) a fear of disease and a conviction that one is sick, leading to "illness-claiming behavior" (a compulsive insistence on being considered a physical cripple); (3) a preoccupation with one's own body; and (4) persistent and unsatisfying pursuit of medical care (doctor shopping) with a history of numerous procedures and surgeries and eventual return of symptoms.[30]

These unfortunate patients manifest both a heightened awareness and an unrealistic interpretation of normal physical signs or sensations, such as bowel habits, heartbeat, sweating, or peristalsis. These sensations are perceived as abnormal, noxious, and alarming, a phenomenon known as *amplification.*[34] These aberrant perceptions result in a chronic morbid preoccupation with bodily functions and a lingering fear of having a disease despite medical reassurance.[11,16,17,30] A distinguishing feature of hypochondriasis is that the patient's symptoms do exist and often are confirmed by physical examination, but the patient exaggerates and misinterprets them.

Hypochondriasis is relatively common. Its prevalence in general medical practice ranges from 4% to 9%.[16] It has a peak incidence among men in their thirties and women in their forties, affecting men and women in about the same proportions.[13,14,24] Hypochondriacs have an increased sense of responsibility for, and place high value on, their personal health and physical appearance. They have an acute sense of body vulnerability and a heightened aversion to death and aging.[34] A milder form of this disorder may be an exaggerated interest in bodily function and health ("health nuts").[49]

The hypochondriac complains at length and in detail, using medical jargon. The complaints focus on the head, neck, and trunk, often in the form of pain. The affected part is displayed to the physician, and the patient typically is unwilling to talk about anything but the symptoms in question. Hypochondriacs often believe they have lost control of their lives and have been characterized as "experts at defeating doctors in order to feel more powerful."[30] Consequently, physicians perceive hypochondriacal patients as more angry and hostile than other patients.[50] The diagnosis may be suggested when the physician feels "frustration, helplessness, or anger associated with a wish to be rid of the patient."[25,30]

Reactive hypochondriasis, or transient hypochondriasis, is an acute response to a psychosocial stress or life crisis, such as an acute myocardial infarction, terminal illness, or recent loss of a family member. In contrast to true hypochondriasis, this form is reversible and does respond to reassurance.[30,49]

DIAGNOSTIC STRATEGIES

Physicians are generally unwilling to consider somatoform disorders in their initial differential diagnosis. The often dramatic presentation of symptoms creates a sense of urgency to take action, a fear of undiscovered medical illness, and a subsequent exhaustive evaluation of every complaint. Repetitive or extensive diagnostic testing rarely excludes organic disease with absolute certainty, however, and may yield false-positive results, prompting further testing. Somatizing patients are more likely to have morbidity from repeated or invasive evaluations than from undiagnosed organic disease.[4,5]

Yielding to the temptation to institute further diagnostic procedures or interventions typically leads to a temporary improvement, closely followed by renewal of symptoms and mutual physician-patient disappointment. This gives rise to inevitable conclusions on the part of the patient ("another quack") and on the part of the physician ("another crock"), leading to an unsatisfactory parting of ways and a perpetuation of the doctor-shopping cycle.[51]

Managed care and capitated reimbursement have created an additional quandary by restricting the supply of care in a time of rising demand for care with a likely simultaneous rise in demand from those patients whose symptoms are relatively minor.[7,19] The most effective diagnostic tool with somatizers is the interview.[5] Evaluation starts with a thorough but focused history and, if available, a review of the patient's medical record. This is followed by a careful problem-oriented physical examination, with meticulous inspection of the area of complaint, and simple or routine diagnostic testing, when appropriate, until attaining a reasonable level of diagnostic certainty.[5,19] Further investigations or hospital admissions should be initiated solely on the basis of new objective signs of disease and only after confirming that the tests have not been performed. One rule of thumb in ordering laboratory tests is to do exactly what would be done if the patient were not a somatizer.[19,25] However, the clinician must resist the impassioned entreaties of the patient when it is clear that further complex or hazardous studies are unlikely to be productive.[13,14,19,52]

Multiple medical and surgical consultations generally prove counterproductive. Hypochondriacs perceive this as a test of their claim to illness and respond simply by propagating and demonstrating symptoms with redoubled zeal.[30]

DIFFERENTIAL CONSIDERATIONS

Distinguishing between the various somatoform disorders is less important than the diagnosis of treatable organic disease or the detection of anxiety and depression, which are both more common and more likely to respond to treatment.[5] Somatoform disorders overlap with depressive and anxiety disorders, and coexistent depression or anxiety disorder should always be considered.[45,53] Patients who have a relatively recent onset of somatization are more likely than patients with long-standing complaints to be exhibiting subtle signs of acute psychosis, organic brain syndrome, grief reaction, depression, or anxiety.

Depression

Approximately 50% to 70% of depressed patients consult their physician for various somatic complaints.[54] Depressed patients may not be aware of a depressed mood or may feel their depression is secondary to the somatic symptoms.[53] As a result, depression is the psychiatric disorder most often mistaken for somatoform disorder.[17]

Although somatoform disorders often coexist with depression, the two conditions must be distinguished. Depression is worse in the morning, better at night, and often associated with a positive family history. The patient is reluctant to describe the symptoms and has vegetative signs of depression (e.g., sleep disturbances, decreased appetite with weight loss).[52,55] Pain is a common symptom, particularly headache and pain involving the back, chest, or pelvic area.[53,54] Somatoform disorders, on the other hand, are worse at the end of the day, and patients have a marked propensity to discuss their symptoms, usually do not have a family history, and show no vegetative signs.[30]

In general, elderly patients do not have more physical symptoms than younger patients. Multiple somatic complaints should not be dismissed as a normal consequence of aging, but rather a symptom of another underlying problem, usually depression or medical disease. Older patients may communicate somatic complaints as a way of expressing anger and provoking guilt among family members.[24]

Anxiety

Patients with acute anxiety often hyperventilate and frequently exhibit physical signs of increased sympathetic activity. They may be hypervigilant and irritable and may show signs of muscular tension.[30] They may offer a history of excessive worrying about their health, feeling "on edge" or irritable, having difficulty relaxing, or sleeping poorly or having trouble falling asleep, and report symptoms of headache, tingling, dizzy spells, and diarrhea.[55]

Physical Illness

A diagnosis of somatization disorder does not confer immunity against physical disease. When patients with this disorder develop true organic disease, they present similar to other patients, with specific complaints, clear chronology, and objective findings that should be appropriately investigated.[31] Unfortunately, subjective reports of distress are often not dependable in these patients, and the emergency physician must rely on more objective evidence, including the physical examination and routine laboratory tests.[25] Multiple physical symptoms starting late in life are frequently the result of physical disease.[11,16] In addition, patients who have a short duration of symptoms are more likely to have organic disease.

Although any organic disease may be mistaken for a somatoform disorder, the occasionally bizarre and atypical manifestations and presentations of the disorders listed in Box 107-3 merit special consideration.[17]

Box 107-3 Organic Diseases Mistaken for Somatoform Disorders

Endocrine disorders: hyperparathyroidism, thyroid disorders, Addison's disease, insulinoma, panhypopituitarism
Guillain-Barré syndrome
Multiple sclerosis
Myasthenia gravis
Poisonings: botulism, carbon monoxide, heavy metals
Porphyria
Systemic lupus erythematosus
Wilson's disease
Uremia

Factitious Disease and Malingering

Patients with somatoform disorders are not deliberately feigning illness; they are exhibiting the result of an unconscious behavior modification. In the past they have unintentionally secured secondary gain from the "sick role" in the form of sympathy, encouragement, attention, support, and relief from responsibilities and challenges without significant loss of self-esteem.[49] In contrast, factitious disorder and malingering both are characterized by the intentional and conscious simulation or production of disease (see Chapter 108). Because such deception is difficult to uncover in the ED, these patients will often be mistaken for having a somatoform disorder.

MANAGEMENT

The symptoms of conversion disorder may provide a protective coping value for the patient, and the physician should be cautious about removing them without first providing adequate psychologic support and treatment. Otherwise, new symptoms may arise to replace previous ones. The external precipitating stress or cause of anxiety should be removed if possible. These patients require psychiatric evaluation and management,[13,14] and psychiatric consultation in the ED can be beneficial.[47]

Recurrence is common, but the prognosis associated with an individual episode of conversion disorder is good, and the likelihood of recovery from symptoms exceeds that of other somatoform disorders.[16,24,42] Factors associated with a good prognosis include (1) good premorbid health, (2) absence of organic illness or concomitant major psychiatric syndromes, (3) acute and recent onset, (4) definite precipitation by a stressful event, and (5) presenting symptoms of paralysis, aphonia, or blindness.[16]

Reassurance

Young patients with no underlying medical or psychiatric illnesses who present with somatization in response to a clear psychosocial stress can often be reassured successfully with an appropriate explanation of their symptoms.[5] Patients with chronic somatization, however, will perceive this as an official denial of their sick role and are almost invariably unwilling to accept reassurance. Because they desire the acknowledgment and recognition that come with the designation of illness, which they feel is rightfully theirs, they are disappointed when no pathologic condition is discovered. Conversely, they are elated when given a diagnosis, but they resist recovery because subconsciously the "specter of cure" poses a threat to their sick role.[49] Accordingly, attempts to cure the condition will be countered with side effects, allergic reactions, and new symptoms. Such patients require another management strategy.[5]

Legitimization of Symptoms

Most patients with chronic somatization interpret a psychologic explanation for their symptoms as an accusation of lying or feeblemindedness. It is critical to convince them that the emergency physician believes in their symptoms and will not try to "talk them out of it." The priority is to listen and truly understand what the patient is feeling and trying to convey. Suffering is always a subjective phenomenon and, in that sense, is genuine in these patients.[25] The emergency physician should convey empathy for the patient's physical discomfort. If the emergency physician acknowledges the legitimacy of the claim to illness and assures the somatizer of ongoing care, limits may be set on the patient's illness behavior.[5,13,14,19,24,30]

Patients should be allowed to tell their story without interruption. Validation of their experiences may be reflected in statements such as, "I can see why you'd feel that way." They should be told that they have an illness that causes them to experience many symptoms, but that these symptoms will not lead to medical deterioration.[4,56] The emergency physician should offer only guarded projections regarding chances for complete "cure" of the condition. Ironically, this may be better received by these patients than overly optimistic assurances because the former serves to safeguard their sick role and shifts the physician away from an adversarial position.[19,52]

Diagnosis

Diagnostic labels are of critical importance for somatizers, but the precise meaning of the term should be clarified for that patient to avoid misinterpretation. Explanations for symptoms that incorporate somatic responses and descriptions such as hyperventilation, tension headache, muscle tension, muscle strain, chest wall muscle spasm, or stress may be better accepted than purely psychiatric diagnoses. This reassures the patient that the emergency physician shares the belief that the symptoms result from socially acceptable ailments, while allowing more in-depth explanations that incorporate the relationship of bodily function to psychologic stress. This in turn serves as a preparation for future psychiatric consultation or psychotropic medication.[5,12-14,52]

At times the best approach may be to share the diagnostic uncertainty with the patient, using such terms as "atypical pain" or "multiple complaints following injury."[5] On a broader scale, managed care organizations must be encouraged to educate their enrollees about the process of somatization, the negative side effects of medications and other interventions, and the range of bodily symptoms in healthy people.[7]

Medications

Patients with somatoform disorder have a high affinity for medications and are reluctant to discontinue drugs, even those with no benefit.[30] The emergency physician should avoid drugs that produce an abstinence syndrome or dependence and those that cannot be safely continued indefinitely.[31] Pain medications, if given, should be prescribed for regular intervals, not "as needed."[30]

Therapy should be kept simple and limited to exercise, diet, physical therapy, and vitamins when possible.[52] Hospitalization and narcotics should be avoided. Benign remedies, such as lotions, nutritional supplements, elastic bandages, and heating pads, may be helpful.[19,25] Drug regimens should be simplified and only the most distressing symptoms addressed. Before starting any type of symptomatic drug treatment, specific target symptoms should be identified. The goal is to restore function and to make the target symptoms tolerable, not to remove them completely. If ED patients request an increase in dosage or a stronger medication, they should be told to review their medications with their regular physician before any changes are made. Insistent patients may be informed that long-term opioid use is associated with significant adverse effects, especially constipation, sedation, impaired cognition, and progressive development of tolerance and addiction.[25]

Mental Health Consultation

Patients with somatoform disorders have difficulty confronting their own emotions, view psychiatric evaluation as threatening to their sick role, and take offense at any suggestion that their fears or beliefs may be unwarranted.[11,15] They usually resist psychiatric consultation and interpret it as an attempt to be "dumped on the psychiatrist."[30] Nevertheless, psychiatric consultation may be appropriate (1) to confirm the diagnosis or discuss medications, (2) when the patient has coexistent manifestations of chronic depression or psychosis, (3) when symptoms suddenly change or become bizarre, (4) when the patient expresses suicidal ideation or severely disruptive behavior, (4) when current management is not working, or (5) when the patient requests psychotherapy.[5,13,14,30] Favorable prognostic indicators include youth, acute onset, concurrent anxiety or depression, and limited medical comorbidity.[57]

Many patients accept psychologic treatment under the rubric of "stress management" as long as it targets physical symptoms and somatic distress.[19] Group therapy techniques presented as education rather than psychotherapy have had some limited success.[58] Patients should be reassured that continuity of care with the primary physician will be provided to avoid the false interpretation that the referral is an abandonment.[5]

Physician Attitudes

Somatizing patients often take over the interview. They may subtly or overtly question the physician's competence or may demand inappropriate tests, stronger medications, or specialty referrals. Emergency physicians caring for these patients predictably react with feelings of uncertainty, helplessness, anger, or guilt. Such feelings may interfere, consciously or unconsciously, with patient care and result in extensive workups and referrals, as well as overmedication or undermedication. Strategies for dealing with these feelings begin with recognition and acknowledgment. Discussing these feelings with colleagues and consultants, sharing with the patient the responsibility for care, and modifying therapeutic expectations are helpful.[5,52]

Treatment Goals

Somatizing patients have a need to be ill. Attaining invalid status enables them to be cared for and nurtured. It offers them a sense of self-importance and respect not otherwise available to them, as well as an honorable release from noxious personal and vocational responsibilities and duties.[41] To attempt a cure poses a threat to this role, and unduly positive projections by physicians are therefore understandably met with disappointment, disbelief, and even thinly veiled reproaches regarding their professional competence.[8,19,52] Thus the goal of therapy must be *control of disability* rather than cure.[24,57] The course of management most likely to prove successful begins with performing a sympathetic and thorough problem-oriented history and physical examination, then offering the patient the paradoxical reassurance that they will probably always be ill. When pain is the dominant feature, the patient should not be promised complete relief; rather, a major task of the patient should be to "learn to live with some pain."[24]

Treatment goals should focus on modification of illness behavior and improvement of functional status.[41] Achievable endpoints include (1) decreased frequency and urgency of medical use, in particular a reduction in ED and unscheduled office visits; (2) avoidance of expensive and hazardous procedures; (3) improved work or school performance; (4) more social activities; and (5) better personal relationships.[5,13,17]

Patients with somatoform disorder have been described as the "least insightful, the least introspective and the least cognitively oriented patients one is likely to encounter."[31] Understanding the link between emotional and somatic distress need not be a treatment goal for these patients, and insight-oriented psychotherapy is neither productive nor cost-effective.[5,19,24,25,31] On the other hand, both the emergency physician and the patient must accept fundamental alterations in the traditional paternalistic physician-patient relationship. Increasing responsibility for health and disease management must be incrementally turned over to the somatizing patient.[24]

DISPOSITION

Appropriate referral for "continued vigilance" should be provided for the patient. Outpatient tests or hospitalization should be avoided unless clear objective signs indicate a need for diagnostic investigation or therapeutic intervention.[24,31]

As a rule, management is best carried out by a single primary care physician who will become the gatekeeper for all medical consultation and care.[4,12-14,17,19,24,30,52,57] The patient should be told that no alarming findings have come to light, that further testing and additional medications are not indicated at this time, and that ongoing care and periodic reassessment are indicated and will be arranged. Patients with chronic somatization should initially be seen every 2 to 4 weeks, even if their symptoms are stable. The visits should be on a time-contingent, not a need-contingent, basis. For the patient, this severs the association between medical contact and the necessity for worsening or additional symptoms and complaints. It also decreases the patient's fear of abandonment by the physician and permits repeated evaluation for early detection of objective signs of organic disease.[5,17,24] The patient seems to value the visit to the physician more highly than any treatment.[31]

KEY CONCEPTS

- The behavior of patients with somatoform disorders is unconsciously driven. They are not "faking" the symptoms or their distress.
- Short-term management should include the legitimization of symptoms, communication of compassion, and assurance that ongoing vigilance of the patient's medical condition will be arranged and maintained.
- Long-term cure of somatization disorder is unlikely. However, a steady state of symptom coping with improved function is an achievable goal. This can only be done in the primary care setting, not in the ED.
- New objective clinical findings should be medically evaluated. Otherwise, laboratory tests, specialty consultations, initiation of medications, and hospitalization should be avoided. Care decisions should be deferred to the patient's primary care physician when possible.

REFERENCES

1. Kessler LG, Cleary PD, Burke JD: Psychiatric disorders in primary care: results of a follow-up study, *Arch Gen Psychiatry* 42:583, 1985.
2. Peterson LG, Cohen LM: Use of psychiatric screening instruments in the ED, *Am J Emerg Med* 3:476, 1985 (editorial).
3. Gold I, Baraff LJ: Psychiatric screening in the emergency department: its effect on physician behavior, *Ann Emerg Med* 18:875, 1989.
4. Zoccolillo MS, Cloninger CR: Excess medical care of women with somatization disorder, *South Med J* 79:532, 1986.
5. Gordon GH: Treating somatizing patients, *West J Med* 147:88, 1987.
6. Schurman RA, Kramer PD, Mitchell JB: The hidden mental health network: treatment of mental illness by nonpsychiatrist physicians, *Arch Gen Psychiatry* 42:89, 1985.
7. Barsky AJ, Borus JF: Somatization and medicalization in the era of managed care, *JAMA* 274:1931, 1995.
8. Gillette RD: Behavioral factors in the management of back pain, *Am Fam Physician* 53:1313, 1996.
9. Woods SM, Natterson J, Silverman J: Medical students' disease: hypochondriasis in medical education, *J Med Educ* 41:785, 1966.
10. Swartz M et al: Somatization symptoms in the community: a rural/urban comparison, *Psychosomatics* 30:44, 1989.
11. *Diagnostic and statistical manual of mental disorders,* ed 3, Washington, DC, 1987, American Psychiatric Association.
12. Lipowski ZJ: Somatization: a borderland between medicine and psychiatry, *CMAJ* 135:609, 1986.
13. Smith RC: A clinical approach to the somatizing patient, *J Fam Pract* 21:294, 1985.
14. Smith RC: Somatization in primary care, *Clin Obstet Gynecol* 31:902, 1988.
15. Stewart DE: The changing faces of somatization, *Psychosomatics* 31:153, 1990.
16. *Diagnostic and statistical manual of mental disorders,* ed 4-TR, Washington, DC, 2000, American Psychiatric Association.
17. Ries RK et al: The medical care abuser: differential diagnosis and management, *J Fam Pract* 13:257, 1981.
18. Göthe CJ, Odont CM, Nilsson CG: The environmental somatization syndrome, *Psychosomatics* 36:1, 1995.
19. Barsky AJ: A 37-year-old man with multiple somatic complaints, *JAMA* 278:673, 1997.
20. Ciccone DS, Just N, Bandilla EB: Non-organic symptom reporting in patients with chronic non-malignant pain, *Pain* 68:329, 1996.
21. Katon W et al: Somatization: a spectrum of severity, *Am J Psychiatry* 148:34, 1991.
22. Escobar JI et al: Somatic symptom index (SSI): a new and abridged somatization construct, *J Nerv Ment Dis* 177:140, 1989.
23. Badura AS et al: Dissociation, somatization, substance abuse, and coping in women with chronic pelvic pain, *Obstet Gynecol* 90:405, 1997.

24. Ford CV: *The somatizing disorders: illness as a way of life,* New York, 1983, Elsevier Biomedical.
25. Servan-Schreiber D, Kolb R, Tabas G: The somatizing patient, *Prim Care* 26:225, 1999.
26. Zwaigenbaum L et al: Highly somatizing young adolescents and the risk of depression, *Pediatrics* 103:1203, 1999.
27. Guze SB: The validity and significance of the clinical diagnosis of hysteria (Briquet's syndrome), *Am J Psychiatry* 132:138, 1975.
28. Epstein RM, Quill TE, McWhinney IR: Somatization reconsidered: incorporating the patient's experience of illness, *Arch Intern Med* 159:215, 1999.
29. McWhinney IR, Epstein RM, Freeman TR: Lingua medica: rethinking somatization, *Ann Intern Med* 126:747, 1997.
30. Dubovsky SL, Weissberg MP: Hypochondriasis. In Dubovsky SL: *Clinical psychiatry in primary care,* ed. 3, Baltimore, 1986, Williams & Wilkins.
31. Murphy GE: The clinical management of hysteria, *JAMA* 247:2559, 1982.
32. Othmer E, DeSouza C: A screening test for somatization disorder (hysteria), *Am J Psychiatry* 142:1146, 1985.
33. DeGruy F et al: Somatization disorder in a university hospital, *J Fam Pract* 25:579, 1987.
34. Barsky AJ, Wyshak G: Hypochondriasis and related health attitudes, *Psychosomatics* 30:412, 1989.
35. Smith GR, Monson RA, Ray DG: Patients with multiple unexplained symptoms: their characteristics, functional health, and health care utilization, *Arch Intern Med* 146:69, 1986.
36. Barsky AJ et al: The clinical course of palpitations in medical outpatients, *Arch Intern Med* 155:1782, 1995.
37. Manu P, Lane TJ, Matthews DA: Somatization disorder in patients with chronic fatigue, *Psychosomatics* 30:388, 1989.
38. Kapoor WN et al: Psychiatric illnesses in patients with syncope, *Am J Med* 99:505, 1995.
39. Coryell W, Norten SG: Briquet's syndrome (somatization disorder) and primary depression: comparison of background and outcome, *Compr Psychiatry* 22:249, 1981.
40. Coryell W: Diagnosis-specific mortality: primary unipolar depression and Briquet's syndrome (somatization disorder), *Arch Gen Psychiatry* 38:939, 1981.
41. Quill TE: Somatization disorder: one of medicine's blind spots, *JAMA* 254:3075, 1985.
42. Kent DA, Tomasson K, Coryell W: Course and outcome of conversion and somatization disorders: a four-year follow-up, *Psychosomatics* 36:138, 1995.
43. Morrison J: Histrionic personality disorder in women with somatization disorder, *Psychosomatics* 30:433, 1989.
44. Orenstein H: Briquet's syndrome in association with depression and panic: a reconceptualization of Briquet's syndrome, *Am J Psychiatry* 146:334, 1989.
45. Rogers MP et al: Prevalence of somatoform disorders in a large sample of patients with anxiety disorders, *Psychosomatics* 37:17, 1996.
46. Ford CV, Folks DG: Conversion disorders: an overview, *Psychosomatics* 26:371, 1985.
47. Dula DJ, DeNaples L: Emergency department presentation of patients with conversion disorder, *Acad Emerg Med* 2:120, 1995.
48. Barnert C: Conversion reactions and psychophysiologic disorders: a comparative study, *Psychiatry Med* 2:205, 1971.
49. Barsky AJ, Klerman GL: Overview: hypochondriasis, bodily complaints, and somatic styles, *Am J Psychiatry* 140:273, 1983.
50. Kellner R et al: Anxiety, depression, and somatization in DSM-III hypochondriasis, *Psychosomatics* 30:57, 1989.
51. Sternbach RA: Varieties of pain games, *Adv Neurol* 4:423, 1974.
52. Lichstein PR: Caring for the patient with multiple somatic complaints, *South Med J* 79:310, 1986.
53. Lipowski ZJ: Somatization and depression, *Psychosomatics* 31:13, 1990.
54. Katon W: Depression: somatization and social factors, *J Fam Pract* 27:579, 1988 (editorial).
55. Goldberg D et al: Detecting anxiety and depression in general medical settings, *BMJ* 297:897, 1988.
56. Johns M: Communicating effectively with a patient who has somatization disorder, *Am Fam Physician* 59:2639, 1999.
57. Barsky AJ: Hypochondriasis: medical management and psychiatric treatment, *Psychosomatics* 37:48, 1996.
58. Kashner TM et al: Enhancing the health of somatization disorder patients: effectiveness of short-term group therapy, *Psychosomatics* 36:462, 1995.

108 Factitious Disorders and Malingering

Thomas B. Purcell

PERSPECTIVE

Patients may present to the ED with symptoms that are intentionally produced or simulated. The inducements that generate this behavior differentiate two distinct varieties: factitious disorders and malingering.

Factitious disorders are characterized by symptoms or signs that are intentionally produced or feigned by the patient in the absence of apparent external incentives.[1,2] These patients constitute approximately 1% of general psychiatric referrals. This is somewhat lower than that seen in emergency medicine and other clinical settings because acceptance of psychiatric treatment is unusual in these patients.[1,3] Among patients referred to infectious disease specialists for fever of unknown origin, 9.3% are factitious.[4] Between 5% and 20% of patients followed in epilepsy clinics have psychogenic seizures, and in some primary care settings the number reaches 44%.[5] Of patients submitting kidney stones for analysis, 2.6% have been found to be fraudulent.[6]

Munchausen's syndrome, the most dramatic and exasperating of the factitious disorders, was originally described in 1951.[7] This fortunately rare syndrome takes its name from Baron Karl F. von Munchausen (1720-1797), a noted raconteur who amused his friends with fantastic and entertaining but untrue personal anecdotes. The diagnosis is appropriately applied to only 10% to 20% of patients with factitious disorders.[1,8] Other names applied include the "hospital hobo syndrome" (patients wander from hospital to hospital seeking admission), peregrinating (wandering) problem patients, hospital addict, polysurgical addiction, laparotomaphilia migrans, Kopenickades syndrome, Ahasuerus syndrome, and hospital vagrant.[3,9,10]

An especially pernicious variant of Munchausen's syndrome involves the simulation or production of factitious disease in children by a parent or caregiver. Also known as Polle syndrome[9] and factitious disorder by proxy,[11] *Munchausen syndrome by proxy* (MSBP) was first described in 1977.[12] The syndrome excludes straightforward physical abuse or neglect and simple failure to thrive; mere lying to cover up physical abuse is not MSBP.[13,14] The key discriminator is motive: the mother is making the child ill so that she can vicariously assume the sick role with all its benefits. Mortality from MSBP is 9% to 31%.[14,15] Children who die are generally under 3 years old, and the most frequent causes of death are suffocation and poisoning.[14] Permanent disfigurement or permanent impairment of function resulting directly from induced disease or indirectly from invasive procedures, multiple medications, or major surgery occurs in at least 8% of these children.[14,16]

Malingering is the simulation of disease by the intentional production of false or grossly exaggerated physical or psychologic symptoms, motivated by external incentives such as avoiding military conscription or duty, avoiding work, obtaining financial compensation, evading criminal prosecution, obtaining drugs, gaining hospital admission (for purposes of obtaining free room and board), or securing better living conditions.[2,17-20] The most common goal among such "patients" presenting to the ED is obtaining drugs, whereas in the office or clinic setting, the gain is more commonly insurance payments or industrial injury settlements.[21] Due to underreporting, the true incidence of malingering is difficult to gauge, but estimates include a 1% incidence among mental health patients in civilian clinical practice, 5% in the military, and as high as 10% to 20% among patients presenting in a litigious context.[19]

CLINICAL FEATURES

Factitious Disorders

In patients with factitious disorder the production of symptoms and signs is compulsive in that the patient is unable to refrain from the behavior even when its risks are known. The behavior is voluntary only in the sense that it is deliberate and purposeful (intentional), but not in the sense that the acts can be fully controlled.[2] The underlying motivation for producing these deceptions, securing the sick role, is primarily unconscious.[8,22,23] Individuals who readily admit that they have produced their own injuries (e.g., self-mutilation) are not included in the category of factitious disorders.[11] The symptoms involved may be either psychologic or physical.

Psychologic Symptoms This disorder consists of the intentional production or feigning of psychologic (often psychotic) symptoms suggestive of a mental disorder. Stimulants may be used to induce restlessness or insomnia, hallucinogens to create altered levels of consciousness, and hypnotics to produce lethargy. The symptoms are often amplified when the patient is aware of being observed. The patient may be extremely suggestible and admit to many additional symptoms proposed by the physician. This condition, seen less often than factitious disorder with physical symptoms, is almost always superimposed on a severe personality disorder.[2,11,17]

Physical Symptoms The intentional production of physical symptoms may take the form of fabrication of symptoms without signs (e.g., feigning abdominal pain), simulation of signs suggesting illness (e.g., fraudulent pyuria, induced anemia), self-inflicted pathology (e.g., producing abscesses by injecting contaminated material under the skin), or genuine complications from the intentional misuse of medications (e.g., diuretics, hypoglycemic agents).[20] These patients are predominantly unmarried women less than 40 years of age. They typically accept their illness with few complaints and are generally responsible workers with moral attitudes and otherwise conscientious behavior.[20,24] Many are in health care occupations, including nurses, aides, and physicians.

These patients are willing to undergo incredible hardship, limb amputation, organ loss, and even death to perpetuate the masquerade.[20] Suggested unconscious incentives include the receipt of nurturing and caring attention and the drama of assuming the patient role. Although multiple hospitalizations often lead to iatrogenic physical conditions, such as postoperative pain syndromes and drug addictions, patients continue to crave hospitalization for its own sake. They typically have a fragile and fragmented self-image and are prone to psychotic, and even suicidal, episodes.[24] Thus, interactions with the health care system and relationships with caregivers serve to provide needed structure that stabilizes the sense of self. The hospital itself may be perceived as a refuge, sanctuary, or womblike environment.[3,20,22,25] Although some patients are motivated by desires for the attention and gratification associated with medical care, others are apparently driven by the conviction that they have a real, but as yet undiscovered, illness. Consequently, artificial symptoms are contrived to convince the physician to continue a search for the elusive disease process.[20]

Munchausen's Syndrome The uncommon patient with true Munchausen's syndrome has a prolonged pattern of "medical imposture," usually years in duration. The behavior usually begins before age 20 and is diagnosed between ages 35 and 39. Twice as many men are affected as women.[3,26] Patients' entire adult life may consist of trying to gain admission to hospitals and then steadfastly resisting discharge. Their career of imposture usually lasts about 9 years but has continued unabated for as long as 50 years.[3] The quest for repeated hospitalizations often takes these patients to numerous and widespread cities, states, and even countries.[17]

These individuals see themselves as very important people, or at least related to such persons, and their life events are depicted as exceptional.[26] They possess extensive knowledge of medical terminology. Frequently there is a history of genuine disease, and the individual may exhibit objective physical findings.[24]

The symptoms presented are "limited only by the person's medical knowledge, sophistication, and imagination."[2] The alleged illnesses involved have been termed *dilemma diagnoses* in that investigators rarely can totally rule out the disorder, clarify the cause, or prove that it did not exist at one time.[3] Common presentations are those that most reliably will result in admission to the hospital, such as abdominal pain, self-injection of a foreign substance,[9,10] feculent urine, bleeding disorders, hemoptysis, paroxysmal headaches, seizures, shortness of breath, asthma with respiratory failure,[3,27] chronic pain,[23] acute cardiovascular symptoms (e.g., chest pain, induced hypertension and syncope),[26] renal colic, and fever of unknown origin (hyperpyrexia figmentatica).[10] Such self-induced conditions themselves may prove highly injurious or even lethal.[9]

The patient usually presents to the ED during evenings or on weekends, so as to minimize accessibility to psychiatric consultants, personal physicians, and past medical records.[10,24] In teaching institutions these patients typically present in July, shortly after the change in resident house officers.[3] They relate their history in a precise, dramatic, even intriguing fashion, embellished with flourishes of pathologic lying and self-aggrandizement (pseudologia fantastica). The history quickly becomes vague and inconsistent, however, when the patient is questioned in detail about medical contacts.[2,25] Attempts to manage the complaint as an outpatient will be adamantly resisted.[23] Once admitted, the patient initially appeals to the physician's qualities of nurturance and omnipotence, lavishing praise on the caregivers. Behavior rapidly evolves, however, as the patient creates havoc on the ward by insisting on excessive attention while ignoring both hospital rules and the prescribed therapeutic regimen.[2] Once the hoax is uncovered and the patient confronted, fear of rejection abruptly changes into rage against the treating physician, closely followed by departure from the hospital against medical advice.[9,10,23]

Munchausen Syndrome by Proxy The diagnosis of MSBP depends on specific criteria (Box 108-1).[14] The presenting complaints typically evade definitive diagnosis and are refractory to conventional therapy for no apparent reason.[14] The symptoms are usually more than five in number, presented in a confused picture, are unusual or serious, and by design, unverifiable, invariably occurring when the mother is alone with the child or otherwise unobserved.[28] In 72% to 95% of cases, simulation or production of illness will occur while the victim is hospitalized.[14]

Simulated illness, faked by the mother without producing direct harm to the child (e.g., adding blood to a urine specimen), is present in 25% of cases. *Produced illness,* which the mother actually inflicts on the child (e.g., injection of feces into an intravenous line), is found in 50% of cases.

Box 108-1 Diagnostic Criteria for Munchausen Syndrome by Proxy

1. Apparent illness or health-related abnormality that the parent or someone who is in *loco parentis* has concocted or produced
2. Presentation of the child for medical treatment, usually persistently
3. Failure by the perpetrator to acknowledge the true etiology or the deception
4. Cessation of the acute symptoms and signs of illness when the child is separated from the perpetrator

Both simulated and produced illness are found in 25% of cases.[14]

The most common presentations of MSBP include factitious bleeding, seizures, central nervous system (CNS) depression, apnea, diarrhea, vomiting, fever, and rash.[14] Reported techniques of simulation or production of disease include administration of drugs or toxins (e.g., chronic arsenic poisoning, ipecac, warfarin, phenolphthalein, hydrocarbons, salt, imipramine, laxatives, CNS depressants), caustics applied to the skin, and nasal aspiration of cooking oil.[12,14-16,24,29] Techniques of asphyxiation include (1) covering the mouth or nose with one or both hands, a cloth, or plastic film and (2) inserting the fingers into the back of the mouth. In such instances even struggling infants may sustain no cutaneous markings.[30] Cases involving seizures are common and may involve third-party witnesses. On personal questioning, however, these witnesses frequently deny the occurrence of seizure activity.[14]

Knowing that another child in the family has been reported to have similar symptoms does not reduce the possibility of MSBP. In a variant of MSBP termed *serial Munchausen syndrome by proxy,* there may be a history of similar strange presentations in multiple siblings, although typically only one child is involved at a time.[15,16,30] In 9% of such cases there is a history of siblings who died under mysterious circumstances.[14]

Perpetrator Characteristics Ninety-eight percent of perpetrators are biologic mothers from all socioeconomic groups.[14] Many have a background in health professions or social work, features of Munchausen's syndrome themselves, or a past history of psychiatric treatment, marital problems, or suicide attempts.[14,15] Depression, anxiety, and somatization are common, but frankly psychotic behavior by the mother is atypical.[14,16] Perpetrators of MSBP have an inherent skill in manipulating health workers and child protection services.[31] They are very pleasant, socially adept, cooperative, and appreciative of good medical care. They often choose to stay in the hospital with their child, cultivate unusually close relationships with hospital staff, and thrive on the staff's attention.[12-14,16,29] This affable relationship with the medical team rapidly changes to excessive anger and denial when confronted with suspicions.[16]

Most of these mothers have had an abusive experience early in life, and they use the health care system as a means to satisfy personal nurturing demands.[28,32] They often cannot distinguish their needs from the child's and will satisfy their own needs first. They derive a sense of purpose from the medical and nursing attention gained when their children are in the hospital.[13,14,16,32] Alternatively, the behavior may enable the mothers to escape from their own physical or psychologic illnesses, marital difficulties, or social problems.[28]

Victim Characteristics Victims of MSBP are equal numbers of male and female children. The mean age at diagnosis is 40 months, and the mean duration from the onset of signs and symptoms to diagnosis is 15 months.[14] The child shows few if any physical signs, and those found are usually incidental to the presenting complaints. A known physical illness that explains part of the symptoms is common among these children.[32] Most have a history of significant failure to thrive and have been hospitalized in more than one institution. Delays in many areas of performance and learning, difficulty with family relationships, attention deficit disorder, or clinical depression may coexist.[16] Victims of MSBP also are found among the elderly population, although this is uncommon.[33]

Malingering

Malingering is frequently found in association with *antisocial personality disorder.* On questioning, malingerers will be vague about prior hospitalizations or treatments. The physicians who previously treated them are usually unavailable. At times, malingerers may be careless about their symptoms and abandon them when they believe no one is watching.[24] In some "patients," such as those seeking drugs, homeless persons seeking hospital admission on a cold night, or prisoners wanting a holiday from incarceration, the secondary gain may be clear. In other persons the external incentive may be obscure.

In contrast to the person with factitious disorders, the malinger prefers *counterfeit mental illness* because it is objectively difficult to verify or disprove. Amnesia is the most common psychologic presentation, followed by paranoia, morbid depression, suicidal ideation, and psychosis.[19]

DIAGNOSTIC STRATEGIES

Factitious Disorders

Identification of factitious disorder is usually made in one of four ways: (1) the patient is accidentally discovered in the act; (2) incriminating items are found; (3) laboratory values suggest nonorganic etiology; or (4) the diagnosis is made by exclusion.[11] Diagnosis may be confounded by genuine medical illnesses predating and coexisting with a factitious disorder. For example, patients with factitious hypoglycemia may have a history of insulin-dependent diabetes mellitus, or factitious skin disorders may be preceded by true dermatologic diseases.[1]

Suspected MSBP requires a detailed description of the event or illness and a search for caregiver witnesses, who should be interviewed personally. Although it is essential to see the child when the symptoms are present, the parents show great ingenuity at frustrating this effort.[32] Additional history of unusual illness in siblings and parents should be sought. Child victims who are verbal should be interviewed in private regarding foods, medicines, and their recollection of the symptoms or events. A careful physical examination should be performed to exclude physical explanations. Prior medical records of the victim and if possible the siblings should be examined, although parents may impede such data gathering.

The major obstacle to early discovery of MSBP is its omission from the differential diagnosis. Once considered, the diagnosis is generally made easily and quickly.[14] A suspected diagnosis may be confirmed through separation of the parent from the child (with consequent cessation of symptoms), covert video surveillance during hospitalization, or toxin screens.[16,28,30] In the majority of cases the caregiver will attempt to induce episodes surreptitiously while in the hospital, often during the first day of admission.[14,28]

Malingering

Malingering should be strongly suspected with any combination of certain factors (Box 108-2).[17,34] A definitive diagnosis of malingering can only be established by securing the patient's confession, a rare circumstance.[35] Because this constitutes criminal behavior, documentation of this diagnosis must be made with care.[19] In the absence of proof of wrongdoing, it is best to assume that the patient is not a malingerer but rather a common somatizer.[35]

Box 108-2 Characteristics of Malingering

1. Medicolegal context of the presentation (e.g., "patient" referred by attorney)
2. Marked discrepancy between the person's claimed stress or disability and objective findings
3. Poor cooperation during the diagnostic evaluation or poor compliance with previously prescribed treatment regimens
4. Signs or history of antisocial behavior

DIFFERENTIAL CONSIDERATIONS

Patients with factitious disorders are distinguished from malingerers because their desired hospitalization or surgery seems to offer no secondary gain other than granting the sick role.[2,9,21] The clinical presentation of the majority of patients with factitious disorders, unlike those with Munchausen's syndrome, is relatively subtle and convincing. The complaints are generally chronic in nature, rather than emergent and precipitous, and there are no obvious associated behavioral aberrations.[20] Malingering is usually associated with less chronicity than factitious disorder, and malingerers are more reluctant to accept expensive, possibly painful, or dangerous tests or surgery.[21]

MANAGEMENT

Treatment options for factitious disorders depend on patient characteristics. Although challenging, management of the more common forms of factitious disorder can be more rewarding, especially with adolescents, than is the case with Munchausen's syndrome.[1,8,22,25] Cases stemming from an underlying depression have a more favorable prognosis than those associated with borderline personalities.[24]

The best approach to patients with factitious disorder, other than Munchausen's syndrome and MSBP, remains an area of controversy. Direct nonaccusatory confrontation has been advocated as "the foundation of effective management," when coupled with the assurance that an ongoing relationship with a physician will be provided.[3,20,21,24] This may be the first step in the acceptance of outpatient therapy.[3]

Others believe that confrontation threatens to undermine a needed psychologic defense. Enforced recognition of external objective reality, while simultaneously disallowing the patient's subjective experience, may generate even more dysfunction to legitimize and maintain symptoms or may place the patient at risk for suicide.[8,11,25,36,37] Some patients may relinquish this defense if they feel safe in doing so and may abandon a claim to disease if some face-saving option is offered. This approach, termed the *therapeutic double bind* or *contingency management,* involves informing the patient that a factitious disorder may exist. The patient is further told that failure to respond fully to medical care would constitute conclusive evidence that their problem is not organic but rather psychiatric. The problem is therefore reframed or redefined in such a way that (1) symptoms and their resolution are both legitimized and (2) the patient has little choice but to accept and respond to a proposed course of action, or seek care elsewhere.[8,37]

Individuals with Munchausen's syndrome typically demonstrate overt sociopathic traits and are demanding and manipulative, especially regarding analgesics.[8] They are difficult to deal with, universally impressing authors on the subject as truculent, noncompliant, hostile, and incorrigible. They have been described as "essentially untreatable," and successful management of this condition is, in fact, considered reportable. Early confrontation or limit setting, especially regarding drug use, is advocated.[8,10,20,23,24] Although Munchausen patients typically do not want to be examined extensively, a thorough physical examination should be performed to rule out physical pathology.

MSBP constitutes a form of child (or elder) abuse, and appropriate action to protect the victim, including notification of welfare services, should take immediate priority.[30,33]

When the diagnosis has been established and the parents confronted, psychiatric care should be made immediately available to the parents, since maternal suicide is a significant risk.[14]

Malingerers do not want to be treated. Since they are "gaming the system" for personal advantage, the last thing they want is an accurate identification of their behavior and appropriate intervention. The emergency physician should maintain clinical neutrality, offering the reassurance that the symptoms and examination are not consistent with any serious disease.

Some authors have characterized patient use of medical resources under false pretenses as criminal behavior, and several states have enacted legislation against the fraudulent acquisition of medical services. Successful prosecution of such behavior has been reported.[38] Conversely, patients with factitious disorders can and do sue. In dealing with such patients, it is advisable to involve hospital administration and risk management. Clandestine searches are inadvisable, and respect for patient confidentiality should be maintained.[11]

DISPOSITION

Patients with factitious disorder should receive primary care follow-up and ongoing care. If acceptable, psychiatric referral should be arranged. Referral to other medical specialists or hospitalization should be avoided when possible.

The manner of presentation and the unavailability of past medical history often allow patients with Munchausen's syndrome to achieve hospital admission. If the patient is discharged from the ED, outpatient primary care follow-up and psychiatric referral should be offered, although both will likely be refused.[23]

Because perpetrators of MSBP will typically induce symptomatic episodes soon after hospitalization, admission of the victims (children or elderly) without taking appropriate precautions may actually place them at increased risk.[14] Visits by the suspected perpetrator should be closely supervised, and no food, drink, or medicines should be brought in by the family. Protective services should be notified. Out-of-home placement of children in established cases of MSBP is advisable, and best outcomes are seen among children taken into long-term care at an early age without access to their mother. Children allowed to return home have a high rate of repeat abuse.[31] In 20% of reported deaths the parents had been confronted and the child sent home to them, subsequently to die.[14]

After courteous but assertive reassurance, suspected malingers should be offered primary care follow-up if the symptoms do not resolve. These individuals may become threatening when they are either denied treatment or overtly confronted.[18]

KEY CONCEPTS

- ED patients who have consciously synthesized symptoms and signs may be divided into two broad diagnostic categories: (1) those with obvious secondary gain (malingering), who control their actions, and (2) those with a motivation of achieving the sick role (factitious disorders), who cannot control their actions.
- ED management of the patient suspected of fabricating disease includes a caring attitude, a search for objective clinical evidence of treatable medical or psychiatric illness, avoidance of unnecessary tests, medications and hospitalizations in the absence of such evidence, and referral for ongoing primary care.
- In cases of suspected Munchausen's syndrome by proxy involving children or elderly persons, protection of the victim takes first priority.

REFERENCES

1. Sutherland AJ, Rodin GM: Factitious disorders in a general hospital setting: clinical features and a review of the literature, *Psychosomatics* 31:392, 1990.
2. *Diagnostic and statistical manual of mental disorders,* ed 4-TR, Washington, DC, 2000, American Psychiatric Association.
3. Burkle FM, Calabro JJ, Parks FB: Munchausen's syndrome presenting as a respiratory failure requiring intubation, *Ann Emerg Med* 16:203, 1987.
4. Aduan RP et al: Factitious fever and self-induced infection: a report of 32 cases and review of the literature, *Ann Intern Med* 90:230, 1979.
5. Riggio S: Psychogenic seizures, *Emerg Med Clin North Am* 12:1001, 1994.
6. Gault MH, Campbell NR, Aksu AE: Spurious stones, *Nephron* 48:274, 1988.
7. Asher R: Munchausen's syndrome, *Lancet* 1:339, 1951.
8. Eisendrath SJ: Factitious physical disorders: treatment without confrontation, *Psychosomatics* 30:383, 1989.
9. Nichols GR, Davis GJ, Corey TS: In the shadow of the baron: sudden death due to Munchausen syndrome, *Am J Emerg Med* 8:216, 1990.
10. Scully RE, Mark EJ, McNeely BU: Weekly clinicopathological exercises, case records of the Massachusetts General Hospital: case 28-1984, *N Engl J Med* 311:108, 1984.
11. Wise MG, Ford CV: Factitious disorders, *Prim Care* 26:315, 1999.
12. Meadow R: Munchausen syndrome by proxy: the hinterland of child abuse, *Lancet* 1:343, 1977.
13. Meadow R: What is, and what is not, "Munchausen syndrome by proxy"? *Arch Dis Child* 72:534, 1995.
14. Rosenberg DA: Web of deceit: a literature review of Munchausen syndrome by proxy, *Child Abuse Negl* 11:547, 1987.
15. Alexander R, Smith W, Stevenson R: Serial Munchausen syndrome by proxy, *Pediatrics* 86:581, 1990.
16. Lacey SR et al: Munchausen syndrome by proxy: patterns of presentation to pediatric surgeons, *J Pediatr Surg* 28:827, 1993.
17. *Diagnostic and statistical manual of mental disorders,* ed 4, Washington, DC, 1994, American Psychiatric Association.
18. Dubovsky SL, Weissberg MP: Hypochondriasis. In Dubovsky SL: *Clinical psychiatry in primary care,* ed 3, Baltimore, 1986, Williams & Wilkins.
19. Mills MJ, Lipian MS: Malingering. In Kaplan HI, Sadock BJ, editors: *Comprehensive textbook of psychiatry,* ed 6, Baltimore, 1995, Williams & Wilkins.
20. Reich P, Gottfried LA: Factitious disorders in a teaching hospital, *Ann Intern Med* 99:240, 1983.

21. Ries RK et al: The medical care abuser: differential diagnosis and management, *J Fam Pract* 13:257, 1981.
22. Eisendrath SJ: Factitious physical disorders, *West J Med* 160:177, 1994.
23. Fishbain DA, Goldberg M, Rosomoff RS, Rosomoff HL: Munchausen syndrome presenting with chronic pain: case report, *Pain* 35:91, 1988.
24. Ford CV: *The somatizing disorders: illness as a way of life*, New York, 1983, Elsevier Biomedical.
25. Spivak H, Rodin G, Sutherland A: The psychology of factitious disorders: a reconsideration, *Psychosomatics* 35:25, 1994.
26. Ludwigs U et al: Factitious disorder presenting with acute cardiovascular symptoms, *J Intern Med* 236:685, 1994.
27. Bernstein JA et al: Potentially fatal asthma and syncope: a new variant of Munchausen's syndrome in sports medicine, *Chest* 99:763, 1991.
28. Samuels MP et al: Fourteen cases of imposed upper airway obstruction, *Arch Dis Child* 67:162, 1992.
29. Fisher GC, Mitchell I: Is Munchausen syndrome by proxy really a syndrome? *Arch Dis Child* 72:530, 1995.
30. Mitchell I et al: Apnea and factitious illness (Munchausen syndrome) by proxy, *Pediatrics* 92:810, 1993.
31. Davis P et al: Procedures, placement, and risks of further abuse after Munchausen syndrome by proxy, non-accidental poisoning, and non-accidental suffocation, *Arch Dis Child* 78:217, 1998.
32. Eminson DM, Postlethwaite RJ: Factitious illness: recognition and management, *Arch Dis Child* 67:1510, 1992.
33. Ben-Chetrit E, Melmed RN: Recurrent hypoglycemia in multiple myeloma: a case of Munchausen syndrome by proxy in an elderly patient, *J Intern Med* 244:175, 1998.
34. Levine SS, Helm ML: An AIDS diagnosis used as focus of malingering, *West J Med* 148:337, 1988.
35. Smith RC: Somatization in primary care, *Clin Obstet Gynecol* 31:902, 1988.
36. Ugurlu S et al: Factitious disease of periocular and facial skin, *Am J Ophthalmol* 127:196, 1999.
37. Teasell RW, Shapiro AP: Strategic-behavioral intervention in the treatment of chronic nonorganic motor disorders, *Am J Phys Med Rehabil* 73:44, 1994.
38. Feldman MD: Factitious disorders and fraud, *Psychosomatics* 36:509, 1995 (letter).

109 Suicide

Stephen A. Colucciello

PERSPECTIVE

Historical Background

Although suicide has occurred in all societies since the beginning of recorded history, attitudes toward suicide have differed dramatically among various eras and cultures. Seneca viewed suicide as the ultimate expression of personal freedom, but later Judeo-Christian religions have routinely condemned it. Shakespeare portrayed suicide sympathetically; the audience had pity or admiration for the victim.[1]

In the United States, suicide is illegal in 49 states, and only since 1994 has assisted suicide of terminally ill patients been sanctioned in Oregon. On the Internet, suicide help groups provide active advice on methods, and numerous bulletin boards condemn them. More than 100,000 sites about suicide now appear on the Internet.[2]

Regardless of personal opinions, two factors are especially relevant to the EP. First, many suicide attempts occur during an acute crisis, such as a personal loss or the exacerbation of an underlying psychiatric disorder. This acute crisis is usually time limited and may be resolvable or treatable. Second, except for the acutely psychotic patient, suicidal patients are ambivalent about dying. The attitude and approach of the EP can help a patient choose crisis resolution rather than death.

Definitions

The term *suicide,* from the Latin *suicidum* (to kill the self), refers to a continuum of thought and action that runs from ideation to completion of the act.[3] *Parasuicide* is used by the British to describe an attempted suicide that is more of a gesture than a serious act. Statistically, there are 10 to 40 suicide attempts for every completed act.[4] *Chronic suicidal behavior* consists of recurrent self-destructive acts, such as heavy drinking in the presence of alcoholic liver disease. *Occult suicide* is applied to self-destructive acts disguised as accidents, such as the intoxicated, depressed driver in an apparently accidental car crash. *Silent suicide* refers to the act of slowly killing oneself by nonviolent means, such as starvation or noncompliance with essential medical treatment. Silent suicide is most common in elderly patients and is frequently unrecognized.

A *suicide pact* involves an agreement between two people who are intimately involved and accounts for 0.6% of all suicides.[5] *Mass suicide* or *group suicide* involves a number of willing and sometimes not-so-willing persons, such as members of an apocalyptic cult.

Epidemiology

Suicidal ideation is common, with as many as one third of people considering suicide during their lifetime.[6] Suicide is the eighth leading cause of death in the United States, claiming more than 31,000 lives annually, with an overall rate of 11.2 per 100,000 population.[7]

Suicide rates vary with age, gender, race, and marital status. Suicides are highest among older individuals, particularly elderly white men. White men commit 73% of all suicides in the United States.[7] Whites and Native Americans are much more likely to commit suicide than African Americans, Hispanics, or Asians. Marriage decreases the likelihood of suicide, but separated or divorced persons have a higher rate of suicide than those who never had a close relationship.

Women attempt suicide three to four times more often than men, whereas men are three to four times more likely to kill themselves. Men have a higher incidence of alcoholism and tend to use more lethal methods, such as firearms. Pregnant women have a significantly lower risk than women of

Box 109-1 Risk Factors for Suicide

Demographics
White men over age 65
Women over age 60
Males ages 15 to 24

Psychiatric Disorders
Major depression
Bipolar disorder
Schizophrenia
Borderline personality disorder
Panic disorder

Substance Abuse
Alcoholism
Drug abuse (especially cocaine)

Medical History
Prior suicide attempts
Chronic pain or illness
Physical or sexual abuse
Recent psychiatric hospital discharge
Terminal illness

Family History
Family violence
Suicide in family

Social Factors
Firearm in home
Living alone
Separated, widowed, or divorced
Unemployed
Recent personal loss
Incarceration

Emotional Factors
Hopelessness
Chronic loneliness
Fixation on death

childbearing age who are not pregnant. Motherhood seems to protect against suicide, except postpartum depression is associated with a higher-than-normal suicide rate.

Most people who attempt suicide have one or more known risk factors (Box 109-1). Individuals with the highest risk include those with psychiatric disorders, alcohol or substance abusers, adolescents, elderly persons, and patients with certain chronic illnesses. A strong association may exist between suicide risk and bisexuality or homosexuality in males.[8]

PATHOPHYSIOLOGY AND ETIOLOGY

Societal, Psychiatric, and Biologic Factors

There are many motivations for attempting suicide. It may be seen as the only escape from a terminal disease or intense chronic pain. It may be an act of revenge or political protest. Most suicide attempts occur in individuals with intense feelings of hopelessness, guilt, or self-hatred, often compounded by the exacerbation of an underlying psychiatric disorder or by the occurrence or perception of a great personal loss. The underlying causes for suicide are similar for adults and adolescents; however, adolescents tend to romanticize suicide, and "copycat" suicides are frequent after the suicide of celebrities or friends. Regardless of the motivation, most suicide attempters are ambivalent, and their attraction to death is usually counterbalanced by a desire to live. This internal conflict is reflected in the high ratio of attempted to completed suicides, and most people consult a physician shortly before their death.

Psychoanalysts explain suicide in terms of psychic forces. Freud believed that suicide stems from aggression, initially directed toward another person, which ultimately turns against the self. Depression and suicide in the freudian model represent internalized anger. Many authorities have recognized this association between aggression and suicide, and in the United States, more than 1000 deaths each year result from murder-suicides. The perpetrators are usually young men with intense sexual jealousy, depressed mothers, or despairing elderly men. Their victims are usually female sexual partners, blood relatives, or young children. The dual risk for suicide and violence is greatest in alcoholics.[9]

The impulses that lead to suicide differ between violent and nonviolent people. "Suicidality" is correlated with anger, fear, and suspiciousness in violent individuals and with feelings of sadness and despair in nonviolent persons. The psychic roots of suicide may arise from childhood trauma. Chronic loneliness during childhood is associated with subsequent suicide attempts during adolescence, and a history of sexual molestation is linked to suicide attempts in women. Current research suggests a biologic basis for depression and suicide involving the serotonergic and dopaminergic systems. People who attempt suicide have altered serotonin receptor function and low serotonin levels.[10,11] These abnormalities may be regulated through serotonergic-related genes in persons with major depression.[12] Other genetic studies report polymorphisms in the tryptophan hydroxylase gene that is involved in the synthesis of serotonin. The genetic susceptibility to suicide, however, may affect individuals only when associated with psychiatric illness or stress.[13]

Depressed patients who attempt suicide excrete less homovanillic acid in their urine and produce less dopamine than depressed patients who have not attempted suicide. Low concentrations of dopamine and serotonin metabolites in the cerebrospinal fluid also correlate with suicidal behavior. Suicide attempts in women vary with estrogen levels, with 42% of attempts occurring during the first week of the menstrual cycle.[14]

Neuroanatomy may also influence suicidality; suicide victims have smaller right-sided parahippocampi than controls.[15] No laboratory tests can identify individuals at increased risk for suicide; however, research holds promise for biologic markers that might be used in the future.

Some drugs, including reserpine, benzodiazepines, and barbiturates, are associated with depression and suicidal behavior, although no relationship exists between any single antidepressant and the occurrence of suicide. Patients who commit suicide shortly after the initiation of antidepressant medications are explained by the "mobilization of energy" theory.[16,17] According to this theory, patients who are profoundly depressed may only develop the energy to attempt suicide as they improve with treatment. Such patients must be monitored very closely during their initial phase of treatment.

Methods of Attempting Suicide

Most completed suicides involve firearms (70%), whereas most attempted suicides involve the ingestion of drugs or poisons (72%).[17] In 1994, for example, 19,750 suicides involved firearms in the United States.[18] Guns are the most common methods of suicide in all victim subgroups, especially among older persons and adolescents, and has increased dramatically in the past decade, recently replacing ingestion as the major cause of suicide among women.[19] The simple presence of a gun in the home represents an independent risk factor for suicide. This is particularly true for adolescents, whose risk for suicide increases 5 to 10 times when there is a gun in the household.[20-22] Suicide by handgun is often associated with drug or alcohol use.[23] In the first week after purchasing a handgun, the rate of gun-related suicide is 57 times higher than the general population.[24]

After gun-related deaths, women are more likely to commit suicide by poisoning, whereas men tend to hang themselves. Antidepressant overdose is the most common cause of suicide by ingestion.[25] Tricyclic antidepressants are associated with more deaths because of their widespread use and high potential for lethality. Most patients hospitalized for self-poisoning have ingested drugs prescribed by their physicians for depression.[26] Selective serotonin-reuptake inhibitors (SSRIs), including fluoxetine (Prozac), sertraline (Zoloft), and paroxetine (Paxil), have replaced many cyclic antidepressants and are less lethal when taken in overdose.

The method that a person chooses to attempt suicide depends on many factors, including psychic issues of self-hate, the desire for a peaceful versus violent death, and the availability of fatal means. Those who jump to their death are more likely single, unemployed, or psychotic. Those who use firearms are more likely to be male, alcoholic, have been arrested, or have an antisocial or borderline personality disorder.[27] Communities with tall buildings and bridges have higher rates of suicide from falls, whereas suicide by gunfire occurs more often in areas where firearms are prevalent.

"Suicide by cop" occurs when a suicidal individual intentionally provokes a police officer by orchestrating a lethal situation where the officer is forced to shoot in self-defense or to protect civilians. This may account for as many as 11% of officer-involved shootings in Los Angeles.[28] These individuals may carry a suicide note; some offer an eerie postmortem apology to the police officer who ultimately kills them.

CLINICAL FEATURES

Psychiatric Illness

Most people who commit suicide have either a diagnosable psychiatric illness or alcoholism. Exceptions include those with mental retardation, dementia, and agoraphobia.[29] Patients with an affective disorder, especially major depression, are at highest risk.[30-32] Approximately 15% to 20% of people with *major depression* commit suicide, usually while under psychiatric care.[33] Individuals who experience hopelessness, anhedonia (loss of ability to experience pleasure), and mood cycling are at highest risk. Approximately 10% of schizophrenic patients will kill themselves. Psychotic patients who commit suicide are most often unmarried Caucasians with high intelligence quotients (IQs).[34] Patients with *borderline personality disorders* are also predisposed to commit suicide. Women with borderline personality disorder who attempt suicide often have a history of childhood sexual abuse and impulsive behavior. The risk is especially high when patients require hospitalization for psychiatric illness and is greatest the first month after discharge from a psychiatric facility.[35,36]

Approximately 40% of patients with *panic disorder* will attempt suicide at some point in their lives. These patients usually have an additional comorbid psychiatric diagnosis (e.g., borderline personality disorder, substance abuse, emotional instability). *Posttraumatic stress disorder,* sustained by military combat personnel and disaster survivors, is also associated with suicide.

Alcoholism and Substance Abuse

Almost 25% of all suicides involve alcoholics, and estimates of the lifetime risk of suicide from chronic alcoholism range from 3% to 25%.[37] Alcoholics who commit suicide usually have multiple risk factors, including major depressive episodes, unemployment, medical illness, and interpersonal loss. In psychiatric patients the use of alcohol increases depression and suicidal behavior.

Substance abuse among mentally ill patients is increasingly common. Patients with the dual diagnoses of substance abuse and a psychiatric disorder are particularly prone to violence in the ED. Psychoactive substance abuse is associated with a greater frequency, repetitiveness, and lethality in suicide attempts than are most other medications.

Nearly one half of all adolescents who attempt suicide use drugs shortly before the attempt, and alcohol intoxication is strongly associated with suicide by firearms.[38] Cocaine use is particularly dangerous; in New York City, 20% of all suicide victims under 61 years of age used cocaine within days of their death. Among young Hispanic men, nearly one half of the suicide victims have toxicologic screens positive for cocaine.[39] In general, cocaine abusers choose violent means of self-destruction, especially firearms.

Adolescents

Among adolescents, suicide has quadrupled during the last 40 years and is now the second leading cause of death (after accidents) between 5 and 19 years of age.[5,9] Although some authorities believe that the rise in adolescent suicide simply corresponds to changing demographics in the United States, others believe that the increase is related to a growing sense of hopelessness, increased economic pressures, and access to firearms.[10] In a survey of high-school students in North Carolina, 24% had seriously considered suicide, 19% had planned suicide, and 9% had actually attempted suicide during a 1-year period.[40]

Adolescent girls are more likely to attempt suicide, whereas adolescent boys are more likely to complete suicide; the ratio of attempted to completed suicides is 25:1 for adolescent girls and 3:1 for boys.[41] Most adolescents who complete suicide have made previous suicide threats.

The majority of youths who kill themselves meet criteria for diagnosable psychiatric disorders, and both alcohol and substance abuse play a significant role in teenage suicide attempts. Adolescents with panic attacks are twice as likely to make suicide attempts than adolescents without panic attacks.[42] Gay, lesbian, bisexual, or "not sure" youths may also be more prone to self-harm.[43]

Nearly 40% of youths in runaway programs admit to prior suicide attempts.[44] Young people may also be influenced by movies or television shows that feature suicide. Teenage suicides increase after television broadcasts on the subject.

From 1989 to 1995, suicide by firearm in young people increased dramatically.[45] The firearm-related suicide rate in U.S. adolescents is 11 times higher than the *combined* rates of 25 other industrialized countries.[46] Having a gun in the home places the troubled adolescent in great danger, and storing the gun in a locked cabinet or separating it from the ammunition does not deter suicide attempts.[47] Surprisingly, up to 23% of adolescents who have attempted suicide report that their families continue to keep firearms and ammunition in the home despite their suicide attempt.

Older Adults

The highest rates of suicide occur in the elderly population. In 1992, suicide was the third leading cause of injury-related deaths among older U.S. residents, after deaths from falls and motor vehicle crashes.[48] Older Americans use highly lethal methods when attempting suicide and, unlike adolescents, rarely stage an attempt that permits rescue. Self-inflicted gunshot wounds account for 88% of elderly suicides.

Caucasian men over age 65 account for approximately 80% of suicide deaths, whereas self-injury among elderly minorities is rare.[49] Suicide among older adults is especially prevalent in those with prior suicide attempts and those with a major depression. Severity of depression is the strongest predictor of suicide in the elderly.[50] Physicians often overlook signs of depression in older patients, even though most who commit suicide see their primary care physician during the month before their death. Elderly persons are also more likely to have chronic illnesses that predispose to suicidal behavior.

Chronic Illness

Patients with terminal illnesses may commit suicide to end their suffering and to reduce the emotional and financial burden on their families. Diseases more highly associated with suicide include cancer, stroke, renal failure, congestive heart failure, and chronic lung disease. A history of cancer is an especially strong risk factor in elderly patients.

The acquired immunodeficiency syndrome (AIDS) epidemic has also increased suicide rates, and the relative risk of suicide in men with AIDS is nearly 37 times higher than in uninfected controls. Patients who are positive for human immunodeficiency virus (HIV) but do not have AIDS-defining conditions are more likely to be suicidal than those with active disease.[51]

History

Recognition of Depression and Suicide Potential

Recognition of suicide potential is relatively straightforward in patients who present shortly after a suicide attempt, as well as in individuals who complain of depression or express suicidal ideation during their evaluation. The potential for suicide should also be addressed in patients with any acute problem related to chronic alcoholism, substance abuse, or any psychiatric disorder. Silent suicide is possible with patients who present to the ED repeatedly because of noncompliance with treatment of their medical disorders. Occult suicide should be suspected in patients who "unintentionally" overdose or have had "accidental" self-inflicted gunshot wounds, lacerated wrists, or falls from heights.

Patients Who Present After a Suicide Attempt or Have Suicidal Ideation Patients in the ED after a suicide attempt with a normal mental status should be queried regarding the specifics of the act after medical evaluation and treatment are initiated. Suicidal patients may give inaccurate histories or may even refuse to speak to the physician. Because most people who attempt suicide communicate their intent to others at some point, an attempt should be made to interview family, friends, police, and paramedics regarding the patient's recent actions and possible motivations. They may also provide information regarding the specifics of the current suicide attempt.

Once the patient is medically stable, the EP should determine the presence of risk factors for successful suicide. Such factors include a history of previous suicide attempts or psychiatric care; a history of excessive alcohol or drug use, both acutely and long term; and signs of depression, including a sense of hopelessness. The patient's marital status and social support are important factors, and the motivation for and the seriousness of the suicide attempt are assessed. If discharge is being considered, patients should be asked whether they would harm themselves if they were released from the ED. Additional demographic information may be helpful (see Box 109-1). The SAD PERSONS mnemonic can be used to document salient points and facilitate subsequent communications with primary care providers or psychiatrists (Table 109-1).

Patients Suspected of Occult or Silent Suicide Attempts Patients who are not overtly depressed or suicidal but who exhibit one or more of the high-risk presentations previously described should be assessed in a sympathetic but direct manner using a "graduated" approach. First, rapport should be established during an assessment of the presenting complaint. This should include a general medical and psychiatric history, as well as an evaluation of the patient's home, work, and social situation, followed by specific questions regarding the signs and symptoms of depression. The EP should ask direct questions regarding suicide, such as, "Have you ever had the thought that life is not worth living?"; "Do you have thoughts of killing yourself now?"; and "What plans, if any, have you made to do this?" Patients who are not depressed or suicidal are not offended by this

Table 109-1. Modified "SAD PERSONS" Scale

Factor	Points assigned
*S*ex (male)	1
*A*ge (<19 or >45)	1
*D*epression or hopelessness	2
*P*revious attempts or psychiatric care	1
*E*xcessive alcohol or drug use	1
*R*ational thinking loss	2
*S*eparated, divorced, or widowed	1
*O*rganized or serious attempt	2
*N*o social supports	1
*S*tated future intent	2

From Hockberger RS, Rothstein RJ: *J Emerg Med* 6:99, 1988.
Five points or less: questionable outpatient treatment; *six or more points:* emergency psychiatric treatment/evaluation; *more than nine points:* psychiatric hospitalization.

Table 109-2. Factors in Differentiating Organic from Functional Psychosis

	Onset	Age of onset	Hallucinations	Orientation
Organic	May be acute	Any age	Often visual	Often disoriented
Functional	Subacute to chronic	14 to 40	Usually auditory	Normal

approach, and it does not place the concept of suicide into the mind of someone who has not been considering it. Patients who are depressed or suicidal are often thankful and relieved for the intervention.

Physical Examination

Suicidal patients should be examined closely for evidence of drug ingestion, trauma, or an associated medical illness. Examination of the patient's mental status, vital signs, pupils, skin, and nervous system is helpful in detecting organic conditions, particularly the toxidromes associated with common ingestions. Patients with altered mentation should be assessed to determine whether their condition is caused by an organic (medical) or functional (psychiatric) cause (Table 109-2). Physical findings associated with chronic disease, alcoholism, and substance abuse should be sought. The physical examination is often overlooked or performed in a cursory manner in patients with psychiatric complaints. Up to 50% of patients with an acute psychiatric presentation may harbor unrecognized medical illnesses.[52]

DIAGNOSTIC STRATEGIES

Routine toxicologic screening tests are unnecessary in the evaluation of suicidal patients. With the exception of acetaminophen, essentially all patients with dangerous overdoses and poisonings demonstrate clinical signs within several hours of ingestion. The EP should consider obtaining an acetaminophen level in overdose patients. An electrocardiogram should be obtained when cyclic antidepressant overdose is suspected and when the history remains unclear. Patients with acute depression, particularly if newly diagnosed, may need screening tests for underlying medical disorders. However, a primary care physician or psychiatrist can safely perform this evaluation during follow-up.

MANAGEMENT

Prehospital Care

The prehospital management must focus on the patient's injuries and potential harm from poisoning or overdose. If the patient refuses to be transported to the hospital or becomes aggressive, emergency medical personnel should involve law enforcement officers. All states give police the right to place individuals into protective custody if they are suspected of being a danger to self or others. The presence of law enforcement officers, or even the threat of calling the police for assistance, usually ensures patient cooperation during transport.

Emergency Department

The clinical assessment of suicide potential requires an empathetic approach. Patients feel more comfortable discussing personal issues when health care personnel are friendly, nonjudgmental, and supportive. Unfortunately, ED staff may be unsympathetic toward patients who attempt suicide because of religious or philosophic beliefs, lack of formal psychiatric training, or inadequate time and personnel to provide appropriate psychiatric evaluation. They may perceive the patient's behavior as abusive or manipulative and may become frustrated regarding ineffective disposition and follow-up options. Failure to anticipate and overcome these factors may result in inadequate patient assessment and reinforce these patients' already low self-esteem.

Medical Clearance The first priority in managing patients is medical stabilization and treatment of injuries, poisoning, or overdose. The second priority is the identification and treatment of associated medical conditions that may cause a patient's altered mental status or violent behavior. Patients with significant injury, poisoning, or other medical problems should be hospitalized, sometimes in an intensive care setting, where their medical problems can be treated while they remain under constant observation. Five to 40 inpatients commit suicide for every 100,000 hospitalizations.[53,54]

Suicide Precautions Most suicide attempts involve minor injury or overdose that can be definitively treated in the ED. These patients must be protected from additional self-harm while in the ED. Suicidal patients who are calm and cooperative should be placed in an area where they can be safely observed by staff. Security personnel should search all potentially suicidal patients. Having the patient change into a hospital gown facilitates removal of weapons and other possessions that might be used to inflict injury, such as belts, neckties, and long shoelaces. The patient's room should be cleared of all potentially harmful objects, including medications, instruments, and glass objects. Someone should accompany the patient when leaving the area to use the restroom. The use of family members as "sitters" may be counterproductive or even dangerous because they may collude with the suicidal patient to leave the ED or may not intervene if the patient attempts to leave. No potentially suicidal patient should be allowed to leave the ED before an evaluation is completed.

Use of Restraints Mechanical and chemical restraint use is based primarily on the physician's impression regarding the immediate risk of elopement or subsequent suicide attempt. Placing a depressed patient in mechanical restraints can impair the EP's rapport with the patient and contribute to the patient's diminished self-esteem. Chemical restraints may calm a violent patient, but may make subsequent psychiatric evaluation more difficult.

Nevertheless, restraints may be *essential* for uncooperative, violent, or psychotic patients and for those at high risk for elopement or self-harm. Restraints may be required for a brief period when ED staffing precludes a high level of observation.

Determination of Risk Once a patient has demonstrated suicidal behavior or ideation, the EP must determine whether the risk is imminent (i.e., within 48 hours), short term (i.e., within days to weeks), or long term.[6] The likelihood of an impending repeat attempt will drive disposition, whether psychiatric hospitalization, emergency psychiatric consultation, or discharge and referral for follow-up.

The EP should determine an individual patient's likelihood for committing suicide if discharged. This assessment is far from an exact science. Scoring systems can help in determining the need for hospitalization, but prospective studies show that most systems cannot predict future attempts at self-harm.[55,56] Nevertheless, the EP should still attempt to determine a patient's immediate risk for self-harm and, when indicated, communicate the assessment to other health care providers.

The SAD PERSONS mnemonic provides a "suicide score" (see Table 109-1). Two points are given for each of four high-risk factors: (1) complaints of depression or hopelessness, (2) existence of an organic brain syndrome or acute psychosis, (3) presence of a well-conceived plan or life-threatening presentation, and (4) expression of determination or ambivalence regarding future suicidal behavior. One point is assigned for other important but less significant factors: male gender; less than 19 or greater than 45 years of age; a history of previous suicide attempts or psychiatric care; stigmata of chronic alcoholism or substance abuse or the history of recent increased use of these substances; a patient who is separated, divorced, or widowed; and the absence of social support systems, such as close family, friends, job, or active religious affiliation.

A SAD PERSONS score of six or more had a sensitivity of 94% and a specificity of 71% compared with formal psychiatric evaluation to identify the need for hospitalization in patients who present immediately after a suicide attempt.[57] A score of less than six has a negative predictive value of 95%. No mortality was noted in patients with low scores evaluated at 6 to 12 months.

Suicide assessment should be based on information obtained from the patient after the metabolism of any drugs or alcohol. Patients who complain of depression or state ambivalence regarding their future intentions to commit suicide while intoxicated may disavow these feelings once they are sober. In addition, the information obtained from a potentially suicidal patient might be confirmed through a family member or friend. Patients who are determined to commit suicide may give false or misleading information.

The crises that precipitate suicide attempts often are time limited, usually lasting from a few hours to a few days. If a crisis has passed or can be adequately addressed, the risk of subsequent suicide is substantially diminished. Hospitalization or emergency psychiatric evaluation should be strongly considered when a patient cannot or will not participate in an evaluation of the current crisis or when the problem is unlikely to be resolved.

Ultimately, the assessment of suicide risk remains a highly individualized process. The crisis that precipitated the suicide event, the patient's current emotional state, and the presence or absence of a supportive home environment must also be considered. When EPs are uncertain regarding the need for hospitalization, they should err on the side of caution and either admit the patient for psychiatric care or request emergency psychiatric evaluation.

A psychiatric social worker or other paraprofessional may assist the EP in gathering information and in making decisions about the need for hospitalization. Even when a psychiatric paraprofessional evaluates the patient, however, the EP still must make an independent judgment about the patient's suicide risk.[58]

Involuntary Commitment

Many patients who are severely depressed or suicidal will agree to be hospitalized for further evaluation and care; however, some may express reticence at being hospitalized. Patients refuse recommended medical treatment usually because of anger or fear. Patients may be angry for being brought to the ED against their wishes or for having to wait for evaluation. Alternatively, they may fear the loss of control associated with hospitalization or the perceived negative stigma associated with a psychiatric disorder. When a patient is reluctant to be hospitalized, the EP should attempt to identify and address the specific concerns. The patient's family and friends may help convince the patient to accept voluntary hospitalization. If these attempts are unsuccessful, involuntary admission is necessary if the physician believes the patient may inflict self-harm.

Controversy surrounds the efficacy of commitment as a long-term preventive measure.[53] Involuntary commitment has not been proven to prevent future suicide and may even precipitate adverse psychiatric consequences (e.g., increased feelings of hopelessness and dependency) or cause rebellion in some patients. Many authorities believe that people who are determined to kill themselves will probably prevail despite the best efforts of family members and health care professionals.[6] Because proven alternatives are lacking, however, involuntary commitment remains a primary intervention when patients are deemed acutely suicidal.

DISPOSITION

Most patients who attempt suicide or have symptoms of depression can be safely managed as outpatients, if the risk for subsequent suicide is judged acceptably low (Box 109-2). Before discharging a patient, the EP should address the crisis that precipitated the suicide attempt. The patient should also be considered low risk for subsequent suicide (e.g., low SAD PERSONS score). Some EPs ask the patient to form a verbal or written "contract" with the EP. This "no harm" agreement usually involves patients vowing not to hurt themselves and agreeing to return to the ED to seek help if the situation worsens before follow-up. Although the "no harm" agreement has not been validated, some believe this is a reasonable approach, whereas others believe that it provides only a false sense of security for the physician.

If the patient is to be discharged, a family member or friend should agree to stay with the patient or to be immediately available to the patient until follow-up is provided. The patient should be discharged to a stable and supportive home environment, which is free of guns and lethal medications.

Adequate disposition may include a conversation with the ongoing provider. If possible, the follow-up appointment should be scheduled within 24 to 48 hours of discharge from

Box 109-2 Factors for Patients at Low Risk for Suicide

1. Few significant risk factors (e.g., low SAD PERSONS score)
2. Stable and supportive home environment
3. Patient agrees to "no harm" contract and will return to ED if situation worsens
4. Family member or friend staying with or available to patient
5. Phone contact with health care provider responsible for follow-up
6. Specific appointment made for follow-up within 24 to 48 hours
7. No gun in home

the ED and should be specific regarding the location and time. This approach maximizes patient compliance with follow-up. Providing a card that indicates how to contact an available physician may be helpful.[59]

DOCUMENTATION

Documentation is important when patients are committed and discharged. If a patient requires involuntary commitment, the EP should document why the patient is a danger to self. If the patient is to be discharged, the record should reflect that the patient is low risk and does not intend self-harm after leaving the ED. Documenting that there is no gun in the home is useful. The use of preformatted charts may improve documentation regarding patients who have attempted self-harm.[60]

PREVENTION

The incidence of suicide parallels the incidence of alcoholism, drug abuse, and psychiatric disease in society. Although most suicide prevention programs have been found to be of questionable value, legislation to control access to lethal drugs and handguns is effective. In Japan, for example, laws requiring prescriptions for all sedative and hypnotic drugs led to a decrease in their use for suicide, with no increase in the use of other methods.[61] In Canada, suicide decreased after gun control laws were tightened.[62]

Despite great interest in the prevention of suicide, uncertainty remains regarding which (if any) interventions are effective to prevent future attempts at self-harm. An insufficient number of patients included in clinical trials may limit conclusions regarding effective therapy.[63] No strong evidence suggests that antidepressants prevent self-harm in patients with prior suicide attempt. However, one small study did show an advantage to depot flupenthixol versus placebo in multiple repeaters.[64] In another small study, dialectic behavior therapy was more effective than standard aftercare in preventing further episodes of self-harm.[65]

Suicide attempts correlate with future suicide. In one study on survivors of self-poisoning, the 5-year mortality from suicide was 65.5 times greater than expected in the female group (compared to a control group who did not attempt self-harm) and 41.5 times greater among males.[66]

KEY CONCEPTS

- Suicide is often provoked by a treatable or reversible short-term crisis.
- Suicidal patients frequently see a physician shortly before their death.
- The most complete information can be elicited with an empathetic approach to the patient and communication with family members, friends, health care providers, and others.
- Suicide precautions include appropriate use of physical and chemical restraints and involuntary commitment.
- The EP should identify risk factors for successful suicide, even though determination of suicide risk is difficult.

REFERENCES

1. Kirkland LR: To end itself by death: suicide in Shakespeare's tragedies, *South Med J* 92:660, 1999.
2. Thompson S: Internet sites may encourage suicide, *Psychiatr Bull* 23:449, 1999; Dobson R: *BMJ* 319:337, 1999.
3. Brent DA et al: Risk factors for adolescent suicide: a comparison of adolescent suicide victims with suicidal inpatients, *Arch Gen Psychiatry* 45:581, 1988.
4. McAlpine DE: Suicide: recognition and management, *Mayo Clin Proc* 62:778, 1987.
5. Brown M: Epidemiology of suicide pacts in England and Wales, *BMJ* 315:286, 1997.
6. Hirschfeld RM, Russell JM: Assessment and treatment of suicidal patients, *N Engl J Med* 337:910, 1997.
7. National Center for Health Statistics et al: Advance report of final mortality statistics, 1994, *Mon Vital Stat Rep* 45(3, suppl), 1996.
8. Remafedi G et al: The relationship between suicide risk and sexual orientation: results of a population-based study, *Am J Public Health* 88:57, 1998.
9. Greenwald DJ, Reznikoff M, Plutchik R: Suicide risk and violence risk in alcoholics: predictors of aggressive risk, *J Nerv Ment Dis* 182:3, 1994.
10. McBride PA et al: The relationship of platelet 5-HT2 receptor indices to major depressive disorder, personality traits, and suicidal behavior, *Biol Psychiatry* 35:295, 1994.
11. Arango V et al: Quantitive autoradiography of alpha 1- and alpha 2-adrenergic receptors in the cerebral cortex of controls and suicide victims, *Brain Res* 630:271, 1993.
12. Mann JJ et al: Possible association of a polymorphism of the tryptophan hydroxylase gene with suicidal behavior in depressed patients, *Am J Psychiatry* 154:1451, 1997.
13. Roy A et al: Genetics of suicide in depression, *J Clin Psychiatry* 60(suppl 2):12, 1999.
14. Fourestie V et al: Suicide attempts in hypoestrogenic phases of the menstrual cycle, *Lancet* 2(8520):1357, 1986 (erratum, 1(8525):176, 1987).
15. Altshuler LL et al: The hippocampus and parahippocampus in schizophrenia, suicide, and control brains, *Arch Gen Psychiatry* 47:1029, 1990 (erratum, 48:422, 1991).
16. Gunnell D, Frankel S: Prevention of suicide: aspirations and evidence, *BMJ* 308:1227, 1994.
17. Birkhead GS et al: The emergency department in surveillance of attempted suicide: findings and methodologic considerations, *Public Health Rep* 108:323, 1993.
18. Zwerling C et al: The choice of weapons in firearm suicides in Iowa, *Am J Public Health* 83:1630, 1993.
19. Meehan PJ, Saltzman LE, Sattin RW: Suicides among older United States residents: epidemiologic characteristics and trends, *Am J Public Health* 81:1198, 1991.
20. Killias M: International correlations between gun ownership and rates of homicide and suicide, *Can Med Assoc J* 148:1721, 1993.
21. Kellerman AL, Reay DT: Protection or peril? An analysis of firearm-related deaths in the home, *N Engl J Med* 314:1557, 1986.
22. Brent DA et al: Firearms and adolescent suicide: a community case-control study, *Am J Dis Child* 147:1066, 1993.
23. Peterson LG et al: Self-inflicted gunshot wounds: lethality of method versus intent, *Am J Psychiatry* 142:228, 1985.
24. Wintemute GJ et al: Mortality among recent purchasers of handguns, *N Engl J Med* 341:1583, 1999.

25. Kapur S, Mieczkowski T, Mann JJ: Antidepressant medications and the relative risk of suicide attempt and suicide, *JAMA* 268:3441, 1992.
26. Prescott LF, Highley MS: Drugs prescribed for self poisoners, *Br Med J Clin Res Ed* 290:1633, 1985.
27. De Moore GM, Robertson AR: Suicide attempts by firearms and by leaping from heights: a comparative study of survivors, *Am J Psychiatry* 156:1425, 1999.
28. Hutson HR et al: Suicide by cop, *Ann Emerg Med* 32:665, 1998.
29. Risk for suicide is increased for most mental disorders where patients require treatment in a hospital setting, *Evidence-Based Med* 2:156, 1997.
30. Henriksson MM et al: Mental disorders and comorbidity in suicide, *Am J Psychiatry* 150:935, 1993.
31. Winokur G, Black DW: Psychiatric and medical diagnoses as risk factors for mortality in psychiatric patients: a case control study, *Am J Psychiatry* 144:208, 1987.
32. Asnis GM et al: Suicidal behaviors in adult psychiatric outpatients. Part I. Description and prevalence, *Am J Psychiatry* 150:108, 1993.
33. Isometsa ET et al: Suicide in major depression, *Am J Psychiatry* 151:530, 1994.
34. Westermeyer JF, Harrow M, Marengo JT: Risk for suicide in schizophrenia and other psychotic and nonpsychotic disorders, *J Nerv Ment Dis* 179:259, 1991.
35. Goldacre M, Seagroatt V, Hawton K: Suicide after discharge from psychiatric inpatient care, *Lancet* 342:283, 1993.
36. Allgulander C: Suicide and mortality patterns in anxiety, neurosis, and depressive neurosis, *Arch Gen Psychiatry* 51:708, 1994.
37. Murphy GE et al: Multiple risk factors predict suicide in alcoholism, *Arch Gen Psychiatry* 49:459, 1992.
38. Rich CL et al: Some difference between men and women who commit suicide, *Am J Psychiatry* 145:718, 1988.
39. Marzuk PM et al: Prevalence of cocaine use among residents of New York City who committed suicide during a one-year period, *Am J Psychiatry* 149:371, 1992.
40. Garrison CZ et al: Aggression, substance use, and suicidal behaviors in high school students, *Am J Public Health* 83:179, 1993.
41. Rosenberg ML et al: The emergence of youth suicide: an epidemiologic analysis and public health perspective, *Annu Rev Public Health* 8:417, 1987.
42. Pilowsky DJ, Wu LT, Anthony JC: Panic attacks and suicide attempts in mid-adolescence, *Am J Psychiatry* 156:1545, 1999.
43. Garofalo R et al: Sexual orientation and risk of suicide attempts among a representative sample of youth, *Arch Pediatr Adolesc Med* 153:487, 1999.
44. Rotheram-Borus MJ: Suicidal behavior and risk factors among runaway youths, *Am J Psychiatry* 150:103, 1993.
45. Cummings P, LeMier M, Keck DB: Trends in firearm-related injuries in Washington State, *Ann Emerg Med* 32:37, 1998.
46. Centers for Disease Control and Prevention: Rates of homicide, suicide, and firearm-related death among children in 26 industrialized countries, *MMWR* 46:101, 1997.
47. Brent DA et al: The presence and accessibility of firearms in the homes of adolescent suicides: a case-control study, *JAMA* 266:2989, 1990.
48. Centers for Disease Control and Prevention: Suicide among older persons-United States, 1980-1992, *MMWR* 45:3, 1996.
49. Casey DA: Suicide in the elderly: a two-year study of data from death certificates, *South Med J* 84:1185, 1991.
50. Alexopoulos GS et al: Clinical determinants of suicidal ideation and behavior in geriatric depression, *Arch Gen Psychiatry* 56:1048, 1999.
51. McKegney FP, O'Dowd MA: Suicidality and HIV status, *Am J Psychiatry* 149:396, 1992.
52. Henneman PL, Mendoza R, Lewis RJ: Prospective evaluation of emergency department medical clearance, *Ann Emerg Med* 24:672, 1994.
53. Robertson WD: Poisonings in the United States, *Am J Emerg Med* 6:544, 1988.
54. Hogarty SS, Rodaitis CM: A suicide precautions policy for the general hospital, *J Nurs Adm* 17:36, 1987.
55. Goldstein RB et al: The prediction of suicide: sensitivity, specificity, and predictive value of a multivariate model applied to suicide among 1906 patients with affective disorders, *Arch Gen Psychiatry* 48:418, 1991.
56. Maris RW: Suicide and life-threatening behavior: introduction, *Suicide Life Threat Behav* 21:1, 1991.
57. Hockberger RS, Rothstein RJ: Assessment of suicide potential by non-psychiatrists using the SAD PERSONS score, *J Emerg Med* 6:99, 1988.
58. Armitage DT, Townsend GM: Emergency medicine, psychiatry and the law, *Emerg Med Clin North Am* 11:869, 1993.
59. Morgan HG, Jones EM, Owen JH: Secondary prevention of non-fatal deliberate self-harm: the green card study, *Br J Psychiatry* 163:111, 1993.
60. Crawford MJ, Turnbull G, Wessely S: Deliberate self harm assessment by accident and emergency staff: an intervention study, *J Accid Emerg Med* 15:18, 1998.
61. Lester D, Abe K: The effect of controls on sedatives and hypnotics on their use for suicide, *J Toxicol Clin Toxicol* 27:299, 1989.
62. Lester D, Leenaars A: Suicide rates in Canada before and after tightening firearm control law, *Psychol Rep* 72:787, 1993.
63. Hawton K et al: Deliberate self-harm: systematic review of efficacy of psychosocial and pharmacological treatment in preventing repetition, *BMJ* 317:441, 1998.
64. Montgomery SA, Roy D, Montgomery DB: The prevention of recurrent suicidal acts, *Br J Clin Pharmacol* 15(suppl 2):183, 1983.
65. Linehan MM et al: Cognitive-behavioral treatment of chronically parasuicidal borderline patients, *Arch Gen Psychiatry* 48:1060, 1991.
66. Rygnestad T: Mortality after deliberate self-poisoning: a prospective follow-up study of 587 persons observed for 5279 person years-risk factors and causes of death, *Soc Psychiatry Psychiatr Epidemiol* 32:443, 1997.

Section IX IMMUNOLOGIC AND INFLAMMATORY DISORDERS

110 Arthritis

Douglas W. Lowery

PERSPECTIVE

Evaluating and managing the inflamed joint remain critical core competencies for emergency physicians (EP). Unfortunately, as the population ages and medical histories become more complex, the typical appearance of a "red hot joint" is becoming more rare. Nevertheless, because of the tremendous pain and disability associated with arthritis, patients with the gamut of arthritic maladies present for emergency evaluation.[1]

History

Rheumatic diseases have been described for thousands of years. Hippocrates wrote of musculoskeletal complaints and joint inflammation. Differences in presentation of joint disease were noted, but distinctions were not made until the 1680s when Sydenham described gout, rheumatism, and chorea. Despite the historical awareness of joint ailments, minimal success in classifying them into recognizable entities occurred until the beginning of the nineteenth century. The phrase *rheumatic fever* was coined in 1808, but not until 1880 was a relationship to streptococcal infection proposed. Similarly, Swediaur noted a relationship between urethritis and arthritis in 1784, but discovery of gonococcal arthritis waited until 1883. Ankylosing spondylitis was first mentioned in 1831, but was not accurately described until the 1930s. In 1876, Garrod postulated that acute gout resulted from monosodium urate deposits in the joints, but the ultimate proof of that hypothesis had to wait until the mid-1900s, when additional technologic advances facilitated the more specific characterization and investigation of many rheumatic conditions.[2]

Heberden described his "nodes" as early as 1802, and Bouchard described his in 1884; but the entity of osteoarthritis was not clearly defined until 1907. In 1819 Brodie described synovitis with its potential to destroy cartilage. This was a basic step toward understanding rheumatoid arthritis. Rheumatoid factor was first measured in the 1940s. The other connective tissue diseases, systemic lupus erythematosus (SLE), systemic sclerosis, and polymyositis were all described in the middle to late 1880s. Reiter's disease was named after the author of a report of the typical joint manifestations occurring after dysentery.[2]

Epidemiology

Maladies affecting the musculoskeletal system are one of the most common human afflictions. Prevalence increases with advancing age, but the arthritides affect all age groups, both genders, all races, and all socioeconomic statuses. Because of their resulting disability and chronic pain, the arthritides bear significant societal costs.[3]

PRINCIPLES OF DISEASE

Anatomy and Physiology

Joints are designed to bear weight and allow motion with as little wear as possible to the components.[4] Three classes of joints are identified: synarthroses (suture lines of the skull), amphiarthroses (fibrocartilaginous unions of the pubic symphysis and the lower third of the sacroiliac joint), and diarthroses (most other joints). The most common type is the diarthrosis or synovial joint, which consists of two ends of subchondral bone (one convex, one concave) almost completely covered by articular cartilage. The cartilage consists of a matrix of collagen fibers and proteoglycans, which are synthesized by the chondrocytes within it. The cartilaginous surfaces are well lubricated and slide against each other. The joint is surrounded by a capsule that is supported by ligaments, tendons, and muscle and is lined with a synovial membrane (Figure 110-1).

Cartilage is deformable, compressible, and lubricated by synovial fluid secreted by cells of the synovial membrane lining the joint space. The synovium is up to three cells thick and consists of two cell types: type A cells, which contain lysosomes, and type B cells, which synthesize the fluid. Both types multiply in synovitis and interact with the vasculature to produce arthritis.[5] Joint fluid has a high viscosity because of its major component, a polysaccharide, hyaluronic acid. The fluid also contains water, glucose, electrolytes, and proteins of low molecular weight.

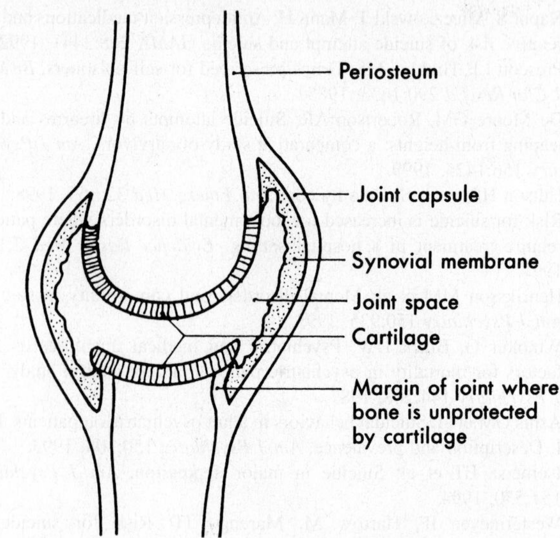

Figure 110-1. **Clinical anatomy of the joint.** ***From Branch WT: Office practice of medicine, ed 2, Philadelphia, 1987, WB Saunders.***

PATHOPHYSIOLOGY

Mechanical trauma to a joint causes a decrease in the number of proteoglycans, probably by causing disequilibrium of anabolism and catabolism.[6] If the trauma is minor and transient, some regeneration of the articular cartilage by the chondrocytes may occur; but if the trauma is persistent, the damage is irreparable.

Marked inflammation of the joint is characterized by predominantly polymorphonuclear cells (PMNs) exuding into the synovial cavity. Viscosity decreases because of decreased hyaluronic acid, the major contributor to synovial fluid viscosity. The trigger for this inflammatory reaction is different with different diseases. In nongonococcal bacterial arthritis, the cells of the synovial lining phagocytize bacteria. In gout and pseudogout, crystals are released from cells lining the synovium by conditions that precipitate an acute attack: minor trauma, ingestion of drugs or foods that raise the uric acid level, and alcohol. The joint inflammation in rheumatoid arthritis, rheumatic fever, and disseminated gonococcal arthritis has an immunologic basis. Reiter's syndrome is probably an immunologic "reactive" arthritis.

PMNs release lysosomal enzymes that elicit a severe inflammatory reaction and ultimately degrade the components of the joint.[7] In rheumatoid arthritis, the "pannus" of proliferating cells erodes into the articular cartilage and bone. Erosions of bone occur in those portions of the joint cavity in which the bone is not covered by cartilage (a portion just distal to the attachment of the capsule). Subchondral bone is resorbed, an effect that is manifested radiologically as juxtaarticular osteoporosis. Figure 110-2 shows the sites at which rheumatic disease occurs.

CLINICAL FINDINGS

Symptoms and Signs

History Pain is the most common complaint of patients with joint problems who come to the ED. The pain may be acute or chronic, or an acute episode in a patient with chronic disease. The patient may have had similar pain before, so it is important to know whether a diagnosis was previously made and what treatment, if any, was instituted.

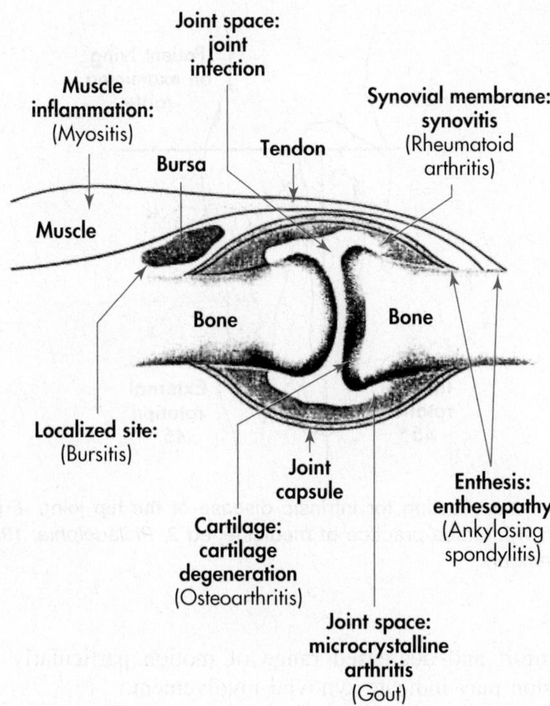

Figure 110-2. **Sites and types of rheumatic disease.** *From Wyngaarden JB, Smith LH, editors:* Cecil textbook of medicine, *ed 18, Philadelphia, 1988, WB Saunders.*

A key determination to make is whether the source of the inflammation or pain is articular or periarticular (outside the joint capsule). True arthritis produces generalized joint pain, warmth, swelling, and tenderness. Discomfort increases with both passive and active motion of the joint because the inflamed synovium is exquisitely sensitive to stretching, and because all parts of the joint are involved in the inflammatory process. By contrast, periarticular inflammation (bursitis, tendinitis, or localized cellulitis) tends to be more focal. Tenderness and swelling do not occur uniformly across the joint, and pain is produced only with certain movements, with the most common being resisted active contraction or passive stretching of the affected muscles or tendons.

If the site of the patient's pain is articular and not periarticular, the next step is to determine whether the arthritis is monarticular or polyarticular. Although certain disease entities (i.e., rheumatoid arthritis, gonococcal arthritis) can be placed in both categories, this basic approach of classification by number of joints involved can assist in narrowing the differential diagnosis (Table 110-1).

If polyarticular, the arthritis may be symmetric (i.e., rheumatoid or drug induced) or asymmetric (i.e., rubella, acute rheumatic fever, or gonococcal). In addition, it may also be migratory (i.e., gonococcal or rubella), subsiding in one area before presenting in another, or additive, remaining in the first joint and progressing to additional joints.

The distribution of joint involvement may give some clues to the disease: the first metatarsophalangeal joint is classically affected in gout; the metacarpophalangeal (MP) joints and proximal interphalangeal (PIP) joints in rheumatoid arthritis; the distal interphalangeal (DIP) joints and first carpometacarpal joint in osteoarthritis; and the knee in septic arthritis, pseudogout, and gout.

Patients with any inflammatory arthritis may have low-grade fever, but high fever with chills is more likely to be septic arthritis. Concomitant renal stones suggest gout, genital ulcerations occur in Reiter's syndrome, and purulent urethral discharge suggests gonococcal arthritis or Reiter's syndrome.

Table 110-1. Causes of Joint Pain

Articular		
Monarticular	**Polyarticular**	**Periarticular**
Osteoarthritis	Rheumatoid arthritis	Bursitis
Septic arthritis	Systemic lupus	Tendinitis
Gout	Viral arthritis	Cellulitis
Pseudogout	Rheumatic fever	
Trauma	Reiter's syndrome	
Hemarthrosis	Lyme disease	
	Serum sickness	
	Drug-induced	

The EP should inquire about what medications a patient is taking. Isoniazid, procainamide, and hydralazine can precipitate lupus, and thiazides can increase the serum uric acid level, leading to gouty arthritis.

Physical Examination

A thorough physical examination should be performed that specifically searches for evidence of particular rheumatic diseases. The skin, eyes, cardiac, pulmonary, and neurologic systems should be examined carefully. Some of the findings may indicate long-standing disease (i.e., tophi in gout, Heberden's nodes in osteoarthritis, swan-neck deformity in rheumatoid arthritis, skin lesions in psoriasis), whereas others may indicate an acute process (i.e., pustular lesions of gonococcemia, mucocutaneous lesions of Reiter's syndrome). Table 110-2 summarizes the findings specific to each type of arthritis.

Joint Examination

Each joint in question should be specifically examined for the following attributes[8]:

1. Warmth and effusion
2. Synovial thickening
3. Deformity
4. Range of motion
5. Pain on motion
6. Tenderness (generalized or localized, articular or periarticular)

The patient should stand, and the vertebral column should be assessed for abnormal curvature or asymmetry. The patient should then bend forward, so that the EP can assess for the limitation of the lumbar spine motion that occurs in ankylosing spondylitis. Sacrum and anterior iliac crests are palpated to elicit pain in the sacroiliac (SI) joints.

A shoulder affected by chronic arthritis or bursitis will have atrophy of the deltoid muscle. Generalized tenderness and pain, both at rest and with active and passive motion, suggest joint involvement. Localized tenderness and pain associated with active movement are more likely to be periarticular in origin. Having the patient place the hands

Table 110-2. Clinical Signs of Rheumatic Diseases

	Findings	Diseases
Scalp, hair	Alopecia, skin lesions	SLE, psoriasis
Skin	Pustular lesions	Gonococcemia
	Malar rash	SLE, dermatomyositis
	Rash on elbows, knees	Psoriasis
	Rash on dorsum of hands	Dermatomyositis
	Tightening of skin	Scleroderma
	Erythema chronicum migrans	Lyme disease
	Hyperkeratotic lesions	Reiter's syndrome
	Rash	Rubella
	Tophi	Gout
	Track marks	Injection drug use
	Erythema marginatum	Rheumatic fever
	Subcutaneous nodules	Rheumatoid arthritis
Eyes	Dryness	Sjögren's syndrome
	Iritis, uveitis	HLA B27 disease
	Conjunctivitis	Reiter's syndrome
	Icterus	Hepatitis
Oral mucosa	Dryness	Sjögren's syndrome
	Ulcerations	SLE, Reiter's syndrome
Pulmonary	Interstitial fibrosis	Scleroderma
	Pleuritis	SLE, rheumatoid arthritis
Cardiac	Friction rubs	Rheumatoid arthritis, SLE
	Murmurs	Endocarditis
		Rheumatoid arthritis
Gastrointestinal examination	Enlarged, tender liver	Hepatitis
Neurologic	Peripheral nerve findings	Vasculitis
Genitalia	Lesions, urethral discharge	Reiter's syndrome, gonococcemia

behind the head and then the back tests for external and internal rotation, respectively.

Early signs of joint inflammation in the elbow are limitation of extension and an increase in the normal angle at which the patient holds the elbow at the side. The hand and wrist provide many clues to the presence of long-standing rheumatic diseases: MP and PIP joints are affected in rheumatoid arthritis, and the first carpometacarpal, PIP, and DIP joints in osteoarthritis. The fingers may be swollen or sausage-like in appearance, an indication of psoriasis or Reiter's syndrome. Subluxation at the MP joints, ulnar deviation, and swan-neck deformities occur in rheumatoid arthritis. The nails may have pitting characteristic of psoriatic arthritis. Although the wrist may not be obviously swollen,

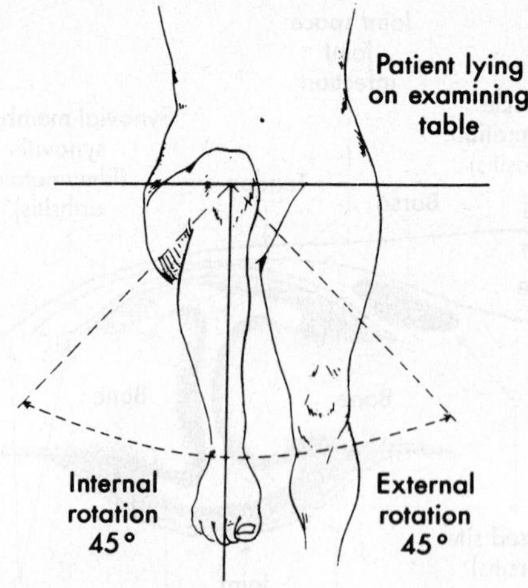

Figure 110-3. **Testing for intrinsic disease of the hip joint.** *From Branch WT:* **Office practice of medicine,** *ed 2, Philadelphia, 1987, WB Saunders.*

discomfort and decreased range of motion particularly on extension may indicate synovial involvement.

Inflammation affecting the hip joint may be reported by the patient as pain in the anterior thigh, knee, or groin. A hip joint effusion will cause the patient to hold the hip partially flexed. An externally rotated and abducted leg in a neonate suggests infection even if the child is afebrile.[9] Range of motion of the hip is most easily tested by flexing the hip, bending the knee at a right angle, and rotating the heel medially and laterally to test for external and internal rotation, respectively (Figure 110-3).[8] Marked irritability and decreased range of movement confirm hip joint involvement.

An effusion of the knee joint is relatively easy to detect when it appears as a ballotable fullness medially and laterally. Small effusions may be detected by examining for a transmitted fluid wave. Fullness of the popliteal fossa may indicate a Baker's cyst. Passive range of motion may elicit crepitus or clicking. Tibiotalar joint effusions produce swelling under the medial malleolus and make it difficult to palpate the extensor hallucis longus tendon. Tenderness, warmth, and swelling of the great toe metatarsophalangeal (MTP) joint occur in gout but can also occur in osteoarthritis and rheumatoid arthritis. Sausage-like swellings of the toes are seen in Reiter's syndrome.

DIAGNOSTIC STRATEGIES

Laboratory Tests

Laboratory tests other than synovial fluid analysis are of limited diagnostic value for evaluating acute arthritis in the ED.[10] The two most general screening tests are a complete blood count (CBC) and an erythrocyte sedimentation rate (ESR). Infective bacterial arthritis usually causes an elevated white blood cell (WBC) count. Many of the chronic rheumatic diseases have a mild associated anemia. The ESR can be used to screen for inflammatory arthritis because the ESR is elevated in almost all such cases. Rheumatoid factor, antinuclear antibody (ANA), antistreptolysin O titers, and Lyme serologies are useful for follow-up but have no role in the acute ED evaluation. The serum uric acid level is not helpful in diagnosing acute gouty arthritis; in the acute phase of the disease, the serum uric level may be normal.

Radiology

Plain radiographs are of more diagnostic help in patients with chronic disease than in those with acute arthritis. The radiograph of a joint should be surveyed using the following systematic approach, summarized by the mnemonic SECONDS:

Soft tissue swelling
Erosions
Calcification
Osteoporosis
Narrowing (joint space)
Deformity
Separation (fractures)[11]

Common findings that help distinguish the different forms of arthritis are set out in Table 110-3. Other radiologic modalities are available but are not usually performed as part of a routine workup in an emergency setting. Ultrasound is useful in evaluating joint effusions and lesions of tendons, ligaments, and skeletal muscle, particularly of the shoulder region.[12]

Computed tomography (CT) scan in the axial plane can detect SI joint disease in difficult cases and is the preferred method for evaluating the sternoclavicular joint.[13] Both sonography and the CT scan have been used to evaluate joint effusions in children with transient synovitis. A magnetic resonance imaging (MRI) scan is excellent for imaging cruciate ligaments of the knee, detecting early edema in periarticular structures, demonstrating fluid collections in tendon sheaths, and determining the extent of cartilage destruction.[14] A contrast MRI scan can differentiate synovitis from synovial fluid and is useful in rheumatoid patients.[15]

Scintigraphy makes use of ^{99m}technetium methylene diphosphonate (^{99m}Tc MDP); thus, a ^{99m}Tc MDP scan can detect osteomyelitis and stress fractures. After intravenous (IV) injection, the radioisotope is absorbed onto hydroxyapatite crystals at the juxtaarticular subchondral cancellous bone, which becomes vascular with inflammation. Gallium scanning is less dependent on blood flow; gallium accumulates where there is a proliferation of serum proteins and leukocytes. Gallium scanning is helpful if searching for infection, especially in the presence of healing fractures or postoperatively, but it is expensive.[12,14,16]

Table 110-3. Common Radiologic Findings in Arthritis

Arthritis	Findings
Acute arthritis (gout, pseudogout, septic arthritis)	Soft tissue swelling
Late septic arthritis (need at least 8-10 days to see changes)	Subchondral bone destruction Periosteal new bone Loss of joint space Osteoporosis Late joint-space narrowing
Late pseudogout (knee, hip, radiocarpal midcarpal, all MP)	Linear calcification in cartilage Asymmetric joint-space narrowing Reactive sclerosis Osteophyte formation Subchondral cyst formation Lack of osteoporosis
Degenerative arthritis (acromioclavicular, first carpometacarpal, first MTP, DIP, knee, hip, cervical spine, lumbosacral spine)	Asymmetric joint-space narrowing Sclerosis of juxtaarticular bone Bone spurs and cysts—adjacent to severe cartilage degeneration No osteoporosis
Tuberculous arthritis (knee, hip, shoulder)	Soft-tissue swelling Marked demineralization Bony rarefaction Little reactive sclerosis Late: bony destruction Joint space preserved
Late rheumatoid arthritis (wrist, MP, PIP, MTP, first IP, foot, atlantoaxial, glenohumeral)	Symmetric joint-space narrowing Osteoporosis of periarticular bone Marginal erosions (no overhanging margins as in gout) Little reactive bone formation

Arthrocentesis

Arthrocentesis is a critical diagnostic adjunct for the emergency department evaluation of acute arthritis. The procedure, which involves puncturing and aspirating a joint space, can be virtually painless, safe, and simple when performed correctly.[17,18] In the ED evaluation of arthritis, arthrocentesis may also be performed for therapeutic reasons, providing substantial relief to patients suffering from hemarthroses, as well as acute and chronic arthritides.[19]

The emergency indications for arthrocentesis in evaluating joint pain include obtaining joint fluid for analysis, draining tense hemarthroses in patients with hemophilia (after the appropriate clotting factor replacement), and for the instillation of analgesics and antiinflammatory agents for acute and chronic arthritis. Emergent arthrocentesis is contraindicated if infection of any kind covers the area to be punctured because of the risk of introducing infection into the joint space. At times, determining whether periarticular tissues are infected or simply inflamed can be quite difficult, and caution is advised in such instances. Arthrocentesis is relatively contraindicated when bleeding diatheses are present or when patients are undergoing anticoagulant therapy, owing to the risk of bleeding in the joint space.[17] Bacteremia is a relative contraindication for arthrocentesis as well. Arthrocentesis of prosthetic joints should only be performed to rule out infection. The primary complications of arthrocentesis are infection in the joint space, bleeding into the joint space, allergic reaction to anesthetic agents, and long-term corticosteroid-related complications. Dry tap, a situation in which no fluid is aspirated after joint puncture, has been reported, but is relatively rare in arthrocentesis of the larger joints. Dry tap is a more common complication in patients with a history of chronic arthritis owing to anatomical abnormalities in the synovium and periarticular tissues.[20]

As with any procedure, careful preparation is the key to success. Position the patient comfortably, providing adequate exposure to the targeted joint and cushioned support for the joint. Muscle tension during the procedure can reduce the joint volume, making the procedure more difficult; thus, every opportunity to provide for the patient's comfort should be met to avoid muscle tension around the joint. Bony landmarks should be carefully palpated. Using aseptic technique, the skin should be prepared with an appropriate surgical scrub. Adequate local anesthesia can be achieved either by use of a vapor coolant or by local infiltration with anesthetic solution such as 1% or 2% lidocaine.[17] Using an 18- to 22-gauge needle attached to a syringe, puncture the joint space and aspirate joint fluid while carefully avoiding abrasion of the articular cartilage. Remove as much fluid as possible before withdrawal of the needle.

Synovial Fluid Examination

Analysis of synovial fluid is especially useful for identifying crystalline and suppurative etiologies of acute arthritis; therefore, synovial fluid should always be analyzed for appearance (color, clarity), cell count, differential, Gram's stain for organisms, and crystal analysis.[21] A positive Gram's stain is diagnostic for septic arthritis, but a Gram's stain that is negative for bacteria does not rule out septic arthritis.

The cell count helps distinguish the noninflammatory fluid of osteoarthritis and traumatic arthritis from the inflammatory fluid that occurs in most other forms of arthritis. A rough estimate can be made in the ED on a wet mount preparation: one to two WBCs per high-power field (hpf) are consistent with a noninflammatory effusion; more than 20 WBC/hpf suggests severe inflammation or infection.[22] Joint fluid in septic arthritis usually has more than 50,000 WBC/mm^3. However, low WBC counts may occur early in infectious arthritis and in partially treated infections; high WBC counts (greater than 50,000/mm^3) can occur in rheumatoid arthritis, gout, and pseudogout. Most of the WBCs in both septic and severe inflammatory arthritis are PMNs. Prediction rules regarding cell count and the likelihood of septic arthritis are common, but are in no way absolute, and cell counts should not be used to rule out a septic etiology.[23] Rather, bacterial cultures should be obtained if there is any suspicion of infection. Fungal and mycobacterial cultures should only be obtained in cases of persistent monarthritis or oligoarthritis, or in immunocompromised patients.[18] Other tests (i.e., synovial fluid glucose, lactic acid, viscosity, mucin clot, and total protein) have limited utility in ruling out infection and are no longer routinely recommended.[17,18,23] Collecting the synovial fluid in the appropriate container is vital for obtaining accurate results. Specimens for cellular analysis should be submitted in tubes with ethylenediaminetetraacetic acid anticoagulant (lavender top), whereas specimens for crystal analysis should be transported in tubes with liquid heparin (green top). Chemical analysis, serology, and viscosity should be analyzed on fluid submitted in a red top tube. Specimens submitted for Gram's stain and culture should be plated as soon as possible, especially if *Neisseria gonorrhoeae* is suspected as the causative organism. Table 110-4 outlines guidelines for synovial fluid interpretation.

Special tests of synovial fluid include analysis for crystals as well as glucose and viscosity. Crystal analysis is best performed using polarizing microscopy of a drop of synovial fluid or postcentrifugation sediment placed on a slide with cover slip.

Monosodium urate crystals are usually needle shaped, negatively birefringent (i.e., yellow when parallel to the compensator and blue when perpendicular), and range in size from 2 to 10 microns. Calcium pyrophosphate crystals, in contrast, are polymorphic, assuming the shape of rhomboids, rods, or even needles. They are positively birefringent (i.e., yellow when perpendicular to the compensator, blue when parallel), and may be as large as 10 microns.[17,18,24] Monosodium urate crystals may persist in synovial fluid even after resolution of a gouty attack.[25] Synovial fluid glucose analysis, when performed, should be evaluated only in the context of concomitant serum glucose. The normal ratio of synovial fluid glucose to serum glucose is 95%. Because severe inflammation decreases synovial fluid glucose, any ratio of synovial fluid to serum glucose less than 50% is suggestive of the severe inflammation of septic arthritis. However, because other arthritides, such as rheumatoid arthritis, can cause severe inflammation, glucose determination is not useful for ruling in or ruling out the diagnosis of septic arthritis. Finally, inflammation causes the loss of hyaluronate, the substance that imparts viscosity to synovial fluid. Thus, inflammatory processes cause a less viscous synovial fluid. By measuring the maximum length of a drop of synovial fluid as it is falls from a syringe, viscosity can be measured. A drop of normal synovial fluid will elongate to 5 cm to 10 cm as it falls away from the syringe, whereas an inflammatory process will result in a much shorter length or even discreet drops.

Electrocardiography

Electrocardiography (ECG) may prove useful in the evaluation of patients with arthritis for whom a diagnosis of acute rheumatic fever is being considered. ECG is indicated for patients with arthritis who have a history of chest pain or complaints that might be related to the heart, or physical examination findings of a new or changing heart murmur, evidence of congestive heart failure, or cardiomegaly. In carditis, prolongation of the P-R interval is the most common finding, and if pericarditis is present, acute diffuse ST segment elevations may be noted. PR prolongation is one of the minor Jones criteria for acute rheumatic fever.[26]

DIFFERENTIAL CONSIDERATIONS

The differential diagnosis of arthritis in the ED is best considered in terms of patterns of the number and distribution of joints involved, as well as the chronicity of the symptoms. Box 110-1 lists the more common causes for consideration in the ED.

MANAGEMENT

The ED approach and management, from diagnosis to treatment, of patients complaining of joint pain vary depending on the number and distribution of joints involved in the patient symptoms. After a diagnosis is made, treatment varies by underlying pathology. Specific entities are discussed here.

Monarticular Arthritis

Septic Arthritis A patient with monarticular arthritis should be considered to have septic arthritis until proven otherwise.

Pathophysiology and Epidemiology Bacterial pathogens reach joint spaces by hematogenous spread, by direct inoculation, and by direct spread from bony or soft tissue infections. The synovium becomes infected before the release of fluid and enzymes that degrade the articular cartilage. In children, hematogenous spread from a remote source is the

Table 110-4. Synovial Fluid Interpretation

Diagnosis	Appearance	WBCs/mm^3	Polymorphonuclear leukocytes (%)	Glucose (% blood level)	Crystals under polarized light	Culture
Normal	Clear	<200	<25	95-100	None	Negative
Degenerative joint disease	Clear	<4000	<25	95-100	None	Negative
Traumatic arthritis	Straw-colored, bloody, xanthochromic, occasionally with fat droplets	<4000	<25	95-100	None	Negative
Acute gout	Turbid	2000-50,000	>75	80-100	Negative birefringence[1]; needle-like crystals	Negative[2]
Pseudogout	Turbid	2000-50,000	>75	80-100	Positive birefringence[1]; rhomboid crystals	Negative
Septic arthritis	Purulent/turbid	5000-50,000	>75	<50	None	Usually positive
Rheumatoid arthritis/seronegative arthritis (Reiter's disease, psoriatic arthritis, ankylosing spondylitis, inflammatory bowel disease)	Turbid	2000-50,000	50-75	~75	None	Negative

From Benjamin GC: Arthrocentesis. In Roberts JR, Hedges JR, editors: *Clinical procedures in emergency medicine,* ed 3, Philadelphia, 1998, WB Saunders.

WBC, White blood cell.

[1]Negative birefringence means that crystals appear yellow when lying parallel to the axis of the slow vibration of light of the first-order red compensator. With the same orientation to the compensator, positive birefringence crystals appear blue. When the crystals lie perpendicular to the axis, the opposite is true—that is, negative birefringence crystals are blue, and positive ones are yellow. A polarizing microscope is necessary for this distinction to be made.

[2]May be coexisting infection.

Box 110-1 Differential Diagnosis of Arthritis in the ED

Monarticular

Septic arthritis
Gout
Pseudogout
Osteoarthritis
Trauma/hemarthrosis
Charcot joint

Polyarticular

Symmetric

Gonococcal arthritis
Viral arthritis
Lyme disease
Drug-induced arthritis
Reiter's syndrome
Rheumatic fever
Seronegative spondyloarthropathies

Asymmetric

Gonococcal
Acute rheumatic fever
Lyme
Systemic lupus erythematosus
Immune complex diseases (viral)
Reiter's syndrome
Reactive

most common cause. Staphylococcal joint infection occurs as a result of trauma or skin infection.[27] Early or delayed postoperative infections occur in up to 10% of patients who have joint surgery and are more common with obese patients, those taking steroids, patients with underlying systemic disease, patients who have had previous procedures, and after long procedures.[14] Spread of infection from osteomyelitis into a joint predominantly occurs in children during the year before growth plate closure. Once in the joint, bacterial growth and invasion can occur essentially unchecked, resulting in a clinical syndrome manifest by the rapid onset of joint pain, swelling, redness, warmth, and decreased range of motion.[28] The resulting septic arthritis, unless rapidly recognized and treated, can result in serious and prolonged morbidity, disability, and even mortality.[29]

Many populations are at increased risk of septic arthritis, including the elderly, patients with prosthetic joints, injection drug users, or immunocompromised patients such as those with human immunodeficiency virus (HIV) or chronic diseases.[28-34] Often the presentations of these special populations are unusual. Septic arthritis in injection drug users usually involves the axial skeleton, but can involve the extremities.

Individuals at risk for nongonococcal septic arthritis are those with poor immune defenses: the old, very young, patients with chronic debilitating disease, patients taking immunosuppressive drugs, and injection drug users, as well as those with prosthetic joints and after arthrocentesis.[28] Septic arthritis often occurs in patients with underlying chronic arthritis, most commonly in patients with rheumatoid arthritis and particularly those taking steroids. It is also seen in those with osteoarthritis and crystal arthritis. The diagnosis of infectious arthritis in a patient with known crystal arthritis can be difficult. An acute flare of pseudogout or gout can cause fever, and crystals may be present in an infected joint.[35,36] Indeed, an acute septic arthritis may cause a high count of crystals, which are released as the articular cartilage is destroyed.[37] Gram's stain and culture must always be done on joint fluid even when a diagnosis of crystal arthritis is made by light microscopy.

Immunocompromised patients pose a challenge in diagnosis and management because of their increased susceptibility to develop suppurative arthritis in multiple joints as well as because of their altered immune response, which alters the clinical constellation of symptoms and signs normally seen in septic arthritis. EPs must maintain a high degree of suspicion when managing joint pain in these special populations. Further, patients prone to noninfectious arthritides, such as hemophilia patients and patients with rheumatoid arthritis, are still at increased risk for septic arthritides, requiring EPs to have a high degree of vigilance in ruling out septic arthritis as the cause of the patients' joint pain as well.[28,31]

The microbiology of septic arthritis has remained fairly constant over time. Overall, *Staphylococcus aureus* is still the most common cause of septic arthritis. The remaining cases of monarthritis are caused by staphylococci, streptococci, gram-negative organisms, and anaerobes in relatively constant proportions.[38] *N. gonorrhoeae* accounts for only 20% of cases of monarticular septic arthritis, whereas it is a more common pathogen in patients presenting with polyarthritis, which is the usual presentation. The microbiology of septic arthritis in several unique populations contrasts with this, although *S. aureus* is the most common pathogen in most populations. Infants younger than 6 months of age are at risk for *Escherichia coli* as well as group B streptococci, and children from 6 to 24 months are at risk for staphylococci, *Kingella kingae*, and in the prevaccination era, *Haemophilus influenzae*.[39] Immunization programs have reduced the incidence of *H. influenzae* by 95%. Pneumococci remain an articular pathogen in the pediatric age group as well.[40] *N. gonorrhoeae* occurs in less than 10% of pediatric patients with monarthritis. Monarthritis in injection drug users usually results from *S. aureus* or gram-negative organisms such *Pseudomonas aeruginosa*, *Enterobacter* organisms, and *Serratia marcescens*.[34]

Infections may complicate arthrocentesis, arthroscopy, and joint replacement procedures.[17,41] The complication rate varies from 0.04% to 4%. Most infectious complications are early, usually within days or weeks. Organisms causing iatrogenic infections after arthrocentesis and arthroscopy are most commonly *S. aureus*, *S. epidermidis*, and gram-negative rods. Intraarticular infection after injection of corticosteroids may be masked by the lingering effects of the antiinflammatory agents themselves, as well as by the underlying arthritides and their associated immunosuppressive medications. Again, a high degree of suspicion for bacterial infection should be exercised in these situations. In the case of prosthetic joints, infections may surface as long as 1 year after the procedure. Presence of any concurrent bacterial infection is a contraindication to joint replacement. *S. aureus* is the most common infecting organism after joint replacement, followed by mixed infections, gram-negative bacteria, and finally, anaerobes.

Clinical Features The clinical features of bacterial arthritis vary based on the host's concurrent medical conditions.

Patients usually complain of pain in the joint, which is often swollen and hot. Typically, infectious arthritis affects a single joint, with the most common joints infected being the knee (40% to 50%), hip (13% to 20%), shoulder (10% to 15%), wrist (5% to 8%), ankle (6% to 8%), elbow (3% to 7%), and the small joints of the hand or foot (5%).[32] In approximately 20% of cases, several joints may be involved at the same time. Even in septic polyarthritis, however, the knees are the most common sites of infection. In addition to joint pain, 80% of patients have a history of fever, though only 20% report shaking chills.[28] Any history of trauma, surgical procedures, or injection drug use should be elicited. Clinically, affected joints in immunocompetent hosts are red, swollen, warm, and exquisitely tender to touch or motion. Most of these patients will also have fever on exam. Laboratory evaluation should include CBC, ESR, and blood cultures. Elevated sedimentation rate is more common than leukocytosis in septic arthritis. Blood cultures will grow the causative organism approximately 50% of the time.[42] Radiographs demonstrate only soft tissue swelling if present; the bony changes of septic arthritis are long-term findings and are not usually present on the initial exam.

The definitive diagnostic test for septic arthritis is arthrocentesis with examination of the synovial fluid. Purulent fluid with elevated WBC counts is typical. However, WBC counts may be low in bacterial arthritis, especially in immunocompromised hosts, and a low WBC alone should not be used to rule out septic arthritis. In fact, WBC count is greater than 50,000 WBC/mm^3 in only 50% to 70% of patients, and less than 50,000 WBC/mm^3 in the remainder. The percentage of polymorphonuclear leukocytes is usually higher than 85%. Gram's stain will show bacteria in 50% to 70% of infected joints.[28] Synovial fluid cultures for both aerobic and anaerobic organisms should be obtained.

Management The key to successful treatment of septic arthritis is rapid diagnosis. Delays in diagnosis directly worsen prognosis. Hospital admission for incision and drainage of the affected joint and administration of intravenous antibiotics is indicated after the diagnosis is made. Empiric antibiotic therapy should be based on Gram's stain or the consideration of likely organisms for the clinical situation. The antibiotic regimen should be adjusted based on final culture results and sensitivities. In the hospital, daily aspirations of the joint fluid, along with irrigation of the joint using a large-bore needle or arthroscopy, should be performed. Failure to respond to therapy in 5 to 7 days, the presence of osteomyelitis, involvement of the hips or shoulders, or involvement of any prostheses usually mandates open arthrotomy for drainage. Parenteral narcotic analgesics and articular immobilization will control pain and discomfort. Antibiotic therapy should continue parenterally for 2 to 4 weeks' duration depending on the response to therapy, and should be followed with 2 to 6 weeks of oral antibiotic therapy at a high dose.[28,38,42,43] The ultimate clinical outcome is determined by the duration of symptoms before treatment, the number of infected joints, age of the patient, immune status of the patient, preceding joint pathology, and the sensitivity and persistence of the causative organism.[28]

Gouty Arthritis

History Greek writers such as Hippocrates described what is now known as gout. Podagra was the foot goddess, a bad-tempered virgin, who attacked victims after they overindulged.[44] For many centuries this disease was thought to be limited to men who had indulged in dietary or sexual excess.[2] Benjamin Franklin's advice was, "Be temperate in wine, in eating, girls and sloth or the gout will seize you and plague you both."[45]

Pathophysiology and Epidemiology Gout is the deposit of uric acid crystals from a supersaturated extracellular fluid. Uric acid can be overproduced in myeloproliferative or lymphoproliferative diseases or underexcreted in the kidney. Risk factors include obesity or weight gain during young adulthood, hypertension, diabetes, alcohol consumption, proximal loop diuretics, and lead exposure.[46,47] During an attack of gouty arthritis, the crystals are ingested by PMNs, resulting in an inflammatory reaction.[46]

Gouty arthritis occurs most commonly in middle-aged men and postmenopausal women. Men often have a history of increased alcohol consumption, dietary excess, or other precipitating event such as stress of illness or surgery.[48] Not all patients, however, with elevated uric acid levels or even crystals present in joint fluid have acute attacks. Women are relatively protected from gouty arthritis until menopause because estrogens increase the renal excretion of uric acid. Postmenopausal women who sustain attacks of gouty arthritis are more often taking diuretic therapy and have a greater degree of renal insufficiency; the attacks often occur in fingers previously involved with osteoarthritis.[48] Increased levels of uric acid (greater than 5.1 in men, 4.0 in women) are usually present for 20 years before the first attack. Gouty attacks have been observed to occur in cardiac intensive care patients on nitroglycerin infusion during or within 12 hours of discontinuation, perhaps from the ethanol that is part of the mixture.[49] Organ transplant recipients have a high incidence of gout related to cyclosporine-induced hyperuricemia. Often, patients with an acute gouty arthritis have a normal uric acid level, possibly because of the uricosuric effect of pain-induced stress hormones.[47]

Clinical Presentation Gouty attacks most commonly occur in the great toe MTP joint (up to 75%), the tarsal joints, the ankle, and the knee. Usually only one joint is involved initially, although up to 40% of patients can experience polyarticular involvement. The pain is excruciating at the onset and the joint is so sensitive that some patients cannot even tolerate the weight of a sheet on the joint. Systemic symptoms may be minimal or absent or the patient may be febrile, mimicking a picture of septic arthritis. Without treatment, the attack is self-limiting, lasting for several days to weeks, and is followed by an intercritical period of weeks to years. Subsequent attacks get closer together, involve more joints, and last longer. Long-term sequelae include renal stones and tophi (foreign body granulomas with the crystals as a nidus), which form in the musculotendinous unit (olecranon bursa, Achilles tendon, ulnar surface of the forearm, hands, knees, feet, toes, fingers, and even the helix of the ear).

The ED patient may either be experiencing a first attack or have a known history of gout with a recurrent episode. Cellulitis and septic arthritis need to be excluded, particularly if the knee is the joint involved; all of these patients may have fever, leukocytosis, and an elevated ESR. A uric acid level is not helpful in diagnosis of gout in the acute setting because it can be normal. Renal function should be checked. During an acute attack, radiographs of the affected joint will only show soft-tissue swelling. Long-standing disease produces asymmetric bone erosions as a result of crystal deposits, with overhanging margins.

The definitive diagnosis of gouty arthritis is made by seeing negative birefringent joint fluid crystals with a polarizing microscope (a yellow crystal against a red background) and having a negative joint fluid culture.

Management The therapy for gout can be separated into treatment of the acute and the chronic phases. Colchicine or nonsteroidal antiinflammatory drugs (NSAIDs) are used to stop the acute gouty attack. Colchicine, which inhibits microtubule formation, is most effective if administered within the first 24 hours of an episode. It inhibits the inflammatory response to crystals in the joint. IV colchicine, more frequently used in the past, is free of the gastrointestinal side effects associated with oral colchicine.[50] The oral dosage regimen is 0.6 mg orally every hour until the pain is controlled, up to a maximum of 4 mg to 6 mg or until side effects supervene. Patients may have severe nausea and vomiting or diarrhea from oral colchicine. After a full course of colchicine is given, no more should be used for a week. Because it is effective for pseudogout and other crystal arthritides, it cannot be used to make the specific diagnosis of gout, although a gratifying therapeutic response does help distinguish crystal arthritis from septic arthritis. Colchicine is contraindicated in patients with hematologic, renal, and hepatic dysfunction.

NSAIDs are very effective for analgesia with an acute attack of gouty arthritis but can have gastrointestinal (GI) and renal side effects. The NSAID most commonly used is indomethacin, in dosages of 75 mg to 200 mg/day for several days with tapering of the dose as the inflammation decreases. One regimen is 50 mg 3 times a day for 2 days, followed by 25 mg 3 times a day for 3 days. NSAIDs are contraindicated in peptic ulcer disease and GI bleeding, and relatively contraindicated in inflammatory bowel disease, congestive heart failure, asthma, and renal insufficiency. They interact with Coumadin, oral hypoglycemics, and anticonvulsants.[51] Ketoprofen may be as effective as indomethacin and has fewer contraindications.[52] Patients who recognize the "twinges" of an impending attack are instructed to start indomethacin, 20 mg 3 times a day; and colchicine, 0.6 mg 3 times a day, to abort a full-blown attack. In resistant cases, oral prednisone (40 mg/day for 3 to 5 days, then tapering by 5 mg/day) or intramuscular (IM) adrenocorticotrophic hormone (ACTH) can be used. ACTH is also recommended for those patients with contraindications to NSAIDs. The dose of ACTH is 40 IU to 80 IU given IM.[50,51,53,54] Uric acid lowering agents should *not* be started during an acute attack.

Long-term therapy of gout is designed to decrease serum uric acid levels either by decreasing production (allopurinol) or increasing excretion (probenecid). Most physicians treat hyperuricemia only in cases of frequent gouty attacks, tophi, joint destruction, or renal stones. Allopurinol is given in doses from 200 mg/day for mild disease to more than 600 mg/day for severe tophaceous disease. It works by decreasing uric acid production through the inhibition of xanthine oxidase. Allopurinol can cause a sometimes-fatal syndrome of exfoliative rash, fever, hepatitis, and renal failure 1 to 6 weeks after initiation of therapy. Those at risk usually have preexisting renal insufficiency or are taking diuretics. Probenecid, a uricosuric agent, may affect the serum levels of many commonly prescribed drugs (i.e., penicillin, ampicillin, and aspirin). Patients already taking uric acid therapy may have an acute gouty attack, which should be managed as outlined previously; the regimen of the uric acid agent should not be changed in the ED for fear of precipitating another acute episode. In patients prone to recurrent acute attacks of gout, colchicine 0.5 mg twice daily reduced the frequency of attacks by 75% to 85%, and attenuated the severity of attacks that did occur.[55] Colchicine may be given prophylactically for 6 to 12 months as a way of suppressing flareups.

Pseudogout Calcium pyrophosphate dihydrate crystal-deposition disease (also called pseudogout) is in the differential diagnosis of monarticular arthritis. It may also appear as asymptomatic calcific deposits in articular hyaline or fibrocartilaginous tissues on radiographs, as pseudorheumatoid arthritis with involvement of multiple symmetric joints, or as systematic symptoms with a gout-like picture: severe monarticular attacks precipitated by illness such as stroke, myocardial infarction, and surgery, separated by asymptomatic intervals.[56] The knee is most commonly involved, followed by the wrist, ankle, and elbow.[57] More than one joint can be involved.

Twenty-five percent of patients with pseudogout present acutely when crystals are shed from cartilaginous tissues into the synovial cavity and then elicit an inflammatory response. The average attack is not as severe as acute gout.[58] In general, these patients are between the sixth and eighth decades who have a previous history of arthritic attacks. Although the most common form is idiopathic, pseudogout specifically occurs in patients with hyperparathyroidism, hemochromatosis, hypothyroidism, hypomagnesemia, hypophosphatemia, and Wilson's disease.[56]

Laboratory testing usually reveals leukocytosis and elevated ESR. Radiographs of the affected joint may show calcification in joints (knee, wrist, and symphysis pubis), tendon insertions, ligaments, and bursae.[59] Joint fluid examination shows the weakly positive birefringent crystals of calcium pyrophosphate dihydrate. The crystals appear rhomboidal on regular light microscopy. The presence of joint fluid crystals and radiographic calcifications is required for a definite diagnosis of pseudogout.[56] The patient's symptoms may mimic septic arthritis, so joint fluid should be Gram's stained and cultured. A serum calcium level may detect unsuspected hyperparathyroidism.

Treatment for an acute attack is similar to the therapy for acute gout: NSAIDs or oral colchicine, although the latter is not as effective as with gout.[60] As in gouty arthritis, colchicine, 0.6 mg twice daily, can be administered prophylactically to prevent subsequent episodes.[61] Aspiration with or without steroid injection can also be used.[56]

A variant form of pseudogout exists in which calcium apatite crystals are present. The arthropathy has a short history and is rapidly progressive and destructive. Shoulders and knees are involved, effusions are cold, and pain is the most common presentation. Radiographs are notable for marked destructive changes and fewer than expected osteophytes.[62] Apatite crystals may be detected by a wet preparation of synovial fluid stained with alizarin red S.[58]

Osteoarthritis (Degenerative Joint Disease) Osteoarthritis (OA or degenerative joint disease) is the most common form of arthritis in the adult population. Patients with osteoarthritis are elderly: men predominate until 60 years of age, then women predominate. The disease is characterized by loss of articular cartilage and reactive changes at the margins of the joint and in subchondral bone.[63] Patients with degenerative joint disease may come to the ED with an acute flare-up in a joint that has long been chronically affected. The initial damage begins in the cartilage, which degenerates; the subchondral bone fractures; and osteophytes are formed in an attempt to repair the damage. Synovitis is more common in advanced disease because of the release of inflammatory mediators by the damaged joint parts, precipitated by trauma or basic calcium phosphate crystals. Articular cartilage that has been lost does not regenerate and may leave the patient with a painful bone-to-bone interface.

The chief complaint in OA is pain. A lack of systemic symptoms helps distinguish these patients from those with rheumatoid arthritis. The hands are predominantly affected in some patients with OA. Bouchard's and Heberden's nodes (osteophyte spurs) are visible and palpable at the PIP and DIP joints, respectively, and are more common in women. The knee has crepitus on active and passive motion. The quadriceps muscle may be atrophied because of disuse. Many patients have involvement of the hip and walk with a limp.[64] The great toe MTP joint is commonly affected (bunion formation).

Results of routine laboratory tests are usually normal. ESR may be elevated. Radiographs of an osteoarthritic joint show asymmetric joint-space narrowing, osteophyte formation at the joint margins, and subchondral cyst formation without osteoporosis. The synovial fluid is generally noninflammatory with fewer than 2000 cells/mm^3 and few PMNs.[65] Occasionally crystals may be seen. A diagnosis of osteoarthritis can be made in patients with knee pain and radiographic evidence of osteophytes and whose age is greater than 50 or who have crepitus or stiffness of more than 30 minutes after nonuse.

Treatment includes judicious exercise for muscle strengthening, relief of muscle spasm, and support for the joint. Analgesics, like acetaminophen, are the drug of first choice. Acetaminophen is comparable to ibuprofen for the short-term treatment of knee OA.[66] If acetaminophen fails to provide relief from symptoms, patients may be started on NSAIDs, although it is not obvious that they are needed for early osteoarthritis. They may be no more efficacious than acetaminophen and the risk of side effects is significant.[67,68] Ultimately those patients with completely denuded cartilage in the hip and knee will need joint replacement.

Polyarthritis

The differential diagnosis of polyarticular arthritis is much broader than monarticular arthritis. It is helpful to divide polyarticular presentations into two groups. Acute presentations (< 6 weeks) include gonococcal arthritis, viral arthritis (e.g., rubella, hepatitis), Lyme disease, Reiter's syndrome, and rheumatic fever. Chronic polyarticular presentations are caused by rheumatoid arthritis, SLE, scleroderma, psoriatic arthritis, dermatomyositis, and other autoimmune diseases. The diseases may be also be distinguished on the basis of symmetric or asymmetric presentations. Rheumatoid arthritis and lupus tend to be symmetric, the others asymmetric. The spondyloarthropathies (ankylosing spondylitis, reactive arthritis, psoriatic arthritis, and the arthropathy of inflammatory bowel disease) involve predominantly larger joints, whereas psoriatic arthritis affects the small joints of the hands.

Gonococcal Arthritis Typically the patient is a young woman (4:1 ratio to men) who has symptoms develop during her menstrual period, in her last two trimesters of pregnancy, or even postpartum.[69] Of the 1 to 3 million patients with gonorrhea in the United States, each year 1% have disseminated infection develop.[28] Clinically the illness begins with fever, chills, and a migratory tenosynovitis and arthralgias that progress to arthritis, predominantly in the knee, ankle, or wrist. The tendon sheaths of the wrists and hands are often involved. The tenosynovitis and arthritis is thought to be an immune-mediated phenomenon. A characteristic rash in two thirds of patients accompanies the tenosynovitis and arthritis—a countable number of hemorrhagic necrotic pustules that have a red surrounding and a pustular center and typically first appear on the distal extremities, including the sides of the fingers. This full clinical spectrum is called the arthritis/dermatitis syndrome. Rarely does the patient complain of cervicitis or urethritis. A similar syndrome has recently been recognized as a result of *N. meningitidis.*[70] The differential diagnosis includes Reiter's syndrome, polyarticular septic arthritis, hepatitis B arthritis, and rheumatic fever.[69]

Blood cultures generally give a poor yield for *N. gonorrhoeae* and do not correlate with positive synovial fluid cultures, which in general are positive for gonococcus in no more than 50% of cases. The Gram's stain is positive more often than the culture.[69] The synovial fluid is inflammatory (30,000 to 100,000 cells/mm^3).[71] Cervical, urethral, rectal, and pharyngeal cultures are positive in up to 75% of cases. For the best yield, all orifices (synovium, blood, cervix, urethra, rectum, pharynx, and skin lesions) should be cultured and plated at the bedside on chocolate agar or Thayer-Martin medium.[28] Cultures take 48 hours to turn positive so the initial diagnosis of gonococcal arthritis is a clinical one; it is the diagnosis to be excluded in any young patient with a fever, migratory polyarthritis, and polytendinitis.

Patients with gonococcal arthritis need to be admitted to the hospital—if unable to comply with treatment—to confirm the diagnosis, rule out endocarditis, and treat purulent synovitis. The current treatment recommendations call for ceftriaxone 1 g IM or IV daily, and for 24 to 48 hours after improvement. Cefixime, 400 mg twice daily, or ciprofloxacin, 500 mg twice daily, is then given orally for a total of 7 days of antibiotics. During treatment, penicillin, amoxicillin, or tetracyclines can be substituted if the *N. gonorrhoeae* strain is found to be susceptible. Beta-lactam-allergic patients can be treated with spectinomycin 2 grams IM every 12 hours.[71]

Viral Arthritis The two viruses that most commonly cause arthritis are rubella and hepatitis B, but arthritis can also occur with mumps, adenoviruses, Epstein-Barr virus, and enteroviruses. The pathophysiology of arthritis in the viral diseases appears to be deposition of soluble immune complexes in the synovium with resultant inflammation. Patients with rubella arthritis often are young women. The characteristic rash has usually appeared several days before, and patients may have just arthritic symptoms. The arthritis is acute, symmetric, and usually polyarticular, but it can occur in only one joint. Generally it resolves within weeks but in some patients lasts months to years.[72] A history of a recent rubella infection or vaccination helps make the diagnosis. The rubella virus can be isolated from synovial fluid, so joint fluid can be sent for viral culture. The joint fluid initially may be noninflammatory, but if the arthritis persists, the fluid may become inflammatory.

The arthritis of hepatitis B usually occurs with or follows

the prodromal syndrome of fever and lymphadenopathy or may be the only presenting symptom. It often precedes the onset of jaundice, seems to occur in conditions of antigen abundance, and clears with the production of antibodies. Immune complexes in the synovial fluid seem to be responsible for the inflammatory, serum-sickness type of reaction. The arthritis may be sudden and severe. The PIP, knee, ankle, and MP joints are most commonly involved. Salicylates may be helpful for the joint complaints. Serologic tests for rheumatoid arthritis are negative.

Lyme Disease Lyme disease is caused by a spirochete, *Borrelia burgdorferi*. It is named for the location of its original discovery in Lyme, Connecticut; its current geographic prevalence is from Massachusetts to Maryland on the East Coast, Wisconsin and Minnesota in the Midwest, and California, Oregon, Utah, and Nevada in the West. The vector for this spirochete is the tick *Ixodes dammini* on the East Coast and in the Midwest and *Ixodes pacificus* in the West. Arthritis is a late manifestation of the disease. The initial illness is seen in the late spring and early summer.[73] A week after a bite from an infected tick, patients may have a characteristic skin lesion, erythema chronicum migrans, develop at the site of the bite. The lesion has a bright red border with central clearing and quickly multiplies, spreading to the thigh, groin, and axilla, and rarely lasts more than 30 days.[73,74] Other early symptoms of the disease are fever, fatigue, severe lethargy, and other viral complaints—arthralgias, myalgias, and headache. Neurologic abnormalities (commonly Bell's palsy and, less commonly, meningitis and radiculoneuritis) or cardiac abnormalities (predominantly fluctuating atrioventricular block sometimes presenting as syncope and often requiring temporary pacing) may develop in the second stage, 4 weeks after the bite.[73,75,76] This stage represents hematogenous dissemination of the spirochetes. At that time, results of serologic testing are more likely to be positive.

Within 6 months of the inoculum, 50% to 60% of patients with untreated disease have frank arthritis develop, asymmetric, most commonly in large joints, particularly the knees.[77,78] Patients have minimal joint pain and usually are afebrile. Large joint effusions are common in the knee.[73,77] Fifty percent may have had preceding intermittent musculoskeletal pain with pain on motion of the affected region without effusions or swelling.[79] The severity of the initial presentation is predictive of the subsequent arthritis.[80] From 10% to 15% of patients can develop recurrent intermittent attacks of monarticular or pauciarticular arthritis, with episodes of tendinitis or bursitis between the attacks.[76] Chronic arthritis is more common in patients who are positive for HLA-DR4.[81] The differential diagnosis consists of gonococcal arthritis and septic arthritis, acute rheumatic fever (ARF), rheumatoid arthritis, and Reiter's syndrome. A history of a previous tick bite or a history of the rash is helpful in making the diagnosis. The joint fluid is an inflammatory one with a predominance of PMNs. Serum immunofluorescent antibody assays are usually negative until approximately 6 weeks, when immunoglobulin M peaks and indicates active disease.[82] Immunoglobulin G (IgG) antibodies are detected when the arthritis presents and peak at 12 months. False-positive titers can be caused by syphilis, but the different clinical presentations should distinguish the diseases. The diagnosis of Lyme disease is a clinical one and serologic testing should be used discriminately to confirm the diagnosis.[76]

In the early stages, treatment is effective in shortening the duration of symptoms and preventing later disease, so if the clinical findings and epidemiology make the disease suspect, medication should be given before the serologic results are available.[81] No evidence seems to recommend prophylactic therapy after a bite even in an endemic area, except perhaps in pregnant patients or with prolonged attachment in small children.[77] Either doxycycline, 100 mg twice daily; amoxicillin, 500 mg 4 times daily; or cefuroxime, 500 mg twice daily, is recommended for the treatment of early Lyme disease. Erythromycin 250 mg 4 times daily and azithromycin, 500 mg on day 1 and 250 mg on following days, are less effective clinically. Treatment is for 20 to 30 days, although the shorter course may not completely eliminate the organism.[73] Amoxicillin is used instead of doxycycline for pregnant and lactating women and for children younger than 8 years of age. The same drugs can be used for cases with mild neurologic and cardiac disease, but their course of therapy needs to be longer. More severe disease needs 20 million units of IV penicillin or 2 g of IV ceftriaxone daily.[81,83] Persistent arthritis requires either 2.4 million units of IM penicillin G benzathine per week for 3 weeks, or 4 million units of IV penicillin G or 2 g of IV ceftriaxone daily for 2 weeks. Treatment failure is most commonly seen in patients who do not have the disease and were mistakenly diagnosed and treated. A patient with chronic complaints and a negative IgG titer does not have Lyme disease and should not be started on antibiotics.

Seronegative Spondyloarthropathies The seronegative spondyloarthropathies share the characteristics of SI involvement, peripheral inflammatory arthropathy, absence of rheumatoid factor, pathologic changes around the enthesis (ligamentous and tendinous insertion into bone), and a genetic component related to the HLA-B27 marker. The most important of these chronic polyarthritic inflammatory diseases are ankylosing spondylitis, reactive arthritis (including Reiter's syndrome), psoriatic arthritis, and the arthropathy of inflammatory bowel disease. Some clinical overlap exists, but each does have its own distinctive features that will help distinguish one from the other. One feature common to all the spondyloarthropathies is the concept of a genetic predisposition that encounters an environmental stimulus.

Patients with ankylosing spondylitis generally have back discomfort with radiologic evidence of sacroiliitis. There is a male predominance. Radiologically, there is a symmetric squaring of the margins of the vertebral bodies, and later the development of a "bamboo spine." The presentation is subacute or chronic—insidious back discomfort of more than 3 months' duration, with morning stiffness that improves with exercise in someone less than 40 years of age. Uveitis is the most common extraarticular manifestation. The peripheral joints are involved in up to 30% of patients with enthesopathic involvement—plantar fasciitis and Achilles tendinitis. The goal of therapy is to control pain, decrease inflammation with NSAIDs, and begin strengthening exercises.[84,85]

Reiter's syndrome represents the clinical manifestation of a reactive arthritis that occurs in genetically susceptible hosts after infection with *Chlamydia trachomatis* in the genitourinary tract, or *Salmonella, Shigella, Yersinia,* or *Campylobac-*

ter organisms in the GI tract. *Salmonella* enteritis leads to reactive arthritis in up to 4% of cases; *Shigella flexneri* is the most common stool isolate causing Reiter's syndrome. Even HIV has been implicated. Reactive arthritis is generally a disease of young men 15 to 35 years of age who have arthritis develop 2 to 6 weeks after an episode of urethritis or dysentery. Because cervicitis is often asymptomatic, the diagnosis is more problematic in women. The syndrome is predominantly polyarticular and asymmetric. The weight-bearing joints of the lower extremities are commonly involved—knees, ankles, and feet, particularly the heels (lover's heel).[86]

Other physical signs appear early and may be gone when the musculoskeletal complaints persist. Patients may have conjunctivitis early in the disease. This ocular component of the illness may progress to iritis, uveitis, or corneal ulceration. In up to 10% of patients, the oral mucosa and tongue may have initially painless lesions that develop into shallow painful ulcers. Similar lesions are seen on the glans penis (balanitis circinata), particularly in uncircumcised men (20% of patients). Penile lesions of circumcised men are more psoriatic in appearance. Fingers and toes may swell and appear sausage-like, a phenomenon that also occurs in psoriatic arthritis. In 10% of patients, hyperkeratotic lesions of keratoderma blennorrhagia (waxy plaques) develop on the palms and soles and look like pustular psoriasis. Patients may have inflammation at the insertion of the Achilles tendon and up to one third of patients have low back pain and have limitation of vertebral movement on range of motion.[86]

Synovial fluid is inflammatory, with a predominance of PMNs. *Chlamydia, Salmonella,* and *Yersinia* antigens have been found in the synovial membrane and even in the joint fluid, but cultures are sterile. The ESR and WBC count are often increased, but these are not specific for the disease. The HLA-B27 antigen occurs in approximately 80% of patients who have the disease. Rheumatoid factor and ANA are typically negative. Early x-ray films show an enthesopathic picture, particularly at the IP joint of the great toe. This finding is related to the changes seen where ligaments attach to bone and occurs at the SI joints, ischial tuberosities, greater trochanter, and Achilles insertion. A fluffy periostitis characteristic for the seronegative arthropathies is seen. An asymmetric sacroiliitis of the vertebral bodies can occur. Ankylosing spondylitis, which may be confused with the spinal lesions of Reiter's syndrome, typically has symmetric and continuous bambooing of the spine.[86]

Patients with reactive arthritis respond well to NSAIDs, particularly indomethacin, up to 250 mg/day. Tetracyclines have improved recovery time for patients with chlamydia-triggered reactive arthritis, but not for that with a GI cause. Patients may have a single episode (the mean length of an episode is 4 to 7 months); may have recurrent bouts of arthritis; or may have a continuous spectrum of disease generally involving the ankles and calcaneus develop. Ankylosing spondylitis and occasionally aortic insufficiency are late complications.[86]

Of patients with inflammatory bowel disease, 20% develop acute migratory, inflammatory polyarthritis of the larger joints of the lower extremities. This generally occurs at the same time as flareups of the bowel disease. Psoriatic arthropathy occurs in up to 20% of patients with psoriasis. Several forms exist; asymmetric oligoarthropathy (with sausage digits), symmetric polyarthropathy, spondylitis (asymmetric as in Reiter's syndrome), DIP involvement, and arthritis mutilans.[86]

Acute Rheumatic Fever Acute rheumatic fever is believed to result from Group A streptococcus pharyngitis, although the exact mechanisms of disease initiation are unclear.[26] The incidence of acute rheumatic fever has been in a long state of decline in developing countries, especially after the discovery of antibiotics. However, reports of outbreaks in developed countries still occur.[87] It is proposed that an abnormal humoral response to streptococcal antigens leads to arthritis, carditis, valvulitis, and chorea in genetically-susceptible individuals, who tend to range from 5 to 20 years of age. The clinical syndrome, then, classically consists of recurring, self-limited episodes of fever associated with polyarthritis, carditis/valvulitis, rash, subcutaneous nodules, or chorea occurring 2 to 3 weeks after an episode of streptococcal pharyngitis.[88] Unchecked advancement of the cardiac manifestations leads to both short- and long-term morbidity and mortality.

Clinically, the diagnosis of acute rheumatic fever is based on the revised Jones criteria. Over the past 50 years, the Jones criteria have undergone several revisions to improve their diagnostic accuracy.[89] The presence of two major, or one major and two minor, criteria in the presence of supporting evidence of prior Group A streptococcal infection is required (Box 110-2).[90] The major manifestations of rheumatic fever include polyarthritis, carditis, chorea, erythema marginatum, and subcutaneous nodules. Migratory arthritis is present in the majority of patients and usually affects the large joints. Owing to the availability and efficacy of antiinflammatory agents, the migratory arthritis is often short-lived and far

Box 110-2 1992 Jones Criteria for Diagnosis of Acute Rheumatic Fever

Major Manifestations	Minor Manifestations
Polyarthritis	Clinical findings
Carditis	Arthralgia
Chorea	Fever
Erythema marginatum	Laboratory findings
Subcutaneous nodules	Elevated acute phase reactants
	Erythrocyte sedimentation rate
	C-reactive protein
	Prolonged PR interval on EKG

Plus:
Supporting evidence of prior Group A streptococcal infection (elevated or increasing streptococcal antibody titer, positive rapid strep test or bacterial throat culture, recent scarlet fever).

Special Writing Group of the Committee on Rheumatic Fever, Endocarditis, and Kawasaki Disease of the Council on Cardiovascular Disease in the Young of the American Heart Association: Guidelines for the diagnosis of rheumatic fever: Jones criteria, 1992 update, *JAMA* 268:2069-2073, 1992. Copyrighted (1992), American Medical Association.

from classic.[88] Rheumatic fever involves the heart in about half of patients, causing both cardiac dysfunction as well as valvular abnormalities. Pericarditis, congestive heart failure, valvular dysfunction, and cardiomegaly all indicate cardiac involvement of acute rheumatic fever. Echocardiography has been recommended even for patients with no clinical evidence of carditis.[87,91] Neurologic dysfunction in acute rheumatic fever can lead to chorea (also known as Sydenham's chorea), weakness, and even behavioral disturbances. Careful neurologic evaluation will demonstrate sparing of sensory functions even in the presence of these other startling findings. The rash of erythema marginatum as well as subcutaneous nodules may also be present in acute rheumatic fever. Erythema marginatum is manifest by the appearance of well-demarcated, pinkish areas of nonpruritic rash, usually on the trunk, but sometimes spreading to the proximal limbs. The plaques demonstrate central clearing and may last only hours. Subcutaneous nodules, on the other hand, are firm, nontender nodules usually located under the skin overlying bony prominences.

The laboratory workup for possible ARF consists of pharyngeal cultures, ESR, C-reactive protein, and antibody to streptolysin O. The latter is helpful in patients with joint involvement as the only clinical manifestation. Anti-DNase B, if available, increases the sensitivity to 95%. The streptozyme test also documents recent streptococcal infection. The synovial fluid is an inflammatory one with an average of 16,000 WBCs, no crystals, and a negative culture.

Poststreptococcal reactive arthritis is a closely related but distinct clinical entity in which patients have some, but not all the diagnostic criteria for acute rheumatic fever. Reactive arthritis is a clinical syndrome characterized by a sterile oligoarthritis associated with bacterial infection in a distant site. In poststreptococcal reactive arthritis, carditis is rare, and the arthritis is often severe. Controversy exists about the relationship and diagnosis of this entity to acute rheumatic fever.[92,93]

Treatment is penicillin G benzathine, 1.2 million U IM or 2 g of oral penicillin V per day for 10 days (erythromycin if the patient is penicillin-allergic). Penicillin can be given as monthly benzathine, 1.2 million U IM or 250 mg orally per day (or 500 mg to 1 g sulfadiazine) through adolescence or up to 5 years from the last episode to prevent recurrences (up to 75% of cases). The arthritis responds well to salicylates, 6 to 8 g/day for adults and 80 to 100 mg/kg/day for children or NSAIDs.[94] They may need to be continued for 2 months or until the ESR is normal. Carditis can be treated with 40 to 60 mg prednisone for 2 weeks to decrease the inflammatory response in the myocardium.[88]

Rheumatoid Arthritis Although rheumatoid arthritis is a chronic disease, at least 20% of patients have an acute presentation and thus rheumatoid arthritis is in the differential diagnosis of polyarticular arthritis.

The disease develops in women 2 to 3 times more often than in men, with a peak incidence between the fourth and sixth decades of life. There appears to be a genetic predisposition related to the HLA-DR4 haplotype. Immune complexes are formed that stimulate PMNs to release the enzymes that ultimately cause joint destruction. The synovial cells increase dramatically in number and produce even more inflammatory substances. A pannus of granulation tissue is formed that ultimately destroys the joint.[95]

Patients commonly see a physician after a prodromal period of fatigue, weakness, and musculoskeletal pain that may last weeks to months. The patient's joints begin to swell in a symmetric and additive pattern, particularly the hands (MP and PIP joints), wrists, and elbows. The foot, however, may be the initial site of involvement and is affected in more than 90% of patients with rheumatoid arthritis, particularly the great and little toe MTP joints. The DIP joints of the fingers are not involved, which helps distinguish rheumatoid arthritis from osteoarthritis, reactive arthritis, and psoriatic arthritis.[96]

Acute presentations may have only warm, tender, swollen joints that may be difficult to distinguish from a viral arthropathy. Tenosynovitis can occur. Acute pericarditis is not related to the duration of disease and also may be an early presentation. In the patient with long-standing rheumatoid arthritis, long-term changes may be observed. These include MP and PIP swelling, ulnar deviation, swan-neck and boutonnière deformities of the hands, and limitation of dorsiflexion of the wrist. The knee is often affected—short term with effusion, long term with muscle atrophy and Baker's cysts.[96] Bursae in the retrocalcaneal region are common complications. Extraarticular complications include subcutaneous nodules (associated with more severe disease), vasculitis of the skin, pulmonary fibrosis, mononeuritis multiplex, and Sjögren's and Felty's syndromes. Patients with long-standing rheumatoid arthritis may have degeneration of the transverse ligament develop that normally keeps the dens of C2 close to the posterior aspect of the anterior part of the C1 ring.

The workup of the patient in whom rheumatoid arthritis is suspected should be directed at excluding other causes of arthritis, such as septic arthritis. Rheumatoid factor, which is an antibody against gamma globulin, is positive in approximately 85% of patients with rheumatoid arthritis but even if negative does not exclude the diagnosis.[96] ESR and C-reactive protein levels may be elevated but are also elevated in other rheumatologic diseases.

Early radiographic features of rheumatoid arthritis are soft-tissue swelling and juxtaarticular osteoporosis leading to uniform joint-space narrowing. The MRI scan is useful early in the disease by demonstrating erosions before they can be seen on conventional x-ray study. Arthrocentesis must be done. The fluid should be evaluated for purulence, crystals, Gram's stain, and culture. The cell count is usually inflammatory, between 4000 and 50,000, with more PMNs (75%) than seen with crystal disease. The joint fluid glucose is usually low.

Excessive movement increases inflammation, so the initial treatment is rest in combination with suppression of the inflammation by medications. The joints should be splinted, the upper extremities for 3 weeks and the lower extremities for 8 weeks. The plan is to decrease the pain, inflammation, and side effects as much as possible.[97]

The mainstay of therapy in the past was the pyramid approach, with salicylates used alone as the first-line medication. Other medications were added only as the disease progressed. Because the first 12 to 18 months are critical in preventing major joint damage, particularly in aggressive disease, salicylates are no longer being used as solo agents.[98] Instead, a "bridge concept" of coadministering different classes of medications has emerged.[98,99] These include steroids, gold, penicillamine, azathioprine, methotrexate, cyclosporine, and sulfasalazine. Oral prednisone, 5 mg to 7.5 mg daily, has been used effectively to control inflammation and methotrexate and sulfasalazine have been used in combination without any increase in the significant side effects of methotrexate alone. For mild disease, most clinicians still use the salicylates or other NSAIDs, which have their GI and renal toxicities related to their inhibition of cyclooxygenase. A scoring system has been used to best predict patients at greatest risk for GI complications, including age, dose, and concurrent steroid use.[97] Acetylsalicylic acid in its original form has GI and platelet toxicity. The enteric-coated form has decreased GI effects but is not as well absorbed, and the nonacetylated form has fewer hypersensitivity reactions, less GI toxicity, and no effect on platelet function. All take up to 2 weeks to reach peak effective serum levels. If NSAIDs are chosen, patients may need to try at least three different types before a reduction in symptoms occurs. In addition, NSAIDs have GI toxicity (a problem in the elderly), change platelet function, and should not be used in patients with renal or cardiac failure.

DISPOSITION

The challenge in the ED management of arthritis is in ruling out septic etiologies. If a patient is diagnosed with nongonococcal septic arthritis based on a positive Gram's stain or culture, or based on strong clinical suspicion even in the face of a negative Gram's stain, the patient should be admitted with emergent orthopedic consultation for parenteral antibiotics and evaluation for possible arthroscopy or arthrotomy. Patients in whom a disseminated gonococcal infection is suspected should be admitted for parenteral antibiotics and orthopedic consultation, except in cases where the patient is well-appearing, the symptomatology is mild, and the patient is able to comply with the daily follow-up plans. Patients with noninfectious etiologies of arthritis may be discharged assuming their pain is controlled.

KEY CONCEPTS

- The number of joints involved and the distribution of joint involvement help pinpoint the most likely cause of arthritis.
- Monarthritis is septic arthritis until proven otherwise.
- The most definitive test for evaluating an inflamed joint for the possibility of bacterial infection is examination of synovial fluid.
- Negative Gram's stain of synovial fluid does not rule out bacterial arthritis.
- Delays in the diagnosis and treatment of septic arthritis worsen outcomes.

REFERENCES

1. Schned ES, Reinertsen JL: The social and economic consequences of rheumatic disease. In Klippel JH, editor: *Primer on the rheumatic diseases,* ed 11, Atlanta, 1997, Arthritis Foundation.
2. Benedek TG: History of the rheumatic diseases. In Klippel JH, editor: *Primer on the rheumatic diseases,* ed 11, Atlanta, 1997, Arthritis Foundation.
3. Felson DT: Epidemiology of the rheumatic diseases. In Koopman WJ, editor: *Arthritis and allied conditions: a textbook of rheumatology.* ed 13, Baltimore, 1997, Williams & Wilkins.
4. Simkin PA: The musculoskeletal system: joints. In Klippel JH, editor: *Primer on the rheumatic diseases,* ed 11, Atlanta, 1997, Arthritis Foundation.
5. Goldring MB: Articular cartilage. In Klippel JH, editor: *Primer on the rheumatic diseases,* ed 11, Atlanta, 1997, Arthritis Foundation.
6. Knudson W, Kuettner KE: Structure: proteoglycans. In Klippel JH, editor: *Primer on the rheumatic diseases,* ed 11, Atlanta, 1997, Arthritis Foundation.
7. Abramson SB: Mediators of inflammation, tissue destruction and repair: cellular constituents. In Klippel JH, editor: *Primer on the rheumatic diseases,* ed 11, Atlanta, 1997, Arthritis Foundation.
8. Cash JM: Evaluation of the patient: history and physical examination. In Klippel JH, editor: *Primer on the rheumatic diseases,* ed 11, Atlanta, 1997, Arthritis Foundation.
9. Middleton DB: Infectious arthritis, *Primary Care* 20:4, 1993.
10. Shmerling RH, Liang MH: Evaluation of the patient: laboratory assessment. In Klippel JH, editor: *Primer on the rheumatic diseases,* ed 11, Atlanta, 1997, Arthritis Foundation.
11. Beachley MC: Radiology of arthritis, *Primary Care* 20:4, 1993.
12. Scott WW: Evaluation of the patient: imaging techniques. In Klippel JH, editor: *Primer on the rheumatic diseases,* ed 11, Atlanta, 1997, Arthritis Foundation.
13. Winalski CS, Shapiro AW: Computed tomography in the evaluation of arthritis, *Rheum Dis Clin North Am* 17:543, 1991.
14. Mitchell M et al: Septic arthritis, *Radiol Clin North Am* 26:1295, 1988.
15. Missenbaum MA, Adams MK: MRI in rheumatology, *Rheum Dis Clin North Am* 20:2, 1994.
16. Lopez-Longo F et al: Primary septic arthritis in heroin users: early diagnosis by radioisotope imaging and geographic variations in the causative agents, *J Rheumatol* 14:991, 1987.
17. Benjamin GC: Arthrocentesis. In Roberts JR, Hedges JR, editors: *Clinical procedures in emergency medicine,* ed 3, Philadelphia, 1998, WB Saunders.
18. Hasselbacher P: Arthrocentesis, synovial fluid analysis, and synovial biopsy. In Klippel JH, editor: *Primer on the rheumatic diseases,* ed 11, Atlanta, 1997, Arthritis Foundation.
19. Schaffer TC: Joint and soft-tissue arthrocentesis, *Primary Care* 20:4, 1993.
20. Roberts WN et al: Dry taps and what to do about them: a pictorial essay on failed arthrocentesis of the knee, *Am J Med* 100:461, 1996.
21. Shmerling RH: Synovial fluid analysis: a critical appraisal, *Rheum Dis Clin North Am* 20:2, 1994.
22. Clayburne G, Baker DG, Schumacher HR: Estimated synovial fluid leukocyte numbers on wet drop prep as a potential substitute for actual leukocyte counts, *J Rheumatol* 19:60, 1992.
23. Javors JM, Weisman MH: Principles of diagnosis and treatment of joint infections. In Koopman WJ, editor: *Arthritis and allied conditions: a textbook of rheumatology,* ed 13, Baltimore, 1997, Williams & Wilkins.
24. Krey PR, Lazaro DM: *Analysis of synovial fluid.* Summit, NJ, 1992, Ciba-Geigy.
25. Pascual E et al: Synovial fluid analysis for diagnosis of intercritical gout, *Ann Int Med* 131:756, 1999.
26. Gibofsky A, Zabriskie JB: Rheumatic fever: etiology, diagnosis, and treatment. In Koopman WJ, editor: *Arthritis and allied conditions: a textbook of rheumatology,* ed 14, Baltimore, 1997, Williams & Wilkins.
27. Barton LL, Dumkle LM, Habib FH: Septic arthritis in childhood, *Am J Dis Child* 141:898, 1987.
28. Mahowald ML: Infectious disorders: septic arthritis. In Klippel JH, editor: *Primer on the rheumatic diseases,* ed 11, Atlanta, 1997, Arthritis Foundation.
29. Baker DG, Schumacher RH: Current concepts: acute monarthritis, *N Engl J Med* 329:1013, 1993.
30. Vassilopoulos D et al: Musculoskeletal infections in patients with human immunodeficiency virus infection, *Medicine* 76:284, 1997.
31. Gilbert MS et al: Long-term evaluation of septic arthritis in hemophiliac patients, *Clin Orth* 328:54, 1996.
32. Dubost J et al: Polyarticular septic arthritis, *Medicine* 72:296, 1993.
33. Sack K: Monarthritis: differential diagnosis, *Am J Med* 102:30S, 1997.
34. Brancos MA et al: Septic arthritis in heroin addicts, *Semin Arth Rheum* 21:81, 1991.
35. Baer PA et al: Coexistent septic and crystal arthritis; report of 4 cases and literature review, *J Rheumatol* 13:604, 1986.
36. Esterhai JL, Gelb I: Adult septic arthritis, *Orthop Clin North Am* 22:3, 1991.

37. Jobanputra P, Gibson T: Case report: diagnosis of pseudogout and septic arthritis, *Br J Rheumatol* 26:379, 1987.
38. Ike RW: Bacterial arthritis. In Koopman WJ, editor: *Arthritis and allied conditions: a textbook of rheumatology,* ed 13, Baltimore, 1997, Williams & Wilkins.
39. Yagupsky P et al: Epidemiology, etiology and clinical features of septic arthritis in children younger than 24 months. *Arch Pediat Adol Med* 149:537, 1995.
40. Bradley JS et al: Pediatric pneumococcal bone and joint infections, *Pediatrics* 102:1376, 1998.
41. Armstrong RW, Bolding F, Joseph R: Septic arthritis following arthroscopy: clinical syndromes and analysis of risk factors, *J Arthro Rel Surg* 8:213, 1992.
42. Mikhail IS, Alarcon GS: Nongonococcal bacterial arthritis, *Rheum Dis Clin North Am* 19:2, 1993.
43. Kim HK, Alman B, Cole WG: A shortened course of parenteral antibiotic therapy in the management of acute septic arthritis of the hip, *J Ped Orth* 20:44, 2000.
44. Cornelius R, Schneider MA: Gouty arthritis in the adult. *Radiol Clin North Am* 26:1267, 1988.
45. Vawter RL, Antonelli MA: Rational treatment of gout, *Postgrad Med J* 91:2, 1992.
46. Terkeltaub RA: Gout: epidemiology, pathology, and pathogenesis. In Klippel JH, editor: *Primer on the rheumatic diseases,* ed 11, Atlanta, 1997, Arthritis Foundation.
47. Edwards NL: Gout: clinical and laboratory findings. In Klippel JH, editor: *Primer on the rheumatic diseases,* ed 11, Atlanta, 1997, Arthritis Foundation.
48. Lally EV, Ho G, Kaplan SR: The clinical spectrum of gouty arthritis in women, *Arch Intern Med* 146:2222, 1986.
49. Shergy WJ, Gilkeson GS, German DC: Acute gouty arthritis and intravenous nitroglycerin, *Arch Intern Med* 148:2505, 1988.
50. Star VL, Hochberg MC: Prevention and management of gout, *Drugs* 45:2, 1993.
51. Pratt PW, Ball GB: Gout: treatment. In Klippel JH, editor: *Primer on the rheumatic diseases,* ed 11, Atlanta, 1997, Arthritis Foundation.
52. Altman RD et al: Ketoprofen versus indomethacin in patients with acute gouty arthritis: a multicenter, double blind comparative study, *J Rheumatol* 15:1422, 1988.
53. Diamond HS: Control of crystal induced arthropathies, *Rheum Dis Clin North Am* 15:557, 1988.
54. Emmerson BT: Drug therapy: the management of gout, *N Engl J Med* 334:445, 1996.
55. Paulus HE et al: Prophylactic colchicine therapy of intercritical gout: a placebo-controlled study of probenecid-treated patients, *Arthritis Rheum* 34:1489, 1991.
56. Ryan LM: Calcium pyrophosphate dihydrate crystal deposition. In Klippel JH, editor: *Primer on the rheumatic diseases,* ed 11, Atlanta, 1997, Arthritis Foundation.
57. Masuda I, Ishikawa K: Clinical features of pseudogout attacks: a survey of 50 cases, *Clin Orthop* 229:173, 1988.
58. Beutler A, Schumacher HR: Gout and pseudogout: when are arthritic symptoms caused by crystal deposition? *Postgrad Med* 95:2, 1994.
59. Bonafede RP: Evaluating CPPD crystal deposition: an important disease of aging, *Geriatrics* 48:59, 1988.
60. Agarwal AK: Gout and pseudogout, *Primary Care* 20:4, 1993.
61. Alvarellos A, Spilberg I: Colchicine prophylaxis in pseudogout, *J Rheumatol* 13:804, 1986.
62. Dieppe P: Apatites and miscellaneous crystals. In Klippel JH, editor: *Primer on the rheumatic diseases,* ed 11, Atlanta, 1997, Arthritis Foundation.
63. Fife RS: Osteoarthritis: epidemiology, pathology, and pathogenesis. In Klippel JH, editor: *Primer on the rheumatic diseases,* ed 11, Atlanta, 1997, Arthritis Foundation.
64. Dearborn JT, Jergesen HE: The evaluation and initial management of arthritis, *Prim Care* 23:215, 1996.
65. Hochberg MC: Osteoarthritis: clinical features and treatment. In Klippel JH, editor: *Primer on the rheumatic diseases,* ed 11, Atlanta, 1997, Arthritis Foundation.
66. Bradley JD et al: Comparison of an inflammatory dose of ibuprofen, an analgesic dose of ibuprofen and acetaminophen in the treatment of patients with osteoarthritis, *N Engl J Med* 325:87, 1991.
67. Brandt KD: Should osteoarthritis be treated with nonsteroidal anti-inflammatory drugs? *Rheum Dis Clin North Am* 19:3, 1993.
68. Brandt KD: Should nonsteroidal anti-inflammatory drugs be used to treat osteoarthritis? *Rheum Dis Clin North Am* 19:1, 1993.
69. Scopelitis E, Martinez-Osuna P: Gonococcal arthritis, *Rheum Dis Clin North Am* 19:2, 1993.
70. Rompalo AM et al: The acute arthritis-dermatitis syndrome, *Arch Intern Med* 147:281, 1987.
71. Goldenberg DL: Gonococcal arthritis and other neisserial infections. In Koopman WJ, editor: *Arthritis and allied conditions: a textbook of rheumatology,* ed 13, Baltimore, 1997, Williams & Wilkins.
72. Naides SJ: Infectious disorders: viral arthritis. In Klippel JH, editor: *Primer on the rheumatic diseases,* ed 11, Atlanta, 1997, Arthritis Foundation.
73. Schoen RT: Identification of Lyme disease, *Rheum Dis Clin North Am* 20:3, 1994.
74. Wright SW, Trott AT: North America tick borne disease, *Ann Emerg Med* 17:964, 1988.
75. Williams DN, Schned ES: Lyme disease: recognizing its many manifestations, *Postgrad Med J* 87:139, 1990.
76. Sigal LH: Lyme disease: testing and treatment: who should be tested and treated for Lyme disease and how? *Rheum Dis Clin North Am* 19:1, 1993.
77. Kalish R: Lyme disease, *Rheum Dis Clin North Am* 19:2, 1993.
78. Steere AC: Musculoskeletal manifestations of Lyme disease, *Am J Med* 98:44S, 1995.
79. Kolstoe J, Messner RP: Lyme disease: musculoskeletal manifestations, *Rheum Dis Clin North Am* 15:649, 1989.
80. Steere AC, Schoen RT, Taylor E: The clinical evolution of Lyme arthritis, *Ann Intern Med* 107:725, 1987.
81. Sigal LH: Infectious disorders: lyme disease. In Klippel JH, editor: *Primer on the rheumatic diseases,* ed 11, Atlanta, 1997, Arthritis Foundation.
82. Magnarelli LA: Lab diagnosis of Lyme disease, *Rheum Dis Clin North Am* 15:735, 1989.
83. Steere AC: *Borrelia burgdorferi.* In Mandell GL, Bennett JE, Dolin R, editors: *Mandell, Douglas, and Bennett's principles and practice of infectious diseases,* ed 5, Philadelphia, 2000, Churchill Livingstone.
84. Taurog JD: Seronegative spondyloarthropathies: epidemiology, pathology, and pathogenesis. In Klippel JH, editor: *Primer on the rheumatic diseases,* ed 11, Atlanta, 1997, Arthritis Foundation.
85. Khan MA: Seronegative spondyloarthropathies: anklyosing spondylitis. In Klippel JH, editor: *Primer on the rheumatic diseases,* ed 11, Atlanta, 1997, Arthritis Foundation.
86. Arnett FC: Seronegative spondyloarthropathies: reactive arthritis (Reiter's syndrome) and enteropathic arthritis. In Klippel JH, editor: *Primer on the rheumatic diseases,* ed 11, Atlanta, 1997, Arthritis Foundation.
87. Veasy LG et al: Resurgence of acute rheumatic fever in the intermountain area of the United States, *N Engl J Med* 316:421, 1987.
88. Gibofsky A, Zabriskie JB: Rheumatic fever. In Klippel JH, editor: *Primer on the rheumatic diseases,* ed 11, Atlanta, 1997, Arthritis Foundation.
89. Shiffman RN: Guideline maintenance and revision: 50 years of the Jones criteria for diagnosis of rheumatic fever, *Arch Ped Adol Med* 149:727, 1995.
90. Special Writing Group of the Committee on Rheumatic Fever, Endocarditis, and Kawasaki Disease of the Council on Cardiovascular Disease in the Young of the American Heart Association: Guidelines for the diagnosis of rheumatic fever: Jones criteria, 1992 update. *JAMA* 268:2069, 1992.
91. Veasy LG: Echocardiography for diagnosis and management of rheumatic fever, *JAMA* 269:2084, 1993.
92. Aviles RJ, et al: Poststreptococcal reactive arthritis in adults: a case series, *Mayo Clin Proc* 75:144, 2000.
93. Jansen TL, Janssen M, VanRiel PL: Acute rheumatic fever or post-streptococcal reactive arthritis: a clinical problem revisited, *Br J Rheumatol* 37:335, 1998.
94. Amigo MC, Martinez-Lavin M, Reyes P: Acute rheumatic fever, *Rheum Dis Clin North Am* 19:2, 1993.
95. Goronzy JJ, Weyand CM: Rheumatoid arthritis: epidemiology, pathology, and pathogenesis. In Klippel JH, editor: *Primer on the rheumatic diseases,* ed 11, Atlanta, 1997, Arthritis Foundation.

96. Anderson RJ: Rheumatoid arthritis: clinical and laboratory features. In Klippel JH, editor: *Primer on the rheumatic diseases,* ed 11, Atlanta, 1997, Arthritis Foundation.
97. Paget SA: Rheumatoid arthritis: treatment. In Klippel JH, editor: *Primer on the rheumatic diseases,* ed 11, Atlanta, 1997, Arthritis Foundation.
98. Healy LA, Wilske KR: Reforming the pyramid: a plan for treating rheumatoid arthritis in the 1990s, *Rheum Dis Clin North Am* 15:615, 1989.
99. Golbus J, Grober JS: New approaches to the treatment of RA; increased use of methotrexate and other remittive agents, *Hosp Formulary* 27, 1992.

111 Tendonitis and Bursitis

Christopher F. Richards
Theodore K. Koutouzis

PERSPECTIVE

Musculoskeletal complaints have been discussed as far back as Hippocrates. Distinctions among various processes of musculoskeletal complaints and joint inflammation were made beginning in the 1680s when Sydenham described gout, rheumatism, and chorea.[1] In the current era, tendon problems represent 30% of all running-related injuries and are present in nearly 40% of tennis players.[2,3] In addition to their incidence, tendon injuries often represent a chronic problem. Many patients have symptoms for months or years in spite of attempted treatment.[4] Emergency management focuses on eliminating other more serious causes of pain such as fractures or joint space infections, discriminating articular from extraarticular sources of pain, identifying the cause of the inflammation, modifying behavior to minimize or eliminate the sources of continuing irritation, and providing antiinflammatory therapy and referral for appropriate follow-up.

PRINCIPLES OF DISEASE

Today's society is more athletically active than ever before. In fact, in all age groups, whether male or female, athletic pursuits and fitness have become an obsession for many. Although physical activity has dramatic health benefits, it also predisposes to significant morbidity and mortality. To this end, overuse syndromes (tendonitis and bursitis) have increased in incidence. Approximately half of all sports participants will be injured at some time, and of those, 25% to 50% will experience tendonitis or bursitis.

Another area of concern is the workplace. The incidence of work-related musculoskeletal disorders is higher in jobs that involve repetitive motions, localized contact stress, awkward positions, vibrations, and forceful exertions.[5] Studies have demonstrated that an improvement in ergonomic design can reduce the incidence of tendonitis and bursitis in the workplace and our daily lives.[5]

Bursae are closed, round, flat sacs lined by synovium that may or may not communicate with the synovial cavity. They occur at areas of friction between skin and underlying ligaments and bone. Bursae also permit the lubricated movement of soft tissues over areas of potential impingement (e.g., subacromial bursa). Many bursae are nameless, and new bursae may form anywhere from frequent irritation. Bursae may become inflamed for many reasons: chronic friction, trauma, crystal deposition, infection, and systemic diseases (rheumatoid arthritis, ankylosing spondylitis, psoriatic arthritis, and gout). The synovial cells of the bursae increase in thickness, and excess fluid accumulates inside and around the affected bursae when inflammation is present.

Tendon sheaths are composed of the same synovial cells as bursae and can become inflamed in a similar manner. Technically, tendonitis refers to inflammation of the tendon only, and tenosynovitis to inflammation of the tendon and its sheath. Inflammatory changes involving the tendon sheath have been well documented in association with tendonitis; however, inflammatory lesions of the tendon alone have not been well documented.[6] Thus, the pathoanatomic distinction of tendonitis and tenosynovitis seems uncertain, and the terms will be used interchangeably here. Because of the similarity of their clinical pictures, tendonitis and bursitis will be discussed together by anatomic regions. These areas are diagrammed in Figure 111-1.

Mechanical overload or repetitive microtrauma to the musculotendinous unit is thought to be the central cause of most tendon problems with extrinsic and intrinsic factors modifying the pathophysiologic state.[7] Intrinsic factors including malalignment, poor muscle flexibility, muscle weakness or imbalance, and others (Box 111-1) may result in excessively high or frequent mechanical loads during normal activity. Extrinsic factors include the ergonomic design of equipment or workplace and excessive duration, frequency, or intensity of activity. Most injuries have a multifactorial etiology. Certain factors may contribute more in one patient than in another. For example, a young athlete may have mechanical overload on the basis of repetitive exercise and poor technique, while in an older patient tendon degeneration and decreased vascularity may be the cause and exercise merely the factor that exposes the problem.

Under most conditions, the musculotendinous units are able to adapt to tension overload. This occurs through an increase in bone mass, hypertrophy of skeletal muscle, increased collagen and mucopolysaccharide content, and collagen cross-linking in tendons. Unfortunately, the virtue of patience is infrequently honored and most patients do not allow sufficient time for this adaptive process to occur. For instance, a runner may increase mileage, intensity, or both too rapidly to allow time for the cellular changes that are required to accommodate the increased stress.

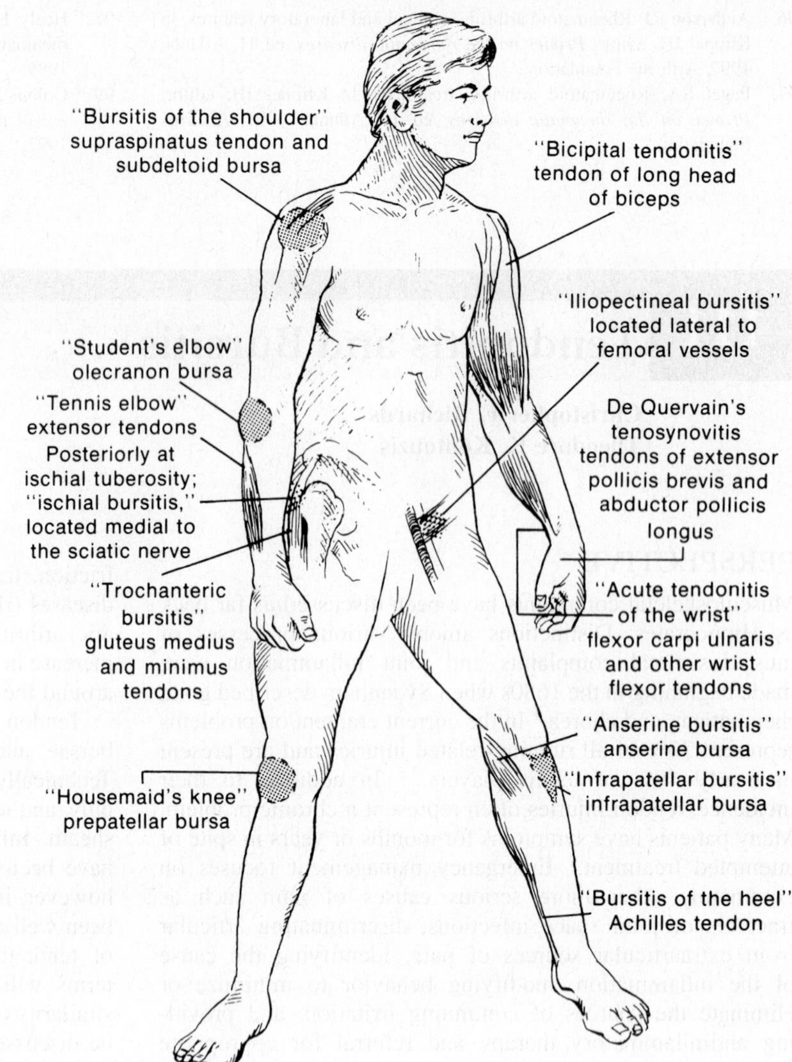

Figure 111-1. **Location of common sites for tendonitis or bursitis.** ***Modified from Branch WT: Office practice of medicine, ed 2, Philadelphia, 1987, WB Saunders.***

Box 111-1 Factors in Chronic Tendon Problems

Intrinsic Factors

Anatomic factors

Malalignment
Muscle weakness or imbalance
Muscle inflexibility
Decreased vascularity

Systemic factors

Inflammatory conditions (SLE, etc.)
Pregnancy
Quinolone-induced tendinopathy

Age-related factors

Tendon degeneration
Increased tendon stiffness
Tendon calcification
Decreased vascularity

Extrinsic Factors

Repetitive mechanical load

Excessive duration
Excessive frequency
Excessive intensity
Poor technique
Workplace factors

Equipment problems

Footwear
Athletic field surface
Equipment factors (i.e., racquet size)
Protective gear

Although the site and mechanism of injury may vary, the ensuing inflammatory response is almost always the same. Immediately following injury, chemotactic and vasoactive chemical mediators are released. This causes vasodilation and cellular edema and attracts increased numbers of polymorphonuclear cells, thus perpetuating the process. If no further injury occurs, this reaction will last from 48 hours to 2 weeks. Repetitive insults will prolong the inflammatory stage. The classic inflammatory signs of pain, warmth, erythema, and swelling will be noted. Following the inflammatory stage, the healing process will proceed through both proliferative and maturation stages. Approximately 6 to 12 weeks following the initial injury, structural organization and collagen cross-linking will have matured to preinjury strength.[8] If the patient continues to exacerbate the inflammatory response, fibrosis with tendon thickening and stenosing tenosynovitis will result.

Table 111-1. Most Common Locations of Tendonitis

Location	Common name
Origin	
Supraspinatus tendon	Rotator cuff tendonitis
Wrist extensor origin	Tennis elbow
Hamstring origin	Hamstring tendonitis
Sheath	
Abductor pollicis longus	De Quervain's disease (trigger finger)
Sheath or tendon	
Achilles tendon	Achilles tendonitis
Wrist flexors	Flexor tendonitis
Insertion	
Achilles calcaneal insertion	Achilles tendonitis, plantar fasciitis

CLINICAL FEATURES

History

The history of patients with tendonitis can be quite variable. A history of repetitive stress can be obtained by inquiring about changes in sports activity, other recreational activities, work activities, or changes in the workplace. Many patients will initially report no such changes, but when prompted to think back over several weeks or months, and to include such things as sports equipment, workplace safety features, protective boots or other features, they will report the offending change or activity. At other times, no cause can be identified for the mechanical overload. A history of pregnancy, quinolone therapy, connective tissue disorders, and systemic illness should also be obtained.

Pain is the most common complaint of patients with joint problems who come to the ED. The pain may be acute or chronic, or an acute episode in a patient with chronic disease. The pain associated with tendonitis and bursitis is frequently more severe after periods of rest. Unlike the pain of morning stiffness associated with arthritis, the pain of tendonitis will resolve quickly after initial movement only to become a throbbing pain after exercise. The patient may have had similar pain before, so it is important to know whether a diagnosis was previously made and what treatment, if any, was instituted.

It is important to determine if the source of inflammation or pain is articular (within the joint capsule) or periarticular (outside the joint capsule). True arthritis produces generalized joint pain, warmth, swelling, and tenderness. Discomfort increases with both passive and active motion of the joint because all parts of the joint are involved In contrast, periarticular inflammation (bursitis, tendonitis, or localized cellulitis) tends to be more localized. Tenderness and swelling do not occur uniformly across the joint, and pain is produced only with certain movements, most commonly resisted active contraction or passive stretching of the affected muscles or tendons. The character and radiation of the pain will vary based on whether the origin, musculotendinous junction, middle substance, sheath, or insertion is affected. Table 111-1 lists the most common sites of tendonitis and the affected part of the tendon.

Physical Examination

In order to eliminate arthritis as a diagnostic possibility, each joint in question should be specifically examined for the following attributes: warmth and effusion, range of motion, deformity, instability, pain on motion, and tenderness (generalized or localized, articular or periarticular). Some tendons, such as the Achilles tendon, are superficial, which facilitates relatively straightforward evaluation and diagnosis. Tendons that are anatomically more inaccessible, such as the supraspinatus tendon, require a more careful approach. Tendinous insertions should be palpated in both tension and laxity, because pain will frequently be absent when the tendon is under tension.

Shoulder A shoulder that is affected by chronic arthritis or bursitis will have atrophy of the deltoid muscle. Generalized tenderness and pain, both at rest and with active and passive motion, suggest an intraarticular process. Localized tenderness and pain associated with active movement are more likely to be periarticular in origin. Having the patient place both hands behind the head and then behind the back tests for external and internal rotation, respectively.

Elbow Early signs of joint inflammation in the elbow are limitation of extension and an increase in the normal angle at which the elbow is held at the side. In olecranon bursitis, localized swelling occurs only over the olecranon. Tenderness of the medial and lateral epicondyles indicates epicondylitis.

Hand and Wrist The hand and wrist provide many clues to the presence of long-standing rheumatic disease: metacarpophalangeal (MCP) and proximal interphalangeal (PIP) joints are affected in rheumatoid arthritis; and the first carpometacarpal, PIP, and distal interphalangeal (DIP) joints in osteoarthritis. Subluxation at the MCP joints, ulnar deviation, and swan-neck deformities occur in rheumatoid arthritis. The nails may have pitting characteristic of psoriatic arthritis. Although the wrist may not be obviously swollen, discomfort and decreased range of motion particularly on extension may indicate synovial involvement.

Hip Inflammation affecting the hip joint may be reported by the patient as pain in the anterior thigh, knee, or groin. A hip joint effusion may cause the patient to hold the hip partially flexed. An externally rotated and abducted leg in a neonate suggests infection, even if the child is afebrile.[9] Range of motion of the hip is most easily tested by flexing the hip, bending the knee at a right angle, and rotating the heel medially and laterally to test for external and internal rotation, respectively[10] (see Figure 111-3). Marked irritability and decreased range of movement confirm hip joint involvement. Lateral hip joint tenderness may indicate trochanteric bursitis, and deep buttock tenderness occurs in ischiogluteal bursitis (Figure 111-2).

Knee An effusion of the knee joint is relatively easy to detect when it appears as a ballotable fullness medially and laterally. Small effusions may be detected by examining for a transmitted fluid wave. Fullness of the popliteal fossa may indicate a Baker's cyst. Passive range of motion may elicit crepitus or clicking. Periarticular involvement is revealed as a fullness above the patella (suprapatellar bursitis), over the lower pole of the patella (prepatellar bursitis), or tenderness at the medial aspect of the knee below the joint margin (anserine bursitis). Tenderness directly over the patellar tendon that decreases when placed under tension is an indicator of patellar tendonitis.

Foot and Ankle Inflammation of the Achilles tendon may occur in Reiter's syndrome; rheumatoid arthritis produces subcalcaneal swelling. Tibiotalar joint effusion produces swelling under the medial malleolus and may make it difficult to palpate the extensor hallucis longus tendon. Tenderness, warmth, and swelling of the great toe metatarsophalangeal (MTP) joint occur in gout but can also occur in osteoarthritis and rheumatoid arthritis.

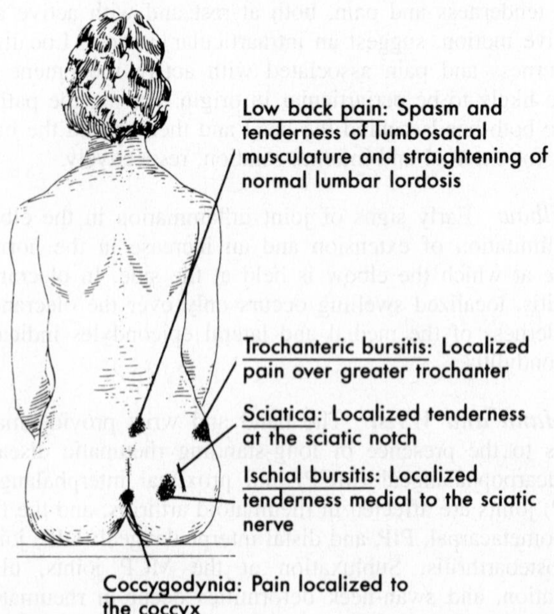

Figure 111-2. Localization of pain and tenderness in conditions causing back and hip pain. *Modified from Branch WT: Office practice of medicine, ed 2, Philadelphia, 1987, WB Saunders.*

SPECIFIC INFLAMMATORY CONDITIONS

Shoulder

Injuries to the shoulder are common. The causes of shoulder pain form a continuum from inflammation of the subacromial bursa, supraspinatus tendonitis, bicipital tendonitis, adhesive capsulitis, and a torn rotator cuff (Figure 111-3). Inflammation of the supraspinatus tendon and bicipital tendon are major causes of a painful shoulder, with inflammation of the supraspinatus being the most common. Inflammation of these tendons results in pain that is reproduced at greater than 60 degrees of passive abduction, at which point the tendon becomes compressed beneath the acromion[11] (Figure 111-4). Occasionally tendonitis of the rotator cuff and biceps occur together.[12]

Supraspinatus Tendonitis The shoulder joint is predisposed to soft tissue injury due to its extensive range of motion and unique anatomic structure. While inherently unstable, the muscles of the rotator cuff, supraspinatus, infraspinatus, teres minor, subscapularis, and the glenohumeral ligaments serve to stabilize the joint. These muscles

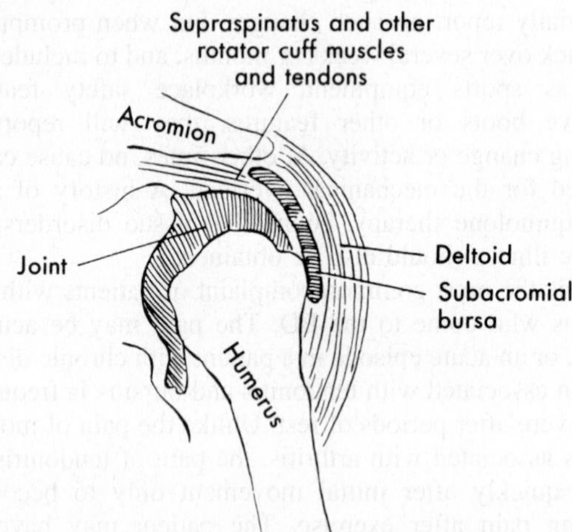

Figure 111-3. Anatomy of the shoulder joint. *Modified from Branch WT: Office practice of medicine, ed 2, Philadelphia, 1987, WB Saunders.*

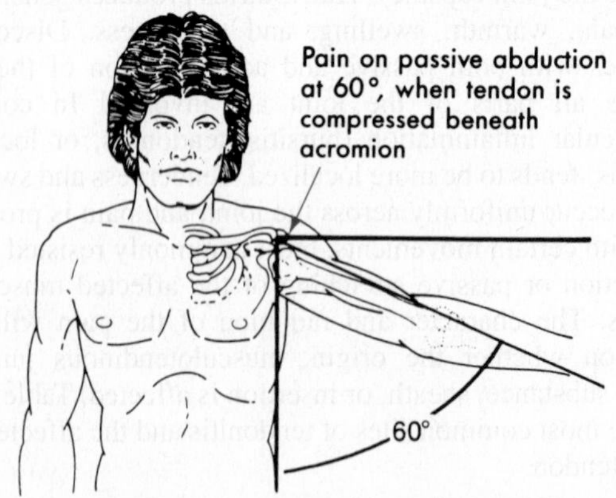

Figure 111-4. Supraspinatus tendonitis. *Modified from Branch WT: Office practice of medicine, ed 2, Philadelphia, 1987, WB Saunders.*

originate from the scapula and insert on the fibrous capsule of the glenohumeral joint through the subacromial space. The long head of the biceps tendon and subacromial bursa is also found in this space. In fact, impingement of these tendons occurs because of their unique position between the humeral head and acromion that confines the area of inflammation and predisposes to chronic tendonitis. The functional arc of the elevated shoulder is forward and in the anterior plane.[13] With this position, the greater tuberosity of the humerus compresses the ligaments of the rotator cuff against the undersurface of the anterior third of the acromion. The mechanism of this tendonitis is overuse of the extremity that leads to microtrauma of the tendinous fibers, along with individual anatomic differences that result from aging, such as osteophytic changes. For instance, older athletes may have an isolated impingement without shoulder joint instability. This is thought to be due to degenerative changes within the joint itself. Neer has classified the impingement syndrome into three progressive stages that may worsen over time.[13] Stage I frequently occurs in patients younger than age 25 who are involved in sports requiring repetitive overhead motions, such as swimming or pitching. It is characterized by edema and hemorrhage within and around the tendon. Flexion and abduction of the arm usually elicit the pain with point tenderness over the greater tuberosity. The patient will characterize the pain as a dull ache, but no weakness or loss of motion should be present.

In stage II, affecting patients between 25 and 40 years of age, the pain becomes constant and usually worsens at night. Active motion will be limited by pain, and almost all motion exacerbates the patient's symptoms. Passive range of motion should be preserved, and on physical exam pain will be more diffuse and intense. As mentioned earlier, the inflammatory response will have ensued and, in addition to tendonitis, fibrosis and thickening of the tendon and bursa will occur.

Partial or complete tears of the rotator cuff, biceps tendon rupture, and osteophytic bony changes herald stage III. The classic test for impingement is performed by raising the patient's humerus in a forced forward flexion while preventing scapular rotation.

Subacromial Bursitis The subacromial bursa, lying between the tendon and the acromion, often becomes secondarily involved. The proximity of these anatomical structures contributes to the spread of the inflammatory response. Thus, subacromial bursitis is thought to be synonymous with supraspinatus tendonitis and typically follows the stages of impingement. Pain and tenderness will be localized to the lateral aspect of the shoulder, and signs of impingement will be noted on physical exam. Although not specific to subacromial bursitis, the painful arc of the subacromial space, which is pain between 70 and 100 degrees of shoulder abduction, will be noted.[11] While rare, primary bursitis may result from rheumatoid arthritis, tuberculosis, gout, and infections.[14]

Calcific Tendonitis Another cause of acute shoulder pain is calcific tendonitis. It appears to affect individuals over the age of 40, and the etiology is unknown. It can affect any tendon of the rotator cuff but seems to have a predilection for the supraspinatus tendon. Most patients are asymptomatic and the finding is noted on routine radiograph. Calcium is deposited within the tendon over time and undergoes spontaneous resorption. The pain associated with this condition is thought to be due to the resorption phase. Acute attacks of calcific tendonitis can develop secondary to crystal release from the tendon, often after trauma. The severe pain is sometimes relieved when the calcific material ruptures into the bursa.[15]

Bicipital Tendonitis With bicipital tendonitis, patients complain of pain in the anterior shoulder, which radiates down the radius. They may also complain of discomfort when rolling on the shoulder at night and when trying to reach a hip pocket or a back zipper.[12] Focal tenderness is elicited in the groove between the greater and lesser tuberosities of the humerus. This discomfort is increased by having the patient resist supination of the wrist with the elbow at 90 degrees and the arm against the body (Yergason's test)[15] (Figure 111-5). Speed's test can also be performed. Pain along the bicipital groove, resulting from resisted forward flexion and forearm supination of an extended elbow, indicates the presence of bicipital tendonitis.

Rotator Cuff Injury An acute rupture of the rotator cuff is diagnosed by having the patient abduct the arm to 90 degrees. Patients with rotator cuff tears cannot perform this maneuver. If the arm is passively abducted to 90 degrees and then released, it will fall back down (drop arm test). Patients with adhesive capsulitis have limitation of passive motion as well as active motion.

Elbow

Lateral Epicondylitis Lateral epicondylitis (tennis elbow) is a common condition that often has an acute onset.[16,17] Although it occurs in many tennis players, less than 5% of those with the syndrome play tennis. Other activities implicated are driving in screws, using a wrench, and working on an assembly line. It often begins as a dull ache on the outer aspect of the elbow that increases with grasping and twisting. It results from inflammation at the insertion of the common extensor tendon (specifically the carpi radialis brevis) onto the lateral epicondyle of the humerus. Resisted active dorsiflexion of the wrist or extension

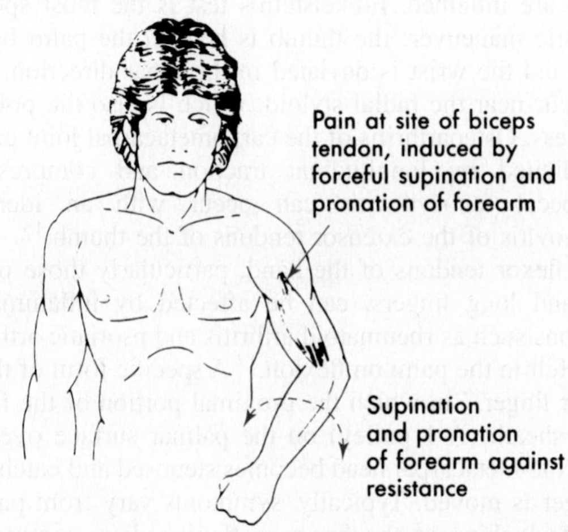

Figure 111-5. **Bicipital tendonitis.** ***Modified from Branch WT: Office practice of medicine, ed 2, Philadelphia, 1987, WB Saunders.***

of the middle finger against resistance can reproduce the pain, with the elbow in extension. Radiographs may be helpful in atypical or prolonged cases to rule out rare pathologic conditions such as bony tumors. Soft-tissue calcifications may be seen. The pain of the less common medial epicondylitis (golfer's, pitcher's, or bowler's elbow) results from inflammation and microtrauma at the site of the insertion of the flexor carpi radialis on the medial epicondyle. An active flexing of the wrist against resistance reproduces pain.

Olecranon Bursitis The olecranon bursa is easily traumatized, resulting in inflammation, pain, and swelling. Gout, rheumatoid disease, pseudogout, and uremia can all produce primary bursal inflammation. Infection can occur locally from puncture wounds or lacerations, or systemically from bacteremia. Sometimes microscopic wounds can introduce infection in the absence of visible trauma. Those at risk are patients with problems of diabetes, chronic alcohol abuse, uremia, and gout.

The treatment of olecranon bursitis remains controversial. Some experts support aspiration and evaluation of the effusion in all cases, even if the area is not red and is only minimally tender. Others feel that aspiration only increases the risk of infection and prefer to treat empirically with antibiotics and NSAIDs or antibiotics alone. Staphylococcal infection is most common, and an antistaphylococcal antibiotic should be chosen if antibiotics are prescribed. A bursal fluid white blood count (WBC) over 5,000/mm^3 suggests bursal fluid infection, even in the presence of a negative Gram's stain. Lastly, some view this process as predominantly inflammatory and believe that only NSAIDs need be administered. Regardless of which treatment is chosen, intrabursal steroids should not be given, and close follow-up to assess the patient's response to treatment should be arranged.[15]

Wrist and Hand

The wrist and hand are comprised of several tendons that pass through thick fibrous retinacular tunnels. This helps prevent subluxation and acts as a pulley system. Overuse syndromes are thought to result from inflammatory changes of the synovial lining between these tendons and the retinaculum. In de Quervain's tendonitis the abductor pollicis longus and extensor pollicis brevis (and sometimes extensor pollicis longus) are inflamed. Finkelstein's test is the most specific diagnostic maneuver; the thumb is held in the palm by the fingers and the wrist is deviated in the ulnar direction. Pain will occur near the radial styloid, which is also the point of tenderness. Osteoarthritis of the carpometacarpal joint causes pain elicited by longitudinal traction and compression. Gonococcal tenosynovitis can occur with an identical tenosynovitis of the extensor tendons of the thumb.[15]

The flexor tendons of the hand, particularly those of the index and long fingers, can be affected by inflammatory conditions such as rheumatoid arthritis and psoriatic arthritis. Pain is felt in the palm on flexion.[17] A specific form of this is "trigger finger," in which the proximal portion of the flexor tendon sheath (A-1 pulley) on the palmar surface over the base of the metacarpal head becomes stenosed and catches as the finger is moved. Typically, symptoms vary from pain to complete locking of the finger in flexion. It is common in middle-aged women.

Conservative treatment with rest, splinting, and antiinflammatory medications may be attempted. Some feel this is inadequate treatment and recommend cortisone injection initially.[8] Cure rates from 84% to 91% have been reported with this treatment.[8] For de Quervain's disease, a thumb spica will be required if cortisone injection provides no improvement. Surgical release of the A-1 pulley may also be performed if the above conservative treatment fails.

Hip

Trochanteric Bursitis Several bursae in the hip region are common sites for inflammation. The trochanteric bursa has both deep and superficial components. The deep bursa is located between the greater trochanter and the tensor fascia lata; the superficial, between the greater trochanter and the skin. Patients are generally middle-aged or older women who complain of acute or chronic pain over the bursal area and lateral thigh. The pain is increased with lying on the hip and with walking. Trochanteric bursitis can occur as a complication of rheumatoid arthritis. The pain of superficial bursitis can be reproduced by hip adduction and that of deep trochanteric bursitis by hip abduction (Figure 111-6). The hip joint itself should appear normal on examination.

Ischial Bursitis Ischial bursitis may develop secondary to trauma or from sitting on a hard surface. Sometimes the pain radiates down the back of the thigh and may mimic sciatic nerve inflammation. The pain can be reproduced by pressure over the ischial tuberosity.

Iliopsoas Bursitis The iliopsoas bursa is the largest bursa around the hip. It lies between the iliopsoas tendon and the lesser trochanter. The pain of iliopsoas bursitis radiates down the medial thigh to the knee and is increased on hip extension.

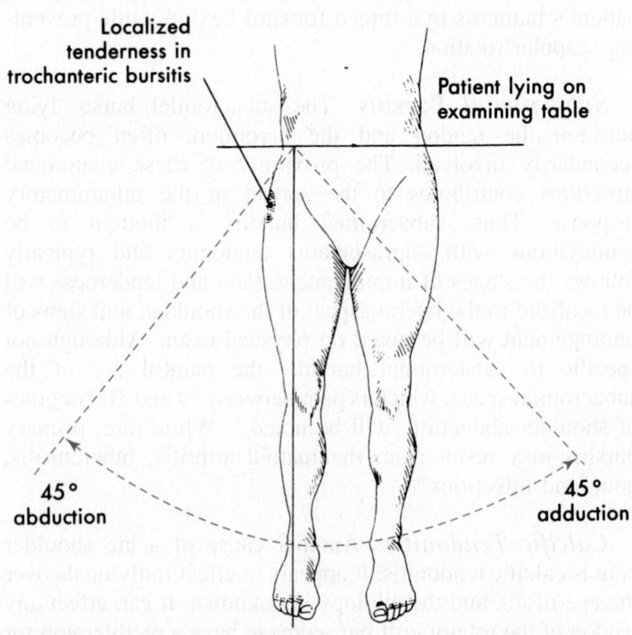

Figure 111-6. **Forced abduction and adduction reproduce pain of trochanteric bursitis.** ***Modified from Branch WT:* Office practice of medicine, *ed 2, Philadelphia, 1987, WB Saunders.***

Knee

Prepatellar Bursitis Prepatellar bursitis causes swelling over the lower pole of the patella, usually as a result of trauma, rheumatoid arthritis, or localized infection. Repetitive microtrauma may produce "housemaid's knee" (i.e., prepatellar bursitis). Repetitive trauma may also produce fibrosis and thickened nodules, thereby requiring excision of the bursa. Pyogenic prepatellar bursitis is thought to be more common in children. This condition will require aspiration, immobilization, and antibiotic coverage. If acute episodes are not resolved within 2 days, incision and drainage should be considered.[17]

Anserine Bursitis Anserine bursitis most commonly occurs in obese older women with large legs and a history of osteoarthritis of the knees. The pain characteristically increases on climbing stairs and can radiate to the inner thigh and midcalf. The area of tenderness is localized to the medial aspect of the knee 2 inches below the joint margin, where the medial hamstrings (sartorius, adductor gracilis, and semitendinosus) attach. The area is usually neither swollen nor warm.

Infrapatellar Bursitis Deep infrapatellar bursitis presents with tenderness on both sides of the tendon, which increases with extreme flexion.[18,19] If signs of infection such as loss of full extension of the knee or resistance to full flexion are present, aspiration of the infrapatellar bursa should be performed along with antibiotic treatment. If infection exists, evaluation for surrounding osteomyelitis is suggested.[17]

Ankle

Achilles Tendonitis Achilles tendonitis is a common overuse syndrome that typically affects male athletes. The tendon arises from the medial and lateral heads of the gastrocnemius muscle and the deep layers of the soleus muscle, and inserts on the calcaneal tuberosity. It is the strongest and largest tendon in the body and can withstand tensile loads of up to eight times the body's weight while running.[20]

The Achilles tendon can be injured from trauma or overuse, or become inflamed as a part of a systemic disease (ankylosing spondylitis, Reiter's syndrome, gout, or pseudogout). However, most causes of Achilles tendonitis are thought to be multifactorial. For instance, an athlete's body mechanics or environmental factors, such as uneven terrain, may apply valgus or varus stress to the tendon. Thus, techniques, environment, equipment, and body mechanics underlie the development of Achilles tendonitis. Additionally, the vascular supply creates a watershed area approximately 2 to 6 cm above the calcaneal insertion and is thought to be responsible for the clinical symptoms and pathological disruption at this site.

Tendonitis will progress through a series of stages, noted below, before final rupture occurs. Initially, the tendon sheath becomes inflamed, and tendon inflammation follows. With repeated stress, scar tissue formation and degeneration of the tendon will occur, thereby reducing its strength. Clinically, the patient will note pain, decreased range of motion, and if chronic, morning stiffness.[20] As with all cases of tendonitis, rest, ice, and nonsteroidal antiinflammatory drugs (NSAIDs) will be the treatment of choice. In order to prevent recurrence, correction of limb malalignment with the use of orthotics or heel wedges may be needed. Changes in the training environment, duration, and intensity may also be modified to eliminate undue stress.

Achilles Tendon Rupture It is possible for untrained athletes to apply excessive force and rupture the Achilles tendon, even in the absence of prior inflammatory changes. Partial and complete rupture may occur, seen traditionally in 30- to 40-year-old men. Complete rupture is more common in the middle-aged recreational athlete. Historically, the patient will note a popping sensation, followed by acute weakness and the inability to continue the exercise or sport. The patient may report a sensation of having been kicked in the back of the ankle. On physical examination, a gap may be appreciated before enough time has elapsed to allow hematoma formation, at which time the area may feel boggy. It is important to note that the ability to plantar flex the foot does not rule out a complete rupture. Muscles such as the posterior tibialis, peroneals, and long toe flexors may remain functional and therefore disguise a complete rupture.[20] Thompson's test is most commonly performed to evaluate for complete rupture. With the patient prone and feet hanging over the edge of the bed, the examiner squeezes the calf muscles and looks for plantar flexion. The absence of plantar flexion is considered a positive test.

Surgery is now the treatment of choice for rupture, especially for the elite athlete. The 10% to 30% rate of return to preinjury activity levels with conservative treatment is unacceptable when compared to approximately 90% for those treated with surgery.[20]

DIAGNOSTIC STRATEGIES

Plain Radiographs

A diagnosis of tendonitis or bursitis is generally made on clinical grounds; however, radiologic studies are sometimes required to confirm the diagnosis by ruling out other causes of pain. Plain radiographs help distinguish extraarticular from articular sources of pain. The radiograph of a joint should be surveyed using a systematic approach. One such approach may be summarized by the mnemonic SECONDS: *S*oft tissue swelling, *E*rosions, *C*alcification, *O*steoporosis, *N*arrowing (joint space), *D*eformity, *S*eparation (fractures).[21]

Ultrasound

Ultrasound (US) is useful in the evaluation of joint effusions and lesions of tendons, ligaments, and skeletal muscles, particularly of the shoulder region. US has been shown to be more sensitive than magnetic resonance imaging and is now considered the gold standard for evaluating tendon involvement with concomitant trauma or rheumatic diseases. US is especially useful when other concurrent conditions (e.g., gouty arthritis) occur and obscure the findings of tendonitis. Currently this modality has limited use in the emergency care setting. However, with the increasing presence and practice of US within the ED, some familiarity will become essential.

In acute or chronic tendonitis, one or more of the following features may be seen: loss of the fibrillar echotexture, focal tendon thickening, diffuse thickening, focal hypoechoic areas, extended hypoechogenicity, irregular and ill-defined borders, microruptures, and peritendinous inflammatory edema.[22] Thickening of the tendon, either focal or diffuse, is another US finding with acute or chronic tendonitis. Hypoechoic areas surrounding tendons provide evidence for surrounding soft tissue inflammation. In addition to tendonitis, tendon tears, both partial and complete, can be delineated by US.

Scintigraphy

Scintigraphy makes use of two isotopes, ^{99m}technetium pertechnetate and phosphonate. After intravenous injection, the isotope binds to plasma protein and concentrates in the joint space, where there is an increase in vascularity from synovitis. A methylene diphosphonate scan can detect osteomyelitis and stress fractures; the radioisotope is absorbed onto hydroxyapatite crystals at the juxtaarticular subchondral cancellous bone, which becomes vascular with inflammation. Gallium scanning is less dependent on blood flow; gallium accumulates where there is a proliferation of serum proteins and leukocytes. Gallium scanning is helpful if searching for infection but is expensive and time consuming. As a result its use in the emergency setting is limited.[23,24]

DIFFERENTIAL CONSIDERATIONS

The most important diagnosis to exclude when a patient has joint pain, warmth, and swelling is septic arthritis. In many cases, the diagnosis is straightforward. The patient has fever and significant joint inflammation associated with decreased range of motion and an effusion. Unfortunately, all cases of septic arthritis aren't clinically obvious. When doubt exists, arthrocentesis should be performed. Patients with exacerbations of preexisting rheumatological conditions may present a similar diagnostic challenge. Arthrocentesis may be necessary to exclude intraarticular involvement. Other conditions that may mimic tendonitis or bursitis include underlying fractures or osteomyelitis. Radiographs and bone scans may be necessary to exclude these conditions.

MANAGEMENT

Most patients with bursitis and tendonitis can be managed conservatively with rest and antiinflammatory medication. The exceptions to this are olecranon bursitis and prepatellar bursitis, which have a moderate risk of being infected, most likely with *Staphylococcus aureus.* Those bursae may require needle aspiration and treatment with antibiotics until culture results are negative. Alternatively, empiric antibiotics may be administered. Most can be managed as outpatients as long as close follow-up can be assured. Patients with prepatellar bursitis who have systemic symptoms may require admission for intravenous antibiotics.[25]

The involved joint should be rested. Shoulders should not be immobilized for more than a few days because of the risk of adhesive capsulitis. Patients with lateral epicondylitis often benefit from a forearm brace. A Jones type of compression dressing, with an elastic bandage to prevent recurrent swelling, may be used in olecranon bursitis. De Quervain's tenosynovitis is immobilized by splinting the wrist and thumb in 20 degrees of dorsiflexion. With Achilles tendonitis, a heel lift or splint in slight plantar flexion is recommended. Absolute rest can be achieved only with casting, but this technique should be left for the consulting orthopedist.

Reduction of inflammation may be assisted by cold treatments (20 minutes at a time every several hours, for the first 24 to 48 hours), changing to heat treatments for the next several days. NSAIDs provide some pain relief in addition to reducing the inflammatory response. Graduated range-of-motion exercises may be useful after the period of immobilization. Tendonitis and bursitis of the shoulder and rotator cuff tears in older patients are treated initially with gravity pendulum range-of-motion exercises, followed by wall climbing with the hand as pain is controlled (Figures 111-7 and 111-8).

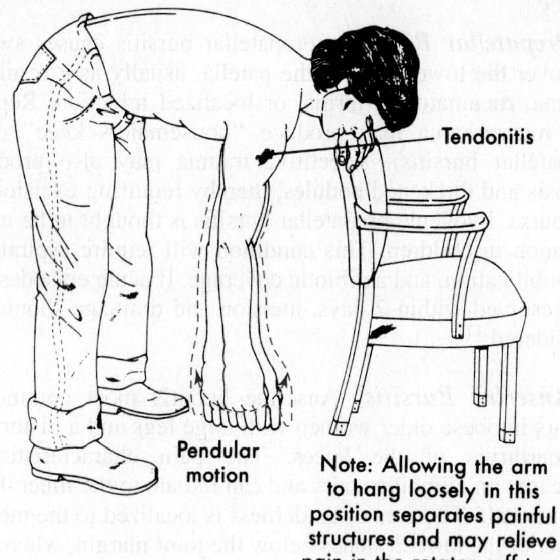

Figure 111-7. **Pendulum exercise.** *Modified from Branch WT: Office practice of medicine, ed 2, Philadelphia, 1987, WB Saunders.*

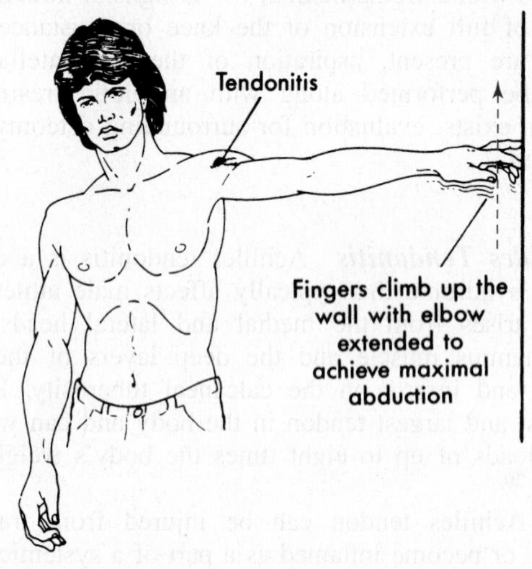

Figure 111-8. **Wall-climbing exercises.** *Modified from Branch WT: Office practice of medicine, ed 2, Philadelphia, 1987, WB Saunders.*

Steroids should not be injected into major tendons—Achilles and patellar—which are at risk for spontaneous rupture if already weakened. Steroids should not be instilled in a bursa if any suspicion of infection exists. Complications of intrabursal injections are infection, local subcutaneous atrophy, bleeding, postinjection flare as a result of release of microcrystals, and tendon rupture.

DISPOSITION

Most patients with tendonitis or bursitis may be safely discharged to home with proper analgesia and immobilization. The exception would be those elderly or disabled patients for whom the tendonitis renders them unable to perform their activities of daily living. Some patients will have complicating medical conditions that contribute to systemic illness and toxicity. Such patients would require admission. These patients include those with diabetes mellitus, immunosuppression, or autoimmune disease. In the vast majority rest, analgesia, and immobilization will provide symptomatic relief. Still, the underlying condition should be sought and evaluated.

KEY CONCEPTS

- Mechanical overload and repetitive microtrauma are the key underlying mechanisms in the development of tendonitis and bursitis.
- Other conditions such as septic arthritis, osteomyelitis, and fractures must be excluded before confirming the diagnosis of tendonitis or bursitis.
- The use of US in the diagnosis of tendonitis, especially in the shoulder, has become widespread and is considered a standard by some. However, its use in emergency medicine is still limited.
- The great majority of patients can be safely treated with conservative measures such as rest, ice, compression, and elevation. Surgical treatment is reserved for selected cases that either have failed conservative treatment or require primary surgical attention, such as rupture of the Achilles tendon.
- Overuse syndromes take at least 6 to 12 weeks to heal. Patients who continue to aggravate the inflammatory response risk fibrous changes and chronic problems.

REFERENCES

1. Benedek TG: History of the rheumatic diseases. In Schumacher HR, editor: *Primer on rheumatic diseases,* Atlanta, 1993, Arthritis Foundation.
2. James SL et al: Injuries to runners, *Am J Sports Med* 6:40-50, 1978.
3. Gruchow HW, Pelletier D: An epidemiologic study of tennis elbow: incidence, recurrence, and effectiveness of prevention strategies, *Am J Sports Med* 7:234-238, 1979.
4. Almekinders LC, Almekinders SV: Outcome in treatment of chronic overuse sports injuries: a retrospective study, *J Orthop Sports Phys Ther* 19:157-161, 1994.
5. Bernacki EJ et al: An ergonomics program designed to reduce the incidence of upper extremity work related musculoskeletal disorders, *J Occup Environ Med* 41:1032-1042, 1999.
6. Kvist M et al: Chronic Achilles paratendonitis in athletes: a histological and histochemical study, *Pathology* 19:1-11, 1987.
7. Archambault JM et al: Exercise loading of tendons and the development of overuse injuries. A review of current literature, *Sports Med* 20:77-89, 1995.
8. Fulcher SM et al: Hand and wrist injuries, *Clin Sports Med* 17:2-19, 1998.
9. Middleton DB: Infectious arthritis, *Primary Care* 20:4, 1993.
10. Gall ED: Evaluation of the patient: history and physical examination. In Schumacher HR, editor: *Primer on rheumatic diseases,* Atlanta, 1993, Arthritis Foundation.
11. Blake R, Hoffman J: Emergency department evaluation and treatment of the shoulder and humerus, *Emerg Med Clin North Am* 17:859-876, 1999.
12. Belzer JP, Durkin RC: Common disorders of the shoulder, *Primary Care* 23:365-388, 1996.
13. Neer C: Anterior acromioplasty for chronic impingement syndrome in the shoulder, *J Bone Joint Surg* 54A:4, 1972.
14. Neviaser RJ: Lesions of the biceps and tendonitis of the shoulder, *Orthop Clin North Am* 11:343, 1980.
15. Neustadt DH: Injection therapy of bursitis and tendinitis. In Roberts JR, Hedges JH, editors: *Clinical procedures in emergency medicine,* Philadelphia, 1991, WB Saunders.
16. Canale: Tendinitis and bursitis. *Campbell's operative orthopedics,* 1998.
17. Chop WM: Tennis elbow, *Postgrad Med J* 36:301, 1989.
18. Gecha SR, Torg E: Knee injuries in tennis, *Clin Sports Med* 7:435-452, 1988.
19. Safran MR, Fu FH: Uncommon causes of knee pain in the athlete, *Orthop Clin North Am* 26:547-559, 1995.
20. Barry N, McGuire J: Musculoskeletal medicine, *Rheum Dis Clin North Am* 22:515-531, 1996.
21. Beachley MC: Radiology of arthritis, *Primary Care* 20:4, 1993.
22. Grassi W et al: Sonographic imaging of tendons, *Arthritis Rheum* 43:1-12, 2000.
23. Mitchell M et al: Septic arthritis, *Radiol Clin North Am* 26:1295, 1988.
24. Lopez-Longo F et al: Primary septic arthritis in heroin users: early diagnosis by radioisotope imaging and geographic variations in the causative agents, *J Rheumatol* 14:991, 1987.
25. Quinn CE: On the trail of septic bursitis, *Emerg Med* 1993.

112 Systemic Lupus Erythematosus and the Vasculitides

Clare T. Sercombe

SYSTEMIC LUPUS ERYTHEMATOSUS

Perspective

Systemic lupus erythematosus (SLE) is a multisystem autoimmune disease with systemic complications, including renal failure and neurologic compromise. Symptoms and clinical courses vary widely, but patients with a known diagnosis of SLE are at risk for certain complications. Use of corticosteroids and immunosuppressive agents for therapy makes these patients challenging when they come to the ED.

Background The disease was originally described by Biett in 1822. The term lupus erythematosus was used by Cazanave to describe the cutaneous manifestations in 1851. Osler first described many of the visceral manifestations in 1904.[1] The term *lupus,* which means "wolf" in Latin, was used to describe the skin lesion, differentiating it from lupus vulgaris. It was not until 1949 that the lupus erythematosus cell was identified, allowing Haserick to describe the autoimmune nature of the disease.[2,3]

Epidemiology The prevalence is 40 per 100,000 people in North America and northern Europe.[4] The highest incidence, for women in their childbearing years, is 1 per 1,000 in white women and 1 per 250 in African-American women.[5] Factors thought to increase the prevalence include familial cases and a lupus-like syndrome caused by certain medications, including hydralazine, isoniazid, and procainamide.

Principles of Disease

In part, the underlying mechanism is an autoimmune response with production of autoantibodies and a failure of the body to suppress them.[6] There is a polyclonal activation of B cells with exaggerated production of autoantibodies. The abnormal cellular and humoral response to the formation of these autoantibodies is modified by genetic, environmental, and hormonal factors. Genetic factors include familial association and relationship to certain human leukocyte antigen (HLA) genotypes. Environmental factors include exposure to sunlight. Autoantibodies are also found in laboratory workers who handle SLE sera. Exposure to certain drugs can also produce an SLE-like syndrome. Hormonal factors include an association to estrogens, which may explain the higher prevalence in women. There may also be a link to Klinefelter's syndrome.[6] The differing manifestations in different patients may reflect the varied autoantibodies produced, the varied organs targeted, and the individual patient's response to the autoantibodies. These autoantibodies may induce immune complex formation or interact directly at the site, binding to tissue, resulting in differing disease manifestations. Pathologic findings are manifestations of the inflammation, inflammatory vasculitis, noninflammatory blood vessel damage, and immune complex deposition.

Clinical Features

The triad of fever, joint pain, and rash in a woman of childbearing age should suggest the diagnosis of SLE; however, the disease ranges from mild illness with cutaneous abnormalities to severe life-threatening complications such as renal failure and lupus cerebritis.

The American Rheumatism Association Revised Criteria for the Classification of Lupus were published in 1982.[7] These criteria consist of 11 conditions that are associated with SLE. Patients must have four criteria present, serially or simultaneously, to be given the diagnosis of SLE (Box 112-1).

Box 112-1 American Rheumatism Association Revised Criteria for the Classification of Lupus*

Malar rash
Discoid rash
Photosensitivity
Oral ulcers
Arthritis
Serositis
  Pleuritis
  Pericarditis
Renal disorders
  Persistent proteinuria
  Cellular casts
Neurologic disorders
  Seizures
  Psychosis
Hematologic disorders
  Hemolytic anemia
  Leukopenia
  Lymphopenia
  Thrombocytopenia
Immunologic disorders
Positive SLE cell preparation
Anti-DNA antibody
Anti-Sm antibody
False positive VDRL or RPR
Antinuclear antibody

*Classification based on 11 criteria. Patient is diagnosed with SLE if any four or more criteria are present, serially or simultaneously, during any interval of observation.

Modified from Tan EM et al: The 1982 revised criteria for the classification of systemic lupus erythematosus, *Arthritis Rheum* 25:1271, 1982.

Rheumatologic Almost all patients with SLE have arthralgias and myalgias at some time during the course of their disease. Like rheumatoid arthritis, the inflammation of the hands, specifically the proximal interphalangeal and the metacarpophalangeal joints, is symmetric. Although the initial presentation can mimic rheumatoid arthritis, joint deformities are less common. Thirty percent of patients develop hitchhiker's thumb, a hyperextension of the interphalangeal joint of the thumb. Tenosynovitis and tendon rupture may also occur, especially in patients taking corticosteroids. Avascular necrosis of the large joints, especially the femoral heads, can also be seen with ischemia caused by the vasculitis, or as a complication of the large doses of corticosteroids used to treat SLE.

Dermatologic The cutaneous manifestations include the characteristic but uncommon malar or butterfly rash of acute cutaneous SLE. The facial eruption may be the first sign of SLE or may accompany flares of the disease. It can be exacerbated by exposure to ultraviolet light. Discoid lupus consists of an erythematous raised plaque with scales usually on the face, head, or neck. This can be associated with alopecia. Only 10% of patients with discoid lupus have SLE, whereas up to 25% of patients with SLE develop skin lesions consistent with discoid lupus.[8] Mucous membrane lesions can be seen with small, shallow ulcerations. Lastly, vasculitic lesions such as ulcerations, purpura, and digital infarcts may occur.

Renal Clinical nephritis, defined as persistent proteinuria, is seen in approximately 50% of patients, although mesangial and glomerular immunoglobulin deposition is seen in almost all patients with SLE. Most patients have no symptoms from their lupus nephritis until it progresses to nephrotic syndrome or frank renal failure. Serum creatinine is an insensitive indicator of early renal disease, because many nephrons must be involved before any elevation is seen. In patients with renal disease, the urinalysis shows hematuria, proteinuria, and red blood cell casts. Patients with active urine sediment may benefit from aggressive therapy with steroids or other immunosuppressive therapy, because mortality for this population is 15% at 5 years and 35% at 10 years.[9]

Indications for treatment include worsening renal failure, decreasing serum complement levels, increasing anti–double-stranded DNA (dsDNA) levels, and nephritic urinary sediment, especially when accompanied by increasing or nephrotic-range proteinuria. Renal biopsy can be useful in making treatment decisions. High-dose corticosteroids with immunosuppressive agents as therapy for renal disease are controversial. Patients who have end-stage SLE renal disease have survival rates similar to other patients on dialysis, approaching 85% at 5 years.[9] Although patients on dialysis experience an improvement of their nonrenal SLE manifestations, they run a high risk of dying from severe SLE or infection in their first year of dialysis. Renal transplantation has been successful in these patients, and recurrent nephritis in the allograft is a rare occurence.[10,11]

Neurologic Nervous system manifestations are varied and include seizures, stroke, psychosis, migraines, and peripheral neuropathies.[12,13] These symptoms may appear early in the course of the disease but are rarely the initial sign of SLE. Central nervous system (CNS) involvement occurs in approximately 50% of patients with SLE.[14] Seizures are the most common manifestation in up to 70% of patients with CNS involvement.[13] Strokes are also common, especially in association with the antiphospholipid antibody syndrome. Frank psychosis can be seen, either as a manifestation of SLE or as a result of corticosteroid use. Lupus cerebritis should be considered in any patient with SLE who exhibits a change in behavior or mental status. Presence of infection should also be considered, especially in patients on immunosuppressive agents. These patients are at risk for bacterial, fungal, and tuberculous infections, in addition to abscesses. Other causes include uremia and hypertensive encephalopathy. Mononeuritis multiplex and peripheral neuropathy have also been described.

A computed tomography (CT) scan is useful in patients with gross focal neurologic deficit, to assess for bleeding or edema associated with an embolic stroke. A magnetic resonance imaging (MRI) scan is much more sensitive for small infarcts, edema, or evidence of vasculitis. Full recovery from neuropsychiatric manifestations is approximately 70% to 85%; however, the mortality from such events is 10% to 15%.[14]

Cardiac Pericarditis is the most common cardiac manifestation of SLE, reported in 30% of patients.[15,16] The diagnosis may be determined on the basis of ECG findings alone, or patients may have signs and symptoms of fever, tachycardia, chest pain, and transient cardiac rubs. Pericarditis is associated with effusion in 20% of patients; however, this rarely progresses to tamponade.[15] Purulent pericarditis due to *Staphylococcus aureus* and tuberculosis has been reported in patients taking steroids. Purulent pericarditis, which is exudative with a high protein and white blood count (WBC),[16] may mimic the effusion seen with SLE, which causes a transudative, serous fluid. Pericarditis in SLE is generally benign and responds well to corticosteroids.

Myocarditis resembling cardiomyopathy is clinically diagnosed in fewer than 10% of patients with SLE, but is found in 40% of patients on autopsy.[17] Some degree of left ventricular dysfunction may be found in a large number of patients with SLE.[18] It may be accompanied by congestive heart failure, ventricular dysrhythmia, tachycardia, or non-specific ECG changes. Severe myocarditis should be treated with large doses of systemic corticosteroids, control of hypertension, and correction of volume overload.

A noninfectious endocarditis, as described by Libman and Sachs, produces vegetative growths on the valves that are usually clinically silent; however, these may be complicated by infection, valvular dysfunction, and rarely, thromboembolism.[19] Libman-Sachs vegetations are seen in up to 10% of patients with SLE.[20] The mitral valve is most commonly involved, although all four valves may have vegetations. Valvular dysfunction may occur independent of vegetations secondary to valvulitis, mucoid degeneration, or aortic dissection. The aortic valve has the highest incidence of hemodynamically significant regurgitation, followed by the mitral valve.

Vasculitis of the coronary arteries or accelerated atherosclerosis due to corticosteroid use may cause coronary ischemia. Coronary vasculitis is best treated with steroids, whereas the atherosclerosis is best treated with conventional methods including aspirin, nitrates, β-blockers, angioplasty, or bypass surgery. Treatment differences make the distinction between the two entities important. The diagnosis can be made by coronary angiography, with evidence of aneurysmal dilatation of the coronary arteries seen in patients with vasculitis.[15] Patients with SLE, hypertension, and hypercholesterolemia are at significantly increased risk for coronary artery disease (CAD).[15]

Patients with SLE tend to have systemic hypertension secondary to lupus nephritis and steroid use, with all of the resultant complications of hypertension. The incidence has been reported in 25% to 50% of patients with SLE. Hypertension is noted in those patients who take high, long-term doses of corticosteroids.

Pulmonary Pleural effusions and pleurisy are common. Pleural effusions, seen in 12% of SLE patients, are usually exudative in nature. Pleural fluid glucose levels are usually similar to serum glucose levels, in contrast to those of rheumatoid arthritis in which the pleural fluid glucose level is very low. Other manifestations include pulmonary infarcts and hemorrhage. Lupus pneumonitis causes diffuse interstitial infiltrates, although patients have usually had the disease for several years before they suffer from pneumonitis. Bacterial, fungal, and opportunistic infections must be considered, especially in those patients taking immunosuppressive agents, before a diagnosis of lupus pneumonitis is given. Patients with SLE are particularly at risk for pneumococcal disease, in part due to autosplenectomy or splenic dysfunction. Patients with SLE may also develop chronic interstitial infiltrates leading to pulmonary fibrosis. These patients need inpatient treatment, and their conditions may progress to chronic hypoxia, pulmonary hypertension, and right-sided heart failure.[21]

Gastrointestinal Gastrointestinal complaints in SLE are common, ranging from oral ulcerations to the much more serious intestinal vasculitis. Oral ulcerations usually accompany disease flares. Esophageal dysmotility is occasionally seen; however it is much less common than in patients with scleroderma. Patients with intestinal pseudoobstruction may have crampy abdominal pain, and a clinical and radiographic picture consistent with obstruction. They should be observed for resolution. Pancreatitis can be seen from either an SLE flare or corticosteroid therapy. Spontaneous bacterial peritonitis is also described. Elevated liver function tests are common, usually the result of the medications given to treat SLE, such as azathioprine; however, infection with cytomegalovirus while on immunosuppressive agents may also occur. Portal hypertension caused by scarring and fibrosis is seen in 4% of patients.[21] The most serious complication is intestinal vasculitis, a syndrome of abdominal pain, bloody diarrhea, and evidence of vasculitis elsewhere. This vasculitis may progress to perforation or gangrene, resulting in peritonitis.

Hematologic Hematologic and vasculitic problems are complex. Anemia, affecting up to 40% of patients, may result from hemolysis or chronic disease. Thrombocytopenia occurs in 25% of patients. Treatment for severe thrombocytopenia is controversial, with some authors advocating use of vinca alkaloids and intravenous γ-globulin.[22] Splenectomy is controversial, with some believing splenectomy exacerbates the disease. Thrombotic thrombocytopenic purpura (TTP) and immune idiopathic thrombocytopenic purpura (ITP) have also been reported in patients with SLE.[12]

Diagnostic Strategies

The diagnosis of SLE is often confirmed with antinuclear antibodies (ANAs). Positive ANAs will occur in more than 95% of the patients with SLE.[4] The degree of positivity of the test is important, with higher titers having a positive predictive value. ANAs may also be positive in elderly patients taking certain medications such as hydralazine and procainamide, with subacute bacterial endocarditis, with infectious hepatitis, and with other immune diseases such as primary biliary cirrhosis. Antibodies to dsDNA and anti-Smith (anti-Sm) antibodies are most specific for SLE. Patients with disease flares may show an increase in their ANA or dsDNA titers. Decreases in complement levels for C3 and C4 also correlate with disease flares in certain patients. The erythrocyte sedimentation rate (ESR) is a very poor index of disease activity. Patients who have an ESR of 50 to 100 mm/hr often show minimal disease activity. C-reactive protein levels often remain low except in the face of concurrent infection. Patients with SLE may have a false positive VDRL or RPR.

A normochromic, normocytic anemia is common in SLE. Leukopenia is common with disease flares as well. Thrombocytopenia occurs in up to 25% of patients. Urinalysis and serum creatinine may be useful tests in patients showing evidence of disease flare, to demonstrate worsening nephritis. Active urine sediment with excretion of red blood cell casts and increasing proteinuria is worrisome.

Management

The treatment of SLE is controversial because the manifestations and severity vary widely among patients. General recommendations include avoidance of stress and fatigue, which can exacerbate symptoms. Approximately one third of patients are photosensitive and should avoid sunlight and use sunscreen. Oral contraceptives may also exacerbate symptoms and only low-estrogen oral contraceptives should be used.

Acetaminophen may be useful for mild to moderate pain control. Drug therapy starts with antiinflammatory agents. Aspirin and nonsteroidal antiinflammatory drugs (NSAIDs) have been used to treat the minor inflammatory complaints such as arthralgias, pleurisy, and pericarditis. Maximally recommended doses of these agents are usually needed. These agents should be avoided in patients with severe gastrointestinal complications or thrombocytopenia. Patients with lupus nephritis should also avoid NSAIDs because the inhibitive effect on prostaglandins may reduce renal function, confusing the clinical picture of worsening renal failure. Some NSAIDs, including ibuprofen, have also been associated with aseptic meningitis with headache, fever, and meningismus.[23] CSF studies in these patients show lymphocytosis, elevated protein levels, and sterile culture.

Corticosteroids are usually the next agent of choice. Topical application controls most cutaneous manifestations. Oral corticosteroids are prescribed in dosages that control disease activity. Minor disease activity (e.g., arthralgias, fatigue, and pleurisy) is usually controlled with 0.5 mg/kg or less in a single daily dose. With minor symptoms, however, antiinflammatory and antimalarial drugs have been advocated to avoid the long-term complications of corticosteroids. Major disease activity (e.g., hemolytic anemia and severe thrombocytopenia) is usually controlled with prednisone 1.0 mg/kg/day. With lupus cerebritis and acute worsening of lupus nephritis, methylprednisolone 1.0 gm IV may be given for several days. Treatment of glomerulonephritis with long-term steroids has not been proven to alter the outcome or course in patients with SLE, and their long-term use remains controversial.[12,24] When tapering, corticosteroids may be changed to an alternate day dosing regimen; however, some patients may experience disease flares at these dosages and come to the ED.

Antimalarial drugs are also effective for the cutaneous and musculoskeletal manifestations of SLE. Hydroxychloroquine and chloroquine are given on an outpatient basis in a loading dose for 4 weeks, followed by maintenance dosing once these symptoms are under control. Withdrawal of the drug may result in disease flare. The antimalarial agents can result in two major ophthalmologic side effects. Corneal deposits, easily seen on slit-lamp examination in patients who complain of floaters in the visual field, are reversible with drug withdrawal or decreased dosage. The second complication, an irreversible retinopathy, is unrelated to the corneal deposits. All patients with SLE who take antimalarial medications should be followed biannually by an ophthalmologist to detect evidence of retinopathy that may lead to blindness. If evidence of retinopathy appears, patients should stop taking the antimalarial medication under a rheumatologist's supervision.

Immunosuppressive agents (e.g., azathioprine and cyclophosphamide) are reserved for patients with severe renal or cerebral disease in whom other therapies have failed, or for patients who have not tolerated corticosteroids.[24] Studies looking at the use of immunosuppressants have shown decreased chronic renal scarring and reduced likelihood of end-stage renal disease, without an increase in mortality.[25] The toxicities of such drugs are numerous and include infections, myelosuppression, and future risk of neoplasms.[24]

Special Considerations

Drug-Induced Lupus Drug-induced lupus was first described in 1954 by Dustan et al and Perry and Schroeder.[26,27] Procainamide was first implicated in 1962 by Ladd.[28] Since then, a large number of agents have been implicated, with hydralazine and procainamide being the most common (Table 112-1). The clinical manifestations vary, with most patients experiencing arthralgias and occasional pleuropericardial

Table 112-1. Drugs Implicated in Lupus-like Syndromes

System	Drug	Risk
Cardiovascular	Procainamide	High
	Quinidine	
	Practolol*	High
Antihypertensive	Hydralazine	High
	Methyldopa	
	Reserpine	
Antimicrobial	Isoniazid	Moderate
	Penicillin	
	Sulfonamides	
	Streptomycin	
	Tetracycline	
	Nitrofurantoin	
Anticonvulsant	Phenytoin	Moderate
	Mephenytoin	Moderate
	Ethosuximide	Moderate
	Primidone	
Antithyroid	Propylthiouracil	Low
	Methylthiouracil	Low
Psychotropic	Chlorpromazine	Low
	Lithium carbonate	
Miscellaneous	D-Penicillamine	High
	Methysergide	Low
	Phenylbutazone	
	Allopurinol	
	Gold salts	
	Aminoglutethimide	

*Removed from market because of lupus-like syndrome.

manifestations. The full manifestations are present in less than 1% of patients taking high-risk drugs, although a positive ANA titer can be found in more than 50% of patients taking high-risk drugs.[29] The patients are usually women, middle-aged or older, and rarely African-Americans, but this may be representative of the group of patients taking these drugs. The condition is usually reversible when the agents are stopped, with resolution within days or weeks; however, manifestations lasting for years have been reported. In patients with significant pleuropericardial disease, a short course of tapered steroids has been used successfully once the implicated medication has been discontinued.

Antiphospholipid Antibody Syndrome The lupus anticoagulant and anticardiolipin antibody are antiphospholipid antibodies that bind to the prothrombin activator complex. This results in a prolongation of the partial thromboplastin time (PTT), but is clinically associated with clotting. This disorder can be seen in patients with SLE, but it occurs also in the normal population, in patients with HIV, in some malignancies, and with drug-induced lupus. The patients without evidence of SLE have a much lower incidence of complications. A prolonged PTT that does not correct when the patient's sample is mixed 50/50 with normal serum suggests the presence of an inhibitor; the lupus anticoagulant and anticardiolipin antibody can then be found with further testing.

The spectrum of the clinical manifestations is wide. Some patients may have repeated episodes of arterial or venous clotting, including recurrent strokes and pulmonary emboli.

Box 112-2 Clinical Manifestations of Antiphospholipid Syndrome

- Arterial occlusion
  - Extremity gangrene
  - Stroke
  - Myocardial infarct
  - Other visceral infarct
  - Aortic occlusion
- Venous occlusion
  - Peripheral venous occlusion
  - Visceral venous occlusion
    - Budd-Chiari syndrome
    - Portal vein occlusion
- Recurrent fetal loss
- Thrombocytopenia
- Coombs' positive hemolytic anemia
- Livedo reticularis
- Neurologic abnormalities
  - Chorea
  - Multiple sclerosis–like syndrome
  - Transient ischemic attacks
- Valvular heart disease
- Sudden multisystem arterial occlusion

Modified from Sammaritano LR et al: Commonly agreed clinical manifestations of antiphospholipid antibody syndrome, *Semin Arthritis Rheum* 20:81, 1990.

Elevated serum creatinine values may be a result of renal vein thrombosis, seen on CT with contrast, mimicking worsening nephritis. Multiple spontaneous abortions have been reported (Box 112-2).

This syndrome may also be associated with thrombocytopenia, with clinically significant bleeding, and with neuropsychiatric disorders believed to be secondary to cerebral ischemia and infarcts.[30] Patients who have evidence of the antiphospholipid syndrome may still undergo surgery, with routine precautions for deep venous thrombosis. Despite the prolonged PTT, there is minimal risk for prolonged bleeding unless thrombocytopenia is also present.

Pregnancy Recurrent spontaneous abortions have been seen in patients with the antiphospholipid syndrome. Subcutaneous heparin with low-dose aspirin throughout pregnancy is currently the treatment of choice to prevent further fetal wastage. As the pregnancy progresses, there is an increased risk of worsening manifestations of SLE and nephritis. These patients are also at risk for pregnancy-induced hypertension. In patients who fail subcutaneous heparin with continued fetal wastage, monthly doses of intravenous γ-globulin can be effective. Corticosteroids in combination with aspirin have shown some benefit. Although they cross the placenta and show little evidence of fetal harm, corticosteroids are a second-line agent due to complications of long-term, high-dose therapy. Other medications, including NSAIDs, antimalarials, and immunosuppressive agents, should be stopped. These patients should be referred to a high-risk obstetrician early in the pregnancy.

Neonatal lupus syndrome is usually diagnosed by dermatologic manifestations of lupus associated with transient anemia and thrombocytopenia. Neonates can also experience congenital complete heart block that may need permanent pacing.[12] The congenital heart block has been associated with transmission of a maternal antibody to anti-SSA (Ro).

Complications of Therapy The complications from SLE itself are many and varied because of the systemic nature of the illness. Treatment of the disease causes further complications. Treatment with NSAIDs can worsen lupus nephritis, either by causing interstitial nephritis or by inhibiting prostaglandins.

Corticosteroids have well-known, long-term complications including steroid-induced diabetes, osteoporosis and resultant fractures, weight gain, pancreatitis, osteonecrosis, accelerated atherosclerosis, and most important, immunosuppression. Patients receiving steroid therapy should be monitored for evidence of infection and should be evaluated for any episode of fever. Patients taking corticosteroids should also be given stress-dose steroids with hydrocortisone 100 mg IV every 8 hours for any systemic infection, surgery, delivery, or obvious stressor.

Patients using antimalarial agents are at risk for the dose-related corneal deposits, which can be managed by outpatient drug discontinuation and rheumatology follow-up. The retinopathy associated with antimalarial agents is irreversible and may progress to blindness. Prompt attention by an ophthalmologist is essential.

Patients taking immunosuppressive agents are also at risk for infection, especially with gram-negative organisms, encapsulated gram-positive organisms, herpes zoster, and opportunistic organisms. Febrile patients who are on azathioprine and cyclophosphamide should be admitted whether a source is evident or not, because gram-negative or streptococcal sepsis occurs in this population. Patients with localized herpes zoster should be admitted for intravenous acyclovir administration to prevent viral dissemination.

Disposition

Because of the systemic and varied nature of the disease, there are no hard and fast rules about admission for complications of SLE. Patients without previous diagnosis of lupus may be admitted for workup and treatment of possible connective tissue disease if they have symptoms that warrant immediate diagnosis (e.g., pericarditis, myocarditis, pleural effusion or infiltrates, evidence of vasculitis, or renal insufficiency). In the patient who has monoarticular or polyarticular arthritis, the joint can be aspirated in the ED if fluid is present. Further workup can be done on an outpatient basis by the primary care physician or a rheumatologist. NSAIDs may alleviate the symptoms.

Patients with known SLE may come to the ED for a flare of their disease, for new systemic complaints, or for fevers. Patients with known disease usually will be able to tell the emergency physician if the problem is consistent with a previous flare versus a new complaint. Patients with worsening disease who take large doses of steroids or immunosuppressive agents should be admitted for consideration of other diagnoses or more aggressive therapy. Patients with known disease and increasing arthritic pain, or mild flare without fever, may be effectively treated with an increase in their NSAID or corticosteroid dosages and prompt follow-up with their rheumatologists.

Patients with evidence of lupus nephritis and worsening renal failure should be admitted for aggressive therapy with steroids or immunosuppressive agents. The serum creatinine level may be elevated, but it is a poor indicator of disease. Proteinuria may be present, or red blood cell casts may be seen on urinalysis. Treatment for lupus nephritis should be done in conjunction with a rheumatologist or nephrologist. Consideration of renal vein thrombosis is necessary in those patients with evidence of antiphospholipid antibody syndrome or nephrotic syndrome.

Mental status changes in the patient with SLE should be approached like any workup for mental status changes, because lupus cerebritis is a diagnosis of exclusion. Laboratory examination for electrolyte imbalances, evidence of hypoxia or hypoglycemia, and a toxicology screen should be performed. A CT scan to assess for hemorrhage, especially in the hypertensive or thrombocytopenic patient, should be performed. Lumbar puncture to evaluate for infection should be performed if the patient is febrile or immunocompromised. MRI may reveal abnormalities with increased signal intensity in the area of involvement. Cerebral ischemia may cause acute mental status changes as a result of a lupus vasculitis or thrombosis associated with antiphospholipid antibody syndrome. Consultation with a rheumatologist is prudent before giving high-dose steroids for lupus cerebritis. Patients with seizures should be treated in the routine manner, and workup of new-onset seizures done with the help of a neurologist.

Patients with cardiac or pulmonary complaints should be admitted for observation or therapy. Those who take corticosteroids are at high risk for CAD. Patients with chest pain should be evaluated for myocardial infarction. If pericarditis is suspected, evaluation of pericardial effusion may be necessary, although tamponade is rare. Patients with myocarditis should be observed for evidence of congestive heart failure and dysrhythmias. Patients taking immunosuppressive agents should be given antibiotic prophylaxis for invasive dental and genitourinary procedures.

Pulmonary complaints are quite difficult to evaluate in the outpatient setting. Patients with fever and infiltrates may have community-acquired pneumonia, especially pneumococcal disease, but opportunistic infection, atypical tuberculosis, and lupus pneumonitis need to be considered. Sputum culture and pulmonary consultation may be appropriate, especially in the hypoxic patient. Hypoxic patients should also be evaluated for pulmonary embolism and for a history of antiphospholipid antibody with thrombosis. Patients with pleural effusions should be admitted to have diagnostic thoracentesis and treatment. Pleural effusions may be complicated by infection, tuberculosis, or malignancy.

Patients with abdominal pain present a diagnostic challenge, because most of them are young women of childbearing age. Workup should include a pelvic examination and pregnancy test. Laboratory examination may not be helpful without baseline values, because many patients are chronically anemic and the WBC may be elevated in those taking corticosteroids. Evidence of an increased anion gap or metabolic acidosis may be indicative of lactic acidosis. Abdominal films may be helpful to show bowel wall thickening or free air. Consultation with a surgeon and overnight observation for serial examinations may be necessary to diagnose vasculitic problems, abscess in immunocompromised patients, or routine causes of abdominal pain. Even if the patient has a common cause of abdominal pain (e.g., pelvic inflammatory disease, pancreatitis, peptic ulcer disease, or biliary colic), admission may be necessary for administration of stress-dose steroids and workup of fever.

SLE predisposes patients to anemia and thrombocytopenia. Patients should be admitted if there is evidence of active hemolysis with decreased hematocrit, or if hemolysis is evident on the blood smear. Patients with thrombocytopenia should be admitted if there is evidence of bleeding or if platelet counts are severely decreased (<50,000/mm^3). If the patient is actively bleeding, platelet transfusion is appropriate; however, rapid destruction of the platelets may occur. Simultaneous administration of intravenous corticosteroids and intravenous γ-globulin will aid in increasing the platelet count and decreasing the amount of platelet destruction.

Patients with evidence of arterial or venous thrombosis should be admitted for anticoagulation and possible embolectomy. Anticoagulation can be achieved acutely with heparin, although large doses are occasionally needed to overcome the antibody effect. The PTT, if not elevated, can be followed to assess for evidence of adequate anticoagulation, with careful observation for bleeding in those patients who are also thrombocytopenic. Otherwise, patients with prolonged PTT and evidence of the lupus anticoagulant can be followed with thrombin times if necessary.

Pregnant patients with SLE should have early follow-up with a high-risk obstetrician. Emergency delivery for the pregnant patient with SLE should include stress-dose steroid administration and close observation of the neonate for congenital complete heart block. Emergent cardiac pacing may be necessary.

Patients experiencing overwhelming sepsis or shock should be given stress-dose steroids in the ED with hydrocortisone 100 mg IV. Broad-spectrum antibiotics may also be given empirically after appropriate cultures are obtained. Adrenal insufficiency from abrupt discontinuation of steroids is another possible cause of shock. If the patient is unstable, admission to the intensive care unit is warranted.

Key Concepts

- Patients with SLE can have multiple and varied symptom complexes; the diagnosis should be considered in patients with fever, rash, or unexplained systemic complaints.
- Patients with deep venous thrombosis without risk factors should be considered for lupus anticoagulant or anticardiolipin antibody.
- Febrile patients with SLE on immunosuppressive therapy should be hospitalized and treated aggressively, because they have a high risk of gram-negative or streptococcal sepsis.
- Patients with worsening renal function or with involvement of the heart, lungs, or CNS should be hospitalized for aggressive treatment to prevent progression of the disease and symptoms.
- Patients with evidence of thrombosis and antiphospholipid syndrome should be anticoagulated and admitted for further workup.

THE VASCULITIDES

Perspective

The vasculitic syndromes are a spectrum of diseases characterized by inflammation and destruction of the blood vessels. The pathophysiology is not well described, and systemic manifestations vary depending on the location, the size of the vessel involved, and whether the vasculitis is a primary or secondary disease state.

Background The first classical description of a vasculitic syndrome was in 1866 by Kussmaul and Maier. It is now known as polyarteritis nodosa.[31] Since then, a number of well-described disease states have been attributed to vasculitic syndromes. In 1952, Zeek presented the first classification system.[32] This system has been revised several times with great difficulty, because of the broad spectrum of disease and large overlap between syndromes (Box 112-3).

Principles of Disease

Vasculitic syndromes are thought to arise because immune complexes are deposited in vessel walls and the complement system is activated.. The complement system then stimulates accumulation of polymorphonuclear cells at the site and release of lysosomal enzymes, resulting in vessel wall damage and necrosis. The clinical manifestations of this process depend on the size of the immune complexes, the mechanics of blood flow through the vessel, the vessel permeability, and the site of deposition.

The relationship between immune complexes and the subsequent development of vasculitis is best studied in the infectious causes of vasculitis. Hepatitis B surface antigen has been demonstrated to be an inciting antigen.[33] Other infectious agents known to be associated with vasculitis include cytomegalovirus, herpes zoster, parvovirus, hepatitis A, hepatitis C, and the human immunodeficiency virus (HIV).[33-36] Malignancies such as hairy cell leukemia, some lymphomas, and the myeloproliferative disorders are also associated. Immune complexes are rarely found in some other vasculitic syndromes, such as polyarteritis nodosa and Wegener's granulomatosis, a phenomenon believed to be the result of rapid clearing of the complexes.

It is important to differentiate thrombosis and vasculitis, because treatments are dramatically different. Antiphospholipid antibody syndrome can mimic vasculitis, especially when present in patients without SLE. Yet in SLE, both vasculitis and thrombosis from antiphospholipid antibody syndrome may be present.

Large Vessel Vasculitides

Temporal Arteritis Temporal or giant cell arteritis (TA) is characterized by granulomatous inflammation with multinucleated giant cells. The distribution is most common in branches of the carotid artery but may involve any large or medium artery. The disease is most commonly seen in women in the sixth and seventh decades of life.

The classic symptoms of TA are consistent with ischemia to the organs fed by branches of the internal and external carotid artery: visual loss in one eye, temporal artery tenderness, and jaw claudication. Some patients will experience central retinal occlusion or transient diplopia. Patients may complain of nonspecific, vague symptoms such as malaise, weight loss, and fever. Headache may be the initial complaint. There is also an association with polymyalgia rheumatica, with patients complaining of early morning shoulder girdle stiffness.

Although the diagnosis is made clinically, helpful laboratory findings include elevated ESR (usually greater than 100

Box 112-3 Classification of Vasculitis

Large Vessel Disease
Arteritis
Temporal (giant cell) arteritis
Takayasu's arteritis
Arteritis associated with Reiter's syndrome, ankylosing spondylitis

Medium and Small Vessel Disease
Polyarteritis nodosa
Primary (idiopathic)
Associated with viruses
- Hepatitis B or C
- Cytomegalovirus
- Herpes zoster
- HIV

Associated with malignancy
- Hairy cell leukemia

Other
- Familial Mediterranean fever

Granulomatous vasculitis
Wegener's granulomatosis
Lymphomatoid granulomatosis

Behçet's disease

Kawasaki disease (mucocutaneous lymph node syndrome)

Predominantly Small Vessel Disease
Hypersensitivity vasculitis (leukocytoclastic vasculitis)
Henoch-Schönlein purpura
Mixed cryoglobulinemia
Serum sickness
Vasculitis associated with connective tissue diseases
- SLE
- Sjögren's syndrome

Vasculitis associated with specific syndromes
- Primary biliary cirrhosis
- Lyme disease
- Chronic active hepatitis
- Drug-induced vasculitis

Churg-Strauss syndrome

Goodpasture's syndrome

Erythema nodosum

Panniculitis

Buerger's disease (thrombophlebitis obliterans)

mm/hr on a Westergren blot), elevated C-reactive proteins, and anemia. The definitive diagnosis is made by temporal artery biopsy.

Most patients are extremely sensitive to glucocorticoids, and treatment should be started for any patient with a high clinical suspicion of TA. The steroids do not significantly change the results of the biopsy and may prevent progression to visual loss. Prednisone should be started at a dosage of 1 mg/kg/day until biopsy can be performed. Patients with severe disease or impending visual loss should be hospitalized and given high-dose steroids until the diagnosis is obtained. Most patients tolerate slow tapering of the steroid dosage, although relapse rates are lower in those who use them longer (1 to 2 years).[37]

Takayasu's Arteritis Takayasu's arteritis (pulseless disease) is a chronic, recurrent, inflammatory vascular disease that affects the aorta, proximal portions of its major branches, and the pulmonary arteries.[38] It is characterized by lymphocytic infiltration and fibrosis of the vessels, resulting in marked thickening of the intima and adventitia, and leading to eventual obstruction of the arteries and ischemic complications. Women are predominantly affected, usually in the second and third decades of life. A high incidence is seen in Japanese females.

In the prepulseless or early phase, the diagnosis is difficult. Fatigue, weight loss, and low-grade fever predominate. Hypertension is frequently seen secondary to aortic or renal artery involvement. With progression of the disease ischemic symptoms appear, with diminished pulses, claudication, retinopathy, and visual loss. Strokes, syncope, subclavian steal syndrome, abdominal pain, and coronary ischemia are also reported.

Early diagnosis is difficult because symptoms are nonspecific. Later, acute phase reactants are elevated and bruits may be auscultated. Definitive diagnosis is made with arteriography and demonstrates stenotic lesions, poststenotic dilation, aneurysms, and increased collateral circulation.

Treatment with prednisone 1 mg/kg/day will induce remission in up to 50% of patients.[39] Other cytotoxic agents such as methotrexate, cyclophosphamide, or azathioprine may be added to achieve remission if relapses occur. Infections may complicate therapy. Hypertension may be treated with calcium channel blockers and angiotensin-converting enzyme inhibitors. Antiplatelet agents may be of benefit. Bypass grafting and endarterectomy are useful in patients with significant disease.

Medium Vessel Vasculitides

Polyarteritis Nodosa and Microscopic Polyangiitis Polyarteritis nodosa (PAN) is characterized by acute inflammation and fibrinoid necrosis of small and medium vessels.[40] The etiology is unknown. Viral hepatitis B or C is associated with a vasculitis identical to PAN but is treated differently.[40] PAN is also linked with drug reactions, serum sickness, and HIV. PAN is more common in men than women. Recently a distinction has been made between PAN and microscopic polyangiitis (MPA). PAN includes vasculitis associated with nerve and gastrointestinal tract involvement, while MPA is associated with nerve, glomerular, and lung tissue. Classic PAN is also perinuclear antineutrophil cytoplasmic antibody (p-ANCA) negative, while MPA is p-ANCA positive, although it is not specific for the disease. Both are excluded if chronic hepatitis B or C is found.

The early clinical picture consists of constitutional symptoms of fever, malaise, arthralgias, and myalgias. PAN then progresses to peripheral neuropathy and bowel ischemia, complicated by hypertension due to renal artery inflammation. MPA is characterized by glomerulonephritis, alveolar hemorrhage, and often rapidly progressing glomerulonephritis.

The diagnosis is made by clinical pattern and histopathology seen on biopsy. After endocarditis and concomitant infections are ruled out as a cause of the vasculitis, biopsy of the involved segment may reveal diagnosis. Abdominal angiography may be useful to demonstrate small berry aneurysms, but these may not be present early in the course of the illness.

Treatment for both PAN and MPA is corticosteroids, especially in cases without organ involvement. Patients with severe disease may need additional therapy with immunosuppressive agents such as cyclophosphamide.[40] Patients with MPA have a higher rate of relapse. Active viral hepatitis, if present, should be treated with antiviral therapy.

Granulomatous Vasculitis Wegener's granulomatosis is a necrotizing granulomatous vasculitis involving the respiratory tract, kidneys, and to variable degrees the medium to small vessels in other organs. The disease is extremely rare, with a slightly increased incidence in men compared with women. The mean age of onset is 45 years.

Patients first complain of upper respiratory tract symptoms with sinusitis, otitis, and nasal ulceration. Destruction of the sinus walls may also occur. Lower respiratory tract symptoms include cough, dyspnea, hemoptysis, and asymptomatic pulmonary infiltrates, occasionally with cavitation. Tracheal stenosis occurs in 13% of patients.[41] Renal involvement is a later finding with glomerulonephritis, which may be aggressive, in 85% of patients.[33,43] Eye involvement includes conjunctivitis and scleritis caused by granulomatous deposition in the sclera. Skin lesions include ulcers, nodules, and granuloma formation. Nervous system involvement, usually a late feature of the disease, is seen in one third of patients and includes cerebral vasculitis, granulomatous deposition in cranial nerves, and peripheral nerve vasculitis resulting in neuropathies.[42] Coronary vasculitis, pericarditis, and conduction defects are rare.[20]

Laboratory examination includes findings of a markedly elevated ESR, normochromic normocytic anemia, and occasionally thrombocytopenia. Urinalysis may show hematuria, active sediment excretion, proteinuria, and red blood cell casts. Recently, antibodies against cytoplasmic components of polymorphonuclear cells (c-ANCA) have been found to be sensitive and specific for a diagnosis of Wegener's granulomatosis.[43] ANAs are usually absent. The chest x-ray study shows multiple sharply demarcated nodular densities, predominantly in the lower lung fields, with pleural effusions in 25% of patients.[41] Lymphadenopathy is rarely seen on radiograph.

Diagnosis of Wegener's granulomatosis is confirmed by an open lung biopsy.

Treatment with corticosteroids alone does little to alter the prognosis, and most patients die from renal disease within a year of diagnosis. Currently, the use of cyclophosphamide and corticosteroids in combination can induce remissions in up to 90% of patients.[41] Complications of this therapy include increased risk of infection, especially disseminated herpes zoster and *Pneumocystis carinii* pneumonia.

Patients with known Wegener's granulomatosis with flares of renal disease should be admitted for intravenous corticosteroid administration. Patients suspected to have Wegener's granulomatosis should be admitted for diagnosis and possible therapy. Renal transplant has been successful in patients who progress to end-stage renal disease.

Lymphomatoid granulomatosis, often confused with Wegener's granulomatosis, is characterized by destructive infiltration of lymphocytoid and plasmacytoid cells. The lower respiratory tract disease is the most prevalent, and upper respiratory tract involvement is rarely seen. Involvement of the kidney with deposition of granulomata is rare; but, in contrast to Wegener's granulomatosis, no vasculitis or glomerulonephritis is present. The spleen, lymph nodes, and bone marrow are usually spared. Malignant lymphoma develops in 50% of patients.[33] There are no specific laboratory findings, although in contrast to Wegener's granulomatosis, the ESR is usually normal or only mildly elevated and the c-ANCA is negative. The chest x-ray study shows multiple nodules similar to those seen in metastatic cancer.

Diagnosis is made by biopsy, usually of lung tissue. Treatment is the same as for Wegener's granulomatosis. Remissions with corticosteroids and cyclophosphamide are seen in 50% of patients, except in those who are also diagnosed with malignant lymphoma, in whom mortality is 90%.[33]

Behçet's Disease Behçet's disease is a chronic relapsing vasculitis characterized by oral ulceration, genital ulceration, and uveitis. The prevalence of Behçet's disease is 1 in 1000 in Japan to 1 in 150,000 in the United States and Europe.[44] It affects men more often than women, mainly young adults. In Japan, it has been linked to histocompatibility antigen HLA-B5.

Recognizing recurrent, painful aphthous ulcers that involve the oral mucosa and genitals makes the clinical diagnosis. Eye involvement includes iritis, uveitis, and optic neuritis, all of which can lead to blindness. The hallmark of Behçet's, a hypopyon uveitis, is seen rarely. CNS vasculitis, resulting in meningoencephalitis, intracranial hypertension, or a multiple sclerosis–like syndrome, can also occur. Gastrointestinal ulceration has been reported in Japanese patients, including ileocecal perforation. Skin lesions including erythema nodosum and cutaneous vasculitis may occur. Cardiac involvement is rare.[20] Nondeforming arthritis involving the knees and ankles has been described. Laboratory examination is nonspecific.

Diagnosis of Behçet's disease is made when a consistent clinical syndrome is associated with nonnecrotizing perivascular infiltrate of lymphocytes and monocytes on biopsy of affected tissue. The disease is well controlled with glucocorticoids at 1 mg/kg/day. Gastrointestinal disease can be controlled with sulfasalazine 2 to 6 gm/day. Eye involvement should be referred to an ophthalmologist. Serious manifestations of uveitis and CNS involvement warrant use of azathioprine or cyclophosphamide, and patients should be admitted to the hospital. Deep venous thrombosis associated with Behçet's rarely results in pulmonary emboli but should be treated with systemic anticoagulation.

Small Vessel Vasculitides

Hypersensitivity Vasculitis Hypersensitivity vasculitis describes a group of clinical syndromes characterized by small vessel vasculitis with a known or presumed inflammatory precipitating antigen, including drugs and infectious organisms, with immune complex deposition. Leukocytoclastic vasculitis describes the pathologic findings in the vessels, primarily the postcapillary venules, with infiltration by polymorphonuclear leukocytes with or without destruction of vessel walls.[33] In later stages red blood cell extravasation and dermal necrosis are seen. The diseases can be seen at any age and have no gender predominance. Common drugs that cause this vasculitis include the penicillins and sulfa drugs.

The syndromes in this category have similar clinical findings. The skin is the most commonly involved organ, with appearance of skin lesions abruptly after exposure to an infectious precipitating antigen, or within 1 to 2 days of taking a drug. The lesions are described as flat, erythematous purpuric papules or palpable purpura, usually on dependent portions such as lower extremities. The lesions may coalesce, forming patches, and may progress to bullae if the destruction is severe. Lower extremity edema is often associated. Burning or pain often is associated with the skin lesions. Other organs may be involved to varying degrees. Systemic symptoms of fever, malaise, and weight loss are common. Laboratory examination is nonspecific, with a mildly elevated ESR and mild leukocytosis.

Several characteristic hypersensitivity vasculitic syndromes have been described.

Henoch-Schönlein Purpura Henoch-Schönlein purpura (HSP) affects mainly the arterioles and capillaries, with peak incidence between 4 and 11 years of age, although adults may also be affected. The syndrome occurs most often in the spring following a viral upper respiratory infection.[33] Other inciting agents associated with HSP include insect stings and drugs.

The rash is accompanied by arthralgias of the lower extremities, most commonly the ankles, with swollen tender joints. Frank arthritis is usually absent. Gastrointestinal complaints, seen in 70% of patients, include abdominal pain, nausea, vomiting, and diarrhea, associated with blood and mucus per rectum.[43] Renal involvement occurs in 50% of patients with hematuria and red blood cell casts; however, it rarely progresses to renal failure.[46] Nervous system involvement is rare, especially in children.[42] The syndrome is relapsing and remitting over several weeks.

The immune complex deposition is immunoglobulin A (IgA), with antigens to drugs, infectious agents, foods, insect bites, and immunizations implicated in the pathogenesis. Most patients do well with supportive care and explanation of the relapsing and remitting nature of the disease. Treatment of the precipitating infection or discontinuation of the drug is necessary, if known. Children with more severe arthralgias and abdominal pain benefit from prednisone at 1 mg/kg/day orally. Adults who have symptoms may be given prednisone 60 mg/day. Prolonged renal impairment occurs in 25% of patients[33]; however, the benefits of steroids on renal prognosis are controversial.

Mixed Cryoglobulinemia Cryoglobulins are immunoglobulins and immune complexes that precipitate in the cold (4° C) and dissolve on rewarming. The syndrome of mixed cryoglobulinemia involves purpura, arthralgias, lymphadenopathy, and demonstration of the presence of cryoglobulins. Middle-aged women are most commonly affected. Precipitating antigens such as hepatitis A, B, and C; cytomegalovirus; or Epstein-Barr virus have been demonstrated (although most precipitants are unknown), resulting in essential mixed cryoglobulinemia.

Clinically, patients have polyarthralgias, purpura, and Raynaud's phenomenon. Hepatomegaly, splenomegaly, and lymphadenopathy are common. Recurrent palpable purpura occurs in virtually all patients.[47] The most serious involvement is renal deposition of the cryoglobulins, resulting in glomerulonephritis. Patients may have fulminant or slowly progressive chronic renal disease. Laboratory examination demonstrates elevated ESR, decreased serum complement levels, and the presence of cryoglobulins.

Diagnosis is made clinically in the presence of cryoglobulins; however, it may be difficult to distinguish from SLE or HSP. Treatment depends on the extent of involvement. Patients with disease limited to the skin may try low-dose steroids, while patients with systemic manifestations usually are started on prednisone 60 mg a day orally. Cyclophosphamide has been helpful in controlling systemic disease and allows for decreasing steroid dosages. Interferon may be useful in treating hepatitis C–related cryoglobulinemia. Patients with underlying diseases such as multiple myeloma and lymphoproliferative disorders should have their underlying disorders treated.

Serum Sickness Serum sickness and serum sickness–like reaction usually occur after ingestion of a known antigen, such as penicillin or sulfa medications. A cutaneous vasculitis is common in the disorder. Usually symptoms start 12 to 36 hours after ingestion if there is a previously immunizing exposure, but may occur up to 10 days after antigen exposure. The manifestations seen in serum sickness are due to immune complex deposition, but not to systemic vasculitis as described in this chapter.

Churg-Strauss Syndrome Churg-Strauss syndrome (allergic granulomatosis and angiitis), first described in 1951 by Churg and Strauss, is characterized by granulomatous vasculitis of multiple organs, with hypereosinophilia in patients with asthma and allergic rhinitis. The vasculitis usually involves the veins and venules of the lower respiratory tract. The exact incidence is unknown, and there is an overlap of pulmonary vasculitides. The mean age is 44 years, with men affected more often than women.

Patients have systemic symptoms of fever, weight loss, and malaise. Pulmonary symptoms are predominant, with a history of asthma for at least 2 years before diagnosis.[45] Skin lesions occur in 60% to 70% of patients, with subcutaneous nodules or palpable purpura present. Pericarditis can lead to constrictive pericarditis. Myocarditis can be seen, manifesting as congestive heart failure.[20] Gastrointestinal symptoms caused by infiltration of the small bowel or stomach walls are associated with infarction, perforation, or bloody diarrhea. Renal disease is much less prominent. The neurologic manifestation is mainly mononeuritis multiplex, found in up to 80% of patients.[42]

Laboratory examination reveals a persistent eosinophilia greater than $1000/mm^3$, often up to an absolute count of $5000/mm^3$ to $20{,}000/mm^3$.[33] Patients may have antineutrophil cytoplasmic antibodies directed against myeloperoxidase (p-ANCA), also seen in polyarteritis nodosa. The chest x-ray study can show patchy, fleeting infiltrates known as Loffler's syndrome, consolidation, or cavitation.

The diagnosis of Churg-Strauss syndrome is made by biopsy, usually of skin or lung tissue. The patient may also have an elevated immunoglobulin E (IgE). Churg-Strauss is extremely responsive to corticosteroids, with usual dosing of prednisone 60 mg/day orally. The prognosis is much improved with treatment, with 5-year survival greater than 50% in contrast to 25% in untreated patients.[33] Cytotoxic agents have no proven benefit.[33]

Goodpasture's Syndrome Goodpasture's syndrome is characterized by glomerulonephritis and pulmonary hemorrhage associated with antibody to glomerular basement membrane. The etiology is unknown, and the disease may occur at any age but primarily affects young men.

Clinically, the patients have cough, dyspnea, and hemoptysis. Initially, the pulmonary hemorrhage may be mild, or it may be severe and life-threatening. Hypoxia is common. Fever, arthralgias, and malaise are also present. The renal manifestations are varied; some patients have normal renal functions, others a rapidly progressing glomerulonephritis. Patients may also have skin involvement with palpable purpura. Laboratory examination is notable for elevated ESR and urinalysis with red blood cell casts. Blood test for antiglomerular basement membrane antibodies (anti-GBM) can be measured, but the level of circulating antibodies does not correlate with the severity of the disease. Complement levels are normal, and in contrast to Wegener's granulomatosis, c-ANCA tests are negative. Chest x-ray study shows hilar pulmonary infiltrates.

Differential diagnosis includes SLE and Wegener's granulomatosis. Diagnosis is made by renal biopsy. Lung tissue shows pulmonary alveolar hemorrhage, with similar linear deposition of antibodies along the alveolar basement membrane.

Management of the airway is the first priority in patients with severe pulmonary hemorrhage. Treatment with methylprednisolone 10 to 15 mg/kg IV is necessary if rapidly progressive glomerulonephritis or severe pulmonary hemorrhage complicates the patient's course. The use of cytotoxic agents like cyclophosphamide, as well as plasmapheresis (2 to 4 L/day of plasma), has been associated with improvement in pulmonary hemorrhage and glomerular lesions if extensive renal damage has not yet occurred.

The prognosis is varied. Some patients have minimal renal involvement and may have occasional flares of pulmonary hemorrhage. These patients should be admitted to the hospital to be observed for airway complications and for development of renal disease. Most patients have renal involvement with development of rapidly progressive glomerulonephritis within weeks, with extremely poor prognosis if untreated. These patients should be admitted for high-dose steroids and renal biopsy, if indicated, to guide management with cytotoxic agents and plasmapheresis. Patients who progress to end-stage renal disease are candidates for transplantation if anti-GBM antibodies return to undetectable levels, otherwise the disease may recur in the transplanted kidney.

Erythema Nodosum Erythema nodosum is a vasculitis of the venules in the subcutaneous layers of the skin. The cause is unclear, but it is usually the result of a hypersensitivity vasculitis from infections, drugs, or a systemic disease. The disease is seen most commonly in spring and fall. Women are more commonly affected than men, with a peak incidence in the third decade of life.[48] The lesions most often appear on the shin. The subcutaneous nodules are initially red, but then have a blue hue as they resolve. Patients may have just the nodules or may have systemic symptoms, including fever and malaise. Arthralgias are seen in 90% of patients at some time during the disease course.[48] Hilar lymphadenopathy may be present.

Patients who have erythema nodosum should be considered for underlying diseases such as viral upper respiratory tract infection, streptococcal infection, sarcoidosis, tuberculosis, and drug exposure. Much rarer causes include inflammatory bowel diseases, histoplasmosis, *Yersinia, Salmonella, Chlamydia,* coccidioidomycosis, psittacosis, and autoimmune diseases such as SLE. Drugs implicated include penicillins, sulfa drugs, aspartame, dilantin, and oral contraceptives. The eruption can last up to 6 weeks. NSAIDs may be useful in controlling the arthralgias. Disposition depends on suspicion of underlying disease but is usually outpatient follow-up.

Panniculitis Subcutaneous nodules manifest vasculitis of the subcutaneous fat layer surrounding the venules. Biopsy of the involved subcutaneous tissue shows fat cell necrosis, infiltration of inflammatory cells with macrophages, and vasculitis. Several forms of panniculitis exist. Diseases associated with panniculitis are erythema nodosum, erythema induratum, lupus profundus, pancreatitis, $<\alpha_1$-antitrypsin deficiency, light-chain paraproteinemia, and C_1 inhibitor deficiency.

Erythema nodosum can exist as a manifestation of systemic disease or as a hypersensitivity to drugs (as discussed previously). Erythema induratum (Bazin's disease) is a vasculitis of the skin of the calf associated with tuberculosis, and is typically seen in girls and young women. The bilateral lesions begin as nodules but then ulcerate and scar. The disease is chronic and recurrent. Mycobacteria are rarely found in the lesions. Therapy is supportive with dressing changes and elevation, unless evidence of active tuberculosis is found elsewhere.[48]

Lupus profundus is inflammation of the subcutaneous fat seen in SLE. It occurs in approximately 2% of patients with SLE.[49] Patients have subcutaneous nodules in the scalp, face, breasts, thighs, and buttocks. The lesions ulcerate and then heal. Of patients with lupus profundus, 50% eventually develop systemic manifestations of SLE.[49] Differential includes erythema nodosum, but in lupus profundus the lesions are usually more chronic and nontender.

Patients with pancreatitis or pancreatic cancer may have disseminated fat necrosis with lesions identical to nodular panniculitis. The fat necrosis is commonly found in periarticular sites. Patients also have fever and arthritis. Sinus tracts may be present with drainage. This form of panniculitis is thought to be due to the release of pancreatic enzymes into the vessels with necrosis at distal sites. Eosinophilia is commonly seen. Prognosis is poor, and the only treatment is to treat the underlying disorder.

Key Concepts

- The diagnosis of systemic vasculitis is difficult and should be considered in patients with rash and pulmonary or renal complaints.
- Consultation with a rheumatologist is helpful for determining management when patients have flares of a known vasculitis.
- Febrile patients on immunosuppressive therapy or corticosteroids have a high risk of sepsis or disseminated viral infections and should be treated aggressively.

REFERENCES

1. Osler W: On the visceral manifestations of the erythema group of skin diseases, *Am J Med Sci* 127:1, 1904.
2. Hargraves MM et al: Presentation of two bone marrow elements: the "tart" cell and the "LE" cell, *Proc Staff Meet Mayo Clin* 24:234, 1949.
3. Haserick JR: Blood factor in acute disseminated lupus erythematosus, *Arch Dermatol* 61:889, 1950.
4. Mills JA: Systemic lupus erythematosus, *N Engl J Med* 330:1871, 1994.
5. Fessel WJ: Systemic lupus erythematosus in the community: incidence, prevalence, outcome and first symptoms; the high prevalence in black women, *Arch Intern Med* 134:1027, 1974.
6. Pisetsky DS: Systemic lupus erythematosus: epidemiology, pathology and pathogenesis. In Klippel JH, editor: *Primer on the rheumatic diseases,* ed 11, Atlanta, 1997, Arthritis Foundation.
7. Tan EM et al: The 1982 revised criteria for the classification of systemic lupus erythematosus (SLE), *Arthritis Rheum* 25:1271, 1982.
8. Gilliam JM: Systemic lupus erythematosus in the skin. In Lahita RG, editor: *Systemic lupus erythematosus,* New York, 1992, John Wiley and Sons.
9. Correia P et al: Why do lupus patients with nephritis die? *BMJ* 290:126, 1985.
10. Nossent HC et al: Systemic lupus erythematosus after renal transplantation: patient and graft survival and disease activity, *Ann Intern Med* 114:183, 1991.
11. Cheigh JS et al: A multicenter study of outcome in systemic lupus erythematosus in patients with end-stage renal disease: long-term follow-up on the prognosis of patients and the evolution of lupus activity, *Am J Kidney Dis* 16:189, 1990.
12. Robinson DR: Systemic lupus erythematosus. In Dale DC, Federman DD, editors. New York, 1996, Scientific American.
13. Futrell N: Connective tissue disease and sarcoidosis of the central nervous system, *Curr Opin Neurol* 7:201, 1994.
14. van Dam AP: Diagnosis and pathogenesis of CNS lupus, *Rheumatol Int* 11:1, 1991.
15. Doherty NE, Siegal RJ: Cardiovascular manifestations of systemic lupus erythematosus, *Am Heart J* 110:1257, 1985.
16. Remetz MS, Matthay RA: Cardiovascular manifestations of connective tissue disease, *J Thorac Imaging* 7:49, 1992.
17. Ansari A et al: Cardiovascular manifestations of systemic lupus erythematosus: current perspective, *Prog Cardiol Dis* 27:421, 1985.
18. Leung WH et al: Cardiac abnormalities in systemic lupus erythematosus: a prospective M-mode, cross-sectional and Doppler echocardiographic study, *Int J Cardiol* 27:367, 1990.
19. Libman E, Sacks B: A hitherto undescribed form of valvular and mural endocarditis, *Arch Intern Med* 33:701, 1924.
20. Remetz MS, Matthay RA: Cardiovascular manifestations of connective tissue disorders, *J Thorac Imaging* 7:49, 1992.
21. Ansari A et al: Vascular manifestations of systemic lupus erythematosus, *Angiology* 37:423, 1986.
22. Gladman DD, Urowitz MB: Systemic lupus erythematosus: clinical and laboratory features. In Klippel JH, editor: *Primer on the rheumatic diseases,* ed 11, Atlanta, 1997, Arthritis Foundation.
23. Wibener HL, Littman BH: Ibuprofen-induced meningitis in systemic lupus erythematosus, *JAMA* 239:1062, 1978.
24. Balow JE: Lupus nephritis: natural history, prognosis, and treatment, *Clin Immunol Allergy* 6:353, 1986.
25. Klippel JH: Systemic lupus erythematosus: treatment. In Klippel JH, editor: *Primer on the rheumatic diseases,* ed 11, Atlanta, 1997, Arthritis Foundation.
26. Dustan HP et al: Rheumatic and febrile syndrome during prolonged hydralazine therapy, *JAMA* 154:23, 1954.
27. Perry HM, Schroeder HA: Syndrome simulating collagen disease caused by hydralazine (Apresoline), *JAMA* 154:670, 1954.
28. Ladd AT: Procainamide-induced lupus erythematosus, *N Engl J Med* 267:1357, 1962.
29. Harmon CE, Portanova JP: Drug-induced lupus: clinical and serological studies, *Clin Rheum Dis* 8:121, 1982.
30. Love PE, Santoro SA: Antiphospholipid antibodies: anticardiolipin and the lupus anticoagulant in systemic lupus erythematosus (SLE) and in non-SLE disorders, *Ann Intern Med* 112:682, 1990.
31. Kussmaul A, Maier K: Uber eine bischer nicht beschreibene eigenthumliche Arterienerkrankung (periarteritis nodosa), die mit Morbus Brightii und rapid fortschreitender allgemeiner Muskellahmung einhergeht, *Disch Arch Klin Med* 1:484, 1866.
32. Zeek PM: Periarteritis nodosa: critical review, *Am J Clin Pathol* 22:777, 1952.
33. Valente RM et al: Vasculitis and related disorders. In Kelly WN et al, editors: *Textbook of rheumatology,* ed 5, Philadelphia, 1997, WB Saunders.
34. Calabrese LH et al: Systemic vasculitis in association with human immunodeficiency virus infection, *Arthritis Rheum* 32:569, 1989.
35. Lehman TJA: Connective tissue disease and nonarticular rheumatism. In Klippel JH, editor: *Primer on the rheumatic diseases,* ed 11, Atlanta, 1997, Arthritis Foundation.
36. Calabrese LH: Vasculitis and infection with the human immunodeficiency virus, *Rheum Dis Clin North Am* 17:131, 1991.
37. Fauci AS et al: The spectrum of vasculitis: clinical, pathologic, immunologic, and therapeutic considerations, *Ann Intern Med* 89:660, 1978.
38. Kerr GS et al: Takayasu's arteritis, *Ann Intern Med* 120:919, 1994.
39. Harris ED: Systemic vasculitis. In Dale DC, Federman DD, editors. New York, 1995, Scientific American.
40. Mandell BF: Systemic vasculitic syndromes. In Dale DC, Federman DD, editors. New York, 2000, Scientific American.
41. Hoffman GS et al: Wegener granulomatosis: an analysis of 158 patients, *Ann Intern Med* 116:488, 1992.
42. Tervaert JWC, Kallenberg C: Neurologic manifestations of systemic vasculitides, *Rheum Dis Clin North Am* 19:913, 1993.
43. Mandell BF: Systemic vasculitis. In Dale DC, Federman DD, editors: New York, 1997, Scientific American.
44. O'Duffy JD: Behçet's disease. In Klippel JH, editor: *Primer on the rheumatic diseases,* ed 11, Atlanta, 1997, Arthritis Foundation.
45. Boulware DW et al: Pulmonary manifestations of rheumatic disease, *Clin Rev Allergy* 3:249, 1985.
46. Koskimies O et al: Renal involvement in Schönlein-Henoch purpura, *Acta Paediatr* 63:357, 1974.
47. Myers AR: Cryoglobulinemia. In Schumacher HR Jr, editor: *Primer on the rheumatic diseases,* ed 9, Atlanta, 1988, Arthritis Foundation.
48. Hurwitz S: *Clinical pediatric dermatology,* ed 2, Philadelphia, 1993, WB Saunders.
49. Foster DW: The lipodystrophies and other rare disorders of adipose tissue. In Isselbacher KJ, Braunwald E, editors: *Harrison's principle of internal medicine,* ed 13, New York, 1994, McGraw-Hill.

113 Allergy, Hypersensitivity, and Anaphylaxis

Robert L. Muelleman
T. Paul Tran

PERSPECTIVE

The human immune system is composed of cellular and protein components interacting in an elegant, interdependent fashion to preserve the self (autologous) and protect the body from harmful nonself (foreign). The goal is to promote survival of the species. The immune system, however, can sometimes overreact, causing allergic reactions and autoimmune diseases. One of the true emergent allergic reactions is anaphylaxis.

In 1902 Portier and Richet[1] discovered—during a Mediterranean cruise—that when an extract of the tentacles of a jellyfish was injected into a dog, it was tolerated the first time but caused death when injected again several weeks later. They coined the term anaphylaxis from Greek (*ana,* against or backwards; *phylax,* guard or protect), meaning "against protection." Today, anaphylaxis refers to a severe systemic allergic reaction in a previously sensitized patient, a syndrome associated with variable clinical features. Although the clinical manifestations of anaphylaxis vary considerably, the distinguishing features are acute respiratory difficulty and vascular collapse, within seconds to minutes after exposure to the offending agent. Other symptoms may include pruritic erythematous rash, urticaria, angioedema, laryngeal edema, rhinitis, conjunctivitis, nausea, vomiting, abdominal pain, palpitations, lightheadedness, and syncope.

Localized allergic reactions refer to other nonsystemic diseases that also result from immune system overactivity. Involved organs commonly include the skin, the airway, and the eye. Urticaria, angioedema, contact dermatitis, certain adverse food reactions, and allergic rhinoconjunctivitis are examples of localized allergic reactions commonly evaluated in the ED. The prototypical urticaria and angioedema are characterized by usually transient, pruritic, red wheals with raised, serpiginous borders. These are caused by edema of the dermis in urticaria and the subcutaneous tissue in angioedema. Pathogenetically, allergic diseases are caused by a variety of mechanisms. Urticaria and angioedema, for example, can be mediated by immunoglobulin E (IgE), the complement system, or via nonimmunologic mechanisms. It is noteworthy that angioedema of the upper airway can be life-threatening due to possible laryngeal obstruction.

Immunopathology

Anaphylaxis is an immediate type hypersensitivity reaction. It is caused by IgE-mediated immunologic release of mediators from mast cells and basophils, with subsequent activation of inflammatory pathways. The term anaphylactoid reaction refers to a syndrome clinically similar to that of anaphylaxis but not mediated by IgE. Although the exact mechanisms are unknown, anaphylactoid reactions seem to result from direct degranulation of mast cells and basophils and may follow a single, first-time exposure to certain agents. Radiopaque contrast media (RCM) reactions and medications such as aspirin and other nonsteroidal antiinflammatory drugs (NSAIDs) are the two most common classes of agents responsible for anaphylactoid-induced fatalities.

Causes and Incidence

The exact incidence of anaphylaxis is not known, but is generally thought to be less than 1% in the general population, and death rarely occurs.[2] Epidemiological data range from 4 cases of anaphylaxis per 10 million in Ontario, Canada, to 9.79 cases per 100,000 in Munich, Germany.[3] A recent retrospective analysis over a 4-month period in Minnesota showed that 17 of 19,122 visits to the ED were for anaphylaxis.[4] In this community (Olmsted, Minnesota) the average annual incidence is 21 per 100,000 person-years.[2]

The cause for anaphylaxis may remain unidentified in as many as two thirds of the cases.[5] In the cases in which a cause can be determined, food is the most frequent causative agent, accounting for approximately one third of anaphylaxis cases.[5,6] Peanuts and shellfish are the most frequent offenders. Next to food, *Hymenoptera* stings, antibiotics, aspirin and NSAIDs, RCM, exercise, and latex are the more common causative agents. Up to 3% of the population is sensitive to insect stings.[7] There are 25 to 50 deaths per year from bee and wasp stings in the United States.[8] Of the antibiotics, penicillin is among the most common causes of anaphylaxis, occurring at a frequency of one to five reactions per 10,000 patient treatments. The other major drug group includes aspirin and NSAIDs. Up to 0.9% of patients taking aspirin experience anaphylaxis,[9] accounting for about 3% of total anaphylactic reactions.[5] Of the 51,797 patients taking NSAIDs, there were 35 cases of shock (not related to gastrointestinal bleeding), 11 cases of angioedema, and 106 cases of urticaria.[10] Another important therapeutic agent that can cause a reaction is RCM. Severe reactions occur in 0.22% of patients given the older hyperosmolar contrast agents and in 0.04% of patients given the newer nonionic agents.[11] Next to medications, exercise is an important cause of anaphylaxis, responsible for 19 of the 266 cases (7%) in one study.[5]

Latex Allergy

The newest, most significant agent causing anaphylaxis is latex, present in latex gloves and latex medical devices. Latex is the natural rubber derived from the commercial rubber tree, *Hevea brasiliensis.* It is widely used in the manufacture of medical products. The functional unit is a rubber particle coated with a layer of protein, lipid, and phospholipid to provide the structural integrity.[12] Although only 0.7% of children in a general population has positive skin-prick test to latex,[13] adults appear to have higher incidences of sensitivity. Up to 2.9% of health care providers in the study by Turjanmaa[14] and 17% in a similar study by Yassin[15] were found to be latex sensitive. The incidence seems to correlate with the expanded use of latex gloves.

Risks for Anaphylaxis

Race, sex, and geographical location generally have no effect on the incidence of anaphylaxis.[3] Adulthood and the parenteral route of administration are more strongly associated with anaphylactic reactions, especially severe ones, than are childhood and the oral route, respectively. Atopy predisposes patients to higher risk of anaphylaxis. Also, the immune memory seems imperfect. Upon reexposure to an antigen, the more remote the first anaphylactic reaction, the less likely the reexposure will result in an anaphylactic reaction.

One interesting aspect of anaphylaxis is the constancy of administration.[3] An anaphylactic reaction may not occur in a susceptible patient as long as a drug is administered regularly. The patient might become more sensitive to the drug and have an anaphylactic reaction if the drug were resumed after an interruption of therapy.

PRINCIPLES OF DISEASE

Development of the Immune System

The two arms of the immune system, the thymus-derived lymphocytes (T cells) and bursa-equivalent lymphocytes (B cells), originally develop from the lymphoid precursor cells. They in turn develop from the pluripotential hematopoietic stem cells in the bone marrow. This common pluripotent stem cell also gives rise to the colony-forming unit for granulocyte, erythroid, myeloid, and megakaryocyte (CFU-GEMM) stem cells, which differentiate into the mast cells, basophils, dendritic cells, neutrophils, platelets, erythrocytes, and macrophages (Figure 113-1).[16]

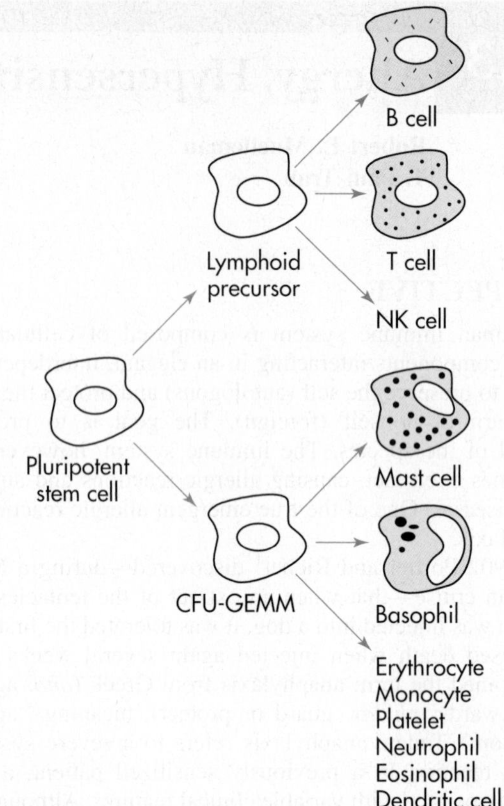

Figure 113-1. **Developmental pathways of the immune and hematopoietic system.** ***After Shearer WT, Fleisher TA. In Middleton E et al, editors:*** **Allergy: clinical and practice,** ***St Louis, 1998, Mosby.***

T Cell Development Lymphoid precursor cells migrate from the bone marrow into the thymus where they progress through ontogeny. Under regulation by cytokines, these precursor cells undergo gene rearrangement, positive and negative selection. In the process T cells acquire the T cell antigen receptors (TCR), various surface markers, and eventuate into two T cell lineages. Using the cluster of differentiation (CD) classification, there are principally two types of mature T cells eventuating out of the thymus: CD_4^+, also called helper T cells, and CD_8^+, also called suppressor T cells. T cells do not interact directly with unprocessed antigens, only with peptides or unfolded proteins that are bound to major histocompatibility complex (MHC) molecules. In general, CD_4^+ T cells recognize exogenously derived antigens (e.g., bacterial proteins) presented in the context of class II MHC molecules. These class II MHC molecules, including the human leukocyte antigens HLA-A, HLA-B, and HLA-C, are found on antigen presenting cells (APCs) such as monocytes, macrophages, B cells, and dendritic cells. CD_4^+ T cells can further be subdivided into Type 1 (Th1) helper T cells and Type 2 (Th2) helper T cells depending on the type of cytokine produced. Th1 cells secrete interferon-γ and interleukin-2 (IL-2). Th2 helper T cells secrete IL-4, IL-5, IL-6, and IL-10. It is the Th2 helper T cells and their cytokines that are involved in the IgE-mediated immediate hypersensitivity anaphylaxis. CD_8^+ T cells recognize antigens in the context of class I MHC molecules. These include HLA-DR, HLA-DQ, and HLA-DP and are found on most somatic cells. The ability of the immune system to recognize antigens in the context of MHC serves as the biological basis for the body to discriminate self from nonself.

B Cell Development and Immunoglobulins B cell ontogeny can be divided into antigen-independent and antigen-dependent stages. During the antigen-independent stage, B cells mature in primary lymphoid organs like the bone marrow and fetal liver. There they undergo gene rearrangement in a stochastic fashion and acquire various surface markers. Later during the antigen-dependent stage, driven by antigen interaction, B cells differentiate into memory B cells and plasma cells, and are ready to secrete immunoglobulins. This step takes places in the secondary lymphoid organs like the lymph nodes and spleen. Immunoglobulins are protein molecules composed of two identical polypeptide heavy chains and two identical polypeptide light chains (see Figure 113-2). The heavy chains (H) have one variable (V) domain, V_H, and three or four constant (C) domains C_H. The light (L) chains have one variable (V) domain V_L and one constant (C) domain C_L. The constant domains of the heavy chains together form the Fc (crystallizable fragment) region of the immunoglobulin molecule, which binds to the surface receptors of effector cells such as mast cells, B cells, or macrophages. The variable domains of the heavy and light chains together form the Fab (antibody-binding fragment) region of the immunoglobulin molecule, which is responsible for antigen binding. The primary role of immunoglobulins is to bind foreign antigens and effect the neutralization or removal of these harmful antigens (e.g., microbes, parasites, toxins) from the body. There are five isotypes or classes of immunoglobulins: IgG, IgA, IgM, IgD, and IgE. Isotype IgE (and IgG subclass 4 [IgG_4]) is, however, the most important antibody in the pathogenesis of anaphy-

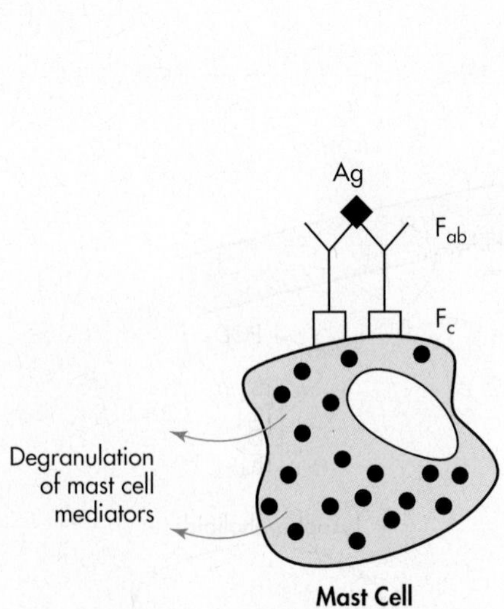

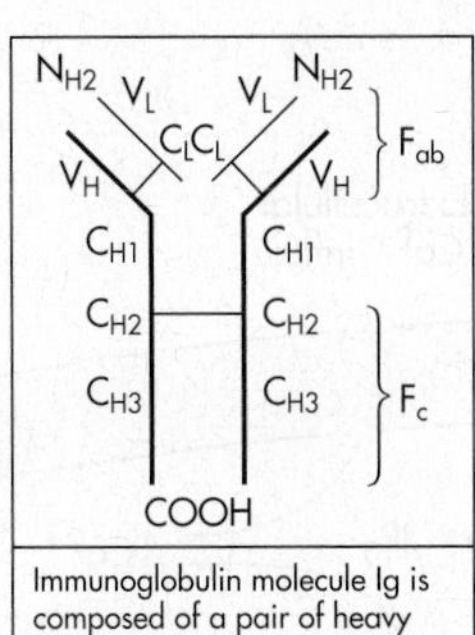

Immunoglobulin molecule Ig is composed of a pair of heavy chains and a pair of light chains with variable (V) and constant (C) domains.

Figure 113-2. **Activation of mast cells with degranulation of mast cell mediators by antigen (Ag) crosslinking adjacent IgE on cell surface.**

laxis. B cell maturation, isotype switching, and immunoglobulin production are driven by cytokines produced by T cells, activated T cells, and bone marrow stromal cells.

Characteristics of the Immune System

Four distinguishing characteristics of the immune system differentiate it from other systems in the body. First, antibodies, found in blood and tissue fluids and on the surface of the B cells themselves, and receptors on T cells are highly specific for antigen; they can bind and distinguish antigens with nearly identical chemical structures. Second, the number of species of antibodies and T cell receptors are enormously diverse. There are up to 10^9 types of antibodies and T cell receptors that are available to bind antigens. Third, besides the brain, the immune system is the only system that has memory. After the first (primary) exposure to an allergen, a subsequent (secondary) challenge—days to years later—can elicit an accelerated and augmented immune response. Both the cellular and humeral arms are activated. The antibody titer is higher, affinity of the antibodies for antigen enhanced, and T cell reactivity increased. Memory response is the basis for prophylactic immunization. And fourth, the immune system is able to discriminate self from nonself.

Classification of Reactions

The original classification of immunopathologic reactions, proposed by Coombs and Gell, lists four types of hypersensitivity reactions. Alternate classifications, such as the Sell classification,[17] have been proposed to reflect our increased understanding of immunopathology. In this chapter, the traditional Coombs and Gell classification is adopted. Type I (immediate hypersensitivity) is IgE- or IgG_4-mediated and accounts for most anaphylactic reactions observed in humans. Type II (cytotoxic) is IgG- or IgM-mediated. IgG or IgM is involved in the binding of circulating antibody to a cell-bound antigen, with possible subsequent activation of the complement cascade and anaphylatoxin production. Anaphylatoxins C3a and C5a stimulate mediator release and may produce the same action as the classic mediators of anaphylaxis at the target tissue level. Type III (immune complex) is IgG or IgM complex-mediated. Circulating soluble antigen-antibody complexes migrate from the circulation to deposit in the perivascular interstitial space, which may activate the complement system. Anaphylactic reactions from blood transfusions or blood component therapy, including serotherapy (immunoglobulin administration), are clinical examples of the overlap of type II and type III reactivity, and have more recently been classified as immune complex–mediated or complement-mediated anaphylaxis. Type IV (delayed hypersensitivity) is T cell–mediated and has no documented relationship to the pathogenesis of anaphylaxis.

PATHOPHYSIOLOGY

Antigens and antigen complexes cause anaphylaxis by activating various pathways of inflammation. The common starting event is the degranulation of mast cells and basophils (Figure 113-2). Classic anaphylaxis is mediated by IgE. Many foods, drugs, insect bites and stings,[3] and some cases of food-dependent, exercise-induced anaphylaxis[18] are mediated through this mechanism. Anaphylactoid reactions involve direct degranulation of mast cells and basophils, independent of IgE. This category includes radiocontrast agents, opioids, biologicals, the majority of idiopathic anaphylaxis (IA), and anaphylaxis caused by physical factors such as sunlight or cold. Radiocontrast agents are also believed to involve other inflammatory pathways.[19] Aspirin and NSAIDs are believed to cause anaphylaxis via abnormal metabolism or arachidonic acid (AA).[3] Immune complex causes anaphylactoid reactions via activation of the complement pathway. Examples include the administration of albumin, dextran, or protamine. Complement activation is also believed to cause cytotoxic anaphylactoid reactions that occur in incompatible blood transfusions, where complement fixes antibodies to formed elements such as red blood cells, platelets, and leukocytes.[3]

Mast cells (and basophils) express surface receptors that have high affinity for the Fc portion of IgE (FcεRI). Sensitization refers to the process of fixation of IgE to mast cells. Subsequent challenge with an appropriate multivalent antigen or immune complex will cause aggregation or cross-linking of surface IgE molecules in a process called activation (see Figure 113-2). A cascade of conformational and biochemical events is then initiated, leading to the exocytosis of preformed mediators and to generation and release of lipid-derived mediators and cytokines. The

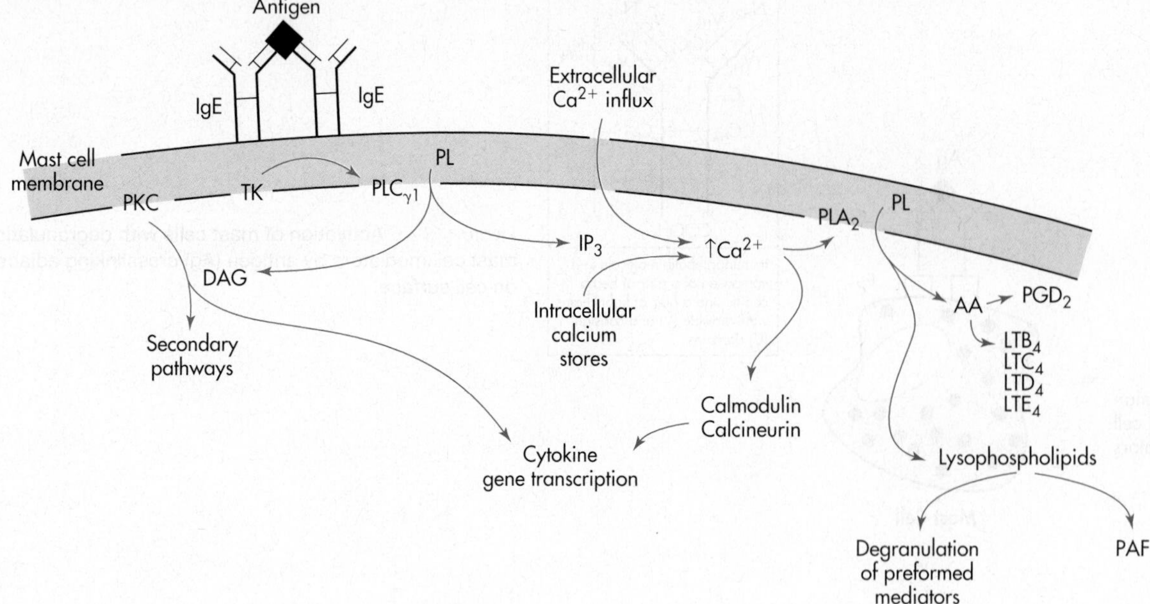

Figure 113-3. **Sequence of events following the crosslinking of adjacent IgE on surface of mast cells. (See text for description.)** ***Modified from McNeil HP, Austen KE. In Frank MM et al, editors:*** **Samter's immunologic diseases,** ***1995, Little Brown.***

mediators and cytokines act on primary target tissues, including the vascular, bronchial, and gastrointestinal smooth muscle, vascular endothelium, and exocrine glands, resulting in the clinical manifestation of allergic reaction and anaphylaxis.

Cascade of Events

The cascade of events (Figure 113-3) during activation starts with phosphorylation of the chains of the IgE receptor by the protein tyrosine kinase (TK), leading to activation of the phospholipase $C\gamma_1$ ($PLC\gamma_1$). $PLC\gamma_1$ then elaborates diacylglycerol (DAG) and inositol triphosphate (IP_3) from membrane phospholipids. DAG in turn activates tyrosine kinase C, which initiates various secondary pathways. IP_3 mobilizes intracellular calcium stores. Increases in intracellular calcium activate the calmodulin and calcineurin pathways, leading to gene expression of cytokines in T cells and mast cells. It is believed that cytokines IL-1, IL-3, IL-4, IL-5, IL-6, INFγ, and GM-CSF are generated. Additionally, increases in intracellular calcium, augmented by formation of calcium channels in cell membrane, also activate phospholipase A_2 (PLA_2). PLA_2 cleaves membrane phospholipids to form lysophospholipids, which like DAG facilitate the fusion of secretory granules with the cell membrane, leading to the exocytosis of the secretory granules. Lysophospholipids are also acetylated to produce platelet-activating factor (PAF). At the same time, PLA_2 mediates the release of AA to serve as substrate in the lipoxygenase and cyclooxygenase pathways. The result of AA metabolism via these two pathways is the generation of mast cell prostanoid PGD_2 and leukotrienes LTC_4, LTD_4, LTE_4, and LTB_4 (Figure 113-4). In human mast cells, LTE_4 is present in much greater quantities than LTB_4.

Mediators of Anaphylaxis

Histamine is the most important of the preformed mediators (Box 113-1). In fact, infusion of histamine has been shown to produce the majority of the clinical features of anaphylaxis

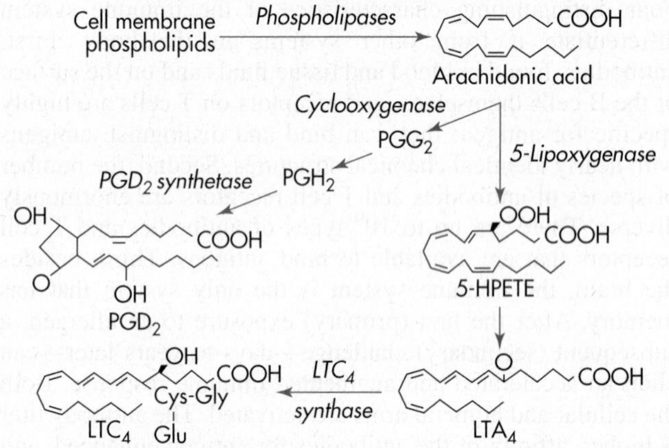

Cell membrane phospholipids → *Phospholipases* → Arachidonic acid (COOH)
Cyclooxygenase → PGG_2 → PGH_2 → *PGD_2 synthetase* → PGD_2 (OH, COOH, OH)
5-Lipoxygenase → 5-HPETE (OOH, COOH) → LTA_4 (COOH)
LTC_4 synthase → LTC_4 (OH, COOH, Cys-Gly, Glu)
LTA_4 hydrolase → LTB_4 (OH, OH, COOH)
LTD_4 (OH, COOH, Cys-Gly, Glu)
LTE_4 (OH, COOH, Cys)

Figure 113-4. **Prostanoid and leukotriene pathways for biosynthesis of lipid-derived mediators in mast cells.** ***Modified from Austen KF. In Harrison TR, Fauci AS, editors:*** **Harrison's principles of internal medicine,** ***ed 14, New York, 1998, McGraw-Hill.***

syndrome.[20] Histamine is produced and stored in preformed granules (pg) in mast cells and basophils, at about 1-2 pg/cell.[21] Not only is histamine an essential mediator in immediate hypersensitivity, it is also an important mediator in inflammation. Three classes of receptors, H_1, H_2, and H_3, mediate the activity of histamine in the body.[22] H_1 receptor

Box 113-1 Preformed Mediators of MAST Cells and Basophils

Preformed Mediators
Histamine
Tryptase
Chymase
Carboxypeptidase A
Cathepsin G
Proteoglycans

Arachidonic Acid Metabolites
LTC_4
LTB_4
LTE_4
PGD_2

Cytokinases and Chemokines
TNF-α
IL-4,5,6,13

stimulation produces bronchial, intestinal, and uterine smooth muscle contraction, increased vascular permeability, nasal mucus production, coronary artery spasm, and increased eosinophil and neutrophil chemokinesis and chemotaxis. H_2 receptor stimulation increases the rate and force of ventricular and atrial contraction, gastric acid secretion, airway mucus production, and vascular permeability, while also causing bronchodilation and inhibition of basophil histamine release.[23] H_3 receptor, found in neurons (in the central nervous system) and peripheral tissues, controls the synthesis and release of histamine.[24] The role of the other preformed mediators in mast cell and basophil degranulation syndrome is not well delineated.

LTC_4, LTD_4, LTE_4 and PGD_2 have similar biologic effects in humans. LTC_4, LTD_4, and LTE_4, also referred to as cysteinyl leukotrienes, were formerly called the slow-reacting substances of anaphylaxis. They are involved in cholinergic-independent bronchial and bronchiolar wall smooth muscle contraction, increased vascular permeability, and increased mucous gland production. These cysteinyl leukotrienes have a slow onset, but are 10 to 1000 times[21] as potent as histamine in causing bronchoconstriction when administered by aerosol. They also have a longer duration of action and potentiate the effects of other bronchoconstrictors such as histamine. It has been postulated that inhibition of cyclooxygenase, and therefore inhibition of prostaglandin, thromboxane, and prostacyclin production, as seen with the use of aspirin and other NSAIDs, results in a shift to the lipoxygenase pathway with a subsequent increase in production of LTC_4, LTD_4, and LTE_4. This may be the explanation for aspirin-induced bronchospasm. Blockage of leukotrienes with experimental antagonists suggests that these leukotrienes may be implicated in the prolonged airway and secondary cardiovascular response of anaphylaxis.[21] PGD_2 is also a potent inhibitor of platelet aggregation.

PAF is an unstored lipid and the most potent compound known to cause aggregation of human platelets with subsequent release of platelet-derived vasoactive mediators. Its other actions include neutrophil activation and chemotaxis, and ileal and parenchymal lung strip smooth muscle contraction. PAF has been demonstrated to produce many of the important clinical manifestations of anaphylaxis, including decreased myocardial contractile force, coronary vasoconstriction, pulmonary edema, and a prolonged increase in total pulmonary resistance with a decrease in dynamic compliance. Blockage of PAF with experimental antagonists suggests that it may be involved in the late cardiac dysfunction and lethality associated with anaphylaxis.[25,26]

Physiologic Effects

The chemical mediators described collectively effect the syndrome of anaphylaxis. Increased vascular permeability can lead to urticaria, angioedema, laryngeal edema, nasal congestion, or gastrointestinal swelling with abdominal cramping and vomiting. Vasodilation can lead to flushing, headaches, reduced peripheral vascular resistance, hypotension, and syncope. Contraction of smooth muscle can lead to bronchospasm, abdominal cramping, or diarrhea. Pulmonary vessel vasoconstriction can lead to pulmonary hypertension, pulmonary edema, and decreased cardiac filling pressures. Coronary vasoconstriction can lead to myocardial ischemia and decreased myocardial contractile force. Changes in atrial chronotropy and ventricular and atrial isotropy can lead to cardiac dysrhythmias. In addition to the direct actions on the target tissues, these preformed mediators, lipid-derived mediators, and cytokines also activate a number of inflammatory pathways, including the complement system, clotting and clot lysis systems, and kallikrein-kinin (contact) system, to contribute to the clinical manifestations of allergy and anaphylaxis.

Classically, cardiovascular collapse in anaphylaxis has been described as a result of peripheral vasodilation, enhanced vascular permeability, leakage of plasma, and intravascular volume depletion. However, hemodynamic reports from humans experiencing anaphylactic shock indicate the explanation may be more complicated. In a variety of clinical settings, hypotension in anaphylaxis has been associated with increased cardiac index, increased cardiac index with decreased peripheral vascular resistance, decreased cardiac index, decreased cardiac index with decreased peripheral vascular resistance, and decreased cardiac index with increased peripheral vascular resistance. In the setting of decreased cardiac index and decreased peripheral vascular resistance a small reduction in oxygen delivery and large reductions in oxygen consumption and oxygen extraction ratios are present, causing reduced organ perfusion and metabolic acidosis.[27]

Pathologic features identified at autopsy of fatal cases of anaphylaxis are most commonly observed in the respiratory and cardiac systems. These include laryngeal edema, pulmonary hyperinflation, peribronchial vascular congestion, intraalveolar hemorrhage, pulmonary edema, increased tracheobronchial secretions, eosinophilic infiltration of the bronchial walls, and varying degrees of myocardial damage. Other autopsy findings include urticarial eruptions, angioedema, visceral congestion, submucosal edema, and hemorrhagic gastritis. Notably, autopsy findings may also be normal after an anaphylactic death.[28]

ETIOLOGY

Numerous agents are known to cause anaphylactic reactions in humans. They can be found in three broad categories of materials: proteins, polysaccharides, and haptens.[19] In this chapter, these agents are, however, categorized according to etiologic and pathogenetic classification: IgE-mediators, immune complex mediators, nonimmunologic activators, or AA modulators (Box 113-2). Reactions without identifiable causative agents have been classified as exercise-induced or IA. The number of substances capable of eliciting an anaphylactic reaction is continuously expanding because of the introduction of new diagnostic and therapeutic agents. The most significant new agent is natural rubber latex.

IgE-Mediated Agents

The diverse group of antigens capable of inducing an anaphylactic response can mechanistically be separated into proteins such as food, haptens such as antibiotics, latex rubber, other therapeutic agents, and *Hymenoptera* stings.

Foods Foods are the major cause, accounting for approximately one third of the cases of anaphylaxis in which a causative agent can be determined.[2,5] A variety of foods ranging from the well-known such as nuts, shellfish, and eggs, to the obscure such as chamomile tea (which may have cross-reactivity with ragweed) have been identified. Shellfish and peanuts are, however, the most common foods that cause anaphylaxis.[5] Even for a person with a known history of food allergy, it may still be difficult to avoid foods that may cause allergic reactions because their identity may be obscured in the processing. It is noteworthy that since allergenic foods are first absorbed transmucosally, symptoms of food anaphylaxis usually are respiratory and localized to the upper airway. On the other hand, when anaphylactic allergens are administered parenterally, symptoms of anaphylaxis tend to be more cardiovascular and systemic. Although allergic reactions to foodstuffs are more common in children (0.3% to 7.5%),[29] the true incidence of food-induced anaphylaxis is much lower.[5,30]

Therapeutic and prophylactic use of large quantities of antibiotics is common in the harvesting of beef cattle, swine, fish, poultry, vegetables, and fruits. Along with antibiotics, sodium and potassium bisulfites and metabisulfites are used as preservatives in foods. Sulfites are antioxidants used in the food and restaurant industry to prevent discoloration of vegetables (e.g., salad bars, avocado dips), fruits, and potatoes, and to preserve fruit and vegetable juices. They are also used to prevent bacterial contamination of wines, beers, and distilled beverages. The sensitivity to ingested sulfites has been well documented, especially among the asthmatic population.[31,32] In August 1986, the Food and Drug Administration (FDA) placed a ban on the use of sulfites in the food and restaurant business in the United States. Establishing a particular foodstuff or preservative as the causative agent responsible for anaphylaxis may be difficult.[33]

Antibiotics Benzylpenicillin, semisynthetic penicillin, and cephalosporins are the most significant antimicrobial anaphylactic agents. The first penicillin-induced anaphylactic fatality was reported in 1949.[34] Because of their low molecular weights, these antimicrobials do not themselves possess antigenic properties. Immunologically, they are haptens, simple chemicals that are not antigenic in themselves but become antigenic after the chemicals or their metabolites form a stable bond with the host protein. Certain binding properties of particular drugs make them more likely to induce sensitization. Although the risk of death from drug-induced anaphylaxis is extremely low (from 1:10,000 to 1:50,000), all drugs must be viewed as potential antigens and should be prescribed only when clinically indicated. This is particularly important for those medications that historically have been identified as inducers of anaphylaxis. Although the frequency of allergic reactions to penicillin varies from 0.7% to 10% in different studies, an anaphylactic response occurs in 0.015% to 0.04%, with a fatality rate of 0.0015% to 0.002%, in patients treated with penicillin. This corresponds to one fatality per 7.5 million injections.[35] Parenterally administered penicillin is responsible for most severe anaphylactic reactions. Only six fatalities from oral penicillin have been well documented.[36] The extensive use of this drug in unsuspected sources, such as foods, in which it is used as a bacteriostatic agent, may make it difficult to ascertain historically that penicillin is the causative agent. Any patient receiving oral penicillin should consider the potential risk for the development of an anaphylactic reaction.[37]

Cephalosporins share the β-lactam ring structure and side chains of the penicillins, and have been incriminated for allergic cross-sensitivity in up to 5% to 16% of patients. It is unclear which epitope is responsible for this cross-reactivity.[38,39] Patients who have urticaria or anaphylactic reactions after taking penicillin are three to four times more likely to have an adverse reaction to cephalosporins. The risks of an anaphylactic reaction in this setting are still low, believed to be less than 2%.[40] Nevertheless, it may be prudent to administer a class of antibiotics other than the cephalosporins when a well-documented significant history of penicillin allergy is obtained. If no other antibiotic choices are available, the first dose of cephalosporin should be administered under medical supervision and observation and should be given orally if possible.

Latex Allergy to natural rubber latex in gloves and other medical products has become a serious health issue for health care providers, patients, and rubber industry workers. Latex antigens are proteins present in raw latex. The antigens can be leached from latex during normal use. For glove wearers, latex antigens are adsorbed onto the cornstarch powder to serve as a contact allergen, or they can become airborne allergens when the gloves are discarded. The prevalence and severity of reactions have rapidly increased in the last decade, probably because of the increased use of latex gloves for barrier protection since the advent of acquired immunodeficiency syndrome (AIDS). The incidence of latex allergy ranges from 0.7% in unselected school-age children,[13] to 3% in atopic children[41] seen at a university hospital allergy clinic, to 17% to 30% in hospital employees.[15,42] Groups at higher risk include spina bifida patients, health care workers, latex industry workers, and patients with a history of atopy or multiple surgical procedures.[43,44] Most common symptoms of latex allergy include allergic urticaria, rhinitis, conjunctivitis, and occupational asthma. There is evidence that patients with specific food allergies are predisposed to latex allergy.[45] Allergy to latex is a type I, immediate, IgE-mediated reaction that can lead to anaphylaxis.[46,47] The true risks of latex-induced anaphylaxis are not known, but in a review of anaphylaxis incidents in 50 children, 27% were due to latex allergy.[48] Diagnostic tools include serological assays and skin-prick testing. There is no effective prophylaxis for latex allergy. In fact, routine use of the H_2 blocker ranitidine for gastroesophageal reflux was reported to increase the risk of a heart conduction block in a case of anaphylaxis caused by

Box 113-2 Etiologic Agents and Pathogenetic Mechanisms of Anaphylaxis

IgE-Mediated Agents

Antibiotics

Penicillin
Cephalosporins
Tetracyclines
Nitrofurantoin
Streptomycin
Vancomycin
Chloramphenicol
Bacitracin
Neomycin
Polymyxin B
Kanamycin
Amphotericin B
Ketoconazole
Sulfonamides

Foreign protein agents

Latex
Heterologous serum
Equine tetanus antitoxin
Equine antivenins
Equine rabies immune serum
Adrenocorticotropic hormone
Insulin
Parathyroid hormone
Asparaginase
Chymotrypsin
Trypsin
Chymopapain
Penicillinase
Relaxin
Seminal plasma
Hymenoptera venom (honeybee, yellow jacket, wasp, hornet)
Fire ant
Kissing bug (triatoma) saliva
Vasopressin
Antilymphocyte globulin
Deerfly venom
Rattlesnake venom
Acacia
Glue
Protamine
Streptokinase
Pollen
Inhalation
Autoinjection (alpine slide)

Endogenous Hormones

Hormonally related (progesterone)
Immune complex– or complement-mediated agents
Whole blood
Cryoprecipitate
Immunoglobulin
Plasma
Radiopaque contrast media (?)*
Local anesthetics (some reaction)

Modulators of Arachidonic Acid Metabolism

Acetylsalicylic acid
NSAIDs
Benzoates (presumed)
Tartrazine (possibly)

Therapeutic Agents

Allergen extracts
Muscle relaxants (some reactions)
Estradiol
Hydrocortisone
Methylprednisolone
Benzylpenicilloyl-polylysine (Pre-Pen)
Procaine (?)*
Tripelennamine
Ethylene oxide gas
Thiopental
Local anesthetics
Esters
Amides
Methylparaben preservative
Human diploid cell rabies vaccine
Thiazides*
Acetaminophen
Mechlorethamine*
Psyllium
Influenza
Egg-based vaccines: measles, mumps, rubella
Yellow fever
Rubber gloves*

Foods

Milk
Egg white
Shellfish
Legumes
Nuts
Citrus fruits
Bananas
Grains
Sunflower seeds
Chocolate
Fish
Beets
Mango
Cottonseed
Corn
Safflower
Chamomile tea
Preservatives
Penicillin
Streptomycin
Bisulfites
Metabisulfites

Direct Histamine-Releasing

Opiates
Curare, *d*-tubocurarine
Radiopaque contrast media
Sodium dehydrocholate (?)*
Sulfobromophthalein (BSP) (?)*
Dextran
Iron-dextran (?)*
Thiamine (?)*

Physical Factors

Exercise
Food independent
Food dependent
Food specific
Food nonspecific

Idiopathic Factors

Modified from Marquardt DL, Wasserman SI: Anaphylaxis. In Middleton E et al, editors: *Allergy: principles and practice,* ed 4, St Louis, 1993, Mosby.
*Precise mechanism not established; this is a presumptive classification.

latex.[49] Avoidance of latex-containing products is currently the recommended approach.[43]

Insect Stings *Hymenoptera* venoms and fire ant stings are responsible for significant anaphylactic morbidity and mortality. The first recorded fatality caused by anaphylaxis was likely the hieroglyphic-documented death of King Menes of Egypt in 2641 BC, when he succumbed to the sting of a wasp or hornet. Stinging *Hymenoptera* insects account for approximately 40 deaths annually in the United States, whereas several more deaths probably go unrecognized and unreported.[8,50,51] Allergic sensitization to *Hymenoptera* has been reported in 0.4% to 4% of the general population.[52,53] The principal offenders (in decreasing order of frequency) are the yellow jackets, honeybees, wasps, and yellow and bald-faced hornets. The imported fire ant has become a very significant pest responsible for anaphylaxis, spreading from the Atlantic and Gulf coasts inland.[54,55]

The *Hymenoptera* venoms are complex mixtures of pharmacologically and biochemically active substances. Honeybee venom has been subjected to the greatest amount of research and contains two major enzymes (hyaluronidase and phospholipase A) and other peptides, including a mast cell–degranulating peptide. Yellow jacket venom not only contains phospholipases A and B and hyaluronidase but also kinins. Hornet venom has, in addition, acetylcholine. Wasp venom has not been extensively studied. Fire ant venom is mostly a nonproteinaceous alkaloid suspension containing phospholipase A and hyaluronidase.

Therapeutic Agents Heterologous sera that were used in diphtheria and tetanus equine antitoxins in the past can act as whole antigenic markers. In fact, until the discovery of penicillin, these two therapeutic agents were the most common iatrogenic causes of anaphylaxis in humans. With the advent of human antisera, a marked reduction in the incidence of anaphylactic reactions from these agents has occurred. In fact, no adverse reactions were noted on repeated immunization using human tetanus antisera in approximately 250 patients who had previous anaphylactic reactions to equine tetanus antisera.[56] Equine antisera is still used in the administration of antilymphocyte serum and in the management of venomous snakebites. Although anaphylactic reactions are rare (1:500,000), the equine antiserum should still be diluted and pretested.

Since the development of heterologous insulin hormone therapy for the management of diabetes mellitus, local and systemic allergic complications have been recognized. A large percentage of local reactions were eliminated with the introduction of purified, single-peak pork insulin. With the introduction of Humulin, an insulin preparation prepared from recombinant DNA, the incidence of anaphylaxis and insulin resistance has declined dramatically.

Allergen extracts are used diagnostically in skin testing and therapeutically for immunotherapy (also known as hyposensitization or desensitization). Exposure to therapeutic pollens, by injection or inhalation, can result in local allergic or systemic anaphylactic reactions.[57,58] Administration of extracts of these allergens is the most probable cause of anaphylaxis in humans, although most of these reactions are mild.[59] High-dose therapy, too frequent administration, or inadvertent intravascular injection increases the risk of anaphylaxis with immunotherapy.

Although corticosteroids are used in the management of anaphylaxis, adverse reactions to these medications have been observed after parenteral administration. Skin testing may demonstrate the specific class of steroids responsible for hypersensitivity, and substitution of a different class should be considered.[60]

Local anesthetics occasionally produce adverse reactions. Most of these reactions are not allergic in nature but are related to a direct effect of the medication.[61] True allergic reactions are rare[62] and are most commonly seen with local anesthetics from the ester family (e.g., procaine, tetracaine, benzocaine). Allergic reactions from local anesthetics belonging to the amide family (e.g., lidocaine, bupivacaine, mepivacaine, dibucaine) are extremely rare if they occur at all. Multidose vials of lidocaine contain the preservative methylparaben, which belongs structurally to the ester family. This preservative has been implicated in allergic reactions in patients with a history of previous lidocaine hypersensitivity.[63] Pure lidocaine is readily available in every ED as 2% cardiac lidocaine (100 mg/5 ml), which contains no methylparaben preservative.

Anaphylactic reactions have occurred after the administration of egg embryo–grown vaccines, including the combined measles, mumps, and rubella (MMR), yellow fever, and influenza vaccines. If the patient is able to tolerate eggs orally, even if the patient has previously experienced anaphylaxis and shows a positive skin test to eggs, it is likely that the patient will tolerate the vaccines.

Immune Complex–Mediated Agents

Anaphylactic-type reactions are uncommon complications after the administration of whole blood and immunoglobulins. This is particularly relevant in IgA-deficient patients exposed to multiple transfusions; these patients may have produced antibodies to IgA present in previous transfusions. With subsequent transfusions, an antigen (IgA)-anti-IgA antibody (IgG) immune complex forms, and subsequent activation of the complement cascade may occur.

Nonimmunologic Activators

Many of the opiate analgesics can be potent agents of histamine release. It is unclear how much cross-sensitivity is present among these agents. Although most of these reactions appear to be a result of direct histamine release, some evidence exists that, rarely, some reactions are true IgE-mediated reactions.[64,65]

RCM commonly cause anaphylactoid reactions. They are hypertonic, water-soluble compounds that are administered by intravascular or intrathecal injection. The older hyperosmolar agents can cause a reaction in up to 5.6% of the patients, with fatalities in up to 0.01%.[66] Subsequent studies put the risks of a serious reaction to high osmolar contrast media at 0.2%, with 11.7 fatalities per million injections.[11,67,68] The newer lower osmolar agents cause allergic reactions much less frequently. The risk of a serious reaction is approximately 0.04%,[11] with an estimated 3.9 fatalities per million injections.[68]

The pathophysiology of RCM reactions is uncertain but is believed to be nonimmunologic. Suggested mechanisms include direct histamine release,[69] alternative complement pathway activation,[70] and activation of the contact system.[71]

Modulators of Arachidonic Acid

Interruption of arachidonic metabolism by aspirin and other NSAIDs has been postulated as the mechanism responsible for anaphylactoid reactions resulting from these agents,[35,72] although AA modulation, anaphylatoxin generation, and direct histamine release may all be partially responsible. The incidence of anaphylactoid reactions to aspirin and NSAIDs varies widely, depending on the population. The incidence of anaphylactoid reactions due to aspirin can range from 0.9% in a normal population to 97% in adults with asthma and rhinosinusitis or nasal polyps.[72] Most aspirin-sensitive patients can tolerate sodium salicylate or acetaminophen as aspirin substitutes.[73] Of note, one of many food additives, tartrazine (foods, drugs, and cosmetics [FD&C] yellow dye Number 5), is a stable azo-coloring agent present in thousands of foods and drugs in the United States.[74] The exact mechanism of tartrazine sensitivity is unknown, although modulation of AA metabolism and several other theories have been proposed.[75]

Exercise-Induced Anaphylaxis

Exercise has been increasingly recognized as a causative factor in certain anaphylactic-like incidents.[76,77] The mechanism remains unclear, but mast cell and basophil mediator release has been demonstrated. These patients are generally dedicated athletes, who may have personal or family atopic history. Exercise-induced anaphylaxis has been demonstrated in some cases to depend on previous food ingestion to which the patient may be subclinically sensitive.[78,79] Provocative foods, if identified, should be avoided. Patients should discontinue the exercise when they experience pruritus. When exercise is continued beyond this point, clinical deterioration is likely in susceptible individuals. Prophylactic treatment with an antihistamine as a single agent or in combination with other agents may be helpful. Avoidance of precipitating factors, modification of exercise, and use of a self-injectable epinephrine kit have been recommended for patients with exercise-induced anaphylaxis.[76]

Idiopathic Anaphylaxis

IA refers to mediator-induced anaphylaxis without a discernible cause. In the United States, it is estimated that 20,000 to 47,000 patients annually see allergists for signs and symptoms of IA.[80] A specific causative agent cannot be found historically, and laboratory studies including a complete blood count (CBC) with differential leukocyte count, erythrocyte sedimentation rate, blood chemistries, complement levels, C1 esterase inhibitor levels, serum and urinary histamine levels, urinalysis, skin testing, and occasionally more specialized tests when clinically indicated are all nondiagnostic. Food diaries and efforts to find systemic disease are often fruitless. Although IA may be life-threatening, it is usually responsive to conventional therapies including antihistamines, sympathomimetics, and steroids.[81] Some cases of IA may be conversion disorders.[82] The overall prognosis for IA is good, but certain patients may experience recurrent IA despite intensive prophylactic administration of antihistamines, sympathomimetics, or steroids.[81,83]

CLINICAL FEATURES

Anaphylaxis in humans primarily affects the cutaneous, respiratory, cardiovascular, and gastrointestinal systems. The clinical expression depends on the degree of hypersensitivity; the quantity, route, and rate of antigen exposure; the pattern of mediator release; and the target organ sensitivity and responsiveness. Most anaphylactic reactions will become clinically evident within seconds to minutes after exposure to the triggering antigen, although a delay of several hours or even days occurs in rare situations. Anaphylactic reactions vary from mild to fatal. In general, the sooner the clinical syndrome manifests after antigenic exposure, the more severe the reaction will be. Anaphylactic reactions after parenteral antigenic exposure are usually more immediate in onset, more rapidly progressive, and more severe in quality than those occurring after topical or oral exposures. Rapid progression from mild urticaria and bronchospasm to shock or asphyxia may occur in minutes. In fact, any systemic manifestation must be considered the forerunner of a potentially lethal process. In fatal cases of anaphylaxis, cardiovascular and respiratory disturbances predominate and usually occur early. Laryngeal edema and circulatory collapse can occur even in the absence of any premonitory warning symptoms or signs. Most fatalities occur within the first 30 minutes after antigenic exposure. The duration of the reaction is variable. Appropriate immediate therapy may terminate the syndrome quickly, or mild systemic manifestations may last up to 24 to 48 hours despite immediate therapy.

The first clinical manifestation of anaphylaxis usually involves the skin; the patient experiences generalized warmth and tingling of the face, mouth, upper chest, palms, soles, or the site of antigenic exposure. Pruritus is a nearly universal feature and may be accompanied by generalized flushing and urticaria, and nonpruritic angioedema may also be evident initially. This may be followed by mild to severe respiratory distress. The patient may describe a cough; a sense of chest tightness, dyspnea, and wheeze from bronchospasm; or throat tightness, dyspnea, odynophagia, or hoarseness associated with laryngeal edema or oropharyngeal angioedema. Hypotension or dysrhythmias may manifest as light-headedness or syncope. Any of these clinical patterns may occur independently of, in combination with, or in association with nasal congestion and sneezing; ocular itching and tearing; cramping abdominal pain with nausea, vomiting, diarrhea, and tenesmus; incontinence; pelvic pain; headache; or a sense of impending doom. The physical examination may reveal tachypnea, tachycardia, and hypotension. Laryngeal stridor, hypersalivation, hoarseness, and angioedema indicate upper airway obstruction, whereas coughing, wheezing, rhonchi, and diminished air flow suggest lower respiratory tract bronchoconstriction. Tachycardia and hypotension suggest circulatory collapse. Commonly observed dysrhythmias include sinus tachycardia, premature atrial and ventricular contractions, nodal rhythm, and atrial fibrillation. Other electrocardiographic (ECG) changes include nonspecific and ischemic ST-T wave changes, right ventricular strain, and intraventricular conduction defects. The patient may have a depressed level of consciousness, but this is rarely due to seizure activity. Urticaria, angioedema, rhinitis, and conjunctivitis may be evident. A summary of the observed clinical manifestations of anaphylaxis along with their related pathophysiology is presented in Table 113-1.

DIFFERENTIAL CONSIDERATIONS

The diagnosis of an anaphylactic reaction depends largely on recognizing the constellation of clinical manifestations that occur abruptly after suspected antigenic exposure. The diagnosis is easy to make in the patient who has urticaria, laryngeal edema, and circulatory collapse 15 minutes after sustaining a bee sting. When only a portion of the full syndrome is present, it may be difficult to recognize the symptoms as an anaphylactic reaction.

Table 113-1. Clinical Manifestations of Anaphylaxis and Related Pathophysiology

Organ system	Reaction	Symptoms	Signs	Pathophysiology
Respiratory tract				
Upper	Rhinitis	Nasal congestion Nasal itching Sneezing	Nasal mucosal edema Rhinorrhea	Increased vascular permeability Vasodilation Stimulation of nerve endings
	Laryngeal edema	Dyspnea Hoarseness Throat tightness Hypersalivation	Laryngeal stridor Supraglottic and glottic edema	As above, plus increased exocrine gland secretions
Lower	Bronchospasm	Cough Wheezing Retrosternal tightness Dyspnea	Cough Wheeze, rhonchi Tachypnea Respiratory distress Cyanosis	As above, plus bronchiole smooth muscle contraction
Cardiovascular system	Circulatory collapse	Light-headedness Generalized weakness Syncope Ischemic chest pain	Tachycardia Hypotension Shock	Increased vascular permeability Vasodilation Loss of vasomotor tone Increased venous capacitance
	Dysrhythmias	As above, plus palpitations	ECG changes: Tachycardia Nonspecific and ischemic ST-T wave changes Right ventricular strain Premature atrial and ventricular contractions Nodal rhythm Atrial fibrillation	Decreased cardiac output Decreased mediator-induced myocardial suppression Decreased effective plasma volume Decreased preload Decreased afterload Hypoxia and ischemia Dysrhythmias Iatrogenic effects of drugs used in treatment Preexisting heart disease
	Cardiac arrest		Pulseless ECG changes: Ventricular fibrillation Asystole	

Skin	Urticaria	Pruritus Tingling and warmth Flushing Hives	Urticaria Diffuse erythema	Increased vascular permeability Vasodilation
	Angioedema	Nonpruritic extremity, periorbital and perioral swelling	Nonpitting edema, frequently asymmetrical	Increased vascular permeability Vasodilation
Eye	Conjunctivitis	Ocular itching Increased lacrimation Red eye	Conjunctival inflammation	Stimulation of nerve endings
Gastrointestinal tract		Dysphagia Cramping abdominal pain Nausea and vomiting Diarrhea (rarely bloody) Tenesmus	Nonspecific	Increased mucus secretions Gastrointestinal smooth muscle contraction
Miscellaneous				
Central nervous system		Apprehension	Anxiety	Secondary to cerebral hypoxia and hypoperfusion
		Sense of impending doom Headache Confusion	Seizures (rarely) Coma (late)	Vasodilation
Hematologic	Fibrinolysis and disseminated intravascular coagulation	Abnormal bleeding and bruising	Mucous membrane bleeding, disseminated intravascular coagulation	Mediator recruitment and activation
			Increased uterine tone Vaginal bleeding	Uterine smooth muscle contraction
Genitourinary		Pelvic pain Vaginal bleeding Urinary incontinence	Urinary incontinence	Bladder smooth muscle contraction

Stridor

In the absence of oropharyngeal angioedema or other clinical manifestations of anaphylaxis, the diagnosis of laryngeal edema should be confirmed by visualization (direct or indirect laryngoscopy) to exclude epiglottitis and supraglottitis, retropharyngeal or peritonsillar abscess, laryngeal spasm, foreign body aspiration, or tumor.

Bronchospasm

Acute asthma may be accompanied by other signs and symptoms of anaphylaxis. Exercise-induced anaphylaxis should be differentiated from exercise-induced asthma, because the former will usually be accompanied by pruritus and other systemic manifestations.

Syncope

Vasovagal syncope is the most common differential diagnosis in the patient arriving with collapse as a result of parenteral administration of an antigen. Classically the patient has bradycardia, hypotension, and pallor as opposed to the tachycardia, hypotension, and diaphoresis usually associated with anaphylaxis. The absence of any other clinical manifestations of anaphylaxis, along with history of stress, pain, and previous episodes of simple faints, helps point toward the diagnosis of vasovagal syncope. Other important causes of syncope such as seizure, hypoglycemia, or cardiac dysrhythmia may need to be ruled out.

Shock

Clinically, septic and spinal shock may be similar to anaphylactic shock if vasodilation is present. Cardiogenic, hypovolemic, or hemorrhagic shock would more likely be seen with cold, clammy skin. Clues from further history or examination will help differentiate these causes. Because anaphylactic shock can progress to cardiogenic shock, measurement of central venous pressures may be necessary.

Angioedema

Angioedema is nonpruritic, well demarcated, localized, nonpitting edema of deep subcutaneous tissue, involving predominantly the periorbital, perioral, and intraoral regions of the face and extremities. Hereditary angioedema (HAE) is an autosomal dominant condition caused by C1 esterase inhibitor deficiency or functional deficiency, which biochemically is confirmed by low levels of C4 and C1 esterase inhibitor activity. The cardinal symptoms and signs of HAE include edema of the airway, face, or extremities and abdominal pain associated with nausea, vomiting, and diarrhea. These clinical manifestations may occur singly or in combination. Trauma and stress are common precipitating factors. Life-threatening acute attacks do not respond satisfactorily to treatment with epinephrine, antihistamines, or steroids. Active airway management is the mainstay of treatment. Fresh frozen plasma contains C1 inhibitor and is effective in abolishing acute attacks. Epinephrine in large doses may be effective, although it should be used with caution.

The angioedema associated with angiotensin-converting enzyme inhibitors has an incidence of 0.1% to 0.2% and a predilection for the tongue, lips, and laryngeal soft tissue.[84,85] The pathophysiology is thought to be prevention of the metabolism of bradykinin and substance P, both of which are potent mediators of tissue inflammation.[86]

Urticaria

Urticaria is discussed in Chapter 114. Important considerations for nonallergic causes of urticaria include occult infections, carcinoid syndrome, mastocytosis, and pheochromocytoma.

MANAGEMENT

Prevention

Spending a few additional minutes with the patient before discharge, obtaining an allergy history, offering environmental modifications, and educating the patient on initiating treatment for recurrence may decrease morbidity and mortality from subsequent episodes of anaphylaxis (Box 113-3). Avoidance of antigens to which the patient is likely to be sensitive is the most important preventive measure a patient can take. Obtaining a thorough personal and family drug allergy and atopic history is crucial before instituting any drug therapy, and all drugs should be correctly identified before being administered. When a drug is prescribed, a definite medical indication must be present. Whenever possible, medications should be administered orally rather than parenterally to decrease the severity of a systemic anaphylactic reaction should the patient react adversely.

Physicians who administer antigenic compounds in their medical practice must be prepared to manage an anaphylactic reaction, and resuscitation equipment should be readily available. Because most anaphylactic reactions that follow parenteral administration begin within 30 minutes, patients should be observed during this period, discharged only if completely asymptomatic, and given a warning to return for subsequent symptoms.[3]

Human antiserum is now available for rabies, tetanus, and

Box 113-3 Prevention of Anaphylaxis and Anaphylactic Death

1. Get thorough drug allergy and atopic history.
2. Check all drugs for proper labeling.
3. Give drug orally rather than parenterally when possible.
4. Give drug in distal extremity if possible when parenteral route necessary.
5. Always have resuscitation equipment available when administering antigenic compounds.
6. Ensure that patients wait in ED 30 minutes after drug administration.
7. Use unrelated drugs when feasible in susceptible population.
8. When antiserum essential, use human if available.
9. If heterologous serum essential, always perform pretest.
10. Predisposed patients should carry warning identification (Medic-Alert, wallet ID).
11. Predisposed patients are taught self-injection of epinephrine, and patients are instructed to carry treatment kit at all times.
12. Patients should avoid known antigens (stinging insects, foods, antibiotics).
13. Perform skin test and consider hyposensitization immunotherapy when appropriate (see section on stinging insect anaphylaxis).
14. Pretreat with antihistamines, steroids if appropriate (see section on RCM reactions).

diphtheria; however, heterologous equine antisera is still used (e.g., for snake bites). Intradermal pretesting should be performed before treatment if time permits, as outlined in the product monographs. However, even pretesting solution can precipitate an anaphylactic reaction.

Predisposed patients who have experienced a moderate or severe anaphylactic reaction should be taught self-administration of an oral antihistamine (e.g., diphenhydramine hydrochloride [Benadryl]) on known exposure, and self-injection of epinephrine (e.g., Epi-Pen, Ana-Kit) at the first indication of allergic symptoms or signs. Epinephrine injection kits have a limited shelf life, which is prolonged by refrigeration. These kits should be readily available at all times; therefore a kit in the home, at work or school, in the patient's purse or briefcase, and in the patient's automobile would be sufficient for most circumstances (Box 113-4). Predisposed patients should be strongly encouraged to carry warning identification stating their hypersensitivity (Medic-Alert bracelet, wallet card).

Pretreatment with antihistamines and steroids significantly decreases the frequency and severity of anaphylactoid reactions in patients who have sustained a prior reaction after injection of RCM. Skin testing and hyposensitization immunotherapy by an allergist are an appropriate way to minimize the frequency and severity of subsequent anaphylactic reactions from bee stings in an appropriately sensitive population.

Prehospital

When a susceptible patient is reexposed to an antigen to which there has been previous reaction, 50 mg of oral diphenhydramine hydrochloride (Benadryl) should be taken if available. At the first signs of any clinical manifestations of anaphylaxis, the patient should self-administer epinephrine if available (adult dose, 0.3 ml of 1:1000 SC; pediatric dose, 0.01 ml/kg of 1:1000 SC). Susceptible patients may even use aerosolized epinephrine via a metered-dose inhaler (e.g., Primatene Mist, Medihaler-Epi) to counteract the effects of laryngeal edema, bronchoconstriction, and other manifestations of anaphylaxis.[87] Multiple inhalations (e.g., 10 to 20 doses, resulting in the inhalation of 1.5 to 3 mg of epinephrine) produce therapeutic plasma levels, with the advantages of ease of administration, rapid absorption, and locally high epinephrine levels in the upper and lower airways. Epinephrine must be used with caution in the elderly and in those with a history of cardiac or hypertensive problems.

Prehospital personnel may be required to resuscitate a moribund patient using basic life support (BLS). Their first priority should be to establish and maintain ventilation.

Local measures to decrease antigen absorption from an extremity include dependent positioning of the extremity, ice to vasoconstrict locally, and application of a loose tourniquet to obstruct the venous and lymphatic circulation. The tourniquet should be released for 1 of every 10 minutes. If an insect stinger remains the wound should not be squeezed, because this may inject more venom into the patient. The stinger should be removed gently with instruments, avoiding disturbance of the venom apparatus.

In addition to usual resuscitative efforts, the early administration of epinephrine is a mainstay of treatment. The clinical situation will determine whether subcutaneous, intramuscular, intravenous, intraosseous, or sublingual administration of epinephrine should be used.

Box 113-4 Epinephrine Injection Kits for Emergency Treatment of Stinging Insect Anaphylaxis

Epi-Pen: delivers 0.3 ml 1:1000 (0.3 mg epinephrine)
Epi-Pen Junior: delivers 0.3 ml 1:2000 (0.15 mg epinephrine)
Ana-Kit: delivers up to 0.6 ml 1:1000, 0.3 ml at one time (total possible: 0.6 mg epinephrine)
The Epi-Pen and Epi-Pen Junior are spring-loaded automatic injectors and are distributed by Center Laboratories (Port Washington, NY). Ana-Kit is capable of delivering fractional doses and is distributed by Hollister Laboratories (Spokane, Wash).

Modified from Valentine MD: Insect sting allergy in children: prevention of future reactions. In Lichtenstein LM, Fauci AS, editors: *Current therapy in allergy and immunology,* Burlington, Ontario, Canada, 1983, BC Decker.

Emergency Department

The goals of treatment should be to slow or reverse the pathophysiologic process in order to prevent or reverse the clinical complications of anaphylaxis (see Table 113-1). Institution of these therapeutic modalities must be initiated quickly and simultaneously when possible. Most anaphylactic fatalities are related to asphyxia from upper respiratory tract obstruction, acute respiratory failure from bronchospasm, or cardiovascular collapse. Attention must therefore be focused on rapidly reversing respiratory and cardiovascular disturbances. Epinephrine and diphenhydramine hydrochloride, as detailed in the following, should be administered early in most anaphylactic cases. All patients should have supplemental oxygen administered, large-bore (14- or 16-gauge) intravenous lines inserted to infuse crystalloid solutions, and continuous cardiac monitoring. A large volume of crystalloid fluid may be required to reverse the hypotension associated with anaphylaxis.

Upper airway obstruction from laryngeal edema or angioedema can progress rapidly. While preparing for more definitive airway management, a chin lift or jaw thrust will help obtain a patent airway. Suctioning the oropharynx of excess secretions may be necessary. A nasopharyngeal or oropharyngeal airway may aid in maintaining a patent airway at this stage. Racemic epinephrine, delivered as a 2.25% solution (0.5 ml placed in a nebulizer in 2.5 ml of normal saline), may be a temporizing measure.

The success rate of intubation will be improved when it is performed early and before soft-tissue swelling progresses. Oral endotracheal intubation is the route of choice, because significant anatomic distortion may be present as a result of edema. Sedation and paralysis should be used with caution, because a distorted airway may preclude intubation after paralysis. Arterial blood gasses play no role in the decision-making process for the patient in acute respiratory distress. Once a patent airway has been obtained and supplemental oxygen delivered, therapy should focus on relieving the patient's bronchospasm.

Epinephrine Drugs used in the treatment of anaphylaxis either inhibit the release of chemical mediators or reverse the effects of mediators on target tissues. Epinephrine, with its combined α- and β-adrenergic agonist actions, is the first drug of choice in the treatment of anaphylaxis. The α-agonist effects of epinephrine increase peripheral vascular resistance and reverse peripheral vasodilation, vascular permeability, and systemic hypotension. The β-agonist effects of epinephrine produce bronchodilatation, cause positive inotropic and chronotropic cardiac activity, and result in an increased production of intracellular cyclic adenosine monophosphate (cAMP).[88] Epinephrine therefore reverses bronchospasm, stimulates increased cardiac output, and inhibits further mediator release. The α- and β-agonist actions of epinephrine can also be potentially dangerous. Excessive α-agonist activity can result in a hypertensive crisis. Excessive β-agonist activity can increase myocardial oxygen consumption caused by increased wall tension, contractility, and chronotropism, and can result in myocardial ischemia or infarction.[89] Increased automaticity and chronotropism can produce hemodynamically significant supraventricular and ventricular tachydysrhythmias.[90,91] Epinephrine should be used with caution in the elderly and in those with known coronary artery disease, and should be avoided in those patients with life-threatening tachydysrhythmias.

The route of administration chosen depends on the severity of the clinical presentation. Subcutaneous epinephrine is usually effective in those situations in which the clinical manifestations are mild and the patient is normotensive. In the patient with diffuse, generalized urticaria, subcutaneous absorption of epinephrine may be slow and unpredictable, so the intramuscular route should be used.

For subcutaneous and intramuscular injections, the initial dose of epinephrine is 0.01 ml/kg of 1:1000 solution, to a maximum of 0.5 ml of 1:1000 solution (0.5 mg). A fraction of the total dose (0.1 to 0.2 ml) should be administered at the site of antigenic exposure if accessible (such as a bee sting or antigen injection in an extremity).

If the patient demonstrates severe upper airway obstruction, acute respiratory failure, or shock (systolic blood pressure less than 80 mm Hg, not associated with a ventricular tachydysrhythmia), intravenous epinephrine should be administered. The risk of supraventricular, accelerated idioventricular, and ventricular tachydysrhythmias; accelerated hypertension; and myocardial ischemia, including the stunned heart syndrome, is increased by using the intravenous route with epinephrine. Because of these risks, dilution and slow administration is recommended. The initial intravenous dose should be 10 ml of a 1:100,000 dilution of aqueous epinephrine over 10 minutes. This would be equivalent to a 100 µg bolus administered at 10 µg/min. If no improvement is seen, a continuous infusion should be set up. Mixing 1 ml of a 1:1000 dilution of epinephrine in 250 ml of D5/W will result in a concentration of 4 µg/ml. This can be started at 1 µg/min and increased to 4 µg/min if needed. In children and infants, an infusion rate of 0.1 µg/kg/min is advised, increasing in increments of 0.1 µg/kg/min to a maximum of 1.5 µg/kg/min. Continuous cardiac monitoring should be used at all times. If a percutaneous intravenous line cannot be established, alternate routes are available. In addition to the subcutaneous and intramuscular routes of administration, intraosseous or sublingual injection or endotracheal nebulization should be considered. The dosage and concentration guidelines for these routes of administration of epinephrine are the same as those for intravenous administration.

Nebulized β-Agonists Bronchospasm refractory to epinephrine may respond to a nebulized β-agonist such as albuterol sulfate (Ventolin, Proventil, Albuterol) or metaproterenol (Alupent 5%), in recommended doses. Continuous nebulization of the β-agonists may be necessary for persistent bronchospasm. The use of anticholinergic therapy with ipratropium bromide (Atrovent) is an additional option in the management of this problem. Anticholinergic medications decrease cyclic guanosine monophosphate (cGMP) levels, thereby decreasing mediator release and reversing the action of mediators on target tissue cells. Nebulized ipratropium bromide is used in a dose of 0.5 mg (2.5 ml of a 0.02% solution).

Antihistamines Antihistamines should be used in all cases, although their role in severe or persistent anaphylaxis is limited. The antihistamines competitively block the action of circulating histamines at target tissue cell receptors but have no role in decreasing mediator release and have no effect on the leukotrienes. Seven classes of H_1 antihistamines exist, and members of the ethanolamine family, such as diphenhydramine hydrochloride, and the alkylamine family, such as chlorpheniramine maleate (Chlor-Trimeton, Chlor-Tripolon), are potent H_1 antagonists. Diphenhydramine hydrochloride is the most commonly used H_1 antihistamine. The typical dose used is 25 to 50 mg every 4 to 6 hours in adults, or 5 mg/kg/day in divided doses for the pediatric population. Diphenhydramine hydrochloride orally or by intramuscular injection may be the only medication required for mild to moderate reactions. A loading dose of 1 to 2 mg/kg IV to a maximum of 100 mg is recommended for severe reactions, although too large a dose or too-rapid administration can result in marked sedation and hypotension. Chlorpheniramine can be administered to children by the same routes at a standard dose of 10 to 20 mg or 0.35 mg/kg/day in divided doses.

Blockade of H_2 receptors may be beneficial with simultaneous H_1 antihistamine therapy.[91-93] H_2 antagonists may inhibit the effect of histamine on myocardial and peripheral vascular tissue.[94] Cimetidine 300 mg IV, followed by outpatient oral administration of cimetidine 300 mg every 6 hours for 2 days, should be considered for patients with persistent symptoms.

Corticosteroids Corticosteroids have an onset of action of approximately 4 to 6 hours after administration and therefore are of limited benefit in the initial treatment of the rapidly deteriorating anaphylactic patient. Their benefit may be realized in persistent bronchospasm or hypotension. Corticosteroids may also blunt the biphasic reaction of anaphylaxis, although their efficacy is not universal.[95-97] Rare cases of deterioration after corticosteroid administration may be the result of anaphylactic sensitivity to this medication.[60,98] An initial intravenous loading dose of hydrocortisone (Solu-Cortef) 250 mg to 1 g, or methylprednisolone (Solu-Medrol) 125 to 250 mg, followed by oral prednisone over 7 to 10 days, is an acceptable regimen after the anaphylactic episode.

Agents to Maintain Blood Pressure In patients with persistent hypotension despite epinephrine and large volumes of intravenous crystalloid administration, the use of isoncotic colloid solutions such as 5% albumin could be considered, because the increased vascular permeability associated with anaphylaxis is usually transient. If the central venous pressure (CVP) is less than 12 mm Hg, crystalloid and colloid fluids should be continued, and dopamine at 5 μg/kg/min should be considered.

If the CVP is greater than 12 mm Hg, dopamine should be started. Causes of elevated filling pressures other than vascular volume or myocardial dysfunction must be kept in mind (i.e., vasopressor administration, increased intraperitoneal and intrathoracic pressures, vasoconstriction, or pulmonary artery hypertension), and a pulmonary artery catheter to monitor wedge pressure and cardiac output may be required. If pulmonary hypertension exists, hyperventilation, hyperoxygenation, and large doses of steroids should be considered. The use of drugs with primarily α-adrenergic activity, such as norepinephrine and metaraminol, could be considered if all of these measures have failed.

Glucagon Glucagon, with positive inotropic and chronotropic cardiac effects mediated independently of α- and β-receptors, may be helpful. Glucagon is thought to enhance cAMP synthesis, which leads to positive isotropy, chronotropy, and smooth muscle relaxation. Glucagon may be considered not only for patients on β-blockers, but also for those patients resistant to traditional therapy.

The initial dose is 1 mg for adults and 0.5 mg for children subcutaneously, intramuscularly, or intravenously, and the patient may require a glucagon infusion of 1 to 5 mg/hr to sustain its therapeutic effect. Side effects include nausea, vomiting, hypokalemia, and hyperglycemia.

DISPOSITION

Most patients with anaphylaxis respond to early aggressive management. A 24- to 48-hour hospital admission should be considered for those patients who have experienced hypotension, upper airway involvement, prolonged bronchospasm, or other indications of a severe reaction. Although the risk of clinical deterioration after apparently complete resolution of a severe anaphylactic reaction is minimal, symptoms will redevelop in a small proportion of patients 24 to 48 hours after the initial systemic reaction.[95,97] This may be related to the high-molecular-weight neutrophil chemotactic factor (HMW-NCF)–mediated late-phase reaction of the biphasic allergic response, which peaks in 4 to 12 hours and lasts up to 48 hours. Patients taking therapeutic doses of β-blocking medications may be susceptible to a similar rebound once the effects of initial therapeutic intervention wane. Patients with mild to moderate anaphylaxis who respond completely to initial treatment are appropriate for discharge after an observation period of 2 to 6 hours. An oral antihistamine, such as diphenhydramine hydrochloride 25 to 50 mg every 6 hours for 48 hours, may prevent possible relapse. These patients should be instructed to return to the ED if their symptoms recur. They should be warned about the sedating side effects of the antihistamines. Oral cimetidine, 300 mg every 6 hours for 48 hours, may be useful, and patients with initially persistent bronchospasm or hypotension who required initial steroid therapy should be continued on oral prednisone for 7 to 10 days. Patients with initially persistent bronchospasm should continue on a metered-dose β-adrenergic bronchodilator inhalant (e.g., albuterol [Ventolin], metaproterenol [Alupent]).

KEY CONCEPTS

- The hallmark of anaphylaxis is urticaria, but deaths from cardiorespiratory compromise can occur without evidence of dermatologic involvement.
- Mild symptoms must be treated aggressively to prevent progression to more serious forms of anaphylaxis.
- Epinephrine is the appropriate immediate drug of choice for the management of anaphylaxis. Prolonged treatment is required for patients with risk factors such as β-adrenergic blockade
- Prevention of subsequent episodes of anaphylaxis should be a priority for the emergency physician before patient discharge.

REFERENCES

1. Portier P, Richet C: De l'action anaphylatique de certain venins, *C Roy Soc Biol* 54:170, 1902.
2. Yocum MW et al: Epidemiology of anaphylaxis in Olmsted County: a population-based study, *J Allergy Clin Immunol* 104:452-456, 1999.
3. Lieberman P: Anaphylaxis and anaphylactoid reactions. In Middelton E et al, editors: *Allergy: principles and practice,* St Louis, 1998, Mosby.
4. Yocum MW, Klein JS: Emergency room incidence of community onset anaphylaxis, *J Allergy Clin Immunol* 93:302, 1994.
5. Kemp SF et al: Anaphylaxis: a review of 266 cases, *Arch Intern Med* 155:1749-1754, 1995.
6. Yocum MW, Khan DA: Assessment of patients who have experienced anaphylaxis: a 3-year survey, *Mayo Clin Proc* 69:16-23, 1994.
7. Golden DB: Epidemiology of allergy to insect venoms and stings, *Allergy Proc* 10:103-107, 1989.
8. Barnard JH: Studies of 400 *Hymenoptera* sting deaths in the United States, *J Allergy Clin Immunol* 52:259-264, 1973.
9. Settipane GA et al: Aspirin intolerance. II. A prospective study in an atopic and normal population, *J Allergy Clin Immunol* 53:200-204, 1974.
10. Strom BL et al: The effect of indication on hypersensitivity reactions associated with zomepirac sodium and other nonsteroidal antiinflammatory drugs, *Arthritis Rheum* 30:1142-1148, 1987.
11. Katayama H et al: Adverse reactions to ionic and nonionic contrast media. A report from the Japanese Committee on the Safety of Contrast Media, *Radiology* 175:621-628, 1990.
12. Yunginger JW: Natural rubber latex allergy. In Middelton E et al, editors: *Allergy: principles and practice,* St Louis, 1998, Mosby.
13. Bernardini R et al: Prevalence and risk factors of latex sensitization in an unselected pediatric population, *J Allergy Clin Immunol* 101:621-625, 1998.
14. Turjanmaa K: Incidence of immediate allergy to latex gloves in hospital personnel, *Contact Dermatitis* 17:270-275, 1987.
15. Yassin MS et al: Latex allergy in hospital employees, *Ann Allergy* 72:245-249, 1994.
16. Shearer WT, Fleisher TA: The immune system. In Middelton E et al, editors: *Allergy: principles and practice,* St Louis, 1998, Mosby.
17. Sell S: Immunopathology. In Rich RR et al, editors: *Clinical immunology: principles and practice,* St Louis, 1996, Mosby.
18. Okazaki M et al: Food-dependent exercise-induced anaphylaxis, *Intern Med* 31:1052-1055, 1992.
19. Austen KF, Metcalfe DD: Anaphylactic syndrome. In Frank MM et al, editors: *Samter's immunologic diseases,* Boston, 1995, Little, Brown and Company.
20. Kaliner M et al: Effects of infused histamine: correlation of plasma histamine levels and symptoms, *J Allergy Clin Immunol* 69:283-289, 1982.
21. Morel DR et al: Leukotrienes, thromboxane A2, and prostaglandins during systemic anaphylaxis in sheep, *Am J Physiol* 261:H782-H792, 1991.
22. Simons FER: Antihistamines. In Middelton E et al, editors: *Allergy: principles and practice,* St Louis, 1998, Mosby.
23. Lieberman P: The use of antihistamines in the prevention and treatment of anaphylaxis and anaphylactoid reactions, *J Allergy Clin Immunol* 86:684-686, 1990.

24. Schwartz LB: Mast cells and their role in urticaria, *J Am Acad Dermatol* 25:190-203, 1991.
25. Lohman IC, Halonen M: The effects of combined histamine and platelet-activating factor antagonism on systemic anaphylaxis induced by immunoglobulin E in the rabbit *Am Rev Respir Dis* 147:1223-1228, 1993.
26. Felix SB et al: Characterization of cardiovascular events mediated by platelet activating factor during systemic anaphylaxis, *J Cardiovasc Pharmacol* 15:987-997, 1990.
27. Fawcett WJ et al: Oxygen transport and haemodynamic changes during an anaphylactoid reaction, *Anaesth Intensive Care* 22:300-303, 1994.
28. Delage C, Irey NS: Anaphylactic deaths: a clinicopathologic study of 43 cases, *J Forensic Sci* 17:525-540, 1972.
29. Castillo R et al: Food hypersensitivity among adult patients: epidemiological and clinical aspects, *Allergol Immunopathol (Madr)* 24:93-97, 1996.
30. Pumphrey RS, Stanworth SJ: The clinical spectrum of anaphylaxis in north-west England, *Clin Exp Allergy* 26:1364-1370, 1996.
31. Wuthrich B: Adverse reactions to food additives, *Ann Allergy* 71:379-384, 1993.
32. Wuthrich B, Huwyler T: [Asthma due to disulfites], *Schweiz Med Wochenschr* 119:1177-1184, 1989.
33. Trevino RJ: Immunology of foods, *Otolaryngol Head Neck Surg* 95:171-176, 1986.
34. Waldbott GL: Anaphylactic death from penicillin, *JAMA* 139:526, 1949.
35. Idsoe O et al: Nature and extent of penicillin side-reactions, with particular reference to fatalities from anaphylactic shock, *Bull World Health Organ* 38:159-188, 1968.
36. Patterson R, Anderson J: Allergic reactions to drugs and biologic agents, *JAMA* 248:2637-2645, 1982.
37. Stark BJ et al: Acute and chronic desensitization of penicillin-allergic patients using oral penicillin, *J Allergy Clin Immunol* 79:523-532, 1987.
38. Miranda A et al: Cross-reactivity between a penicillin and a cephalosporin with the same side chain, *J Allergy Clin Immunol* 98:671-677, 1996.
39. Sastre J et al: Clinical cross-reactivity between amoxicillin and cephadroxil in patients allergic to amoxicillin and with good tolerance of penicillin, *Allergy* 51:383-386, 1996.
40. Anderson JA: Cross-sensitivity to cephalosporins in patients allergic to penicillin, *Pediatr Infect Dis J* 5:557-561, 1986.
41. Novembre E et al: The prevalence of latex allergy in children seen in a university hospital allergy clinic, *Allergy* 52:101-105, 1997.
42. Hunt LW et al: An epidemic of occupational allergy to latex involving health care workers, *J Occup Environ Med* 37:1204-1209, 1995.
43. Woods JA et al: Natural rubber latex allergy: spectrum, diagnostic approach, and therapy, *J Emerg Med* 15:71-85, 1997.
44. Theissen U et al: IgE-mediated hypersensitivity to latex in childhood, *Allergy* 52:665-669, 1997.
45. Kim KT, Hussain H: Prevalence of food allergy in 137 latex-allergic patients, *Allergy Asthma Proc* 20:95-97, 1999.
46. Warshaw EM: Latex allergy, *J Am Acad Dermatol* 3:1-24, 1998.
47. Kurup VP et al: Latex antigens induce IgE and eosinophils in mice, *Int Arch Allergy Immunol* 103:370-377, 1994.
48. Dibs SD, Baker MD: Anaphylaxis in children: a 5-year experience, *Pediatrics* 99:E7, 1997.
49. Patterson LJ, Milne B: Latex anaphylaxis causing heart block: role of ranitidine, *Can J Anaesth* 46:776-778, 1999.
50. Johansson B et al: Human fatalities caused by wasp and bee stings in Sweden, *Int J Legal Med* 104:99-103, 1991.
51. Benecke M, Seifert B: [Forensic entomology exemplified by a homicide. A combined stain and postmortem time analysis], *Arch Kriminol* 204:52-60, 1999.
52. Fernandez J et al: Epidemiological study of the prevalence of allergic reactions to *Hymenoptera* in a rural population in the Mediterranean area, *Clin Exp Allergy* 29:1069-1074, 1999.
53. Novembre E et al: Epidemiology of insect venom sensitivity in children and its correlation to clinical and atopic features, *Clin Exp Allergy* 28:834-838, 1998.
54. Rhoades RB et al: Survey of fatal anaphylactic reactions to imported fire ant stings. Report of the Fire Ant Subcommittee of the American Academy of Allergy and Immunology, *J Allergy Clin Immunol* 84:159-162, 1989.
55. deShazo RD, Soto-Aguilar M: Reactions to imported fire ant stings, *Allergy Proc* 14:13-16, 1993.
56. Jacobs RL et al: Adverse reactions to tetanus toxoid, *JAMA* 247:40-42, 1982.
57. Yeates DB et al: Bronchial and alveolar allergen-induced anaphylaxis and the stimulation of bronchial mucociliary clearance in ragweed-sensitized dogs, *Proc Assoc Am Physicians* 109:440-452, 1997.
58. Lang GM et al: Potential therapeutic efficacy of allergen-monomethoxypolyethylene glycol conjugates for in vivo inactivation of sensitized mast cells responsible for common allergies and asthma, *Int Arch Allergy Immunol* 113:58-60, 1997.
59. Patterson R, Valentine M: Anaphylaxis and related allergic emergencies including reactions due to insect stings, *JAMA* 248:2632-2636, 1982.
60. McNamara RM: Anaphylaxis after intravenous corticosteroid administration, *J Emerg Med* 4:213-215, 1986.
61. Aldrete JA, Johnson DA: Allergy to local anesthetics, *JAMA* 207:356-357, 1969.
62. Fisher MM, Bowey CJ: Alleged allergy to local anaesthetics, *Anaesth Intensive Care* 25:611-614, 1997.
63. Kajimoto Y et al: Anaphylactoid skin reactions after intravenous regional anaesthesia using 0.5% prilocaine with or without preservative—a double-blind study, *Acta Anaesthesiol Scand* 39:782-784, 1995.
64. Fisher MM et al: Anaphylactoid reactions to narcotic analgesics, *Clin Rev Allergy* 9:309-318, 1991.
65. Harle DG et al: Anaphylaxis following administration of papaveretum. Case report: implication of IgE antibodies that react with morphine and codeine, and identification of an allergenic determinant, *Anesthesiology* 71:489-494, 1989.
66. Shehadi WH: Adverse reactions to intravascularly administered contrast media: a comprehensive study based on a prospective survey, *Am J Roentgenol Radium Ther Nucl Med* 124:145-152, 1975.
67. Mishkin MM: Contrast media safety: what do we know and how do we know it? *Am J Cardiol* 66:34F-36F, 1990.
68. Henry DA et al: The safety and cost-effectiveness of low osmolar contrast media. Can economic analysis determine the real worth of a new technology? *Med J Aust* 154:766-772, 1991.
69. Pinet A et al: Evaluation of histamine release following intravenous injection of ionic and nonionic contrast media, *Invest Radiol* 23:S174-S177, 1988.
70. Siegle RL et al: Iodinated contrast material: studies relating to complement activation, atopy, cellular association, and antigenicity, *Invest Radiol* 15:S13-S17, 1980.
71. Freyria AM, Lasser EC: Primers of contact system activity in asthmatic patients and contrast material reactors, *Invest Radiol* 23:S197-S199, 1988.
72. Manning ME: Reactions to aspirin and other nonsteroidal anti-inflammatory drugs, *Allergy Clin North Am* 12:611-631, 1992.
73. Mathison DA et al: Precipitating factors in asthma. Aspirin, sulfites, and other drugs and chemicals, *Chest* 87:50S-54S, 1985.
74. Dipalma JR: Tartrazine sensitivity, *Am Fam Physician* 42:1347-1350, 1990.
75. Anderson JA: Milestones marking the knowledge of adverse reactions to food in the decade of the 1980s, *Ann Allergy* 72:143-154, 1994.
76. Volcheck GW, Li JT: Exercise-induced urticaria and anaphylaxis, *Mayo Clin Proc* 72:140-147, 1997.
77. Hough DO, Dec KL: Exercise-induced asthma and anaphylaxis, *Sports Med* 18:162-172, 1994.
78. Caffarelli C et al: Food related, exercise induced anaphylaxis, *Arch Dis Child* 75:141-144, 1996.
79. Caffarelli C: Exercise-induced anaphylaxis related to cuttlefish intake, *Eur J Pediatr* 155:1025-1026, 1996.
80. Patterson R et al: Idiopathic anaphylaxis: an attempt to estimate the incidence in the United States, *Arch Intern Med* 155:869-871, 1995.
81. Krasnick J et al: Idiopathic anaphylaxis: long-term follow-up, cost, and outlook, *Allergy* 51:724-731, 1996.
82. Choy AC et al: Undifferentiated somatoform idiopathic anaphylaxis: nonorganic symptoms mimicking idiopathic anaphylaxis, *J Allergy Clin Immunol* 96:893-900, 1995.
83. Patterson R et al: Algorithms for the diagnosis and management of idiopathic anaphylaxis, *Ann Allergy* 71:40-44, 1993.
84. Slater EE et al: Clinical profile of angio-edema associated with ACE inhibition, *JAMA* 260:967, 1988.

85. Roberts JR, Wuerz RC: Clinical characteristics of angiotensin converting enzyme inhibitor-induced angioedema, *Ann Emerg Med* 20:555, 1991.
86. Anderson MW, deShazo RD: Studies of the mechanism of ACE inhibitor associated angioedema: the effect of an ACE inhibitor on cutaneous response to bradykinin, codeine, and histamine, *J Allergy Clin Immunol* 85:856, 1990.
87. Heilborn H et al: Comparison of subcutaneous injection and high-dose inhalation of epinephrine: implications for self-treatment to prevent anaphylaxis, *J Allergy Clin Immunol* 78:1174, 1986.
88. Horach A et al: Severe myocardial ischemia induced by intravenous adrenaline, *BMJ* 286:519, 1983.
89. Sullivan TJ: Cardiac disorders in penicillin-induced anaphylaxis: association with intravenous epinephrine therapy, *JAMA* 248:2161, 1982.
90. Fischer MM: Clinical observations on the pathophysiology and treatment of anaphylactic cardiac collapse, *Anaesth Intensive Care* 14:17, 1986.
91. Dimlich RVW: Histamine antagonists in the treatment of shock hyperglycemia in the rat, *Ann Emerg Med* 14:91, 1985.
92. Runge JW et al: Histamine antagonists in the treatment of acute allergic reactions, *Ann Emerg Med* 21:237, 1992.
93. Lieberman P: The use of antihistamines in the treatment of anaphylaxis and anaphylactoid reactions, *J Allergy Clin Immunol* 86:684, 1990.
94. Schellenberg RR et al: H_2 antagonist inhibits increases in heart rate and norepinephrine by histamine (abstract), *J Allergy Clin Immunol* 83:309, 1989.
95. Popa VT, Lerner SA: Biphasic systemic anaphylactic reactions: three illustrative cases, *Ann Allergy* 53:151, 1984.
96. Stark BJ, Sullivan TJ: Biphasic and protracted anaphylaxis, *J Allergy Clin Immunol* 78:76, 1986.
97. Douglas DM et al: Biphasic systemic anaphylaxis: an inpatient and outpatient study, *J Allergy Clin Immunol* 93:977, 1994.
98. Baumgartner TG et al: Suspected anaphylaxis methylprednisolone injection: case report and literature review, *Am J Clin Nutr* 10:44, 1983.

114 Dermatologic Presentations

Rita K. Cydulka
Mary H. Stewart

PERSPECTIVE

Skin conditions and complaints account for an estimated 4% to 12% of all ED visits.[1,2] In addition to medical and family history, three factors are particularly important: onset and evolution of the skin problem, symptomatology, and prior treatment. To perform an adequate physical examination, the patient must be undressed and adequate lighting must be present. The scalp, mouth, and nails must be thoroughly examined. Although the examination depends largely on inspection, the skin should be palpated to assess the texture, consistency, and tenderness of the lesions.

Skin lesions may be divided into growths and rashes. Growths are subdivided into epidermal, pigmented, and dermal or subcutaneous proliferative processes. Rashes may be divided into two groups depending on whether the epidermis is involved. Lesions and rashes with epidermal involvement include eczematous rashes, scaling, vesicular, papular, pustular, and hypopigmented rashes. Rashes without epidermal involvement include erythema, purpura, and induration. The diagnosis is aided by the configuration of the lesions and distribution on the body's surface. Occasionally a configuration is specific for a disease; however, the morphology of the primary lesion is usually given more diagnostic weight (Table 114-1). Finally, many skin diseases have preferential areas of involvement, so the location of the eruption may aid in diagnosis.

Cutaneous eruptions can be manifestations of either dermatologic disease or underlying systemic illness. The former is by no means less significant than the latter. The fact that a disease is limited to the skin does not mean it cannot present a life threat.

SCALES, PLAQUES, AND PATCHES

Fungal Infection

Principles of Disease The dermatophytoses are superficial fungal infections that are limited to the skin. A variety of lesions may occur, but the most common are scaling, erythematous papules, plaques, and patches, which often have a serpiginous or wormlike border.[3] Dermatophytes generally grow best in excessive heat and moisture and grow only in the keratin or outer layer of the skin, nails, and hair. Keratin tends to accumulate in body folds, such as between toes, in the inguinal area, the axilla, and the inframammary areas. With the exception of tinea capitis, dermatophyte infections are not markedly contagious.[3]

Any eruption thought to be a dermatophyte infection can be examined under the microscope in a potassium hydroxide (KOH) preparation. The specimen is examined for the characteristic branching hyphae of the dermatophytes or the short, thick hyphae and clustered spores of tinea versicolor.[4] Affected hair, nail, or scales may be cultured using Sabouraud agar incubated at room temperature for 2 to 3 weeks.[5]

Tinea Capitis

Clinical Features Tinea capitis is a fungal infection of the scalp. Although primarily regarded as a disease of preschool children, tinea capitis is becoming increasingly recognized in adults, infants, and neonates. It is more common among African Americans than among other racial groups, but the reasons for this are unknown.[6] The current epidemic in the United States caused by *Trichophyton tonsurans* differs from the epidemic of the 1940s and 1950s caused by *Microsporum audouinii* in that many patients have seborrheic-like scaling in the absence of alopecia.[6] Clinically, "black dots,"

Table 114-1. Definitions of Skin Lesions

Lesion	Appearance
Macule	Flat, color differs from surrounding skin
Patch	A macule with surface changes (i.e., scale or wrinkling)
Papule	Elevated skin lesion <0.5 cm in diameter
Plaque	Elevated skin lesion >0.5 cm in diameter; without substantial depth
Nodule	Elevated skin lesion >0.5 cm in diameter and depth
Cyst	Nodule filled with expressible material
Vesicle	Blisters <0.5 cm in diameter filled with clear fluid
Bullae	Blisters >0.5 cm in diameter filled with clear fluid
Pustule	Vesicle filled with cloudy or purulent fluid
Crust	Liquid debris that has dried on the skin surface; usually moist and yellowish-brown
Scale	Visibly thickened stratum corneum; usually white
Lichenification	Epidermal thickening characterized by visible and palpable skin thickening and accentuated skin markings
Induration	Dermal thickening that *feels* thick and firm
Wheal	Papule or plaque of dermal edema; often with central pallor and irregular borders
Erythema	Red appearance of skin caused by vasodilatation of dermal blood vessels; blanchable
Purpura	Red appearance of skin caused by blood extravasated from disrupted dermal blood vessels; nonblanchable
Macular purpura	Flat, nonpalpable
Papular purpura	Elevated, palpable

Modified from Lookingbill DP, Marks JG: *Principles of dermatology,* ed 2, Philadelphia, 1993, WB Saunders.

representing hair broken off near the scalp, may be noted.[7,8] Hair loss occurs because hyphae grow within the shaft, rendering it fragile, so that the hair strands break off 1 to 2 mm above the scalp. Circular patches of partial baldness may result. The disease may be transmitted by close child-to-child contact and contact with household pets, hats, combs, barber's shears, and similar items. Complications include lymphadenitis, bacterial pyoderma, tinea corporis, pigmenting pityriasis alba, "id" reaction after treatment, secondary bacterial infection, and scarring alopecia.[6]

Differential Considerations The differential diagnosis of tinea capitis includes alopecia areata, atopic dermatitis, nummular eczema, bacterial infection, psoriasis, seborrheic dermatitis, "tinea" amiantacea, trichotillomania (hair pulling), and Langhans' cell histiocytosis.

Diagnostic Strategies A KOH preparation is not helpful in the case of kerion or if no alopecia exists, and a fungal culture should be obtained.[9] A bacterial culture should be considered in the case of kerion to exclude superinfection.[5,9] A toothbrush, Papanicolaou smear cytology brush,[10] or moistened cotton swab[11] is helpful for obtaining quick, painless sampling of large areas of the scalp.[10-12]

Management Systemic therapy is required for tinea capitis. Treatment usually begins with griseofulvin 20 mg/kg/day, taken as a single dose with a fat-containing food for a minimum of 6 weeks, or 2 weeks after clinical resolution of inflammation.[5,9] Patients should be referred for monthly follow-up evaluation. Higher dosages may be needed. Alternative therapy includes fluconazole 200 mg/day (adults) or 3 to 5 mg/kg per day (children); itraconazole 200 mg daily (adults) and 3 to 5 mg/kg per day (children) for 4 to 6 weeks, oral terbinafine at 3 to 6 mg/kg per day for 4 to 6 weeks, or terbinafine cream once a day for 8 weeks.[5,9,13,14] Selenium sulfide shampoo 250 mg twice weekly decreases shedding of spores.[9] Family members should be evaluated.

Kerion A kerion is a dermatophytic infection, usually of the scalp, that appears as an indurated, boggy inflammatory plaque studded with pustules.[3] It is commonly confused with bacterial infections. Kerions should be treated as tinea capitis, with the addition of prednisone 1 mg/kg/day for 1 to 2 weeks, to help decrease the inflammatory reaction and subsequent scarring.[6,15,16] If bacterial superinfection exists, oral cephalexin or dicloxacillin can be added for the first week of treatment.[9]

Tinea Corporis

Clinical Features Tinea corporis is the classic "ringworm" infection. It affects the arms, legs, and trunk and is classically a sharply marginated, annular lesion with raised or vesicular margins and central clearing (Figure 114-1). Lesions may be single or multiple, the latter occasionally being concentric. Tinea cruris, which involves the groin, is similar in appearance and may also include the perineum, thighs, and buttocks, but the scrotum is characteristically spared.

Differential Considerations The differential diagnosis of tinea cruris includes granuloma annular psoriasis, intertrigo with secondary candidiasis, and erythrasma.[17]

Management Infections of the body, groin, and extremities usually respond to topical measures alone.[17] A number of effective topical antifungal agents are available, including clotrimazole (Lotrimin), haloprogin (Halotex), miconazole (Micatin), tolnaftate (Tinactin), terbinafine, naftifine, and griseofulvin 1%. Two or three daily applications of the cream form of any of these preparations result in healing of most superficial lesions in 1 to 3 weeks.[5,9,18-20] Acute inflammatory lesions displaying oozing or blisters should be treated additionally (four times a day) with open, wet compresses of Burow's solution—an aluminum acetate solution that is useful as a soothing wet dressing for inflammatory skin conditions. There is often involvement of the feet and toenails.[5]

Tinea Pedis Tinea pedis, or athlete's foot, appears with scaling, maceration, vesiculation, and fissuring between the toes and on the plantar surface of the foot. In extensive cases, the entire sole may be involved. A secondary bacterial infection may occur. The vesicular pustular form of tinea pedis should be considered when vesicles and pustules on the instep are noted. The differential diagnosis includes contact dermatitis and dyshidrotic eczema. A KOH preparation should help differentiate between these processes. Treatment is similar to that of tinea corporis.[21]

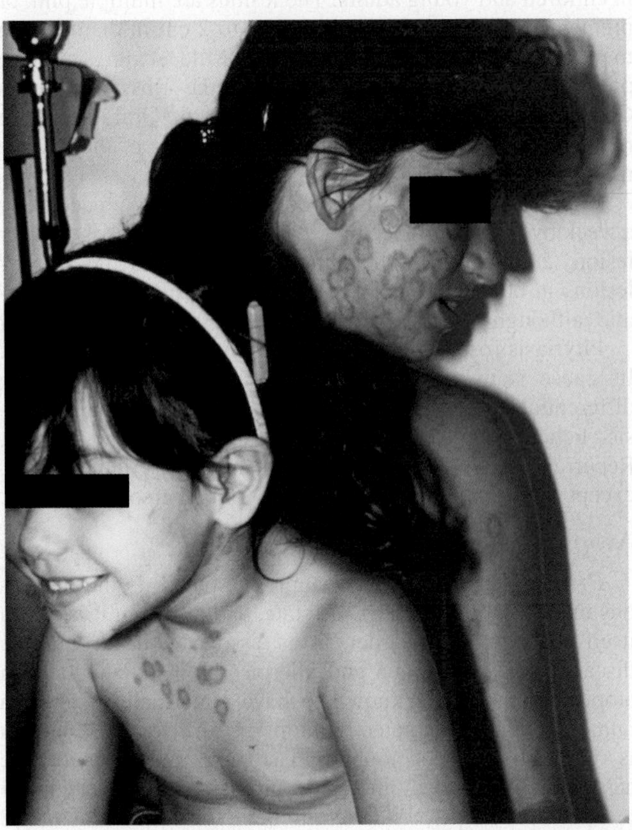

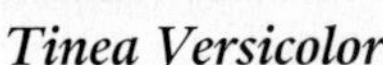

Figure 114-1. **Tinea corporis.** *Photo courtesy David Effron, MD.*

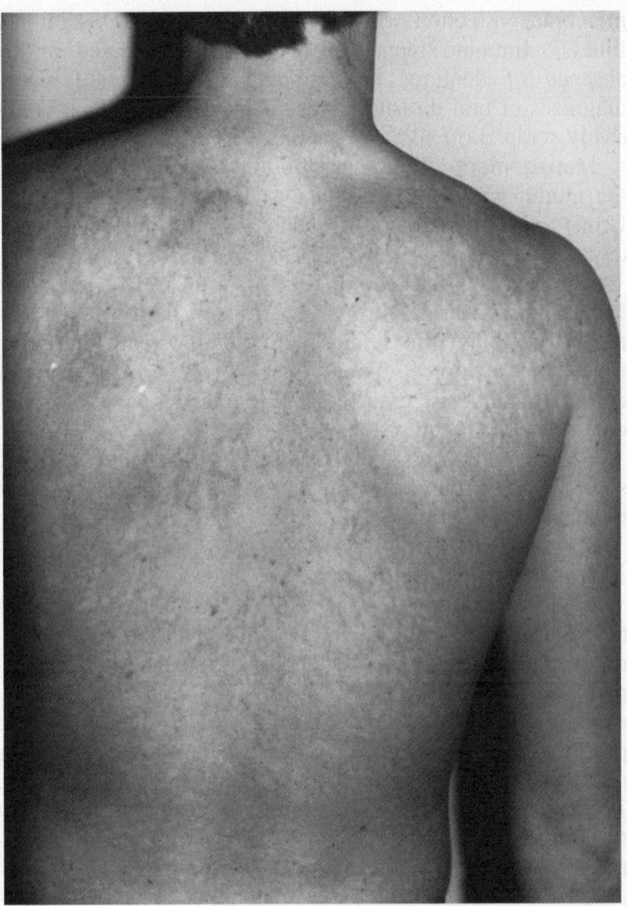

Figure 114-2. **Tinea versicolor.** *Photo courtesy David Effron, MD.*

Tinea Versicolor

Clinical Features Tinea versicolor is a superficial yeast infection caused by *Pityrosporum ovale.*[22] Superficial scaling patches occur mainly on the chest and trunk but may extend to the head and limbs. As the name implies, lesions can be a variety of colors including pink, tan, or white.[3] The disease may be associated with pruritus, but medical care is often sought because the spots do not tan. On physical examination, a fine subtle scale is noted that may appear hypopigmented (Figure 114-2). Pale yellow or orange fluorescence under Wood's light is sometimes present. The differential diagnosis includes vitiligo and seborrheic dermatitis. A KOH preparation reveals short hyphae mixed with spores ("chopped spaghetti and meatballs").

Management Tinea versicolor is treated with 2.5% selenium sulfide shampoo, imidazole creams, or oral ketoconazole as a single 400 mg dose or 200 mg daily for 3 to 5 days.[5,22-24] Recurrence rates vary from 15% to 50% and are considered the rule rather than the exception.[22] Monthly prophylaxis with propylene glycol and water, selenium shampoo, or azole creams can help prevent recurrences.[9,22] Pigmentation may not return to normal for months.

Tinea Unguium

Clinical Features Tinea unguium results in nails that are opaque, thickened, cracked, and crumbled. Subungual debris is present, and the nail may contain yellowish longitudinal streaks. The nail of the great toe is most commonly involved. Involvement of all of the nails of the hands and feet is rare.

Management Topical therapy of the nails alone rarely results in a cure because penetration into the nail keratin is poor. Fingernails typically respond more rapidly to therapy than toenails. Oral griseofulvin and ketoconazole require prolonged courses with high relapse rates and numerous side effects.[24] Newer agents such as itraconazole, fluconazole, and terbinafine are safer and more effective. They also offer shorter treatment periods, thus improving compliance.[24] The infection may be resistant to this regimen as well, however, and surgical removal of the nail is occasionally required.[17] Recurrence is common.

Candidiasis

Perspective Infection by *Candida albicans* can occur in infancy, old age, persons with acquired immunodeficiency syndrome (AIDS), pregnancy, obesity, malnutrition, persons with diabetes and other endocrine imbalances, malignancy, and those with other debilitating illnesses. Patients treated with corticosteroids, immunosuppressive agents, and antibiotics are also prone to cutaneous fungal infections.

Oral Thrush

Clinical Features Oral thrush is the most common clinical expression of *Candida* infection.[25] Thrush is most common in newborns, with one third being affected by the first week of life. The appearance is that of patches of white or gray friable material covering an erythematous base on the buccal mucosa, gingiva, tongue, palate, or tonsils. Fissures or crust at the corners of the mouth may be present. Oral mucous membrane infection with *C. albicans* is an AIDS-defining illness.[9] Immunosuppression should be considered in the absence of dentures or antibiotic use. The differential diagnosis of oral thrush includes lichen planus, which is not easily scraped off like *C. albicans.*

Management Treatment of oral thrush involves painting the mouth with 1 ml of oral nystatin suspension (100,000 U/ml) four times a day for infants or 4 to 6 ml four times a day swish and swallow for older children and adults. Treatment should be continued for 5 to 7 days after the lesions disappear. Clotrimazole troches dissolved in the mouth two to five times daily is a preferable treatment option for adults.[3] If topical therapy is not effective or in cases of chronic candidosis, oral ketoconazole, itraconazole, or fluconazole may be prescribed.[25]

Patients with oral candidiasis because of dentures should soak their dentures overnight in dilute (1:10) sodium hypochlorite solution.[3]

Cutaneous Candidiasis

Clinical Features Cutaneous candidiasis favors the moisture and maceration of the intertriginous areas—the interdigital web spaces, groin, axilla, and intergluteal and inframammary folds. Lesions appear as moist, bright-red macules rimmed with a collarette of scale, which represents the pustule roof with scalloped borders. Small satellite papules or pustules are just peripheral to the main body of the rash. These satellite lesions are the most typical indicators of a *Candida* infection. Intertriginous lesions are prone to bacterial superinfection.

Candidal onychia and paronychia are occupational conditions in those whose hands are frequently immersed in hot water. These infections also occur with thumb sucking by children who have thrush. The paronychial area becomes red and swollen and the nails thick and brittle, with transverse ridging. Destruction of the nail plate may occur.

Differential Considerations and Diagnostic Strategies The differential diagnosis of cutaneous candidiasis includes contact dermatitis, tinea cruris, intertrigo, malaria, or folliculitis. Candidiasis, however, is less sharply demarcated than tinea cruris, and brighter red than intertrigo. A KOH preparation taken from a pustule and roof of the lesion will reveal hyphae and pseudohyphae.

Management Treatment of intertriginous lesions requires the removal of excessive moisture and maceration. Lesions should be exposed to circulating air from a fan several times a day. Inflammatory lesions should be soaked in or covered with compresses of cool water or Burow's solution. Topical imidazole creams, such as clotrimazole and miconazole, should be applied sparingly to affected areas. Prescription creams, such as econazole, ketoconazole, or sulconazole, are also effective.

Protecting the hands from water is an integral part of the treatment of candidal paronychia. Prolonged immersion should be avoided and contact with water prevented by gloves with cotton liners. Nystatin or clotrimazole cream should be applied frequently to the nail folds for 6 to 8 weeks. A search for underlying immunocompromise should begin in patients with chronic, recurrent candidiasis.

SCALY PAPULES

Fungal lesions are typically scaly, as are lesions of secondary syphilis. Additional scaly diseases are discussed next.

Pityriasis Rosea

Pityriasis rosea is a mild skin eruption predominantly found in children and young adults. The lesions are multiple pink or pigmented oval papules or plaques 1 to 2 cm in diameter on the trunk and proximal extremities. Mild scaling may be present. The lesions are parallel to the ribs, forming a Christmas tree–like distribution on the trunk. Oral lesions are rare. In children, papular or vesicular variants of the disease may occur.[3]

In half the cases, the generalized eruption is preceded by a week by the appearance of a "herald patch." This is a larger lesion, 2 to 6 cm in diameter, that resembles the smaller lesions in other respects. The eruption is usually asymptomatic, although pruritus may be present.

Pityriasis rosea is self-limited, resolving in 8 to 12 weeks. Its cause is unknown, although a virus is suspected. The differential diagnosis includes tinea corporis, guttate psoriasis, lichen planus, drug eruption, and secondary syphilis. Recurrences are rare. Treatment is usually unnecessary, except for symptomatic alleviation of bothersome pruritus.

Atopic Dermatitis

Principles of Disease Atopic dermatitis is the cutaneous manifestation of an atopic state, and although it is not in itself an allergic disorder, it is associated with allergic diseases such as asthma and allergic rhinitis. Patients with atopic dermatitis are known to have abnormalities of both humoral and cell-mediated immunity.[26] The exact mechanism is unclear, but eosinophil, mast cell, and lymphocyte activation triggered by increased production of interleukin-4 by specific T-helper cells seem to be involved. Increased IgE levels are found in most but not all patients with atopic dermatitis, but there is a poor correlation between the severity of the dermatitis and the serum immunoglobulin (Ig)E level.[26] The course of atopic dermatitis involves remissions and exacerbations.

Clinical Features Skin lesions appear as inflammatory thickened, papular, or papulovesicular lichenification and hyperpigmentation.[27] The skin is typically dry and may be scaly, but in the acute phase, it may also be vesicular, weeping, or oozing. The distribution of lesions varies with the age of the patient. In infants, inflammatory exudative plaques are seen on the cheeks, extensor surfaces, and in the diaper area. Older children and adults have lesions in the antecubital and popliteal flexion areas, neck, face, and upper chest. Infantile atopic dermatitis usually begins in the fourth to sixth month of life and improves by the third to fifth year of life. The childhood form occurs between 3 and 6 years of age and resolves spontaneously or continues into the adult form.[27]

Intense pruritus is a hallmark of atopic dermatitis. The itching may be focal or generalized, is worse during the winter, and is triggered by increased body temperature and emotional stress. It may be particularly annoying at night. Excoriations may be prominent, and secondary bacterial infection of excoriated lesions is common. Repeated scratching and rubbing produce lichenification, a condition of hyperpigmentation, thickening of the skin, and accentuation of skin furrows. Lichenification is a common feature of chronic atopic dermatitis.

Differential Considerations The differential diagnosis of infantile atopic dermatitis includes histiocytosis X,

Wiskott-Aldrich syndrome, chronic seborrheic dermatitis, phenylketonuria, Bruton's X-linked agammaglobulinemia, psoriasis, and scabies. Fixed-drug eruptions and contact dermatitis round out the differential diagnosis regardless of age.[26,27] Complications of atopic dermatitis include pyogenic skin infections, otitis externa, cataracts, keratoconus, retinal detachment, and cutaneous viral infections.

Management Treatment should be aimed at controlling inflammation, dryness, and itching. Skin dryness may be treated by the application of lubricating ointments such as Vaseline or 10% urea in Eucerin cream (not lotion). Treatment of exudative areas includes the application of wet dressings. Such dressings are useful for their moisturizing, antiinflammatory, and antipruritic actions. Two to three layers of gauze soaked in Burow's solution should be applied for 15 to 20 minutes four times a day. Antihistamines may be helpful in reducing the pruritus and are also useful for their sedative and soporific effects.

Topical corticosteroids are the cornerstone of therapy and should be prescribed in ointment form. When the dermatitis is severe, a fluorinated corticosteroid ointment such as half-strength betamethasone valerate should be applied to affected areas of the body three times a day. Fluorinated corticosteroids should not be used on the face because they can produce permanent cutaneous atrophy. Milder corticosteroid preparations such as 0.025% triamcinolone ointment may be used on the face and intertriginous areas. Patients with extremely severe disease may require systemic steroids. Ultraviolet B treatment is moderately effective, although its mechanism of action is not well understood.[26]

Cyclosporine and other immunosuppressant agents are being used with some promising benefit. Further studies are needed to determine ideal dosing and safety profiles for these agents.[26]

PUSTULES

Impetigo

Principles of Disease Impetigo is a slowly evolving pustular eruption, most common in preschool children. Currently, *Staphylococcus aureus* is the most common pathogen, with Group A streptococcus a distant second.[28] Poor health and hygiene, malnutrition, and various antecedent dermatoses, especially atopic dermatitis, predispose individuals to impetigo.

Clinical Features *Streptococcal impetigo* is found most often on the face and other exposed areas. The eruption often begins as a single pustule, but develops into multiple lesions. It begins as 1- to 2-mm vesicles with erythematous margins. When these break, they leave red erosions covered with a golden yellow crust. Lesions may be pruritic but usually are not painful. Regional lymphadenopathy is commonly present. Lesions are very contagious among infants and young children and less so in older children and adults. Postpyodermal acute glomerulonephritis is a recognized complication of streptococcal impetigo.

Staphylococcal impetigo may be differentiated from streptococcal impetigo (ecthyma) by little surrounding erythema in the staphylococcal infection that is more superficial.[3] Other diagnostic considerations are herpes simplex virus (HSV) and inflammatory fungal infections. A Gram stain obtained from the weepy erosion after removing the crust will reveal gram-positive cocci.

Bullous impetigo is caused by staphylococci infected by phage group 2. This form is seen primarily in infants and young children. The initial skin lesions are thin-walled, 1- to 2-cm bullae. When these rupture, they leave a thin serous crust and collarette-like remnant of the blister roof at the rim of the crust. The face, neck, and extremities are most often affected. The differential diagnosis is contact dermatitis, HSV infection, superficial fungal infections, and pemphigus vulgaris. A Gram stain of the fluid from a bulla reveals gram-positive cocci. Cultures are positive 95% of the time.

Management Both systemic and topical therapy is equally successful in treating impetigo.[28-30] For more extensive lesions, systemic treatment should be used. There is no evidence, however, that systemic antibiotics prevent the development of acute glomerulonephritis.[28,31] The efficacy of topical mupirocin 2% ointment three times a day and oral erythromycin, 250 mg four times a day to 10 days in adults or 30 mg/kg/day in children, or cephalexin 30 to 40 mg/kg/day three times for 7 to 10 days are similar.[9,28-31]

Therapy for bullous impetigo consists of an oral penicillinase-resistant semisynthetic penicillin such as dicloxacillin, 250 mg four times a day for 5 to 7 days for adults, or erythromycin, 250 mg four times a day in adults or 30 to 50 mg/kg/day in children. If the infection is limited to a small area, mupirocin 2% ointment three times a day may be applied. Without treatment, impetigo heals within 3 to 6 weeks.[28-31]

Folliculitis

Clinical Features Folliculitis is an inflammation in the hair follicle, usually caused by *S. aureus.* It appears as a pustule with a central hair. The lesions are usually on the buttocks and thighs, occasionally in the beard or scalp, and may cause mild discomfort. Differential diagnosis includes acne, keratosis pilaris, and fungal infection. Gram-negative folliculitis with *Pseudomonas aeruginosa* occurs with infected hot tubs and swimming pools or in individuals taking antibiotics for acne and can be differentiated from staphylococcal folliculitis by a Gram stain of the lesion.

Management Treatment with an antiseptic cleanser such as povidone-iodine or chlorhexidine every day or every other day for several weeks is usually adequate. For patients with extensive involvement, a 10-day course of erythromycin, 250 mg four times a day, or dicloxacillin, 250 mg four times a day, may be added.[3,31,32]

Hidradenitis Suppurativa

Hidradenitis suppurativa affects the apocrine sweat glands. Recurrent abscess formation in the axillae and groin resembles localized furunculosis. The condition tends to be recurrent and may be extremely resistant to therapy. Hidradenitis suppurativa may be treated with drainage of abscesses. Antistaphylococcal antibiotics are useful if administered early and for a prolonged period.[9] Many cases do not respond, however, and eventually require local excision and skin grafting of the involved area. Antiandrogen therapy may be considered if antibiotics do not produce improvement.[9]

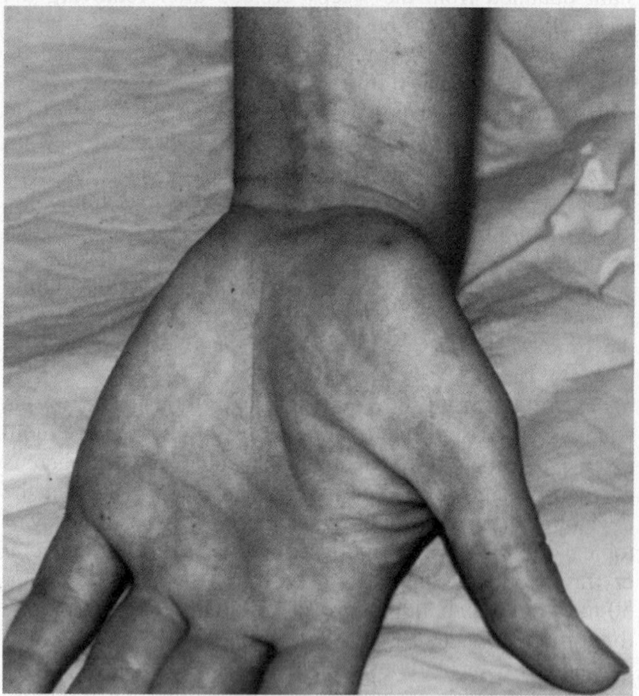

Figure 114-3. **Typical skin lesions of disseminated gonococcal disease.** ***Photo courtesy David Effron, MD.***

Carbuncle

A carbuncle is a large abscess that develops in the thick, inelastic skin of the back of the neck, back, or thighs. Carbuncles produce severe pain and fever. Septicemia may accompany the lesions. The diagnosis of skin abscess, furuncle, or carbuncle is usually made clinically.

Local heat should be applied to furuncles and carbuncles, which should be incised and drained when fluctuant. Antibiotics are unnecessary with incision and drainage unless cellulitis or septicemia is present.

Gonococcal Dermatitis

Clinical Features The arthritis-dermatitis syndrome is the most common presentation of disseminated gonococcal disease.[33,34] It occurs in 1% to 2% of patients with gonorrhea, affecting women primarily.[33] Fever and migratory polyarthralgias commonly accompany the skin lesions. The lesions are often multiple and have a predilection for periarticular regions of the distal extremities.[33]

The lesions begin as erythematous or hemorrhagic papules that evolve into pustules and vesicles with an erythematous halo (Figure 114-3). They closely resemble the lesions of meningococcemia at this stage. They are tender and may have a gray necrotic or hemorrhagic center. Healing with crust formation usually occurs within 4 to 5 days, although recurrent crops of lesions may appear even after antibiotics have been started.[33]

Diagnostic Strategies The lesions usually have a negative culture for gonococci, and the Gram stain only occasionally reveals the organisms. A more reliable diagnostic technique is immunofluorescent antibody staining of direct smears from pustules.[33] This method indicates that the lesions may be the result of hematogenous dissemination of nonviable gonococci.[33]

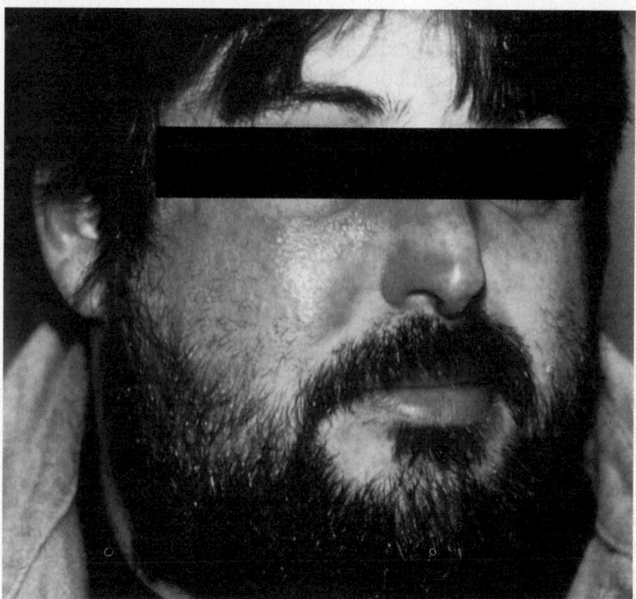

Figure 114-4. **Facial cellulitis.** ***Photo courtesy David Effron, MD.***

Management Current treatment of disseminated gonococcal infection is ceftriaxone, 1 g IM or IV every 24 hours, or ceftizoxime or cefotaxime, 1 g IV every 8 hours. Patients allergic to β-lactam antibiotics may be treated with spectinomycin 2 g IM every 12 hours. A total of 7 days of antibiotic therapy is required, with the remaining course of cefixime, 400 mg twice a day, cefuroxime or ciprofloxacin, 500 mg twice a day, or ofloxacin, 400 mg twice a day. Ciprofloxacin and ofloxacin are not recommended for pregnant women or children under 17 years old.[33,34] Hospitalization is recommended for patients in whom the diagnosis is uncertain and for those who have septic arthritis, meningitis, or endocarditis.

ERYTHEMA

Cellulitis is an infection of the skin tissue denoted by erythema, swelling, and local tenderness (Figure 114-4).[35-39] Erysipelas is a streptococcal infection of the skin and subcutaneous tissue. The involved area is red, indurated, and edematous.[40] These disorders are covered in Chapter 131.

RED MACULES

Drug Eruption

Principles of Disease A given drug can produce a skin eruption of a different appearance in different patients or a different appearance in the same patient on different occasions. The most common eruptions are urticaria (hives) (Figure 114-5) and more commonly morbilliform rashes (Figure 114-6).

Drug reactions tend to appear within a week after the drug

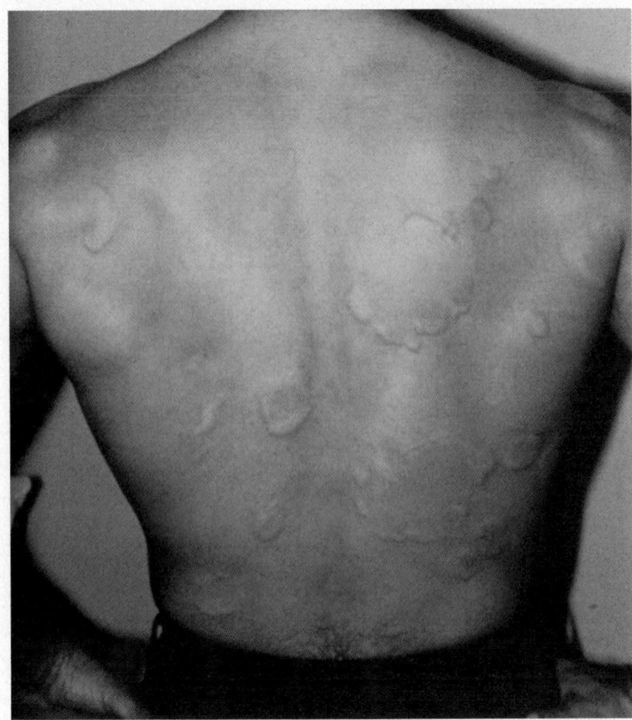

Figure 114-5. **Urticaria (hives).** ***Photo courtesy David Effron, MD.***

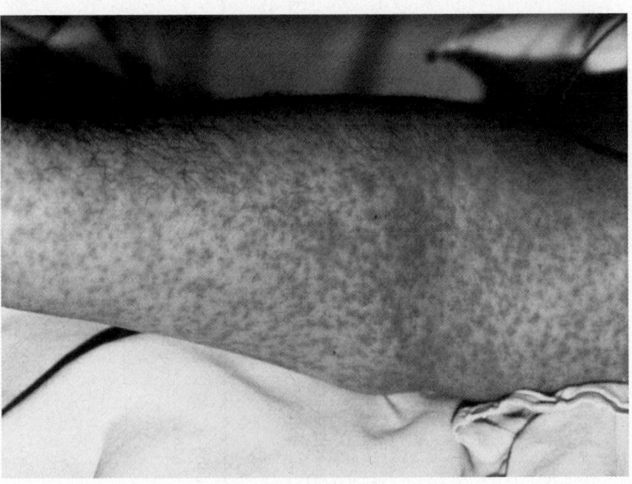

Figure 114-6. **Morbilliform drug eruption.** ***Photo courtesy David Effron, MD.***

is taken, with the exception of reactions to semisynthetic penicillins, which commonly occur later. Skin lesions may appear after a drug has been discontinued and may worsen if the drug or its metabolites persist in the system. Special note should be made of penicillin because it is the most common cause of drug reaction. Serum sickness and urticaria are the most common manifestations of penicillin allergy. Atopic patients and those with a history of hay fever, asthma, or eczema are at special risk.

On the other hand, a number of drugs in common use rarely produce eruptions. Among these are acetaminophen, aluminum hydroxide (Maalox), codeine, digoxin, erythromycin, ferrous sulfate, meperidine (Demerol), morphine, and prednisone.

Clinical Features Some of the more common skin reactions produced by commonly used drugs are listed in Table 114-2. *Exanthematous drug eruptions* resemble the skin manifestations of various viral or bacterial infections and are usually widespread symmetric maculopapular eruptions. Severe cases may progress to exfoliative dermatitis.

Eczematous drug rashes resemble those of contact dermatitis but are generally more extensive. They begin as erythematous or papular eruptions that may become vesicular. Prior sensitization to a topical medication is common in cases of this type of eruption.

Vasculitic lesions begin as erythematous papules or nodules but may ulcerate and become gangrenous. Purpuric drug eruptions may be the result of bone marrow suppression, platelet destruction, or vasculitis (Figure 114-7). In severe cases inpatient management with systemic corticosteroid administration, platelet transfusion, plasmapheresis, or splenectomy may be necessary.

Photosensitive drug reactions require the presence of sunlight and are seen most commonly on sun-exposed areas of skin. This class of reactions is commonly divided into phototoxic and photoallergic. Phototoxic reactions are more common. Sulfonamides, sulfonylureas, thiazide diuretics, and tetracyclines are common causes (see Figure 114-7). This type of reaction does not primarily involve immunologic mechanisms and occurs in any person taking an adequate quantity of the drug and exposed to sunlight. The lesions usually have the appearance of a severe sunburn but may be bullous or papular. Pruritus is typically minimal or absent.[41]

Photoallergic reactions are the result of antigen formation that results in the formation of sensitized lymphocytes. These reactions therefore represent a delayed immunologic response. A photoallergic reaction occurs only in sensitized individuals, usually 2 weeks or longer after exposure to the drug and sunlight. Its occurrence is not dose related, and the eruption usually appears eczematous and intensely pruritic. Chlorpromazine, promethazine, and chlordiazepoxide are common sensitizers of photoallergic reactions.[41]

Patients who develop photoallergic reactions should be withdrawn from inciting drugs. Patients who are subject to photosensitive drug eruptions may be required to avoid prolonged sunlight exposure. Sunscreen containing 5% aminobenzoic acid (PABA) should be used during any such exposure.

Fixed-drug eruptions appear and recur at the same anatomic site after repeated exposure to the same drug. The lesions are usually sharply marginated and round or oval. They may be pigmented, erythematous, or violaceous. Pruritus may be prominent.

Differential Considerations The differential diagnosis of drug eruptions includes viral exanthem, chronic exfoliative erythroderma caused by psoriasis or atopic dermatitis, malignancy, scarlet fever, staphylococcal scarlatiniform eruptions, and Kawasaki syndrome.[9,41]

Management Treatment of drug eruptions should begin with discontinuation of the inciting agent. Patients should be warned that drug eruptions clear *slowly* after discontinuation of the offending agent. Itching may be treated with the application of a drying antipruritic lotion such as calamine. Cool compresses, tepid water baths with colloidal oatmeal (Aveeno) emollient or cornstarch, and diphenhydramine

Table 114-2. Types of Lesions Characteristically Caused by Commonly Used Drugs

	Type of eruption									
Therapeutic agents	**Exanthematous**	**Urticarial***	**Erythema multiforme†**	**Toxic epidermal necrolysis**	**Eczematous**	**Erythema nodosum**	**Vasculitis**	**Purpura**	**Photosensitive**	**Fixed**
Anovulatory drugs		X				X			X	X
Aminophylline					X					
Barbiturates	X	X	X	X				X		X
Bromides		X	X			X				
Chloramphenicol		X					X			
Insulin	X	X								
Iodides		X	X			X	X	X		
Isoniazid	X	X								
Meprobamate	X	X			X			X		X
Penicillin	X	X	X	X	X	X	X	X		
Phenacetin										X
Phenolphthalein		X	X	X						X
Phenothiazines	X	X	X		X			X		X
Phenylbutazone	X	X		X			X	X		X
Quinine	X	X								
Quinidine	X	X	X				X		X	X
Salicylates	X	X	X			X				X
Sulfonamides	X	X	X	X	X	X	X		X	X
Tetracycline	X	X		X			X		X	X
Thiazides	X		X		X				X	
Others	Chloral hydrate	Opiates	Tolbutamide, phenytoin	Tolbutamide	Diphenhydramine ephedrine, thiamine, methyldopa		Antimalarial drugs, guanethidine		Antimalarial drugs, chlordiazepoxide, reserpine	Diazepam, indomethacin

*Most common causes of drug-induced urticaria are aspirin and penicillins.
†The long-acting sulfonamides have been linked to Stevens-Johnson syndrome.

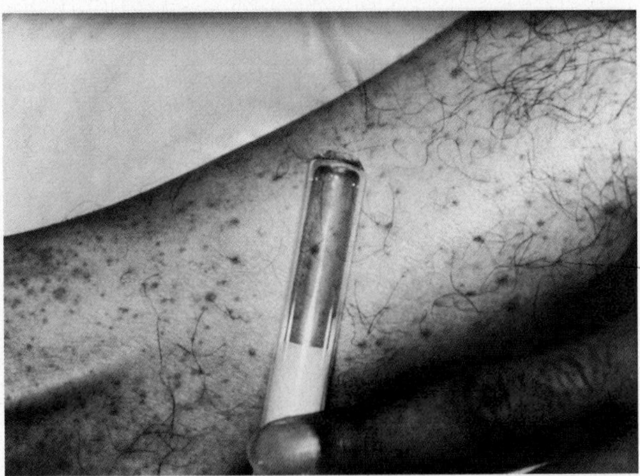

Figure 114-7. **Purpuric lesions.** ***Photo courtesy David Effron, MD.***

(Benadryl) 50 mg (5 mg/kg/24 hr in children) every 6 hours are likely to be beneficial.

Staphylococcal Scalded Skin

Clinical Features Staphylococcal scalded skin syndrome generally occurs in children 6 years of age or younger. It is caused by an infection with phage group 2 exotoxin-producing staphylococci. The illness begins with erythema and crusting around the mouth. The erythema then spreads down the body, followed by bulla formation and desquamation. Mucous membranes are usually not involved, but minimal involvement is occasionally seen. After desquamation occurs, the lesions dry up quickly, with clinical resolution in 3 to 7 days.

Management Most group 2 toxin-producing organisms are penicillin resistant. Although most patients will recover without antibiotic treatment, IV therapy with 50 to 100 mg/kg of nafcillin daily or oral cloxacillin 50 mg/kg/day or dicloxacillin is recommended.[9,42,43]

Toxic Epidermal Necrolysis

Principles of Disease The main feature of nonstaphylococcal-induced toxic epidermal necrolysis (TEN), or Lyell's disease, is the separation of large sheets of epidermis from underlying dermis. The full thickness of epidermis is involved. The two conditions are easily histologically distinguishable with a skin biopsy (Figure 114-8). A mortality rate of 15% to 20% is expected with this condition.[41]

Drugs including the long-acting sulfa drugs, penicillin, aspirin, barbiturates, phenytoin, carbamazepine, allopurinol, and nonsteroidal anti-inflammatory drugs are an important cause of TEN. TEN has occurred after vaccination and immunization against poliomyelitis, measles, smallpox, diphtheria, and tetanus. It has also been found in association with lymphoma.

Clinical Features Mucosal lesions may precede the cutaneous involvement. Patients have a positive Nikolsky's sign at the site, where minor rubbing results in desquamation of underlying skin, including the pigment. This is contrary to staphylococcal scalded skin syndrome, in which substantial pigment remains. The onset is usually on the face, and

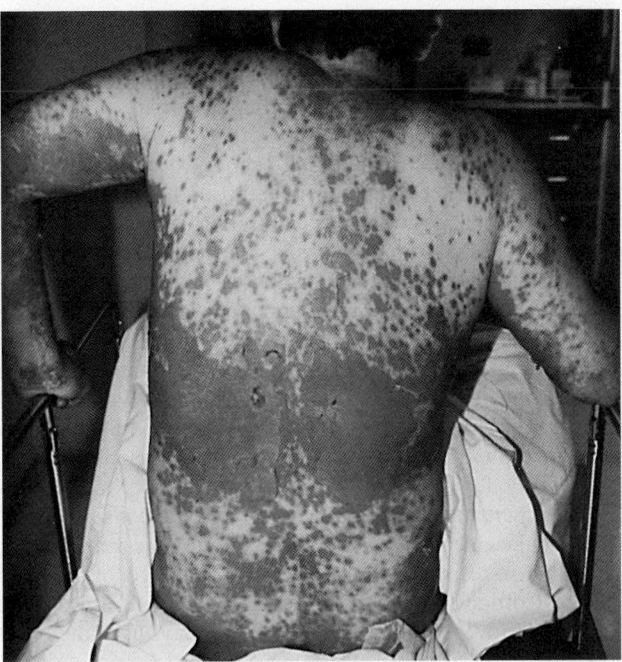

Figure 114-8. **Toxic epidermal necrolysis.** ***Photo courtesy David Effron, MD.***

mucous membrane involvement is the rule. Involvement of the eyes may be particularly troublesome, even resulting in permanent injury. The erythema usually precedes loosening of the epidermis.

Management The treatment of TEN includes discontinuation of the offending agent, fluid replacement, and aggressive infection control.[9,41] Administration of systemic corticosteroids is controversial.[41] They have little effect on the disease and may mask signs of impending sepsis. Plasmapheresis is considered experimental.[44] The mainstay of treatment is excellent supportive care, prevention of secondary infection, and expert wound management. This is usually best accomplished in a center with burn expertise.

Toxic Shock Syndrome

Principles of Disease Toxic shock syndrome (TSS) is an acute febrile illness characterized by a diffuse desquamating erythroderma. Classically composed of high fever, hypotension, constitutional symptoms, multiorgan involvement, and rash, the syndrome gained notoriety in the early 1980s because of association with tampon use. However, it is also well known in men and children. Its appearance has often been linked to exotoxin-producing *S. aureus*. Most cases of nonmenstrual TSS occur in the postoperative setting. TSS has also been associated with various staphylococcal and streptococcal infections, including empyema, osteomyelitis, fasciitis, septic abortion, peritonsillar abscess, sinusitis, burns, and subcutaneous abscess.[43]

TSS is associated with severe group A β-hemolytic streptococcal infections. It has been reported in previously healthy patients, immunocompromised patients, and elderly patients. Fatigue, localized pain, and nonspecific symptoms herald the onset of this disease, followed by septic shock and multisystem organ failure.[43,45,46]

Clinical Features Diagnosis of TSS requires the presence of (1) fever of at least 38.9° C; (2) hypotension, with a systolic blood pressure of 90 mm Hg or less; (3) skin rash; and (4) involvement of at least three organ systems.[9,43] Systemic involvement may include the gastrointestinal (GI) tract, muscular system, or central nervous system (CNS) and laboratory evidence of renal, hepatic, or hematologic dysfunction. Headache, myalgias, arthralgia, alteration of consciousness, nausea, vomiting, and diarrhea may be present.

The rash is typically a diffuse, blanching, macular erythroderma. Accompanying nonexudative mucous membrane inflammation is common. Pharyngitis, sometimes accompanied by a "strawberry tongue," conjunctivitis, or vaginitis may be seen. As a rule, the rash fades within 3 days of its appearance. This is followed by a full-thickness desquamation, most commonly involving the hands and feet.

Management Initial treatment of TSS consists of IV fluid replacement, ventilatory support, pressor agents, penicillinase-resistant antibiotics, and drainage of infected sites.[43] Corticosteroids reduce the severity of illness and duration of fever if initiated within 2 to 3 days after the onset of illness.[47]

Urticaria

Principles of Disease Approximately 15% to 20% of the population experience urticaria during their lifetime. Acute urticaria is seen in both sexes and is more likely to have an allergic cause. Chronic urticaria is more common in women in their 40s and 50s. Half of all patients with chronic urticaria have the disease for 5 years, and one fourth for 20 years.[48]

Various mediators, including histamine, bradykinin, kallikrein, and acetylcholine, are thought to play a role in urticaria production. Urticaria may be initiated by immunologic or nonimmunologic mechanisms. Hives found in anaphylaxis and serum sickness represent an immunologic reaction. Nonimmunologic urticaria may be produced by degranulation of mast cells, which may be caused by a number of foods and drugs, including aspirin and narcotics.

Substances that can cause urticaria by contact with the skin include foods, textiles, animal dander and saliva, plants, topical medications, chemicals, and cosmetics.[48,49] The role of drugs in the production of urticaria is discussed in the section on drug eruption. Almost any drug may produce urticaria, although penicillin and aspirin are the most common. Traces of penicillin may be present in dairy products, as well as in medications. The mechanism of production of urticaria by aspirin is unknown but is probably nonimmunologic, and the effects of aspirin may persist for a number of weeks after ingestion.[48,49]

A variety of food allergies, such as fish, eggs, or nuts, may result in urticaria. In addition, foods such as lobster and strawberries can release histamine through a nonimmunologic mechanism. Hereditary forms of urticaria include familial cold urticaria and hereditary angioneurotic edema.

Infections are an uncommon cause of urticaria, except in children in whom viral infections often cause hives. Occult infections with *Candida,* the dermatophytes, bacteria, viruses, and parasites may trigger hives. Viral infections that produce urticaria include hepatitis, mononucleosis, and coxsackievirus infections.

The inhalation of pollens, mold, animal dander, dust, plant products, and aerosols may produce urticaria. Respiratory symptoms may accompany the dermatosis, and a seasonal pattern of occurrence may be present. Stings and bites of insects, arthropods, and various marine animals may also produce an urticarial eruption.

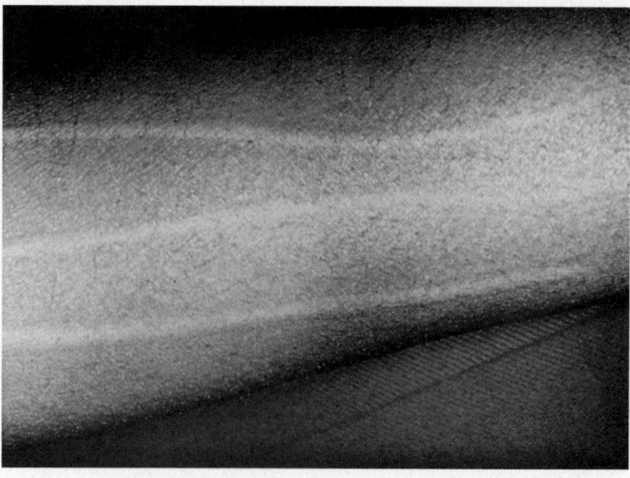

Figure 114-9. **Dermatographism.** ***Photo courtesy David Effron, MD.***

Occasionally, patients with systemic lupus erythematosus, lymphoma, carcinoma, hyperthyroidism, rheumatic fever, and juvenile rheumatoid arthritis develop an urticarial eruption. The association is uncommon enough that it is not necessary for an urticaria workup to include a search for malignancy in most cases.

A number of physical agents produce urticaria. Dermatographism is present when firm stroking of the skin produces an urticarial wheal within 30 minutes (Figure 114-9) and is the most common form of physical urticaria. Pressure urticaria is distinct from dermatographism in that the onset of urticaria is delayed by 4 to 8 hours after the application of physical pressure. There is no other particular significance to this form of urticaria.

Cold urticaria may be either familial or, more commonly, acquired. Cold urticaria may also be associated with underlying illness, such as cryoglobulinemia, cryofibrinogenemia, syphilis, and connective-tissue disease.[48,49] Cyproheptadine, 2 to 4 mg two or three times a day, is useful in the suppression of primary cold urticaria.[50] Side effects of this drug include drowsiness and an increased appetite.[50] Antihistamines 30 to 60 minutes before cold exposure may be helpful. Doxepin is also useful; begin at 10 mg at bedtime and gradually increase to 10 to 25 mg three times a day.[50]

Cholinergic urticaria is induced by exercise, heat, or emotional stress. It may be associated with pruritus, nausea, abdominal pain, and headache.[48,50] The lesions of cholinergic urticaria are wheals 1 to 3 mm in diameter surrounded by extensive erythematous flares and occasionally satellite wheals. Cholinergic urticaria responds better to hydroxyzine than do other physical urticarias.[50]

Heat is a rare cause of hives. Solar urticaria, also uncommon, is confined to sun-exposed areas of skin and clears rapidly when the light stimulus is removed. Extensive sun exposure may cause wheezing, dizziness, and syncope in a susceptible individual.[50] Sunscreens have not been proven to be effective for the prevention of solar urticaria.[50]

The cause of chronic urticaria in adults is often not

determined, although the etiologic factors responsible for urticaria in children are more readily identifiable.[51]

Clinical Features Urticaria appears as edematous plaques with pale centers and red borders and is easily recognizable (see Figure 114-5). Individual hives are transient, lasting less than 24 hours, although new hives may continuously develop, which represent localized dermal edema produced by transvascular fluid extravasation.

Differential Considerations The differential diagnosis of urticaria includes erythema multiforme, erythema marginatum, and juvenile rheumatoid arthritis.

Management Treatment of urticaria involves the removal of the inciting factor, when applicable, and the administration of antihistamines or other antipruritics. Hydroxyzine (Atarax, Vistaril) in a dose of 10 to 25 mg (2 mg/kg/24 hr in children) is usually effective in providing symptomatic relief. Alternatives are nonsedating antihistamines, such as terfenadine 60 mg twice a day, astemizole 10 mg daily, or fexofenadine 60 mg twice a day.[52] Prednisone is also effective, but the urticaria can rebound, making cessation of prednisone sometimes difficult. For chronic urticaria, long-term therapy with antihistamines may be needed.

EXANTHEMS

Principles of Disease

An exanthem is defined as a skin eruption that occurs as a symptom of a general disease. Approximately 30 enteroviruses, predominantly the coxsackievirus and echovirus groups, and four types of adenoviruses are known to produce exanthems. Other viruses may do so as well. The exanthems of the coxsackievirus and echovirus are most thoroughly documented. Most viral exanthems are maculopapular, although scarlatiniform, erythematous, vesicular, and petechial rashes are occasionally seen. The eruptions are variable in their extent, are nonpruritic, and do not desquamate. Oropharyngeal lesions may be present.

Infection with echovirus type 9 may be accompanied by meningitis and a petechial exanthem resembling meningococcemia, although the exanthem also occurs without meningeal involvement. Infections caused by echovirus type 16 (Boston exanthem) and coxsackievirus group B, type 5, may resemble roseola infantum but are more likely to occur in adults.

Infections caused by coxsackievirus group A, type 16, cause a distinctive syndrome of vesicular stomatitis and 1 to 4 mm oral vesicles involving the dorsa of the hands and lateral borders of the feet. Disease caused by coxsackievirus group A, type 9, has been the most extensively studied. It may be associated with meningoencephalitis or interstitial pneumonia. The rash is usually maculopapular, begins on the face or trunk, and spreads to the extremities. A vesicular eruption resembling varicella may occur.

The classic viral exanthems are rubeola (measles), rubella (German measles), herpes virus 6 (roseola), parvovirus B19 (erythema infectiosum, or fifth disease), and the enteroviruses (ECHO and coxsackie).[3,9] Widespread immunization programs have reduced the incidence of rubeola and rubella.

Measles

Clinical Features Measles is a highly contagious viral illness spread by contact with infectious droplets, with an incubation period of 10 to 14 days. Patients are contagious from 1 to 2 days before onset of symptoms up to 4 days after the appearance of the rash.[53] Symptoms begin with fever and malaise. The fever usually increases daily in a stepwise fashion until it reaches approximately 40.5° C on the fifth or sixth day of the illness. Cough, coryza, and conjunctivitis begin within 24 hours of the onset of symptoms.

On the second day of the illness, Koplik's spots, which are pathognomonic of the disease, appear on the buccal mucosa as small, irregular, bright red spots with bluish-white centers. Beginning opposite the molars, Koplik's spots spread to involve a variable extent of the oropharynx.

The cutaneous eruption of measles begins on the third to fifth day of the illness. Maculopapular erythematous lesions involve the forehead and upper neck and spread to involve the face, trunk, arms, and finally the legs and feet. Koplik's spots begin to disappear coincident with the appearance of the rash. By the third day of its presence, the rash begins to fade, doing so in the order of its appearance, and the fever subsides.

Complications include otitis media, encephalitis, and pneumonitis. Otitis media is the most common complication. Encephalitis occurs in approximately 1 in 1,000 cases of measles and carries a 15% mortality. Measles pneumonia may also be life-threatening.

Management If bacterial invasion occurs with otitis or pneumonia, the use of antibiotics is indicated. Otherwise treatment is supportive. Isolation of infected children is of limited value because exposure usually occurs before the appearance of the rash and the presence of Koplik's spots render the disease diagnosable. Measles is not contagious after the fifth day of the presence of the rash. Infection confers lifelong immunity.

The illness can be modified or prevented by the administration of human immune serum globulin (ISG) in a susceptible person within 6 days of exposure. The recommended dose of ISG is 0.25 ml/kg IM in children. Live measles virus vaccine given within 72 hours of exposure may be effective in preventing measles.[53] Some authors suggest vitamin A shortly after exposure. The incidence of measles has decreased since the resurgence seen in 1989 to 1991.[54] The patterns observed during outbreaks include a shift from preschool-aged children to older adults and among groups who do not routinely obtain vaccination such as immigrants.

Rocky Mountain Spotted Fever

Principles of Disease Rocky Mountain spotted fever is caused by *Rickettsia rickettsii,* an organism harbored by a variety of ticks. The organism is transmitted to humans through tick saliva at the time of a tick bite or when the tick is crushed while in contact with the host. Although originally described in the Rocky Mountain region, this disease occurs in other portions of North, South, and Central America. Most reported cases are from the southeastern United States.

Clinical Features The onset of the illness is usually abrupt, with headache, nausea and vomiting, myalgias, chills, and a fever spiking to 40° C. Occasionally the onset is more gradual, with progressive anorexia, malaise, and fever. The disease may last 3 weeks and may be severe with prominent CNS, cardiac, pulmonary, GI, renal, and other organ involvement; disseminated intravascular coagulation (DIC); or shock.

The rash develops on the second to fourth day or occasionally as late as the sixth day of the illness. It begins with erythematous macules that blanch on pressure, appearing first on the wrists and ankles. These macules spread up the extremities and to the trunk and face in a matter of hours. They may become petechial or hemorrhagic. Lesions on the palms and soles are particularly characteristic. Increased capillary fragility and splenomegaly may be present.

Diagnostic Strategies The Weil-Felix reaction is the best known serologic diagnostic test, but the development of Weil-Felix agglutinins in cases of Rocky Mountain spotted fever is not constant, and more specific immunofluorescent procedures have been developed.[55] Treatment should not await the result of such tests, however, but should begin as soon as the disease is suspected on clinical grounds.

Management Tetracycline (25 to 30 mg/kg/day in divided doses) is the antibiotic of choice. If the patient is unable to take oral medications, tetracycline may be administered IV, with a 15 mg/kg loading dose followed by a maintenance dosage of 15 mg/kg/day. Doxycycline may be used as well in a dosage of 4.4 mg/kg/day divided every 6 hours followed by 1.1 mg/kg twice a day, up to 30 mg/day. Chloramphenicol may be used for patients allergic to tetracycline and in children younger than 9 years of age. A usual course is 6 to 10 days and should continue for 72 hours after defervescence.[55] Sulfa drugs should be avoided, as they can exacerbate the illness. Rickettsiae are routinely resistant to penicillins, cephalosporins, aminoglycosides, and erythromycin.[55]

Roseola Infantum

Roseola infantum, otherwise known as *exanthem subitum* or sixth disease, is a benign illness caused by human herpes virus 6 and characterized by fever and a skin eruption. A roseola-like illness has occasionally been associated with other illnesses.[53] Ninety-five percent of cases are seen in children 6 months to 3 years of age, and most of these are in infants younger than 2 years. A febrile seizure may occur. The fever typically has an abrupt onset, rising rapidly to 39° to 41° C, and is present consistently or intermittently for 3 to 4 days, at which time the temperature drops precipitously to normal.

The rash appears with defervescence. The lesions are discrete pink or rose-colored macules or maculopapules 2 to 3 mm in diameter, which blanch on pressure and rarely coalesce. The trunk is involved initially, with the eruption typically spreading to the neck and extremities. Occasionally, the eruptions are limited to the trunk. The rash clears over 1 to 2 days without desquamation.

Despite the presence of a high fever, the infant usually appears well. Encephalitis is a very rare complication.[53] The prognosis is excellent, and no treatment is necessary.

Rubella

Rubella, or German measles, is a viral illness characterized by fever, skin eruption, and generalized lymphadenopathy. It is spread by droplet contact, and peak incidence is in the winter and early spring. The incubation period is typically 14 to 21 days, and the rash heralds the onset of the illness in children. The maximum time of communicability is in the few days before and 5 to 7 days after the onset of the rash.[53] Infants with congenital rubella can shed virus for more than a year.[53] In adults, a 1 to 6 day prodrome of headache, malaise, sore throat, coryza, and low-grade fever precedes the rash. These symptoms generally disappear within 24 hours after the appearance of the skin eruption.

The rash of pink to red maculopapules appears first on the face and spreads rapidly to the neck, trunk, and extremities. Those on the trunk may coalesce, but lesions on the extremities do not. The rash remains for 1 to 5 days, classically disappearing at the end of 3 days. Although clearing may be accompanied by fine desquamation, this sign is usually absent.

Lymphadenopathy may begin as early as a week before the rash. Although this is generalized, the nodes most apparent are the suboccipital, postauricular, and posterior cervical groups. Palpable adenopathy may be apparent several weeks after other signs and symptoms have subsided.

The major complications of rubella include encephalitis, arthritis, and thrombocytopenia. The most severe complication is fetal damage. A total of 24% of infected fetuses have a congenital defect. A maternal infection may be determined by obtaining serum for hemagglutination inhibition antibody determinations, acutely and in 2 weeks. A fourfold rise in the titer is diagnostic of rubella infection. The routine use of postexposure prophylaxis of rubella in an unvaccinated woman in early pregnancy is *not* recommended.

No treatment is required in many cases of rubella. Antipyretics are usually adequate for the treatment of headache, arthralgias, and painful lymphadenopathy.

Erythema Infectiosum

Erythema infectiosum, or fifth disease, is caused by parvovirus B19 infection. It is characterized by mild systemic symptoms, fever in 10% to 15% of patients, and a characteristic rash. Arthralgia and arthritis occur commonly in adults, but rarely in children. The rash is intensely red on the face and gives a "slapped-cheek" appearance with circumoral pallor. A maculopapular lacelike rash, which may be noted on the arms, moves caudally to the trunk, buttocks, and thighs. The rash may recur with changes in temperature and exposure to sunlight. The incubation period is usually between 4 and 14 days.[53,56]

Parvovirus B19 infection may also result in asymptomatic infection, upper respiratory infection, atypical rash, and arthritis without rash.

Rarely, it has been reported to cause hapatitis.[56] Infected immunodeficient patients may experience chronic anemia as a result of this disease. Patients with sickle cell disease or other hemolytic anemias may develop an aplastic crisis lasting 7 to 10 days.[56] Parvovirus B19 infection during pregnancy can cause fetal hydrops and death.[56] No congenital anomalies have been reported. No treatment is required.

Scarlet Fever

Clinical Features The incidence of scarlet fever has declined in recent years. The illness has an abrupt onset with fever, chills, malaise, and sore throat followed within 12 to 48 hours by a distinctive rash that begins on the chest and spreads rapidly, usually within 24 hours. Circumoral pallor may be noted. The skin has a rough sandpaper-like texture because of the multitude of pinhead-size lesions. The pharynx is injected, and there may be erythematous lesions or petechiae on the palate. After the resolution of symptoms,

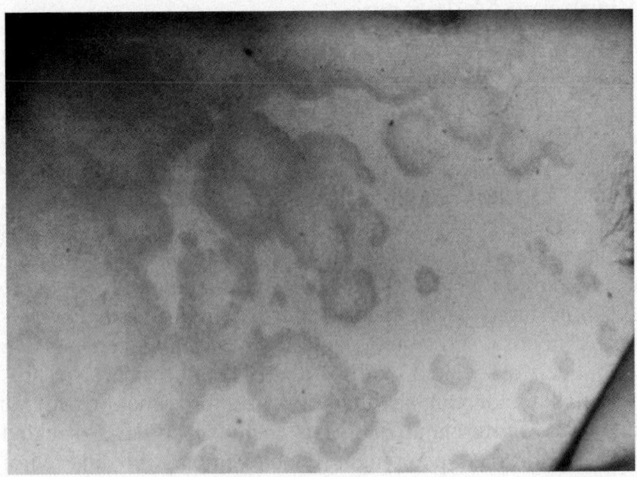

Figure 114-10. **Erythema marginatum associated with rheumatic fever.** *Photo courtesy David Effron, MD.*

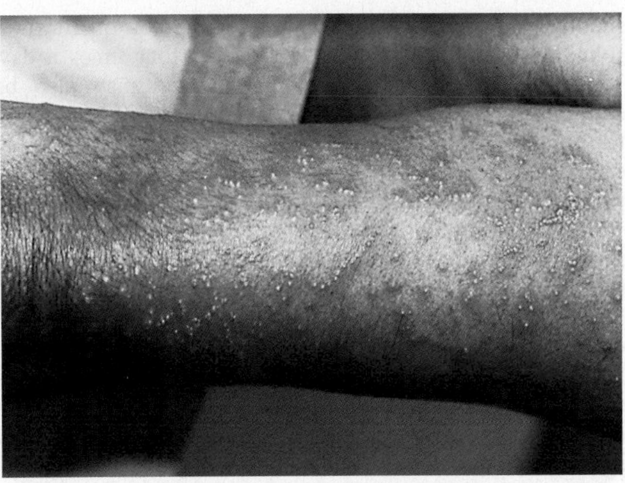

Figure 114-11. **Contact dermatitis secondary to nickel.** *Photo courtesy David Effron, MD.*

desquamation of the involved areas occurs and is characteristic of the disease.

Complications include the development of a streptococcal infection of lymph nodes, tonsils, the middle ear, and the respiratory tract. Late complications include rheumatic fever and acute glomerulonephritis (Figure 114-10).

Management Treatment is aimed at providing adequate antistreptococcal blood antibiotic levels for at least 10 days. Oral penicillin VK 50 mg/kg/day (40,000 to 80,000 units) in four divided doses in children or 250 mg four times a day in adults is administered. Intramuscularly, benzathine penicillin (given as Bicillin CR) is given. In patients weighing less than 30 pounds, 300,000 units of benzathine penicillin is used. In patients weighing 31 to 60 pounds, 600,000 units benzathine is used; in patients weighing 61 to 90 pounds, 900,000 units benzathine is used; and in those weighing more than 90 pounds, 1.2 million units benzathine is used. In patients allergic to penicillin, 250 mg of erythromycin four times a day or 40 mg/kg/day should be given orally for 10 days. Other macrolides and certain other cephalosporins may also be used.

PAPULAR LESIONS

Contact Dermatitis

Principles of Disease Contact dermatitis is an inflammatory reaction of the skin to a chemical, physical, or biologic agent. The inducing agent acts as an irritant or allergic sensitizer. Allergic contact dermatitis is a form of delayed hypersensitivity mediated by lymphocytes sensitized by the contact of the allergen to the skin. It is less common than irritant contact dermatitis.[57] Caustics, industrial solvents, and detergents are common causes of irritant dermatitis. Dermatitis may result from brief contact with a potent caustic or from repeated or prolonged contact with milder irritants.

Clothing, jewelry, soaps, cosmetics, plants, and medications contain allergens that commonly cause allergic contact dermatitis. The most common allergens include rubber compounds, plants of the *Rhus* genus (poison ivy, oak, and sumac), nickel (often used in jewelry alloys), paraphenyldenediamine (an ingredient in hair dyes and industrial chemicals), and ethylenediamine (a stabilizer in topical

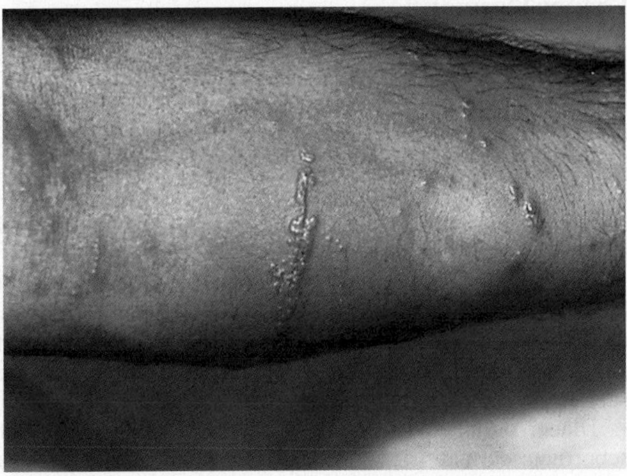

Figure 114-12. **Typical linear lesions of contact dermatitis secondary to poison ivy.** *Photo courtesy David Effron, MD.*

medications).[58] Sensitization to poison ivy results in sensitization to other plants in this family such as cashew, mango, lacquer, and ginkgo trees.[59]

Clinical Features The primary lesions of contact dermatitis are papules, vesicles, or bullae on an erythematous bed. Of the allergens, *Rhus* species are the most likely to cause bullous eruptions. Oozing, crusting, scaling, and fissuring may be found, along with lichenification in chronic lesions. The distribution of the eruption depends on the specific contactant and may be localized, asymmetric linear, or unilateral (Figures 114-11 and 114-12). Mucous membranes are usually spared unless directly exposed to the inciting agent. A history of exposure is the most significant factor favoring the diagnosis. If doubt exists about the diagnosis, the patient should be referred for allergic patch testing.

Management Treatment of contact dermatitis includes avoidance of the irritant or allergen and treatment of secondary bacterial infection. Oozing or vesiculated lesions should be treated with cool wet compresses of Burow's solution applied for 15 minutes three or four times a day. Topical baths, available over the counter, may also be comforting. A course of systemic corticosteroids is often necessary.[58] Prednisone in a dosage of 30 to 80 mg/day (depending on the severity of involvement) should be prescribed initially. This should be tapered over at least 10 to 14 days, and 21 days for poison ivy. The long, slow taper is needed to prevent rebound of the disease. The treatment may be discontinued when a daily dose of 10 mg is reached. Systemic antihistamines, such as hydroxyzine or diphenhydramine, may help control pruritus.[9,58,59]

The patient should also be counseled to wash all clothes that might have contacted the plant, since the irritant plant oil can persist. Once the offending agent is reliably removed from the skin and clothes, ongoing outbreak is attributable to the initial contact, not spread from the serous fluid from the bullae. The patient is not contagious to others unless there is direct contact with the plant oil in persons who are sensitized.

Diaper Dermatitis

Clinical Features Diaper dermatitis is a common disorder. The condition is exacerbated by heat, moisture, friction, and the presence of urine and fecal material. Occlusive clothing in infants tends to foster all of these. Lesions begin as erythematous plaques in the genital, perianal, gluteal, and inguinal areas. More severe involvement results in moist, eroded lesions that may extend beyond the primary areas of appearance.

Infection with *C. albicans* and fecal bacterial flora is an important contributory factor to the development of diaper dermatitis. Lesions infected with *Candida* are moist, red patches with well-demarcated borders. Papular or pustular satellite lesions are also present.

Diaper dermatitis may reflect the presence of atopic or seborrheic dermatitis in the infant. The presence of lesions elsewhere on the body, particularly on the face, in cases of atopic dermatitis, or the scalp, in cases of seborrhea, alerts the physician to these possibilities. Ammonia and bacterially produced putrefactive enzymes produce dermatitis as contact irritants. Such rashes are accompanied by characteristic odors. The existence of diaper dermatitis as a true allergic contact dermatitis is rare.

Management Treatment consists primarily of altering the physical environment in which diaper dermatitis thrives. Excess clothing should be removed, and occlusive plastic or rubber diaper covers should not be used. Diapers should be changed frequently and left off for prolonged periods if possible. Sterilized cloth diapers are preferred.

If exudative lesions are present, treatment with topical cool wet compresses of saline or Burow's solution is indicated for 2 to 3 days. Continuous air exposure of the area should be attempted.[58] Zinc oxide (Desitin) may dry the area. Severe contact or seborrheic dermatitis may require short-term treatment with topical corticosteroids, such as 1% hydrocortisone in a cream base.[58] Ointment-based topical medications for treatment of diaper dermatitis should be avoided because their occlusive nature enhances moisture retention. Nystatin cream or powder should be applied to lesions infected with *Candida*.

Erythema Multiforme

Principles of Disease The most common precipitating factors in erythema multiforme are exposure to drugs and HSV infection. Other causes include other viral infections, especially hepatitis and influenza A. Less common causes include fungal diseases such as dermatophytosis, histoplasmosis, and coccidioidomycosis, and bacterial infections, especially streptococcal infections and tuberculosis. Various collagen vascular disorders have been known to precipitate erythema multiforme, particularly rheumatoid arthritis, systemic lupus erythematosus, dermatomyositis, and periarteritis nodosa. Pregnancy and various malignancies have also been associated with erythema multiforme. No provocative factor can be identified in approximately half of all cases. Differential diagnosis includes urticaria, scalded skin syndrome, pemphigus, and pemphigoid and viral exanthems.

Clinical Features Erythema multiforme is an acute, usually self-limiting disease precipitated by a variety of factors. It is characterized by the sudden appearance of skin lesions that are erythematous or violaceous macules, papules, vesicles, or bullae. Their distribution is often symmetrical, most commonly involving the soles and palms, the backs of the hands or feet, and the extensor surfaces of the extremities. The presence of lesions of the palms and soles is particularly characteristic.[60]

The target lesion with three zones of color is the hallmark of erythema multiforme. It is a central, dark papule or vesicle that is surrounded by a pale zone, a halo of erythema (Figure 114-13), and is commonly found on the hands or wrist.

Stevens-Johnson syndrome, a severe form of erythema multiforme, is occasionally fatal. It is characterized by bullae, mucous membrane lesions, and multisystem involvement (Figure 114-14). The patient may be toxic, complaining of chills, headache, and malaise, and displaying fever, tachycardia, and tachypnea. Systemic involvement may occur, with renal, GI, or respiratory tract lesions, resulting in hematuria, diarrhea, bronchitis, or pneumonia. Purulent conjunctivitis may be severe enough to cause the eyes to swell shut. Death results from infection and dehydration.

Management Treatment should begin with a search for the underlying cause. Mild forms resolve spontaneously in 2 to 3 weeks. Severe cases may last up to 6 weeks and may require hospital admission for IV hydration, local skin care, systemic analgesia, and systemic corticosteroid therapy, which should consist of 80 to 120 mg of prednisone daily in divided doses. Bullous lesions should be treated with the application of wet compresses soaked in a 1:16,000 solution of potassium permanganate or a 0.05% silver nitrate solution several times a day. The major complications of Stevens-Johnson syndrome are infection and fluid loss. Renal involvement and pneumonia are rare. Severe conjunctivitis may result in corneal scarring and blindness. Reported mortality rates for Stevens-Johnson syndrome range from 0 to 15%.[3,15]

Pediculosis

Clinical Features The diagnosis is made by the identification of nits or adult lice with the microscopic examination of hairs plucked from the symptomatic area. Nits are

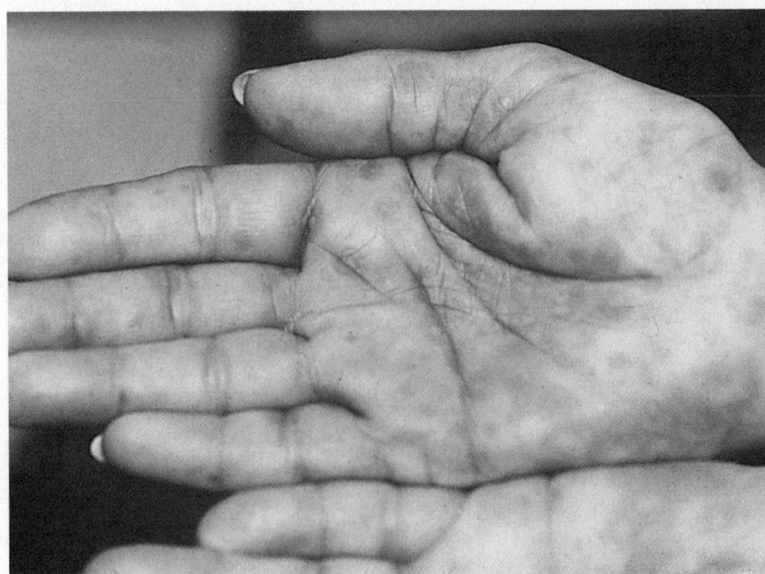

Figure 114-13. **Erythema multiforme.** *Photo courtesy David Effron, MD.*

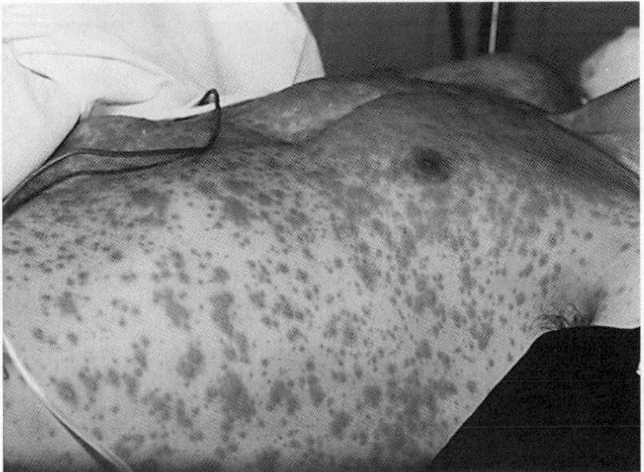

Figure 114-14. **Stevens-Johnson syndrome.** *Photo courtesy David Effron, MD.*

relatively more common than the adult louse form. Nits attach to the bases of hair shafts, appearing as white dots (Figure 114-15). Adult forms look like blue or black grains. The patient complains of intense itching and scratching. A secondary infection may result from the latter.

The organisms causing pediculosis corporis reside in the seams of clothing and bedding materials while they feed on the human host. Except with heavily infested individuals, the parasites are absent from the body itself. Erythematous macules or wheals may be present, along with intense pruritus. The treatment consists of laundering or boiling clothing and bed linen. If nits are found in the body hair, a treatment with lindane lotion may be instituted, but this is not necessary is most cases (Figures 114-16 and 114-17).

Pediculosis capitis is seen more commonly in small children than in adults. Pruritus is the major symptom and may be confined to the occipital or postauricular scalp. Excoriations commonly result in secondary bacterial infections and regional lymphadenopathy.

Diagnostic Strategies The diagnosis is made by the identification of nits cemented to hairs at the hair-scalp junction (see Figure 114-15).

Management Lindane (Kwell) lotion or cream is no longer the preferred prescription topical treatment.[61] Permethrin (Nix) is the recommended treatment. It remains active for 2 weeks. Crème rinses and conditioning shampoos should not be used during this period because they coat the hairs and protect the lice from the insecticide. Permethrin is applied to the scalp after the hair is shampooed and dried. It is rinsed out with water after 10 minutes. It must be applied when the hair is dry because lice can close down their respiratory airways for up to 30 minutes when immersed in water.[61] Higher cure rates are achieved if the dose is repeated 1 week after the initial usage.

Because the condition may be spread by sexual contact, sexual partners should also be treated. Other uninfested household members need not undergo a course of therapy. Underclothing, pajamas, and sheets and pillow cases should be machine washed (hot water) and dried, laundered and ironed, or boiled. Pruritus that persists after the course of therapy may result from an irritation of the skin by the pediculicide, sensitization, or patient anxiety.

For treatment of pediculosis capitis, treatment is with permethrin. A single dose of oral ivermectin, 200 μg/kg repeated in 10 days, has been shown to eradicate head lice.[61] Lindane should be reserved for treatment failures. Household contacts should be examined for involvement, but uninfected persons need not be treated.

Scabies

Clinical Features Scabies is a mite infestation characterized by severe itching, which usually worsens at night. The areas of the body most commonly involved are the interdigital web spaces, flexion areas of the wrists, axillae, buttocks, lower back, penis, scrotum, and breasts (Figure 114-18). The infestation tends to be more generalized in infants and children than in adults. The typical lesions are reddish papules or vesicles surrounded by an erythematous

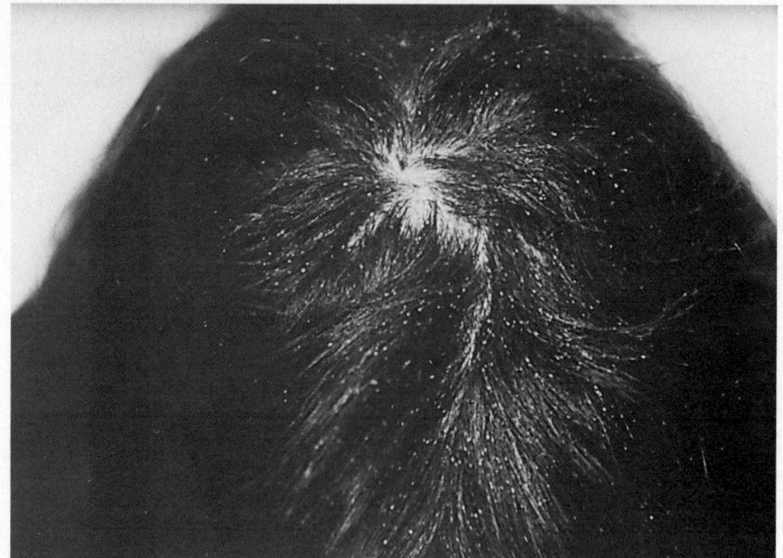

Figure 114-15. **Nits as seen in head lice.** *Photo courtesy David Effron, MD.*

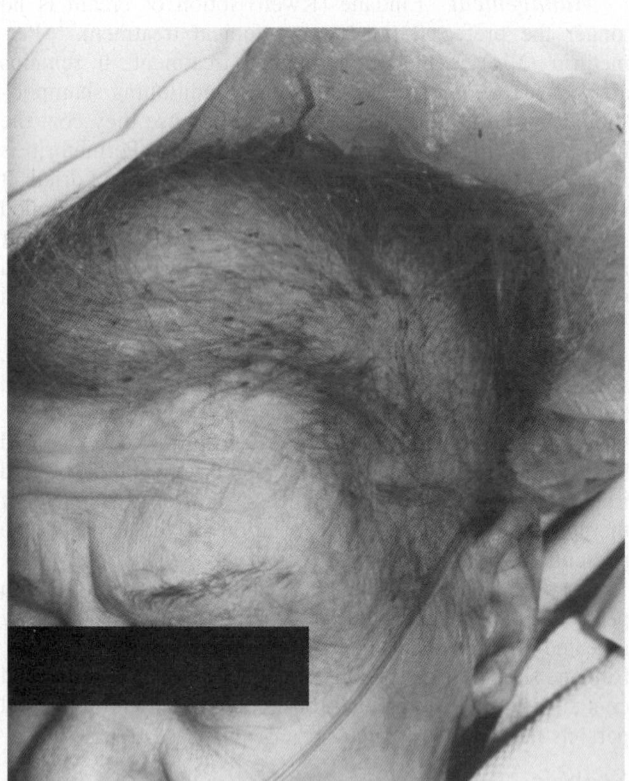

Figure 114-16. **Body lice.** *Photo courtesy David Effron, MD.*

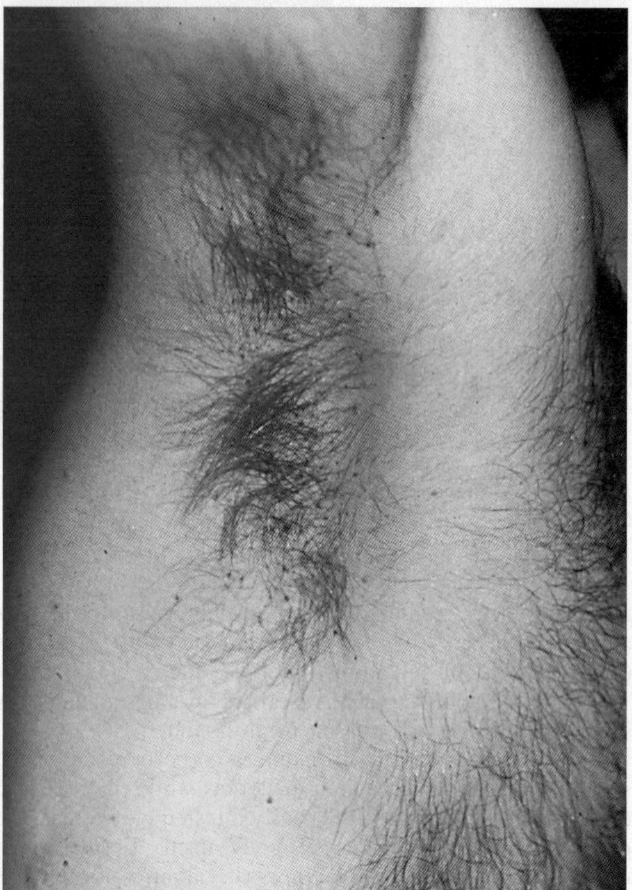

Figure 114-17. **Body lice.** *Photo courtesy David Effron, MD.*

border and scratch marks. Scabies in infants and young children often have generalized skin involvement, including the face, scalp, palms, and soles. In infants, the most common presenting lesions are papules and vesiculopustules.[62]

Immunosuppressed patients may develop Norwegian scabies, which is manifested by extensive hyperkeratosis and crusting of the hands, feet, and scalp. It is highly contagious because of excessive mite proliferation.[63,64] Secondary infections of these lesions are common.

Close personal contact is involved in transmission of

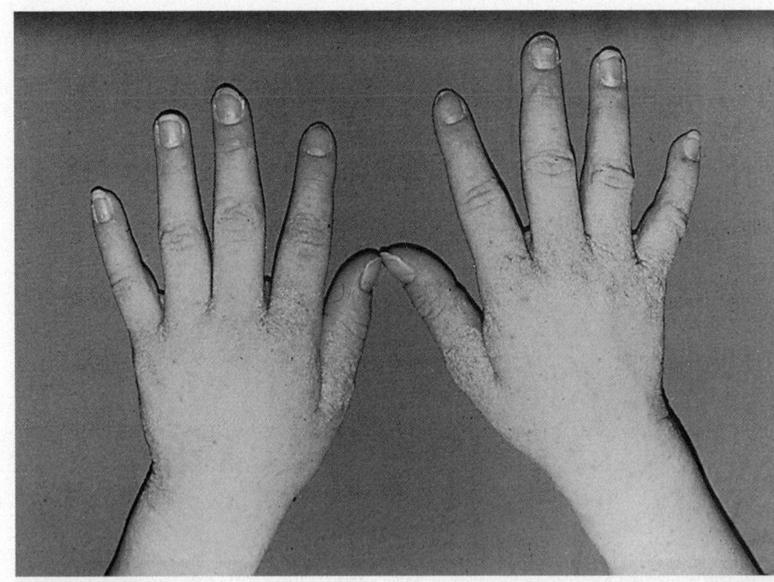

Figure 114-18. **Scabies.** ***Photo courtesy David Effron, MD.***

scabies. Multiple family members are likely to become infested. The infestation is also transmitted with sexual contact.

Management Treatment options include crotamiton (Eurax) lotion and cream, or permethrin 5% cream (Elimite). Lindane is no longer the preferred treatment. Patients in whom the former treatment fails may respond to the latter. Permethrin 5% cream (Elimite) applied overnight once weekly for 2 weeks over the entire body is the treatment of choice for infants and small children. It is more effective than crotamiton (Eurax) in eliminating the mite, in reducing secondary bacterial infection, and in reducing pruritus. Postscabietic nodules and pruritus may persist for months, even after successful treatment.[61,62,65,66]

Treatment of Norwegian scabies may require repeated treatment with scabicides and sometimes sequential use of several agents.[66]

All family members and sexual contacts also should be treated. Intimate articles of clothing and sheets and pillow cases should be washed and dried by machine (hot water), laundered and ironed, or boiled.

It may take several weeks after therapy for the signs and symptoms to abate. A hypersensitivity state or anxiety may prolong symptoms long after the mites have been destroyed.

Syphilis

Clinical Features Syphilis is transmitted only by direct contact with an infectious lesion. The causative organism is the spirochete *Treponema pallidum.* After an incubation period of 10 to 90 days, the primary lesion appears, which lasts from 3 to 12 weeks and heals spontaneously. In 6 weeks to 6 months after exposure, the disease enters the secondary stage, which involves a variety of mucocutaneous lesions. These lesions also heal spontaneously in 2 to 6 weeks as the disease enters the latent phase. Either a prolonged latent phase or tertiary syphilis follows. Of untreated patients, 25% display at least one relapse of mucocutaneous lesions of the oral cavity or anogenital region.

The chancre is the dermatologic manifestation of primary syphilis. Chancres usually appear as single lesions but may be multiple. They appear at the site of spirochete inoculation, usually the mucous membranes of the mouth or genitalia. The chancre begins as a papule and characteristically develops into an ulcer approximately 1 cm in diameter with a clean base and raised borders. The chancre is painless unless secondarily infected, and it may be accompanied by painless lymphadenopathy.

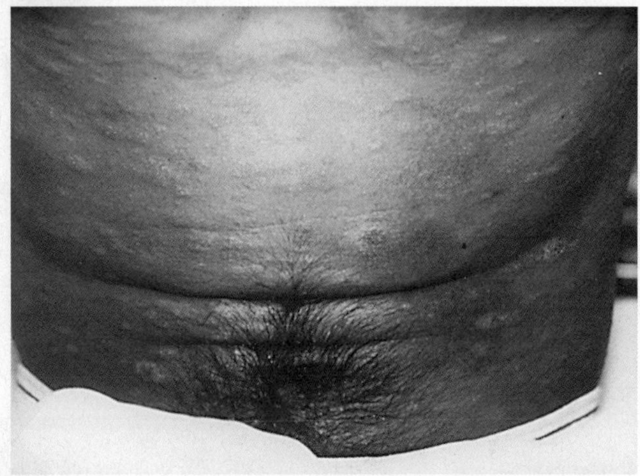

Figure 114-19. **Secondary syphilis.** ***Photo courtesy David Effron, MD.***

The secondary stage usually follows the primary stage by 6 weeks or more but rarely overlaps primary syphilis. There are a number of cutaneous manifestations of secondary syphilis. Lesions may be erythematous or pink macules or papules, usually with a generalized symmetrical distribution (Figure 114-19). Pigmented macules and papules classically appear on the palms and soles (Figures 114-20 and 114-21). The lesions may be scaly but are rarely pruritic.

Papular, annular, and circinate lesions are more common in nonwhites. Generalized lymphadenopathy and malaise accompany the skin lesions. Irregular, patchy alopecia may be seen. Moist, flat, verrucous condyloma latum may appear in the genital area. These lesions are highly contagious.

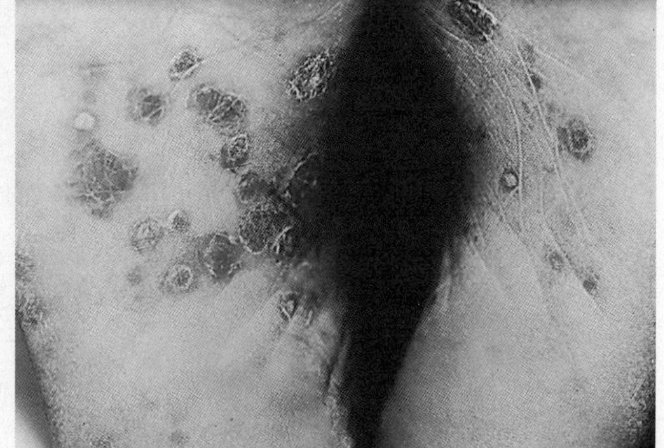

Figure 114-20. **Cutaneous manifestation of secondary syphilis on soles of feet.** ***Photo courtesy David Effron, MD.***

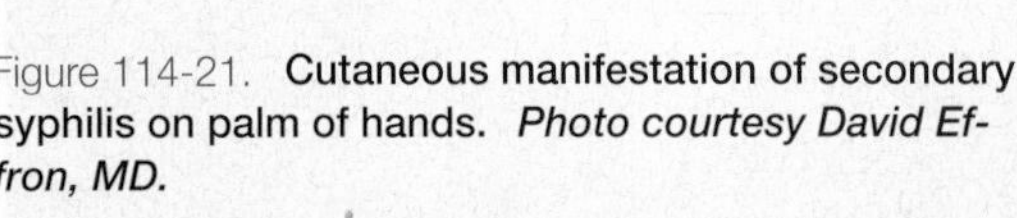

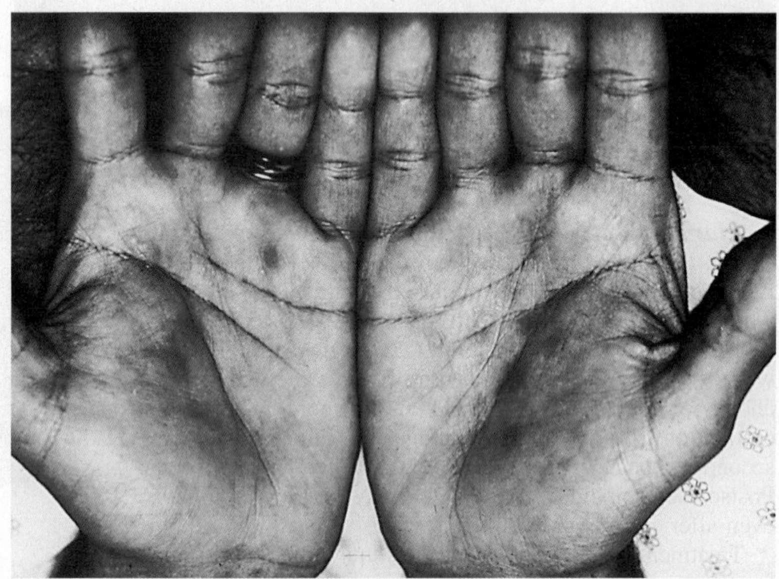

Figure 114-21. **Cutaneous manifestation of secondary syphilis on palm of hands.** ***Photo courtesy David Effron, MD.***

Diagnostic Strategies The diagnosis of primary syphilis is made primarily by the identification of spirochetes with darkfield microscopy. Because a darkfield microscope is often not available to the EP, the diagnosis of primary syphilis must be suspected on clinical grounds and the patient referred to a dermatologist or appropriate public agency for diagnosis and treatment. The Venereal Disease Research Laboratory (VDRL) test, the most commonly used diagnostic serologic test, is positive in approximately three fourths of patients with primary syphilis, but the test tends to be negative early in the course of the disease.[34]

The VDRL test is invariably positive in cases of secondary syphilis, usually in titers of 1:16 or greater. The darkfield examination of moist lesions may also be positive, but the diagnosis in this stage is based on a positive serologic test. The most specific and sensitive serologic test is the fluorescent treponemal antibody-absorption (FTA-ABS) test.[34]

A biologic false-positive serologic test for syphilis is defined as a positive VDRL test with a negative FTA-ABS test. This situation is seen acutely after vaccination or infections, especially mycoplasmal pneumonia, mononucleosis, hepatitis, measles, varicella, malaria, and in pregnancy. Chronic biologic false-positive reactions (i.e., those lasting longer than 6 months) may occur with systemic lupus erythematosus, thyroiditis, lymphoma, narcotic addiction, or in elderly patients. Most false-positive reactions are in low titer ranges of 1:1 to 1:4.

Management Incubating syphilis, the stage before the appearance of primary lesions, may be treated with 4.8 million units of procaine penicillin IM after 1 g of probenecid orally. Primary and secondary syphilis is treated with benzathine penicillin G in a dose of 2.4 million units IM. Patients allergic to penicillin should be treated with doxycycline, 100 mg twice a day, tetracycline, 500 mg four times a day, or erythromycin, 500 mg four times a day for 14 days.[34] HIV-infected patients require more intensive therapy.

Treatment may be administered in the ED if the diagnosis can be made on clinical, microscopic, or serologic grounds. If this cannot be done, a serologic sample should be drawn and the patient referred for treatment. The VDRL test may be expected to return to nonreactive in 6 to 12 months after the treatment of primary disease or 1 to 1½ years after the

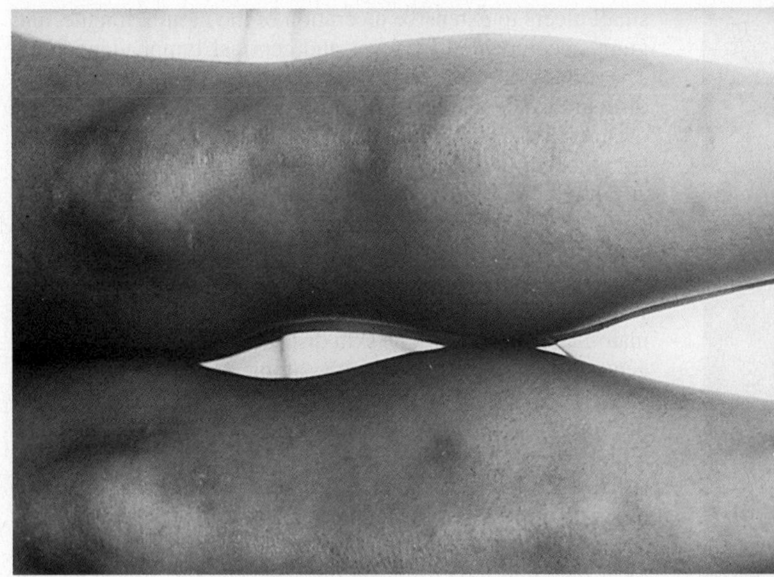

Figure 114-22. **Erythema nodosum.** *Photo courtesy David Effron, MD.*

treatment of secondary disease. Patients with tertiary syphilis who are adequately treated may nevertheless retain a positive serologic result. Within 12 hours of receiving therapy, patients may experience a febrile reaction and diffuse rash called the Jarisch-Herxheimer reaction. The reaction resolves spontaneously, usually within 24 hours.

NODULAR LESIONS

Erythema Nodosum

Clinical Features Erythema nodosum is an inflammatory reaction of the dermis and adipose tissue that is seen with painful red to violet nodules. Nodules are elevated lesions located deep in the skin over which the skin, on palpation, can be moved. These painful nodules occur most commonly over the anterior tibia but may also be seen on the arms or body. Fever and arthralgia of the ankles and knees may precede the rash.[3,9] As the lesions evolve, they may turn yellow-purple and resemble bruises (Figure 114-22). Women are affected three times more often than men, with the highest incidence being in the third to fifth decades of life.[67]

A number of underlying conditions produce erythema nodosum: tuberculosis, sarcoidosis, coccidioidomycosis, histoplasmosis, ulcerative colitis, regional enteritis, pregnancy, infections with streptococci, *Yersinia enterocolitica,* and *Chlamydia.* As with erythema multiforme, many cases of erythema nodosum are idiopathic. The relationship of drugs to erythema nodosum is noted in the earlier section on drug eruption. Oral contraceptive agents are a leading cause of drug-induced cases. The differential diagnosis includes traumatic bruises and subcutaneous fat necrosis.

Management When an underlying condition can be determined, this should be treated as indicated. Chest radiograph may be considered to rule out sarcoidosis, tuberculosis, or deep fungal infection. Bed rest, elevating the legs, and wearing elastic stockings reduce pain and edema. Aspirin in a dosage of 600 mg every 4 hours or nonsteroidal antiinflammatory agents may also afford some relief.[9,67] Erythema nodosum is a self-limited process that usually resolves in 3 to 8 weeks.[9] Patients with severe pain may be treated with 360 to 900 mg of potassium iodide daily for 3 to 4 weeks. Stopping therapy before this time may result in a relapse. Potassium iodide may act through an immunosuppressive mechanism mediated via heparin release from mast cells.[9,67]

VESICULAR LESIONS

Perspective

Vesicles are elevated lesions that contain clear fluid. Vesicles greater than 1 cm are known as bullae. Vesicles may sometimes be associated with red papular lesions, as in contact dermatitis or erythema multiforme.

Pemphigus Vulgaris

Clinical Features Pemphigus vulgaris is an uncommon, but important, dermatologic disorder. The mortality rate before the use of steroids was approximately 95%. The current mortality rate is 10% to 15%, related more to steroid-induced complications than to the disease. Pemphigus is a bullous disease, affecting both sexes equally, and is most common in patients 40 to 60 years of age.[68] The typical skin lesions are small, flaccid bullae that break easily, forming superficial erosions and crusted ulcerations. Any area of the body may be involved. Nikolsky's sign is present and characteristic of the disease. Blisters may be extended or new bullae may be formed by firm tangential pressure of a finger on the intact epidermis.

Before the appearance of the skin involvement, mucous membrane lesions occur; 50% to 60% of patients have oral lesions. The oral lesions typically antedate the cutaneous lesions by several months.[9,68] The most common site is in the mouth, especially the gums and vermilion borders of the lips. Oral lesions are bullous but commonly break, leaving painful, denuded areas of superficial ulceration.

The cause of pemphigus is unknown, although studies suggest an autoimmune mechanism. The development of pemphigus has been associated in a few instances with the use of medications, most notably penicillamine and captopril.[9] A positive Tzanck cytologic test suggests the diagnosis (i.e., finding acantholytic cells, degenerated, rounded epithelial cells with amorphous nuclei). Acantholytic cells are not specific for pemphigus, however, and the diagnosis

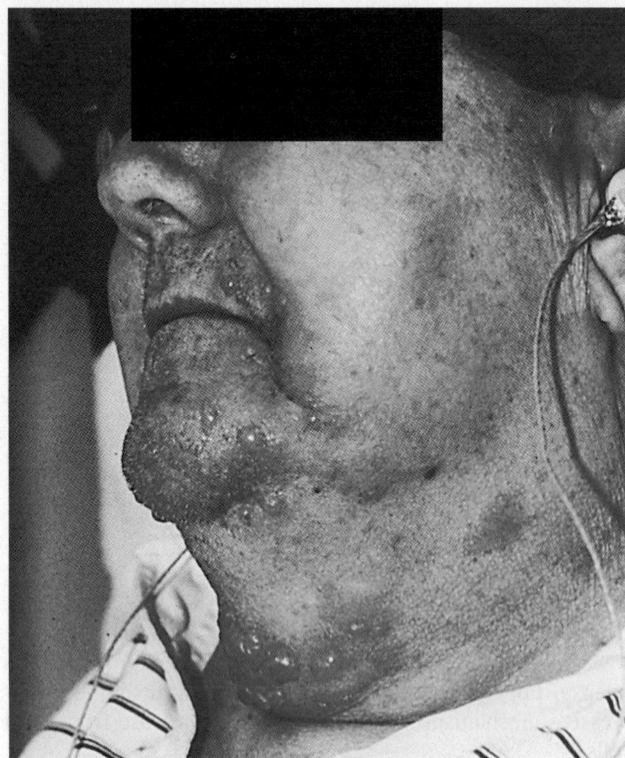

Figure 114-23. **Bullous pemphigus.** *Photo courtesy David Effron, MD.*

must be confirmed by serum immunofluorescence. The differential diagnosis includes bullous pemphigoid, epidermolysis, dermatitis herpetiformis, toxic epidermal necrolysis, bullous scabies, and bullous systemic lupus erythematosus (Figure 114-23).[9,68-71]

Management Pain control and local wound care are essential components of therapy. Once the diagnosis is made, treatment with oral glucocorticoids in initial doses of 100 to 300 mg of prednisone, or an equivalent drug, should be instituted in conjunction with a dermatologist. Other immunosuppressant drugs may also be used. Despite the condition's localization to the skin and mucous membranes, death was the rule before treatment with steroids, and the mortality rate continues to be substantial.[9] Deaths are related to an uncontrolled spread of the disease, secondary infection, dehydration, and thromboembolism. Other medical illness, as well the side effects of high-dosage corticosteroids, also contribute to mortality.

Herpes Simplex

Perspective Two known variants of HSV cause human infection: HSV-1 and HSV-2. The former primarily affects nongenital sites, whereas lesions caused by the latter are found predominantly in the genital area and are transmitted primarily by venereal contact.

Clinical Features The mouth is the most common site of HSV-1 infections. Children are affected more commonly than adults.[9] Small clusters of vesicles appear but are soon broken, leaving irregularly shaped, crusted erosions. The severity of gingivostomatitis varies from the presence of small ulcers to extensive ulceration of the mouth, tongue, and gums accompanied by fever and cervical lymphadenopathy. The infection may be so severe that oral fluid intake is difficult, and dehydration may result. Healing typically occurs in 7 to 14 days, unless a secondary infection with streptococci or staphylococci occurs.

The hallmark of skin infection with HSV is painful, grouped vesicles on an erythematous base. Those above the waist are usually caused by HSV-1, whereas those below the waist generally result from HSV-2 (Figures 114-24 and 114-25). The lesions are usually localized in a nondermatomal distribution. The skin distribution may become more generalized in patients with atopic eczema and other dermatoses. Adults with HSV infection should avoid contact with children with atopic dermatitis, especially in the first 3 to 5 days of infection.

HSV-2 infections in men are seen with either single or multiple vesicles on the shaft or glans penis. Fever, malaise, and regional adenopathy may be present.[34] A prodrome of local pain and hyperesthesia may precede the appearance of the cutaneous lesions. The vesicles erode after several days, become crusted, and heal in 10 to 14 days. Infections in women involve the introitus, cervix, or vagina. Vesicles may be grouped or confluent. Herpetic cervicitis or vaginitis may be the cause of severe pelvic pain, dysuria, or vaginal discharge.[9,34] Recurrence is common, but recurrent episodes tend to be less severe. A correlation has been discovered between HSV-2 reproductive tract infections and carcinoma of the cervix, based on serologic epidemiologic data.[9,34]

Management Recommended treatment for a first clinical episode of genital herpes is with acyclovir (Zovirax), 200 mg orally five times a day for 7 to 10 days, famciclovir, 125 mg twice a day, or valacyclovir, 500 mg three times a day or until clinical resolution occurs. These agents reduce the duration of viral shedding, accelerate healing, and shorten the duration of symptoms, but they have not succeeded in preventing recurrent episodes.[9] Prophylactic administration of acyclovir may be effective in ameliorating the severity of recurrent genital herpes, but the effects of long-term administration are unknown.[9] Although many episodes of recurrent herpes infection do not benefit from acyclovir therapy, 200 mg five times a day may be given orally for recurrences at the beginning of the prodrome. Famciclovir, 125 mg twice a day for 5 days, or valacyclovir, 500 mg three times a day for the same duration are equally effective.[9]

Severe initial attacks of genital herpes have been successfully treated with the IV infusion of acyclovir. Admission to the hospital is required, however, because such treatment is necessary for several days, especially for the immunocompromised patient. A mucocutaneous herpes infection in such patients is potentially fatal, having a propensity for generalization and dissemination to the internal organs.

Supportive care is important and pain control is a major concern. Systemic analgesics and topical anesthetic agents may be useful. Patient education regarding the prevention or spread of the disease during sexual contact and the birth process is imperative.

Varicella

Clinical Features Varicella, or chickenpox, is an infection caused by the varicella-zoster virus. After an incubation period of 14 to 21 days, the illness begins with a low-grade

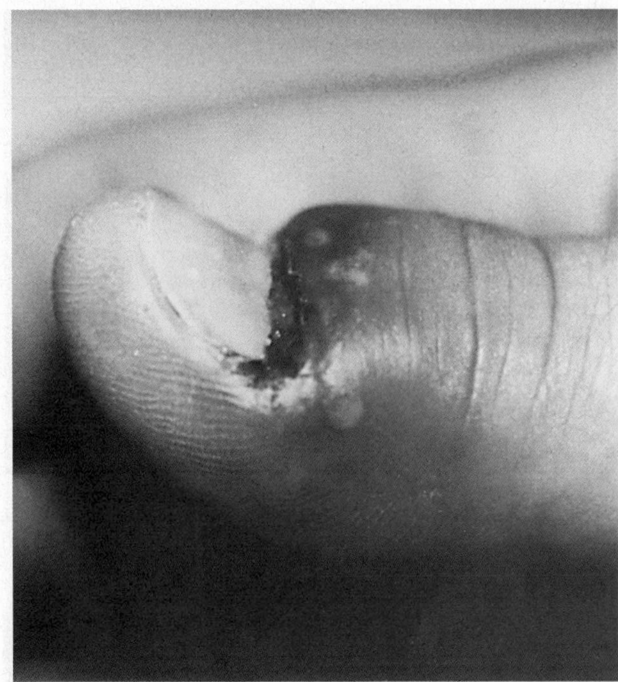

Figure 114-24. **HSV-1 infection.** ***Photo courtesy David Effron, MD.***

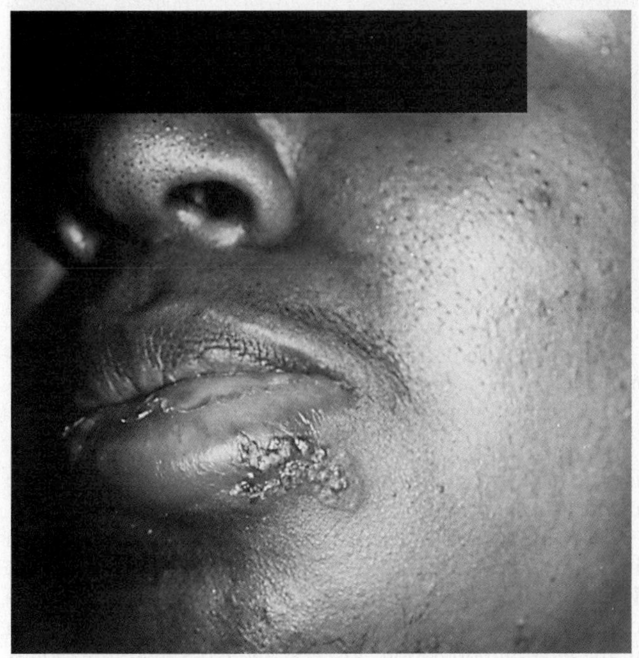

Figure 114-25. **Herpetic whitlow.** ***Photo courtesy David Effron, MD.***

fever, headache, and malaise. The exanthema coincides with these symptoms in children and follows them by 1 to 2 days in adults.

The skin lesions rapidly progress from macules to papules to vesicles to crusting, sometimes within 6 to 8 hours. The vesicle of varicella is 2 to 3 mm in diameter and surrounded by an erythematous border (Figure 114-26). An unusual form of varicella presents with larger bullae (Figure 114-27). The drying of the vesicle begins centrally, producing umbilication. The dried scabs fall off in 5 to 20 days.

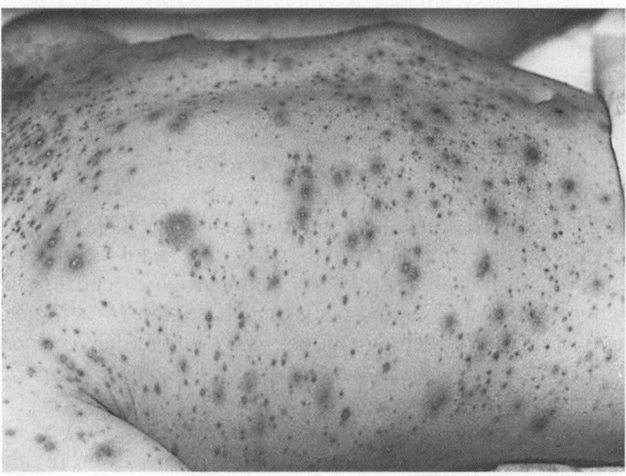

Figure 114-26. **Chickenpox.** ***Photo courtesy David Effron, MD.***

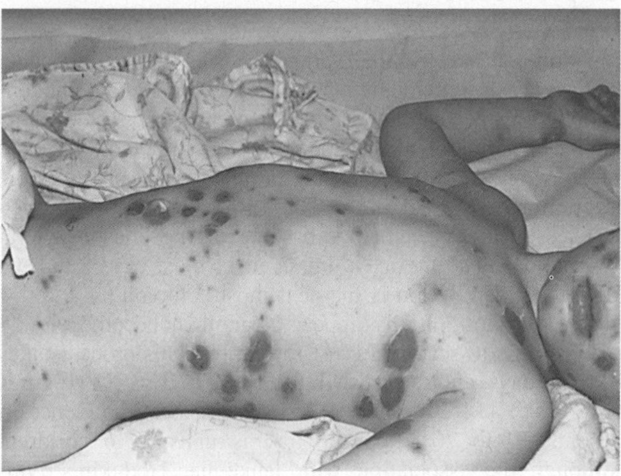

Figure 114-27. **Bullous chickenpox.** ***Photo courtesy David Effron, MD.***

Lesions appear in crops on the trunk, where they are seen in the highest concentration, and on the scalp, face, and extremities. The hallmark of varicella is the appearance of lesions in all stages of development in one region of the body. Extensive eruptions are often associated with a high and prolonged fever.

Complications of chickenpox include encephalitis or meningitis, pneumonia, and staphylococcal or streptococcal cellulitis, thrombocytopenia, arthritis, hepatitis, and glomerulonephritis.[53] Varicella pneumonia occurs more commonly in adults than in children.

Management The illness is self-limited, and treatment is symptomatic only. Salicylates should be avoided in patients with chickenpox to minimize the risk of subsequent Reye syndrome. Oral acyclovir may be effective if it can be started within 24 hours of development of rash for patients with chronic respiratory or skin disease. Some studies report a diminution in duration and magnitude of fever and number and duration of lesions with the early use of acyclovir.[72]

The isolation of infected patients is often futile because the disease may be transmitted before the diagnosis is clinically evident. Because the disease has the potential to be contagious until all vesicles are crusted and dried, infected persons should be kept at home until this stage is reached.

Varicella-zoster and varicella titers should be checked in pregnant women and immunocompromised patients who are exposed to chickenpox and, if negative, varicella-zoster immune globulin should be administered within 96 hours of exposure.[74] Fetal infection after maternal varicella in the first or early second trimester of pregnancy may result in varicella embryopathy, characterized by limb atrophy, scarring on extremities, and CNS and ocular manifestations.[53,73] Maternal varicella that occurs between 5 days before delivery and 2 days after delivery may result in disseminated herpes in the newborn.[74]

A vaccine against chickenpox was recently approved by the Food and Drug Administration. It appears to be highly efficacious and very safe. In addition, the incidence of zoster occurring after vaccination appears to be lower than in naturally acquired disease.[73]

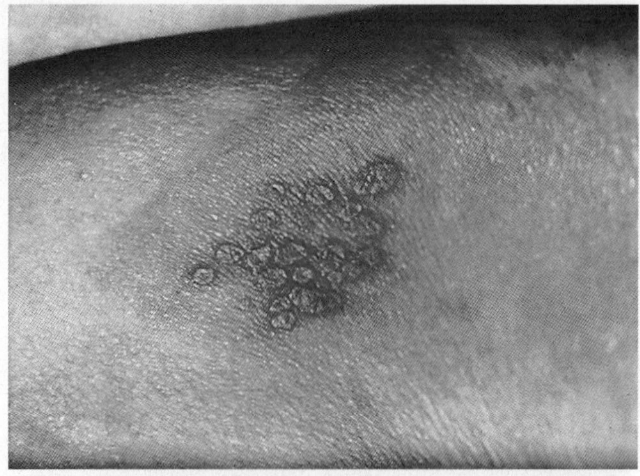

Figure 114-28. **Herpes zoster.** ***Photo courtesy David Effron, MD.***

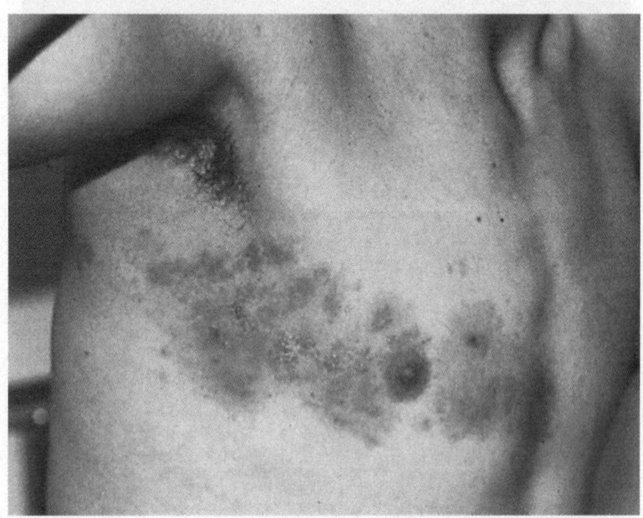

Figure 114-29. **Herpes zoster infection.** ***Photo courtesy David Effron, MD.***

Herpes Zoster

Clinical Features Herpes zoster, or shingles, is an infection caused by the varicella-zoster virus. It occurs exclusively in individuals who have previously had chickenpox. Before the rash appears, the patient typically develops pain in a dermatomal distribution. This pain is of variable intensity; sharp, dull, or burning in quality; and precedes the eruption by 1 to 10 days. The rash consists of grouped vesicles on an erythematous base involving one or several dermatomes. The thorax is involved in most cases, and the trigeminal distribution is the next most common.[73]

The vesicles initially appear clear, then become cloudy and progress to scab and crust formation. This process takes 10 to 12 days, and the crusts fall off in 2 to 3 weeks (Figures 114-28 and 114-29). Herpes zoster has a peak incidence in patients 50 to 70 years old and is unusual in children. Although the association with leukemia, Hodgkin's lymphoma, and other malignancies is well known, rarely does the appearance antedate the diagnosis of such disease. Most cases of herpes zoster occur in healthy individuals.[73]

Herpes zoster may be transmitted from patients with chickenpox to susceptible individuals. Chickenpox may also be acquired by contact with shingles, although this is less common.[75] It is generally believed, however, that herpes zoster is caused by a reactivation of latent varicella-zoster virus present since the initial infection with chickenpox. During the latent period between the two illnesses, the virus is thought to reside in dorsal root ganglion cells.[9,73]

Herpes zoster has a very low mortality rate and is rarely life threatening even when dissemination to the visceral organs occurs. Complications include CNS involvement, ocular infection, and neuralgia. Meningoencephalitis, myelitis, and peripheral neuropathy have been reported.

Ocular complications occur in 20% to 70% of the cases involving the ophthalmic division of the trigeminal nerve. The severity varies from mild conjunctivitis to panophthalmitis, which threatens the eye.[73] Eye involvement produces anterior uveitis, secondary glaucoma, and corneal scarring. There is a close correlation between eye involvement and vesicles located at the tip of the nose.

Postherpetic neuralgia, pain that persists after the lesions have healed, occurs more commonly in elderly and immunosuppressed patients.[73,76] It may last a number of months and is often resistant to treatment with standard analgesic medications.

Herpes zoster generally tends to be more severe in immunosuppressed patients, especially those with AIDS, Hodgkin's disease, or other lymphomas.[73,76] Cutaneous dissemination occurs more commonly in these patients than in the general population. Visceral and CNS dissemination is also more likely to occur in those patients; therefore they should be considered for hospitalization.

Management Treatment other than analgesia is rarely necessary. Burow's solution compresses diluted 1:20 to 1:40 in water may be applied to hasten drying. Early systemic corticosteroid therapy may shorten the duration of postherpetic neuralgia but does not lessen the severity of pain or the rate of the healing of the lesions.[73] Antiviral chemotherapy, with acyclovir, famciclovir, vidarabine, foscarnet, valacyclovir, and interferon alpha have been shown to be effective for immunocompromised patients.[73] Postherpetic neuralgia is a complicated problem with few satisfactory solutions.

Capsaicin cream has met with some success but cannot be applied to inflamed or eroded skin.[9]

Intravenous acyclovir may be of some benefit in the treatment of severe ocular herpes zoster. Treatment includes mydriasis and the application of topical corticosteroids. Unlike with herpes simplex conjunctivitis, eye involvement caused by herpes zoster does not appear to be exacerbated by corticosteroids.

SKIN LESIONS ASSOCIATED WITH SYSTEMIC DISEASE

Numerous systemic illnesses have cutaneous manifestations (Table 114-3). Some of the most common illnesses include AIDS, diabetes mellitus, connective tissue diseases, and endocrine disorders.

CLINICAL FEATURES OF LESIONS ASSOCIATED WITH INTERNAL MALIGNANCY

Cutaneous lesions most directly indicative of an internal malignancy arise from the extension of the tumor to the skin or by hematogenous or lymphatic metastasis. The neoplasms that most commonly produce such a cutaneous extension are lymphomas, leukemias, and carcinomas of the breast, GI tract, lung, ovary, prostate, uterus, and bladder. Skin metastases generally signify a poor prognosis.[67]

Acanthosis Nigricans

Acanthosis nigricans is associated with internal malignancy, despite the fact that most cases do not have tumors.[77] Benign cases may be familial or related to endocrine disease or obesity. The term *malignant acanthosis nigricans* is used to designate the form associated with neoplastic disease. This phrasing is misleading because acanthosis nigricans is only a marker of the underlying disease and is never infiltrated with malignant cells.

The lesion appears as a hyperpigmented verrucous, velvet-like hyperplasia and hypertrophy of the skin accompanied with accentuation of the skin markings. The chief sites of involvement are the body folds, especially the axillae, antecubital fossae, neck, and groin.

More than 90% of cases of "malignant" acanthosis nigricans are associated with intraabdominal malignancies, of which two thirds are adenocarcinomas of the stomach.[77,78] Carcinomas of the colon, ovary, pancreas, rectum, and uterus make up the majority of the rest.[77] Regardless of the tumor type, acanthosis nigricans is associated with tumors that usually are highly malignant and metastasize early.[67,78] The mechanism of this dermatosis in cases of internal malignant disease is postulated to be a result of tumor products that bind to and stimulate insulin-like growth factors in the skin.[77]

Dermatomyositis

The incidence of dermatomyositis with malignant disease ranges from 6% to 55% and is generally higher in older patients. In younger individuals the appearance of dermatomyositis does not necessarily call for a tumor workup. Tumors commonly associated with dermatomyositis are carcinomas of the breast, ovary, and GI and female genital tracts. Polymyositis occurring alone without the accompanying skin findings is rarely associated with malignancies.[67,82]

Erythema Multiforme

Erythema multiforme may be associated with acute forms of leukemia. It is seen with acute monocytic, lymphocytic, and granulocytic forms and is also found in chronic leukemias and Hodgkin's disease.[9,83]

Erythema Nodosum

Erythema nodosum is another reaction found in association with leukemia and Hodgkin's lymphoma, as well as with metastatic carcinoma, and as previously described, with inflammatory bowel disease.[78,83]

Erythroderma

Generalized erythroderma is almost pathognomonic for Hodgkin's disease; however, it is also a common skin manifestation of lymphocytic leukemia. Although less common, it is also seen with other forms of leukemia, carcinoma, and mycosis fungoides. The appearance of erythroderma may precede the diagnosis of internal malignant disease by many years. The skin eruption is invariably accompanied by intractable pruritus.[83]

Acquired Ichthyosis

Acquired ichthyosis is a skin condition manifested as generalized dryness of the skin, scaling, and superficial cracking, or as hyperkeratosis of the palms and soles. Hodgkin's disease is the most common malignant disease associated with the nonfamilial form of ichthyosis. Non-Hodgkin's lymphoma and carcinomas of the breast, lung, colon, and cervix have also been associated with acquired ichthyosis.[67]

Pruritus

Itching may be an important indicator of Hodgkin's disease, leukemia, adenocarcinoma or squamous cell carcinoma of various organs, carcinoid syndrome, multiple myeloma, and polycythemia vera. It may appear years before the underlying malignancy is identified.[67,83] In cases of Hodgkin's disease, the itching is usually continuous and may be accompanied by a severe burning sensation. Although usually generalized, pruritus commonly begins in the feet and may be limited to the lower extremities. It may be intractable and associated with urticaria, erythroderma, excoriation, or lichenification.

The pruritus of leukemia and systemic carcinoma is generally less severe than that found with Hodgkin's disease. Nevertheless, itching associated with internal malignant disease may be difficult to control. Conventional anti-H_1 antihistamines, cimetidine, cholestyramine, and cyproheptadine have each been used with variable results.[79] Occasionally, only the suppression of the tumor is beneficial.

Purpura

Purpura is the most common manifestation of acute granulocytic and monocytic leukemia. It may also be associated with myeloma, lymphoma, and polycythemia vera. Although the most common cause of purpura in these conditions is thrombocytopenia secondary to bone marrow infiltration, in some instances the platelet count is normal and the causative mechanism obscure.[9] Purpura is caused by vascular abnormalities, thrombocytopenia, or other coagulation defects. A variety of diseases and conditions may be the underlying cause, and the treatment should be directed toward this cause whenever possible (Boxes 114-1 and 114-2).[84] Thrombocytopenic and nonthrombocytopenic forms are

Text continued on p. 1662

Table 114-3. Skin Lesions Associated with Systemic Disease

Disease	Lesions	Comments
AIDS[3,9,74]	Chronic ulcerative herpes simplex	
	Kaposi's sarcoma (Figures 114-30 and 114-31)	Diagnostic for AIDS
	Severe herpes zoster	
	Oral hairy leukoplakia	
	Genital warts	
	Molluscum contagiosum (Figure 114-32)	
	Seborrheic dermatitis 2 Pityrosporum	
	Recurrent staphylococcal abscesses	
	Mycobacterial papules, nodules, abscesses	
	Oral and rectal squamous cell carcinoma	
	Lymphoma	
	Severe psoriasis	
	Acquired ichthyosis	
	Folliculitis	
	Human papillomavirus infection	
	Lichenoid photoeruptions	
Diabetes mellitus[67]	Diabetic dermopathy	Most common
	Necrobiosis lipoidica diabeticorum	Most characteristic
	Cellulitis (Figure 114-33)	Control of diabetes does not affect presence
	Vascular ulceration (Figure 114-34)	
	Acanthosis nigricans	
	Bullosis diabeticorum	
	Diabetic thick skin	
	Scleroderma	
Dermatomyositis[78]	Heliotrope discoloration and edema of eyelids	Skin lesions may precede muscle disease
	Scaly erythema of malar prominences	Symmetric proximal weakness, remissions and exacerbations
	Erythematous dermatitis over joint exterior surfaces, especially hands (Figure 114-35)	Increased creatine phosphokinase aldolase with active disease
	Raynaud's phenomenon	
Systemic lupus erythematosus[79]	Discoid lesions	Patients with cutaneous discoid lupus generally have benign diseases
	Malar erythema (Figure 114-36)	
	Hypertrophic or verrucous palm and sole lesions	
	Lupus panniculitis	
	Oral ulcers	
	Raynaud's phenomenon	
Rheumatoid arthritis[80]	Rheumatoid nodules and necrobiosis	
	Vasculitic lesions	
	Pyoderma gangrenosum	
	Urticaria	Still's disease
Hyperthyroidism[67,81]	Fine, velvety, smooth skin	
	Increased sweating	
	Hyperpigmentation or hypopigmentation	
	Pretibial edema	
	Alopecia	
	Onchyrosis	
	Urticaria	
Hypothyroidism[67,81]	Dry, coarse	
	Myxedema (Figure 114-37)	
	Carotene color	
	Pruritus	
	Atopic dermatitis	
	Ichthyosis	
	Erythema nodosum	
	Easy bruising	
	Alopecia (lateral one third of eyebrows)	
Ulcerative colitis[77]	Pyoderma gangrenosum	Associated with state of disease
	Erythema nodosum	
	Aphthous stomatitis	

Box 114-1 Causes of Purpura

Thrombocytopenic	Nonthrombocytopenic
Aplastic anemia	Drugs
Drug-induced	Infection (meningococcemia, Rocky Mountain spotted fever)
Idiopathic	Qualitative platelet defect
Malignant disease	Vasculitis
Sarcoidosis	
Splenomegaly	
Systemic lupus erythematosus	
Thrombotic	
Tuberculosis	

Box 114-2 Commonly Used Drugs Associated with Purpura

Amitriptyline	Isoniazid
Aspirin	Meprobamate
Cephalothin	Methyldopa
Chloramphenicol	Penicillin
Chlorpromazine	Phenacetin
Chlorpropamide	Phenobarbital
Diazoxide	Phenylbutazone
Digitoxin	Quinidine
Furosemide	Rifampin
Hydrochlorothiazide	Sulfonamides
Indomethacin	Tolbutamide

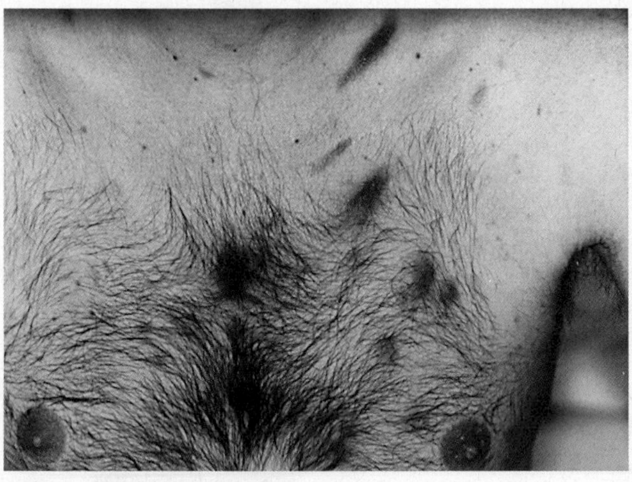

Figure 114-30. **Kaposi's sarcoma associated with AIDS.** ***Photo courtesy David Effron, MD.***

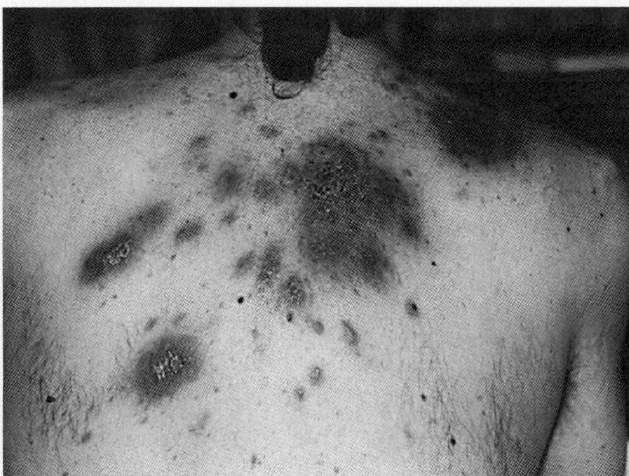

Figure 114-31. **Kaposi's sarcoma in an AIDS patient.** ***Photo courtesy David Effron, MD.***

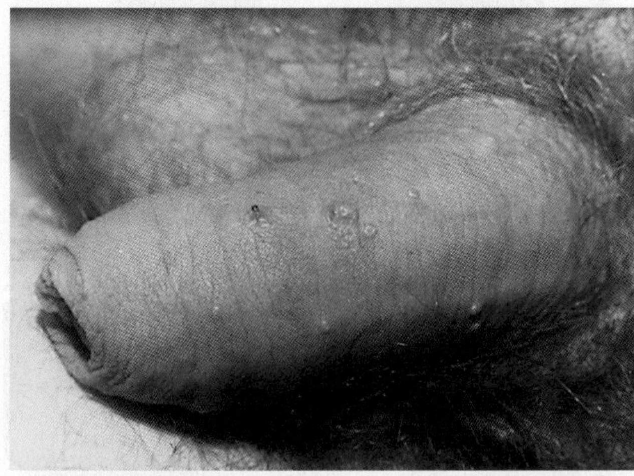

Figure 114-32. **Molluscum contagiosum caused by a virus is more prevalent with AIDS.** ***Photo courtesy David Effron, MD.***

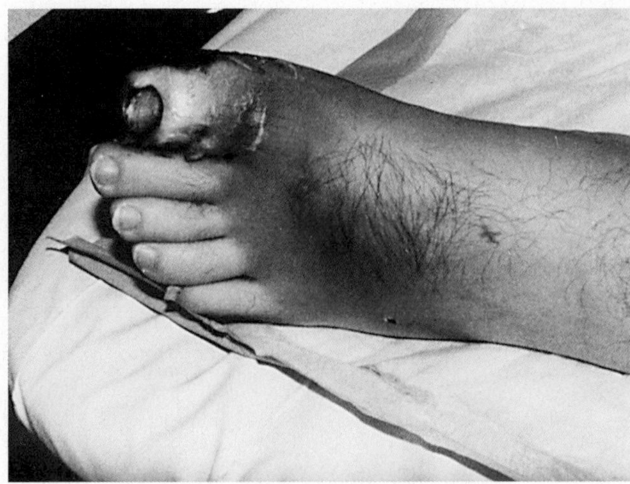

Figure 114-33. **Gangrene of the toe with cellulitis in a diabetic patient.** ***Photo courtesy David Effron, MD.***

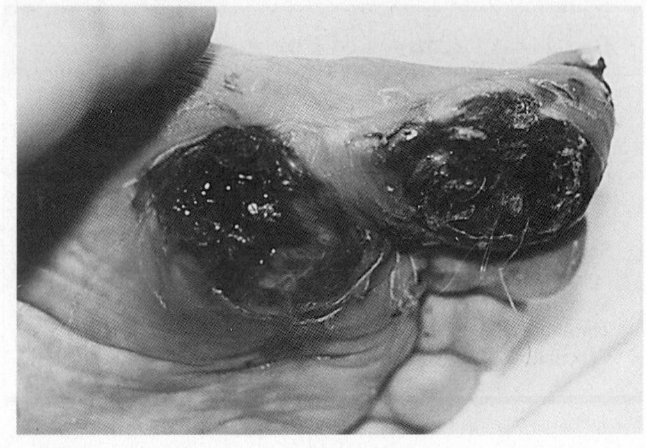

Figure 114-34. **Vascular ulceration secondary to diabetes.** ***Photo courtesy David Effron, MD.***

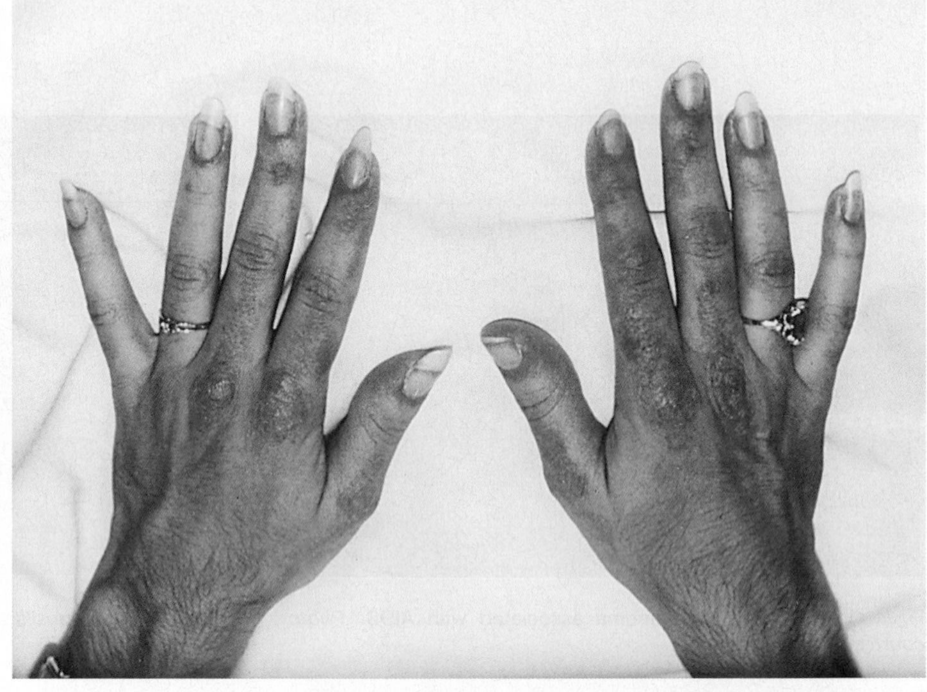

Figure 114-35. **Erythematous dermatitis over joint extensor surfaces, dermatomyositis.** ***Photo courtesy David Effron, MD.***

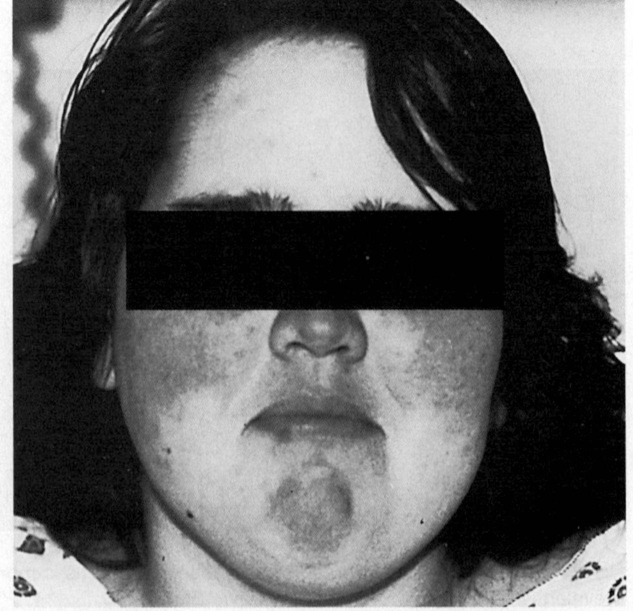

Figure 114-36. **Malar erythema in a patient with systemic lupus erythematosus.** ***Photo courtesy David Effron, MD.***

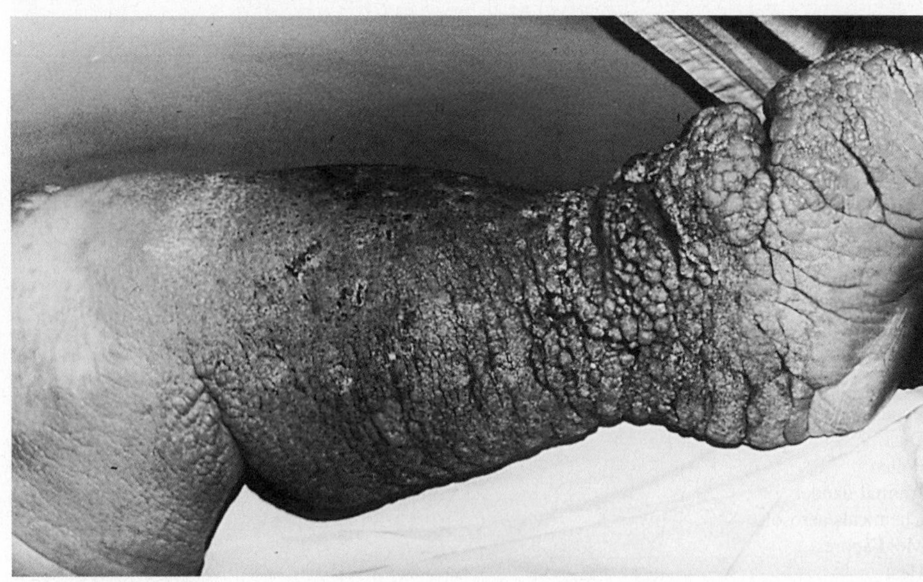

Figure 114-37. **Severe myxedema in a hypothyroid patient.** *Photo courtesy David Effron, MD.*

Table 114-4. Common Causes of Urticaria[9,48,49]

Cause	Common responsible factors
Bacterial infection	*Streptococcus*
	Staphylococcus
	Yersinia
	Mycobacterium
Viral infection	Herpes simplex virus
	Epstein-Barr virus
	Cytomegalovirus
	Hepatitis viruses (especially B)
	Many acute viral syndromes (adenovirus, enterovirus)
Other infections	Parasites
	Coccidioidomycosis
	Histoplasmosis
	Rickettsia
	Spirochete (Lyme disease)
Envenomation	Bees
	Wasps
	Scorpions
	Spiders
	Jellyfish
	Fleas
	Mites
Drugs	Penicillin
	Sulfa
	Cephalosporins
	Salicylates
	Morphine, codeine, other opiates
	Nonsteroidal antiinflammatory drugs
	Barbiturates
	Amphetamines
	Blood and blood products

Continued

Table 114-4. Common Causes of Urticaria[9,48,49]—cont'd

Cause	Common responsible factors
Foods	Nuts Shellfish Eggs Strawberries Tomatoes Milk, cheese Chocolate
Contacts	Chemicals Cosmetics Topical medications Plants Textiles Foods
Inhalants	Dust Pollen Animal dander Chemicals/aerosols Mold spores
Physical agents	Heat Cold Light Pressure (dermatographism) Water
Diseases	Collagen vascular disease Lupus, juvenile rheumatoid arthritis, polyarteritis nodosa, dermatomyositis, Sjögren syndrome, rheumatic fever Inflammatory bowel disease Crohn's disease, ulcerative colitis Malignancy Carcinoma, leukemia, lymphoma Miscellaneous Serum sickness, thyroiditis, aphthous stomatitis, Behçet's disease

differentiated by the results of the patient's platelet count. Serious bleeding seldom occurs if the platelet count is greater than $50,000/mm^3$. If the platelet count is less than $10,000/mm^3$ or serious bleeding is encountered, platelet transfusion should be initiated. Because of the short circulating half-life of infused platelets, transfusion should be used as a short-term measure only.

Urticaria

Urticaria is occasionally found in Hodgkin's disease and more rarely in leukemia and internal carcinoma. Cold urticaria may occur with multiple myeloma (Table 114-4).

CLINICAL FEATURES OF LESIONS ASSOCIATED WITH NARCOTIC ADDICTION

Individuals who inject opiates and other drugs parenterally develop characteristic skin lesions secondary to such use.[85] Skin lesions have been most extensively described in heroin addicts. Skin tracks, or indurated linear hyperpigmented streaks, are produced by repeated IV injection (Figure 114-38). They follow the course of the superficial veins used in the injection, most commonly in the antecubital fossae and the dorsa of the hands.

Subcutaneous injection results in round or oval hyperpigmented atrophic depressed scars 1 to 3 cm in diameter (Figure 114-39). Abscesses, which often require drainage, commonly precede the development of such scars. Hypertrophic scarring and keloid formation may also occur.

Increased pigmentation may occur in sun-exposed areas and at the site of tourniquet applications.

KEY CONCEPTS

- Infection with *Candida albicans* can occur normally in infancy, in obese people, during pregnancy, and in old age. In other patients, the following underlying problems should be considered: AIDS and other immunodeficiency states, diabetes and other endocrine imbalances, malignancy, malnutrition, and other debilitating illnesses.
- Rashes that are associated with mucosal lesions, blisters, or desquamating skin are often caused by significant soft tissue infections, drug eruptions, or immune disorders.
- Purpura result from blood leaking from vessels into the skin and do not blanch when pressure is applied. Purpura less than 3 mm in diameter are called petechiae. Nonpalpable purpura are often caused by coagulation defects (usually platelet abnormalities), while palpable purpura are usually a sign of vasculitis.
- Diffuse pruritus in the absence of a skin rash may be a sign of underlying malignancy.

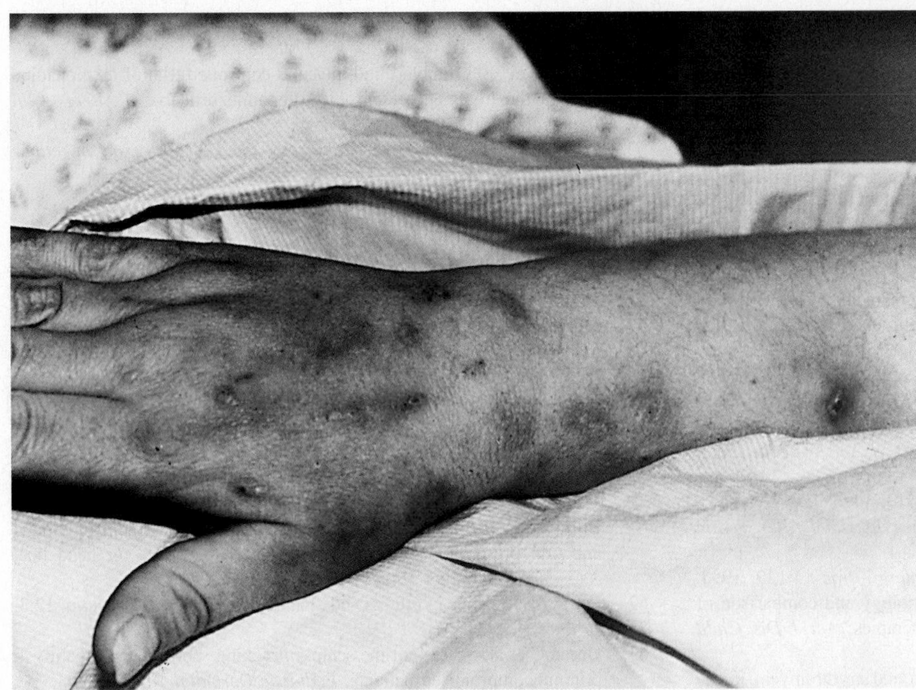

Figure 114-38. **Tracks secondary to IV heroin abuse.** ***Photo courtesy David Effron, MD.***

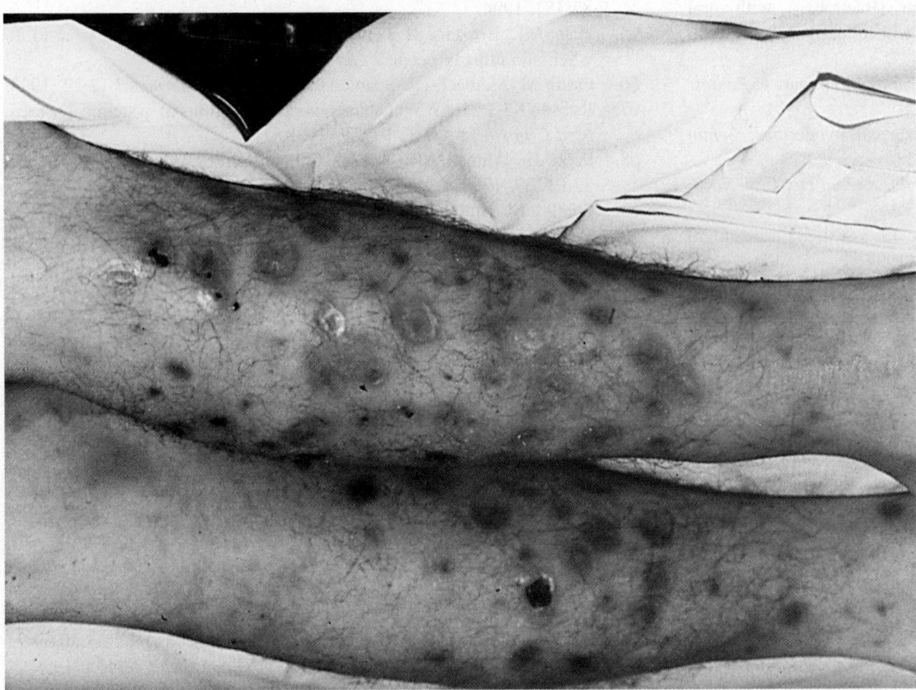

Figure 114-39. **Scars from subcutaneous illicit drug injection.** ***Photo courtesy of David Effron, MD.***

REFERENCES

1. Shivaram V, Christoph RA, Hayden GF: Skin disorders encountered in a pediatric emergency department, *Pediatr Emerg Care* 9:202, 1993.
2. Little JM, Hall MN, Pettice YJ: Teaching dermatology: too dependent on dermatologists? *Fam Med* 25:92, 1993.
3. Lookingbill DP, Marks JG: *Principles of dermatology,* ed 2, Philadelphia, 1993, WB Saunders.
4. Babel DE: How to identify fungi, *J Am Acad Dermatol* 6:S108, 1994.
5. Stein D: Tineas: superficial dermatophyte infections, *Pediatr Rev* 19:368, 1998.
6. Frieden IJ, Howard R: Tinea capitis: epidemiology, diagnosis, treatment and control, *J Am Acad Dermatol* S42:44-48, 1994.
7. Stevenson L, Brooke DS: Tinea capitis, *J Pediatr Health Care* 8:189, 1994.
8. Hayes AG: Black dot tinea capitis in a man, *Int J Dermatol* 32:740, 1993.
9. Edwards L: *Dermatology in emergency medicine,* New York, 1997, Churchill Livingstone.
10. Hubbard TW, deTriquet JM: Brush-culture method for diagnosing tinea capitis, *Pediatrics* 90:416, 1993.
11. Friedlander S, Pickering B, Cunningham B: Use of the cotton swab method in diagnosing tinea capitis, *Pediatr* 104:277-279, 1999.
12. Aly R: Ecology, epidemiology and diagnosis of tinea capitis, *Pediatr Infect Dis J* 18:180, 1999.
13. Legendre R, Escola Macre J: Itraconazole in the treatment of tinea capitis, *J Am Acad Dermatol* 23:559, 1990.
14. Maroon TS et al: A randomized double-blind, comparative study of terbinatone vs. griseofulvin in tinea capitis, *J Dermatol Treat* 3:25, 1992.

15. Pomeranz AJ, Fairley JA: Management errors leading to unnecessary hospitalization for kerion, *Pediatrics* 93:986, 1994.
16. Honig PJ et al: Treatment of kerions, *Pediatr Dermatol* 11:69, 1994.
17. Commens CA: Superficial mycoses: a practical approach, *Med J Aust* 158:470, 1993.
18. Aly R et al: Topical griseofulvin in the treatment of dermatophytoses, *Clin Exp Dermatol* 19:43, 1994.
19. Smith EB: Topical antifungal drugs in the treatment of tinea pedis, tinea cruris, and tinea corporis, *J Am Acad Dermatol* S24:129-136, 1993.
20. Chren M: Costs of therapy for dermatophyte infections, *J Am Acad Dermatol* S103:57-65, 1993.
21. Savin R et al: Efficacy of terbinafine 1% cream in the treatment of moccasin-type tinea pedis: results of placebo-controlled multicenter trials, *J Am Acad Dermatol* 30:663, 1994.
22. Assaf R, Weil M: The superficial mycoses, *Dermatol Clin* 14:57, 1996.
23. Borelli D, Jacobs PH, Nall L: Tinea versicolor: epidemiologic, clinical, and therapeutic aspects, *J Am Acad Dermatol* 25:300, 1991.
24. Scher R: Onychomycosis: therapeutic update, *J Am Acad Dermatol* 40:S21, 1999.
25. Hay R: Yeast infections, *Dermatol Clin* 14:113, 1996.
26. Harrigan E, Rabinowitz L: Atopic dermatits, *Immunol Allergy Clin North Am* 19:383, 1999.
27. Berstein J, Zeiss CR: Atopic dermatitis, *Allergy Proc* 14:129, 1993.
28. Demidovich CW et al: Impetigo: current etiology and comparison of penicillin, erythromycin and cephalexin therapies, *Am J Dis Child* 144:1313, 1990.
29. Britton JW et al: Comparison of mupirocin and erythromycin in the treatment of impetigo, *J Pediatr* 117:827, 1990.
30. McLinn S: A bacteriologically controlled, randomized study comparing the efficacy of 2% mupirocin ointment (Bactroban) with oral erythromycin in the treatment of patients with impetigo, *J Am Acad Dermatol* 22(5, pt 1):883, 1990.
31. Jain A, Daum R: Staphylococcal infections in children: part 1, *Pediatr Rev* 20:186, 1999.
32. Feingold DS: Staphylococcal and streptococcal pyodermas, *Semin Dermatol* 12:331, 1993.
33. Cucurull E, Espinoza L: Gonococcal arthritis, *Rheum Dis Clin North Am* 24:305-322, 1998.
34. Centers for Disease Control and Prevention: 1998 sexually transmitted disease treatment guidelines, *MMWR* 47:1, 1998.
35. Salzman M: Meningococcemia, *Infect Dis Clin North Am* 10:709, 1996.
36. Hacker SM: Common infections of the skin, *Postgrad Med* 96:43, 1994.
37. Schwartz G, Wright S: Changing bacteriology of periorbital cellulitis, *Ann Emerg Med* 28:617, 1996.
38. Sadow KB, Chamberlain JM: Blood cultures in the evaluation of children with cellulitis, *Pediatrics* 101:E4, 1998.
39. McCollough M: Progress toward eliminating *Haemophilus influenzae* type b disease among infants and children—United States 1987-1997 [commentary], *Ann Emerg Med* 34:110, 1999.
40. Sigurdsson AF et al: The etiology of bacterial cellulitis as determined by fine-needle aspiration, *Scand J Infect Dis* 21:537, 1989.
41. Beltrani V: Cutaneous manifestations of adverse drug reactions, *Immunol Allergy Clin North Am* 18:867, 1998.
42. Pollack S: Staphylococcal scalded skin syndrome, *Pediatr Rev* 17:1996.
43. Manders S: Toxin-mediated streptococcal and staphylococcal disease, *J Am Acad Dermatol* 39:383,386, 1998.
44. Egan C et al: Plasmapheresis as an adjunct in toxic epidermal necrolysis, *J Am Acad Dermatol* 40:458, 1999.
45. Cohen-Abbo A, Harper MB: Case report: streptococcal toxic shock syndrome presenting as septic thrombophlebitis in a child with varicella, *Pediatr Infect Dis J* 12:1033, 1993.
46. Soravia C et al: Group A betahaemolytic streptococcus septicaemia: the toxic strep syndrome. Report of our cases-developing septic shock and multiple organ failure, *Intensive Care Med* 19:53, 1993.
47. Todd JK et al: Corticosteroid therapy for patients with toxic shock syndrome, *JAMA* 252:3399, 1984.
48. Westo WL, Badgett JT: Urticaria, *Pediatr Rev* 19:240, 1998.
49. Tharp MD: Chronic urticaria: pathophysiology and treatment approaches, *J Allergy Clin Immunol* 98:S325, 1996.
50. Beltrani VS: Urticaria and angioedema, *Dermatol Clin* 14:171, 1996.
51. Srabani G, Kanwar AJ, Kaur S: Urticaria in children, *Pediatr Dermatol* 10:107, 1993.
52. Finn AF et al: A double-blind, placebo-controlled trial of fexofenadine HCl in the treatment of chronic idiopathic urticaria, *J Allergy Clin Immunol* 104:1077, 1999.
53. Peter G, editor: Red Book: *Report of the Committee on Infectious Diseases,* St Louis, 1997, American Academy of Pediatrics.
54. Measles, *MMWR* 43:673, 1994.
55. Akinbami L, Cheng T: Rocky Mountain spotted fever, *Pediatr Rev* 19:171, 1998.
56. Resnick S: New aspects of exanthematous diseases of childhood, *Dermatol Clin* 15:257, 1997.
57. Martini MC, Marks JG: Contact dermatitis and contact urticaria. In Sams WM, Lynch PJ, editors: *Principles and practice of dermatology,* New York, 1990, Churchill Livingstone.
58. Friedlander SF: Contact dermatitis, *Pediatr Rev* 19:166, 1998.
59. Lawrence R: Poisonous plants: when they are a threat to children, *Pediatr Rev* 18:164, 1997.
60. Dotson RL, Zurowski S, Walker KD: Erythema multiforme, *Missouri Med* 90:221, 1993.
61. Burkhart CG, Burkhart CN, Burkhart KM: An assessment of topical and oral prescription and over-the-counter treatments for head lice, *J Am Acad Dermatol* 38:979, 1998.
62. Paller AS: Scabies in infants and small children, *Semin Dermatol* 12:3, 1993.
63. Duran C et al: Scabies of the scalp mimicking seborrheic dermatitis in immunocompromised patients, *Pediatric Dermatol* 10:136, 1993.
64. Schlesinger I, Oelrich DM, Tyring SK: Crusted (Norwegian) scabies in patients with AIDS: the range of clinical presentations, *South Med J* 87:352, 1994.
65. Haag ML, Brozena SJ, Fenske NA: Attack of the scabies: what to do when an outbreak occurs? *Geriatrics* 48:45, 1993.
66. Orkin M, Maibach HI: Scabies therapy, *Semin Dermatol* 12:22, 1993.
67. Robson KJ, Piette WW: Cutaneous manifestations of systemic diseases, *Med Clin North Am* 82:P1359, 1998.
68. Scott JE, Ahmed AR: The blistering diseases, *Med Clin North Am* 82:P1239, 1998.
69. Shatley M: Bullous pemphigoid, *Missouri Med* 90:274, 1993.
70. Warren SD, Lesher JL: Cicatricial pemphigoid, *South Med J* 86:461, 1993.
71. Said S et al: Localized bullous scabies, *Am J Dermatol* 15:590, 1993.
72. Dunkle LM et al: A controlled trial of acyclovir for chicken pox in normal children, *N Engl J Med* 325:1539, 1991.
73. McCrary ML, Severson J, Tyring SK: Varicella zoster virus, *J Am Acad Dermatol* 41:1, 1999.
74. Stewart M: Treatment of varicella in pregnancy. In *Critical decisions in emergency medicine,* vol 9, Dallas, 1995, American College of Emergency Physicians.
75. Grossman KL, Rasmussen JE: Recent advances in pediatric infectious disease and their impact on dermatology, *J Am Acad Dermatol* 24:379, 1991.
76. McCross IN, Wung D: HIV related skin disease, *Med J Aust* 158:179, 1993.
77. Kim NY: Pigmentary diseases, *Med Clin North Am* 82:185, 1998.
78. Katz SK, Gordon KH, Roenigk HH: The cutaneous manifestations of gastrointestinal disease, *Prim Care Clin Office Pract* 23:455, 1996.
79. Callen J: Lupus erythematosus in dermatological signs of internal disease. In Callen JP, editor: *Clinical dermatology,* Philadelphia, 1988, WB Saunders.
80. Greer KE: Cutaneous disease and arthritis in dermatological signs of internal disease. In Callen JP, editor: *Clinical dermatology,* Philadelphia, 1988, WB Saunders.
81. Greer KE: Thyroid and the skin in dermatological signs of internal disease. In Callen JP, editor: *Clinical dermatology,* Philadelphia, 1988, WB Saunders.
82. Sigurgeirsson B et al: Risk of cancer in patients with dermatomyositis or polymyositis: a population-based study, *N Engl J Med* 326:363, 1992.
83. Dermatological signs of internal disease. In Callen JP, editor: *Clinical dermatology,* Philadelphia, 1988, WB Saunders.
84. Macaione AS: An approach to purpura, *Cutis* 12:41, 1973.
85. Sternbach GL, Moran JF, Elistram M: Heroin addiction: acute presentation of medical complications, *Ann Emerg Med* 9:161, 1980.

115 Anemia, Polycythemia, and White Blood Cell Disorders

Glenn C. Hamilton
Timothy G. Janz

ANEMIA

Perspective

Anemia is an absolute decrease in the number of circulating red blood cells (RBCs). The diagnosis is made when laboratory measurements fall below accepted normal values (Table 115-1).

In emergency medicine, anemia may be divided into two broad categories: emergent, having immediate life-threatening complications, and nonemergent, with less imminent patient danger. Factors other than absolute number of circulating RBCs may place the patient in one category or another (e.g., rate of onset, underlying hemodynamic reserve of patient).[1,2] Both groups necessitate a sound diagnostic approach, but emergent anemia may require supportive therapy concomitant with or in advance of the definitive diagnosis. The urgency depends predominantly on the patient's hemodynamic tolerance of the anemia.[3]

Principles of Disease

The major function of the RBC is oxygen transport from the lung to the tissue and carbon dioxide transport in the reverse direction. Oxygen transport is influenced by the amount of hemoglobin, its oxygen affinity, and blood flow. An alteration in any of the major components usually results in compensatory changes in the other two. For example, a decrease in hemoglobin from anemia is compensated by both inotropic and chronotropic cardiac changes, resulting in increased blood flow and decreased hemoglobin affinity at the tissue level and allowing more oxygen release. These compensatory responses may collapse because of disease severity or underlying pathologic conditions. The result is tissue hypoxia and eventual cell death.[4]

Anemia often stimulates the compensatory mechanism of erythropoiesis controlled by the hormone erythropoietin. Erythropoietin is a glycoprotein produced in the kidney (90%) and liver (10%). It regulates the production of RBCs by controlling the differentiation of the committed erythroid stem cell. It is stimulated by tissue hypoxia and products of RBC destruction during hemolysis. Erythropoietin levels are elevated in many types of anemia.[5,6]

The bone marrow contains pluripotent stem cells that can differentiate into erythroid, myeloid, megakaryocytic, and lymphoid progenitors. Erythropoietin enhances the growth and differentiation of the erythroid progenitors. When the late normoblast extrudes its nucleus, it still contains a ribosomal network, which identifies the reticulocyte. The reticulocyte retains its ribosomal network for about 4 days, of which 3 are spent in the bone marrow and 1 in the peripheral circulation. The red blood cell matures as the reticulocyte loses its ribosomal network and circulates for 110 to 120 days. The erythrocyte is then removed by macrophages that detect senescent signals.

Under steady state conditions, the rate of red blood cell production equals the rate of destruction. Red blood cell mass remains constant as an equal number of reticulocytes replace the destroyed, senescent erythrocytes during the same period.[5]

Common sites of blood loss in trauma include the pleural, peritoneal, and retroperitoneal spaces. In nontraumatic circumstances the gastrointestinal (GI) tract, uterus, and adnexa must be considered.

Causes other than blood loss may be responsible for severe anemia of rapid onset. Certain rare hemolytic conditions can cause a rapid intravascular destruction of RBCs (Box 115-1). More common is the patient with chronic compensated hemolytic anemia (e.g., sickle cell disease), who decompensates with an acute-onset anemia as a result of decreased erythrocyte production triggered by a viral infection.

Beyond red cell destruction, the status of hemoglobin function must be considered. Impaired hemoglobin transport of oxygen is seen in cases of carbon monoxide poisoning. Methemoglobinemia from nitrates and sulfhemoglobinemia resulting from hydrogen sulfide may severely decrease functional hemoglobin. These patients often have fatigue, altered mental status, shortness of breath, and other manifestations of hypoxia without signs of RBC loss or volume depletion.[7,8]

Clinical Features

The clinical presentation of anemia depends on the rapidity of its development and the patient's ability to compensate for and tolerate the insult. The most common cause of clinically severe anemia is blood loss.

Clinical signs and symptoms include tachycardia, decreased blood pressure, postural hypotension, increased heart rate, and increased respiratory rate. Complaints of thirst, altered mental status, and decreased urine output may accompany this picture.

The patient's age, concomitant illness, and underlying hematologic, cerebral, and cardiovascular status tremendously influence the clinical findings. Children and young adults may tolerate a significant blood loss with unaltered vital signs until a precipitant hypotensive episode occurs. Elderly patients commonly have underlying disease states that compromise their ability to compensate for blood loss.[9]

Pertinent elements of the history and physical examination of patients with acute anemia are listed in Box 115-2.[10]

Emergent Anemia

Diagnostic Strategies The stabilization of emergent anemia commonly runs parallel to the assessment. If the signs

Table 115-1. Hemogram Normal Values

Age	Hemoglobin (g/dl)	Hematocrit (ml/dl)	Red blood cell count ($\times 10^6$)
3 mo	10.4-12.2	30-36	3.4-4.0
3-7 yr	11.7-13.5	34-40	4.4-5.0
Adult man	14.0-18.0	40-52	4.4-5.9
Adult woman	12.0-16.0	35-47	3.8-5.2

Box 115-1 Causes of Rapid Intravascular Red Blood Cell Destruction

Mechanical hemolysis associated with disseminated intravascular coagulation
Massive burns
Toxins (e.g., some poisonous venoms—brown recluse spider, cobra)
Infections such as malaria or *Clostridium* sepsis
Severe glucose-6-phosphate dehydrogenase deficiency exposed to oxidant stress
ABO incompatibility transfusion reaction
Cold agglutinin hemolysis (e.g., *Mycoplasma* organisms, infectious mononucleosis)
Paroxysmal nocturnal hemoglobinuria exacerbated by transfusion
Immune complex hemolysis (e.g., quinidine)

and symptoms suggest potential life-threatening conditions, intravenous (IV) lines are placed and samples for the following initial laboratory tests are drawn:

1. Complete blood count (CBC) and peripheral smear
2. Blood sample for type and crossmatch
3. Prothrombin time
4. Partial thromboplastin time
5. Electrolyte levels
6. Glucose level
7. Creatinine level
8. Urinalysis for free hemoglobin
9. Clotted and unclotted blood samples for further studies

If possible, an initial hematocrit is obtained and measured in the ED. Although it may take hours before the hematocrit correctly reflects the degree of blood loss, the initial value is useful in determining the patient's baseline level. Occasionally, this value reveals an underlying anemia with the acute blood loss superimposed. Depending on severity, a blood sample is sent for type and crossmatch. Peripheral smear interpretation is done on pretreatment blood samples.

Measurements of coagulation status, electrolytes, glucose, blood urea nitrogen, and creatinine are useful in the diagnosis of underlying disease processes that may relate to the patient's anemia. Studies for folate, B_{12}, iron, total iron-binding capacity, reticulocytes, and direct antiglobulin (Coombs') test are altered by transfusion. Therefore pretreatment samples are saved for the consultant.[11,12]

Box 115-2 History and Physical Examination for Clinically Severe Anemia

History

General

Prehospital status, therapy, and response to therapy
Bleeding diathesis
Previous blood transfusion
Underlying diseases, including allergies
Current medications, especially those causing platelet inhibition

Trauma

Nature and time of injury
Blood loss at scene

Nontrauma

Skin: petechiae, ecchymoses
Gastrointestinal: hematemesis, hematochezia, melena, peptic ulcer
Genitourinary: last menstruation, menorrhagia, metrorrhagia, hematuria

Physical Examination

Vital signs measured serially

Blood pressure, pulse, respiratory rate
Orthostatic blood pressure and pulse (contraindicated with severe hypotension)
Level and content of consciousness
Skin
Pallor
Diaphoresis
Jaundice
Cyanosis
Purpura, ecchymoses, petechiae
Evidence of penetrating wounds

Cardiovascular

Murmurs, S_3, S_4
Quality of femoral and carotid pulses

Abdomen

Hepatosplenomegaly
Pain, guarding, rebound on palpation
Rectal and pelvic examination
Masses
Stool hemoglobin testing

Nonemergent Anemia

Clinical Features Nonemergent anemias are usually seen in ambulatory patients complaining of fatigue and feeling "washed out." Other voiced complaints include irritability, headache, postural dizziness, angina, decreased exercise tolerance, shortness of breath, or decreased libido. The history and physical examination are more detailed than in the patient with clinically severe anemia (Box 115-3). Most of these patients do not need immediate stabilization and can be further evaluated as outpatients.

Diagnostic Strategies The initial laboratory evaluation includes a CBC with leukocyte differential, reticulocyte

Box 115-3 History and Physical Examination for Nonemergent Anemia

History

Symptoms of anemia

Chest pain, exercise tolerance, dyspnea
Weakness, fatigue, dizziness, syncope

Bleeding diathesis

Bleeding after trauma, injections, tooth extractions
Spontaneous bleedings, such as epistaxis, menorrhagia
Spontaneous purpura and petechiae

Sites of blood loss

Respiratory: epistaxis, hemoptysis
Gastrointestinal: hematemesis, hematochezia, melena
Genitourinary: abnormal menses, pregnancies, hematuria
Skin: petechiae, ecchymoses

Intermittent jaundice, dark urine

Dietary history

Vegetarianism
Poor nutrition

Drug use and toxin exposure, including alcohol

Racial background, family history

Underlying disease

Uremia, liver disease, hypothyroidism
Chronic disease states, such as cancer, rheumatic or renal disease
Previous surgery
Miscellaneous

Prior treatment for anemia

Weight loss

Back pain

Physical Examination

Skin

Pallor
Purpura, petechiae, angiomas
Ulcerations

Eye

Conjunctival jaundice, pallor
Funduscopic hemorrhage, petechiae

Oral

Tongue atrophy, papillary soreness

Cardiopulmonary

Heart size, murmurs, extra cardiac sounds
Wheezing rales, other signs of pulmonary edema

Abdomen

Hepatomegaly, splenomegaly
Ascites
Masses

Lymph nodes

Neurologic

Altered positions or vibratory sense
Peripheral neuritis

Rectal and pelvic

count, peripheral smear (Figure 115-1), and RBC indices, including mean corpuscular volume, mean corpuscular hemoglobin, and mean corpuscular concentration.

Reasonable criteria for the admission of patients with nonemergent anemia are found in Box 115-4.[12]

Differential Considerations The differential diagnosis of anemia is facilitated by classifying the anemia into one of three groups: decreased RBC production, increased RBC destruction, and blood loss.[13] A complementary approach uses the RBC morphology and indices.[14] This is illustrated in Figure 115-2 as an algorithmic summary.

Decreased Red Blood Cell Production Anemias caused by decreased RBC production have a natural history of insidious onset and an associated decreased reticulocyte count. A subclassification of anemias caused by decreased RBC production by indices is listed in Box 115-5. RBC indices and morphology manifested in the peripheral smear are useful in securing the diagnosis. The definitive diagnosis may require a bone marrow examination. Appropriate diagnostic tests may be initiated, but replacement therapy of iron, B_{12}, or folate without proof of cause is unnecessary and unwise.

RBC indices are useful in classifying production deficit anemias. Their calculation and normal ranges are provided in Table 115-2. The mean corpuscular volume (MCV) is a measure of RBC size. Decreases and increases reflect microcytosis and macrocytosis, respectively. The mean corpuscular hemoglobin (MCH) value incorporates both the RBC size and hemoglobin concentration. It is influenced by both and is the least helpful of the indices. The MCH concentration is a measure of hemoglobin concentration (MCHC). Low values represent hypochromia. High values are noted only when decreased cell membrane relative to cell volume exists, such as in spherocytosis. An additional index is the RBC distribution width (RDW). It is a measure of the homogenicity of the RBCs measured. It is automatically calculated as the standard deviation of the MCV divided by the MCV multiplied by 100. A normal RDW is 13.5% + 1.5%. It is useful in differentiating iron deficiency from thalassemia.[15]

Microcytic anemias The hypochromic microcytic anemias can be subdivided into deficiencies of the three building blocks of hemoglobin: iron (iron deficiency anemia), globin (thalassemia), and porphyrin (sideroblastic anemia and lead poisoning). Anemia of chronic disease, a secondary iron abnormality, rounds out the differential diagnosis. Not all microcytic anemias are the result of iron deficiency, and routine iron therapy for a patient with a low MCV and MCHC is inappropriate.

Iron deficiency anemia Iron deficiency is a common cause of chronic anemia seen in the ED. It is the most common

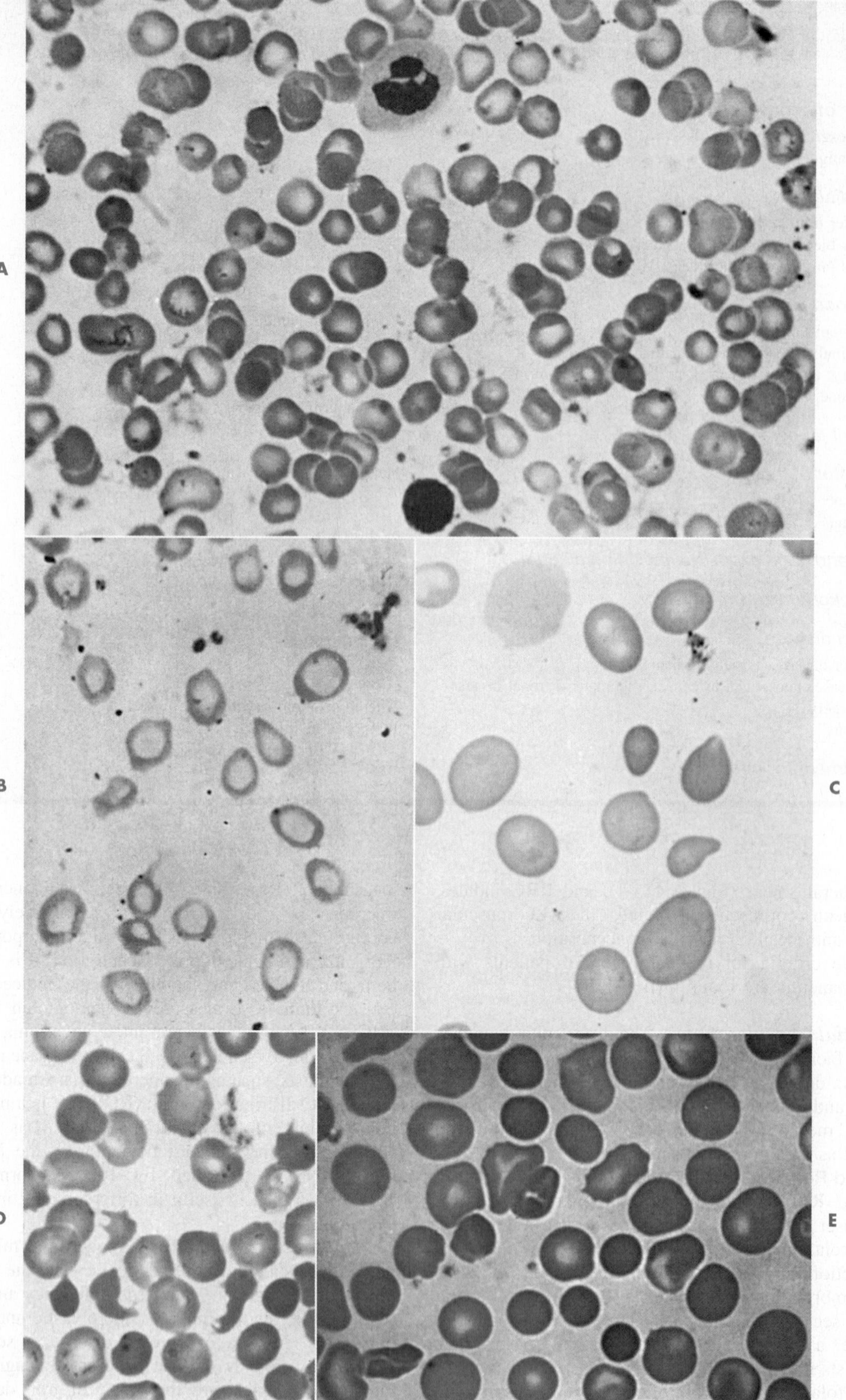

Figure 115-1. **Blood smears. A,** Normal smear. **B,** Iron deficiency anemia. **C,** Macrocyte. **D,** Schizocyte. **E,** Microspherocytes. **A, G,** *and* **H** *from Dougherty WB:* Introduction to hematology, *ed 2, St Louis, 1976, Mosby;* **B** *to* **F** *from Miale JB:* Laboratory medicine: hematology, *ed 6, St Louis, 1982, Mosby.*

Continued

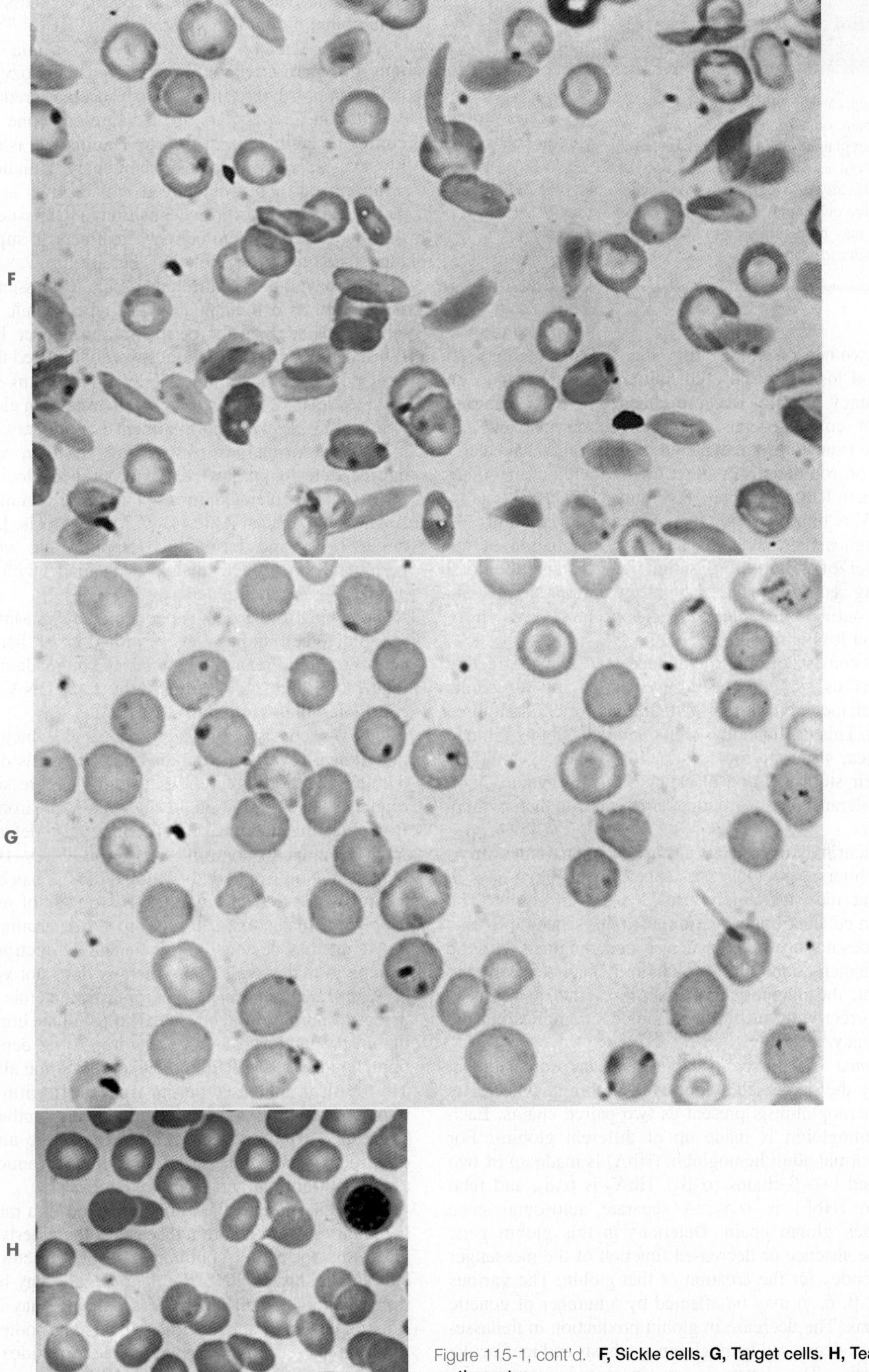

Figure 115-1, cont'd. **F, Sickle cells. G, Target cells. H, Teardrop erythrocytes.**

Box 115-4 Admission Criteria for Nonemergent Anemia

Developing cardiac symptoms, such as shortness of breath or chest pain, or neurologic symptoms
Initial unexplained hemoglobin value less than 8 to 10 g/dl or hematocrit less than 25% to 30%
Major difficulty in patient home-to-hospital transportation if extensive evaluation is necessary (the definition of "difficulty" may be determined by the patient, private physician, and insurance carrier)

anemia in women of childbearing age. In older patients, an occult blood loss, especially GI, initially may appear as an iron deficiency anemia. Because changes in RBC size and hemoglobin content occur only after bone marrow and cytochrome iron stores are depleted, a patient may have early symptoms of iron deficiency (e.g., fatigue) without manifesting changes in RBC structure (see Figure 115-1, *B*). Actually, a low MCV is relatively rare in iron deficiency anemia.

The diagnosis is made by laboratory evaluation of the fasting level of serum iron, serum ferritin, and the total iron-binding capacity. The laboratory interpretation and pitfalls are outlined in Table 115-3. A concentrated search for occult blood loss is mandatory.

Therapy consists of oral iron replacement. A cost-effective form is ferrous sulfate. The dosage is 325 mg for adults (60 mg of elemental iron) or 100 to 200 mg for children three times a day. This medication is well tolerated, although it may cause nausea, vomiting, or constipation. Patients should be warned their stools will be blackened. In rare patients with poor oral tolerance or absorption, parenteral iron therapy may be necessary.

The patient may experience a sense of improvement in as little as 24 hours. Reticulocytosis appears over 3 to 4 days in children but may take more than 1 week in adults. The hemoglobin concentration rises on a similar schedule. If this response does not occur, the patient is noncompliant with the iron supplementation, the blood loss may exceed the replacement, the diagnosis is incorrect, or the diagnosis is partially correct with an additional process complicating the iron deficiency.[15-18]

Thalassemia Thalassemia is a genetic autosomal defect reflected by the decreased synthesis of globin chains.[19] The globin in hemoglobin is present as two paired chains. Each type of hemoglobin is made up of different globins. For example, normal adult hemoglobin (HbA) is made up of two α-chains and two β-chains ($\alpha_2\beta_2$). HbA_2 is $\alpha_2\delta_2$, and fetal hemoglobin (HbF) is $\alpha_2\gamma_2$. A separate autosomal gene controls each globin chain. Deletions in this globin gene result in the absence or decreased function of the messenger RNA that codes for the creation of that globin. The various globins (α, β, δ, γ) may be affected by a number of genetic combinations. The decrease in globin production in thalassemia results in decreased hemoglobin synthesis and ineffective erythropoiesis. The latter is an increased intramarrow hemolysis with the destruction of RBCs before they are released. Normal erythropoiesis has a 10% to 20% ineffective release incidence, with associated intramarrow RBC destruction. This number may double or triple in cases of thalassemia. The cause is believed to be excess chains of the uninhibited globin precipitating in the RBCs.[19,20]

Although many variations in thalassemia are possible, only three are commonly considered. Homozygous β-chain thalassemia (thalassemia major) occurs predominantly in Mediterranean populations. It represents one of the most common single gene disorders. The disease is characterized by severe anemia, hepatosplenomegaly, jaundice, abnormal development, and premature death. Patients are transfusion dependent and die of iron deposition in the tissue, particularly the myocardium, or infection. Treatment is supportive with transfusion and iron chelating therapy.[21]

Heterozygous β-chain thalassemia (thalassemia minor) is manifested as a mild microcytic hypochromic anemia with target cells seen on the peripheral smear (see Figure 115-1, *G*), an MCV commonly more severely lowered than with iron deficiency anemia, a normal level of serum iron, and an elevated level of HbA_2 ($\alpha_2\delta_2$) on hemoglobin electrophoresis (2% to 5%). Usually no treatment is necessary.

α-Thalassemia has a spectrum from an asymptomatic carrier state to prenatal death. Four gene loci control this range. In the tolerated forms it is more commonly seen in Asians and African-Americans. Microcytosis, hypochromia, target cells, and basophilic stippling are noted on the peripheral smear. The diagnosis is made with hemoglobin electrophoresis and genetic testing.

Screening for carriers is performed by measurement of the red blood cell indices and estimation of hemoglobin A_2 concentration. Prenatal diagnosis can be made by analysis of fetal blood and, more recently, by fetal DNA, obtained by chorionic-villus sampling.

Therapy consists of blood transfusions, which are based on the clinical severity of the anemia. The goals of transfusion therapy include correction of anemia, suppression of erythropoiesis, and inhibition of increased GI iron absorption. Iron-chelating therapy, most commonly deferoxamine, is often required to control excess iron stores. Bone marrow transplantation from HLA-identical donors has been successful in disease-free survival in 60% to 90% of recipients, but its role in thalassemia has yet to be determined. Although much interest centers on permanent correction of genetic deficits in thalassemia, gene therapy does not yet exist.[22]

Sideroblastic anemia Sideroblastic anemia involves a defect in porphyrin synthesis. The resultant impaired hemoglobin production causes excess iron to be deposited in the mitochondria of the RBC precursor, but some also circulates. The result is increased serum iron and ferritin levels, with transferrin saturation. The defective heme synthesis results in ineffective erythropoiesis, mild to moderate anemia, and a dimorphic peripheral smear with hypochromic microcytes along with normal and macrocytic cells.[23]

Sideroblastic anemia, although found in a rare sex-linked hereditary form, is more a disease of the elderly. Indeed, the idiopathic form is a common type of refractory anemia in elderly patients. Pallor and splenomegaly may be noted, and iron staining of the peripheral smear may demonstrate iron-containing Pappenheimer inclusion bodies in RBCs. Some of these patients are deficient in pyridoxine (vitamin B_6) and respond to treatment with 100 mg of pyridoxine three times a day. Most remain anemic, but a 1- to 2-month pyridoxine trial is acceptable treatment. These patients can have an iron overload develop, particularly if long-term transfusion therapy is necessary, but may respond to iron

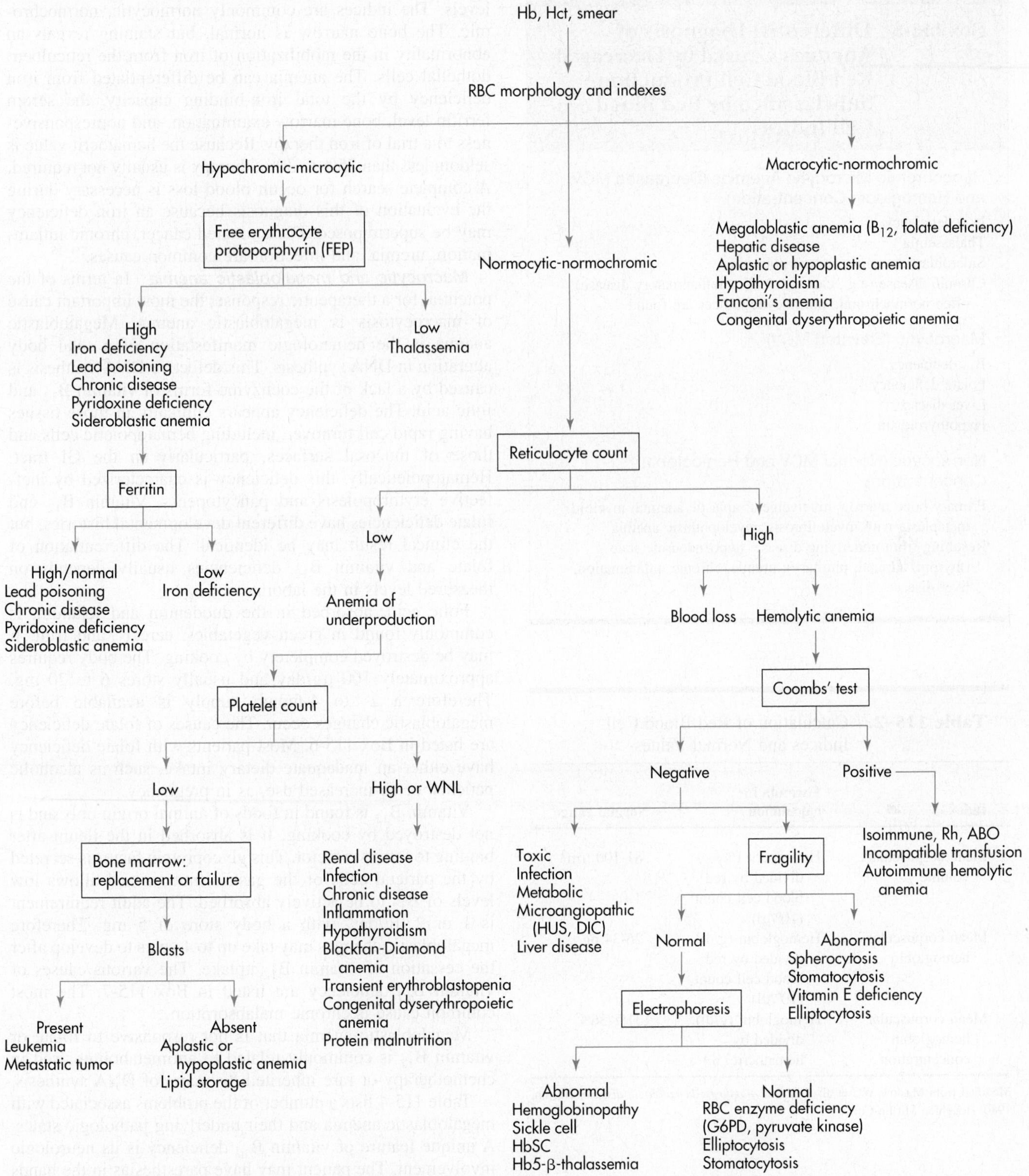

Figure 115-2. **Evaluation of anemia.** ***From Barkin RM, Rosen P:*** **Emergency pediatrics: a guide to ambulatory care, *ed 4, St Louis, 1994, Mosby.***

chelation therapy. Idiopathic sideroblastic anemia is considered a preleukemic state. Approximately 20% of these patients have acute myelogenous leukemia develop.

Secondary causes of sideroblastic anemia include toxins such as chloramphenicol, isoniazid, and cycloserine, as well as diseases including hemolytic and megaloblastic anemia, infection, carcinoma, leukemia, and rheumatoid arthritis. The exact mechanisms of these causative agents and diseases are unknown. Lead poisoning is one reversible cause of sideroblastic anemia. It may be suggested by the appearance

Box 115-5 Differential Diagnosis of Anemias Caused by Decreased Red Blood Cell Production Subclassified by Red Blood Cell Indices

Hypochromic Microcytic Anemias (Decreased MCV and Hemoglobin Concentration)

Iron deficiency
Thalassemia
Sideroblastic anemia or lead poisoning
Chronic disease (e.g., cancer, renal or inflammatory disease), often normochromic normocytic indices are found

Macrocytic (Elevated MCV)

B_{12} deficiency
Folate deficiency
Liver disease
Hypothyroidism

Normocytic (Normal MCV and Hemoglobin Concentration)

Primary bone marrow involvement: aplastic anemia, myeloid metaplasia with myelofibrosis, myelophthisic anemia
Resulting from underlying disease: hypoendocrine state (thyroid, adrenal, pituitary), uremia, chronic inflammation, liver disease

Table 115-2. Calculation of Red Blood Cell Indices and Normal Values

Index	Formula for calculation	Normal range
Mean corpuscular volume	Hematocrit (%) divided by red blood cell count ($10^6/\mu l$)	81-100 μm^3
Mean corpuscular hemoglobin	Hemoglobin (g/dl) divided by red blood cell count ($10^6/\mu l$)	26-34 pg
Mean corpuscular hemoglobin concentration	Hemoglobin (g/dl) divided by hematocrit (%)	31%-36%

Modified from Maslow WC et al: *Practical diagnosis: hematologic disease,* Boston, 1980, Houghton Mifflin Co.

of RBC basophilic stippling on the peripheral smear. Elevated blood lead levels are diagnostic. Alcohol abuse may also result in disordered heme synthesis, which can be corrected by alcohol cessation or by parenteral pyridoxal phosphate in cases of continued abuse. Oral pyridoxine may be ineffective because of an impaired conversion to the active form in alcoholic patients.[23]

Anemia of chronic disease The anemia of chronic disease is common. It is characterized by low serum iron levels, a low total iron-binding capacity, and normal or elevated ferritin levels. The indices are commonly normocytic, normochromic. The bone marrow is normal, but staining reveals an abnormality in the mobilization of iron from the reticuloendothelial cells. The anemia can be differentiated from iron deficiency by the total iron-binding capacity, the serum ferritin level, bone marrow examination, and nonresponsiveness to a trial of iron therapy. Because the hematocrit value is seldom less than 25% to 30%, therapy is usually not required. A complete search for occult blood loss is necessary during the evaluation of this diagnosis because an iron deficiency may be superimposed. Disseminated cancer, chronic inflammation, uremia, and infection are common causes.[24-26]

Macrocytic and megaloblastic anemia In terms of the potential for a therapeutic response, the most important cause of macrocytosis is megaloblastic anemia. Megaloblastic anemia is the hematologic manifestation of a total body alteration in DNA synthesis. This defective DNA synthesis is caused by a lack of the coenzyme forms of vitamin B_{12} and folic acid. The deficiency appears clinically in those tissues having rapid cell turnover, including hematopoietic cells and those of mucosal surfaces, particularly in the GI tract. Hematopoietically, this deficiency is characterized by ineffective erythropoiesis and pancytopenia. Vitamin B_{12} and folate deficiencies have different developmental histories, but the clinical result may be identical. The differentiation of folate and vitamin B_{12} deficiencies usually depends on measured levels in the laboratory.

Folic acid, absorbed in the duodenum and jejunum, is commonly found in green vegetables, cereals, and fruit. It may be destroyed completely by cooking. The body requires approximately 100 µg/day and usually stores 6 to 20 mg. Therefore a 2- to 4-month supply is available before megaloblastic changes occur. The causes of folate deficiency are listed in Box 115-6. Most patients with folate deficiency have either an inadequate dietary intake, such as alcoholic patients, or an increased use, as in pregnancy.

Vitamin B_{12} is found in foods of animal origin only and is not destroyed by cooking. It is absorbed in the ileum after binding to intrinsic factor. This glycoprotein factor is secreted by the parietal cells of the gastric mucosa and allows low levels of B_{12} to be actively absorbed. The adult requirement is 1 or 2 µg/day, with a body store of 5 mg. Therefore megaloblastic changes may take up to 4 years to develop after the cessation of vitamin B_{12} uptake. The various causes of vitamin B_{12} deficiency are listed in Box 115-7. The most common cause is chronic malabsorption.

Megaloblastic anemia that is not responsive to folate or vitamin B_{12} is commonly related to antimetabolites used in chemotherapy or rare inherited disorders of DNA synthesis.

Table 115-4 lists a number of the problems associated with megaloblastic anemia and their underlying pathologic states. A unique feature of vitamin B_{12} deficiency is its neurologic involvement. The patient may have paresthesias in the hands and feet, decreased proprioception, or decreased vibratory sense. The insidiously developing classic neurologic complex includes loss of proprioception, weakness and spasticity of the lower extremities with altered reflexes, and variable mental changes such as depression, paranoid ideation, irritability, and forgetfulness. The latter two complaints have also been noted with folic acid deficiency. These patients have some of the lowest hemoglobin levels seen in any disease state.[27]

Macrocytic anemia is suggested when the MCV is greater

Table 115-3. Diagnostic Tests for Iron Deficiency Anemia

Test	Normal result	Iron deficiency level	Interpretation
Fasting serum iron	60-180 μg/dl	<60 μg/dl	Diurnal variation (draw in morning); increased by hepatitis, hemochromatosis, hemolytic anemia, and aplastic anemia; decreased in infection
Total iron-binding capacity	250-400 μg/dl	>400 μg/dl	Increased in late pregnancy or hepatitis, decreased in infection
Percentage of saturation (serum iron) of total iron-binding capacity	15%-45%	<15%	
Serum ferritin	10-10,000 mg/ml	<10 mg/ml	Reflects iron stores; may increase as an acute-phase reactant in infection
Bone marrow stainable iron	Hemosiderin granules in reticuloendothelial cells	Absent	Standard for iron stores assessment

Box 115-6 Causes of Folate Deficiency

Inadequate Dietary Intake

Poor diet or overcooked or processed food diet
Alcoholism

Inadequate Uptake

Malabsorption with sprue and other chronic upper intestinal tract disorders, drugs such as phenytoin and barbiturates, or blind loop syndrome

Inadequate Use

Metabolic block caused by drugs such as methotrexate or trimethoprim
Enzymatic deficiency, congenital or acquired

Increased Requirement

Pregnancy
Increased RBC turnover: ineffective erythropoiesis, hemolytic anemia, chronic blood loss
Malignancy: lymphoproliferative disorders

Increased Excretion or Destruction or Dialysis

Box 115-7 Causes of Vitamin B_{12} Deficiency

Inadequate Dietary Intake

Total vegetarianism: no eggs, milk, or cheese
Chronic alcoholism (rare)

Inadequate Absorption

Absent, inadequate, or abnormal intrinsic factor, as seen in patients with pernicious gastrectomy and anemia. In the latter, autoimmune antibodies act against the gastric parietal cells and intrinsic factor. Abnormal ileum, as can occur in sprue and inflammatory bowel disease.

Inadequate Use

Enzyme deficiency
Abnormal vitamin B_{12}-binding protein

Increased Requirement by Increased Body Metabolism

Increased Excretion or Destruction

than 100 μm^3 on the RBC indices. Other criteria must be met for megaloblastosis to be the cause of macrocytic anemia. On the peripheral smear, large oval red cells (macroovalocytes) and hypersegmented polymorphoneutrophils are believed to be diagnostic (see Figure 115-1, *C*). A bone marrow aspirate may reveal morphologic changes consistent with megaloblastic erythropoiesis. Other potentially useful laboratory tests include vitamin B_{12} and folate levels, red cell folate, and lactate dehydrogenase (LDH). The laboratory techniques, values, and interpretations are listed in Table 115-5. Once megaloblastic anemia is diagnosed and a folate or vitamin B_{12} deficiency determined, standard diagnostic regimens are followed to determine the precise origin of the deficiency.

Because one deficiency may cause GI absorptive changes that beget other deficiencies, the emergency physician may be forced to initiate therapy before the final diagnosis is made. However, the emergency physician is cautioned to obtain necessary laboratory specimens before pursuing this course. The usual dosage for patients with folate deficiency megaloblastic anemia is 1 mg of oral folic acid per day. Parenteral administration is usually unnecessary because most cases are dietary deficiencies. Because malabsorption is the most common cause of vitamin B_{12} deficiency, parenteral therapy is 1 to 10 μg/day for the first 7 to 10 days. Thereafter, only monthly 100 μg doses are necessary. The response is often dramatic, with reticulocyte counts rising up to 30% to 50% and normalization of the RBC, white blood cell (WBC), and platelet counts in 6 to 8 weeks. The use of vitamin B_{12} or folate supplements in undiagnosed anemia is to be discouraged. The use of routine B_{12} injections in the elderly has decreased but is still a too common practice.[27,28]

Macrocytic anemias unassociated with megaloblastic changes are often seen. Liver disease, often associated with alcoholism, is the most common cause. Macrocytic target cells may be seen on the peripheral smear in conjunction with this disorder. Hypothyroidism and hemolysis may also be seen as macrocytic anemia. The screening tests to differentiate between megaloblastic anemia and macrocytic anemia of other causes include a peripheral smear for macroovalocytes, hypersegmented polymorphonucleophils, and the LDH level.[27,29]

Normochromic and normocytic anemias The origins of normochromic and normocytic anemias caused by decreased production are not as obvious because the macrocytic and microcytic anemias give clues to their origin by alterations in the RBC indices. One hematologic parameter that can aid in the diagnosis of normocytic anemia associated with hypoproduction is the corrected reticulocyte count. Reticulocytes reflect RBC production in bone marrow. RBCs are released from the bone marrow every 1 to 3 days and contain residual RNA that can be detected by supravital staining. Reticulocytes have an MCV of 160 mm^3 and in sufficient numbers can increase the MCV of the total erythrocyte count. The reticulocyte count is expressed as a percentage of the total RBC population and must be related ("corrected") to the RBC count of the patient. Thus the corrected reticulocyte count is equal to the measured percentage of reticulocytes times the patient's hematocrit (%) divided by 45% (taken as the normal hematocrit). The normal range is 1% to 3%.

Normocytic anemias may be classified as primary bone marrow involvement or secondary marrow response to underlying disease.

Aplastic anemia is rare but may be severe in its presentation. It is suspected in anemic patients with normal indices, a low reticulocyte count, and a history of exposure to certain drugs or chemicals (Table 115-6). It is related to drug or chemical exposure in 50% of the cases. Viral hepatitis, radiation, and pregnancy have been associated with aplastic anemia. Another group of patients is considered to have "autoimmune" origin.

The aplastic state may extend to all cell lines and results from destruction by immune-stimulated lymphocytes or failure of the marrow stem cell. Occasionally, only one cell line fails, as in RBC aplasia. This represents injury occurring at a later stage of cellular differentiation. The precise diagnosis necessitates a bone marrow examination, but the causative factor may be difficult to determine.

The general treatment of aplastic anemia includes removal of suspected marrow toxins from the environment, aspirin avoidance, oral hygiene, and suppression of menses. Transfusions are given in life-threatening circumstances only. Bone marrow or peripheral blood stem cell transplantation from a histocompatible sibling can cure the bone marrow failure with survival rates of 77% to 90%. However, since 30% of patients have suitably matched sibling donors, only a small number undergo allogenic transplantation. Immunosuppression with antithymocyte globulin, antilymphocyte, and other cytotoxic chemotherapy globulin is used in the majority of patients that are not stem cell transplantation candidates. Unrelated donors are preferred to avoid sensitization of the patient against non-HLA antigens that are present in family donor bone marrow. The disease has a wide range of severity, the overall 5-year survival rate being 30% to 40%. Even with supportive therapy, up to 80% of patients with severe aplastic anemia still die. Bone marrow transplantation before blood product sensitization has resulted in an 80% 5-year survival rate. This is usually combined with immunosuppressive therapy, antilymphocyte globulin. Difficulties are still encountered in finding the correct immunologic match.[30,31]

Myelophthisic anemia is a bone marrow failure resulting

Table 115-4. Clinicopathologic Correlation of Megaloblastic Anemia Manifestations

Presentation	Pathologic condition
Lemon yellow skin	Combination of pallor with low-grade icterus from ineffective erythropoiesis
Petechiae, mucosal bleeding	Thrombocytopenia
Infection	Leukopenia
Fatigue, dyspnea on exertion, postural hypotension	Anemia
Sore mouth or tongue	Megaloblastosis of mucosal surfaces
Diarrhea and weight loss	Malabsorption from mucosal surface change
Paresthesias and ataxia	Related to myelin abnormality in vitamin B_{12} deficiency only

Table 115-5. Serum Tests for Diagnosis and Differentiation of Megaloblastic Anemia

Test	Technique	Value	Interpretation
Vitamin B_{12}	Microbiologic or radioisotope	Normal: 300-900 µg/L Deficient: <200 µg/L	Although clinically they may overlap, vitamin B_{12} is usually normal in folate deficiency
Folate	Microbiologic or radioisotope	Deficient: <3 µg/L	Vitamin B_{12} deficiency may elevate folate by blocking transfer of serum folate to RBCs; hemolysis may elevate folate level
Red cell folate	Calculated	Normal: 200-700 µg/L Folate deficiency: <140 µg/L	Index of tissue folate is less influenced by diet and is increased in vitamin B_{12} deficiency because of block
LDH	Spectrophotometric	Normal: 95-200 IU Megaloblastic anemia: 4-50 times normal	Normal in other macrocytic anemias; elevated 2 to 4 times normal in hemolytic anemias; isoenzymes may be helpful

from replacement by an invading tumor, leukemia, lymphoma, or rarely granuloma. A more basic defect or inhibitor may complicate the problem because the degree of anemia cannot always be correlated with the extent of bone marrow invasion. Any patient with oncologic disease may have this type of anemia develop. Useful clues are signs of extramedullary hematopoiesis, such as hepatosplenomegaly and a leukoerythroblastic peripheral smear that demonstrates immature WBCs, nucleated RBCs, and poikilocytosis (teardrop-shaped red cells) (see Figure 115-1, *F*). The final diagnosis is made by bone marrow examination. Therapy is directed at the underlying disorder.[30,31]

Myelofibrosis of unknown origin is the usual cause of a primary bone marrow failure associated with extramedullary hematopoiesis. This myeloid metaplasia occurs in the liver and spleen and involves a blood picture similar to that of myelophthisic anemia. The diagnosis may be made by bone marrow examination. Treatment is supportive, although a splenectomy or the use of alkylating agents may be necessary to treat complications of the extramedullary blood cell production, such as hepatosplenomegaly.

The hypoplastic anemias of secondary origin are commonly seen as mild chronic anemias with low reticulocyte counts. They have a normal MCV and RDW. Their diagnosis is made by exclusion. Anemia of chronic disease may have microcytic or normocytic indices. It is associated with chronic inflammation (e.g., rheumatoid arthritis, chronic infections such as tuberculosis and osteomyelitis, and malignancy). Hypoendocrinism caused by hypothyroidism, hypoadrenalism, or hypopituitarism results in a hypometabolic state in which the bone marrow responds poorly to erythropoietin.[32] Erythropoietin levels may be low. The anemia of chronic renal failure is considered to be caused by a number of factors. Decreased erythropoietin production, hemolysis, suppression by dialyzable factors, and increased blood loss caused by platelet abnormalities combine to cause a mild to moderate anemia. If necessary, it may be corrected by erythropoietin replacement therapy.[32]

Increased Red Blood Cell Destruction The hemolytic anemias are defined by a shortened life span of the erythrocyte. In their acute form, hemolytic anemias can be devastating and require rapid diagnosis and intervention (see Box 115-1). Fortunately, they are relatively rare compared with the chronic hemolytic conditions. Chronic disorders may be related to primary blood disorders (e.g., sickle cell anemia) or may be a result of other disease states (e.g., chronic renal failure). These disorders may present as an acute hemolytic anemia if the tenuous balance between red cell production and destruction is upset. If the patient can be shown to have a normal hematocrit and reticulocyte count at the same time, a differentiation between acquired and inherited hemolytic anemia is possible.[33]

Clinical features The clinical signs and symptoms of hemolytic anemias can be categorized as being generated by intravascular or extravascular processes. Although this is not a precise representation of the underlying pathophysiologic condition, the division assists in the differential approach in the ED.

Intravascular hemolysis is usually associated with an acute process and has a dramatic appearance. Large numbers of RBCs may lyse within the circulation. Pathologically, it primarily involves the handling of released hemoglobin and a compensatory response to an acute decrease in oxygen-carrying capability. Free hemoglobin initially binds to haptoglobin and hemopexin. This complex is transported to the liver, converted to bilirubin, conjugated, and excreted. When this binding and transport system is overwhelmed, free hemoglobin may appear in the blood. Hemoglobin is a large molecule that remains in serum and may tint it pink.

In contrast, myoglobin is a small molecule that is rapidly cleared from the serum. An examination of spun whole blood shows clear serum in myoglobinemia, pink serum with free hemoglobin from intravascular hemolysis, and yellow serum from extravascular hemolysis with increased bilirubin production. In severe cases the latter mechanism may also result in free hemoglobin.

The clinical appearance of intravascular hemolysis may vary from mild chronic anemia, as seen in cases of mechanical hemolysis, to prostration, fever, abdominal and back pain, and mental changes, seen with transfusion reactions. Jaundice, brown to red urine, and oliguria associated with hemoglobin's complex-induced acute renal failure can also occur.

Extravascular hemolysis is more common and usually better tolerated. The splenic blood flow slows as the RBCs travel in the sinusoids close to the reticuloendothelial system, the latter being uniquely designed for removing older or damaged cells. Primary splenic overactivity, antibody-mediated changes, or RBC membrane abnormalities may cause this normal splenic function to increase to a pathologic degree. Hemolysis may also occur within the bone marrow. Normal erythropoiesis is ineffective 10% to 20% of the time. This percentage increases when abnormal RBCs are produced, as in cases of thalassemia, megaloblastic anemia, and some hemolytic anemias.[33,34]

After hemoglobin is disassembled in the reticuloendothelial cell, globin returns to the amino acid pool, iron is transported via transferrin to the bone marrow or iron stores, and the pyrrole ring is converted to bilirubin. The unconjugated bilirubin circulates to the liver and is transformed. It is excreted in the urine as conjugated bilirubin. The clinical picture of extravascular hemolysis is usually mild to moderate anemia, mild and intermittent jaundice, and enlargement of the spleen. The signs and symptoms vary with the severity and chronicity of the hemolysis.

Ancillary evaluation Once hemolysis is suspected, the history and laboratory tests have a diagnostic precedence over

Table 115-6. Aplastic Anemia Caused by Drugs or Chemicals

Cause	Relative incidence (%)
Chloramphenicol	61
Phenylbutazone	19
Anticonvulsants	4
Insecticides	4
Solvents	4
Sulfonamides	3
Gold	3
Benzene	2

From Silver BM, Zuckerman KS: *Med Clin North Am* 64:609, 1980.

Box 115-8 Pertinent History and Physical Examination for Hemolytic Anemia

History

Alteration of color in urine or feces
- Association with drugs, cold, sleep
- Early or recent onset anemia history with symptoms

Ethnic background
Family history of anemia or jaundice
Drug or toxic exposure
Disease states associated with hemolysis, such as systemic lupus erythematosus, renal failure, lymphoma, infectious mononucleosis, prosthetic heart valve

Physical Examination

Jaundice
Hepatosplenomegaly
Ulcerations, particularly in the lower extremities
Enlarged lymph nodes

Box 115-9 Diagnostic Tests for Hemolysis

Peripheral blood smear
Corrected reticulocyte index or reticulocyte production index
Haptoglobin levels
Plasma free and urine hemoglobin
Lactic dehydrogenase level
Fractionated bilirubin level
Direct and indirect Coombs' test
RBC membrane stability (osmotic fragility)

the physical examination. Important historical and physical examination points are listed in Box 115-8.[33,34]

Laboratory assessment The important diagnostic tests for hemolysis are found in Box 115-9.

The blood smear is often more diagnostic than the bone marrow examination. The typical cell seen in intravascular hemolysis is the schizocyte (see Figure 115-1, *D*). The classic cell of extravascular hemolysis is the spherocyte (see Figure 115-1, *E*). It may be seen in congenital spherocytosis but more commonly indicates splenic activity against an antibody-coated RBC membrane. An increase in macrocytes reflects the younger cells associated with reticulocytosis. The specific diagnosis may be made with the blood smear, as with sickled cells or Heinz bodies in cases of glucose-6-phosphate-dehydrogenase (G6PD) deficiency.[34,35]

Haptoglobin binds hemoglobin on a molecule-for-molecule basis. Its absence implies saturation and degradation after binding with hemoglobin and is an early finding in hemolysis. It has a normal range of 40 to 180 mg/ml, is decreased in hepatic failure, and increases as an acute-phase reactant. After haptoglobin is bound, hemoglobin binds with hemopexin, transferrin, and albumin before circulating in its free form. Plasma-free hemoglobin levels are determined in suspected cases of intravascular hemolysis. The result is considered positive if the level is greater than 40 to 50 mg/dl. Hemoglobin is excreted by the kidney and may be found as a smoky red pigment that is orthotoluidine positive with no associated RBCs. Prussian blue staining granules of hemosiderin may be found intracellularly in renal tubule cells excreted in the urine during chronic hemolytic states.[35]

LDH is released when the RBC is broken down peripherally or in the marrow. It is elevated in hemolytic, thalassemic, sideroblastic, and megaloblastic anemias. It may also be seen in cases of uremia, polycythemia vera, and erythroleukemia. Normal levels of LDH range from 95 to 200 IU and may be fractionated.[34,35]

In extravascular hemolysis, bilirubin is often delivered to the liver faster than the conjugating mechanism can handle it. Normal total levels are less than 1.5 mg/dl, and the indirect component constitutes less than 0.5 mg/dl. Conjugated or indirect bilirubin may rise as high as 4 to 5 mg/dl even with normal liver function. Higher levels connote some degree of underlying hepatic insufficiency.[34,35]

The direct antiglobulin (Coombs') test detects antibody or complement on human RBC membranes. It is an essential test in the evaluation of hemolysis. Approximately 90% of patients with autoimmune hemolytic anemia have a positive direct Coombs' test. The indirect test measures antibody titers in serum. The key to the direct antiglobulin test is the reagent. It contains an antihuman immunoglobulin (Ig)G that is produced in rabbits. This antihuman IgG in its broad-spectrum form reacts with IgG, IgM, or C_3 proteins that may coat RBCs. The reaction causes an agglutination of RBCs that is graded from 0 to 4. Agglutinating properties depend on immunoglobulin size. IgM is a large antibody form that can bridge the distance between cells, cause agglutination, and fix complement. The direct antiglobulin test is limited in diagnosing IgM-mediated hemolysis. It is best in determining IgG or complement on the RBC surface. IgG is not large enough to cause agglutination, and the antihuman globulin attaches to RBC-bound IgG, which allows agglutination. C_3 is detected in a similar manner. Both represent possible immunologic causes of hemolysis. This form of hemolysis is usually mediated extravascularly through the spleen because IgG is a poor initiator of the complement system. The direct antiglobulin test evaluates the RBC surface for immunologic markers. The indirect test assumes the IgG or C_3 is in the serum and tests for serum antibody activity against RBCs. Positive tests for immunologic markers do not correlate agglutination activity with the severity of hemolysis.[36]

Differential diagnosis Hemolytic anemias may be classified as congenital or acquired, Coombs positive or Coombs negative, or caused by processes intrinsic or extrinsic to the cell membrane. The last method gives a useful differential classification of hemolysis (Box 115-10).

Intrinsic enzyme defects From 85% to 90% of the membrane-sustaining energy production of the erythrocyte is through the anaerobic glycolytic pathway. At least eight known enzyme deficiencies are associated with this pathway. The most common is pyruvate kinase. It is seen as hemolytic jaundice and is usually diagnosed in infancy.[37]

The remaining 10% to 15% of RBC glycolysis occurs by way of the hexose monophosphate shunt. This bypass mechanism occurs in the early stages of the glycolytic pathway and generates nicotinamide-adenine dinucleotide phosphate (NADPH), which is important in maintaining

Box 115-10 Classification of Hemolytic Anemia

Intrinsic

A. Enzyme defect
 1. Pyruvate kinase deficiency
 2. G6PD deficiency
B. Membrane abnormality
 1. Spherocytosis
 2. Elliptostomatocytosis
 3. Paroxysmal nocturnal hemoglobinuria
 4. Spur cell anemia
C. Hemoglobin abnormality
 1. Hemoglobinopathies
 2. Thalassemias (anemias)
 3. Unstable hemoglobin
 4. Hemoglobin M

Extrinsic

A. Immunologic
 1. Alloantibodies
 2. Autoantibodies
B. Mechanical
 1. Microangiopathic hemolytic anemia
 2. Cardiovascular, such as prosthetic heart valve disease
C. Environmental
 1. Drugs
 2. Toxins
 3. Infections
 4. Thermal
D. Abnormal sequestrations, as in hypersplenism

reduced glutathione. Glutathione is essential in the protection of hemoglobin from oxidant injury. A deficiency of the first enzyme in this pathway, G6PD, occurs in 11% of African-American men. In this form the enzyme deteriorates with age, and older RBCs are subject to hemolysis by oxidant stresses. G6PD is sex linked and has a wide range of severity. The most common form in African Americans is self-limited because as the bone marrow responds, younger cells with more normal levels of G6PD predominate and can handle the oxidant stress. The variants in Sicilians, Greeks, and Arabs can be particularly devastating. The clinical presentation is usually an acute hemolytic episode that may be both intravascular and extravascular in appearance. It occurs 24 to 48 hours after the ingestion of an oxidant drug (Box 115-11) or after acute infections, such as viral hepatitis. The anemia induced by oxidant drugs is dose related. The older cells lyse at certain drug levels. The oxidant creates forms of activated oxygen, such as peroxide, that either denature the hemoglobin or destroy cell membranes. The former process produces Heinz bodies, which are clumps of denatured hemoglobin found in RBCs early during an episode. These cells are removed by the spleen. The diagnosis is made by enzymatic screening for G6PD. This test cannot be performed immediately after the hemolytic episode. A 3-week delay avoids a false-negative result caused by a predominance of young cells. Treatment includes volume and RBC support as necessary. Oxidant drug avoidance is the only prevention.[38,39]

Box 115-11 Drugs Associated with Hemolysis in G6PD Deficiency

Analgesics and antipyretics: acetanilid, aspirin, phenacetin
Antimalarials: primaquine, quinacrine, quinine
Nitrofurans
Sulfa drugs: sulfamethoxazole, sulfacetamide, sulfones
Miscellaneous: naphthalene, fava beans, methylene blue, phenylhydrazine, nalidixic acid

Intrinsic membrane abnormality Abnormalities appear in a number of ways. An altered shape is the main feature of the autosomal dominant hereditary spherocytosis or elliptocytosis. The spleen sequesters these abnormal cells. Clinical sequelae range from compensated asymptomatic anemias to severe life-threatening acquired aplastic crises. The diagnosis is made by reviewing the family history, blood smear, and osmotic fragility testing. Splenectomy is the treatment of choice for those cases requiring therapeutic intervention.[37,40]

Paroxysmal nocturnal hemoglobinemia is a stem cell defect causing an abnormal erythrocyte, neutrophil, and platelet sensitivity to complement. It is most often seen as a chronic hemolysis, hemosiderinuria, leukopenia, and thrombocytopenia. The peripheral smear is normal and the direct Coombs' test is negative. Its major complication is thrombosis, with a predilection for the hepatic vein. Normal activation of complement using sucrose or acid hemolysis (the Ham test) is diagnostic. Transfusion can be a life-threatening hazard in patients with this disease because RBC lysis is caused by donor complement. Because of this danger, only washed packed cells should be used.[40]

Intrinsic hemoglobin abnormality More than 350 types of abnormal hemoglobins have been documented. Problems that may be seen include unstable hemoglobins that appear as a Heinz body–position anemia, M hemoglobins that fix iron in its ferric or methemoglobin state, and hemoglobins with an increased oxygen affinity that result in tissue hypoxia and erythrocytosis.

Sickle cell disease is the most important hemoglobinopathy for the emergency physician. In hospitals serving a large African-American population, it is seen on an almost daily basis. Even physicians who treat the problem often are at risk for overlooking the major complications of this disease. They may err because of complacency and the tendency to react automatically when a too-well-known "sickler" arrives. Physicians with less experience may fail to recognize the complexity of an unfamiliar problem.

Sickle cell disease is genetically determined. An abnormal allele at the gene loci for hemoglobin β-chains produces an altered messenger RNA that in turn results in valine replacement of glutamic acid at the sixth position from the N-terminal end of the β-chain. On the molecular level this change causes an interlocking of the affected chain with adjacent hemoglobin in the deoxygenated state. This connection causes the formation of bundles of parallel rods called *tactoids.* These polymers grow to form a *p*-crystalline gel, then a crystal. This gel formation is facilitated by a low pH level and reduced by the presence of other hemoglobins, such as HbF. The result is a sickled cell that is less deformable, causes an increase in the viscosity and sludging tendency of blood, and is sequestered in and destroyed by the spleen and liver. These changes may occur when smaller amounts of polymer do not result in a sickled cell and are associated with a RBC membrane leak. The clinical complex of vasoocclusive events, chronic hemolysis, thrombosis, and organ injury is derived from this pathologic process.[41-49]

The globin in hemoglobin is made up of two pairs of identical polypeptide chains. In normal hemoglobin variants and most clinically significant hemoglobinopathies, the β-chains are constant. The gene loci for β-chains result in HbA (α_2, β_2). They may have a normal allelic substitution, such as δ-chains, resulting in the HbA_2 (α_2, δ_2), or abnormal substitution as noted in HbS. Each person has two non-sex–linked gene foci for β-chains, one from each parent. The alleles appearing at these loci are both expressed in the formation of RBC hemoglobin. This fact explains the basis for the various HbS syndromes. In sickle cell trait disease (HbAs), the patient is heterozygous and only one parent contributes the abnormal S allele. In each cell, 50% of the hemoglobin is normal HbA. Sickle disease (HbSS) is homozygous, and all hemoglobin is HbS. A parent may contribute alleles other than S; thus a wide number of variants can exist. Two clinically important S variants are sickle thalassemia and sickle cell hemoglobin C disease. Therefore all hemoglobinopathies that cause sickling are not HbS.[42,50]

In addition, HbSS is not limited to the African-American population. Up to 10% of patients with various sickling disorders identify themselves as non–African-American.[41-43]

Sickle cell trait is found in 8% to 10% of African Americans. It is usually asymptomatic, although it may manifest as decreased urine-concentrating ability, spontaneous hematuria, and rare vasoocclusive crises with an increased incidence of splenic infarction at high altitudes. No added risk occurs during general anesthesia. The diagnosis is usually made after sickle cell screening (Sickledex Screen) and a characteristic hemoglobin electrophoresis. Genetic counseling is useful for these patients.[42,44]

Sickle cell disease can be a recurrent, painful, and frustrating problem for both patients and physicians. It is estimated that fewer than 10% of a sickle cell population are recurrent ED users. The setting is usually that of a large urban hospital caring for a predominantly African-American population. The patients are seen in what is considered a vasoocclusive crisis. Preceding infection, cold exposure, and stress such as trauma are all potential precipitating factors in these crises. Many of these episodes are considered to be spontaneous in their onset. The emotional component of these crises is not well understood, but the possibility of narcotic abuse does exist. The painful crisis is believed to have its origin in tissue ischemia caused by increased viscosity, sludging, and microvascular obstruction, resulting from irreversible sickled cells. Sludging and vascular blockage cause stasis, deoxygenation, and local acidosis, which promote the vicious circle of continued sickling. The pain is commonly deep and aching and is most often found in the abdomen, chest, back, and extremities. The disease may mimic an acute abdomen (e.g., cholecystitis), pulmonary embolus, renal colic, or other painful problems. Unfortunately, HbSS may also contribute to these same problems. A directed history that relates this pain pattern to previous sickling episodes, a careful repeated physical examination, and specific organ-related laboratory tests are all the physician has to differentiate the "uncomplicated" crisis from a more serious pathologic condition. Children may be seen more often with skeletal crises, leading to bone deformities. In these cases osteomyelitis and bone infarct must be differentiated.[44-48]

Acute chest syndrome (ACS) is a leading cause of death, accounting for 25% of premature deaths associated with sickle cell disease. ACS is a common cause of hospitalization in sickle cell disease, second only to vasoocclusive crisis. Patients with the ACS present with fever, cough, chest pain, dyspnea, and new infiltrates on the chest radiograph. The pathophysiology of ACS is not well understood but suggests that it may be a specific form of acute lung injury. The injury is postulated to be related to pulmonary microvascular sludging, infarction of pulmonary parenchyma, and bone marrow fat embolization from infarcted bone. Macrovascular pulmonary embolism and infection may also have a pathogenetic role. The differential diagnosis of ACS includes pneumonia, pulmonary embolism, congestive heart failure, and adult respiratory distress syndrome. No definitive diagnosis or therapy is currently available for ACS. Management is supportive and consists of hydration, analgesia, assuring adequate oxygenation and ventilation, and empiric antibiotics.[51,52]

Although most of the diagnostic and therapeutic problems of sickle cell disease are related to vasoocclusive crises, other serious complications must be anticipated. Sickle cell disease is a chronic hemolytic state with reasonably compensated hematocrit values in the 20% to 30% range and elevated reticulocyte counts. This compensated balance may be disrupted by a rare iron deficiency or more commonly a folate deficiency. A potentially life-threatening aplastic crisis may be seen with an acute postinfectious or folate deficiency suppression of erythropoiesis. This aplastic condition is suspected when the hemoglobin level falls 2 g/dl or more from previous stable levels, and the reticulocyte count remains low (< 2%). Finally, children may have an acute splenic sequestration syndrome. This syndrome involves acute splenic enlargement from increased intrasplenic sickling and obstruction. The child may have lassitude and be in shock. Each of these may result in a rapidly falling RBC count and progressive symptoms of anemia. Patients with HbSS are also subject to all other causes of anemia, such as hemolysis from G6PD deficiency.[47] An increased susceptibility to infection is a well-documented phenomenon with HbSS. In infancy an increased incidence of sudden death may be related to pneumococcal sepsis and meningitis. All febrile children with sickle cell anemia should have a WBC count done and blood cultures obtained. Those less than 2 years old with temperatures of 39.5° C or higher and WBC counts greater than 20,000/mm^3 should be given IV antibiotics immediately. Adults with fever require a careful evaluation and laboratory assessment, including appropriate cultures. Early institution of appropriate antibiotics is necessary in those patients with a discernible source of infection. In children and adults, *Staphylococcus* and *Pneumococcus* species and *Haemophilus influenzae* are particularly common. An increased incidence of *Salmonella* osteomyelitis also occurs. The origin of this related immunologic deficiency is believed to be multifactorial, with functional asplenia, poorly migrating neutrophils, and decreased opsonin production as contributors.[48]

The potential for chronic organ damage in patients with sickle cell anemia is almost unlimited. A cross-section of these problems is listed in Table 115-7. These should be quickly reviewed each time a patient with sickle cell anemia enters the ED. The leading causes of death in HbSS are cardiopulmonary disease, chronic renal failure, stroke, and infection.[49]

Diagnostically, most patients with HbSS seen in the ED are well known with defined pain patterns. Because of a slow, but longer, growth period caused by the delayed onset of puberty, adult patients with HbSS have a youthful appearance and long, thin extremities. In a patient with suspected sickle cell disease, an inquiry should be made into the family history, previous pain episodes, and symptoms relative to chronic anemia, infection susceptibility, and ischemic organ damage. Table 115-7 suggests an outline to follow for the physical examination.

All patients should have a CBC, and present blood levels should be compared with those of previous visits. Other laboratory tests are selected on the basis of potential organ complications. Unfortunately, no test is available that detects whether a patient is in a crisis. At present, this difficult task is based on inadequate clinical grounds. In new presentations, the peripheral smear may show sickled cells, and the sickle cell screening test with Sickledex may help, particularly if drug-motivated malingering is suspected (see Figure 115-1, *H*). The definitive diagnosis is aided by hemoglobin electrophoresis.[42,44,49]

At present, the antisickling agent hydroxyurea reduces the frequency of painful crises in adults with a history of three or more crises annually. The beneficial effects of hydroxyurea in

Table 115-7. Organ Damage Seen in Hemoglobin Sickle Cell Disease

Organ or system	Injury
Skin	Stasis ulcer
Central nervous system	Cerebrovascular accident
Eye	Retinal hemorrhage, retinopathy
Cardiac	Congestive heart failure
Pulmonary	Intrapulmonary shunting, embolism, infarct, infection
Vascular	Occlusive phenomenon at any site
Liver	Hepatic infarct, hepatitis resulting from transfusion
Gallbladder	Increased incidence of gallstones caused by bilirubin
Spleen	Acute sequestration
Urinary	Hyposthenuria, hematuria
Genital	Decreased fertility, impotence, priapism
Skeletal	Bone infarcts, osteomyelitis, aseptic necrosis
Placenta	Insufficiency with fetal wastage
Leukocytes	Relative immunodeficiency
Erythrocytes	Chronic hemolysis

sickle cell disease are assumed to be due to the induction of hemoglobin F, but other mechanisms may be operative. Other agents, including clotrimazole, magnesium 5-azacitidine, erythropoietin, and butyric acid, may have a future role in therapy.[53-57] Bone marrow transplantation offers the only current cure for sickle cell disease. Despite survival rates greater than 90% and disease-free survival between 80% and 90%, the role of bone marrow transplantation in sickle cell disease remains uncertain.[58,59]

Present therapies are directed toward symptomatic relief and attempts to stop the cycle of deoxygenated sickling and intravascular sludging. These include rest, adequate nutrition, hydration, oxygenation, analgesia, transfusion, and therapy for infection. Most patients with sickle cell anemia are mildly dehydrated because of urine-concentrating difficulties. Fluid replacement can be oral or IV, and the emergency physician should be aware of the potential for congestive heart failure in patients past their second decade. A satisfactory starting solution is 5% dextrose in half-normal saline begun at a rate of 150 to 200 ml/hr.[60]

Oxygen through a nasal cannula at 2 to 4 L/min may help hypoxic patients and may be given to any patient with HbSS as a low-risk treatment modality with potential benefit. Oxygenation has recently been shown to decrease erythropoietin levels and the number of irreversibly sickled cells.

Analgesia is both the major benefit and bane of sickle cell crisis treatment. Many emergency physicians caring for large sickle cell patient populations have developed protocols for establishing better physician-patient rapport and lessening the chance of narcotic addiction and manipulation. One protocol for severe pain is the following: patients are evaluated, treated with oxygen and hydration, and given IV morphine sulfate, 5 mg, then a constant infusion at 5 mg/hr plus diphenhydramine or hydroxyzine, 25 to 50 mg, on admission. Another approach consists of intravenous bolus doses of morphine sulfate (0.15 mg/kg/dose up to 10 mg/dose). At 6 hours the patient is allowed to decide whether inpatient or outpatient therapy is desired. Outpatient therapy includes 4 to 6 days of an effective oral analgesic. A 60-mg dose of oral morphine sulfate is given 1 to 2 hours before stopping the infusion. This protocol brings uniformity to the patient's expectations for care and the physician's decisions on therapy and admission. Its major disadvantage has been the tendency to treat the patient automatically, rather than closely considering the potential acute complications of sickle cell disease.

No standard pain management exists for sickle cell disease. The emergency physician may choose from a variety of analgesics (nonsteroidal anti-inflammatory, mixed opioid agonist-antagonists, opiates), dosages, and timing intervals. The most important aspect of pain management in these patients is a consistent, thorough, and attentive approach that offers true pain relief. Blood transfusion has a well-accepted role in sickle cell anemia. Very selected use can decrease the chronic transfusion problems of antigen sensitization, iron overload, and hepatitis. Aplastic or splenic sequestration crises may necessitate transfusion. Serial hemoglobin values and reticulocyte counts must be obtained during hospitalization. Priapism may improve with transfusion, although urologic drainage procedures should be considered. Exchange transfusions are recommended for patients, particularly children, with cerebrovascular accidents. Acute symptoms may be reversed and the frequency of recurrence decreased with a regulated 3- to 4-week transfusion program. The goal is to suppress reticulocytosis and decrease the HbS level less than 25%. Rarely, transfusions are given for control of bony or visceral crises. This is not an ED procedure and is considered only after hematologic consultation. Prophylactic transfusions to dilute HbS levels are also recommended in pregnancy and before major surgery.[61,62]

A number of other therapies are being tested for both prophylaxis and crisis management, including supplemental zinc, induced hyponatremia, gelation inhibitors, membrane active agents, and gene manipulation. Careful examination, analgesic protocol, and compassion remain the basis for management. A reason for a painful crisis should always be sought.

The general prognosis of sickle cell patients has improved because of an improvement in their care and the rapid use of antibiotics for potential infections.

Sickle cell-β-thalassemia is seen most commonly in persons of Mediterranean descent. The severity of the disease relates to the concentration of HbS in the RBCs and a decrease in the MCHC. It should be considered in a patient with a low MCV and a positive sickle preparation. It is generally a milder form than homozygous sickle cell disease. HbSC disease falls between HbSS and HbS thalassemia in terms of severity. In addition to many of the complications of HbSS, HbSC disease has an increased incidence of eye hemorrhage and pregnancy complications and may cause splenomegaly. The peripheral smear demonstrates a combination of sickled cells and normocytic target cells.[42,50]

Extrinsic alloantibodies Alloantibodies are formed in response to foreign RBC antigens. In the case of the ABO system these antibodies are preformed. The ABO system is one of the most important RBC wall antigens. ABO incompatibility resulting in donor cell destruction by the recipient's alloantibodies can be a life-threatening reaction. These antibodies are IgM immunoglobulins and can act as a hemolysin, both agglutinating RBCs and fixing complement, causing intravascular hemolysis.

The Rh system is another set of antigens on the RBC. This system is unique in that individuals do not have antibodies that correspond to antigens in the Rh system unless they have been sensitized by a previous exposure to antigens they lack. The antibodies produced are IgG in nature, and they accelerate extravascular destruction of RBCs by the spleen and liver. Most autoimmune antibodies are directed toward antigens in the Rh system.[63]

Extrinsic autoantibodies The evaluation of autoimmune hemolysis is as complex as its origin. The major feature of autoimmune hemolysis is the production of an IgG or IgM antibody to an antigen present on the RBC membrane. Why the body responds in this manner is still unknown. The IgM antibodies can agglutinate, fix complement, and act as intravascular hemolysins. The IgG antibodies may fix complement to the cell but usually do not complete the hemolysis process. These IgG- or C_3-labeled cells undergo an accelerated extravascular destruction. The direct antiglobulin test is useful in revealing these labeled cells.[64]

Autoimmune hemolytic anemias are acquired disorders, of which 40% to 50% are idiopathic. The remainder are associated with a number of diseases, which are listed in Box 115-12. The classification of autoimmune hemolytic anemias is based on the optimal temperature at which the antibody reacts with the RBC membrane. Therefore there are warm-reacting (>37° C) and cold-reacting (<37° C) antibodies.[64]

Box 115-12 Diseases Associated with Autoimmune Hemolytic Anemia

Neoplasms

Malignant: chronic lymphocytic leukemia, lymphoma, myeloma, thymoma, chronic myeloid leukemia
Benign: ovarian teratoma, dermoid cyst

Collagen Vascular Disease

Systemic lupus erythematosus
Periarteritis nodosa
Rheumatoid arthritis

Infections

Mycoplasma
Syphilis
Malaria
Bartonella
Virus: mononucleosis, hepatitis, influenza, coxsackievirus, cytomegalovirus

Miscellaneous

Thyroid disorders, ulcerative colitis
Drug immune reactions

The warm-reacting antibodies are characterized by a higher incidence in younger patients (30 to 60 years of age), predominance in women, variable complement fixation, and a positive direct antiglobulin test for IgG. The cold-reacting antibodies, or cold agglutinins, are seen predominantly in men and in older patients (50 to 80 years of age) and with IgM complement fixation. They may also be found in infectious mononucleosis and *Mycoplasma* infections, as well as lymphoma. Hemolysis may be intravascular and extravascular, and the direct antiglobulin test is positive for complement.[64]

Clinically, the patient with immune hemolytic anemia has the signs and symptoms of anemia and often of splenomegaly. Spherocytosis and reticulocytosis are noted in the blood smear. The direct antiglobulin test is positive in 90% of cases. The strength of the direct antiglobulin test does not correlate with the severity of the hemolysis because the Coombs' reaction is a different antibody function than hemolysis or stimulation of reticuloendothelial sequestration. In patients with newly diagnosed reticulocytopenic or severe hemolytic anemia, the emergency physician may need to institute transfusion therapy. Compatible blood may be almost impossible to find because the antibody can react with almost all donors. The most compatible donor cells using the ABO and Rh systems should be transfused with the knowledge that they will be no more compatible than the patient's own blood cells. Prednisone in a dose of 60 to 100 mg should be given orally or intravenously. It is believed to produce an improvement in 60% of patients with warm antibody reactions. Splenectomy and immunosuppressive therapy are also effective in treating these reactions. Cold agglutinin hemolytic anemia may be self-limited, as after infectious

Box 115-13 Drugs Associated with Immune Hemolytic Anemia

Hapton type with antibodies to the drug
1. Complement-fixing antibody: quinidine, quinine, phenacetin, ethacrynic acid, p-amino salicylate, sulfa drugs, and oral hypoglycemic agents
2. Noncomplement-fixing antibody: penicillin dosages greater than 20 million units per day

Autoimmune type with antibodies to RBC membrane: D-methyldopa, L-dopa, mefenamic acid, and chlordiazepoxide

Cephalosporins at dosages greater than 4 g/day may cause hemolysis by direct membrane injury

mononucleosis. Other forms respond well to cold avoidance, variably to immunosuppressive agents, but poorly to steroids and splenectomy. Deaths commonly result from uncontrolled hemolysis, the underlying primary disorder, and pulmonary embolism.[63,64]

Drug-induced hemolytic anemias may be difficult to diagnose. The emergency physician should know the drugs most often associated with this Coombs' positive phenomenon and realize this test is sometimes positive only in the drug's presence. Common drugs and mechanisms of action are listed in Box 115-13.[65]

Extrinsic mechanical causes Hemolysis may be caused by trauma to the RBC. The peripheral smear may demonstrate schizocytes or fragmented cells, which should immediately raise the suspicion of traumatic injury (see Figure 115-1, *D*). Microangiopathic hemolytic anemia, cardiac trauma, and "march" hemoglobinemia are the most commonly encountered forms of traumatic hemolysis.

Microangiopathic hemolytic anemia is a form of microcirculatory fragmentation by threads of fibrin deposited in the arterioles (Figure 115-3). An underlying disease is inevitably present. It may be found in renal lesions, such as malignant hypertension and preeclampsia, vasculitis, thrombotic thrombocytopenic purpura, disseminated intravascular coagulation, and vascular anomalies. Signs and symptoms are those of intravascular hemolysis. Treatment is directed at the causative disease.

Cardiac trauma to RBCs results from increased turbulence. It may be found in prosthetic valves, atraumatic arteriovenous fistula, aortic stenosis, and other left-sided heart lesions. Surgical correction may be necessary. Supportive therapy with an iron supplement is usually required.

March hemoglobinemia is a form of trauma caused by the breaking of intravascular RBCs by repetitive pounding. Soldiers, marathon runners, and anyone else with repetitive striking against a hard surface may incur this problem. Reassurance and a change in the patient's pattern of activity are the recommended therapy.[35,66]

Environmental causes Hemolysis may be seen in cases of severe burns, freshwater drowning, and hyperthermia. Toxic causes of hemolysis have been documented to be of animal origin, such as brown recluse spider and some snake bites; vegetable origin, such as castor beans and certain mushrooms; and mineral origin, such as copper. Certain infections are associated with hemolytic states. Malaria, *Bartonella,* and *Clostridium* sepsis are three well-known causes.

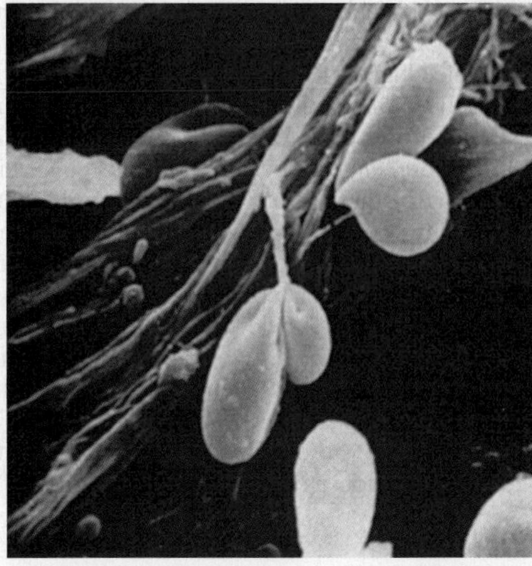

Figure 115-3. **Hanged red cell. Dense fibrin band in background formed from accumulations of finer strands, some of which are still evident. It is only these denser, more amorphous structures that typically persist postmortem. (In vitro model, scanning electron microscope, ×5,200.)** *From Bull BS, Kuhn IN:* **Blood** *35:104, 1970.*

Abnormal sequestration Hypersplenism may be caused by any disease that enlarges the spleen or stimulates the reticuloendothelial system. This can set up an unfortunate cycle in which the enlarged spleen traps more blood components and grows larger. It is usually seen as splenomegaly with pancytopenia and marrow hyperactivity.[51] Cr-labeled RBCs may demonstrate increased trapping in the spleen. The therapy for symptomatic or severe disease is splenectomy. Adults usually tolerate a splenectomy well, but children should be approached conservatively because the risk of postsplenectomy life-threatening sepsis is increased significantly.[67]

POLYCYTHEMIA

Definition

Polycythemia is a term commonly used for erythrocytosis (i.e., increased numbers of RBCs). This disorder is seen occasionally in emergency medicine but rarely in a life-threatening manner that requires emergency intervention.

Pathophysiology

Erythropoiesis is controlled by the kidney-produced glycoprotein hormone erythropoietin. It is activated in the liver and regulates the committed erythropoietic stem cell. Its major stimulant is tissue hypoxia. Neoplastic dysfunction of the bone marrow also may result in an elevated absolute RBC count.

The major complication of polycythemia relates to the increase in blood viscosity associated with increased RBC numbers. As the hematocrit rises past 60%, the viscosity increases almost exponentially. This condition increases the possibility of reduced tissue flow, thrombosis, and hemorrhage. This hazard is usually blunted to a degree by an associated increase in blood volume and some viscosity-reducing vascular dilation.[68,69]

Clinical Features

The history may range from only mild headaches to a full-blown syndrome of hypervolemia (vertigo, dizziness, blurred vision, headache), hyperviscosity (venous thrombosis), and platelet dysfunction (epistaxis, spontaneous bruising, and GI bleeding).

On physical examination, the skin and mucous membrane manifestations of the elevated RBC count are often readily observed. Plethora, engorgement, and venous congestion are commonly noted. Other systems to be examined include the fundus for venous congestion, the abdomen for evidence of splenomegaly, and the cardiopulmonary system for signs of congestive heart failure. Uterine, central nervous system, renal, and hepatic tumors should be sought. All are associated with secondary polycythemia. Laboratory testing defines the disorder with an elevated RBC count, usually greater than the hematocrit. This results in a low MCV, usually related to low serum iron and iron stores. Specific laboratory testing is discussed in the section on the differential diagnosis.[69]

Differential Diagnosis

Polycythemia is classified as apparent primary or secondary (Box 115-14).

Apparent polycythemia is a decrease in plasma volume such as is found with dehydration. The RBC volume does not exceed the upper limit of normal. Although a questionable diagnostic entity, "stress" polycythemia is a tendency for an elevated hematocrit value found in overweight, hypertensive, overstressed middle-aged men. Increased cigarette smoking with its associated increased carboxyhemoglobin level is considered to be partially responsible. The symptoms are minimal, and the treatment is confined to moderation, weight loss, and blood pressure control. The risk of vascular occlusive complications is minimal. The hematocrit is usually less than 60% and RBC mass measurements are normal.[70,71]

Primary polycythemia vera is a myeloproliferative disorder found predominantly in middle-aged or older patients. It may manifest with all of the clinical components of polycythemia. Initial symptoms are reported in up to 30% of patients. The most common problems are thrombotic episodes (cerebrovascular accident, myocardial infarction, deep vein thrombosis), bleeding, and bruising. Primary polycythemia vera is a disease that involves all cell lines—hematopoietic stem, erythroid, granulocytic, and megakaryocytic. The diagnostic criteria used by the Polycythemia Vera Study Group are listed in Box 115-15.

Polycythemia vera may be satisfactorily treated with phlebotomy as necessary. The reduced hematocrit improves some symptoms, but neither the leukocyte nor the platelet count is decreased. Maintaining the hematocrit less than 55% is recommended to decrease hypervolemia and hyperviscosity. Complications necessitating additional therapy include hyperuricemia, refractory increased RBC mass, severe pruritus, excessive splenomegaly, or thrombocytosis. Additional therapy may consist of hydroxyurea, busulfan, chlorambucil, interferon-α, anagrelide, or radioactive phosphorus (^{32}P). Recent studies suggest no improvement in long-term survival with the addition of these treatments. The natural history of the disease is that it burns out over 15 to 20 years. However, myelofibrosis with myeloid metaplasia may develop. In 10% of cases, acute leukemia develops with a rapid and poorly responsive downhill course. The median survival beginning from treatment to death ranges from 9 to 14 years.[72-74] The most common causes of death are thrombosis (29%), hematologic malignancies (23%), nonhematologic malignancies (16%), hemorrhage, and myelofibrosis with myeloid metaplasia.[75]

Box 115-14 Classification of Polycythemia

A. Apparent polycythemia
B. Primary polycythemia vera
C. Secondary polycythemia
   1. Appropriately increased erythropoietin caused by tissue hypoxia
      a. Right-to-left shunt congenital heart disease
      b. Pulmonary disease (e.g., bronchial-type chronic obstructive pulmonary disease)
      c. Carboxyhemoglobinemia
      d. High-altitude acclimatization
      e. Decreased tissue oxygen release from high oxygen-affinity hemoglobinopathies
   2. Inappropriate autonomous erythropoietin production
      a. Renal origin: carcinoma, hydronephrosis, cyst
      b. Other lesions: uterine fibroids, hepatoma of adrenal origin, cerebellar hemangioma
      c. Congenital overproduction
D. Pure or essential erythrocytosis
E. AIDS and zidovudine treatment

Box 115-15 Diagnostic Criteria for Polycythemia Vera*

Category A

Increased RBC mass
   In men: >36 ml/kg
   In women: >32 ml/kg
Normal arterial oxygen saturation (>92%)
Splenomegaly

Category B

Thrombocytosis: platelets >400,000/mm^3
Leukocytosis: WBC count >12,000/mm^3 (with no fever or infection)
Leukocyte alkaline phosphatase score >100
B_{12} > 900 pg/ml, unbound vitamin B_{12}-binding capacity <2200 pg/ml

For polycythemia vera to be diagnosed, either all three criteria in category A or the first two criteria in category A along with any two criteria in category B must be present.

The secondary polycythemias are classified first according to appropriate erythropoietin response to abnormal tissue oxygen levels. This group of disorders may be ruled out by normal measured arterial oxygen saturation. Second, inappropriate autonomous erythropoietin production is considered. This condition can be assessed with an erythropoietin assay. Because of the strong associations with renal pathologic conditions, a patient with a suspected inappropriate erythropoietin response should have an IV pyelogram or computed tomography scan. Most patients with secondary polycythemia have no central nervous system symptoms or splenomegaly. Because erythropoietin stimulates only the red cell pathway, these patients have normal WBC and platelet counts.[76]

Management

Emergency treatment of any form of symptomatic polycythemia is phlebotomy. Usually not more than 500 ml of blood is slowly removed as the volume is replaced with a comparable amount of saline. No hemodynamic compromise should occur if this procedure is carried out slowly. In true emergencies, up to 1 to 1.5 L of blood may be removed over a 24-hour period. The initial goal is to lower the hematocrit level toward 60%. The final goal is a level less than 55%.

Disposition

A number of patients with known polycythemia may be managed with outpatient phlebotomies. Any newly diagnosed or symptomatic patient should be admitted to the hospital for full evaluation.

WHITE BLOOD CELL DISORDERS

The WBC count and accompanying differential are the most common laboratory tests ordered in the ED. It is essential that the basic physiology, pathophysiology, and clinical evaluation of WBCs be understood.

Physiology and Pathophysiology

The series has three morphologically indistinguishable cell types: B cells (humoral immunity), T cells (cellular immunity), and null cells. Because lymphocytes can freely leave and return to the circulation, the storage pools are less well defined. Only 5% of the total body lymphocytes are in the circulation. No marginal pool exists.[77]

Leukocytes primarily function extravascularly. The primary function of each series is closely integrated with the other. The WBCs reach their site of action through the circulation. The rate new cells enter the circulation is usually in equilibrium with the rate of loss in the tissues.

Abnormal cell counts are due to changes in production, the marginal pool, or the rate of tissue destruction. Just as in anemia or platelet count abnormalities, the differential diagnosis of increased (leukocytosis) or decreased (leukopenia) WBC counts can be organized by processes altering production, destruction, loss, and sequestration. This chapter focuses primarily on quantitative, rather than qualitative, disorders.[77]

The granulocytic and lymphocytic series are the two cell lines of WBCs. The granulocytic series is primarily involved in phagocytic activity. Its origin is the pluripotential stem cells located in the bone marrow. A subset of these cells differentiates and matures into the phagocytic cell lines, which include neutrophils, monocytes, basophils, and eosinophils. Granulocytes are maintained in a series of developmental and storage pools. The most important is the postmitotic storage pool for neutrophils, which represents 15 to 20 times the circulating population. This pool contains metamyelocytes, band neutrophils, and mature neutrophils (polymorphonuclear neutrophils). The pool can be drawn on as a ready reserve during rapid consumption of granulocytes. Circulating neutrophils are subdivided equally into the circulating neutrophil pool and the marginal pool. The latter consists of mature cells adherent to the blood vessel wall. These cells can rapidly enter the circulating pool and cause a substantial increase, even doubling, of the WBC count. This involvement does not alter the maturity pattern of the differential count.[77] The lymphocytic series matures in lymphoid tissues located in bone marrow, thymus, spleen, lymph nodes, and elsewhere. They are involved in the immune response against a foreign substance.

Table 115-8. Normal Ranges for Blood Leukocyte Count (cells/mm^3)

Age	Average	95% range (average value ± 2 SD)
1 wk	12,200	5,000-21,000
6 mo	11,900	6,000-17,500
12 mo	11,400	6,000-17,500
4 yr	9,100	5,500-15,500
8 yr	8,300	4,500-13,500
Adults	7,400	4,500-11,000

Modified from Miale JB: *Laboratory medicine: hematology,* ed 6, St Louis, 1982, Mosby.

Normal Values and Influences

One unique problem in WBC disorders is the wide variability of normal values and the multiple factors influencing them. WBC counts are usually performed automatically using electrical impedance or optical diffraction techniques. Differential counts are commonly performed by direct examination of 100 to 500 cells using the oil immersion lens of the microscope. Automated techniques for all differential counts are becoming more popular. The normal values for the WBC count are listed in Table 115-8. The "normal" count is age dependent until childhood and may be shifted upward by exercise, gender (women), smoking, and pregnancy. Decreases in total WBC count between 1,000 and 1,200 cells/mm^3 have been noted in African Americans. Laboratory errors may be caused by improper sample preparation, nucleated RBCs, or platelet clumping. The blood smear differential count may also be influenced by small sample size, improper cell identification, and age group (children). Differential ranges are listed in Table 115-9. One common but easily corrected error in laboratory reporting is giving the results in terms of the percentage of cell type. Absolute counts for each cell type are more accurate and useful in assessing infection risk.[78,79]

Abnormal Values

Because of the wide range of normal values, all abnormal WBC counts should be interpreted in the context of the patient presentation. A careful history and physical examination, absolute cell counts, and a review of the peripheral smear differential count are the starting points for determining the origins of quantitative WBC disorders.

Leukocytosis

Most cases of leukocytosis are caused by increases in the neutrophil or lymphocyte cell lines. Neutrophil leukocytosis (neutrophilia) is an absolute neutrophil count greater than 7,500 cells/mm^3 and is commonly associated with infection or inflammation (Box 115-16). Because increased neutrophil destruction is associated with both these pathologic processes, the bone marrow stores are drawn on, and the usual ratio of 1 band to 10 neutrophils increases. This manifests as a "left shift" in the differential count and represents immature neutrophils from the postmitotic pool moving into the circulation.

Table 115-9. Normal Percentage Ranges for Leukocyte Differential Count in Blood*

Age	Segmented neutrophils	Band neutrophils	Lymphocytes	Monocytes	Eosinophils	Basophils
1 wk	34 ± 15 (4,100)	11.8 ± 4 (1,420)	41 ± 5 (5,000)	9.1 (1,100)	4.1 (500)	0-4 (50)
6 mo	23 ± 10 (2,710)	8.8 ± 3 (1,000)	61 ± 15 (7,300)	4.8 (480)	2.5 (300)	0-4 (50)
12 mo	23 ± 10 (2,680)	8.1 ± 3 (990)	61 ± 15 (7,000)	4.8 (550)	2.6 (300)	0-4 (50)
4 yr	34 ± 11 (3,040)	8.0 ± 3 (730)	50 ± 15 (4,500)	5.0 (450)	2.8 (250)	0-6 (50)
8 yr	45 ± 11 (3,700)	8.0 ± 3 (660)	39 ± 15 (3,300)	4.2 (350)	2.4 (200)	0-6 (50)
Adult	51 ± 15 (3,800)	8.0 ± 3 (620)	34 ± 10 (2,500)	4.0 (300)	2.7 (200)	0-5 (40)

Modified from Miale JB: *Laboratory medicine: hematology,* ed 6, St Louis, 1982, Mosby.
*Numbers in parentheses indicate the average number of cells per cubic millimeter.

Box 115-16 Causes of Leukocytosis

Neutrophils (Absolute Count >7500 Cells/mm³)

Inflammation: rheumatoid arthritis, gout
Infection: bacterial most common
Tissue necrosis: cancer, burns, infarctions
Metabolic disorders: diabetic ketoacidosis, thyrotoxicosis, uremia
Rapid RBC turnover: hemorrhage, hemolysis
Myeloproliferative disorders: chronic myeloid leukemia, polycythemia vera
Malignancy (e.g., GI cancers)
Stress: exercise, pain, surgery, hypoxia, seizures, trauma
Drugs: epinephrine, corticosteroids, lithium, cocaine
Pregnancy
Heredity or idiopathic disease
Laboratory error: automated counters, platelet clumping, precipitated cryoglobulin

Lymphocytosis (Absolute Count >9000/mm³, Ages 1 to 6; 7000/mm³, Ages 7 to 16; 4000/mm³, Adults)

Viral infection (primary cause): mononucleosis, rubeola, rubella, varicella, toxoplasmosis
Bacterial infection: pertussis, tuberculosis, hepatitis, cytomegalovirus
Lymphoproliferative: acute or chronic lymphocytic leukemia
Immunologic response: immunization, autoimmune diseases, graft rejection
Endocrine: hypothyroidism
Relative lymphocytosis associated with granulocytopenia

Modified from Miale JB: *Laboratory medicine: hematology,* ed 6, St Louis, 1982, Mosby.

WBC counts can increase without a "left shift" or increase in band forms by demarginating neutrophils from the vessel walls. It is often seen as a response to stress, exercise, or epinephrine. Severe stress can raise the WBC count to 18,000 to 20,000 cells/mm³.[78,80,81]

Chronic Myeloid Leukemia One of the myeloproliferative causes of a neutrophilic leukocytosis is chronic myeloid leukemia (CML). Although it is the least common of the major leukemias (60% acute, 31% chronic lymphocytic leukemia, 15% CML), it must be considered in neutrophilia. Patients with CML are usually older than 40 years of age and have WBC counts greater than 50,000 cells/mm³. The differential count has elevated polymorphoneutrophil and metamyelocyte counts. Less often the basophil and eosinophil count are increased. CML is a stem cell disorder in which the WBC count is elevated and the differential is normal. Mature and intermediate granulocytes are overproduced. Platelets also may be increased, but RBC production is down, resulting in anemia. The patient often complains of fatigue, anorexia, sweating, and weight loss. Physical findings include pallor, sternal tenderness, and splenomegaly (90% of patients). In the laboratory, decreased leukocyte alkaline phosphatase and increased vitamin B_{12} levels are found. This helps differentiate CML from other causes of neutrophilia. The Philadelphia chromosome (Ph^1) is almost always associated with the disease. The chronic phase of CML is treated with an alkylating agent (e.g., busulfan) or an antimetabolite (e.g., hydroxyurea). Selected patients may benefit from a bone marrow transplantation.[82,83]

The need for urgent therapy in CML is usually related to hyperuricemia and renal injury or severe anemia, causing angina or heart failure. Rarely, hyperleukocytosis occurs, but the more mature, "less sticky" cells in CML usually do not cause problems unless the count exceeds 500,000 cells/mm³. A higher cell count may cause leukostasis and result in deafness, visual impairment, pulmonary ventilation-perfusion abnormalities, and priapism. Treatment involves hydration, leukapheresis, transfusion as necessary, allopurinol to prevent severe hyperuricemia, and specific chemotherapy (hydroxyurea). Late problems in the natural history of CML involve progressive loss of cell differentiation and response to therapy. The term *blastic crisis* represents the sudden appearance of an acute form of leukemia, which is a rare substage of the evolving deterioration.[82-84] This condition may present in lymphoid or myeloid forms. Blast counts greater than 50,000 cells/mm³ may predispose the patient to the complications of leukostasis.

Leukemoid Reaction The leukemoid reaction is a nonleukemic reactive granulocytic leukocytosis that resembles CML but has no associated Ph^1 chromosome, no absolute increase in basophils and eosinophils, and an increase in leukocyte alkaline phosphatase. It is difficult to distinguish from CML in the ED, and both must be considered as a potential diagnosis in granulocytic leukocytosis. WBC counts are usually greater than 50,000 cells/mm³. A leukemoid reaction may be seen in tuberculosis, Hodgkin's disease, sepsis, and metastatic tumor, particularly bronchogenic, gastric, and renal carcinoma.[81]

Lymphocytic Leukocytosis Lymphocytic leukocytosis (lymphocytosis) is an age-dependent definition: 9,000 cells/mm^3, ages 1 to 6; 7,000 cells/mm^3, ages 6 to 16; 4,000 cells/mm^3, adults. It is seen in a variety of disorders, primarily infections and lymphoproliferative disease.[85]

In the past *acute* and *chronic* were descriptive terms applied to lymphocytic neoplasma with respect to patient survival time before present therapy was available. The terms *acute* and *chronic* are currently used to describe the cell maturity, the rapidity of onset, and the aggressiveness of therapy.

Chronic Lymphocytic Leukemia Chronic lymphocytic leukemia (CLL) is primarily a B cell disorder and is the most common type of leukemia in the 50-year and older population. Patients initially complain of fatigue, weight loss, increased susceptibility to infection, skin rashes, and easy bruising. The lymph nodes are nontender and smooth and may appear in only one or two areas. Splenic and hepatic enlargement occurs in more than 50% of patients. Laboratory support of the diagnosis is an absolute lymphocyte count of greater than 5,000 cells/mm^3 in adults. Anemia, thrombocytopenia, and neutropenia are often found. Autoimmune hemolytic anemias, a positive direct antiglobulin test, and other altered immune system problems are seen. Early therapy may be directed toward complications of anemia, thrombocytopenia, impaired or accentuated immune response, or enlarged lymph nodes or spleen. Leukostasis is seldom seen in CLL, but therapy is considered when the total count rises over 200,000/mm^3.[86]

Acute Lymphocytic Leukemia Acute lymphocytic leukemia (ALL) is most commonly diagnosed in children less than 10 years of age. It is the most common malignancy in children less than 15 years of age. In ALL the potential for leukostasis increases when the blast count rises above 50,000 cells/mm^3. Oncologic therapy is based on clinical staging and includes chemotherapy or radiation. Aggressive therapy has improved childhood survival rates from 1 to 15 years or more. This response to treatment has not been found to the same degree in adults.[87,88]

Leukopenia

In adults, leukopenia is defined as an absolute blood cell count of less than 4,000 cells/mm^3. Leukopenia is commonly associated with a reduction in one cell type, the neutrophil, and this decrease has the greatest clinical significance. The absolute neutrophil count is calculated by multiplying the WBC by the combined percentage of band and segmented neutrophils. The absolute neutrophil count can be classified as mild (1,000 to 1,500 cells/mm^3), moderate (500 to 1,000 cells/mm^3), and severe (<500 cells/mm^3) risk levels for infection. The latter is a potentially life-threatening state because the patient is markedly susceptible to overwhelming infection. The physical signs of infection may be minimal in severe neutropenia because there are too few cells to generate a substantial inflammatory or purulent response. Neutropenia may be caused by decreased production, increased destruction, or movement of circulating neutrophils into marginal or tissue pools. Until recently, it was most often caused by a decrease in bone marrow production (Table 115-10). Autoimmune neutropenia is also becoming more commonly diagnosed because it is considered to have a role in acquired immunodeficiency syndrome.[81,89,90]

Table 115-10. Linkage of Leukopenia to Phases of Neutrophil Maturation

Mechanism	Example
Proliferation in bone marrow	Aplastic anemia, leukemia, cancer chemotherapy (cyclophosphamide, azathioprine, methotrexate, chlorambucil)
	Drugs: phenothiazines, phenylbutazone, indomethacin, propylthiouracil, phenytoin, cimetidine, semisynthetic penicillins, sulfonamides, postviral infection, tuberculosis sepsis
Maturation in bone marrow	Folate or B_{12} deficiency, chronic idiopathic neutropenia
	Starvation
Distribution	Hypersplenism: sarcoidosis, portal hypertension, malaria
Increased use	Infection: viral most common (mononucleosis, rubella, rubeola), *Rickettsia* organisms, overwhelming bacterial infection
	Autoimmune disease: systemic lupus erythematosus, AIDS, Felty's syndrome
Laboratory error	Leukocyte clumping, long delay in running test

A thorough medical history must be taken in all patients found to have neutropenia. A prior history of neutropenia, a review of recent infection, and family history are sought. Review of systems will focus on bleeding problems, fatigue, sweats, weight loss, and autoimmune symptoms. Physical examination is directed toward sites of infection, lymphadenopathy, hepatosplenomegaly, and underlying disease. In patients with severe neutropenia and fever, a full radiologic and direct examination of commonly involved areas, such as the chest and urine, should be done, and sputum, urine, and blood cultures obtained. Basic isolation techniques, early admission, and consultation with a specialist are recommended. Specific therapies may be started after cultures and consultation are completed. A number of empiric antibiotic regimens are recommended for febrile patients with neutropenia.[91] Human granulocyte colony-stimulating factor is often used in the setting of neutropenia, but is best done in consultation with a hematologist.[92,93] Patients with a clear reversible source or without significant clinical findings and mild to moderate levels of neutropenia may have outpatient follow-up monitoring arranged, preferably after discussion with their physician.

RATIONALE FOR SELECTION OF WBC AND DIFFERENTIAL COUNTS

The WBC count has not proved to be a highly specific test in the diagnosis of a variety of disease entities.[94] For example, recent studies evaluating the WBC count in the diagnosis of abdominal pain find it a useful confirming test or helpful in selecting patients for observation. In evaluating the bacterial versus viral infectious potential in febrile children, the WBC and differential counts have shown limited usefulness, except in children less than 2 years of age in whom counts greater than 15,000 cells/mm^3 have an increased correlation with bacteremia.[94,95]

Box 115-17 Agents and Conditions That Elevate the WBC Count

Acetylcholine	Lithium
Acidosis	Menstruation
Adrenergic drugs	Myocardial infarction
Alcohol	Neonatal asphyxia
Allergic reactions	Neoplasm
Bacterial infection	Normal pregnancy
Blood donation	Pain
Burns	Polyarteritis nodosa
Competitive running	Prednisone
Crying in infants	Pulmonary infarction
Fever	Seizures
Gout	Snake bite
Hemolysis	Supraventricular tachycardia
Heparin	Surgery
Histamine	Trauma
Hypoxia	Uremia
Iron overdose	Viral infection
Juvenile rheumatoid arthritis	Vomiting
Lead and other toxins	

In addition to the nonspecificity of the WBC count, the differential count provides additional helpful information in less than 1% of cases. The absolute leukocyte count or the differential cannot reliability distinguish between viral and bacterial infection. The test should be viewed as having limited screening value in the acute care setting. Multiple agents and conditions increase the WBC count (Box 115-17), making the test less specific for infection than previously assumed.

KEY CONCEPTS

- Anemia in the elderly population often presents as an exacerbation of preexisting, comorbid diseases.
- One of the most important, but often overlooked, studies in the evaluation of suspected hemolytic anemia is the peripheral blood smear.
- Studies for folate, B_{12}, iron, total iron-binding capacity, reticulocytes, and direct antiglobulin (Coombs') test are altered by transfusion.
- Acute chest syndrome is a common cause of death among patients with sickle cell disease and should be suspected when patients present with chest pain and shortness of breath.
- The white blood cell determination in the ED is overused and has limited clinical value.

REFERENCES

1. Williams MD, Wheby MS: Anemia in pregnancy, *Med Clin North Am* 76:631, 1992.
2. Izaks GJ, Westendorp RG, Knook DL: The definition of anemia in older person, *JAMA* 281:1714, 1999.
3. Mansouri A, Lipschitz DA: Anemia in the elderly patient, *Med Clin North Am* 76:619, 1992.
4. Spivak JL, Eichner ER: *The fundamentals of clinical hematology,* ed 3, Baltimore, 1993, Johns Hopkins University Press.
5. Hillman RS, Ault KA: Normal erythropoiesis. In Hillman RS, Ault KA, editors: *Hematology in clinical practice,* ed 2, New York, McGraw-Hill, 1998.
6. Bayless PA: Selected red cell disorders, *Emerg Med Clin North Am* 11:481, 1993.
7. Barber AE: Cell damage after shock, *New Horiz* 4:151, 1996.
8. Rodgers KG: Cardiovascular shock, *Emerg Med Clin North Am* 13:793, 1995.
9. Longstreth GF: Epidemiology of hospitalization for acute upper gastrointestinal hemorrhage: a population-based study, *Am J Gastroenterol* 90:206, 1995.
10. Strobach RS, Anderson SK, Doll DC, Ringenberg QS: The value of the physical examination in the diagnosis of anemia, *Arch Intern Med* 148:831, 1988.
11. Jain R: Use of blood transfusion in management of anemia, *Med Clin North Am* 76:727, 1992.
12. Hillman RS, Ault KA: Clinical approach to anemia. In Hillman RS, Ault KA, editors: *Hematology in clinical practice,* ed 2, New York, 1998, McGraw-Hill.
13. Welborn JL, Meyers FJ: A three-point approach to anemia, *Postgrad Med* 89:179, 1991.
14. Bessman JD, Gilmer PR, Gardner FH: Improved classification of anemias by MCV and RDW, *Am J Clin Pathol* 80:322, 1988.
15. Fairbanks VR: Laboratory testing for iron status, *Hosp Pract* 26:17, 1991.
16. Brown RG: Determining the cause of anemia: general approach, with emphasis on microcytic hypochromic anemias, *Postgrad Med* 89:161, 1991.
17. Andrews NC: Disorders of iron metabolism, *N Engl J Med* 341:1986, 1999.
18. Brittenham GM: Disorders of iron metabolism: iron deficiency and overload. In Hoffman R et al, editors: *Hematology: basic principles and practice,* ed 2, New York, 1995, Churchill Livingstone.
19. Olivieri NF: The β-Thalassemias, *N Engl J Med* 341:99, 1999.
20. Giardina PJ, Hilgartner MW: Update on thalassemia, *Pediatr Rev* 13:55, 1992.
21. Brittenham GM et al: Efficacy of deferoxamine in preventing complications of iron overload in patients with thalassemia major, *N Engl J Med* 31:567, 1994.
22. Lucarelli G, Giardini C, Angelucci E: Bone marrow transplantation in the thalassemia. In Winter JN, editor: *Blood stem cell transplantation,* Boston, 1997, Kluwer Academic.
23. Beutler E: Hereditary and acquired sideroblastic anemias. In Beutler E et al, editors: *Williams hematology,* ed 5, New York, 1995, McGraw-Hill.
24. Damon LE: Anemias of chronic disease in the aged: diagnosis and treatment, *Geriatrics* 47:47, 1992.
25. Lipschitz DA: The anemia of chronic disease, *J Am Geriatr Soc* 38:1258, 1990.
26. Means RT, Krantz SB: Progress in understanding the pathogenesis of the anemia of chronic disease, *Blood* 80:1639, 1992.
27. Hoffbrand V, Provan D: ABC of clinical hematology. Macrocytic anaemias, *BMJ* 314:430, 1997.
28. Stabler SP, Allen RH, Savage DG, Lindenbaum J: Clinical spectrum and diagnosis of cobalamin deficiency, *Blood* 76:871, 1990.
29. Babior BM: The megaloblastic anemias. In Beutler E et al, editors: *Williams hematology,* ed 5, New York, 1995, McGraw-Hill.
30. Young NS, Maciejewski J: The pathophysiology of acquired aplastic anemia, *N Engl J Med* 336:1365, 1997.
31. Young NS: Acquired aplastic anemia, *JAMA* 282:271, 1999.
32. Humphries JE: Anemia of renal failure: use of erythropoietin, *Med Clin North Am* 76:711, 1992.
33. Santhosh-Kumar CR, Kolhouse JF: Hemolytic anemias. In Wood ME, Bunn RA, editors: *Hematology/oncology secrets,* Philadelphia, 1999, Hanley Belfus.
34. Leonard KA, Klein HG: Acute hemolytic disorders. In Bell WR, editor: *Hematologic and oncologic emergencies,* New York, 1993, Churchill Livingstone.
35. Tabbara IA: Hemolytic anemias: diagnosis and management, *Med Clin North Am* 76:649, 1992.
36. Nydegger UE, Kazatchkine MD, Mieschner PA: Immunopathologic and clinical features of hemolytic anemia due to cold agglutinins, *Semin Hematol* 28:66, 1991.
37. Jacobasch G, Rapoport SM: Hemolytic anemias due to erythrocyte enzyme deficiencies, *Mol Aspects Med* 17:143, 1996.
38. Valentine WN, Paglia DE: Erythroenzymopathies and hemolytic anemia, *J Lab Clin Med* 115:12, 1990.

39. Beutler E: Glucose-6-phosphate dehydrogenase deficiency. In Beutler E et al, editors: *Williams hematology,* ed 5, New York, 1995, McGraw-Hill.
40. Palek J, Jarolim P: Hereditary spherocytosis, elliptocytosis, and related disorders. In Beutler E et al, editors: *Williams hematology,* ed 5, New York, 1995, McGraw-Hill.
41. Bunn HF: Pathogenesis and treatment of sickle cell disease, *N Engl J Med* 337:762, 1997.
42. Embury SH: Sickle cell disease. In: Hoffman R et al, editors: *Hematology. Basic principles and practice,* ed 2, New York, 1995, Churchill Livingstone.
43. *Sickle cell disease: Screening diagnosis, management and counseling in newborns and infants,* AHCPR Publication 93-0562, USDHHS, Rockville, Md, 1993.
44. Chenh C: *Resource manual for hemoglobinopathies,* Columbus, 1992, Division Maternal and Child Health, Ohio Department of Health.
45. Platt OS et al: Mortality in sickle cell disease, *N Engl J Med* 330:1639, 1994.
46. Platt OS et al: Pain in sickle cell disease: rates and risk factors, *N Engl J Med* 325:11, 1991.
47. Serjaent GR: *Sickle cell disease,* ed 2, Oxford, England, 1992, Oxford University Press.
48. Kravis E, Fleisher G, Ludwig S: Fever in children with sickle cell hemoglobinopathies, *Am J Dis Child* 16:1075, 1992.
49. Steingart R: Management of patients with sickle cell disease, *Med Clin North Am* 76:669, 1992.
50. Nagel RL, Lawrence C: The distinct pathobiology of sickle cell-hemoglobin C disease: therapeutic implications, *Hematol Oncol Clin North Am* 5:433, 1991.
51. Hargis CA, Claster S: Acute chest syndrome in sickle cell disease, *Crit Decisions Emerg Med* 11:1, 1997.
52. Gladwin MT et al: The acute chest syndrome in sickle cell disease, *Am J Respir Crit Care Med* 159:1368, 1999.
53. Brugnara C et al: Therapy with oral clotrimazole induces inhibition of the Gardos channel and reduction of erythrocyte dehydration in patients with sickle cell disease, *J Clin Invest* 97:1227, 1996.
54. de Franceschi L et al: Oral magnesium supplements reduce erythrocyte dehydration in patients with sickle cell disease, *J Clin Invest* 100:1847, 1997.
55. Charache S, Terrin ML, Moore RD: Effect of hydroxyurea on the frequency of painful crisis in sickle cell anemia, *N Engl J Med* 332:1317, 1995.
56. Nagel RL et al: F reticulocyte response in sickle cell anemia treated with recombinant human erythropoietin: a double-blind study, *Blood* 81:9, 1993.
57. Perrine SP et al: Sodium butyrate enhances fetal globin gene expression in erythroid progenitors of patients with Hb SS and beta thalassemia, *Blood* 74:454, 1989.
58. Walters MC et al: Collaborative multicenter investigation of marrow transplantation for sickle cell disease: current results and future directions, *Biol Blood Marrow Transplant* 3:310, 1997.
59. Vermylen C, Cornu G: Hematopoietic stem cell transplantation for sickle cell anemia, *Curr Opin Hematol* 4:377, 1997.
60. Charache S, Koshy M, Milner PF: Care of patients with sickle cell anemia in the adult emergency department. In Bell WR, editor: *Hematologic and oncologic emergencies,* New York, 1993, Churchill Livingstone.
61. Wayne AS, Kevy SW, Nathan DG: Transfusion management of sickle cell disease, *Blood* 81:1109, 1993.
62. Vichinsky EP et al: A comparison of conservative and aggressive transfusion regimens in the perioperative management of sickle cell disease, *N Engl J Med* 333:206, 1995.
63. Kickler TS, Ness PM: Blood component therapy. In Bell WR, editor: *Hematologic and oncologic emergencies,* New York, 1993, Churchill Livingstone.
64. Engelfriet CP, Overbeeke MA, von dem Borne AE: Autoimmune hemolytic anemia, *Semin Hematol* 29:3, 1992.
65. Salama A, Mueller-Eckardt C: Immune-mediated blood cell dyscrasias related to drugs, *Semin Hematol* 29:54, 1992.
66. Eichner ER: The anemia of athletes, *Phys Sports Med* 14:122, 1986.
67. Erslev AJ: Hypersplenism and hyposplenism. In Beutler E et al, editors: *Williams hematology,* ed 5, New York, 1995, McGraw-Hill.
68. Hinshelwood S, Bench AJ, Green AR: Pathogenesis of polycythemia vera, *Blood Rev* 11:224, 1997.
69. Landaw SA: Polycythemia vera and other polycythemic states, *Clin Feb Med* 10:85, 1990.
70. Messinezy M, Pearson TC: Apparent polycythemia: diagnosis, pathogenesis, and management, *Eur J Haematol* 51:125, 1993.
71. Djulbegovic B, Habley T, Joseph G: A new algorithm for the diagnosis of polycythemia, *Am Fam Phys* 41:113, 1991.
72. Conley CL: Polycythemia vera, *JAMA* 263:2481, 1990.
73. Beutler E: Polycythemia vera. In Beutler E et al, editors: *Williams hematology,* ed 5, New York, 1995, McGraw-Hill.
74. Wehmeier A et al: Incidence and clinical risk for bleeding and thrombotic complications in myeloproliferative disorders, *Ann Hematol* 63:101, 1991.
75. Berk PD et al: Treatment of polycythemia vera: a summary of clinical trials conducted by the Polycythemia Vera Group. In Wasserman LR, Berk PD, Berlin NI, editors: *Polycythemia vera and the myeloproliferative disorders,* Philadelphia, 1995, WB Saunders.
76. Erslen AJ: Secondary polycythemia (erythrocytosis). In Beutler E et al, editors: *Williams hematology,* ed 5, New York, 1995, McGraw-Hill.
77. Hillman RS, Ault KA: Normal myelopoiesis. In Hillman RS, Ault KA, editors: *Hematology in clinical practice,* ed 2, New York, 1998, McGraw-Hill.
78. Werman HA, Brown CG: White blood cell and differential counts, *Emerg Med Clin North Am* 4:41, 1986.
79. Shapiro MF, Greenfield S: Complete blood counts and leukocyte differential counts, *Ann Intern Med* 105:65, 1987.
80. McCarthy DA et al: Leukocytosis induced by exercise, *BMJ* 295:636, 1987.
81. Dale DC: Neutrophilia. In Beutler E et al, editors: *Williams hematology,* ed 5, New York, 1995, McGraw-Hill.
82. Faderl S et al: The biology of chronic myeloid leukemia, *N Engl J Med* 341:164, 1999.
83. Savage DG, Szydlo RM, Goldman JM: Clinical features at diagnosis in 430 patients with chronic myeloid leukemia seen at a referral centre over a 16-year period, *Br J Haematol* 96:111, 1997.
84. Bunin N, Pui CH: Differing complications of hyperleukocytosis in children with acute lymphoblastic or acute nonlymphoblastic leukemia, *J Clin Oncol* 3:1590, 1985.
85. Kipps TJ: Lymphocytosis and lymphocytopenia. In Beutler E et al, editors: *Williams hematology,* ed 5, New York, 1995, McGraw-Hill.
86. Cheson BD et al: National Cancer Institute-sponsored Working Group guidelines for chronic lymphocytic leukemia: revised guidelines for diagnosis and treatment, *Blood* 87:4990, 1996.
87. Pui CH: Childhood leukemia, *N Engl J Med* 332:1618, 1995.
88. Mauer AM: Acute lymphocytic leukemia. In Beutler E et al, editors: *Williams hematology,* ed 5, New York, 1995, McGraw-Hill.
89. Frontiera M, Myers AM: Peripheral blood and bone marrow abnormalities in the acquired immunodeficiency syndrome, *West J Med* 147:157, 1987.
90. Groopman JE: Management of the hemolytic complications of human immunodeficiency virus infection, *Rev Infect Dis* 12:931, 1990.
91. Hughes WT et al: Guidelines for the use of antimicrobial agents in neutropenic patients with unexplained fever, *J Infect Dis* 161:381, 1990.
92. Maher DW et al: Filgrastin in patients with chemotherapy-induced febrile neutropenia: a double-blind placebo-controlled trial, *Ann Intern Med* 121:492, 1994.
93. American Society of Clinical Oncology Recommendations for the Use of Hematopoietic Colony-Stimulating Factors: Evidence-based clinical practice guidelines, *J Clin Oncol* 12:2471, 1994.
94. Badgett RG, Hansen CJ, Rogers CS: Clinical usage of the leukocyte count in emergency department decision making, *J Gen Intern Med* 5:198, 1990.
95. Da Silva O, Ohlsson A, Kenyon C: Accuracy of leukocyte indices and C-reactive protein for diagnosis of neonatal sepsis: critical review, *Pedatr Infect Dis J* 14:362, 1995.

116 Disorders of Hemostasis

Timothy G. Janz
Glenn C. Hamilton

PERSPECTIVE

Hemostasis is the process of blood clot formation that represents a coordinated response to vessel injury. This requires an orchestrated response from platelets, the clotting cascade, blood vessel endothelium, and fibrinolysis. Thrombin-stimulated clot formation and plasmin-induced clot lysis are closely related and regulated. The dynamic process is often viewed in phases: platelet plug formation, coagulation cascade propagation, clot formation, and clot fibrinolysis.

Most hemostatic abnormalities are acquired and result from drugs (e.g., aspirin or Coumadin), from associated disease (e.g., hepatic insufficiency), or from iatrogenic causes (e.g., multiple transfusions).

PRINCIPLES OF DISEASE

Hemostasis depends on the normal function and integration of the vasculature, platelets, and the coagulation pathway.

Vasculature

Vascular integrity is maintained by a lining of nonreactive overlapping endothelial cells supported by a basement membrane, connective tissue, and smooth muscle. These cells are important in maintaining a barrier to macromolecules and, when injured, in contributing to the metabolic response and local vasoconstriction. The vascular wall is an important contributor to hemostasis.[1]

The endothelium contributes to both clot formation and regulation by producing substances such as von Willebrand factor, antithrombin III, heparin sulfate, prostacyclin, nitric oxide, and tissue factor pathway inhibitor.

Platelets

Platelets have multiple and ever-expanding roles in our understanding of hemostasis. They are complex cytoplasmic fragments released from bone marrow megakaryocytes under the control of thrombopoietin. The platelets contain lysosomes, granules, a trilaminar plasma membrane, microtubules, and a canalicular system. The granules are an important component of hemostasis and contain platelet factor 4, adhesive and aggregation glycoproteins, coagulation factors, and fibrinolytic inhibitors. Each participates in the process of coagulation. The platelet role is termed primary hemostasis and it serves as the initial defense against blood loss. A fibrin clot, incorporating coagulation factors, usually reinforces a platelet clot. Platelet activity is summarized in Box 116-1. Any of the listed steps may be absent, altered, or inhibited by inherited or acquired disorders.[2-6]

Coagulation Pathway

The coagulation pathway is a complex system of checks and balances. The result is the controlled formation of a fibrin clot. Factors have been given standard Roman numerals matching their order of discovery and are listed in Box 116-2.[7]

A simplified version of the coagulation pathway is given in Figure 116-1. The clotting cascade is traditionally depicted as consisting of intrinsic and extrinsic pathways. The intrinsic pathway is initiated by the exposure of blood to a negatively charged surface (e.g., glass surface in the aPTT clotting time). The extrinsic pathway is activated by tissue factor exposed at the site of vessel injury or thromboplastin. Both pathways converge to activate factor X, which then activates prothrombin to thrombin. The primary physiologic event that initiates clotting is the exposure of tissue factor at the injured vessel site. Tissue factor is a critical cofactor that is required for activation of factor VII. The activated factor VII activates factor X directly, and indirectly by activating factor IX.

Because of limited amounts of tissue factor and the rapid inactivation by tissue factor pathway inhibitor, the extrinsic pathway initiates the clot process. Sustained generation of thrombin and clot formation depends on the intrinsic pathway by the activation of factor IX by activated factor VII. This helps explain the bleeding problems associated with hemophilia.[7,8] Intrinsic, extrinsic, and common pathways must function normally for hemostasis to occur, and each may be evaluated with laboratory tests.[1,7] The clinically important groups of coagulation factors are as follows:

1. Thrombin-sensitive factors contributing to the metabolic response and local vasoconstriction: I, V, VIII, XIII
2. Vitamin K–sensitive factors: II, VII, IX, X
3. Sites of heparin activity: IIa, IXa, Xa (major site), XIa, platelet factor 3

The thrombin-sensitive factors are activated by thrombin and may give rise to a bleeding disorder if defective synthesis occurs. The vitamin K–sensitive factors may also cause bleeding from defective synthesis, as occurs with liver disease and Coumadin anticoagulants. Heparin in combination with antithrombin III affects the coagulation pathway at multiple sites.[9-12]

Coagulation Control

All the components of the coagulation reaction are necessary to prevent excessive bleeding. Hemostasis is a balance between the excessive bleeding state and thrombosis. Once coagulation is initiated, controls are necessary to prevent local or generalized thrombosis. These controls include the following:[11,13-18]

1. Removal and dilution of activated clotting factors caused by blood flow, which also mechanically opposes growth of the hemostatic plug
2. Modulation of platelet activity by endothelial-generated nitric oxide and prostacyclin
3. Removal of activated coagulation components by the reticuloendothelial system

Box 116-1 Role of Platelets in Hemostasis

Adhesion to subendothelial connective tissue: collagen, basement membrane, and non-collagenous microfibrils, serum factor VIII (von Willebrand) permits this function, adhesion creates the initial bleeding arrest plug
Release of adenosine diphosphate, the primary mediator and amplifier of aggregation; release of thromboxane A, another aggregator and potent vasoconstrictor; release of calcium, serotonin, epinephrine, and trace thrombin
Platelet aggregation over the area of endothelial injury
Stabilization of the hemostatic plug by interaction with the coagulation system:
- Platelet factor 3, a phospholipid that helps accelerate certain coagulation system steps
- Platelet factor 4, a protein that neutralizes heparin
- Pathway initiation and acceleration by thrombin production
- Possible secretion of active forms of coagulation proteins

Stimulation of limiting reactions of platelet activity

Box 116-2 Coagulation Factors

I. Fibrinogens
II. Prothrombin
III. Tissue thromboplastin
IV. Calcium
V. Labile factor (proaccelerin)
VI. Not assigned
VII. Proconvertin
VIII. Antihemophilic A factor
IX. Antihemophilic B factor (plasma thromboplastin component, Christmas factor)
X. Stuart-Prower factor
XI. Plasma thromboplastin antecedent
XII. Hageman factor (contact factor)
XIII. Fibrin stabilizing factor

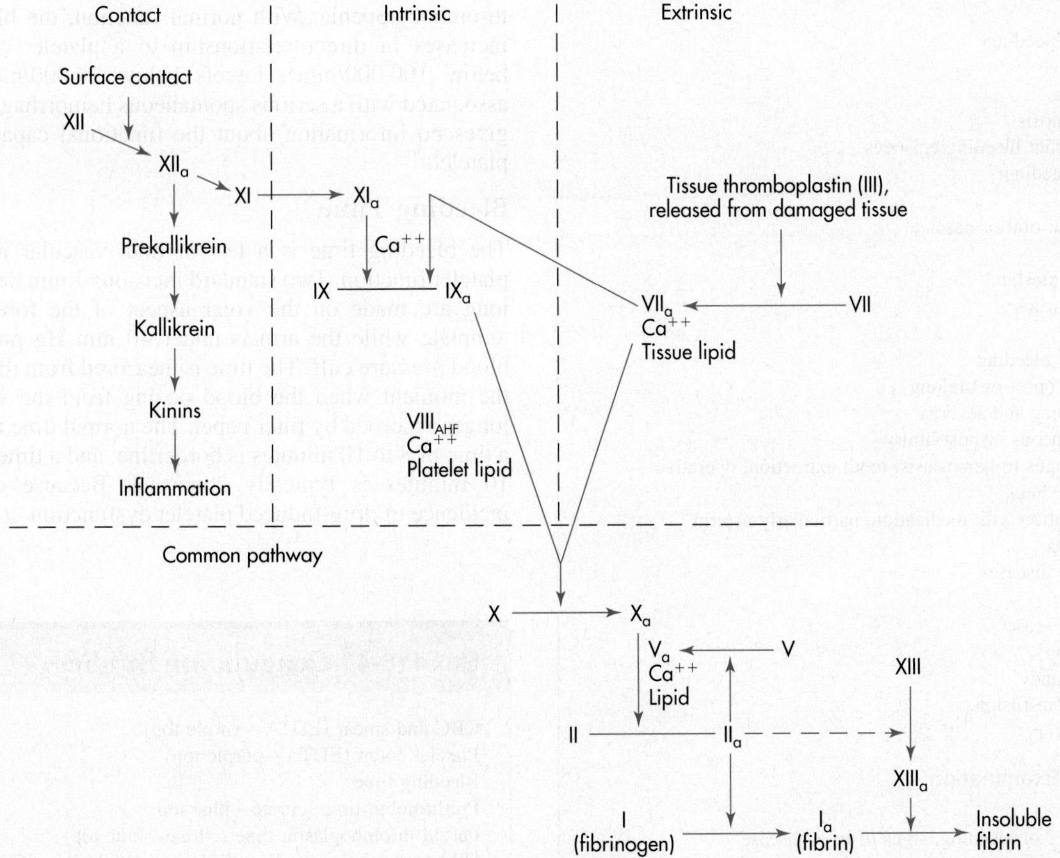

Figure 116-1. **Coagulation pathway.**

4. Regulation of clotting cascade by antithrombin III, protein C, protein S, and tissue factor pathway inhibitor
5. Activation of the fibrinolytic system

CLINICAL FEATURES

Prehospital

The prehospital treatment of bleeding problems has no special concerns. Local pressure and volume repletion are the mainstays of blood loss therapy. The prehospital team must be aware that inherited coagulopathies may complicate any medical or traumatic problems and that acquired forms can develop rapidly. Patients who do not respond rapidly to the usual measures of hemostasis either in the field or in the ED should be considered as having a potential bleeding disorder.

History and Physical Examination

An outline of the history and physical examination is given in Box 116-3. The history alone may be useful in differentiating between platelet and coagulation factor abnormalities. Platelet disorders usually occur as acquired petechiae, purpura, or mucosal bleeding and are more common in women. Coagulation problems are commonly congenital, present with delayed deep muscle or joint bleeding, and are seen more often in men.

Box 116-3 Clinical Evaluation of Bleeding Patient

History

- Nature of bleeding
  - Petechiae
  - Purpura
  - Ecchymosis
  - Significant bleeding episodes
- Sites of bleeding
  - Skin
  - Mucosa: oral or nasal
  - Muscle
  - Gastrointestinal
  - Genitourinary
  - Joints
- Patterns of bleeding
  - Recent onset or lifelong
  - Frequency and severity
  - Spontaneous or post-injury
  - Challenges to hemostasis: tooth extraction, operative procedures
  - Association with medication, particularly aspirin
- Medications
- Associated diseases
  - Uremia
  - Liver disease
  - Infection
  - Malignancy
- Previous transfusion
- Family history

Physical Examination

- Vital signs
- Skin: nature of bleeding, signs of liver disease
- Mucosa: oral or nasal
- Lymphadenopathy
- Abdomen: liver size and shape, splenomegaly
- Joints: signs of previous bleeding
- Other sites of blood loss: pelvic, rectal, urinary tract

DIAGNOSTIC STRATEGIES

The definitive diagnosis depends on the laboratory evaluation. Tests pertinent to the ED are discussed in the following sections and listed in Box 116-4.

Complete Blood Count and Blood Smear

The complete blood count (CBC) assesses the degree of anemia associated with the bleeding episode. Reductions in hemoglobin and hematocrit values often lag behind the actual loss of red blood cells (RBCs) in acute hemorrhage because of a slow equilibration time. The peripheral blood smear may demonstrate schistocytes or fragmented RBCs in disseminated intravascular coagulation (DIC). Teardrop-shaped or nucleated RBCs may reflect myelophthisic disease. A characteristic WBC morphologic condition is seen with thrombocytopenia associated with infectious mononucleosis, folate or B_{12} deficiency, or leukemia.[19]

Platelet Count

The platelet count may be estimated from the smear. Normally one platelet is present per 10 to 20 RBCs. Often the count is automated, the normal range being 150,000 to 400,000/mm^3. Platelet counts less than 100,000/mm^3 define thrombocytopenia. With normal function, the bleeding time increases in direct relationship to a platelet count falling below 100,000/mm^3. Levels below 20,000/mm^3 may be associated with a serious spontaneous hemorrhage. The count gives no information about the functional capability of the platelet.[20]

Bleeding Time

The bleeding time is a test of both vascular integrity and platelet function. Two standard incisions 1 mm deep and 1 cm long are made on the volar aspect of the forearm with a template while the arm is under 40 mm Hg pressure via a blood pressure cuff. The time is measured from the incision to the moment when the blood oozing from the wound is no longer absorbed by filter paper. The normal time is 8 minutes, a time of 8 to 10 minutes is borderline, and a time longer than 10 minutes is typically abnormal. Because of the high incidence of drug-induced platelet dysfunction, it is important

Box 116-4 Coagulation Studies

- CBC and smear (EDTA—purple top)
- Platelet count (EDTA—purple top)
- Bleeding time
- Prothrombin time (citrate—blue top)
- Partial thromboplastin time (citrate—blue top)
- Other coagulation studies: fibrinogen level, thrombin time, clot solubility, factor levels, inhibitor screens
- As necessary: electrolytes, glucose, BUN, creatinine, type and cross-match

BUN, Blood urea nitrogen; *CBC,* complete blood count.

to ask the patient about medications, particularly aspirin. The test is independent of the coagulation pathways.[20,21] As mentioned previously, the bleeding time is prolonged below platelet counts of 100,000/mm^3, but does not represent platelet dysfunction. However, prolonged bleeding times associated with platelet counts greater than 100,000/mm^3 suggest impaired function.

Prothrombin Time

The prothrombin time (PT) tests the factors of the extrinsic and common pathways. The patient's anticoagulated plasma is combined with calcium and tissue factor prepared from rabbit or human brain tissue. Sensitivity to factor deficiencies depends on the source of tissue factor. Prothrombin time detects deficiencies in fibrinogen, prothrombin, factor V, factor VII, and factor X. It is typically used to test the extrinsic pathway. A normal control sample is simultaneously run, and the clotting times of both are recorded. The time in seconds is usually given over the normal control time, for example, 12.5/11.5. A PT 2 seconds or more over the control time can be considered significant. Results are usually reported using the international normalized ratio (INR). The test is useful in monitoring the use of coumarin anticoagulants, and the time may be prolonged in liver disease and other abnormalities of vitamin K–sensitive factors.[22]

Partial Thromboplastin Time

The partial thromboplastin time (PTT) tests the components of the intrinsic and common pathways, that is, essentially all factors but VII and XIII in the entire clotting cascade. In this test a phospholipid source and a contact-activating agent (kaolin) are added to anticoagulated citrate plasma. After an incubation period allowing factor XII to become activated, calcium is added and the clotting time is recorded. A normal control sample is run simultaneously. Normal ranges may vary according to the hospital laboratory. The typical normal time is 25 to 29 seconds. Factor levels must usually be less than 40% before the PTT is prolonged. The test may be altered by clotting factor inhibitors of external origin (e.g., heparin) or internal origin (e.g., anti-VIII antibody). Inappropriately high values may occur if the plasma is too turbid or icteric. The aPTT is most sensitive to abnormalities in the sequence of the coagulation cascade that precedes the activation of factor X.[23-25]

Fibrinogen

Fibrinogen is present in sufficient concentration to be measured directly. Because it is the final coagulation substrate, its level reflects the balance between production and consumption. It may be decreased by hypoproduction, as in severe liver disease, or by overconsumption, as in cases of DIC. Low levels or altered functions increase the PT, PTT, and thrombin clotting time. Since fibrinogen is an acute phase reactant, certain conditions, including malignancy, sepsis, inflammation, and pregnancy, may alter the interpretation of the test result.

Thrombin Time

The measurement of thrombin clotting time bypasses the intrinsic and extrinsic pathways by directly converting fibrinogen to fibrin. It is a useful screening test of both qualitative and quantitative abnormalities of fibrinogen and inhibitors such as heparin or fibrin split products.[26]

Clot Solubility

The result of clot solubility testing may be the only abnormality in disorders involving factor XIII deficiencies and some abnormal fibrinogen. A washed clot is incubated in acetic acid or urea. If the clot is not properly cross-linked, it dissolves.[12]

Factor Level Assays

Factor levels are determined either by bioassays in which the ability of the sample of plasma to normalize controlled substrate-deficient plasma is evaluated or by an immunologic assay. Inhibitor screening tests reveal antibodies in plasma that prolong the normal plasma clotting when mixed.[9,18,24]

DIFFERENTIAL CONSIDERATIONS AND MANAGEMENT

When a bleeding disorder is diagnosed or suspected, the assessment initially includes stabilization and may necessitate volume, RBC, and coagulation factor replacement. If the disorder is known, clinical complications associated with its underlying pathophysiologic condition must be considered. If the disorder is unknown, a rapid differential diagnosis must be made. A clinically useful scheme approaches bleeding disorders in terms of three constituents: vascular integrity, platelets, and coagulation factors. This differential diagnostic approach can be further divided into inherited and acquired disorders.

Vascular Disorders

The vascular disorders are seen with signs and symptoms similar to those of thrombocytopenic states. The inherited forms are rare. The acquired forms are usually associated with connective tissue changes or endothelial damage. The differential diagnosis of vascular disorders is listed in Box 116-5.[27]

Platelet Disorders

General Approach Most platelet abnormalities occur in women and are acquired. The bleeding source is usually

Box 116-5 Differential Diagnosis of Vascular Disorders

Inherited

Disorders of connective tissue
- Pseudoxanthoma elasticum
- Ehlers-Danlos syndrome
- Osteogenesis imperfecta

Disorders of blood vessels
- Hemorrhagic telangiectasia

Acquired

Scurvy (vitamin C deficiency)
Simple or senile purpura
Purpura secondary to steroid use
Vascular damage
- Infection (meningococcemia)
- Azotemia (hemolytic-uremic syndrome)
- Hypoxemia
- Thrombotic thrombocytopenic purpura
- Snake bite
- Dysproteinemic purpura

capillary, with resultant cutaneous and mucosal petechiae or ecchymosis. Epistaxis, menorrhagia, and gastrointestinal (GI) bleeding are common presenting symptoms. The bleeding is usually mild and occurs immediately after surgery or dental extractions. Preceding trauma does not usually cause the bleeding incident. Petechiae and purpura may be noted on physical examination. Superficial ecchymoses may be found around a venipuncture site. Deep muscle hematomas and hemarthroses are not aspects of the clinical picture. The bleeding time is prolonged, and the platelet count may be low, normal, or high. The differential diagnosis of platelet disorders is listed in Box 116-6.

Thrombocytopenia

Decreased Production Thrombocytopenia from decreased bone marrow production is usually caused by the effects of chemotherapeutic drugs, myelophthisic disease, or direct bone marrow effects of alcohol or thiazides.

Splenic Sequestration Splenic sequestration is rare and is seen primarily with hypersplenism resulting from hematologic malignancy, portal hypertension, or disorders of increased splenic RBC destruction, such as hereditary spherocytosis or autoimmune hemolytic anemia.[28]

Increased Destruction

Immune thrombocytopenia Thrombocytopenia associated with an increased peripheral destruction of platelets and shortened platelet survival caused by an antiplatelet antibody is seen in a number of diseases. In most cases a cause is identifiable.

Collagen vascular diseases, particularly systemic lupus erythematosus (SLE), may cause an antiplatelet antibody-related platelet decrease. Similar associations have been noted with leukemia and lymphoma, particularly lymphocytic lymphoma. All evaluations of suspected immune thrombocytopenia should include a CBC, peripheral smear, antinuclear antibody test, and bone marrow examination.[29] A number of drugs have been associated with thrombocytopenia of immunologic origin. Quinine and quinidine are common offenders that affect platelets through an "innocent bystander" mechanism. The platelet is coated with a drug-antibody complex, complement is fixed, and intravascular platelet lysis occurs. Because of its relatively high frequency, heparin is an important cause of drug-induced thrombocytopenia in hospitalized patients. Platelets are activated by the formation of an IgG-heparin complex. Low-molecular-weight heparin may be associated with less thrombocytopenia than standard, unfractionated heparin; however, both forms of heparin have cross-reactivity.[30,31] Digitoxin, sulfonamides, phenytoin, heparin, and aspirin can also cause adverse platelet effects, usually within 24 hours of ingestion. An idiopathic thrombocytopenic purpura (ITP) type of syndrome has been reported in intravenous cocaine users.[32] Clinical trials with platelet GPIIb-IIIa (glycoprotein) antagonists suggest that intravenous GPIIb-IIIa inhibitors may have an increased risk of associated thrombocytopenia, independent of heparin therapy.[33] The platelet count may fall below 10,000/mm^3 and be complicated by serious bleeding. Laboratory testing may confirm the presence of antibody, especially in the cases of quinine and quinidine. After stopping the drug, the platelet count improves slowly over 3 to 7 days. A short course of corticosteroid therapy such as prednisone in a dose of 60 mg with rapid tapering may facilitate recovery.[34-36]

Postinfectious immune thrombocytopenia is usually associated with viral diseases such as rubella, rubeola, and varicella. Although many cases associated with sepsis are of a mechanical origin, some immune mechanisms have been reported.[34]

Posttransfusion thrombocytopenia is a rare disorder that causes a precipitous fall in platelets approximately 1 week after the transfusion. In 90% of cases, it is linked to a PLAI antigen on the platelet. The platelet count often precipitously falls below 10,000/mm^3, with a significant risk for major bleeding. Intracranial hemorrhage occurs in approximately 10% of cases. Patients are usually middle-aged women with a history of pregnancy, who may have been previously sensitized to the PLAI antigen during pregnancy. About 98% of the population carry this antigen. Despite the fact that 2% of blood recipients are mismatched in respect to this antigen, it is a fortunately rare occurrence. Plasma exchange therapy is a potential antidote.[34,37]

Idiopathic thrombocytopenic purpura ITP should be considered after other causes have been excluded. It is associated with an immunoglobulin (Ig)G antiplatelet anti-

Box 116-6 Differential Diagnosis of Platelet Disorders

Thrombocytopenia

- Decreased production
  - Decreased megakaryocytes secondary to drugs, toxins, or infection
  - Normal megakaryocytes with megaloblastic hematopoiesis or hereditary origin
- Platelet pooling and splenic sequestration
- Increased destruction
  - Immunologic
    - Related to collagen vascular disease, lymphoma, leukemia
    - Drug related
    - Infection
    - Posttransfusion
    - Idiopathic (autoimmune) thrombocytopenic purpura
  - Mechanical
    - Disseminated intravascular coagulation
    - Thrombotic thrombocytopenic purpura
    - Hemolytic-uremic syndrome
  - Vasculitis
- Dilutional secondary to massive blood transfusion

Thrombocytopathy

- Adhesion defects such as von Willebrand's disease
- Release defects: acquired and drug-related
- Aggregation defects such as in thrombasthenia

Thrombocytosis

- Autonomous (primary thrombocythemia)
- Reactive (secondary thrombocythemia)
  - Iron deficiency
  - Infection/inflammatory
  - Trauma
  - Nonhematologic malignancy
  - Postsplenectomy
  - Rebound from alcohol, cytotoxic drug therapy, folate/vitamin B_{12} deficiency

body that has proved difficult to detect. The two clinically important forms are acute and chronic.[29,34,38]

The acute form is seen most often in children 2 to 6 years old. A viral prodrome is common, usually within 3 weeks of the onset. The platelet count falls, usually to less than 20,000/mm^3. The course is self-limited, with a greater than 90% rate of spontaneous remission. Morbidity and mortality are low, although full recovery may take several weeks. Treatment is supportive, and steroid therapy does not alter the disease course.[34,38]

The more chronic form of ITP is primarily an adult disease found three times more often in women than men. Its onset is insidious, without prodrome, and presents as easy bruising, prolonged menses, and mucosal bleeding. The patient may have petechiae or purpura, and platelet counts between 30,000/mm^3 and 100,000/mm^3 are common. Splenomegaly is unusual. Bleeding complications are of unpredictable frequency and severity, although the long-term mortality rate is approximately 1%.[38,39] The course is one of waxing and waning severity, and spontaneous remission is rare.

Associated diseases, such as lymphoma and SLE, must be ruled out before the diagnosis can be made. Quantitative laboratory tests of antiplatelet antibody may differentiate between patients who will favorably respond to therapy and those who will not. Hospitalization is recommended during the initial evaluation because the differential diagnosis is complex and the bleeding risk is significant. Treatment usually includes corticosteroids, splenectomy, and in refractory cases, immunosuppressive therapy such as with cyclophosphamide, azathioprine, or vincristine. Plasmapheresis, androgens, gammaglobulin, anti-Rh(D), danazol, and colchicine have all met with varied success. Platelet transfusions are used only to control life-threatening bleeding because of increased antiplatelet antibody titers and short-lived hemostatic effect. The care otherwise is supportive. The use of all nonessential drugs should be stopped, particularly those that might inhibit platelet function, such as aspirin.[34,38-41]

A similar pattern of thrombocytopenic purpura has been reported in sexually active homosexual men. Although the clinical presentation and response to therapy mimic ITP, the mechanism is believed to be nonspecific deposition of immune complexes and complement, rather than antiplatelet IgG.[42]

Nonimmune thrombocytopenia Nonimmune platelet destruction is usually consumptive or mechanical. Consumption occurs as part of the process of intravascular coagulation, although it may be seen at sites of significant endothelial loss. Thrombotic thrombocytopenic purpura, hemolytic-uremic syndrome, and vasculitis all initiate platelet destruction through endothelial damage.[43,44] The most striking differences between the first two are the age of onset and the prognosis.

Thrombotic thrombocytopenic purpura The pathologic state of thrombotic thrombocytopenic purpura (TTP) is the result of subendothelial and intraluminal deposits of fibrin and platelet aggregates in capillaries and arterioles. Hemolytic uremic syndrome (HUS) is similar to TTP; however, HUS is associated with less central nervous system (CNS) and more renal involvement than TTP. Although the initiating event is unclear, prostacyclin and abnormal platelet aggregation are believed to play a central role in the pathogenesis of the disease. The disease may affect patients of any age or sex, but the majority are 10 to 40 years old, and 60% of cases occur in women. It is classically seen as the constellation of thrombocytopenic purpura, microangiopathic hemolytic anemia, fluctuating neurologic symptoms, renal disease, and fever. However, only 40% of cases present with the classic pentad.

The platelet count ranges from 10,000/mm^3 to 50,000/mm^3, and generalized purpura and bleeding complaints are common. Anemia is universal, with hematocrit levels commonly less than 20%. The hemolysis may cause jaundice or pallor, and the blood smear characteristically contains numerous schistocytes and fragmented red blood cells. The neurologic symptoms include stroke, seizures, paresthesias, altered levels of consciousness, and coma, all of which characteristically fluctuate in severity. The renal component varies from hematuria and proteinuria to acute renal failure. Fever is present in 90% of patients.

Untreated, the disease follows a progressive and fatal course, with 80% mortality 1 to 3 months after diagnosis. Therapy has included corticosteroids, splenectomy, anticoagulation, exchange transfusion, and dextran. However, plasma exchange with fresh frozen plasma (plasmapheresis) is the current treatment of choice. Over the last several years, the aggressive use of plasma exchange has reduced the mortality rate from 90% to 17%. In addition to plasma exchange, initial therapy may also include steroids such as prednisone and antiplatelet agents such as aspirin and dipyridamole (Persantine). Splenectomy, gammaglobulin, vincristine, and other therapies may have a role in resistant cases. With the exception of life-threatening bleeding, platelet transfusion should be avoided because platelets may cause additional thrombi in the microcirculation.[43-47]

Situations Dilutional thrombocytopenia occurs in cases of massive transfusion, exchange transfusion, or extracorporeal circulation. Volume replacement with stored bank blood is platelet poor because platelets have a life span of only 9 days. The number of transfusions directly correlates with the degree of thrombocytopenia. The current transfusion practice is to monitor platelet counts for every 10 units of red blood cells and transfuse once the platelet count approaches 50,000/mm^3.[48]

Thrombocytopathy Knowledge of abnormal platelet function as a clinical disorder has grown rapidly in recent years. The drug-induced form may be one of the most commonly seen causes of abnormal bleeding.[49] Defects may occur at any level of platelet function, including adhesion, release, and aggregation.

Adhesion Defects The representative adhesion disorder is von Willebrand's disease, which is more a factor VIII problem than platelet deficiency. The platelets are normal in terms of their morphologic condition, number, release, and aggregation. The abnormal adhesion results not from the platelet but from endothelium-based plasma deficiency of a factor VIII component (von Willebrand's factor) that permits platelet adhesion.[50,51]

Release Defects The release defects include "storage pool" syndromes in which the release is normal, but the amounts of adenosine diphosphate, calcium, and serotonin are decreased. Release defects may be congenital or acquired, as in SLE, alcoholism, or lymphoma. Drugs induce the most common release problem. Aspirin and related drugs block the enzyme cyclooxygenase, which participates in thromboxane A_2 formation. The decreased release of thromboxane A_2 results in decreased aggregation and less local vasoconstriction. Both may contribute to an increased bleeding risk. Testing for this risk has been suggested by the development of the postaspirin bleeding time as a screening test for hemostatic disorders. Aspirin is unique in that it permanently poisons this reaction for the life of the platelet in dosages of only 300 to 600 mg. Phenylbutazone and indomethacin affect function only while measurably circulating. A similar problem may occur in uremia or dysproteinemia and as a rare inherited form.[5,6,52]

Aggregation Defects Primary aggregation defects are associated with the rare recessive trait thrombasthenia. This is a platelet membrane abnormality that may be discovered by the lack of clot retraction during a 2-hour clot retraction test.[21]

Platelet Transfusions Most platelet function disorders are not treated with platelet transfusion because efficacy is questionable and alloimmunization may occur. Platelet transfusions are commonly indicated for primary bone marrow disorders (e.g., aplastic anemia or acute leukemia). Assessing the risk of spontaneous bleeding using platelet counts is an imprecise science. Less mature platelets associated with peripheral consumption or sequestration are less likely to allow spontaneous hemorrhage than those associated with primary bone marrow involvement. An estimate of functionality is combined with the platelet count for a better predictor of primary hemostasis potential. At counts below 50,000/mm^3 a variable degree of risk exists, especially associated with trauma, ulcers, or invasive procedure. At over 50,000/mm^3, hemorrhage caused by platelet deficiency is unlikely. Spontaneous bleeding in the absence of surgery, trauma, or other risk factors may develop in platelet counts less than 10,000/mm^3.[53]

Thrombocytosis Thrombocytosis may be discovered in the ED. The reactive form is considered benign. The differential diagnosis (see Box 116-6) should be considered when confronted by a platelet count over 600,000 to 1,000,000/mm^3. The primary or autonomous state may be associated with bleeding or thrombosis. It is often an associated finding in cases of polycythemia vera, myelofibrosis, or chronic myelogenous leukemia. Suspected autonomous thrombocytosis requires a full hematologic evaluation.[1,54]

Disorders of the Coagulation Pathway

The coagulation system accomplishes secondary hemostasis through a complex enzymatic cascade. The clinically significant disorders have a number of characteristic features that help differentiate them from the platelet disorders. They include the following[18]:

1. The bleeding source is often an intramuscular or deep soft tissue hematoma from small arterioles.
2. The congenital form of the disease occurs predominantly in men, often as a sex-linked inheritance.
3. Bleeding may occur after surgery or trauma but is delayed in onset up to 72 hours.
4. Epistaxis, menorrhagia, and GI sources of bleeding are rare, whereas hematuria and hemarthrosis are common in severe cases.
5. The bleeding time is normal except in cases of von Willebrand's disease.

The PT and PTT are the basic laboratory diagnostic tools used in the evaluation of coagulation disorders and can be used to organize the approach to their diagnosis.[18]

Abnormal Prothrombin Time and Other Tests Normal An elevated PT reflects an extrinsic pathway abnormality via factor VII deficiency. The hereditary form is a rare autosomal recessive gene. The acquired form is commonly seen as a manifestation of vitamin K deficiency, coumarin use, or liver disease. Because factor VII has the shortest half-life (3 to 5 hours) of the coagulation factors, it is the first to manifest a deficiency when its active form is under-produced. The PT is a sensitive gauge of hepatic function and the efficacy of coumarin administration. INRs calculate the prothrombin ratio raised to the power of a sensitivity index (151) for specific thromboplastin reagents. Most warfarin therapy is recommended to maintain the INR between 2.0 and 3.0.[55-57]

Abnormal Partial Thromboplastin Time and Other Tests Normal Two groups of inherited disorders manifest an isolated elevation in the PTT. The first group is the contact factors (e.g., XII [Hageman factor]), prekallikrein (Fletcher factor), and high-molecular-weight kininogen. They cause a benign disorder in which the PTT is elevated but the patient has no bleeding diathesis. These deficiencies exist as isolated laboratory abnormalities, and thus they should not be invoked as a cause of the patient's bleeding problem. They may be specifically assayed when precise diagnosis is necessary.[11,17]

The second group causes significant bleeding problems resulting from deficiencies of factors within the intrinsic coagulation system. They are the most common inherited abnormalities of the entire clotting system. Factor VIII, IX, and XI deficiencies account for 99% of inherited bleeding disorders. Patients with active life-threatening bleeding who are suspected of having a congenital bleeding disorder can be supported with fresh frozen plasma, 15 ml/kg, while diagnostic studies are being done. The risk of viral transmission of hepatitis B or C or the human immunodeficiency virus must be considered.

In the patient with a prolonged PTT and a lifelong history of bleeding, the most important test in initiating the differential diagnosis is a factor VIII assay. This test measures the ability of the patient's plasma to correct the prolonged PTT of plasma deficient in factor VIII. This ability is compared with that of normal plasma and is given as a percentage of normal. The test measures the procoagulant activity of factor VIII but does not discriminate between abnormal activity resulting from an abnormal factor VIII or low levels of normal factor VIII. The two forms of this deficiency are hemophilia A and von Willebrand's disease.[9,58]

Hemophilia A Hemophilia A is caused by a variant form of factor VIII that is present at normal levels but lacks a clot-promoting property. The incidence is 60 to 80 persons per million population. Of cases, 70% have been found to be of a sex-linked recessive nature; that is, the disease is carried on the X chromosome at location Xq28. Factor VIII circulates in the plasma in very low concentrations and is normally bound to von Willebrand factor. The source of factor VIII production is uncertain, but the liver is considered to be a significant source since hemophilia A can be corrected by liver transplantation. A female carrier mating with a normal man would be predicted to pass the disease on to half her sons. Likewise, a male hemophiliac would have all normal sons and all carrier daughters. The remaining 25% to 30% of cases of the disease are believed to result from a spontaneous genetic abnormality. The familial form has a remarkable consistency of severity from generation to generation, although the degree of severity has considerable variation. This severity may be directly related to the level of factor VIII coagulant (factor VIII:C) activity. Cases with less than 1% activity are severe, with a tendency toward spontaneous bleeding. Cases with 1% to 5% activity are moderate, with rare spontaneous bleeding but increased problems with surgery or trauma. Cases with 5% to 10% activity and above are considered mild, with little risk of spontaneous bleeding but still with hazards after trauma and surgery. A number of hemophiliacs may have activity above 10% but have few problems unless stressed. The PTT may lack sensitivity for this group because it is significantly prolonged only at factor VIII:C levels less than 35% to 40%.[9,59-62]

The disease is seen as a disorder of secondary hemostasis with a characteristic pattern of bleeding. Bleeding can occur anywhere, but deep muscles, joints, the urinary tract, and intracranial sites are the most common. Recurrent hemarthrosis and progressive joint destruction are major causes of morbidity in hemophilia. Intracranial bleeding is the major cause of death for all age groups of hemophiliacs. Mucosal bleeding such as epistaxis and oral bleeding or menorrhagia is rare unless the disease is associated with von Willebrand's disease or platelet inhibition, such as with aspirin use. GI bleeding is rare unless peptic ulcer disease is also present. Trauma is a common initiator of bleeding in all stages of severity. This potential hazard must be viewed expectantly with all hemophiliacs because late bleeding, usually by 8 hours but up to 1 to 3 days after trauma, may occur.[60-62]

Management of hemophilia A The total therapy of hemophilia involves a team effort of physicians, specialized nurses, physical therapists, social workers, the patient, and the patient's family. The therapeutic responsibility of the emergency physician consists of three areas: preparation for and identification of the problem, initial evaluation, and admission of new bleeders; replacement therapy for bleeding episodes; and the anticipation of potential life threats and the admission of known bleeders for observation in selected circumstances. At one time the treatment of hemophilia-associated bleeding was a relatively common emergency medicine activity, but since 1975, hemophilia home therapy has increasingly been instituted. Therefore many hemophiliacs now come to the ED only with complicated problems or trauma-related difficulties, and most are knowledgeable about their disease.[60-63]

Preparation In preparing for the problem, the emergency physician should have updated information covering disease processes and current therapy. A cooperative effort should be made between the ED and the hematology service to generate a file of known hemophiliacs in the area who are followed at the hospital. The file should include the primary physician, diagnosis, factor VIII activity level, blood type, presence of antihemophilia factor antibodies, and time of last hospitalization. A protocol should be developed for ordering and administering factor VIII.

Replacement therapy The accepted therapy for hemophilia A is factor VIII replacement using cryoprecipitate or factor VIII:C concentrates. These concentrates are exposed to heat treatment or solvent-detergent mixtures to decrease transmission of hepatitis B, hepatitis C, and human immunodeficiency virus. In the past the concentrate was made from fractionated freeze-dried antihemophilic factor and contained 250 to 1,500 IU of factor VIII:C in a reconstituted volume. Factor VIII is also produced by recombinant DNA techniques and is considered by some to be the replacement product of choice. Recombinant-derived factor VIII is comparable to plasma-derived factor VIII in terms of characteristics and control of bleeding, but with no discernible side effects. Factor VIII:C concentrates are commonly used in severe hemophilia and for home use. Cryoprecipitate is the cold precipitable protein fraction derived from fresh frozen plasma thawed at 1° to 6° C. It was once the mainstay of hemophilia A therapy. It may be used when noninfectious factor VIII concentrates are not available.[63-67]

Replacement therapies have some hepatitis C and hepatitis B risk. Persistent hepatitis B surface antigen occurs in the blood of 5% of hemophiliacs, whereas the anti-B surface antigen is found in 80%. This problem has been overshadowed by the association of acquired immunodeficiency syndrome with hemophilia. The association is related to blood product use, and although the total number is low, the incidence is high—3.6/1,000 hemophilia A patients.[64,65]

The therapy for a bleeding episode includes a number of considerations: the circumstances in which factor VIII is given, the dosage, the timing of maintenance, the duration of dosage, the presence of antibodies, and the means of gauging effectiveness. Tables 116-1 and 116-2 include guidelines for the recommended treatment in a variety of circumstances. Most important, the emergency physician should believe patients who say they are bleeding and institute early therapy.[61,63]

The response to therapy can be monitored by clinical improvement, a decreasing PTT, and optimally, serial factor VIII: C activity levels. The infusion of one unit of factor VIII per kilogram increases factor VIII levels by 2%. The lack of a response to factor VIII administration should raise the question of circulating antibodies. All hemophiliacs should be screened for the development of these antihemophilic factor antibodies when they are given in-hospital therapy or if they become refractory to home therapy. The 7% to 20% of patients who develop these IgG immunoglobulins usually have a severe deficiency, necessitating multiple factor VIII transfusions. The treatment may be complex, and hospitalization is necessary. A variety of therapies have been considered, including "overwhelming" factor VIII doses, exchange plasmapheresis, immunosuppressive therapy, and the infusion of prothrombin complexes containing activated clotting factors. Other recommended therapies include porcine factor VIII, which has less cross-reactivity with the human product, and in the likely future, recombinant activated factor VII.[63,68-70] Acquired IgG antihemophilic factor antibodies may exist in nonhemophiliac patients. They can occur in the postpartum period, as immunologic reactions to penicillin or phenytoin, and in association with SLE, rheumatoid arthritis, or inflammatory bowel disease. The diagnosis is made by the occurrence of an acquired hemophilia-like syndrome with positive-antibody titers in the appropriate setting.

The "lupus anticoagulant" is unique in that it may be associated with an increased risk of thrombosis, as well as a hemorrhagic diathesis.[61,71]

Desmopressin acetate (DDAVP) has been shown to increase levels of factors VIII:C and VIII:Ag in patients with hemophilia A and in some with von Willebrand's disease. It is given IV in a 0.3 μg/kg/dose. Benefits are primarily noted in patients with mild to moderate disease and last for 4 to 6 hours.[72]

Table 116-1. Recommended Factor VIII Therapy for Specific Problems in Hemophilia

Type of bleeding	Initial dosage	Duration	Comment
Skin			
Abrasion	None	None	Treat with local pressure and topical thrombin
Laceration Superficial	Usually none; if necessary treat as minor	None	Local pressure and anesthetic with epinephrine may benefit; watch 4 hours after suturing, reexamine in 24 hours
Deep	Minor bleed (12.5 mg/kg)	Single-dose coverage	May need hospitalization for observation; repeat may be necessary for suture removal
Nasal epistaxis			
Spontaneous	Usually none; may need to be treated as mild bleed	None	Uncommon; consider platelet inhibition; treat in usual manner
Traumatic	Moderate bleed (25 mg/kg)	Up to 5-7 days	Trauma-related bleed can be significant
Oral			
Mucosa or tongue bites	Usually none; treat as minor if persists	Single dose	Commonly seen
Traumatic (laceration) or dental extraction	Moderate (25 U/kg) to severe (50 U/kg)	Single dose; may need more	Saliva rich in fibrin lytic activity; oral ε-aminocaproic acid (Amicar) may be given 100 mg every 6 hours for 7 days to block fibrinolysis; check contraindications; hospitalize patients with severe bleeds
Soft tissue/muscle hematomas	Moderate (25 U/kg) to severe (50 U/kg)	2-5 days	May be complicated by local pressure on nerves or vessels (e.g., iliopsoas, forearm, calf)
Hemarthrosis			
Early	Mild (12.5 U/kg)	Single dose	Treat as earliest symptom (pain); knee, elbow, ankle more common
Late or unresponsive cases of early	Mild to moderate (25 U/kg)	3-4 days	Arthrocentesis rarely necessary and only with 50% level coverage; immobilization is critical point of therapy
Hematuria	Mild (12.5 U/kg)	2-3 days	Urokinase, the fibrinolytic enzyme, is in urine; with persistent hematuria an organic cause should be ruled out
Major bleeding GI severe bleeding Neck/sublingual Retroperitoneal Intraabdominal Major trauma Head injury (see text) Central nervous system bleed (see text) Surgical procedure	Major bleed (50 U/kg)	7-10 days or 3-5 days after bleeding ceases	In head trauma, therapy should be given prophylactically; early CT scan of head recommended for all

Table 116-2. Dosage of Factor VIII_{AHF}

Bleeding risk	Desired factor VIII level (%)	Initial dose (U/kg)
Mild	5-10	12.5
Moderate	20-30	25
Severe	50 or greater	50

Standard calculation

1. Patient's plasma volume (50 ml/kg × weight in kg) × (Desired level of factor VIII in percent) – (Present level of factor VIII in percent) = Number of units for initial dose
2. In emergency therapy, the present level of factor VIII is assumed to be zero.
3. One unit is the activity of the coagulation factor present in 1 ml of normal human plasma.
4. Because the half-life of factor VIII is 8 to 12 hours, the desired level is maintained by giving half the initial dose every 8 to 12 hours.
5. Cryoprecipitate is assumed to have 80 to 100 units of factor VIII:C per bag; factor VIII:C concentrates list the units per bottle on the label.

Anticipation of life threats The anticipation of delayed bleeding in patients with hemophilia may necessitate admission and observation for a variety of trauma-related injuries. Patients with deep lacerations; patients with soft tissue injuries in areas where the pressure from a developing hematoma could be destructive such as in the eye, mouth, neck, back, and spinal column; and patients with a history of major trauma forces without injury are all candidates for prophylactic admission. Head trauma is potentially life-threatening to hemophiliacs, and CNS bleeding is the major cause of death for patients in all age groups. Studies found a 3% to 13% risk of intracranial hemorrhage, yet no patient given replacement therapy within 6 hours had an intracranial bleed. It is recommended that head trauma patients have factor VIII therapy initiated to a 50% activity level and be admitted for 24 hours of observation. All patients with anything but the most trivial head trauma should have a head computed tomography (CT) scan. Any patient with an altered level of consciousness or focal neurologic signs should be started immediately on factor VIII therapy and have a CT scan obtained. Obviously all of these patients are treated in joint consultation with their primary physician and hematologist.[73,74]

Gene therapy represents potential development in the treatment of hemophilia. With cloning of the genes encoding factor VIII, the possibility exists for either a partial or complete cure of hemophilia. Although genetic testing and counseling are currently available, no genetic therapies for hemophilia A currently exist.[59,62,63]

von Willebrand's Disease To understand von Willebrand's disease, it is helpful to review the nomenclature used to refer to factor VIII in some centers. Factor VIII has at least three activities. First is the antihemophilic, or coagulant, activity, VIII:C. All references to factor VIII in this chapter thus far have been to this activity. A second activity supports platelet adhesion and in vitro aggregation with the antibiotic ristocetin; it is called *von Willebrand factor activity,* or VIII/vWF. A third component reacts with rabbit antibodies to factor VIII. It is termed the factor VIII antigen, or VIII:Ag, and relates to the measured plasma level rather than the activity of factor VIII. The antigen and cofactor activity for platelet function are structurally related.[51,75] Von Willebrand's disease has both a decreased factor VIII:Ag level and a decreased VIII:C activity secondary to underproduction. The patient's platelets are normal in number, morphologic condition, and other functions, but in the absence of circulating factor VIII/vWF, their adhering properties are diminished. Von Willebrand's disease is the most common hereditary bleeding disorder, with an estimated prevalence of 1%. The disease occurs in 5 to 10 persons per million population as an autosomal dominant trait with a variable penetrance pattern. A rare X-linked inheritance has been described.[51,75-77]

The disease presentation is usually milder and less crippling than that of hemophilia. The factor VIII:C level is in the 6% to 50% range. Bleeding sites are predominantly mucosal (e.g., epistaxis) and cutaneous. Hemarthroses are rare, but menorrhagia and GI bleeding are common. The laboratory differentiation from hemophilia A includes an abnormal bleeding time, a decreased level of factor VIII:Ag, and abnormal platelet aggregation with ristocetin.[78] In patients with severe disease, replacement therapy with factor VIII in the form of cryoprecipitate is the method of choice. Because the VIII/vWF content of each bag is unavailable, the standard dose is 1 bag of cryoprecipitate per 10 kg of body weight. It has large amounts of VIII:C and a factor influencing VIII/vWF. A unique response to the transfusion of plasma components in patients with von Willebrand's disease is the stimulation of a progressive increase in VIII:C activity lasting 12 to 40 hours. After the initial dose, fewer units are necessary, and longer dosage schedules may be followed by a clinical response and a combination of factor VIII:C activity and serial bleeding times.

In extreme circumstances, without alternatives, fresh frozen plasma may be used. A factor VIII concentrate (Humate-P, Armour, Kankakee, Ill) has also demonstrated sufficient VIII/vWF to treat the disease.[53,79] Drug therapy with desmopressin has benefit in patients with mild to moderately severe von Willebrand's disease. It is most useful in a specific type of the disease and should not be given without prior consultation with a hematologist.[72]

Hemophilia B (Christmas Disease) Hemophilia B is a deficiency of factor IX activity. Its genetic pattern and clinical presentation are indistinguishable from those of hemophilia A, but its incidence is only one fifth that of hemophilia A. Factor IX is a vitamin K–dependent glycoprotein. Its deficiency is diagnosed by a factor IX assay, usually after the factor VIII:C assay is found to be normal. Its replacement schedule is similar to that of hemophilia A, but a purified factor IX concentrate or recombinant factor IX preparation is used. The plasma prothrombin complex (factors II, VII, IX, and X) and fresh frozen plasma are also useful, but they have higher risks of viral transmission and venous or arterial thrombosis. The maintenance dosage schedule is increased to every 24 hours because of the longer half-life of factor IX.[63,80]

Similar to hemophilia A, gene testing and counseling are available. Gene therapy in animals has shown promising results, and preliminary results from a human study suggest that the severity of hemophilia B can be altered and improved by gene manipulation.[59,81,82]

Miscellaneous Coagulation Disorders These laboratory and other findings may be caused by any deficiency of the common coagulation pathway. An altered fibrinogen level or abnormal function is a relatively common cause. In cases of this deficiency the thrombin time is also abnormal. The inherited forms are rare. The acquired forms have been related to fibrin-blocking substances and hypofibrinogenemia, which are found most often in cases of DIC and dysfibrinogenemia associated with macroglobulinemia, multiple myeloma, and hepatomas. In the context of emergency medicine, fibrinogen's most important role relates to its activity in DIC.

The other components of the common pathway (factors II, V, and X) have rare inherited deficiencies. The acquired forms are far more common and relate to vitamin K deficiency (decreased factor II, VII, IX, and X activity), Coumadin use (same factors as with vitamin K deficiency), hepatic insufficiency (potentially all factors except VIII), and massive transfusion of stored blood (low in factors V, VIII, and platelets).

Disseminated Intravascular Coagulation DIC is a relatively common acquired coagulopathy. Its ubiquitous nature, multiple origins, and potentially devastating sequelae, balanced by an effective mode of therapy, make the early diagnosis of this hematologic process critical. It is most often encountered in the critical care setting. Hemostasis is a fine

Table 116-3. Laboratory Diagnosis of Disseminated Intravascular Coagulation

Test	Finding	Pathophysiology
Peripheral smear	Low platelets, schistocytes, RBC fragments	RBC fragmentation on fibrin strands; schistocytes not always seen
Platelet count	Low (usually <100,000/mm^3)	Consumed in clotting; lower numbers are reflected in bleeding time
PT	Prolonged	Factors II and IV consumed
PTT	Prolonged	Factors II, V, and VIII consumed
Thrombin time	Prolonged	Decrease in factor II and fibrin degradation products
Fibrinogen level	Low	Factor II consumed; may be difficult to interpret because this is an acute-phase reactant
Fibrin degradation products	Zero to large	Dependent on amount of secondary fibrinolysis
Serum creatinine or urinalysis	May be abnormal	Functional assessment of organ most commonly injured by fibrin deposition

RBC, Red blood cell; *PT,* prothrombin time; *PTT,* partial thromboplastin time

balance between procoagulants and inhibitors, thrombus formation, and lysis. The balance may be disturbed by pathologic processes that result in an out-of-control coagulation and fibrinolytic cascade within the systemic circulation. The following occurs in this abnormal clotting sequence:

1. Platelets and coagulation factors are consumed, especially fibrinogen, V, VIII, and XIII.
2. Thrombin is formed, overwhelming its inhibitor system and acting to accelerate the coagulation process and directly activate fibrinogen.
3. Fibrin is deposited in small vessels in multiple organs.
4. The fibrinolytic system by means of plasmin may lyse fibrin and impair thrombin formation.
5. Fibrin degradation products are released and affect platelet function and inhibit fibrin polymerization.
6. Coagulation inhibition levels (e.g., antithrombin III, protein C, and tissue factor pathway inhibitor) are decreased.

The clinical consequence of these processes is the life-threatening combination of a bleeding diathesis from loss of platelets and clotting factors, fibrinolysis, and fibrin degradation product interference; small vessel obstruction and tissue ischemia from fibrin deposition; and RBC injury and anemia from fibrin deposition. The condition must be suspected in any patient who in the appropriate clinical setting develops purpura, a bleeding tendency, and signs of organ injury, particularly the CNS or kidney. This broad description is further confused clinically by the variable acuteness and intensity of intravascular clotting, the effectiveness of fibrinolysis, and other systemic manifestations of the initiating disease.[83-86]

The clinical diagnosis is necessarily supported by laboratory tests. The tests recommended in Table 116-3 usually confirm the presence of DIC. Other tests (e.g., specific degradation products of fibrin and fibrinogen) can confirm the diagnosis. These are rarely available in the ED.

Two conditions that may simulate DIC are severe liver disease and primary fibrinolysis. Liver disease of this severity usually is manifested with clinical jaundice and splenomegaly. Primary fibrinolysis is a rare disorder that affects fibrinogen and fibrin but usually leaves the coagulation components (platelet, factor V, and factor VIII) in the low normal range. The paracoagulation test is negative, and the euglobulin lysis time is rapid.[83,84]

When planning therapy, the emergency physician must remember that defibrination is always secondary to serious underlying pathologic process. Once the diagnosis is confirmed, the initial treatment is toward reversing the triggering mechanism. Many episodes of DIC are self-limited, such as in a transfusion reaction, or compensated, such as associated with a tumor mass, and do not require intervention other than support.[83-86]

Replacement therapy is usually instituted simultaneously with attempts to control the primary process. The goal is to avoid depletion of clotting factors. The therapy is partially based on which of the two major pathologic components of DIC dominates the clinical picture. If active bleeding is present, replacement therapy with platelets, coagulation factors found in fresh frozen plasma or cryoprecipitate (I, V, VIII), and blood is recommended. Selective replacement therapy can be based on the laboratory and clinical response. The retardation of bleeding, decrease in fibrin degradation products, and rise in platelet counts and fibrinogen level are useful monitors. Normalization of clotting times is too late to be of value in monitoring.[84-86]

Heparin has selective use in the treatment of DIC when fibrin deposition and thrombosis dominate the pathologic picture. Certain disease states are more associated with fibrin deposition, in which case heparin therapy should be considered. Examples include purpura fulminans, retained dead fetus before delivery, giant hemangioma, and acute promyelocytic leukemia. Heparin therapy is of little benefit in cases of meningococcemia, abruptio placentae, severe liver disease, and trauma. Low doses of heparin (300 to 500 U/hour) as a continuous infusion are currently recommended. Low-molecular-weight heparin may also be used instead of unfractionated heparin. Continuous monitoring of the clinical response, heparin levels, and bleeding status is necessary. Other therapeutic agents (e.g., antithrombin III, protein C, and tissue factor inhibitors) remain under investigation.[87-90]

The goals of emergency care in cases of DIC include initial suspicion, aggressive diagnostic pursuit, understanding of potential life-threatening complications, and only rarely, initiation of therapy.

DISPOSITION

All patients with bleeding disorders of unknown cause or of a significant degree should be admitted for further evaluation.

The circumstances in which a patient with a known bleeding disorder may be discharged for home care are discussed in earlier sections on individual disease states. Transferring these patients may be necessary, particularly if hematologic consultation is not readily available. The standard criteria of hemodynamic stability, appropriate monitoring, and full knowledge and understanding on the part of the family and accepting physician should be met before transfer. Because of the delayed bleeding pattern in hemophiliacs, it may be especially hazardous to transfer them over long distances. Therefore the importance of advance knowledge and preparation is reemphasized. Outpatients are usually managed under the auspices of the hematologic consultant. Early notification and appropriate follow-up arrangements should be made with these specialists.

KEY CONCEPTS

- Although hemostatic disorders are confirmed by specific patterns of laboratory tests, a careful history and focused physical examination are often the keys to the diagnosis of hematologic diseases.
- The PT is a sensitive gauge of hepatic function (i.e., synthesis of factor VII) and the efficacy of coumarin administration.
- Persons with hemophilia often understand their disease and its treatment quite well Early consultation with a hematologist, as well as the patient, should be considered part of the management plan.
- Serious platelet dysfunction can occur at normal platelet counts. For example, antiplatelet therapy and renal disease can alter platelet function without reducing blood counts.
- Factor VIII, IX, and XI deficiencies account for 99% of inherited bleeding disorders.
- Patients with active life-threatening bleeding who are suspected of having a congenital bleeding disorder can be supported with fresh frozen plasma, 15 ml/kg, while diagnostic studies are being done.

REFERENCES

1. Rogers GM: Endothelium and the regulation of hemostasis. In Lee GR et al, editors: *Wintrobe's clinical hematology,* ed 10, Baltimore, 1999, Williams & Wilkins.
2. Coughlin SR: Protease-activated receptors and platelet function, *Thromb Haemost* 82:353, 1999.
3. Sixma JJ et al: Platelet adhesion to collagen: an update, *Thromb Haemost* 78:434, 1997.
4. Shattil SJ, Kashiwagi H, Pampori N: Integrin signaling: the platelet paradigm, *Blood* 91:2645, 1998.
5. Lefkovits J, Plow EF, Topol EJ: Platelet glycoproteins IIb/IIIa receptors in cardiovascular medicine, *N Engl J Med* 332:1553, 1995.
6. Parise LV et al: Platelets in hemostasis and thrombosis. In Lee GR et al, editors: *Wintrobe's clinical hematology,* ed 10, Baltimore, 1999, Williams & Wilkins.
7. Greenberg CS, Orthner CL: Blood coagulation and fibrinolysis. In Lee GR et al, editors: *Wintrobe's clinical hematology,* ed 10, Baltimore, 1999, Williams & Wilkins.
8. Rapaport SI, Rao LV: The tissue factor pathway: how it has become a "prima ballerina," *Thromb Haemost* 74:7, 1995.
9. Jesty J, Nemerson Y: The pathways of blood coagulation. In Beutler E et al, editors: *Williams hematology,* ed 5, New York, 1995, McGraw-Hill.
10. Broze GJ: Tissue factor pathway inhibitor and the revised theory of coagulation, *Annu Rev Med* 46:103, 1995.
11. Bauer KA, Rosenberg RD: Control of coagulation reactions. In Beutler E et al, editors: *Williams hematology,* ed 5, New York, 1995, McGraw-Hill.
12. Moesson MW: The roles of fibrinogen and fibrin in hemostasis and thrombosis, *Senior Hematol* 29:177, 1992.
13. Perry DJ: Antithrombin and its inherited deficiencies, *Blood Rev* 8:37, 1994.
14. Esmon CT: The role of protein C and thrombomodulin in the regulation of blood coagulation, *J Biol Chem* 264:4743, 1989.
15. Baugh RJ, Broze GJ, Krishnasawamy S: Regulation of extrinsic pathway factor Xa formation by tissue factor pathway inhibitor, *J Biol Chem* 273:4378, 1998.
16. Moncada S, Higgs A: The L-arginine-nitric oxide pathway, *N Engl J Med* 329:2002, 1993.
17. Rosenberg RU: Regulation of the hemostatic mechanism. In Stamatoyannopoulos G et al, editors: *Molecular basis of blood diseases,* ed 3, Philadelphia, 2000, WB Saunders.
18. Bennett JS: Blood coagulation and coagulation tests, *Med Clin North Am* 68:557, 1985.
19. Clodfelter RL: The peripheral smear, *Emerg Med Clin North Am* 4:59, 1986.
20. Miletich J: Bleeding time. In Beutler E et al, editors: *Williams hematology,* ed 5, New York, 1995, McGraw-Hill.
21. Rodgers RPC, Levin J: A critical reappraisal of the bleeding time, *Semin Thromb Hemost* 16:1, 1990.
22. Miletich J: Prothrombin time. In Beutler E et al, editors: *Williams hematology,* ed 5, New York, 1995, McGraw-Hill.
23. Angelos MA, Hamilton GC: Coagulation studies, *Emerg Med Clin North Am* 4:95, 1986.
24. Kessler CM, Bell WR: Coagulation factors. In Spivak JL, Eichner ER, editors: *The fundamentals of clinical hematology,* ed 3, Baltimore, 1993, John Hopkins University Press.
25. Miletich J: Activated partial thromboplastin time. In Beutler E et al, editors: *Williams hematology,* ed 5, New York, 1995, McGraw-Hill.
26. Bovill E, Tracy R: Methods for the determination of the plasma concentration of fibrinogen. In Beutler E et al, editors: *Williams hematology,* ed 5, New York, 1995, McGraw-Hill.
27. Schneiderman P: The vascular purpuras. In Beutler E et al, editors: *Williams hematology,* ed 5, New York, 1995, McGraw-Hill.
28. Hill-Zobel RL et al: Organ distribution and the fate of human platelets: studies of asplenic and splenomegalic patients, *Am J Hematol* 23:231, 1986.
29. Goebel RA: Thrombocytopenia, *Emerg Med Clin North Am* 11:445, 1993.
30. Warkentin TE et al: Heparin-induced thrombocytopenia in patients treated with low-molecular weight or unfractionated heparin, *N Engl J Med* 332:1330, 1995.
31. Warkentin TE, Chong BH, Greinacker A: Heparin-induced thrombocytopenia: towards consensus, *Thromb Haemost* 79:1, 1998.
32. Burdy MJ, Martin SE: Cocaine-associated thrombocytopenia, *Am J Med* 91:656, 1992.
33. Gingliano RP, Hyatt RR: Thrombocytopenia with GPIIIa/IIb inhibitors: a meta-analysis, *J Am Coll Cardiol* 31:185A, 1998.
34. Kovachy RJ: Immune thrombocytopenic purpura. In Wood ME, Bunn PA, editors: *Hematology/oncology secrets,* ed 2, Philadelphia, 1999, Hanley Belfus.
35. Kaufman DW et al: Acute thrombocytopenic purpura in relation to the use of drugs, *Blood* 82:2714, 1993.
36. Warkentin T, Kelton JG: Heparin and platelets, *Hematol Oncol Clin North Am* 4:243, 1990.
37. Waters AW: Post-transfusion purpura, *Blood Rev* 3:83, 1989.
38. Nugent DJ: Immune thrombocytopenic purpura. In Bell WR, editor: *Hematologic and oncologic emergencies,* New York, 1993, Churchill Livingstone.
39. Bussel J: Autoimmune thrombocytopenic purpura, *Hematol Oncol Clin North Am* 4:179, 1990.
40. George JN, El-Harake MA, Raskob GE: Chronic idiopathic thrombocytopenic purpura, *N Engl J Med* 331:1207, 1994.
41. George JN et al: Idiopathic thrombocytopenic purpura: a practice guideline developed by explicit methods for the American Society of Hematology, *Blood* 88:3, 1996.
42. Walsh C et al: Thrombocytopenia in homosexual patients, *Ann Intern Med* 103:542, 1985.
43. Hassell K: Thrombotic thrombocytopenic purpura and hemolytic uremic syndrome. In Wood ME, Bunn PA, editors: *Hematology/oncology secrets,* ed 2, Philadelphia, 1999, Hanley Belfus.

44. George JN, El-Harake M: Thrombocytopenia due to enhanced platelet destruction by nonimmunologic mechanisms. In Beutler E et al, editors: *Williams hematology,* ed 5, New York, 1995, McGraw-Hill.
45. George JN et al: Thrombotic thrombocytopenic purpura-hemolytic uremic syndrome: diagnosis and management, *J Clin Apheresis* 13:120, 1998.
46. Rock G et al: Laboratory abnormalities in thrombotic thrombocytopenic purpura: Canadian apheresis group, *Br J Haematol* 103:1031, 1998.
47. Bell WR et al: Improved survival in thrombotic thrombocytopenic purpura-hemolytic uremic syndrome: clinical experience in 108 patients, *N Engl J Med* 325:398, 1991.
48. George JN: Thrombocytopenia: pseudothrombocytopenia, hypersplenism and thrombocytopenia associated with massive transfusion. In Beutler E et al, editors: *Williams hematology,* ed 5, New York, 1995, McGraw-Hill.
49. Bennett JS, Kolodzik MA: Disorders of platelet functions, *Dis Mon* 38:577, 1992.
50. Ruggeri A, Zimmerman T: Review: von Willebrand factor and von Willebrand's disease, *Blood* 70:895, 1987.
51. Bloom AL: Von Willebrand factor: clinical features of inherited and acquired disorders, *Mayo Clinic Proc* 66:743, 1991.
52. Bick RL: Acquired platelet function defects, *Hematol Oncol Clin North Am* 5:1203, 1992.
53. College of America Pathologists: Practice parameter for the use of fresh frozen plasma, cryoprecipitate, and platelets, *JAMA* 271:777, 1994.
54. Buss DH, Stuart JJ, Lipscomb GE: The incidence of thrombotic and hemorrhagic disorders in association with extreme thrombocytosis, *Am J Hematol* 20:365, 1985.
55. Hirsh J et al: Oral anticoagulants: mechanism of action, clinical effectiveness, and optimal therapeutic range, *Chest* 114:445S, 1998.
56. Mammen EF: Coagulation abnormalities in liver disease, *Hematol Oncol Clin North Am* 6:1287, 1992.
57. Erban SB, Kinnar JL, Schwartz SJ: Routine use of the prothrombin and partial thromboplastin times, *JAMA* 262:2428, 1989.
58. Hultin M: Coagulation factor assays. In Beutler E et al, editors: *Williams hematology,* ed 5, New York, 1995, McGraw-Hill.
59. DiMichele D, Neufeld EJ: Hemophilia: a new approach to an old disease, *Hematol Oncol Clin North Am* 12:1315, 1998.
60. Bell B, Canty D, Audet M: Hemophilia: an updated review, *Pediatr Rev* 16:290, 1995.
61. Hoyer LW: Hemophilia A, *N Engl J Med* 330:38, 1994.
62. Cahill MR, Colvin BT: Haemophilia, *Postgrad Med J* 73:201, 1997.
63. The United States Pharmacopeial Convention, Inc: Hemophilia management, *Transfus Med Rev* 12:128, 1998.
64. Pierce GF et al: The use of purified clotting factor concentrates in hemophilia: influence of vial safety, cost, and supply on therapy, *JAMA* 261:3434, 1989.
65. Bray GL et al: The Recombinate Study Group: a multicenter study of recombinant factor VIII (Recombinate): safety, efficacy, and inhibitor risk in previously treated patients with hemophilia A, *Blood* 83:2428, 1994.
66. Serenetis S et al: Human recombinant DNA-derived antihemophilic factor (factor VIII) in the treatment of hemophilia A: conclusion of a 5-year study of home therapy, *Haemophilia* 5:9, 1999.
67. Berntorp E: Second generation, B-domain deleted recombinant factor VIII, *Thromb Haemost* 78:256, 1997.
68. Ehrenforth S et al: Incidence of development of factor VIII and factor IX inhibitors in haemophiliacs, *Lancet* 339:594, 1992.
69. Yee TT et al: Factor VIII inhibitors in haemophiliacs: a single-center experience over 34 years, 1964-1997, *Br J Haematol* 104:909, 1999.
70. Hedner U, Glazer S, Falch J: Recombinant activated factor VII in the treatment of bleeding episodes in patients with inherited and acquired bleeding disorder, *Transfus Med Rev* 7:78, 1993.
71. Gastineau DA et al: Lupus anticoagulant: an analysis of the clinical and laboratory features of 219 cases, *Am J Hematol* 19:265, 1985.
72. Rose EH, Aledort LM: Nasal spray desmopressin (DDAVP) for mild hemophilia A and von Willebrand disease, *Ann Intern Med* 114:563, 1991.
73. Andes WA, Wulff K, Smith WB: Head trauma in hemophilia: a prospective study, *Arch Intern Med* 144:1981, 1984.
74. Dietrich AM et al: Head trauma in children with congenital coagulation disorders, *J Pediatr Surg* 29:28, 1994.
75. Miller J: Von Willebrand disease, *Hematol Oncol Clin North Am* 4:107, 1990.
76. Rodeghiero F, Castaman G, Dini E: Epidemiological investigation of the prevalence of von Willebrand's disease, *Blood* 69:454, 1987.
77. Sadler JE, Gralnick HR: A new classification for von Willebrand's disease, *Blood* 84:676, 1994.
78. Triplett DA: Laboratory diagnosis of von Willebrand disease, *Mayo Clin Proc* 66:832, 1991.
79. Berntorp E, Nilsson IM: Use of a high severity factor VIII concentrate (Humate-P) in von Willebrand disease, *Vox Song* 56:212, 1989.
80. Roberts HR, Eberst ME: Current management of hemophilia B, *Hematol Oncol Clin North Am* 7:1269, 1993.
81. Wang L et al: Sustained correction of bleeding disorder in hemophilia B mice by gene therapy, *Proc Natl Acad Sci U S A* 30:3906, 1999.
82. Kay M: Gene therapy for the hemophiliacs, *Proc Natl Acad Sci U S A* 31:9973, 1999.
83. Lankiewicz MW, Bell WR: Disseminated intravascular coagulation. In Bell WR, editor: *Hematologic and oncologic emergencies,* New York, 1993, Churchill Livingstone.
84. Seligsohn U: Disseminated intravascular coagulation. In Beutler E et al, editors: *Williams hematology,* ed 5, New York, 1995, McGraw-Hill.
85. Matsuda T: Clinical aspects of DIC-disseminated intravascular coagulation. *Pol J Pharmacol* 48:73, 1996.
86. Levi M, ten Cate H: Disseminated intravascular coagulation, *N Engl J Med* 341:586, 1999.
87. Eisele B et al: Antithrombin III in patients with severe sepsis: a randomized, placebo-controlled, double-blind multicenter trial plus a meta-analysis on all randomized, placebo-controlled, double-blind trials with antithrombin III in severe sepsis, *Intensive Care Med* 24:663, 1998.
88. Baudo F et al: Antithrombin III replacement therapy in patients with sepsis and/or postsurgical complications: a controlled double-blind, randomized, multicenter study, *Intensive Care Med* 24:336, 1998.
89. Smith OP et al: Use of protein-C concentrate, heparin, and haemodiafiltration in meningococcus-induced purpura fulminans, *Lancet* 350: 1590, 1997.
90. Bergum P et al: The potent, factor X (a)-dependent inhibition by rNAPc2 of factor X (a) (FVIIa)/tissue factor involves the binding of its cofactor to an exosite on FVII, followed by occupation of the active site, *Blood* 92:669, 1998.

117 Selected Oncologic Emergencies

Neil Schamban
Marc Borenstein

PERSPECTIVE

In 1998, cancer was the second leading cause of death in the United States. In that year alone, more than 1 million cases were diagnosed, with more than 550,000 deaths.[1] More than 20 million patient-physician contacts ranging from routine follow-up visits to ED encounters with patients in extremis took place. Oncologic emergencies include fever and neutropenia, superior vena cava syndrome (SVCS), acute tumor lysis syndrome, hyperviscosity syndrome, hyperuricemia, hypercalcemia, neoplastic cardiac tamponade, spinal cord compression, and raised intracranial pressure (ICP). The accurate diagnosis and appropriate treatment of oncologic emergencies can improve the quality of life dramatically in patients with cancer. In addition, a reversible life-threatening emergency can occur in a patient with an underlying malignancy that is otherwise highly treatable or even curable, thus making identification and management of the oncologic emergency a potentially life-saving action.

Changing trends in cancer that have produced an increased number of ED visits secondary to cancer and its complications include:

- Increased number of elderly patients receiving chemotherapy
- More aggressive chemotherapy regimens
- Broader use of chemotherapy for cancer treatment
- Increasing use of bone marrow transplantation
- More effective treatment options, increasing cure and survival rates

FEVER

Principles of Disease

Fever, a common problem in the cancer patient, can be caused by inflammation, transfusions, antineoplastics, antimicrobials, and tumor necrosis. Although fever can be secondary to malignancy with a significant tumor burden, most fevers (55% to 70%) occurring in cancer patients have an infectious etiology. Granulocytopenia, defined as polymorphonuclear leukocytes fewer than 500/mm^3, predisposes the patient to an increased risk of infection. There is an added increased risk for patients with polymorphonuclear leukocyte levels below 200/mm^3.

Cancer patients with significant fever (defined by the Infectious Disease Society of America as a single oral temperature ≥ 38.3° C [101° F] or an elevation of 38° C [100.4° F] for at least 1 hour) and a polymorphonuclear leukocyte count less than 500/mm^3 should be presumed to have an infectious etiology. Antimicrobial therapy should be started immediately after appropriate cultures have been obtained.[2,3]

Predisposing factors to infection and sepsis in the neutropenic cancer patient include:

- Clinical debilitation, prolonged bed rest
- Nutritional compromise
- Disruption of mucous membranes and skin barriers
- Indwelling catheters
- Central nervous system (CNS) dysfunction secondary to cancer, sedatives, opiates, or psychotropic medications

With the onset of granulocytopenia, the host's inflammatory response is markedly altered, thus impairing the ability to detect the presence of infection; an undetected and untreated infection can be rapidly fatal in this patient population. Infection is the number one cause of cancer death, and untreated infections have a 20% to 50% 48-hour mortality.[3-5] The EP can have a major impact on these patients and their ultimate survival if he or she institutes aggressive management early and effectively.

Clinical Features

Because fever is often the first—and occasionally the only—sign of infection in the granulocytopenic cancer patient, the EP must take a deliberate history and perform a meticulous physical examination. In the absence of granulocytes, traditional markers of inflammation such as erythema, warmth, and pyuria may be absent or minimal, making it essential to search for and not minimize subtle signs of inflammation. There is no predictable pattern, severity, or incidence of infectious complications in the neutropenic host; therefore, broad-spectrum empiric antibiotic therapy should be initiated promptly in all febrile, granulocytopenic patients.

Diagnostic Strategies

Before empiric antimicrobial therapy is begun, the patient should have a chest radiograph, complete blood count (CBC), differential cell count, platelet count, prothrombin time, partial thromboplastin time, blood chemistries, urinalysis, and aspiration or biopsy of any accessible sites suggestive of infection. Two sets of blood cultures should be obtained for aerobic, anaerobic, and fungal growth. Urine should be sent for culture, even in the absence of pyuria. However, the use of sputum culture and Gram's stain, although still recommended, has become controversial because of inconsistencies in collection and preparation that have led to false-negative and false-positive results. An indwelling nasogastric tube predisposes the neutropenic patient to sinusitis. Sinus films are difficult to interpret, however, and when sinusitis is suspected, computed tomography (CT) scanning is preferred. A lumbar puncture, preceded by head CT scanning, is indicated when symptoms point to the CNS. Some authorities have recommended surveillance cultures of the stool, nose, and throat; this recommendation is not universally accepted and is generally not indicated in patients with solid tumors. Despite an intensive and comprehensive evaluation, an infectious cause is initially substantiated in only 50% to 70% of febrile, granulocytopenic patients. Nuclear, gallium citrate, and indium 111 scans do not have a place in the emergency diagnosis and management of these patients, but may be useful in the definitive evaluation.

Differential Considerations

Overall, approximately 85% of the initial pathogens are bacterial, and 50% of infections are caused by gram-negative pathogens, although fungal, viral, and parasitic infections are also important primary or secondary complications. Overall, 67% of adults and 30% of children with leukemia who are febrile and granulocytopenic from their illness or combination chemotherapy have documented bacterial infections, and approximately 8% have fungal infections.[3,4] The gram-negative organisms, especially *Pseudomonas aeruginosa, Klebsiella* species, and *Escherichia coli,* are the most predominant bacterial pathogens, although *P. aeruginosa* had been declining in incidence, most probably because of empiric antibiotic regimens and protocols. In some centers, gram-positive organisms have again become the predominant isolates, including *Staphylococcus aureus* and *S. epidermidis.* Once believed to be a contaminant, *S. epidermidis* has arisen as a major pathogen and may be resistant to antistaphylococcal penicillins and cephalosporins. Fungal infections, especially *Candida albicans,* can be a major problem in granulocytopenic febrile patients who are treated with broad-spectrum antibiotics for protracted periods. Although significant institutional variation has been noted, histoplasmosis, *Cryptococcus, Aspergillus,* and *Phycomycetes* are additional fungal pathogens encountered in the compromised host. In contrast to patients with acquired immunodeficiency syndrome, parasitic infections are not a common source of infection in patients with solid tumors. *Pneumocystis carinii,* however, may be seen when corticosteroid use or hematologic malignancy has resulted in lymphocyte dysfunction. Herpes simplex, herpes varicella zoster, and cytomegalovirus are common viral pathogens. The compromised host is at risk for a large number of individual pathogenic agents, thus further complicating the diagnosis and management of these complex patients.[3,6]

Occasionally fever is without a source and is believed to be secondary to the underlying disease. However, it is impossible to differentiate patients with bacteremia-induced fever from those with unexplained fever on clinical and demographic factors such as their age, sex, underlying malignancy, or the types of therapeutic modalities or invasive diagnostic procedures they had received. In addition, the absence of physical findings indicative of infection does not exclude a potentially life-threatening septic event because at least 50% of septic patients lack any distinct physical findings. Despite the potential for few physical findings, a meticulous physical examination should be conducted, including the fundi (looking for *Candida* endophthalmitis), rectum, perineum and groin (for perirectal abscess), skin and mucous membranes (for any lesions suggesting malignancy or cellulitis), axillae, and catheters.[5,7]

Management

Patients should be admitted to an isolation room. Potentially neutropenic patients should receive high priority for care. If an isolation room is not available, any setting removed from potentially infectious patients can be used to expedite care. Hand washing and reverse isolation techniques should be practiced. Cultures on all febrile, neutropenic patients should be obtained quickly and appropriate broad-spectrum antibiotics prescribed without delay. The absence of signs of infection must not dissuade the EP from instituting empiric therapy because the responses that mark the infection site in noncompromised hosts (i.e., erythema infiltrates and exudate) may be so impaired in the febrile, neutropenic patient that the source of fever is obscured.

In the initial evaluation and management of the febrile cancer patient, one must take into account the particular underlying malignancy, prior use of antimicrobial therapy, and how the degree of treatment has affected the host's immunologic compromise. For example, in acute leukemia normal circulating neutrophils and monocytes are largely replaced by blast cells, which do not function well in the phagocytizing and killing of bacterial and fungal agents. Chemotherapeutic agents and irradiation exacerbate or potentiate the underlying defect in already compromised host defenses. Corticosteroids impair granulocyte and mononuclear cell mobilization in leukemic patients. The individuals who should be most aggressively treated in the ED are those with severely compromised host defenses and in whom fever is accompanied by an increased respiratory rate, a change in mental status, agitation or apprehensiveness, and hemodynamic instability.

The optimal antimicrobial regimen should be synergistic, broad spectrum, and bactericidal with a low potential for toxicity and chosen for efficacy against the most likely causes of systemic and rapidly progressing infection: *P. aeruginosa, E. coli, Klebsiella* species, and *S. aureus.* A two-drug regimen is usually selected because historical studies from the 1980s disclosed a greater survival rate with gram-negative bacteremia when the isolate was sensitive to and treated with two antibiotics in a combined regimen as compared to when the isolate was sensitive to only one of two antibiotics used in a combined regimen.

In the past 10 years there have been significant advances in the antimicrobial armamentarium with development of broad-spectrum single agents such as the carbapenems (imipenem/cilastatin, meropenem) and the third to fourth generation cephalosporins (ceftazidime, cefepime). These agents when investigated as monotherapy for granulocytopenic, febrile patients have been found to be as effective as a dual-drug combination of an anti-pseudomonal penicillin (ticarcillin, carbenicillin, or piperacillin) plus an aminoglycoside (gentamicin or tobramycin) in clinical trials.[3,6,8,9]

Use of initial empiric vancomycin is included as first-line therapy at institutions where there has been a significant incidence of methicillin-resistant *S. aureus.* Amikacin is generally reserved as a second-line aminoglycoside for isolates that demonstrate aminoglycoside resistance.

Current recommendations for antimicrobial therapy of fever in neutropenic cancer patients include the following[2-4,7,10]:

- an antipseudomonal penicillin + an aminoglycoside ± vancomycin
- ceftazidime ± an aminoglycoside
- ceftazidime ± vancomycin
- cefepime ± vancomycin
- imipenem/cilastatin
- meropenem

SUPERIOR VENA CAVA SYNDROME

Perspective

SVCS is an acute or subacute process caused by the obstruction of the superior vena cava (SVC) secondary to compression, infiltration, or thrombosis. Malignancy currently accounts for 85% to 95% of SVC obstruction and is encountered as a complication in 3% to 8% of patients with cancer of the lung or lymphoma.[11,12] Small-cell and squamous cell lung cancers exceed all other causes of malignant SVC obstruction and are causal in 65% of all cases. It is noteworthy, however, that breast and testicular cancer produce 10% to 15% of SVC obstruction. Forty to fifty years ago, benign etiologies accounted for up to two thirds of SVC obstruction. Thoracic aortic aneurysm alone accounted for up to 40% of cases, mostly related to the high incidence of luetic aneurysm, which Hunter first described in 1757.[13,14] Gradually, benign causes for SVCS have decreased, composing 10% to 25% of the reported cases of SVCS. Other common nonmalignant etiologies include goiter, pericardial constriction, primary thrombosis, idiopathic sclerosing aortitis, tuberculous mediastinitis, fibrosing mediastinitis (histoplasmosis and methysergide treatment), arteriosclerotic or (rarely) luetic aneurysm, and indwelling central venous catheters.[12,15] In contrast to the adult population SVCS in pediatric patients is most often iatrogenic secondary to indwelling catheters, ventriculoperitoneal shunts, and complications of cardiovascular surgical procedures.

Clinical Features

A knowledge of the unique anatomic relationship of the SVC in the anterior superior mediastinum is crucial to understanding the clinical presentation of SVC obstruction. The SVC is easily compressed by any of its bounding contiguous structures (trachea, heart, aorta, azygos vein, and paratracheal and bronchial lymph nodes). This compression can produce a constellation of symptoms that reveal the exact site of the pathophysiologic process (Figure 117-1). The SVC arises from the innominate veins, which in turn arise from the internal jugular and subclavian veins. The azygos vein, the last main auxiliary vessel of the SVC, drains blood from the chest wall. As a consequence of this anatomic relationship, if the SVC is blocked above or at the entrance of the azygos, blood may bypass and decompress the obstruction through the chest wall collateral vessels and rejoin the SVC via the azygos. If the obstruction falls below or at the entrance of the azygos, blood must traverse in a retrograde manner down the azygos and other chest wall veins to reach the drainage area of the inferior vena cava, which subsequently causes more prominent symptoms and further embarrassment to the patient.[11]

Because the clinical features of the SVCs are characterized by venous hypertension within the area ordinarily drained by the SVC, many of the findings are more noticeably evident in the recumbent or stooped-over position. Early signs may include periorbital edema, conjunctival suffusion, and facial swelling, which will be most evident in the early morning hours and subside by midmorning. The differential diagnosis also includes the nephrotic syndrome, although a history of lower extremity–dependent edema will also be elicited. In one study the most common symptom is shortness of breath (>50%), with swelling of the face, trunk, and upper extremities observed in approximately 40% of patients. Cough, dysphagia, and chest pain are less commonly reported, each occurring in approximately 20% of patients. With increasing impedance to blood flow, the full-blown syndrome begins to manifest itself with thoracic and neck vein distention (67% and 59%), facial edema (56%), tachypnea (40%), tightness of the shirt collar (the Stoke sign), plethora of the face, edema of the upper extremities, and cyanosis.[11,16] The severity of the syndrome is also related to the pace of the obstruction; the more gradual the onset of obstruction, the longer the time for development of collateralization with less severe symptomatology.

Early reports of severe SVCS describe patients with

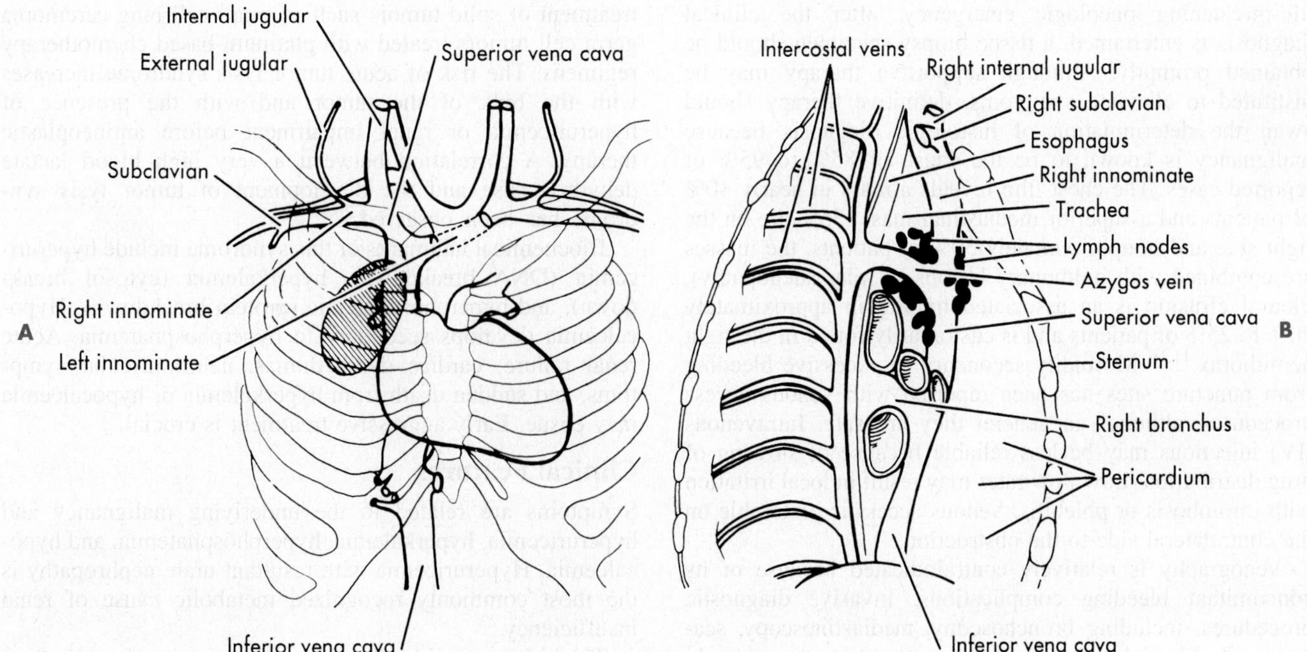

Figure 117-1. **Frontal (A) and sagittal (B) sections of the thorax showing the relationship of the azygos vein to the superior vena cava (SVC), coalescence of innominates to form the SVC at the right second rib, and encasement of the SVC by nodal structures. Shaded area indicates classic site of obstruction.** *From Lokich JL, Goodman R:* JAMA *231:58, 1975.*

increased ICP resulting in headache, blurred vision, altered mental status, coma, seizures, cerebral hemorrhage, and papilledema. In rare cases, death from cerebral edema was noted.[17] Portacaval shunts resulting from portal venous hypertension were reported to give rise to esophageal varices and tortuous collateral vessels on the chest and abdomen, mimicking the caput medusae of a patient with cirrhosis, although the direction of flow is caudad (i.e., from cava to portal) in this instance. Airway obstruction and cardiac complications were reported. Without appropriate intervention, prolonged SVC obstruction was believed to lead to irreversible thrombosis and death.[13,14,17]

Important concepts have changed since these early reports. Seizures do not occur in the absence of intracranial metastases and airway obstruction does not occur in the absence of tracheal compression by extrinsic tumor. Overall, little evidence in the current literature substantiates the notion of untreated SVC obstruction as life-threatening except when it occurs with tracheal compression.[11,18]

SVCS can occur in conjunction with spinal cord compression (the Rubin syndrome). Venous obstruction usually develops before the spinal cord compression, which is localized in most instances to the low cervical or upper thoracic spinal cord. This syndrome is most commonly found with malignancies of lymphoma and lung cancer. Patients with venous obstruction and back pain should be evaluated with magnetic resonance imaging (MRI) of the vertebral spine.

Diagnostic Strategies

The clinical diagnosis of SVC obstruction should be apparent but is mimicked by a few other clinical entities—most noteworthy are pericardial tamponade and heart failure, which can usually be excluded by physical examination. Mild and early cases can be difficult to differentiate clinically. Ultrasound can be used to exclude pericardial effusion. Because SVCS usually does not represent an immediately life-threatening oncologic emergency, after the clinical diagnosis is entertained, a tissue biopsy specimen should be obtained promptly. Although supportive therapy may be instituted to alleviate symptoms, definitive therapy should await the determination of histologic diagnosis because malignancy is known to be the cause of 85% to 95% of reported cases. The chest film reveals a mass in nearly 10% of patients and a superior mediastinal mass (75% are on the right side and in approximately 50% of patients, the masses are combined with pulmonary lesions or hilar adenopathy). Pleural effusion is an associated finding in approximately 20% to 25% of patients and is customarily found in the right hemithorax.[11,16] Morbidity secondary to excessive bleeding from puncture sites has been reported with venous access procedures, although in general they are safe. Intravenous (IV) injections may be less reliable because of slowing of drug distribution. Low flow rates may result in local irritation with thrombosis or phlebitis. Venous access is preferable on the contralateral side to the obstruction.

Venography is relatively contraindicated because of its concomitant bleeding complications. Invasive diagnostic procedures, including bronchoscopy, mediastinoscopy, scalene node biopsy, and limited thoracotomy, are commonly used to establish the diagnosis and extent of the disease. After SVC obstruction is suspected, the appropriate consulting services should be contacted and plans for immediate diagnosis undertaken.[11,16]

Management

Historically, radiation therapy has been emphasized as the primary treatment for SVC compression. Current treatment uses chemotherapy because of the increased incidence of tumor sensitivity to newer antineoplastic agents. However, temporizing measures that would alleviate symptoms related to vascular compression should be immediately instituted.

Elevation of the head of the bed has been shown to be an immediately effective measure. Diuretics have been used with transient symptomatic relief, although they must be used judiciously because overzealous administration can result in hypovolemia and further slowing of blood flow. Steroids have been shown to be of limited effectiveness but may be useful in the presence of respiratory compromise.[16] Current management approaches include percutaneous transluminal stent placement.[19]

The prognosis for patients treated for SVCS depends on the tumor type, with better survival with lymphoma than with bronchogenic carcinoma. The overall survival is approximately 25% at 1 year and 10% at 30 months after treatment.

Although SVCS occurs in only 3% to 8% of patients with cancer of the lung and lymphoma, if keyed into the early and late manifestations of the disease process, the EP can have a tremendous effect on the immediate and long-term survival of this patient population.

ACUTE TUMOR LYSIS SYNDROME

Perspective

Acute tumor lysis syndrome most commonly occurs within 1 to 5 days of instituting chemotherapy or radiation therapy of rapidly growing tumors that are extremely sensitive to antineoplastic drugs. This syndrome is most commonly seen after chemotherapy of hematologic malignancies, including acute leukemias and lymphomas, particularly Burkitt's lymphoma, in which the growth fraction often exceeds 90%.[20-22] With advances in the effectiveness of chemotherapy, acute tumor lysis syndrome has been described after treatment of solid tumors such as small-cell lung carcinoma germ cell tumors treated with platinum-based chemotherapy regimens. The risk of acute tumor lysis syndrome increases with the bulk of the tumor and with the presence of hyperuricemia or renal impairment before antineoplastic therapy. A correlation between a very high blood lactate dehydrogenase and the development of tumor lysis syndrome has been observed.[20,22]

Biochemical hallmarks of this syndrome include hyperuricemia (DNA breakdown), hyperkalemia (cytosol breakdown), and hyperphosphatemia (protein breakdown). Hypocalcemia develops secondary to hyperphosphatemia. Acute renal failure, cardiac dysrhythmias, neuromuscular symptoms, and sudden death from hyperkalemia or hypocalcemia may ensue. Early aggressive treatment is crucial.

Clinical Features

Symptoms are related to the underlying malignancy and hyperuricemia, hyperkalemia, hyperphosphatemia, and hypocalcemia. Hyperuricemia with resultant urate nephropathy is the most commonly recognized metabolic cause of renal insufficiency.[22]

The kidney provides the primary mechanism for excretion of uric acid, potassium, and phosphate. Rapid proliferation of tumor cells may exceed the removal rate of the respective substances, resulting in increased levels of uric acid, potassium, and phosphate. In fact, increased quantities of these substances have been observed in patients undergoing rapid lysis of chemosensitive tumors.

The integrity of renal function is a critical factor in determining the degree of metabolic derangements. In patients with preexisting renal insufficiency, the metabolic derangements of acute tumor lysis are more likely to be severe; however, even when renal function appears normal at the start of treatment, the rapid lysis of certain tumors may overwhelm the excretory capacity of the kidney. Similar to hyperuricemia, hyperphosphatemia may also cause renal failure. A possible mechanism is precipitation of calcium phosphate within the kidney.[22]

Hyperkalemia, along with a contributing hypocalcemia, may result in life-threatening ventricular dysrhythmias.[20] Hypocalcemia may also cause neuromuscular instability with muscle cramps and occasionally tetany. Confusion and convulsions also have been described in case reports.[22]

Management

Because of the life-threatening complications associated with acute tumor lysis, patients at high risk for developing this syndrome should be treated with prophylactic measures as soon as possible. Chemotherapy should be delayed, if possible, until metabolic disturbances, especially prerenal azotemia and hyperuricemia, are corrected. Initial management is aimed at controlling preexisting hyperuricemia with hydration, allopurinol, and alkalinization of the urine to a pH greater than 7. Diuretics are added if necessary, and frequent monitoring of electrolytes, calcium, and phosphorus is essential.

Most articles agree that it is wise to alkalinize the urine as a prophylactic measure against hyperuricemia, but caution is advised should hyperphosphatemia and hypocalcemia develop. Under these circumstances, alkali therapy may aggravate manifestations of hypocalcemia such as tetany.[22,23] Although alkalinization increases the solubility of uric acid, the primary means of uric acid control is hydration and diuresis to maintain adequate urinary flow.[22]

If tumor lysis syndrome develops, hemodialysis should be considered as early as possible as a potentially life-saving measure. This therapy is effective in lowering uric acid, potassium, and phosphate levels, as well as in controlling uremic symptoms. See the suggested criteria for instituting hemodialysis in Box 117-1.

The prognosis is good in the absence of renal failure. If renal failure exists and hemodialysis of 5 to 7 days is necessary, the prognosis is grave. With aggressive management, the incidence of renal and metabolic complications of cytoreductive therapy may be decreased.

Box 117-1 Criteria for Instituting Hemodialysis

Serum potassium > 6 mEq/L (6 mmol/L)
Serum uric acid > 10 mg/dl (590 μmol/L)
Serum creatinine > 10 mg/dl (880 μmol/L)
Serum phosphorus > 10 mg/dl (phosphate > 3.2 mmol/L) or rapidly rising
To reduce volume overload
Symptomatic hypocalcemia

Modified from Cohen LF et al: *Am J Med* 64:486, 1980.

HYPERVISCOSITY SYNDROME

Perspective

Viscosity is the resistance that a liquid exhibits to the flow of one layer over another. Excessive elevations in certain paraproteins, marked leukocytosis, or erythrocytosis can result in elevated serum viscosity and the development of significant sludging, decreased perfusion of the microcirculation, and vascular stasis. The outcome of these pathophysiologic events leads to the development of hyperviscosity syndrome (HVS). HVS deserves urgent medical therapy to forestall or reverse the effects of sludging in the microcirculation of the CNS, visual system, and cardiopulmonary system.[24]

The most common causes of HVS include the dysproteinemias. The most common is Waldenström's macroglobulinemia, which accounts for 85% to 90% of all HSV cases. Multiple myeloma, the next most common cause, is responsible for 5% to 10% of cases. Other etiologies include cryoglobulinemia, a benign hyperglobulinemia of the immunoglobulin M–immunoglobulin G (IgG) type, and leukemias.[24-26]

The blastic phase of chronic myelogenous leukemia, chronic granulocytic leukemia, and the blast cell crisis of acute lymphoblastic and nonlymphoblastic leukemias also commonly cause HVS.[24,25] Other more benign causes include leukemoid reaction, polycythemia vera, and the accumulation of abnormal hemoglobins in sickle cell disease. The incidence of HVS in Waldenström's macroglobulinemia is found to be approximately 20%, in IgG myeloma approximately 4.2%, and in IgA myeloma as high as 25%.[25]

The inherent physiochemical properties of the dysproteinemias, along with extremely high concentrations of these proteins, seem to predispose to the development of hyperviscosity. Paradoxically, HSV also has been reported in kappa light chain disease owing to a greater tendency to form unstable, highly polymerized circulating aggregates. The etiologic factor most responsible for HVS in the leukemias appears to be leukocytosis with white blood cell (WBC) counts in excess of 100,000/mm^3, usually accompanied by blast forms exceeding 100,000/mm^3 in the peripheral smear. The clinical manifestations of HVS become most apparent when the serum viscosity relative to water is greater than 4 to 5, normal serum viscosity relative to water being 1.4 to 1.8.[24-26]

Clinical Features

A symptomatic triad of bleeding, visual disturbances, and neurologic manifestations is a classic presentation of HSV. Visual disturbances, and on occasion visual loss, may occur with retinopathy characterized by venous engorgement (e.g., "sausage-link" or "boxcar" segmentation), which is also seen in the bulbar conjunctiva, microaneurysms, hemorrhages, exudates, and occasionally papilledema. Persistent bleeding diatheses from mucosal surfaces, especially nasal mucosa, the gastrointestinal (GI) tract, and sites of minor surgery or trauma, even in the face of a normal platelet count, are common. Other clinical findings encompass myriad neurologic disturbances, including headache, dizziness, jacksonian and generalized seizures, somnolence, lethargy, coma, auditory disturbances (including hearing loss), and hypotension. Constitutional symptoms of fatigue, anorexia, and weight loss that are nonspecific early on are commonly associated with the underlying malignancy or with numerous electrolyte disturbances related to the underlying malignant process. Cardiopulmonary findings, including acute respiratory failure and hypoxemia, congestive heart failure, myocardial infarction, and valvular abnormalities, have all been reported. Renal insufficiency and failure may be a complication of the syndrome and will exacerbate existing clinical findings secondary to the expanded plasma volume.[24,25]

The laboratory evaluation of the patient with suspected HVS should include coagulation, renal, electrolyte, and differential white count profiles. Serum and urine protein electrophoresis should be done with all suspected dysproteinemias, with the diagnosis supported by a large spike on the serum electrophoresis. A clue to the presence of hyperviscosity may be the inability of the laboratory to perform chemical tests on the blood because of the serum stasis and increased viscosity that clogs analyzers. In multiple myeloma, significant hypercalcemia may also occur, and with high M-protein fractions, a factitious hyponatremia may be present. The diagnosis may be also entertained when a patient is brought to the ED in a stupor or coma and anemia and rouleaux formation are found on the peripheral smear.[27]

Because HVS is often a presenting characteristic of dysproteinemias and leukemias with blastic transformation and because a history of previously documented disease is often absent, this syndrome must be considered in patients with unexplained somnolence and coma.

Management

Emergency leukapheresis or plasmapheresis is the definitive treatment for HVS. Temporizing measures provided by the EP should focus on adequate rehydration and diuresis. An immediate temporizing measure in a patient with frank coma and an established dysproteinemia is a 2-U phlebotomy with replacement of the patient's red blood cells with physiologic saline.[24-27] After plasmapheresis or leukapheresis has adequately alleviated the clinical findings, chemotherapeutic modalities can be used.

HYPERURICEMIA

Perspective

Hyperuricemia is a serious and well-known consequence of certain malignant disorders, which, if recognized early, can result in a significant decrease in morbidity of the cancer patient. Hyperuricemia's major source is cell breakdown and its major excretory pathway is renal. The pathogenesis of hyperuricemia results from either increased production or decreased excretion of uric acid or both. Increased production of uric acid commonly results from rapid dissolution of neoplastic tissues after chemotherapy or radiation therapy of undifferentiated lymphomas or lymphoblastic lymphomas and with acute lymphoblastic leukemias. In addition, hyperuricemia may be seen with multiple myeloma and occasionally with disseminated metastatic carcinoma. With massive release of precursors, uric acid levels rise precipitously and may reach levels as high as 15 to 20 mg/dl. As a result, uric acid crystals form in the highly concentrated and acidified urine of the distal tubules. Intrarenal obstruction follows, and acute renal failure ensues.[22,28]

Chronic, moderately elevated levels of the serum uric acid may result in renal colic, obstructive uropathy, or chronic renal failure. Either uric acid renal calculi or interstitial deposits of sodium urate develop. This situation is associated with neoplastic overproduction of uric acid precursors. Polycythemia vera, myeloid metaplasia, mast cell disease, and chronic granulocytic leukemia are often associated with this type of hyperuricemia.

Decreased excretion may be a result of underlying renal insufficiency or a consequence of precipitation of urates in the renal tubules, parenchyma, or ureters with subsequent development of renal insufficiency and further reduction in excretion of uric acid. Three types of renal diseases are attributable to hyperuricemia: acute hyperuricemic nephropathy, uric acid nephrolithiasis, and gouty nephropathy.

Clinical Features

Hyperuricemia can occur with or without symptoms. Symptoms may be associated with the underlying malignancy. Hyperuricemia precipitated or aggravated by therapy of these diseases may occur as an isolated metabolic disturbance or may be accompanied by other manifestations of the tumor lysis syndrome (see previous discussion). If an underlying neoplastic disease has been diagnosed, hyperuricemia should be sought and treated before renal damage develops. In patients with urate stones and hyperuricemia, examination of the peripheral blood may provide evidence of an underlying myeloproliferative disorder. Acute oliguria after chemotherapy or radiation therapy suggests hyperuricemia, and the uric acid level in the blood often far exceeds that associated with acute renal failure.

A number of benign diseases are associated with hyperuricemia that may coexist with neoplasia. These include hereditary gout, hyperparathyroidism, psoriasis, sarcoidosis, and renal failure of any cause. From a therapeutic standpoint, however, the finding of hyperuricemia obviates the importance of the primary cause; the therapy is the same. The long-term administration of certain drugs may lead to elevated serum uric acid levels. Various diuretics, including thiazides and furosemide, are important examples.[22,29]

Management

When possible, hyperuricemia should be treated before chemotherapy or radiation therapy, especially with bulky tumors or if the serum uric acid level is borderline or increased. If a uric acid elevation of more than 9 mg/dl is found, allopurinol, fluids, and alkalinization of the urine should be initiated. If possible, this regimen should be started a day or two before chemotherapy or radiation treatment is initiated. Patients with histories of gouty arthritis should also receive colchicine, 0.6 mg orally twice a day, to avoid the acute attacks that can be associated with allopurinol administration. Patients should be kept well hydrated. Alkalinization of the urine with oral sodium bicarbonate may help prevent nephropathy. In patients with acute distal tubular uric acid obstruction, management includes administering allopurinol together with the fluid and electrolyte management used in other forms of acute renal failure.

If hyperuricemia is secondary to malignancy, cytolytic therapy should be stopped. Allopurinol in dosages of 300 to 600 mg/day will usually decrease uric acid level in the serum in approximately 3 days, so its administration should be started 2 or 3 days before cytolytic therapy, if time permits. Hydration is vital in maintaining a urine output above 2 L/day. Alkalinization to keep the urine pH above 7 can be accomplished by administering sodium bicarbonate, 9 to

12 g/day. Diuretics are to be used as needed. Acetazolamide (Diamox) in doses of 1 g/day will usually alkalinize the urine temporarily until allopurinol becomes effective. If oliguria occurs, mannitol may be started with 12.5 g of a 20% solution given intravenously over 3 minutes to keep urine output more than 250 ml/hr. The dose of mannitol is limited to 100 g every 24 hours to avoid clinical features resembling water intoxication. If these measures fail, peritoneal dialysis or hemodialysis or flushing the ureters via retrograde catheters may be considered. Clearly, prevention of this complication is far better than treatment. The cancer patient who comes to the ED with renal colic warrants careful evaluation for hyperuricemia. The prognosis depends on the underlying malignancy and degree of renal failure.[22,28]

HYPERCALCEMIA

Perspective

Hypercalcemia occurs in approximately 20% to 40% of cancer patients and is the most common life-threatening metabolic disorder associated with cancer.[30] It affects multiple organ systems and induces a variety of pathophysiologic events that may be more immediate threats to life than the cancer itself.

Two mechanisms have been proposed to explain the development of hypercalcemia associated with malignancy. The first mechanism involves patients with metastatic bone involvement. The hypercalcemia is most likely associated with the release of calcium and phosphate caused by associated osteolysis. The second mechanism involves those patients with no bone disease. A variety of tumor-produced hormonelike substances have been associated with hypercalcemia development, including parathyroid hormone, prostaglandins, and peptides, all of which affect bone turnover.

Hypercalcemia is a common feature of many malignancies but most often complicates cancer of the breast, lung, head, and neck, as well as multiple myeloma and leukemia. Bony metastases are not a prerequisite for hypercalcemia and when present do not necessarily cause hypercalcemia. In patients who are hypercalcemic from squamous cell lung cancer, only one in six has bone metastases. In small-cell lung carcinoma, hypercalcemia is almost never seen despite the presence of bone marrow metastases in 20% to 50% of cases. A complex interaction of various substances (parathyroid hormone, prostaglandins, peptides, steroids, osteoclastic factors) appears to be the result of both increased bone synthesis and degradation. The exception is multiple myeloma, in which bone destruction is accompanied by minimal bone synthesis. Other entities that cause hypercalcemia are listed in Box 117-2.[31,32]

Clinical Features

The development of symptoms of hypercalcemia is nonspecific. There is little correlation between serum calcium levels and the presence and severity of symptoms. Acute hypercalcemia results in marked CNS effects ranging from personality changes (depression, paranoia, lethargy, somnolence) to coma. With chronic hypercalcemia, symptoms include a history of anorexia, nausea, vomiting, constipation, polyuria, polydipsia, memory loss, and a shortened QT interval on the electrocardiogram. The symptoms, signs, and complications of hypercalcemia are summarized in Box 117-3.

In patients with carcinoma, any of the symptoms listed previously should suggest the diagnosis of hypercalcemia, but the EP should be particularly suspicious of hypercalcemia in any cancer patient with lethargy or a change in mental status. Many patients may also have electrolyte abnormalities such as hypokalemia and dehydration. Evaluation of serum electrolytes therefore should accompany measurements of serum calcium, phosphorus, albumin, and alkaline phosphate. In general, a serum calcium level higher than 14 mg/dl constitutes a medical emergency. In chronic hypercalcemia, the EP may see patients with blood calcium levels as high as 15 mg/dl with only mild symptoms. With an acute onset, the EP can see patients comatose at a level of only 12 to 13 mg/dl.[22,28-30]

Many benign conditions can result in hypercalcemia. The most common are hyperparathyroidism and Paget's disease of bone. Clinical features include a long history of hypercalcemia symptoms, particularly renal stones. Chronic changes on

Box 117-2 Nonneoplastic Causes of Hypercalcemia

Hyperparathyroidism
Hyperthyroidism
Renal insufficiency (diuretic phase of acute renal failure, after transplantation, secondary hyperparathyroidism)
Drugs (thiazide diuretics, lithium, and calcium carbonate)
Hypervitaminosis (A and D)
Acute adrenal insufficiency
Immobilization (Paget disease, fracture, paraplegia)
Acromegaly
Myxedema
Milk-alkali syndrome
Sarcoidosis
Benign monoclonal gammopathy
Rarer still are factitious hypercalcemia, idiopathic hypercalcemia of infancy (with elfin facies), familial hypocalciuric hypocalcemia, and hypercalcemia from pheochromocytoma or periostitis

Box 117-3 Common Signs and Symptoms of Hypercalcemia in Malignancy

General
Itching

Neurologic
Fatigue, muscle weakness, hyporeflexia, lethargy, apathy, disturbance of perception and behavior, stupor, coma

Renal
Polyuria, polydipsia, renal insufficiency

Gastrointestinal
Anorexia, nausea, vomiting, constipation, abdominal pain

Cardiovascular
Hypertension, dysrhythmias, digitalis sensitivity

bone films, such as subperiosteal reaction and cysts or a "ground-glass" appearance of the skull, suggest hyperparathyroidism. Diagnosis of Paget's disease rests in biopsy results. Vitamin D excess, milk-alkali syndrome, and adrenal insufficiency are other common causes in the differential diagnosis of hypercalcemia.[22,28]

The acute onset of severe hypercalcemia or chronic exposure of the renal tubules to elevated calcium levels may reduce the glomerular filtration rate and renal blood flow, resulting in acute renal failure.[22]

Management

The therapeutic modalities used in the treatment of hypercalcemia are numerous, but they should always be used in conjunction with therapy of the underlying malignant disease. The exception to this is breast cancer, when hormone therapy should be stopped until hypercalcemia is regulated.

The treatment for hypercalcemia will depend on the clinical status of the patient and on the calcium level in his or her blood, but the general principles of treatment include treating the cancer when possible, encouraging ambulation, correcting dehydration, increasing calcium excretion, decreasing calcium removal from bone, and reducing calcium intake.

If serum calcium levels are below 14 mg/dl, oral rehydration and ambulation may suffice. Normal saline solution can be administered if the oral intake is not sufficient. If the serum phosphate level is not elevated, oral phosphates may be used cautiously. Phospho-Soda, 5 ml by mouth, 2 or 3 times daily, is usually tolerated with mild to no diarrhea.

Mithramycin given as 25 μg/kg intramuscularly (IM) once every 4 to 5 days is not generally part of the initial emergency management of hypercalcemia and has been supplanted in most cases by the bisphosphonates. Prednisone, 60 to 80 mg/day, or other corticosteroids, may be effective within a few days to a week. This drug is more useful for long-term treatment than for acute control. Corticosteroids are particularly valuable in breast carcinoma, myeloma, and lymphoma. They should not be initiated without oncologic consultation because they are chemotherapeutic agents for these malignancies.

If the serum calcium level is greater than 14 mg/dl or significant symptoms are present, a more aggressive management should be undertaken. Continuous cardiac monitoring in the ED is necessary and central venous or pulmonary artery pressure monitoring may be required. Intravenous phosphates, although able to effectively lower the serum calcium level through precipitation of inorganic calcium phosphate salts in bone, are not recommended in view of their serious complications, which include widespread visceral calcifications, shock, and renal failure.

Saline rehydration and diuresis stimulates renal tubular excretion of calcium and is the most important initial component of hypercalcemia emergency management. Dehydration should be corrected within 1 to 2 hours with normal saline solution. When urine flow is adequate, furosemide, 40 to 60 mg IV, may be given to increase excretion of calcium. Although the calciuric effect of furosemide is modest, it is also useful in preventing fluid overload in patients predisposed to cardiac failure. Careful attention to fluid input and output ensures that the patient remains euvolemic. Calcitonin may be effective in doses of 4 to 8 IU/kg IM. This treatment, although relatively safe when renal function is normal, is not generally part of the initial emergency management of hypercalcemia. If prostaglandin production is suspected, as in renal cancer, indomethacin or aspirin may be given, although their theoretic appeal exceeds their practical values. Fifty percent of hypercalcemic cancer patients also have hypokalemia. Serum potassium levels should be monitored every 4 hours and potassium chloride (20 to 40 mEq/L) supplemented intravenously or orally as necessary to prevent severe hypokalemia.[22,28,30,31]

In the past 5 years after approval by the U.S. Food and Drug Administration, bisphosphonates have become the treatment of choice for managing cancer-induced hypercalcemia, supplanting all other pharmacologic approaches except corticosteroids. Several agents are now available including clodronate, pamidronate, and ibandronate, with other more potent bisphosphonates in development. Pamidronate, 90 mg, given as an infusion over 4 to 24 hours effectively and safely achieves normocalcemia within a few days (mean 4 days) in more than in 90% to 95% of patients.[32-35]

NEOPLASTIC CARDIAC TAMPONADE

Perspective

Although cardiac tamponade resulting from neoplasm is rarely seen in the ED, it is an important clinical problem because it can occur abruptly and result in the death of a patient with a tumor that may be responsive to treatment with a resultant complete remission or significantly prolonged partial remission. The decompensated state of cardiac function results from a marked rise in intrapericardial pressure, which is caused by fluid accumulating within the pericardial sac, a result of malignancy or pericardial thickening with scar formation. This results in a thick constrictive neoplastic encasement. If not recognized and decompressed promptly, neoplastic cardiac tamponade can lead to circulatory compromise and death. Signs and symptoms will partially be affected by the rapidity of development. In the era before diagnostic ultrasound this medical and oncologic emergency was often unrecognized. In one early series before ultrasound, the first physician missed the diagnosis in 11 of 17 patients, and a number of times the diagnosis was missed by more than a single examiner.[36]

In most instances, pericardial effusion is accompanied by signs and symptoms that presage the development of the clinical picture of tamponade, including dyspnea, apprehension, anxiety, and chest pain. In rare instances, tamponade may be the first manifestation of the malignancy, solid tumor, or leukemia. Any patient in the ED with a history of cancer, shortness of breath, and hypotension should be suspected of having pericardial tamponade. The diagnoses of pulmonary embolism, congestive heart failure, and anxiety can be mistakenly made in this setting.

Principles of Disease

The most common cause of neoplastic pericardial tamponade is malignant pericardial effusion, often associated with postirradiation pericarditis, fibrosis, and effusion. Only rarely does a tumor or radiation fibrosis cause a neoplastic constrictive pericarditis with resultant tamponade. In most reported cases, cardiac tamponade represents a clinical progression of neoplastic or postirradiation pericarditis.

Neoplastic pericarditis can result from any number of

benign, malignant, primary, or secondary tumors of the pericardium or mediastinum.[37-39] The most common benign tumors of the pericardium or mediastinum are fibromas, angiomas, and teratomas. Pericardial mesothelioma can have a clinical course characterized by rapid accumulation of massive quantities of bloody pericardial fluid, eventually leading to tamponade. Secondary involvement of the pericardium may result from either direct invasion from structures or metastases from a distant primary tumor. These metastases are usually multiple rather than solitary lesions. The tumors most commonly associated with pericardial involvement include those of the lung and breast, leukemia, Hodgkin's and non-Hodgkin's lymphomas, melanomas, GI primary tumors, and sarcomas.[39,40] Clinically recognizable symptoms or signs of pericardial disease are difficult to appreciate before death. Less than 30% of patients with autopsy-proven malignant pericardial disease were diagnosed antemortem.[39,40]

Radiation pericarditis has been a well-known complication of radiotherapy since the introduction of modern megavoltage techniques. The cardiac effects of radiotherapy may manifest themselves immediately with acute pericarditis or be delayed for months to years, although the majority of patients develop effusion within the first year. The acute forms of pericarditis are inflammatory or effusive, usually self-limited, and subside without residual constriction; the chronic effusive and constrictive types may lead to tamponade and death.[41]

Neoplastic constrictive pericarditis, although rare, may be caused directly by metastatic lesions invading the pericardium or indirectly from radiation therapy complications with resultant fibrous thickening of the pericardium. Each of these entities can progress to cardiac tamponade because of thickening by tumor or radiation fibrosis—resulting in a decrease in the distensibility of the pericardium—thus reaching the critical point of cardiopulmonary decompensation earlier, despite smaller volumes of slowly accumulating effusion.

The symptoms and signs of neoplastic and radiation pericarditis mimic pericarditis from other causes, and because of the usual insidious onset of the effusion of fibrous pericardial thickening, the condition might be attributed to the underlying malignancy and not suspected until the full-blown picture of cardiac tamponade develops.

The severity of cardiac tamponade and eventual cardiopulmonary decompensation depend on the rate of development of pericardial fluid accumulation, the fluid volume, and the tempo of compression of the heart. Clinically the progressive elevation of intracardial pressure interferes with ventricular expansion and results in decreased cardiac volume. There is a rapid rise of intracardial chamber pressures with subsequent transmission of this pressure peripherally in pulmonary and vena caval beds. In an effort to maintain cardiac output, various compensatory mechanisms come into play (tachycardia, peripheral vasoconstriction, decreased renal flow with resultant increased blood volume because of sodium and water retention), all to maintain arterial pressure and venous return. When these compensatory mechanisms fail to maintain cardiac output, ventricular end diastolic pressure increases and subsequent circulatory collapse is impending. The signs and symptoms parallel these pathophysiologic changes. The most common symptoms include extreme anxiety and apprehension, a precordial oppressive feeling, or actual retrosternal chest pain with dyspnea of varying degrees. True orthopnea and paroxysmal nocturnal dyspnea are uncommon, but when they occur the patient assumes a variety of positions to get relief from the chest pain and the dyspnea. Other prominent symptoms include cough, hoarseness, hiccups, and occasional GI manifestations such as dysphagia, nausea, vomiting, and epigastric or right upper quadrant abdominal pain that is probably the result of visceral congestion.[16,39,40,42]

Clinical Features

Patients with severe tamponade are acute ill and may appear ashen, pale, or markedly diaphoretic with an impaired consciousness ranging from mildly confused to unresponsive. Rapid, shallow, and occasionally labored breathing may be present along with peripheral cyanosis and distended jugular veins. Seizures have been reported. Striking facial plethora and a full neck secondary to edema (Stokes collar) have also been seen in SVCS. Pulses are soft and easily compressible. The systolic blood pressure is usually low, with a decreased pulse pressure, although normal systolic, diastolic, and pulse pressures have been reported with moderate degrees of tamponade. Kussmaul's signs (quiet heart sounds, an enlarged cardiomediastinal silhouette, tachycardia, and most notably pulsus paradoxus) are extremely useful findings in the physical evaluation of tamponade. The ED must remember that with significant hypovolemia, atrial septal defect, and aortic insufficiency, pulsus paradoxus may be absent and an unreliable finding. Ascites, hepatomegaly, peripheral edema, and mottling are other findings that reflect elevated venous pressure and decreased cardiac output.[16,39,40,43]

Diagnostic Strategies

Low voltage and the nonspecific findings of pericardial effusion, sinus tachycardia, ST elevation, and nonspecific ST-T wave changes may occur. Electrical alternans with 1:1 total atrial-ventricular complexes has been considered almost pathognomonic of cardiac tamponade. Approximately two thirds of the reported cases of pulsus alternans were in patients with tamponade caused by massive pericardial effusion in neoplastic pericarditis. The alternation customarily disappears soon after removal of a small volume of fluid, but it can also disappear spontaneously or be observed in attendance with a fluid increase.[40]

Radiographic signs of tamponade suggestive of pericardial effusion include an enlarged cardiac silhouette with clear lung fields and normal vascular pattern, although a normal chest radiograph does not exclude tamponade. The typical "water-bottle" appearance of the heart on a plain radiograph is often present. Echocardiography is the simplest and most sensitive of diagnostic tests and can be done at the bedside immediately to confirm pericardial effusion (Figure 117-2). Therapeutic intervention with echocardiographic equipment can then guide the pericardiocentesis. Thoracic CT scanning has also become important in diagnosing pericardial effusions.[40,41]

The diagnosis of cardiac tamponade should be suspected in any cancer patient with dyspnea. Highly suggestive symptoms include clouded sensorium, thready pulse, pulsus paradoxus exceeding 50% of the pulse pressure, low systolic pressure, engorged neck veins with a rising peripheral venous pressure above 130 mm H_2O, a falling pulse pressure below 20 mm Hg, and electrical alternans. This is an uncommon yet pathognomonic sinusoidal variation in QRS size secondary to the pendular effect of the heart swinging in the fluid medium

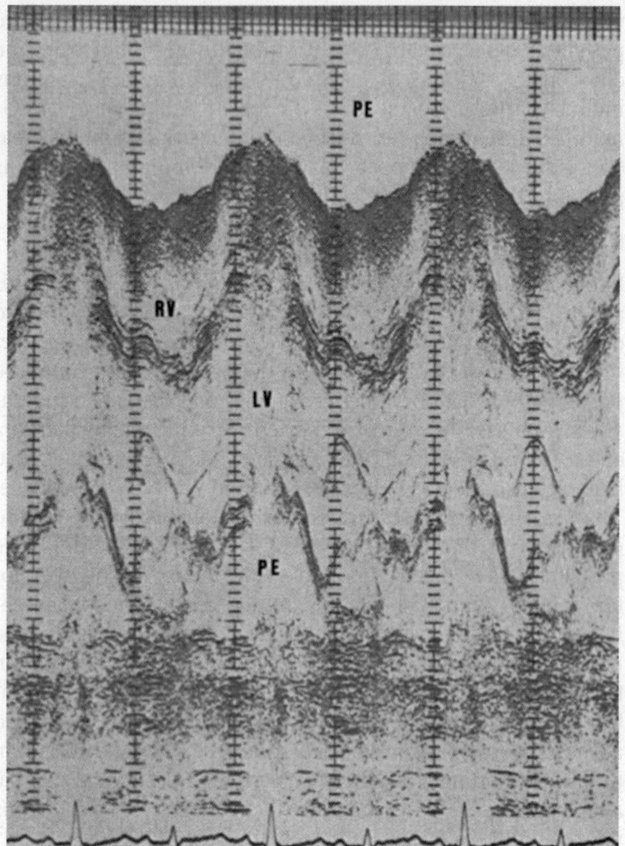

Figure 117-2. **M-mode echocardiogram. Large pericardial effusion (*PE*) is noted anteriorly and posteriorly. Entire heart shows pendular motion with anterior swing coinciding with large QRS complex and posterior swing coinciding with small QRS complex. *RV,* Right ventricle; *LV,* left ventricle. *From Agarwal SK:* J Med Soc NJ *80:198, 1983.***

of the pericardial sac.[43] In this setting, sudden death may occur and pericardiocentesis should be performed as soon as possible.

Management

In the ED, the only effective life-saving treatment for tamponade is immediate removal of the pericardial effusion via pericardiocentesis. The procedure carries some risk, including induction of cardiac dysrhythmias and hemorrhage from an injured coronary vessel. Aspiration of as little as 50 to 100 ml of fluid has been shown to temporarily alleviate the pathologic process.[16,39,40] Removal of the maximum amount of fluid is advisable, along with inserting of an indwelling catheter, during the first pericardiocentesis because fluid may reaccumulate during the first 24 hours. After pericardial fluid has been obtained, it must be sent for biochemical and cytologic analysis. Other types of supportive therapy may be needed during the evaluation process while preparing for pericardiocentesis, such as intravenous hydration with normal saline and oxygen therapy.

After the patient has been stabilized, additional therapeutic interventions should be planned and initiated by the appropriate admitting services because reaccumulation of effusion in neoplastic tamponade is not easily managed on a short-term basis. Pericardial windows, radiotherapy, intrapericardial chemotherapy, and pericardiectomy may be justified.[16,39,40]

The prognosis of neoplastic cardiac tamponade is dependent on the underlying type and extent of cancer. The presence of total electrical alternans is an adverse prognostic sign, even when the alternans disappears with pericardiocentesis. Despite a poor prognosis for patients with cancers such as melanoma or non–small-cell lung cancer, some patients with treatment-responsive lymphomas have had long-term survival after neoplastic cardiac tamponade.

NEUROLOGIC EMERGENCIES

Perspective

Of all patients with cancer, 15% to 20% have neurologic complications.[45] Neurologic symptoms are occasionally the presenting complaint in patients with systemic cancer, but more often symptoms develop in patients known to have cancer. In both settings it is necessary to initiate both an appropriate workup and emergency intervention. Neurologic emergencies in cancer patients include cerebral herniation, seizures, epidural spinal cord compression, CNS infections, and reversible toxic or metabolic encephalopathies. Treatment is needed within minutes to hours after the patient arrives at the ED to prevent permanent neurologic dysfunction or death.

Cerebral Herniation

Principles of Disease Cerebral herniation occurs when the ICP increases locally within the skull from an expanding mass lesion. This produces a shift of brain substance in the direction of least resistance caudally through the tentorial opening and the foramen magnum. Causes of cerebral herniation in cancer patients commonly include primary or metastatic brain tumors and intracerebral hemorrhage. Less common causes include subdural hematoma, brain abscess, acute hydrocephalus, and radiation-induced brain necrosis.[46] Primary brain tumors account for approximately one half of intracranial tumors. Metastatic brain tumors are seen most commonly in lung, breast, colon, kidney, and testicular cancer and in patients with choriocarcinoma and malignant melanoma.[45,47]

Clinical Features Three distinct herniation syndromes have been described: *uncal, central,* and *tonsillar* herniation. In uncal herniation a lateral mass displaces the temporal lobe, which compresses the upper brain stem. A rapid loss of consciousness is seen in conjunction with unilateral pupillary dilatation and ipsilateral hemiparesis. Central herniation usually results from slowly expanding, multifocal lesions that cause a downward and lateral shift of the diencephalon and upper pons. A slowly decreasing level of consciousness, small reactive pupils, and Cheyne-Stokes respiration, without focal signs, are seen clinically. Central herniation is sometimes mistaken for toxic or metabolic encephalopathy because of the lack of focal signs. A history of headache or focal neurologic complaints or any lateralizing findings mandates the acquisition of a CT scan to rule out a herniating mass lesion before lumbar puncture. Tonsillar herniation is produced by a large posterior fossa mass that pushes the cerebellar tonsils through the foramen magnum, compressing the medulla and resulting in a rapidly decreasing level of consciousness, occipital headache, vomiting, hiccups, hypertension, meningismus, and abrupt changes in the respiratory pattern.[45-48]

Management After the clinical diagnosis of cerebral herniation is made, emergency management is mandatory before the cause can be established. Intubation with hyperventilation to a Pco_2 of 25 to 30 mm Hg will lower the ICP by producing cerebral vasoconstriction and may be necessary for brief periods of neurologic deterioration. Excessive or prolonged hyperventilation may cause paradoxic vasodilatation and should be avoided. Mannitol, 1 g/kg IV, should be given and may be repeated in 4 to 6 hours. Dexamethasone, 12 to 24 mg IV, has not been shown to improve outcome or reduce ICP acutely in severe head injury,[49,50] but is often administered in patients with raised ICP or impending herniation caused by CNS malignancy resulting from the effect of corticosteroids on reducing cerebral edema associated with the neoplastic process. A CT scan of the brain should be obtained as soon as emergency stabilization is accomplished. Epidural or subdural hematoma and hydrocephalus usually require surgery, whereas abscess and metastases are usually managed with antibiotics and antineoplastics or radiation, respectively. After stabilization and an initial diagnosis have been made, neurologic or neurosurgical consultation and prompt admission to an intensive care unit (ICU) are mandatory.[45,46]

Seizures

Principles of Disease Seizures are common in patients with cancer. Their immediate management is necessary to prevent physical injury, increased ICP, and risk of aspiration. Seizures increase the brain's metabolic requirements and lead to increased cerebral blood flow. This may precipitate increased ICP in susceptible patients. Seizures may result from brain metastases, toxic or metabolic disturbances (usually hyponatremia or uremia), vascular problems (especially intracerebral hemorrhage or subdural hematomas), and infections. Diagnostic laboratory studies should include a complete blood count, electrolytes, glucose level, blood urea nitrogen (BUN) level, calcium and magnesium levels, liver function tests, arterial blood gas (ABG) counts, coagulation studies, and appropriate cultures. A head CT scan should be done and followed by a lumbar puncture, when indicated.[45,46]

Management The therapy for seizures depends on the specific cause and the patient's clinical status. For example, a single hypoglycemic or hypoxic seizure usually requires only correction of the underlying metabolic defect. Patients with a single seizure whose workup reveals a chronic problem (e.g., a cerebral metastasis) will require anticonvulsants and therapy specific for the malignancy. A loading dose of phenytoin (15 to 18 mg/kg IV) may be given and followed by oral maintenance. Prolonged single seizures or repetitive seizures require more aggressive treatment, including diazepam, 5 to 10 mg IV, or lorazepam, 1 to 2 mg IV, followed by IV phenytoin. Active airway and ventilatory management is essential. A bedside fingerstick glucose level should be obtained immediately. Thiamine and naloxone are not routinely indicated. In addition, when repetitive seizures have occurred, management of the underlying cause should be initiated rapidly and the patient admitted to an ICU.[45,46]

Epidural Spinal Cord Compression

Principles of Disease Epidural spinal cord compression from metastatic cancer is common, serious, and potentially treatable. It is most often caused by lymphoma, lung, breast, or prostate carcinoma. With the exception of lymphoma, which extends through the intervertebral foramina from paravertebral lymph nodes, these tumors metastasize to the vertebral body and extend into the spinal canal to compress the spinal cord. Less common causes of spinal cord compression in patients with cancer include melanoma, myeloma, renal cell carcinoma, vertebral subluxation, spinal epidural hematomas, and intramedullary metastasis. Acute myelopathy in patients with cancer may also be caused by radiation, paraneoplastic necrotizing myelitis, ruptured intervertebral disk, and meningeal carcinomatosis with spinal cord involvement. Most cases (68%) of epidural cord compression occur in the thoracic spine, 15% occur in the cervical spine, and 19% in the lumbosacral spine.[51]

Clinical Features Back pain, either local or radicular, is the initial symptom in 95% of patients with epidural metastasis. It may be acute in onset or develop insidiously over weeks to months and usually predates other symptoms. The pain may increase during physical examination with spinal percussion, neck flexion, Valsalva maneuver, or straight leg raising, and is usually located at the level of the tumor.[51-53] Other symptoms are usually present at the time of diagnosis and may include weakness (75% of patients) and autonomic or sensory symptoms (50% of patients). Fifty percent of patients are not ambulatory at the time of diagnosis. The neurologic examination will usually reveal symmetric weakness with either flaccidity and hyporeflexia (if the diagnosis is made very early) or spasticity and hyperreflexia (if the diagnosis is made later).

Diagnostic Strategies Plain radiographs of the spine should be obtained in any patient with known or suspected cancer who has back pain, either alone or with symptoms of nerve root or spinal cord injury.[45,51,52] Plain radiographic films will show evidence of a tumor in the vertebral body in 70% to 90% of patients with vertebral metastases.[45,53] Immediate myelography or MRI is indicated if the plain films are abnormal, regardless of whether the neurologic examination is abnormal or is consistent with spinal cord compression or what the findings on plain x-ray films are. In cases with questionable findings on plain films of the spine, tomograms, coned-down views, or a CT scan may reveal bony metastases not otherwise appreciated. Myelography can demonstrate a complete or near-complete obstruction of contrast dye flow at the level of vertebral body involvement. MRI has emerged as the procedure of choice for intramedullary metastases and has replaced myelography, which is associated with significant morbidity resulting from lumbar puncture and dye insertion at multiple levels (including cisternal puncture) to demonstrate the length of the compression or skip lesions along the spinal cord.[48,53]

Management

Because minimal weakness at the time of presentation may progress to profound, irreversible weakness over several hours, treatment should be started immediately. In the ED, a loading dose of dexamethasone, 10 to 100 mg IV followed by 4 to 24 mg every 6 hours for 3 days (to reduce cord edema) is initiated at the time of diagnosis and immediate oncology and radiation oncology consultations are obtained. Although corticosteroids are routinely administered to patients with suspected spinal cord compression, high-dose corticosteroids have been associated with complications, and their use is controversial.[53] Radiation treatment is the usual therapy and can be initiated after steroid treatment. The prognosis depends on the radiosensitivity of the tumor, the location of the compression, the pretreatment performance status, and the rate of decompensation. Surgery is indicated only if the diagnosis is in doubt, if a tissue diagnosis is required, if the spine is unstable, or when radiation to the involved area has already been given in maximal doses.[45,47,52]

Intramedullary metastases are similar in presentation and treatment to epidural cord compression but are associated with a very poor prognosis. Epidural hematomas have been described in patients with thrombocytopenia or a coagulopathy as a complication of lumbar puncture. A rapidly progressive paraparesis and back pain are seen. MRI or myelography can establish the diagnosis; the treatment is surgical decompression. Platelet transfusions may limit progression in the ED.[45,52]

Central Nervous System Infections

Principles of Disease Patients with cancer are susceptible to a variety of CNS infections because they may have impaired immune responses secondary to their underlying disease or as a consequence of treatment with steroids, chemotherapy, splenectomy, or irradiation. Most CNS infections occur in patients with leukemia, lymphoma, or head and neck cancer. Patients with head and neck cancer are susceptible (in addition to the reasons discussed previously) because of fistula formation and tumor invasion, which allows organisms access to the CNS. Important CNS infections include meningitis, brain abscess, and encephalitis. These often have similar presentations, making their differentiation in the ED difficult.

Clinical Features Meningitis is characterized by fever, headache, and altered mental status. Meningismus is often absent. The diagnosis of meningitis in patients with cancer is often delayed because the manifestations of the disease are attributed to other processes: fever to systemic infection, headache to cerebral metastases, and altered mental status to a toxic or metabolic encephalopathy.

Diagnostic Strategies All cancer patients with fever and an altered mental status require a lumbar puncture, which should be preceded by a head CT scan if cerebral metastases are suspected.[46,54] In addition, thrombocytopenia and coagulopathy should be considered and either ruled out or treated appropriately with platelet transfusions or fresh frozen plasma, respectively, before a lumbar puncture is done. The fluid obtained should be sent for a cell count and differential cell count, Gram's stain, India ink stain, protein and glucose levels, bacterial and fungal cultures, cryptococcal antigen level, and cytologic examination. The absence of WBCs in the CSF does not rule out meningitis, especially in neutropenic patients. The likely organisms responsible for meningitis vary with the underlying disease and the peripheral WBC count.

Differential Considerations Brain abscess is usually seen in patients with leukemia or head and neck tumors and accounts for 30% of CNS infections in cancer patients.[46] Patients have symptoms of elevated ICP (headache, vomiting, and papilledema), lateralizing findings, and a source of infection.[47,54] Fever is usually present. Head CT scanning will characteristically demonstrate an ill-defined mass early in the course of an abscess with the classic well-defined mass with a low-density center and a contrast-enhancing ring seen later. Edema and mass effect are common. A lumbar puncture is not helpful in making the diagnosis and may precipitate cerebral herniation. Organisms that cause abscess include gram-negative rods, *Aspergillus* and *Phycomycetes* species, and *Toxoplasma gondii.* Emergency management includes high-dosage antibiotics. If herniation develops, immediate steps to reduce the ICP, followed by emergency surgery, are indicated.

Encephalitis is rare in patients with cancer and is most often caused by herpes zoster or *T. gondii.* The presenting complaints are usually headache, fever, and altered mental status. The CT scan is commonly normal, but may show diffuse edema, whereas the lumbar puncture may show pleocytosis with an elevated protein level but no demonstrable organism. It is difficult to distinguish encephalitis from meningitis in the ED, but the overall clinical picture in both diseases mandates hospital admission for further evaluation.

Management When a CNS infection is suspected, broad-spectrum antibiotic coverage should be promptly initiated. A third-generation cephalosporin (ceftriaxone or ceftazidime) and vancomycin is a proper choice. Ampicillin may be added when there is suspicion of *Listeria.* Ceftazidime with or without an aminoglycoside is generally selected when the likelihood of infection with *Pseudomonas* is high. Neutropenic patients (polymorphonuclear WBC count $<1000/mm^3$) with either leukemia or lymphoma usually have a gram-negative infection (often with *P. aeruginosa*). Patients with lymphoma and a normal WBC count are commonly infected with *Listeria monocytogenes, S. pneumoniae,* or *C. neoformans.* Infections with *Haemophilus influenzae* and *Neisseria meningitidis* are uncommon. Patients with head and neck tumors may develop staphylococcal infection.[45-47]

Encephalopathy

Toxic and metabolic encephalopathy should be actively sought when patients with cancer have an acute or subacute altered mental status in the absence of fever or headache. Toxic and metabolic causes should be routinely excluded even when infection or a metastatic complication is suspected. Signs of encephalopathy include confusion, aberrant behavior, and a decreased level of consciousness. These may develop acutely or insidiously over days to weeks. Patients with cancer are particularly susceptible to toxic and metabolic encephalopathy because their disease can have multiple-organ involvement and can cause electrolyte and nutritional abnormalities, and encephalopathy can result from the drugs used to treat the disease (especially chemotherapeutic agents and narcotics).[45,47] In the ED, encephalopathic patients first should be evaluated carefully for a possible infection or mass lesion. The metabolic workup should include electrolytes; BUN, creatinine, glucose, and calcium levels; ABG levels; and liver function tests. Toxicology screens should be considered in possible ingestions and in patients who are unable to give a history. Naloxone and 50% dextrose should be given while the workup is proceeding. Specific treatment is indicated for any abnormalities found during the workup. Hospital admission is usually required unless the cause is easily and rapidly reversible and is unlikely to recur.

KEY CONCEPTS

- Hypercalcemia secondary to malignancy is unrelated to bony metastases in 20% of patients and is associated with a poor prognosis independent of therapeutic response. Hydration and use of bisphosphonates (such as pamidronate) have become the mainstays of initial treatment.
- Spinal cord compression presents as back pain in greater than 95% of patients. If ambulatory at the time of diagnosis, 80% of patients will maintain the ability to ambulate. MRI has become the diagnostic modality of choice, and high-dose dexamethasone is given to all patients and is followed by radiation therapy in most cases.
- Superior vena caval obstruction is rarely life threatening and requires tissue diagnosis. Although caused by malignancy in 70% to 80% of cases, thrombosis secondary to indwelling central lines is increasing as an etiology. Stenting of the SVC has become the approach to SVC obstruction unresponsive to chemotherapy or radiation therapy.
- Fever and neutropenia in the cancer patient represent a true medical emergency requiring rapid diagnosis, cultures, and treatment with broad-spectrum, bactericidal, synergistic antimicrobials. An aminoglycoside plus an extended-spectrum penicillin or third-generation cephalosporin with or without vancomycin remain the standard combinations in patients without penicillin allergy.
- Neoplastic pericardial effusion can present insidiously with symptoms such as apprehension, anxiety, dyspnea, and weakness. Bedside ultrasound has become a rapid, safe imaging modality for establishing the diagnosis before the development of a critically ill patient in clinically apparent tamponade.
- Acute tumor lysis syndrome, previously limited to hematologic malignancies, is now being described in patients receiving chemotherapy for solid tumors. It can present with dyspnea, mental status changes, cardiac dysrhythmia, or seizures. Treatment includes urinary alkalinization and emergency hemodialysis in cases complicated by acute renal failure.

REFERENCES

1. Landis SH et al: Cancer statistics, *CA Cancer J Clin* 48:6-29, 1998.
2. Hughes WT et al: 1997 guidelines for the use of antibiotic agents in neutropenic patients with unexplained fever: the Infectious Disease Society of America, *Clin Infect Dis* 25:551, 1997.
3. Friefeld AG, Walsh TJ, Pizzo PA: Fever and neutropenia. In DeVita VT et al, editors. *Cancer: principles and practice of oncology,* ed 5, Philadelphia, 1997, Lippincott-Raven.
4. Chanock SJ, Pizzo PA: Fever in the neutropenic host, *Infect Dis Clin North Am* 10:777, 1996.
5. Pizzo PA: Management of fever in patients with cancer and treatment-induced neutropenia, *N Engl J Med* 328:1323, 1993.
6. Klastersky J: Empiric therapy for bacterial infections in neutropenic patients, *Cancer Treat Res* 79:101, 1995.
7. Alexander SW, Pizzo PA: Current considerations in the management of fever and neutropenia, *Curr Clin Top Infect Dis* 19:160, 1999.
8. Friefeld AG: Infectious complications in the immunocompromised host, the antimicrobial armamentarium, *Hematol Oncol Clin North Am* 7:813, 1993.
9. Kibber CC: Neutropenic infections: strategies for empirical therapy, *J Antimicrob Chemother* 36(suppl B):107, 1995.
10. EORTC International Antimicrobial Therapy Cooperative Group and the National Cancer Institute of Canada Clinical Trials Group: Vancomycin added to empirical combination antibiotic therapy for fever in granulocytic cancer patients, *J Infect Dis* 163:951, 1991.
11. Yahalom, Yoachim: Superior vena caval syndrome. In DeVita VT et al, editors: *Cancer: principles and practice of oncology* ed 5, Philadelphia, 1997, JB Lippincott-Raven.
12. Parish JM: Etiologic considerations in superior vena cava syndrome, *Mayo Clin Proc* 56:407, 1981.
13. Hunter W: History of aneurysm of the aorta with some remarks on aneurysm in general, *M Obser Aug (London)* 1:323, 1957.
14. Schecter MM: The superior vena cava syndrome, *Am J Med Sci* 227:46, 1954.
15. Adar R, Rosenthal T, Moyes M: Vena cava obstruction: some epidemiological observations in 76 patients, *Angiology* 25:433, 1974.
16. Keefe DL: Cardiovascular emergencies in the cancer patient, *Semin Oncol* 27:244, 2000.
17. Lokich JJ, Goodman RL: Superior vena cava syndrome, *JAMA* 231:58, 1975.
18. Schraufragel DE et al: Superior vena cava obstruction, is it a medical emergency? *Am J Med* 70:1169, 1981.
19. Jackson JE, Brooks DM: Stenting of superior vena cava obstruction, *Thorax* 50 (suppl. 1):531, 1995.
20. Cohen LF et al: Acute tumor lysis syndrome: a review of 37 patients with Burkitt's lymphoma, *Am J Med* 68:486, 1980.
21. Kalemkerian GP, Darwish B, Varterasian ML: Tumor lysis syndrome in small cell lung carcinoma and other solid tumors, *Am J Med* 103:363, 1997.
22. Warrell RP: Metabolic emergencies. In DeVita VT et al, editors: *Cancer: principles and practice of oncology,* ed 5, Philadelphia, 1997, Lippincott-Raven.
23. Pimentel L: Medical complications of oncologic disease, *Emerg Med Clin North Am* 11:407, 1993.
24. Kwaan HC, Bongu A: The hyperviscosity syndromes, *Semin Thromb Hemost* 25:199, 1999.
25. Gertz MA, Kyle RA: Hyperviscosity syndrome, *J Intensive Care Med* 10:128, 1995.
26. Gertz MA, Fonseca R, Rajkumar SV: Waldenstrom's macroglobulinemia, *Oncologist* 5:63, 2000.
27. Anderson KC, Hamblin TJ, Traynor A: Management of multiple myeloma today, *Semin Hematol* 36:3, 1999.
28. Flombaum CD: Metabolic emergencies in the cancer patient, *Semin Oncol* 27:322, 2000.
29. Thomas CR et al: Common emergencies in cancer medicine, *J Nat Med Assoc* 83:815, 1991.
30. Mundy GR, Guise TA: Hypercalcemia of malignancy, *Am J Med* 103:134, 1997.
31. Barri YM, Knochei JP: Hypercalcemia and electrolyte disturbances in malignancy, *Hematol Oncol Clin North Am* 10:775, 1996.
32. Theriault RL: Hypercalcemia of malignancy: pathophysiology and implications for treatment, *Oncology* 7:47, 1993.
33. Body JJ: Hypercalcemia: current and future directions in medical therapy, *Cancer* 88:3054, 2000.
34. Nussbaum SR et al: Single-dose intravenous therapy with pamidronate for the treatment of hypercalcemia of malignancy: comparison of 30-, 60-, and 90-mg doses, *Am J Med* 95:297, 1993.
35. Purohit OP et al: A randomized double-blind comparison of intravenous pamidronate and clodronate in the hypercalcemia of malignancy, *Br J Cancer* 72:1289, 1995.
36. Williams C, Soutter L: Pericardial tamponade: diagnosis and treatment, *Arch Intern Med* 94:571, 1954.
37. Silkey S, Reyes CV: Cardiac tamponade in lung cancer, *J Surg Oncol* 28:201, 1985.
38. Fraser RS, Viloria JB, Wans NS: Cardiac tamponade as a presentation of extracardiac malignancy, *Cancer* 45:1697, 1980.
39. Helms SR, Carlson MD: Cardiovascular emergencies, *Semin Oncol* 16, 1989.
40. Pass HI: Malignant pleural and pericardial effusions. In DeVita VT et al, editors: *Cancer: principles and practice of oncology,* ed 5, Philadelphia, 1997, JB Lippincott.
41. Martin RG et al: Radiation-related pericarditis, *Am J Cardiol* 35:216, 1975.
42. Vaitkus PT, Herrmann HC, LeWinteer MM: Therapy of malignant pericardial effusion, *JAMA* 272:59, 1994.
43. Maguire WM: Mechanical complications of cancer, *Emerg Med Clin North Am* 11:421, 1993.

44. Johnson FE et al: Unsuspected malignant pericardial effusion causing cardiac tamponade: rapid diagnosis by computed tomography, *Chest* 4:501, 1982.
45. DeAngelis LM, Posner JB: Neurologic complications. In Holland JF et al, editors: *Cancer medicine,* ed 4, Baltimore, 1997, Williams and Wilkins.
46. Cascino TL: Neurologic complications of systemic cancer, *Med Clin North Am* 77:265, 1993.
47. Quinn JA, DeAngelis LM: Neurologic emergencies in the cancer patient, *Semin Oncol* 27:311, 2000.
48. Jeyapalan SA, Batchelor TT: Diagnostic evaluation of neurologic metastases, *Cancer Invest* 18:381, 2000.
49. Braakman R et al: Megadose steroids in severe head injury, *J Neurosurg* 58:326, 1983.
50. Dearden NM et al: Effect of high-dose dexamethasone on outcome from severe head injury, *J Neurosurg* 64:81, 1986.
51. Rodichock LD et al: Early diagnosis of spinal epidural metastases, *Am J Med* 70:1181, 1981.
52. Daw HA, Markman M: Epidural spinal cord compression in cancer patients: diagnosis and management, *Cleve Clin J Med* 67:497, 2000.
53. Byrne TN: Spinal cord compression from epidural metastases, *N Engl J Med* 327:614, 1992.
54. Quadri TL, Brown AE: Infectious complications in the critically ill patient with cancer, *Semin Oncol* 27:335, 2000.

Section XI METABOLISM AND ENDOCRINOLOGY

118 Acid-Base Disorders

Jeff D. Disney

Lowry and Brönsted first introduced the concept of an acid-base pair. They defined an *acid* as a substance that can donate a proton (hydrogen ion, H^+) and a *base* as a substance that can accept a proton. Mathematically, an equation can express this relationship as follows:

$$\text{Acid} \leftrightarrow H^+ + \text{Base} \qquad (1)$$

If we rewrite this equation with HA representing the acid and A^- the corresponding base, we obtain the following:

$$HA \leftrightarrow H^+ + A^- \qquad (2)$$

We can further refine this equation and apply a dissociation constant to obtain the Henderson-Hasselbalch equation, as follows:

$$pH = pK_a + \log \frac{[HA]}{[A\bar{v}]} \qquad (3)$$

The Henderson-Hasselbalch equation relates the concentrations of the acid-base pair to the pH. As the pH changes, so does the concentration. Because the equation is based on the logarithm, subtle changes in the serum pH can cause large and often significant alterations in the concentration of the acid-base pair. Clinically, this equation dictates how drugs will disperse, enzymes will react, and medications will bind at a given serum pH.

In humans, H^+ concentration is extremely low (approximately 4×10^{-12} mEq/L) and strictly regulated. This is vitally important because protein and enzyme systems function properly only within a narrow pH spectrum.

Normally, blood is slightly alkalemic relative to water (pH 7.0) with a pH that ranges from 7.36 to 7.44. *Acidemia* is defined as a serum pH of less than 7.36. Conversely, *alkalemia* is defined as a pH of greater than 7.44.

PRINCIPLES OF DISEASE

Changes in serum pH are dealt with by three compensatory systems: (1) the physiologic buffers, (2) the lungs, and (3) the kidneys. One or more of these systems may be involved in the normalization of serum pH.

Physiologic Buffers

Physiologic buffers, defined as a weak acid and its salt, oppose marked changes in pH after the addition of an organic acid or a base, as follows:

$$H^+ + \text{Buffer}^- Na^+ \leftrightarrow \text{Buffer}^- H^+ + Na^+ \qquad (4)$$

The human body uses three important physiologic buffers to minimize surges in pH: (1) the bicarbonate–carbonic acid system (primarily located in red blood cells), (2) intracellular protein buffers, and (3) phosphate buffers located within bone.[1] Patients with malnutrition or chronic disease, and thus low albumin and bone density, and anemic patients have an ineffective buffering capability.

Bicarbonate–Carbonic Acid Buffer System The bicarbonate–carbonic acid buffer system is unique among physiologic buffering systems. The system is open ended; continual removal of organic acid is made possible by the exhalation of carbon dioxide (CO_2). In equilibrium the equation is as follows:

$$H^+ + HCO_3^- \leftrightarrow H_2CO_3 \leftrightarrow H_2O + CO_2 \qquad (5)$$

This buffer system, catalyzed by carbonic anhydrase, is abundant and serves as the major contributor to maintenance of acid-base balance.[2] Clinically, its importance is in the transient buffering of serum and interstitial fluid. It is the primary system to handle the acute load of organic acidemia.

Intracellular Blood Protein Buffers Many protein buffers in blood are effective in maintaining acid-base homeostasis. The most important blood buffer is *hemoglobin,* which can buffer large amounts of H^+, preventing significant changes in the pH.[3] If hemoglobin did not exist, venous blood would be 800 times more acidic than arterial

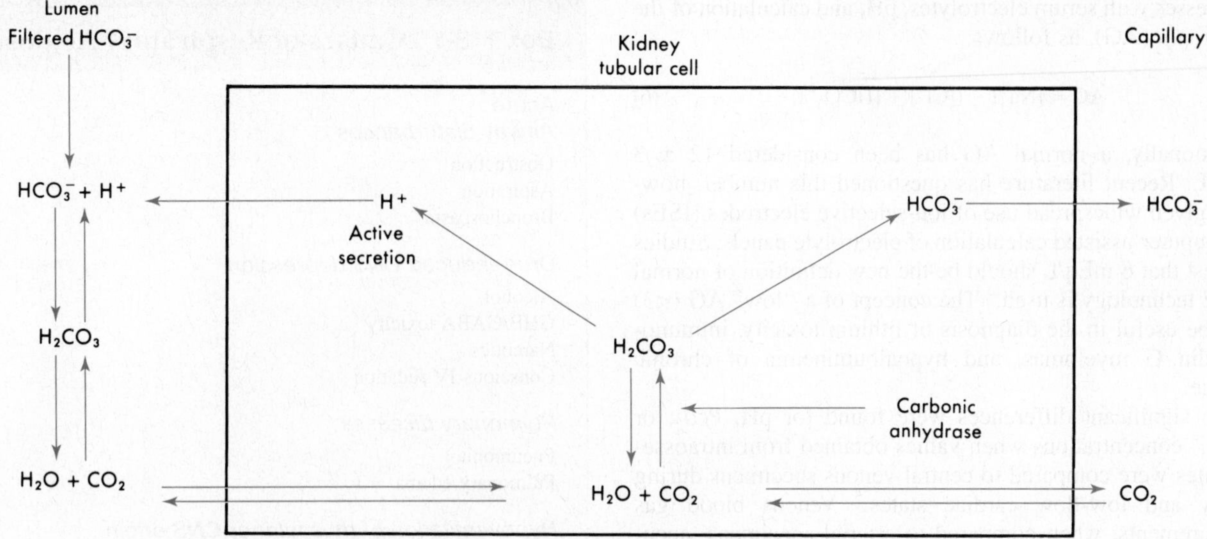

Figure 118-1. **Renal tubular bicarbonate (*HCO_3^-*) and active hydrogen ion (*H^+*) secretion. *H_2CO_3*, carbonic acid.**

blood, circulating at a pH of 4.5 instead of the normal venous pH of 7.37.

Bone as Buffer Bone contains a large reservoir of bicarbonate and phosphate and can buffer a significant acute acid load (see Equations 4 and 5).

Pulmonary Compensation

The second compensatory system for pH changes involves a relationship between the peripheral chemoreceptors, located in the carotid bodies, and central chemoreceptors, located in the medulla oblongata. Both these receptors influence respiratory drive and can initiate changes in minute ventilation. A drop in pH stimulates the respiratory center, resulting in increased minute ventilation. This in turn lowers the partial pressure of arterial carbon dioxide ($Paco_2$), driving the pH toward the normal range. Conversely, an increase in pH decreases ventilatory effort, which increases $Paco_2$ and lowers the pH back toward normal (see Equation 5).

A diabetic patient in ketoacidosis will hyperventilate to compensate for the organic acidemia and would be expected to have a low $Paco_2$. This compensatory response is the expected reaction to a fall in serum pH. In general, compensatory processes will return the pH toward normal but not fully normalize it.

Renal Compensation

The kidneys play little role in the acute compensation of acid-base disorders. More than 6 to 12 hours of sustained acidosis will result in active excretion of H^+ (predominantly in the form of ammonium, NH_4^+) with retention of bicarbonate, HCO_3^-. Conversely, more than 6 hours of alkalemia will stimulate renal excretion of bicarbonate with retention of H^+ in the form of organic acids, resulting in near-normalization of pH (Figure 118-1).

In metabolic acidosis there is either an excess production or infusion of H^+ (e.g., lactic acid production, ketoacid production) or an excessive loss of anion (HCO_3^-) and accompanying sodium and potassium cations (Na^+, K^+) (e.g. diarrhea). In general the kidney attempts to preserve Na^+ by exchanging it for excreted H^+ or K^+. The quantity of potassium excreted depends on the level of acidosis and the serum K^+ level. In the presence of an H^+ load, hydrogen ions move from the extracellular fluid (ECF) into the intracellular fluid. For this to occur, potassium moves outside the cell into the ECF to maintain electroneutrality. In severe acidosis, significant overall depletion of total body K^+ stores can occur despite serum hyperkalemia. Clinically, this is the rationale for initiating intravenous (IV) potassium in the patient with diabetic ketoacidosis, despite an often-elevated serum K^+ level.

In metabolic alkalosis there is a shift of H^+ extracellularly, accompanied by an electroneutral shift of serum Na^+ and K^+ intracellularly. Renal excretion of K^+ also occurs in an attempt to preserve H^+. If the alkalosis continues, the renal compensation may be unable to keep pace, especially if hypokalemia ensues. With excessive excretion of potassium, the kidney paradoxically begins to excrete H^+ in an attempt to retain K^+.

Clinically, an aciduria often exists with a serum alkalosis. This paradoxical aciduria is a clinical clue to the magnitude of hypokalemia. Renal compensation is unable to correct for alkalosis until potassium levels are restored.

Conditions that change serum potassium will also alter serum pH. Excessive diuresis, occurring without potassium supplementation, will generate a mild alkalemia, as H^+ is shifted intracellularly to support the extracellular osmotic movement of K^+. Conversely, excessive administration of potassium can cause H^+ to shift extracellularly, which may produce a mild acidosis.

DIAGNOSTIC STRATEGIES

A stepwise clinical approach to acid-base disorders starts with a good history and physical examination. Particular attention should be paid to the patient's past medical history, current medication or chance of toxic ingestion, occurrence of vomiting or diarrhea, level of consciousness on admission, respiratory rate, skin turgor, and urine output. Evaluation progresses with serum electrolytes, pH, and calculation of the *anion gap* (AG), as follows:

$$AG = [Na^+] - ([Cl^-] + [HCO_3^-]) \quad (6)$$

Traditionally, a normal AG has been considered 12 ± 3 mEq/L. Recent literature has questioned this number, however, given widespread use of ion-selective electrodes (ISEs) in computer-assisted calculation of electrolyte panels. Studies suggest that 6 mEq/L should be the new definition of normal if ISE technology is used.[4] The concept of a "low" AG (<3) may be useful in the diagnosis of lithium toxicity, immunoglobulin G myelomas, and hypoalbuminemia of chronic disease.

No significant differences were found for pH, P_{CO_2}, or HCO_3^- concentrations when values obtained from intraosseous sites were compared to central venous specimens during steady and low-flow cardiac states.[5] Venous blood gas measurements, when compared to arterial specimens, accurately demonstrate the degree of acidosis in adult ED patients presenting with organic acidemia.[6] In infants, capillary tube blood gases are as reliable as formal arterial blood gases (ABGs) in determining hypercarbia or acidosis.[7]

Trauma centers have also been utilizing acid-base calculations to predict the utilization of blood products. The *base deficit* (BD) on admission can be a valuable indicator of shock and the efficacy of resuscitation.[8] In a retrospective analysis of 2954 patients admitted to a level 1 trauma center, blood transfusions within 24 hours of admission were required in 72% of patients with an admission BD less than −6 versus 18% of patients with a BD greater than −6.[9] Some recommend that patients with a BD less than −6 should undergo costly type and crossmatch rather than economical type and screen. Patients with BD greater than −2 should have a specimen drawn but only held.

The *delta gap* (ΔG = deviation of AG from normal − deviation of HCO_3^- from normal) can be calculated to help resolve the possibility of a mixed acid-base disorder or further differentiate an elevated-AG metabolic acidosis.[10] Mathematically refined and with normal values substituted, the equation follows:

$$\Delta G = (\text{Calculated AG} - 12) - (24 - \text{Measured } HCO_3^-) \quad (7)$$

Values greater than +6 equate to either simultaneous metabolic alkalosis or respiratory acidosis. Values less than −6 imply a greater loss of HCO_3^-, suggesting concurrent respiratory alkalosis or rarely a low-AG state.

RESPIRATORY ACIDOSIS

Respiratory acidosis is characterized by increased Pa_{CO_2} and decreased pH. In the acute state the serum HCO_3^- concentration is normal. The transition from acute to chronic respiratory acidosis is defined as the point at which renal compensation manifests as HCO_3^- retention.[11]

Clinical Features

Respiratory acidosis is caused by any disorder that results in a decrease in minute ventilation and thus CO_2 retention. Common causes include pulmonary pathology and conditions that influence respiratory drive (Box 118-1). The clinical picture depends on the severity and chronicity of the process, as well as the underlying disease. Patients with acute respiratory acidosis may have CO_2 narcosis, characterized by headache, asterixis, weakness, tremors, blurred vision, confusion, and somnolence. If prolonged, signs of intracranial pressure elevation with papilledema are manifested.

Box 118-1 Causes of Respiratory Acidosis

Acute

Airway disturbances

Obstruction
Aspiration
Bronchospasm

Drug-induced CNS depression

Alcohol
GHB/GABA toxicity
Narcotics
Conscious IV sedation

Pulmonary diseases

Pneumonia
Pulmonary edema

Hypoventilation of muscular or CNS origin

Myasthenia gravis
CNS injury
Guillain-Barré syndrome

Chronic

Lung diseases

Chronic bronchitis
Chronic obstructive pulmonary disease

Neuromuscular disorders

Poliomyelitis
Myasthenia gravis

Obesity with decreased alveolar ventilation

CNS, Central nervous system; *GHB/GABA,* gamma-hydroxybutyrate/gamma-aminobutyric acid; *IV,* intravenous.

Physiologic Compensation

In acute respiratory acidosis the only effective buffers are the intracellular proteins (Figure 118-2). The HCO_3^- formed by intracellular buffering diffuses out of the cell into the ECF, increasing about 1 mEq/L for every 10–mm Hg rise in the Pa_{CO_2}. In acute situations this HCO_3^- compensation is insignificant and has only minimal effect on the prevailing pH. Profound acidemia develops quickly if ventilation is not improved.

In chronic respiratory acidosis, such as chronic obstructive pulmonary disease (COPD), renal retention of HCO_3^- plays a significant role in acid buffering. The initial response occurs beyond the first 6 to 12 hours and takes several days to reach maximal contribution. Chloride is excreted to maintain electrical neutrality. This results in the characteristic hypochloremia of a chronic respiratory acidosis. Plasma HCO_3^- concentration increases approximately 3.5 mEq/L for every 10–mm Hg increase in the Pa_{CO_2}. This provides excellent compensation and normalizes the pH.

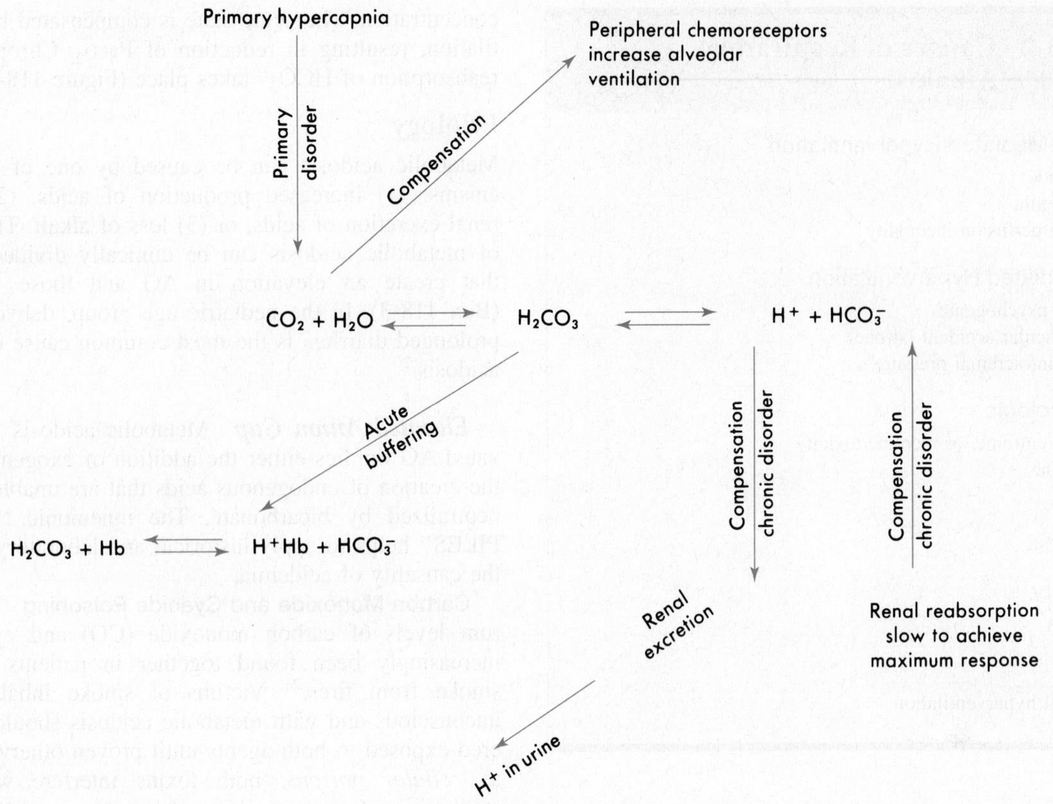

Figure 118-2. **Respiratory acidosis and regulation.**

Management

Therapy of acute respiratory acidosis is directed toward correction of minute ventilation, returning the $Paco_2$ to normal. This may entail establishment of a definitive airway, initiation of artificial respiration, or treatment of an underlying toxic or neurologic condition.

Likewise, improving ventilation treats chronic respiratory acidosis. Bronchodilators (e.g., β_2-agonists, ipratropium), postural drainage, and antibiotics for infection are used to manage the underlying cause. Sensitivity of the respiratory center progressively decreases with prolonged exposure to acidosis and hypercapnia. Consequently, ventilatory drive becomes dependent on relative hypoxemia. Administration of oxygen to these patients will reduce their hypoxic drive and minute ventilation, creating potential CO_2 narcosis. Oxygen must therefore be given with caution to patients with chronic respiratory acidosis. If the patient has severe hypoxemia, however, the EP should be prepared to actively manage airway and ventilation. If assisted ventilation is required, the $Paco_2$ should be lowered slowly to avoid posthypercapneic metabolic alkalosis.[12]

Transient respiratory acidosis is often seen in postictal patients. Respiratory acidosis is the most common acid-base disorder seen acutely in the seizure patient.[13] Treatment centers on control of the seizure activity and assisted ventilation if required. IV bicarbonate use is not recommended because these patients often resolve their acid-base disorder with return of spontaneous ventilation.

In patients with known coronary artery disease, research suggests that acute respiratory acidosis leads to direct vasodilation of coronary vasculature. This is believed to be an instinctive attempt to maintain myocardial blood flow.[14]

RESPIRATORY ALKALOSIS

Increased minute ventilation is the primary cause of respiratory alkalosis, characterized by decreased $Paco_2$ and increased pH. Patients with uncompensated acute respiratory alkalosis have normal plasma HCO_3^- concentration. In chronic respiratory alkalosis, eventual renal compensation results in decreased plasma HCO_3^- concentration.

Etiology

Conditions that lead to respiratory alkalosis are central nervous system (CNS) diseases, anxiety, hysteria, hypermetabolic states, toxicity states, hepatic insufficiency, and assisted ventilation (Box 118-2). Alkalemia of pregnancy (pH 7.46 to 7.50) is primarily respiratory in origin. This change occurs early and is sustained throughout the gestation. A Pco_2 of 31 to 35 mm Hg is considered normal in the antepartum period. Therefore a Pco_2 of 40 in the pregnant woman would represent hypercapnia. Renal compensation leads to an excretion of HCO_3^-. A serum bicarbonate level of 18 to 22 mEq/L in these women is normal.[15]

Respiratory alkalosis may also be a clue to transcutaneous salicylate toxicity.[16] Salicylate poisonings are almost exclusively seen in patients with underlying skin conditions, such as psoriasis and ichthyosis, for which the salicylic acid is used as a keratolytic agent.

Clinical Features

Symptoms vary according to the degree and chronicity of the alkalosis and the associated symptoms caused by the underlying disorder. The symptoms of alkalosis result from irritability of the central and peripheral nervous systems and from increased resistance in the cerebral vasculature. Symp-

Box 118-2 Causes of Respiratory Alkalosis

Hypoxia-Mediated Hyperventilation
High altitude
Severe anemia
Ventilation/perfusion inequality

CNS-Mediated Hyperventilation
Voluntary, psychogenic
Cerebrovascular accident (stroke)
Increased intracranial pressure

Pharmacologic
Salicylate, caffeine, or nicotine toxicity
Progesterone
Pressors

Septicemia

Pulmonary
Pneumonia
Embolism
Edema
Mechanical hyperventilation

toms include paresthesias of the lips and extremities, lightheadedness, dizziness, muscle cramps, and carpopedal spasms identical to those seen with hypocalcemia.[17]

Physiologic Compensation

Acute Alkalosis After the onset of respiratory alkalosis, H^+ ions are secreted from within the cell to the ECF. These H^+ ions reduce the plasma HCO_3^- concentration, attempting to offset the acute alkalosis. During the acute state the plasma HCO_3^- concentration is lowered approximately 2 mEq/L for each 10–mm Hg decrease in the $Paco_2$.[18]

Chronic Alkalosis With persistently low Pco_2, renal H^+ secretion is decreased. Mild hypokalemia often occurs as potassium shifts into the cells while H^+ enters the ECF. Renal secretion of HCO_3^- occurs, and chloride is retained to maintain electroneutrality. This creates the hypokalemia and hyperchloremia characteristic of a chronic respiratory alkalosis. During the first 7 to 9 days, compensation is insufficient to normalize the pH, and alkalemia prevails.[19] Beyond 2 weeks, patients with a chronic respiratory alkalosis will have a normal pH.

Management

Treatment of respiratory alkalosis is directed toward the underlying cause. In the patient with tetany or syncope caused by psychogenic hyperventilating, a rebreathing mask or paper bag allows for CO_2 retention and acid-base normalization. This should be used cautiously and only when other serious conditions (e.g., hypoxia, toxicity, intracranial event) have been eliminated from the differential diagnosis.

METABOLIC ACIDOSIS

Metabolic acidosis is defined as acidemia created by a primary increase in H^+ concentration or a reduction in HCO_3^- concentration. The acute state is compensated by hyperventilation, resulting in reduction of $Paco_2$. Chronically, renal reabsorption of HCO_3^- takes place (Figure 118-3).

Etiology

Metabolic acidosis can be caused by one of three mechanisms: (1) increased production of acids, (2) decreased renal excretion of acids, or (3) loss of alkali. The etiologies of metabolic acidosis can be clinically divided into those that create an elevation in AG and those that do not (Box 118-3). In the pediatric age group, dehydration from prolonged diarrhea is the most common cause of metabolic acidosis.[20]

Elevated Anion Gap Metabolic acidosis with an elevated AG implies either the addition of exogenous acids or the creation of endogenous acids that are unable to be fully neutralized by bicarbonate. The mnemonic "CAT MUD PILES" helps to apply historical and laboratory findings to the causality of acidemia.

Carbon Monoxide and Cyanide Poisoning Elevated serum levels of carbon monoxide (CO) and cyanide have increasingly been found together in patients exposed to smoke from fires.[21] Victims of smoke inhalation found unconscious and with metabolic acidosis should be considered exposed to both agents until proven otherwise. Known as *cellular poisons,* both toxins interfere with cellular respiration at the cytochrome/electron transfer stage. The result is anaerobic metabolism and the generation of organic acidemia.

Acute Alcohol Intoxication and Alcoholic Ketoacidosis Acute alcohol intoxication results in a significant number of ED encounters. Chemically, ethyl alcohol donates its hydrogen ion under physiologic pH. This results in an acute hydrogen ion load and mild metabolic acidosis. When combined with respiratory acidosis due to alcohol's centrally mediated respiratory depression, it becomes evident why many patients with acute ethanol ingestion can present with moderate acidemia.

Alcoholic ketoacidosis (AKA) is a syndrome first described more than 50 years ago.[22] Clinically, AKA presents similar to DKA; however, hyperglycemia and glycosuria are traditionally absent. The onset of AKA is preceded by prolonged, massive ingestion of ethyl alcohol, abruptly terminated because of abdominal pain and vomiting. There is also a component of malnutrition and dehydration. Patients present with AGs in the range of 30 to 35 mEq/L and hypocapnia secondary to compensatory hyperventilation. The ratio of β-hydroxybutyrate to acetoacetate is higher in AKA (approximately 6:1) than in DKA (about 3:1).[23]

Toluene Ingestion Traditionally used as a solvent, toluene has become an inhalational agent abused by teenagers for its euphoric effect.[24] Toluene produces a profound AG acidosis that is further complicated by distal renal tubular damage.[25]

Methanol, Ethylene Glycol, and Paraldehyde The toxic effects of methanol (methyl or wood alcohol) result from the formation of its metabolite, formaldehyde, which is converted to formic acid, contributing to the metabolic acidosis. Ethylene glycol's toxic metabolites are oxalates, aldehydes, and lactic acid; oxalates result in significantly elevated AGs and increased mortality. Paraldehyde poisoning is rare; its use is now restricted to hospitalized patients and patients under

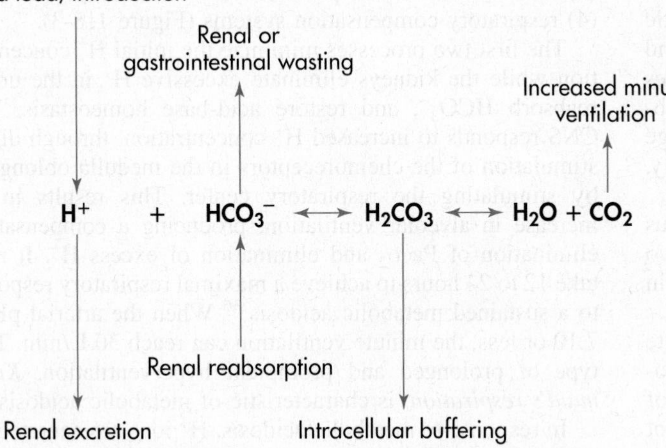

Figure 118-3. Metabolic acidosis and regulation.

Box 118-3 Causes of Metabolic Acidosis

Elevated Anion Gap ("CAT MUD PILES")

Carbon monoxide/Cyanide exposure
Acute alcohol intoxication/Alcoholic ketoacidosis
Toluene exposure
Methanol intoxication
Uremia
Diabetic ketoacidosis
Paraldehyde ingestion
Isoniazid (INH)/Iron intoxication
Lactic acidosis
Ethylene glycol intoxication
Salicylate intoxication

Normal Anion Gap

Gastrointestinal loss of HCO_3^-

Diarrhea
Enterostomy
Ureteroenterostomy

Renal loss of HCO_3^-

Renal tubular acidosis
Acetazolamide

Hyperalimentation

close medical supervision. Ingestion leads to the creation of acetic and chloracetic acids.

Uremia The acidosis in uremic patients results from a failure by the kidney to excrete acids. Hydrogen ion elimination is a direct secretory function of the renal tubules. The ability to excrete NH_4^+, HSO_4^-, and HPO_4^{-2}, however, varies directly with glomerular filtration rate (GFR). Any pathologic process affecting the GFR will increase HSO_4^- and HPO_4^{-2}, resulting in an increased AG. In pure uremia the AG rarely exceeds 25 mEq/L. In the patient with chronic renal failure, increased-AG metabolic acidosis is common. In acute renal failure, however, hyperchloremic, non-AG metabolic acidosis is more common.

In pyelonephritis or obstructive uropathy the acidosis is not related to increased AG because tubular function is affected more than GFR. Increased-AG metabolic acidosis in the patient with elevated serum blood urea nitrogen (BUN) and creatinine levels suggests renocortical disease.

Diabetic Ketoacidosis DKA presents clinically as a triad: hyperglycemia (usually >200 mg/dl), ketonemia (>1:2 dilutions) and acidemia (pH <7.3). DKA can be caused by any condition that reduces insulin availability or activity or that increases glucagon. DKA occurs most often in type I diabetic patients with little or no endogenous insulin; however, its occurrence in type II patients, particularly obese African-Americans, is not as rare as once thought.[26] Increased lipolysis, resulting in the breakdown of free fatty acids, leads to production of ketoacids. Precipitating events usually include infections, surgery, and emotional or physical stressors.

Isoniazid and Iron Toxicity Isoniazid (INH) is a common and potentially lethal medication currently in standard use for the treatment of tuberculosis. EPs must be aware that ingestions of greater than 30 mg/kg pose a danger of not only recurrent seizures but also life-threatening metabolic acidosis.[27] Treatment involves pyridoxine administration to control seizures and hemodialysis to reduce both intravascular drug concentration and acidemia.

Elevated-AG metabolic acidosis from iron ingestion is a direct result of mitochondrial poisoning and uncoupled oxidative phosphorylation. Metabolic acidosis is typically appreciated in phase I of toxicity, usually within 6 hours of ingestion. It becomes quite apparent in phase III, signaling impending hepatic failure and shock. Effective treatment depends on early recognition and administration of deferoxamine.

Lactic Acidosis Lactic acidosis is a marker of hypoperfusion and ongoing shock.[28] A product of anaerobic metabolism, lactic acidosis develops when an imbalance exists between lactic acid production and subsequent conversion by the liver and kidney. Pyruvic acid is metabolized aerobically into CO_2 and H_2O or anaerobically to lactic acid. Lactic acid is then buffered by HCO_3^-, forming lactate. The liver converts 80% of lactate into CO_2 and H_2O and 20% to glucose. This reaction regenerates HCO_3^- in the process and balances the acid-base status.

There are two forms of lactic acid. The "L" form is most common and the traditional form measured when obtaining serum lactate levels. The "D" form has recently gained attention because of an increasing number of patients with small-bowel resection or gastric bypass surgery.[29] D-Lactic acidosis is characterized by episodes of encephalopathy and acidemia. Development of *short-gut syndrome* requires ingestion of a large carbohydrate load, carbohydrate malabsorption with increased delivery of carbohydrates to the large bowel, prominent lactobacilli, diminished colonic motility, and impaired D-lactic acid metabolism.

New medications for human immunodeficiency virus (HIV) have also been shown to induce lactic acidosis. Two patients taking zidovudine developed fatal lactic acidosis in the setting of early hepatic disease.[30]

Initial measurement of metabolic acidosis (serum lactate levels), compared with the traditional carboxyhemoglobin (COHb) levels, might better indicate the severity of COHb toxicity and better predict hyperbaric treatment requirements.[31]

Recent studies support the clinical experience of metformin-induced lactic acidosis. A popular hypoglycemic agent, *metformin* is believed to induce lactic acidosis, especially in the patient with renal insufficiency, by reducing pyruvate dehydrogenase activity and enhancing anaerobic metabolism. The exact mechanism, however, remains unclear.[32]

Treatment of lactic acidosis necessitates elucidation of the underlying cause and initiation of case-specific resuscitation.

Salicylates Salicylates' first toxic effect on acid-base balance results from direct stimulation of the respiratory center, increasing minute ventilation and inducing hypocapnia. In the early presentation of salicylate toxicity, respiratory alkalosis is often the only acid-base disturbance appreciated.[33]

Salicylates may also cause metabolic acidosis by uncoupling oxidative phosphorylation and inhibiting the dehydrogenase enzymes of the Krebs cycle.

Normal Anion Gap Metabolic acidosis with a normal AG is caused by either an excessive loss of HCO_3^- or an inability to excrete H^+ (see Box 118-3). Any condition that causes excessive loss of intestinal fluid distal to the stomach may cause metabolic acidosis. Diarrhea, tube drainage, and skin fistulas, with loss of HCO_3^- rich intestinal, biliary, or pancreatic fluids, are common causes. Ureterosigmoidostomy (surgical insertion of ureters into the sigmoid colon) produces a hyperchloremic acidosis because of loss of HCO_3^- in exchange for the reabsorption of Cl^-.

Patients with renal failure develop an inability to excrete their dietary H^+ load; the severity is proportional to the degree of reduction in the GFR. Those with renal tubular acidosis (RTA) type 1 are unable to secrete H^+ at the *distal* tubule, whereas impairment of HCO_3^- reabsorption at the *proximal* tubule is the defect in RTA type 2. Recent literature suggests that calculation of the *urinary anion gap* (UAG = $[Na^+ + K^+] - Cl^-$) may be helpful.[34] A negative UAG suggests gastrointestinal loss of bicarbonate, whereas a positive UAG suggests altered urinary acidification.

Other causes of normal-AG metabolic acidosis include medications such as pentamidine, amphotericin B, and rifampin. All three can induce renal tubular damage and resultant RTA.[35]

Physiologic Compensation

The body responds to acidemia by utilizing four buffering systems: (1) extracellular bicarbonate–carbonic acid system, (2) intracellular blood protein system, and (3) renal and (4) respiratory compensation systems (Figure 118-3).

The first two processes minimize the initial H^+ concentration while the kidneys eliminate excessive H^+ in the urine, reabsorb HCO_3^-, and restore acid-base homeostasis. The CNS responds to increased H^+ concentration, through direct stimulation of the chemoreceptors in the medulla oblongata, by stimulating the respiratory center. This results in an increase in alveolar ventilation, producing a compensatory elimination of $Paco_2$ and elimination of excess H^+. It may take 12 to 24 hours to achieve a maximal respiratory response to a sustained metabolic acidosis.[36] When the arterial pH is 7.10 or less, the minute ventilation can reach 30 L/min. This type of prolonged and prominent hyperventilation, *Kussmaul's respiration,* is characteristic of metabolic acidosis.

In response to metabolic acidosis, H^+ ions are excreted by the kidney while HCO_3^- is reabsorbed. The rate-limiting reaction (the synthesis of H_2CO_3 from CO_2 and H_2O) is catalyzed by carbonic anhydrase (see Figure 118-1). Therefore, inhibitors of this enzyme can create a metabolic acidosis by preventing the renal excretion of H^+.

The excretion of H^+ requires buffering with HPO_4^- or NH_3, with ammonium playing the largest role. This buffering is called *titratable acidity.* The kidney responds to an increased H^+ load by the augmentation of cellular NH_3 production and consequently NH_4^+ excretion.

In summary, H^+ ions are acutely buffered by extracellular and intracellular mechanisms. However, these mechanisms are not potent enough to correct acidosis sufficiently. Acidemia will stimulate the CNS ventilatory center, and the $Paco_2$ will be reduced secondary to Kussmaul's respiration. With continued and chronic acidemia, the kidneys will secrete H^+ (as NH_4^+ and $H_2PO_4^-$) and reabsorb HCO_3^- in an attempt to neutralize the acidosis.

Management

Initiation of therapy begins with stabilization of the airway, breathing, and circulation (ABCs). In treating patients with metabolic acidosis, primary efforts should be directed at restoring their homeostatic mechanisms. The EP must treat the *patient,* using laboratory markers only as a guide.

Active correction of the pH depends on the severity of the acid-base imbalance, the etiology, the patient's compensatory capabilities, and the potential harm caused by the EP's therapy. Most patients with metabolic acidosis do not require aggressive attempts at pH manipulation. For many the causality is easily discernible, and treatment involves stabilization of homeostatic mechanisms. For example, metabolic acidosis after a seizure resolves within approximately 15 minutes. Rather than administration of sodium bicarbonate ($NaHCO_3$), immediate treatment would involve termination of the seizure activity, maintenance of the airway, and provision for acid-base normalization by ventilatory loss of CO_2.

If IV infusion of an alkaline solution is necessary for the acute management of acidosis, $NaHCO_3$ is the form traditionally chosen. Lactated Ringer's solution, synthetic buffers, sodium citrate, and other solutions have also been used.

Therapy with $NaHCO_3$ has some inherent complications. Bicarbonate penetration into the CNS across the blood-brain barrier is very slow; consequently, intravenous HCO_3^- therapy alkalinizes the plasma much faster than the CNS. As the serum pH increases, the peripheral chemoreceptors will decrease minute ventilation, raising Pco_2 in an attempt to normalize the serum pH. CO_2, which rapidly diffuses across the blood-brain barrier, will rise intracerebrally, and the CNS will become more acidotic despite alkalinization of the plasma. This inverse reaction is referred to as *paradoxical CNS acidosis.* Much discussion surrounds this phenomenon and IV bicarbonate use. Buffer therapy during out-of-hospital cardiac arrest had little to no benefit in one study, regardless of the arterial pH.[37] The only prospective, randomized, controlled study failed to demonstrate any difference between the bicarbonate and control groups.[38]

Because $NaHCO_3$ imparts a significant sodium load on the patient, several low-sodium buffers have been developed. *THAM,* or tris(hydroxymethyl)aminomethane (tromethamine), is a weak organic base with a significantly less sodium load. *Tribonate* is a mixture of THAM, acetate, phosphate, and $NaHCO_3$ and has only one-third the sodium content of normal sodium bicarbonate. Neither agent, however, has proved to be clinically more efficacious than $NaHCO_3$.[39]

Rapid $NaHCO_3$ replacement can result in paradoxical CNS intracellular acidosis, impaired oxygen delivery, hypokalemia, or hypocalcemia. Other complications include "overshoot" alkalosis, hypernatremia, and hyperosmolality. Several bedside formulas are available to assist the EP in determining the adequate dose, such as the following:

$$NaHCO_3 \text{ (mEq)} = 25 - (\text{Measured } HCO_3) \times (\text{Weight [kg]}/2) \quad (8)$$

Once this dose has been ascertained, the EP should replace one-half the calculated $NaHCO_3$ dose initially. Another rule of thumb is to treat patients who have a pH less than 7.1 with 1 mEq/kg.[40] Further $NaHCO_3$ therapy should be determined by patient response and laboratory parameters.

METABOLIC ALKALOSIS

Metabolic alkalosis is produced by conditions that increase HCO_3^- or reduce H^+. This usually requires either the loss of H^+ or the retention of HCO_3^-. The diagnosis requires knowledge of the $Paco_2$ because elevation of the plasma HCO_3^- may be secondary to renal compensation of a chronic respiratory acidosis.

Etiology

Metabolic alkalosis is usually caused by an increase in HCO_3^- reabsorption secondary to volume, potassium, or chloride loss (Box 118-4). Loss of H^+ and Cl^- from aggressive vomiting and nasogastric suctioning can also lead to HCO_3^- retention. Renal impairment of HCO_3^- excretion, especially in the setting of alkali therapy, can lead to a significant metabolic alkalosis.

ECF volume reduction can increase the plasma HCO_3^- concentration when combined salt and water losses occur, typically in patients using diuretics. This state forces a contraction of the ECF around a constant plasma HCO_3^-, creating a relative excess in HCO_3^- concentration; this is known as *contraction alkalosis.*

Metabolic alkalosis can be caused by hypokalemia as H^+ is shifted intracellularly in exchange for the osmotic movement of K^+ extracellularly. There is also an increase in renal H^+ secretion and HCO_3^- reabsorption. The net effect is ECF alkalosis with paradoxical intracellular acidosis, which is easily reversed with potassium therapy.

Primary hyperaldosteronism, hyperreninism, licorice ingestion, Cushing's syndrome, and congenital adrenal hyperplasia are associated with mineralocorticoid excess. This leads to an increased Na^+ reabsorption in the distal tubule with its accompanying H^+ and K^+ secretion to maintain electroneutrality.

Box 118-4 Causes of Metabolic Alkalosis

Volume Contracted (Saline Responsive)

Vomiting
Diuretics
Ion-deficient baby formula
Colonic adenomas

Normal Volume/Volume Expanded (Saline Resistant)

Primary aldosteronism
Exogenous mineralocorticoids
Adenocarcinoma
Bartter's syndrome
Cushing's disease
Ectopic adrenocorticotropic hormone (ACTH)

In patients with chronic respiratory acidosis (e.g., COPD), renal compensation leads to an elevated serum bicarbonate. Acutely correcting the $Paco_2$ by increasing minute ventilation produces posthypercapneic alkalosis and can lead to severe neurologic disorder.[41]

Physiologic Compensation

Although somewhat less predictable, acute compensation of metabolic alkalosis involves the respiratory center, and chronic compensation involves the renal system. Chemoreceptors controlling ventilation respond to an increased pH by inducing hypoventilation, increasing $Paco_2$, and forming H^+. A $Paco_2$ of greater than 55 mm Hg is unlikely to be caused by simple respiratory compensation of metabolic alkalosis.[42] This value should alert the EP to a ventilation disorder complicating the picture.

The kidney has the ability to excrete excess HCO_3^- in the urine. In patients with renal failure, impairment in renal HCO_3^- excretion can sustain metabolic alkalosis.

Management

An EP can easily treat the simple loss of H^+ from aggressive vomiting or nasogastric suction. For more complicated etiologies, however, management can be directed by measurement of the urinary chloride, which helps classify metabolic alkalosis into saline responsive or saline resistant.[43]

Saline-Responsive Alkalosis (Urinary Chloride <10 mEq/L) Treatment is directed toward correcting the urinary excretion of HCO_3^-. Administration of NaCl and KCl suppresses both renal acid excretion and renal HCO_3^- excretion. NaCl and KCl should be considered for patients with mild to moderate saline-responsive alkalosis. In patients who are severely volume depleted, consultation for admission and administration of IV mineral acids (e.g., arginine monohydrochloride) may be necessary. In edematous states for which saline therapy may be contraindicated, acetazolamide will increase the excretion of $NaHCO_3$, treating both the alkalosis and the edema. In renal failure patients, severe metabolic alkalosis should be treated with dialysis.

Saline-Resistant Alkalosis (Urinary Chloride >10 mEq/L) In mineralocorticoid excess, hypokalemia and increased secretion of aldosterone lead to excessive renal excretion of H^+ and a reabsorption of HCO_3^-. Treatment can be successful with potassium replacement by reversing the intracellular shift of H^+. This reduction of cellular H^+ also enhances HCO_3^- excretion. Additional therapy can be directed toward reducing mineralocorticoid activity (e.g., administering spironolactone, an aldosterone antagonist).

MIXED ACID-BASE DISORDERS

Double and triple acid-base disturbances are common. Traditionally, mixed disorders have been difficult to evaluate in the ED.[44] However, recent literature provides some guidelines for ascertaining the mixed disorder and its causes.

Clues to the presence of a mixed acid-base disturbance can either be historical (e.g., polydrug ingestion) or clinical, with varied chemistry and ABG findings that differ from those anticipated. Using the ΔG concept, the EP can determine the mixed disorder, as follows:

$$\Delta G = \Delta AG - \Delta HCO_3^- \quad (9)$$

where

$$\Delta AG = \text{Observed AG} - \text{Upper normal value of AG}$$

$$\Delta HCO_3^- = \text{Lower normal value of } HCO_3^- - \text{Observed } HCO_3^-$$

Values for the ΔG are all gaussian, and therefore the mean value should be near zero.[45] An expected normal range for the ΔG would be 0 ± 6. A positive ΔG (+6 or greater) is almost always caused by high-AG acidosis and a primary metabolic alkalosis. DKA/AKA with severe vomiting, lactic acidosis in the setting of chronic diuretic use, or renal disease with vomiting are clinical examples.

A negative ΔG (−6 or less), on the other hand, can be of varied clinical representation. Most often there is either a mixed high-AG and normal-AG acidosis, or high-AG acidosis with chronic respiratory alkalosis and a compensating hyperchloremic acidosis. Clinically, these patients often have severe underlying metabolic disease with ongoing toxic ingestion (e.g., profound hypermagnesemia, hyponatremia, or hypercalcemia in patients with lithium toxicity)[46] or chronic lung disease, acute lactic acidosis, and furosemide use.[47]

Other algorithms and relationships in these disorders can also assist in rapid interpretation of mixed acid-base disturbances (Box 118-5).

Box 118-5 Relationships in Acid-Base Disturbances

Respiratory Acidosis

Acute

1. HCO_3^- increases 1 (range: 0.25 to 1.75) mEq/L for every 10–mm Hg increase in Pco_2.
2. pH drops 0.08 for every 10-mEq/L rise in HCO_3^-.

Chronic (>5 days of hypercapnia)

HCO_3^- increases 4 mEq/L for every 10–mm Hg increase in Pco_2 (±4).

Limit of compensation: bicarbonate will rarely exceed 45 mEq/L.

Metabolic Acidosis

Note: It may take 12 to 24 hours for maximal respiratory response to develop.

1. $Paco_2 = (1.5 \times HCO_3^-) + 8 \pm 2$.
2. $Paco_2$ is equivalent to last two digits of pH (i.e., if Pco_2 is 20, pH should be 7.20).
3. $\Delta Pco_2 = 1 - [1.3 \times (\Delta HCO_3^-)]$.
4. For pure anion gap acidosis, rise in anion gap should be equal to the fall in bicarbonate concentration (i.e., Δgap should equal 0).
5. For pure non–anion gap (hyperchloremic) acidosis, fall in bicarbonate should be equal to rise in chloride concentration (i.e., Δbicarb = −Δchloride).
   Limit of compensation: $Paco_2$ will not fall below 10 to 15 mm Hg.

Respiratory Alkalosis

Acute

HCO_3^- drops 1 to 3.5 mEq/L for every 10–mm Hg drop in Pco_2.

Limit of compensation: bicarbonate is rarely below 18 mEq/L.

Chronic (renal compensation starts within 6 hours and is usually at a steady state by 1½ to 2 days)

HCO_3^- drops 2 to 5 mEq/L for every 10–mm Hg drop in Pco_2.

Limit of compensation: bicarbonate is rarely below 12 to 14 mEq/L.

Metabolic Alkalosis

1. $Pco_2 = 0.9(HCO_3^-) + 9$
2. Pco_2 increases 0.6 mm Hg for each mEq/L increase in HCO_3^-.
   Limit of compensation: Pco_2 rarely exceeds 55 mm Hg.

KEY CONCEPTS

- Traditionally, a normal AG has been considered 12 ± 3 mEq/L. Recent data suggest that 6 mEq/L should be considered normal if the latest laboratory technology is used.
- The magnitude of the *base deficit* (BD) can be a valuable indicator of shock and the efficacy of resuscitation.
- During acute alkalosis, the plasma HCO_3^- concentration is lowered approximately 2 mEq/L for each 10–mm Hg decrease in the $Paco_2$.
- Contraction alkalosis can result from extracellular volume reduction, with a consequent increase in the plasma HCO_3^- concentration, when combined salt and water losses occur. This typically occurs in patients using diuretics.
- The body responds to acidemia by utilizing four buffering systems: (1) extracellular bicarbonate–carbonic acid system, (2) intracellular blood protein system, and (3) renal and (4) respiratory compensation systems.
- Metabolic acidosis can be caused by one of three mechanisms: (1) increased production of acids, (2) decreased renal excretion of acids, or (3) loss of alkali. The etiologies of metabolic acidosis can be clinically divided into those that create an elevation in the anion gap and those that do not.

REFERENCES

1. Williamson JC: Acid-base disorders: classification and management strategies, *Am Fam Pract* 52:584, 1995.
2. Narins RG, Emmett M: Simple and mixed acid-base disorders: a practical approach, *Medicine* 59:161, 1980.

3. Peters JP, Van Slyke DD: *Hemoglobin and oxygen: carbonic acid and acid-base balance,* Baltimore, 1931, Williams & Wilkins.
4. Jurado R et al: Low anion gap, *South Med J* 91:624, 1998.
5. Kissoon N et al: Comparison of the acid-base status of blood obtained from intraosseous and central venous sites during steady and low-flow states, *Crit Care Med* 21:1765, 1993.
6. Brandenburg MA: Comparison of arterial and venous blood gas values in the initial emergency department evaluation of patients with diabetic ketoacidosis, *Ann Emerg Med* 31:459, 1998.
7. Harrison AM et al: Comparison of simultaneously obtained arterial and capillary blood gases in pediatric intensive care unit patients, *Crit Care Med* 25:1904, 1997.
8. Davis JW, Shackford SR, Hollbrook TL: Base deficit as a sensitive indicator of compensated shock and tissue oxygen utilization, *Surg Gynecol Obstet* 173:473, 1991.
9. Davis JW et al: Admission base deficit predicts transfusion requirements and risk of complications, *J Trauma* 41:769, 1996.
10. Salem MM, Mujais SK: Gaps in the anion gap, *Arch Intern Med* 152:1625, 1992.
11. Narins RG, Emmett M: Simple and mixed acid-base disorders: a practical approach, *Medicine* 59:161, 1980.
12. Kassirer JP: Serious acid-base disorders, *N Engl J Med* 291:773, 1974.
13. Wijdicks EF, Hubmayr RD: Acute acid-base disorders associated with status epilepticus, *Mayo Clin Proc* 69:1044, 1994.
14. Kazmaier S et al: Effects of respiratory alkalosis and acidosis on myocardial blood flow and metabolism in patients with coronary artery disease, *Anesthesiology* 89:831, 1998.
15. Landon M: Acid-base disorders during pregnancy, *Clin Obstet Gynecol* 37:16, 1994.
16. Chiaretti A et al: Salicylate intoxication using a skin ointment, *Acta Paediatr* 86:330, 1997.
17. Saltzman H, Heyman A, Seigker HO: Correlation of clinical and physiological manifestations of sustained hyperventilation, *N Engl J Med* 268:1431, 1963.
18. Arbus GS et al: Characterization and clinical application of the "significance band" for acute respiratory alkalosis, *N Engl J Med* 280:117, 1969.
19. Gledhill N, Beirne GJ, Dempsey JA: Renal response to short-term hypocapnia in man, *Kidney Int* 8:376, 1975.
20. Chabli R: Diagnostic use of anion and osmolal gaps in pediatric emergency medicine, *Pediatr Emerg Care* 13:204, 1997.
21. Baud FJ et al: Elevated blood cyanide concentrations in victims of smoke inhalation, *N Engl J Med* 325:1761, 1991.
22. Cooperman MT et al: Clinical studies of alcoholic ketoacidosis, *Diabetes* 23:433, 1974.
23. McGarry JD, Foster DW: Diabetic ketoacidosis. In Rifkin H, Raskin P, editors: *Diabetes Mellitus,* American Diabetic Association. 5:185, 1981.
24. Ellenhorn M et al, editors: Inhalant abuse. In *Medical toxicology: diagnosis and treatment of human poisoning,* ed 2, Baltimore, 1997, Williams & Wilkins.
25. Kamijima M et al: Metabolic acidosis and renal tubular injury due to pure toluene inhalation, *Arch Environ Health* 49:410, 1994.
26. Kitabchi A, Wall BM: Management of diabetic ketoacidosis, *Am Fam Physician* 60:455, 1999.
27. Romero J, Kuczler F: Isoniazid overdose: recognition and management, *Am Fam Physician* 57:749, 1998.
28. Bernardin G et al: Blood pressure and arterial lactate levels are early indicators of short-term survival in human septic shock, *Intensive Care Med* 22:17, 1996.
29. Uribarri J, Oh MS, Carrol HJ: D-lactic acidosis: a review of clinical presentation, biochemical features and pathophysiologic mechanisms, *Medicine* 77:73, 1998.
30. Sundar K et al: Zidovudine induced fatal lactic acidosis and hepatic failure in patients with acquired immunodeficiency syndrome: a case report of two patients, *Crit Care Med* 25:1425, 1997.
31. Turner M, Esaw M, Clark RJ: Carbon monoxide poisoning treated with hyperbaric oxygen: metabolic acidosis as a predictor of treatment requirements, *J Accid Emerg Med* 16:96, 1999.
32. Hulisz DT, Bonfiglio MF, Murray RD: Metformin associated lactic acidosis, *J Am Board Fam Pract* 11:233, 1998.
33. Kreisberg RA, Wood BC: Drug and chemical induced metabolic acidosis, *Clin Endocrinol Metab* 12:391, 1983.
34. Batlle DC et al: The use of the urinary anion gap in the diagnosis of hyperchloremic metabolic acidosis, *N Engl J Med* 318:594, 1988.
35. Perazella M, Brown E: Electrolyte and acid-base disorders associated with AIDS, *J Gen Intern Med* 9:232, 1994.
36. Pierce NF et al: The ventilatory response to acute base deficit in humans: time course during development and correction of metabolic acidosis, *Ann Intern Med* 72:633, 1970.
37. Dybvik T, Strand T, Steen PA: Buffer therapy during out-of-hospital cardiopulmonary resuscitation, *Resuscitation* 29:89, 1995.
38. Levy MM: An evidence-based evaluation of the use of sodium bicarbonate during cardiopulmonary resuscitation, *Crit Care Clin* 14:457, 1998.
39. Offenstandt G: Alkali therapy in the treatment of acute metabolic acidosis, *Minerva Anestesiol* 65:202, 1999.
40. Cummins R et al: *Advanced cardiac life support, 1997-1999,* Dallas, 1997, Scientific Publishing.
41. Rotherman EB Jr, Safar P, Robin ED: CNS disorder during mechanical ventilation in chronic pulmonary disease, *JAMA* 189:993, 1964.
42. Weinberger SE, Schwartzstein RM, Weiss JW: Hypercapnia, *N Engl J Med* 321:1223, 1989.
43. Schrier RW, editor: *Renal and electrolyte disorders,* ed 4, Boston, 1992, Little, Brown.
44. Schreck DM, Zacharias D, Grunau CF: Diagnosis of complex acid-base disorders: physician performance versus the microcomputer, *Ann Emerg Med* 15:164, 1986.
45. Wrenn K: The delta gap: an approach to mixed acid-base disorders, *Ann Emerg Med* 19:1310, 1990.
46. Emmett M, Narins RG: Clinical use of the anion gap, *Medicine* 56:38, 1977.
47. Turino GM, Golding RM, Heinemann HO: Renal response to mechanical ventilation in patients with chronic hypercapnia, *Am J Med* 56:151, 1974.

119 Electrolyte Disturbances

Michael A. Gibbs
Allan B. Wolfson
Vivek S. Tayal

PERSPECTIVE

Abnormalities of serum electrolyte levels generally cannot be diagnosed by the history and physical examination alone. Severe electrolyte disturbances can be fatal, however, and some disorders may produce no symptoms or nonspecific clinical manifestations until life-threatening effects occur.

SODIUM

Normal Physiology

Water makes up approximately 60% of body weight and is distributed in three compartments: the intracellular space (ICS), the interstitial space (ISS), and the intravascular space (IVS). The ICS makes up approximately two thirds of total body water, with the remaining one third in the ISS and IVS. The concentration of sodium, the predominant extracellular cation, governs the movement of water among these three compartments. When the extracellular sodium concentration decreases, water shifts to the ICS to restore osmotic equilibrium. When the extracellular sodium concentration rises, water shifts out of the ICS. Under normal conditions sodium leaks passively into cells down a concentration gradient and is transported back out of the cell by the sodium-potassium, adenosine triphosphatase (Na^+-K^+ ATPase) pump.

Sodium homeostasis and water balance are under the hormonal regulation of the renin-angiotensin system and antidiuretic hormone, respectively. *Renin,* an enzyme produced by the kidney, is released in response to decreases in circulating intravascular volume. Renin catalyzes the production of *angiotensin I,* which is then converted to angiotensin II in the lung. *Angiotensin II* stimulates the production of aldosterone, a mineralocorticoid hormone produced by the zona glomerulosa of the adrenal glands. *Aldosterone* enhances sodium reabsorption and potassium excretion in the distal nephron.

Antidiuretic hormone (ADH, vasopressin, arginine vasopressin) is synthesized in the hypothalamus and secreted from the posterior pituitary. ADH is released primarily in response to rises in serum osmolality, but also to decreases in intravascular volume or arterial pressure. Volume depletion is the most potent stimulus for ADH production, and with decreases in plasma volume, ADH may be secreted even in the face of hypotonicity. ADH enhances renal water reabsorption by increasing tubular water permeability. Other factors that may stimulate ADH release include angiotensin, catecholamines, opiates, caffeine, stress, hypoglycemia, and hypoxia.

Hyponatremia

Principles of Disease Hyponatremia is defined as a serum sodium concentration of less than 135 mEq/L. Hyponatremia can be classified into three categories based on the patient's clinical volume status: (1) hypovolemic hyponatremia, (2) euvolemic hyponatremia, and (3) hypervolemic hyponatremia (Box 119-1). When assessing the patient with a low serum sodium, it is also important to consider the possibility of sampling errors (e.g., phlebotomy from a venous site proximal to an infusion of hypotonic solution), as well as pseudohyponatremia and redistributive hyponatremia.

Pseudohyponatremia Pseudohyponatremia refers to a falsely low serum sodium measurement in patients whose plasma contains excessive protein or lipid. Relative percentage of water in plasma is reduced. Flame photometry, which determines sodium content per unit of plasma, shows an artifactually low sodium level, although both the total sodium content and serum osmolarity remain within the normal range. Measurement of the serum sodium by direct potentiometry avoids this problem.[1]

Redistributive Hyponatremia Redistributive hyponatremia is caused by osmotically active solutes in the extracellular space that draw water from the cell, diluting the serum sodium concentration. Common situations causing such hyperosmolar states include hyperglycemia (e.g., diabetic keotoacidosis) and parenteral administration of mannitol or glycerol for the management of intracranial hypertension or glaucoma. The measured serum sodium in patients with hyperglycemia can be corrected by adding approximately 1.6 mEq/L for every 100-mg/dl rise in the serum glucose over 100 mg/dl.

Hypovolemic Hyponatremia Hypovolemic hyponatremia results from the loss of water and sodium with a greater relative loss of sodium. Typical causes include vomiting, diarrhea, gastrointestinal (GI) suction or drainage tubes, fistulas, and "third spacing" of fluids (e.g., burns, intraabdominal sepsis, bowel obstruction, pancreatitis). Causes specifically attributable to renal losses include diuretic use, mineralocorticoid deficiency, renal tubular acidosis, and salt-wasting nephropathy. When sodium losses are sufficient to decrease glomerular filtration rate (GFR) significantly, the amount of filtrate delivered to the loop of Henle (where free water is generated) is decreased, and little free water appears in the urine. Also, because ADH is released in response to intravascular volume deficits despite hypotonicity, hyponatremia may be maintained even in patients whose GFR would otherwise be adequate to excrete excess free water. Hypovolemic hyponatremia can also be worsened when fluid losses are replaced with hypotonic fluids.

Euvolemic Hyponatremia The many causes of euvolemic hyponatremia include the *syndrome of inappropriate secretion of ADH* (SIADH), defined as the secretion of ADH in the absence of an appropriate physiologic stimulus. Its hallmark is an inappropriately concentrated urine despite the presence of a low serum osmolality and a normal circulating blood volume. Causes of SIADH include central nervous

Box 119-1 Causes of Hyponatremia

Sampling Error

Pseudohyponatremia
Hyperlipemia
Hyperproteinemia

Redistributive Type
Hyperglycemia
Mannitol

Hypovolemic Type
Renal losses
GI losses
Third-space losses
Excessive sweating
Addison's disease

Euvolemic Type
SIADH
Psychogenic polydipsia

Hypervolemic Type
Congestive heart failure
Hepatic cirrhosis
Nephrotic syndrome

SIADH, Syndrome of inappropriate secretion of antidiuretic hormone.

system (CNS) disorders, pulmonary disease, drugs, stress, pain, and surgery (Box 119-2). Before the diagnosis of SIADH can be confirmed, other potential causes of euvolemic hyponatremia (e.g., hypoadrenalism, hypothyroidism, renal failure) should be ruled out. *Psychogenic polydipsia* is a rare cause of euvolemic hyponatremia. This is most often seen in patients with psychiatric disorders who consume large volumes of water, usually in excess of 1 L/hr, overwhelming the capacity of the kidneys to excrete free water in the urine.[2] In contrast to SIADH, the urine in patients with psychogenic polydipsia is maximally dilute.

Hypervolemic Hyponatremia Hypervolemic hyponatremia results when sodium is retained but retention of water exceeds that of sodium. This is seen in edematous states such as congestive heart failure (CHF), hepatic cirrhosis, and renal failure. In these conditions, decreased effective renal perfusion causes the secretion of both ADH and aldosterone. This leads to increased tubular reabsorption of both sodium and water, decreased delivery of water to the distal nephron, and inability to produce hypotonic urine.

Clinical Features The signs and symptoms of hyponatremia depend on the rapidity with which the serum sodium concentration declines, as well as on its absolute level. The acutely hyponatremic patient is almost always symptomatic when the serum sodium falls below 120 mEq/L, whereas patients with chronic hyponatremia may tolerate much lower levels. Very young and very old patients typically develop symptoms with lesser decreases in the serum sodium level.

The primary symptoms of hyponatremia are related to the CNS, including lethargy, apathy, confusion, disorientation, agitation, depression, and psychosis. Focal neurologic deficits, ataxia, and seizures have been reported.[3] Other nonspecific signs and symptoms include muscle cramps, anorexia, nausea, and weakness.

Box 119-2 Causes of SIADH

CNS Disease
Brain tumor, infarction, injury, or abscess
Meningitis
Encephalitis

Pulmonary Disease
Pneumonia
Tuberculosis
Lung abscess
Pulmonary aspergillosis

Drugs
Exogenous vasopressin
Diuretics
Chlorpropamide
Vincristine
Thioridazine
Cyclophosphamide

Diagnostic Strategies The urinary sodium concentration can be a useful tool in the assessment of the patient with hyponatremia. Patients with hypovolemic hyponatremia caused by renal sodium wasting typically have an inappropriately high urinary sodium concentration (>20 mEq/dl); those with extrarenal sodium wasting and intact renal sodium-conserving mechanisms have a low urinary sodium concentration (<10 mEq/L). Patients with euvolemic hyponatremia generally have a urinary sodium concentration greater than 20 mEq/L. Patients with hypervolemic hyponatremia caused by CHF or cirrhosis typically have a concentration below 10 mEq/L, and those with renal failure have a concentration above 20 mEq/L.[4]

Management Because tolerance for hyponatremia is highly variable, treatment should be guided by the severity of symptoms, the estimated duration of illness, and the patient's volume status rather than by the serum level alone. Severe neurologic dysfunction and seizures are an indication for immediate treatment. Patients with signs of shock or symptomatic fluid overload also require rapid intervention. Because individuals with acute hyponatremia typically develop more prominent symptoms than those with chronic hyponatremia and are more tolerant of rapid correction of sodium deficits, aggressive treatment is a reasonable goal in these patients. In contrast, patients with chronic hyponatremia are usually less symptomatic and are more susceptible to complications when the serum sodium is corrected rapidly, making aggressive treatment both less necessary and less desirable.

Hypovolemic Hyponatremia Patients with hypovolemic hyponatremia should have volume deficits corrected with isotonic NaCl (0.9%). Isotonic saline is hypertonic compared with the hyponatremic patient's serum and will therefore cause a modest elevation of the serum sodium concentration.

Euvolemic Hyponatremia Patients with hyponatremia and a normal total circulating volume can usually have free water intake restricted while the etiology of the hyponatremia is determined and specific treatment for the underlying disorder is begun. Significantly, patients with SIADH who are given normal saline may actually experience a further decrease in the serum sodium as free water is retained and a hypertonic urine is excreted. Lithium and demeclocycline, which inhibits the action of ADH, can also be used in the treatment of SIADH.

Hypervolemic Hyponatremia The cornerstone of therapy for patients with hypervolemic hyponatremia is fluid restriction, which is effective in most patients. The addition of diuretics may accelerate water excretion, although this approach should be used with caution because sodium excretion is also enhanced. Dialysis may be required to remove large amounts of water in patients with advanced renal failure.

Symptomatic Hyponatremia Patients with severely symptomatic hyponatremia may require administration of 3% NaCl (513 mEq of Na^+/L). The rate of correction of hyponatremia should be dictated by the rapidity of its onset. Acute hyponatremia may be corrected at rates of up to 1 to 2 mEq/L/hr, and chronic hyponatremia should be corrected at a rate not greater than 0.5 mEq/L/hr. In general the serum sodium should not be corrected to above 120 mEq/L or increased by more than 10 mEq/L in a 24-hour period. Hypertonic saline should be administered through a controlled intravenous (IV) infusion, with careful attention to fluid input and output and frequent assessment of serum electrolytes. The approximate required dose of hypertonic saline can be calculated with the following formula:

$$(\text{Desired } [Na^+] - \text{Measured } [Na^+]) \times (0.6)\ (\text{Weight in kilograms}) = \text{mEq } [Na^+] \text{ administered}$$

Overaggressive correction of the serum sodium may have serious consequences. *Central pontine myelinolysis* (CPM), also known as cerebral demyelination, involves the destruction of myelin in the pons and is thought to result from rapid elevation of the serum sodium. Patients may develop cranial nerve palsies, quadriplegia, or coma. CPM is more likely to occur in patients with chronic hyponatremia than in those with acute hyponatremia. Most cases have been associated with rapid correction of serum sodium in alcoholic, malnourished, and elderly patients, although it has also been described in otherwise healthy patients.

Hypernatremia

Principles of Disease Hypernatremia is defined as serum sodium concentration above 145 mEq/L. Patients at the extremes of age and those with chronic disorders are particularly vulnerable.[5] Hypernatremia is most often the result of a decrease in free water, because of either reduced water intake or increased water loss. Less often, hypernatremia is caused by an increase in total sodium (Box 119-3). This classification scheme helps in identifying the underlying cause and guiding therapy.

Reduced water intake may be the result of limited access, inability to tolerate oral fluids, defective thirst mechanisms, or depressed mentation.

Increased water loss may occur through several different organ systems, including the GI tract, skin, respiratory tract, or kidney. GI losses may occur from protracted diarrhea, vomiting, nasogastric tube suction, or third spacing. Renal causes of water loss include osmotic diuresis (e.g., hyperglycemia, mannitol administration) and renal tubular concentrating defects. *Diabetes insipidus* (DI) results in the loss of large amounts of dilute urine from the loss of concentrating ability in the distal nephron. DI may be *central* (lack of ADH secretion from the pituitary) or *nephrogenic* (lack of responsiveness to circulating ADH) (Box 119-4). Central DI is seen with CNS disease or surgery involving the hypothalamus and pituitary. Common mechanisms include stroke, infection, tumor, trauma, and systemic diseases. Nephrogenic DI may be caused by congenital disease, renal failure, sickle cell anemia, hypercalcemia, hypokalemia, and certain drugs, including lithium, cisplatin, amphotericin B, aminoglycosides, and demeclocycline. With a normal thirst mechanism and access to water, DI patients are generally able to maintain near-normal serum levels.[6,7] However, they quickly become hypernatremic when removed from a water source, and any sodium-containing IV fluids will exacerbate the problem.

Excessive sodium intake, accidentally, intentionally, or iatrogenically, may cause hypernatremia in the absence of corresponding intake of water. Because the kidney can usually excrete an increased sodium load effectively, most cases are seen in patients with renal insufficiency. Examples include hypertonic enteral or parenteral nutritional fluids, saline absorption, administration of large amounts of sodium

Box 119-3 Causes of Hypernatremia

I. Reduced water intake
   - A. Disorders of thirst perception
   - B. Inability to obtain water
     1. Depressed mentation
     2. Intubated patient

II. Increased water loss
   - A. Gastrointestinal
     1. Vomiting, diarrhea
     2. Nasogastric suctioning
     3. Third spacing
   - B. Renal
     1. Tubular concentrating defects
     2. Osmotic diuresis (e.g., hyperglycemia, mannitol)
     3. Diabetes insipidus
     4. Relief of urinary obstruction
   - C. Dermal
     1. Excessive sweating
     2. Severe burns
   - D. Hyperventilation

III. Gain of sodium
   - A. Exogenous sodium intake
     1. Salt tablets
     2. Sodium bicarbonate
     3. Hypertonic saline solutions
     4. Improper formula preparation
     5. Salt water drowning
     6. Hypertonic renal dialysate
   - B. Increased sodium reabsorption
     1. Hyperaldosteronism
     2. Cushing's disease
     3. Exogenous corticosteroids
     4. Congenital adrenal hyperplasia

Box 119-4 Causes of Diabetes Insipidus

Central
Idiopathic
Head trauma
Suprasellar/infrasellar tumors (e.g., craniopharyngioma)
Cerebral hemorrhage
CNS infections (e.g., meningitis, encephalitis)
Granulomatous disorders (e.g., tuberculosis, sarcoid, Wegener's, histiocytosis)

Nephrogenic
Congenital renal disorders
Obstructive uropathy
Renal dysplasia
Polycystic disease

Systemic Disease with Renal Involvement
Sickle cell disease
Sarcoidosis
Amyloidosis

Drugs
Amphotericin B
Phenytoin
Lithium
Aminoglycosides
Methoxyflurane

bicarbonate, seawater drowning, and salt ingestion.[6] The administration of ticarcillin and carbenicillin, which contain large amounts of sodium chloride, is another potential cause.

Clinical Features In hypernatremia, free water is lost in excess of sodium, so patients may be significantly dehydrated before signs of volume depletion are evident. Total free water deficits are often underestimated in this setting. Common symptoms include anorexia, nausea, vomiting, fatigue, and irritability.[3] Physical findings may include lethargy, confusion, stupor, coma, muscle twitching, hyperreflexia, spasticity, tremor, ataxia, or focal findings such as hemiparesis or extensor plantar reflexes.

Management

Hypovolemic Hypernatremia The primary goals in the emergency management of hypovolemic hypernatremia are to restore volume deficits and to maintain organ perfusion. Treatment should be initiated with an infusion of isotonic solution (0.9% NaCl). Once the patient is hemodynamically stable, the remaining free water deficits can be replaced.

Euvolemic Hypernatremia Euvolemic hypernatremic patients may have had either hypotonic fluid losses (e.g., with DI) or hypertonic fluid losses from increased insensible fluid loss. Patients with DI generally have a low urine specific gravity (<1.005) and low urine osmolality. The DI is usually the result of a previously recognized disorder, and patients can usually maintain their serum osmolality if they have access to water. Treatment is with oral fluids or 0.45% saline. Patients with central DI require parenteral or intranasal vasopressin. The response to vasopressin may be monitored by checking urine osmolality, urine specific gravity, and serum electrolytes.[7]

Hypervolemic Hypernatremia The treatment of hypervolemic hypernatremia should focus on increasing renal sodium excretion while maintaining free water intake. A strategy of diuretic administration (e.g., furosemide) followed by infusion of hypotonic fluids will gradually restore the serum sodium to the normal range. Dialysis may be needed for patients with renal failure.

Symptomatic Hypernatremia Patients with acute hypernatremia usually tolerate rapid correction of free water deficits. On the other hand, aggressive treatment of chronic hypernatremia with hypotonic fluids may result in life-threatening complications. It is recommended that in this setting free water deficits be corrected over at least a 48-hour period. When hypernatremia develops over days, brain cells produce osmotic substances (*idiogenic osmoles*) that hold water in the cell and help maintain cellular volume and tonicity.[6] Overzealous administration of hypotonic fluids may cause rapid shifts of water into brain cells, cellular swelling, and cerebral edema.

Assuming only loss of free water, the free water deficit can be calculated as follows:

$$\text{Water deficit} = \text{Normal total body weight}$$
$$(\text{Normal }[Na^+]/\text{Measured }[Na^+] - 1)$$

POTASSIUM

Normal Physiology

The relative concentrations of potassium in the intracellular fluid and extracellular fluid are the major determinants of the normal osmotic and electrochemical gradient of all living cells. Precisely controlled transcellular movement of potassium in excitable tissues is required for neuronal transmission, cardiac conduction, and excitation-contraction coupling. Potassium is also important for acid-base balance; the exchange of potassium ions (K^+) and hydrogen ions (H^+) across the cell membrane serves as a first-line buffering system during acute acidosis and alkalosis. Potassium is also required for intracellular glucose metabolism, oxidative phosphorylation, and protein synthesis.[8]

The adult human body contains between 2500 and 3500 mmol of potassium, 98% of which is found in the intracellular compartment. For this reason the serum potassium level is not an accurate indicator of total potassium stores. The normal range of the serum potassium concentration is 3.5 to 5.0 mEq/L.[9]

Ingested potassium is absorbed in the small intestine through passive transport mechanisms. Renal excretion is the major route of potassium elimination; less than 8% of losses occur in the feces and sweat. In the kidneys, 90% of the filtered load of potassium is reabsorbed in the proximal tubule, and potassium balance is determined by the handling of the cation in the distal nephron. The Na^+-K^+ ATPase pump transports potassium from the serum into distal tubular cells against a concentration gradient. Potassium then moves passively into the tubular lumen in exchange for sodium and is excreted in the urine. When the serum potassium level increases, pump activity increases and renal potassium excretion increases. When the serum potassium level falls, the pump is less active and excretion decreases. *Aldosterone* also controls potassium homeostasis. Increased aldosterone release causes retention of sodium and excretion of potassium at the distal tubule. Decreased aldosterone release or inhibition of aldosterone (by drugs such as angiotensin-converting enzyme [ACE] inhibitors or spironolactone) promotes potassium retention. Acidosis and alkalosis also affect renal potassium handling. Acidosis promotes secretion of H^+ into the distal tubule, with retention of potassium, and alkalosis tends to favor renal potassium excretion.[10]

The serum potassium level depends on the distribution of potassium between the serum and cells, as well as the balance between potassium intake and excretion. Acute decreases in the plasma pH cause potassium to shift out of the cell in exchange for H^+. Conversely, alkalosis promotes movement of extracellular potassium into the cell in exchange for intracellular H^+. In general a change of 0.1 pH units causes an inverse change of approximately 0.6 mEq in the serum potassium. Respiratory acid-base disturbances affect serum potassium in the same manner as metabolic changes, but not as predictably. Potassium levels are also influenced by hormones and hormone receptor stimulation. *Insulin* increases cellular potassium uptake by means of the Na^+-K^+ ATPase pump. Insulin release is stimulated by hyperkalemia, and hypokalemia inhibits insulin release. α-Adrenergic stimulation promotes hyperkalemia, and β-stimulation causes uptake of potassium into cells.[9]

Hypokalemia

Principles of Disease Hypokalemia is relatively common, although life-threatening hypokalemia is much less common.[10] Hypokalemia may be the result of decreased potassium intake, increased potassium excretion, or transcellular potassium shifts (Box 119-5).

Hypokalemia resulting from decreased dietary intake is rare. However, when poor intake is combined with other factors (e.g., vomiting or diarrhea, high insulin or aldosterone levels), severe hypokalemia may result. Patients suffering from prolonged starvation may become hypokalemic when they are fed because insulin secretion and increased cellular uptake cause potassium to move into cells.

Pronounced renal or GI potassium losses may result in hypokalemia. *Diuretic therapy,* the most common cause of hypokalemia in clinical practice, increases sodium delivery to the distal tubule, promoting potassium excretion. Associated volume depletion and high levels of aldosterone cause K^+ and H^+ excretion and may worsen hypokalemia. In addition, alkalosis from H^+ excretion promotes cellular potassium uptake, further lowering the serum potassium.[10]

Other disorders can cause significant renal potassium loss. These include osmotic diuresis, high mineralocorticoid states, magnesium depletion, and high urinary concentrations of anions such as penicillin. Intrinsic renal causes of potassium

Box 119-5 Causes of Hypokalemia

I. Decreased intake
  A. Decreased dietary potassium
  B. Impaired absorption of potassium
  C. Clay ingestion
  D. Kayexalate
II. Increased loss
  A. Renal
    1. Hyperaldosteronism
      a. Primary
        1. Conn's syndrome
        2. Adrenal hyperplasia
      b. Secondary
        1. Congestive heart failure
        2. Cirrhosis
        3. Nephrotic syndrome
        4. Dehydration
      c. Bartter's syndrome
    2. Glycyrrhizic acid (licorice, chewing tobacco)
    3. Excessive adrenocorticosteroids
      a. Cushing's syndrome
      b. Steroid therapy
      c. Adrenogenital syndrome
    4. Renal tubular defects
      a. Renal tubular acidosis
      b. Obstructive uropathy
      c. Salt-wasting nephropathy
    5. Drugs
      a. Diuretics
      b. Aminoglycosides
      c. Mannitol
      d. Amphotericin B
      e. Cisplatin
      f. Carbenicillin
  B. Gastrointestinal
    1. Vomiting
    2. Nasogastric suction
    3. Diarrhea
    4. Malabsorption
    5. Ileostomy
    6. Villous adenoma
    7. Laxative abuse
  C. Increased losses from skin
    1. Excessive sweating
    2. Burns
III. Transcellular shifts
  A. Alkalosis
    1. Vomiting
    2. Diuretics
    3. Hyperventilation
    4. Bicarbonate therapy
  B. Insulin
    1. Exogenous
    2. Endogenous response to glucose
  C. β_2-Agonists (albuterol, terbutaline, epinephrine)
  D. Hypokalemic periodic paralysis
    1. Familial
    2. Thyrotoxic
IV. Miscellaneous
  A. Anabolic state
  B. IV hyperalimentation
  C. Treatment of megaloblastic anemia
  D. Acute mountain sickness

loss include renal tubular acidosis (RTA), chronic interstitial disease, and drugs that affect tubular potassium reabsorption. RTA type 1 is caused by a defect in H^+ secretion in the *distal* tubule, and RTA type 2 is associated with a similar defect in the *proximal* tubule. In both cases, increased potassium excretion at the distal tubule is the result. Other causes of increased renal potassium loss include hypercalcemia; toxins (e.g., cisplatin, amphotericin B, aminoglycosides), leukemia, interstitial nephritis, and postobstructive diuresis.

Primary hyperaldosteronism (Conn's syndrome), which is typically caused by adrenal adenoma, is characterized by hypertension and hypokalemia.[11] *Secondary hyperaldosteronism,* due to increased renin release, causes hypokalemia in the face of volume depletion as potassium is exchanged for sodium at the distal tubule. In *Bartter's syndrome,* a disorder causing hyperplasia of the juxtaglomerular apparatus and hyperreninism, patients typically have weakness and hypokalemia.

GI losses of potassium occur in patients with protracted vomiting and diarrhea. Vomiting itself does not cause potassium loss; rather, hypokalemia results from hypovolemia, secondary hyperaldosteronism, and alkalosis. Diarrhea can cause hypokalemia from losses in the stool and secondary hyperaldosteronism. Patients with villous adenomas classically have tremendous losses of potassium from diarrheal fluid.

Loss of potassium from the skin in sufficient quantities to cause hypokalemia is unusual unless the patient has experienced extreme sweating or is a victim of extensive burns or toxic epidermal necrolysis.[10]

Hypokalemia may result from transcellular potassium shifts, most often because of alterations in acid-base balance. As mentioned, acidosis causes potassium to move out of the cell in exchange for H^+, and the reverse is true for alkalosis. Although acidosis is typically associated with hyperkalemia, acidosis may also be associated with hypokalemia in the presence of increased urinary potassium losses (e.g., diabetic ketoacidosis). β-Receptor stimulation is another common cause of hypokalemia resulting from transcellular shifts. In the ED this is most likely to occur in the patient receiving large doses of β-agonists for the treatment of asthma or chronic obstructive pulmonary disease.[12,13]

The periodic paralyses are associated with varying serum potassium levels, including hypokalemia. They often are associated with thyroid disease and are distinguished by symmetric proximal weakness.[14]

Clinical Features Hypokalemia may affect the neuromuscular, cardiovascular, GI, and renal systems, as well as acid-base balance. Signs and symptoms of neuromuscular dysfunction usually occur when the serum potassium level is less than 2.5 mEq/L.[15] CNS signs may include lethargy, depression, irritability, and confusion. Peripheral manifestations include paresthesias, depressed deep tendon reflexes, fasciculations, myalgias, and prominent muscle weakness. Muscular paralysis may occur with serum levels below 2.0 mEq/L.

Patients with severe hypokalemia may develop *rhabdomyolysis* because of impaired energy metabolism, membrane pump dysfunction, and local muscle ischemia.[16] Potassium is released from injured muscle, so the responsible hypokalemia may not be clinically evident, with serum levels normal or even elevated.

Cardiovascular manifestations of hypokalemia include palpitations, postural hypotension, ectopy, and dysrhythmias. First- and second-degree heart block, atrial fibrillation, paroxysmal ventricular contractions, ventricular fibrillation, and asystole have all been reported. The electrocardiogram (ECG) shows flattening of T waves, ST-segment depression, and the appearance of U waves.[16]

Hypokalemia impairs intestinal smooth muscle activity and may cause nausea, vomiting, and abdominal distention. Severe hypokalemia may produce paralytic ileus.[10] The renal manifestations of hypokalemia include polyuria, polydipsia, and impaired ability to concentrate urine or excrete an acid load.

The effect of hypokalemia on acid-base balance is to promote *metabolic alkalosis.* In response to a low serum potassium level, potassium moves out of the cell in exchange for H^+, causing an extracellular alkalosis and an intracellular acidosis. In response to the drop in intracellular pH, renal tubular cells excrete H^+, leading to paradoxical aciduria and exacerbating the extracellular alkalosis.

Management Because potassium is an intracellular cation, a low serum potassium level reflects a much greater total potassium deficit. In the absence of acute shifts caused by acid-base disturbances, a decrease of the serum potassium by 1.0 mEq/L may reflect a 370-mEq deficit of total potassium. Because up to 50% of administered potassium is excreted in the urine, correction of large deficits may require several days.

Whenever possible, oral therapy is preferable to IV therapy because the risk of hyperkalemia is significantly less. However, patients with prominent symptoms (e.g., dysrhythmias) and those who are unable to tolerate oral supplements should receive IV potassium replacement. IV potassium is usually given at a rate of 10 to 20 mEq/hr, but larger doses can be given to patients with severe depletion or severely symptomatic hypokalemia (e.g., respiratory muscle weakness). Doses greater than 20 mEq/hr should be given in a monitored setting through a large-bore peripheral venous catheter or a central venous access site.[17]

Burning at the infusion site is the most common side effect of IV potassium administration. Slowing the rate of infusion will usually decrease venous irritation. The most important potential risk of IV potassium administration is acute hyperkalemia, which is most likely in patients with renal insufficiency. If dysrhythmias (e.g., frequent premature ventricular contractions [PVCs], heart block, tachycardia, widening of the QRS complex) develop, the potassium infusion should be discontinued immediately.

Oral potassium is preferred for mild hypokalemia. Several oral preparations are available in liquid or tablet form. Although liquid preparations are typically better absorbed, matrix tablets are often better tolerated. Hypokalemia can be effectively corrected with oral supplements, and large amounts of oral potassium can be given to increase serum levels rapidly.

Potassium can be given as the chloride salt in most patients. Potassium phosphate, rather than potassium chloride, may be given if there is associated hypophosphatemia (e.g., in diabetic ketoacidosis). Patients with distal RTA should be treated with potassium bicarbonate, potassium citrate, or potassium gluconate, which provide both potassium and base equivalents. The hypokalemia of proximal

RTA may be better treated with potassium chloride because the administered base cannot be reabsorbed well proximally and can obligate potassium loss when it reaches the distal tubule.

Hyperkalemia

Principles of Disease Hyperkalemia may be the result of increased potassium intake, enhanced potassium absorption, impaired potassium excretion, or shifts of potassium out of cells into the serum (Box 119-6).

When faced with a report of a high serum potassium level, the EP should first consider the possibility of laboratory error. Hemolysis during phlebotomy, as may occur when blood is obtained with a small needle or sampled in a high-vacuum tube, releases potassium into the sample and causes a spuriously high potassium level to be measured. Laboratory technicians usually note the presence of pink serum, indicating hemolysis. Pseudohyperkalemia may also occur when potassium is released from platelets in patients with severe thrombocytosis or from leukocytes in patients with extreme leukocytosis.[18]

Hyperkalemia rarely results from increased potassium intake. This is more common when potassium supplements are inadvertently taken by patients with renal insufficiency or in those taking a potassium-sparing diuretic or an ACE inhibitor.[18] Parenteral medications such as penicillin and carbenicillin, as well as transfused blood, also contain significant amounts of potassium and may precipitate hyperkalemia.

Renal insufficiency (i.e., decreased GFR), defects in tubular potassium secretion, or hypoaldosteronism can cause hyperkalemia. As GFR decreases to approximately 5 to 15 ml/min, excretion of the normal daily potassium load is impaired. Defects in tubular potassium excretion are associated with a number of conditions. Hypoaldosteronism may be the result of causes as varied as RTA type 4, Addison's disease, nonsteroidal antiinflammatory drugs (NSAIDs), and ACE inhibitors.

Transcellular potassium shifts (e.g., acute acidosis, β-receptor antagonism) are another major cause of hyperkalemia. Periodic paralysis is an inherited disorder characterized by hyperkalemia caused by cellular efflux of potassium associated with stressors such as exercise, infection, and diet. Drugs may also be the cause of transcellular potassium shifts. Digitalis poisons the Na^+-K^+ ATPase pump, with resultant hyperkalemia in severe cases. Succinylcholine causes transient potassium efflux because of depolarization of the muscle cell membrane. High-dose trimethoprim-sulfamethoxazole has also been implicated in hyperkalemia, especially with concomitant renal insufficiency.[19,20]

Life-threatening hyperkalemia may result when large amounts of potassium are released from damaged cells. Rhabdomyolysis, tumor cell necrosis, and hemolysis are important causes.[15] Acute renal failure that may be associated with these conditions impairs potassium excretion, further exacerbating endogenous hyperkalemia.

Clinical Features Cardiovascular and neurologic dysfunction are the primary manifestations of hyperkalemia.[18] Patients may have a variety of dysrhythmias, including second- and third-degree heart block, wide-complex tachycardia, ventricular fibrillation, and even asystole. The ECG can provide valuable clues to the presence of hyperkalemia. As potassium levels rise, peaked T waves are the first characteristic manifestation. Further rises are associated with progressive ECG changes, including loss of P waves and widening and slurring of QRS complex. Eventually the tracing assumes a sine-wave appearance, followed by ventricular fibrillation or asystole. Concomitant alkalosis, hypernatremia, or hypercalcemia antagonizes the membrane effects of hyperkalemia and may delay or diminish the characteristic ECG findings.

Neuromuscular signs and symptoms of hyperkalemia include muscle cramps, weakness, paralysis, paresthesias,

Box 119-6 Causes of Hyperkalemia

I. Pseudohyperkalemia
  A. Hemolysis of sample
  B. Thrombocytosis
  C. Leukocytosis
  D. Laboratory error
II. Increased potassium intake and absorption
  A. Potassium supplements (oral and parenteral)
  B. Dietary—(salt substitutes)
  C. Stored blood
  D. Potassium-containing medications
III. Impaired renal excretion
  A. Acute renal failure
  B. Chronic renal failure
  C. Tubular defect in potassium secretion
    1. Renal allograft
    2. Analgesic nephropathy
    3. Sickle cell disease
    4. Obstructive uropathy
    5. Interstitial nephritis
    6. Chronic pyelonephritis
    7. K-sparing diuretics
    8. Miscellaneous (lead, systemic lupus erythematosus, pseudohypoaldosteronism)
  D. Hypoaldosteronism
    1. Primary (Addison's disease)
    2. Secondary
      a. Hyporeninemic hypoaldosteronism (renal tubular acidosis type 4)
      b. Congenital adrenal hyperplasia
      c. Drug induced
        i. Nonsteroidal antiinflammatory drugs
        ii. ACE inhibitors
        iii. Heparin
        iv. Cyclosporine
IV. Transcellular shifts
  A. Acidosis
  B. Hypertonicity
  C. Insulin deficiency
  D. Drugs
    1. β-blockers
    2. Digitalis toxicity
    3. Succinylcholine
  E. Exercise
  F. Hyperkalemic periodic paralysis
V. Cellular injury
  A. Rhabdomyolysis
  B. Severe intravascular hemolysis
  C. Acute tumor lysis syndrome
  D. Burns and crush injuries

tetany, and focal neurologic deficits, but these are rarely specific enough to suggest the diagnosis in themselves.[15,16]

Management The treatment of hyperkalemia includes cardiovascular monitoring, administration of calcium chloride or gluconate to treat hemodynamic instability, initiation of measures to lower serum potassium, and correction of the underlying cause.

All patients with suspected hyperkalemia should be on a cardiac monitor with attention to the morphology of the T waves and QRS complex. Peaked T waves, loss of P waves, slurring of the QRS, and second- or third-degree heart block all suggest hyperkalemia and are indications for immediate therapy. Treatment of the hyperkalemic patient is directed toward antagonism of the membrane effects of hyperkalemia, promotion of transcellular potassium shifts, and removal of potassium from the body.

Calcium Chloride or Gluconate Immediate antagonism of potassium at the cardiac membrane is achieved with IV administration of calcium chloride or gluconate. This is indicated in patients with unstable dysrhythmia or hypotension. Several ampules of calcium (10 ml of 10% solution) may be required.[16,18] Because of the brief duration of action (approximately 20 to 40 minutes), other measures should also be instituted promptly.[18]

Sodium Bicarbonate Sodium bicarbonate infusion promotes a shift of potassium into cells. One ampule (44 mEq) should be given by slow IV push over 5 to 15 minutes. The duration of action is approximately 2 hours. Sodium bicarbonate should be used with caution when hypertonicity, volume overload, or alkalosis poses a risk to the patient. Bicarbonate therapy is less efficacious than insulin or albuterol.[21,22]

Glucose and Insulin Cellular uptake of potassium can also be induced with a regimen of IV glucose and insulin. Regular insulin (10 to 20 U) may be given by bolus infusion. Dextrose should be administered to euglycemic and diabetic patients with blood glucose below 250 mg/dl to prevent hypoglycemia. This combination lasts 4 to 6 hours.[18] Rapid infusion of hypertonic glucose solution may transiently exacerbate hyperkalemia by its osmotic effect on cells.

β_2-Agonists The known effect of β_2-agonists to cause movement of potassium into cells may be harnessed to lower the serum potassium level acutely. Treatment with nebulized albuterol (5 to 20 mg) lowers the serum potassium level for at least 2 hours.[22,23]

Exchange Resins Definitive treatment for hyperkalemia remains the removal of potassium from the body. Exchange resins (e.g., sodium polystyrene sulfonate [Kayexalate]) and hemodialysis are two such options. Given orally or rectally, each gram of Kayexalate can remove approximately 1.0 mEq of potassium. An oral dose of 20 g of Kayexalate in a sorbitol produces effects in 1 to 2 hours. Rectal enemas of 50 g of Kayexalate, retained for 30 minutes, work in approximately 30 minutes. Kayexalate should be used with caution in patients with poor cardiovascular reserve because of the potential to exacerbate volume overload.

Dialysis Hemodialysis corrects hyperkalemia rapidly, and consultation with a nephrologist is indicated in the unstable hyperkalemic patient with newly diagnosed or chronic renal failure. Hyperkalemia resulting from severe rhabdomyolysis is difficult to treat with the usual measures and also mandates consultation for emergency dialysis. Dialysis removes potassium from the blood only, and subsequent shifts of intracellular potassium may cause rebound hyperkalemia. Dialysis can be effective in treating hyperkalemia-induced cardiac arrest.[24]

Underlying Cause Treatment of any underlying causative disorder should be initiated at the same time as therapy for hyperkalemia. This may include the treatment of rhabdomyolysis with fluids and bicarbonate; treatment of Addison's disease with corticosteroids, IV fluids, and glucose; treatment of digitalis toxicity with digoxin-binding antibodies; or discontinuation of drugs that may have precipitated hyperkalemia.

Patients with hyperkalemia should be admitted to a monitored bed, with care provided by a clinician skilled in the treatment of electrolyte disorders.

CALCIUM

Normal Physiology

Hundreds of enzymatic reactions are mediated by changes in intracellular calcium. Cellular growth and reproduction, membrane integrity, receptor activation, neurotransmission, glandular secretion, enzyme activation, muscle contraction, cardiac contractility, platelet aggregation, and immune function all depend on the precise regulation of free calcium. Evidence also indicates that cellular injury and ultimately cell death are mediated by changes in free intracellular calcium.[25]

The adult human body contains approximately 1200 g of calcium, with more than 99% in the mineral component of bone. The remaining 1% is distributed in three different plasma fractions: (1) approximately 50% is bound to serum proteins, primarily albumin; (2) 10% is complexed with serum anions (phosphate, bicarbonate, citrate, lactate); and (3) 40% is in the free ionized state. *Ionized calcium* is the physiologically active form, and concentrations are tightly regulated by the endocrine system.

Dietary calcium is absorbed in the proximal intestine through both active and passive processes. Absorption is enhanced by the action of vitamin D. In the kidneys, 99% of the filtered load of calcium is reabsorbed. Approximately 90% of calcium reabsorption occurs passively in the proximal tubule and loop of Henle. The remaining 10% occurs in the distal tubule under the control of *parathyroid hormone* (PTH, parathormone). A fall in free serum calcium stimulates the release of PTH, which in turn increases reabsorption. PTH also mediates the hydroxylation of vitamin D to its active form, 1,25-dihydroxycholecalciferol (1,25-DHCC).

The skeleton acts as a calcium pool that buffers acute changes in serum concentration. When the serum calcium falls, PTH stimulates an increase in bone turnover and the release of calcium into the serum. A rise in serum calcium suppresses PTH production and causes the release of calcitonin. *Calcitonin* decreases osteoclastic activity and enhances skeletal deposition of calcium.

The serum calcium level reflects the net outcome of several processes. On one hand, intestinal absorption and bone resorption add calcium to the blood; on the other, calcium is lost from the blood by renal excretion, skeletal uptake, or abnormal deposition in soft tissues. A decrease in the serum ionized calcium activates the PTH–vitamin D system to increase the entry of calcium into the blood from the bone and GI tract. A rise in the serum calcium suppresses the PTH–vitamin D system and increases the release of calcitonin, which decreases calcium entry into the blood.

Most hospital laboratories measure *total* serum calcium concentrations. Normal values range from 8.5 to 10.5 mg/dl. However, the total serum calcium is often a poor indicator of the ionized calcium status. Several factors may influence the measurement of the total serum calcium, regardless of the ionized calcium. Alterations in serum protein concentrations (primarily albumin) affect the total calcium. A decrease in albumin concentration will lower the measured serum calcium, and an increase will raise it. Physiologically this change is not of significance because the ionized calcium remains unchanged. A corrected serum calcium that accounts for changes in serum albumin concentrations can be calculated as follows:

$$\text{Corrected calcium} = \text{Serum calcium (mg/dl)} + 0.8[4 - \text{Serum albumin (g/dl)}]$$

This formula is only an estimate, and the ionized calcium should be measured whenever hypocalcemia is suspected. Blood gas analyzers can measure ionized calcium from a sample of blood or serum. The normal range is 1.00 to 1.15 mmol/L.

Changes in acid-base status influence the ratio of bound to ionized calcium without altering the total measured calcium. Acidosis decreases calcium binding to albumin, and alkalosis increases binding. Thus acute changes in blood pH may have important physiologic effects by changing the ionized calcium even when the total serum calcium remains unchanged.[25]

Box 119-7 Causes of Hypocalcemia

I. Parathyroid hormone insufficiency
   A. Primary hypoparathyroidism
      1. Congenital syndromes
      2. Maternal hyperparathyroidism
   B. Secondary hypoparathyroidism
      1. Neck surgery
      2. Metastatic carcinoma
      3. Infiltrative disorders
      4. Hypomagnesemia, hypermagnesemia
      5. Sepsis
      6. Pancreatitis
      7. Burns
      8. Drugs (chemotherapeutics, ethanol, cimetidine)

II. Vitamin D insufficiency
   A. Congenital rickets
   B. Malnutrition
   C. Malabsorption
   D. Liver disease
   E. Renal disease
      1. Acute and chronic renal failure
      2. Nephrotic syndrome
   F. Hypomagnesemia
   G. Sepsis
   H. Anticonvulsants (phenytoin, primidone)

III. Parathyroid hormone resistance states (pseudohypoparathyroidism)

IV. Calcium chelation
   A. Hyperphosphatemia
   B. Citrate
   C. Free fatty acids
   D. Alkalosis
   E. Fluoride poisoning

Hypocalcemia

Principles of Disease The causes of ionized hypocalcemia are numerous (Box 119-7) and can be divided into disorders causing PTH insufficiency, vitamin D insufficiency, PTH resistance states, and calcium chelation.

Parathyroid Hormone Insufficiency PTH insufficiency may be caused by either primary or secondary hypoparathyroidism. *Primary hypoparathyroidism* is rare and is usually congenital. Maternal hyperparathyroidism may result in fetal parathyroid hypoplasia and transient hypoparathyroidism.

Secondary hypoparathyroidism is more common and is most often iatrogenic, resulting from inadvertent removal of the parathyroid glands or disruption of the vascular supply during parathyroid, thyroid, or carotid surgery. Permanent hypocalcemia is the usual consequence. Excision of a functional parathyroid adenoma, leaving only the chronically suppressed but otherwise unaffected parathyroid tissue, causes hypocalcemia that usually resolves over several days. Metastatic carcinoma or infiltrative disorders (e.g., hemochromatosis, sarcoidosis, Wilson's disease) may destroy parathyroid tissue and cause hypocalcemia. Both severe hypomagnesemia and severe hypermagnesemia may impair PTH release. Drugs that may suppress parathyroid function include chemotherapeutic agents, cimetidine, and ethanol.

Vitamin D Deficiency Vitamin D deficiency may result in hypocalcemia because of decreased GI calcium absorption. Nutritional vitamin D deficiency is rare in the United States because of the fortification of milk but can occur when exposure to sunlight is limited, especially in elderly, chronically ill, and debilitated patients. Children of mothers with vitamin D deficiency may be born with congenital rickets. Characteristic findings include hypocalcemia, hypophosphatemia, and specific radiographic findings (widening of the distal radius and ulna, craniotabes). Vitamin D insufficiency resulting from intestinal malabsorption may occur in patients with small-bowel or biliary disease or pancreatic exocrine failure. Cholestyramine may also prevent adequate vitamin D absorption. Once absorbed, vitamin D is hydroxylated in the liver and kidney to its active form, 1,25-DHCC. Hepatic disease and renal disease may lead to inadequate activation of the vitamin. Hypercatabolism of vitamin D may occur in association with agents that stimulate the hepatic microsomal oxidase system, such as the anticonvulsants phenytoin and primidone.

Parathyroid Hormone Resistance States PTH resistance states are termed *pseudohypoparathyroidism.* These rare familial syndromes are characterized by renal unresponsiveness to PTH and resultant parathyroid hyperplasia.[26] Differentiation from hypoparathyroidism is based on elevated PTH levels and a lack of increase in urinary cyclic adenosine monophosphate (cAMP) after PTH administration.

Hypocalcemia is common in patients with chronic renal failure. This results from vitamin D deficiency, impaired responsiveness to PTH, and phosphate retention. Generally these patients are asymptomatic, possibly because of a protective effect of systemic acidosis. However, rapid correction of metabolic acidosis with exogenous sodium bicarbonate may precipitate severe hypocalcemia, often causing tetany and seizures.

Calcium Chelation Calcium complexes with several different substances in serum, including proteins, fatty acids, and anions. Increases in the concentration of these substances may thus result in ionized hypocalcemia. Citrate is used as a blood preservative and anticoagulant. The citrate load associated with massive blood transfusion (>6 U) causes hypocalcemia in up to 94% of patients.[27] Hypocalcemia is usually short-lived, and ionized calcium levels return to normal shortly after transfusion. Because citrate is metabolized by temperature-dependent enzymes in tissues and excreted by the liver, hypothermia and hepatic failure are important risk factors for protracted hypocalcemia after blood transfusion. Citrate is also a constituent of radiocontrast material, and hypocalcemia has been associated with the administration of these agents.

Exogenous administration of phosphate and endogenous hyperphosphatemia (e.g., with acute renal failure, rhabdomyolysis, or tumor lysis syndrome) are well-known causes of hypocalcemia.[28] Exogenous bicarbonate also complexes with calcium and may cause symptomatic hypocalcemia. Alkalosis, either metabolic or respiratory, enhances the binding of calcium to serum proteins, resulting in ionized hypocalcemia. Free fatty acids liberated in various conditions (e.g., acute pancreatitis, hyperadrenergic states, acute ethanol ingestion) can chelate free calcium to form calcium soaps. Fluoride poisoning may also cause hypocalcemia. This may occur after exposure to hydrofluoric acid or ammonium bifluoride, components of many household cleaners and rust removers. These compounds release free fluoride ion, a direct cellular toxin that binds calcium, forming calcium fluoride. Numerous cases of severe hypocalcemia, cardiac dysrhythmias, and death have been reported after ingestion, inhalation, or cutaneous exposure to these products.

Clinical Features The clinical manifestations of hypocalcemia depend not only on the serum level but also on the rapidity with which it declines. Although the signs and symptoms of hypocalcemia are numerous (Box 119-8), the effects on neuromuscular function predominate.

A declining serum calcium level is associated with progressive neuromuscular hyperexcitability. CNS manifestations may include depression, irritability, confusion, and focal or generalized seizures. Peripheral nervous system manifestations include perioral paresthesias, muscle weakness and cramps, fasciculations, and tetany.[25] Latent tetany can often be demonstrated by eliciting Chvostek's or Trousseau's sign. *Chvostek's sign* is elicited by tapping over the facial nerve and causing twitching of the ipsilateral facial muscles. *Trousseau's sign* describes carpal spasm in response to inflation of an arm blood pressure cuff to 20 mm Hg above systolic blood pressure for 3 minutes.

Severe hypocalcemia causes a decrease in myocardial contractility and rarely bradycardia, hypotension, and symptomatic CHF. Patients with preexisting cardiac dysfunction and those taking digoxin or diuretics are especially at risk. The ECG may demonstrate QT prolongation, and an inverse relationship exists between the serum calcium level and the QT interval. However, the ECG is a poor predictor of hypocalcemia and should not be used to rule in or rule out this disorder.

Bronchospasm and laryngeal spasm occur rarely. Symptoms and signs ranging from anxiety and depression to psychosis and dementia may be seen.

Box 119-8 Clinical Features of Hypocalcemia

Neuromuscular

Paresthesias
Muscle weakness
Muscle spasm
Tetany
Chvostek's and Trousseau's signs
Hyperreflexia
Seizures

Cardiovascular

Bradycardia
Hypotension
Cardiac arrest
Digitalis insensitivity
QT prolongation

Pulmonary

Bronchospasm
Laryngeal spasm

Psychiatric

Anxiety
Depression
Irritability
Confusion
Psychosis
Dementia

Management In patients with suspected hypocalcemia or a documented low total serum calcium level, the first step in management should be the verification of true ionized hypocalcemia. When hypocalcemia is the presumed cause of tetany, seizures, hypotension, or dysrhythmias, it may be appropriate to initiate treatment before the ionized calcium level is available. All patients with symptomatic hypocalcemia should be treated with parenteral calcium. Two different formulations are readily available in most EDs: (1) 10-ml ampules of 10% calcium chloride, which contain 360 mg of elemental calcium, and (2) 10-ml ampules of 10% calcium gluconate, which contain 93 mg of elemental calcium. For the adult patient the recommended initial dose is 100 to 300 mg of elemental calcium given as calcium chloride or calcium gluconate. This dose of calcium will increase the serum ionized calcium for only a short time (1 to 2 hours) and should be followed by repeated doses or an infusion at a rate of 0.5 to 2 mg/kg/hr.[25] For neonates, infants, and children the recommended initial dose is 0.5 to 1.0 ml/kg of 10% calcium gluconate over 5 minutes.[26]

The most common side effects of IV calcium administration are hypertension, nausea, vomiting, and flushing. Bradycardia and heart block occur in rare cases. Patients receiving IV calcium should be placed on a cardiac monitor, and administration should be discontinued if bradycardia ensues. Calcium should be administered with extra caution in patients taking digoxin because it may precipitate (or exacerbate) digoxin-induced cardiotoxicity. Because calcium may cause severe tissue irritation and necrosis if it extravasates, it should always be given through a well-functioning catheter. Whenever possible, calcium chloride should be diluted in 5% dextrose in water (D5W).[25,26]

Symptoms refractory to appropriate doses of calcium may be caused by coexisting hypomagnesemia. In patients with normal renal function, administration of 2 to 4 g of 10% magnesium sulfate should be considered.

Patients with asymptomatic hypocalcemia may be treated with oral calcium supplements. Available preparations include calcium ascorbate, calcium gluconate, and calcium lactate. Most patients require 1 to 4 g of elemental calcium daily in divided doses.

Hypercalcemia

Principles of Disease Hypercalcemia is a relatively common medical disorder. Routine laboratory screening can be expected to detect hypercalcemia in 0.1% to 1.0% of patients, depending on the population being screened.[29-31] Hypercalcemia is usually mild (<12 mg/dl) and asymptomatic and rarely requires emergency treatment. Nevertheless, hypercalcemia may be an important clue to a serious underlying medical disorder. *Hypercalcemic crisis* occurs in a subset of patients who have severe hypercalcemia (usually >14 mg/dl) and is generally associated with prominent signs and symptoms. In this situation, immediate measures to lower the serum calcium are indicated.

Although hypercalcemia has many causes, more than 90% of cases result from primary hyperparathyroidism or malignancy (Box 119-9).[32]

Primary hyperparathyroidism is the most common cause of hypercalcemia in outpatients, representing 25% to 50% of cases.[33] This may result from parathyroid adenoma (80%), parathyroid hyperplasia (15%), or parathyroid carcinoma (5%).[34] Hyperparathyroidism may also occur in association with other endocrine tumors as part of one of the familial syndromes of multiple endocrine adenomatosis. In primary hyperparathyroidism, PTH is elevated in more than 90% of cases; the remainder of patients have high-normal PTH levels that are inappropriate for the degree of hypercalcemia. An elevated PTH level leads to increased bone resorption, a relative decrease in renal calcium excretion, and increased intestinal calcium absorption. Patients typically develop hypercalcemia, phosphaturia, hypophosphatemia, and a hyperchloremic metabolic acidosis.

Malignancy is the most common cause of hypercalcemia in hospitalized patients, and hypercalcemia is the most common paraneoplastic complication of cancer. The reported prevalence of hypercalcemia in patients with cancer ranges from 15% to 60%.[35,36] A multitude of solid tumors may cause hypercalcemia, including cancers of breast, lung, colon, stomach, cervix, uterus, ovary, kidney, bladder, and head and neck. Hypercalcemia is also seen with hematologic malignancies such as multiple myeloma and lymphoma. Hypercalcemia in patients with cancer can result from several different mechanisms, including production of parathyroid hormone–related protein (PTHRP) by the tumor.[37,38] This polypeptide is homologous to PTH in its first 13 *N*-terminal amino acids and binds to the PTH receptor, mimicking all the actions of the hormone. PTHRP is secreted by solid malignancies and their metastases and is not subject to normal feedback control mechanisms.[39] Assays for PTHRP are available to confirm this cause of cancer-related hypercalcemia.[40] Less often, hypercalcemia may result from the production of other bone-resorbing substances by the tumor (e.g., transforming growth factor-α) or the local effects of osteolytic skeletal metastasis. Virtually all patients with cancer-associated hypercalcemia have low concentrations of PTH, readily distinguishing this cause of hypercalcemia from primary hyperparathyroidism.

Thiazide diuretics are associated with up to 20% of cases of hypercalcemia. These agents can increase the reabsorption of calcium in the distal convoluted tubule by as much as 70%. Hypercalcemia is typically mild, although it may be exaggerated in patients with dehydration.

Granulomatous disorders (e.g., sarcoidosis, tuberculosis, coccidioidomycosis, histoplasmosis, leprosy) can cause hypercalcemia. In these conditions, activated macrophages convert 25-hydroxyvitamin D to its active form (1,25-DHCC), resulting in enhanced intestinal calcium absorption, hypercalcemia, and hypercalciuria.[41] Certain lymphomas may cause severe hypercalcemia by a similar mechanism. Interestingly, hypercalcemia in patients with sarcoidosis may occur as a seasonal event in patients who live in the Northern Hemisphere, presumably because of increased production of vitamin D in the skin during longer exposure to the summer sun.[42]

Box 119-9 Causes of Hypercalcemia

Primary Hyperparathyroidism

Malignant Disease

Parathyroid hormone–related protein
Ectopic production of 1,25-dihydroxyvitamin D
Other bone-resorbing substances
Osteolytic bone metastasis

Medications

Thiazide diuretics
Lithium
Estrogens
Vitamin D toxicity
Vitamin A toxicity
Calcium ingestion

Granulomatous Disorders

Sarcoidosis
Tuberculosis
Coccidioidomycosis
Beryliosis
Histoplasmosis
Leprosy

Nonparathyroid Endocrine Disorders

Hyperthyroidism
Adrenal insufficiency
Pheochromocytoma
Acromegaly
Vasoactive intestinal polypeptide–producing tumor

Miscellaneous

Milk-alkali syndrome
Immobilization
Idiopathic hypocalcemia of infancy
Physiologic (in the newborn)

Acute vitamin A intoxication is an uncommon but well-recognized cause of hypercalcemia, resulting from an increase in osteoclastic activity. This usually occurs after an accidental massive ingestion of a preparation containing vitamin A. Chronic hypervitaminosis A can occur in patients using large doses of the vitamin for a variety of dermatologic conditions (e.g., acne vulgaris). Because vitamin A is highly lipophilic, toxicity may take several weeks to resolve after discontinuation of the vitamin. Increased exogenous vitamin D intake may also result in hypercalcemia.

Milk-alkali syndrome is caused by excessive ingestion of calcium and absorbable antacids such as milk or calcium carbonate and is characterized by hypercalcemia, alkalosis, and renal failure. The disorder is less common since nonabsorbable antacids and H_2-receptor antagonists became available for the treatment of peptic ulcer disease.

Lithium therapy for bipolar (manic-depressive) disorders can put patients at increased risk for developing hypercalcemia. Clinical and in vitro studies suggest that lithium alters the release of PTH by shifting the set-point for inhibition of hormone secretion by circulating calcium.

Thyroid hormone causes hypercalcemia by increasing bone turnover through direct stimulation of osteoclastic bone resorption. In most cases the symptoms of hyperthyroidism predominate, and hypercalcemia does not become apparent until hyperthyroidism is managed. Hypercalcemia may also be seen in patients after renal transplantation or in the early phase of acute tubular necrosis.

Clinical Features The clinical manifestations of hypercalcemia are nonspecific and vary widely from patient to patient (Box 119-10). Severity of symptoms depends on both the level of serum calcium and the rapidity of its rise.

Hypercalcemia decreases neuronal conduction and in general causes CNS depression. Symptoms range from fatigue, weakness, and difficulty concentrating to confusion, lethargy, stupor, and even coma.

Hypercalcemia has several effects on the cardiovascular system. The volume depletion with which hypercalcemia is typically associated may result in hypotension. Because hypercalcemia causes an increase in vascular tone, however, the blood pressure may be misleadingly normal. Characteristic ECG changes include shortening of the QT interval and to a lesser degree prolongation of the PR interval and QRS widening. Rarely, severe hypercalcemia causes sinus bradycardia, bundle branch block, high-degree atrioventricular block, and even cardiac arrest. Calcium potentiates the action of digoxin, and the side effects of digoxin are accentuated when hypercalcemia is present.[34]

An acute rise in the serum calcium impairs the reabsorption of fluid and electrolytes in the renal tubule, promoting the development of dehydration, which is worsened by vomiting and poor fluid intake. This may lead to a vicious cycle of volume depletion, reduced GFR and calcium excretion, intensified hypercalcemia, and further dehydration, culminating in oliguric renal failure, coma, and death. Chronically, hypercalcemia and associated volume depletion predispose the patient to renal calculi, nephrocalcinosis, and calcium-induced interstitial nephritis.

Anorexia, nausea, vomiting, and abdominal pain are common but nonspecific symptoms of hypercalcemia. Hypercalcemia decreases smooth muscle tone and may lead to constipation or intestinal ileus. An increased serum calcium enhances the release of hydrochloric acid, gastrin, and pancreatic enzymes. Chronic hypercalcemia has been associated with an increased risk of peptic ulcer disease and pancreatitis.

Box 119-10 Clinical Features of Hypercalcemia

Neurologic

Fatigue, weakness
Confusion, lethargy
Ataxia
Coma
Hypotonia, diminished deep tendon reflexes

Cardiovascular

Hypertension
Sinus bradycardia, atrioventricular block
ECG abnormalities (short QT, bundle branch block)
Ventricular dysrhythmias
Potentiation of digoxin toxicity

Renal

Polyuria, polydipsia
Dehydration
Loss of electrolyte
Prerenal azotemia
Nephrolithiasis
Nephrocalcinosis

Gastrointestinal

Nausea, vomiting
Anorexia
Peptic ulcer disease
Pancreatitis
Constipation, ileus

Management Treatment should be initiated at once in patients with evidence of significant dehydration, alteration of consciousness, or symptomatic dysrhythmias. Patients with severe hypercalcemia (>14 mg/dl) require immediate treatment regardless of symptoms. The four basic goals of therapy are (1) restoration of intravascular volume, (2) enhancement of renal calcium elimination, (3) reduction of osteoclastic activity, and (4) treatment of the primary disorder (Box 119-11). Although it may not be realistic to expect to achieve these goals in the ED, it is important for the EP to initiate therapy and involve the appropriate consultants as early as possible.

Fluid Administration The administration of isotonic saline is the first step in the management of severe hypercalcemia. Once the intravascular volume has been restored to normal, the serum calcium will usually have decreased by 1.6 to 2.4 mg/dl, although hydration alone rarely leads to complete normalization. The expansion of intravascular volume increases renal calcium clearance by increasing GFR and sodium delivery to the distal tubules. The rate of fluid administration should be based on the severity of hypercalcemia, the degree of dehydration, and the patient's cardiovascular tolerance of acute volume expansion. In elderly patients and those with poor left ventricular function, central

Box 119-11 Management of Hypercalcemia

I. Restoration of intravascular volume
   A. Correct dehydration with isotonic solution
   B. Correct associated electrolyte abnormalities
II. Enhancement of renal calcium elimination
   A. Saline diuresis
   B. Loop diuretics (e.g., furosemide)
   C. *Avoid* thiazide diuretics
III. Reduction of osteoclastic activity
   A. Biphosphonates
      1. Etidronate, 7.5 mg/kg over 24 hr
      2. Pamidronate, 60 to 90 mg over 24 hr
   B. Plicamycin, 25 μg/kg over 4 hr
   C. Calcitonin, 4 IU/kg every 12 hr
   D. Hydrocortisone, 200 to 300 mg/day
   E. Gallium nitrate, 200 mg/m^2
IV. Treatment of primary disorder
   A. Parathyroidectomy for hyperparathyroidism
   B. Withdrawal of causative medications
   C. Treatment of nonparathyroid endocrine disorders

venous pressure monitoring may be used to adjust fluid administration rates. Two to five liters per day is often required. Coexisting electrolyte deficiencies should also be corrected.

Furosemide Loop diuretics such as furosemide inhibit the resorption of calcium in the thick ascending loop of Henle, increasing the calciuric effect of hydration. Volume expansion must precede the administration of furosemide, however, because the drug's effect depends on the delivery of calcium to the distal nephron. IV doses of 10 to 40 mg every 6 to 8 hours are usually sufficient. Thiazide diuretics should *not* be used because they enhance distal absorption of calcium and may worsen hypercalcemia.

Osteoclast Inhibitors Therapy for severe hypercalcemia should also include agents that reduce the mobilization of calcium from bone. Drugs that inhibit osteoclast-mediated bone resorption include the bisphosphonates, plicamycin, calcitonin, glucocorticoids, and gallium nitrate.

The *bisphosphonates* act by inhibiting osteoclastic bone resorption and decreasing the viability of osteoclasts.[43] Etidronate and pamidronate have similar efficacy and a reasonable adverse effect profile.[44-47] *Etidronate* is administered at 7.5 mg/kg over 4 hours daily for 3 to 7 days. Serum calcium concentrations reach normal levels in 60% to 100% of patients. Reported side effects include transient rises in serum creatinine and serum phosphate. *Pamidronate* is administered in a single 24-hour IV infusion of 60 to 90 mg. Adverse effects are limited to mild hyperpyrexia, transient leukopenia, and hypophosphatemia.

Plicamycin (*mithramycin*) inhibits ribonucleic acid (RNA) synthesis in osteoclasts and is an effective agent in the treatment of hypercalcemia. It is administered intravenously over 4 hours in a dose of 25 μg/kg. Serum calcium levels decrease within 12 hours, typically reaching a nadir within 48 to 72 hours. Side effects such as phlebitis, nephrotoxicity, hepatotoxicity, and thrombocytopenia limit the use of plicamycin in the treatment of hypercalcemia.

Calcitonin is a naturally occurring hormone that lowers serum calcium when given in doses of 4 IU/kg subcutaneously every 12 hours. Among the anticalcemic agents available, calcitonin has the most rapid onset of action, although it causes only a modest reduction in the serum calcium.[48] Side effects include mild nausea, abdominal cramping, flushing, and rare allergic reactions. When hypercalcemia is severe and the need to lower the serum calcium is urgent, it is reasonable to administer a dose of calcitonin in combination with a more potent agent such as a bisphosphonate.

The *glucocorticoids* act by inhibiting the actions of vitamin D. They may be effective calcium-lowering agents in patients with hypercalcemia caused by hematologic malignancies, granulomatous disorders, or vitamin D intoxication. Hydrocortisone 200 to 300 mg/day or the equivalent dose of another glucocorticoid is recommended.

Underlying Cause Pharmacologic therapy does not permanently normalize the serum calcium concentration. The underlying cause of the hypercalcemia needs to be treated as well. Primary hyperparathyroidism is definitively managed by parathyroidectomy. In the hands of experienced surgeons, more than 90% of patients are cured. When hypercalcemia is caused by malignancy, treatment must be directed at the underlying tumor because normocalcemia is difficult to sustain without successful treatment of the underlying cause. Hypercalcemia caused by medication responds to discontinuation of the offending agent. Hypercalcemia caused by nonparathyroid endocrine disease responds to treatment of the underlying disorder.

MAGNESIUM

Normal Physiology

Magnesium is the second most abundant intracellular cation. It is a cofactor in hundreds of enzymatic reactions, including all those involving adenosine triphosphate (ATP). Magnesium is essential for the production and use of energy, deoxyribonucleic acid (DNA) and protein synthesis, ion channel gating, hormone receptor binding, neurotransmission, cardiac excitability, and muscle contraction.[49]

The adult human body contains approximately 2000 mEq of magnesium. One half of total magnesium is in the mineral component of bone, and 40% to 50% is found in the intracellular compartment. Only 1% to 2% of the body's magnesium is present in the extracellular fluid, so the serum magnesium is often a poor reflection of the total magnesium content. One third of the serum magnesium is bound to albumin, with the rest in the biologically active ionized form. The normal range for serum magnesium is 1.8 to 3.0 mg/dl. A balance between GI absorption and renal excretion maintains magnesium homeostasis.

Dietary sources of magnesium include green vegetables, meats, fish, beans, nuts, and grains. Absorption of ingested magnesium occurs in the small intestine through both active and passive transport mechanisms. In the kidney, 95% of the filtered load of magnesium is reabsorbed in the proximal tubule and loop of Henle.[50] In deficiency states, magnesium resorption is enhanced in the distal convoluted tubule under the influence of PTH. In hypermagnesemic states, renal excretion of magnesium increases.

Hypomagnesemia

Principles of Disease Hypomagnesemia is one of the most common electrolyte deficiencies in clinical practice.[49]

Approximately 10% to 20% of hospitalized patients and 50% to 60% of patients admitted to the intensive care unit are hypomagnesemic.[51] Despite the high prevalence of hypomagnesemia, several factors can make the diagnosis a challenge. First, the clinical manifestations of hypomagnesemia are nonspecific, so the disorder is often overlooked. Second, the serum magnesium is not measured as part of the "routine" electrolyte panel.[52] Third, the serum magnesium level is an insensitive indicator of magnesium deficiency. Although a low serum magnesium is indicative of a magnesium deficit, patients with a normal magnesium level may still have a severe deficiency. Fourth, hypomagnesemia often coexists with and may be masked by other electrolyte deficiency states.

Numerous studies have demonstrated the high prevalence of hypomagnesemia in patients with *hypokalemia.*[53] Because magnesium is required for the normal functioning of the Na^+-K^+ ATPase pump, hypomagnesemia may result in refractory hypokalemia that is not correctable by the administration of potassium alone. Magnesium replacement enhances potassium retention and decreases the amount of supplemental potassium required to achieve a net positive balance.[54] Magnesium is also required for the normal synthesis and release of PTH. Patients with hypomagnesemic *hypocalcemia* typically have inappropriately low levels of PTH and target organ resistance to the hormone, which are corrected by magnesium administration. A high prevalence of *hypophosphatemia* in patients who are hypomagnesemic has also been described.

Because the kidneys normally conserve magnesium efficiently, significant hypomagnesemia usually occurs only when there is renal magnesium wasting or when intestinal losses exceed dietary intake and absorption (Box 119-12). In the ED, hypomagnesemia is most often associated with the use of diuretics and with alcohol abuse.

Diuretics Patients taking diuretics for the treatment of hypertension, CHF, or both are at significant risk for hypomagnesemia. Both the thiazide and the loop diuretics promote renal magnesium loss and may cause severe magnesium deficiency.[55] In one study, typical diuretic doses increased urinary magnesium excretion by 25% to 50%. Some authors recommend that all patients receiving diuretics be considered candidates for magnesium supplementation. The use of a potassium-sparing diuretic in conjunction with a conventional diuretic is less likely to cause hypomagnesemia because these agents also have a magnesium-sparing effect.

Alcoholism The reported prevalence of hypomagnesemia in alcoholic patients varies widely, from 30% to 80%.[56,57] Hypomagnesemia in the alcoholic patient is multifactorial; potential causes include poor nutrition, increased urinary excretion, GI losses from vomiting and diarrhea, and pancreatic insufficiency.

Renal, Gastrointestinal, and Endocrine Disorders Hypomagnesemia can also result from renal magnesium wasting or from decreased production of (or end-organ responsiveness to) PTH.[58] Magnesium wasting may be seen in some patients with postobstructive diuresis, acute tubular necrosis, chronic glomerulonephritis, chronic pyelonephritis, or interstitial nephropathy, as well as after renal transplantation. The decreased magnesium excretion typically found with acute and chronic renal failure, however, generally results in these patients tending to be *hyper*magnesemic.

GI causes of hypomagnesemia include short-bowel syndrome, protein-calorie malnutrition, bowel fistula, continuous nasogastric suctioning, chronic diarrhea, and administration of total parenteral nutrition.[58] Patients with acute pancreatitis typically have an intracellular magnesium deficiency despite normal serum concentrations. This is most likely in patients who are also hypocalcemic.

Box 119-12 Causes of Hypomagnesemia

Alcoholic Abuse

Diuretic Use

Renal Losses

Acute and chronic renal failure
Postobstructive diuresis
Acute tubular necrosis
Chronic glomerulonephritis
Chronic pyelonephritis
Interstitial nephropathy
Renal transplantation

Gastrointestinal Losses

Chronic diarrhea
Nasogastric suctioning
Short-bowel syndrome
Protein-calorie malnutrition
Bowel fistula
Total parenteral nutrition
Acute pancreatitis

Endocrine Disorders

Diabetes mellitus
Hyperaldosteronism
Hyperthyroidism
Hyperparathyroidism
Acute intermittent porphyria

Pregnancy

Drugs

Aminoglycosides
Amphotericin
β-Agonists
Cisplatin
Cyclosporine
Diuretics
Foscarnet
Pentamidine
Theophylline

Congenital Disorders

Familial hypomagnesemia
Maternal diabetes
Maternal hypothyroidism
Maternal hyperparathyroidism

Hypomagnesemia is the most common electrolyte abnormality in ambulatory diabetic patients and is also a common finding in patients with diabetic ketoacidosis. Excessive urinary loss associated with glycosuria and transcellular shifts of the cation are the proposed mechanisms. The clinical consequences of magnesium deficiency include impairment of insulin secretion and peripheral insulin resistance. Hypomagnesemia also may play a role in the development of retinopathy, hypertension, and the abnormal platelet function often observed in diabetic patients. Other endocrine and metabolic causes of hypomagnesemia include primary and secondary aldosteronism, hyperthyroidism, primary hyperparathyroidism, and acute intermittent porphyria.

Pregnancy Pregnancy is marked by a state of hypomagnesemia. Serum levels usually decline in the third trimester. Patients with preterm labor are more likely to have a significantly depressed serum magnesium level.[59]

Drugs Hypomagnesemia has also been associated with a number of drugs.[60] This may be caused by renal magnesium wasting (e.g., aminoglycosides, amphotericin B, cisplatin, diuretics, foscarnet, pentamidine) or transcellular magnesium shifts (e.g., β-agonists, cyclosporine, theophylline).[61]

Congenital Disorders Congenital disorders causing hypomagnesemia include primary infantile hypomagnesemia and familial hypomagnesemia. Maternal diabetes, maternal hyperparathyroidism, and maternal hypothyroidism may also be associated with hypomagnesemia in the newborn.

Clinical Features The clinical manifestations of hypomagnesemia are nonspecific and can easily be confused with those caused by other metabolic abnormalities. Symptoms are inconsistent, variable in severity, and not well correlated with a specific serum magnesium level. However, patients are usually symptomatic at serum levels of 1.2 mg/dl or less. The clinical manifestations of hypomagnesemia most likely to be prominent in the emergency setting involve the neuromuscular and cardiovascular systems.

Neuromuscular manifestations may include muscle weakness, tremor, hyperreflexia, tetany, and a positive Chvostek's or Trousseau's sign. CNS findings range from apathy, irritability, and dizziness to seizures, papilledema, and coma. Focal neurologic findings have also been described.

Dysrhythmia is the most common cardiovascular manifestation of hypomagnesemia. A number of studies demonstrate an increased incidence of supraventricular dysrhythmias (atrial fibrillation, multifocal atrial tachycardia, paroxysmal supraventricular tachycardia) and ventricular dysrhythmias (PVCs, ventricular tachycardia, torsades de pointes, ventricular fibrillation) in patients who are magnesium deficient.[62] Patients taking diuretics for the treatment of CHF are particularly vulnerable. Digitalis-induced dysrhythmias are also more likely in the presence of hypomagnesemia. Because magnesium is an essential cofactor for the Na^+-K^+ ATPase pump that is inhibited by digitalis, hypomagnesemia typically worsens the manifestations of digitalis toxicity.

Hypomagnesemia has been associated with a wide range of ECG findings, including prolongation of the PR, QRS, and QT intervals; ST-T-segment abnormalities; flattening and widening of the T wave; and presence of U waves. These findings, however, are nonspecific and may be at least partly caused by associated hypokalemia. Thus the ECG should not be used to rule out magnesium disturbances.

The relationship between hypomagnesemia and ischemic heart disease is controversial. Hypomagnesemia is common in ED patients with chest pain and in those admitted to the coronary care unit.[62] Patients who "rule in" for myocardial infarction (MI) are more likely to be hypomagnesemic than those who do not. This finding has been shown to be independent of concomitant diuretic use. Serum magnesium levels decline transiently after acute MI, increasing the risk of dysrhythmia.[63,64] Proposed mechanisms include transcellular shifts of the cation and chelation with free fatty acids released after acute MI. Although several studies demonstrate a benefit of empiric magnesium administration after acute MI, the largest trial to date, the International Study of Infarct Survival (ISIS IV), failed to confirm a significant benefit.[65]

Management Because it is often an inaccurate reflection of total magnesium stores, the serum magnesium level should not be used alone to guide therapy. However, magnesium administration is appropriate in patients with a low serum level (<1.2 mg/dl), as well as in those with a normal serum magnesium level and symptoms suggestive of hypomagnesemia. For life-threatening conditions (dysrhythmias, seizures) in which hypomagnesemia is the suspected cause, parenteral magnesium should be given. In patients with normal renal function, 2 to 4 g of 50% magnesium sulfate (16.6 to 33.3 mEq) is a reasonable initial dose. This should be diluted in saline or dextrose and given over 30 to 60 minutes. More rapid administration may result in venous irritation and phlebitis. Bolus administration should be avoided because this may cause bradycardia and varying degrees of heart block, as well as hypotension. Magnesium should be administered with caution, if at all, in patients with atrioventricular block or renal insufficiency. Most administered magnesium is promptly excreted in the urine. Total magnesium repletion therefore requires administration of more than a single dose, generally over days.

Several different oral magnesium formulations are available. Preparations of magnesium gluconate, magnesium carbonate, magnesium oxide, and magnesium chloride each provide different doses of elemental magnesium. Large doses of magnesium salts may cause diarrhea. Magnesium as the chloride salt or as enteric-coated tablets (e.g., Slow-Mag) is usually better tolerated.

Hypermagnesemia

Principles of Disease Hypermagnesemia is a fairly rare disorder. Under normal circumstances the kidneys increase magnesium excretion as the magnesium load increases. A healthy adult can excrete more than 6 g of magnesium daily. For this reason, clinically significant hypermagnesemia is encountered almost exclusively in the setting of *renal insufficiency* (Box 119-13). Serum magnesium levels rise as the creatinine clearance falls below 30 ml/min and typically reach approximately 2.5 mEq/L as renal function nears zero. Although severe renal failure alone may cause symptomatic hypermagnesemia, this is more likely when a patient with preexisting renal failure is challenged with an exogenous magnesium load. Clinically significant hypermagnesemia can

Box 119-13 Causes of Hypermagnesemia

Impaired Renal Magnesium Excretion

Exogenous Magnesium Administration

Antacids
Laxatives
Cathartics
Dialysate
Parenteral

Impaired Magnesium Elimination

Anticholinergics
Narcotics
Chronic constipation
Bowel obstruction
Gastric dilation
Colitis

Miscellaneous

Rhabdomyolysis
Tumor lysis syndrome
Adrenal insufficiency
Hyperparathyroidism
Hypothyroidism
Lithium therapy

be produced even by usual therapeutic doses of magnesium-containing preparations in patients with renal insufficiency. Elderly patients misusing over-the-counter medications are particularly at risk.

Iatrogenic hypermagnesemia may result from parenteral magnesium administration, excessive magnesium in dialysate solutions, or ingestion of magnesium-containing antacids or laxatives.[66] Severe hypermagnesemia may rarely occur in the patient with normal renal function, but only when such massive magnesium loads are administered that magnesium absorption exceeds the normal renal excretory capacity. IV magnesium infusion for the treatment of preeclampsia and eclampsia is a common cause of hypermagnesemia but leads to problems only when excessive doses are given or when renal function is compromised. Another situation particularly relevant to the EP is multidose administration of magnesium-containing cathartics during overdose management. Although several case reports document severe hypermagnesemia in this setting, clinically significant hypermagnesemia is rare in the absence of preexisting renal insufficiency.[67] A review of 102 patients receiving multiple doses of magnesium citrate during overdose management (mean dose 9.22 g) reported only modest rises in serum magnesium, with no clinically significant side effects.[68]

Decreased GI motility may cause an increase in the absorption of magnesium-containing substances and result in toxicity. This may occur after the ingestion of certain drugs (e.g., anticholinergics, narcotics) or in patients with hypomotility disorders (e.g., chronic constipation, colitis, bowel obstruction, gastric dilation). Although symptomatic hypermagnesemia is more likely in patients with preexisting renal insufficiency, it has been reported in patients with normal renal function.[69]

Other, less common causes of hypermagnesemia include rhabdomyolysis, tumor lysis syndrome, adrenal insufficiency, hyperparathyroidism, hypothyroidism, and lithium therapy.

Clinical Features The clinical manifestations of hypermagnesemia generally correlate well with the serum level. Early signs of hypermagnesemia, including nausea, vomiting, weakness, and cutaneous flushing, usually appear at serum levels of approximately 3 mg/dl. As levels rise above 4 mg/dl, hyporeflexia is seen, and deep tendon reflexes are eventually lost. Hypotension and ECG changes (e.g., QRS widening, QT and PR prolongation, conduction abnormalities) are seen at serum levels of 5 to 6 mg/dl. Levels greater than 9 mg/dl are associated with respiratory depression, coma, and complete heart block.[70] Asystole, cardiac arrest, and death have been reported in patients with serum magnesium levels of 10 to 15 mg/dl.[71,72] Although hypermagnesemia may decrease the anion gap, numerous cases of hypermagnesemia with a normal anion gap have been reported.

Management The first step in the management of hypermagnesemia is to discontinue all exogenous magnesium. Further treatment depends on the clinical presentation, the degree of hypermagnesemia, and the patient's underlying renal function. Patients with mild symptoms and normal renal function may require only observation. If more prominent symptoms are present, hydration with isotonic fluids and administration of IV furosemide can be used to accelerate magnesium elimination. If these measures are used, the serum potassium level should be closely monitored.

Patients with severe hypermagnesemia should receive IV calcium. Calcium directly antagonizes the membrane effects of hypermagnesemia and reverses respiratory depression, hypotension, and cardiac dysrhythmias. For life-threatening manifestations of hypermagnesemia, 100 to 200 mg of calcium, as either 10% calcium gluconate (93 mg calcium per ampule) or 10% calcium chloride (360 mg calcium per ampule), is a reasonable dose. Repeat boluses or a continuous infusion (2 to 4 mg/kg/hr) may be required to sustain the effect while measures to increase magnesium elimination are instituted. Dialysis should be considered in patients with coma, respiratory failure, or hemodynamic instability and in those with severe hypermagnesemia associated with renal failure.

PHOSPHORUS

Normal Physiology

Phosphorus is located primarily in the cell complexed with oxygen and hydrogen as *phosphate*. In this form, phosphate is an important component of nucleic acids (RNA and DNA) and of the phospholipid cell membrane. Phosphate is an essential component of ATP, the energy currency of all living cells, and of erythrocyte 2,3-diphosphoglycerate (2,3-DPG), which promotes the release of circulating oxygen at the tissue level. Phosphate also binds with calcium to form hydroxyapatite, the major salt of bone matrix.[73]

In the serum, phosphate is an important acid-base buffer. In the presence of acidosis, divalent phosphate (HPO_4^{-2}) binds excess hydrogen ion, shifting to the monovalent form ($H_2PO_4^-$). The reverse occurs when the extracellular fluid becomes alkalotic.

The normal adult human body contains approximately 700 g of phosphate, 80% of which is contained in the mineral component of bone. Phosphate balance is maintained by three different organs: intestine, kidney, and bone. PTH and vitamin D are the major hormonal regulators of plasma phosphate concentration, although these hormones are released in response to changes in ionized calcium rather than phosphate. Normal serum phosphate levels range from 3 to 4.5 mg/dl.

Dietary sources of phosphate include fruits, vegetables, meats, and dairy products. Absorption of ingested phosphate occurs through active and passive transport in the small intestine. Vitamin D enhances the absorption of both phosphate and calcium.

In the kidneys, 90% of the filtered load of phosphate is reabsorbed in the proximal tubule. Renal reabsorption increases in deficiency states. When serum phosphate levels increase, renal reabsorption decreases. PTH acts at the proximal and distal tubules to inhibit phosphate resorption. In the absence of normal renal function, PTH cannot increase phosphate excretion and may actually increase serum phosphate levels because of its effect on intestine and bone.[74] Thyroid hormone and growth hormone both increase renal phosphate resorption.

The release and uptake of phosphate by bone are primarily determined by the mechanisms governing calcium metabolism. When the serum calcium level falls, both calcium and phosphate are released into the extracellular space by the action of PTH. When serum calcium levels rise, bone formation increases, and phosphate and calcium shift from the serum into bone.[73]

Hypophosphatemia

Principles of Disease Hypophosphatemia has traditionally been classified as mild (2.5 to 2.8 mg/dl), moderate (1.0 to 2.5 mg/dl), or severe (<1.0 mg/dl). The incidence of hypophosphatemia in hospitalized patients is 2% to 3% and as high as 30% in those admitted to the intensive care unit. Severe hypophosphatemia is seen in up to 0.5% of hospitalized patients. Important risk factors include diabetic ketoacidosis, malnutrition, diuretic or antacid therapy, sepsis, and alcoholism. The many causes include (1) disorders that result in increased renal excretion, (2) disorders that are associated with decreased GI absorption, and (3) disorders in which phosphate shifts from the serum into cells (Box 119-14).[75]

Renal phosphate loss is most often the result of diuretic therapy. The thiazides, loop diuretics, and acetazolamide promote renal phosphate wasting.[74-76] Hypophosphatemia may also be seen in patients with acute renal failure, renal transplantation, and long-term peritoneal dialysis, although renal insufficiency is typically associated with hyperphosphatemia rather than hypophosphatemia.[77] In hyperparathyroidism, high levels of circulating PTH increase renal phosphate excretion and may cause hypophosphatemia.

Diabetic ketoacidosis is an important cause of hypophosphatemia. Metabolic acidosis and insulin deficiency mobilize intracellular phosphate stores, and in the setting of an ongoing osmotic diuresis, urinary losses increase. Because of a shift of phosphate from cells to the blood, serum levels may be normal in the face of a profound total deficit. Treatment of diabetic ketoacidosis with insulin causes phosphate to move back into cells and may result in a sharp decline in the serum level.[78] The benefit of routine phosphate replacement in diabetic ketoacidosis is unproven, although patients with low serum phosphate levels in the face of acidosis should be presumed to have a severe deficiency. Because these patients are often hypokalemic, replacement with potassium phosphate salts is a reasonable approach.

Decreased phosphate intake and impaired intestinal phosphate absorption are other causes of hypophosphatemia. Up to 50% of alcoholics are hypophosphatemic. Increased renal excretion and decreased intake are the proposed mechanisms. Hypophosphatemia may be exacerbated when glucose-containing solutions are administered because these cause phosphate to shift from the serum into cells.

Because phosphate is ubiquitous in most food sources, starvation and chronic malnutrition are relatively uncommon causes in the developed world, although low-birth-weight infants are particularly vulnerable. Decreased intestinal phosphate absorption occurs in malabsorptive syndromes, chronic diarrhea, and vitamin D deficiency. Phosphate-binding antacids (calcium carbonate, aluminum hydroxide, aluminum carbonate) prevent the absorption of dietary phosphate, and long-term therapy can lead to hypophosphatemia.

Transcellular shifts of phosphate from the extracellular space into cells is the third mechanism of hypophosphatemia. Respiratory alkalosis is a common cause of hypophosphatemia. Reduction of intracellular carbon dioxide tension increases the activity of phosphofructokinase, the rate-limiting enzyme of glycolysis, and phosphorylation of glucose precursors increases cellular uptake of serum phosphate, causing hypophosphatemia. Hyperventilation-induced hypophosphatemia may occur in the setting of sepsis, heatstroke, salicylate poisoning, neuroleptic malignant syndrome, hepatic encephalopathy, alcohol withdrawal, and acute panic disorders.

Box 119-14 Causes of Hypophosphatemia

- I. Renal loss
  - A. Diuretic therapy
  - B. Renal tubular dysfunction
  - C. Hyperosmolar states
    - 1. Diabetic ketoacidosis
    - 2. Hyperosmolar hyperglycemic nonketotic coma
  - D. Hyperparathyroidism
  - E. Aldosteronism
  - F. Glucocorticoid administration
- II. Insufficient intestinal absorption
  - A. Decreased dietary intake
  - B. Starvation/malnutrition
  - C. Phosphate-binding antacids
  - D. Vitamin D deficiency
  - E. Chronic diarrhea
  - F. Nasogastric suctioning
- III. Transcellular shift
  - A. Respiratory alkalosis
    - 1. Sepsis
    - 2. Heatstroke
    - 3. Salicylate poisoning
    - 4. Neuroleptic malignant syndrome
    - 5. Hepatic encephalopathy
    - 6. Alcohol withdrawal
  - B. Hyperglycemia
  - C. Insulin administration

The administration of glucose-containing solutions to chronically malnourished patients can precipitate the so-called refeeding syndrome, in which insulin release increases cellular phosphate uptake, decreasing the serum concentration. This can be prevented by adding supplemental phosphate to the diet. β-Receptor agonists used in the management of acute asthma stimulate cellular uptake of phosphate and may precipitate hypophosphatemia.[79-80] Administration of catecholamines and sodium bicarbonate also shifts phosphate into the cell. Increased metabolic demands in postoperative patients increase cellular phosphate uptake and can cause a deficiency state. Certain rapidly growing malignancies (e.g., leukemia, Burkitt's lymphoma, histiocytic lymphoma) also take up enough phosphate to cause hypophosphatemia.

Clinical Features The signs and symptoms of hypophosphatemia result from impaired production of ATP and inadequate energy metabolism. Virtually every organ system can be affected (Box 119-15). Mild or moderate hypophosphatemia is usually asymptomatic, and major clinical sequelae are usually seen only in severe hypophosphatemia. With severe phosphate depletion, myocardial depression is seen, and hypotension, impaired pressor responsiveness, and left ventricular dysfunction have been reported.[81] Hypophosphatemia also reduces the threshold for ventricular dysrhythmias.

Respiratory insufficiency is common among severely

Box 119-15 Clinical Features of Hypophosphatemia

Cardiovascular
Decreased contractility
Hypotension
Dysrhythmias
Cardiomyopathy

Pulmonary
Respiratory failure
Ventilator dependence

Skeletal Muscle
Weakness
Myalgias
Rhabdomyolysis

Hematologic
Decreased tissue oxygen delivery
Hemolysis
Leukocyte dysfunction
Platelet dysfunction

Neurologic
Paresthesias
Seizures
Coma

hypophosphatemic patients. Decreased energy substrate leads to respiratory muscle weakness, depressed diaphragmatic contractility, hypoxia, and respiratory acidosis. Rapid correction of chronic respiratory acidosis with assisted ventilation may decrease the serum phosphate level further by shifting the anion into the cell. Inability to wean a ventilated patient may be an important consequence of hypophosphatemia.

The effects of hypophosphatemia on skeletal muscle are also related to depletion of intracellular ATP. Symptoms include muscle weakness, myalgias, and fatigue.[82] Hypophosphatemia may cause rhabdomyolysis. This may be asymptomatic, manifested only by increased serum muscle enzyme levels, or may cause severe muscle pain and weakness and acute renal failure. Rhabdomyolysis may be precipitated by acute alcohol withdrawal, by the treatment of diabetic ketoacidosis, and in hypophosphatemic patients by hyperalimentation. Significant rhabdomyolysis results in the release of phosphate from muscle cells, and serum phosphate levels may be normal or even high despite intracellular hypophosphatemia.

Hypophosphatemia results in impaired production of 2,3-DPG in the erythrocyte, causing a leftward shift of the oxyhemoglobin dissociation curve and decreased tissue oxygen delivery. In the absence of adequate ATP stores, the erythrocyte is unable to maintain membrane integrity and the ability to deform and alter its shape as it passes through capillaries. This may result in hemolysis and increased destruction in the spleen. Hypophosphatemia is also associated with leukocyte dysfunction with impaired chemotaxis, phagocytosis, and opsonization, increasing the susceptibility to infection.

Neurologic manifestations of severe hypophosphatemia

Box 119-16 Causes of Hyperphosphatemia

I. Pseudohyperphosphatemia
  A. Paraproteinemia
  B. Hyperlipidemia
  C. Hemolysis
  D. Hyperbilirubinemia
II. Renal
  A. Acute and chronic renal failure
  B. Increased renal tubular reabsorption
    1. Hypoparathyroidism
    2. Thyrotoxicosis
    3. Excess vitamin D administration
III. Cellular injury
  A. Rhabdomyolysis
  B. Tumor lysis syndrome
  C. Hemolysis
IV. Increased intake
  A. Phosphate enemas or laxatives
  B. Intravenous or oral phosphate administration

include weakness, confusion, seizures, and coma. Peripheral neuropathy and an ascending motor paralysis resembling Guillain-Barré syndrome have been reported.

Management The treatment of hypophosphatemia depends both on the serum level and on the severity of symptoms. Mild or moderate hypophosphatemia can usually be treated with oral supplements such as potassium phosphate. Severe hyperphosphatemia should be treated with IV phosphate. Two preparations are available: potassium phosphate and sodium phosphate. Because hypophosphatemia and hypokalemia can coexist in some disorders (e.g., diabetic ketoacidosis, alcoholism), replacement with the potassium salt is most appropriate.[83,84]

Complications of IV phosphate administration include acute hypocalcemia and hyperphosphatemia. Patients should be monitored for signs of hypocalcemia, such as tetany. Phosphate should be administered with particular caution in patients with renal dysfunction.[73,74]

Hyperphosphatemia

Principles of Disease Hyperphosphatemia (>5.0 mg/dl) is rare in patients with normal renal function because the kidneys readily excrete an excess phosphate load. True hyperphosphatemia can result from decreased phosphate clearance, an increased endogenous phosphate load, or an increased exogenous load (Box 119-16).

Pseudohyperphosphatemia represents a spurious elevation of inorganic phosphate measurements caused by interference with analytical methods. Causes include paraproteinemia (e.g., multiple myeloma), hyperlipidemia, hemolysis, and hyperbilirubinemia.

Renal failure is the most common cause of hyperphosphatemia.[74] The serum phosphate typically remains normal until the creatinine clearance falls below 30 ml/min.[85] Hyperphosphatemia is usually mild unless an exogenous phosphate load is given. Hyperphosphatemia may also occur in patients with normal renal function when renal phosphate resorption is increased, as occurs with PTH deficiency, and in the setting of thyrotoxicosis or excessive vitamin D administration.

Hyperphosphatemia can also occur with large endogenous phosphate loads, as with extensive cell damage, which causes phosphate to be released into the extracellular space. This may occur in the setting of rhabdomyolysis, tumor lysis syndrome, or hemolysis.[86] Patients with these disorders often develop renal failure, impairing phosphate excretion and further increasing serum levels.

Hypophosphatemia may also result from exogenous loads, as with IV, oral, or rectal phosphate administration. Infants, elderly persons, and patients with preexisting renal insufficiency are particularly vulnerable.[87-90]

Clinical Features The clinical signs of hyperphosphatemia reflect the associated hypocalcemia that results when excess serum phosphate binds with calcium and precipitates in tissues. Signs of neuromuscular hyperexcitability (e.g., paresthesias, hyperreflexia, tetany, seizures) and myocardial depression (e.g., hypotension, bradycardia, left ventricular dysfunction) predominate. Tissue deposition of calcium phosphate may result in acute heart block and death.

Management The emergency treatment of hyperphosphatemia involves supportive care and treatment of symptomatic hypocalcemia. In patients with normal renal function, infusion of isotonic saline increases phosphate clearance. The administration of dextrose and insulin drives phosphate into cells, temporarily lowering the serum level.

Aluminum-containing antacids are the mainstay of the prevention of hyperphosphatemia in patients with chronic renal failure.[91] Although these are usually not administered in the ED, their use is reasonable in the management of hyperphosphatemia after a large overdose of exogenous phosphate. When hyperphosphatemia poses a threat to life, hemodialysis or peritoneal dialysis should be considered, especially in patients with renal failure.

KEY CONCEPTS

- The primary symptoms of *hyponatremia* are related to the central nervous system, including lethargy, apathy, confusion, disorientation, agitation, depression, and psychosis.
- Treatment of *hyponatremia* is based on severity of symptoms, estimated duration of illness, and patient's volume status. Patients with acute hyponatremia are usually symptomatic (e.g., severe weakness, diminished consciousness, seizures) when the serum sodium falls below 120 mEq/L, whereas patients with chronic hyponatremia may tolerate much lower levels.
- Acute *hyponatremia* may be corrected at rates of up to 1 to 2 mEq/L/hr, and chronic hyponatremia should be corrected at a rate not greater than 0.5 mEq/L/hr. In general the serum sodium should not be increased by more than 10 mEq/L in a 24-hour period.
- Oral therapy for *hypokalemia* is preferable to IV therapy because of the risk of inducing hyperkalemia through the IV route. However, patients with prominent symptoms (e.g., dysrhythmias) and those who are unable to tolerate oral supplements should receive IV potassium replacement.
- The ECG can provide valuable clues to the presence of *hyperkalemia* (e.g., peaked T waves, loss of P waves, QRS widening).
- Treatment of *hyperkalemia* includes cardiovascular monitoring, administration of calcium for hemodynamic instability, lowering of serum potassium, and correction of the underlying disorder.
- Treatment of *hypercalcemia* (IV fluids, furosemide, osteoclastic inhibitors such as bisphosphonates [etidronate, pamidronate], plicamycin, calcitonin, glucocorticoids, and gallium nitrate) should be initiated in patients with significant symptoms (e.g. severe dehydration, alteration of consciousness, dysrhythmias) or when the calcium level is above 14 mg/dl. The goals of therapy are normalization of volume status, enhancement of renal calcium elimination, diminution of osteoclastic activity, and treatment of the underlying disorder.
- In *hypomagnesemia,* although the serum magnesium level often inaccurately reflects total body stores, magnesium supplementation should be considered when the level is less than 1.2 mg/dl. IV magnesium therapy should be instituted for patients with significant symptoms (e.g., seizures, dysrhythmias).

REFERENCES

1. Weisberg LS: Pseudohyponatremia: a reappraisal, *Am J Med* 86:315, 1989.
2. Illowsky BP, Kirch DG: Polydipsia and hyponatremia in psychiatric patients, *Am J Psychiatry* 145:675, 1988.
3. Riggs JE: Neurologic manifestations of fluid and electrolyte disturbances, *Neurol Clin* 7:509, 1989.
4. Chung SM et al: Clinical assessment of extracellular fluid volume in hyponatremia, *Am J Med* 83:905, 1987.
5. Snyder NA, Feigal DW, Arieff AI: Hypernatremia in elderly patients: a heterogenous morbid entity, *Ann Intern Med* 107:309, 1987.
6. Conley S: Hypernatremia, *Pediatr Clin North Am* 37:365, 1990.
7. Buoncore CM, Robinson AG: The diagnosis and management of diabetes inspidus during medical emergencies, *Endocrinol Metab Clin North Am* 22:411, 1993.
8. Brown RS: Potassium homeostasis and clinical implications, *Am J Med* 77:3, 1994.
9. Brem AS: Disorders of potassium homeostasis, *Pediatr Clin North Am* 37:419, 1990.
10. Zull DN: Disorders of potassium metabolism, *Emerg Med Clin North Am* 7:771, 1989.
11. Young WF et al: Primary aldosteronism: diagnosis and treatment, *Mayo Clin Proc* 65:96, 1996.
12. Salmeron M et al: Nebulized versus intravenous albuterol in hypercapnic acute asthma: a multicenter, double-blind, randomized study, *Am J Respir Crit Care Med* 149:1466, 1994.
13. Bodenhamer J et al: Frequently nebulized β-agonists for asthma: effects on serum electrolytes, *Ann Emerg Med* 21:1337, 1992.
14. Capobianco DJ: Hyperthyroidism and periodic paralysis, *J Fla Med Assoc* 77:884, 1990.
15. Riggs JE: Neurologic manifestations of fluid and electrolyte disturbances, *Neurol Clin* 7:509, 1989.
16. Weisberg LS, Szerlap HM, Cox M: Disorders of potassium homeostasis in critically ill patients, *Crit Care Clin* 3:835, 1987.
17. Hamill RJ et al: Efficacy and safety of potassium infusion therapy in hypokalemic critically ill patients, *Crit Care Med* 19:694, 1991.
18. Williams ME, Rosa RM, Epstein FH: Hyperkalemia, *Adv Intern Med* 31:265, 1986.
19. Alappan R, Peerazella MA, Buller GK: Hyperkalemia in hospitalized patients treated with trimethoprim-sulfamethoxazole, *Ann Intern Med* 124:316, 1996.
20. Mimh LB, Rathburn RC, Resman-Targoff BH: Hyperkalemia associated with high dose trimethoprim-sulfamethoxazole in a patient with the acquired immunodeficiency syndrome, *Pharmacotherapy* 15:793, 1995.
21. Allon M: Hyperkalemia in end-stage renal disease: mechanisms and management, *J Am Soc Nephrol* 6:1135, 1995.

22. Allon M, Shanklin N: Effect of bicarbonate administration in plasma potassium in dialysis patients: interactions with insulin and albuterol, *Am J Kidney Dis* 28:508, 1996.
23. Allon M. Dunlay R, Copkney C: Nebulized albuterol for acute hyperkalemia in-patients on hemodialysis, *Ann Intern Med* 110:426, 1989.
24. Lin JL et al: Outcomes of severe hyperkalemia in cardiopulmonary resuscitation with concomitant hemodialysis, *Intensive Care Med* 20:287, 1994.
25. Reber PM, Heath H III: Hypocalcemic emergencies, *Med Clin North Am* 79:93, 1995.
26. Kainer G, Chan JCM: Hypocalcemic and hypercalcemic disorders in children, *Curr Probl Pediatr* 10:497, 1989.
27. Wilson RF et al: Electrolyte and acid-base changes with massive blood transfusions, *Am Surg* 58:535, 1992.
28. Crain JC, Hodson EM, Martin HC: Phosphate enema poisoning in children, *Med J Aust* 160:347, 1994.
29. Potts JT: Management of asymptomatic hyperparathyroidism, *J Clin Endocrinol Metab* 70:1489, 1990.
30. Consensus Development Conference Panel: Diagnosis and management of asymptomatic primary hyperparathyroidism, *Ann Intern Med* 114:593, 1991.
31. Palmer M et al: Prevalence of hypercalcemia in a healthy survey: a 14-year follow up study of serum calcium values, *Eur J Clin Invest* 18:39, 1988.
32. Bilezikian JP: Etiologies and therapy of hypercalcemia, *Endrocrinol Metab Clin North Am* 18:389, 1989.
33. Rizzoli R, Bonjour JP: Management of disorders of calcium homeostasis, *Baillieres Clin Endocrinol Metab* 6:129, 1992.
34. Kaye TB: Hypercalcemia: how to pinpoint the cause and customize therapy, *Postgrad Med* 97:153, 1995.
35. Pimentel L: Medical complications of oncologic disease, *Emerg Med Clin North Am* 11:407, 1993.
36. Walls J, Bundred N, Howell A: Hypercalcemia and bone resorption in malignancy, *Clin Orthop* 312:51, 1995.
37. Broadus AE et al: Humoral hypercalcemia of cancer: identification of a novel parathyroid hormone–like peptide, *N Engl J Med* 319:556, 1988.
38. Kao PC et al: Parathyroid hormone–related peptide in plasma of patients with hypercalcemia and malignant lesions, *Mayo Clin Proc* 65:1399, 1990.
39. Budayr AA et al: Increased serum levels of a parathyroid hormone–like protein in malignancy-associated hypercalcemia, *Ann Intern Med* 111:807, 1989.
40. Burtis WJ et al: Immunocytochemical characterization of circulating parathyroid hormone–related protein in patients with humoral hypercalcemia of cancer, *N Engl J Med* 322:1106, 1990.
41. Rizzato B, Fraioli P, Montemurro L: Nephrolithiasis as a presenting feature of chronic sarcoidosis, *Thorax* 50:555, 1995.
42. Connin CC et al: Precipitation of hypercalcemia in sarcoidosis by foreign sun holidays: report of four cases, *Postgrad Med J* 66:307, 1990.
43. Sato M, Grasser W: Effect of diphosphonates on isolated rat osteoclasts as examined by reflected light microscopy, *J Bone Miner Res* 5:31, 1991.
44. Singer FR et al: Treatment of hypercalcemia of malignancy with intravenous etidronate: a controlled multicenter study, *Arch Intern Med* 151:471, 1991.
45. Singer FR: Role of the bisphosphonate etidronate in the therapy of cancer-related hypercalcemia, *Semin Oncol* 17:34, 1990.
46. Fitton A, McTavish D: Pamidronate: a review of its pharmacological properties and therapeutic efficacy in resortive bone disease, *Drugs* 41:289, 1991.
47. Gucalp R et al: Comparative study of pamidronate disodium and etidronate disodium in the treatment of cancer-related hypercalcemia, *J Clin Oncol* 10:134, 1992.
48. Levine MM, Kleeman CR: Hypercalcemia: pathophysiology and treatment, *Hosp Pract* 22(7):73, 1987.
49. Whang R, Ryder KW: Frequency of hypomagnesemia and hypermagnesemia, *JAMA* 263:3063, 1990.
50. Olinger ML: Disorders of calcium and magnesium metabolism, *Emerg Med Clin North Am* 7:795, 1989.
51. Martin BJ, Black J, McLelland AS: Hypomagnesemia in elderly hospital admission: a study of clinical significance, *Q J Med* 78:177, 1991.
52. Whang R, Hampton EM, Whang DD: Magnesium homeostasis and clinical disorders of magnesium deficiency, *Ann Pharmacother* 28:220, 1994.
53. Ryan MP: Interrelationship of magnesium and potassium homeostasis, *Miner Electrolyte Metab* 19:290, 1993.
54. Hamill-Ruth RJ, McGory R: Magnesium repletion and its effect on potassium homeostasis in critically ill adults: results of a double-blind, randomized, controlled study, *Crit Care Med* 24:38, 1996.
55. Ramsey LE, Yeo WW, Jackson PR: Metabolic effects of diuretics, *Cardiology* 2:48, 1994.
56. Elisaf M et al: Acid-base and electrolyte abnormalities in alcoholic patients, *Miner Electrolyte Metab* 20:274, 1994.
57. Ragland G: Electrolyte abnormalities in the alcoholic patient, *Emerg Med Clin North Am* 8:761, 1990.
58. Al-Ghamdi SM, Cameron EC, Sutton RA: Magnesium deficiency: pathophysiologic and clinical overview, *Am J Kidney Dis* 24:737, 1994.
59. Kurzel RB: Serum magnesium levels in pregnancy and preterm labor, *Am J Perinatol* 8:119, 1991.
60. Cameron JD: Serum magnesium as affected by drugs, *Clin Chem* 35:506, 1989.
61. Shah GM, Kirschenbaum MA: Renal magnesium wasting associated with therapeutic agents, *Miner Electrolyte Metab* 17:58, 1991.
62. Millane TA, Ward DE, Camm AJ: Is hypomagnesemia arrhythmogenic? *Clin Cardiol* 15:103, 1992.
63. Salem M et al: Hypomagnesemia is a frequent finding in the emergency department in patients with chest pain, *Arch Intern Med* 151:2185, 1991.
64. Rasmussen JS et al: Magnesium deficiency in patients with ischemic heart disease with and without acute myocardial infarction uncovered by an intravenous loading test, *Arch Intern Med* 148:329, 1988.
65. ISIS IV Collaborative Group: ISIS IV: randomized factorial trial assessing early oral captopril, oral mononitrate, and intravenous magnesium sulfate in 58,050 patients with suspected acute myocardial infarction, *Lancet* 345:669, 1995.
66. Quereshi TI, Melonakos TK: Acute hypermagnesemia after laxative use, *Ann Emerg Med* 28:552, 1996.
67. Gerald SK, Hernadez C, Khayam-Bashi H: Extreme hypermagnesemia caused by an overdose of magnesium-containing cathartics, *Ann Emerg Med* 17:728, 1988.
68. Woodard JA et al: Serum magnesium concentration after repetitive magnesium cathartic administration, *Am J Med* 8:297, 1990.
69. Clark BA, Brown RS: Unsuspected morbid hypermagnesemia in elderly patients, *Am J Nephrol* 12:336, 1992.
70. Mosseri M et al: Electrocardiographic manifestations of combined hypercalcemia and hypermagnesemia, *J Electrocardiol* 23:235, 1990.
71. Ferdinandus J, Pederson JA, Whang R: Hypermagnesemia as a cause of refractory hypotension, *Ann Intern Med* 141:669, 1991.
72. Zwerling H: Hypermagnesemia-induced hypotension and hypoventilation, *JAMA* 266:2374, 1991.
73. Yucha CB, Toto KH: Calcium and phosphorus derangements, *Crit Care Clin* 6:747, 1994.
74. Peppers MP, Gehelo M, Desai H: Hypophosphatemia and hyperphosphatemia, *Crit Care Clin* 7:201, 1991.
75. Thatte L et al: Review of the literature: severe hyperphosphatemia, *Am J Med Sci* 310:167, 1995.
76. Itescu S, Haskell LP, Tannenberg AM: Thiazide-induced clinically significant hypophosphatemia, *Clin Nephrol* 27:161, 1987.
77. Kurtin P, Kouba J: Profound hypophosphatemia in the course of acute renal failure, *Am J Kidney Dis* 10:346, 1987.
78. Bohannon NJ: Large phosphate shifts with treatment for hyperglycemia, *Arch Intern Med* 149:1423, 1989.
79. Brady HR et al: Hypophosphatemia complicating bronchodilator therapy for acute severe asthma, *Arch Intern Med* 10:2367, 1989.
80. Laaban JP et al: Hypophosphatemia complicating management of acute severe asthma, *Ann Intern Med* 112:68, 1990.
81. Davis SV, Olichwier KK, Chakko SC: Reversible depression of myocardial performance in hypophosphatemia, *Am J Med Sci* 295:183, 1988.

82. Gravelyn TR et al: Hypophosphatemia-associated respiratory muscle weakness in a general inpatient population, *Am J Med* 84:870, 1988.
83. Lentz RD, Brown DM, Kjellstrand CM: Treatment of severe hypophosphatemia, *Ann Intern Med* 89:941, 1989.
84. Lloyd CW, Johnson CE: Management of hypophosphatemia, *Clin Pharm* 7:123, 1988.
85. Sirmon MD, Kirkpatrick WG: Acute renal failure: what to do until the nephrologist comes, *Postgrad Med* 87:55, 1990.
86. Vachvanichsanong P et al: Severe hyperphosphatemia following acute tumor lysis syndrome, *Med Pediatr Oncol* 24:63, 1995.
87. Biarent D et al: Acute phosphate intoxication in seven infants under parenteral nutrition, *J Parenter Enteral Nutr* 16:558, 1992.
88. Fass R, Do S, Hixson LJ: Fatal hyperphosphatemia following Fleet Phospho-Soda in a patient with colonic ileus, *Am J Gastroenterol* 88:929, 1993.
89. Korzets A et al: Life-threatening hyperphosphatemia and hypocalcemic tetany following the use of Fleet enemas, *J Am Geriatr Soc* 40:620, 1992.
90. DiPalma JA et al: Biochemical effects of oral sodium phosphate, *Dig Dis Sci* 41:749, 1996.
91. Ghazali A et al: Management of hyperphosphatemia in patients with renal failure, *Curr Opin Nephrol Hypertens* 2:566, 1993.

120 Diabetes Mellitus and Disorders of Glucose Homeostasis

Rita K. Cydulka
Jonathan Siff

PERSPECTIVE

Diabetes mellitus is the most common endocrine disease. It comprises a heterogenous group of hyperglycemic disorders characterized by high serum glucose and disturbances of carbohydrate and lipid metabolism. Acute complications include hypoglycemia, diabetic ketoacidosis, and hyperglycemic hyperosmolar nonketotic coma. Long-term complications include disorders of the microvasculature, the cardiovascular system, eyes, kidneys, and nerves. Despite the discovery of insulin more than 75 years ago by Banting and Best,[1] the incidence of severe debilitating complications, including arteriosclerosis, renal failure, retinopathy, and neuropathy, remains high. The Diabetes Control and Complications Trial proved that tight blood glucose control reduces the risk of these late sequelae.[2] Patients with diabetes mellitus incur ED costs three times higher and are admitted to the hospital four times more often than nondiabetic patients.[3,4]

PRINCIPLES OF DISEASE

Normal Physiology

Maintenance of the plasma glucose concentration is critical to survival because plasma glucose is the predominant metabolic fuel used by the central nervous system (CNS). The CNS cannot synthesize glucose, store more than a few minutes' supply, or concentrate glucose from the circulation. Brief hypoglycemia can cause profound brain dysfunction, and prolonged severe hypoglycemia may cause cellular death. Glucose regulatory systems have evolved to prevent or correct hypoglycemia.[5]

The plasma glucose concentration is normally maintained within a relatively narrow range, between 60 and 150 mg/dl, despite wide variations in glucose that occur after meals and exercise. Glucose is derived from three sources: intestinal absorption from the diet; *glycogenolysis,* the breakdown of glycogen; and *gluconeogenesis,* the formation of glucose from precursors, including lactate, pyruvate, amino acids, and glycerol. After glucose ingestion, the plasma glucose concentration increases as a result of glucose absorption. Endogenous glucose production is suppressed. Plasma glucose then rapidly declines to a level below the baseline.

Insulin Insulin receptors on the beta cells of the pancreas sense elevated blood glucose and trigger insulin release into the blood. For incompletely understood reasons, glucose taken by mouth evokes more insulin release than parenteral glucose. Certain amino acids induce insulin release, even causing hypoglycemia in some patients. Sulfonylurea oral hypoglycemic agents are effective in part by stimulating the release of insulin from the pancreas.

The number of receptor sites helps determine the sensitivity of the particular tissue to circulating insulin. The number and sensitivity of receptor sites are also the primary factors in the long-term efficacy of the sulfonylurea oral hypoglycemic agents. Receptor sites are increased in glucocorticoid deficiency and may be relatively decreased in obese patients.

Under normal circumstances, degradation of insulin is rapid through the liver and kidney. The half-life of insulin is 3 to 10 minutes in the circulation. Whereas insulin is the major *anabolic* hormone pertinent to the diabetic disorder, glucagon plays the role of the major *catabolic* hormone in disordered glucose homeostasis.

Although most tissues have the enzyme systems required to synthesize glycogen and to hydrolyze glycogen, only the liver and kidneys contain *glucose-6-phosphatase,* the enzyme necessary for the release of glucose into the circulation. The liver is essentially the sole source of endogenous glucose production. Renal gluconeogenesis and glucose release contribute substantially to the systemic glucose pool only during prolonged starvation.

The hepatocyte does not require insulin for glucose to cross the cell membrane. However, insulin augments both the hepatic glucose uptake and the hepatic glucose storage needed for the process of energy generation and glycogen and fat synthesis. Insulin inhibits hepatic gluconeogenesis and glycogenolysis.[6]

Muscle can store and use glucose, primarily through glycolysis to *pyruvate,* which is reduced to lactate or transaminated to form alanine. *Lactate* released from muscle is transported to the liver, where it serves as a gluconeogenic precursor. *Alanine* may also flow from muscle to liver. During a fast, muscle can reduce its glucose uptake, oxidize fatty acids for its energy needs, and through proteolysis, mobilize amino acids for transport to the liver as gluconeogenic precursors. Adipose tissue can also use glucose for fatty acid synthesis for oxidation to form triglycerides. During a fast, adipocytes can also decrease their glucose use and satisfy energy needs through the β-oxidation of fatty acids. Other tissues do not have the capacity to decrease glucose use on fasting and therefore produce lactate at relatively fixed rates.

Glucose transport across the fat cell membrane also requires insulin. A large percentage of the adipocyte glucose is metabolized to form α-glycerophosphate, required for the esterification of fatty acids to form triglycerides. Although most insulin-mediated fatty acid synthesis occurs in the liver, a very small percentage occurs in fat cells, using the acetyl coenzyme A generated by glucose metabolism. Very low levels of insulin are required to inhibit intracellular lipolysis while stimulating the extracellular lipolysis required for circulating lipids to enter the fat cell.

Glucose Regulatory Mechanisms Maintenance of the normal plasma glucose concentration requires precise matching of glucose use and endogenous glucose production of dietary glucose delivery. The regulatory mechanisms that maintain systemic glucose balance involve hormonal, neurohumoral, and autoregulatory factors. Glucoregulatory hormones include insulin, glucagon, epinephrine, cortisol, and growth hormone. Insulin is the main glucose-lowering hormone. Insulin suppresses endogenous glucose production and stimulates glucose use. Insulin is secreted from the beta cells of the pancreatic islets into the hepatic portal circulation and has important actions on the liver and the peripheral tissues. Insulin stimulates glucose uptake, storage, and use by other insulin-sensitive tissues such as fat and muscle.[5]

Counterregulatory hormones include glucagon, epinephrine, norepinephrine, growth hormone, and cortisol. When glucose is not getting into the cells because of either a lack of food intake or lack of insulin, the body perceives a "fasting state" and releases *glucagon,* attempting to provide the glucose necessary for brain function. In contrast to the fed state, in the fasted state the body metabolizes protein and fat. Glucagon is secreted from the alpha cells of the pancreatic islets into the hepatic portal circulation. Glucagon lowers hepatic levels of fructose 2,6-biphosphate, resulting in decreased glycolysis and increased gluconeogenesis, an effect that may be enhanced by ketosis.[7] Glucagon increases the activity of adenyl cyclase in the liver, thereby increasing glycogen breakdown to glucose and further increasing hepatic gluconeogenesis. Glucagon acts to increase ketone production in the liver. Thus, whereas insulin is an anabolic agent that reduces blood glucose, glucagon is a catabolic agent that increases blood glucose. Glucagon is released in response to hypoglycemia, as well as to stress, trauma, infection, exercise, and starvation. It increases hepatic glucose production within minutes, although transiently.

Epinephrine both stimulates hepatic glucose production and limits glucose use through both direct and indirect actions mediated through both α- and β-adrenergic mechanisms. Epinephrine also acts directly to increase hepatic glycogenolysis and gluconeogenesis. It acts within minutes and produces a transient increase in glucose production but continues to support glucose production at approximately basal levels thereafter. *Norepinephrine* exerts hyperglycemic actions by mechanisms similar to those of epinephrine, except that norepinephrine is released from axon terminals of sympathetic postganglionic neurons.

Growth hormone initially has a plasma glucose–lowering effect. Its hypoglycemic effect does not appear for several hours. Thus growth hormone release is not critical for rapid glucose counterregulation; this is also true for *cortisol.* Over the long term, both growth hormone and cortisol may also increase glucose production.

Classification

The National Diabetes Data Group (NDDG) defines four major types of diabetes mellitus: type 1 diabetes mellitus, type 2 diabetes mellitus, gestational diabetes, and impaired glucose tolerance/impaired fasting glucose (Box 120-1).[8] The 1997 NDDG report discontinues the use of the terms "insulin-dependent diabetes mellitus" and "non-insulin-dependent diabetes mellitus" because they are confusing and clinically inaccurate. The group also recommends that Arabic numerals 1 and 2 be used to replace roman numerals I and II in the designation of types "one" and "two."[8]

Type 1 Diabetes Mellitus Type 1 (or I) diabetes is characterized by an abrupt critical onset, insulinopenia,

Box 120-1 Classification of Diabetes Mellitus and Other Categories of Glucose Intolerance

Diabetes Mellitus

Type 1 (or type I, formerly "insulin-dependent")
- Immune mediated
- Idiopathic

Type 2 (or type II, formerly "non–insulin-dependent")

Other specific types
- Genetic defects of beta-cell function
- Genetic defects in insulin action
- Diseases of exocrine pancreas
- Endocrinopathies
- Drug or chemical induced
- Infections
- Uncommon forms of immune-mediated diabetes
- Other genetic syndromes sometimes associated with diabetes

Gestational Diabetes Mellitus

Impaired Glucose Tolerance

Impaired fasting glucose

From American Diabetes Association: *Diabetes Care* 20:1183, 1997.

tendency to ketosis even in the basal state, and dependency on parenteral insulin to sustain life. From 85% to 90% of patients with type 1 diabetes demonstrate evidence of one or more autoantibodies implicated in the cellular-mediated autoimmune destruction of the beta cells of the pancreas. There are also strong human leukocyte antigen (HLA) associations found in type 1 diabetes. The autoimmune destruction has multiple genetic predispositions and may be related to undefined environmental insults.[8]

Type 2 Diabetes Mellitus Patients with type 2 (or II) diabetes may remain asymptomatic for long periods and show low, normal, or elevated levels of insulin because of insulin resistance. Ketosis is rare in type 2. Patients have a high incidence of obesity. No association exists with viral infections, islet cell autoantibodies, or HLA expression. Hyperinsulinemia may be related to peripheral tissue resistance to insulin because of defects in the insulin receptor.[9] Defects in muscle glycogen synthesis have an important role in the insulin resistance that occurs in type 2. A subgroup of patients who develop type 2 before 25 years of age have a mutation in the glucokinase gene and on chromosome 7.[10]

Gestational Diabetes Gestational diabetes "mellitus" (GDM) is characterized by an abnormal oral glucose tolerance test (OGTT) that occurs during pregnancy and either reverts to normal during the postpartum period or remains abnormal. The clinical pathogenesis is thought to be similar to that of type 2. Clinical presentation is usually nonketotic hyperglycemia during pregnancy.

Impaired Glucose Tolerance A fourth category of diabetes mellitus as defined by the NDDG is impaired glucose tolerance (IGT) and its analog, *impaired fasting glucose* (IFG). This group is composed of persons whose plasma glucose levels are between normal and diabetic and are at increased risk for the development of future diabetes and cardiovascular disease. The pathogenesis is thought to be related to insulin resistance.[8] Presentations of IGT/IFG include nonketotic hyperglycemia, insulin resistance, hyperinsulinism, and often obesity.

IGT/IFG differs from the other classes in that it is not associated with the complications of diabetes mellitus. Many of these patients even spontaneously develop normal glucose tolerance. The EP, however, should not be complacent about the patient with IGT because the decompensation of this group into the category of diabetes mellitus is 1% to 5% per year.[11]

Epidemiology

The prevalence of diabetes is difficult to determine because many standards have been used in diagnosis. The NDDG, using the 75-g OGTT as the diagnostic criterion, estimates prevalence at 6.6%, with 11.2% of the population having IGT.[5] These figures are probably too high because most subjects diagnosed with IGT or diabetes by OGTT never develop diabetes.[5] The true prevalence of the disease is probably closer to 1% to 2%.[12] One fourth of these patients have type 1, and three fourths have type 2.[5] Some groups have a much higher rate of diabetes, such as the Pima Native Americans who have a 40% rate of type 2; however, diabetes mellitus is significantly more prevalent in whites than in nonwhites.[13]

The peak age of onset of type 1 diabetes is 10 to 14 years. Approximately one of every 600 schoolchildren has this disease. In the United States the prevalence of type 1 is approximately 0.26% by age 20 years, and the lifetime prevalence approaches 0.4%. The annual incidence among persons from birth to 16 years of age in the United States is 12 to 14 per 1 million population. The incidence is age dependent, increasing from near-absence during infancy to a peak occurrence at puberty and another small peak at midlife.[14]

The morbidity of diabetes is related mostly to its vascular complications. A mortality of 36.8% has been related to cardiovascular causes, 17.5% to cerebrovascular causes, 15.5% to diabetic comas, and 12.5% to renal failure.

Pathophysiology and Etiology

Type 1 diabetes results from a chronic autoimmune process that usually exists in a preclinical state for years.[6] The classic manifestations of type 1, hyperglycemia and ketosis, occur late in the course of the disease, an overt sign of beta-cell destruction.

The most striking feature of longstanding type 1 diabetes is the near-total lack of insulin-secreting beta cells and insulin, with the preservation of glucagon-secreting alpha cells, somatostatin-secreting delta cells, and pancreatic polypeptide–secreting cells.

Although the exact cause of diabetes remains unclear, research has provided many clues. First, studies of the pathogenesis of diabetes mellitus have demonstrated that the cause of the disordered glucose homeostasis varies from individual to individual[15,16] This cause may determine the presentation in each patient. Individual patients are currently not studied for the source of their disease, except on an experimental basis. The goals of the work in progress, however, are to identify who is susceptible to the development of diabetes and to prevent diabetic emergencies and sequelae or to prevent expression of the disease.

A genetic basis for diabetes is suggested by the association of type 1 with certain HLA markers and by the findings of numerous twin and family studies.[6,17] Families who move from areas with low frequency of type 1 diabetes to areas with high frequency have an incidence of disease similar to that in the areas where they reside; this suggests an environmental basis for diabetes. An autoimmune cause has been clearly demonstrated in many type 1 diabetic patients. Islet cell amyloid also has been associated with diabetes.[18] In both types a variety of viruses have been implicated, most notably congenital rubella, Coxsackie B virus, and cytomegalovirus.[19]

Research has identified two groups of cellular carbohydrate transporters in cell membranes. Sodium-linked glucose transporters are found primarily in the intestine and kidney. The glucose transporter (GLUT) proteins are found throughout the body and transport glucose by facilitated diffusion down concentration gradients. The GLUT-4 transporter, found primarily in muscle, is insulin responsive, and a signaling defect in the protein may be responsible for insulin resistance in some diabetic patients.[20]

CLINICAL FEATURES

Type 1

The patient with type 1 diabetes is usually lean, less than 40 years of age, and ketosis prone. Plasma insulin levels are absent to low; plasma glucagon levels are high but suppressible with insulin, and patients require insulin therapy once symptoms appear. Onset of symptoms may be abrupt, with polydipsia, polyuria, polyphagia, and weight loss developing rapidly. In some cases the disease is heralded by ketoacidosis.[5] A myriad of problems related to type 1 diabetes may prompt an ED visit, including acute metabolic complications such as DKA to late complications such as cardiovascular or circulatory abnormalities, retinopathy, nephropathy, neuropathy, foot ulcers, severe infections, and various skin lesions.

Type 2

The patient with type 2 diabetes is usually middle aged or older, overweight, with normal to high insulin levels. Insulin levels are lower than would be predicted for glucose levels, however, leading to a relative insulin deficiency, probably because of an insulin secretory defect.[5] All type 2 patients demonstrate impaired insulin function related to poor insulin production, failure of insulin to reach the site of action, or failure of end-organ response to insulin.

As with type 1 diabetes, research suggests distinct subgroups of patients under the classification of type 2 diabetes. Although most adult patients are obese, 20% are not. Nonobese patients form a subgroup with a different disease, more similar to type 1. Another subgroup comprises young persons with maturity-onset diabetes.[10] They have an autosomal dominant inheritance of their disease, are usually not obese, and have a relatively mild course of disease.

Symptoms tend to begin more gradually in type 2 diabetes than in type 1. The diagnosis of type 2 is often made because of an elevated blood glucose found on routine laboratory examination. Glucose may be controlled by dietary therapy, oral hypoglycemic agents, or insulin, depending on the individual. Decompensation of disease usually leads to hyperosmolar nonketotic coma rather than ketosis.

DIAGNOSTIC STRATEGIES

Serum Glucose

As a rule, any random plasma glucose level greater than 200 mg/dl, a fasting plasma glucose concentration greater than 140 mg/dl, or a 2-hour postload OGTT is sufficient to establish the diagnosis of diabetes. In the absence of hyperglycemia with metabolic decompensation these criteria should be confirmed by repeat testing on a different day.[8] Some authors believe that a value of 150 mg/dl more accurately distinguishes diabetic from nondiabetic patients. Formal OGTTs are unnecessary, except during pregnancy or in patients suspected of diabetes who do not meet the criteria for a particular classification. The World Health Organization (WHO) and NDDG protocols for the OGTT are not in the realm of the EP's practice.

Glycosylated Hemoglobin

The most important test in the assessment of diabetic control is probably the measurement of glycosylated hemoglobin (HbA_{1c}). In vivo there is a slow, progressive, irreversible binding of glucose to the *N*-terminal valine of the hemoglobin β-chain. HbA_{1c} measures the quality of glycemic control over time. Given the long half-life of red blood cells, the percentage of HbA_{1c} is an index of glucose concentration of the preceding 6 to 8 weeks, with normal values approximately 4% to 6% of total hemoglobin, depending on the assay used.[21] Levels in poorly controlled patients may reach 10% to 12%. Measurement of glycated albumin can be used to monitor diabetic control over 1 to 2 weeks because of its short half-life but is rarely used clinically. The American Diabetes Association (ADA) recommends at least biannual measurements of HbA_{1c} for the follow-up of all types of diabetes.[21] The ADA currently sets an HbA_{1c} of less than 7% as a treatment goal.[22]

Urine Glucose

Urine glucose measurement methods are basically of two types: reagent tests and dipstick tests. The *reagent tests* (e.g., Clinitest) are copper reduction tests. They may be affected by many substances, are somewhat more cumbersome and expensive than dipstick methods, and use tablets that are very caustic and dangerous if accidentally ingested (Box 120-2).

Dipstick tests generally use glucose oxidase, which may also be affected by different substances (Box 120-3). Dipsticks are inexpensive and convenient but may vary in their sensitivity and strength of reaction to a given concentration of glucose. Dipstick interpretation can vary significantly, depending on the observer and the type of lighting. Both falsely high and falsely low urine glucose readings also can occur.[23] With the "plus" system, one-plus, two-plus, three-plus, and four-plus have different implications about

Box 120-2 Substances Interfering with Copper Reduction Tests (False-Positive Results)

Ascorbic acid
Cephaloridine
Cephalothin
Dilute urine
Gentisic acid (aspirin)
Glucuronic acid conjugates
Homogentisic acid
Isoniazid
Lactose in pregnant women
Levodopa
Metaxalone (Skelaxin) metabolite
Methyldopa
Penicillin
Probenecid (Benemid)
Reducing sugars
Salicylates
Streptomycin

From *Contemp Pharm Pract* 3:224, 1980.

Box 120-3 Substances Interfering with Glucose Oxidase Tests

False-Positive Results
Chloride glucose hypochlorite
Glutathione
Homogentisic acid
Hydrogen peroxide
Peroxide

False-Negative Results
Ascorbic acid
Aspirin
Bilirubin
Catalase
Catechol
Cysteine
3,4-Dihydroxyphenylacetic acid
Epinephrine
Ferrous sulfate (Feosol)
Gentisic acid
5-Hydroxyindole acetic acid
5-Hydroxytryptamine
5-Hydroxytryptophan
L-Dopamine
Levodopa
Meralluride injection
Methyldopa (Aldomet)
Sodium bisulfate
Tetracycline (with vitamin C)
Uric acid

From *Contemp Pharm Pract* 3:224, 1980.

urine glucose concentrations, depending on the brand of dipstick. Using reflectance colorimeters to read dipsticks increases accuracy. Urine glucose tests must be interpreted loosely because many factors can affect their results.

Urine Ketones

Urine ketone dipsticks use the nitroprusside reaction, which is a good test for acetoacetate but does not measure β-hydroxybutyrate. Although the usual acetoacetate/β-hydroxybutyrate ratio in diabetic ketoacidosis is 1:2.8, it may be as high as 1:30, in which case the urine dipstick does not reflect the true level of ketosis. When ketones are in the form of β-hydroxybutyrate, the urine ketone dipsticks may infrequently yield negative reactions in patients with significant ketosis.

Dipstick Blood Glucose

Dipsticks for testing blood glucose are clearly a more accurate way of monitoring blood glucose than urine dipsticks but also may be inaccurate. Hematocrits below 30% or above 55% cause unduly high or low readings, respectively, and a number of the strips specifically disclaim accuracy when used for neonates. Sensitivity of dipsticks to a variety of factors varies with the particular brand. The largest errors are in the hyperglycemic range. Dipstick readings rarely err more than 30 mg/dl when actual concentrations are below 90 mg/dl. Although specific glucose concentrations may not be accurately represented, blood glucose dipsticks are useful in estimating the general range of the glucose value.

Reflectance meters increase the accuracy of the dipstick blood glucose determination. If maximum accuracy is desired, however, the EP should normally order a laboratory blood glucose determination.

HYPOGLYCEMIA

Hypoglycemia is a common problem in patients with type 1 diabetes, especially if tight glycemic control is practiced, and may be the most dangerous acute complication of diabetes. The estimated incidence of hypoglycemia in diabetic patients is nine to 120 episodes per 100 patient-years.[24-27] As aggressive efforts continue to keep both fasting and postprandial glucose within normal range, the incidence of hypoglycemia may increase. The most common cause of coma associated with diabetes is an excess of administered insulin with respect to glucose intake. Hypoglycemia may be associated with significant morbidity and mortality. Severe hypoglycemia is usually associated with a blood sugar below 40 to 50 mg/dl and impaired cognitive function.[28]

Principles of Disease

Protection against hypoglycemia is normally provided by cessation of insulin release and mobilization of counterregulatory hormones, which increase hepatic glucose production and decrease glucose use (see earlier discussion). Diabetic patients using insulin are vulnerable to hypoglycemia because of insulin excess and failure of the counterregulatory system.[5]

Hypoglycemia may be caused by missing a meal, increasing energy output, or increasing insulin dosage. It can also occur in the absence of any precipitant (Box 120-4). Oral hypoglycemic agents have also been implicated in causing hypoglycemia, both in the course of therapy and as an agent of overdose.

Box 120-4 Precipitants of Hypoglycemia in Diabetic Patients

Addison's disease
Akee fruit
Anorexia nervosa
Antimalarials
Decrease in usual food intake
Ethanol
Factitious hypoglycemia
Hepatic impairment
Hyperthyroidism
Hypothyroidism
Increase in usual exercise
Insulin
Islet cell tumors
Malfunctioning, improperly adjusted, or incorrectly used insulin pump
Malnutrition
Old age
Oral hypoglycemics
Overaggressive treatment of diabetic ketoacidosis and hyperglycemic hyperosmolar nonketotic-coma
Pentamidine
Phenylbutazone
Propranolol
Recent change of dose or type of insulin or oral hypoglycemic
Salicylates
Sepsis
Some antibacterial sulfonylureas
Worsening renal insufficiency

Hypoglycemia without warning, or *hypoglycemia unawareness,* is a dangerous complication of type 1 diabetes probably caused by previous exposure to low blood glucose concentrations.[28] Even a single hypoglycemic episode can reduce neurohumoral counterregulatory responses to subsequent episodes.[29,30] Other factors associated with *recurrent* hypoglycemic attacks include overaggressive or intensified insulin therapy, longer history of diabetes, autonomic neuropathy, and decreased epinephrine secretion or sensitivity.[28]

The *Somogyi phenomenon* is a common problem associated with iatrogenic hypoglycemia in the type 1 diabetic patient. The phenomenon is initiated by excessive insulin dosage, which results in an unrecognized hypoglycemic episode that usually occurs in the early morning while the patient is sleeping. The counterregulatory hormone response produces *rebound hyperglycemia,* evident when the patient awakens. Often the patient and even the EP interpret this hyperglycemia as an indication to increase the insulin dosage, which exacerbates the problem.[31,32] Instead, the insulin dosage should be lowered or the timing changed.

Clinical Features

Symptomatic hypoglycemia occurs in most adults at a blood glucose level of 40 to 50 mg/dl. The rate at which glucose decreases, however, as well as the patient's age, gender, size, overall health, and previous hypoglycemic reactions, also contribute to symptoms. Signs and symptoms of hypoglycemia are caused by excessive secretion of epinephrine and CNS dysfunction and include sweating, nervousness, tremor, tachycardia, hunger, and neurologic symptoms ranging from bizarre behavior and confusion to seizures and coma.[24] In patients with hypoglycemia unawareness the prodrome to marked hypoglycemia may be minimal or absent. These individuals may rapidly become unarousable without warning. They may have a seizure or show focal neurologic signs, which resolve with glucose administration.

Box 120-5 Summary of Treatment for Hypoglycemia

1. Suspect hypoglycemia.
   Check serum glucose; obtain sample before treatment.
   If clinical suspicion of hypoglycemia is strong, proceed before laboratory results are available.
2. Correct serum glucose.
   If patient is awake and cooperative, administer sugar-containing food or beverage PO.
   If patient is unable to take PO:
   - 25-75 g glucose as D50W (1-3 ampules) IV
   - Children: 0.5-1 g/kg glucose as D25W IV (2-4 ml/kg)

   Neonates: 0.5-1 g/kg glucose (1-2 ml/kg) as D10W
   If unable to obtain IV access:
   - 1-2 mg glucagon IM or SC; may repeat q20min
   - Children: 0.025-0.1 mg/kg SC or IM; may repeat q20min

Box 120-6 Causes of Hypoglycemia

Postprandial
- Alimentary hyperinsulinism
- Fructose intolerance
- Galactemia
- Leucine sensitivity

Fasting

Underproduction of glucose
- Hormone deficiencies
  - Hypopituitarism
  - Adrenal insufficiency
  - Catecholamine deficiency
  - Glucagon deficiency
- Enzyme defects
- Substrate deficiency
  - Malnutrition
  - Late pregnancy
- Liver disease
- Drugs

Overuse of glucose
- Hyperinsulinism
  - Insulinoma
  - Exogenous insulin
  - Sulfonylureas
  - Drugs
  - Shock
- Tumors

Diagnostic Strategies

The cardinal laboratory test for hypoglycemia is blood glucose. It should be obtained, if possible, before therapy is begun. As noted, dipstick readings are very helpful in permitting rapid, reasonably accurate blood glucose estimates before therapy.

Laboratory testing should address any suspected cause of the hypoglycemia, such as ethanol or other drug ingestion. If factitious hypoglycemia is suspected, testing for insulin antibodies or low levels of C peptide may be helpful.

Management

In alert patients with mild symptoms, consumption of sugar-containing food or beverage orally (PO) is often adequate (Box 120-5). In other patients, after blood is drawn for glucose determination, one to three ampules of 50% dextrose in water (D50W) should be administered intravenously (IV) while the ABCs (airway, breathing, circulation) of resuscitation are being completed. Augmentation of the blood glucose level by administering an ampule of D50W may range from less than 40 mg/dl to more than 350 mg/dl.[33] These therapeutic steps are appropriately performed in the field if prehospital care is available. If alcohol abuse is suspected, thiamine should also be administered. D50W should not be used in infants or young children because venous sclerosis can lead to rebound hypoglycemia. In a child less than 8 years of age it is advisable to use 25% (D25W) or even 10% dextrose (D10W). D25W may be prepared by diluting D50W 1:1 with sterile water. The dose is 0.5 to 1 g/kg body weight or, using D25W, 2 to 4 ml/kg.

If the EP is unable to obtain intravenous (IV) access rapidly, 1 to 2 mg of glucagon may be given intramuscularly (IM) or subcutaneously (SC).[34] The onset of action is 10 to 20 minutes, and peak response occurs in 30 to 60 minutes. It may be repeated as needed. Glucagon may also be administered IV; 1 mg has an effect very similar to that of one ampule of D50W. Glucagon is ineffective in causes of hypoglycemia where glycogen is absent, notably alcohol-induced hypoglycemia.

Families of type 1 diabetic patients often are taught to administer intramuscular (IM) glucagon at home. Of those families so instructed, only 9% to 42% actually inject the glucagon when indicated.[35] Intranasal glucagon may become more widely accepted.[36] Prehospital care providers and EPs should seek a history of glucagon administration because it will alter initial blood glucose readings.

All patients with severe hypoglycemic reactions require aspiration and seizure precautions. Although the response to IV glucose generally is rapid, older patients may require several days for complete recovery.

Overdoses of oral hypoglycemic agents pose special problems because the hypoglycemia induced tends to be prolonged and severe. The hypoglycemia may be delayed in onset by as much as 24 hours and may recur as late as or later than 72 hours. Chlorpropamide is particularly troublesome in this respect. Thus it is imperative that patients with overdose of oral hypoglycemic agents have a minimum observation period of 24 hours, and more if hypoglycemia is recurrent. Patients with overdose of oral hypoglycemic agents often require constant infusion of D10W to maintain a normal serum glucose.

Once therapy for hypoglycemia has been given, the EP must take a careful history to determine the cause.

Disposition

Type 1 diabetic patients with brief episodes of hypoglycemia uncomplicated by other disease may be discharged from the ED if a cause of the hypoglycemia can be found and corrected by instruction or medication. All patients should be given a meal before discharge to ensure the ability to tolerate oral feedings and to begin to replenish glycogen stores in glycogen-deficient patients. If the patient may be sent home, follow-up instructions and arrangements based on the cause of the hypoglycemia are imperative.

Nondiabetic Patient

Hypoglycemia in the nondiabetic patient may be classified as postprandial or fasting (Box 120-6). The most common cause of *postprandial hypoglycemia* is alimentary hyperinsulinism, such as that seen in patients who have undergone gastrectomy, gastrojejunostomy, pyloroplasty, or vagotomy. *Fasting hypoglycemia* is caused when there is an imbalance between glucose production and use. The causes of inadequate glucose production include hormone deficiencies, enzyme defects, substrate deficiencies, severe liver disease, and drugs. Causes of overuse of glucose include the presence of an insulinoma, exogenous insulin, sulfonylureas, drugs, endotoxic shock, extrapancreatic tumors, and a variety of enzyme deficiencies.

Emergency treatment is similar to that of hypoglycemia in the diabetic patient. Patients should be referred to their primary care physician for workup of the underlying cause.

DIABETIC KETOACIDOSIS

Principles of Disease

Pathophysiology Diabetic ketoacidosis (DKA) is a syndrome in which insulin deficiency and glucagon excess combine to produce a hyperglycemic, dehydrated, acidotic patient with profound electrolyte imbalance (Figure 120-1).[37] All derangements producing DKA are interrelated and are based on insulin deficiency. DKA may be caused by cessation of insulin intake or by physical or emotional stress despite continued insulin therapy.

The effects of insulin deficiency may be mimicked in peripheral tissues by a lack of either insulin receptors or insulin sensitivity at receptor or postreceptor sites. When the hyperglycemia becomes sufficiently marked, the renal threshold is surpassed and glucose is excreted in the urine. The hyperosmolarity produced by hyperglycemia and dehydration is the most important determinant of the patient's mental status.[38]

Glucose in the renal tubules draws water, sodium, potassium, magnesium, calcium, phosphorus, and other ions from the circulation into the urine.[39] This osmotic diuresis combined with poor intake and vomiting produces the profound dehydration and electrolyte imbalance associated with DKA (Table 120-1). Exocrine pancreatic dysfunction closely parallels endocrine beta-cell dysfunction, producing malabsorption that further limits the body's intake of fluid and exacerbates electrolyte loss.

In 95% of patients with DKA the total sodium level is normal or low. Potassium, magnesium, and phosphorus deficits are usually marked.[40,41] As a result of acidosis and dehydration, however, the initial reported values for these electrolytes may be high. Hypokalemia may further inhibit insulin release.

The cells, unable to receive fuel substances from the circulation, act as they do in starvation from other causes. They decrease amino acid uptake and accelerate proteolysis

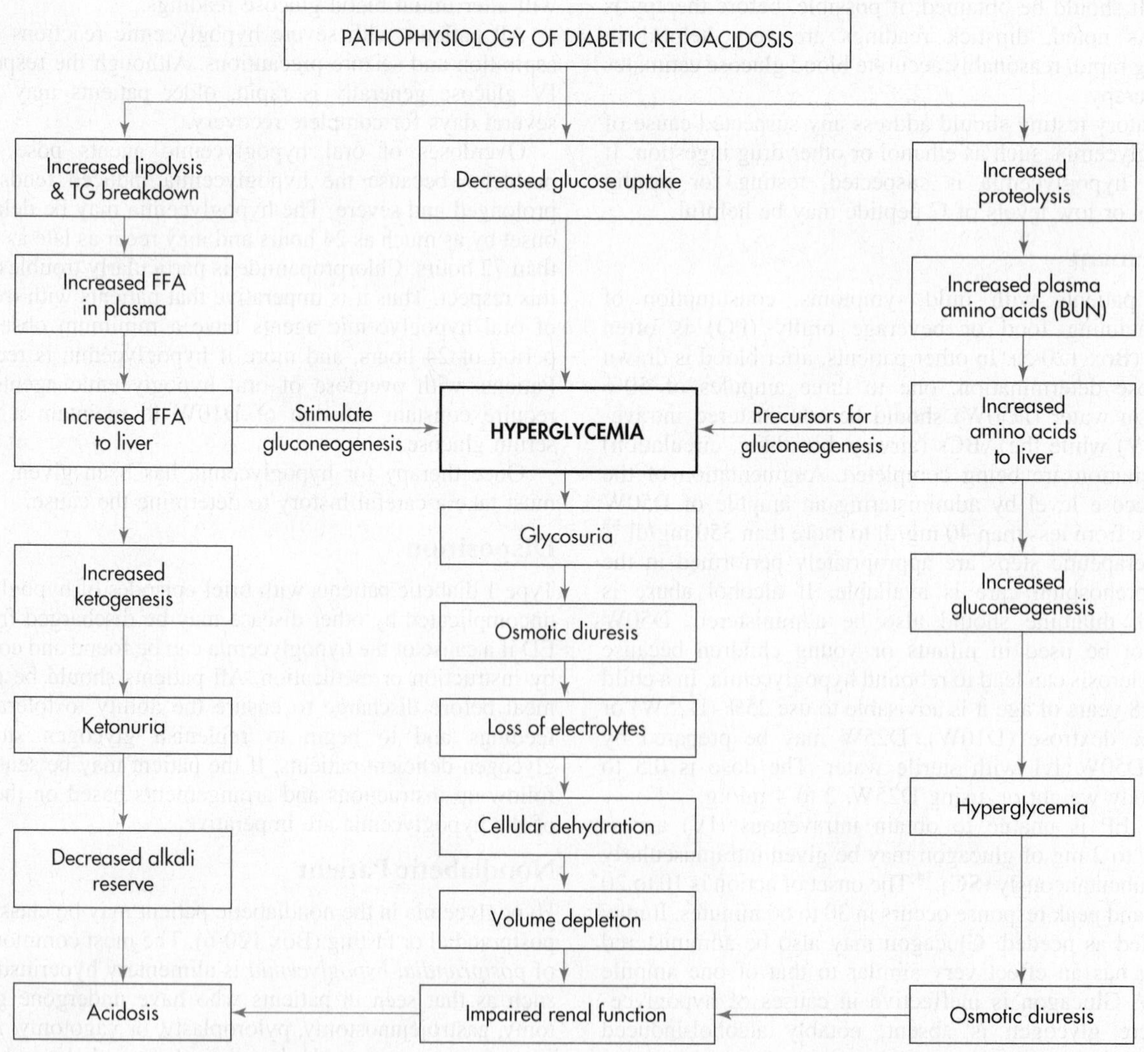

Figure 120-1. **Syndrome of diabetic ketoacidosis (DKA).** ***TG,*** **Total glucose concentration;** ***FFA,*** **free fatty acids;** ***BUN,*** **blood urea nitrogen.**

such that large amounts of amino acids are released to the liver and converted to two-carbon fragments.

Adipose tissue in the patient with DKA fails to clear the circulation of lipids. Insulin deficiency results in activation of a hormone-sensitive lipase that increases circulating free fatty acid (FFA) levels. Long-chain FFAs, now circulating in abundance as a result of insulin deficiency, are partially oxidized and converted in the liver to acetoacetate and β-hydroxybutyrate. This alteration of liver metabolism to oxidize FFAs to ketones rather than the normal process of reesterification to triglycerides appears to correlate directly with the altered glucagon/insulin ratio in the portal blood. Despite the pathologic glucagon-mediated increased production of ketones, the body acts as it does in any form of starvation, to decrease the peripheral tissue's use of ketones as fuel. The combination of increased ketone production with decreased ketone use leads to ketoacidosis.

The degree of ketosis has been related to the magnitude of release of the counterregulatory hormones epinephrine, glucagon, cortisol, and somatostatin. Glucagon is elevated fourfold to fivefold in DKA and is the most influential ketogenic hormone. It is believed to affect ketogenesis by reducing the concentration of malonyl coenzyme A and by inhibiting glycolysis. Epinephrine, norepinephrine, cortisol, growth hormone, dopamine, and thyroxin have all been shown to enhance ketogenesis indirectly by stimulating lipolysis. Because propranolol and metyrapone can block the effect of counterregulatory hormones, they have been successfully used to inhibit the development of DKA in patients with frequent episodes not otherwise treatable.

Acidosis plays a prominent role in the clinical presentation of DKA. The acidotic patient attempts to increase lung ventilation and rid the body of excess acid with Kussmaul's respiration. Bicarbonate (HCO_3^-) is used up in the process. Current evidence suggests that acidosis compounds the effects of ketosis and hyperosmolality to directly depress mental status.

Acidemia is not invariably present, even with significant ketoacidosis. *Ketoalkalosis* has been reported in diabetic patients vomiting for several days and in some with severe dehydration and hyperventilation.[42] The finding of alkalemia, however, should prompt the consideration of alcoholic ketoacidosis, where this finding is much more common.[43]

Etiology Most often, DKA occurs in the patient with type 1 diabetes and is associated with inadequate administration of insulin, infection, or myocardial infarction (MI). DKA can also occur in type 2 patients and may be associated with any type of stress, such as sepsis or gastrointestinal (GI) bleeding. Approximately 25% of all episodes of DKA occur in patients whose diabetes was previously undiagnosed.[7,44]

Diagnostic Strategies

History Clinically, most patients with DKA complain of a recent history of polydipsia, polyuria, polyphagia, visual blurring, weakness, weight loss, nausea, vomiting, and abdominal pain. Approximately one half of these patients, especially children, report abdominal pain, which may mimic acute inflammation of the abdomen. In children this pain usually is idiopathic and probably is caused by gastric distention or stretching of the liver capsule; it resolves as the metabolic abnormalities are corrected. In adults, however, abdominal pain more often signifies true abdominal disease.

Physical Examination Physical examination may or may not demonstrate depressed sensorium. Typical findings include tachypnea with Kussmaul's respiration, tachycardia, frank hypotension or orthostatic blood pressure changes, the odor of acetone on the breath, and signs of dehydration.[45] An elevated temperature is rarely caused by DKA itself and suggests the presence of sepsis.

Laboratory Tests Initial tests allow for preliminary confirmation of the diagnosis and immediate initiation of therapy (Table 120-2). Subsequent tests are made to determine more specifically the degree of dehydration, acidosis, and electrolyte imbalance and to reveal the precipitant of DKA.

On arrival to the ED, serum and urine glucose and ketones, electrolytes, and arterial blood gases (ABGs) should be checked. *Glucose* is usually elevated above 350 mg/dl; however, euglycemic DKA (blood glucose < 300 mg/dl) has been reported in up to 18% of patients.[5] ABGs demonstrate a low pH. Venous pH is not significantly different from arterial pH in patients with DKA, and some researchers consider the use of venous blood superior to repeated arterial puncture. *Metabolic acidosis* with anion gap is secondary to elevated plasma levels of acetoacetate and β-hydroxybutyrate, although lactate, FFAs, phosphates, volume depletion, and several medications also contribute to this condition.[5] Rarely, a well-hydrated patient with DKA may have a pure hyperchloremic acidosis and no anion gap. If an immediate *potassium* level is not available via ABG, an electrocardiogram (ECG) may indicate potassium levels. Despite initial potassium levels that are normal to high, a total potassium deficit of several hundred milliequivalents results from potassium and hydrogen shifts.

Other tests may include complete blood count (CBC) with differential, magnesium, calcium, amylase, blood urea nitrogen (BUN), creatinine, phosphorus, ketone, and lactate level determinations. A complete urinalysis helps in assessment of infection or renal disease. Elevated urine-specific gravity, BUN, and hematocrit suggest dehydration. Appropriate

Table 120-1. Average Fluid and Electrolyte Deficits in Severe Diabetic Ketoacidosis (per Kilogram Body Weight)

Weight	Water (ml/kg)	Sodium (mEq/L)	Potassium (mEq/L)	Chloride (mEq/L)	Phosphorus (mEq/L)
<10 kg	100-120	8-10	5-7	6-8	3
10-20 kg	80-100	8-10	5-7	6-8	3
>20 kg	70-80	8-10	5-7	6-8	3

Table 120-2. Typical Laboratory Values in Diabetic Ketoacidosis (DKA) and Hyperglycemic Hyperosmolar Nonketotic Coma (HHNC)

	DKA	HHNC
Glucose (mg/dl)	>350	>700
Sodium (mEq)	low 130s	140s
Potassium (mEq)	~4.5-6.0	~5
Bicarbonate (mEq)	<10	>15
BUN (mg/dl)	25-50	>50
Serum ketones	Present	Absent

cultures should be dictated by clinical findings. A patient with mild DKA or with recurrent episodes receives testing as deemed appropriate by the EP.

The serum *sodium* value is often misleading in DKA. Sodium is often low in the presence of significant dehydration because it is strongly affected by hyperglycemia, hypertriglyceridemia, salt-poor fluid intake, and increased GI, renal, and insensible losses. When *hyperglycemia* is marked, water flows from the cells into the vessels to decrease the osmolar gradient, thereby creating dilutional hyponatremia. Lipids also dilute the blood, thereby further lowering the value for sodium. Newer autoanalyzers remove triglycerides before assay, thus eliminating this artifact.

Hypertriglyceridemia is common in DKA because of impaired lipoprotein lipase activity and hepatic overproduction of very-low-density lipoprotein.[5] In the absence of marked lipemia, the true value of sodium may be approximated by adding 1.3 to 1.6 mEq/L to the sodium value on the laboratory report for every 100 mg/dl glucose over the norm. Thus, if the laboratory reports a serum sodium value of 130 mEq/L and a blood glucose value of 700 mEq/L, the total serum sodium value is more accurately assessed to be between 137.8 and 139.6 mEq/L.

Acidosis and the hyperosmolarity induced by hyperglycemia shift *potassium, magnesium,* and *phosphorus* from the intracellular to the extracellular space. Dehydration produces hemoconcentration, which contributes to normal or high initial serum potassium, magnesium, and phosphorus readings in DKA, even with profound total deficits. The EP may correct for the effect of acidosis on the serum potassium determination by subtracting 0.6 mEq/L from the laboratory potassium value for every 0.1 decrease in pH noted in the ABG analysis.[46] Thus, if the potassium is reported as 5 mEq/L and the pH is 6.94, the corrected potassium value would be only 2 mEq/L, representing severe hypokalemia. While insulin is administered and the hydrogen ion (H^+) concentration decreases, the patient needs considerable potassium replacement. Finally, hyperglycemia and the anion gap have significant effects on plasma potassium concentration, independent of acidosis.[38] No conversion factor has been developed for estimating true magnesium levels, although initial values may be high.

All laboratory determinations must be interpreted with caution. Serum creatinine determinations made by autoanalyzer may be falsely elevated.[37] Leukocytosis more closely reflects the degree of ketosis than the presence of infection. Only the elevation of band neutrophils has been demonstrated to indicate the presence of infection, with a sensitivity of 100% and a specificity of 80%.[47] The diagnosis of pancreatitis is confounded by the usually elevated urine and serum amylase levels in DKA. Typically, this is salivary amylase, but most laboratories are not equipped to make this distinction. A serum lipase determination will help distinguish pancreatitis from elevated salivary amylase levels.

Differential Considerations

Alcoholics, especially those who have recently abstained from drinking, with Kussmaul's respiration, a fruity odor to the breath, and acidotic ABG values may have *alcoholic ketoacidosis.*[43,48] These patients may be euglycemic or hypoglycemic, and a large part of their acidosis is often caused by the unmeasured β-hydroxybutyric acid.[43] Alcoholic ketoacidosis accounts for approximately 20% of all cases of ketoacidosis.

Ketoacidosis can also develop with fasting in the third trimester of pregnancy and in nursing mothers who do not eat.[49]

Other entities that may manifest with various combinations of altered mental status, acidosis, and abdominal pain include hypoglycemia, cerebrovascular accident (stroke), trauma, sepsis, hyperglycemic hyperosmolar nonketotic coma, postictal states, lactic acidosis, uremic acidosis, and abdominal emergencies. Intoxications by ethanol, salicylates, methanol, isopropyl alcohol, chloral hydrate, paraldehyde, ethylene glycol, and cyanide all share some features of DKA.

Management

General Measures The approach to the DKA patient in extremis is the same as for any patient in extremis. The comatose patient, especially if vomiting, requires intubation. The patient in hypovolemic shock requires aggressive fluid resuscitation with 0.9% saline solution rather than pressors. Other types of shock are possible and must be sought. Close monitoring of vital signs is essential. In the patient whose therapy may precipitate fluid overload caused by cardiac compromise or renal failure, a central venous pressure line or Swan-Ganz line should be inserted.

The diagnosis of DKA is generally simple: once hyperglycemia, ketosis, and acidosis have been established, fluid, electrolyte, and insulin therapy should begin (Box 120-7).

Insulin DKA cannot be reversed without insulin, so insulin therapy should be initiated as soon as the diagnosis is certain. In the past, very high dosages of insulin were administered to diabetic patients in DKA because they were thought to be extremely insulin resistant. However, low-dosage insulin therapy has proved as effective as high-dosage therapy.[7] The rate of decrease in blood sugar is equal or only slightly more gradual. The overall potassium requirement is less. High dosages of insulin have potentially harmful effects, including a greater incidence of iatrogenic hypoglycemia and hypokalemia.[37]

The exact amount of insulin administered varies. Many start therapy with a bolus of 10 units of regular insulin IV. This initial bolus may produce certain problems, however, and makes no significant difference in therapy.[50] The current therapy of choice is regular insulin infused at 0.1 U/hr up to 5 to 10 U/hr, mixed with the IV fluids. Regular insulin, 10 to 20 U/hr, administered IM accomplishes similar effect but

Box 120-7 Summary of Treatment for Diabetic Ketoacidosis

Identify DKA: serum glucose, electrolytes, ketones, and ABG; also draw CBC with differential; urinalysis; chest x-ray film and ECG, if indicated.

1. Supplement insulin.
   - ± Bolus: 0.1 U/kg regular insulin IV
   - Maintenance: 0.1 U/kg regular insulin IV
   - Change IV solution to D5W 0.45% normal saline when glucose ≤300 mg/dl.
2. Rehydrate.
   - 1-2 L normal saline IV over 1-3 hours
   - Children: 20 ml/kg normal saline over first hour
   - Follow with 0.45% normal saline
3. Correct electrolyte abnormalities.
   - Sodium
     - Correct with administration of normal saline and 0.45% normal saline.
   - Potassium
     - Ensure adequate renal function.
     - Add 20-40 mEq KCl to each liter of fluid.
   - Phosphorus
     - Usually unnecessary to replenish
   - Magnesium
     - Correct with 1-2 g $MgSO_4$ (in first 2 L if magnesium is low).
4. Correct acidosis.
   - Add 44-88 mEq/L to first liter of IV fluids only if pH ≤7.0.
   - Correct to pH 7.1.
5. Search and correct underlying precipitant.
6. Monitor progress and keep meticulous flow sheets.
   - Vital signs
   - Fluid intake and urine output
   - Serum glucose, K^+, Cl^-, HCO_3^+, CO_2, pH
   - Amount of insulin administered
7. Admit to hospital or intensive care unit.
   - Consider outpatient therapy in children with reliable caretaker *and*
     - Initial pH >7.35
     - Initial HCO_3^- ≥20 mEq/L
     - Can tolerate PO fluids
     - Resolution of symptoms after treatment in ED
     - No underlying precipitant requiring hospitalization

subjects the patient to repeated painful injections. In theory, IM insulin may accumulate at a poorly perfused administration site, failing to enter the systemic circulation in a timely manner.

In children the IV dosage of regular insulin may be calculated at 0.1 U/kg. Children are more likely than adults to develop cerebral edema in response to a rapid lowering of plasma osmolarity. Thus reduction of glucose levels in children should be gradual.[51]

Because the half-life of regular insulin is 3 to 10 minutes, IV insulin should be administered by constant infusion rather than by repeated bolus. Once the blood glucose has dropped to 250 to 300 mg/dl, dextrose should be added to the IV fluids to prevent iatrogenic hypoglycemia and cerebral edema. In patients with euglycemic DKA, dextrose should be added to the IV fluids at the start of insulin therapy.

Insulin adheres to the walls of glass and polyvinyl bottles and tubing, making it uncertain as to the exact amount of insulin being administered.[52] Running approximately 10 units of the insulin infusion through the tubing accomplishes adherence without altering the delivered concentration of the remainder of the infusate.

Insulin resistance occurs rarely in diabetic patients and requires an increase in dosage to obtain a satisfactory response. Resistance may be caused by obesity or accelerated insulin degradation.[5]

Two general categories of insulin resistance are described.[53] *Postreceptor-binding resistance* is the more common type. It is a mild-to-moderate resistance probably caused by defects in intracellular metabolism. It takes only a small amount of insulin to fill the receptors. Once they are filled, administration of additional insulin produces no additional effect. The second type, *prereceptor-receptor resistance,* is rare. This severe resistance may be caused by insulin antibodies, high concentrations of stress hormones, antireceptor antibodies, or any combination of these.[54]

Dehydration The severely dehydrated patient has a fluid deficit of 3 to 5 L. No uniformly accepted formula exists for the administration of fluid in this disorder.[55]

If the patient is in hypovolemic shock, the EP should administer fluids as rapidly as possible in the adult, or in 20-ml/kg boluses in the child, until a systolic pressure of 80 mm Hg is obtained. In the adult who has marked dehydration and does not have clinical shock or heart failure, 1 L may be administered in the first hour. In general, 2 L of normal saline (NS) over the first 1 to 3 hours is followed by a slower infusion of half-NS solution. Patients with DKA without extreme volume depletion may be successfully treated with a lower volume of IV fluid replacement.[44] NS solution at 20 ml/kg over the first hour is the usual fluid resuscitation therapy for a child. Thereafter, fluid rate should be adjusted according to age, cardiac status, and degree of dehydration to achieve a urine output of 1 to 2 ml/kg/hr. Whereas some authors advocate half-NS or colloid solution, most evidence and practice favor initial resuscitation with 0.9% NS solution.[51]

Fluid resuscitation alone may help to lower hyperglycemia. Because even in DKA a low level of circulating insulin may be present, increased perfusion may transport insulin to previously unreached receptor sites. In addition, a large volume of glucose may be cleared by the kidneys in response to improved renal perfusion. The mean plasma glucose concentration has been noted to drop 18% after administration of saline solution without insulin.[7]

Acidosis also decreases after fluid infusion alone. Increased perfusion improves tissue oxygenation, thus diminishing formation of lactate. Increased renal perfusion promotes renal H^+ loss, and the improved action of insulin in the better-hydrated patient inhibits ketogenesis.

Some authors believe that the rapid decrease of the hyperosmolarity of DKA caused by the administration of 0.45% NS solution may precipitate cerebral edema, one of the most dangerous complications associated with the patient in DKA, especially children.[56-58]

Potassium Potassium replacement is invariably needed in DKA. The initial potassium level is often normal or high despite a large deficit because of severe acidosis. Potassium levels often plummet with correction of acidosis and administration of insulin. Potassium should be administered with the fluids while the laboratory value is in the upper half of the normal range. Renal function should be monitored. In patients with low serum potassium at presentation, hypokalemia may become life threatening when insulin therapy is administered. IV potassium should be aggressively administered in concentrations of 20 to 40 mEq/L as required.

Some administer a portion of the potassium as the phosphate salt. In DKA, phosphate falls from a mean value of 9.2 mg/dl to 2.8 mg/dl within 12 hours of therapy, reflecting an average total deficit of 0.5 to 1.5 mmol/kg.[53,59] This may result in a decreased level of 2,3-diphosphoglycerate (2,3-DPG) and subsequent poor oxygen delivery to red blood cells (RBCs). Other problems associated with the hypophosphatemia are depressed myocardial and respiratory muscle performance, hemolysis, impaired phagocytosis, thrombocytopenia, platelet dysfunction, confusion, and disorientation.[7] The only caveat with phosphorus administration is that its magnesium- and calcium-lowering properties may induce symptomatic hypomagnesemia and hypocalcemia. Despite theoretic benefits, no clinical benefit from the routine administration of phosphorus in DKA has been shown.[7,60]

Magnesium Magnesium deficiency is a common problem in patients with DKA without renal disease. Both the initial pathophysiology and the therapy for DKA induce profound magnesium diuresis. Magnesium deficiency may exacerbate vomiting and mental changes, promote hypokalemia and hypocalcemia, or induce fatal cardiac dysrhythmia. The normal person requires 0.30 to 0.35 mEq/kg/day. Thus it is reasonable to include 0.35 mEq/kg of magnesium in the fluids of the first 3 to 4 hours, with further replacement dependent on blood levels and the clinical picture. This amounts to 2.5 to 3 g of magnesium sulfate in the 70-kg patient.

Acidosis Bicarbonate therapy may be indicated in severely acidotic patients (pH ≤7.0).[7] The use of bicarbonate is not warranted in less ill patients for several reasons. First, bicarbonate worsens the inhibition of oxygen release from RBCs caused by the 2,3-DPG deficiency seen in phosphorus-depleted patients with DKA. Second, overly rapid correction of acidosis is contraindicated because the blood-brain barrier (BBB) is much more permeable to carbon dioxide than to bicarbonate. Thus the correction of intravascular acidosis terminates Kussmaul's respiration, further augmenting the blood carbon dioxide available to cross the BBB. Slowly, sufficient bicarbonate crosses the BBB to provide adequate buffering. In the short term, however, as the blood acidosis is corrected, the acidity of the fluid surrounding the brain increases, causing paradoxical cerebrospinal fluid (CSF) acidosis. The clinical significance of an acid CSF pH is controversial.

Third, the administration of bicarbonate increases the potassium requirement, both immediately by driving potassium into the cell and more gradually by affecting the kidney, thereby making iatrogenic hypokalemia more likely. When bicarbonate is used, serum potassium levels need to be followed even more closely.

Fourth, the overaggressive use of bicarbonate may produce alkalosis, which induces dysrhythmias largely through its effect on the distribution of electrolytes. Alkalemia occurring late in the course of therapy is more common in patients who have received bicarbonate because ketones are metabolized to carbon dioxide, water, and bicarbonate.

Fifth, evidence suggests that lowered pH produces a feedback mechanism that directly inhibits ketogenesis. Bicarbonate can increase ketonuria and delay the fall in serum ketones when compared with saline infusion alone.

Finally, patients treated with bicarbonate fare no better and possibly worse than patients treated without bicarbonate. It is possible to manage patients who have severe DKA with fluids and insulin alone. When this is done, pH normalization is similar to that in a bicarbonate control group.

When bicarbonate therapy is deemed necessary, the pH should not be corrected above 7.1.[55] Response to therapy should be followed initially with hourly vital signs; fluids should be administered and urine output measured; insulin should be given; and glucose, pH, and anion gap measurements should be determined. Plasma bicarbonate may remain low even while pH increases and anion gap narrows because of the hyperchloremia that develops from rapid saline infusion, loss of bicarbonate in the urine as ketones, and exchanges with intracellular buffers.

Complications

The precipitating causes of DKA may have associated morbidity and mortality equal to or worse than those of DKA itself. These include iatrogenic causes, as well as infection and MI. Morbidity in DKA is largely iatrogenic: (1) hypokalemia from inadequate potassium replacement, (2) hypoglycemia from inadequate glucose monitoring and failure to replenish glucose in IV solutions when serum glucose drops below 250 to 300 mg/dl, (3) alkalosis from overaggressive bicarbonate replacement, (4) congestive heart failure from overaggressive hydration, and (5) cerebral edema probably caused by too-rapid osmolal shifts. DKA is responsible for 70% of diabetes-related deaths in children. The mortality of treated DKA decreased from approximately 38% between 1930 and 1959 to about 5% to 7% in the 1980s. The primary causes of death remain infection (especially pneumonia), arterial thromboses, and shock. The decrease in mortality demonstrates that appropriate therapy can make a difference.

Cerebral edema should be suspected when the patient remains comatose or lapses into coma after the reversal of acidosis. It generally occurs 6 to 10 hours after the initiation of therapy. There are no warning signs or clinical predictors, and the mortality is currently 90%. Subclinical cerebral edema in children is probably very common.[61] Furthermore, subclinical cerebral edema may either precede or follow the onset of therapy, thus raising the question of whether this entity is caused by therapy or is simply a manifestation of the basic pathophysiology of DKA.

Because clinically evident cerebral edema does not usually occur unless the blood sugar level is below 250 mg/dl and insulin is being used, insulin may directly antagonize the brain's defenses against fluid shifts while the plasma glucose level approaches normal values. Other theories attribute the formation of cerebral edema to (1) "idiogenic osmols" developed in the brain as a result of insulin therapy, (2) the rate of fluid administration, and (3) the rate of correction of the acidosis. Other less common causes have been suggested.[62] Several authors recommend the administration of mannitol, 0.25 to 2 mg/kg, at the first sign of altered mental status in children being treated for DKA.[58] Steroids are ineffective treatment for cerebral edema secondary to DKA and may worsen DKA.

An unusual infection associated with DKA is *mucormycosis.* Acute gastric dilation and myonecrosis are other rare complications of DKA. Poor prognostic signs include hypotension, azotemia, coma, and underlying illness.[63]

Disposition

Most patients require hospital admission, often to the intensive care unit. All pregnant diabetic patients in DKA require admission and consultation with an endocrinologist and obstetrician specializing in the care of high-risk pregnancies. Some children (initial pH >7.35, bicarbonate ≥20 mEq/L) with resolution of findings who can tolerate oral fluids after 3 or 4 hours of treatment may be discharged home with a reliable caregiver.[64] Patients who have mild DKA may be treated on an outpatient basis if (1) the patient or parent is reliable, (2) the underlying causes do not require inpatient therapy, and (3) close follow-up is pursued.

HYPERGLYCEMIC HYPEROSMOLAR NONKETOTIC COMA

Hyperglycemic hyperosmolar nonketotic coma (HHNC) represents a syndrome of acute diabetic decompensation characterized by marked hyperglycemia, hyperosmolarity and dehydration, and decreased mental functioning that may progress to frank coma. Ketosis and acidosis are generally minimal or absent. Focal neurologic signs are common. DKA and HHNC may occur together; some even consider HHNC and DKA to be at two ends of a spectrum, with many patients in the middle.[7,65]

Principles of Disease

Pathophysiology As with DKA, the pathophysiology of HHNC varies with the particular patient. Because most patients with HHNC are elderly, decreased renal clearance of glucose produced by the decline of renal function with age often contributes to the illness. As with DKA, decreased insulin action results in glycogenolysis, gluconeogenesis, and decreased peripheral uptake of glucose. The hyperglycemia pulls fluid from the intracellular space into the extracellular space, transiently maintaining adequate perfusion. Soon, however, this fluid is lost in a profound osmotic diuresis, limited finally by hypotension and a subsequent drop in the glomerular filtration rate (GFR). The urine is extremely hypotonic, with urine sodium concentration between 50 and 70 mEq/L, compared with 140 mEq/L in extracellular fluid. This hypotonic diuresis produces profound dehydration, leading to hyperglycemia, hypernatremia, and associated hypertonicity. Often the patient is prevented from taking in adequate fluids by stroke, Alzheimer's disease, or other diseases, greatly exacerbating the dehydration of renal origin.

The reason for the absence of ketoacidosis in HHNC is unknown. FFA levels are lower than in DKA, thus limiting substrates needed to form ketones. The most likely reason for the blunted counterregulatory hormone release and lack of ketosis seems to be that these patients continue to secrete the tiny amount of insulin required to block ketogenesis.[66]

Etiology HHNC is a syndrome of severe dehydration that results from a sustained hyperglycemic diuresis under circumstances in which the patient is unable to drink sufficient fluids to offset the urinary losses. The full-blown syndrome does not usually occur until volume depletion has progressed to the point of decreased urine output.

Box 120-8 Precipitants of Hyperglycemic Hyperosmolar Nonketotic Coma

External Insult
- Trauma
- Burns
- Dialysis
- Hyperalimentation

Drugs
- Antimetabolites
- L-Asparaginase
- Chlorpromazine
- Chlorpropamide
- Cimetidine
- Diazoxide
- Didanosine
- Ethacrynic acid
- Furosemide
- Glucocorticoids
- Immunosuppressants
- Phenytoin
- Propranolol
- Thiazides

Disease Process
- Cushing's syndrome and other endocrinopathies
- Hemorrhage
- Myocardial infarction
- Renal disease
- Subdural hematoma
- Cerebrovascular accident
- Infection
- Down syndrome

HHNC is most common in elderly patients with type 2 diabetes but has been reported in children with type 1 diabetes.[67] Box 120-8 lists the broad range of predisposing factors.[6,68] HHNC may occur in patients who are not diabetic, especially after burns, parenteral hyperalimentation, peritoneal dialysis, or hemodialysis.[69]

Clinical Features

The prodrome for HHNC is significantly longer than that of DKA. Clinically, extreme dehydration, hyperosmolarity, volume depletion, and CNS findings predominate.[66] If awake, patients may complain of fever, thirst, polyuria, or oliguria. Approximately 20% of patients have no known history of type 2 diabetes. The most common associated diseases are chronic renal insufficiency, gram-negative pneumonia, GI bleeding, and gram-negative sepsis. Of these patients, 85% have underlying renal or cardiac impairment as a predisposing factor. Arterial and venous thromboses often complicate the picture.

The patient often exhibits orthostatic hypotension or frank hypotension, tachycardia, and fever with signs of marked dehydration. On the average, the HHNC patient has a 24% fluid deficit, or 9 L in the 70-kg patient. The depression of the sensorium correlates directly with the degree and rate of development of hyperosmolarity. Some patients have normal mental status. Seizures are usually associated with neurologic findings, especially epilepsia partialis continua (continuous focal seizures) and intermittent focal motor seizures.[70] Stroke and hemiplegia are also common. Less common neurologic findings include choreoathetosis, ballism, dysphagia, segmental myoclonus, hemiparesis, hemianopsia, central hyperpyrexia, nystagmus, visual hallucinations, and acute quadriplegia.

Diagnostic Strategies

Laboratory findings usually reveal a blood glucose level greater than 600 mg/dl and serum osmolarity greater than

350 mOsm/L.[31] The BUN concentration is invariably elevated (see Table 120-2). Although patients with HHNC do not have a ketoacidosis caused by diabetes, they may have a metabolic acidosis secondary to some combination of lactic acidosis, starvation ketosis, and retention of inorganic acids attributable to renal hypoperfusion.

The patient with HHNC typically manifests more profound electrolyte imbalance than with DKA. Levels of potassium, magnesium, and phosphorus may seem initially high, even in the presence of marked total deficit. In the absence of acidemia, however, the discrepancy between the initial electrolyte reading and body stores is less than that of DKA. Initial serum sodium readings will be inaccurate because of hyperglycemia.

Differential Considerations

The differential diagnosis of HHNC is identical to that of DKA. In addition, diabetic patients receiving chlorpropamide are subject to water intoxication with dilutional hyponatremia, which may manifest as coma without acidosis that is clinically indistinguishable from HHNC. The patient with HHNC who has a sharply depressed sensorium may not be initially distinguishable from the patient with profound hypoglycemia. When blood glucose cannot be rapidly checked, the immediate administration of one ampule of D50W will minimally worsen HHNC and may be lifesaving for patients with hypoglycemia.

Management

The fluid, electrolyte, and insulin regimens for the initial resuscitation of HHNC are subject to the same controversies as the therapies for DKA (Box 120-9). Whereas some physicians use half-NS solution rapidly infused, most use NS solution, switching to half-NS later in the resuscitation. Just as in DKA, overly rapid correction of serum osmolarity may predispose to the development of cerebral edema in children. There are few reports of cerebral edema complicating HHNC in adults.

Dehydration Under central venous or pulmonary artery pressure monitoring, rapid administration of NS in a similar fashion to initial therapy for DKA is generally safe. After the initial shock and drastic extracellular fluid deficits are ameliorated by rapid administration of the first 2 to 3 L of NS, 0.45% NS solution should be substituted. In patients with concomitant congestive heart failure, sterile water has been successfully administered via central venous line at a rate of 500 ml/hr, with no detectable hemolysis or other complications. Glucose should be added to resuscitation fluids when the blood glucose level drops below 300 mg/dl.

Electrolytes The guidelines for the administration of potassium, magnesium, and phosphorus are similar to those for DKA.

Insulin Low-dosage insulin, such as that administered in the patient with DKA, is generally effective and safe once the restoration of volume has been instituted.

Other Considerations A vigorous search for the underlying precipitant for HHNC must be pursued. Response to therapy should be followed in the manner described for patients in DKA. *Phenytoin* (Dilantin) is contraindicated for the seizures of HHNC because it is often ineffective and may impair endogenous insulin release. Phenytoin-induced HHNC even occurs in nondiabetic patients. Low-dosage subcutaneous *heparin* may be indicated to lessen the risk of thrombosis, which is increased by the volume depletion, hyperviscosity, hypotension, and inactivity associated with HHNC.

Box 120-9 Summary of Treatment for Hyperglycemia Hyperosmolar Nonketotic Coma

Identify HHNC, then treatment is the same as initial DKA treatment.

1. Supplement insulin.
   - ± Bolus: 0.05-0.1 U/kg regular insulin IV
   - Maintenance: 0.05-0.01 U/kg regular insulin IV
   - **Caution:** serum glucose rapidly corrects with fluid administration alone; monitor glucose to avoid hypoglycemia.
   - Change IV solution to D5W 0.45% normal saline when glucose ≤300 mg/dl.
2. Rehydrate.
   - Rapid administration of 2-3 L normal saline over first several hours
   - CVP or Swan-Ganz monitoring may be necessary in patients with history of heart disease
   - Correct one half of fluid deficit in first 8 hours, remainder over 24 hours
3. Correct electrolyte abnormalities.
   - Sodium
     - Correct with administration of normal saline and 0.45% normal saline.
   - Potassium
     - First ensure adequate renal function.
     - Add 20-40 mEq KCl to each liter of fluid.
   - Phosphorus
     - Usually unnecessary to replenish
   - Magnesium
     - Correct with 1-2 g $MgSO_4$ (in first 2 L if magnesium is low).
4. Correct acidosis.
   - Add 44-88 mEq/L to first liter of IV fluids *only* if pH ≤7.0.
   - Correct to pH 7.1.
5. Search and correct underlying precipitant.
6. Monitor progress and keep meticulous flow sheets.
   - Vital signs
   - Fluid intake and urine output
   - Serum glucose, K+, Cl^-, HCO_3^-, CO_2, pH, ketones
   - Amount of insulin administered
7. Admit to hospital or intensive care unit

Complications

Reasons for high morbidity and mortality rates are not always clear, but many patients with HHNC are elderly and have underlying cardiac and renal disease. Pediatric HHNC differs from adult HHNC in that children have a much higher incidence of fatal cerebral edema.[67] Other causes for morbidity and mortality are similar to those described for DKA. The mortality rate of treated HHNC patients has been 40% to 70% in the past but now ranges from 8% to 25%.[71]

Disposition All patients with HHNC must be hospitalized.

LATE COMPLICATIONS OF DIABETES

Late complications of diabetes cause significant morbidity and mortality. They develop approximately 15 to 20 years after the onset of overt hyperglycemia. The Diabetes Control and Complications Trial showed that tight glycemic control significantly reduces the risk of microvascular disease, such as microalbuminuria (the earliest sign of nephropathy), neuropathy, and retinopathy, but at the expense of greatly increasing the risk of recurrent hypoglycemia.[72-74]

Vascular Complications

Diabetes is associated with increased risk for atherosclerosis and thromboembolic complications, which are a major cause of morbidity and premature death.[75] The cause for accelerated atherosclerosis is unknown, although it is probably related to oxidated low-density lipoprotein and increased platelet activity. Atherosclerotic lesions are widespread, causing symptoms in many organ systems. Coronary artery disease and stroke are common. Diabetic patients have an increased incidence of "silent" MI, complicated MIs, and congestive heart failure.[8,76,77] Peripheral vascular disease is noted clinically by claudication, nonhealing ulcers, gangrene, and impotence.

Diabetic Nephropathy Renal disease is a leading cause of death and disability in diabetic patients. Approximately one half of end-stage renal disease in the United States is caused by diabetic nephropathy.[78] Diabetic nephropathy involves two pathologic patterns: diffuse and nodular. Clinical renal dysfunction does not correlate well with the histologic abnormalities. Disease usually progresses from enlarged kidneys with elevated GFR to the appearance of microalbuminuria, to macroproteinuria with hypertension, reduced GFR, and renal failure.[79] The appearance of microalbuminuria correlates with the presence of coronary artery disease and retinopathy.[80]

Azotemia generally does not begin until 10 to 15 years after the diagnosis of diabetes is made. Progression of renal disease is accelerated by hypertension. Meticulous control of diabetes can reverse microalbuminuria and may slow the progression of nephropathy.[2,21,72-74] Hypertension should be aggressively managed. Angiotensin-converting enzyme (ACE) inhibitors are effective in controlling hypertension and lowering microalbuminuria.[81] Chronic hemodialysis and renal transplantation are unfortunate endpoints for many diabetic patients with renal disease.

Retinopathy Diabetes is a leading cause of adult blindness in the United States. Approximately 11% to 18% of all diabetic patients have treatable diabetic retinopathy ranging from mild to severe and manifesting in many forms. The severity of diabetic retinopathy is clearly related to the quality of glycemic control.[77,82]

Background (simple) *retinopathy* is found in most diabetic patients who have prolonged disease. Background retinopathy is characterized by microaneurysms, small vessel obstruction, cotton-wool spots or soft exudates (microinfarcts), hard exudates, and macular ischemia.[79] The characteristics of *proliferative retinopathy* are new vessel formation and scarring. Complications of proliferative retinopathy are vitreal hemorrhage and retinal detachment, which may ultimately cause unilateral vision loss. Treatment for diabetic retinopathy is photocoagulation.

Maculopathy is background retinopathy with macular involvement. It results primarily in a deficit of central vision. As with proliferative retinopathy, it is vital that the patient be under the care of an ophthalmologist. Laser therapy in the early stages can dramatically alter the course of this disabling disease.

The diabetic patient may enter the ED with complaints ranging from acute blurring of vision to sudden unilateral or even bilateral blindness. Less often, diabetic patients have more gradual vision loss caused by the common senile cataract or the "snowflake" cataract, which may disappear as hyperglycemia is corrected. The associated hyperlipidemia of diabetes may lighten the color of retinal vessels, producing lipemia retinalis. Anterior ischemic optic neuropathy has been reported.

The EP should refer diabetic patients with retinopathy to an ophthalmologist. Even in those with normal vision, ophthalmologic procedures may limit visual loss or prevent crises such as neovascular glaucoma.

Neuropathy Both autonomic and peripheral neuropathy are well-known complications of diabetes. The prevalence of peripheral neuropathy ranges from 15% to 60%.[5] The cause of the neuropathy is not clearly understood, but evidence suggests several factors in its development. Neuropathy may result from the effects of diabetic vascular disease on the vasa nervorum. Myoinositol, the polyol pathway, and nonenzymatic glycosylation of protein may have roles. All these factors are related to elevated blood glucose level. Neurologic manifestations of diabetes may regress with improved glycemic control. Pathologically, segmental demyelinization occurs with loss of both myelinated and unmyelinated axons, particularly those affecting the distal part of the peripheral nerve.

Several distinct types of neuropathy have been recognized in diabetes. *Peripheral symmetric neuropathy* is a slowly progressive, primary sensory disorder manifesting bilaterally with anesthesia, hyperesthesia, or pain. The pain is often severe and worse at night. It affects upper and lower extremities, although lower extremities and the most distal sections of the involved nerves are most often affected. There may be a motor deficiency as well. Pain is very difficult to control. Simple pain medications, amitriptyline (75 mg at bedtime), and fluphenazine (1 mg three times daily) have been effective for some patients.[84]

Mononeuropathy, or *mononeuropathy multiplex,* affects both motor and sensory nerves, generally one nerve at a time. The onset is rapid, with wasting and tenderness of the involved muscles. Clinically, sudden onset of wristdrop, footdrop, or paralysis of cranial nerves III, IV, and VI is noted.

Diabetic truncal mononeuropathy occurs rapidly in a radicular distribution. In contrast to other mononeuropathies, it is primarily, if not exclusively, sensory. If it causes pain, it may mimic an MI or acute abdominal inflammation. Similar to diabetic mononeuropathy, it may be most bothersome at night and generally resolves in a few months. Whereas diabetic mononeuropathy often is the first clue of diabetes, truncal mononeuropathy is more often found in known diabetic patients.

Autonomic neuropathy presents in many forms. Neuropathy of the GI tract is manifested by difficulty swallowing, delayed gastric emptying, constipation, or nocturnal diarrhea. Impotence and bladder dysfunction or paralysis may occur. Orthostatic hypotension, syncope, and even cardiac arrest have resulted from autonomic neuropathy. Diabetic diarrhea responds to diphenoxylate and atropine, loperamide, or clonidine. Orthostatic hypotension is treated by sleeping with the head of the bed elevated, avoidance of sudden standing or sitting, and the use of full-length elastic stockings.

The Diabetic Foot

Approximately 20% of hospitalizations in diabetic patients are related to foot problems. Sensory neuropathy, ischemia, and infection are the principal contributors to diabetic foot disease. Loss of sensation leads to pressure necrosis from poorly fitting footwear and small wounds going unnoticed. The most common cause of injury is pressure on plantar bony prominences. All neuropathic foot ulcers should be assessed for infection and debrided of devitalized tissue, with radiographs for the presence of foreign bodies, soft tissue gas, or bony abnormalities. Weight bearing must be eliminated by total-contact casting.[84]

Not all ulcers are infected. Infection is suggested by local inflammation or crepitation. Conversely, some uninflamed ulcers are associated with underlying osteomyelitis. Most mild infections are caused by gram-positive cocci, such as *Staphylococcus aureus* or streptococci, and may be treated with oral antibiotics, a strict non-weight-bearing regimen, meticulous wound care, and daily follow-up. This may not be possible in an ED where patients are not reliable, do not have good home support, or do not have excellent follow-up care easily available.[85]

Deeper, limb-threatening infections—as evidenced by full thickness ulceration, cellulitis greater than 2 cm in diameter with or without lymphangitis, bone or joint involvement, or systemic toxicity—are usually polymicrobial and caused by aerobic gram-positive cocci, gram-negative bacilli, and anaerobes. These patients require hospitalization and, after culture, IV empiric antimicrobial therapy with ampicillin-sulbactam, ticarcillin-sulbactam, cefoxitin, imipenem, or a fluoroquinolone and clindamycin; strict non-weight-bearing status; tight glycemic control; early surgical intervention for debridement; drainage; and meticulous wound care.[84,86] Occult osteomyelitis should be considered in all cases of neuropathic ulceration. Up to one third of patients must undergo amputation.

Infections

Diabetic patients are more prone to complications of infections because of their inability to limit microbial invasion with effective polymorphonuclear leukocytes and lymphocytes.[5] They have an increased incidence of extremity infections and pyelonephritis compared with the general population. In addition, they are particularly susceptible to certain other infections such as tuberculosis, mucocutaneous candidiasis, intertrigo, mucormycosis, soft tissue infections, nonclostridial gas gangrene, osteomyelitis, and malignant *Pseudomonas* otitis externa.[5] Treatment for diabetic patients with infection include rapid culture and antibiotics, glycemic control, and generally hospitalization.

Cutaneous Manifestations

Dermal hypersensitivity refers to pruritic, erythematous indurations that occur at insulin injection sites. The declining prevalence of this condition has paralleled the improved purification of insulin. Insulin *lipoatrophy* likewise seems to be a result of insulin impurities and is manifested as subcutaneous depressions at injection sites. Although lipoatrophy is now more common than dermal hypersensitivity, its prevalence has also declined sharply because insulin preparations have improved. Insulin *lipohypertrophy* is manifested by raised areas of subcutaneous fat deposits at insulin injection sites. These lesions generally reflect the failure of the patient to rotate injections sites adequately. They resolve spontaneously over months if insulin injection is avoided in the affected areas and sites are properly rotated.

Insulin pumps are often associated with localized skin problems, usually a reaction to the tape securing the tubing and needles. Occasionally, sensitivity to the catheters is seen. Skin infections at the site of injection are the most common complication of insulin pumps. Changing the patient to buffered pure-pork from unbuffered beef-pork insulin is the only intervention that seems to reduce the rate of infection. A few patients have been noted to develop hard nodules at the injection site. The cause of these nodules is uncertain.

Diabetic patients who use oral hypoglycemic agents may develop rashes associated with these medications. After consuming ethanol, approximately 38% of type 2 patients taking chlorpropamide exhibit a "flush" consisting of redness of the face and neck and a sense of warmness or burning. Patients may demonstrate urticaria in response to both insulin and oral hypoglycemics.

Diabetic skin conditions include fungal infections, acanthosis nigricans, necrobiosis lipoidica diabeticorum, xanthoma diabeticorum, bullosis diabeticorum, and diabetic dermopathy. *Acanthosis nigricans* is characterized by a velvety brown-black thickening of the keratin layer, most often in the flexor surfaces. It is the cutaneous marker for a group of endocrine disorders with insulin resistance.[9] *Necrobiosis lipoidica diabeticorum* begins as erythematous papular or nodular lesions, usually in the pretibial area, but in other areas as well. The early lesions may contain telangiectasias. These lesions spread and frequently form a single pigmented area of atrophic skin, often with a yellow and sometimes ulcerated center and an erythematous margin. A history of previous trauma is sometimes found.

The three forms of diabetic thick skin are (1) scleroderma-like skin changes of the fingers and dorsum of the hand associated with stiff joints and limited mobility, (2) clinically inapparent but measurable thick skin, and (3) "scleroderma adultorum," or increased dermal thickness on the back and posterior upper neck in middle-age, overweight patients with type 2 diabetes.[87]

Xanthoma diabeticorum is evidence of the hyperlipidemia associated with diabetes. It is similar to the xanthoma found in nondiabetic hyperlipidemic patients. Xanthomas have an erythematous base and a yellowish hue.

Bullosis diabeticorum is a rare occurrence. Bullae are usually filled with a clear fluid and are most often found on the extremities, especially the feet. The fluid is occasionally slightly hemorrhagic. The bullae usually heal spontaneously without scarring.

Diabetic dermopathy, or "skin spots," is the most common finding in diabetes.[87] It presents as discrete, depressed, and brownish lesions generally less than 15 mm in diameter and found in the pretibial area.

Resistant, aggressive *impetigo* or *intertrigo* should suggest diabetes.

Insulin Allergy

Insulin allergy is mediated by immunoglobulin E and is manifested by local itching or pain and delayed brawny edema, urticaria, or anaphylaxis. Systemic reactions are usually seen in patients who have previously discontinued insulin and then resumed therapy. Mild reactions may be treated with antihistamines, whereas anaphylaxis must be treated with epinephrine. Patients with significant reactions must be admitted for desensitization.[5]

DIABETES IN PREGNANCY

Before the discovery of insulin in 1922, diabetes in pregnancy was associated with a fetal death rate of 60% to 72% and maternal morbidity of approximately 30%. In 1977, a linear relationship between glycemic control and perinatal mortality was discovered. Strict metabolic control is now a goal of all diabetic pregnancies.[49,88]

Pregnant patients should be watched extremely closely and aggressively treated for impending or actual DKA. For a variety of reasons, pregnant women have a special predisposition to both glucose intolerance and excess ketone production. Although uncommon, DKA may cause perinatal asphyxia and reduce fetal oxygen delivery.[49,88,89] Intellectual deficits in offspring have been associated with maternal ketonuria from any cause.

Pregnancy is associated with progression of *retinopathy* for unknown reasons.[90] Whether pregnancy worsens diabetic nephropathy or hastens the progression to end-stage renal disease is controversial.[91] Although *nephrotic syndrome* develops in 71% of pregnancies, blood pressure and proteinuria eventually return to first-trimester values. *Diabetic nephropathy* is associated with an increased risk of preterm labor, stillbirth, neonatal death, fetal distress, and intrauterine growth retardation; otherwise, literature is sparse on the effect of pregnancy on diabetic neuropathy. *Autonomic neuropathy,* particularly gastroparesis, makes adequate nutrition difficult for both mother and fetus. Pregnant women should be referred for parenteral feedings if conservative therapy fails to control vomiting.[49]

Hypoglycemia is common in pregnancy in part because of intensive insulin treatment to maintain euglycemia.[92] Hypoglycemic unawareness is not uncommon. The effects of hypoglycemia on the fetus are unclear. *Ketoacidosis* is associated with a 50% to 90% fetal mortality rate.[49,93]

ORAL HYPOGLYCEMIC AGENTS

The widespread availability of a variety of oral medications for hyperglycemia, some with serious side effects, require the EP to be familiar with these drugs. *Sulfonylureas,* developed in the 1940s, continue to be the mainstay of oral diabetes treatment. These drugs increase insulin secretion by binding to specific beta-cell receptors.[94] This class of drugs works best in patients with early onset of type 2 diabetes and fasting glucose less than 300 mg/dl.[95] This class of drugs is contraindicated in patients with known allergy to sulfa agents.

Metformin works by decreasing hepatic glucose output, leading to decreased insulin resistance and lower blood glucose. Used alone, metformin does not cause hypoglycemia, but it is contraindicated in patients with renal insufficiency and metabolic acidosis. Metformin should be withheld for 48 hours before administration of iodinated contrast media due to the risk of acidosis. Metformin must be used with caution in patients with hypoxemia, liver compromise, and alcohol abuse. These patients are at increased risk of developing lactic acidosis, which carries a 50% mortality rate.[95,96]

The *thiazolidinediones* reduce insulin resistance and are especially useful in patients who require large amounts of insulin and still lack adequate glucose control. Because of a rare case of hepatic toxicity, troglitazone is now limited to use only with other agents.[96] Pioglitazone and rosiglitazone are approved for monotherapy. Liver function should be monitored for at least 1 year after the initiation of therapy with thiazolidinediones.

α-Glucosidase inhibitors delay intestinal monosaccharide absorption and prevent complex carbohydrate breakdown.[95] They must be titrated to minimize GI side effects and should not be used in patients with certain GI disorders. Liver function monitoring is required due to dose-dependent hepatotoxicity.

Repaglinide is similar to the sulfonylureas in action and mechanism. It has a more rapid onset of action, carries less risk of hypoglycemia, and is suitable for patients allergic to sulfa.[96] Care should be used in patients with renal or hepatic dysfunction.[95]

NEW-ONSET HYPERGLYCEMIA

Patients often present to the ED with typical diabetic symptoms such as polyuria, polydipsia, and polyphagia. Many have serum glucose greater than 200 mg/dl but are not ketotic. These patients with normal electrolytes may be treated with IV hydration alone or with insulin, often reducing the glucose to 150 mg/dl. In reliable patients whose initial glucose is greater than 400 mg/dl, initiation of oral hypoglycemic therapy may be appropriate, with lifestyle modification. An HbA_{1c} value should be sent before initiation of therapy to help evaluate treatment. Initial therapy with sulfonylureas is appropriate; glyburide or glipizide, 10 mg once daily, is recommended. In obese patients or those in whom sulfonylureas are contraindicated, metformin may be an alternative.

NEW TRENDS

Recent changes in the therapy of diabetes include greater use of human insulin, which has prevented some of the adverse reactions to beef and pork products. Unfortunately, some patients demonstrate sensitivity reactions even to subcutaneously injected human insulin.[97] More physicians are teaching their type 1 patients and families how to administer glucagon to treat severe hypoglycemia. Initiation of immunosuppressive therapy at the initial diagnosis of type 1 diabetes can prolong the patient's ability to secrete insulin. However, this beneficial effect, whether achieved by azathioprine or cyclosporine, is not usually sustainable.[98] The potential side effects of immunosuppressive agents have precluded large trials in patients early in their disease.[99] Prophylactic insulin therapy, nicotinamide, oral insulin, or glutamate decarboxylase and avoidance of cow's milk may prevent or delay the onset of type 1 diabetes in patients at risk.[6]

Glycemic control now involves improved technology and more widespread individual monitoring. More patients alter their insulin dosages daily in response to their findings. Diabetic patients with tight glycemic control benefit by limiting the progression of microvascular disease: neuropathy, renal disease, and certain types of retinopathy. However, they are more likely than other diabetic patients to experience hypoglycemic episodes.

EPs and prehospital care providers are encountering patients with insulin pumps. Many insulin pumps are available, each having a pump mechanism, a reservoir for insulin, tubing, and indwelling subcutaneous needles. They are attached, usually with tapes, to the patient's body and administer insulin at a regular adjustable rate. Most pumps also allow the patient to administer additional boluses of insulin as necessary. These pumps support tight glycemic control and are acceptable to some patients. However, motivated patients can achieve equivalent control by adjusting daily injections. Insulin pumps are associated with a variety of complications (e.g., iatrogenic hypoglycemia).

Because glucose rotates the polarization of light waves, new fiberoptic technology has been developed to determine blood glucose noninvasively. This technology may be applied to the insulin pumps in the future.

The basic concepts of the diabetic diet remain unchanged, although many studies emphasize foods and medications that alter glucose absorption. Various high-fiber diets have improved glycemic control. The mostly beneficial but occasionally deleterious effects of exercise have also been elaborated.[94]

Newer therapies include pancreatic and pancreatic beta-cell transplants. Solid-organ pancreatic transplantation remains controversial among both diabetologists and transplant surgeons. Transplantation ameliorates many secondary complications of diabetes, such as nephropathy, neuropathy, gastroparesis, retinopathy, and microvascular changes. The percentage of grafts functioning after 1 year and the 1-year patient survival rate are greater than 75% in selected medical centers.[100] Rejection, posttransplant pancreatitis, and graft thrombosis, as well as other vascular and immunosuppression problems, continue to plague transplant recipients.

Research into peptides involved in glucose regulation offers an additional avenue for future treatments. These peptides include glucagon-like peptide (GLP-1), amylin, and insulin-like growth factor I (IGF-I).[94] Advances in understanding the genetics of diabetes may allow identification of persons at risk for its development and prevention of its phenotypic expression.[6]

KEY CONCEPTS

- Hypoglycemia may be associated with significant morbidity and mortality. Once the diagnosis is suspected and, if possible, confirmed by laboratory evaluation, treatment should be immediately initiated.
- Hypoglycemia caused by oral hypoglycemic agents may be prolonged. Patients should be observed for an extended period or hospitalized.
- The essentials of treatment of diabetic ketoacidosis are restoration of insulin, correction of dehydration, correction of potassium, correction of acidosis, and treatment of the underlying cause.
- Hyperglycemic hyperosmolar nonketotic coma is often associated with focal neurologic signs that resolve with treatment. The essentials of treatment are correction of profound dehydration, correction of electrolytes, and treatment of the underlying cause.

REFERENCES

1. Banting FG, Best CH: Pancreatic extracts, *J Lab Clin Med* 7:464, 1922.
2. Diabetes Control and Complications Trial Research Group: The effect of intensive treatment of diabetes on the development and progression of long-term complications in insulin-dependent diabetes mellitus, *N Engl J Med* 329:977, 1993.
3. Smith DM et al: Unexpected hospital admissions among patients with diabetes mellitus, *Arch Intern Med* 143:41, 1983.
4. Smith DM, Weinberger M, Katz BP: Predicting nonelective hospitalization: a model based on risk factors associated with diabetes mellitus, *J Gen Intern Med* 2:168, 1987.
5. Unger RH, Foster DW: Diabetes mellitus. In Wilson JD, Foster DW, editors: *Williams' textbook of endocrinology,* ed 8, Philadelphia, 1992, Saunders.
6. Atkinson MA, MaClaron NK: Mechanisms of disease: the pathogenesis of insulin-dependent diabetes mellitus, *N Engl J Med* 21:1428, 1994.
7. Umpierrea GE, Khajavi M, Kitabchi AE: Review: Diabetic ketoacidosis and hyperglycemic hyperosmolar nonketotic syndrome, *Am J Med Sci* 311(5):225, 1996.
8. American Diabetes Association: Report of the Expert Committee on the Diagnosis and Classification of Diabetes Mellitus, *Diabetes Care* 20:1183, 1997.
9. Perez MI, Kohn SR: Cutaneous manifestations of diabetes mellitus, *Am Acad Dermatol* 30:519, 1994.
10. Froguel PH et al: Familial hyperglycemia due to mutations in glucokinase, *N Engl J Med* 328:697, 1993.
11. Birmingham Diabetes Survey Working Party: Ten-year follow-up report on Birmingham Diabetes Survey, *BMJ* 2:35, 1976.
12. Bingly PJ et al: Can we really predict IDDM? *Diabetes* 42:213, 1993.
13. Knowler WC et al: Diabetes incidence and prevalence in Pima Indians: a 19-fold greater incidence than in Rochester, Minnesota, *Am J Epidemiol* 108:497, 1978.
14. Krolewski AS et al: Epidemiologic approach to the etiology of type I diabetes mellitus and its complications, *N Engl J Med* 317:1390, 1987.
15. MaClaren N, Schatz D, Drash A: Initial pathogenic events in IDDM, *Diabetes* 38:534, 1989.
16. Atkinson MA et al: 64,000 MR_4 autoantibodies are predictive of insulin-dependent diabetes, *Lancet* 225:1357, 1990.
17. Gianani R et al: Prognostically significant heterogeneity of cytoplasmic islet cell antibodies in relative of patients with type I diabetes, *Diabetes* 41:347, 1992.
18. Johnson KH et al: Islet amyloid, islet-amyloid polypeptide, and diabetes mellitus, *N Engl J Med* 321:513, 1989.
19. Gamble DR: A possible virus etiology for juvenile diabetes. In Creutzfeldt W, Kobberling J, Nee JV, editors: *The genetics of diabetes mellitus,* New York, 1982, Academic Press.
20. Shepherd PR, Kahn BB: Glucose transporters and insulin action, *N Engl J Med* 341:248, 1999.
21. American Diabetes Association: Clinical practice recommendations, *Diabetes Care* 16:5, 1993.
22. American Diabetes Association: Standards of medical care for patients with diabetes mellitus (position statement), *Diabetes Care* 20(suppl 1):S5, 1997.
23. James GP, Bee DE: Glucosuria: accuracy and precision of laboratory diagnosis by dipstick analysis, *Clin Chem* 25:966, 1979.
24. Bell DS, Cutter G: Characteristics of severe hypoglycemia in the patient with insulin-dependent diabetes, *South Med J* 87:616, 1994.
25. DCCT Research Group: Epidemiology of severe hypoglycaemia in the Diabetes Control and Complications Trial, *Am J Med* 90:450, 1991.
26. Potter J et al: Insulin-induced hypoglycemia in an accident in the emergency department: the tip of an iceberg, *BMJ* 285:1180, 1982.
27. Mulhausser I, Berger M, Sonnenberg G: Incidence and management of severe hypoglycemia in 434 adults with insulin-dependent diabetes mellitus, *Diabetes Care* 8:274, 1985.
28. Cranston I et al: Restoration of hypoglycaemia awareness in patients with long-duration insulin-dependent diabetes, *Lancet* 344:283, 1994.
29. Heller SR, Cryer PE: Reduced neuroendocrine and symptomatic responses to subsequent hypoglycemia in non-diabetic humans, *Diabetes* 40:223, 1991.
30. Widom B, Simonson DC: Effect of intermittent hypoglycemia on counter regulatory hormone secretion, *Diabetologia* 33:84, 1990.

31. Bolli GB et al: Abnormal glucose counterregulation after subcutaneous insulin in insulin-dependent diabetes mellitus, *N Engl J Med* 310:1706, 1984.
32. Bolli GB et al: Glucose counterregulation and waning insulin in the Somogyi phenomenon (posthypoglycemic hyperglycemia), *N Engl J Med* 311:1214, 1984.
33. Adler PM: Serum glucose changes after administration of 50% dextrose solution: pre- and in-hospital calculations, *Am J Emerg Med* 4:504, 1986.
34. Collier A et al: Comparison of intravenous glucagon and dextrose in treatment of severe hypoglycemia in an accident and emergency department, *Diabetes Care* 10:712, 1987.
35. Daneman D et al: Severe hypoglycemia in children with insulin-dependent diabetes mellitus: frequency and predisposing factors, *J Pediatr* 115:681, 1989.
36. Pontiroli AE et al: Intranasal glucagon as remedy of hypoglycemia: studies in healthy subjects and type I diabetic patients, *Diabetes Care* 12:604, 1989.
37. Kitabchi AE, Wall BM: Diabetic ketoacidosis, *Med Clin North Am* 79:9, 1995.
38. Adrogué HJ et al: Determinants of plasma potassium levels in diabetic ketoacidosis, *Medicine* 65:163, 1986.
39. Fulop M, Tannenbaum H, Dreyer N: Ketotic hyperosmolar coma, *Lancet* 2:635, 1973.
40. Bohannon NJ: Large phosphate shifts with treatment for hyperglycemia, *Arch Intern Med* 149:1423, 1989.
41. Vincor F et al: Hyperamylasemia in diabetic ketoacidosis: sources and significance, *Ann Intern Med* 91:200, 1979.
42. Zonszein J, Baylor P: Diabetic ketoacidosis with alkalemia: a review, *West J Med* 149:217, 1988.
43. Fulop M: Alcoholism, ketoacidosis, and lactic acidosis, *Diabetes Metab Rev* 5:365, 1989.
44. Lebovitz HE: Diabetic ketoacidosis, *Lancet* 345:767, 1995.
45. Holmes L: The patient with chronic endocrine disease. In Herr, Cydulka RK, editors: *Emergency care of the compromised patient,* Philadelphia, 1994, Lippincott.
46. Adrogué HJ, Madias NE: Changes in plasma potassium concentration during acute acid-base disturbances, *Am J Med* 71:456, 1981.
47. Slovis CM et al: Diabetic ketoacidosis and infection: leukocyte count and differential as early predictors of serious infection, *Am J Emerg Med* 5:1, 1987.
48. Fulop M, Ben-Ezra J, Bock JL: Alcoholic ketosis, *Alcohol Clin Exp Res* 10:610, 1986.
49. Reece EA, Homko CJ: Diabetes-related complications of pregnancy, *J Natl Med Assoc* 85:537, 1993.
50. Lindsay R, Bolte RG: The use of an insulin bolus in low-dose insulin infusion for pediatric diabetic ketoacidosis, *Pediatr Emerg Care* 5:55, 1989.
51. Ionescu-Tirgoviste C et al: Study of plasma osmolarity during the treatment of diabetic ketoacidosis, *Med Intern* 17:67, 1979.
52. Weisenfeld S et al: Adsorption of insulin to infusion bottle and tubing, *Diabetes* 17:766, 1968.
53. Foster DW, McGarry JD: The metabolic derangements and treatment of diabetic ketoacidosis, *N Engl J Med* 309:159, 1983.
54. Filer JS, Kahn CR, Roth J: Receptor, antireceptor antibodies and mechanism of insulin resistance, *N Engl J Med* 300:413, 1979.
55. Adrogué HJ, Barrero J, Eknoyan G: Salutary effects of modest fluid replacement in the treatment of adults with diabetic ketoacidosis: use in patients without extreme volume deficit, *JAMA* 262:2108, 1989.
56. Duck SC et al: Cerebral edema complicating therapy for diabetic ketoacidosis, *Diabetes* 25:111, 1976.
57. Duck SC, Kohler E: Cerebral edema in diabetic ketoacidosis, *J Pediatr* 98:674, 1981.
58. Duck SC, Wyatt DT: Factors associated with brain herniation in the treatment of diabetic ketoacidosis, *J Pediatr* 113:10, 1988.
59. Kebler R, McDonald FD, Cadnapaphornchai P: Dynamic changes in serum phosphorus levels in diabetic ketoacidosis, *Am J Med* 79:571, 1985.
60. Fisher JN, Kitabchi AE: A randomized study of phosphate therapy in the treatment of diabetic ketoacidosis, *J Clin Endocrinol Metab* 57:177, 1983.
61. Krane EJ et al: Subclinical brain swelling in children during treatment of diabetic ketoacidosis, *N Engl J Med* 312:1147, 1985.
62. Van der Meulen JA, Klip A, Grinstein S: Possible mechanism for cerebral oedema in diabetic ketoacidosis, *Lancet* 2(8554):306, 1987.
63. Kent LA, Grill GV, Williams G: Mortality and outcome of patients with brittle diabetes and recurrent ketoacidosis, *Lancet* 844:778, 1994.
64. Bonadio WH: Pediatric diabetic ketoacidosis: pathophysiology and potential for outpatient management of selected children, *Pediatr Emerg Care* 8:287, 1992.
65. Cahill GF Jr: Hyperglycemic hyperosmolar coma: a syndrome almost unique to the elderly, *J Am Geriatr Soc* 31:103, 1983.
66. Siperstein MD: Diabetic ketoacidosis and hyperosmolar coma, *Endocrinol Metab Clin North Am* 21:915, 1992.
67. Vernon DD, Postellon DC: Nonketotic hyperosmolal diabetic coma in a child: management with low-dose insulin infusion and intracranial pressure monitoring, *Pediatrics* 77:770, 1986.
68. Munshi MN, Martin RE, Fonseca VA: Hyperosmolar nonketotic diabetic syndrome following treatment of human immunodeficiency virus infection with didanosine, *Diabetes Care* 17:316, 1994.
69. Levine SN, Sanson TH: Treatment of hyperglycaemic hyperosmolar non-ketotic syndrome, *Drugs* 38:462, 1989.
70. Venna N, Sabin TD: Tonic focal seizures in non-ketotic hyperglycemia of diabetes mellitus, *Arch Neurol* 38:512, 1981.
71. Wachtel TJ, Silliman RA, Lamberton P: Prognostic factors in the diabetic hyperosmolar state, *J Am Geriatr Soc* 35:737, 1987.
72. Zimmerman BR: Glycaemia control in diabetes mellitus towards the normal profile, *Drugs* 47:611, 1994.
73. Hadden DR: The Diabetes Control and Complications Trial (DCCT): what every endocrinologist needs to know, *Clin Endocrinol* 40:293, 1994.
74. Clarke WL: The Diabetes Control and Complications Trial: new challenges for the primary physician, *Va Med Q* 121:185, 1994.
75. Winocour PD: Platelets, vascular disease, and diabetes mellitus, *Can J Physiol Pharm* 72:295, 1994.
76. Brownlee M, Cahill GH: Diabetic control and vascular complications. In Paoletti R, Gotto AM, editors: *Atherosclerosis review,* vol 4, New York, 1979, Raven.
77. Stephenson J, Fuller JH: Microvascular and acute complications in IDDM patients: the EURODIAB IDDM complications study, *Diabetologia* 37:278, 1994.
78. Woodrow G, Brownjohn AM, Turney JH: Acute renal failure in patients with type 1 diabetes mellitus, *Postgrad Med J* 70:192, 1994.
79. Konen JC, Shihabi ZK: Microalbuminuria and diabetes mellitus, *Am Fam Physician* 48:1421, 1993.
80. Chavers BM et al: Relationship between retinal and glomerular lesions in IDDM patients, *Diabetes* 43:441, 1994.
81. Hamet P: Hypertension and diabetes, *Clin Exp Hypertens* 15:1327, 1993.
82. Engerman RL: Pathogenesis of diabetic retinopathy, *Diabetes* 38: 1203, 1989.
83. Davis JL et al: Peripheral diabetic neuropathy treated with amitriptyline and fluphenazine, *JAMA* 238:2291, 1977.
84. Caputo GM et al: Assessment and management of foot disease in patients with diabetes, *N Engl J Med* 330:854, 1994.
85. Lipsky BA, Pecoraro RE, Wheat LJ: The diabetic foot: soft tissue and bone infection, *Infect Dis Clin North Am* 4:409, 1990.
86. Pliskin MA, Todd WF, Edelson GW: Presentations of diabetic feet, *Arch Fam Med* 3:273, 1994.
87. Bernstein JE: Cutaneous manifestations of diabetes mellitus, *Curr Concepts Skin Dis* 1:3, 1980.
88. Steel JM et al: Insulin requirements during pregnancy in women with type I diabetes, *Obstet Gynecol* 4:83:253, 1994.
89. Berk MA, Miodovnik M, Mimouni F: Impact of pregnancy on complications of insulin-dependent diabetes mellitus, *Am J Perinatol* 5:359, 1988.
90. Klein BEK, Moss SE, Klein R: Effect of pregnancy on progression of diabetic retinopathy, *Diabetes Care* 13:34, 1990.
91. Kitzmiller JL, Combs CA: Maternal and perinatal implications of diabetic nephropathy, *Clin Perinatology* 20:561, 1993.
92. Diamond MP et al: Impairment of counter-regulatory hormone secretion in response to hypoglycemia in pregnant women with insulin dependent diabetes mellitus, *Am J Obstet Gynecol* 166:70, 1993.
93. Kitzmiller JL: Diabetic ketoacidosis and pregnancy, *Contemp Obstet Gynecol* 20:141, 1982.

94. Mahler RJ, Adler ML: Clinical review 102: type 2 diabetes mellitus, update on diagnosis, *J Clin Endocrinol Metab* 84:1165, 1999.
95. Florence JA, Yeager BF: Treatment of type 2 diabetes mellitus, *Am Fam Physician* 59:2835, 1999.
96. Abramowicz M, editor: Rosiglitazone for type 2 diabetes mellitus, *Med Lett Drugs Ther* 41:71, 1999.
97. Grammer LC, Metzger BE, Patterson R: Cutaneous allergy to human (recombinant DNA) insulin, *JAMA* 251:1459, 1984.
98. Bougneres PF et al: Limited duration of remission of insulin dependency in children with recent overt type I diabetes treated with low-dose cyclosporine, *Diabetes* 39:1264, 1990.
99. Fathman CG, Myers BD: Cyclosporine therapy for autoimmune disease, *N Engl J Med* 326:1693, 1992.
100. Sussman KE: Diabetes—the road ahead, *Am J Med* 85:166, 1988.

121 Rhabdomyolysis

Laura J. Bontempo

PERSPECTIVE

Rhabdomyolysis is a clinical syndrome caused by injury to skeletal muscle that results in release of its contents into the extracellular fluid and the circulation. The injury may be reversible or irreversible, and the diagnosis rests on measurement of these released substances in either plasma or urine. The earliest reference to rhabdomyolysis occurs in the Old Testament, from the Book of Numbers.[1] During the Exodus the Israelites consumed large amounts of quail, and many became ill and died from an illness involving intense muscle pain and weakness. The quail ingested by the Israelites may have fed on hemlock seeds during their westward migration to the Sinai Peninsula. This theory is supported by reports of severe muscle pain and even muscle paralysis after consuming quail that had fed on hemlock seeds. In the late nineteenth century a clinical syndrome of muscle pain, weakness, and brown urine was called "Meyer-Betz disease" in the German literature.[2]

In 1941, Bywaters and Beall[3] described the clinical course of four victims with crush injuries to the limbs after air raids during World War II. They noted the link between muscle injury and renal dysfunction in their classic monograph, as follows:

> The patient has been buried for several hours with pressure on a limb. On admission he looks in good condition except for swelling of the limb, some local anesthesia and whealing. The hemoglobin, however, is raised and a few hours later despite vasoconstriction made manifest by pallor, coldness and sweating, the blood pressure falls. This is restored to the pre-shock level by (often multiple) transfusions of serum, plasma, or occasionally, blood. Anxiety may now arise concerning the circulation in the injured limb, which may show diminution of arterial pulsation distally, accompanied by all the changes of incipient gangrene. Signs of renal damage soon appear, and progress even though the crushed limb be amputated. The urinary output, initially small, owing perhaps to the severity of the shock, diminishes further. The urine contains albumin and many dark brown or black granular casts. These later decrease in number. The patient is alternately drowsy and anxiously aware of the severity of his illness. Slight generalized edema, thirst, and incessant vomiting develop, and the blood pressure often remains slightly raised. The blood urea and potassium, raised at an early stage, become progressively higher, and death occurs comparatively suddenly, frequently within a week. Necropsy reveals necrosis of muscle and in the renal tubules, degenerative changes and casts containing brown pigment.

The relationship between traumatic muscle injury and kidney failure was aptly described and has been reviewed extensively in the past 60 years. In the mid-1970s the first references were made to nontraumatic rhabdomyolysis.[4,5] Since then the number of known causes for this syndrome has greatly increased.

Acute renal failure (ARF) is one of the most serious complications of rhabdomyolysis. Approximately 5% to 15% of patients hospitalized with ARF in the United States have rhabdomyolysis as the etiology.[6,7] Other studies report an incidence of 1% to 20%. Well-designed prospective studies of rhabdomyolysis and its complications are lacking, so the true incidence of ARF in this setting is unknown.

PRINCIPLES OF DISEASE

Anatomy and Physiology

Skeletal muscle is the largest organ in the human body. Functioning of muscle cells is critically dependent on a healthy cell membrane, the sarcolemma, which maintains cellular ionic gradients and ensures proper metabolic functioning. The sarcolemma contains sodium-potassium pumps, calcium protein-carrier pumps, and other channels and structures.[8] The sodium-potassium pump moves sodium out of the cell's sarcoplasm and potassium into the sarcoplasm. More sodium is transported than potassium, which creates a net negative charge to the interior of the cell. In addition, a concentration gradient is created between intracellular and extracellular sodium ions. Normally the concentration of intracellular sodium ions is very low, approximately 10 mEq/L, when compared with the extracellular fluid.[8]

The calcium pumps work to maintain a low intracellular fluid calcium concentration. Located in the sarcolemma, the pumps move calcium from the sarcoplasm to the outside of the cell. Additional pumps help to move calcium into the muscle cell's internal structures, the sarcoplasmic reticulum and the mitochondria. As sodium ions move down the electrochemical gradient (i.e., return into the cell), calcium ions are able to move out from the cell into the extracellular fluid[8] (Figure 121-1).

With the exception of the sodium-calcium exchange, all these pumps rely on active transport and use adenosine triphosphate (ATP) as their energy source.[8]

Myoglobin is also found in a cell's sarcoplasm. It is the major heme protein that supplies oxygen to skeletal and

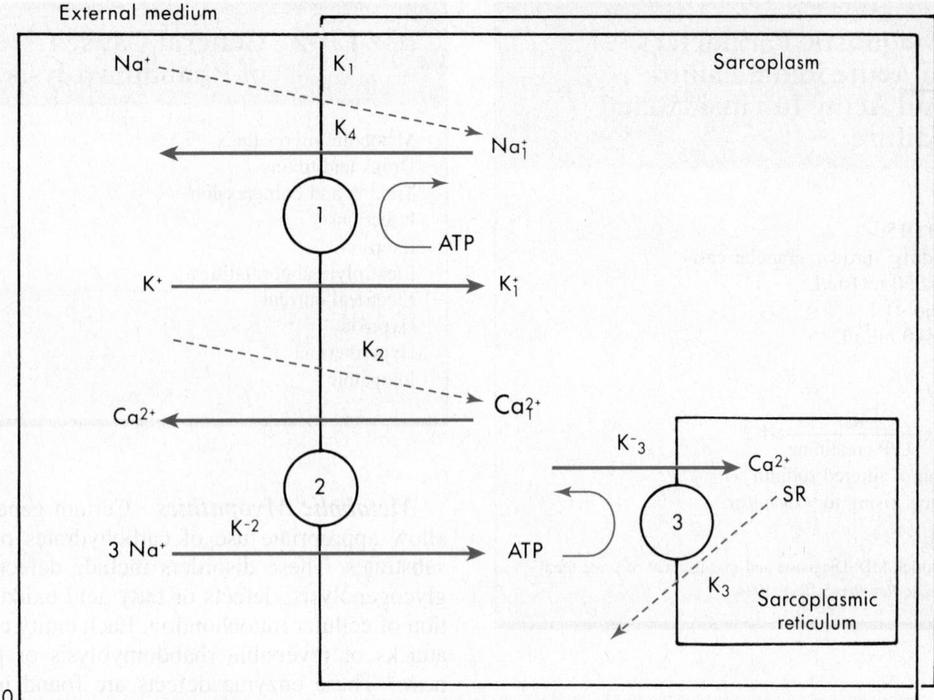

Figure 121-1. **Normal membrane ionic pump function of skeletal muscle cell. When this function is ineffective, calcium stores will increase in the cell, which may initiate a series of outputs leading to cellular injury.** *From Balustein MP:* Am J Physiol *232:C165, 1977.*

cardiac muscle. Myoglobin has a higher affinity than hemoglobin for oxygen, which causes influx of oxygen into muscle cells.[9] Cell damage results in myoglobin release, which produces the classic dark-colored urine of rhabdomyolysis.

Skeletal muscle cells contain, in their cytoplasm, proteases and other proteolytic enzymes that have low activity in the cell's normal physiologic state. These enzymes decompose myofibrillar proteins so that they may be recycled. The activity level of these enzymes appears to depend on intracellular calcium levels; the greater the concentration of calcium, the more disinhibited or active the enzymes become. With significant elevation of intracellular calcium, their activity level is raised to a point at which enzymes become destructive to the cell.[10]

Pathophysiology

Despite the large number of specific diseases causing rhabdomyolysis, the final common pathway of injury involves *damage to the sarcolemma with loss of its intrinsic functions.* The damage results in an influx of calcium and a subsequent rise in the intracellular calcium concentration, as well as liberation of intracellular contents, such as myoglobin, aldolase, aspartate transaminase, lactate dehydrogenase, creatine kinase, potassium, uric acid and phosphorus.[11]

Loss of function of the cell membrane results in loss of the ionic gradients created by the sodium-potassium and calcium pumps. This causes extracellular hypocalcemia and a rise in intracellular calcium.[12] Elevated intracellular calcium leads to greater activity of intracellular proteases, phospholipases, and other proteolytic enzymes. These enzymes then cause further cell damage and destruction.[9,13]

Intracellular calcium can accumulate secondary to direct membrane damage (i.e., crush injury) or through ATP depletion. Membrane damage from direct trauma makes the sarcolemma more permeable to calcium, which follows the electrochemical gradient and travels into the cell.[10,14] In atraumatic rhabdomyolysis, lack of adequate energy, in the form of ATP, can cause the ion pumps to stop functioning, with calcium accumulation in a muscle cell.[9,10] The ATP depletion can result from a mismatch between energy supply and demand (e.g., vigorous or prolonged exercise) or a defect in energy use (e.g., McArdle's syndrome, or absence of muscle phosphorylase).[9]

Once destruction of the myocyte has begun, myoglobin is released. As the levels of free plasma myoglobin increase, excess myoglobin is filtered by the kidneys and enters the urine.[15] Myoglobin accumulation, coupled with hypovolemia and acidosis, can precipitate and cause blockage to renal tubular flow.[16] Myoglobin may also be directly toxic to the renal tubular cells.[6,9,17]

The most common cause of rhabdomyolysis-induced ARF is acute intrinsic renal failure (AIRF), formerly known as acute tubular necrosis (ATN). AIRF is defined as a decrease in the glomerular filtration rate (GFR) caused by a toxic or ischemic event that is not reversed on discontinuation of the insult. AIRF is invariably associated with some degree of tubular injury and has a characteristic urine profile of low specific gravity (~1.010), brown casts and a fractional excretion of sodium greater than 1% (Box 121-1).

The role of myoglobin in the nephrotoxicity of this syndrome has been well studied. Bywaters and Beall[3] first noticed the association of renal failure with the excretion of acid urine. They studied the effect of myoglobin infusions on renal function in the rabbit and concluded that hypovolemia

Box 121-1 Diagnostic Parameters in Acute Renal Failure and Acute Intrinsic Renal Failure

Odorless urine
Specific gravity <1.015
Urine sediment: "dirty" brown, granular casts
Urine osmolarity <350 mOsm/L
U/P osmolarity ratio <1.1
Urine sodium >20-40 mEq/L
U/P urea <4
U/P creatinine <20
Renal failure index: $\frac{U_{Na}}{U/P\ creatinine} > 1\text{-}2$
Fractional excretion of filtered sodium >1%-2%
Free water clearance: rising to >15 ml/hr

U/P, Urinary to plasma.
Modified from McGoldrick MD: Diagnosis and management of acute renal failure: part I, *Cardiovasc Rev Rep* 5:1031, 1984.

and an acid urine were required for this substance to cause renal injury.[3,18] Myoglobin infusions in normovolemic rabbits with urine pH above 6 had no deleterious effect on kidney function.[18]

Other studies have demonstrated that myoglobin dissociates into its two components, globin and ferrihemate, with pH values at 5.6 or less.[18] Infusions of the globin component have no effect on renal function even in the presence of hypovolemia and acidic urine. Ferrihemate may be the toxic subunit of myoglobin.[19]

Tubular obstruction by myoglobin, uric acid, and other muscle breakdown products may also be causative in the development of ARF. Tubular obstruction, although universally present, may not be the primary event in the development of AIRF associated with rhabdomyolysis.[7]

Compartment syndromes may be a cause or a complication of rhabdomyolysis. A compartment syndrome exists when the circulation to tissues within a closed space is compromised by increased pressure within that space.[20,21] The excessive pressure may occur as a result of a decrease in the size of the compartment, an increase in the size of the contents of the compartment, or a combination of both. Once established, a compartment syndrome tends to be self-sustaining because (1) capillaries become occluded as a result of the increased pressure; (2) venous pressure increases, further decreasing perfusion pressure; and (3) arteriolar vasospasm leads to tissue ischemia, swelling, and edema, causing progressive increases in the compartmental pressure. In 2 to 4 hours, ischemic skeletal muscle may develop functional deficits, which may become irreversible after 10 hours.[20] Within 30 minutes, nerve tissue undergoing vascular compromise may exhibit reversible deficits, which may become fixed within 12 to 24 hours.[21] Therefore it is critical that the diagnosis of rhabdomyolysis be made as early as possible.

Etiology

Exercise, alcohol, drugs, infections, trauma, and seizures are the leading causes of rhabdomyolysis.[10] Multiple causes have been found in a significant number of cases (Box 121-2).

Box 121-2 General Causes of Rhabdomyolysis

Metabolic myopathies
Drugs and toxins
Trauma and compression
Infections
Exertion
Electrolyte abnormalities
Electrical current
Hypoxia
Hyperthermia
Idiopathic

Metabolic Myopathies Certain genetic defects do not allow appropriate use of carbohydrates or lipids as energy substrates. These disorders include defects in glycolysis or glycogenolysis, defects of fatty acid oxidation, and dysfunction of cellular mitochondria. Each entity can cause recurrent attacks of reversible rhabdomyolysis or progressive weakness.[9] These enzyme defects are found in 23% to 47% of adult patients with rhabdomyolysis.[22,23] Such inappropriate use of carbohydrates and lipids causes an imbalance between the energy demand and supply of the muscle cell.

Trauma and Compression Most information regarding rhabdomyolysis from trauma and compression has been obtained from mass-casualty incidents.[24-26] Muscle injury from trauma and compression is multifaceted. Initially there is direct mechanical injury to the sarcolemma, and its homeostatic functions are disrupted.[14] Sodium and calcium travel down their concentration gradients into the intracellular fluid. This causes an abrupt rise in the intracellular calcium concentration as well as an influx of water.[9] The elevated calcium then activates enzymes destructive to the cell, as previously discussed. The water influx contributes to intravascular volume depletion.[10,14,27]

When circulation is reestablished, the damaged cell is reperfused and the extruded intracellular contents, including myoglobin, are brought into the general circulation.[10,28] Also, reperfusion is associated with an influx of neutrophils, which can occlude the microcirculation and cause further muscle ischemia.[9,10]

Of 200 patients admitted to a trauma unit in South Africa after sustaining injuries from beatings, 26 were in a prerenal state, and 21 developed renal failure.[29] In addition to overt trauma, traumatic rhabdomyolysis can be seen in anesthetized surgical patients and comatose patients who remain in a given position for a prolonged time.[9,30]

Exertion Rhabdomyolysis can result from prolonged or strenuous exercise and is seen in both trained and untrained athletes.[31-33] Eccentric exercise (work done by a muscle during lengthening) is more damaging to muscle fibers, as evidenced by higher creatine kinase levels, than concentric exercise (work done by a muscle during shortening).[11] Hot conditions contribute to the incidence of exertional rhabdomyolysis because of increased dehydration or increased activity of heat-sensitive degradative enzymes.[33,34] With prolonged exercise the sarcolemmic ion pumps can also fail from depletion of cellular energy sources, specifically ATP.[9] These factors can lead to elevated intracellular calcium and rhabdomyolysis, which, coupled with dehydration and acidosis from lactic acid production, can cause ARF.[10,33,35]

Exertional rhabdomyolysis is not always the result of voluntary muscle exertion. The same pathophysiology is seen in patients with status epilepticus, myoclonus, dystonia, chorea, tetanus, and mania.[9,36-38]

Electrical Current Rhabdomyolysis occurs in approximately 10% of patients who initially survive a high-voltage electrical injury or lightning strike.[39] Rhabdomyolysis from electrical current appears to be a result of both the heat generated by the electrical current and the direct effects of the current in disrupting the sarcolemma.[40]

Hyperthermia Multiple disorders can raise the core body temperature and result in sarcolemma disruption. Neuroleptic malignant syndrome (fever in patients treated with phenothiazines or haloperidol), malignant hyperthermia (rapid rise in body temperature after anesthesia with halogenated hydrocarbons or succinylcholine), and both classic and exertional heat stroke are some of the most common etiologies.[16,41,42] In hyperpyrexic syndromes, cellular energy demands outstrip available energy supplies causing membrane dysfunction and cellular injury.[43]

Hypothermia may also cause rhabdomyolysis, most likely through direct injury to components of the sarcolemma, which cannot maintain structural integrity below certain temperature levels.[44]

Drugs and Toxins Drugs in almost every class of medication have been implicated as a cause of rhabdomyolysis.[9] Common offenders include ethanol, cocaine and other illicit drugs, lipid-lowering agents, carbon monoxide, and biologic toxins.

Ethanol Ethanol appears to be directly toxic to the skeletal muscle cell membrane, and this toxicity appears to be potentiated by starvation.[10] For this reason, ethanol-induced rhabdomyolysis is often seen in patients who are "binge drinkers." Electrolyte abnormalities also play a role. Chronic alcohol abusers often have hypokalemia, hypophosphatemia, and hypomagnesemia.[16] These deficiencies, coupled with ethanol's direct sarcolemmic toxic effects, make the ethanol abuser more susceptible to rhabdomyolysis.[10]

Ethanol is also a sedative-hypnotic, which can induce obtundation and lead to immobilization of a body part with external compression of its blood supply. In addition, excessive motor activity from seizures or delirium tremens can induce rhabdomyolysis.

Cocaine The incidence of rhabdomyolysis in patients who use cocaine varies from 5% to 30% in published reports.[41] It is unclear why cocaine causes rhabdomyolysis. Hypotheses include cocaine-induced vasospasm with resultant muscle ischemia, excessive energy demands placed on the sarcolemma and direct toxic effects on myocytes.[45-47] Seizures, agitation, trauma, and hyperpyrexia may also play a role.[9] In general the severity of the rhabdomyolysis parallels the severity of the cocaine intoxication, and those patients with very high creatine kinase levels tend to have the most severe complications from this disease.[45,48] Intravenous cocaine use may be associated with a higher incidence of rhabdomyolysis-induced ARF compared with smoking cocaine.[45]

Other Illicit Drugs Agents such as phencyclidine hydrochloride (PCP), amphetamines, and "ecstasy" (3,4-methylenedioxymethamphetamine) may also cause this syndrome.[9,49] These drugs may raise the energy demands of a normal muscle cell to a level that cannot be met by available energy supplies.[50]

Lipid-Lowering Agents The 3-hydroxy-3-methylglutaryl coenzyme A (HMG-CoA) reductase inhibitor, lipid-lowering agents (e.g., lovastatin, simvastatin) have been associated with rhabdomyolysis, as have the branched-chain fatty esters that inhibit liver triglyceride synthesis (e.g., clofibrate, gemfibrozil).[9,51,52] The mechanisms of action are unclear. These agents may precipitate rhabdomyolysis when used alone or with other drugs. Patients with preexisting renal dysfunction may be more susceptible.[53] Rhabdomyolysis has occurred in many patients taking HMG-CoA reductase inhibitors along with gemfibrozil.[51,54,55]

Carbon Monoxide Rhabdomyolysis is a known complication of carbon monoxide poisoning.[56,57] The pathophysiology is unknown, but hypoxia, coma resulting in muscle compression, and direct myocyte toxic effects may play a role.[56]

Biologic Toxins Some snake envenomations cause rhabdomyolysis through direct myocyte injury resulting in the release of intracellular contents to the extracellular circulation. Species known to do this include the European adder, Australian tiger snake, Australian king brown snake, sea snakes, North and South American rattlesnakes, and the death adder. Multiple myocyte toxins may be present in a single venom.[9]

Stings from Africanized bees and honeybees ("killer bees") can also cause rhabdomyolysis. This is also mediated through direct myotoxins.[9,58,59]

Infections Bacterial, viral, and parasitic infections have been associated with rhabdomyolysis.[60] Influenza viruses A and B are the most frequently cited viral etiologies.[61,62] The influenza virus may be directly toxic to myocytes, but this has not been proven.[10,63] Rhabdomyolysis associated with human immunodeficiency virus (HIV) has been reported in many patients. However, the independent role of HIV in causing the disease is unclear because many patients were also taking multiple medications and some had concurrent infections.[64,65]

Legionella is the most common known bacterial etiology of rhabdomyolysis. Its myotoxic effects are mediated through an endotoxin.[10,66,67] *Salmonella* and *Streptococcus* also can induce rhabdomyolysis through both direct myocyte invasion and inhibition of glycolytic enzymes.[10,66,68]

Electrolyte Abnormalities Hypophosphatemia is believed to cause membrane injury by severe depletion of ATP. Hypokalemia has also been shown to cause rhabdomyolysis. Potassium is a vasodilator of the microcirculation for a metabolically active muscle cell when its extracellular concentration is high enough. Hypokalemia may prevent local vasodilation and lead to focal muscle ischemia.[6,10] Both hyponatremia and hypernatremia have been associated with rhabdomyolysis.[9] Case reports of the former primarily involve patients with hyponatremia induced by psychogenic polydipsia.[69]

Hypoxia Any condition causing tissue hypoxia will promote cellular injury and may lead to this syndrome.

Intrinsic vascular injury or obstruction, hypotension, or external compression of the blood supply to a muscle group may all cause tissue hypoxia and rhabdomyolysis.[7] Certain blood disorders (e.g., sickle cell anemia) may cause vascular thrombosis, resulting in tissue hypoxia and subsequent muscle injury.[12,70]

Idiopathic Cause Some patients develop rhabdomyolysis, at times recurrently, without obvious cause. Whether such patients have a genetic defect requires further study.

CLINICAL FEATURES

Patients with rhabdomyolysis classically present with complaints of muscle weakness, swelling, and pain. The myalgias may be focal or diffuse depending on the underlying etiology of the disease. The patient may also note dark- or cola-colored urine. However, a high clinical suspicion for rhabdomyolysis must be maintained in patients at risk because up to 50% of those with serologically proven rhabdomyolysis do not complain of myalgias or muscle weakness.[71]

History The history can be extremely helpful in making the diagnosis. For example, if a patient is brought to the ED with an overdose of a sedative-hypnotic drug, information about the patient's body position and length of time immobilized is useful. Unfortunately, many patients with rhabdomyolysis from this etiology are unable to give an adequate history because of altered mental status. The history should include any recent trauma or compression, excessive exertion, envenomations, infections, electrical shock, or temperature extremes. Other areas are use of prescription medications, over-the-counter drugs, and alcohol or illicit drugs; known medical conditions; and family history of muscle dysfunction or disease.

Physical Examination Physical examination may reveal motor weakness with tenderness to palpation of the affected muscle groups. The overlying skin may be discolored. With trauma or compression the affected area may have sensory and motor losses that do not follow one nerve distribution.[14] Unfortunately, such physical signs are present in only 4% to 15% of patients.[71] Absence of characteristic physical findings does not rule out rhabdomyolysis.

The patient may appear clinically dehydrated from the reduced extracellular fluid volume. The patient must also be examined closely for any signs of trauma.

Some patients with severe rhabdomyolysis show respiratory insufficiency, presumably caused by diffuse muscle injury resulting in weakened respiratory efforts. In addition, some patients may develop hepatic insufficiency, which occasionally leads to hepatic failure requiring liver transplantation.

Compartment syndromes are relatively common complications of rhabdomyolysis. Some studies have reported persistent peripheral nerve deficits in 10% to 20% of patients with compartment syndrome.[72]

DIAGNOSTIC STRATEGIES

Myoglobin

The most reliable method of diagnosing rhabdomyolysis is laboratory evaluation. In the past the diagnosis rested on the demonstration of myoglobin in the serum. Unfortunately, serum myoglobin is an unreliable marker for rhabdomyolysis for several reasons. The half-life of myoglobin in plasma is 1 to 3 hours, and it may disappear completely from plasma within 6 hours of injury. The amount of myoglobinuria depends on plasma concentration of myoglobin, GFR, extent of myoglobin binding in plasma, and urine flow rate. For example, a given patient with moderate muscle injury and a normal GFR who is excreting very concentrated urine may have a significant amount of myoglobin in the urine. On the other hand, a patient with a much larger amount of muscle injury but a low GFR and very dilute urine would have much less myoglobin in the urine.

Urinalysis typically shows brown urine with a large amount of blood on dipstick evaluation but few if any red blood cells (RBCs) on microscopic evaluation. This occurs because the various dipstick tests cannot distinguish myoglobinuria from hematuria or hemoglobinuria.[73] Brown casts and renal tubular epithelial cells may also be found.[9]

Methods used to measure urine myoglobin include immunodiffusion, radioimmunoassay, and dipstick tests. The dipstick tests involve use of reagents (e.g., guaiac, or *o*-toluidine) and are only slightly less sensitive than radioimmunoassay, which is the best method available.[73] Because of the rapid excretion of myoglobin from the urine, however, a significant number of patients with rhabdomyolysis will have false-negative dipstick results.[71]

Creatine Kinase

Measurement of creatine kinase levels (CK; formerly CPK, creatine/creatinine phosphokinase) is a more sensitive method than myoglobin testing to detect rhabdomyolysis. CK is an excellent marker for this disease because it is easily measured, is present in the serum immediately after muscle injury, and is not rapidly cleared from serum. In general, peak CK levels occur within 24 to 36 hours of muscle injury and diminish approximately 39% per day (Figure 121-2).[42] Failure of levels to decrease in this manner suggests ongoing muscle injury.

Rhabdomyolysis cannot be defined by a specific CK level. In general, however, a CK level greater than five times normal is diagnostic, and levels as high as several hundred thousand have been reported.[11,35,46,64] A clear relationship exists between CK level and severity of disease, although patients may have significant morbidity with only moderately elevated CK levels.[46,74,75] For this reason, even modest elevations of CK must be taken seriously, particularly early in the disease process. The CK subtype present in skeletal muscle is MM, but when considerable skeletal muscle injury occurs, a small amount of CK-MB also is present in the serum. This fraction rarely exceeds 3% to 5% of the total CK in the absence of coincident myocardial infarction.

Other Tests

Electrolyte evaluation may show hyperkalemia, hyperphosphatemia, hypocalcemia, hyperuricemia, and hypoalbuminemia. An elevated anion gap is characteristically present.[76] Hyperkalemia (>5.5 mEq/L) has been reported on initial laboratory studies in 20% to 40% of patients.[71] It is caused by a combination of intracellular potassium release from muscle necrosis and decreased renal excretion.[7] Hyperphosphatemia associated with this syndrome is caused by a leakage of phosphorus from injured muscle. Levels usually do not exceed 7 mg/dl.

Hypocalcemia is the most common metabolic abnormality and occurs early in the course of rhabdomyolysis. In one

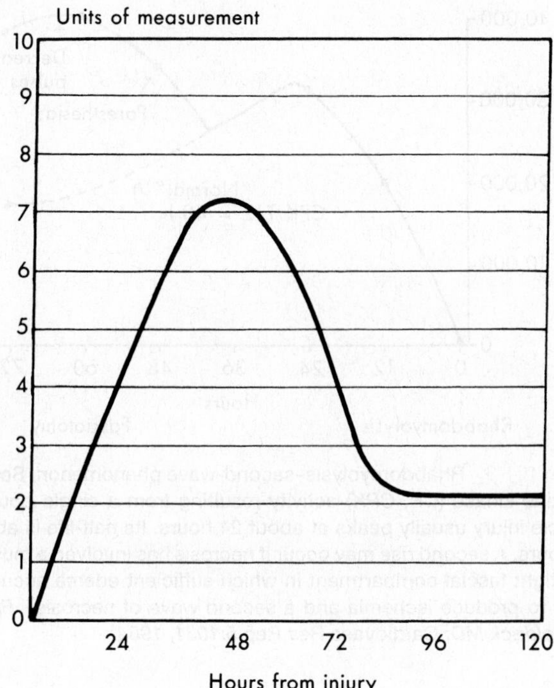

Figure 121-2. **Typical creatine kinase (CK) elimination curve.**

series of 76 patients, hypoglycemia was present in 63%.[77] Hypercalcemia often develops later in this syndrome, and most hypercalcemic patients also experience ARF.[71] Although the exact cause of hypercalcemia in this setting is unknown, it is hypothesized that calcium is mobilized from damaged muscle, and parathyroid hormone and 1,25-dihydroxycholecalciferol levels are increased during recovery from rhabdomyolysis.[10]

The combination of elevated serum phosphate and calcium may result in precipitation of calcium phosphate ($CaPO_4$) in soft tissue, blood vessels, and eyes.[9]

For reasons related to increased muscle mass, hyperuricemia is particularly likely to occur in well-trained athletes with exertional rhabdomyolysis. Hypoalbuminemia may result from leakage of protein from injured vessels and proteinuria.

Many patients with acute rhabdomyolysis demonstrate evidence of disseminated intravascular coagulation (DIC). Thrombocytopenia, hypofibrinogenemia, and increased fibrin split products in serum or urine with prolongation of prothrombin time may be seen. The coagulopathy is a result of muscle necrosis and liberation of activating substances (e.g., thromboplastin) from injured cells.

Some patients have elevated levels of aspartate transaminase (AST), alanine transaminase (ALT), and lactate dehydrogenase (LDH) from muscle injury alone. Occasionally a patient may be misdiagnosed as having hepatic injury when, in fact, all enzyme elevations are caused only by muscle injury.

DIFFERENTIAL CONSIDERATIONS

The history, physical examination, and laboratory evaluation of patients presenting with rhabdomyolysis are unique to this disease entity. On initial presentation, however, the patient must be fully evaluated and alternate diagnoses considered.

Pigmenturia has a variety of causes (Box 121-3). Patients with pigmenturia must be differentiated into those with myoglobinuria and those with hematuria, through microscopic identification of RBCs in the urine; patients cannot be differentiated by dipstick testing alone. Patients with hemoglobinuria will have a positive dipstick test for blood but no RBCs on microscopic analysis. It is differentiated from rhabdomyolysis by checking for plasma discoloration. With hemoglobinuria, but not with myoglobinuria, the plasma will also be discolored.[16] Hematuria and hemoglobinuria have lengthy differential diagnoses of their own. Hematuria can be present with rhabdomyolysis if there was associated renal trauma.

Box 121-3 Differential Diagnosis of Pigmenturia

Hemoglobinuria
Hemolysis

Hematuria
Renal causes
Trauma

Acute Intermittent Porphyria

Bilirubinuria

Food
Beets

Drugs
Vitamin B_{12}
Rifampin
Phenytoin
Laxatives

Pigmenturia can be associated with acute intermittent porphyria. These patients generally have a very different clinical presentation from acute rhabdomyolysis, and the urine will contain porphobilinogen.[9] Bilirubin, a degradation product of heme, will also cause pigmenturia when present in the urine; the urine should test positive for urobilinogen. Pigmenturia can also be a direct drug or food effect; the urine should test negative for blood, and few or no RBCs are seen on microscopic evaluation.

In crush injury the motor weakness and possible paralysis may mimic spinal injury.[78] All trauma patients must be treated with spinal precautions, and laboratory-proven rhabdomyolysis does not rule out concurrent spinal injury. With rhabdomyolysis, however, motor function will often improve as the disease is treated.

Myocardial infarction must be considered in patients with an elevated CK level and pain, especially if the pain is localized to the chest.

MANAGEMENT

Saline Infusion

The mainstay of therapy for rhabdomyolysis is the administration of large volumes of saline very early in the course of the disease. In patients with trauma or compression, saline resuscitation should begin in the field.[79] Early intervention has decreased the incidence of AIRF.[10] Resuscitation should be undertaken with half-isotonic saline. Potassium-containing fluids should be avoided due to the risk of rhabdomyolysis-associated hyperkalemia. High-volume infusions should be started as soon as possible and infusion rates titrated for a urine output of 200 to 300 ml/hr.[15]

Patients may require up to 20 L fluid in the first 24 hours to achieve urine flow rates of 200 to 300 ml/hr. Cardiac, pulmonary, and electrolyte status should be carefully monitored.

Urine Alkalinization

Urine alkalinization may help with renal myoglobin clearance by increasing myoglobin's solubility. Alternatively, elevated serum myoglobin levels may not be nephrotoxic unless accompanied by intravascular volume depletion and acidosis.[18] The goal is to keep the urine pH greater than 6.5. Although the use of large fluid volumes and bicarbonate early in rhabdomyolysis seems very effective, prospective randomized studies using these agents have not been performed. Volume expansion alone may be effective therapy for these patients.

Mannitol

Mannitol may have many beneficial effects in the treatment of rhabdomyolysis. It acts as an osmotic diuretic, an intravascular volume expander, a renal vasodilator, and possibly a free radical scavenger. As a diuretic, mannitol increases urine flow, which may help prevent obstruction from myoglobin casts. Renal vasodilation increases renal blood flow and GFR and may decrease tubular obstruction. As a volume expander, mannitol draws fluid from the interstitial space, decreasing intravascular dehydration and potentially reducing muscular swelling.[9,16,80] In cases of early ARF, mannitol may convert oliguric renal failure to nonoliguric renal failure, which has a somewhat better prognosis.[7] Loop diuretics (e.g., furosemide) can acidify the urine and should not be used.[15]

Chelation Therapy

A potential role for iron chelators is under investigation. Chelation therapy reduces renal injury in animal models, but this is not yet validated for humans.[81]

General Measures

Electrolyte Abnormalities Concurrent with the previous treatments, electrolyte abnormalities must be monitored and managed. Hyperkalemia is a potentially life-threatening complication of rhabdomyolysis and should be treated following the usual medical regimen. Hyperkalemia coupled with hypocalcemia can predispose to malignant cardiac dysrhythmias. Intravenous calcium may be ineffective as a treatment for hyperkalemia if given to a patient with hyperphosphatemia. The calcium and phosphate can combine and precipitate.[9] Dialysis may be required.

The use of calcium for asymptomatic hypocalcemic patients should be avoided because it may raise intracellular calcium levels, promoting further muscle injury. Symptomatic hypercalcemia generally requires only volume expansion and diuretic therapy.

For patients with a rising or elevated potassium level, persistent acidosis, or oliguric renal failure with fluid overload, dialysis may be necessary.[9,10] Dialysis with supportive care should effectively limit the morbidity and mortality from ARF associated with rhabdomyolysis.

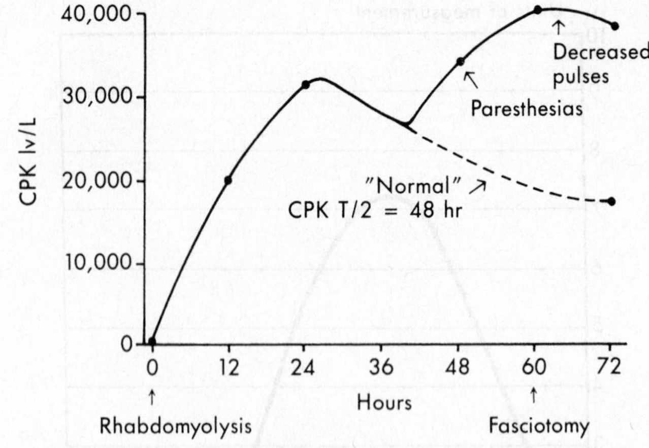

Figure 121-3. **Rhabdomyolysis–second-wave phenomenon. Serum creatine kinase (CK, *CPK*) activity resulting from a single bout of muscle injury usually peaks at about 24 hours. Its half-life is about 48 hours. A second rise may occur if necrosis has involved a muscle in a tight fascial compartment in which sufficient edema accumulates to produce ischemia and a second wave of necrosis.** *From McGoldrick MD:* Cardiovasc Rev Rep *5:1031, 1984.*

Coagulopathy Therapy for the coagulopathy associated with this syndrome is directed at treatment of the underlying disease process. DIC usually resolves spontaneously after several days, but if hemorrhagic complications occur, therapy with platelets, vitamin K, and fresh frozen plasma may be necessary.

Compartment Syndrome Clinicians should routinely monitor compartmental pressures in the patient with suspected or existing compartment syndrome. When compartmental pressure exceeds 35 mm Hg, fasciotomy should be strongly considered, although the decision to perform a fasciotomy must be decided on a case-by-case basis.[82] The failure of CK levels to decline should suggest ongoing muscle injury from a compartment syndrome (Figure 121-3).

DISPOSITION

No good prospective studies support a standardized approach to disposition of the patient with rhabdomyolysis. The high risk for renal failure, however, mandates close monitoring of renal function, electrolytes, and hydration status, which usually requires admission to the hospital, where CK levels can be assessed for ongoing muscle injury. Also, unless the patient is a victim of trauma or compression injury, the underlying etiology of the rhabdomyolysis requires investigation to prevent recurrences.

KEY CONCEPTS

- Rhabdomyolysis classically presents in patients complaining of muscle weakness, swelling and pain. Because only half of patients have all these physical findings, however, the EP should suspect the syndrome in all patients at risk, particularly when they present with an altered sensorium.
- In patients with rhabdomyolysis, urine dipstick testing is strongly positive for blood, without or with very few red blood cells. The diagnosis is confirmed by an elevated serum creatine kinase (CK) level.
- Early fluid resuscitation resulting in a urine output of 200 to

300 ml/hr is key in reducing the risk of rhabdomyolysis-induced renal failure.

- Hyperkalemia with hypocalcemia can precipitate malignant cardiac dysrhythmias and must be treated aggressively.
- CK level that continues to rise beyond 48 hours may indicate continued muscle injury. The patient requires careful evaluation for compartment syndromes or other etiologies.

REFERENCES

1. Book of Numbers 11:31-35.
2. Meyer-Betz F: Beobachtungen an einem eigenartigen mit: Muskellahmungen verbunden Fall von Hamoglobinurie, *Dtsch Arch Klin Med* 101:85, 1911.
3. Bywaters EGL, Beall D: Crush injuries with impairment of renal function, *BMJ* 1:427, 1941.
4. Koffler A, Friedler RM, Massry SG: Renal failure due to non-traumatic rhabdomyolyis, *Ann Intern Med* 85:23, 1976.
5. Grossman RA et al: Nontraumatic rhabdomyolysis and acute renal failure, *N Engl J Med* 291:807, 1974.
6. Zager RA: Rhabdomyolysis and myohemoglobinuric acute renal failure, *Kidney Int* 49:314, 1996.
7. McGoldrick MD: Acute renal failure following trauma. In *Anesthesiology,* Philadelphia, 1989, JB Lippincott.
8. *Textbook of medical physiology,* ed 7, Philadelphia, 1986, WB Saunders.
9. David WS: Myoglobinuria, *Neurol Clin* 18:215, 2000.
10. Visweswaran P, Guntupalli J: Environmental emergencies: rhabdomyolysis, *Crit Care Clin* 15:415, 1999.
11. Hemer R: When exercise goes awry: exertional rhabdomyolysis, *South Med J* 90:548, 1997.
12. Lopez JR et al: Myoplasmic calcium concentration during exertional rhabdomyolysis, *Lancet* 345:424, 1995.
13. Reddy MK et al: Removal of Z-lines and actinin from isolated myofibrils by a calcium activated neutral protease, *J Biol Chem* 250:4278, 1975.
14. Gans L, Kennedy T: Management of unique clinical entities in disaster medicine, *Emerg Med Clin North Am* 14:312, 1996.
15. Slater MS, Mullins RJ: Rhabdomyolysis and myoglobinuric renal failure in trauma and surgical patients: a review, *J Am Coll Surg* 186:693, 1998.
16. Vanholder R et al: Rhabdomyolysis, *J Am Soc Nephrol* 11(8), 2000.
17. Holt S, Moore K: Pathogenesis of renal failure in rhabdomyolysis: the role of myoglobin, *Exp Nephrol* 8:72, 2000.
18. Bywaters EGL, Stead JK: The production of renal failure following injection of solutions containing myohemoglobin, *Q J Exp Physiol* 33:53, 1944.
19. Braun SR et al: Evaluation of the renal toxicity of heme proteins and their derivatives: a role in the genesis of acute tubule necrosis, *J Exp Med* 131:443, 1970.
20. Edlich RF, Edgerton MT, McLaughlin RE: Compartment syndrome. In *Current emergency therapy,* Rockville, Md, 1985, Aspen.
21. Heppenstall RB et al: The compartment syndrome: an experimental and clinical study of muscular energy metabolism using phosphorus nuclear magnetic resonance spectroscopy, *Clin Orthop* 226:138, 1988.
22. Lofberg M et al: Metabolic causes of recurrent rhabdomyolysis, *Acta Neurol Scand* 98:268, 1998.
23. Tonin P et al: Metabolic causes of myoglobinuria, *Ann Neurol* 27:181, 1990.
24. Collins AJ: Renal dialysis treatment for victims of the Armenian earthquake, *N Engl J Med* 320:1291, 1989.
25. Sheng ZY: Medical support in the Tangshan earthquake: a review of the management of mass casualties and certain major injuries, *J Trauma* 27:1130, 1987.
26. Shimazu T et al: Fluid resuscitation and systemic complications in crush syndrome: 14 Hanshin-Awaji earthquake patients, *J Trauma* 42:641, 1997.
27. Poels PJE, Gabreels FJM: Rhabdomyolysis: a review of the literature, *Clin Neurol Neurosurg* 95:175, 1993.
28. Rubinstein I et al: Involvement of nitric oxide in experimental muscle crush injury, *J Clin Invest* 101:1325, 1998.
29. Knottenbelt JD: Traumatic rhabdomyolysis from severe beating—experience of volume diuresis in 200 patients, *J Trauma* 37:214, 1994.
30. Bildsten SA et al: The risk of rhabdomyolysis and acute renal failure with the patient in the exaggerated lithotomy position, *J Urol* 152:1970, 1994.
31. Sinert R et al: Exercised-induced rhabdomyolysis, *Ann Emerg Med* 23:1301, 1994.
32. Teitjen DP, Guzzi LM: Exertional rhabdomyolysis and acute renal failure following the Army Physical Fitness Test, *Mil Med* 154:23, 1989.
33. Knochel JP: Catastrophic medical events with exhaustive exercise: "white collar rhabdomyolysis," *Kidney Int* 38:700, 1990.
34. Zager RA, Aultschuld R: Body temperature: an important determinant of severity of ischemic renal injury, *Am J Physiol* 251:F87, 1986.
35. Line RL, Rust GS: Acute exertional rhabdomyolysis, *Am Fam Physician* 52:502, 1995.
36. Sato T et al: Recurrent reversible rhabdomyolysis associated with hyperthermia and status epilepticus, *Acta Paediatr* 84:1083, 1995.
37. Manji H et al: Status dystonicus: the syndrome and its management, *Brain* 121:243, 1998.
38. Jankovic J: Myoglobinuric renal failure in Huntington's chorea, *Neurology* 36:138, 1986.
39. Slater MS, Mullins RJ: Rhabdomyolysis and myoglobinuric renal failure in trauma and surgical patients: a review, *J Am Coll Surg* 186:693, 1998.
40. Brumback RA, Feeback DL, Leech RW: Rhabdomyolysis following electrical injury, *Semin Neurol* 15:329, 1995.
41. Abraham B et al: Malignant hyperthermia susceptibility: anaesthetic implications and risk stratification, *Q J Med* 90:13, 1997.
42. Winston T et al: Rhabdomyolysis and myoglobinuric acute renal failure associated with classic heat stroke, *South Med J* 88:1065, 1995.
43. Levenson JL: Neuroleptic malignant syndrome, *N Engl J Med* 313:163, 1985.
44. *Harrison's principles of internal medicine,* ed 11, New York, 1987, McGraw-Hill.
45. Singhal PC et al: Rhabdomyolysis and acute renal failure associated with cocaine abuse, *Clin Toxicol* 28:321, 1990.
46. Welch RD, Todd K, Krause GS: Incidence of cocaine-associated rhabdomyolysis, *Ann Emerg Med* 20:154, 1991.
47. Roth D et al: Acute rhabdomyolysis associated with cocaine intoxication, *N Engl J Med* 319:673, 1988.
48. Counselman FL et al: Creatine phosphokinase elevation in patients presenting to the emergency department with cocaine-related complaints, *Am J Emerg Med* 15:221, 1997.
49. Henry JA, Jeffreys KJ, Dawling S: Toxicity and deaths from 3,4-methylenedioxymethamphetamine (ecstasy), *Lancet* 2:384, 1992.
50. Richards JR et al: Methamphetamine abuse and rhabdomyolysis in the ED: a 5-year study, *Am J Emerg Med* 17:681, 1999.
51. Pierce LR, Wysowski DK, Gross TP: Myopathy and rhabdomyolysis associated with lovastatin-gemfibrozil combination therapy, *JAMA* 264:71, 1990.
52. Hino I et al: Pravastatin-induced rhabdomyolysis in a patient with mixed connective tissue disease, *Arthritis Rheum* 39:1259, 1996.
53. Biesenbach G et al: Myoglobinuric renal failure due to long-standing lovastatin therapy in a patient with pre-existing chronic renal insufficiency, *Nephrol Dial Transplant* 11:2059, 1996.
54. Duell PB, Connor WE, Illingworth DR: Rhabdomyolysis after taking atorvastatin with gemfibrozil, *Am J Cardiol* 81:368, 1998.
55. Tal A, Rajeshawari M, Isley W: Rhabdomyolysis associated with simvastatin-gemfibrozil therapy, *South Med J* 90:546, 1997.
56. Florkowski CM et al: Rhabdomyolysis and acute renal failure following carbon monoxide poisoning: two case reports with muscle histopathology and enzyme activities, *Clin Toxicol* 30:443, 1992.
57. Shapiro AB et al: Carbon monoxide and myonecrosis: a prospective study, *Vet Hum Toxicol* 31:136, 1989.
58. Kolecki P: Delayed toxic reaction following massive bee envenomation, *Ann Emerg Med* 33:114, 1999.
59. Hiran S et al: Rhabdomyolysis due to multiple honey bee stings, *Postgrad Med J* 70:937, 1994.
60. Friedman BI, Libby R: Epstein-Barr virus infection associated with rhabdomyolysis and acute renal failure, *Clin Pediatr* 25:228, 1986.
61. Goebel J et al: Acute renal failure from rhabdomyolysis following influenza A in a child, *Clin Pediatr* 36:479, 1997.

62. Singh U, Scheld WM: Infectious etiologies of rhabdomyolysis: three case reports and review, *Clin Infect Dis* 22:642, 1996.
63. Kagan H et al: Formation of ion permeable channels by tumor necrosis factor-alpha, *Science* 255:1427, 1995.
64. Chariot P et al: Acute rhabdomyolysis in patients infected by human immunodeficiency virus, *Neurology* 44:1692, 1994.
65. Del Rio C et al: Acute human immunodeficiency virus infection temporally associated with rhabdomyolysis, acute renal failure and nephrosis, *Rev Infect Dis* 12:282, 1990.
66. Byrd RP Jr, Roy TM: Rhabdomyolysis and bacterial pneumonia, *Respir Med* 92:359, 1998.
67. Malvy D et al: Legionnaire's disease and rhabdomyolysis, *Intensive Care Med* 18:132, 1992.
68. Abdulla AJ, Moorehead JF, Sweeny P: Acute tubular necrosis due to rhabdomyolysis and pancreatitis associated with *Salmonella enteritidis* food poisoning, *Nephrol Dial Transplant* 8:672, 1993.
69. Korzets A et al: Severe hyponatremia after water intoxication: a potential cause of rhabdomyolysis, *Am J Med Sci* 312:92, 1996.
70. Devereuz S, Knowles SM: Rhabdomyolysis and acute renal failure in sickle cell anemia, *BMJ* 290:1707, 1985.
71. Gabow PA, Kaehny WD, Kellener SP: The spectrum of rhabdomyolysis, *Medicine* 61:141, 1982.
72. Kunkel JM: Thigh and leg compartment syndrome in the absence of lower extremity trauma following MAST application, *Am J Emerg Med* 5:2, 1987.
73. Loun B et al: Adaptation of a quantitative immunoassay for urine myoglobin: predictor in detecting renal dysfunction, *Clin Chem* 105:479, 1996.
74. Ward MM: Factors predictive of acute renal failure in rhabdomyolysis, *Arch Intern Med* 148:1553, 1988.
75. Brody SL et al: Predicting the severity of cocaine-associated rhabdomyolysis, *Ann Emerg Med* 19:1137, 1990.
76. Oster JR et al: Metabolic acidosis with extreme elevation of anion gap: case report and literature review, *Am J Med Sci* 317:38, 1999.
77. Bank WJ et al: A disorder of muscle lipid metabolism and myoglobinuria: absence of carnitine palmityl transferase, *N Engl J Med* 292:443, 1975.
78. Michaelson M et al: Crush syndrome: experience from the Lebanon war, 1982, *Isr J Med Sci* 20:305, 1984.
79. Pretto EA et al: An analysis of prehospital mortality in an earthquake, *Prehosp Disaster Med* 9:260, 1994.
80. Odeh M: The role of reperfusion-induced injury in the pathogenesis of the crush syndrome, *N Engl J Med* 324:1417, 1991.
81. Paller MS: Hemoglobin and myoglobin-induced renal failure in rats: role of iron in nephrotoxicity, *Am J Physiol* 255:F539, 1988.
82. Owen CA et al: Intramuscular pressure with limb compression: clarification of the pathogenesis of the drug-induced compartment syndrome/crush syndrome, *N Engl J Med* 5:2, 1987.

122 Selected Endocrine Disorders

John M. Wogan

The three conditions described in this chapter—hyperthyroidism, hypothyroidism, and adrenal insufficiency—are similar in several respects. They advance in a slow, insidious fashion, expressing nonspecific signs and symptoms over months to years, and then are acutely precipitated by intercurrent stress. Each is relatively uncommon. EPs may not have the clinical experience to facilitate ready diagnosis. The characteristic symptom complexes are subtle and may be difficult to recognize, especially in their early stages. All three conditions are potentially lethal if untreated, and in their extreme manifestations, these endocrine disorders may constitute medical emergencies. No confirmatory laboratory studies are immediately available. Therefore it is often necessary to initiate treatment on the basis of clinical judgment alone.

HYPERTHYROIDISM

Perspective

Historical Background Although Parry recognized the association of exophthalmos, goiter, and cardiovascular hyperactivity as early as 1786, Graves and von Basedow are commonly credited with the initial descriptions (in 1835 and 1840) of the diseases that bear their names.[1] Trosseau accidentally administered tincture of iodine rather than tincture of digitalis to a hyperthyroid patient and astutely recognized its therapeutic value.[2] The usefulness of sympathetic blockade was initially demonstrated when postoperative thyrotoxic patients were successfully treated with procaine spinal anesthesia.[3] Canary and Ramey demonstrated the efficacy of peripheral pharmacologic adrenergic block.[4,5]

The terms *hyperthyroidism, thyrotoxicosis, thyrotoxic crisis,* and *thyroid storm* do not have precise, consensual definitions. They refer to the continuum of disease that results from thyroid hyperfunction. Hyperthyroidism and thyrotoxicosis are designations for the milder forms of disease. Thyroid storm and thyrotoxic crisis refer to the heightened and life-threatening manifestations of thyroid hyperactivity, including high fever and cardiovascular, neurologic, and gastrointestinal dysfunction.[6-8]

Whereas hyperthyroidism is common, true thyroid storm is rare. From 1% to 2% of patients with hyperthyroidism may progress to thyroid storm, which usually supervenes on a long history of uncomplicated hyperthyroidism.[6-8] Six to 8 months of symptoms are usual, and hyperthyroidism may have been present for as long as 2½ to 5 years.[8-11]

A number of stresses may precipitate thyroid storm (Box 122-1). The transition from simple thyrotoxicosis to thyroid storm may be abrupt, coincident with the acute precipitant.[9]

Etiology Hyperthyroidism and thyrotoxicosis have many causes (Box 122-2). Most cases of thyroid storm are secondary to *toxic diffuse goiter* (*Graves' disease*) and therefore, as with the underlying disease, occur in women in their third and fourth decades of life. *Toxic multinodular goiter* may produce thyroid storm, usually in women in their

Box 122-1 Precipitants of Thyroid Storm

Medical	Drug Related
Infection	^{131}Iodine therapy
Vascular accidents	Premature withdrawal of antithyroid therapy
Pulmonary embolism	Ingestion of thyroid hormone
Visceral infarction	Contrast radiographic studies
Surgery	Drug reaction (thioridazine hydrochloride [Mellaril], iothiouracil [Itrumil])
Burns	
Trauma	
Emotional stress	
Endocrine	
Hypoglycemia	
Diabetic ketoacidosis	
Hyperosmolar nonketotic coma	

Box 122-2 Etiologic Factors of Thyrotoxicosis

Toxic diffuse goiter (Graves' disease)
Toxic multinodular goiter
Toxic uninodular goiter
Factitious thyrotoxicosis
T_3 toxicosis
Thyrotoxicosis associated with thyroiditis
  Hashimoto's thyroiditis
  Subacute (de Quervain's) thyroiditis
Graves' or Basedow's disease
Metastatic follicular carcinoma
Malignancies with circulating thyroid stimulators
TSH-producing pituitary tumors
Struma ovarii with hyperthyroidism
Hypothalamic hyperthyroidism

T_3, Triiodothyronine; *TSH*, thyroid-stimulating hormone.

fourth through seventh decades. Thyroid storm from *toxic uninodular goiter* is uncommon and less severe.

Factitious hyperthyroidism results from an exogenous source of thyroid hormone and may be difficult to diagnose.[12,13] It occurs most often in the settings of acute intoxication or fad dieting; full-blown thyroid storm in this setting is rare.[14]

Amiodarone, an iodine-rich antidysrhythmic indicated for the treatment of ventricular and supraventricular dysrhythmias, has complex effects on thyroid physiology. Asymptomatic changes in thyroid hormone levels are common. Clinically relevant thyrotoxicosis has been reported in 1% to 24% of patients receiving amiodarone.[15]

Hyperthyroidism secondary to *thyroiditis,* either Hashimoto's or subacute, rarely causes thyroid storm, and is usually but not always mild.[13] Other causes of hyperthyroidism (see Box 122-2) are even less likely to cause thyroid storm.

Principles of Disease

The pathophysiologic mechanisms underlying both thyrotoxicosis and the shift from uncomplicated hyperthyroidism to thyroid storm are not entirely clear. Many of the signs and symptoms are those of adrenergic hyperactivity.[16] However, neither catecholamine sensitivity nor serum catecholamine levels appear to be elevated. The concept of catecholamine hyperfunction is useful, however, and adrenergic blockade forms the cornerstone of therapy.

Thyroid hormone has direct inotropic and chronotropic effects on the heart, but these effects do not explain the clinical spectrum of thyroid storm.[17] In addition, thyroid levels are not necessarily acutely elevated when the transition from uncomplicated thyrotoxicosis to thyroid storm occurs.[6] Thyroid storm probably reflects the addition of adrenergic hyperactivity, induced by a nonspecific stress, into the setting of untreated or undertreated hyperthyroidism.[18]

Clinical Features

"Signal" symptoms of hyperthyroidism include agitation, nervousness, palpitations, and weight loss. Typical signs are fever, tachycardia, ophthalmopathy, goiter, and heart failure. Women in their fourth through sixth decades are at greatest risk.

A wide variety of laboratory studies of thyroid function are available, but only a few are typically necessary to corroborate the diagnosis. The free thyroxine assay and the free thyroxine index are especially useful.

Treatment depends on the severity of thyroid hyperactivity and end-organ dysfunction. Toxic patients require emergency intervention with a β-blocker, a thioamide, iodine, and dexamethasone, as well as good supportive therapy.

The manifestations of thyroid storm are protean. Fever is common, as are cardiovascular and neurologic sequelae. In patients with Graves' disease, exophthalmos and goiter may be signal findings.

Lahey[19,20] recognized that two distinct clinical presentations are possible with thyroid hyperactivity. He designated these syndromes as "activated thyroidism" and "unactivated thyroidism." The distinction proved clinically useful, and Lahey's syndromes are currently referred to as hyperthyroidism and apathetic hyperthyroidism, respectively. Hyperthyroidism occurs in younger patients, and its signs and symptoms, typically with multiple organ involvement, probably reflect the end-organ responsiveness to thyroid hormone in this group. Apathetic hyperthyroidism occurs in older patients in whom end-organ responsiveness is attenuated compared with younger patients, and in whom the clinical picture is dominated by depressed mental function and cardiac complications.

Signs and symptoms of hyperthyroidism may be distinctive (Box 122-3). Weight loss is common and may be dramatic.[6,8,11] For this reason, thyroid hormone is inappropriately prescribed as part of many fad diets. Between one fourth and one half of patients coming to the ED in thyroid storm report a weight loss of more than 40 pounds.[8,11]

Fever is often present in thyroid storm, may be quite high, and may herald the onset of thyrotoxic crisis in previously uncomplicated disease.[11] Heat intolerance is common and reflects the underlying hypermetabolic state.

Cardiovascular manifestations of thyrotoxicosis are dramatic and characterized by a hyperdynamic, electrically excitable state. Common symptoms include palpitations, dyspnea, and chest pain.[2,9,11] Enhanced contractility produces elevations in systolic blood pressure and the pulse pressure, leading to a dicrotic or water-hammer pulse.[2] Unless there is

Box 122-3 Signs and Symptoms of Thyrotoxicosis

Symptoms

Common

Weight loss (20 to 40+ lb)
Palpitations
Nervousness
Tremor

Less common

Chest pain
Dyspnea
Edema
Psychosis
Disorientation
Diarrhea/hyperdefecation
Abdominal pain

Signs

Common

Fever
Tachycardia (100 to 170+ beats/min)
Wide pulse pressure (40 to 100 mm Hg)
Congestive heart failure
Thyromegaly
Tremor
Hyperhidrosis
Thyrotoxic stare/lid retraction

Less common

Weakness
Shock
Psychosis
Somnolence/obtundation/coma
Infiltrative ophthalmopathy
Jaundice
Tender liver
Pretibial myxedema

underlying hypertensive heart disease, the diastolic pressure is usually not elevated.[21] A systolic flow murmur is often present, which resolves with treatment of the thyrotoxicosis.[2,22] Either sinus tachycardia or less often atrial tachydysrhythmia is usually present.[11,21] Sinus tachycardia is seen independent of congestive heart failure (CHF) and out of proportion to fever.[10] Hyperthyroid atrial fibrillation may occur either with or without underlying heart disease, is typically refractory to digitalis therapy, and reverts in 20% to 50% of cases after antithyroid therapy.[10,21,23] Atrial premature contractions and atrial flutter may also occur in thyrotoxicosis.[21]

For many years the existence of "thyrocardiac" disease (i.e., CHF caused by thyrotoxicosis without any concomitant heart lesion) was controversial. Most sources now agree that thyrocardiac heart failure is a real phenomenon.[10,24] Thyrocardiac disease may be accompanied by an increased sympathetic tone; it occurs primarily in elderly patients and can usually be treated by digitalis, possibly in combination with β-blocker therapy (although β-blockers can exacerbate preexisting heart failure in rare cases); it is ameliorated by antithyroid treatment.[24,25]

When hyperthyroidism results from Graves' disease, ophthalmopathy may be seen. Indeed, eye findings may be valuable clues to the existence of underlying thyroid disease. The severity of ophthalmopathy does not necessarily parallel the magnitude of thyroid dysfunction but reflects the responsible autoimmune process.[26] The manifestations of ophthalmopathy include upper-lid retraction, staring, lid lag (Graefe's sign), exophthalmos, and extraocular muscle palsies.[1,27,28]

Behavior is characterized by agitation, anxiety, and restlessness. Wide mood swings are typical. Fear and even frank paranoia occur. Careless examination might lead to incorrect ED triage to psychiatric evaluation rather than appreciation of the medical nature of the disease. In more severe cases, agitation may lead to seizures and even coma.

Proximal myopathy is common, particularly in elderly patients. Dyspnea with minimal exertion secondary to respiratory muscle weakness has been demonstrated.[29] β-Blockers have been used with questionable success to treat myopathy.[30] Other neuromuscular abnormalities, including bulbar palsy, myasthenia gravis, periodic paralysis, and flaccid quadriplegia, have been reported to be associated (although rarely) with thyrotoxicosis.[12,31,32]

A number of nonspecific gastrointestinal disturbances are possible. Hyperphagia, diarrhea, nausea, vomiting, and abdominal pain have all been noted but are not usually signal symptoms of the disease. Hepatic dysfunction, either with or without CHF, is possible.[6,9,33] When jaundice occurs as a primary hepatic sign, it is primarily unconjugated, mild, and probably from the unmasking of occult liver disease (e.g., Gilbert's disease). Treatment of the thyrotoxicosis is sufficient to resolve jaundice.[33]

With respect to dermatologic manifestations, the thyrotoxic patient is typically flushed with warm, moist skin; hair is fine and straight; and 60% to 97% of patients with underlying Graves' disease will have an appreciable goiter.[34,35] Hyperpigmentation, vitiligo, or alopecia may occur, especially when an autoimmune mechanism is responsible for the disease. Pretibial myxedema may be present in 5% of cases.

Diagnostic Strategies

The clinical suggestion of thyrotoxicosis must be confirmed by laboratory studies. Pituitary and hypothalamic causes of hyperthyroidism are unusual. Primary thyroid glandular hyperfunction is the rule, and serum levels of various thyroidal hormones reflect this fact. Thyroxine (T_4) and triiodothyronine (T_3) levels are elevated, whereas the thyrotropin (thyroid-stimulating hormone [TSH]) level is depressed. Various measures are used to assess each of these hormones.

Total serum T_4 comprises a component bound to circulating plasma proteins, primarily *thyroxine-binding globulin* (TBG), and a portion that circulates freely. The latter is referred to as *free T_4* (FT_4) and is the metabolically active form of T_4. Abnormalities in TBG levels can affect assays of total T_4 and T_3. The thyroid gland will attempt to maintain appropriate physiologic levels of free hormone regardless of the amount of bound hormone. High or low TBG levels result in high or low levels of bound thyroid hormone, respectively. Assays of total T_4 or T_3 may thus appear to be abnormal, despite normal FT_4 levels and a clinically euthyroid state because of abnormalities in TBG (Box 122-4).

Serum levels of both total circulating T_4 and FT_4 are available. In an analogous fashion, total circulating T_3 and *free T_3* (FT_3) may also be measured. Typically, T_4, FT_4, T_3, and FT_3 levels are measured with radioimmunoassay (RIA) techniques.

In the *T_3 resin uptake* (T_3RU) test, radiolabeled T_3 is passed over a resin column to which thyroid hormone may bind and over which the patient's serum has already been passed. The resin uptake of the radiolabeled T_3 will be inversely proportional to the amount of thyroid hormone in the patient's serum. Because only free thyroid hormone is available to bind to the resin column, changes in TBG levels will lead to directly proportional changes in the T_3RU

Box 122-4 Factors that Affect Thyroid-Binding Globulin (TBG) Levels

Depression of TBG	Elevation of TBG
Androgen therapy	Estrogen therapy
Dilantin therapy	Pregnancy
Large doses of salicylates	Oral contraceptives
Nephrotic syndrome	Congenital elevation
Congenital depression	

test. The product of the total T_4 level and the T_3RU is the *free T_4 index* (FT_4I). The FT_4I is a good estimate of the serum free T_4 level.

TSH levels are typically low in primary hyperthyroidism and are usually of little assistance in the diagnosis of thyrotoxic crisis. TSH assays are valuable in distinguishing secondary and tertiary causes of hypothyroidism, as in the rare case of a TSH-producing tumor.

Newer serum TSH assays, unlike prior assays, are sensitive enough to discriminate the low-normal TSH level, sometimes seen in a euthyroid state, from the very low TSH level associated with primary hypothyroidism.[36] These sensitive TSH assays may be too expensive to be used as a routine screening study.

The best screening tests to identify hyperthyroidism are the T_4 RIA and the FT_4I.[36] Each has sensitivity and specificity of approximately 90%. If the T_4 level is normal but the patient has signs and symptoms of hyperthyroidism, a T_3 RIA level might be useful because of the well-described situation of T_3 toxicosis, in which only T_3 levels are high.[12,37] T_3 toxicosis may be seen in Graves' disease (particularly in iodine-deficient areas), toxic multinodular goiter, and autonomous adenoma and may herald early disease or the return of disease after surgical therapy.[37-40]

In summary, a good screen for hyperthyroidism is the T_4 RIA or the FT_4I. If these initial thyroxine assays do not confirm hyperthyroidism but clinical evidence is very strong, a T_3 RIA and a sensitive TSH assay should be ordered.

If a patient appears to be remarkably thyrotoxic and a more complete characterization of thyroid function is desired, a diagnostic panel including T_4 RIA, T_3 RIA, TSH, and TBG will be helpful. However, none of these studies is typically available on an immediate basis in the ED.

Electrolytes, glucose, calcium, bilirubin, hematocrit, and liver function tests should be checked in addition to thyroid function tests (TFTs). Laboratory abnormalities in thyroid storm are multiple, mild, and nonspecific.

Hyperglycemia is present in 30% to 55% of patients.[9] Possible explanations for hyperglycemia include insulin resistance, decreased insulin secretion, increased glycogenolysis, and rapid intestinal absorption of glucose.[11]

Hypercalcemia is fairly common, occurring in at least 10% of cases, and is usually mild and asymptomatic. A normocytic, normochromic anemia is common, as is leukocytosis. Either *hypernatremia* or *hyponatremia* is possible but is rarely abnormal enough to cause symptoms. Depressed cholesterol levels are often noted. Minimal elevations in liver function studies, even in the absence of CHF, are seen.[9,33]

Table 122-1. Comparison of Activated and Apathetic Thyrotoxicosis

Parameter	Activated	Apathetic
Age	4th decade	7th decade
Duration of symptoms	8 mo	26 mo
Weight loss	10 lb	40 lb
Thyroid weight	70 gm	45 gm
Eye findings	Frequent	Rare
Congestive heart failure	Common	Common
Atrial fibrillation	One third	Three fourths
Depression/apathy	Uncommon	Common

Differential Considerations

The differential diagnosis is crucial because a number of serious illnesses, including other endocrine diseases, can show similar symptoms. Differential possibilities include sepsis and intoxication with anticholinergic and adrenergic agents, notably cocaine and amphetamines. *Hypoglycemia* and several withdrawal syndromes (e.g., from ethanol, narcotics, and sedative-hypnotics) may produce a picture of adrenergic hyperfunction with altered mental status, which might be mistaken for hyperthyroidism. *Heat stroke,* with its characteristic hyperpyrexia and disturbed sensorium, might appear similar to thyrotoxicosis but is usually distinguished by its clinical setting. Patients with psychiatric illness may show signs similar to thyroid hyperactivity. Other endocrine abnormalities, especially hypothyroidism, may mimic some of the symptoms of apathetic hyperthyroidism.

Apathetic Hyperthyroidism In 1931, Lahey[20] called attention to a second form of thyrotoxicosis, "nonactivated" or "apathetic" thyroidism. Signs and symptoms of this condition are few and subtle, and the initial appearance of disease may be single organ failure (e.g., CHF), producing diagnostic confusion by pointing to diagnoses other than thyrotoxicosis.[41]

The cause of apathetic hyperthyroidism is usually multinodular goiter rather than Graves' disease, and the patients are therefore typically older (in their seventh or eighth decades), have small multinodular or nonpalpable goiters, and lack autoimmune ophthalmopathy.[42,43] Cardiovascular symptoms, especially CHF and atrial fibrillation, are prominent, as might be expected from the advanced age of patients. Weight loss is significant, averaging 40 pounds in one study.[43] Depressed mental function, ranging from a placid demeanor to frank coma, is common but may alternate with tremor and hyperactivity. Apathetic thyrotoxicosis usually occurs in elderly patients but has been reported in most age groups, including children[42,44] (Table 122-1).

Management

Mild hyperthyroidism does not require emergency therapy, and the hyperthyroid patient may be referred to an outpatient setting for further evaluation. Thyroid storm, on the other hand, requires immediate therapy. Treatment has five

Box 122-5 Treatment of Thyroid Storm

1. If the diagnosis of thyroid storm is highly likely (on the basis of clinical criteria) and the patient is toxic, immediate therapy, as below, is indicated. If immediate therapy is not needed, draw diagnostic studies and refer for further evaluation.
2. Block synthesis: PTU 150 mg PO/NG q6hr
   Block release: SSKI 3-5 drops PO/NG q8hr
   Block peripheral effects:
   T_4 conversion: Dexamethasone 2 mg PO/NG q6hr
   β-Blockade: Propranolol 1-2 mg IV q15min prn
   Supportive care: Treat fever with Tylenol
   Treat heart failure with digitalis and diuretics
   Identify and treat precipitating factors
   Rehydrate
   Hydrocortisone 100 mg IV q8hr

PTU, Propylthiouracil; *SSKI,* potassium iodide; *PO,* orally; *NG,* by nasogastric tube; *IV,* intravenously.

goals: (1) inhibit hormone synthesis, (2) block hormone release, (3) prevent peripheral conversion of T_4 to T_3, (4) block the peripheral effects of thyroid hormone, and (5) provide general support (Box 122-5).

Inhibition of Hormone Synthesis Thioamides, including *propylthiouracil* (PTU) and *methimazole,* inhibit thyroidal peroxidase, thereby preventing hormone synthesis. PTU is generally preferred over methimazole because it has the additional minor effect of inhibiting peripheral conversion of T_4 to T_3. PTU is given in an initial dose of 600 to 1000 mg by mouth (PO) or by nasogastric (NG) tube, followed by 200 to 250 mg every 4 to 6 hours. Further organification of iodine will be blocked within 1 hour of PTU administration, but the drug should be continued for several weeks while the hyperthyroidism is brought under control.

Blockage of Hormone Release Because preformed T_4 and T_3 are stored in the thyroid colloid, release of hormone can occur for weeks despite synthesis inhibition. Thus prevention of colloid hormone release is the second goal of therapy. Both iodine and lithium can inhibit thyroid hormone release. Lithium is not generally used because it can be difficult to titrate the dose, and toxic effects are common. Thioamides should be given at least 1 hour before iodine therapy to prevent organification of the iodine. *Lugol's iodine solution,* 30 drops per day in 3 to 4 divided doses PO or by NG tube; *potassium iodide* (SSKI), 5 drops every 6 hours PO or by NG tube; or *sodium iodide,* 1 g slow intravenous (IV) drip every 8 to 12 hours, is acceptable.

Prevention of Peripheral Hormone Conversion The peripheral conversion of T_4 to T_3, which is responsible for perhaps 85% of T_3 present in the circulation, may be blocked by PTU, propranolol, or dexamethasone.[45,46] For PTU and propranolol, this effect is probably not quantitatively significant. *Dexamethasone,* however, is effective through this mechanism and should be given as 2 mg intravenously (IV) every 6 hours.[47] If hydrocortisone is given, dexamethasone is probably unnecessary.

Peripheral Adrenergic Blockade Blockade of the peripheral adrenergic hyperactivity of thyroid crisis may be the most important factor in reducing morbidity and mortality. Initial attempts at blockade were surgical.[3] β-Blockade is currently the method of choice for staunching the peripheral manifestations of thyroid storm. *Propranolol* can reduce dysrhythmias, hyperpyrexia, tremor, palpitations, restlessness, anxiety, and perhaps myopathy.[48,49] Propranolol is effective IV in slow 1-mg to 2-mg boluses, which may be repeated every 10 to 15 minutes until the desired effect is achieved.[50] Effective oral propranolol therapy usually begins at 20 to 120 mg/dose or 160 to 320 mg/day in divided doses.[51,52]

The contraindications to β-blockade (reactive airway disease, diabetes mellitus, CHF, pregnancy) are the same as for other medical conditions. High-output CHF and heart failure associated with tachydysrhythmias may respond to β-blocker therapy. In rare cases, β-blockers have been associated with worsening of CHF, usually in patients with preexisting, nonthyroid cardiac disease. Therefore the clinical response to these agents should be monitored carefully. The complicated patient with both a tachydysrhythmia and CHF might be managed with a judicious combination of β-blockade and digitalis.

Supportive Care Supportive care addresses several areas. First, hyperpyrexia should be treated aggressively with acetaminophen. Aspirin should not be used because it displaces thyroid hormone from thyroglobulin, thus theoretically increasing the pool of metabolically active hormone. Ice packs and hypothermia blankets may also be used.

Second, CHF should be managed with digitalis, diuretics, and oxygen. Third, dehydration is a common complication of fever, diarrhea, and vomiting and requires appropriate fluid replacement.

Corticosteroids are uniformly used (in stress dosages of 300 mg/day of hydrocortisone equivalent administered IV) but with little scientific justification.

Vigorous attempts should be made to identify and treat factors that might have precipitated thyroid storm. Precipitants are usually of a medical rather than a surgical nature[11,18,41] (see Box 122-1). In about 50% of cases, no acute precipitant will be identified.[9]

With appropriate therapy, fever, tachycardias, tremor, and altered sensorium should all show improvement in the first 12 to 24 hours. Indeed, sinus tachycardia should respond within minutes of IV propranolol injection. CHF may not revert for weeks. Neuromuscular manifestations resolve slowly over weeks to months.

HYPOTHYROIDISM

Perspective

Historical Background As early as the fourth century AD, a condition resembling myxedema was reportedly treated with ground sheep thyroid.[53] Paracelsus, in the sixteenth century, and Platter, in the early seventeenth century, called attention to the association of cretinism and endemic goiter.[1] Curling[54] described two cretins with absent thyroids. In 1874, Gull[55] recognized a syndrome that resembled childhood cretinism in adult women. Ord[56] described five more cases in 1879. He was struck by the nonpitting, gelatinous nature of the generalized edema and coined the term *myxedema.* He also correlated the thyroid atrophy found at autopsy with the clinical state of myxedema. Murray[57] described an effective treatment of myxedema in 1891 using ground sheep thyroid extract.

Epidemiology Hypothyroidism, as with hyperthyroidism, has a broad spectrum of clinical findings. It includes subclinical presentations (detectable only by an elevated TSH level) and full-blown myxedema coma, characterized by hypothermia, mental obtundation, and myxedema.[58]

Hypothyroidism occurs 3 to 10 times more often in women than in men.[59-61] This fact reflects the increased prevalence of autoimmune thyroid disease in women. The peak incidence is in the seventh decade; however, hypothyroidism can occur at any age.[61,62] About 50% of cases of myxedema become evident after admission to a hospital.[63]

Because hypothyroidism deprives the body of calorigenic ability, patients are unable to deal with low ambient temperatures. Consequently, most cases of hypothyroidism become manifest during the winter months.[61,64]

Principles of Disease

Thyroid failure may occur from disease of the thyroid (primary hypothyroidism), pituitary (secondary), or hypothalamus (tertiary). Secondary failure accounts for 4% or fewer of cases.[63] Tertiary failure is even less common. The two major causes of primary hypothyroidism are autoimmune destruction of the gland and iatrogenic failure after surgical or other ablation of the gland[59,60] (Box 122-6).

The many complex effects of iodine-rich amiodarone on thyroid physiology may lead to asymptomatic abnormalities of thyroid hormone levels, including an elevated TSH, as well as clinically relevant hypofunction of the thyroid gland. Hypothyroidism has been estimated to occur in 1% to 32% of patients taking amiodarone.[15]

Clinical Features

As in many other endocrine conditions, hypothyroidism usually follows an indolent course. A 4-year delay may occur between the appearance of symptoms and diagnosis.[59] Many hypothyroid patients consult more than one physician before their disease is discovered. Patients with mild hypothyroidism may develop dramatic clinical presentations, even myxedema coma when physiologically stressed by one of several factors (Box 122-7). Precipitating factors other than exposure to cold can be identified in less than one half of patients. In one study, fewer than 10% of patients had not been exposed to cold.[62] Infection is difficult to identify. Signs and symptoms, such as fever, tachycardia, sweating, and leukocytosis, may not develop in hypothyroid patients.[41] Prognosis and extent of intervention are determined by the severity of hypothyroidism.

As with hyperthyroidism, the diagnosis of hypothyroidism should be sought when signal symptoms and signs are present, especially in a high-risk demographic group. Typical symptoms include fatigue, cold intolerance, and paresthesias. Suggestive signs are pseudomyotonic deep tendon reflexes, hypothermia, dry skin, and depressed mental function. Elderly women are at high risk.

Box 122-6 Etiologic Factors of Hypothyroidism

Primary

Autoimmune hypothyroidism
Idiopathic
Postsurgical thyroidectomy
External radiation therapy
Radioiodine therapy
Inherited enzymatic defect
Iodine deficiency
Antithyroid drugs
Lithium, phenylbutazone

Secondary

Pituitary tumor
Infiltrative disease (sarcoid) of pituitary

Box 122-7 Precipitants of Myxedema Coma

Exposure to cold
Infection (usually pulmonary)
Congestive heart failure
Trauma
Drugs: phenothiazines, phenobarbital, narcotics, anesthetics, benzodiazepines, lithium
Iodides
Cerebrovascular accident
Hemorrhage (especially gastrointestinal)
Hypoxia
Hypercapnia
Hyponatremia
Hypoglycemia

The signs and symptoms of hypothyroidism have varying frequencies (Table 122-2). It is often difficult to distinguish, solely on clinical grounds, primary disease from secondary disease[65] (Box 122-8). Definitive discrimination of primary failure from secondary failure is based on laboratory parameters.

The significant life threats that accompany profound hypothyroidism are respiratory insufficiency, hypotension, and coma. These elements are more characteristic of myxedema coma in its dramatic extreme than of simple hypothyroidism, but they are described first because they pose the greatest danger to the patient.

Myxedema coma is a poorly defined but readily recognizable syndrome that represents hypothyroidism in its dramatic extreme. It is coma that results from either hypothyroidism or one of the causes or complications of hypothyroidism (Box 122-9).[59,62,63,66,67] The readily treatable conditions should be considered before attributing coma solely to hypothyroidism.

Hypothyroid coma is rare and not well understood.[41] In one series, it occurred in only 0.1% of all patients with hypothyroidism. It is extremely rare in the under-50 age

Table 122-2. Prevalence of Clinical Features of Hypothyroidism

Clinical feature	Frequency (%)
Symptoms	
Paresthesias	92
Loss of energy	79
Intolerance to cold	51
Muscular weakness	34
Muscle and joint pain	31
Inability to concentrate	31
Drowsiness	30
Constipation	27
Forgetfulness	23
Emotional lability	15
Depressed auditory acuity	15
Headaches	14
Dysarthria	14
Blurred vision	8
Fullness in throat	81
Signs	
Pseudomyotonic reflexes	95
Change in menstrual pattern	86
Hypothermia	80
Dry scaly skin	79
Puffy eyelids	70
Hoarse voice	56
Weight gain	41
Dependent edema	30
Sparse axillary and pubic hair	30
Pallor	24
Thinness of eyebrows	24
Yellow skin	23
Loss of scalp hair	18
Abdominal distention	18
Goiter	16
Decreased sweating	10
Weight loss	6
Unsteady gait	5

From Bloomer H, Kyle LH: *Arch Intern Med* 104:234, 1959.

group. Behavioral disturbances varying from confusion to frank psychosis are usually present before coma supervenes. Milder degrees of hypothyroidism may be manifested by mental slowing, depression, dementia, or lethargy.

Drug-induced coma is particularly noteworthy. Metabolism of tranquilizers, sedatives, and anesthetics is reduced in hypothyroidism.[41] The effects of these agents are thus potentiated and prolonged. The often-cited case of myxedema coma that occurs after hospitalization or surgery is usually drug induced.

Cold intolerance is a complaint in about one half of patients.[59,62] Weight gain, seldom more than 15 pounds and usually 7 to 8 pounds, is usually not associated with increased appetite.[59] Nonspecific symptoms, including decreased energy, weakness, inability to concentrate, and poor memory, are common.[59,62] Constipation is reported in one fourth of patients.[59]

Hypothermia is present in approximately 80% of patients with myxedema.[62,63] Temperatures as low as 24° C (75.2° F) have been recorded in myxedema coma.[63] Loss of the calorigenic action of thyroid hormone may be exacerbated by the absence of shivering.[68] Hypothermia is so common in myxedema that a normal temperature, present in up to 25% of patients, should suggest an underlying infection. Hypother-

Box 122-8 Primary versus Secondary Hypothyroidism

Primary (Thyroid)

Previous thyroid surgery
Obese
Hypothermia more common
Increased serum cholesterol
Voice coarse
Pubic hair present
Sella turcica normal
Plasma cortisol normal
Skin dry and coarse
Heart increased in size
Normal menses and lactation
No response to TSH
Good response to levothyroxine without steroids
Serum TSH increased

Secondary (Pituitary)

No prior thyroid surgery
Less obese
Hypothermia less common
Normal serum cholesterol
Voice less coarse
Pubic hair absent
Sella turcica may be increased in size
Plasma cortisol decreased
Skin fine and soft
Heart usually normal
Traumatic delivery, no lactation, amenorrhea
Good response to TSH
Poor response to levothyroxine without steroids
Serum TSH decreased

From Senior RM, et al: *JAMA* 217:61, 1971.
TSH, Thyroid-stimulating hormone.

Box 122-9 Causes and Complications in Myxedema Coma and Hypothyroidism

Hypothyroidism
Hypercapnic narcosis
Hypoxia
Hypothermia
Hypotension
Hypoglycemia
Hyponatremia
Sepsis
Drugs: sedatives, hypnotics, anesthetics, tranquilizers
Adrenal insufficiency

mia may contribute to abnormal mental function in myxedema coma. If used, mercury thermometers must be shaken down well so as not to elevate the patient's temperature falsely into the normal range. Automated hypothermia thermometers are preferable. Hypothyroid habitus, absence of shivering, and pseudomyotonic reflexes may help distinguish myxedematous from accidental hypothermia. Fewer than 15% of hypothyroid patients survive temperatures below 32.2° C (90° F).[69]

The primary pulmonary abnormality is depression in respiratory drives, both hypoxic and hypercapnic.[70,71] Hypoxia is correctable with hormone replacement, but hypercapnia is only partially correctable.[70-72] Carbon dioxide narcosis is a prime cause of altered sensorium in myxedema coma.[73] Pulmonary function studies reveal normal volumes and flow rates with disordered neuromuscular function.[74] Other respiratory problems include upper airway obstruction from glottic edema, vocal cord edema, and glossomegaly. Pleural effusions are demonstrable in one third of cases.[70-72]

The blood pressure may be elevated, normal, or low. Diastolic hypertension is described.[61] Of patients in full myxedema coma, 50% initially exhibit clinical shock, with systolic pressure less than 100 mm Hg, but another third may have a blood pressure greater than 120/80 mm Hg.[62] *Sinus bradycardia* is the most common dysrhythmia seen in myxedema. Patients receiving thyroid replacement therapy are sensitive to catecholamines, but ventricular tachycardia is an extremely rare complication of replacement therapy.[73] In myxedema the capillaries are "leaky."[75] Transudation produces pleural and pericardial effusions. These effusions characteristically accumulate slowly, are very unlikely to produce tamponade, and resolve with thyroid replacement therapy in 6 months to 1 year.[76,77] Ascites is present in less than 4% of hypothyroid patients.[78] Ascitic fluid has a high protein content. The ascites resolves with thyroid replacement.[79]

Generalized nonpitting edema, particularly in a periorbital distribution, is typical. The edema is secondary to hyaluronic acid deposition and characteristically not initially found in dependent areas.[80,81] The skin is smooth, doughy, dry, and cool. It has been described as yellow or sallow, a change secondary to decreased conversion of carotene to vitamin A. The hair is dry and coarse. The eyebrows may be thinned or absent, especially in their lateral extent. Exophthalmopathy or pretibial myxedema may suggest previous Graves' disease. A goiter or thyroidectomy scar should be sought. Goiter is uncommon.[41] In most patients, no gland is appreciable on palpation.[62] The typical husky, deep voice of the hypothyroid patient is not neurologic but rather secondary to mucopolysaccharide infiltration of the vocal cords.[82]

Pseudomyotonic, or "hung up," *deep tendon reflexes* are observed in 58% to 92% of patients.[59,64] Characteristically, a prolonged relaxation phase may be discovered by testing the Achilles reflex while the patient kneels on a chair.[59] The relaxation phase of the deep tendon reflex is usually at least twice as long as the contraction phase.[83] Pseudomyotonic reflexes have also been described in other conditions, including diabetes, localized edema, hypothermia, and pernicious anemia.[60]

Paresthesias are present in 80% of cases.[60,84] The most common involvement is a mononeuropathy, particularly of the median nerve in *carpal tunnel syndrome.* Up to 5% of patients with carpal tunnel syndrome have hypothyroidism.[85,86]

Cerebellar symptoms were recognized in the original descriptions of myxedema; approximately 40% of patients described an unsteady gait.[87] A positive Romberg's sign, ataxic gait, adiadochokinesia, intention tremor, and nystagmus have been described.[74,87,88] The pathophysiology of these changes, although not completely understood, may be related more to increased muscle tone and prolonged muscle contraction than to a primary cerebellar dysfunction. Resolution usually occurs after thyroid replacement therapy.[87]

Decreased auditory acuity and tinnitus may occur and resolve with thyroid replacement therapy.[59,60,64] An atypical facial neuralgia, vertigo, and a subjective report of blurred vision without objective evidence of optic neuritis or retinal involvement are possible.[64]

The initial signs of hypothyroidism may be primarily *rheumatic.*[89] Findings attributable to hypothyroidism include joint effusions, synovial and capsular swelling, generalized weakness, stiffness, arthralgias, and myalgias.[89-91] Effusions typically have a high volume, normal protein, normal cell count, and high viscosity. They are presumably transudates and resolve with thyroid replacement therapy.[89]

Chondrocalcinosis has been reported in association with hypothyroidism and offers one explanation for joint pain. A myopathy, with nonspecific electromyogram findings and occasionally elevated creatine kinase levels, may be present.[92]

Decreased peristalsis in myxedema can lead to constipation, abdominal distention, and even a clinical picture consistent with an acute abdomen.[67]

Menorrhagia and irregular menses may be seen.

Diagnostic Strategies

The most sensitive diagnostic test to detect primary hypothyroidism is the serum TSH assay. Because the signs and symptoms of hypothyroidism are initially subtle, objective measurement of thyroid function is necessary to confirm clinical observation. In addition, certain laboratory abnormalities may be associated with hypothyroidism.

In patients believed to have hypothyroidism, the relevant thyroid function studies are the TSH and FT_4, which will be elevated and depressed, respectively. Early in the course of hypothyroidism, a physiologic compensatory elevation in TSH levels may maintain normal FT_4. Therefore a high TSH level may be the only laboratory abnormality in hypothyroidism. T_4 levels may be spuriously depressed or elevated in hypothyroidism because of alterations in TBG levels previously listed. Conditions that depress these levels are associated with a low T_4 level even if the patient has a normal FT_4 level and is clinically euthyroid. Elevated TBG levels can cause "normal" thyroxine levels when clinical hypothyroidism exists.

Knowledge of the T_3 level is not very helpful because it may be normal in patients with overt hypothyroidism. In addition, a low T_3 level is not necessarily an indication of thyroid disease. Depression of T_4 5′-deiodinase activity decreases peripheral T_4 conversion to T_3 and is associated with an increase in reverse T_3 (rT_3) levels. These patients are physiologically euthyroid but have low T_3 levels, the so-called sick euthyroid state. Factors that decrease T_4 5′-deiodinase activity are chronic disease (cardiac, hepatic, pulmonary, renal), diabetes, malignancy, amiodarone therapy,[15] chronic articular disease, infections, myocardial infarction, acute starvation, chronic malnutrition, propranolol, iopanoic acid, other cholecystographic agents, seizures, and glucocorticoid therapy.

In secondary or tertiary hypothyroidism, both the FT_4 and the TSH levels are low.

Hyponatremia occurs often and is usually mild. Levels as low as 110 mEq/dl have been seen.[69] The mechanism is thought to be syndrome of inappropriate secretion of antidiuretic hormone (SIADH), and thyroid replacement therapy reverses the abnormality.[93-95] *Hypoglycemia* is unusual and typically mild; its correction usually does not materially affect the clinical symptoms.[61,96] The presence of hypoglycemia should suggest hypothalamic-pituitary involvement because it is more characteristic of secondary than primary hypothyroidism. *Hypercalcemia* is rare, mild when present, and of uncertain cause.[97] Cholesterol levels are typically elevated, are rarely less than 250 mg/dl, and in 86% of cases are greater than 290 mg/dl.[59] A mild normocytic, normochromic anemia without reticulocytosis may be present. Creatine kinase may be elevated if a myopathy coexists.

Arterial blood gas (ABG) measurements may reflect a respiratory acidosis secondary to hypoventilation.

A chest x-ray study may reveal an enlarged cardiac silhouette from either pericardial effusion or cardiomyopathy. Pleural effusions may also be present. Pericardial effusions demonstrated by echocardiography may be present in 30% of patients.[76] Chest x-ray studies and electrocardiograms (ECGs) are fallible techniques to establish the presence of pericardial effusion.[76,98] Chest x-ray studies have a 30% false-negative rate and a nearly 40% false-positive rate in detection of hypothyroid pericardial effusions.[76] Effusions are often present without an enlarged cardiac silhouette.[77] Conversely, a high cardiothoracic ratio may simply reflect cardiomyopathy and not effusion.[76] ECG evidence of a pericardial effusion (e.g., low-voltage, diffuse ST-T changes) is present in only 50% of patients with an effusion and in as many as 20% without an effusion.[76]

Differential Considerations

The habitus of the myxedematous patient is characteristic and usually recognizable. Hypothermia and depressed mental acuity are seen in other conditions, which may be mistaken for hypothyroidism. Sepsis and accidental hypothermia, for example, may mimic hypothyroidism. Nephrotic syndrome with renal failure may initially be confused with myxedema coma.

The demeanor of a patient with either apathetic hyperthyroidism or clinical depression may be similar to that associated with hypothyroidism. Hyperglycemic states and intoxication with drugs such as sedative-hypnotics and barbiturates may be seen with acute lethargy and hypothermia.

Management

Thyroid replacement, in the form of thyroxine, is the cornerstone of treatment for hypothyroidism. Coma in the patient with myxedema is typically multifactorial, with inadequate ventilation especially important. Four areas should be addressed in treating myxedema: (1) immediate thyroid replacement therapy, (2) identification and treatment of precipitating factors, (3) reversal of metabolic abnormalities, and (4) general supportive care.

Thyroid Replacement The magnitude of hypothyroidism dictates the route and dose of thyroid replacement therapy. Mild cases may be treated with oral thyroid hormone replacement, adjusting the dosage over a period of weeks. Myxedema coma should be treated much more aggressively and on clinical grounds alone because laboratory confirmation will not be immediately available. The most important factor in survival may be prompt IV administration of significant doses of thyroid hormone. Because thyroid replacement therapy may lead to dysrhythmias or cardiac ischemia, the appropriate dose has been controversial.[41,66,77] Many patients with atheromatous disease have tolerated the doses of thyroid hormone needed to ensure survival. The efficacy of thyroid replacement therapy appears to be dose related.[62]

Levothyroxine (T_4) is generally preferred over triiodothyronine (T_3) because it has a more gradual onset of action.[41] The chance of cardiac complication is thus presumably reduced.[99] Even though oral and intramuscular formulations of T_4 may have erratic and unpredictable absorption, excellent clinical responses to oral doses of T_4 have been reported, even in the presence of myxedema ileus.[100] IV T_4 preparations would still ensure hormonal availability.[62] A dose of 500 μg of T_4, administered PO or IV on day 1, is followed by 100 μg/day.[100] Patients should receive cardiac monitoring and periodic ECGs. If signs of ischemia or dysrhythmias are observed, the dose of thyroxine may be reduced by 25% and continued. Bradycardia generally improves in 24 to 48 hours.[100]

Precipitating Factors An active search for precipitating factors is crucial. CHF and infection, especially pulmonary infection, are the two most common stresses.[62] Infection may be subtle in its presentation because many of the typical signs of infection will be masked by the hypothyroidism.[41] Exposure to cold is almost always present[63] (see Box 122-9).

Along with diagnostic TFTs (FT_4, TSH, TBG), electrolytes, glucose, calcium, and ABGs should be checked. A chest x-ray study and ECG should also be obtained.

Metabolic Abnormalities *Hypoventilation* and *hypoglycemia* are the two immediately serious metabolic abnormalities of myxedema. ABGs may be the only indication that significant hypercapnia and respiratory acidosis exist. An elevated serum carbon dioxide partial pressure may be seen in nearly one third of patients with myxedema coma, and ventilator support can immediately reverse this cause of coma.[62] Serious hypoglycemia is unusual and is less characteristic of primary hypothyroidism than of secondary hypothyroidism.[61,62,96] If present, hypoglycemia can contribute to coma, although seizures may be a more likely outcome.[62,68] Patients should receive 5% dextrose in water (D5W), and serum glucose should be monitored.

Hyponatremia is usually mild and responds to water restriction.[66,73,95] Indications for hypertonic saline (sodium level <110 to 115 mEq/L, mental status changes, seizures) are the same as in other medical conditions. *Hypercalcemia* is rarely significant.[96]

Signs of CHF, ischemia, dysrhythmias, and pleural or pericardial effusions may be sought on chest x-ray studies and ECGs. Tamponade is a rare complication of myxedematous pericardial effusion.[77,98] Thyroid replacement therapy and expectant observation are usually sufficient.[76,77]

Supportive Care General supportive care should focus on maintenance of blood pressure, ventilatory support when necessary, and avoidance of sedatives, narcotics, and anesthetics when possible.

Hypotension, along with hypoventilation and hypothermia, is an acute, life-threatening complication of myxedema. A fluid challenge should be the first line of therapy; however, pressors are often necessary.[65] The response to vasopressor therapy is uniformly poor until thyroid therapy has begun.[96] The action of pressors is augmented by thyroid hormone.[101]

The approach to *hypothermia* is less aggressive. Active rewarming is not only unnecessary, but it also can theoretically be harmful.[63] Hormone replacement and blankets are usually adequate measures. There are few data on active core rewarming of extremely low temperatures in conjunction with thyroid therapy of patients with hypothyroidism and hyperthermia.

Stress dosages of corticosteroids, such as 300 mg of hydrocortisone IV followed by 100 mg IV every 6 to 8 hours, are routinely given to patients in myxedema coma. Steroids are given because myxedema may be either a manifestation of panhypopituitarism or a coexisting condition with primary adrenal failure.

Untreated, myxedema coma is lethal. With aggressive treatment, mortality rates of 0% to approximately 50% have been reported.[62,66]

ADRENAL INSUFFICIENCY

Perspective

Adrenocortical insufficiency, first recognized by Addison in 1844, is an uncommon, potentially life-threatening, readily treatable condition. Production of glucocorticoids, primarily cortisol, inadequate to meet the metabolic requirements of the body is the hallmark of the condition. The protean clinical presentations of hypocortisolism are well described and detailed in the following section.

The clinical features of adrenal insufficiency vary according to the locus of the lesion producing the disease (primary or secondary adrenal failure) and the duration of the condition (acute or chronic adrenal insufficiency).

Principles of Disease

In primary adrenal insufficiency, or *Addison's disease,* the adrenal gland itself cannot produce cortisol, aldosterone, or both. Absence of glucocorticoids produces a compensatory elevation of adrenocorticotropic hormone (ACTH) and melanocyte-stimulating hormone (MSH). Likewise, lack of aldosterone leads to a reflex increase in renin production. In *secondary adrenal failure* the locus of failure is the hypothalamic-pituitary axis. Secondary adrenal failure is usually characterized by depressed ACTH secretion and blunted cortisol production, but aldosterone levels remain appropriate because of stimulation by both the renin-angiotensin axis and hyperkalemia.[102] A special case, often called *functional adrenal insufficiency,* occurs when administration of exogenous corticosteroids leads to depression of ACTH secretion. When exogenous steroids are discontinued, the clinical picture of secondary adrenal failure may follow (Box 122-10).

Acute Adrenal Insufficiency Acute adrenal insufficiency is probably a rare condition. It may represent either an exacerbation of longstanding disease or a de novo case.

Box 122-10 Etiologic Factors of Adrenocortical Insufficiency

I. Primary adrenal failure
  A. Idiopathic
    1. Autoimmune
    2. True idiopathic
  B. Infectious
    1. Granulomatous
      a. Tuberculosis
    2. Protozoal and fungal
      a. Histoplasmosis
      b. Blastomycosis
      c. Coccidioidomycosis
      d. Candidiasis
      e. Cryptococcosis
    3. Viral
      a. Cytomegalovirus
      b. Herpes simplex
  C. Infiltration
    1. Sarcoidosis
    2. Neoplastic (metastatic)
    3. Lymphoma/leukemia
    4. Hemochromatosis
    5. Adrenoleukodystrophy
    6. Amyloidosis
    7. Iron deposition
  D. Postadrenalectomy
  E. Hemorrhage
  F. Congenital adrenal hyperplasia
  G. Congenital unresponsiveness to ACTH
II. Secondary adrenal failure
  A. Pituitary insufficiency
    1. Infarction (Sheehan's syndrome)
    2. Hemorrhage
    3. Pituitary or suprasellar tumor
    4. Isolated ACTH deficiency
    5. Infiltration disease
      a. Sarcoidosis
      b. Histiocytosis X
      c. Hemachromatosis
  B. Hypothalamic insufficiency
  C. Head trauma
III. Functional disease: glucocorticoid administration

Chronic disease is more prevalent and probably accounts for most cases of acute adrenal insufficiency seen in EDs.

The most common cause of adrenal insufficiency is hypothalamic-pituitary-adrenal (HPA) axis suppression from long-term exogenous glucocorticoid administration. When adrenal failure represents a rapid worsening of chronic adrenal failure, both the cause of the underlying failure and the precipitant of abrupt decompensation should be identified.

Acute precipitating stresses include surgery, anesthesia, psychologic stresses, alcohol intoxication, hypothermia, myocardial infarction, diabetes mellitus, intercurrent infection, asthma, pyrogens, and hypoglycemia[103-108] (Box 122-11).

Acute adrenal insufficiency occurring in a previously normal HPA axis is unusual and is produced by either pituitary or adrenal hemorrhage or infarction.

Adrenal hemorrhage is a rare condition[109] (Box 122-12). Not all cases of adrenal hemorrhage lead to glandular failure.

Box 122-11 Precipitants of Acute Adrenal Insufficiency

Stimulators

Surgery
Anesthesia
Volume loss
Trauma
Asthma
Hypothermia
Alcohol
Myocardial infarction
Pyrogens
Hypoglycemia
Pain
Psychotic break
Depressive illness

Inhibitors

Morphine
Reserpine
Chlorpromazine
Barbiturates

Box 122-12 Causes of Adrenal Hemorrhage

Overwhelming septicemia (Waterhouse-Friderichsen syndrome)
Birth trauma
During pregnancy
Idiopathic adrenal vein thrombosis
During seizures
Anticoagulant therapy
After venography
After trauma or surgery

Only 10% of cases of adrenal hemorrhage may produce clinical insufficiency.[109] This is not surprising because more than 90% of the gland must be destroyed before signs of adrenal insufficiency develop.[110] Adrenal failure that does develop from adrenal hemorrhage is lethal.[111] It would be unusual to see a case of hemorrhagic adrenal failure in the ED. De novo cases in otherwise healthy persons are rare. The typical patient has a severe illness (e.g., myocardial infarction, systemic infection, burn) and is often receiving anticoagulant therapy.[109] Attention to the possibility of adrenal hemorrhage in a high-risk patient may lead to early diagnosis and therapy, with significant improvement in survival.[112] Adrenal hemorrhage associated with sepsis (acute fulminating meningococcemia, or Waterhouse-Friderichsen syndrome) may lead to adrenal failure that may contribute to shock and death.[111]

The most common cause of acute adrenal insufficiency is *functional,* from exogenous glucocorticoid administration. Many medical indications exist for glucocorticoid therapy (Box 122-13). The probability of HPA axis suppression depends on the frequency, strength, and schedule, as well as on the duration of steroid therapy.[113-116] The degree of suppression cannot be predicted accurately even with consideration of these factors. Recovery of the HPA axis after discontinuation of therapy may take up to 1 year.[113] In addition to the oral route, glucocorticoids can produce HPA suppression when administered nasally or via inhalation.[117,118]

Box 122-13 Nonendocrine Disorders with Glucocorticoid Therapy

1. Rheumatoid arthritis
2. Psoriatic arthritis
3. Gouty arthritis
4. Bursitis and tenosynovitis
5. Systemic lupus erythematosus
6. Acute rheumatic carditis
7. Pemphigus
8. Erythema multiforme
9. Exfoliative dermatitis
10. Mycosis fungoides
11. Allergic rhinitis
12. Bronchial asthma
13. Atopic dermatitis
14. Serum sickness
15. Allergic conjunctivitis
16. Uveitis
17. Retrobulbar neuritis
18. Sarcoidosis
19. Löffler's syndrome
20. Berylliosis
21. Idiopathic thrombocytopenic purpura
22. Autoimmune hemolytic anemia
23. Lymphomas
24. Immune nephritis
25. Tuberculous meningitis
26. Urticaria
27. Chronic active hepatitis
28. Ulcerative hepatitis
29. Regional enteritis
30. Nontropical sprue
31. Dental postoperative inflammation
32. Cerebral edema
33. Subacute nonsuppurative thyroiditis
34. Malignant exophthalmos
35. Hypercalcemia
36. Trichinosis
37. Myasthenia gravis
38. Organ transplantation
39. Alopecia areata

From Liddle G. In Williams R, editor: *Textbook of endocrinology,* Philadelphia, 1981, Saunders.

Chronic Adrenal Insufficiency The major cause of primary chronic adrenal insufficiency is *idiopathic,* representing 66% to 75% of cases. Idiopathic adrenal failure encompasses two distinct clinical entities: autoimmune adrenal failure and true idiopathic disease. Adrenal antibodies are found in 51% to 63% of cases of idiopathic disease. Antibodies to other organs can be demonstrated.[119] Autoimmune diseases of other organs, including diabetes mellitus, primary ovarian failure, Hashimoto's thyroiditis, Graves' disease, pernicious anemia, and hypoparathyroidism, are associated in 53% of cases.[120,121]

Metastasis from malignant carcinoma to the adrenal glands is not unusual, but adrenal insufficiency from metastatic disease is rare.[122] The usual primary malignancies are lung, gastrointestinal system, and breast.[122,123]

Tuberculous Addison's disease, once the most common cause of adrenal insufficiency in the United States, is now unusual.[124] Adrenal calcifications are a possible radiographic finding (see Box 122-11).

Clinical Features

Signal symptoms for adrenal insufficiency include weakness, fatigue, nausea, vomiting, and weight loss. Hypotension is typically present. These symptoms are obviously nonspecific and common, making diagnosis difficult. When primary adrenal glandular failure is chronic, patients have a characteristic hyperpigmented appearance.

Recognition of patients at risk for adrenal failure facilitates diagnosis. The most common cause of adrenal insufficiency in ED patients is suppression of the HPA axis as a result of long-term glucocorticoid therapy. An exacerbation of chronic primary glandular failure is also possible but usually is not a diagnostic dilemma. True acute, de novo adrenal insufficiency is rare.

The acute life threats in adrenal insufficiency are hypotension and hypoglycemia. Hypotension responds well to glucocorticoid replacement with IV hydration and hypoglycemia to IV administration of D5W.

The signs and symptoms of adrenal insufficiency have varying frequencies (Table 122-3). Lethargy is generalized. In severe cases, weakness can be severe enough to make talking difficult. The hyperkalemia of adrenal failure is rarely severe enough to produce frank muscular paralysis.[125]

The mortality and major morbidity produced by adrenal insufficiency are usually secondary to either hypotension or hypoglycemia.

Hypotension, with systolic blood pressures of less than 110 mm Hg, is often present. In one study only 3% of addisonian patients initially exhibited systolic pressures greater than 125 mm Hg.[124] Orthostatic symptoms are common. Several mechanisms produce hypotension. Cortisol deficiency, even in the presence of normovolemia, can lead to hypotension by directly depressing myocardial contractility.[126] Responsiveness to catecholamines is also reduced. If aldosterone deficiency coexists, sodium wasting can lead to hypovolemia. Volume deficits are greater in primary than in secondary adrenal insufficiency. Elevations in renin-angiotensin function and ADH secretion are seen and partially compensate for the relative or absolute hypovolemia present.[127,128] Understandably, response to pressors is poor, to volume replacement better, and to volume plus corticosteroids best.[126]

Nonspecific gastrointestinal symptoms, including nausea and vomiting, are present in 56% to 87% of cases.[124,129] The patient may be in severe pain, and the clinical picture may include an acute abdomen. Anorexia is universally present and is one mechanism leading to the weight loss that always accompanies chronic adrenal insufficiency. Dehydration and sodium wasting can lead to a craving for salt.

More than three fourths of patients with Addison's disease have *mucocutaneous hyperpigmentation.*[124,129] The mechanism is compensatory ACTH and MSH secretion. No hyperpigmentation is seen in secondary adrenal insufficiency. The melanin deposits are usually in areas of trauma and friction (flexion creases of the palms and soles, elbows, knees, and buccal mucosa) and in old scars. Bluish black discolorations may be present on the lips and gums.

Table 122-3. Prevalence of Clinical Features of Adrenal Insufficiency

Clinical feature	Frequency (%)
Weakness and fatigue	99-100
Hyperpigmentation (skin)	92-97
Hyperpigmentation (mucous membranes)	71-82
Weight loss	97-100
Nausea, vomiting	56-87
Anorexia	98-100
Hypotension (110/70)	82-91
Abdominal pain	34
Salt craving	22
Diarrhea	20
Constipation	19
Syncope	12-16
Vitiligo	4-9
Musculoskeletal complaints	6
Lethargy	—
Confusion	—
Psychosis	—
Auricular calcification	—

Hyperpigmentation usually develops over months of relative adrenal insufficiency. Vitiligo may be present in some patients, usually when adrenal failure is autoimmune in origin.[129]

Nonspecific, diffuse musculoskeletal complaints are present in 6% of cases. Patients may have a generalized loss of body hair and hardening of the auricular cartilage.

Changes in mental functioning may occur. Lethargy and an organic brain syndrome picture may be the initial evidence of adrenal insufficiency, especially in elderly patients. Depression, manic psychosis, and generalized seizures have also been described.

Two thirds of patients with adrenal failure have associated *hypoglycemia.*[124,129] The symptoms are characteristic of hypoglycemia: perspiration, tachycardia, weakness, nausea, vomiting, headache, convulsions, and coma. The glucose levels are less than 45 mg/dl. The pathophysiology is decreased gluconeogenesis and increased peripheral glucose use secondary to lipolysis.

Electrolyte abnormalities are common. Hyponatremia is present in 88% of cases, hyperkalemia in 64%, either hyponatremia or hyperkalemia in 92%, and hypercalcemia in 6% to 33%.[124,129-131]

Hyponatremia, seldom less than 120 mEq/L, has several possible causes. Elevated ADH levels, either secondary to decreased circulating blood volume or decreased cortisol, lower serum sodium levels.[128] A decreased glomerular filtration rate (GFR) causes decreased fluid to be delivered to the distal renal tubules, leading to diminished sodium reabsorption. Finally, if aldosterone deficiency coexists with hyponatremia, it can lead to urinary losses of sodium. On a high-sodium diet, aldosterone deficiency usually leads to no overt symptoms, but when salt intake is decreased, volume depletion can become clinically evident.

Hyperkalemia is usually in the 4.5-mEq/L range and seldom greater than 7.0 mEq/L.[125] Muscle paralysis, of the

Landry type of ascending flaccid quadriplegia, is possible but rare.[126] Hyperkalemic dysrhythmias should also be considered but are rare.[132] Hyperkalemia in adrenal insufficiency is produced by acidosis, aldosterone deficiency, and depressed GFR.[125]

Hypercalcemia is relatively common.[130,131] Its pathophysiology is not entirely clear but may be related to either increased protein binding or volume depletion with associated facilitation of renal tubule reabsorption. Total calcium, but not ionized calcium, is increased.

Other metabolic abnormalities include azotemia and elevated hematocrit levels, both referable to hypovolemia. A mild metabolic acidosis may be present.

Diagnostic Strategies

The diagnosis of acute adrenal insufficiency is initially clinical, and therapy should often begin before laboratory values confirm the clinical impression. In some patients the condition is suggested by a history of chronic adrenal failure or glucocorticoid therapy. This facilitates diagnosis, and the task is to identify the intercurrent stress that has precipitated symptomatic adrenal failure. However, the patient may be too ill to give a history of chronic adrenal insufficiency. Alternatively, the case may represent de novo acute adrenal insufficiency. Laboratory abnormalities (e.g., hyponatremia, hyperkalemia, hypoglycemia) may help confirm the clinical impression.

Adrenal failure may be considered when a patient complains of severe anorexia or weakness, especially when accompanied by weight loss. Hypotension of unclear cause may indicate adrenal insufficiency. Changes in mental status may also be signal symptoms of impending adrenal insufficiency, especially in elderly patients.

Once suggested, the diagnosis of adrenal failure should proceed concomitant with treatment. The diagnosis is based on a failure of the adrenals to respond to exogenous ACTH with cortisol production, the *ACTH stimulation test.* Several ACTH stimulation protocols have been developed. In perhaps the simplest and quickest protocol, 0.25 mg of cosyntropin (synthetic ACTH, Cortrosyn) is administered at time zero. For cortisol determination, serum samples are drawn at time zero, 1 hour, and at 6- to 8-hour intervals thereafter. Normal adrenals will respond with an increase in cortisol of at least 10 mg/dl or to three times baseline level. A 24-hour urine sample is obtained for 17-hydroxysteroid determination to confirm the diagnosis suggested by the serum cortisol levels.

A 48-hour ACTH stimulation test can confirm the diagnosis of adrenal insufficiency and differentiate primary from secondary causes. Whereas rapid ACTH stimulation tests have excellent sensitivity, they may occasionally make an erroneous diagnosis of adrenal failure in patients with normal adrenal function.

Management

The goals in treating adrenal insufficiency are (1) glucocorticoid replacement, (2) correction of electrolyte and metabolic abnormalities as well as hypovolemia, and (3) treatment of the event precipitating abrupt decompensation.

Glucocorticoid Replacement If the diagnosis of adrenal failure is unconfirmed, *dexamethasone phosphate,* 4 mg IV every 6 to 8 hours, is the corticosteroid replacement that should be used while an ACTH stimulation test is performed. Dexamethasone is approximately 100 times more potent than cortisol, and this amount of dexamethasone will not factitiously elevate serum cortisol determinations. Replacement with hydrocortisone could confound interpretation of serum cortisol determinations.

If the patient is known to have adrenal failure, 100 mg of *hydrocortisone hemisuccinate* IV every 6 to 8 hours should be used.[103] If IV access cannot be maintained, *cortisone acetate,* 100 mg intramuscularly every 6 to 8 hours, may be used, but its absorption is erratic and not as reliable as the IV route. The dose of glucocorticoid is tapered over the next several days and eventually converted to an oral preparation.

Supportive Care If salt and water replacement is adequate, mineralocorticoid replacement is usually not necessary. Subsequent to the addisonian crisis, patients may require titration with mineralocorticoid preparations such as *fludrocortisone acetate* (Florinef); 100 mg of hydrocortisone has the salt-retaining effect of 0.1 mg of Florinef. If dexamethasone is used, Florinef should be added to prevent salt loss.

Addisonian patients are often up to 20% volume depleted. Unless specifically contraindicated by the patient's cardiovascular status, correction of hypovolemia should be aggressive. One liter of normal saline may be infused over the first hour; D5W is usually added to treat accompanying hypoglycemia. Up to a total of 3 L may be required over the first 8 hours. Optimal correction of hypotension requires both glucocorticoid and volume replacement.

Treatment of hypoglycemia should be immediate. For symptomatic hypoglycemia or extremely low serum levels, IV glucose (50 to 100 ml of D50W) is preferable. If IV access is impossible, subcutaneous glucagon (1 to 2 mg) may be attempted, although a 10- to 20-minute period of latency should be anticipated.

Electrolyte abnormalities are usually corrected with saline rehydration. Special attention must be given to the potassium level. Symptomatic hyperkalemia in adrenal insufficiency should be treated with the same agents as hyperkalemia from any other medical illness (e.g., bicarbonate, insulin, calcium).

Precipitating Factors The intercurrent stress causing abrupt loss of adrenal integrity should be identified and treated. Drug ingestion and psychiatric history should be elicited. Symptoms referable to myocardial infarction, asthma, or an infection must be noted. Appropriate cultures should be obtained, and if infection is suspected, antibiotics should be started.

KEY CONCEPTS

- Signs and symptoms of hyperthyroidism include agitation, nervousness, palpitations, weight loss, fever, tachycardia, ophthalmopathy, goiter, and heart failure.
- Severely hyperthyroid patients require emergency intervention with a β-blocker, a thioamide, iodine, and dexamethasone, as well as supportive therapy.
- Patients with mild hypothyroidism may develop dramatic clinical presentations, even myxedema coma when physiologically stressed.

- The most sensitive diagnostic test to detect primary hypothyroidism is the serum thyroid-stimulating hormone (TSH) assay.
- "Signal" symptoms of adrenal insufficiency include weakness, fatigue, nausea, vomiting, and weight loss. Hypotension is typically present.
- If adrenal insufficiency is unconfirmed, dexamethasone is optimal because it will not falsely elevate serum cortisol. If the patient has adrenal failure, hydrocortisone hemisuccinate is indicated.

REFERENCES

1. Major RH: *Classic descriptions of disease,* Springfield, Ill, 1978, Thomas.
2. Ginsburg AM: The historical development of the present conception of cardiac conditions in exophthalmic goiter, *Ann Intern Med* 5:505, 1931.
3. Knight RA: The use of spinal anesthesia to control sympathetic hyperactivity in hyperthyroidism, *Anesthesiology* 6:225, 1945.
4. Canary JJ et al: Effects of oral and intramuscular administration of reserpine in thyrotoxicosis, *N Engl J Med* 257:435, 1957.
5. Ramey ER, Bernstein H, Goldstein MS: Effect of sympathetic blocking agents on the increased oxygen consumption following administration of thyroxine, *Fed Proc* 14:118, 1955.
6. Roizen M, Becker CE: Thyroid storm: a review of cases at University of California, San Francisco, *Calif Med* 115:5, 1971.
7. Nelson NC, Becker WF: Thyroid crisis: diagnosis and treatment, *Ann Surg* 170:263, 1969.
8. McArthur JW et al: Thyrotoxic crisis: an analysis of the thirty-six cases seen at the Massachusetts General Hospital during the past twenty-five years, *JAMA* 134:868, 1947.
9. Waldstein SS et al: A clinical study of thyroid storm, *Ann Intern Med* 52:626, 1960.
10. Griswold D, Keating JH Jr: Cardiac dysfunction in hyperthyroidism, *Am Heart J* 38:813, 1949.
11. Mazzaferri EL, Skillman TG: Thyroid storm, *Arch Intern Med* 124:684, 1969.
12. Hamilton CR, Maloof F: Unusual types of hyperthyroidism, *Medicine* 52:195, 1973.
13. Gorman CA, Wahner HW, Tauxe WN: Metabolic malingerers: patients who deliberately induce or perpetuate a hypermetabolic or hypometabolic state, *Am J Med* 48:708, 1970.
14. Schottstaedt ES, Smoller M: "Thyroid storm" produced by acute thyroid hormone poisoning, *Ann Intern Med* 64:847, 1966.
15. Harjai KJ, Licata AA: Effects of amiodarone on thyroid function, *Ann Intern Med* 126:63, 1997.
16. Levey GS: Catecholamine sensitivity, thyroid hormone and the heart, *Am J Med* 50:413, 1971.
17. Levey GS, Epstein SE: Myocardial adenyl cyclase: activation by thyroid hormone and evidence for two adenyl cyclase systems, *J Clin Invest* 48:1163, 1969.
18. Rosenberg IN: Thyroid storm, *N Engl J Med* 283:1052, 1970.
19. Lahey FH: The crisis of exophthalmic goiter, *N Engl J Med* 199:255, 1928.
20. Lahey FH: Non-activated (apathetic) type of hyperthyroidism, *N Engl J Med* 204:747, 1931.
21. Sandler G, Wilson GM: The nature and prognosis of heart disease in thyrotoxicosis, *Q J Med* 28:347, 1959.
22. Graettinger JS et al: A correlation of clinical and hemodynamic studies in patients with hyperthyroidism with and without congestive heart failure, *J Clin Invest* 38:1316, 1959.
23. Lawrence JR et al: Digoxin kinetics in patients with thyroid dysfunction, *Clin Pharmacol Ther* 22:7, 1977.
24. Likoff WB, Levine SA: Thyrotoxicosis as the sole cause of heart failure, *Am J Med Sci* 206:425, 1943.
25. Ikran H: Haemodynamics of beta-adrenergic blockade in hyperthyroid patients with and without heart failure, *BMJ* 1:1505, 1977.
26. Solomon DH et al: Identification of subgroups of euthyroid Graves' ophthalmopathy, *N Engl J Med* 296:181, 1977.
27. Werner SC: Classification of the eye changes in Graves' disease, *Am J Ophthalmol* 68:646, 1969.
28. Werner SC: Modification of the classification of eye changes in Graves' disease, *Am J Ophthalmol* 83:725, 1977.
29. Massey DG et al: Circulatory and ventilatory response to exercise in thyrotoxicosis, *N Engl J Med* 276:1104, 1967.
30. Pimstone N, Marine N, Pimstone B: Beta adrenergic blockade in thyrotoxic myopathy, *Lancet* 2:1219, 1968.
31. Kammer GM, Hamilton CR: Acute bulbar muscle dysfunction and hyperthyroidism, *Am J Med* 56:464, 1974.
32. Kusakabe T, Joshida M, Nishikawa M: Thyrotoxic periodic paralysis: a peculiar case with unusual dystonic behavior and variable relations of paralysis to serum potassium levels, *J Clin Endocrinol Metab* 43:730, 1976.
33. Greenberger NJ et al: Jaundice and thyrotoxicosis in the absence of congestive heart failure, *Am J Med* 36:840, 1964.
34. Odell WD et al: Symposium on hyperthyroidism, *Calif Med* 113:35, 1970.
35. Hegedus L et al: Thyroid size and goitre frequency in hyperthyroidism, *Danish Med Bull* 34:121, 1987.
36. De los Santos ET, Starich GH, Mazzaferri EL: Sensitivity, specificity, and cost-effectiveness of the sensitive thyrotropin assay in the diagnosis of thyroid disease in ambulatory patients, *Arch Intern Med* 149:526, 1989.
37. Hollander CS et al: Clinical and laboratory observations in cases of triiodothyronine toxicosis confirmed by radioimmunoassay, *Lancet* 1:609, 1972.
38. Hollander CS et al: Hypertriidothyronaemia as a premonitory manifestation of thyrotoxicosis, *Lancet* 2:731, 1971.
39. Jacobs HS et al: Total and free triiodothyronine and thyroxine levels in thyroid storm and recurrent hyperthyroidism, *Lancet* 2:263, 1973.
40. Hollander CS et al: T_3 toxicosis in an iodine-deficient area, *Lancet* 2:1276, 1972.
41. Urbanic RC, Mazzaferri EL: Thyrotoxic crisis and myxedema coma, *Heart Lung* 7:435, 1978.
42. McGee RR, Whittaker RL, Tulius IF: Apathetic thyroidism: review of the literature and report of four cases, *Ann Intern Med* 50:1418, 1959.
43. Thomas FB, Mazzaferri EL, Skillman TG: Apathetic thyrotoxicosis: a distinctive clinical and laboratory entity, *Ann Intern Med* 72:679, 1970.
44. Grossman A, Waldstein SS: Apathetic thyroid storm in a ten year old child, *Pediatrics* 28:447, 1961.
45. Schimmel M, Utiger RD: Thyroidal and peripheral production of thyroid hormones: review of recent findings and their clinical importance, *Ann Intern Med* 87:760, 1977.
46. Oppenheimer JH, Schwartz HL, Jurks ML: Propylthiouracil inhibits the conversion of 1-thyroxine to 1-triiodothyronine: an explanation of the antithyroxine effects of PTU and evidence supporting the concept that T_3 is the active thyroid hormone, *J Clin Invest* 51:2493, 1972.
47. Croxson M, Hall TD, Nicoloff JJ: Combination drug therapy for treatment of hyperthyroid Graves' disease, *J Clin Endocrinol Metab* 45:623, 1977.
48. Zonazein J et al: Propranolol therapy in thyrotoxicosis: a review of 84 patients undergoing surgery, *Am J Med* 66:411, 1979.
49. Turner P, Granville-Grossman KL, Smart JV: Effect of adrenergic receptor blockade on the tachycardia of thyrotoxicosis and anxiety state, *Lancet* 2:1316, 1965.
50. Das G, Krieger M: Treatment of thyrotoxic storm with intravenous administration of propranolol, *Ann Intern Med* 70:985, 1969.
51. Hellman R et al: Propranolol for thyroid storm, *N Engl J Med* 297:671, 1977.
52. Mackin JF, Canary JJ, Pittman CS: Thyroid storm and its management, *N Engl J Med* 291:1396, 1974.
53. Lewis NDG, Davies GR: Correlative study of endocrine imbalance and mental disease, *J Nerv Ment Dis* 54:385, 1921.
54. Curling TB: Two cases of absence of the thyroid bodies, *Med Chir Trans Lond* 33:303, 1850.
55. Gull WW: On a cretinoid state supervening in adult life in women, *Trans Clin Soc Lond* 7:180, 1873.

56. Ord WM: On myxedema, a term proposed to be applied to an essential condition in the "cretinoid" affection occasionally observed in middle-aged women, *Med Chir Trans Lond* 61:57, 1877.
57. Murray GR: Note on the treatment of myxedema by hypodermic injections of an extract of the thyroid gland of a sheep, *BMJ* 2:796, 1891.
58. Mayberry WE et al: Radioimmunoassay for human TSH: clinical value in patients with normal and abnormal thyroid function, *Ann Intern Med* 74:471, 1971.
59. Bloomer H, Kyle LH: Myxedema: a reevaluation of clinical diagnosis based on eighty cases, *Arch Intern Med* 104:234, 1959.
60. Swanson JW, Kelly JJ, McConahey WM: Neurologic aspects of thyroid dysfunction, *Mayo Clin Proc* 56:504, 1981.
61. Nickerson JF et al: Fatal myxedema, with and without coma, *Ann Intern Med* 53:475, 1960.
62. Forester CF: Coma in myxedema: report of a case and review of the world literature, *Arch Intern Med* 111:734, 1963.
63. Senior RM et al: The recognition and management of myxedema coma, *JAMA* 217:61, 1971.
64. Nickel SN, Frame B: Neurologic manifestation of myxedema, *Neurology* 8:511, 1958.
65. Curtis RH: Hyponatremia in primary myxedema, *Ann Intern Med* 44:376, 1956.
66. Nichols AB, Hunt WB: Is myxedema coma respiratory failure? *South Med J* 69:945, 1976.
67. Royce PC: Severely impaired consciousness in myxedema: a review, *Am J Med Sci* 261:46, 1971.
68. Malden M: Hypothermic coma in myxedema, *BMJ* 2:764, 1955.
69. Hyams DE: Hypothermic myxedema coma, *Br J Clin Pract* 1:1, 1963.
70. Zwillich CW et al: Ventilatory control in myxedema and hypothyroidism, *N Engl J Med* 292:662, 1975.
71. Massumi RA, Winnacker JL: Severe depression of the respiratory center in myxedema, *Am J Med* 36:876, 1964.
72. Wilson WR, Bedell GN: The pulmonary abnormalities in myxedema, *J Clin Invest* 39:42, 1960.
73. Winawer SJ, Rosen SM, Cohn H: Myxedema coma with ventricular tachycardia, *Arch Intern Med* 111:647, 1963.
74. Greene JA: Comparison or symptoms, physical and laboratory findings of myxedema and pernicious anemia: with a report of three cases, *Ann Intern Med* 10:622, 1936.
75. Lange K: Capillary permeability in myxedema, *Am J Med Sci* 208:5, 1944.
76. Kerber RE, Sherman B: Echocardiographic evaluation of pericardial effusion in myxedema: incidence and biochemical and clinical correlations, *Circulation* 52:823, 1975.
77. Smolar EN et al: Cardiac tamponade in primary myxedema and review of the literature, *Am J Med Sci* 272:345, 1976.
78. Watanakunakorn C, Hodges RE, Evans TC: Myxedema: a study of 400 cases, *Arch Intern Med* 116:183, 1965.
79. De Castro F et al: Myxedema ascites: report of two cases and review of the literature, *J Clin Gastroenterol* 13:411, 1991.
80. Goldberg RC, Chaikoff IL: Myxedema in the radiothyroidectomized dog, *Endocrinology* 50:115, 1952.
81. Aikawa JK: The nature of myxedema: alterations in the serum electrolyte concentrations and radiosodium space and the exchangeable sodium and potassium content, *Ann Intern Med* 44:30, 1956.
82. Ritter FN: The effects of hypothyroidism on the ear, nose and throat: a clinical and experimental study, *Laryngoscope* 77:1427, 1967.
83. Maclean D, Taig DR, Emslie-Smith D: Achilles tendon reflex in accidental hypothermia and hypothermic myxedema, *BMJ* 2:87, 1973.
84. Sanders V: Neurologic manifestations of myxedema, *N Engl J Med* 266:547, 1962.
85. Doyle JR, Carroll RE: The carpal tunnel syndrome: a review of 100 patients treated surgically, *Calif Med* 108:263, 1968.
86. Phalen GS: The carpal tunnel syndrome: seventeen years experience in diagnosis and treatment of six hundred and fifty-four hands, *J Bone Joint Surg* 48A:211, 1966.
87. Cremer GM, Goldstein NP, Paris J: Myxedema and ataxia, *Neurology* 19:37, 1969.
88. Jellinek EH, Kelly RE: Cerebellar syndrome in myxoedema, *Lancet* 2:225, 1960.
89. Bland JH, Frymoyer JW: Rheumatic syndromes of myxedema, *N Engl J Med* 282:1171, 1970.
90. Wilson J, Walton JN: Some muscular manifestations of hypothyroidism, *J Neurol Neurosurg Psychiatry* 22:320, 1959.
91. Crevasse LE, Logue RB: Peripheral neuropathy in myxedema, *Ann Intern Med* 50:1433, 1959.
92. Mace BEW, Mallya RK, Staffurth JS: Myxoedema presenting with chondrocalcinosis and polymyositis, *J R Soc Med* 73:887, 1980.
93. Holvey DN et al: Treatment of myxedema coma with intravenous thyroxine, *Arch Intern Med* 113:89, 1964.
94. Goldberg M, Reivich M: Studies on the mechanism of hyponatremia and impaired water excretion in myxedema, *Ann Intern Med* 56:120, 1962.
95. Pettinger WA, Taylor L, Ferris TF: Inappropriate secretion of antidiuretic hormone due to myxedema, *N Engl J Med* 272:362, 1965.
96. Perlmutter M, Cohn H: Myxedema crisis of pituitary or thyroid origin, *Am J Med* 36:883, 1964.
97. Lowe CE, Bird ED, Thomas WC: Hypercalcemia in myxedema, *J Clin Invest* 39:42, 1960.
98. Kurtzman RS, Otto DL, Chepey JJ: Myxedema heart disease, *Radiology* 84:624, 1965.
99. Ibbertson K, Fraser R, Alldis D: Rapidly acting thyroid hormones and their cardiac action, *BMJ* 2:52, 1959.
100. Arlot S et al: Myxedema coma: response of thyroid hormones with oral and intravenous high-dose L-thyroxine treatment, *Intensive Care Med* 17:16, 1990.
101. Brewster WR Jr et al: The hemodynamic and metabolic interrelationships in the activity of epinephrine, norepinephrine and thyroid hormone, *Circulation* 13:1, 1956.
102. Williams GH et al: Studies of the control of plasma aldosterone concentration in normal man, *J Clin Invest* 51:1731, 1972.
103. Ichikawa Y: Plasma corticotropin (ACTH), growth hormone (GH) and II-OHCS (hydroxycorticosteroid) response during surgery, *J Lab Clin Med* 78:882, 1971.
104. Von Werder K et al: Adrenal function during long-term anesthesia in man, *Proc Soc Exp Biol Med* 135:854, 1970.
105. Sachar EJ et al: Disrupted 24-hour patterns of cortisol secretion in psychotic depression, *Arch Gen Psychiatry* 28:19, 1973.
106. Bellet S et al: Effect of acute ethanol intake on plasma II-hydroxycorticosteroid levels in accidental hypothermia, *Lancet* 1:324, 1970.
107. Sprunt JG, Maclean D, Browning MCK: Plasma corticosteroid levels in accidental hypothermia, *Lancet* 1:324, 1970.
108. Jacobs HS, Nabarro JDN: Plasma II-hydroxycorticosteroid and growth hormone levels in acute medical illnesses, *BMJ* 2:595, 1969.
109. Xarli VP et al: Adrenal hemorrhage in the adult, *Medicine* 57:211, 1978.
110. Rosenthal FD, Davies MK, Burden AC: Malignant disease presenting as Addison's disease, *BMJ* 1:1591, 1978.
111. Bosworth DC: Reversible adrenocortical insufficiency in fulminant meningococcemia, *Arch Intern Med* 139:823, 1979.
112. Anderson KC, Kuhajda FP, Bell WR: Diagnosis and treatment of anticoagulant-related adrenal hemorrhage, *Am J Hematol* 11:379, 1981.
113. Danowski TS et al: Probabilities of pituitary-adrenal responsiveness after steroid therapy, *Ann Intern Med* 51:11, 1964.
114. Graber AL et al: Natural history of pituitary-adrenal recovery following long-term suppression with corticosteroids, *J Clin Endocrinol Metab* 25:11, 1965.
115. Ackerman GL, Nolan GM: Adrenocortical responsiveness after alternate-day corticosteroid therapy, *N Engl J Med* 278:405, 1968.
116. Streck WF, Lockwood DH: Pituitary adrenal recovery following short-term suppression with corticosteroids, *Am J Med* 66:910, 1979.
117. Heroman WM et al: Adrenal suppression and cushingoid changes secondary to dexamethasone nose drops, *J Pediatr* 96:500, 1980.
118. Vaz R et al: Adrenal effects of beclomethasone inhalation therapy in asthmatic children, *J Pediatr* 100:660, 1982.
119. Blizzard RM, Chee D, Davis W: The incidence of adrenal and other antibodies in the sera of patients with idiopathic adrenal insufficiency (Addison's disease), *Clin Exp Immunol* 2:19, 1967.
120. Blizzard RM, Kyle M: Studies of the adrenal antigens and antibodies in Addison's disease, *J Clin Invest* 42:1653, 1963.
121. Genant HK, Hoagland HC, Randall RV: Addison's disease and hypothyroidism (Schmidt's syndrome), *Metabolism* 16:189, 1967.
122. Sheeler LR et al: Adrenal insufficiency secondary to carcinoma metastatic to the adrenal gland, *Cancer* 52:1312, 1983.

123. Glomset DA: The incidence of metastasis of malignant tumors to the adrenal, *Am J Cancer* 32:57, 1938.
124. Nerup J: Addison's disease—clinical studies: a report of 108 cases, *Acta Endocrinol* 76:127, 1974.
125. Bell H, Hayes W, Vosbrugh J: Hyperkalemic paralysis due to adrenal insufficiency, *Arch Intern Med* 115:418, 1965.
126. Webb WR et al: Cardiovascular responses in adrenal insufficiency, *Surgery* 58:273, 1965.
127. Schwartz J et al: Role of vasopressin in blood pressure regulation during adrenal insufficiency, *Endocrinology* 112:234, 1983.
128. Ahmed ABJ et al: Increased plasma arginine vasopressin in clinical adrenocortical insufficiency and its inhibition by glucosteroids, *J Clin Invest* 46:111, 1967.
129. Dunlop D: Eighty-six cases of Addison's disease, *BMJ* 2:887, 1963.
130. Jorgensen H: Hypercalcemia in adrenocortical insufficiency, *Acta Med Scand* 193:175, 1973.
131. Walser M, Robinson BHB, Duckett JW: The hypercalcemia of adrenal insufficiency, *J Clin Invest* 42:456, 1963.
132. Somerville W, Levine HD, Thorn GW: Electrocardiogram in Addison's disease, *Medicine* 30:43, 1951.

Section XII INFECTIOUS DISEASE

123 Bacteria

Madonna Fernández-Frackelton
Thomas W. Turbiak

DIPHTHERIA

Perspective

History In the fifth century BC, Hippocrates described a disease characterized by sore throat, membrane formation, and death through suffocation. In 1826 the French physician Bretonneau named the condition "diphtherite," from the Greek word for "leather," because the membrane resembled leather.[1] Klebs observed the *Corynebacterium diphtheriae* microorganism on smears obtained from patients' membranes in 1883, and 1 year later Loeffler isolated *Corynebacterium* organisms in pure cultures. Loeffler subsequently demonstrated that diphtheria was a localized infection and postulated that its systemic effects were caused by an elaborated toxin.

In 1890 Behring and Kitasato first demonstrated diphtheria immunization. One year later they administered the first dose of antitoxin to a human with diphtheria. Schick developed the skin test for diphtheria immunity in 1913. During the 1930s and 1940s, toxoid immunization (formalin and heat-treated toxin) was routinely used. In the 1950s Freeman found that only bacteria infected with the B-phage produced toxin. Subsequent studies elucidate the toxin genome and the mechanism of toxin activity at the cellular level.[1]

Epidemiology *C. diphtheriae* is spread primarily by person-to-person contact via nasopharyngeal secretions or by direct contact with skin lesion exudate. Transmission is associated with crowded indoor living conditions. Fomites and foods have been implicated but probably do not represent a major route of transmission. Humans are the only known reservoir for *C. diphtheriae* and may transmit the infection while actively ill, as asymptomatic carriers, or in the convalescent stage after an acute infection.[1]

Immunization against diphtheria is highly effective. Before widespread immunization programs began in the United States, the incidence of diphtheria was well in excess of 100 cases/100,000 population. By 1988 the Centers for Disease Control and Prevention (CDC) reported only several cases per year nationwide. When diphtheria had a high incidence, it most often affected children; currently, the sporadic cases include adults, many of whom are not adequately immunized. Patients who have received three or more doses of toxoid have a lower death rate than unimmunized persons.[2]

Between 1991 and 1996 more than 145,000 cases of diphtheria and 4000 deaths were reported in the Newly Independent States of the Former Soviet Union (NISFSU). This marked the first large-scale epidemic of diphtheria in an industrialized country in three decades. Factors contributing to this outbreak include decreased childhood immunizations, a large population of susceptible adults, poor socioeconomic conditions, and high population movement.[3] Three urban outbreaks of predominantly cutaneous diphtheria occurred in Seattle between 1972 and 1982 among a population of urban alcohol abusers. Outbreaks are associated with poor hygiene, crowding, season, underlying skin disease, contaminated fomites, pyoderma, and the appearance of new *C. diphtheriae* strains.[1]

A substantial portion of the U.S. population is not adequately protected against diphtheria, and most recent outbreaks in the United States have occurred in unimmunized or underimmunized adults in urban and poor rural areas.[1,4] Even in industrialized nations where childhood vaccination rates are high, more than 50% of adults older than age 40 lack protective antibodies.[5] In the prevaccine era, 80% of people acquired natural immunity against diphtheria by age 15 and recurrent exposure to the toxigenic strains of the bacteria acted as a booster. Because childhood immunization nearly eliminates the toxigenic strains in a given population, adult immunity wanes; thus a high number of adults in industrialized nations are susceptible to diphtheria.[5]

The World Health Organization reports a decreasing incidence of diphtheria that is attributed to vaccination. Diphtheria is still endemic in Africa, Asia, Eastern Europe (Poland and NISFSU), Central America, and South America.[6] The ease of international travel and the recent epidemic of diphtheria in eastern Europe underscore the importance of aggressively continuing childhood immunizations and reimmunization of adults.

Etiology Diphtheria is caused by *C. diphtheriae,* an unencapsulated, club-shaped gram-positive bacillus named for its shape ("korynee" for club) and for its characteristic clinical appearance ("diphtheria" for "hide," a reference to the leatherlike appearance of the membrane). When viewed on stained smears, the bacteria look like Oriental characters.[1]

Principles of Disease

Localized infection by *C. diphtheriae* occurs at various sites of the respiratory tract or the skin. Respiratory tract diphtheria includes faucial (pharyngeal or tonsillar), nasal, and laryngeal (tracheobronchial) types, named for the primary location. Cutaneous diphtheria may be a primary skin infection or may occur as a secondary infection of a preexisting wound.

The *C. diphtheriae* bacterium produces an exotoxin that contributes to formation of the diphtheritic membrane; the toxin is transported via the circulation to other parts of the body, where its effects are manifested.[7] The degree of toxicity depends on the location and extent of membrane formation. Pharyngeal diphtheria generally has the greatest toxicity and cutaneous diphtheria the least toxicity.

The diphtheritic membrane—composed of leukocytes, erythrocytes, fibrin, epithelial cells, and bacteria—forms as a result of necrosis caused by the local effect of the exotoxin. The membrane begins with localized erythema that progresses to grayish-white patches, which then coalesce. The membrane is accompanied by surrounding edema and cervical adenitis. The initial white, filmy appearance changes to a thick, grayish-black membrane with sharply defined borders. This membrane is adherent, and bleeding occurs if removal is attempted.[1]

The *C. diphtheriae* exotoxin is a protein with a molecular weight of 62,000 produced by bacterial strains lysogenized by the Corynephage B Tox+.[7] The exotoxin inhibits protein synthesis in the cell, and circulating exotoxin most profoundly affects the nervous system, heart, and kidneys.[1]

Systemic effects of diphtheria are caused by the exotoxin's action on the cardiovascular and nervous systems. The exotoxin's disruption of cellular protein synthesis produces a peripheral neuropathy manifested by muscle weakness. About 20% of all patients with symptomatic respiratory infection have polyneuritis, but 75% of patients with severe disease develop some form of neuropathy.[7] The muscles of the palate are usually the first to become paralyzed. Less commonly, the spinal cord, other cranial nerves, and peripheral nerves may be affected. Degenerative lesions develop in the dorsal root and ventral horn ganglia of the spinal cord and in the cranial nerve nuclei, whereas cortical cells are spared. Proximal muscle groups are affected first.[1] In severe cases, paralysis may develop in the first few days of illness. Generally the paralysis does not last more than 10 days, and complete function returns.[1]

The extent of cardiac problems correlates with the degree of infection and membrane formation at the local infection site. Signs of cardiac dysfunction usually appear 1 to 2 weeks after the onset of illness; the earlier in the course of the illness, the more severe the disease. Diphtheria toxin injures the heart muscle cells directly, producing myocarditis. Electrocardiographic (ECG) changes suggestive of myocarditis occur in up to two thirds of patients; clinical signs of myocarditis are less common (10% to 25%).[1]

Clinical Features

History and Physical Examination The incubation period of respiratory tract diphtheria is usually 2 to 4 days but may range from 1 to 8 days. The signs and symptoms are often indistinguishable from those of other upper respiratory tract infections. In a series of 676 patients, fever and sore throat were the most frequent presenting complaints (79% and 69%, respectively). Weakness (42%), dysphagia (35%), headache (20%), change of voice (15%), and loss of appetite (10%) were also common. Cough, shortness of breath, nasal discharge, and neck edema occurred in less than 10% of patients. Of note, however, shortness of breath and neck edema were present in approximately 40% of patients who died of the disease.[8]

Fever is usually low grade. Cervical adenopathy is present in approximately one third of patients, and a diphtheritic membrane is observed in more than half of all patients.[8]

In patients with faucial diphtheria, the extent of the membrane usually parallels the clinical toxicity. If the membrane is limited to the tonsils, the disease may be mild; if the membrane covers the entire pharynx, the onset of illness is usually abrupt and the severity high. Swelling of the cervical lymph nodes and infiltration of tissues of the neck may be so extensive that the patient has a "bull-neck" appearance. Patients with this form of "malignant diphtheria" usually have high fever, severe muscle weakness, vomiting, diarrhea, restlessness, and delirium. Death occurs from respiratory tract obstruction or cardiac failure resulting from myocarditis.

Nasal diphtheria presents with unilateral or bilateral serous or serosanguinous discharge from the anterior portions of the nares. The diphtheritic membrane may be visible. These patients do not usually develop constitutional symptoms. Treatment is important to prevent a persistent carrier state.

Laryngeal (tracheobronchial) diphtheria may begin in the larynx or spread downward from a more cephalad primary site. Patients may develop respiratory tract edema with subsequent upper airway obstruction.

Cutaneous diphtheria is reported mostly in the tropics. It occurs in temperate climates, alcohol abusers, and socioeconomically disadvantaged populations.[1] Patients with cutaneous diphtheria generally do not display systemic toxicity. The skin characteristically has an ulcer with a grayish membrane. Wounds from which *C. diphtheriae* is cultured are indistinguishable from other chronic skin conditions.

Complications The most serious complications of diphtheria are airway obstruction (resulting from membrane formation and edema), congestive heart failure, cardiac conduction disturbances, and muscle paralysis. Mortality in two recent large series ranged from 2.3% to 3% overall but was up to 7% in patients with myocarditis and 25.7% in patients with the toxic form of the disease (with neck swelling).[9]

Although systemic infection is rare, endocarditis, mycotic aneurysms, osteomyelitis, and septic arthritis have been described in immunocompromised hosts.[1]

Diagnostic Strategies

When diphtheria is the suspected pathogen, the laboratory should be notified because "routine cultures" will not identify *C. diphtheriae.* For respiratory diphtheria, throat or nasopharyngeal swabs should be obtained. If present, membranous material should be examined. For cutaneous disease, samples should be obtained from any skin lesions. Specimens should be transported to the laboratory immediately for rapid inoculation onto culture media.[10] The specimen must be collected before antibiotic therapy is initiated. The laboratory should culture the specimen on tellurite media. Immunofluorescent staining of a 4-hour culture may provide a rapid diagnosis,[1] but direct staining is frequently unreliable. Isolates of *C. diphtheriae* should be tested for virulence. Polymerase chain reaction (PCR) can be used to detect the diphtheria toxin structural gene.[10] A positive culture for group A β-hemolytic streptococcus does not exclude diphtheria because up to 30% of patients with diphtheria test positive for streptococcal infection. A leukocytosis is common. The platelet count may be decreased, and there may be proteinuria. A baseline ECG is of value in the event that myocarditis develops.

Differential Considerations

In the absence of a diphtheritic membrane, it may be difficult to differentiate diphtheria from many conditions, especially in the early phase of infection (Box 123-1). Generally, the diphtheritic membrane is darker, grayer, more fibrous, and more firmly attached to the underlying tissues than the other conditions that have a membrane-like appearance. Vincent's angina involves the gingivae, which are not affected in diphtheria. Acute epiglottitis generally has a much more rapid onset than diphtheria; indirect laryngoscopy clearly differentiates the two conditions.

Cutaneous diphtheria may have an appearance similar to that of other ulcerated acute and chronic skin conditions. Other primary conditions often coexist because cutaneous diphtheria may be a secondary infection.

Management

The goals of therapy are to limit the activity of already produced toxin and to eliminate future toxin production by terminating the growth of *C. diphtheriae*. Although the likelihood of a patient in the United States developing airway obstruction from diphtheria is remote, the management is identical to that for other forms of airway obstruction. Circulation may be compromised by dehydration caused by fever and decreased oral intake caused by neurologic impairment. The toxin's effect on the myocardium may result in congestive heart failure or dysrhythmias. No data support the use of steroids.[1]

Equine serum diphtheria antitoxin should be administered promptly after the clinical diagnosis of respiratory diphtheria. Antitoxin can be obtained by contacting the CDC. The size and location of the membrane, the duration of illness, and the patient's overall degree of toxicity determine the dosage of antitoxin. The Committee on Infectious Diseases of the American Academy of Pediatrics (AAP) recommends 20,000 to 40,000 U for pharyngeal or laryngeal involvement of 48 hours' duration, 40,000 to 60,000 U for nasopharyngeal lesions, and 80,000 to 100,000 U for extensive disease of 3 or more days' duration or for diffuse swelling of the neck.[11] After conjunctival or intradermal sensitivity skin testing, the antitoxin is administered intravenously (IV). If the patient exhibits sensitivity to the antitoxin, desensitization should be performed. Active immunization against diphtheria should also be initiated because clinical infection does not necessarily confer immunity.[11]

In addition to antitoxin therapy, antibiotics should be administered for 14 days. Erythromycin, 40 to 50 mg/kg/day (up to 2 g) IV or orally in divided doses; intramuscular (IM) aqueous crystalline penicillin, 100,000 to 150,000 U/kg/day in four divided doses; or procaine penicillin, 25,000 to 50,000 U/kg/day in two divided doses for 14 days given IM every 12 hours is acceptable.[11] More treatment failures are reported with penicillin than with erythromycin. The newer macrolides, azithromycin and clarithromycin, have similar activity to erythromycin in vitro and may encourage better compliance. These agents, however, have not been adequately tested in this setting. An equivalent daily oral therapy may be substituted when the patient is able to swallow. Three negative cultures should be documented after treatment.[11]

Vigorous cleansing of the lesion and a course of antibiotics are recommended for cutaneous diphtheria. Administration of antitoxin for cutaneous infection is of questionable value; however, some experts recommend 20,000 to 40,000 U of antitoxin.[11]

Carriers of *C. diphtheriae* should receive oral penicillin G or erythromycin for 7 days or IM benzathine penicillin G (600,000 U for those less than 30 kg and 1,200,000 units for those over 30 kg). In addition, active immunization should be provided for the unimmunized and partially immunized carriers. At least 2 weeks after therapy is completed, cultures should be obtained. If the cultures are positive, 10 additional days of erythromycin therapy is recommended.[11]

Individuals who have been in close contact with the patient should have cultures taken and be kept under surveillance for 7 days. Previously immunized close contacts should receive a booster of diphtheria toxoid if the last booster was more than 5 years earlier. (The booster should be diphtheria, tetanus, and pertussis [DTP], diphtheria-tetanus [DT], or tetanus-diphtheria with a lower dose of diphtheria toxoid [Td] as appropriate for age according to the recommended immunization schedule.) Close contacts who are not immunized or whose immunization status is unknown should receive the same antimicrobial therapy as carriers (as previously described), should have cultures taken before and after therapy, and should have active immunization initiated. Close contacts who cannot be kept under surveillance should receive benzathine penicillin IM (to ensure compliance) and a diphtheria toxoid booster (as appropriate for age and

Box 123-1 Differential Diagnosis of Respiratory Diphtheria

Streptococcal or viral pharyngitis
Tonsillitis
Vincent's angina
Acute epiglottitis
Mononucleosis
Laryngitis
Bronchitis
Tracheitis
Monilial infection
Rhinitis

immunization history). Some practitioners treat this group with 5000 to 10,000 U antitoxin IM (at a site separate from the toxoid booster) after sensitivity testing. This is generally not recommended, however, because of the risk of horse serum allergy.[11]

A universal program of primary immunization along with regular diphtheria boosters every 10 years is the most effective control measure for diphtheria. For this reason, EDs should routinely administer diphtheria toxoid along with tetanus toxoid for wound management.

A patient with clinically suspected or proven diphtheria should be isolated and hospitalized. Close observation for progression of the disease (airway, cardiac, or neurologic problems) is recommended. Close contacts of the patient need to be located and treated. Staff members should also review their own immunization status and the degree of patient contact.

PERTUSSIS

Perspective

History *Pertussis* means "violent cough," which is the hallmark of the disease. It is also called *whooping cough* because of the progressive, repetitive, and severe episodes of coughing that are followed by a forceful inspiration, which create the characteristic whooping sound. Pertussis has been described since 1500. In the prevaccination era, pertussis was responsible for more infant deaths than measles, scarlet fever, diphtheria, and poliomyelitis combined.[12] The organism was identified in 1906 by Bordet and Gengon.[13] A vaccine was developed in the 1940s. Although pertussis still remains a significant cause of morbidity and mortality, worldwide vaccination programs have decreased the overall incidence of the disease.[14]

Epidemiology Pertussis remains prevalent worldwide. In the United States, pertussis rates have been steadily rising and appear to have peaked in 1996.[14,15] Growth of a susceptible adult population may be the primary contributing factor. Also, a decreased acceptance of the vaccine occurred when a 1991 report found evidence of a causal relationship between the whole-cell pertussis vaccine and acute encephalopathy.[16] The acellular pertussis vaccine has been approved in the United States since 1991 and is now the recommended vaccine.

Although pertussis can occur at any age, it is predominantly a pediatric illness. The age-specific attack rates are highest in children younger than 1 year of age. The incidence of pertussis has been increasing in all age groups, and the greatest percentage increase is occurring in people 15 years of age or older. The attack rate, morbidity, and mortality is greater in women than men for unclear reasons.[13] There appears to be a seasonal variation; 50% of cases in the United States occur from June through September.

The incubation period of pertussis is approximately 7 to 10 days, although the time from exposure to the onset of illness may range from less than 1 week to more than 3 weeks.[15] Pertussis is very contagious. From 50% to 100% of susceptible people develop pertussis when exposed to a symptomatic household member.[13] Transmission is by exposure of airborne droplet particles from infected people. Neither vaccination against pertussis nor natural immunity from disease produces lifelong protection. Attack rates are greater than 50% in adults exposed 12 years after completion of a vaccination series.

Etiology Pertussis is caused by organisms of the *Bordetella* genus, which are nonmotile, small, gram-negative coccobacilli that appear singly or in pairs. There are four species of this genus. *B. pertussis* and *B. parapertussis* are responsible for disease in humans. *B. bronchiseptica* causes illness in animals, including kennel cough, and rarely may cause pertussis in immunocompromised humans. *B. avium* causes turkey coryza but is not known to infect humans.[13]

Principles of Disease

The *Bordetella* organism adheres to ciliated respiratory epithelial cells. Although *B. pertussis* does not invade beyond the layer of epithelium in the respiratory tract and is almost never recovered in the bloodstream, it does produce toxins that act locally and systemically. These toxins include pertussis toxin, dermonecrotic toxin, adenylate cyclase toxin, tracheal cytotoxin, and endotoxin.[17]

Local tissue damage consists of inflammatory changes of the mucosal lining of the respiratory tract, primarily congestion and cellular infiltration with lymphocytes and granulocytes. As the infection progresses, secondary pneumonia or otitis media may occur. Systemic effects of the toxins include sensitization to histamine and increased secretion of insulin.[17]

Clinical Features

History and Physical Examination Pertussis exists in three distinct sequential clinical stages: the *catarrhal phase,* the *paroxysmal phase,* and the *convalescent phase.*[18] The catarrhal phase begins after an incubation period of approximately 7 to 10 days. Symptoms are indistinguishable from those of a nonspecific upper respiratory tract infection with cough, low-grade fever, rhinitis, and anorexia. During this stage of illness, patients are usually not diagnosed as having pertussis. Infectivity is greatest during the catarrhal phase, which lasts approximately 1 to 2 weeks.

The paroxysmal phase begins as the cough increases and the fever subsides. The frequent paroxysms of coughing occur 40 to 50 times per day. The patient coughs repeatedly in short exhalations. After 10 to 15 coughs, the patient inhales forcefully. The single, sudden, forceful inhalation produces the whoop. Many patients never develop this characteristic whoop. During the paroxysm of coughing, the patient may exhibit cyanosis, bulging of the eyes, protrusion of the tongue, salivation, and lacrimation. After the inspiratory gasp, the patient may choke, vomit, or become briefly apneic. Infants may be physically exhausted after a typical paroxysm. Between episodes of coughing, patients do not appear acutely ill. This phase subsides after 2 to 4 weeks.

The convalescent phase is characterized by a residual cough that lasts for several weeks to months. Paroxysms of coughing may be triggered by an unrelated upper respiratory infection or by exposure to a respiratory irritant. This recurrence of coughing does not represent recurrence of pertussis infection.

Atypical presentations may occur in young infants who have cough, nasal congestion, apnea cyanotic episodes, bradycardia, and tachypnea.[12] Older children and adults who have partial protection from vaccination (or previous illness) may have long-lasting intractable dry cough that is frequently misdiagnosed as bronchitis.[13,19]

Tachypnea is variably present and may be related to the degree of pulmonary involvement. Low-grade fever is common during the catarrhal phase. The presence of fever during other stages of illness suggests secondary infection. Conjunctival injection and rhinorrhea occur during the catarrhal phase. Chest examination may reveal rhonchi or clear lung fields; the presence of rales suggests pneumonia.

Complications The major complications of pertussis are superinfection with pneumonia, central nervous system (CNS) sequelae, otitis media, and complications related to the paroxysm of coughing.[19]

Pneumonia complicating pertussis is a leading cause of death, especially in infants and young children.[13] Aspiration of gastric contents and respiratory secretions may occur during the paroxysm of coughing, whooping, and vomiting. Secondary pulmonary infection may also be a consequence of decreased respiratory tract clearance related to the actions of the *Bordetella* organism and toxins on bronchial and lung mucosa. Organisms causing pneumonia as a complication of pertussis include *Streptococcus pneumoniae, S. pyogenes, Haemophilus influenzae,* and *Staphylococcus aureus.* Viral superinfections (respiratory syncytial virus, cytomegalovirus, and adenoviral) can also complicate pertussis infections. A fever should alert the physician to a possible superinfection.

CNS complications include seizures (3%), encephalopathy (0.9%), and intracerebral hemorrhage.[13] The mechanisms may include hypoxia, a toxin, or secondary infection by neurotropic viruses. CNS hemorrhages may occur as a consequence of the increased cerebral vascular pressures generated during the paroxysm of coughing and whooping. Sudden increases in intrathoracic and intraabdominal pressures can cause a multiplicity of other complicating conditions (Box 123-2).

Bradycardia, hypotension, and cardiac arrest can occur in neonates and young infants with pertussis[19]; intensive care monitoring is recommended for these patients.

Diagnostic Strategies

Pertussis is often inaccurately diagnosed because of a lack of knowledge of the disease, atypical presentation of illness, and an overestimation of the degree of protection provided by vaccination.[15] The diagnosis should be considered in any patient with prolonged cough with paroxysms, whoops, or posttussive vomiting. Up to 25% of adults with prolonged cough in the United States have serologic evidence of pertussis.[20]

Ancillary studies are of limited value in the ED. During the paroxysmal phase a marked leukocytosis is often present, with a white blood cell (WBC) count of 25,000 to 50,000/mm^3 and a characteristic lymphocytosis. Adults with pertussis frequently do not have the characteristic elevated WBC count with lymphocytosis, and infants and immunocompromised hosts may not be able to mount this response.[19] The chest radiograph may show peribronchial thickening, atelectasis, or pulmonary consolidation.[13]

Laboratory confirmation of diagnosis is made by nasopharyngeal culture; cough specimens and throat swabs are not adequate. The *Bordetella* organism is fastidious, and isolation requires Bordet-Gengou medium to which antibiotics have been added (to reduce overgrowth of competing bacteria) for up to 7 days. A synthetic culture medium is also available. Even under ideal laboratory conditions, only 80% of suspected cases are culture positive. Direct fluorescent antibody techniques are available to identify *B. pertussis* in nasopharyngeal specimens and are a particularly useful screening tool in outbreak investigation.[13]

Adults generally come to medical attention late in the disease, and cultures are rarely positive (3.6%). PCR is much more likely to identify the organism (38.1% of cases) but is not widely available. Serologic testing may also be useful in the future but is generally only available in the research laboratory.[20]

Differential Considerations

The differential diagnosis includes acute viral upper respiratory tract infections, various pneumonias, bronchiolitis, cystic fibrosis, tuberculosis, exacerbation of chronic obstructive pulmonary disease, and foreign bodies of the respiratory tract. The marked leukocytosis may suggest the diagnosis of leukemia.

Management

Acute Treatment The most important aspects of the treatment of acute illness are supportive oxygenation, suctioning, maintenance of hydration and nutrition, and avoidance of respiratory irritants. All severely ill patients and any child younger than 1 year of age should be hospitalized.[18] Neonates with pertussis should be admitted to an intensive care unit.[19] Any patient with suspected pertussis and associated pneumonia, hypoxia, or CNS complications or those experiencing severe paroxysms should also be admitted.

Antibiotics are indicated but may not alter the severity or duration of illness when initiated after the catarrhal phase of illness. Erythromycin is the drug of choice at 50 mg/kg/day (maximum dose 2 g) in four divided doses for 14 days.[12,19] The antibiotic reduces infectivity and carriage. Corticosteroids, especially in infants, may reduce the severity and course of illness, and β_2-adrenergic agonists may reduce the frequency and severity of the paroxysmal coughing episodes.[19] Early clinical trials with pertussis immune globulin have shown significant improvement in lymphocytosis and paroxysmal coughing in infants. This may be a useful

Box 123-2 Pertussis Complications

- Periorbital edema
- Subconjunctival hemorrhage
- Petechiae
- Epistaxis
- Hemoptysis
- Subcutaneous emphysema
- Pneumothorax
- Pneumomediastinum
- Diaphragmatic rupture
- Umbilical and inguinal hernias
- Rectal prolapse

treatment for very ill patients in the future.[21] Standard cough suppressants and antihistamines are ineffective.[13]

Patients without significant complications may be managed as outpatients and advised of the potential complications.[18] The patient should be strictly isolated for 7 days and erythromycin prescribed to limit the spread of infection. Erythromycin should also be prescribed for any unimmunized person or partially immunized infant with a history of significant exposure to the index case.[19,20] Adults who will come in close contact with susceptible children should also take erythromycin prophylaxis.[22]

Vaccination

Pertussis vaccine is available as a whole-cell vaccine and as an acellular vaccine. Both are distributed in combination with diphtheria and tetanus toxoids as DPT or diphtheria, tetanus, and acellular pertussis (DTaP). The acellular pertussis vaccines contain inactivated pertussis toxin and may contain one or more other bacterial components.[23] Adverse reactions occur more commonly from the pertussis component of the DPT vaccine than from any of the other vaccines commonly administered to children. Most recipients develop fever, irritability, behavioral changes, and local discomfort at the site of inoculation. Moderately severe reactions are uncommon but include fever of 40° C or greater, persistent crying, high-pitched crying, and seizures. Severe neurologic complications (prolonged seizures, encephalopathy) occur rarely but led to the decreased use of the whole-cell form of the vaccine and the development of DTaP. Both vaccines are highly effective; however, the new acellular vaccine has fewer side effects than the older whole-cell vaccine. DTaP has replaced DPT for childhood immunizations, and whole-cell pertussis vaccines are recommended only for use in the United States when the acellular vaccine is not available.[13,15,17]

Pertussis immunity wanes significantly 10 years after immunization, causing an increasing incidence of the disease in people over 15 years of age. The acellular pertussis vaccine is safe and effective in adolescents and adults, but routine booster immunization is not currently recommended. It may be useful for the control of pertussis during outbreaks and in patients at high risk for exposure to pertussis (parents, health care workers, and child care workers); more data are needed to define the impact of pertussis in these groups.[17]

TETANUS

Perspective

History Tetanus is a toxin-mediated disease characterized by severe uncontrolled skeletal muscle spasms. The major risk to life is related to spasms of the muscles of respiration, which can lead to hypoxia and death. Despite a progressive decrease in the number of cases of tetanus in the United States, the mortality rate among unimmunized and inadequately immunized individuals remains high.

Generalized tetanus is a spectacular disease that has inspired the descriptive powers of physicians since the early Greeks. Hippocrates described a case as follows[24]:

> The master of a large ship smashed the index finger of his right hand with the anchor. Seven days later, a somewhat foul discharge appeared; then trouble with his tongue—he complained he could not speak properly. The presence of tetanus was diagnosed, his jaws became pressed together, his teeth were locked, then symptoms appeared in his neck: on the third day opisthotonus appeared with sweating. Six days after the diagnosis was made, he died.

The modern history of tetanus is a case study in medical science and in the development of immunizations.[24] In 1884 Carle and Rattone produced tetanus in rabbits by injecting material from an acne pustule that came from an infected human. In the same year, Nicolaier showed that bacteria were the causative agents by producing tetanus in animals from injection of soil samples. In 1889 Kitasato obtained pure cultures of spore-forming bacteria that caused tetanus when introduced into animals. One year later, Faber proved that tetanus was a toxin-mediated disease when he induced the illness by injecting animals with bacteria-free filtrates of *Clostridium tetani* cultures. The discovery of antitoxin in immune animals by Behring and Kitasato in 1890 led to the development of commercial antitoxin.[25]

Epidemiology *C. tetani* bacteria and spores are ubiquitous, and tetanus is endemic throughout the world. It is more common in warm, damp climates and relatively rare in cold regions. Most cases occur in developing countries, especially in Africa, Asia, and South America. The worldwide incidence is estimated to be 500,000 to 1 million cases annually, with a mortality rate of 45%.[26,27] Most cases in economically deprived areas occur in neonates and children and are related to inadequate immunization standards and poor hygiene.[25]

In the United States, the incidence of tetanus has steadily declined from 0.2 to 0.15 cases/1 million population. From 1995 to 1997, 124 cases were reported, giving an annual average of 41 cases; this is the lowest annual average since national tetanus surveillance began in 1947 (Figure 123-1).[28] Approximately 60% of patients are age 20 to 59, and only one case of neonatal tetanus was reported. Case fatality is much higher for patients more than 60 years of age (18%) compared with that for patients younger than 39 years of age (2.3%) (Figure 123-2).[28]

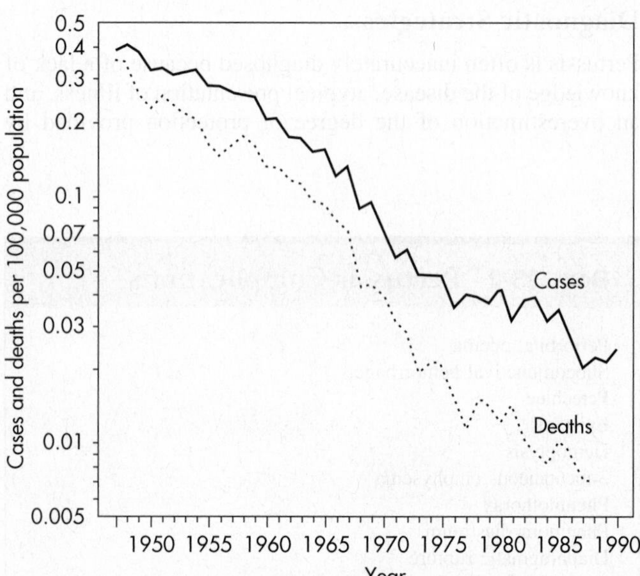

Figure 123-1. **Reported incidence of tetanus and tetanus-related deaths—United States, 1947 to 1997. *From* MMWR *47(SS-2):1-13, 1998.***

More than 70% of tetanus cases occur after an acute injury causes a break in the skin. The most common portals of entry for the organism are puncture wounds, lacerations, and abrasions. Chronic wounds such as skin ulcers, abscesses, or gangrene can also serve as sources of infection. Postoperative tetanus has been reported in patients who have undergone intestinal operations and abortions.[26] In these cases the source of bacteria may be endogenous because up to 10% of humans harbor *C. tetani* in the colon. The disease is also common in IV narcotic addicts, perhaps because of additives such as quinine, which lower the redox potential at the site of injection.[26] In 10% to 30% of cases, no wound or condition is identified that could have served as a portal of entry for the organism. Therefore lack of a wound does not exclude the diagnosis of tetanus.

Most cases of tetanus in the United States occur in individuals with no documented history of adequate immunization. Cases are reported in patients who have been fully vaccinated, but of those 16 patients from 1995 to 1997, no deaths occurred.[28] As tetanus vaccination of children has improved, older people have accounted for an increasing percentage of all cases.

Etiology *C. tetani* is an anaerobic, motile, spore-forming, gram-positive, slender, rod-shaped organism. The bacillus can form a single spherical terminal endospore that swells the end of the organism and produces a characteristic drumstick appearance. The ubiquitous organism is found in soil, dust, and the feces of animals and humans. The bacterium exists in its sporulative form in the environment. Vegetative forms are highly susceptible to heat and other adverse environmental conditions, but spores are hardy and can survive in soil for months to years. Spores are resistant to heating and chemical disinfectants. Only the vegetative forms produce neurotoxins.[26]

Principles of Disease

The development of clinical tetanus requires a portal of entry for the infecting spores because *C. tetani* is a noninvasive organism. Conditions that promote germination of the spores, growth of the organism, and toxin production must exist in the infected tissue in the immunologically susceptible host.[25]

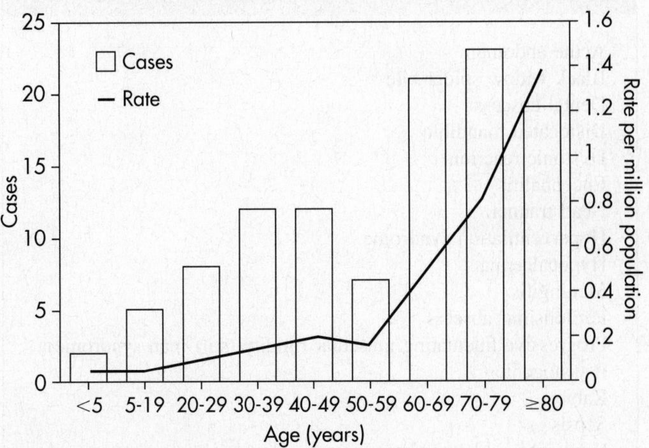

Figure 123-2. **Reported tetanus cases and incidence rates by age group—United States, 1995 to 1997.** ***From*** **MMWR** ***47(SS-2):1-13, 1998.***

Predisposing wound conditions include the presence of damaged or devitalized tissue, foreign bodies, or other bacteria. These conditions reduce the oxidation-reduction potential of the tissue and allow spores to revert to the vegetative form of the bacteria. In this state, the bacilli can produce the toxins that cause the clinical illness. Germination and replication of *C. tetani* can occur without clinical signs of a local wound infection. Adequate immunization and the presence of antibody protection prevent the growth of the organism at the site of entry.

C. tetani produces three exotoxins: tetanospasmin, tetanolysin, and nonconvulsive neurotoxin.[25] Tetanospasmin causes the symptoms and signs of clinical tetanus; tetanolysin and nonconvulsive neurotoxin are of no known clinical significance. Tetanospasmin travels from the site of infection by hematogenous and axonal spread to the spinal cord, brain, motor end plates of skeletal muscle, and sympathetic nervous system. This interferes with the release of inhibitory neurotransmitters and causes disinhibition of motor groups. This disinhibition results in excessive, uncontrolled muscle activity. Simultaneous spasm of agonist and antagonist muscle groups occurs. Tetanospasmin may also cause autonomic nervous system dysfunction by its effect on the brainstem and autonomic interneurons. The clinical manifestations include dysrhythmias and wide fluctuations in blood pressure.[29] The binding of the toxin at the synapse is irreversible. Recovery occurs at the neuromuscular junction only when a new axonal terminal is produced.[25]

Clinical Features

History and Physical Examination A history of injury is present in more than 70% of patients who present with tetanus. The majority of patients have inadequate immunization to tetanus. The incubation period for tetanus is generally from 3 to 14 days but can range from 1 day to several months.[25] A shorter incubation period is associated with a worse prognosis.[30] The duration of the incubation period is not useful in making the diagnosis of tetanus because many patients have no history of an antecedent wound. Four types of clinical tetanus have been defined: generalized, cephalic, localized, and neonatal.

Generalized tetanus is the fully developed state of skeletal muscle hypertonicity and is the most common and severe form of the disease.[25] Trismus is the presenting symptom in most patients and is caused by increased masseter muscle tone. Patients may complain of lockjaw and present to a dentist or oral surgeon. As the other facial muscles become involved, the characteristic sardonic smile (risus sardonicus) appears. Other early symptoms include irritability, weakness, myalgia, muscle cramps, dysphagia, hydrophobia, and drooling. The muscle rigidity increases as the disease progresses. The time from an initial symptom to the first muscle spasm is called the *onset period.* A shorter onset period is predictive of a poorer prognosis.

In the most severe form of tetanus, muscle rigidity becomes generalized and reflex muscle spasms may be precipitated by external stimuli (noise, light, touch) or occur spontaneously. Opisthotonos develops because posterior trunk and extremity muscles are stronger than anterior muscle groups. Spasm of laryngeal and respiratory muscles can lead to ventilatory failure and death. Autonomic dysfunction is manifested by tachycardia, hypertension, temperature elevation, cardiac dysrhythmias, vasoconstriction, and diaphoresis.

Throughout the course of these dramatic symptoms, the patient usually remains lucid.

The illness is progressive, with an increase in manifestations over the first 3 days, persistence of symptoms for an additional 5 to 7 days, and reduction of spasms after 10 days. If the patient survives, recovery is complete after 4 weeks or more.

Cephalic tetanus is manifested by trismus plus cranial nerve palsies.[26] Cephalic tetanus is rare, accounting for 1% to 3% of all tetanus cases. Most of these cases occur after facial trauma or otitis media. Patients develop trismus and palsies of cranial nerve III, IV, VII, IX, X, or XII ipsilateral to the site of local infection. The most commonly involved cranial nerve is the facial nerve (VII). The clinical course is variable. In one third of cases, resolution of symptoms is complete. Two thirds of these cases progress to generalized tetanus.

Localized tetanus is a form of the disease characterized by persistent muscle spasms in proximity to the site of inoculation. Symptoms may be mild or severe. Although local tetanus may progress to generalized disease, most cases do not. This form of illness may be present for weeks to months before resolution.

Neonatal tetanus is a form of generalized tetanus that occurs almost exclusively in underdeveloped countries, where maternal immunization is inadequate and contaminated material is used to cut and dress the umbilical cords. The incubation period is short, with symptoms beginning during the first week of life. Early clinical manifestations include irritability and poor sucking and swallowing.[24]

Complications Acute respiratory failure is the main cause of morbidity and mortality in tetanus. Asphyxia results from the hypertonicity of muscles of the upper airway and diaphragm. Inability to clear secretions can lead to atelectasis or bronchiolitis. Cardiovascular complications are related to hyperactivity of the sympathetic nervous system and include dysrhythmias, vasomotor instability, hypertension, tachycardia, myocarditis, and pulmonary edema.[25]

Muscle spasms produce subluxations and fractures of the spine, long bone fractures, and dislocations of the shoulder and temporomandibular joints. Rhabdomyolysis occasionally produces myoglobinuria and acute renal failure. Renal failure may also result from dehydration and sympathetic nervous system overactivity. Renal vein thrombosis is another cause of renal failure in neonatal tetanus.

Infection may occur in the initial inoculating wound or secondary to invasive treatment modalities. Hyperthermia is caused by muscle spasms and sympathetic hyperactivity. Stasis can lead to venous thrombosis and pulmonary embolism. Gastrointestinal (GI) complications include peptic ulcer, ileus, intestinal perforation, and constipation. The syndrome of inappropriate secretion of antidiuretic hormone occurs in a small number of patients. Hemolysis has also been reported.

The overall mortality rate for generalized tetanus ranges from zero to 50%. Mortality is a function of the previous immunization status, incubation period, severity of illness, age (with the greatest mortality at the extremes of life), underlying disease, and the sophistication of medical treatment available.[28,30] Death is a result of respiratory failure, dysrhythmia, pneumonia, pulmonary embolus, or secondary infections. Long-term complications in survivors are relatively few. The most common problem may be the psychologic trauma after recovery.[25]

Diagnostic Strategies

Because wound cultures for *C. tetani* are positive in only one third of cases, they are of limited value as a diagnostic tool. Tetanus is essentially a clinical diagnosis.[26,27] In 1990 the CDC adopted a clinical case definition for the public health surveillance of generalized tetanus: "acute onset of hypertonia or painful muscular contractions (usually of the muscles of the jaw and neck without other apparent medical cause as reported by a health care professional)."[28]

Lumbar puncture may be indicated to exclude meningitis when the diagnosis of tetanus is uncertain. A computed tomography scan is helpful in determining the presence of an intracranial pathologic condition. A serum calcium level may be needed to exclude the diagnosis of hypocalcemia. Electromyography may be useful if the diagnosis of cephalic or localized tetanus is in doubt.

Differential Considerations

Because the diagnosis of tetanus is clinically based, it is important to consider other more common conditions with clinical similarities to tetanus (Box 123-3). Trismus is most commonly caused by intraoral infections. These disorders can be excluded with careful history and physical examination of the oral cavity and teeth. Mandibular dislocation can be ruled out with appropriate radiographs of the mandible and temporomandibular joints. Dystonic reactions can be differentiated from tetanus by the medication history and the symptoms being alleviated by benztropine or diphenhydramine. Patients with encephalitis usually exhibit an altered sensorium. Meningitis can be excluded by examining the cerebrospinal fluid (CSF). Rabies must be considered when there are symptoms of brainstem dysfunction, including dysphagia and respiratory muscle dysfunction. A history of exposure to secretions of an infected animal is the most helpful historical point. In addition, rabies does not cause trismus.

Strychnine poisoning is similar to tetanus in that the patient develops opisthotonos while remaining awake.

Box 123-3 Differential Diagnosis of Tetanus

Acute abdomen
Black widow spider bite
Dental abscess
Dislocated mandible
Dystonic reaction
Encephalitis
Head trauma
Hyperventilation syndrome
Hypocalcemia
Meningitis
Peritonsillar abscess
Progressive fluctuating muscular rigidity (stiff-man syndrome)
Psychogenic
Rabies
Sepsis
Subarachnoid hemorrhage
Status epilepticus
Strychnine poisoning
Temporomandibular joint syndrome

Strychnine is suggested by a history of toxin ingestion and by muscle rigidity alternating with periods of relaxation. Also, trismus is a later finding. Treatment of the two conditions is similar, and toxicologic studies can confirm the presence of strychnine.

Cephalic tetanus is especially difficult to diagnose when the cranial nerve palsy precedes trismus. The differential diagnosis of cephalic tetanus also includes Bell's palsy, cranial nerve palsies, and facial cellulitis with facial nerve compression and ophthalmoplegia. The diagnosis of tetanus is made on clinical grounds. No other disease fully mimics classical generalized tetanus.

Management

Acute Treatment Four basic principles guide the treatment of tetanus: aggressive supportive care, administration of antitoxin, elimination of toxin production, and active immunization.[26] Cardiac and respiratory status should be monitored closely. An aggressive approach to airway support should be maintained. If any sign of airway compromise develops, the patient should be intubated.[25,31] All intubated patients should be considered for tracheostomy because reflex spasms may be less likely with a tracheostomy than with an endotracheal tube.

Patients should be handled gently to minimize reflex muscle spasm. Muscle spasms should be treated to maintain patient comfort and prevent complications. Benzodiazepines given IV as intermittent boluses or by continuous infusion reduce muscle spasms and are also sedatives and anxiolytics.[31] Large doses may be needed. If benzodiazepines are not effective in reducing the spasms, nondepolarizing neuromuscular blocking agents can be used. Pancuronium, atracurium, or vecuronium can be used for this purpose.[26] Patients remain lucid and must be sedated during neuromuscular blockade. Dantrolene is a direct muscle relaxant without CNS activity. It has been recommended as an adjunctive muscle relaxant in tetanus, but its exact role is not well defined. Barbiturates and chlorpromazine have also been recommended as muscle relaxants.

Autonomic instability requires monitoring and treatment. Sympathetic overactivity can be treated with combined α- and β-adrenergic agents such as labetalol. The use of β-agonists alone can lead to unopposed α-activity resulting in severe hypertension. If β-blockers are necessary, a short-acting agent such as esmolol should be used.[26] Bradydysrhythmia should be treated with temporary pacing instead of atropine or sympathomimetic drugs. Acute hypertension can be treated with a titratable agent with a short half-life, such as sodium nitroprusside. Magnesium sulfate has been recommended for treating symptoms of autonomic dysfunction in severe tetanus.[25] Narcotics may also be a useful adjunct in this situation. Continuous spinal anesthesia has been reported to be useful in treating severe tetanus associated with autonomic instability.[32] Intrathecal baclofen has been shown to decrease contractures, maintain respiratory drive, decrease the need for mechanical ventilation, and consequently decrease the mortality rate.[30,33]

Human tetanus immunoglobulin (TIG) and tetanus toxoid should be administered to all patients with suspected tetanus.[25] TIG does not neutralize toxin already present in the nervous system, nor does it treat any existent symptoms. TIG neutralizes any circulating extraneuronal toxin or toxin at the site of production and reduces the mortality rate. TIG should be administered as early as possible at a site separate from the toxoid. Dosage recommendations vary, with most authors advising the administration of 3000 to 6000 U TIG IM.[26] Some sources report equal effectiveness with doses of 500 U.[25] If the larger doses are used, the antitoxin should be given in divided doses, including administration of a portion of the dose proximal to the site of inoculation. Local injection of TIG into the wound is of no value. Protective antibody levels are achieved 48 to 72 hours after administration of TIG. Because the half-life of TIG is 25 days, repeat doses are not needed. The preparation of TIG available in the United States is not licensed for intrathecal administration, which is of no proven benefit.[34]

Toxin production is eliminated by treatment of *C. tetani* infection. Because surgical care and antibiotic use can cause a transient release of tetanospasmin, the EP should consider delaying these measures until after the antitoxin has been administered.[25,35] The wound should be debrided and cleansed, and foreign bodies should be removed. Penicillin, tetracycline, erythromycin, and metronidazole are all effective against *C. tetani.* Most references recommend penicillin G, 10 to 24 million U per day IV in divided doses in adults (for pediatrics, use 100,000 U/kg/day in divided doses) for 10 to 14 days. Doxycycline 100 mg IV every 12 hours is an alternative.[36] Metronidazole (500 mg orally every 6 hours) may have greater efficacy than penicillin.[37]

Aggressive intensive care can markedly reduce the mortality rate of this disease. When transfer is necessary, the patient with suspected airway or ventilatory compromise should be intubated. Cardiac dysrhythmias should be stabilized and acute alterations in blood pressure treated. Muscle spasms should be controlled to reduce the likelihood of further complications and to maintain patient comfort.[13,26]

Vaccination Tetanus immunity is often lacking in ED patients and is as low as 50% in U.S. patients older than 65 years of age.[38] Patient memory of the immunization history does not reliably correlate with an adequate immunization status. A significant percentage of elderly patients lack protective levels of tetanus antibody, and many of these patients fail to seroconvert after receiving tetanus boosters. Furthermore, poor compliance exists with published guidelines for tetanus immunoprophylaxis in wound care.[39]

Adults with uncertain histories of a complete primary immunization series should receive a primary series. To ensure adequate protection of an individual, it has been recommended that booster doses of Td be given routinely at mid-decade ages (e.g., 15 years, 25 years).[40] The standard vaccination program consists of a primary series of three tetanus toxoid doses, followed by booster doses every 10 years. Age-specific guidelines for tetanus prophylaxis have been developed by the Immunization Practices Advisory Committee and published by the CDC (Tables 123-1 to 123-3).[40]

Tetanus prophylaxis should be updated for all patients who come to the ED for management of a wound. Patients with an unknown or uncertain immunization status should be considered to have no previous tetanus immunization. Patients younger than 7 years of age should receive diphtheria-tetanus or DTaP. Patients 7 years of age or older should receive Td instead of DT because adverse reactions from larger doses of diphtheria toxoid are more common in older individuals.

After complete primary immunization has been accomplished, booster immunizations need to be given only every 10 years if wounds are clean and minor. Antibodies to

Table 123-1. Routine Diphtheria, Tetanus, and Pertussis Vaccination Schedule for Children <7 Years of Age—United States, 1997

Dose	Customary age	Age/interval	Product
Primary 1	2 months	6 wk or older	DTaP or DTP*
Primary 2	4 months	4-8 wk after first dose†	DTaP or DTP*
Primary 3	6 months	4-8 wk after second dose†	DTaP or DTP*
Primary 4	15 months	6-12 mo after third dose†	DTaP or DTP*
Booster	4-6 years, not needed if fourth vaccination administered after fourth birthday		DTaP or DTP*
Additional booster	Every 10 years after last dose		Td

Modified from MMWR 46(02):35-39, 1997.
*DTaP is preferred; DTP is an acceptable alternative.
†Prolonging the interval does not require restarting the series.

Table 123-2. Routine Diphtheria and Tetanus Vaccination Schedule Summary for Persons >7 Years of Age—United States, 1991

Dose	Age/interval	Product
Primary 1	First dose	Td
Primary 2	4-8 wk after first dose*	Td
Primary 3	6-12 mo after second dose*	Td
Booster	Every 10 yr after last dose	Td

Modified from *MMWR Morb Mortal Wkly Rep* 40(RR-10):1, 1991.
*Prolonging the interval does not require restarting series.

Table 123-3. Summary Guide to Tetanus Prophylaxis in Routine Wound Management, 1991

History of absorbed tetanus toxoid (doses)	Clean, minor wounds		All other wounds*	
	Td(†)	TIG	Td(†)	TIG
Unknown or < three	Yes	No	Yes	Yes
≥ Three(‡)	No(§)	No	No(‖)	No

Modified from *MMWR Morb Mortal Wkly Rep* 40(RR-10):1, 1991.
*Such as, but not limited to, wounds contaminated with dirt, feces, soil, and saliva; puncture wounds; avulsions; and wounds resulting from missiles, crushing, burns, and frostbite.
†For children <7 years old; DPT (DT, if pertussis vaccine is contraindicated) is preferred to tetanus toxoid alone. For persons ≥7 years of age, Td is preferred to tetanus toxoid alone.
‡If only three doses of *fluid* toxoid have been received, then a fourth dose of toxoid, preferably an adsorbed toxoid, should be given.
§Yes, if >10 years since last dose.
‖Yes, if >5 years since last dose. (More frequent boosters are not needed and can accentuate side effects.)

antitoxin develop rapidly in people who have previously received at least two doses of tetanus toxoid. The speed of antibody response after revaccination may be slower with increasing intervals from the time of primary vaccination.[40] This finding may explain how rare cases of tetanus have occurred despite primary vaccination and emergency booster immunizations.

For inadequately immunized patients of any age, referral should be made to ensure that the patient receives the remainder of the immunizations required. TIG is recommended for unimmunized patients with wounds at high risk for tetanus. The dose of TIG in wound prophylaxis is 250 U IM. When tetanus toxoid and TIG are given concurrently, separate injection sites should be used. The only contraindication to tetanus and diphtheria toxoids is a history of a neurologic or severe hypersensitivity reaction after a previous dose. Adverse reactions to tetanus toxoid and tetanus-diphtheria toxoids occur commonly and may be the result of the preservative thiomersal. The most common side effects are minor: local swelling, pain, erythema, pleuritis, fever, nausea, vomiting, malaise, and nonspecific rash.[41] Serious anaphylactic reactions rarely occur. Local reactions do not preclude future use of toxoid. If a patient who requires immunoprophylaxis gives a history suggestive of a neurologic or severe anaphylactic reaction after a previous dose, only TIG should be administered. This will protect the patient from developing tetanus from the present injury but will not confer active immunity. Such patients should be referred to an allergist for measurement of antibody levels and antitoxin desensitization and immunization if needed.[42] No evidence exists that tetanus or diphtheria toxoids are teratogenic. TIG is not contraindicated in pregnancy.

BOTULISM

PERSPECTIVE

History Botulism is a rare, life-threatening paralytic illness caused by neurotoxins produced by *Clostridium botulinum.* The disease usually occurs in one of five forms: food-borne botulism, infant botulism, wound botulism, unclassified botulism, and inadvertent botulism.

Botulism received its name from *botulus,* Latin for sausage, because many of the early cases resulted from ingestion of contaminated sausages. Kerner studied a number of outbreaks of botulism in Germany in the nineteenth century, and for a time, botulism was known as *Kerner's disease.* Van Ermengem investigated an epidemic of botulism in a group of musicians at a funeral in 1896 in Belgium. He isolated the organism, discovered the toxin, and determined that the illness is toxin mediated.[43]

The disease first received attention in the United States during the World War I era, when housewives were encouraged to preserve fruits and vegetables. The recommended methods for home canning did not destroy the spores of *C. botulinum.* Because these foods were often not adequately heated, epidemics of botulism occurred. Meyer described the circumstances favoring toxin production and the conditions necessary to destroy spores during food processing. In 1950 the CDC began surveillance of this disease. In 1976 Pickett reported the syndrome of infant botulism, which is now the most common form of the illness.[44]

Epidemiology Fewer than 100 cases of botulism are reported in the United States annually.[45,46] Of these, one third are food-borne botulism and two thirds are infant botulism.[43]

C. botulinum spores are found throughout the United States. The highest incidences of botulism are reported from Alaska, Washington, Oregon, and California. Toxin type A and B spores are widely distributed in soil. Type A is more prevalent west of the Mississippi, and type B is more common in the eastern states.[47]

Toxin type E spores are found in mud and sand at the bottom of oceans in northern latitudes, accounting for the prevalence of type E toxin in cases of fish-borne botulism. Typical food-borne botulism results from the ingestion of preformed heat-labile toxin, not the ingestion of either spores or the live bacteria. Food-borne botulism usually results from exposure to home-canned foods that are inadequately preserved and undercooked. Occasionally, larger outbreaks occur after the ingestion of contaminated food at restaurants or from commercial sources. Restaurant and commercial food epidemics, although less common, have the potential of causing major epidemics. A variety of preserved foods has been implicated, and botulism has also been reported to result from ingestion of improperly prepared and stored fresh foods.[45-47]

Infant botulism is the most common form of the illness. It occurs in children younger than 1 year of age. Most cases occur from 1 week to 11 months of age, with a peak incidence at 2 to 4 months. No sex or racial preference is described. In contradistinction to food-borne botulism in adults, infant botulism is caused by the ingestion of spores with in vivo production of toxin. Honey and, to a lesser extent, corn syrup have been implicated as sources of *C. botulinum* spores that cause infant botulism.[48] For this reason it has been recommended to avoid feeding honey to any child under 12 months of age.

The environment (dust, soil) probably accounts for the major source of ingested botulinum spores. Type A and B botulinum toxins have been responsible for all infant cases. Some investigators have explored a possible relationship between infant botulism and the sudden infant death syndrome,[44] but a 10-year prospective study of 248 infants diagnosed with sudden infant death syndrome revealed no cases attributable to *C. botulinum.*[49]

Wound botulism once accounted for approximately one case per year, but the increased use of black tar heroin has resulted in a dramatic increase in cases. In 1994, 11 of the 53 adult botulism cases reported to the CDC were wound botulism. All occurred among injection drug users in California.[50] Toxin types A and B are the causative agents.

Unclassified, or hidden botulism, is a rare illness. Between 1976 and 1984, 31 cases were reported to the CDC. Toxin types A, B, and F were identified in these patients. This form may be analogous to infant botulism in which the *Clostridium* bacterium produces its toxin in vivo.[47] Patients with compromise of gastric acidity, disturbances of GI motility, or abnormal GI bacterial flora may be susceptible to in vivo production of botulinum toxin.[44] The mortality rate is highest in this form of botulism.

Inadvertent botulism is an iatrogenic form of botulism that occurs in patients who have been treated with injections of botulinum toxin for dystonic and other movement disorders.[44]

The potential exists for botulinum toxin to be used as an offensive biologic weapon. It is highly potent and easy to produce. In 1995, Iraq revealed that, during the Gulf War, it had 11,200 L of botulinum toxin loaded into SCUD missile warheads. The Aum Shinrikyo, responsible for the 1995 sarin attack on the Tokyo subway, had also produced botulinum toxin.[47]

Etiology *C. botulinum* is a strictly anaerobic, gram-positive, rod-shaped organism. It forms spores that germinate under certain environmental conditions. The bacteria may then produce a potent exotoxin that is responsible for the disease.[51] Seven strains of *C. botulinum* exist; five of these (A, B, E, F, and G) are known to be responsible for human disease. Most human cases are caused by strains A, B, and E.

Each strain of *C. botulinum* produces a specific toxin type. Botulinum toxins are the most potent biologic toxins known. They are 15,000 to 100,000 times more toxic than sarin, the organophosphate used in the Tokyo subway terrorist attack.[47] Doses as small as 0.05 to 0.1 μg can cause death in humans.[44] The toxins are heat labile. Heating at 100° C for 10 minutes or 80° C for 30 minutes will destroy any botulism toxin. Consequently, heating toxin-contaminated food just before ingestion will prevent food-borne botulism. Spores are highly heat resistant and can survive at a temperature of 120° C.[51]

Principles of Disease

Botulism results from the action of the neurotoxin produced by *C. botulinum.* The neurotoxin blocks presynaptic acetylcholine release. Food-borne botulism results from ingesting food that contains preformed toxin. Toxin-contaminated food may have normal appearance and taste or exhibit signs of food spoilage caused by proteolytic enzymes produced by types A and B strains. Because of the tremendous potency of the toxin, one taste can provide enough toxin to cause clinical illness. Digestive enzymes do not destroy preformed toxin.[51]

Despite the ubiquitous nature of botulinum spores, the incidence of disease is low. This is explained by the cascade of requirements for toxin production and action within the human body. For optimal growth, *C. botulinum* requires an acidic environment, and a lack of competition from other bacteria.[51]

After toxin has entered the body, three steps must occur before clinical illness can occur.[43] First, the toxin must be transported from the GI tract or wound to the neuron. Second, the toxin must bind to the presynaptic nerve membrane and become internalized within the neuron. Finally, the toxin must block the release of acetylcholine, resulting in neuromuscular blockade. This interference with neurotransmission occurs predominantly at the cholinergic synapses of the cranial nerves, autonomic nerves, and neuromuscular junction. Clinically, cranial nerve palsies, parasympathetic blockade, and a descending, flaccid paralysis occur.

Clinical Features

History and Physical Examination *Food-borne botulism* is the prototype for understanding the clinical signs and symptoms of all forms of botulism. Symptoms begin approximately 18 to 36 hours (range, 2 hours to 14 days) after the ingestion of toxin-containing food.[51] A shorter incubation period is associated with a more severe form of illness. Early symptoms include weakness, malaise, lightheadedness, nausea, vomiting, and constipation. These symptoms are generally not severe and occur in fewer than half of the patients.

Neurologic symptoms may begin at the same time or be delayed in onset for several days. The cranial nerves are first affected. Patients experience diplopia, blurred vision, and photophobia. Dysphonia, dysphagia, and dysarthria occur because bulbar nerves are involved.[43,44] Vertigo is also a common symptom. Next, a symmetric descending muscular weakness occurs, involving the upper and lower extremities and the muscles of respiration.[44] Blockade of the cholinergic fibers of the autonomic nervous system leads to a variety of symptoms. Decreased salivation causes a dry mouth, which may be so severe that the patient complains of a painful tongue and sore throat. GI symptoms from an ileus and urinary retention may also occur. In one ED series of patients with food-borne botulism, all had at least three of the following four symptoms: weakness, dry mouth, double vision, and difficulty speaking. This constellation of symptoms should prompt the EP to inquire about the ingestion of home-canned or improperly prepared food or the presence of similar symptoms in family members or friends.

The patient with botulism is usually alert and is afebrile unless secondary infection is present. Postural hypotension may be present. Ocular signs are prominent and include ptosis, extraocular palsies, and markedly dilated and fixed pupils. The absence of ocular abnormalities does not exclude the diagnosis. Dryness of the mouth, tongue, and pharynx leads to a red, dry appearance of the mucous membranes.[43] The gag reflex is depressed or absent.

Muscle weakness is usually present but varies from mild to severe. Neck muscles are often weak. Upper extremity muscles are more affected than those of the lower extremity. Proximal muscles are weaker than distal muscles. Deep tendon reflexes may be normal, symmetrically decreased, or absent. Sensory examination is normal. The abdomen may be distended with hypoactive or absent bowel sounds. Bladder distention may signify urinary retention. Respirations may be tachypneic and shallow or normal. In advanced illness, signs of respiratory failure may be present.[43]

Atypical presentations of food-borne botulism have been reported, and certain serotypes produce distinct variations in the pattern of symptoms. Type A disease may be more severe and is more commonly associated with bulbar findings and upper extremity weakness. Type B illness may cause a depression in mental status. Types B and E may be associated with a greater incidence of GI and autonomic symptoms.[43,51]

Infant botulism is different in its clinical presentation because of the manifestations of neurologic findings in infants. The onset of illness is at 1 week to 11 months of age. Constipation is a common presenting symptom.[47,52] Several days to weeks later, the infant develops a weak suck, feeble cry, depressed gag reflex, and pooling of secretions and food in the oral cavity. Generalized weakness, hypotonia, and loss of head control occur. Deep tendon reflexes are depressed. Cranial nerve involvement causes alterations in facial expression, ptosis, and extraocular palsies. Signs of respiratory failure may be present. Fever is absent unless secondary infection is present.

Wound botulism causes some notable differences from food-borne botulism. The incubation period is longer, averaging about 10 days, because the toxin must be produced at the site of the wound.[51] If the wound is infected, the patient may be febrile. GI symptoms are absent in wound botulism.

The clinical presentation of *unclassified botulism* is similar to that of food-borne botulism, although the mortality of the former is significantly greater.

Recovery from botulism is slow, and survivors are hospitalized for several weeks to months.[48]

Complications Complications from botulism relate to respiratory failure and the problems expected from intensive supportive care. The major cause of death from botulism is respiratory failure resulting from weakness of the respiratory musculature. Aspiration of oral secretions and gastric contents from loss of protective airway reflexes may occur. Overall, the mortality rate has decreased from 60% to less than 10% with modern intensive care.[48] In patients who recover, muscle strength and endurance may not return to normal for up to 1 year, and persistent psychologic problems are common.[43]

Diagnostic Strategies

The initial diagnosis of botulism is clinical. Routine laboratory studies are of no value in the diagnosis. If a lumbar puncture is performed, the CSF in patients with botulism is normal or may show a slight elevation of protein.[48]

Confirmation of the diagnosis is made by detecting botulinus toxin in the patient's blood; botulinus toxin or *C. botulinum* in the gastric contents, stool, or wound of the patient; or toxin or organisms in the suspected food source. Because most hospital laboratories are unable to process such specimens, the CDC should be contacted. Serial measurements of vital capacity are helpful in recognizing deteriorating ventilatory function.

Electromyography can detect electrophysiologic abnormalities consistent with the diagnosis of botulism.[53] Electromyography may also be useful in differentiating botulism from other paralytic illnesses. The electromyographic signature of botulism is a decreased amplitude of the compound muscle action potential in response to a supramaximal stimulus and facilitation of the muscle action potential with repetitive nerve stimulation. A normal test result does not exclude the diagnosis.

Differential Considerations

The differential diagnosis of *adult botulism* includes a wide variety of illnesses.[43] Commonly, the first presenting case is misdiagnosed. This is because early symptoms may suggest diagnoses such as pharyngitis or gastroenteritis, both of which can affect several members of a single household. Only after one or more cases progress to classic botulism is the diagnosis usually suspected.

Botulism must be differentiated from other illnesses that cause paralysis. In Guillain-Barré syndrome, weakness usually starts distally and ascends, paresthesias may be present, and the cerebrospinal protein is elevated. Tick paralysis is associated with an ascending paralysis, lack of bulbar involvement, and presence of a tick. In myasthenia gravis, eye signs are also prominent, but pupillary response is preserved, no autonomic symptoms are present, and weakness responds to the administration of edrophonium. Of note, minimal improvement in weakness after the administration of edrophonium has been reported in botulism.[43] Poliomyelitis causes fever, asymmetric neurologic signs, and CSF abnormalities. Diphtheria can be distinguished by the prolonged interval between pharyngitis and neurologic symptoms. Eaton-Lambert syndrome does not usually involve bulbar muscles. Cerebrovascular accidents of the brainstem have an acute onset and neuroanatomically localizing signs and symptoms.

Certain toxins must also be considered in the differential diagnosis of botulism. Anticholinergics (atropine, belladonna, jimson weed) cause pupillary dilation and dry, red mucous membranes but also cause delirium with abnormal mentation. Organophosphate insecticides cause a characteristic odor, fever, and altered mental status. Dystonic reactions are self-limited and respond to diphenhydramine or benztropine. Neuromuscular blockade from the administration of aminoglycosides is distinguished by the history. Heavy metal poisoning produces changes in mental status. In paralytic shellfish poisoning, paresthesias occur prominently, a history of shellfish ingestion is present, and recovery occurs within 24 hours.

Infant botulism has a broader differential diagnosis. Common illnesses that mimic the presentation of infant botulism include sepsis, various viral illnesses, dehydration, encephalitis, meningitis, and failure to thrive. Neurologic illnesses such as Guillain-Barré syndrome, myasthenia gravis, and poliomyelitis should also be considered. Hypothyroidism, hypoglycemia, Reye's syndrome, diphtheria, and toxin exposures are on the list of differential diagnoses, as are less common conditions such as inborn disorders of metabolism, congenital muscular dystrophy, and cerebral degenerative diseases.

Management

The principal treatment of botulism consists of supportive care and specific treatment with antitoxin and other medications to block the effects of the toxin.

All patients with suspected botulism should be admitted to the hospital and placed in a monitored setting.[51] The ventilatory status must be closely monitored because respiratory failure may develop rapidly and insidiously. When signs of ventilatory failure develop, early endotracheal intubation should be performed. A decrease in vital capacity to less than 30% of predicted is a standard criterion mandating mechanical ventilation. Ileus should be treated with nasogastric suction, and urinary retention with an in-dwelling urinary catheter.

Saline enemas and cathartics have been recommended to cleanse the GI tract of residual toxin. Cathartics should not be given if an ileus is present. Magnesium-containing cathartics should be avoided because magnesium can exacerbate muscle weakness. Special care must be taken when using GI clearance in infants with botulism. Because the source of toxin is outside the GI tract in wound botulism, bowel decontamination is not indicated.

Antitoxin should be administered as soon as possible after appropriate laboratory specimens have been obtained. The antitoxin currently available is a botulism equine trivalent antitoxin preparation that can be obtained by contacting the CDC.[47] One vial should be given IV and one IM. Antitoxin neutralizes only circulating toxin and has no effect on bound toxin. Botulinus antitoxin is derived from horse serum, so testing for hypersensitivity should be done before administering the drug; hypersensitivity reactions occur in approximately 9% of patients of patients.[48] Antitoxin is generally not recommended in infant botulism because efficacy has not been demonstrated and because of the risk of anaphylaxis to horse serum.[51] A human antitoxin is available in the United States exclusively for the treatment of infant botulism under a treatment investigational new drug protocol. (The California Department of Health can be called at 510-540-2343 24 hours a day.) The use of prophylactic antitoxin may be appropriate in certain exposed persons without symptoms.[54]

Antibiotics are not currently recommended for food-borne botulism. Antibiotics may increase cell lysis and promote toxin release. In wound botulism, because the source of toxin is related to in vivo production within an infected wound, debridement and antibiotic administration should be *considered* only after antitoxin has been administered; their value is unproved in wound botulism.[36] Otherwise, the use of antibiotics should be limited to treating secondary infections (e.g., aspiration pneumonia) that may develop. Although antibiotic treatment of both infant and wound botulism is unproved,[52] if an agent is used, the currently recommended agent is amoxicillin.[36] Aminoglycoside antibiotics may prolong the neuromuscular blockade and should therefore be avoided.[51]

Guanidine hydrochloride may enhance the release of acetylcholine from terminal nerve fibers. For this reason, it has been recommended as an experimental component of botulism therapy.[43,51]

After the clinical suspicion of botulism exists, the CDC should be contacted for assistance. (The CDC can be contacted by calling 404-639-3311 [day] and 404-639-2888 [nights, weekends, and holidays]). State and local health departments may also be helpful in investigating and preventing major epidemics. Area EDs should be alerted so that subsequent cases will be suspected and diagnosed.

PNEUMOCOCCEMIA

Perspective

History More than a century after the identification of *S. pneumoniae* as a pathogen in human disease and more than 50 years after the discovery of antibiotics, pneumococcus remains a significant cause of morbidity and mortality worldwide. Pneumococcemia is the presence of *S. pneumoniae* in the blood. The clinical presentation ranges from a mild illness to a fulminant, life-threatening, systemic syndrome. *S. pneumoniae* also causes localized infection such as otitis media, pneumonia, and meningitis. Pneumococcal endocarditis, septic arthritis, and peritonitis occur less commonly.

The *S. pneumoniae* bacterium was discovered in 1880 by Sternberg when he inoculated rabbits with his own saliva. Later that year, Pasteur identified the organism when he inoculated rabbits with the saliva of a child who had died of hydrophobia (rabies). In 1884 Friedlander described pneumococcemia. In 1902 Cole published the first case reports of pneumococcemia, including a patient who had meningitis and arthritis without pneumonia. Wandel presented evidence that strongly suggested that *S. pneumoniae* migrated from the lung to the blood by way of the lymphatic system. In 1964,

Austrian described a second pathway by which pneumococcemia develops: bacteria pass directly from the upper respiratory tract (middle ear or sinus) to the subarachnoid space, then through the arachnoid villa and into the venous sinus.[55] In 1967 Belsey observed *S. pneumoniae* bacteremia in young children with no previous or subsequent focus of pneumococcus infection.[56]

An immunizing vaccine against *S. pneumoniae* was initially developed in the 1940s but was not produced commercially because of the availability of penicillin. The first vaccine was not licensed for use in the United States for more than 30 years. The 14-valent pneumococcal vaccine that was licensed in 1977 was replaced in 1983 by a 23-valent vaccine for use in people older than 2 years of age.[57] A new 7-valent conjugate vaccine—PVC7—is now available and licensed for use in infants younger than 2 years of age and for other high-risk patients.[57,58]

Epidemiology *S. pneumoniae* remains a substantial cause of serious illness despite the availability of antibiotics and vaccine. Pneumococcal infection appears sporadically in normal individuals and in patients with impaired host defense mechanisms. Epidemics of pneumococcal infection rarely occur, although bacterial serotypes may cluster by geographic area. Most cases of pneumococcal infections are community acquired and have a peak incidence in winter.

The precise incidence of pneumococcemia is unknown because it is not a reportable disease and blood cultures are often not performed on patients with uncomplicated focal pneumococcal infections. The estimated incidence of pneumococcemia in the United States is 15 to 30 cases/100,000 population annually for all people, 50 to 83 cases/100,000 population annually for those older than 65 years of age, and 160 cases/100,000 population annually for children younger than 2 years of age.[58] Certain populations, such as Native Alaskans and Native Americans (Apache), have a substantially higher incidence of infection. Studies demonstrate a higher incidence of pneumococcemia in men than in women. Pneumococcemia occurs in 20% to 25% of cases of pneumococcal pneumonia.[59]

People at higher risk for pneumococcemia include those with chronic respiratory or cardiovascular disease, chronic alcohol abuse, cirrhosis, diabetes mellitus, absent or functionally impaired spleen (splenectomy or sickle cell disease), chronic renal failure, nephrotic syndrome, organ transplantation, lymphoma, Hodgkin's disease, multiple myeloma, and acquired immunodeficiency syndrome (AIDS).[57-59] Widespread outbreaks of pneumococcal infection have been uncommon since antibiotics became available. Several outbreaks have occurred in jails, shelters for the homeless, and military training camps. Pneumococcemia may be the first clinical manifestation of human immunodeficiency virus (HIV) infection.[58] Although it is uncommon, relapsing and recurrent pneumococcal infection with an identical strain of *S. pneumococcus* occurs in immunocompromised patients, including those with asplenia, complement deficiency, and hypogammaglobulin deficiency.[60]

The fatality rate for pneumococcemia is approximately 15% to 20% for all cases, with a substantially higher mortality rate in the elderly (30% to 40%), people with underlying disease, and those with localized infections such as meningitis.[58] The case fatality rate is significantly lower for children (1% to 7%).[60] The mortality rate from pneumococcal infection is likely to increase because of the increasing number of elderly and AIDS patients and the emergence of antibiotic-resistant strains.[61]

Etiology Pneumococcemia is caused by *S. pneumoniae,* an encapsulated, lancet-shaped, gram-positive coccus. The microorganism is a facultative anaerobe that is often observed in pairs (hence its former name *Diplococcus pneumoniae*). Antigenic differences in the polysaccharides capsule separate *S. pneumoniae* into 90 serotypes.[62] Approximately 10 capsular types account for 62% of invasive disease worldwide, with certain types being more virulent than others.[57] In the United States, the seven serotypes present in the PCV7 vaccine account for 80% of infection in blood and CSF of children younger than 6 years of age and 50% of isolates in people 6 years of age or older.[57]

Principles of Disease

S. pneumoniae enters the blood by spreading from the lung to the mediastinal lymph nodes into the thoracic duct and then into the circulation via the cervical lymph nodes. This occurs as a sequel to upper respiratory tract colonization or by spreading from the upper respiratory tract to the subarachnoid space via the arachnoid villa to the venous sinus and into the blood (with or without meningeal involvement).

S. pneumoniae bacteremia causes a clinical picture that ranges from a minor febrile illness to life-threatening septic shock. The different capsules that surround different *S. pneumoniae* serotypes confer varying levels of resistance to phagocytosis, resulting in a variation in virulence among serotypes. The shaking chills and fever that occur with pneumococcemia are believed to be caused by a toxin. Research directed toward identifying the exogenous and endogenous mediators of sepsis and shock holds promise for new treatment modalities.

The diversity in individual clinical reactions to pneumococcemia is not well understood. The patients who demonstrate substantial host resistance are able to develop active immunity. Pediatric studies demonstrate that young children can spontaneously recover from blood culture–proven pneumococcemia without antibiotics.[63] In patients with pneumococcal infections, immunity develops within several days of onset of infection because antibodies specific to the capsule serotype develop in the patient. This is similar to the response to the pneumococcal vaccine.

Clinical Features

History and Physical Examination The clinical presentation of pneumococcemia ranges from mild illness to fulminant disease culminating in death within several hours. Occult bacteremia presents as a febrile illness in which the only direct indication of pneumococcemia is a positive blood culture (most often 24 to 48 hours) subsequent to the clinical evaluation. Sepsis is the systemic response to infection, manifested by two or more of the following: (1) temperature greater than 38° C or less than 36° C; (2) heart rate greater than 90 beats/min; (3) respiratory rate greater than 20 breaths/min or PA_{CO_2} less than 32 mm Hg; and (4) WBC count greater than 12,000/mm^3, less than 4000/mm^3, or greater than 10% immature (band) forms.[64] Toxicity is the clinical appearance of the patient with sepsis. It includes lethargy, poor perfusion, cyanosis, and hypoventilation or hyperventilation. Either bacteremia or sepsis can occur in conjunction with localized infection.

The history should include medical history; recent use of antibiotics; a description of symptoms, including fever, chills, cough, shortness of breath, headache, and skin rash; and a review of systems. There should be an assessment of the patient's social situation, including availability of caregivers, transportation to medical care, and the ability to comply with discharge instructions.

In children, the clinical presentation of pneumococcemia is similar to that of other common febrile illnesses with the exception of a higher incidence of febrile seizures.[65] Although signs of focal infection such as pneumonia may be present, often the only indications of pneumococcemia are fever or other signs of bacterial toxicity.

Most adult patients have fever. Cough, rigors, pleuritic pain, and GI symptoms occur in approximately one third of adult patients. Many patients complain of vague, nonspecific constitutional symptoms similar to those of common viral syndromes. Fever (>38.5° C) occurs in 90% of younger patients but in fewer than 60% of those older than 65 years of age.[59] Findings on physical examination vary with the site, if any, of localized infection. Patients with signs of sepsis have an increased risk of a fulminant course with rapid deterioration.

Diagnosis of bacteremia in an elderly patient may be quite challenging; elevated temperature and elevated WBC may not be present.[59] Other than a localized focus of infection and subtle behavioral changes, the diagnosis may substantially depend on laboratory test results.

Complications Cardiovascular collapse can occur with fulminant pneumococcal sepsis. Patients who develop severe illness from pneumococcemia may have end-organ damage (secondary to inadequate perfusion), disseminated intravascular coagulopathy (DIC), septic emboli, and other complications. These include respiratory failure, hypothermia, GI bleeding, hepatic coma, renal failure, and myocardial infarction.[59]

Pneumococcemia occasionally results in hematogenous seeding, which causes peritonitis, arthritis, endocarditis, and cellulitis.[65] Patients with asplenia (postsurgical) or inadequate splenic function (as occurs in sickle cell disease) may develop a fulminant type of pneumococcemia termed *overwhelming postsplenectomy infection (OPSI),* which is characterized by septic shock, adrenal hemorrhage, and DIC.[66] Although the true incidence of OPSI is unknown, studies demonstrate that it is substantial and that the risk for it does not decrease over time after splenectomy. Most invasive pneumococcal infections occur in the first 2 years after splenectomy, and about two thirds occur between 5 and 20 years. OPSI may initially present with symptoms indistinguishable from those of common viral illnesses.[66]

Diagnostic Strategies

Ancillary testing of adults with suspected bacteremia should include a complete blood count (CBC) with differential count; blood cultures; urine culture and sensitivity; electrolyte, glucose, serum creatinine, and blood urea nitrogen tests; chest radiograph; Gram's stain and culture and sensitivity testing of sputum (if pneumonia is suspected); and antigen testing of body fluids. If the patient appears to be toxic or has signs of respiratory compromise, arterial blood gas and a coagulation profile should be obtained. If signs of meningitis are present, a lumbar puncture should be performed. The WBC count is usually elevated. A normal or low WBC count is prognostic of more serious disease, as are hypoxemia and hypercarbia.[59] Musher demonstrated a higher mortality rate in patients with serum creatinine levels higher than 2.0 mg/dl, bilirubin levels higher than 1.5 ng/dl and albumin levels less than 2.5 g/dl.[59]

Differential Considerations

Pneumococcemia in its more benign presentation must be differentiated from other febrile illnesses, such as viral infections. The combination of clinical findings and culture results enable the EP to make the distinction between bacteremia and sepsis of other origins. The presence of fever and shock, with or without a distinct rash, suggests the possibility of sepsis caused by *H. influenzae, Neisseria meningitidis,* and other streptococcus types.

Management

Acute Treatment Managing pneumococcemia consists of stabilizing life-threatening conditions, eradicating the infection, and treating predisposing or coexisting conditions. The decision to initiate antibiotic therapy for pneumococcemia is often made with limited objective data, which include the clinical findings, the patient's age group, underlying condition(s), and preliminary laboratory studies.

Although the mediators of *S. pneumoniae* toxicity are not elucidated, eliminating the bacterial organism by prompt initiation of antibiotics is essential for reducing the morbidity and mortality of pneumococcal infection. Antibiotic administration should begin in the ED. To simplify selection of a treatment strategy, patients can be divided into three general groups:

1. *Bacteremia or sepsis is suspected on the basis of clinical findings; however, the organism has not been identified.* The patient in this group is given broad-spectrum antibiotics initially, with the selection based on factors that include the most likely organism(s), the patient's age (neonate, child, adult, or elderly) and immune status, the presence of coexisting disorders, and local patterns of antibiotic resistance. The antibiotic regimen is changed to a narrower-spectrum drug subsequent to positive identification of the organism and its sensitivities.
2. S. pneumoniae *growth is reported from blood cultures drawn (usually 1 to 2 days) previously.* The treatment regimen for "occult bacteremia" is guided by the patient's age, history, physical examination, general appearance, and ancillary tests. Often, the antibiotic selected on the initial visit for a localized infection (e.g., amoxicillin) is sufficient to treat the pneumococcal bacteremia subsequently identified by the laboratory. The patient should be reevaluated promptly. The decision to admit a child for inpatient care is based on the findings at the time of reevaluation. In a survey of pediatric EPs, 76% indicate that they admit all patients with occult *S. pneumoniae* bacteremia.[67]
3. *Bacteremia or sepsis is suspected and* S. pneumoniae *is identified from a site of local infection, such as a Gram's stain of sputum.* The antibiotic regimen is focused narrowly.

The adult patient with laboratory-proven pneumococcemia

is treated with penicillin G, 6 to 12 million U/day in divided doses every 4 hours IV. If the organism is susceptible, pneumococcemia with meningitis is treated with up to 24 million U of penicillin G per day. In children, the dosage for meningitis is 250,000 U/kg/24 hours in divided doses every 4 hours IV up to a maximum of 20 million U. When meningitis is present, the drug selected must penetrate the CSF and attain acceptable concentrations.

IM ceftriaxone is commonly administered to children with suspected bacteremia who are treated as outpatients while culture results are pending. Ceftriaxone (initial dose of 100 mg/kg IV, followed by daily dosage of 100 mg/kg in divided doses every 12 hours, up to a maximum of 4 g) and cefotaxime (200 mg/kg/day in divided doses every 6 hours IV, up to a maximum of 12 g) offer the advantage of being excellent antibiotics for *N. meningitidis* and *H. influenzae*. Alternatives for the treatment of pneumococcemia in a penicillin-allergic patient include cefotaxime, ceftriaxone, vancomycin, or chloramphenicol. The decision to use cephalosporins or one of the other drugs is based on the type of allergic reaction to penicillin reported by the patient.[67] Chloramphenicol has the associated risk of toxicity and interaction with anticonvulsant medications.

S. pneumoniae resistance to penicillin has emerged in recent years.[56,62] Other drugs that can be used to treat pneumococcemia are ceftriaxone, cefotaxime, and vancomycin. *Penicillin intermediate resistance* is defined as a mean inhibitory concentration (MIC) greater than 0.1 μg/ml, and high-level resistance is defined as MIC greater than 2.0 μg/ml.[68] CDC surveillance has found penicillin resistance in 15% to 40% of sterile site isolates recovered during 1995 and 1996 in patients 65 and older.[68] Overall in the United States, 28% of isolates are intermediate resistance, and 16% are highly resistant to penicillin.[62] There are substantial geographic variations in the prevalence of pneumococcal serotypes and resistance.[68] A total of 16.4% of the isolates are resistant to one or more of the following drugs: penicillin, cephalosporins, macrolides, chloramphenicol, and trimethoprim-sulfamethoxazole. Macrolide resistance is present in 30% of *S. pneumoniae* isolates, but in 67% of isolates that are highly resistant to penicillin.[68]

The development of resistance is a stepwise process, with successive genetic mutations; however, resistant strains may spread rapidly when transported to geographically distant areas by infected persons. The recommended IV dosages of penicillin and other β-lactam antibiotics generally achieve serum concentrations many times greater than the MICs for *S. pneumoniae* of intermediate resistance and, in some cases, even for highly resistant strains. For suspected high-level penicillin-resistant strains, it is recommended that vancomycin, imipenem, or extended-spectrum cephalosporins (with MICs < 8.0 μg/ml) be selected. Treatment of meningitis caused by penicillin-resistant *S. pneumoniae* presents a unique problem because of the high level of antibiotic concentration required to sterilize the CSF. Ceftriaxone and cefotaxime are preferred for empiric treatment of suspected pneumococcal meningitis; however, treatment failures have been reported. In areas where resistance to extended-spectrum cephalosporins is prevalent, empiric therapy with vancomycin plus cefuroxime or cefotaxime should be considered. Susceptibility testing should guide antibiotic selection. The patient with pneumococcemia may not have an obvious response to treatment for the first 24 to 48 hours of therapy. This may be attributed to the normal course of the disease, an incorrect diagnosis, underlying illness, or an antibiotic regimen that does not sufficiently treat the infection.

Disposition of the patient depends on three factors: the patient's age, his or her overall clinical condition, and the presence of coexisting illnesses. Patients of any age who appear to be toxic should be treated with antibiotics promptly and admitted to the hospital. Patients with underlying or coexisting conditions and those with an unclear course of illness should also be admitted.

Children who are afebrile and appear to be well at the time of the initial examination are unlikely to have serious sequelae develop[63]; however, they may occasionally develop serious complications, including meningitis.[69] As a result, for the febrile child who appears well enough to be discharged, close follow-up is important. The decision to discharge should be based on clinical findings, medical history, ability of the parents to follow the discharge instructions, and availability of close follow-up.

Vaccination The pneumococcal vaccine is effective in preventing infection; the currently available 23-valent vaccine contains the purified polysaccharide antigens of the serotypes that cause 85% to 90% of pneumococcemia infections in the United States.[58] Although the overall protective efficacy of the vaccine is only 56% to 57%, it is safe, inexpensive, and of substantial value for well-defined groups at risk.[58] Unfortunately, the 23-valent pneumococcal vaccine has limited immunogenicity in children younger than 2 years of age. The 7-valent conjugate vaccine links the polysaccharide to proteins, resulting in improved immunogenic response in children younger than 2 years of age.[57]

The CDC recommends the 23-valent vaccine for the following patients[57]:

1. Immunocompetent adults with chronic illnesses (e.g., cardiovascular or pulmonary disease, diabetes mellitus, alcoholism, cirrhosis, or CSF leaks) or those 65 years of age or older.
2. Immunocompromised adults (e.g., splenic dysfunction or asplenia, Hodgkin's disease, lymphoma, leukemia, multiple myeloma, chronic renal failure, nephrotic syndrome, or organ transplantation associated with immunosuppression).
3. Adults and children older than 2 years with asymptomatic HIV infections.
4. Children older than 2 years with chronic illness (e.g., anatomic or functional asplenia [including sickle cell disease], nephrotic syndrome, CSF leak, and conditions associated with immunosuppression). The vaccine is not indicated for children having only recurrent upper respiratory tract disease, such as otitis media and sinusitis.
5. Persons living in special environments or social settings with an identified increased risk (e.g., certain Native American populations).

The CDC and AAP recommend the 7-valent vaccine for the following people[57,70]:

1. All children ages 2 to 23 months at 2, 4, 6, and 12 to 15 months.
2. Children age 24 to 59 months who are at high risk of pneumococcal disease (sickle cell disease, HIV infection, and other immunocompromising medical condi-

tions.) This should be followed by the 23-valent vaccine 2 months after the 7-valent vaccine is given.
3. Consider for all children 24 to 59 months with priority given to the following:
   a. those aged 24 to 35 months
   b. Alaskan natives, Native Americans, and African Americans
   c. Children who attend day care

The Immunization Practices Advisory Committee on pneumococcal vaccine recommends that revaccination be strongly considered at 6 years or older for people who are most likely to have a rapid decline of pneumococcal antibodies (e.g., renal failure, transplant recipients, and patients with nephrotic syndrome) and for those at risk for fatal infection (e.g., asplenia). Children 10 years of age or younger with nephrotic syndrome, sickle cell anemia, or asplenia should be considered for revaccination after 3 to 5 years. Patients who have received the old 14-valent vaccine should not be routinely vaccinated with the newer 23-valent vaccine.

Other preventive measures for pneumococcemia include passive immunization with immunoglobulins of patients with congenital or acquired immunodeficiency diseases and daily antibiotic prophylaxis of children with functional or anatomic asplenia.[11]

MENINGOCOCCEMIA

Perspective

History Few clinical situations in emergency medicine produce feelings of greater fear, stress, or awe than meningococcal infection. Virtually all veteran ED staff have had a patient who appeared relatively well at the time of initial examination, only to be moribund and in critical condition with fulminant infection several hours later.

"Cerebro-spinal fever" was initially described in 1805 by Vieusseux in Geneva. Weichselbaum identified the causative microbial agent in 1887.[71] Throughout the nineteenth and first half of the twentieth centuries, epidemics occurred periodically in most regions of the world. "Serum therapy" was introduced in France in 1907 and the in United States in 1913 as the first direct treatment of meningococcal disease. Beginning in 1937, sulfonamide therapy replaced serotherapy with an apparent improvement in disease outcome and eradication of the carrier state, especially in crowded military populations. In the 1940s sulfonamide resistance began to emerge, and in 1963 an outbreak of resistant strains occurred in the United States, which spurred efforts to develop vaccines to protect against infection.[71,72]

Epidemiology The incidence of meningococcal disease increases in the spring and fall in industrialized countries such as the United States. During nonepidemic periods, children younger than 5 years of age have the highest incidence of infection. During epidemics, the incidence increases among children ages 5 to 9, an observation that may be of value in predicting the beginning of an epidemic. The incidence of meningococcal disease is several times higher among military recruits than the general public, but the risk of disease diminishes after several weeks of military housing. Military recruits demonstrate an increased incidence of carrier state in the first few weeks of service and produce antibodies to the *N. meningitidis* that persist for several months.[72] Other groups considered to be at higher risk for meningococcal disease than the general population include close patient contacts, patients with complement deficiency, those with properdin deficiency, those with chronic alcohol abuse, and those exposed to both active and passive smoking.[72,73]

The incidence of meningococcal infection in the United States is 0.8 to 1.3 cases per year per 100,000 population.[73] Of the more than 13 serogroups, groups A, B, C, Y, and W-135 cause most of the infections. Groups B and C are the most common serogroups in the United States.[74] Although grouping is important for tracking the disease, all groups are capable of causing the same spectrum of clinical disease.

The mortality rate of meningococcal septicemia without meningitis is 20% to 60%, compared with 5% for cases of meningitis alone.[72]

Etiology Meningococcal disease is caused by *N. meningitidis,* an aerobic, gram-negative diplococcus. *N. meningitidis* is classified into at least 13 serogroups on the basis of agglutination tests using antibodies to capsular antigens.

Principles of Disease

N. meningitidis enters the body via the nasopharynx and may either remain there, causing an asymptomatic carrier state, or produce mild symptoms of an upper respiratory tract infection. In certain patients the bacteria enter the bloodstream and cause symptoms and signs of bacteremia, sepsis, fulminant infection, or localized infection. The precise host and microorganism characteristics that determine whether clinical disease develops are not fully elucidated. Complement deficiency in the host may play a role in the host's inability to fight this infection.[73] The release of lipooligosaccaride endotoxin by lysis of the *N. meningitidis* cell is the initial event in the development of meningococcal sepsis. The exogenous mediators appear to stimulate the release of endogenous mediators, including tumor necrosis factor, interleukin-1, and the host's complement system. The complement-activating products and other chemical mediators contribute to multiple organ failure.[75]

After exposure to *N. meningitidis,* protective antibodies develop. Immunity in children is conferred initially by maternal antibodies that pass through the placenta and later by the development of antibodies after exposure to the bacteria. In children the incidence of meningococcal disease is inversely proportional to the levels of antibody active against *N. meningitidis.*[76]

Clinical Features

History and Physical Examination The clinical presentation of meningococcemia ranges from a mild illness to fulminant disease.[74] Occult bacteremia presents as a febrile illness in which the only direct indication of meningococcemia is a positive blood culture report obtained (most often 24 to 48 hours) subsequent to the clinical evaluation. Toxicity is the clinical appearance of the patient with sepsis. It includes lethargy, poor perfusion, cyanosis, and hypoventilation or hyperventilation.

In its mildest form, meningococcal bacteremia cannot be readily distinguished from more benign infections. Occasionally children with "occult" or "unsuspected" bacteremia who initially have fever but no other signs specific of meningococcal infection are later found to have blood cultures positive for *N. meningitidis.*[67] Initial diagnoses in these cases include common childhood infections such as otitis media, acute viral upper respiratory infections, and gastroenteritis. Some patients have resolution of their illness after treatment with an oral regimen of antibiotics. In one study, three patients who were initially bacteremic had spontaneous resolution without antibiotic treatment. On the other hand, despite the total absence of clinical clues for meningococcal infection on the initial visit, some untreated patients subsequently deteriorate rapidly.[74]

The duration of symptoms usually ranges from less than 12 hours to 14 days. An elevated temperature is present in 71% to 89% of cases, and hypothermia is present in 4% of cases. Although skin lesions are present in 71% of cases, petechiae, or purpura, are present in only 49% of cases. Shock occurs in 42% of patients, arthritis in 8%, and seizures in 8%. Other findings include irritability, lethargy, emesis, diarrhea, cough, and rhinorrhea. Only 60% of patients have the classic signs of meningococcal infection: fever and petechiae or purpura. Meningitis is diagnosed in 55% of cases, although lumbar punctures are not performed in some unstable patients. The classic symptoms and signs of meningitis may not be present. Infants or children may experience only fever, irritability, and vomiting.

The skin should be carefully examined for the presence of lesions that may be the only clue of meningococcemia. Petechiae are present in 50% to 60% of cases, but macular and maculopapular lesions are also common. The rash structure may also be faint papules, maculopapular combinations, nodules, isolated petechiae, and extensive coalescent areas of ecchymosis, occasionally with vesicle formation.[74] The maculopapular rash is often present initially, with the petechial rash appearing within 24 hours. The petechiae may be at any location on the skin or mucous membranes, but they are most common on the trunk and extremities, especially at pressure points such as under elastic underwear or socks. The skin manifestations of severe cases of meningococcemia can include purpura fulminans. This condition is characterized by rapidly spreading ecchymoses and gangrene of the extremities. Purpura fulminans occurs most often in children and is often associated with DIC infection. Herpes labialis commonly occurs within 2 days of the onset of illness.[72]

The most dreaded manifestation is fulminant meningococcemia, the Waterhouse-Friderichsen syndrome. It occurs in 10% to 20% of patients with meningococcal disease and is characterized by extreme severity and rapid clinical deterioration, including vasomotor collapse and shock.[72] This is an overwhelming disease in which the patient rapidly develops severe toxicity strongly suggestive of an endotoxin-mediated process. Usually a diffuse petechial and purpuric rash is present with extensive intracutaneous hemorrhage. Shock results from both intravascular volume loss and congestive heart failure, probably because of myocarditis. DIC develops with hemorrhage or thrombi formation and arterial embolization. Renal failure, coma, and bilateral adrenal hemorrhage often occur.

Chronic meningococcemia is a syndrome characterized by fever, rash, and joint complaints of longer than 1 week in conjunction with a positive blood culture for *N. meningitidis.* Headache and upper respiratory symptoms are often present. It is the rarest form of meningococcal disease, accounting for 1% to 2% of cases.[72]

Complications Some patients become acutely ill and may develop myocarditis with congestive heart failure or conduction abnormalities, myopericarditis, acute respiratory failure, DIC, renal failure, or purulent arthritis.[75] If CNS infection accompanies the meningococcemia, cranial nerve dysfunction may occur acutely, with residual effects in some cases. Vasculitis in severe cases of meningococcal septicemia may result in skin lesions that necessitate plastic surgery, and loss of digits or limbs that result from gangrene.[72]

In fatal meningococcal infections, the heart, CNS, skin, mucous and serous membranes, and adrenal glands are most commonly damaged.[77] The most common abnormality is myocarditis associated with acute congestive heart failure. Meningitis, mucocutaneous bleeding, and visceral hemorrhages are also common. After the acute phase of infection, inflammatory reactions can include nonsuppurative arthritis, pericarditis, and vasculitis.[71,72]

Poor prognostic indicators in meningococcemia include seizures on presentation, hypothermia, hyperpyrexia, a total peripheral WBC count of less than 500/mm^3, a platelet count of less than 100,000/mm^3, the development of purpura fulminans, the onset of petechiae within 12 hours of admission, an absence of meningitis, the presence of shock, a low sedimentation rate, and extremes of age.[74] In one study, all patients who developed organ system failure had one or more of the following at the time of initial presentation: circulatory insufficiency (hypotension or shock), peripheral WBC count less than 10,000 cells/mm^3, or a coagulopathy.

Diagnostic Strategies

The tentative diagnosis of meningococcemia is based on clinical findings and is confirmed by blood cultures, by antigen detection tests, or from a Gram's stain of a peripheral blood buffy-coat specimen, petechial scraping, or pleural or pericardial fluid.[72]

The WBC count is usually elevated, sometimes as high as 65,000/mm^3, with a left shift in the differential cell count. A low or normal sedimentation rate may predict a poor prognosis, as may a low WBC count.[71] The symptoms and signs of CNS infection may be nonspecific in the infant and child younger than age 2. If meningitis is present, the CSF pressure is usually elevated, the protein level is increased, and the glucose level is decreased. Usually a pleocytosis is present, with a predominance of polymorphonuclear leukocytes. Gram-negative diplococci may be seen on microscopy. Early in the disease, the CSF may be free of inflammatory cells. Other, normally sterile body fluids (e.g., synovial fluid) may be purulent and culture positive for *N. meningitidis.* Immunoassays may be particularly useful in patients in whom antibiotics have been administered. PCR of the CSF is about 90% sensitive and specific for *N. meningitidis* and, if available, may also be useful in these cases.[72]

Differential Considerations

It is difficult to distinguish the clinical signs of meningococcemia from bacteremia caused by *S. pneumoniae,* other streptococcal groups, *H. influenzae,* and *N. gonorrhoeae.* Localized infection may enable the EP to focus the differential diagnosis.

The differential diagnosis of meningococcemia also includes viral exanthems, Rocky Mountain spotted fever, typhus, typhoid fever, endocarditis, vasculitis syndromes (polyarteritis nodosa and Henoch-Schönlein purpura), toxic shock syndrome, acute rheumatic fever, drug reactions, Henoch-Schönlein purpura, Kawasaki syndrome, and idiopathic thrombocytopenic purpura.[74]

In one study of 319 patients hospitalized with fever and petechiae, 26 patients (8.2%) had culture-proven *N. meningitidis,* 13 (4%) had sepsis from other bacterial causes, and 68 (21.3%) had other bacterial infections without sepsis. The remainder had viral or other etiologies.[78]

Management

Acute Treatment The keys to reducing morbidity and mortality in meningococcemia are prompt recognition and immediate initiation of antibiotic therapy. Delays in initiating therapy for the completion of diagnostic studies or admission to the inpatient unit should be avoided. To simplify selection of a treatment strategy, EPs can divide patients into three general groups:

1. *Bacteremia or sepsis is suspected based on clinical findings; however, the organism has not been identified.* The patient in this group should receive broad-spectrum antibiotics, with selection based on factors that include the most likely organism(s), the patient's age and immune status, the presence of coexisting disorders, and local patterns of antibiotic resistance. A narrower-spectrum agent is selected after positive identification of the organism and its sensitivities.
2. *N. meningitidis growth is reported from prior blood cultures.* The treatment regimen for occult bacteremia is guided by the patient's age, history, physical examination, general appearance, and ancillary tests. The antibiotic selected at the time of the initial visit may be sufficient to treat the meningococcal bacteremia subsequently identified by the laboratory. The decision to hospitalize the child is based on the findings at the time of reevaluation and the risk of sequelae. In a survey of pediatric emergency specialists, 76% indicate that they admit all patients with *N. meningitidis* bacteremia.[67]
3. *Bacteremia or sepsis is suspected and N. meningitidis is identified from a site of local infection, such as a Gram's stain of CSF.* The antibiotic regimen is focused narrowly.

The standard antibiotic regimen for laboratory-proven meningococcemia is penicillin G, 24 million U/day in divided doses every 2 to 4 hours IV for adults, and penicillin, 250,000 U/kg/day in divided doses every 2 to 4 hours IV for children up to a maximum of 20 million U, or ampicillin, 200 to 400 mg/kg/day in four divided doses IV.[72]

Acceptable alternatives to penicillin include cefotaxime (200 mg/kg/day in divided doses every 6 hours IV up to a maximum of 12 g) and ceftriaxone (initial dose of 100 mg/kg IV, followed by daily dosage of 100 mg/kg in divided doses every 12 hours up to a maximum of 4 g). The cephalosporins offer the advantage of safety with a rapid onset of action. Chloramphenicol is also acceptable. Ceftriaxone IM is commonly administered to children with suspected bacteremia who are treated as outpatients while culture results are pending. Ceftriaxone and cefotaxime offer the advantage of being excellent antibiotics for *S. pneumoniae* and *H. influenzae.* Alternatives for treating meningococcemia in a penicillin-allergic patient include cefotaxime, ceftriaxone, or chloramphenicol. The decision to use cephalosporins or one of the other alternate drugs is based on the type of allergic reaction to penicillin reported by the patient.[67]

Several reports have demonstrated the efficacy of ceftriaxone, 80 to 100 mg/kg IV in a single daily dose; however, twice-a-day dosing remains the standard recommendation at this time. In addition to the obvious advantage of extended dosing intervals, ceftriaxone-treated patients have a more rapid sterilization of the CSF and a lower incidence of hearing loss than conventionally treated patients.

IV fluid replacement and inotropic support with dopamine (2 to 10 μg/kg/min) or dobutamine (1 to 10 μg/kg/min) should be initiated promptly in hypotensive patients to maintain systemic arterial pressure.[72] Electrolyte and acid-base abnormalities should be corrected. If patient are oliguric or anuric, hemodialysis may be necessary to correct these abnormalities.[72]

The role of corticosteroids in the treatment of meningococcal infection without meningitis remains controversial. Although corticosteroids were once widely recommended for the treatment of the adrenal insufficiency associated with fulminant meningococcemia, more recent studies demonstrate that adrenal function is not impaired in all patients. In the absence of well-controlled studies, some EPs may empirically administer replacement levels to massive doses of corticosteroids for treating fulminant meningococcemia.

Some studies of corticosteroid use in treating bacterial meningitis demonstrate decreased duration of fever, decreased levels of endogenous CNS mediators, short-term differences in neurologic findings, and a reduction in the incidence of sensorineural hearing loss; however, a meta-analysis of studies published before 1989 concluded that the demonstrated benefit may be limited to a reduction of sensorineural hearing loss in *H. influenzae* meningitis in children. Subsequent to this report, a placebo-controlled double-blind trial of dexamethasone therapy in infants and children demonstrated that administration of the corticosteroids before the initiation of antibiotic (cefotaxime) therapy resulted in a significant reduction in CNS inflammation and neurologic and audiologic sequelae.[79] It has become common practice to administer corticosteroids (dexamethasone 0.15 mg/kg) 15 to 20 minutes before antibiotics for presumed bacterial meningitis, but the data are controversial.

Plasmapheresis has been reported to be beneficial in several cases of fulminant meningococcemia. Improvement correlates with the reduction of plasma concentrations of interleukin-1 and tumor necrosis factor, two of the likely mediators of toxicity in meningococcemia.[80] Patients with meningococcemia may deteriorate rapidly. In acutely ill patients, hemodynamic monitoring with a Swan-Ganz catheter may be necessary.

Virtually all patients with meningococcemia have DIC, but routine heparinization in these patients has failed to improve outcome and is not recommended. In patients with peripheral gangrene, there may be a benefit from low-dose heparin (10 U/kg/h) with fresh frozen plasma.[72]

Future therapeutic adjuncts to antibiotic therapy may include the development of monoclonal antibodies to the bacterial pathogens, as well as to the endotoxins and endogenous mediators of sepsis.[79]

Antibiotic Prophylaxis and Vaccination To limit the risk to others from the patient with meningococcemia, isolation should be maintained, and close contacts should receive antibiotic prophylaxis. Household, nursery school, and day care center contacts should receive prophylaxis promptly. Intimate contacts (e.g., those who kiss or share food with the patient) and health care workers with intimate exposure (e.g., mouth-to-mouth resuscitation, intubation, or suctioning) should receive rifampin, 10 mg/kg (up to 600 mg) orally every 12 hours for four doses. The dose for infants younger than 1 month of age is 5 mg/kg. Patients should be warned that rifampin will discolor their urine, and contact lenses should be removed to avoid permanent staining. Ceftriaxone IM (125 mg for children younger than 12 years of age and 250 mg for those older than 12 years of age) is effective against group A strains. This is an alternative for pregnant women and for cases in which compliance with an oral regimen cannot be ensured. Ciprofloxacin (500 mg orally) is also an alternative for adults.[11,73]

If the meningococcus is sensitive to sulfonamides, sulfisoxazole may be used. The dosages are 1 g orally every 12 hours for those older than 12 years, 500 mg orally every 12 hours for children 1 to 12 years old, and 500 mg orally every day for infants younger than 1 year. Each age group should receive 2 days of sulfisoxazole therapy.[11] Nasopharyngeal cultures are not of value when assessing who should receive prophylaxis.[11]

Meningococcal vaccine should be considered as an adjunct to prophylaxis in epidemics and for close contacts in sporadic cases if one of the serotypes contained in the vaccine is identified as the causative agent. The currently available vaccine is a quadrivalent vaccine containing purified capsular polysaccharides for group A, C, Y, and W-135. Unfortunately, the polysaccharides other than A are poor immunogens for children younger than 2 years of age. In addition, no vaccine exists for group B, the most prevalent serogroup that causes meningococcal infection in the United States. The quadrivalent vaccine is not recommended for routine use but should be administered to children 2 years and older in high-risk groups, such as those with asplenia (functional or surgical) and those with terminal complement deficiency.[73] The vaccine is currently administered to U.S. military recruits. Consideration should be given to vaccinating persons traveling to areas of the world with hyperendemic or epidemic meningococcal disease, such as sub-Saharan Africa.[76]

KAWASAKI DISEASE

Perspective

History Kawasaki disease (KD) is an acute vasculitis that occurs primarily in infants and children. The precise cause of the disease is not well understood, and no definitive diagnostic test has been developed.

KD, previously named *mucocutaneous lymph node syndrome,* was first recognized in Japan by Kawasaki in 1967. In 1971 Melish reported a similar syndrome in the United States.[81,82] During the past 20 years, numerous microorganisms and environmental conditions have been implicated as the putative etiologic agent(s). Although no definitive treatment exists for KD, it was observed in the mid-1980s that certain pharmacologic regimens can reduce the morbidity.[82,83]

Epidemiology The incidence of KD is highest in Japanese children or children of Japanese ancestry. In the United States, whites have a lower incidence than other groups. Peak incidence occurs in the spring and winter. The disease appears to have a higher incidence in children of middle and upper socioeconomic classes. More than 80% of cases occur in children younger than 5 years, with the highest incidence occurring in children between 1 and 2 years of age. Fewer than 40 cases of KD have been reported in adults, and controversy remains regarding whether all the cases are actually KD.[84]

Cases of KD may occur sporadically or during outbreaks. No evidence exists, however, for person-to-person spread among household, school, or daycare contacts. Community-wide outbreaks have been observed to occur in cycles of 2 to 4 years.

There are 5000 to 6000 cases a year of KD in Japan (120 to 150/100,000 population), and it is estimated that there are at least 3000 cases per year in the United States. KD has replaced acute rheumatic fever as the leading cause of acquired heart disease in children.[83] In children younger than 5 years of age, the annual incidence is approximately 4 to 15/100,000 population.[85] Multiple outbreaks in the continental United States and Hawaii have been reported but, for unclear reasons, epidemics are not observed in Japan.[86] In Hawaii, active surveillance in a limited geographic area finds an annual incidence rate of 135 cases/100,000 children younger than age 5, a rate similar to that reported in Japan. The mortality rate for KD in children is estimated at 0.3% to 2.3%.[84]

Etiology The etiology of KD is unclear despite 30 years of extensive research. An infectious agent is suggested by the following observations of KD: KD has a seasonal peak in winter and spring; epidemics occur with a clear epicenter; the peak age group is toddlers with a few rare cases in infants, suggesting a role for transplacental antibodies in protection; and KD has many clinical manifestations similar to known infectious diseases (e.g., scarlet fever, measles).[82]

Three risk factors appear to have an association with KD: respiratory illness within 30 days, shampooing or spot-cleaning rugs within 30 days (possibly caused by house dust mite contact or a transmitted microbe), and living near a body of water that might contain an arthropod vector or animal reservoir.[86] The precise relationship among the various host factors, environmental factors, and the infectious agent remains to be explained.

Principles of Disease

During the acute phase of the illness, marked immune system activation is present, with a decreased number of CD8 cells, an increase in the number of activated helper T cells, monocytes, and polyclonal B-cells (which produce immunoglobulin G and M antibodies). In addition, increased levels of circulating cytokines, including tumor necrosis factor-α, interleukin-1, and interferon-α, are present. The antibodies are cytotoxic to human vascular endothelial cells.[83,87] The precise link between this mechanism of vascular injury and immune system activation is the subject of ongoing research. The clinical findings and laboratory abnormalities are similar to those observed in diseases caused by bacterial toxins, including streptococcal and staphylococcal toxic shock syndrome, scarlet fever, and staphylococcal scalded-skin syndrome. It is postulated that KD may be caused by a toxin acting like a "superantigen" from a yet undefined bacterium.[83]

Autopsy findings at both the microscopic and gross anatomic levels correlate with the clinical findings and immune system activity. During the first 11 days of the illness (acute phase), perivasculitis and vasculitis of the small blood vessels and inflammation of the intima of medium and large arteries occur. In most cases, only the inflammation in the coronary arteries is clinically significant. During this period, myocarditis is the most common cause of death. From days 11 to 20 (subacute phase), the myocarditis is less pronounced, but aneurysms form with associated thrombi and stenosis of medium-sized arteries, and perivasculitis and vessel-wall edema occur. In this phase, myocardial infarction, aneurysm rupture, and myocarditis are the usual causes of death. From days 21 to 60 (convalescent phase), vascular inflammation decreases; death may occur from myocardial infarction resulting from thrombosis. The chronic phase begins at 61 days and may last for life. During this period, scar formation and intimal thickening occur in the coronary arteries—changes that may contribute to ischemic heart disease.[86]

Clinical Features

History and Physical Examination Patients with KD experience fever in association with at least four of the following five features: bilateral conjunctival injection, rash, cervical lymphadenopathy, mucous membrane changes, and extremity findings. Each of the clinical criteria, with the exception of the cervical adenopathy, is found in approximately 90% of cases.

Cervical adenopathy is present in 50% of cases, and is frequently the most prominent feature. Nodes are firm and tender but not fluctuent.[86] The fever is generally high and spiking in pattern, with an average duration of 1 to 2 weeks. Generally the fever does not last more than 4 weeks. The conjunctival injection generally involves the bulbar conjunctivae more than the palpebral conjunctivae, is not associated with an exudate, and persists for 1 to 2 weeks. A mild uveitis is often detected by slit-lamp examination. The mucous membrane changes are not associated with ulcerations.[86]

The patient's hands and feet are often so erythematous and indurated that fine motor movements are impaired. A child may be unwilling to stand or walk because of the pain. Between 10 and 20 days after the onset of fever, desquamation of the fingers and toes begins. Beau's lines (transverse grooves of the nails) may appear 1 to 2 months after the onset of fever. The rash, which usually appears within 5 days of the onset of fever, is highly variable. The primary lesion may include scarlatiniform erythroderma, an urticarial exanthem with large erythematous plaques, or a morbilliform maculopapular rash with or without target lesions (resembling erythema multiforme). The rash usually involves the trunk and extremities with prominence in the perineal area. Fine pruritic vesicles may be present, but bullae and pustular lesions are not seen. Desquamation may occur, especially in the perineal region.[83,86,88]

Other signs and symptoms include arthritis and arthralgias, irritability, aseptic meningitis, urethritis with sterile pyuria, myositis and myalgia, hepatitis, diarrhea, pneumonia, and hydrops of the gallbladder, with or without obstructive jaundice.[88]

KD is the most common cause of acquired pediatric heart disease in the United States.[83] The earliest cardiac complications are myocarditis associated with congestive heart failure, pericarditis, pericardial effusions, mitral and aortic insufficiency, and cardiac dysrhythmias; these complications may occur 10 days after the onset of illness, and many resolve within several weeks. Approximately 20% of patients develop coronary artery abnormalities, including aneurysms. Most fatalities occur within this period and result from myocardial infarction from thrombosis or (less commonly) coronary artery aneurysm rupture. Many of the aneurysms eventually resolve, but arterial stenosis may remain permanently.[83,88] The likelihood that an aneurysm will resolve is related to the size of the aneurysm, with the larger aneurysms having the worst prognosis. Patients with asymptomatic coronary artery stenosis may seek emergency care of cardiovascular symptoms many years later. It is important to inquire about childhood illness such as KD when evaluating young patients with acute cardiovascular symptoms.

The clinical course of KD is divided into three phases. The *acute phase* lasts 1 to 2 weeks and is characterized by fever, myocarditis, pericardial effusion, and the other diagnostic signs described previously. In addition to these diagnostic signs, some patients may have an accompanying aseptic meningitis, hepatic dysfunction, or diarrhea. The *subacute phase* lasts approximately 10 days to 1 month after the onset of illness. During this period, the fever, rash, and lymphadenopathy resolve, but conjunctivitis, anorexia, and the extreme irritability often persist. Desquamation of fingers and toes, arthritis, arthralgias, myocardial dysfunction, and thrombocytosis most often occur in this phase. The risk of sudden death is greatest during this phase. The *convalescent phase* begins when most other clinical findings are resolved and continues until the sedimentation rate is normal, usually 6 to 8 weeks after the onset of illness.[86]

Complications The most grave complication of KD is coronary aneurysms that occur in 20% to 25% of untreated patient and 3% to 5% of patients treated with IV immunoglobulin (IVIG) and aspirin (see management).[82] Myocardial infarction occurs in 39% of patients with persistent aneurysms, with a 50% mortality rate.[83] Sudden death occurs in 1% to 2% of untreated patients.[82] Congestive heart failure secondary to myocarditis or myocardial infarction is more common in patients younger than 6 months and older than 9 years of age.[89] Rare complications include aneurysmal rupture with hemopericardium and distal extremity thrombosis secondary to cardiogenic shock or aneurysms in other vessels.[86]

Poor prognostic indicators for KD include a low platelet count, fever lasting more than 16 days, recurrent fever after an afebrile period of more than 48 hours, dysrhythmias other than first-degree block, age younger than 1 year or older than 9 years, and a low hematocrit or albumin on presentation.[86]

Diagnostic Strategies

The diagnosis of KD is based on clinical findings. The CDC case definition of KD is fever lasting 5 days or more without another more reasonable explanation and at least four of the following five criteria[88]:

1. Bilateral conjunctival injection without exudate
2. At least one of the following mucous membrane changes: injected or fissured lips, injected pharynx, or "strawberry" tongue
3. At least one of the following extremity changes: erythema of palms or soles, edema of the hands or feet, or generalized or periungual desquamation
4. Rash
5. Cervical lymphadenopathy (at least one lymph node 1.5 cm or greater in diameter)

These diagnostic criteria are useful in preventing overdiagnosis but may lead to the misdiagnosis of atypical or incomplete KD. This is especially important in children younger than 6 months of age in whom the clinical diagnosis is difficult. This younger age group is at greater risk for coronary artery aneurysms.[89] Some patients with fever of unknown origin and fewer than four of the five criteria have coronary artery disease develop and are considered to have atypical KD.[86]

Although no definitive test exists, the EP may identify certain characteristically abnormal test results, establish a baseline for subsequent comparison, and exclude other disease entities. All patients with suspected KD should have an ECG and echocardiogram to define baseline cardiac conduction, left ventricular function, and coronary artery anatomy. Coronary arteriography may be indicated when persistent echocardiogram abnormalities or signs of myocardial ischemia are present.

All patients should have a CBC (including platelet count), C-reactive protein determination, sedimentation rate, and serum transaminase and bilirubin tests. Typical laboratory findings in patients with KD include an elevated WBC count with a left shift, a normochromic normocytic anemia (during the acute phase), and an elevated platelet count (which peaks in the third or fourth week of illness). Serum transaminase levels may be elevated. The sedimentation rate becomes elevated during the acute phase and remains elevated after the fever resolves, a finding that may help distinguish KD from viral syndromes.

Patients with suspected KD should also have a urinalysis, blood culture, chest radiography, antistreptolysin-O titer, and throat culture for group A streptococcus (GAS) to exclude other illnesses with similar clinical findings. Because 20% to 25% of children may carry GAS in their throats, many children with KD have positive cultures.[86] The urinalysis may show proteinuria and sterile pyuria.

In difficult cases, it may be necessary to order viral cultures, Epstein-Barr viral titers, rickettsial titers, leptospirosis titers, liver function tests, rheumatoid factor, and blood and urine mercury levels. If neurologic signs suggesting meningitis are present or insufficient findings exist to explain the high fever and rash, a lumbar puncture is necessary. A slit-lamp examination to look for uveitis may be a helpful adjunct.

Differential Considerations

Many cases fit the classical case criteria definition. In atypical cases, the diagnosis of KD is difficult. The differential diagnosis includes measles, toxic shock syndrome, scarlet fever, leptospirosis, Stevens-Johnson syndrome, staphylococcal scalded-skin syndrome, influenza, Rocky Mountain spotted fever, juvenile rheumatoid arthritis, drug reaction, other viral infections, and mercury toxicity.[86,88] The commonly observed head and neck manifestations of KD may lead to misdiagnosis of retropharyngeal abscess or other infections of the neck, measles, and GAS infections.

Laboratory studies that may be useful in differentiating KD from alternative diagnoses include hemoglobin concentration, sedimentation rate, and serum alanine aminotransferase level. Patients with KD do not have Koplik's spots, exudative conjunctivitis, or severe cough, as is present in patients with measles.[86]

Management Management of KD includes supportive and symptomatic care along with administration of gammaglobulin and high-dose aspirin. Aspirin is administered for its antiinflammatory and antithrombolytic effects; gammaglobulin is given for its antiinflammatory effect. Treatment should be instituted as soon as possible in the course of the illness, preferably within 10 days of the onset of fever.

The recommended gammaglobulin regimen is 2 g/kg IV as a single infusion over 12 hours. Retreatment with gammaglobulin should be considered for patients with persistent or return of fever or other signs of inflammation 24 hours after completion of therapy.[11] Aspirin is recommended in a dosage of 80 to 100 mg/kg/day in four divided doses during the acute phase of the illness until the patient is afebrile. Children with KD manifest decreased absorption and increased clearance of aspirin; most do not achieve therapeutic salicylate levels despite high-dose aspirin. For this reason, it is not necessary to monitor aspirin levels.[88] After the acute symptoms are controlled, aspirin is reduced to 3 to 5 mg/kg (up to 80 mg/day maximum) in a single daily dose. This is continued for 6 to 8 weeks. A cost-effectiveness analysis of aspirin and gammaglobulin demonstrates that this regimen results in both lower costs and lower rates of coronary artery dilation than aspirin alone or low-dose gammaglobulin.[90]

If coronary artery abnormalities exist, therapy is continued for a longer interval. In cases judged to be at high risk for thrombosis, dipyridamole (2 to 3 mg/kg 2 to 3 times a day) may be added to the therapeutic regimen.[86] Coumadin or heparin along with the described antiplatelet therapy may be used in some patients with severe coronary disease.[86]

The IV gammaglobulin plus aspirin regimen has been demonstrated to reduce the incidence of coronary artery abnormalities.[82,86] Other therapy may be necessary on a case-by-case basis to treat the myocarditis and related congestive heart failure (e.g., digoxin and diuretics), conduction abnormalities, dysrhythmias, or coronary artery thrombosis.

In the acute phase, patients with KD should be hospitalized to confirm the diagnosis, to stabilize complications (e.g., myocarditis, pericarditis, and congestive heart failure), and to initiate therapy. Cardiac complications may necessitate admission for monitoring and treatment of congestive heart failure or management of coronary artery thrombosis with fibrinolytic therapy.

TOXIC SHOCK SYNDROME

Perspective

History In 1978 Todd and colleagues published a report of a series of seven children (8 to 17 years of age) who had high fever, rash, headache, confusion, conjunctival injection, edema, vomiting, diarrhea, renal failure, hepatic dysfunction, DIC, and shock.[91] *S. aureus* was cultured from various body sites but not the blood in five of the seven cases.

In 1979 and 1980 several investigators reported clusters of similar cases in young menstruating women.[92] The term *toxic shock syndrome (TSS)* was coined to describe the constellation of signs and symptoms. They noted the onset of TSS during or immediately after menstruation, association with tampon use, positive vaginal cultures for *S. aureus,* recurrence of illness during subsequent menses, and the value of antistaphylococcal antibiotics in preventing recurrences. In response to the growing concern about TSS, changes were made to reduce the absorbency and composition of tampons.[92] Nonmenstrual cases were also recognized in both men and women as a result of a variety of predisposing conditions.[93,94]

In the late 1980s, several reports described GAS infection associated with shock and multisystem organ failure. This has been called *streptococcal toxic shock syndrome (strep*

TSS) because is shares so many features with staphylococcal TSS.[95]

Epidemiology The peak incidence of TSS occurred in 1980, with 2.4 to 16 cases/100,000 population.[92,94] Since then, the reduction in cases of the menstrual form of TSS has followed an active effort to decrease certain known risk factors. It is recognized that most cases of TSS are associated with the use of high-absorbency tampons during menses.[92] Since 1985, polyacrylate-containing tampons have been removed from the market.[94]

Staphylococcal TSS is described at all ages, but the largest number of cases occur in women in the 15- to 34-year age range. The age and sex distribution reflects this association with menses. The mortality rate from TSS has declined over the past 10 years. The case fatality rate has progressively decreased from 10% before 1980 to less than 1% in 1989.

Nonmenstrual TSS occurs in people of all ages in both sexes; despite the decreased incidence of menstrual cases, the incidence of nonmenstrual TSS remains constant. Thus the proportion of reported nonmenstrual cases has increased from 7% in 1980 to approximately 50% of all cases in recent years. This form of TSS has been reported secondary to a wide variety of surgical procedures, focal infections, and various other predisposing factors (Box 123-4).[93,96]

Streptococcal TSS is also described in all ages, with most cases occurring in patients 20 to 50 years of age. Both genders are equally affected, and the disease is usually associated with an identifiable infectious source. Unlike staphylococcal TSS, the morbidity rate of streptococcal TSS remains extremely high at 30% to 70%.[94,97]

Etiology

Colonization or infection with *S. aureus* must occur for staphylococcal TSS to develop. *S. aureus* has been detected in virtually all cases of both forms of the illness. *S. aureus* has been isolated from the vagina or cervix in 98% of women with menstrual TSS compared with a colonization rate of less than 10% of normal women.[98] *S. aureus* has also been identified in almost all cases of nonmenstrual TSS. Because the organism is often not invasive, the blood cultures are often negative. Streptococcal TSS is caused by infection with group A streptococci.[94]

Principles of Disease

S. aureus produces exotoxins that are mediators of the clinical syndrome. Certain local factors favor production of these toxins. Toxic shock syndrome toxin (TSST-1) and other exotoxins are associated TSS development.[92–94] TSST-1 is identified in more than 90% of menstrual cases and 60% of nonmenstrual cases. Other toxins also may play a role in nonmenstrual TSS. GAS produces streptococcal pyrogenic exotoxin A (SPEA) and B (SPEB). These exotoxins are absorbed into the bloodstream through inflamed or traumatized mucous membranes or from areas of focal infection. Absorbed toxins induce mononuclear cells to produce cytokines, tumor necrosis factor-α and interleukins with begin the cascade of systemic vasculitis and multisystem manifestations of the disease. Host immune factors are important in the pathogenesis of TSS. Patients with TSS have low levels of antibodies to TSST-1, whereas controls have high antibody levels.[94]

Box 123-4 Sources of Nonmenstrual Toxic Shock Syndrome

Surgical Procedures

Amputations
Arthrodesis
Arthroscopy
Breast surgery (augmentation, reduction, removal of prosthesis)
Bladder suspension
Cholecystectomy
Cyst enucleation
Dilatation and curettage
Episiotomy
Exploratory laparotomy
External fixators
Herniorrhaphy
Hysterectomy
Hip surgery
Lipoma removal
Loop electrosurgical excision
Lumbar sympathectomy
Orchiectomy
Osteoplasty
Peritoneal lavage
Pleurectomy
Salpingo-oophorectomy
Septorhinoplasty
Shoulder repair
Sinus surgery
Skin grafting
Spinal fusion
Suction lipectomy
Subtotal thyroidectomy
Tubal ligation
Uretero lithotomy
Varicose vein ligation

Focal Infections

Abrasions
Abscesses
Adenitis
Bites (animal, human, insect)
Bronchitis
Burns
Bursitis
Cellulitis
Cysts
Empyema
Endocarditis
Furuncle
Heroin injection site
Hydradenitis suppurativa
Laryngotracheitis
Mastitis
Osteomyelitis
Perirectal abscess
Pharyngitis
Prostatitis
Septic arthritis
Subcutaneous insulin pump

Vaginal (Nonmenstrual)

Childbirth (vaginal or cesarean)
Abortion (spontaneous or induced)
Vaginal infections
Pelvic inflammatory disease
Barrier contraception (sponge, diaphragm, cervical cap)

Other

AIDS
Influenza
Nasal packing for epistaxis
Tympanic membrane drainage tube
Unknown

Clinical Features

History and Physical Examination Some patients have a prodromal illness consisting of fever, chills, and myalgias that progresses to the systemic syndrome. Others become abruptly symptomatic within hours.

The major symptoms of TSS are fever, rash, tachycardia, and hypotension.[99] The fever is usually abrupt in onset with a high temperature. The classic rash is a nonpruritic, diffuse, blanching, macular erythroderma. Initially, the subtle rash may be faint and evanescent and may be mistaken for the flush associated with a fever.[96] It then progresses to a more distinct exanthem. The rash is usually diffuse but may be localized to the trunk, extremities, or perineum. After 5 to 12 days, a fine flaking desquamation occurs on the face and trunk, and there is a full-thickness peeling of skin involving the palms, soles, and fingers. Hypotension results from an absolute or relative hypovolemia.[93,94]

Table 123-4. Comparison of Staphylococcal and Streptococcal Toxic Shock Syndrome

Feature	Staphylococcal	Streptococcal
Age	Primarily 15-35 years	Primarily 20-50 years
Sex	Greatest in women	Either
Severe pain	Rare	Common
Hypotension	100%	100%
Erythroderma rash	Very common	Less common
Renal failure	Common	Common
Bacteremia	Low	60%
Tissue necrosis	Rare	Common
Predisposing factors	Tampons, packing, NSAID use?	Cuts, burns, bruises, varicella, NSAID use?
Thrombocytopenia	Common	Common
Mortality rate	<3%	30%-70%

NSAID, Nonsteroidal antiinflammatory drug.

Because TSS involves virtually every organ system, a wide constellation of signs and symptoms may be seen. GI involvement is manifested by vomiting, diarrhea, and severe abdominal pain. Hepatomegaly may be present, and myalgias and arthralgias commonly occur. Edema of the face and eyelids, and hyperemia of the pharynx, tongue, and conjunctiva may be seen. An intense headache occurs in almost all cases. Alterations in mental status, including confusion, somnolence, agitation, and combativeness are present in 55% of patients and are out of proportion to hypotension.[96] Possible genital findings include hyperemia of the vulva and vagina, vaginal ulcerations, a purulent cervical discharge, and tenderness of the external genitalia and adnexa.[93-96]

Comparisons between staphylococcal and streptococcal TSS are presented in Table 123-4.

Complications Complications of TSS include acute respiratory distress syndrome, shock, gangrene, DIC, renal failure, and a constellation of neuropsychiatric symptoms.[100] Less common findings in staphylococcal TSS include rhabdomyolysis, seizures, pancreatitis, pericarditis, and cardiomyopathy. Women with the menstrual form of TSS may experience one or more recurrent episodes; recurrences of the nonmenstrual form are rare.

In streptococcal TSS, rhabdomyolysis occurs in up to 63% of patients and is usually related to the underlying soft tissue infection.[99]

Diagnostic Strategies

The revised case definitions for the TSSs are given in Boxes 123-5 and 123-6. According to these criteria, the patient must have fever, rash, desquamation, and hypotension. Furthermore, three of the major organ systems must be involved. It is not required that specific tests be performed to exclude other diseases; but if such tests are obtained, the results of these studies must be negative. The case definition does not require a positive culture for *S. aureus,* but does for *Streptococcus* organisms. These case definitions are useful to the clinician, but they are not specific or foolproof.[93,94]

There are not specific laboratory changes associated with TSS, but many abnormalities are common. Either leukocytosis or leukopenia can occur, but a marked bandemia (40% to 50%) is very common.[94,95,97] Elevated creatinine levels occur in 40% to 89% of patients.[99] Hypoalbuminemia and life-threatening hypocalcemia are prominent initially and persist throughout the course of the disease.[94] Other abnormalities include anemia, thrombocytopenia, hyperbilirubinemia (76%), elevated transaminase levels (50% to 75%), and sterile pyuria.[99]

Box 123-5 Case Definition of Toxic Shock Syndrome (Revised)

Fever: temperature ≥38.9° C (102° F)
Rash: diffuse macular erythroderma
Desquamation 1 to 2 weeks after onset of illness, particularly of palms and soles
Hypotension: systolic blood pressure ≤90 mm Hg for adults or below fifth percentile by age for children less than 16 years of age, orthostatic drop in diastolic blood pressure ≥15 mm Hg from lying to sitting, orthostatic syncope, or orthostatic dizziness
Multisystem involvement—*three* or more of the following:
- Gastrointestinal: vomiting or diarrhea at onset of illness
- Muscular: severe myalgia or creatine phosphokinase level at least twice the upper limit of normal for laboratory
- Mucous membrane: vaginal, oropharyngeal, or conjunctival hyperemia
- Renal: BUN or creatinine at least twice the upper limit of normal for laboratory or urinary sediment with pyuria (≥5 leukocytes per high-power field) in the absence of urinary tract infection
- Hepatic: total bilirubin, AST,* ALT† at least twice the upper limit of normal for laboratory
- Hematologic: platelets ≤100,000/mm³
- CNS: disorientation or alterations in consciousness without focal neurologic signs when fever and hypotension are absent

Negative results on the following tests, if obtained:
- Blood, throat, or CSF cultures (blood culture may be positive for *S. aureus*)
- Rise in titer to Rocky Mountain spotted fever, leptospirosis, or rubeola

*AST (SGOT) denotes serum aspartate transaminase.
†ALT (SGPT) denotes serum alanine transaminase.

Box 123-6 Case Definition for Streptococcal Toxic Shock Syndrome

1. Isolation of group A streptococcus from:
   A. A sterile body site
   B. A nonsterile body site
2. Clinical signs of severity
   A. Hypotension AND
   B. Clinical and laboratory abnormalities (requires two or more of the following):
      Renal impairment
      Coagulopathy
      Liver abnormalities
      Acute respiratory distress syndrome
      Extensive tissue necrosis (i.e., necrotizing fasciitis)
      Erythematous rash

Definite Case: 1A + 2(A + B)
Probable Case: 1B + 2(A + B)

Group A Streptococcal Necrotizing Fasciitis

Definite:
1. Necrosis of soft tissue with involvement of fascia **PLUS**
2. Serious systemic disease including one or more of the following:
   A. Death
   B. Shock (systolic blood pressure <90 mm Hg)
   C. Disseminated intravascular coagulopathy
   D. Failure of organ system (respiratory failure, liver failure, renal failure) **PLUS**
3. Isolation of GAS from normally sterile body site

Suspected:
1 + 2 + serologic diagnosis of GAS (antistreptolysin O or DNAse B)
1 + 2 + histologic confirmation of gram-positive cocci in a necrotic soft tissue infection

Differential Considerations

The diagnosis of TSS is made on a clinical basis after ancillary testing and consideration of the differential diagnosis. Other diseases to consider include KD, staphylococcal scalded-skin syndrome, scarlet fever, drug reactions such as Stevens-Johnson syndrome, Rocky Mountain spotted fever, leptospirosis, meningococcemia, atypical measles, and viral illnesses.

KD occurs predominantly in children, usually does not progress to shock, lacks the multisystem involvement, exhibits a protracted fever, and is associated with thrombocytosis later in its course. Staphylococcal scalded-skin syndrome presents with a desquamating rash acutely, whereas the desquamation of TSS occurs in the convalescent phase. Staphylococcal scalded-skin syndrome does not progress to shock, is not associated with multisystem illness, and lacks mucous membrane involvement. Scarlet fever differs in its clinical course by a lack of shock and multisystem involvement, positive cultures for GAS, and a rise in the convalescent titer. Stevens-Johnson syndrome usually occurs after drug administration, has characteristic mucous membrane lesions, and lacks desquamation. Rocky Mountain spotted fever occurs after a tick bite, does not present with hypotension, has a distinctive rash, and is associated with a severe headache without an altered mental status. Leptospirosis occurs in endemic areas and may be distinguished by positive serologic studies and cultures. The rash of meningococcemia is characterized by petechiae and purpura occurring anywhere on the skin.[93]

Management

The initial therapy of TSS is supportive. Hypotension often responds to large volumes of isotonic crystalloids (10 to 20 L/day), although hemodynamic monitoring and vasopressors may be necessary. Most patients should be managed in an intensive care setting.[93-96]

The source of bacteria, such as tampons, nasal packs, and other foreign bodies, must be removed. Areas of infection and surgical wounds should be incised and drained promptly. If specimens are sent for culture, the laboratory should be informed of the suspected diagnosis.

Antibiotics may not affect the clinical course of staphylococcal TSS, but are probably beneficial if the patient has bacteremia or occult areas of infection. They are recommended in streptococcal TSS because there is typically an obvious source of infection.

For septic patients without an identified organism, broad-spectrum antibiotics should be administered as soon as possible. Although penicillin has been the mainstay of treatment for streptococcal infection, treatment failures occur commonly in severe disease. For both staphylococcal and streptococcal TSS, most clinicians recommend clindamycin as a first-line agent.[93-96] Clindamycin is a potent suppresser of bacterial toxin synthesis; it also facilitates phagocytosis of streptococci and has a longer postantibiotic effect than the β-lactams. The dose is 600 to 900 mg every 8 hours. (The pediatric dose is 20 to 40 mg/kg/day divided every 6 to 8 hours.) Clindamycin and erythromycin have also been shown to decrease monocyte synthesis of tumor necrosis factor-α.[93-96]

Patients who do not respond to massive fluid resuscitation, antibiotics, and pressors should be considered for IVIG treatment, especially if pulmonary edema develops and requires mechanical ventilation. Pooled immune globulin has high titers for antibodies to TSS-1 and other exotoxin, and significant improvement has been reported with its use. The recommended dose is 400 mg/kg administered over several hours.[93,96]

The value of corticosteroids in TSS is still unresolved, but they are not currently recommended for treating staphylococcal or streptococcal TSS.[94]

KEY CONCEPTS

- All patients appearing septic should be treated with broad-spectrum antibiotics as soon as possible, even before a definitive diagnosis is made.
- A surgeon should be consulted immediately for patients with sepsis and a debridable source of infection.
- Immunity to diphtheria, tetanus, and pertussis wanes significantly in adults. Pertussis should always be considered as a cause of persistent cough in adults. A tetanus vaccination history should always be obtained from patients with trauma or infection. When there is doubt about the history, the age-appropriate vaccine according to CDC guidelines is administered.
- Neonates with suspected pertussis should be admitted to an intensive care setting.

- Botulism should be kept in the differential for the infant with failure to thrive, constipation, or decreased muscle tone and for the IV drug user with neurologic symptoms
- IV gammaglobulin should be administered as soon as a diagnosis of Kawasaki syndrome is made.

REFERENCES

1. MacGregor RR: Corynebacterium diphtheria. In Mandell GL, Douglas RG, Bennett JE, editors: *Principles and practice of infectious disease,* ed 5, Philadelphia, 2000, Churchill Livingstone.
2. Centers for Disease Control: Summary of notifiable diseases, United States, *MMWR* 37:20, 1989.
3. Vitek CR, Wharton M: Diphtheria in the former Soviet Union: reemergence of a pandemic disease, *Emerging Infect Dis* 4:1-17, 1998.
4. Alagappan K et al: Antibody protection to diphtheria in geriatric patients: need for ED compliance with immunization guidelines, *Ann Emerg Med* 30:455-458, 1997.
5. Galazka A: The changing epidemiology of diphtheria in the vaccine era, *J Infect Dis* 181(suppl 1):S2-S9, 2000.
6. World Health Organization: Expanded programme on immunization, *Weekly Epidemiol Rec* 68:137, 1993.
7. Hadfield TL et al: The pathology of diphtheria, *J Infect Dis* 181(suppl 1):S116-S120, 2000.
8. Kadirova R, Kartoglu Ü, Strebel PM: Clinical characteristics and management of 676 hospitalized diphtheria cases, Kyrgyz republic, 1995, *J Infect Dis* 181:S110-S115, 2000.
9. Rakhamanova AG et al: Diphtheria outbreak in St. Petersburg: clinical characteristics of 1,860 adult patients, *Scan J Infect Dis* 28;37-40, 1996.
10. Efstratiou A et al: Current approaches to the laboratory diagnosis of diphtheria, *J Infect Dis* 181:S138-S145, 2000.
11. American Academy of Pediatrics: *Report of the committee on infectious diseases,* ed 23, Elk Grove Village, Ill, 1994, The Academy.
12. Pasternack M: Pertussis in the 1990s: diagnosis, treatment, and prevention, *Curr Clin Top Infect Dis* 17:24-36, 1997.
13. Hewlett EL: *Bordetella* species. In Mandell GL, Douglas RG, Bennett JE, editors: *Principles and practice of infectious diseases,* ed 5, Philadelphia, 2000 Churchill Livingstone.
14. Centers for Disease Control and Prevention: Pertussis—United States, January 1992-June 1995, *MMWR* 44:525-529, 1995.
15. Decker MD, Edwards KM: Acellular pertussis vaccines, *Ped Clin North Am,* 47:309-335, 2000.
16. Braun MM et al: Infant immunization with acellular pertussis vaccines in the Unites States: assessment of the first two years' data from the vaccine adverse event reporting system, *Pediatrics* 106:E51, 2000.
17. Keitel WA, Edwards KM: Acellular pertussis vaccine in adults, *Inf Dis Clin North Am* 13:83-94, 1999.
18. Watkins WF: Pertussis. In Harwood-Nuss A, editor: *The clinical practice of emergency medicine,* Philadelphia, 1996, JB Lippincott.
19. Hoppe JE: Neonatal pertussis, *Pediatr Infect Dis* 19:244-247, 2000.
20. Wright SW: Pertussis infection in adults, *South Med J* 91:702-708, 1998.
21. Bruss JB et al: Treatment of severe pertussis: a study of the safety and pharmacology of intravenous pertussis immunoglobulin, *Pediatr Infect Dis* 18:505-511, 1999.
22. Dodhia H, Miller E: Review of the evidence for the use of erythromycin in the management of persons exposed to pertussis, *Epidemiol Infect,* 120:143-149, 1998.
23. Centers for Disease Control and Prevention: Pertussis vaccination: use of acellular pertussis vaccines among infants and young children. Recommendations of the Advisory Committee on Immunizations Practices (ACIP), *MMWR* 46(RR-7):1-25, 1997.
24. Stoll BJ: Tetanus, *Pediatr Clin North Am* 26:415-431, 1979.
25. Bleck TP: *Clostridium tetani.* In Mandell GL, Douglas RG, Bennett JE, editors: *Principles and practice of infectious diseases,* ed 5, Philadelphia, 2000, Churchill Livingstone.
26. Abrutyn E: Tetanus. In Fauci AS et al, editors: *Harrison's principles of internal medicine,* ed 14, New York, 1998, McGraw-Hill.
27. Loscalzo IL et al: Tetanus: a clinical diagnosis, *Am J Emerg Med* 13:489-490, 1995.
28. Centers for Disease Control and Prevention: Tetanus Surveillance—United States, 1995-1997, *MMWR* 47(SS-2):1-13, 1998.
29. Lipman J et al: Autonomic dysfunction in severe tetanus: magnesium sulfate as an adjunct to deep sedation, *Crit Care Med* 15:987-988, 1987.
30. Toh HC, Tiam AP: Severe tetanus in a patient with ulcerating inflammatory breast carcinoma, *Acta Oncologica* 36:94-96, 1997.
31. Ernst ME et al: Tetanus: pathophysiology and management, *Ann Pharmacother* 31:1507-1513, 1997.
32. Shibuya M et al: The use of continuous spinal anesthesia in severe tetanus, *J Trauma* 29:1423-1429, 1989.
33. Konstanzer DJ, Weinzierl FX, Klinggelhofer J: Intrathecal baclofen in tetanus: four cases and a review of the reported cases, *Intensive Care Med* 23:896-902, 1997.
34. Abrutyn E, Berlin JA: Intrathecal therapy in tetanus: a meta-analysis, *JAMA* 266:2262, 1991.
35. Tobias JD: Anesthetic implications of tetanus, *South J Med* 91:384-387, 1998.
36. Gilbert DN, Moellering RC, Sande MA, editors: *Sanford guide to antimicrobial therapy,* ed 30, Hyde Park, Vt, 2000, Antimicrobial Therapy Inc.
37. Ahmadsyah I, Salim A: Treatment of tetanus: an open study to compare the efficacy of procaine penicillin and metronidazole, *BMJ* 291:648-650, 1985.
38. Alagappan K, Rennie W, Kwiatkowski T: Seroprevalence of tetanus antibodies among adults older than 65 years, *Ann Emerg Med* 28:18-21, 1996.
39. Giangrasso J, Smith RK: Misuse of tetanus immunoprophylaxis in wound care, *Ann Emerg Med* 14:573-579, 1985.
40. Centers for Disease Control and Prevention: Diphtheria, tetanus and pertussis: recommendations for vaccine use and other preventive measures, *MMWR* 40 (RR-10):1, 1991.
41. Centers for Disease Control and Prevention: Update: vaccine side effects, adverse reactions, contraindications, and precautions—recommendations of the Advisory Committee on Immunization Practice (ACIP), *MMWR* 45(RR-12):1-31, 1996.
42. Lindsey D: Tetanus prophylaxis: do our guidelines assure adequate protection? *J Trauma* 24:1063-1064, 1984.
43. Bleck T: *Clostridium botulinum* (botulism). In Mandell GL, Douglas RG, Bennett JE, editors: *Principles and practice of infectious diseases,* ed 5, Philadelphia, 2000, Churchill Livingstone.
44. Cherington M: Clinical spectrum of botulism, *Muscle Nerve* 21:701-710, 1998.
45. Centers for Disease Control and Prevention: Food-borne botulism—Oklahoma, 1994. *MMWR* 44:200-202, 1995.
46. Centers for Disease Control and Prevention: Food-borne botulism from eating home-picked eggs—Illinois, 1997, *MMWR* 49:778-780, 2000.
47. Shapiro RL, Hatheway C, Swerdlow DL: Botulism in the United States: a clinical and epidemiologic review, *Ann Intern Med* 129:221-228, 1998.
48. Centers for Disease Control and Prevention: Botulism in the United States 1899-1996. In *Handbook for epidemiologists, clinicians and laboratory workers,* Atlanta, 1998, US Department of Heath and Human Services.
49. Byard RW et al: *Clostridium botulinum* and sudden infant death syndrome: a 10-year prospective study, *J Pediatr Child Health* 28:156-157, 1992.
50. Passare DJ, Werner SB, McGee J: Wound botulism associated with black tar heroin injecting drug users, *JAMA* 279:859-863, 1998.
51. Abrutyn E: Botulism. In Fauci AS et al, editors: *Harrison's principles of internal medicine,* ed 14, New York, 1998, McGraw-Hill.
52. Urdaneta-Carruyo E, Suranyi A, Milano M: Infantile botulism: clinical and laboratory observations of a rare neuroparalytic disease, *J Pediatr Child Health* 36:193-195, 2000.
53. Maselli RA, Bakshi N: AAEM case report 16: botulism. American Association of Electrodiagnostic Medicine, *Muscle Nerve* 23:1137-1144, 2000.
54. Rubenstein E: Food poisoning. In Rubenstein E, Federman DD, editors: *Scientific American medicine,* New York, 1990, Scientific American.

55. Austrian R: The pneumococcus at Hopkins: early portents of future developments, *John Hopkins Med J* 144:192-201, 1979.
56. Ball P: Therapy for pneumococcal infection at the millennium: doubt and certainties, *Am J Med* 107(suppl 1A):77S-82S, 1999.
57. Centers for Disease Control and Prevention: Preventing pneumococcal disease among infants and young children: recommendations of the Advisory Committee on Immunizations Practices (ACIP), *MMWR* 49(RR09):1-38, 2000.
58. Centers for Disease Control and Prevention: Preventing pneumococcal disease: recommendations of the Advisory Committee on Immunizations Practices (ACIP), *MMWR* 46(RR-8):1-24, 1997.
59. Musher DM et al: Bacteremic and nonbacteremic pneumococcal pneumonia, *Medicine* 79:210-220, 2000.
60. Totapally BR, Walsh WT: Pneumococcal bacteremia in children: a 6-year experience in a community hospital, *Chest* 113:1207-1214, 1998.
61. Butler JC, Schuchat A: Epidemiology of pneumococcal infections in the elderly, *Drugs Aging* 15:11-19, 1999.
62. Harwell JI, Brown RB: The drug-resistant pneumococcus, *Chest* 117:530-541, 2000.
63. Korones DN, Shapiro ED: Occult pneumococcal bacteremia: what happens to the child who appears well at reevaluation? *Pediatr Infect Dis J* 13:382-386, 1994.
64. The ACCP/SCCM Consensus Conference Committee: Definitions for sepsis and organ failure and guidelines for the use of innovative therapies in sepsis, *Chest* 101:1644-1655, 1992.
65. Rosenberg N, Cohen SN: Pneumococcal bacteremia in pediatric patients, *Ann Emerg Med* 11:2-6, 1982.
66. Kobel D-E et al: Pneumococcal vaccine in patients with absent or dysfunctional spleen, *Mayo Clin Proc* 75:749-753, 2000.
67. Ros SP, Herman BE, Beissel J: Occult bacteremia: is there a standard of care? *Pediatr Emerg Care* 10:264-267, 1994.
68. Butler JC, Cetron MS: Pneumococcal drug resistance: the new "special enemy of old age," *Clin Infect Dis* 28:730-735, 1999.
69. Dershewitz RA et al: A comparative study of the prevalence, outcome, and prediction of bacteremia in children, *J Pediatr* 103:352-358, 1983.
70. Overturf GD: Technical report: prevention of pneumococcal infections, including the use of pneumococcal conjugated and polysaccharide vaccines and antibiotic prophylaxis, *Pediatrics* 106:367-376, 2000.
71. Apicella MA: *Neisseria meningitidis.* In Mandell GL et al, editors: *Principles and practice of infectious disease,* ed 5, Philadelphia, 2000, Churchill Livingstone.
72. Solberg CO: In Fauci AS et al *Harrison's principles of internal medicine,* ed 14, New York, 1998, McGraw-Hill.
73. Centers for Disease Control and Prevention: Prevention and control of meningococcal disease: recommendations of the Advisory Committee on Immunization Practice (ACIP), *MMWR* 49(RR07):1-10, 2000.
74. Salzman MB, Rubin LG: Meningococcemia, *Infect Dis Clin North Am* 10:709-725, 1996.
75. de Kleijn ED et al: Pathophysiology of meningococcal sepsis in children, *Eur J Pediatr* 157:869-880, 1998.
76. Riedo FX, Plikaytis BD, Broome CV: Epidemiology and prevention of meningococcal disease, *Pediatr Infect Dis* 14:643-657, 1995.
77. Hardman JM: Fatal meningococcal infections: the changing pathologic picture of the '60s, *Mil Med* 133:951-964, 1968.
78. Van Nguyen OV, Nguyen EA, Weiner LB: Incidence of invasive bacterial disease in children with fever and petechiae, *Pediatrics* 74:77-80, 1984.
79. Odio CM et al: The beneficial effects of early dexamethasone administration, *N Engl J Med* 324:1525-1531, 1991.
80. Drapkin MS et al: Plasmapheresis for fulminant meningococcemia, *Pediatr Infect Dis J* 8:399-400, 1989.
81. Kawasaki T et al: A new infantile acute febrile mucocutaneous lymph node syndrome (MLNS) prevailing in Japan, *Pediatrics* 54:271-276, 1974.
82. Burns JC, Kushner HI, Bastian JF: Kawasaki disease: a brief history, *Pediatrics* 106:E27, 2000.
83. Saulsbury FT: Kawasaki syndrome In Mandell GL et al, editors: *Principles and practice of infectious diseases,* ed 5, Philadelphia, 2000, Churchill Livingstone.
84. Jackson JL et al: Adult Kawasaki disease: report of two cases treated with intravenous gamma globulin, *Arch Intern Med* 154:1398-1405, 1994.
85. Centers for Disease Control: Multiple outbreaks of Kawasaki syndrome—United States, *MMWR* 34:33-35, 1985.
86. Rowley AH, Shulman ST: Kawasaki syndrome, *Clin Microbiol Rev* 11:405-414, 1998.
87. Leung DYN, Schlievert PM, Meissner HC: The immunopathogenesis and management of Kawasaki syndrome, *Arthritis Rheum* 41:1538-1547, 1998.
88. Rowley AH, Shulmen ST: Kawasaki syndrome, *Pediatr Clin North Am* 46:313-329, 1999.
89. Momenah T et al: Kawasaki disease in older children, *Pediatrics* 102:E7, 1998.
90. Sato N et al: Selective high dose gamma-globulin treatment in Kawasaki disease: assessment of clinical aspects and cost effectiveness, *Pediatr Int* 41:1-7, 1999.
91. Todd J et al: Toxic-shock syndrome associated with phage-group-I staphylococci, *Lancet* 2:1116-1118, 1978.
92. Centers for Disease Control and Prevention: Toxic-shock syndrome—United States, *MMWR* 48(LMRK):60-70, 1999.
93. Parsonnet J: Nonmenstruating toxic-shock syndrome: new insights into diagnosis, pathogenesis, and treatment, *Curr Clin Top Infect Dis* 16:1-20, 1996.
94. Stevens DL: The toxic shock syndromes, *Infect Dis Clin North Am* 10:727-746, 1996.
95. Wessels MR: Streptococcal and enterococcal infections. In Fauci AS et al, editors: *Harrison's principles of internal medicine,* ed 14, New York, 1998, McGraw-Hill.
96. Deresiewicz RL, Parsonnet J: Staphylococcal infections. In Fauci AS et al, editors: *Harrison's principles of internal medicine,* ed 14, New York, 1998, McGraw-Hill.
97. Salandy D, Brenner B: *Toxic shock syndrome,* eMedicine.com/emerg/topic600/htm, 1999.
98. Guinan ME et al: Vaginal colonization with staphylococcus aureus in healthy women, *Ann Intern Med* 96(part 2): 944-947, 1982.
99. Hauser AR: Another toxic shock syndrome: streptococcal infection is even more dangerous than the staphylococcal form, *Postgraduate Med* 104:31-43, 1998.
100. Rosene KA et al: Persistent neuropsychiatric sequelae of toxic shock syndrome, *Ann Intern Med* 96:865-870, 1982.

124 Viruses

Michael Alan Polis
Tenagne Haile-Mariam

Most viral infections present as benign, self-limited upper respiratory tract or gastrointestinal infections, and therapy is most often directed at control of symptoms. The exact identification of the causative virus is usually not required. For several viral diseases that have specific therapy or postexposure prophylaxis, recognizing the disease and promptly instituting therapy or prevention may prevent permanent sequelae or death. Examples of how prompt recognition and therapy can change the outcome of potentially fatal viral illness are the early institution of acyclovir in the treatment of herpes simplex virus (HSV) encephalitis and the appropriate use of rabies vaccine and immunoglobulin in exposed patients.

CLASSIFICATION

Viruses were first distinguished from other microorganisms by their ability to pass through filters of small pore size. Initial classifications of viruses were based on the pathologic properties (e.g., enteroviruses) or epidemiologic features (e.g., arboviruses) of the viruses. More recently, classification has been based on the genetic relationships of the viruses. The constituents of the current classification are the type and structure of the viral nucleic acid, the type of symmetry of the virus capsid, and the presence or absence of an envelope (Table 124-1).

The genetic information of viruses is encoded in nucleic acids, either DNA or RNA, that can be either single- or double-stranded and circular (closed ended) or linear (open ended). The genomes of the smallest viruses may encode for only three or four proteins, whereas those of the largest viruses encode for several hundred proteins. A protein coat, called the *capsid,* is composed of a repeating series of protein subunits, called *capsomeres.* The viral nucleic acid and the surrounding protein coat are jointly referred to as the *nucleocapsid.* The use of repeating protein structures limits the shape of the capsid. All but the most complex viruses are either helically symmetric or icosahedral. Finally, some virus nucleocapsids are surrounded by a lipid envelope acquired by the virus as it buds from the cell cytoplasm, nuclear membranes, or endoplasmic reticulum. Some virally encoded proteins may be inserted into this lipid envelope.

VIRAL IMMUNIZATIONS

Whereas treatment strategies against most bacterial diseases have focused on treating and eradicating bacteria from the host after disease has developed, the most successful strategies against viral diseases have concentrated on immunization. The history of immunization against viral diseases began in 1796 when Jenner injected pustular material from the lesions of cowpox into a child to prevent smallpox.[1] The term *vaccination* is derived from *vaccinia,* the virus once used as a smallpox immunization, originally meaning "inoculation to render a person immune to smallpox." Currently, the terms *vaccination* and *immunization* are used interchangeably to mean the administration of any vaccine. *Immunization* is a broader term that includes administering immunobiologics such as immune globulins.

Viral vaccines are suspensions of live, attenuated, or inactivated whole viruses or parts of viruses that are administered to induce immunity. Some vaccines, such as the surface antigen of hepatitis B, are highly defined; others, such as live, attenuated viruses, are complex. Immune globulin is an antibody preparation obtained from large pools of human blood plasma. It is given intramuscularly for passive immunization against measles and hepatitis A, and intravenously (IV) as replacement therapy for antibody-deficiency disorders. Specific immune globulins are preparations of monoclonal antibodies or are prepared from special donor pools preselected for high antibody titers against specific antigens such as hepatitis B, varicella-zoster, or rabies. None of the immune globulin preparations, when properly prepared, can transmit infectious viruses such as hepatitis B virus or human immunodeficiency virus (HIV).

The modern era of immunization began in 1885, when Louis Pasteur and colleagues injected the first of 14 daily doses of rabbit spinal cord suspensions containing progressively inactivated rabies virus into 9-year-old Joseph Meister, who had been bitten by a rabid dog 2 days earlier.[2] The introduction of the inactivated poliomyelitis vaccine in 1955 and the attenuated live oral polio vaccine in 1962 has virtually eliminated the threat of paralytic poliomyelitis in the United States and other developed countries.[3,4] Vaccines against measles, mumps, rubella, influenza, and hepatitis B have greatly reduced morbidity and mortality associated with these diseases. The worldwide eradication of smallpox in 1977 is a testament to the advances made against viral diseases.[5] Currently, a massive World Health Organization campaign to eradicate polio worldwide is underway.

Administration of an immunobiologic agent does not automatically confer adequate immunity. Some products require more than one dose to produce an adequate antibody response or periodic boosters to maintain protection. The simultaneous administration of immune globulin with a live virus vaccine may result in diminished antibody response to the vaccine. Deviation from the recommended volume or number of doses of any vaccine is strongly discouraged. Significant problems also remain in developing countries that cannot afford vaccines or have problems delivering vaccines to their at-risk populations. Table 124-2 summarizes currently available viral vaccines, their indications, and recommended uses.[6-10]

ANTIVIRAL CHEMOTHERAPY

Because most viral illnesses are self-limited, treatment is generally targeted at ameliorating symptoms. The revolution in molecular biology has unlocked pathophysiologic mecha-

Table 124-1. Classification of Viruses

Family	Example(s)	Representative diseases
DNA viruses		
Poxviridae	Variola	Smallpox
	Orf	Contagious pustular dermatitis
Herpesviridae	Herpes simplex 1 and 2	Mucocutaneous ulcers, herpes encephalitis
	Cytomegalovirus	Pneumonitis in immunocompromised patients
	Varicella-zoster virus	Chickenpox, shingles
	Human herpes virus 6	Roseola infantum
	Epstein-Barr virus	Mononucleosis
Adenoviridae	Adenovirus (50+ species)	Upper respiratory tract infections, diarrhea
Papillomavirinae	Papillomavirus (80+ species)	Warts (e.g., plantar, genital)
Polyomavirinae	JC virus	Progressive multifocal leukoencephalopathy
Hepadnaviridae	Hepatitis B	Hepatitis
Parvoviridae	Parvovirus B19	Aplastic anemia
RNA viruses		
Reoviridae	Colorado tick fever	Fever and rash
	Rotavirus	Gastroenteritis
Togaviridae	Eastern equine encephalitis	Epidemic encephalitis
	Rubella	German measles
Flaviviridae	Yellow fever	Hemorrhagic fever
	Dengue	Dengue hemorrhagic fever
	Hepatitis C	Chronic hepatitis
Coronaviridae	Coronavirus	Upper respiratory tract infections
Paramyxoviridae	Respiratory syncytial virus	Bronchiolitis
	Measles	Measles (rubeola), subacute sclerosing panencephalitis
	Parainfluenza	Croup
Rhabdoviridae	Rabies	Rabies
Filoviridae	Ebola	Hemorrhagic fever
Orthomyxoviridae	Influenza A or B	Influenza
Bunyaviridae	La Crosse	Encephalitis
	Hantaan	Hemorrhagic fevers, adult respiratory distress syndrome
Arenaviridae	Lassa	Hemorrhagic fever
	Lymphocytic choriomeningitis virus	Meningoencephalitis
Retroviridae	Human immunodeficiency virus	Acquired immunodeficiency syndrome
Picornaviridae	Poliovirus	Polio
	Coxsackie B	Myocarditis
	Hepatitis A	Enteric hepatitis
	Rhinovirus (115+ species)	Upper respiratory infections
Caliciviridae	Norwalk virus	Gastroenteritis
	Hepatitis E	Enteric hepatitis
Unclassified viruses		
Subviral agents		
Satellites	Delta virus	Hepatitis
Prions	—	Kuru, Creutzfeldt-Jakob disease

nisms of viral diseases and opened up the field of viral chemotherapy. The initial therapeutic armamentarium for viral diseases has been aimed at illnesses associated with significant mortality (e.g., ribavirin for Lassa fever, acyclovir for herpes simplex encephalitis) or those associated with significant end-organ damage (e.g., ganciclovir for cytomegalovirus [CMV] retinitis, acyclovir for ophthalmic zoster) (Table 124-3).

Amantadine and Rimantadine

Amantadine (Symmetrel) and rimantadine (Flumadine) are effective in preventing and treating influenza A, but have no activity against influenza B. They prevent or greatly reduce the uncoating of the viral RNA of influenza A after attachment and endocytosis by host cells.[11] When initiated before exposure to influenza A, amantadine, 200 mg a day orally, is effective in preventing illness in 50% to 90% of subjects. When begun within 2 days after the onset of symptoms of influenza A, amantadine has reduced the duration of fever and systemic symptoms by 1 to 2 days. The drug is generally well tolerated, with the most common therapy-limiting toxicities being central nervous system (CNS) effects, such as nervousness, light-headedness, difficulty concentrating, insomnia, and decreased psychomotor

Table 124-2. Viral Vaccines

Virus	Vaccine	Type	Indication	Recommended schedule
Smallpox	Vaccinia	Live	None	None
Polio	Oral polio vaccine (OPV, Sabin)	Live	During outbreaks Unvaccinated travelers	IPV preferred in almost all cases
	Inactivated polio vaccine (IPV, Salk)	Inactivated	All children	2, 4, 12-18 months, and at 4-6 years
Measles	Measles, mumps, rubella (MMR)	Live	All normal children	12 to 15 months and 4 to 6 years
Mumps	MMR	Live	All normal children	Same as for measles
Rubella	MMR	Live	All normal children	Same as for measles
Hepatitis A	HAV vaccine	Inactivated	People at risk (e.g., travelers, people living in areas of high prevalence)	2 doses, 6 months apart Immunoglobulin should be given if travel is imminent
Hepatitis B	HBV vaccine	Inactivated or recombinant	All children People at risk of exposure (e.g., health care workers)	At birth, 1-4, and 6-18 months Hepatitis B immune globulin should be given in addition in case of high-risk exposure
Influenza A	Influenza vaccine	Inactivated	People at high risk for complications (e.g., elderly) or those capable of transmitting influenza to high-risk patients (e.g., health care workers)	One dose yearly in the fall or winter
Rabies	Human diploid cell vaccine (HDCV) Rabies vaccine absorbed (RVA) Purified chick embryo cell (PCEC)	Inactivated Inactivated Inactivated	Postexposure prophylaxis Preexposure prophylaxis in high-risk groups (e.g., veterinarians)	HDCV, RVA, or PCEC 1.0 ml IM in the deltoid region on days 0, 3, 7, 14, and 28 Rabies immune globulin (RIG), 20 IU/kg should be administered around the wound site, as possible, with the remainder given IM at an anatomically distant site
Yellow fever	17D virus strain	Live	People older than 6 months traveling to endemic areas	Boosters every 10 years
Varicella	Varicella	Live	All healthy children At-risk adults	People 1 to 12 years old: receive 1 dose People older than 13: 2 doses 4 to 8 weeks apart

Table 124-3. Drugs for the Treatment of Viral Illnesses

Virus	Disease	Drug of choice	Alternate treatment	Prophylaxis or suppressive	Comments
Cytomegalovirus (CMV)	Retinitis	Ganciclovir, 5 mg/kg IV *bid* for 14 to 21 days, then 5 mg/kg IV *qd*	Foscarnet, 90 mg/kg IV bid for 14 to 21 days, then 90 to 120 mg/kg IV *qd* Cidofovir, 5 mg/kg *q* wk IV for 2 weeks, then 5 mg/kg *q* 2wks Ganciclovir implant Ganciclovir, foscarnet, or cidofovir intraocular injections	—	—
	Colitis, esophagitis	Same as for retinitis, but need for maintenance not established	Foscarnet, as above	—	—
	Pneumonitis	Ganciclovir, as above, with or without IV immune globulin, but need for maintenance not established	—	—	—
Hepatitis B virus	Chronic hepatitis	Interferon alfa, 5 million U SC or IM *qd* or 10 million U SC or IM 3 times/week for 16 to 24 weeks	Lamivudine 100 mg PO *qd* for 1 to 3 years	Hepatitis B immune globulin (HBIG)	—
Hepatitis C virus	Chronic hepatitis	Interferon alfa, 3 million units SC or IM 3 times/week with ribavirin 600 mg PO bid for 24 weeks	Peginterferon, 1 μg/kg SC once a week for 48 weeks	—	—
Herpes simplex virus (HSV)	Genital, primary	Acyclovir, 200 mg PO 5 times/day or 400 mg PO *tid* for 7 to 10 days Famciclovir, 250 PO *tid* for 5 to 10 days Valacyclovir, 1 g PO *bid* for 7 to 10 days	—	Acyclovir, 200 to 400 mg PO *bid* Valacyclovir, 500 to 1,000 mg PO *qd* Famciclovir, 250 mg PO *bid*	Acyclovir 5 mg/kg *q*8h
	Encephalitis	Acyclovir, 10 to 15 mg/kg IV *q*8h for 14 to 21 days	—	—	—
	Mucocutaneous disease in the immunocompromised host	Acyclovir, 5 mg/kg *q*8h for 7 to 14 days	Foscarnet, 40 to 60 mg IV q8h (for acyclovir-resistant HSV)	—	—
	Neonatal	Acyclovir, 20 mg/kg IV *q*8h for 14 to 21 days	—	—	—
	Keratoconjunctivitis	Trifluridine, 1% ophthalmic solution, 1 drop topically, *q*2h, up to 9 drops daily for 10 days	—	—	—

Continued

Table 124-3. Drugs for the Treatment of Viral Illnesses—cont'd

Virus	Disease	Drug of choice	Alternate treatment	Prophylaxis or suppressive	Comments
Human Immunodeficiency virus (HIV)	—	Combination therapy with: Zidovudine Didanosine Zalcitabine Lamivudine Stavudine Abacavir Saquinavir Ritonavir Indinavir Nelfinavir Amprenavir Lopinavir Nevirapine Delavirdine Efavirenz	See Chapter 126 for dosing and therapeutic combination therapy	—	See Chapter 126 for dosing and therapeutic combination therapy
Influenza A virus	Influenza A	Oseltamivir, 75 mg PO bid for 5 days Rimantadine, 200 mg PO qd for 5 days	Zanamivir, 2 inhalations bid for 5 days Amantadine, 100 mg PO bid for 5 days	—	—
Influenza B virus	Influenza B	Oseltamivir, 75 mg PO bid for 5 days	Zanamivir, 2 inhalations bid for 5 days	—	—
Lassa fever virus	Lassa fever	Ribavirin, 1 g IV *q*6h for 4 days, then 500 mg IV *q*8h for 6 days	—	—	Treatment for Lassa fever is investigational
Papillomavirus	Condyloma acuminatum	Interferon alfa-2b, 1 million U/0.1 ml intralesional injection in up to 5 warts *tiw* for 3 weeks Imiquimod 5%, topical application to warts 3 times/week	—	—	—
Respiratory syncytial virus (RSV)	Severe bronchiolitis or pneumonia in infants and children	Ribavirin aerosol, 12 to 18 hours daily for 3 to 7 days with a 20 mg/ml concentration reservoir	—	RSV immune globulin can be used for prophylaxis in young children Palivizumab, a monoclonal antibody, can be given monthly to premature infants	—
Varicella-zoster virus (VZV)	Varicella (chickenpox)	Acyclovir, 20 mg/kg, up to 800 mg, PO *qid* for 5 days	—	—	—
	Herpes zoster (shingles)	Valacyclovir, 1 g PO *tid* for 7 days Famciclovir, 500 mg PO *tid* for 7 days	Acyclovir 800 mg PO 5 times/day for 7 to 10 days	—	—
	Varicella or zoster in an immunocompromised host	Acyclovir, 10 mg/kg IV *q*8h for 7 days	Foscarnet, 40 mg/kg IV *q*8h for 10 days (for acyclovir-resistant VZV)	—	—

performance. These reactions occur particularly in older patients who have impaired renal function; they should receive no more than 100 mg of amantadine daily. Rimantadine is mostly metabolized before renal excretion and has a lower incidence of CNS toxicity than amantadine. Other side effects include nausea and loss of appetite. Overdose is associated with an anticholinergic syndrome.

Prophylaxis with daily amantadine or rimantadine is indicated for the duration of the influenza season in people at high risk for contracting influenza in which the influenza vaccine is contraindicated. When influenza A is reported in a community, appropriate management is to administer the influenza vaccine and give amantadine for 2 weeks while antibody production is induced. Adults having an acute onset of fever, cough, headache, and myalgias may be treated with 200 mg of amantadine followed by 100 mg for 5 to 7 days. Resistance to amantadine and rimantadine may emerge when these drugs are used to treat influenza A.[12]

Zanamivir and Oseltamivir

Zanamivir (Relenza) and oseltamivir (Flumadine) were approved in 1999 for the treatment of influenza A and B. Both medications act by inhibiting the activity of neuraminidase, an enzyme involved in the release of viral progeny from infected cells.[13] They have been shown to decrease the duration of moderate or severe symptoms of influenza by about 1 day. Either medication should be started within 2 days of onset of symptoms if efficacy is to be expected. These neuraminidase inhibitors are not approved for prophylactic use.[14] Zanamivir is administered by inhalation through a novel device *(Diskhaler)* and is approved for use in patients older than 12 years of age. The dose is 2 inhalations twice a day for 5 days. Most of the inhaled dose is deposited in the respiratory tract and cleared unchanged in the urine or stool. The most common side effect is bronchospasm in predisposed patients. Such patients should be given a fast-acting inhaled bronchodilator before receiving zanamivir.

Oseltamivir is an oral medication approved for patients older than 18. The dose is 75 mg twice daily for 5 days. It is cleared by renal secretion, and reduction of the dose to 75 mg daily is recommended for patients with a creatinine clearance of less than 30 ml/min.

Acyclovir

Acyclovir (Zovirax) is one of the drugs of choice for serious infections caused by HSV or varicella-zoster virus (VZV). Only 15% to 30% of the oral formulation is absorbed, so the IV form is required to treat HSV encephalitis, disseminated or ophthalmic zoster, or extensive HSV or VZV in the immunocompromised patient. Oral acyclovir has some use in treating primary HSV infections and in suppressing frequent HSV recurrences.[15] In general, the more immunocompromised the patient, the higher the likelihood he or she would require IV acyclovir therapy. Acyclovir is rarely associated with gastrointestinal upset, reversible renal dysfunction, or encephalopathy. Acyclovir-resistant isolates have been found in immunocompromised patients receiving multiple courses of therapy for HSV and VZV infections. These isolates may be less virulent and may remain sensitive and respond to treatment with foscarnet.[16,17]

Famciclovir and Valacyclovir

Famciclovir[18] (Famvir) and valacyclovir[19] (Valtrex) are analogs of acyclovir that inhibit herpesvirus DNA synthesis. They are much more bioavailable than acyclovir and can be given less frequently. Both are available only as oral formulations.

Ganciclovir

Ganciclovir (Cytovene) is used to treat life- or sight-threatening CMV infections in immunocompromised patients.[20] Patients with acquired immunodeficiency syndrome (AIDS) and CMV colitis or esophagitis may also improve with ganciclovir.[21] Ganciclovir is also effective against HSV, but isolates resistant to acyclovir are also resistant to ganciclovir.[16,17] Some CMV isolates in immunocompromised patients have been found to be or may become resistant to ganciclovir.[22] The most common therapy-limiting toxicities of ganciclovir are granulocytopenia and thrombocytopenia, which are usually reversible when therapy ceases.

Cidofovir

Cidofovir (Vistide) is a nucleotide agent used to treat CMV retinitis in people with HIV infection and for acyclovir-resistant HSV infections. It is only administered parenterally, but has a long half-life, making weekly or less frequent administration possible.[23] The most common toxicity is renal insufficiency, which is usually reversible on discontinuation of the drug.

Foscarnet

Foscarnet (Foscavir, Trisodium Phosphonoformate Hexahydrate, Phosphonoformic Acid) is an antiviral agent with activity against the human herpesviruses and HIV-1. It has been shown to be effective against CMV retinitis in AIDS patients and in acyclovir-resistant HSV and VZV infections.[16,17,24,25] The main limiting toxicity of foscarnet is renal insufficiency, which is usually reversible after the drug is discontinued. Other toxicities include malaise, headache, fatigue, nausea, vomiting, anemia, hypomagnesemia, hypophosphatemia, hyperphosphatemia, and hypocalcemia.

Vidarabine

IV vidarabine (Vira-A, Adenine Arabinoside, Ara-A) can be effective for life-threatening HSV and VZV infections, but because of its toxicities, acyclovir and foscarnet have largely replaced it.[26]

Trifluridine

Trifluridine 1% ophthalmic solution (Viroptic, Trifluorothymidine) is effective for treating primary keratoconjunctivitis and recurrent epithelial keratitis caused by HSV. Treatment of ocular infections should be undertaken in consultation with an ophthalmologist. Duration of treatment depends on the lesions' response to the medication.

Interferon Alfa, Recombinant

Interferons are naturally occurring proteins with both antiviral and immunomodulating properties that are produced by host cells in response to an inducer. Injected intralesionally, interferon alfa (Intron A, Roferon A, Interferon alfa-2a, Interferon alfa-2b, peg-Intron) is effective in treating refractory condyloma acuminatum.[27] High-dosage interferon alfa injected subcutaneously has induced remission in cases of Kaposi's sarcoma associated with HIV-1 infection.[28] Patients with chronic hepatitis B who have lost hepatitis B e antigen with interferon therapy have better long-term outcome with lower rates of end-stage liver disease and its complications.[29]

Interferon alfa-2b combined with ribavirin has been shown to induce virologic and histologic response in patients with chronic hepatitis C infection.[30] Therapy is discontinued because of side effects in about 20% of patients. Although there is a higher incidence of response with this combination therapy than with interferon alone, fewer than one fourth of patients who are nonresponders to interferon therapy can be expected to respond to combination therapy.[30,31] The toxicities of interferon therapy include fever, malaise, headache, fatigue, alopecia, and bone marrow suppression. Recent data suggest that the response of hepatitis C may be improved with the use of new interferon products bound to polyethylene glycol (pegylated interferon, peg-Intron).[31a] Use of this agent in combination with ribavirin is currently in clinical trials.

Therapy for HIV Infection

There are currently three classes of 15 antiretroviral drugs available for the treatment of HIV infection. The nucleoside reverse transcriptase inhibitors include zidovudine, didanosine, zalcitabine, stavudine, lamivudine, and abacavir. The nonnucleoside reverse transcriptase inhibitors include delavirdine, nevirapine, and efavirenz. The protease inhibitors include saquinavir, indinavir, ritonavir, nelfinavir, amprenavir, and lopinavir. The treatment of HIV infection is highly specialized. Treatment usually requires the administration of at least three of the antiretroviral agents. Treatment of HIV infection is covered in Chapter 126.

SPECIFIC VIRAL DISEASES

DNA Viruses

Poxviridae The elimination from the natural environment of variola, the virus that causes smallpox, at one time the most devastating worldwide pestilence, is one of the great medical and public health accomplishments of this past century.[5] Other human poxvirus diseases include monkeypox, vaccinia, molluscum contagiosum, orf, and paravaccinia. The poxviruses are the largest pathogenic viruses, consisting of complex, brick-shaped capsids and double-stranded DNA.

Variola (Smallpox), Monkeypox, Vaccinia, and Cowpox Viruses Within the Poxviridae family, the orthopoxvirus genus contains at least nine homogeneous viruses including variola, vaccinia, cowpox, and monkeypox. The last naturally acquired case of smallpox occurred in Somalia in October 1977.[5] Two cases occurred in 1978 in Birmingham, England, related to a research laboratory. Because there were neither nonhuman reservoirs nor human carriers of variola and because of the availability of rapid diagnostic techniques and an effective vaccine, the elimination of smallpox from the natural environment was a feasible goal. Global eradication was certified by the World Health Organization in 1980.

Vaccinia virus The origin of the vaccinia virus is not well established. Edward Jenner, in his "An Inquiry into the Causes and Effects of the Variolae Vaccinae" in 1798, observed that the pustular material from the lesions of cowpox, when inoculated into humans, protected them from infection with smallpox.[1]

Cowpox virus Cowpox causes vesicular lesions on the udders and teats of cows. Human disease is manifested as vesicular lesions on the hands. Generalized infection is rare.

Monkeypox virus The disease of monkeypox is clinically similar to that of smallpox. Most cases have occurred in west and central Africa. The case fatality rate is 12% to 16%, and the secondary attack rate is approximately 10%. Most identified cases were in children younger than 16 years, possibly because of the lack of smallpox immunity in the pediatric population.[35]

Parapoxviruses, Molluscum Contagiosum, and Tanapox Viruses Other viruses within the Poxviridae family that cause disease in humans include the parapoxviruses (paravaccinia and bovine pustular stomatitis virus), the molluscum contagiosum, and tanapox viruses. The milker's node virus, or paravaccinia, produces vesicular lesions on the udders or teats in cattle and is transmitted to humans by direct contact. Milker's nodules that develop on the fingers or hands are small, watery, painless nodules occasionally associated with lymphadenopathy. The lesions generally resolve completely within 3 to 8 weeks.

Bovine pustular stomatitis, ecthyma contagiosum, or orf virus causes papillomatous lesions on the mucous membranes and corneas of sheep. Single lesions generally develop in infected humans at the site of an abrasion.

Molluscum contagiosum is a generally benign human disease characterized by multiple small, painless, pearly, umbilicated nodules. They appear on epithelial surfaces, commonly in anogenital regions, and may be spread through close contact or autoinoculation. In immunocompetent people, the lesions may clear rapidly or persist for up to 18 months. The infection is often seen in people with HIV infection in which the lesions are often not restricted to the genital area and may increase in size and number.[33] Curettage or other forms of local ablation might be helpful in such recalcitrant cases.

Herpesviridae There are at least eight known human herpesviruses. Herpes simplex 1 and 2 (HSV-1 and HSV-2) are the agents of herpes genitalis, labialis, and encephalitis. VZV is the agent of chickenpox and herpes zoster. Epstein-Barr virus (EBV) is the agent of infectious mononucleosis and is associated with nasopharyngeal carcinoma, Burkitt's lymphoma, and other lymphoproliferative syndromes. CMV is associated with heterophile-negative infectious mononucleosis and invasive disease in immunocompromised patients. Human herpesvirus-6 (HHV-6) is associated with *roseola infantum.*[34] The role of HHV-7 has not been completely elucidated. HHV-8 is associated with Kaposi's sarcoma,[35] body-cavity-based lymphomas, and multicentric Castleman's disease. In addition, a closely related monkey virus, herpesvirus simiae or herpes B virus, has been shown to cause a fatal encephalitis in humans.

Herpes Simplex Virus

Principles of disease A localized primary lesion, latency, and a tendency for local recurrence characterize infections with HSV-1 and HSV-2 (Herpesvirus hominis). The primary lesion with HSV-1 may be mild and inapparent and may occur during childhood. Reactivation of latent HSV-1 infection usually results in herpes labialis (cold sores, fever blisters). Neurologic involvement is not uncommon with HSV-1. Although it usually occurs in association with a primary infection, neurologic signs may appear after a recrudescence and may manifest as encephalitis. Though uncommon, HSV-1 encephalitis is one of the most common causes of encephalitis in the United States, with estimates of several hundred to several thousand cases occurring yearly. HSV-2 is most commonly associated with genital herpes, although either HSV-1 or HSV-2 may infect any mucous membrane, depending on the route of inoculation. HSV-2 is commonly associated with aseptic meningitis rather than meningoencephalitis. The incubation period for primary herpes infection is 2 to 12 days.[36]

On contact with abraded skin or mucous membranes, HSV replicates locally in epithelial cells, which lyse and cause a local inflammatory response. Thin-walled vesicles on an erythematous base are the characteristic lesions of superficial HSV infection. Multinucleated giant cells with ballooning degeneration and intranuclear inclusions may be seen on a Tzanck preparation of a smear of the base of these vesicles. After primary infection, HSV may become latent within sensory nerve ganglia. Emotional stress, sunlight, fever, or local trauma may trigger reactivation of the virus. HSV encephalitis usually involves the temporal lobes, resulting in a necrotizing, hemorrhagic encephalitis.

Clinical features

Oropharynx Primary HSV-1 is often asymptomatic but may appear as pharyngitis and gingivostomatitis in children younger than 5 years of age. Associated with fever, pharyngeal edema, erythema, cervical adenopathy, and multiple small vesicles that ulcerate and multiply, the disease generally lasts from 10 to 14 days. Recurrences occur in 60% to 90% of people after primary infection but are generally milder than the primary infection. Vesicles generally recur on the vermilion border, are usually small, and crust within 48 hours.

Eyes Herpes simplex infections of the eye are most often caused by HSV-1. Primary infections present as follicular conjunctivitis, blepharitis, or corneal epithelial opacities, which usually heal completely within 2 to 3 weeks. Recurrences may result in keratitis. Branching dendritic ulcers, detectable with fluorescein staining, are diagnostic and may result in diminished visual acuity. Deep stromal involvement may result in corneal scarring.

Hands Primary herpetic finger infections, or herpetic whitlow, are generally caused by HSV-1 among medical or dental personnel and by HSV-2 among the general population. The lesions are associated with intense pain and itching but generally resolve in 2 to 3 weeks. Recurrent whitlow with severe local neuralgia may occur.

Genital area Primary genital herpes is generally seen in the sexually active population and is caused by HSV-2 in 70% to 95% of cases. The lesions usually involve the shaft or glans of the penis in men and the vulva, perineum, buttocks, cervix, and vagina in women. Primary infection may be associated with fever, malaise, anorexia, and inguinal adenopathy. Vaginal discharge is common. Urethral involvement resulting in urinary retention is not uncommon in women. Herpetic sacral radiculomyelitis is uncommon but may also lead to urinary retention, myalgias, and obstipation. The lesions may last for several weeks before completely clearing. Recurrences of genital herpes are generally shorter and milder than the primary episodes and may be preceded by a prodrome of tenderness, itching, or tingling. Healing of recurrent lesions generally is complete in 6 to 10 days.

Perianal area Primary perianal and anal herpes is common among people who engage in anal intercourse and may be especially prolonged and severe among HIV-1 infected persons.

Neonatal infection Neonatal infection occurs in 1 in 2500 to 10,000 births and is caused by the transmission of the virus at the time of delivery. The rate of infection is estimated to be 40% to 50% after a primary maternal infection and less than 10% after a recurrence.[37] Infection may present after several days to weeks with vesicles or conjunctivitis, but neurologic involvement, with seizures, cranial nerve palsies, lethargy, and coma, is common. Untreated disseminated or CNS disease is fatal in more than 70% of patients.

Encephalitis Encephalitis caused by HSV is uncommon, but it is the most common acute, nonepidemic encephalitis in the United States. Cases do not have a seasonal distribution. Other than in the neonate, HSV-1 is the usual pathogen. The clinical disease begins acutely, with fever and focal neurologic signs, often localized to the temporal lobe. The patient may complain of a bad odor not perceived by anyone else (temporal lobe hallucination). Headache, meningeal signs, lethargy, confusion, stupor, or coma is often present. Cerebrospinal fluid (CSF) findings are nonspecific, with a moderate mononuclear pleocytosis. Culture of the CSF is generally negative for HSV. Localization of the encephalitis within the temporal lobes via electroencephalogram (EEG), magnetic resonance imaging (MRI), or computed tomography (CT) scan increases the likelihood of a diagnosis of HSV encephalitis. The diagnosis of HSV encephalitis can be made reliably only with a biopsy of the lesion and subsequent isolation or detection of the virus by culture or direct fluorescent antibody tests. The early diagnosis of HSV encephalitis may be improved by using the polymerase chain reaction to amplify HSV DNA in CSF.[38] The mortality rate of untreated patients approaches 80%, and fewer than 10% of patients are left without neurologic sequelae.[26] Treatment with acyclovir appears to reduce mortality and decrease the neurologic sequelae more effectively than treatment with vidarabine.[39]

Considerations The superficial lesions of HSV are indistinguishable from those of VZV. Pharyngitis and gingivostomatitis in children may mimic streptococcal or diphtheritic pharyngitis, herpangina, aphthous stomatitis, Stevens-Johnson syndrome, Vincent's angina, and infectious mononucleosis. Primary genital herpes may mimic the appearance of chancroid, syphilis, candidiasis, or Behçet's syndrome. In the neonate, in the absence of vesicles, congenital HSV infection may mimic disease caused by rubella, CMV, or *Toxoplasma* organisms. Encephalitis caused by HSV may be clinically indistinguishable from other viral encephalitides, tuberculous and fungal meningitis, brain abscesses, brain tumors, and cerebrovascular accidents.

Management Oral acyclovir (200 mg 5 times daily), oral valacyclovir (1 g twice daily), or IV acyclovir (5 mg/kg 3 times daily) is recommended for treating primary genital herpes or mucocutaneous herpes in the immunocompromised host, although some authorities use higher dosages in these patients.[40] Because of the safety and efficacy of oral acyclovir, there is little indication for using acyclovir ointment. In people with severe or frequent recurrences, acyclovir, 200 mg 3 to 5 times daily, can be used as an effective suppressive regimen. Both famciclovir and valacyclovir are approved for suppressive therapy and offer a more convenient dosing regimen than acyclovir.

In the immunocompromised host, acyclovir is effective in both the treatment and prophylaxis of recurrent mucocutaneous herpes. Foscarnet has been shown to be effective in the host in the treatment of mucocutaneous herpes that is resistant to acyclovir.[17,25] IV acyclovir, 10 mg/kg IV every 8 hours, is the treatment of choice for HSV encephalitis in adults and children. Vidarabine, 30 mg/kg/day IV, is also effective in neonatal encephalitis.[39]

Disposition Patients with cutaneous HSV infections can generally be managed easily. The diagnosis often carries with it a great deal of stigma and guilt that must be dealt with carefully. Assurance as to the generally benign nature of the infection is helpful. Counseling should include cautions about the transmissibility of the virus, even during asymptomatic periods. Women of childbearing age should discuss management of HSV during pregnancy and delivery with their obstetricians.

Encephalitis caused by HSV is a treatable medical emergency. Prompt recognition and institution of appropriate therapy in the ED before a definitive diagnosis has been made may decrease the high mortality rate and neurologic sequelae associated with this disease. When HSV encephalitis is suspected, because of the minimal toxicity and demonstrable efficacy of acyclovir, empiric initiation of IV acyclovir is indicated in the ED.

Varicella-Zoster Virus VZV, or human (alpha) herpesvirus 3, is the agent of both chickenpox and herpes zoster, or shingles.

Clinical features

Chickenpox Chickenpox is an acute, generalized viral disease with sudden onset of fever, malaise, and a skin eruption that is initially maculopapular and then vesiculated for several days before a granular scab is left. Lesions occur in crops, with several stages present at the same time. Lesions may appear anywhere on the skin and mucous membranes. There may be few lesions and mild, inapparent infections. Most cases occur in children younger than 9 years of age, but adults with the disease may have high fevers and severe constitutional symptoms. Children with acute leukemia are at increased risk of disseminated disease, which has a case fatality rate of greater than 5%. Neonates developing varicella before 10 days of age and mothers who develop the disease in the perinatal period are at increased risk for generalized disease. Fatal disease in adults, although uncommon, is usually associated with pneumonic involvement of the virus. In children, fatal disease is usually associated with septic complications and encephalitis.

Herpes zoster Herpes zoster is a reactivation infection of VZV that has been latent in a dorsal root ganglion. Often preceded by tingling or hypesthesia, multiple vesicles on an erythematous base appear in crops along nerve pathways supplied by sensory nerves of a single or associated group of dorsal root ganglia. The distribution is usually unilateral and dermatomal. Zoster occurs predominantly in older adults but has been seen in younger people when associated with HIV infection.[41] The lesions are often extremely painful. Postherpetic neuralgia is common in the elderly, may last for months or years, and is refractory to treatment. Involvement of the ophthalmic branch of the trigeminal nerve may lead to corneal ulceration.

Differential considerations The diagnoses of chickenpox and herpes zoster are clinical. Laboratory tests are generally not required. Multinucleated giant cells may be seen on Tzanck preparations from the base of a lesion, but these can also occur in herpes simplex lesions. Scrapings can also be submitted for antibody-linked fluorescent microscopy testing, which will yield rapid results and differentiate between HSV and VZV.

Management

Chickenpox Using acyclovir for uncomplicated chickenpox in children is safe but relatively expensive and only modestly effective. Parents of children with chickenpox should be cautioned not to give their children aspirin or aspirin-containing compounds because of the strong association between this practice and the development of Reye's syndrome.[42] The association of Reye's syndrome with other nonsteroidal antiinflammatory agents is unknown. Acetaminophen may be used as an antipyretic. Because adults are more likely to suffer morbidity and mortality from chickenpox, one might opt to treat otherwise healthy adults with acyclovir. Famciclovir or valacyclovir are probably as effective and easier to administer, although they are not approved for the treatment of chickenpox. Patients with pneumonitis or other severe illness should be treated with IV acyclovir. In immunocompromised patients, varicella-zoster immunoglobulin (VZIG) and IV acyclovir have been shown to decrease morbidity.

A live, attenuated vaccine has shown a high degree of protection of both normal children and children with leukemia and was licensed in the United States in 1995. It is recommended for immunocompetent people older than 12 months of age. In those older than 12 years, two doses of vaccine are to be administered 4 to 8 weeks apart. It is also recommended for use as postexposure prophylaxis in the nonimmune host. The vaccine is most effective in preventing or attenuating illness in these circumstances if it is administered within the first 3 to 5 days after exposure.[43] The vaccine is a live attenuated virus and is not recommended for immunocompromised patients.

Herpes zoster Uncomplicated herpes zoster is generally treated with supportive measures, especially pain control, and acyclovir, famciclovir, or valacyclovir.[44] Disseminated disease and complicated zoster, involving more than one dermatome or the ophthalmic branch of the trigeminal nerve, should be treated with IV acyclovir. Foscarnet is useful for acyclovir-resistant VZV in immunocompromised patients.[16] Famciclovir may decrease the duration of postherpetic neuralgia. Susceptible immunocompromised patients exposed to infected individuals should receive VZIG within 72 hours to prevent or modify clinical illness.[43] Using corticosteroids to decrease the incidence of postherpetic neuralgia is controversial.

Disposition Chickenpox and herpes zoster are highly contagious. Although the diseases are generally benign, patients should be warned to avoid situations that may put them in contact with steroid-treated or immunocompromised persons. The incubation period is most commonly 13 to 17 days, and the period of communicability may be from 5 days before to 5 days after the appearance of the vesicles. Susceptible people should be considered potentially infectious from 10 to 21 days after exposure. Susceptible health care workers should not care for people with varicella or zoster. Health care workers without a well-documented history of chickenpox or herpes zoster should have their antibody levels checked before they begin their employment to determine their susceptibility to subsequent infection definitively.

Cytomegalovirus

Principles of disease CMV, or human herpesvirus-5, is commonly associated with heterophile-negative infectious mononucleosis, which is clinically and hematologically similar to EBV mononucleosis. More severe infections with CMV occur in the perinatal period and among immunocompromised patients. Severe CMV infections are also found in transplant recipients when organs from CMV-seropositive donors are transplanted into CMV-seronegative recipients.

Primary infection with CMV is often associated with a vigorous T-lymphocyte response. CMV persists indefinitely, probably within multiple cell types in various organs. Reactivation leading to CMV-associated disease may occur in response to a variety of external stimulants.

Clinical features CMV infection in immunocompetent older children and adults is generally subclinical but may be similar to that of EBV mononucleosis. It is characterized by fever, lymphadenopathy, exudative pharyngitis, and peripheral lymphocytosis with atypical lymphocytes present on peripheral blood smears. The acute infection resolves in 2 to 4 weeks, but malaise and viral excretion may persist for months. In the perinatal period, severe, generalized infection occurs and is associated with lethargy, convulsions, jaundice, petechiae, hepatosplenomegaly, chorioretinitis, and pulmonary infiltrates. Survivors may have varying degrees of neurologic impairment. Fetal infection may occur after primary or reactivated maternal infections, with primary infections carrying a much higher risk. Among immunocompromised people, severe, generalized disease may occur, often associated with severe end-organ disease such as colitis, esophagitis, pneumonitis, retinitis, and adrenalitis. Retinitis caused by CMV is the most common cause of blindness among people with AIDS.[20] CMV can cause a polyradiculopathy, as well as other, less common, neurologic manifestations, in patients with AIDS that manifests as ascending lower extremity weakness with incontinence and loss of deep tendon reflexes. Therapy with ganciclovir and foscarnet is indicated, but treatment results may be disappointing.[45]

Differential considerations Mononucleosis caused by CMV may be clinically indistinguishable from syndromes caused by EBV or toxoplasmosis. In the perinatal period, infants with generalized infections require evaluation for other common perinatal infections, such as toxoplasmosis, rubella, syphilis, and HSV. Recipients of organ transplants and other immunocompromised patients with fever and other signs and symptoms of generalized infection require intensive evaluation for bacterial and viral causes of infection. Diagnosis of CMV infection depends on viral isolation, detection of CMV pp65 antigen, or the demonstration of a fourfold rise in antibody to viral antigens.

Management Only supportive care is indicated for immunocompetent adults and children. Ganciclovir, foscarnet, and cidofovir have been approved for treating CMV retinitis in immunocompromised people.[20,23,24,40] Concurrent use of IV immune globulins with ganciclovir may decrease the mortality rate associated with CMV pneumonitis in bone marrow recipients.[49]

Immunocompetent adults and older children can be managed at home. Suspected CMV infections in the perinatal period or in immunocompromised patients can be life threatening and generally require hospitalization for aggressive evaluation, monitoring, and specialized care.

Epstein-Barr Virus (Infectious Mononucleosis)

Principles of disease EBV, or human herpesvirus-4, is most commonly associated with infectious mononucleosis, an acute viral syndrome characterized by fever, exudative pharyngotonsillitis, lymphadenopathy, and peripheral lymphocytosis with atypical lymphocytes. EBV also has been strongly implicated in the pathogenesis of African Burkitt's lymphoma and nasopharyngeal carcinoma. Acute immunoblastic sarcoma, involving a polyclonal expansion of EBV-infected B lymphocytes, may occur in people with an X-linked immunoproliferative disorder. Hodgkin's disease and other lymphomas in immunocompromised patients, such as renal transplant recipients or people with AIDS, have also been associated with EBV infection. A chronic form of the disease has been implicated as one of the causes of the chronic fatigue syndrome, but the true association of EBV with the majority of people with this syndrome is probably very unlikely.[47]

EBV infects and transforms B lymphocytes. Infection is common and widespread in early childhood in developing countries, where it is usually mild or asymptomatic. In developed countries, infectious mononucleosis usually presents in older children and young adults, commonly among high school and college students. It is transmitted via the oropharyngeal route, often by kissing. The incubation period may be as long as 4 to 6 weeks and pharyngeal excretion may persist for 1 year or more.

Clinical features The syndrome is usually mild in children, but 95% of young adults will have abnormal transaminases and 4% will have jaundice. Hepatosplenomegaly is common. Severe exudative pharyngitis, fevers, lymphadenopathy, and fatigue are characteristic of infectious mononucleosis. The disease generally resolves in 1 to 3 weeks, but malaise and fatigue may rarely persist for several months. Occasionally, tonsillar swelling may cause respiratory compromise. Splenic rupture is rare, but must be considered in patients with left upper quadrant pain and a falling hematocrit level. Neurologic complications, including encephalitis, aseptic meningitis, transverse myelitis, Guillain-Barré syndrome, optic neuritis, and peripheral neuropathies, occur in less than 1% of patients.

Diagnostic strategies and differential considerations Laboratory diagnosis is based on the finding of lymphocytosis greater than 50% or an elevation in heterophile antibodies (Monospot). Heterophile antibodies are sensitive and specific antibodies that usually appear early in the illness. Other virus-specific antibodies are available but are rarely needed to diagnose mononucleosis because 90% of cases are heterophile positive.

In the absence of immediate availability of heterophile antibody testing, a presumptive diagnosis can be made by the finding of significant cervical lymphadenopathy, particularly posterior cervical, and exudative pharyngitis coupled with a lymphocytosis and the presence of atypical lymphocytes on a blood smear. HHV-6, CMV, and toxoplasmosis may cause syndromes that are clinically and hematologically similar to infectious mononucleosis.

Management Treatment is entirely supportive, except when rare complications of organ compromise are present. The use of corticosteroids in uncomplicated illness is controversial. They are generally used for impending airway obstruction, hemolytic anemia, or severe thrombocytopenia. The infection confers a high degree of resistance to reinfection. Patients should be cautioned about potential communicability to previously uninfected people.

Human Herpesvirus-6

Principles of disease HHV-6 has been implicated as the causative agent of roseola infantum (exanthem subitum).

HHV-6 was isolated from the blood of four patients with roseola infantum who subsequently seroconverted 2 weeks after the rash.[34]

Clinical features Roseola infantum is the most common exanthem of children younger than 2 years of age and occurs most often at about 1 year of age. The illness begins abruptly with the acute onset of fever, often as high as 41° C, lasting 3 to 5 days. Despite the fever, the child usually remains active and alert. A fine, evanescent, rose-colored maculopapular rash appears on the trunk after lysis of the fever, which may last for 1 to 2 days. The rash may spread to the face and extremities. Most cases are self-limited, although febrile convulsions may occur in conjunction with the fever. Although secondary cases occur with an incubation period of approximately 10 days, most cases of roseola occur without known exposure.

Differential considerations The disease may appear similar to other childhood exanthems. The child generally will look well despite the high fever.

Management Acetaminophen may reduce the fever. Routine supportive measures should be used if febrile seizures occur.

Human Herpesvirus-7 HHV-7 has been associated with a clinical presentation similar to that of HHV-6, but its role in disease has not yet been fully elucidated.[48]

Human Herpesvirus-8 (Kaposi's Sarcoma–Associated Herpesvirus, KSHV) HHV-8 genomic sequences can be isolated from almost all Kaposi's sarcomas regardless of the HIV status of the affected patients.[49] In addition, KSHV can be propagated in vitro from Kaposi's sarcoma.[50] Mechanisms of disease pathogenesis as well as epidemiology of transmission for this virus remain unclear and continue to be actively investigated.[48]

Herpes B Virus

Principles of disease Herpes B virus, or herpesvirus simiae, a close relative of human herpes simplex, is enzootic in macaques and most commonly associated with Rhesus, cynomolgus, or African green monkeys. Like human herpes simplex, herpes B virus produces mild disease in monkeys that is characterized by intermittent reactivation and shedding, particularly during times of stress, such as during handling. Among monkey handlers and those exposed to the animals' saliva or tissues, including kidney cell cultures, monkey B virus is a serious occupational hazard. Of 23 symptomatic human infections, 18 resulted in a progressive mucocutaneous disease and fatal encephalitis.[51]

Clinical features After a penetrating bite or scratch from an infected monkey, herpetiform vesicles form at the site of the injury. Giant cells may be seen on a Tzanck preparation. An acute febrile illness with headache and lymphocytosis may follow as long as 3 weeks after the injury. An ascending myelitis ensues, leading to death from respiratory paralysis or encephalomyelitis within 3 weeks of the onset of symptoms. The incidence of asymptomatic infection is unknown.

Differential considerations The initial skin lesions appear similar to that of herpes simplex. In the context of any exposure to monkey tissues and the appearance of a herpetiform lesion, the diagnosis of herpes B virus infection must be considered because of the high mortality rate associated with monkey B virus infections.

Treatment Suspected B virus infection is a medical emergency. There have been anecdotal reports of successful prevention of disease progression with IV acyclovir.[52] The apparent response of the infection to treatment emphasizes the need for early recognition and treatment of this disease.

Adenoviridae

Adenovirus

Principles of disease Adenoviruses are the most clinically important viruses because of their capacity to cause upper respiratory tract infections, conjunctivitis, and gastroenteritis. Nevertheless, no drugs or therapeutic measures are available specifically for adenoviral infections.

Clincial features Adenoviruses cause respiratory diseases ranging from pharyngitis and tracheitis to fulminant bronchiolitis and pneumonia. Cough, fever, sore throat, and rhinorrhea are the most common symptoms and generally last only a few days. Pneumonitis with interstitial infiltrates may occasionally be seen with some strains. Upper respiratory findings may be associated with conjunctivitis (pharyngoconjunctival fever). Adenoviruses, usually types 8, 19, and 37, may cause an epidemic keratoconjunctivitis, which in severe cases may be associated with conjunctival scarring. Other syndromes associated with adenoviruses include hemorrhagic cystitis, infantile diarrhea, intussusception, encephalitis, and meningoencephalitis.

Differential considerations Other pathogens causing similar atypical pneumonia syndromes include influenza and parainfluenza viruses and *Mycoplasma pneumoniae*. Diarrheal syndromes may be similar to those caused by rotaviruses.

Management Treatment for adenovirus infections is supportive.

Papillomaviridae

Principles of Disease Human papillomaviruses (HPV) cause a variety of cutaneous and mucous membrane lesions, including common warts, anogenital or venereal warts (condyloma acuminatum), and respiratory or laryngeal papillomas.

More than 70 types of HPVs have been identified. Laryngeal papillomas (most commonly HPV types 6 and 11) and genital warts (most commonly HPV types 16 and 18) may undergo malignant transformation.[56,57]

Clinical Features Common warts are generally well-circumscribed, hyperkeratotic, painless papules most commonly occurring on the extremities and transmitted by close personal contact. Plantar warts, found on the soles of the feet, may be very painful. Venereal warts, found on the internal or external genitalia or perianal region, are hyperkeratotic, exophytic papules, either sessile or pedunculated, and are sexually transmitted. Laryngeal papillomas in children are presumably acquired during passage through the birth canal. Malignant transformation may occur, particularly in patients receiving radiation therapy.

Differential Considerations The diagnosis of warts is usually made clinically. Condyloma acuminatum must be distinguished from condyloma latum caused by syphilis. Diagnosis of cervical HPV infections can be made during colposcopy with prior application of a 3% to 5% acetic acid solution to the internal genital tract. Flat condylomata appear as shiny white patches with ill-defined borders and irregular surfaces. Acetowhitening can also reveal subclinical vulvar or penile warts.

Management Warts generally regress spontaneously within months or years, but because of the possibility of malignant transformation of genital or laryngeal warts, they should be removed. Freezing with liquid nitrogen is effective for most accessible lesions. Salicylic acid plasters and curettage are useful for plantar warts. Podophyllin as a 10% solution in tincture of benzoin is useful for accessible genital warts. Laryngeal warts require surgery or laser therapy. Interferon alfa has been effective in the intralesional treatment of genital warts.[27] Imiquimod (Aldara) has been approved for the topical self-treatment of genital warts.[55]

All patients with genital warts should be screened for other sexually transmitted diseases. Because of the potential for malignant transformation, people with internal genital warts should be referred to a qualified specialist for treatment and follow-up care.

Polyomaviridae

Principles of Disease JC virus (JCV) and BK virus (BKV) are human polyomaviruses that cause ubiquitous but asymptomatic infection in populations worldwide. Progressive multifocal leukoencephalopathy (PML) is a rare, slowly progressive, demyelinating disease of the CNS, which become large plaques, seen mostly in severely immunocompromised patients, that is associated with JCV.[56] Similarly, BKV viruria is relatively common in immunosuppressed or pregnant people. Rare, symptomatic infection may present as urethral stenosis in renal transplant patients and hemorrhagic cystitis in bone marrow transplant patients.

Clinical Features Initial presentations of PML in immunocompromised patients include paresis, personality changes, and impaired higher cortical functioning. The disease is generally rapidly progressive, usually progressing to death within 2 to 4 months of the initial neurologic symptom. PML is commonly seen in people with advanced AIDS.[56]

Differential Considerations The differential diagnosis includes other causes of progressive neurologic disease in immunocompromised patients, including toxoplasmic encephalitis, primary CNS lymphoma, HIV encephalopathy, tuberculous meningitis, and vascular disease. The lack of contrast enhancement on CT and MR scans is helpful in making the diagnosis. The use of polymerase chain reaction coupled with such radiologic findings has increased the ability to narrow the differential diagnosis of such progressive brain lesions.[57]

Management No specific treatment for PML is available; the disease is generally rapidly progressive; ultimate transfer to appropriate nursing care facilities is often necessary. Recently, there have been reports of significant improvements in patients who have been placed on potent antiretroviral (anti-HIV) therapy.[58]

Hepadnaviridae

Hepatitis B Virus and Hepatitis Delta Virus A description of hepatitis B and delta hepatitis can be found in Chapter 85.

Parvoviridae

Parvoviruses (Erythema Infectiosum, Aplastic Crisis)

Principles of disease Parvovirus B19 has been implicated as the causal agent in several epidemics of erythema infectiosum, or fifth disease. It is also associated with transient aplastic crisis in patients with chronic hemolytic disease, particularly with sickle cell disease.[59] Fetal infection also has been recognized, and infections during pregnancy have been associated with hydrops fetalis and spontaneous abortion.[60]

Clinical features

Erythema infectiosum Erythema infectiosum is a mild, usually nonfebrile disease of children between 4 and 10 years of age, characterized by a striking erythema of the cheeks, a "slapped-cheek" appearance. The rash usually appears after an incubation period of 4 to 14 days without a prodrome. A total of 1 to 4 days later, an erythematous rash on the extremities may be seen spreading to the trunk in a lacelike pattern. The rash generally fades within a week but may persist for several weeks and may be precipitated by skin trauma or sunlight exposure. Constitutional symptoms are generally mild in children, but adults with the disease commonly have associated arthralgias and arthritis. Rare cases of encephalitis and pneumonia have been reported.

Aplastic crisis Parvovirus B19 has a propensity for attacking and causing a marked reduction in erythroid cell precursors and has been established as a cause of transient aplastic crisis in patients with chronic hemolytic anemia. Recovery is associated with reappearance of reticulocytes in the peripheral smear 7 to 10 days after their disappearance. In patients with AIDS and other immunosuppressive illnesses, parvovirus B19 infection can manifest as chronic anemia. These patients often have persistent parvovirus infection without an appropriate immunoglobulin response.[61]

Differential considerations In children, erythema infectiosum may resemble other viral exanthems. The "slapped-cheek" appearance of the rash is characteristic.

Management Erythema infectiosum is generally a mild disease, and no treatment is required. Patients with parvovirus B19–associated aplastic crisis may require blood transfusions. Therapy with immunoglobulin can decrease the need for transfusions in immunosuppressed patients with chronic anemia.[62] Women who develop parvovirus infection during pregnancy should be followed closely for the development of fetal hydrops fetalis. The role of intrauterine blood transfusions in the treatment of this disorder remains controversial.[60]

Although the disease is probably transmitted via respiratory secretions, patients are probably no longer infectious by the time the rash appears.[62]

RNA Viruses

Reoviridae

The family Reoviridae (from respiratory enteric orphans) includes three viruses causing human disease: orthoreovirus, orbivirus (including the virus of Colorado tick fever), and rotavirus. The reoviruses commonly infect humans but infrequently cause human disease. Upper respiratory infections, exanthems, pneumonia, hepatitis, encephalitis, gastroenteritis, and biliary atresia have on occasion been associated with these viruses.

Colorado Tick Fever

Principles of disease Colorado tick fever, or mountain fever, is a tickborne disease transmitted to humans by the hard-shelled wood tick *Dermacentor andersoni.* It occurs primarily in the western United States, but a serotype has been isolated from the *Ixodes ricinus* tick in Germany and the dog tick, *Dermacentor variabilis,* from Long Island. Illness generally occurs in late spring through summer.

Clinical findings and features The incubation period for Colorado tick fever is 3 to 6 days, and a history of tick exposure is elicited in 90% of patients. The disease generally occurs in people engaged in activities that bring them into contact with ticks. The fever is biphasic or "saddle-backed," with the patient initially acutely experiencing chills, lethargy, prostration, headache, ocular pain, photophobia, abdominal pain, and severe myalgias. The initial fever of 2 to 3 days breaks for a similar period and is followed by a second fever of approximately 3 days. Rash, occasionally petechial, is an uncommon finding, occurring in 5% to 10% of patients. Meningoencephalitis is an uncommon serious complication in children.[63] Convalescence may last 1 to 3 weeks; half of infected persons are viremic 4 weeks after the onset of illness.[63]

Differential considerations Colorado tick fever is commonly misdiagnosed as Rocky Mountain spotted fever. Patients with fever and rash after tick bites in endemic areas should be treated for Rocky Mountain spotted fever. Confirmation of the diagnosis of Colorado tick fever is by mouse inoculation or fluorescent staining of erythrocytes.

Management Treatment is supportive and symptomatic.

Orbivirus Other than Colorado tick fever, six other viruses have been implicated in human disease. Changuinola virus transmitted from *Phlebotomus* flies; lebombo and orungo viruses from mosquitoes; and kemerovo, lipovnik, and tribec viruses from ticks have been associated with febrile illnesses and rarely, encephalitis.

Rotavirus

Principles of Disease Rotaviruses derive their name from their wheel-like appearance when seen by transmission electron microscopy. They cause severe gastroenteritis in infants and young children, particularly between the ages of 6 months and 2 years; the gastroenteritis is manifested by severe diarrhea and vomiting, which often lead to dehydration and occasionally, death.[64] In temperate climates, illness occurs mainly in the winter, is commonly associated with nosocomial infection, and is spread primarily person to person by the fecal-oral route. The incubation period is approximately 2 days.

Clinical Features Mucosal epithelial cells of the small intestine appear to be infected, selectively leading to shortening of villi and decreased absorption of salt and water. A secretory diarrhea is produced with impaired D-xylose absorption. The clinical disease ranges from asymptomatic to severe, fatal diarrhea and dehydration. The illness is abrupt in onset with nausea, vomiting, watery diarrhea, low-grade fevers, headache, and myalgias. The course of the disease is generally 3 to 9 days. Fatalities are common in developing countries but rare in the developed world. In newborns, rotavirus has been associated with neonatal necrotizing enterocolitis.[65] Infections in adults are usually asymptomatic.

Differential Considerations Rotavirus enteritis should be suspected in any child with watery diarrhea in the cooler months of the year. Fecal leukocytes and erythrocytes are not generally seen in rotaviral diarrhea. Other enteric viruses can produce a clinical syndrome similar to that of the rotavirus. Definitive diagnosis can be made by visualizing the virus in the stool by electron microscopy, but radioimmunoassays, enzyme immunoassays, and latex agglutination methods for detecting antigen are highly reliable and available at most hospital laboratories.

Management Specific treatment for rotaviral infections is not currently available. IV fluids are established as effective therapy, but when the patient is able to take oral fluids, oral rehydration using the standard World Health Organization formula of sugar and electrolytes can be used in the outpatient setting for mild to moderate dehydration.

In August 1998, an oral vaccine against rotavirus was licensed for use in the United States but postlicensure surveillance revealed an increased incidence of intussusception in immunized infants. The Centers for Disease Control and Prevention (CDC) no longer recommends that the vaccine be administered.[66]

Togaviridae

Alphavirus (Group A Arbovirus)

Principles of disease Arboviruses (from *ar*thropod-*bo*rne *vir*uses) are transmitted to humans by an arthropod vector, with humans usually being an unimportant host in the reproductive cycle of the virus. Most arboviruses are mosquito borne, but ticks, sandflies, gnats, and midges may serve as important vectors for some diseases. The alphaviruses and flaviviruses are the most common arboviruses causing disease in humans, but some bunyaviruses, reoviruses, rhabdoviruses, filoviruses, arenaviruses, and orthomyxoviruses also are transmitted via arboviral vectors.

The alphaviruses are transmitted by the bite of a mosquito. The three alphaviruses that cause human disease in the United States are the agents of eastern equine encephalitis (EEE), western equine encephalitis (WEE), and Venezuelan equine encephalitis (VEE). Other important alphaviruses include chikungunya (Africa, Southeast Asia, Philippines), Mayaro (South America), O'nyong (Africa), Ross River (Australia, South Pacific), and Sindbis (Africa, Asia, Soviet Union, Australia, and Scandinavia).

Clinical features These arboviruses can cause outbreaks of encephalitis in various parts of the United States.[67] The few cases of EEE in the United States occur predominantly near freshwater swamps of the Eastern seaboard. Although more than 95% of cases are subclinical, cases presenting with encephalitis have a mortality rate approaching 50%. Infections occur most commonly in children younger than 10 years of age or in the elderly. The onset of symptoms is often fulminant, with headache, fevers, convulsions progressing rapidly to decreasing level of consciousness, and death. Focal neurologic symptoms may also occur. WEE is present throughout the United States but occurs mostly in the western and central parts of the nation. Children younger than 1 year of age and the elderly are most often affected. More than 99% of cases are inapparent, and the encephalitis is usually mild with a mortality rate of approximately 3%. VEE is predominantly found in Central and South America, but the disease has been seen in Texas and Florida. VEE usually presents as an influenza-like illness, with only approximately one third of patients having encephalitis, with a mortality rate of less than 1%, predominantly in children.

Differential considerations Other viral causes of encephalitis in the United States include HSV, HIV, St. Louis encephalitis (a flavivirus), California (La Crosse) encephalitis (a bunyavirus), and the recently encountered West Nile–like encephalitis (a flavivirus).[68,69] Other viruses, such as mumps, rabies, polio, and other enteroviruses, may also present as encephalitides. The WBC count in the CSF of persons with EEE may be very high, and the diagnosis of meningoencephalitis must be considered. Diagnoses can be confirmed by a rise in antibody titers.

Management Management is entirely supportive. For people with expected intensive exposure to these viruses, an investigational vaccine may be available from the U.S. Army Medical Research Institute for Infectious Diseases in Fort Detrick, Maryland.

Rubella Virus (German Measles)

Clinical features Rubella is a mild febrile illness associated with a diffuse maculopapular rash, fever, malaise, headache, and postauricular, occipital, and posterior cervical lymphadenopathy.

Transmission of rubella is via contact with respiratory secretions. The incubation period of rubella ranges from 12 to 23 days. Accompanied by viremia, the rash usually lasts 3 to 5 days. The disease is highly communicable from about 1 week before to 4 days after the onset of the rash. The most common complications of rubella are arthropathies, or frank arthritis, predominantly affecting the fingers, wrists, and knees; the arthropathies may persist for several months. Encephalitis and thrombocytopenia are rare complications.

Although the disease is generally a mild, febrile illness in children and adults, the consequences of rubella occurring during pregnancy (congenital rubella syndrome) may be tragic. Severe consequences include fetal death, premature delivery, and a variety of congenital defects, including hearing loss, cataracts, retinopathy, mental retardation, and a variety of cardiac abnormalities. The younger the fetus at the time of a maternal infection, the more likely the fetus will be affected. During the first 2 months of pregnancy, the fetus has approximately a 90% chance of being affected, approximately an 80% chance of being affected from an infection during the third month, and a 66% chance during the fourth month. No congenital defects were found in the 106 children born to mothers after laboratory-proven maternal infection contracted after the seventeenth week of pregnancy.[70]

Differential considerations The rash associated with rubella ("third disease") is one of the classic common exanthems of childhood. It may be similar to the rash of measles (rubeola, or "first disease"), scarlet fever ("second disease"), a variant of scarlet fever or toxin-producing staphylococcal disease ("fourth disease"), erythema infectiosum ("fifth disease"), and roseola (exanthem subitum, or "sixth disease").[71]

Management Rubella control is required to prevent birth defects in the offspring of women who develop the disease during pregnancy. Vaccination to prevent rubella in the United States is recommended for all children at the age of 15 months. Vaccination results in a greater than 95% seroconversion rate. Because of the production of a transient viremia, pregnancy should be delayed for 3 months after a susceptible woman has been vaccinated. No cases of the congenital rubella syndrome attributable to rubella vaccine have occurred in more than 800 women inadvertently vaccinated during pregnancy who carried their infants to term.[72] There is no evidence of decreasing immunity with age. Persons with rubella should be cautioned to avoid contact with susceptible women. Because of an increasing failure to vaccinate susceptible people, a moderate resurgence of rubella and a major increase in the congenital rubella syndrome in the United States occurred in 1990.[73]

Flaviviridae

Flavivirus (Group B Arbovirus)

Principles of disease More than 60 flaviviruses have been identified, with more than 20 causing human disease. Three of the most common, all transmitted to humans via a mosquito vector, are the agents of yellow fever, dengue, and St. Louis encephalitis. The West Nile virus has recently been reported in New York City.[69]

Clinical features *Yellow fever* is present in tropical South America and Africa. Fever, chills, headache, nausea, and vomiting follow a 3- to 6-day incubation period.[74] The disease may be biphasic, with fever, jaundice, hemorrhage, and characteristic "black vomit" (from the coagulopathy secondary to an affected liver) occurring after a brief period of remission. The case fatality rate is 5%.

Dengue occurs in tropical areas worldwide. There are several reports of dengue transmission within the United States, but these cases have been limited to Texas.[75] Classic dengue fever (breakbone fever) is a nonfatal disease characterized by fever, headache, arthralgias, weakness, nausea, and anorexia after an incubation period of 5 to 10 days. Patients may experience severe bone pain. A generalized macular rash that occasionally desquamates may be seen. The fever lasts 5 to 7 days, but recovery may be prolonged. Dengue hemorrhagic fever, characterized by increased vascular permeability and bleeding associated with thrombocytopenia, has a mortality rate of less than 5% in people who receive good medical care but a mortality rate of up to 50% in those left untreated.[76]

St. Louis encephalitis occurs in the summer in most areas of the Western Hemisphere. After an incubation period of 4 to 21 days, infection with the St. Louis encephalitis virus may produce a simple fever and headache, aseptic meningitis, or encephalitis. The mortality rate associated with the encephalitis may approach 10%. The disease commonly affects the elderly.

The first cases of *West Nile virus encephalitis* in the Western Hemisphere were reported in New York City in 1999. Several cases affecting the elderly were fatal.[68] By 2001, it had been found in birds and mosquitoes as far south as Maryland and Virginia.

Differential considerations The differential diagnosis of yellow fever is wide and includes hepatitis, malaria, typhoid, dengue, and other viral hemorrhagic fevers in endemic areas. Viral antigen detected in the blood by enzyme-linked immunoadsorbent assay provides for a rapid diagnosis. The differential diagnosis for dengue is similar to that for yellow fever. Diagnosis is made by viral isolation or serology. St. Louis encephalitis may present like other causes of meningoencephalitis. In the elderly, it may be misdiagnosed as stroke. Diagnosis is made by serologic tests.

Management Treatment for these viral diseases is supportive. The diseases are not contagious through person-to-person contact, but the virus is generally transmissible to the mosquito during the clinical illness. Control of epidemics is achieved by reducing the mosquito vector populations and limiting access of mosquitoes to infected hosts. Persons traveling to endemic areas should be vaccinated for yellow fever.[77]

Hepatitis C Hepatitis C, a flavivirus, is an important cause of morbidity and mortality throughout the world. In the United States, hepatitis C had been associated with most cases of posttransfusion (non-A, non-B) disease. As a result of testing the blood supply, the incidence of transfusion-related hepatitis C has decreased. Yet the prevalence of infection remains high in certain populations, such as IV drug users. In the United States, it is estimated that 3.9 million people have hepatitis C infection.[78] Globally, more than 170 million people are infected.[79]

Chronic hepatitis C infection has been associated with cirrhosis and hepatocellular carcinoma. Estimates of the rate of long-term morbidity and mortality resulting from chronic hepatitis C vary. The likelihood of developing cirrhosis ranges from 5% to 25% in different studies.[80] Interferon alfa-2b is used to treat chronic infections. More recently, the addition of ribavirin is recommended, especially in patients who are initially nonresponsive to interferon monotherapy.[81] Early data on the use of pegylated interferon have been promising.[31a,31b]

The recognition that about 20% of the cases of transfusion-related non-A, non-B hepatitis could not be explained by infection with hepatitis C or any other known infectious hepatitis led investigators to look for agents of "not A–E" hepatitis. Modern molecular biology techniques have led to the cloning of HGV/GBV-C/hepatitis G virus (HGV). Although HGV/GBV-C appear to have a prevalence of 1% to 4% in eligible blood donors, the relationship between these viruses and acute or chronic hepatitis remains to be elucidated. Other novel viruses may be implicated as possible causes of transfusion-related hepatitis and chronic liver disease.[85]

Coronaviridae

Coronavirus

Clinical features Coronaviruses are agents of the common cold in adults and lower respiratory tract disease in children. More recently they have been implicated in diarrheal disease in children.

Coronaviruses primarily cause upper respiratory tract disease in adults. Lower respiratory tract infections caused by coronaviruses occur uncommonly in adults and more commonly in children. They appear to cause diarrheal disease in children younger than 1 year of age, but the association is less clear.

Differential considerations Coronaviruses probably account for 15% of adult colds. Rhinoviruses account for most of the rest, with parainfluenza viruses, influenza viruses, respiratory syncytial viruses, adenoviruses, and enteroviruses also causing upper respiratory infections and colds. Rotaviruses, Norwalk viruses, and enteroviruses cause most viral cases of gastroenteritis in children.

Management Treatment is entirely supportive.

Paramyxoviridae

Parainfluenza Viruses

Clinical features The parainfluenza viruses are the most common causes of croup in children and, along with the respiratory syncytial virus (RSV), are the most common causes of lower respiratory tract infections that require hospitalization in infants.[83]

The virus is passed via the respiratory route, and hand-to-mucous membrane transmission is likely. The incubation period is most often from 1 to 4 days and results in a febrile illness lasting approximately 4 days.

Infection with the parainfluenza viruses does not confer lasting immunity. Parainfluenza virus type 1 is the predominant cause of croup, or laryngotracheobronchitis, occurring during the autumn months in children under 3 years of age. Parainfluenza virus type 2 is also associated with croup, causes less morbidity than type 1, and often occurs in alternate years with type 1. Parainfluenza type 3 infections occur in the spring and are associated with bronchiolitis and pneumonia in infants younger than 1 year of age, similar to RSV. Parainfluenza type 3 is also associated with croup in children younger than 3 years of age and with tracheobronchitis in older children. Parainfluenza type 4 is recovered less often, but appears to be associated with mild respiratory illness. Severe croup or bacterial superinfection of laryngotracheitis may lead to respiratory compromise.

Differential considerations Viruses causing upper respiratory tract infection similar to that caused by the parainfluenza viruses include adenoviruses, rhinoviruses, influenza virus, RSV, echoviruses, coxsackieviruses, and coronaviruses. Identification of parainfluenza viral infection can be made by a fourfold rise in antibody titer between acute and convalescent serum.

Management Croup may be worse at night; mist inhalation is often helpful. Treatment with nebulized racemic epinephrine may be used to treat severe croup, but the relief it affords can be short lived, and return to pretreatment state can be seen within 2 hours of therapy. Intramuscular steroids have been shown to be helpful, and their use has been associated with a decreased requirement for hospitalization of children with croup.[83] The parainfluenza viruses can reinfect individuals within months of primary infection, so prevention of infection is unlikely.

Principles of disease Infections with RSV occur worldwide mostly in midwinter to late spring. Infants with pneumonia show marked inflammation in the interstitial tissue and alveoli of the lungs, whereas infants with bronchiolitis show less alveolar involvement but may have marked changes in the bronchioles. Severe disease may result in obstruction of bronchioles with evidence of peripheral airway obstruction or emphysema. Transmission is via respiratory secretions and probably by hand to nose or eye droplet inoculation.

Respiratory Syncytial Virus Infections caused by RSV account for the largest number of hospitalizations for respiratory infections in infants. Bronchiolitis and pneumonia, the most severe manifestations of RSV infection, commonly occur in children under 6 months of age. Children older than 1 year of age are less likely to have lower respiratory tract infection.[84] Older children and adults commonly have colds and cough, but elderly patients may have severe disease.

Clinical features The average incubation time of RSV infections is 2 to 8 days. The most common manifestations are bronchiolitis and pneumonia in infants; tracheobronchitis, croup, and otitis media in young children; and upper respiratory infections in older children and adults. Bronchiolitis in infancy may lead to an increased risk of asthma and the development of chronic obstructive airway disease in later life. Fatal disease may occur in immunocompromised infants.

The diagnosis of RSV infection may be made definitively by culturing the virus or detecting RSV antigens from respiratory secretions, nasal washes, or nasopharyngeal or throat swabs.

Differential consideration The syndromes associated with RSV infections overlap those of other upper and lower respiratory tract pathogens and include rhinovirus, parainfluenza and influenza viruses, echoviruses, coxsackieviruses, and coronaviruses. RSV may be presumptively diagnosed in an infant with pneumonia or bronchiolitis when no bacterial pathogens are noted. Noninfectious causes for hypoxemia in infants such as foreign-body aspiration and asthma must also be considered.

Management Therapy of RSV is largely supportive. For infants sick enough to be hospitalized, aerosolized ribavirin has been shown to shorten the duration of illness and improve hypoxemia in normal infants.[85] Corticosteroids have not been shown to be beneficial. During the winter, high-risk infants can be protected against RSV infection with monthly infusions of human RSV immunoglobulin or with monthly intramuscular injections of a monoclonal anti-RSV antibody preparation.[86] Severe disease may occur in immunocompromised infants, and respiratory precautions need be adopted to prevent transmission from patient to patient and staff to patient.[87]

Mumps Virus

Principles of disease Mumps, or infectious parotitis, is an acute viral illness characterized by fever, swelling, and tenderness of the salivary glands, with the parotid gland most commonly involved. Mumps occurs most commonly in the winter and spring and since the advent of widespread pediatric immunization, mostly in older children. The virus is spread via the respiratory tract and by direct contact with the saliva of infected people. The incubation period is 2 to 4 weeks, and the disease is communicable from 1 week before to 9 days after the onset of parotitis, with a period of maximal infectiousness approximately 2 days before the onset of illness. One third of cases are asymptomatic.

Clinical features Nonsuppurative parotid swelling is the hallmark of mumps; the swelling may be unilateral. Trismus is sometimes seen. In the first 3 days, the temperature may range between normal and 40° C. The most important, but less common, manifestations are epididymoorchitis and meningitis. Orchitis occurs in 15% to 25% of postpubertal men and is usually unilateral. Although some testicular atrophy generally occurs, the incidence of sterility is very low, especially when the orchitis is unilateral.[88] More than 50% of patients with mumps have a lymphocytic pleocytosis in the CSF, and hypoglycorrhachia is common, but symptomatic meningitis occurs in fewer than 10% of cases. Encephalitis is uncommon, occurring in 1 in 6000 cases, and is the major determinant of mortality. Congenital infection is rare but may result in fetal loss if it occurs in the first trimester.[89] Rare complications of mumps include hydrocephalus, deafness, transverse myelitis, Guillain-Barré syndrome, pancreatitis, mastitis, oophoritis, myocarditis, and arthritis.

Differential considerations In children, the diagnosis of mumps is made by a history of exposure and the presence of parotid swelling and tenderness in association with constitutional symptoms. Laboratory confirmation is generally not required. The differential diagnosis includes other viral infections and other causes of parotid swelling and tenderness such as bacterial parotitis or sarcoidosis.

Management Treatment is supportive and should include an analgesic and antipyretic agent. No data support the use of steroids to prevent complications of or ameliorate the symptoms of orchitis in postpubertal men.

Contacts who have had no history of mumps or of previous vaccination should be immunized. Because there is no risk in vaccinating those who are already immune, serologic screening to identify susceptible people is unnecessary. More than 95% of recipients of the vaccine develop long-lasting immunity. Previously infected people, including those with asymptomatic cases, have long-lasting, and possibly lifelong, immunity.

Measles Virus (Rubeola)

Principles of disease Measles is a highly communicable viral illness acquired as an infection of the respiratory tract. Generally, all susceptible people exposed to an active case will acquire infection. After multiplication in the respiratory mucosa, the virus spreads to regional lymphoid cells and then via the bloodstream to leukocytes in the reticuloendothelial system. The clinical manifestations appear after a second viremic phase.

Before the availability of an effective vaccine in 1963, measles was a ubiquitous disease. It is now uncommon in countries where routine infant vaccination is practiced but persists in epidemics in countries without such practices and accounts for 2 million deaths per year.

Clinical features The incubation period of measles is 10 to 14 days. Cough, coryza, conjunctivitis, and fever precede a rash by 2 to 4 days. Pinpoint grayish spots surrounded by bright red inflammation (Koplik's spots) are characteristically found on the lateral buccal mucosa before the appearance of the rash and are considered pathognomonic for measles. Discrete red macular and papular lesions begin on the head and progress downward over 3 days to cover the entire body. Laryngitis, tracheobronchitis, bronchiolitis, and pneumonitis may accompany the disease. Bacterial superinfections may occasionally delay recovery. An acute encephalomyelitis, which has a mortality rate of 25%, may rarely complicate recovery. Unlike rubella, measles acquired during pregnancy is not teratogenic but may result in stillbirth or premature delivery.

Infants and malnourished children generally develop more severe disease. Deaths from pneumonia and diarrhea may occur in up to 10%. Measles may exacerbate vitamin A deficiency and lead to blindness.

Measles may present with atypical findings in people who were vaccinated with the inactivated vaccine before its removal from the market in the United States in 1968. An atypical rash, predominantly on the extremities, may accompany pneumonitis, pleural effusion, and peripheral edema. The current vaccine is a live, attenuated strain available as a single antigen or in combination with rubella vaccine or with mumps and rubella vaccines.[90]

Differential considerations The diagnosis is made primarily from clinical characteristics. Other viral exanthems may at times present with a similar rash.

Management Treatment of the primary disease is supportive. Immunocompromised children and infants younger than 1 year of age who are susceptible and have been exposed to measles may be given passive immunization within 6 days of exposure. Healthy infants should receive 0.25 ml/kg of immune globulin intramuscularly, and immunocompromised children should be given 0.5 ml/kg intramuscularly, up to 15 ml.

Routine vaccination has led to a decrease in the number of measles cases reported in the United States by greater than 99%. Since 1983 there had been an increase in cases among babies younger than 15 months of age and in nonimmunized inner-city preschool children.[91] Outbreaks have occurred among the 2% to 5% of people who fail to seroconvert after a single dose of vaccine, notably on college campuses.[90] Because a second dose converts 95% of those initial failures, the current recommendation is for a two-dose measles vaccination program, with the first dose given at 15 months of age and the second on school entry. People should also be revaccinated if they are entering educational institutions after high school or entering hospital service and have not had either a documented case of measles or this two-dose regimen. These new recommendations have resulted in a decrease in cases of measles since the resurgence of 1989 to 1991.

Measles is a reportable disease in most states, and the local health authority should be contacted. Children should be kept out of school for at least 4 days after the appearance of the rash.

Subacute Sclerosing Panencephalitis

Principles of disease Subacute sclerosing panencephalitis (SSPE) is a degenerative disease of the brain caused by measles virus or a defective variant that persists in the CNS after primary measles. SSPE has virtually disappeared in the United States since the 1970s, approximately 10 years after measles vaccination began.

Clinical features SSPE is a subacute encephalitis involving both the white and the gray matter of the cerebral hemispheres and brainstem and follows 1 in 100,000 cases of measles. A total of 5 to 10 years after a generally uncomplicated case of primary measles that may have occurred at a younger than average age, SSPE presents with myoclonus and variable focal neurologic deficits. Personality changes and intellectual deterioration occur early in the disease. Progressive neurologic degeneration ensues, and death usually occurs within months to years of diagnosis.

Differential considerations The disease may present like other degenerative neurologic disorders, but characteristic EEG changes and the findings of measles antibodies in the CSF and markedly elevated serum antibodies to measles confirm the diagnosis.

Management Treatment is entirely supportive.

Rhabdoviridae

Within the Rhabdoviridae family of viruses are two genera, Lyssavirus, containing the rabies and rabies-like viruses, and Vesiculovirus, containing the vesicular stomatitis and related viruses. Lyssavirus contains six viruses, but only the rabies, duvenhage, and Mokola viruses are known to cause disease in humans.

Vesicular Stomatitis Virus and Related Viruses

Vesicular stomatitis virus (VSV) commonly infects wild and domestic animals and occasionally infects humans. Transmission is believed to be from insect bites. VSV-New Jersey and VSV-Indiana produce an influenza-like febrile illness 1 to 2 days after exposure and last 4 to 7 days. Oral vesicular lesions have occasionally been noted.[92] The disease is nonspecific. Diagnosis can be made serologically. Treatment is supportive.

Filoviridae

Marburg and Ebola Viruses

Principles of disease Marburg and Ebola viruses cause bleeding and shock, which are associated with thrombocytopenia, in a high percentage of infected people. Although the viruses have infected African green monkeys and cynomolgus monkeys, respectively, the infection is fatal to the monkeys, and the natural reservoir is unknown. Monkey-to-human and human-to-human transmission via contaminated tissues or materials has been documented. Aerosol transmission has not been documented.

Marburg and Ebola viruses produce systemic febrile illnesses (African hemorrhagic fever) associated with gastrointestinal bleeding and a high mortality rate.

Clinical features The illness is of sudden onset 7 to 10 days after exposure to infected tissue or contact with contaminated materials. Headache, fever, myalgias, arthralgias, and lethargy are early signs. The cardinal sign of these infections is gastrointestinal bleeding. Reported cases of Marburg virus and Ebola virus disease have a mortality rate of 25% and 90%, respectively. An outbreak of Ebola viral hemorrhagic fever in Zaire in 1995 had a case fatality rate of greater than 90%.[93]

Differential considerations Marburg and Ebola virus diseases may appear clinically similar to other African hemorrhagic fevers, particularly Rift Valley fever, Lassa fever, and yellow fever. Diagnosis is made by isolation of the virus from blood or demonstrating rising antibody titers.

Management No vaccine exists; treatment is supportive.[94]

Orthomyxoviridae

Influenza Virus

Principles of disease Influenza is generally a self-limited infection of the upper respiratory tract associated with fever, cough, coryza, sore throat, and malaise.[11] Three types of influenza are recognized. Type A has been associated with most widespread epidemics and pandemics and is associated with most mortality caused by influenza. Influenza B causes regional or widespread epidemics every 2 to 3 years. Influenza C is associated with sporadic cases.

Clinical features The usual clinical disease caused by influenza begins 1 to 4 days after exposure to aerosol respiratory secretions. Fevers ensue and are accompanied by myalgias, coryza, and conjunctivitis; headache; and a nonproductive cough. Patchy infiltrates may be seen on chest radiograph. Symptoms generally last only a few days, but fatigue and malaise may persist for weeks. The most common serious complications of influenza, particularly among the elderly and people with chronic diseases, are pneumonia caused by influenza itself and pneumonia attributable to secondary bacterial infections. Rare complications of influenza infection include aseptic meningitis, pericarditis, and a postinfectious neuritis that resembles the Guillain-Barré syndrome.

Viral cultures remain the gold standard for the laboratory diagnosis of influenza, but results are often not timely enough to aid the clinician in initiating therapy. Commercially available point-of-care tests that promise results within minutes may be more relevant with the availability of the neuraminidase inhibitors.

Differential considerations The diagnosis of influenza is made on clinical grounds during the appropriate season.

Serologic confirmation is rarely required, but definitive diagnosis can be made by serologic testing or by isolation of the virus from nasal secretions. The syndromes produced by the influenza viruses overlap with those produced by other viruses such as the parainfluenza viruses, RSV, adenoviruses, coronaviruses, and echoviruses.

Management General supportive measures ameliorate the symptoms of influenza. The neuraminidase inhibitors zanamivir and oseltamivir have been approved for treating both Influenza A and B. The dose of oseltamivir should be decreased to 75 mg *bid* in patients with a creatinine clearance of less than 30 ml/min. Zanamivir or oseltamivir should be administered within 2 days of the onset of symptoms if efficacy is to expected.[13,14] Amantadine, 100 mg twice a day, is effective in the treatment and prophylaxis of clinical disease caused by influenza A but not influenza B.[95] Confusion is a common side effect of amantadine, particularly in the elderly, so the dosage should be decreased accordingly. Amantadine should be used with caution in patients with renal failure. Vaccination is recommended yearly for people who are at high risk of significant morbidity or mortality from influenza; these include immunosuppressed patients or those with chronic illnesses, people older than 65 years of age, and women in the second or third trimester of pregnancy. Vaccination is also recommended for service personnel who may transmit the infection to others or who provide vital services, such as health care workers, police, or fire fighters. Aspirin and aspirin-containing products should be avoided, especially among children and adolescents, particularly during influenza epidemics because of the association between the use of aspirin during a bout of influenza and the subsequent development of Reye's syndrome.[42]

Bunyaviridae

California Encephalitis and Bunyavirus Hemorrhagic Fevers

Pathophysiology and clinical findings California encephalitis viruses, including the La Crosse and Johnson Canyon viruses, are transmitted by mosquito bite, predominantly in the northern United States in the summer and fall months. Approximately 100 cases are reported yearly. Infection is mostly asymptomatic, but the mortality rate of the encephalitis is approximately 1%.[96]

Hantaviruses cause a hemorrhagic fever with renal syndrome. Rodents carry the agents, and the virus is transmitted via aerosols infected from rodent urine. More than 100,000 cases occur in Asia and Europe, and the mortality rate is approximately 6%.[97]

In 1994, a previously unknown hantavirus was found to cause a pulmonary syndrome associated with tachypnea, hemoconcentration, thrombocytopenia, and leukocytosis.[98] Cases occurred predominantly in the southwestern United States, were associated with a mortality rate higher than 50%, and were believed to have been transmitted from the deer mouse, *Peromyscus maniculatus.* The virus has been named the *Muerto Canyon* or *Sin Nombre virus.*

Rift Valley fever virus is carried by a mosquito and generally produces a nonspecific febrile disease. Up to 100,000 cases occur yearly in Africa. Some patients develop a severe retinitis that may lead to blindness.

Congo-Crimean hemorrhagic fever is a severe, rare, tick-transmitted disease that occurs in Africa and Asia and has a mortality rate approaching 50%.[94]

Management Treatment of all these diseases is supportive. The CDC provides IV ribavirin for investigational use.

Arenaviridae

Lymphocytic Choriomeningitis Virus, Lassa Virus, and Arenaviral (Hemorrhagic Fever) Viruses

Principles of disease The arenaviruses are carried by parasites of rodents and probably are passed to humans from contact with infected rodent urine. Four arenaviruses are known to cause human disease: lymphocytic choriomeningitis (LCM) virus causes a meningoencephalitis that may be severe but is rarely fatal; Junin and Machupo viruses, from Argentina and Bolivia, respectively, and the Lassa virus, from Africa, all cause severe and often fatal hemorrhagic fevers.

Clinical features *Lassa virus* is also commonly transmitted from person to person. LCM occurs in the Americas, Europe, and Asia and is usually passed from house mice, pet hamsters, or laboratory animals.[104] Influenza-like symptoms follow a 1- to 3-week incubation period and are generally followed by complete recovery. Meningitis may ensue, but even severe cases are associated with good recovery. Orchitis and parotitis may accompany the disease. LCM is believed to account for only a small percentage of the cases of aseptic meningitis in the United States.

Lassa fever is a highly contagious disease occurring in West Africa with a case fatality rate of 15% in hospitalized patients.[94,100] A gradual onset of fever and malaise begins after an incubation period of 7 to 18 days. Retrosternal chest pain, vomiting, and diarrhea accompany severe headache and pharyngitis. Pneumonitis and respiratory distress may develop. Early lymphopenia followed by neutrophilia and elevated transaminases are associated with a poor prognosis.

Argentine hemorrhagic fever (AHF), caused by the Junin virus, causes a skin rash and petechiae and is more likely to be hemorrhagic than Lassa fever. The disease presents after a 7- to 10-day incubation period with fever, malaise, anorexia, and myalgias. Petechiae and gastrointestinal bleeding occur between days 4 and 6, and shock may follow. Case fatality rates range up to 30%. Bolivian hemorrhagic fever (BHF), caused by Machupo virus, is similar to AHF but occurs much less commonly.[101]

Differential considerations LCM may resemble other viral causes of meningitis or encephalitis. The diagnosis of arenaviral infections requires a fourfold rise in antibody titer.

Management Supportive care only is required for LCM. Ribavirin has been used effectively to treat Lassa fever and can result in a fivefold decrease in the mortality rate.[102] AHF and possibly BHF may be successfully treated with convalescent plasma from a recovered patient. Prevention of arenaviral infections can best be accomplished by controlling the infected vectors. Special care must be taken to prevent person-to-person spread of Lassa fever.

Retroviridae Three subfamilies are described in family Retroviridae, the type C oncoviruses (HTLV-I, HTLV-II), the lentiviruses (HIV-1, HIV-2), and the spumaviruses. Only the oncoviruses and lentiviruses have been shown to cause disease in humans.

Type C Oncoviruses The demonstration that RNA could be transcribed into DNA by the reverse transcriptase in RNA tumor viruses laid the groundwork for the discovery of human retroviruses.[103] Human T-cell leukemia virus type 1 (HTLV-1) was isolated in 1980.[104] Approximately 1% of people infected in childhood with HTLV-1 develop adult T-cell leukemia-lymphoma as adults. HTLV-1 has also been associated with tropical spastic paraparesis, also known as *HTLV-I-associated myelopathy.* HTLV-II was isolated in 1982 and found to be associated with a T-cell variant of hairy cell leukemia.[105]

Human Immunodeficiency Virus HIV is a slow virus, or lentivirus, related to animal viruses such as visna and feline leukemia virus. A full description of HIV and AIDS is found in Chapter 126.

Picornaviridae The family Picornaviridae is derived from "pico," or very small, and "RNA," their nucleic acid type. Picornaviridae contains two viruses that infect humans, the enterovirus, containing 67 recognized species—including the polioviruses, coxsackieviruses, echoviruses, and hepatitis A virus—and the rhinovirus, with more than 100 human species.

Poliovirus

Principles of disease Poliomyelitis is an acute viral infection that ranges from an inapparent infection to a nonspecific febrile illness to aseptic meningitis to severe paralysis and death. Since the introduction of vaccination in the United States, only a handful of cases of paralytic poliomyelitis has been diagnosed each year, and most of these cases are either imported or vaccine associated.[106]

Poliovirus types 1, 2, and 3 can all cause paralytic poliomyelitis, with type 1 the most common isolate and type 2 the least common. Poliovirus is transmitted during close contact; transmission by both the fecal-oral route and via respiratory secretions has been documented. Susceptibility to poliovirus is universal, but paralytic infections are rare, increasing in incidence with age at the time of infection. At least 95% of infections are inapparent or asymptomatic.

Clinical features Paralytic poliomyelitis usually occurs after an incubation period of 7 to 14 days. The disease in children is usually biphasic, with a brief viremic phase lasting 1 to 3 days. After recovery for 2 to 5 days, an abrupt onset of headache, fever, malaise, vomiting, and CSF pleocytosis ensues. This meningitic phase lasts for 1 to 2 days before the beginning of weakness and flaccid paralysis. Bulbar paralytic poliomyelitis involves paralysis of the muscle groups innervated by the cranial nerves. The most important complications of paralytic poliomyelitis are respiratory, especially respiratory failure caused by paralysis of the respiratory muscles, aspiration pneumonia, and pulmonary embolism. Myocarditis may rarely occur. Muscular paralysis usually extends for only 1 to 3 days after its onset. A postparalytic paralysis syndrome has been described, in which neuromuscular weakness recurs several decades after the acute poliovirus infection.[107]

Differential considerations Paralytic poliomyelitis can usually be recognized on clinical presentation. Other enteroviruses can cause a similar syndrome. Guillain-Barré syndrome and postencephalitic syndromes may resemble paralytic poliomyelitis. The differential diagnosis of nonparalytic poliomyelitis includes any of the causes of bacterial and viral meningitis and encephalitis. The definitive diagnosis is made by isolation of the virus from fecal material or respiratory secretions.

Management Specific antiviral treatment for poliomyelitis is not available. Management is supportive, and reporting to local health authorities is mandatory. In the acute phase of paralytic poliomyelitis, patients require hospitalization.

Routine vaccination in the United States has dramatically reduced the number of cases of paralytic poliomyelitis. The Salk inactivated poliovirus vaccine (IPV) is recommended for most indications in the United States. IPV has the advantage of preventing paralytic disease, but it does not protect susceptible contacts by secondary spread. The Sabin oral polio vaccine (OPV) protects susceptible contact, but it is associated with vaccine-associated cases of paralytic disease.[108] As of January 1, 2000, the CDC recommended that all U.S. children should receive 4 doses of IPV at age 2 months, 4 months, 6-18 months, and 4-6 years, and that OPV be used only in special situations such as the control of an outbreak or if an unvaccinated child is to travel to an endemic region.[4]

Coxsackieviruses, Echoviruses, and Other Enteroviruses

Principles of disease The enteroviruses are spread from person to person via the fecal-oral route. As with poliovirus, inapparent infections greatly outnumber symptomatic cases.

All enteroviruses enter the body through the oropharynx and multiply in the tissues around the oropharynx. The viruses are stable in acid conditions and are capable of passing through the stomach to the intestines.

Clinical features Most enteroviral infections are inapparent. The most common clinical manifestation is that of a nonspecific febrile illness. Young children may be admitted to hospitals with enteroviral fevers that simulate bacterial sepsis. Coxsackie B virus and some of the echoviruses may cause severe perinatal infection associated with fever, meningitis, myocarditis, and hepatitis.

Febrile diseases with rashes are often associated with enteroviruses. Exanthems resembling rubella occurring during the summer months have been seen with the echoviruses and coxsackie A viruses. Vesicular lesions are seen, such as with the hand-foot-and-mouth syndrome caused by some coxsackie A and B viruses. Herpangina, a specific disease characterized by a vesicular rash on the cheeks and soft palate and associated with fever, sore throat, and severe pain on swallowing, is caused by the coxsackie A virus. Roseola-like exanthems and petechial exanthems are also associated with coxsackievirus and echovirus infections.

The enteroviruses are the most common causes of viral meningitis. The course is generally benign but often can be confused with a bacterial process, particularly in the acute phase of the infection when CSF may show a neutrophil predominance.

Coxsackie B viruses are strongly associated with myocarditis, although echoviruses and coxsackie A viruses can also cause the disease. Severe cases may lead to dysrhythmias, heart failure, or death.

Enteroviruses cause upper respiratory tract infections similar to other etiologies of the common cold. Interstitial pneumonias may also occur. Pleurodynia (Bornholm disease, the devil's grip) is generally associated with the coxsackie B viruses. This disease involves the intercostal muscles and may last for several weeks.

Other proven or suggested associations with the enteroviruses and disease include enterovirus 70 and acute hemorrhagic conjunctivitis, coxsackieviruses, and echoviruses with diarrhea and gastroenteritis; coxsackieviruses and echoviruses with hemolytic-uremic syndrome; and enteroviruses with acute myositis. Other suggested disease associations include chronic cardiomyopathy, aortitis, hepatitis, pancreatitis, orchitis, diabetes mellitus, lymphadenopathy, a mononucleosis-like syndrome, and infectious lymphocytosis. A progressive, dementing, chronic meningitis associated with enteroviruses has been reported in individuals with common variable immunodeficiency syndrome.

Management No specific treatments for the enteroviruses exist. Care is supportive. Vaccines exist for poliovirus and hepatitis A, and immune serum globulin may also prevent the acquisition of hepatitis A infection.

Hepatitis A Virus The hepatitis A virus has recently been isolated and classified among the picornaviruses.

Rhinovirus

Principles of disease Rhinoviruses are the most common cause of the common cold. More than 100 strains exist. Rhinovirus transmission generally occurs primarily via hand contact and inoculation of the eye or nasal mucosa and less commonly via aerosolization of respiratory secretion. Viral replication probably occurs on the epithelial surface of the nasal mucosa.

Clinical features After a 1- to 4-day incubation period, usual symptoms of rhinoviral infection include nasal obstruction, sneezing, sore throat, cough, and malaise. Severe tracheobronchitis and pneumonia may rarely occur. Fever and lower respiratory tract infections are more common in children with rhinovirus infections than in adults.

Differential considerations Other respiratory pathogens such as coronaviruses, RSV, parainfluenza viruses, influenza viruses, adenoviruses, and enteroviruses may produce clinical syndromes similar to those produced by the rhinoviruses. The rhinoviruses, in general, cause less morbidity than do the parainfluenza viruses and RSV. Definitive diagnosis is made by the demonstration of a rise in antibody titer.

Management Treatment is aimed at relieving symptoms. Routine vaccination appears unlikely because of the number of serotypes. Because hand-to-face inoculation appears to be the predominant means of transmission, frequent handwashing during epidemic periods may decrease the spread of rhinovirus infections.

Caliciviridae

Caliciviruses and Astroviruses

Principles of disease Caliciviruses and astroviruses are small RNA viruses implicated in outbreaks of gastroenteritis, predominantly in children. The Norwalk virus has recently been included among the caliciviruses. The Norwalk virus has been found in the stools from patients with acute gastroenteritis. These viruses have not yet been grown in vitro, but the clinical syndromes associated with them appear to be widespread.[109]

Features The incubation period is probably 1 to 4 days, and the disease lasts from 1 to 3 days. The disease is generally mild and accompanied by low-grade fever. Vomiting appears to be less common with astroviral disease than with caliciviruses. One third of outbreaks of gastroenteritis can be attributed to a Norwalk-like agent. Diarrhea induced by these agents is associated with transient fat malabsorption. Outbreaks have occurred in schools and other institutions and through the ingestion of inadequately cooked shellfish.[110] The mode of transmission is unknown but is probably via the fecal-oral route. Vomiting and diarrhea occur with myalgias, malaise, headache, and low-grade fever. Diarrheal stools are moderate and nonbloody.

Differential considerations Other causes of gastroenteritis causing a similar syndrome include adenoviruses, enteroviruses, and coronaviruses. Electron microscopy can make the definitive diagnosis.

Management Treatment is supportive. The gastroenteritis is generally self-limited and resolves without specific treatment. Oral rehydration solutions are generally adequate; rarely, IV therapy is required.

Unclassified Viruses

Hepatitis E Virus Hepatitis E virus is an RNA virus that has been identified as a cause of enterically transmitted hepatitis. It has been implicated as a cause of fulminant hepatitis in pregnant women.

Prions

Principles of disease *Prion* is the term coined from *pro*teinaceous *in*fectious particles, the transmissible agent putatively responsible for a group of chronic neurodegenerative disorders sharing certain pathologic features. Prions have not been found to contain nucleic acid.[111,112] Other terms for these agents included *unconventional virus* and *virino.* The group of diseases, also referred to as *slow virus infections* or simply *slow infections,* includes Creutzfeldt-Jakob disease (CJD), kuru, and the Gerstmann-Sträussler syndrome. Bovine spongiform encephalopathy (BSE), or new-variant CJD, occurred primarily in the United Kingdom in the early 1990s, probably related to a change in the practice of offal rendering.[113] By 2001, a few cases had been found elsewhere in Europe but not in the United States.

A characteristic feature of these diseases is the lack of any inflammatory response. A reactive astrocytosis to the presence of the virus occurs in the CNS accompanied by neuronal vacuolation resulting in spongiform encephalopathy.

Findings CJD is a rare disease, usually presenting in late middle age with a progressive dementia combined with ataxia and myoclonic jerking. Distribution is worldwide and sporadic. CJD has been transmitted from person to person via direct inoculation, including corneal transplants and dura mater grafts. Kuru and the Gerstmann-Sträussler syndrome present as cerebellar syndromes, with dementia occurring late in the course of the disease. Kuru has been associated with cannibalism confined to a few primitive tribes in the highlands of New Guinea.[114] Progression of CJD and kuru is rapid, with death usually occurring in less than 1 year. The Gerstmann-Sträussler syndrome follows a more slowly progressive course of up to 10 years.

Differential considerations CJD can be confused with Alzheimer's disease or other slowly dementing diseases. Other diseases to be considered include multiinfarct dementia, nutritional deficiency syndromes, or primary brain tumors. CT and MR scans are usually nondiagnostic, but EEG may often show changes characteristic of CJD.

Management Treatment for these diseases is entirely supportive.

KEY CONCEPTS

- *Influenza:* People should receive an influenza vaccine annually. Patients with symptoms of influenza may have the course of their illness shortened by 1 to 2 days if treatment with amantadine, rimantadine, or neuraminidase inhibitors is initiated within 48 hours after symptom onset.

- *Herpes simplex infection:* Patients who have primary genital herpes or severe or frequent recurrences of infection and patients who are immunosuppressed and have continuous infections should receive treatment with acyclovir, famciclovir, or valacyclovir. The treatment of herpes simplex encephalitis is a medical emergency requiring rapid diagnosis and treatment with intravenous acyclovir.
- *Herpes zoster infection:* Patients with herpes zoster that is disseminated or that involves more than one dermatome or the ophthalmic branch of the trigeminal nerve should be treated with IV acyclovir.
- *Rabies:* Immediate postexposure treatment with both rabies vaccine and rabies immunoglobulin should be administered after exposure (contact of infected secretions with abraded skin or mucous membranes) to a skunk, raccoon, fox, and most other carnivores and bats.

REFERENCES

1. Jenner E: *An inquiry into the causes and effects of the variolae vaccinae,* Birmingham, Ala, 1978, The Classics of Medicine Library.
2. Centers for Disease Control: A centennial celebration: Pasteur and the modern era of immunization, *MMWR* 34:389, 1985.
3. Salk JE et al: Studies in human subjects on active immunization against poliomyelitis. I. A preliminary report of experiments in progress, *JAMA* 151:1081, 1953.
4. Centers for Disease Control and Prevention: Poliomyelitis prevention in the United States: updated recommendations of the Advisory Committee on Immunization Practices (ACIP), *MMWR* 49(RR-5):1, 2000.
5. Fenner F: Global eradication of smallpox, *Rev Infect Dis* 4:916, 1982.
6. Centers for Disease Control and Prevention: Recommended childhood immunization schedule—United States, 1999, *MMWR* 48:12-16, 1999.
7. Centers for Disease Control: Diphtheria, tetanus, and pertussis: recommendations for vaccine use and other preventive measures: recommendations of the Immunization Practices Advisory Committee (ACIP), *MMWR* 40(RR-10):1, 1991.
8. Centers for Disease Control: Update on adult immunization: recommendations of the Immunization Practices Advisory Committee (ACIP), *MMWR* 40(RR-12):1, 1991.
9. Centers for Disease Control and Prevention: Prevention of hepatitis A through active or passive immunization: recommendations of the Advisory Committee on Immunization Practices (ACIP), *MMWR* 48(RR-12):1, 1999.
10. Centers for Disease Control and Prevention: Prevention and control of influenza: recommendations of the Advisory Committee on Immunization Practices (ACIP), *MMWR* 48(RR-3):1, 1999.
11. Cox N, Subbarao K: Influenza, *Lancet* 354:1277, 1999.
12. Hayden FC et al: Emergence and apparent transmission of rimantadine-resistant influenza A virus in families, *N Engl J Med* 321:1696, 1989.
13. Hayden FG et al: Efficacy and safety of the neuraminidase inhibitor zanamivir in the treatment of influenza virus infections, *N Engl J Med* 337:874, 1997.
14. Centers for Disease Control and Prevention: Neuraminidase inhibitors for treatment of influenza A and B infections, *MMWR* 48(RR-14):1, 1999.
15. Whitley RJ, Gnann JW Jr: Acyclovir: a decade later, *N Engl J Med* 327:782, 1992.
16. Safrin S et al: Foscarnet therapy in five patients with AIDS and acyclovir-resistant varicella-zoster virus infection, *Ann Intern Med* 115:19, 1991.
17. Chatis PA et al: Successful treatment with foscarnet of an acyclovir-resistant mucocutaneous infection with herpes simplex virus in a patient with acquired immunodeficiency syndrome, *N Engl J Med* 320:297, 1989.
18. Tyring S et al: Famciclovir for the treatment of acute herpes zoster: effects on acute disease and postherpetic neuralgia: a randomized, double-blind, placebo-controlled trial, *Ann Intern Med* 123:89, 1995.
19. Beutner KL et al: Valacyclovir compared with acyclovir for improved therapy for herpes zoster in immunocompetent adults, *Antimicrob Agents Chemother* 39:1546, 1995.
20. Drew WL: Cytomegalovirus infection in patients with AIDS, *Clin Infect Dis* 14:608, 1992.
21. Goodgame RW: Gastrointestinal cytomegalovirus disease, *Ann Intern Med* 119:924, 1993.
22. Erice A et al: Progressive disease due to ganciclovir-resistant cytomegalovirus in immunocompromised patients, *N Engl Med* 320:289, 1989.
23. Polis MA et al: Anticytomegaloviral activity and safety of cidofovir in patients with human immunodeficiency virus infection and cytomegalovirus viruria, *Antimicrob Agents Chemother* 39:882, 1995.
24. Palestine AG et al: A randomized, controlled trial of foscarnet in the treatment of cytomegalovirus retinitis in patients with AIDS, *Ann Intern Med* 115:665, 1991.
25. Safrin S et al: A controlled trial comparing foscarnet with vidarabine for acyclovir-resistant, thymidine kinase deficient herpes simplex virus, *J Infect Dis* 325:551, 1991.
26. Whitley RJ et al: Adenine arabinoside therapy of biopsy-proved herpes simplex encephalitis, *N Engl J Med* 297:289, 1977.
27. Eron LJ et al: Interferon therapy for condylomata acuminata, *N Engl J Med* 315:1059, 1986.
28. Lane HC et al: Anti-retroviral effects of interferon alfa in AIDS-associated Kaposi sarcoma, *Lancet* 2:1218, 1988.
29. Niederau C et al: Long-term follow-up of HBeAg positive patients treated with interferon alfa for chronic hepatitis B, *N Eng J Med* 334:1422-1427, 1996.
30. McHutchison JG et al: Interferon Alfa-2b alone or in combination with ribavirin as initial treatment for chronic hepatitis C, *N Engl J Med* 339:1485-1492, 1998.
31. Poynard T et al: Randomised trial of interferon alfa-2b plus ribavirin for 48 weeks or for 24 weeks versus interferon alfa-2b plus placebo for 48 weeks for treatment of chronic infection with hepatitis C virus, *Lancet* 352:1426-1432, 1998.

31a. Zeuzem S et al: Peginterferon alfa-2a in patients with chronic hepatitis C, *N Engl J Med* 343:1666-1672, 2000.

31b. Heathcote E et al: Peginterferon alfa-2a in patients with chronic hepatitis C and cirrhosis, *N Engl J Med* 343:1673-1680, 2000.

32. Centers for Disease Control and Prevention: Human monkeypox—kasai oriental, Democratic Republic of Congo, February 1996–October 1997, *MMWR* 46:1168, 1997.
33. Kaplan MH et al: Dermatologic findings and manifestations of acquired immunodeficiency syndrome (AIDS), *J Am Acad Dermatol* 16:485, 1987.
34. Hall CB et al: Human herpesvirus-6 infection in children: a prospective study of complications and reactivation, *N Engl J Med* 331:432, 1994.
35. Chang Y et al: Identification of herpesvirus-like DNA sequences in AIDS-associated Kaposi's sarcoma, *Science* 266:1865, 1994.
36. Whitley RJ, Kimberlin DW, Roizman B: Herpes simplex viruses, *Clin Infect Dis* 26:541, 1998.
37. Brown AZ et al: Effects on infants of a first episode of genital herpes during pregnancy, *N Engl J Med* 317:1246, 1987.
38. Aurelius E et al: Rapid diagnosis of herpes simplex encephalitis by nested polymerase chain reaction assay of cerebrospinal fluid, *Lancet* 1:189, 1991.
39. Whitley R et al: A controlled trial comparing vidarabine with acyclovir in neonatal herpes simplex virus infections, *N Engl J Med* 324:444, 1991.
40. Balfour H: Drug therapy: antiviral drugs, *N Engl J Med* 340:1255-1268, 1999.
41. Buchbinder SP: Herpes zoster and human immunodeficiency virus infection, *J Infect Dis* 166:1153, 1992.
42. Hurwitz ES et al: National surveillance for Reye's syndrome: a five-year review, *Pediatrics* 70:895, 1982.
43. Centers for Disease Control and Prevention: Prevention of varicella: updated recommendations of the Advisory Committee on Immunization Practices (ACIP), *MMWR* 48:1, 1999.

44. Cohen J et al: Recent advances in varicella-zoster virus infection, *Ann Intern Med* 130:922, 1999.
45. McCutchan JA: Cytomegalovirus infections of the nervous system in patients with AIDS, *Clin Infect Dis* 20:747, 1995.
46. Emmanuel D et al: Cytomegalovirus pneumonia after bone marrow transplantation successfully treated with the combination of ganciclovir and high-dose intravenous immune globulin, *Ann Intern Med* 109:777, 1988.
47. Fukuda K et al: The chronic fatigue syndrome: a comprehensive approach to its definition and study, *Ann Intern Med* 121:953, 1994.
48. Levy JA: Three new human herpes viruses (HHV 6, 7, and 8), *Lancet* 349:558, 1997.
49. Moore PS, Chang Y: Detection of herpesvirus-like DNA sequences in Kaposi's sarcoma in patients with and without HIV infection, *N Engl J Med* 332:1181, 1995.
50. Foreman K et al: Propagation of a human herpesvirus from AIDS-associated Kaposi's sarcoma, *N Engl J Med* 336:163, 1997.
51. Palmer AE: B-virus, herpesvirus simiae: historical perspective, *J Med Primatol* 16:99, 1987.
52. Centers for Disease Control: B-virus infection in humans—Pensacola, Florida, *MMWR* 36:289, 1987.
53. Steinberg BM, Abramson AL: Laryngeal papillomas, *Clin Dermatol* 3:130, 1985.
54. Campion MJ et al: Progressive potential of mild cervical atypia: prospective cytological, colposcopic, and virological study, *Lancet* 2:237, 1986.
55. Beutner K et al: Imiquimod, a patient-applied immune response modifier for treatment of external genital warts, *Antimicrob Agents Chemother* 42:789, 1998.
56. Chaisson RE, Griffin DE: Progressive multifocal leukoencephalopathy in AIDS, *JAMA* 264:79, 1990.
57. Antinori A et al: Diagnosis of AIDS-related focal brain lesions: a decision-making analysis based on clinical and neuroradiologic characteristics combined with polymerase chain reaction assays in CSF, *Neurology* 48:687, 1997.
58. Baqi M, Kucharczyk W, Walmsley SL: Regression of progressive multifocal encephalopathy with highly active antiretroviral therapy, *AIDS* 11:1526-1527, 1997.
59. Adler SP et al: Risk of human parvovirus B19 infections among school and hospital employees during endemic periods, *J Infect Dis* 168:361, 1993.
60. Fairley CK, Smoleniec JS, Caul OE: Observational study of effect of intrauterine transfusions on outcome of fetal hydrops after parvovirus B19 infection, *Lancet* 346:1335, 1995.
61. Abkowitz JL et al: Clinical relevance of parvovirus B19 as a cause of anemia in patients with human immunodeficiency virus infection, *J Infect Dis* 176:269, 1997.
62. Frickhofen N et al: Persistent B19 parvovirus infection in patients infected with human immunodeficiency virus type 1 (HIV-1): a treatable cause of anemia in AIDS, *Ann Intern Med* 113:926, 1990.
63. Goodpasture HC et al: Colorado tick fever: clinical, epidemiologic, and laboratory aspects of 228 cases in Colorado in 1973-1974, *Ann Intern Med* 88:303, 1978.
64. Centers for Disease Control: Viral agents of gastroenteritis: public health importance and outbreak management, *MMWR* 39(RR-5), 1990.
65. Rotbart HA et al: Neonatal rotavirus associated necrotizing enterocolitis: case control study and prospective surveillance during an outbreak, *J Pediatr* 112:87, 1988.
66. Centers for Disease Control and Prevention: Intussusception among recipients of rotavirus vaccine—United States, 1989-1999. *MMWR* 48:577-581, 1999.
67. Centers for Disease Control and Prevention: Arbovirus disease—United States, 1993, *MMWR* 43:385, 1994.
68. Centers for Disease Control and Prevention: Outbreak of West Nile–like viral encephalitis—New York 1999, *MMWR* 48:845-849, 1999.
69. Asnis DS et al: The West Nile virus outbreak of 1999 in New York: the Flushing Hospital experience, *Clin Infect Dis* 30:413, 2000.
70. Munro ND et al: Temporal relations between maternal rubella and congenital defects, *Lancet* 2:201, 1987.
71. Shapiro L: The numbered diseases: first through sixth, *JAMA* 194:680, 1971.
72. Centers for Disease Control: Rubella vaccination during pregnancy, 1976-1986, *MMWR* 36:457, 1987.
73. Centers for Disease Control: Increase in rubella and congenital rubella syndrome—United States, 1988-1990, *MMWR* 40:93, 1991.
74. Monath TP: Yellow fever: a medically neglected disease: report on a seminar, *Rev Infect Dis* 9:165, 1987.
75. Rawlings JA et al: Dengue surveillance in Texas, 1995, *Am J Trop Med Hyg* 59:95, 1998.
76. Halstead SB: Pathogenesis of dengue: challenges to molecular biology, *Science* 239:476, 1988.
77. Centers for Disease Control: Yellow fever vaccine: recommendations of the Immunization Practices Advisory Committee (ACIP), *MMWR* 39(RR-6), 1990.
78. Alter MJ et al: The prevalence of hepatitis C virus infection in the United States, 1988 through 1994, *N Engl J Med* 341:556, 1999.
79. World Health Organization: Hepatitis C: global prevalence, *Wkly Epidem Rec* 72(46):341-344, 1997.
80. Seefe LB: Natural history of hepatitis C, *Hepatology* 26:21S, 1997.
81. Gish RG: Standards of treatment in chronic hepatitis C, *Semin Liver Dis* 19(suppl 1):35, 1999.
82. Naoumov NV et al: Presence of a newly described human DNA virus (TTV) in patients with liver disease, *Lancet* 352:195, 1998.
83. Johnson DA et al: A comparison of nebulized budesonide, intramuscular dexamethasone, and placebo for moderately severe croup, *N Engl J Med* 339:498, 1998.
84. Glezen WP et al: Risk of primary infection and reinfection with respiratory syncytial virus, *Am J Dis Child* 140:543, 1986.
85. Hall CB et al: Aerosolized ribavirin treatment of infants with respiratory syncytial viral infection, *N Engl J Med* 308:1443, 1983.
86. Simoes E: Respiratory syncytial virus infection, *Lancet* 354:847, 1999.
87. Snydman DR et al: Prevention of nosocomial transmission of respiratory syncytial virus in a newborn nursery, *Infect Control Hosp Epidemiol* 9:105, 1988.
88. Candel S: Epididymitis in mumps, including orchitis: further clinical studies and comments, *Ann Intern Med* 34:20, 1951.
89. Siegel M, Fuerst HT, Peress NS: Comparative fetal mortality in maternal virus diseases: a prospective study on rubella, measles, mumps, chickenpox and hepatitis, *N Engl J Med* 274:768, 1966.
90. Centers for Disease Control and Prevention: Measles—United States, first 26 weeks, 1994, *MMWR* 43:673, 1994.
91. Gustafson T et al: Measles outbreak in a fully immunized secondary-school population, *N Engl J Med* 316:771, 1987.
92. Fields BN, Hawkins K: Human infection with the virus of vesicular stomatitis during an epizootic, *N Engl J Med* 277:989, 1967.
93. Centers for Disease Control and Prevention: Outbreak of Ebola viral hemorrhagic fever—Zaire, 1995, *MMWR* 44:381, 1995.
94. Centers for Disease Control: Management of patients with suspected viral hemorrhagic fever, *MMWR* 37:1, 1988.
95. Dolin R et al: A controlled trial of amantadine and rimantadine in the prophylaxis of influenza A infection, *N Engl J Med* 307:580, 1982.
96. Centers for Disease Control and Prevention: La Crosse encephalitis in West Virginia, *MMWR* 37:79, 1988.
97. Chen HX et al: Epidemiological studies on hemorrhagic fever with renal syndrome in China, *J Infect Dis* 154:394, 1986.
98. Centers for Disease Control and Prevention: Hantavirus pulmonary syndrome—Northeastern United States, 1994, *MMWR* 43:54, 1994.
99. Biggar RJ et al: Lymphocytic choriomeningitis outbreak associated with pet hamsters: fifty-seven cases from New York State, *JAMA* 232:494, 1975.
100. McCormick JB et al: A case-control study of the clinical diagnosis and course of Lassa fever, *J Infect Dis* 155:445, 1987.
101. MacKenzie RB: Epidemiology of Machupo virus infection. I. Pattern of human infection, San Joaquin, Bolivia, 1962-1964, *Am J Trop Med Hyg* 14:808, 1985.
102. Huggins JW et al: Prospective, double-blind, concurrent, placebo-controlled clinical trial of intravenous ribavirin therapy of hemorrhagic fever with renal syndrome, *J Infect Dis* 164:1119, 1991.
103. Temin HM, Mizutani S: RNA-dependent DNA polymerase in virions of Rous sarcoma virus, *Nature* 226:1211, 1970.
104. Poiesz BJ et al: Detection and isolation of type C retrovirus particles from fresh and cultured lymphocytes of a patient with cutaneous T-cell lymphoma, *Proc Natl Acad Sci* (USA) 22:7415, 1980.

105. Kalyanaraman VS et al: A new subtype of human T-cell leukemia virus (HTLV-II) associated with a T-cell variant of hairy cell leukemia, *Science* 218:571, 1982.
106. Strebel PM et al: Epidemiology of poliomyelitis in the United States one decade after the last reported case of indigenous wild virus–associated disease, *Clin Infect Dis* 14:568, 1992.
107. Dalakas MC et al: A long-term follow-up study of patients with post-poliomyelitis neuromuscular symptoms, *N Engl J Med* 314:959, 1986.
108. Hull HF et al: Paralytic poliomyelitis: seasoned strategies, disappearing disease, *Lancet* 343:1331, 1994.
109. Blacklow NR, Greenberg HB: Viral gastroenteritis, *N Engl J Med* 325:252, 1991.
110. Morse DL et al: Widespread outbreaks of clam and oyster associated gastroenteritis: role of Norwalk virus, *N Engl J Med* 314:678, 1986.
111. Prusiner SB: Molecular biology of prion disease, *Science* 252:1515, 1991.
112. Johnson RT: Prion disease, *N Engl J Med* 326:486, 1992.
113. Tan L et al: Risk of transmission of bovine spongiform encephalopathy to humans in the United States: a report of the Council on Scientific Affairs. American Medical Association, *JAMA* 281:342, 1999.
114. Gajdusek DC: Unconventional viruses and the origin and disappearance of kuru, *Science* 197:943, 1977.

SUGGESTED READINGS

Fields BN et al, editors: *Fields virology,* ed 3, Philadelphia, 1996, Lippincott-Raven.
Mandell GL, Bennett JE, Dolin R, editors: *Principles and practice of infectious diseases,* ed 5, New York, 2000, Churchill Livingstone.
Richman DD, Whitley RJ, Hayden FG, editors: *Clinical virology,* New York, 1997, Churchill Livingstone.

125 Rabies

Ellen J. Weber

Rabies is probably the oldest infection known to man. The term *rabies* comes from the Sanskrit "rabhas," which means "to do violence." The Eshmuna Code of Babylon, from the twenty-third century BC, contains one of the earliest regulations regarding rabies: a fine of 40 shekels was issued to the owner of a dog that killed another man through a rabid bite.[1,2]

Today, rabies is a huge public health problem in the Third World; it is estimated that 35,000 to 60,000 people die from the disease each year.[3,4] In the United States, human rabies is extremely rare; on average, two cases per year are reported. This is the result of a successful vaccination program for domestic animals that began in 1947; before that time, there were 40 human cases a year.[5]

EPIDEMIOLOGY

Worldwide, dogs are the most commonly infected animal and cause more transmission of rabies to humans than any other species. Dogs are the primary reservoir of rabies in Asia, Mexico, and many developing countries of Africa and Latin America.[3] In the United States more than 90% of all rabies occurs in wild animals; the principal reservoirs are raccoons, skunks, foxes, and bats.[6] In Europe, Canada, and the Arctic and sub-Arctic regions, the principal carrier is the fox, and in Puerto Rico, the mongoose. Jackals are the main wildlife reservoir of rabies in Africa.

In the United States, rabies in terrestrial animals occurs in discrete geographic regions where the virus is primarily transmitted among members of a single species (Figure 125-1). Each species and location is associated with a distinctive variant of the rabies virus. Along the Eastern seaboard, rabies is endemic in raccoons, which carry a unique strain of the rabies virus; a different strain of virus is carried by skunks in the North Central states, yet another by the skunks in the South Central states, and another viral strain is carried by the rabid skunks endemic to California. Arctic and red foxes in Alaska carry another rabies variant; as a result of their migration across Canada, the same rabies virus variant is found in the red foxes of New England. Two additional gray fox reservoirs with unique rabies virus variants are in Arizona and in Texas. Finally, there is a unique rabies virus strain associated with the dogs and coyotes of Southern Texas, the result of a long-standing interaction between unvaccinated dogs and coyotes at the Texas-Mexico border. Rabid animals outside the United States also carry unique variants of rabies virus associated with their species and location.

In all of these areas, other wild carnivores or domestic animals may become infected by contact with the endemic species and will carry the viral variant of the endemic species (spillover). The increase in skunk rabies in New England is largely attributable to the raccoon epizootic that has occurred there, although some of the skunk rabies has resulted from spillover from foxes. Using monoclonal antibody characterization, rabies virus isolates from skunks in that area have been shown to be of raccoon or fox origin.[6,7]

Rabid bats account for 14% of all cases of rabies in animals.[6] They are ubiquitous throughout the United States and North America, and different species of bats carry distinct viral variants (Figure 125-2). Rabid bats are capable of infecting terrestrial animals in any area of the country, as well as humans. Thus the only state in the United States that remains rabies-free is Hawaii, where there are no rabid bats or rabid terrestrial animals.[6]

The association of a unique rabies virus variant with a particular species and locale makes it possible to determine the source of rabies in areas or species that were previously rabies-free.[8] Additionally, antigenic typing permits identification of the source of human infections when the animal contact is unknown.[9]

Wild and Domestic Animal Rabies

Since the 1950s, rabies in U.S. domestic animals has significantly decreased, but the population of wild animals

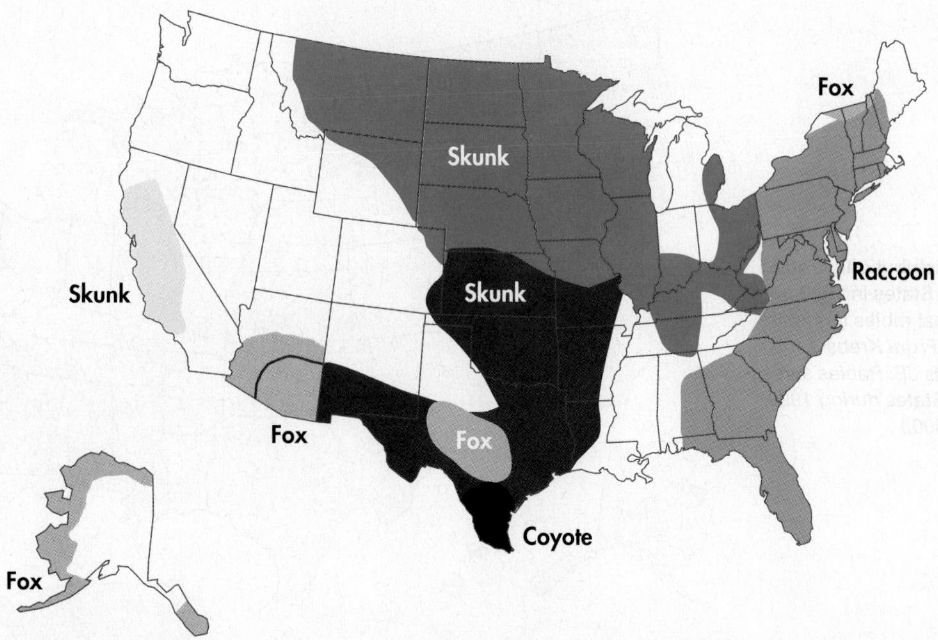

Figure 125-1. **Distribution of antigenically distinct rabies viruses and their predominant terrestrial wildlife species in the United States.** ***Krebs J, Rupprecht CE, Childs JE: Rabies surveillance in the United States during 1999, JAVMA 217:1799, 2000.***

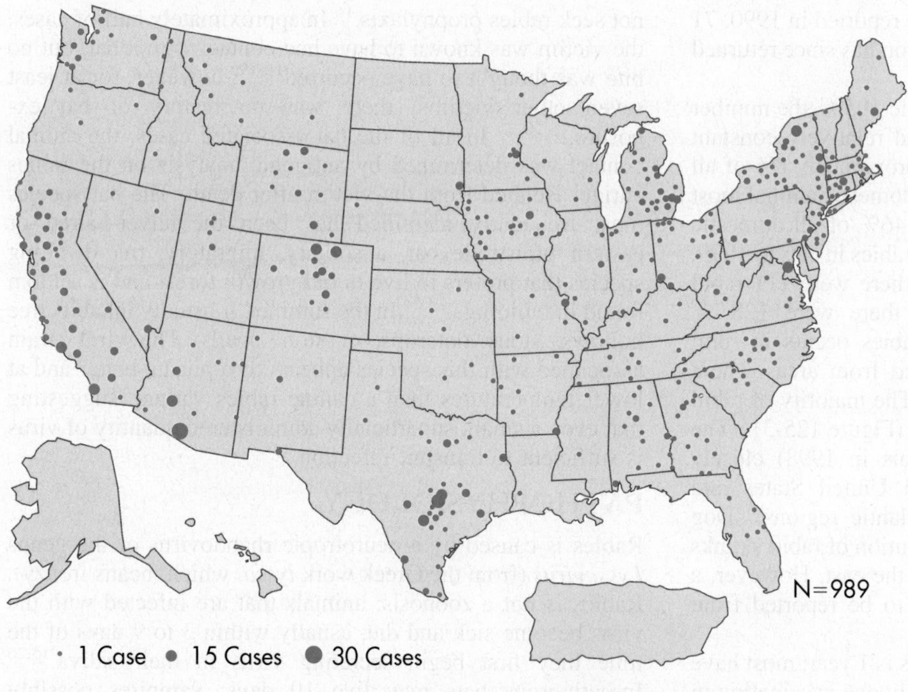

Figure 125-2. **Rabid bats have been identified in all states except Hawaii.** ***Krebs J, Rupprecht CE, Childs JE: Rabies surveillance in the United States during 1999, JVMA 217:1799, 2000.***

has actually increased. In 1999 the total wild animal population was 7067 compared with 4742 cases in 1988.[6,10] In the 1960s and 1970s, the majority of wildlife rabies was found in skunks in the United States. However, in the late 1970s, an epizootic among raccoons began in the mid-Atlantic states and spread north and south to cover the entire Eastern seaboard; now the majority of wildlife rabies in the United States is attributable to raccoons. The source of this epizootic appears to be the inadvertent translocation of rabid raccoons from the southeastern states to the mid-Atlantic region to stock the area for hunting. This determination was based on the fact that the raccoons first seen in the mid-Atlantic states, and now along the entire east coast, carry the same antigenic variant as those in the southeastern states.[6,11] Although the total number of rabid raccoons appears to have peaked, the population continues to spread geographically north and westward. The epizootic reached Maine in 1994 and Ohio in 1996.[12] The first rabid raccoon in

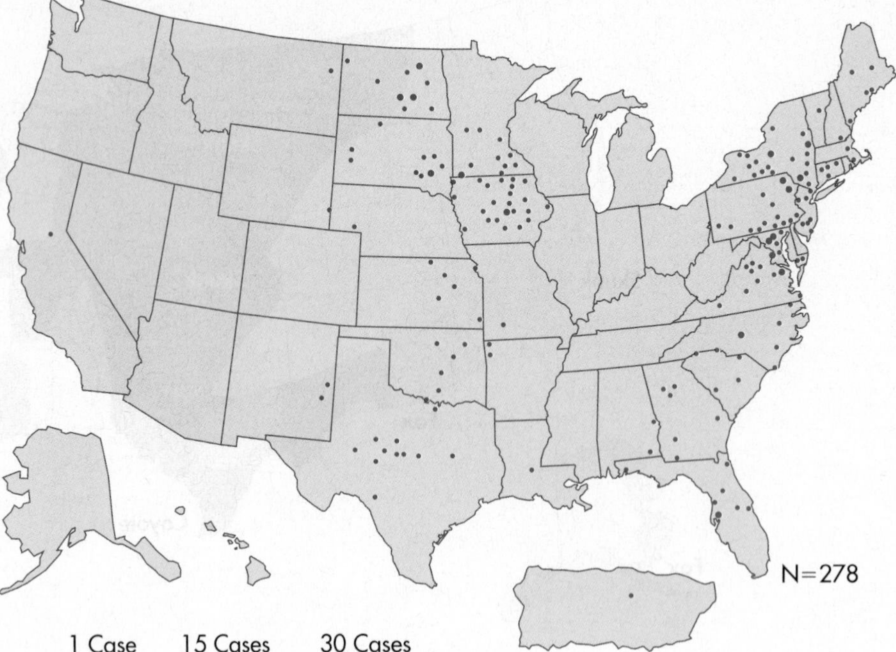

Figure 125-3. **The distribution of rabies in cats in the United States in 1999 parallels that of wild animal rabies (compare with Figure 125-1).** *From Krebs J, Rupprecht CE, Childs JE: Rabies surveillance in the United States during 1999, JAVMA 217:1799, 2000.)*

Canada was found in Ontario in July 1999.[6] A smaller epizootic of coyotes began in the early 1990s in southern Texas; whereas three rabid coyotes were reported in 1990, 71 were found in 1993,[13,14] but the population has since returned to low levels.[6]

Having declined dramatically since the 1950s, the number of rabid domestic animals has remained relatively constant for the last decade and accounts for approximately 8% of all rabies in the United States. Cats are the domestic animal most frequently reported rabid, representing 46% of all domestic animal rabies.[6] There were 278 cases of rabies in cats in 1999, compared with 192 in 1988. In 1999, there were 111 rabid dogs in the United States; in 1988, there were 128.[6,10] Approximately 80% of cat and dog rabies occurs in rural areas, and almost all cases are reported from areas where rabies is enzootic in wildlife species.[15] The majority of rabid cats are found in the mid-Atlantic states (Figure 125-3).[6] The distribution of rabid cattle (116 animals in 1998) closely follows that of skunks in the central United States and raccoons in the Northeast and mid-Atlantic regions.[6] Dog rabies also appears to parallel the distribution of rabid skunks in the central states and of raccoons in the east. However, a large number of rabid dogs continues to be reported from Texas.[6]

The median age of rabid cats and dogs is 1 year; most have not been vaccinated or have received only one vaccination in their lifetime.[15] Rabid dogs are usually pets, whereas rabid cats are more likely to be strays. Most owners are unaware of their pets' exposure to wild animals that may carry rabies.

Rabies in Humans

Human cases of rabies in the United States remain infrequent. Between 1990 and 2000, 31 cases of human rabies were diagnosed in the United States and 25 of these cases are presumed to have been acquired in the United States.[6] Twenty-three of these cases were associated with bats, whereas only two were associated with the dog and coyote populations of Texas. In two or three cases of bat-acquired rabies was a bite known to have occurred, and the victim did not seek rabies prophylaxis.[16] In approximately half of cases, the victim was known to have had contact with a bat, but no bite was thought to have occurred[16-19]; however, for at least seven other victims, there was no history of bat exposure.[16,20-22] In all of the bat-associated cases, the animal contact was determined by antigenic analysis on the rabies variant isolated from the victim after death. The bat species most frequently identified has been the silver-haired or eastern pipistrelle bat, a solitary, migratory, tree-dwelling species that prefers to live in old growth forest and is seldom found in buildings.[23,24] In the summer, it usually inhabits tree hollows, stony outcrops, or stone walls. The viral strain associated with this species appears to replicate better and at lower temperatures than a canine rabies variant, suggesting that even a small, superficially administered quantity of virus is sufficient to transmit infection.[25]

PATHOPHYSIOLOGY

Rabies is caused by a neurotropic rhabdovirus of the genus *Lyssavirus* (from the Greek work *lyssa,* which means frenzy). Rabies is not a zoonosis; animals that are infected with the virus become sick and die, usually within 3 to 9 days of the time they first begin secreting virus in their saliva.[15,26] Insectivorous bats may live 10 days; vampires possibly longer.[27,28] There has been some suggestion that dogs can become asymptomatic carriers, but transmission of disease from such an animal to humans has never been documented.[9,29,30] A survey of rabid dogs in the United States in 1988 found that all died within 8 days of becoming ill; the median time until death was 3 days.[15]

Animals are capable of transmitting rabies once they start secreting virus in saliva. Most animals with rabies will be sick before excretion of virus but some may not become ill for several days after virus can be found in their saliva.[26] The classic picture of a mangy dog foaming at the mouth and wildly running through town is not often seen; clinical signs are invariably present but frequently more subtle. Indeed, less than half of cases of rabies in domestic animals are initially recognized by veterinarians.[15] The animal may display aggressive behavior, ataxia, irritability, anorexia, lethargy, or excessive salivation; cats are more likely to demonstrate aggressive or irritable behavior than dogs. In a wild animal, however, what may be most apparent is a change in instinctive behavior: for instance, a nocturnal animal boldly walking through downtown in broad daylight.[31] An unprovoked bite from a domestic animal may be a sign of rabies; however, humans—especially children—often inadvertently provoke a pet by cornering it or competing with it for its natural prey.

Rabies is transmitted when the virus is introduced into bite wounds or open cuts in skin or onto mucous membranes.[16] Almost all documented cases of rabies have been transmitted by a bite. The risk of transmission by a bite is about 50 times that of a scratch[32]; however, one dog owner contracted rabies after his Doberman scratched him on the lip.[33] Rabies has also been contracted by recipients of corneal transplants from infected donors and people who were exposed to bat aerosol in a cave or aerosolized rabies virus in a laboratory.[5,34] Experimentally, rabies has been transmitted by aerosol, by virus in contact with open wounds or mucous membranes, and by ingestion of virus.[5,34] In wild animals, rabies may be transmitted transplacentally.[34] Other than through corneal transplants, human-to-human transmission has never been confirmed, although two possible cases in family members of rabies victims in Ethiopia that were not laboratory-confirmed have been described.[35] Rabies virus has never been isolated from blood.

The virus replicates in muscle cells near the site of the bite, then ascends to the central nervous system along peripheral nerves, traveling at a rate of 8 to 20 mm per day.[11] The incubation period from bite to disease in humans ranges from 30 to 90 days. Although claims of incubation periods as long as 19 years exist, antigenic analysis has now confirmed latency periods of up to 7 years.[9] The risk of developing rabies after a bite ranges from 5% to 80%; the biting animal, the severity of the exposure, and the location of the bite all contribute to the ultimate mortality in unvaccinated victims.[32,36] Bites on the head and neck have a shorter incubation period (as short as 15 days) than those on the trunk or lower extremity, most likely because of the rich peripheral nerve supply in the head and neck area.[28] Mortality is lower in victims with lower-extremity bites.[36,37]

CLINICAL FEATURES

The prodrome of the disease in humans is nonspecific and is usually misdiagnosed in areas where human rabies is rare.[38] Patients may present with headache, fever, runny nose, sore throat, myalgias, and gastrointestinal symptoms. Back pain and spasms are frequent.[39-41] Agitation and anxiety may result in a diagnosis of psychosis or drug intoxication.[39,40,42] Paresthesias or pain at the bite site may be the first neurologic symptom and progress to what appears to be a polyradiculitis until the encephalitis occurs.[38]

Full-blown rabies occurs in two forms: the "furious" or encephalitic form is manifested by agitation, hydrophobia, and extreme irritability; the hydrophobia, so named because of patients' inability to swallow, appears to result from an exaggerated respiratory tract protective reflex that results in a violent, jerky contraction of the diaphragm and accessory muscles of inspiration when the patient attempts to swallow liquids.[38] Overwhelming terror accompanies the phenomenon and may generalize to the sight of water or having water touch the face.[11] The less common paralytic or "dumb" form of rabies resembles Guillain-Barré syndrome; consciousness is initially spared. The two forms can overlap or progress from one to the other. Ultimately, coma and death occur.

MANAGEMENT

Once manifested, rabies is usually fatal within 3 to 10 days; with intensive care unit support, survival times are as long as 4 months, but the outcome remains dismal.[5,38] No specific or effective rabies treatment currently exists; pooled human rabies immune globulin given intrathecally, ribavirin, and interferon have all been administered after onset of symptoms without success.[5,11,27,38,43] Only three patients are known to have survived clinical rabies; all had received some form of preexposure or postexposure prophylaxis.[5]

POSTEXPOSURE PROPHYLAXIS ASSESSMENT

Despite the fact that human rabies is extremely rare in the United States, from 20,000 to 40,000 people a year receive postexposure prophylaxis (PEP), at a cost of about $1600 per series.[44] From 30% to 60% of these treatments are probably inappropriate. In 60% of cases, the animal is not rabid.[45] Thus it is imperative that practitioners understand the indications for prophylaxis and recommended treatment measures. The clinical scenario should be discussed with public health officials; such consultations are estimated to reduce unnecessary prophylaxis fivefold.[45] Local or state agencies should be contacted first because they are most familiar with the animals in the area. If immediate consultation is required and local agencies are unavailable, emergency physicians can call the Division of Viral and Rickettsial Diseases at the Centers for Disease Control and Prevention (CDC) at 404-639-1050 during business hours and at 404-639-2888 on nights, weekends, and holidays.[16]

The decision about whether to begin postexposure prophylaxis after a bite depends on a number of factors: the type of exposure, the location of the incident, and the biting animal (Table 125-1). Treatment decisions may be modified if the animal is available for testing or observation.

Exposure

Bites are considered significant exposures; nonbite exposures that involve contamination of either a mucous membrane or an open wound (one that has bled within 24 hours) with saliva may also require prophylaxis. Petting a rabid animal and contact with its blood, urine, or feces are not considered exposures.[16] Skunk spray does not require prophylaxis. Dry virus is not infectious.

Biting Animal

In the United States, high-risk animals are raccoons, skunks, foxes, bats, and coyotes. Dogs along the U.S.-Mexico border and those in developing countries are also high risk. Wild carnivores in areas where rabies is endemic may be infected with rabies; the risk of transmission of rabies to humans from the bites of these animals is about 10 times lower than the risk from the predominant reservoir but high enough to warrant prophylaxis.[32] Therefore bites of high-risk animals, or of

Table 125-1. Guidelines for Determining Need for Rabies Prophylaxis

Animal type	Evaluation and disposition of animal	Postexposure prophylaxis recommendations
Dogs, cats, and ferrets	Healthy and available for 10 days observation	Persons should not begin prophylaxis unless animal develops clinical signs of rabies*
	Rabid or suspected rabid	Immediately vaccinate
	Unknown (e.g., escaped)	Consult public health officials
Skunks, raccoons, foxes, and most other carnivores; bats	Regarded as rabid unless animal proven negative by laboratory tests†	Consider immediate vaccination
Livestock, small rodents, lagomorphs (rabbits and hares), large rodents (woodchucks and beavers), and other mammals	Consider individually	Consult public health officials Bites of squirrels, hamsters, guinea pigs, gerbils, chipmunks, rats, mice, other small rodents, rabbits, and hares almost never require antirabies postexposure prophylaxis

From CDC: Human rabies prevention—United States, 1999: recommendations of the Advisory Committee on Immunization Practices (ACIP), *MMWR* 48:1, 1999.

Note: For consultation, contact local health officials; if unavailable, call the Division of Viral and Rickettsial Diseases at the Centers for Disease Control at 404-639-1050 during business hours; 404-639-2888 nights, weekends and holidays.

*During the 10-day observation period, begin postexposure prophylaxis at the first sign of rabies in a dog, cat, or ferret that has bitten someone. If the animal exhibits clinical signs of rabies, it should be euthanized immediately and tested.

†The animal should be euthanized and tested as soon as possible. Holding for observation is not recommended. Discontinue vaccine if immunofluorescence test results of the animal are negative.

other wild carnivores in areas where rabies is endemic, require prophylaxis. Significant nonbite exposures to these animals should also be treated. Treatment should be started immediately. If a high-risk animal is caught, it should be euthanized and tested immediately, regardless of whether it appears ill. Postexposure prophylaxis for the victim may be discontinued if the animal is proven not to be rabid.

Transmission of rabies from bats appears to have occurred from seemingly unimportant or unrecognized bites. As a result, the threshold for treating bat exposures is exceedingly low. The CDC recommends that "... postexposure prophylaxis should be considered when direct contact between a human and a bat has occurred, unless the exposed person can be certain bite, scratch or mucous membrane exposure did not occur."[16] Postexposure prophylaxis is recommended when a bat is found indoors in the same room as a person who might be unaware that a bite or direct contact had occurred (such as a sleeping individual, an unattended child, or a mentally disabled person) and rabies cannot be ruled out by testing the bat. Prophylaxis would not be recommended for other household members unless contact with the bat had occurred.

Small rodents (squirrels, gophers, rats, chipmunks, and guinea pigs) and lagomorphs (rabbits and hares) are very unlikely to carry rabies and thus are low risk. However, in areas where raccoon rabies is endemic, groundhogs (woodchucks) have been found to be rabid in significant numbers. Woodchucks accounted for 93% of the 371 cases of rabies in rodents reported to the CDC between 1990 and 1996 and 40 of the 45 cases among rodents and lagomorphs in 1999.[6,16] Current recommendations are to consult state or local health departments before initiating PEP for cases involving rodents.[16] Bites from rodents outside the United States should receive prophylaxis.

Bites from livestock should be considered individually, and public health officials should be consulted.[16]

Domestic animals, and particularly urban cats and dogs, in the United States are generally low risk, with the exception of dogs at the U.S.-Mexico border. However, domestic animals in endemic areas may be at somewhat higher risk. Domestic animals (dogs, cats, and ferrets) should be observed for 10 days, and PEP should be withheld unless the animal becomes ill. In nonendemic areas, PEP is usually withheld even if the animal is not available. Rabies has rarely been diagnosed in vaccinated domestic animals; this phenomenon appears to be restricted to animals that had received only one vaccination in their lifetime.[15,46] Bites from dogs in developing countries should always be considered high risk, and prophylaxis should be given without waiting for test results.[47]

Biting Incident

Animals who are behaving oddly, or who bite without provocation, have a higher risk of carrying rabies. However, the circumstances of the bite should be taken into consideration only when evaluating a bite from an otherwise low-risk animal, such as a dog or cat.

Animal in Captivity

Wild animals that have been caught should be sacrificed immediately and the head sent under refrigeration to an appropriate laboratory for rabies fluorescent antibody testing. Unless the risk of transmission is low, the victim should begin prophylaxis, which may be discontinued when the results of the test are known. Domestic animals in the United States that are apparently healthy should be observed for 10 days; if the animal does not become ill, the victim does not require treatment. If the animal appears sick, is stray or unwanted, or the exposure was particularly severe—such as a bite to the face or neck—it should be sacrificed and tested immediately and the victim treated accordingly.[48,49]

POSTEXPOSURE PROPHYLAXIS

Prophylaxis consists of three steps: wound care, passive immunization, and active immunization. No step in this treatment should be omitted. When prophylaxis appears to be indicated, treatment should be begun immediately.[16] Discussions with local public health officials will decrease unnecessary treatment, and advice is available from either state health officials or the CDC 24 hours a day. It is not known whether, or for how long, it is safe to delay treatment, nor is this recommended.[50] On the other hand, if prophylaxis is indicated, it should be administered regardless of the length of the delay because evidence exists that the incubation period of rabies can be more than a year.

Wound Care

Rabies is easily killed by sunlight, soap, or drying. Experimental studies have shown that scrubbing and flushing the wound with benzalkonium chloride, 20% soap solution, or Ivory soap was nearly 100% protective when performed within 3 hours of inoculation of virus.[51] Povidone-iodine, which is virucidal, has not been tested. Although wound care should never be relied on as the only preventive measure, it is an *essential* part of postexposure rabies prevention, especially because there have been rare cases in which a patient developed rabies despite what was thought to be appropriate immunoprophylaxis. Furthermore, wound treatment may be the only prevention available for a victim out in the wild who is days or weeks away from medical care.

Current CDC recommendations for wounds in which rabies transmission is of concern are immediate and thorough washing with soap and water and a virucidal agent such as povidone-iodine (Box 125-1).[16] Wounds should be scrubbed or swabbed, not simply flushed.[52] After treatment, the wound should be thoroughly rinsed with water or saline.

Box 125-1 Rabies Wound Treatment

Early treatment essential (less than 3 hours)
Scrub wound and edges with soap and water
If puncture, swab deeply in wound and around edges
Follow with virucidal agent:
1% or 2% benzalkonium chloride
or
povidone-iodine*

*Povidone-iodine never tested but recommended by CDC.

Immunoprophylaxis

Rabies immunoprophylaxis requires both passive immunization with antibody (immune globulin) and active immunization with vaccine (Box 125-2). It is essential that both parts of this treatment be given, even when treatment is delayed. Human rabies immune globulin (HRIG) 20 IU/kg should be administered as soon after the bite as possible. If anatomically feasible, the entire dose of HRIG should be infiltrated into and around the wound(s); any remaining volume should be injected intramuscularly at a site distant from the vaccine.[16]

Human diploid cell vaccine (HDCV) is the vaccine most widely available in the United States. The first dose should be administered on the day of the bite; four subsequent injections are required. The vaccine should be administered in the deltoid, rather than the gluteal, region to avoid accidental administration into fat, which will prevent antibody formation.[43,53] HRIG and HDCV should be given in different anatomical sites and never mixed in the same syringe. All known treatment failures that have occurred since 1980 have resulted from a deviation from the recommended regimen. Patients either did not have their wounds cleansed with soap and water, did not receive rabies vaccine in the deltoid area, or did not receive RIG at the wound site.[16,43,47,53]

Local reactions (itching, erythema, pain, or swelling) occur in 30% to 74% of PEP recipients; systemic reactions including headache, myalgia, and nausea occur in 5% to 40% of recipients, usually those who receive frequent vaccine boosters.[16] Anaphylaxis has occurred in 0.1% of cases; three cases of Guillain-Barré syndrome have occurred after millions of doses given.[16,54] An immune-complex type of reaction involving urticaria, arthralgia, arthritis, angioedema, nausea, and vomiting occurs in about 6% of patients who receive boosters of HDCV; it is uncommon in those receiving primary vaccination.[16] Two alternative vaccines, rabies vaccine adsorbed (RVA) and purified chick embryo culture (PCEC) vaccine, are also available. Both appear to be associated with fewer hypersensitivity reactions in patients receiving boosters.[24,55] Although HDCV may be administered intradermally for preexposure prophylaxis, neither RVA nor PCEC vaccine is approved for intradermal use.

Box 125-2 Rabies Immunoprophylaxis

Human Rabies Immune Globulin (HRIG) 20 IU/kg
If anatomically feasible, infiltrate full dose into and around wound; remainder given intramuscularly
and
Human Diploid Cell Vaccine (HDCV) 1 ml IM (deltoid) days 0, 3, 7, 14, 28
If previously vaccinated, do not give HRIG; give HDCF 1 ml IMM days 0 and 3

Patients requiring rabies immunoprophylaxis when outside the United States may receive a different regimen and different vaccines than those used in the United States. Some countries still use vaccines derived from nerve tissue. The World Health Organization (WHO) has approved a variety of treatment regimens that reduce cost, including those that administer rabies immune globulin only in severe bites or use fewer vaccine doses.[24,47] These abbreviated regimens are not approved in the United States.[32] Some countries, such as Thailand, use an intradermal route for postexposure prophylaxis; the WHO cautions that such injections should be administered only by staff who have been trained in this technique.[24] Thus bite victims traveling abroad may require additional treatment when they return to the United States. Public health officials should be contacted for advice.

Prophylaxis, including both passive and active immunization, given during pregnancy does not result in an increase in fetal wastage, congenital defects, or side effects.[56] and should not be withheld when indicated. Corticosteroids, antimalarials, and other immunosuppressives can interfere with the development of active immunity and should be withheld during the course of treatment if possible. Otherwise, rabies antibody response should be checked.[16] Similarly, patients with immunosuppressive illnesses should be monitored for antibody response.[16,47] Patients with histories of hypersensitivity should nevertheless be cautiously given

Table 125-2. Rabies Preexposure Prophylaxis Guide

Risk category	Nature of risk	Typical populations	Preexposure recommendations
Continuous	Virus present continuously, often in high concentrations Specific exposures likely to go unrecognized Bite, nonbite, or aerosol exposure	Rabies research laboratory workers;* rabies biologics production workers	Primary course Serologic testing every 6 months; booster vaccination if antibody titer is below acceptable level†
Frequent	Exposure usually episodic, with source recognized, but exposure also might be unrecognized Bite, nonbite, or aerosol exposure	Rabies diagnostic laboratory workers,* spelunkers, veterinarians and staff, and animal-control and wildlife workers in rabies-enzootic areas	Primary course Serologic testing every 2 years; booster vaccination if antibody titer is below acceptable level†
Infrequent (greater than population at large)	Exposure nearly always episodic with source recognized Bite or nonbite exposure	Veterinarians and animal-control and wildlife workers in areas with low rabies rates Veterinary students Travelers visiting areas where rabies is enzootic and immediate access to appropriate medical care including biologics is limited	Primary course No serologic test or booster vaccination
Rare (population at large)	Exposure always episodic with source recognized Bite or nonbite exposure	U.S. population at large, including persons in rabies-epizootic areas	No vaccination necessary

From CDC: Human rabies prevention—United States, 1999: recommendations of the Advisory Committee on Immunization Practices (ACIP). *MMWR* 48:1, 1999.
*Judgment of relative risk and extra monitoring of vaccination status of laboratory workers are the responsibilities of the laboratory supervisor.
†Minimum acceptable antibody level is complete virus neutralization at a 1:5 serum dilution by the rapid fluorescent focus inhibition test. A booster dose should be administered if the titer falls below this level.

immunoprophylaxis in a controlled setting, with antihistamines and epinephrine available.[16] Rabies developed in a patient who was sensitive to equine antirabies immune globulin and was not given passive immunization.[33]

PREEXPOSURE PROPHYLAXIS

For people with frequent exposures to rabies, preexposure prophylaxis may be indicated.[16] These people include laboratory personnel working with live rabies virus, veterinarians, animal handlers, and those spending long periods in countries in which rabies is endemic and medical care difficult to obtain (Table 125-2). Preexposure prophylaxis guarantees protection for individuals who have continuous and inapparent exposures (i.e., lab workers); it also allows protection when postexposure therapy may be delayed (e.g., in remote areas). After an exposure, patients who have had preexposure prophylaxis do not require HRIG; vaccine is only given on days 0 and 3 (see Box 125-2).

KEY CONCEPTS

- The epidemiology of rabies in the United States has undergone a major evolution, with the primary source of this disease now in wild animals rather than in domestic animals.
- Despite an increase in the numbers of terrestrial wild animals with rabies, the predominant threat to humans in the United States appears to be contact with bats.
- PEP is indicated for victims of bites or significant nonbite exposures from wild carnivores in endemic areas and bat contact where a bite cannot be ruled out or the bat cannot be tested. In most cases in the United States, domestic animals should be observed before starting PEP.
- Discussion with public health officials is highly recommended to guide decisions about PEP and reduce the number of unnecessary treatments.
- PEP involves three important components: local wound care with soap and water and a virucidal agent, passive immunization with rabies immune globulin, and active immunization with vaccine. The regimen should be adhered to precisely because treatment failures have occurred when it was not followed.

REFERENCES

1. Fisher DJ: Resurgence of rabies: a historical perspective on rabies in children, *Arch Pediatr Adolesc Med* 149:306, 1995.
2. Koprowski H: Visit to an ancient curse, *Sci Am* May/June:48, 1995.
3. Chomel BB: The modern epidemiological aspects of rabies in the world, *Comp Immunol Microbiol Infect Dis* 16:11, 1993.
4. Haupt W: Rabies—risk of exposure and current trends in prevention of human cases, *Vaccine* 17:1742, 1999.
5. Anderson L, Nicholson K, Tauxe R: Human rabies in the U.S., 1960-79, *Ann Int Med* 100:728, 1984.
6. Krebs J, Rupprecht CE, Childs JE: Rabies surveillance in the United States during 1999, *JAVMA* 217:1799, 2000.
7. Krebs JW, Strine TW, Childs JE: Rabies surveillance in the United States during 1992 [published erratum appears in *JAVMA* 204:423, 1994], *JAVMA* 203:1718, 1993.
8. Translocation of coyote rabies—Florida, 1994, *MMWR* 44:580, 587, 1995.

9. Smith JS et al: Unexplained rabies in three immigrants in the United States: a virologic investigation, *N Engl J Med* 324:205, 1991.
10. Eng TR et al: Rabies surveillance, United States, 1988, *MMWR CDC Surveill Summ* 38:1, 1989.
11. Case records of the Massachusetts General Hospital. Weekly clinicopathological exercises. Case 21-1998. A 32-year-old woman with pharyngeal spasms and paresthesias after a dog bite [clinical conference], *N Engl J Med* 339:105, 1998.
12. Centers for Disease Control and Prevention: Update: raccoon rabies epizootic—United Sates, 1996, *MMWR* 45:1117, 1997.
13. Reid-Sanden F et al: Rabies surveillance in the United States during 1989, *JAVMA* 197:1571, 1990.
14. Krebs J et al: Rabies surveillance in the United States during 1993, *JAVMA* 205:1695, 1994.
15. Eng T, Fishbein D: Epidemiologic factors, clinical findings, and vaccination status of rabies in cats and dogs in the United States in 1988: National Study Group on Rabies, *JAVMA* 197:201, 1990.
16. Human rabies prevention—United States, 1999. Recommendations of the Advisory Committee on Immunization Practices (ACIP), *MMWR* 48:1, 1999.
17. Centers for Disease Control and Prevention: Human Rabies—Washington, *MMWR* 44:625, 1995.
18. Centers for Disease Control and Prevention: Human Rabies—Texas and New Jersey, 1997, *MMWR* 46:1, 1998.
19. Centers for Disease Control and Prevention: Human Rabies—California, 1995, *MMWR,* 1996.
20. Centers for Disease Control and Prevention: Human rabies—Montana and Washington, 1997, *MMWR* 46:770, 1997.
21. Centers for Disease Control and Prevention: Human rabies—California, *MMWR* 43:455, 1994.
22. Centers for Disease Control and Prevention: Human rabies—New York, 1993, *MMWR* 42:799, 1994.
23. Centers for Disease Control and Prevention: Human Rabies—Connecticut, 1995, *MMWR* 45:207, 1996.
24. Dreesen DW: A global review of rabies vaccines for human use, *Vaccine* 15 Suppl:S2, 1997.
25. Fu ZF: Rabies and rabies research: past, present and future, *Vaccine* 15 Suppl:S20, 1997.
26. Sikes E: Pathogenesis of rabies in wildlife. 1. Comparative effect of varying doses of rabies virus inoculated into foxes and skunks, *Am J Vet Res* 23:1041, 1962.
27. Roine R et al: Fatal encephalitis caused by a bat-borne rabies-related virus: clinical findings, *Brain* 111:1505, 1988.
28. Sikes R: Rabies. In Hubbert W, McCulloch W, Schnurrenberger P, editors: *Diseases transmitted from animals to man,* ed 6, Springfield, Ill, 1975, Charles C Thomas.
29. Fishbein DB: Latent rabies (letter), *N Engl J Med* 324:1891, 1991.
30. Hemachudha T et al: Latent rabies (letter), *N Engl J Med* 324:1890, 1991.
31. Marin Co: *Thirteenth rabid animal incident of the year,* County of Marin, Calif, 1986.
32. Fishbein D, Robinson L: Rabies, *N Engl J Med* 329:1632, 1993.
33. Udwadia Z, Udwadia F, Katrak S: Human rabies: clinical features, diagnosis, complications, and management, *Crit Care Med* 17:834, 1989.
34. Afshar A: A review of non-bite transmission of rabies virus infection, *Br Vet J* 135:142, 1979.
35. Fekadu M et al: Possible human-to-human transmission of rabies in Ethiopia, *Ethiop Med J* 34:123, 1996.
36. Baer G: Animal models in the pathogenesis and treatment of rabies, *Rev Inf Dis* 10:S739, 1988.
37. Shah U, Jaswal G: Victims of a rabid wolf in India: effect of severity and location of bites on development of rabies, *J Infect Dis* 134:25, 1976.
38. Warrell D, Warrell M: Human rabies and its prevention: an overview, *Rev Infect Dis* 10:S726, 1988.
39. Centers for Disease Control and Prevention: Human rabies—California, 1987, *MMWR* 37:305, 1988.
40. Centers for Disease Control and Prevention: Human rabies—West Virginia, 1994, *MMWR* 44:86, 1995.
41. Centers for Disease Control and Prevention: Human rabies—Miami 1994, *MMWR* 43:773, 1994.
42. Centers for Disease Control and Prevention: Human rabies—Texas and California, 1993, *MMWR* 43:93, 1994.
43. Shill M, Baynes R, Miller S: Fatal rabies encephalitis despite appropriate post-exposure prophylaxis, *N Engl J Med* 316:1257, 1987.
44. Krebs JW, Long-Marin SC, Childs JE: Causes, costs, and estimates of rabies postexposure prophylaxis treatments in the United States, *J Public Health Manag Pract* 4:56, 1998.
45. Helmick C: The epidemiology of human rabies postexposure prophylaxis, 1980-1981, *JAMA* 250:1990, 1983.
46. Kappus K: Canine rabies in the U.S. 1971-73: a study of reported cases with reference to vaccination history, *Am J Epidem* 103:242, 1976.
47. Wilde H et al: Failure of rabies postexposure treatment in Thailand, *Vaccine* 7:49, 1989.
48. Centers for Disease Control and Prevention: Rabies Prevention—United States, 1991, *MMWR* 40, RR-3:1, 1991.
49. Fishbein D, Baer G: Animal rabies: implications for diagnosis and human treatment, *Ann Int Med* 109:935, 1988.
50. McQuiston J: Personal communication, April, 2000.
51. Dean D, Baer G, Thompson W: Studies on the local treatment of rabies-infected wounds, *Bull WHO* 28:477, 1963.
52. Kaplan M, Cohen D, Koprowski H: Studies on local treatment of wounds for the prevention of rabies, *Bull WHO* 26:765, 1962.
53. Lumbiganon P, Bunyahotra V, Pairojkul C: Human rabies despite treatment with rabies immune globulin and human diploid cell rabies vaccine—Thailand, *JAMA* 259:25, 1988.
54. Knittel T et al: Guillain-Barré syndrome and human diploid cell vaccine (letter), *Lancet* 1334, 1989.
55. Centers for Disease Control: Rabies vaccine, adsorbed: a new rabies vaccine for use in humans, *MMWR* 37:217, 1988.
56. Chutivongse S et al: Postexposure rabies vaccination during pregnancy: effect on 202 women and their infants, *Clin Infect Dis* 20:818, 1995.

126 AIDS and HIV

Richard E. Rothman
Catherine A. Marco
Gabor D. Kelen

PERSPECTIVE

History

The first cases of AIDS came to light in 1981, when reports of Kaposi's sarcoma (KS) and *Pneumocystis carinii* pneumonia (PCP) in previously healthy homosexual men appeared in the literature. Shortly thereafter, it was recognized that these patients shared the common characteristic of a defect in cell-mediated immunity, leading to naming the clinical disease acquired immunodeficiency syndrome, or AIDS. In 1983, an RNA retrovirus coined human immunodeficiency virus, or HIV, was identified as the causative agent for the syndrome. The development of an antibody assay in 1985 permitted serologic diagnosis, allowing researchers to track the HIV epidemic and identify the principal modes and risk factors for disease transmission.

Epidemiology

Most epidemiologic data regarding HIV infection are derived from patients who meet the definition of AIDS, which is a reportable disease in all states. The most up-to-date definition of AIDS, published in 1993 by the Centers for Disease Control and Prevention (CDC), is shown in Box 126-1.[1] Case definitions include either the presence of one or more AIDS-indicator conditions, or laboratory evidence of severe immunosuppression as evidenced by a CD4 T lymphocyte count of less than 200 cells/mm[3].

Worldwide estimates indicate that 33.6 million adults and 1.2 million children were living with HIV at the end of 1999.[2] Cumulative HIV-related deaths totaled 16.3 million. Approximately 95% of HIV-infected persons live in the developing world. Sub-Saharan Africa has the highest levels of infection, with over 23 million persons living with disease and 13.6 million deaths attributed to HIV-related illnesses since the start of the epidemic. The medical and economic impacts of HIV and AIDS are expected to continue to devastate these areas, because these populations have the least access to the medical, social, and economic resources that might prevent new disease or delay the progression of HIV-related illnesses.

In developed countries significant progress has been made in controlling the HIV epidemic. In 1996, for the first time since HIV was recognized, there was a decline in the incidence of AIDS and the number of AIDS-related deaths.[3] This remarkable trend has been attributed primarily to the availability of new antiretroviral therapies. Unfortunately, the rates of decline in AIDS cases and AIDS deaths have slowed over the past several years.[4] In North America there were 44,000 new cases of HIV reported in 1999 and an estimated 920,000 persons living with HIV or AIDS.

Within the United States, HIV-positive persons are concentrated primarily in large urban settings. Until 1987 New York, Newark, Miami, San Francisco, and Los Angeles accounted for nearly 50% of AIDS cases. Although these cities still represent high intensity pockets of infection, the majority of new cases now occur outside these epicenters, with the most significant increases seen in smaller metropolitan areas.

Eighty-three percent of AIDS cases have occurred in adult men, 16% in adult women, and just over 1% in children.[2,4] The proportion of adult women among those infected with HIV has increased over the past 5 years, with adult women now representing 23% of those living with AIDS.[2,4] Nearly half of all people who acquire HIV in the United States become infected before they turn 30, and the vast majority will die well before their 45th birthdays. There is a disproportionate rate of infection among minority groups, with African Americans and Hispanics making up an ever-increasing proportion of new HIV cases and persons living with AIDS. Among women, African Americans and Hispanics account for 80% of reported AIDS cases; among men, African Americans and Hispanics account for 61% of cases.

The primary risk factors associated with an increased likelihood of acquiring HIV infection include homosexuality or bisexuality, intravenous drug use (IVDU), heterosexual exposure to a partner at risk, blood transfusion prior to 1985, and vertical and horizontal maternal-neonatal transmission. A greater number of risk factors are associated with a greater likelihood of infection.[5]

United States HIV surveillance data demonstrate significant changes in the distribution of newly acquired HIV cases over the past several years. There has been a relative decrease in newly acquired HIV in homosexual and bisexual men, and a relative increase in incidence of HIV among intravenous drug users and heterosexual contacts.

The change in the distribution of AIDS cases by mechanism of transmission since the start of the HIV epidemic is shown in Table 126-1. During the past several years, the greatest percentage increase in reported AIDS cases has occurred among women (attributed principally to heterosexual exposure from an infected partner), minority populations, and children. Because these populations often lack access to primary health services and are frequently underinsured, there has been a trend toward increasing use of ED services by patients with HIV and AIDS. Recent surveillance data from centers located in Baltimore, Chicago, Atlanta, and New York report HIV seroprevalence of 2% to 11%.[6]

PRINCIPLES OF DISEASE

Pathophysiology

HIV is a cytopathic human retrovirus that belongs to the lentivirus subfamily. There are two major subtypes of HIV, HIV-1 and HIV-2. HIV-1 is the predominant subtype worldwide and is the cause of AIDS. HIV-2 causes a similar immune syndrome but is rarely seen in the United States, restricted primarily to western Africa.

The HIV virion is composed of a central single-stranded RNA molecule and the enzyme reverse transcriptase. These are surrounded by a core protein and a lipid bilayer envelope that contain virally encoded transmembrane proteins critical for recognition and attachment to target host lymphocytes (predominantly CD4 cells). HIV-1 has been isolated from a variety of body fluids including blood, serum, semen, vaginal secretions, urine, cerebrospinal fluid (CSF), tears, breast milk, bone marrow, alveolar fluid, synovial fluid, amniotic fluid, and saliva. Only a few modes of transmission have been proven: semen, vaginal secretions, blood or blood products, breast milk, and transplacental transmission in utero. There have been no instances of casual transmission, although there is one case report of possible salivary transmission.[7] The HIV virion is extremely labile and easily neutralized by heat and common disinfecting agents such as 50% ethanol, 35% isopropyl alcohol, 0.3% hydrogen peroxide, disinfectant (Lysol), or a 1:10 solution of household bleach.

Box 126-1 Indicator Conditions for Case Definitions of AIDS

Esophageal candidiasis
Cryptococcosis
Cryptosporidiosis
Cytomegalovirus retinitis
Herpes simplex virus
Kaposi's sarcoma
Brain lymphoma
Mycobacterium avium complex
Pneumocystis carinii pneumonia
Progressive multifocal leukoencephalopathy
Brain toxoplasmosis
Human immunodeficiency virus (HIV) encephalopathy
HIV wasting syndrome
Disseminated histoplasmosis
Isosporiasis
Disseminated *Mycobacterium tuberculosis* disease
Recurrent *Salmonella* septicemia
CD4 T lymphocyte <200 cells/mm^3*
Pulmonary tuberculosis*
Recurrent bacterial pneumonia*
Invasive cervical cancer*

*Added in 1993.

HIV selectively attacks cells within the immune system (primarily T4 helper cells, but macrophages and monocytes may also be involved), a characteristic that accounts for much of the immunodeficiency it produces in affected individuals. HIV-1 transmembrane proteins gp41 and gp120 play a critical role in recognition and attachment of HIV virions to receptors on host lymphocytes. Following infection, viral RNA is reverse transcribed into DNA by reverse transcriptase, one of the critical enzymes required for HIV replication. The viral genome thus becomes permanently integrated into the host's genome. Once integrated, retroviral DNA may lie dormant, or it may be actively transcribed and translated to produce virally encoded proteins and new HIV virions. HIV protease is another critical retroviral enzyme in the life cycle of the virus, responsible for activation of viral protein precursors into the functional enzymes required for virion infectivity.

Primary HIV exposure is characterized by a transient viremia and a decrease in CD4 cell counts, followed by establishment of equilibrium between virus and host immunity. A persistent latent period, during which time the virus lies dormant in the host genome, can last for years. The "set point" or steady state viral load level in the blood of the patient allows prediction of long-term clinical outcomes. Lower levels of viremia correlate with longer clinical latency periods. In the later stages of HIV, there is a sudden increase of viremia that correlates with a dramatic decrease in CD4 T lymphocytes. This is followed by the appearance of opportunistic infections, or malignancies, and ultimately death.

HIV-1 is highly heterogeneous. Multiple genetic subtypes exist in a variety of geographic and sociologic settings. Further genetic diversity exists within individual hosts due to the highly mutable character of the virus. High error rates, which occur in reverse transcription, ensure extensive viral diversity, a critical factor in the pathogenesis and ongoing emergence of drug-resistant phenotypes.[8]

Tests for HIV

HIV infection is most commonly established by HIV serology, or detection of antibodies to the virus. Testing

Table 126-1. Distribution of AIDS Cases by Mechanism of Transmission in the United States

	Percentage of cases (%)			
Primary risk factor	**1981-1987**	**1988-1992**	**1993-1995**	**1996-1998***
Male homosexual contact	64.0	54.6	50.8	45.9
Intravenous drug use (IVDU)	17.2	24.2	27.3	28.4
Male homosexuality and IVDU	8.3	7.0	5.6	6.3
Heterosexual contact	2.5	6.1	10.1	15.6
Transfusion recipient	2.6	1.9	1.0	0.8
Perinatal transmission	1.2	1.5	1.0	N/A
Hemophilia	1.0	0.9	0.8	0.7
No risk reported	3.2	3.9	4.6	0.6

Modified from CDC: AIDS and HIV infection the United States: 1995 update, *MMWR* 44:849, 1995; and US Department of Health and Human Services: HIV/AIDS Surveillance Report, *CDC* 11:1, 1999.

*Refers to estimated percentages.

involves sequential use of an enzyme-linked immunoassay (EIA) and a Western blot (WB) assay. Criteria for positive results are a repeatedly positive EIA followed by a positive WB. EIA detects the binding of specific serum antibodies to HIV antigens that are adherent to a microtiter plate. The WB technique detects electrophoretically separated viral antigens in the patient's serum. A positive WB requires detection of two of the following: p24, gp41, and gp120/160. Final HIV serology results are reported as positive, negative, or indeterminate. Overall sensitivity and specificity of HIV serology is >99.9%.[9]

False-negative HIV tests are accounted for primarily by testing performed during the "window period" (usually the first several months) of acute infection, after viral transmission but before the appearance of antibodies. Ninety-five percent of these become positive by 3 months and 98% by 6 months.[10] Less common explanations of false-negative results include seroreversion, which may occur in late-stage disease or in patients on highly active antiretroviral therapies (HAART), atypical strains of HIV-1, or HIV-2 infection.[11-13] False-positive test results may occur in several clinical circumstances: (1) recipients of blood transfusions containing the HIV antibody; (2) children less than 6 months of age in whom a positive test result may be caused by transplacentally acquired antibodies; (3) patients with cross-reacting antibodies (e.g., antihepatitis A immunoglobulin M [IgM], anti-hepatitis B core IgM, antinuclear, anti–smooth muscle, anti-parietal cell, and anti–mitochondrial antibodies); and (4) patients with cross-reactive human lymphocyte antigens (HLAs) from the H9 cell line or other human retroviruses.[14] In populations with a low prevalence of true-positive results (e.g., heterosexual men or women in low seroprevalence areas) the frequency of false-positive tests (both positive EIA and WB) is increased.[15] This fact is often cited as one of the principal reasons for not offering indiscriminate HIV screening in the ED.

Indeterminate results most often occur with a positive EIA and a single band (rather than two or three) on WB. The most important factor to consider when evaluating an indeterminate WB is the patient's risk profile. Low-risk patients with indeterminate results are rarely infected with HIV-1 or HIV-2, and repeat testing usually shows persistence of one band with the cause rarely established. Referral to an infectious disease specialist and follow-up serology at 3 months are indicated. Patients in higher risk groups with indeterminate results usually are found to have definitively positive WB assays 3 or 6 months later.[16]

Other methods for detection of HIV infection include detection of viral specific antigens and assays for HIV nucleic acid. Neither of these techniques is considered superior to routine serology in terms of accuracy, and should only be used in patents with confusing serologic results requiring clarification. The quantitative plasma HIV ribonucleic acid (RNA) assay is most commonly employed, and is also now used routinely for HIV staging and monitoring of response to retroviral therapy. Tests results are reported as copies per milliliter, with survival time directly correlated to viral burden.

There are a variety of novel HIV tests that are not routinely used in clinical care but are relevant to emergency physicians. The single use diagnostic system (SUDS) assay is analogous to EIA screening tests, and can be performed in less than 1 hour. This test is now routinely employed in the management of occupational exposures to help guide decisions in the use of postexposure prophylaxis (PEP).[17] Sensitivity is sufficient to report negative test results; positive test results require confirmation with routine serology. Recently, the SUDS test has been advocated for use in inner-city EDs, which have high seroprevalence rates and where follow-up visits may be impractical or difficult to achieve.[18,19] Other experimental tests that may be relevant for ED use include a saliva test, which can be developed in under 30 minutes. Potential advantages of this test include ease of specimen collection, reduced costs, rapid availability of results, and improved compliance with testing.

Traditionally it has been thought that serologic testing of patients for HIV in the ED is not indicated. This perception was based principally on logistical issues including difficulties with obtaining proper informed consent, providing appropriate counseling, maintaining confidentiality, and ensuring appropriate follow-up for test results. More recently the concept of ED testing for HIV has been reexamined, since it is well established that early recognition of HIV (and early therapeutic intervention) can significantly delay progression of disease, reduce risk of opportunistic infections, and lead to decreased morbidity and mortality. One recent study using a rapid serologic testing model demonstrated that follow-up among newly tested HIV-positive patients was nearly 75%, with a cost of $40 per patient enrolled and counseled, and $600 to $1100 per infection detected.[19] Recommendations from studies such as this and a forthcoming review from the Society for Academic Emergency Medicine Public Health Task Force Committee suggest that screening for HIV in the ED may be indicated under appropriate circumstances (i.e., populations in which HIV prevalence is at least 1%, sufficient resources are in place to ensure appropriate pretest and posttest counseling, and expeditious referral can be made for patients whose test results are positive). If HIV screening programs are to be further developed, it is likely that identification of high-risk subgroups will also be required to ensure cost-effectiveness.[6,19,20] Meanwhile for those individual cases in whom HIV is suspected, the emergency physician should provide referral for voluntary testing and counseling.

Testing of patients for HIV in the ED to determine which patients require special infection control precautions is not recommended. Such practice has not been shown to alter rates of health care worker exposure to HIV-infected blood and detracts attention from other significant blood-borne infections. Furthermore, patients with undiagnosed HIV infection may have a wide range of clinical conditions and no identifiable risk factors.

CLINICAL FEATURES

The broad spectrum of disease states for HIV-related disorders ranges from asymptomatic seropositive cases to severe, life-threatening complications of AIDS. It includes a wide variety of opportunistic infections, malignancies, and other HIV-related diseases. Nearly every organ system may be affected by HIV. Because the differential diagnosis is so broad for many ED patients, this chapter addresses a clinical approach, as well as some focused information on some of the more commonly seen disorders, to provide an overview of the rapidly evolving diagnoses and therapeutic modalities available.

Initial Evaluation and Management

The initial evaluation and management of the HIV-infected patient must determine stability. Airway, breathing, and circulation must be rapidly assessed and appropriate interventions initiated. For unstable patients intravenous access, cardiac monitoring, and oxygen administration are typically indicated. Following initial stabilization, the remainder of the history and physical may be conducted.

The history must include information relevant to the chief complaint, including duration, location, qualities, characteristics, level of distress, and relieving or inciting factors. Existence of similar problems should be solicited. Medical history should include any relevant medical problems, time of diagnosis of HIV infection, previous AIDS-defining conditions, recent hospitalizations, surgical history, current medications, and allergies. Information regarding potential risk factors for HIV infection may be relevant in the evaluation of many ED patients, particularly in endemic areas. The infection rate may be surprisingly high, even for patients with complaints not associated with HIV.[8] Furthermore, inquiries about risk factors help in the medical evaluation, remind physicians of the potential for occupational exposure to the virus, and afford the opportunity to offer referral for testing and counseling to those who engage in high-risk behavior. Many cases of early HIV infection may not be detected during ED evaluation because of a low clinical suspicion of the disease, particularly in areas where AIDS is not prevalent. Although inquiries regarding risk factors may be offensive to some patients, this may often be averted by tactful inquiries about previous HIV testing or risk factors, presented as questions routinely asked of patients.

The existence of an advanced directive may be important historical information. Many HIV-infected patients have expressed opinions about the level of intervention desired in various clinical settings, particularly in critical care settings and at the end of life.

Following initial stabilization and gathering of historical information, a focused physical examination should be conducted. Elements of the examination relevant to the chief complaint should be performed, with special attention given to the identification of potentially treatable disorders.

The emergency physician must be able to rapidly and effectively assess the patient, identify potentially life-threatening disorders, administer urgent interventions, generate an appropriate differential diagnosis, and initiate therapy, consultation, and disposition.

Several methods of classification and staging of HIV infection have been developed. The Walter Reed classification system[21] is based on clinical and immunologic features. Other classifications are based on CD4 lymphocyte counts.[22,23] The 1993 CDC case definition of AIDS incorporated CD4 lymphocyte counts of less than 200 cells/mm^3.[1,21] Box 126-1 illustrates selections of AIDS-defining illnesses.

Acute HIV syndrome (acute seroconversion syndrome) commonly follows primary exposure by 2 to 6 weeks and may cause nonspecific symptoms including fever, adenopathy, fatigue, pharyngitis, diarrhea, weight loss, and rash.[24] Additional symptoms such as myopathy, peripheral neuropathy, or other neurologic or immunologic manifestations are less commonly present.[25] These relatively nonspecific symptoms may be present for 1 to 3 weeks, and many patients do not seek medical attention during this phase of illness.

Disease progression is widely variable among individuals and groups, depending in part on the mode of transmission. The median time from the initial HIV infection to the diagnosis of AIDS has been estimated at 11 years. Some long-term nonprogressors have remained free of AIDS-defining conditions for over 20 years.[26] Both clinical and laboratory predictors of disease progression have been identified. Clinical predictors of more rapid development of clinically significant immunodeficiency include oral candidiasis, oral hairy leukoplakia, dermatomal varicella, lymphadenopathy, and constitutional symptoms.[27] The best predictor of immunologic susceptibility to opportunistic infection is the CD4 cell count.[28] Other laboratory markers predictive of disease progression include β_2-microglobulin levels, p24 antigenemia, neutropenia, and plasma HIV-1 RNA determinations.[29-32] After the diagnosis of AIDS is established, the average survival time is estimated to be between 16 and 24 months. Improved antiretroviral and HIV-prophylactic treatments have extended the disease-free interval in HIV-infected individuals.[33]

Complications

Fever and Other Systemic Symptoms Systemic symptoms such as fever, weight loss, and malaise are common among ED patients. The differential diagnosis is lengthy and includes a variety of infectious causes, malignancies, and drug reactions (Table 126-2 and Box 126-2). Fever is a common complaint in patients with AIDS. When it is caused by primary HIV infection, it tends to occur in the afternoon or evening and is generally responsive to antipyretics. Evidence of an infectious cause or other reason for fever should be sought by careful history and physical examination. Laboratory investigation of fever may include a complete blood count (CBC), electrolyte values, erythrocyte sedimentation rate, liver function tests, serologic test for syphilis, urinalysis and culture, blood cultures (aerobic, anaerobic, and fungal), blood tests for cryptococcal antigen, serologic tests for *Toxoplasma* and *Coccidioides,* and chest radiography. Stool culture, stool examination for ova and parasites, urine culture for fungus and mycobacteria, and sputum smear and culture for fungus and mycobacteria may yield additional important clues to diagnosis. If there are neurologic signs or symptoms or if no other source of fever is identified, lumbar puncture (LP) should be performed after a cranial computed tomography (CT) scan has been done.

Atypical mycobacterium, *Mycobacterium avium* complex (MAC), causes disseminated disease in up to 50% of patients with AIDS. It is usually associated with severe weight loss, diarrhea, and constitutional symptoms such as fever, malaise, and anorexia. It only rarely causes significant pulmonary disease in patients with HIV. Ziehl-Neelsen (acid-fast) stain of stool or other body fluids commonly yields positive findings, and the organism can also be cultured from blood. Infection with MAC may be treated with triple therapy consisting of clarithromycin (1000 mg twice daily), ethambutol (15 mg/kg daily), and rifabutin (300 to 450 mg daily). Treatment often reduces the degree of bacteremia and symptomatology but does not typically eradicate the organism. Rifabutin, clarithromycin, or azithromycin may be used as prophylaxis in patients with CD4 counts below 50 to 75 cells/mm^3.[34]

Cytomegalovirus (CMV) is a common cause of opportunistic infection. Disseminated disease is common. It is the most common cause of retinitis in HIV-infected patients.[35] Colitis and esophagitis may also result from CMV infection. Treatment with ganciclovir or foscarnet is indicated, and oral ganciclovir may be used for prophylaxis.

Many patients with fever or other systemic symptoms may be managed as outpatients if adequate follow-up observation

Table 126-2. Common Drug Reactions in HIV-Infected Persons

	Fever	Rash	N/V	Diarrhea	H/A	ΔMS	Neuropathy	↑LFT	↓WBC	↓Hct	↓plt	Other
Acyclovir		X	X	X								Vertigo
Amphotericin	X		X		X				X	X	X	Nephrotoxicity
Atovaquone	X	X	X	X	X				X	X		
Azithromycin		X	X	X	X							
Clarithromycin			X	X	X							
Clindamycin		X										
Clotrimazole			X	X								
Dapsone	X	X	X		X				X	X		Hepatitis
Didanosine		X	X	X	X	X	X					Pancreatitis
Fluconazole		X	X	X	X			X				
Foscarnet	X		X	X						X		Nephrotoxicity, seizures
Ganciclovir	X		X	X					X	X		
Ibuprofen		X	X	X				X	X	X		
Indinavir		X	X		X							Nephrolithiasis
Isoniazid	X	X	X				X	X	X	X	X	Hepatitis
Itraconazole		X	X	X	X			X				
Ketoconazole			X	X				X				
Lamivudine	X		X	X	X		X					Cough
Narcotics			X			X						
Pentamidine		X							X	X		Metallic taste
Pyrimethamine									X	X		
Rifabutin		X	X					X	X		X	Skin discoloration
Ritonavir			X	X	X							Paresthesias
Saquinavir		X	X	X								
TMP-SMX	X	X	X					X	X		X	Hepatotoxicity, ↓K
Zalcitabine	X	X	X	X	X		X					
Zidovudine	X	X	X	X	X	X			X	X		

*This table represents only a partial list of adverse drug reactions. An authoritative source should be consulted whenever adverse drug reactions are suspected.

Box 126-2 Causes of Systemic Symptoms in HIV-Infected Patients

Infections, Including:
Primary human immunodeficiency virus (HIV) infection
(e.g, acute retroviral syndrome, HIV wasting syndrome)

Protozoal Infections:
Pneumocystis carinii pneumonia
Toxoplasmosis
Cryptosporidiosis

Bacterial Infections:
Streptococcus pneumoniae
Haemophilus influenzae
Pseudomonas aeruginosa
Salmonellosis
Bacteremia (any organism)

Atypical Bacterial Infections:
Mycobacterium avium-intracellulare (MAI)
Mycobacterium tuberculosis (TB)

Fungal Infections:
Histoplasmosis
Cryptococcosis
Coccidioidomycosis

Viral Infections:
Herpes simplex virus
Herpes zoster virus
Cytomegalovirus
Hepatitis viruses

Adverse Drug Reactions

Neoplasms, Including:
Kaposi's sarcoma
Lymphoma
Hodgkin's disease

and home assistance are available. Indications for hospital admission include toxic appearance, neutropenia with fever, active bleeding, or other need for urgent diagnosis and treatment.

Pulmonary Involvement

Pulmonary manifestations of HIV are among the most common reasons for ED visits among patients with AIDS. The differential diagnosis of respiratory involvement is broad and includes such causes as bacterial infections (e.g., *Streptococcus pneumoniae, Haemophilus influenzae, Chlamydia pneumoniae, Pseudomonas aeruginosa, Staphylococcus aureus, Mycobacterium tuberculosis, Mycobacterium avium-intracellulare* [MAI]), protozoal infections (e.g., *P. carinii, Toxoplasma gondii*), viral infections (e.g., CMV, adenovirus), fungal infections (e.g., *Cryptococcus neoformans, Histoplasma capsulatum, Aspergillus fumigatus, Blastomyces dermatitides*), malignancies (e.g., KS, carcinoma, lymphoma), and others (e.g., lymphocytic interstitial pneumonitis, pulmonary hypertension).

Patients with fever and productive cough are likely to have a bacterial pneumonia, whereas a nonproductive cough is more likely to accompany PCP, fungal infection, or neoplasm. Hemoptysis is often associated with pneumococcal pneumonia and tuberculosis (TB).

Diagnostic evaluation of patients with HIV infection and pulmonary complaints may include CBC, chest radiography, and arterial blood gas (ABG) analysis. Hypoxia may be more pronounced after exercise with *Pneumocystis* infection. Other tests may be indicated in certain situations, such as serum lactic dehydrogenase (LDH), sputum culture, Gram's stain, and special stains (Gomori, Giemsa, acid-fast). Obtaining blood cultures in the ED can prevent delays in initiating appropriate antimicrobial therapy.

Although radiographic findings of many pulmonary complications may be nondiagnostic, certain patterns may be suggestive of specific disorders. A focal infiltrate on plain chest radiography suggests bacterial pneumonia. A diffuse infiltrative process on chest radiography, especially in the absence of leukocytosis, is associated with PCP. PCP is suggested by increased serum LDH and hypoxia, which may be more severe than expected from radiographic findings. Hilar adenopathy with diffuse pulmonary infiltrates suggests cryptococcosis, histoplasmosis, mycobacterial infection, or neoplasm. KS can cause cough, fever, and dyspnea, and the chest radiograph may mimic that seen with PCP. Table 126-3 lists common radiographic findings and associated conditions in the HIV-infected patient.

As with all disease processes, ED management of pulmonary complications must first include evaluation and management of the airway, breathing, and circulation. Definitive airway management may be indicated in severe cases. Volume repletion and pressors may be indicated for hypotension. Other treatment measures, such as volume repletion, oxygen administration, and pressors, may be indicated for initial stabilization. If the diagnosis can be ascertained or is strongly suspected, specific treatment can be instituted while the patient is in the ED, particularly if PCP is suspected. If the symptoms are of new onset or there has been a change from previous status, admission should be considered. Decisions regarding patients with known pulmonary involvement are based on comparison with baseline status, the effectiveness of ongoing or previous treatment, and the individual's ability to obtain outpatient follow-up observation (see Disposition).

Pneumocystis carinii *Pneumonia* PCP is the most common opportunistic infection in AIDS. More than 80% of patients with AIDS acquire PCP at some time during their illness, and it is the initial opportunistic infection in 60% of cases.[36] Although traditionally classified as a protozoan, it has been suggested that its morphology more closely resembles a fungus.[37] A determined investigation of new or subtle symptoms may lead to an early diagnosis. The chest radiograph commonly shows a diffuse interstitial infiltrate, but may also reveal normal findings, asymmetry, nodules, cavitation, or bullae.[38] Gallium scanning of the chest commonly yields positive findings even with negative radiograph results, but false-positive results may occur up to 50% of the time.[39] Although bronchoscopy (bronchoalveolar lavage, brush biopsy, transbronchial biopsy) has been the mainstay of establishing the diagnosis,[40] examination of induced sputum by indirect immunofluorescent staining using monoclonal antibodies has been shown to be an easy and

Table 126-3. Chest Radiographic Abnormalities: Differential Diagnosis in the Patient With AIDS

Finding	Potential causes
Diffuse interstitial infiltration	*Pneumocystis carinii*
	Cytomegalovirus (CMV)
	Mycobacterium tuberculosis
	Mycobacterium avium complex (MAC)
	Histoplasmosis
	Coccidioidomycosis
	Lymphoid interstitial pneumonitis
	Mycoplasma pneumoniae
Focal consolidation	Bacterial pneumonia
	Mycoplasma pneumoniae
	P. carinii
	M. tuberculosis
	MAC
Nodular lesions	Kaposi's sarcoma (KS)
	M. tuberculosis
	MAC
	Fungal lesions
	Toxoplasmosis
Cavitary lesions	*P. carinii*
	M. tuberculosis
	Bacterial infection
	Fungal infection
Pleural effusion	KS
	(Small effusion may be associated with any infection)
Adenopathy	KS
	Lymphoma
	M. tuberculosis
	Cryptococcus
Pneumothorax	KS
Normal radiograph	Histoplasmosis (40%)
	P. carinii (20%)
	M. tuberculosis
	Cryptococcosis

effective method of diagnosing PCP.[41] The differential diagnosis includes viral, bacterial, mycobacterial, fungal, and protozoal pneumonias, as well as malignancies. The more common causes to be considered in the differential diagnosis are shown in Box 126-2. Differentiation of these entities in the ED may be difficult, if not impossible.

Establishment of a definitive diagnosis is not necessary prior to the initiation of treatment. Treatment should be initiated as early as possible, with 15 to 20 mg/kg/day of trimethoprim and 75 to 100 mg/kg/day of sulfamethoxazole (TMP-SMX), given either orally or intravenously for a total of 21 days[42] (e.g., two Bactrim DS tablets every 8 hours). Other therapeutic options include pentamidine isethionate, dapsone, clindamycin plus primaquine, atovaquone, or trimetrexate. In addition, steroid treatment (prednisone 40 mg PO twice daily with a tapering dosage over 3 weeks) is recommended for patients with a Pao_2 less than 70 mm Hg, or an A-a gradient greater than 35.[43,44] Most (60% to 80%) respond to therapy, although *Pneumocystis* persists in the lungs of two thirds of patients. The optimal duration of therapy has not been definitively established, but 3 weeks of treatment is commonly recommended.

Adverse effects of TMP-SMX occur in up to 65% of patients with AIDS and are 20 times more common than in the general population (see Table 126-2). However, 75% of patients are able to tolerate a full course of therapy. Adverse effects generally become apparent after 7 to 14 days of therapy. The most common are nausea, vomiting, rash, fever, neutropenia, thrombocytopenia, hyponatremia, and hepatitis. Pentamidine can cause nausea, vomiting, diarrhea, neutropenia, hypoglycemia, hyperglycemia, renal impairment, hepatic toxicity, and orthostatic hypotension.[45] Because sterile abscesses may develop at the injection site, intravenous infusion is preferred. Prophylaxis against PCP may be an important step in preventing reinfection and is recommended for patients with CD4 cell counts below 200 cells/mm^3.[46] Preferred therapeutic agents include TMP-SMX (one double strength (DS) tablet PO once or twice daily), pentamidine, pyrimethamine plus sulfadoxine, dapsone, or pyrimethamine plus dapsone.[47]

Mycobacterium tuberculosis The incidence of *M. tuberculosis* (MTB) in HIV-infected patients has increased dramatically from a low point reached in 1985, particularly in socioeconomically disadvantaged groups, including prisoners[48] and intravenous drug users.[49] The increase in TB among the HIV-infected population is thought to be secondary to a number of factors, including increased risk of reactivation of latent infection, high rates of infection after exposure, overlap in at-risk groups, and rapid progression to clinically significant disease.[50] TB may be a very early manifestation of AIDS. Fever, cough, and hemoptysis are common symptoms. Radiographic abnormalities may vary considerably. Radiographic features may be alveolar infiltrates, interstitial infiltrates, cavitation, pleural effusions, mediastinal adenopathy, and alveolar opacities.[51] Extrapulmonary disease involving the CNS, bone, viscera, skin, pericardium, eye, pharynx, and lymph nodes may occur in up to 75% of cases.

The diagnosis of TB is based on a number of factors including risk of infection, clinical picture, direct examination of patient specimens, and identification of mycobacteria from cultures. Purified protein derivative (PPD) skin testing is often helpful, particularly in advanced stages of immunosuppression. Additionally, the use of a nucleic acid amplification test, in conjunction with clinical stratification, may have important diagnostic value.[52] Negative PPD test results are common among those infected.[53] Attempts to diagnose TB by stain and culture of sputum may not be fruitful; bronchoscopy or biopsy of affected organs (e.g., lymph nodes, liver, brain) is often required.

Multidrug-resistant TB remains an issue of concern, particularly among the HIV-infected population. Outbreaks involving organisms resistant to multiple pharmacologic agents, including isoniazid and rifampin, have occurred.[54,55] Treatment of suspected cases should be determined in conjunction with an infectious disease specialist, taking into consideration local resistance as well as individual susceptibility tests. AIDS patients with TB should receive a four-drug regimen with isoniazid, rifampin, pyrazinamide, and either ethambutol hydrochloride or streptomycin. Second-line agents may include ciprofloxacin, ofloxacin, kanamycin, amikacin, capreomycin, ethionamide, cycloserine, and para-aminosalicylic acid (PAS).[56] All HIV-infected patients with positive PPD findings should receive prophylaxis with a regimen of isoniazid plus pyridoxine or rifampin plus pyrazinamide.[9,34] Steps toward prevention of TB and its spread include early identification, initiation of multidrug therapy, respiratory isolation, and the use of personal respiratory protection devices.

Neurologic Involvement

Neurologic diseases are the initial manifestation of AIDS in 10% to 20% of patients. The frequency of neurologic complications increases over the course of HIV infection, with cross-sectional studies showing a 75% to 90% prevalence of neurologic disorders in patients with AIDS.[57] Neurologic disease may be caused by a variety of opportunistic infections, neoplasms, or direct effects of HIV infection on the CNS. In the early stages of HIV infection aseptic meningitis, herpes zoster radiculitis, and inflammatory demyelinating polyneuropathy are common. Later stages of HIV are associated with cognitive dysfunction, dementia, opportunistic infections, cancers, and sensory neuropathies. The most common AIDS-defining neurologic complications are HIV encephalopathy (dementia), *C. neoformans,* toxoplasmosis, and primary CNS lymphoma.

Less common CNS infections that should be considered in the presence of neurologic symptoms include bacterial meningitis, histoplasmosis (usually disseminated), CMV, progressive multifocal leukoencephalopathy (PML), herpes simplex virus (HSV), neurosyphilis, and TB. Noninfectious CNS processes include CNS lymphoma, cerebrovascular accidents, and metabolic encephalopathies.

Clinical pictures in patients with serious neurologic complications can be nonspecific, making diagnosis and disposition challenging. The most common symptoms indicative of CNS pathology are seizures, meningismus, focal neurologic deficits, altered mental status, and headache (new or persistent). Infection accounts for the vast majority of neurologic disorders and is most often accompanied by fever.

Patients with CD4 cell counts >200 cells/mm^3, who present with fever and meningismus in the absence of focal neurologic deficits, should have an immediate LP performed. For those with focal deficits or new seizures, immediate neuroimaging is recommended, followed by LP if neuroimaging is unrevealing. Diagnostic evaluation of patients with altered mental status or headache should proceed as in the non–HIV-infected population, with neuroimaging and LP reserved for those cases in which another cause for the symptoms is not identified. For those patients with CD4 cell counts of <200 cells/mm^3 a more aggressive approach is advocated, with any of the findings described above demanding emergent imaging, usually followed by LP (Figure 126-1).[58]

The choice of imaging modality in the ED varies. Generally speaking, for those CNS processes that require immediate identification, CT without contrast is considered adequate.[59] If the entire ED evaluation is unrevealing, more advanced diagnostic imaging should be pursued immediately if the patient's symptoms are severe. For all other cases, close follow-up is indicated with the patient's primary provider, since it has been demonstrated that more subtle lesions may be identified by CT with contrast or magnetic resonance imaging (MRI).[60] CSF analysis should include opening and closing pressures, cell count, glucose, protein, Gram's stain, bacterial culture, viral culture, fungal culture, toxoplasma and cryptococcal antigens, and coccidioidomycosis titer.

HIV Encephalopathy HIV encephalopathy, or AIDS dementia complex, occurs in up to one third of patients with HIV.[57] It is a progressive process caused by direct HIV infection and is commonly heralded by impairment of recent memory or subtle cognitive deficits, such as difficulty concentrating. Early stages of dementia may be confused with depression, the effects of psychoactive substances, or anxiety disorders. Deficits become more debilitating in later stages of disease and can include more obvious changes in mental status, seizures, frontal release signs, and hyperactive deep tendon reflexes. It is important to recognize that AIDS dementia is a diagnosis of exclusion. Thus, even among patients with AIDS coming to the ED with an established diagnosis of dementia, the appearance of progressive signs or symptoms requires immediate further evaluation to rule out other CNS processes. Neuroimaging findings in patients with HIV encephalopathy typically show atrophy and diffuse deep matter hyperintensities. LP findings are typically normal.

Cryptococcus neoformans *C. neoformans* may be seen in up to 10% of patients with AIDS and may cause either focal cerebral lesions or diffuse meningoencephalitis.[61] The most common initial symptoms are fever and headache, often accompanied by nausea and vomiting. Less common are visual changes, dizziness, seizures, and cranial nerve deficits.[62] The diagnosis depends on identifying organisms in CSF. Cryptococcal antigen in the CSF is nearly 100% sensitive and specific; less definitive are India ink staining (60% to 80% sensitive), fungal culture (95% sensitive), and serum cryptococcal antigen (95% sensitive). Treatment of cryptococcal meningitis requires admission for intravenous amphotericin B (0.7 mg/kg/day); flucytosine (100 mg/kg/day) may be added to this regimen. A response can be expected approximately 60% of the time.[61] The initial course of therapy lasts 8 to 10 weeks, and because of the high relapse rate (approximately 50%) chronic suppressive therapy with lower doses of oral fluconazole should be continued after successful treatment. The most clinically significant adverse effect of treatment for cryptococcal meningitis is bone marrow suppression.

Toxoplasma gondii *T. gondii* is the most common cause of focal encephalitis in patients with AIDS.[57] Common symptoms include headache, fever, altered mental status, and seizures. Focal neurologic deficits are found in up to 80% of cases.[64] Serologic testing is not useful in making or excluding the diagnosis because antibody to *T. gondii* is prevalent in the general population. The presence of antibody to *T. gondii* in the CSF is helpful, although there is a high rate of false-positive results. Diagnosis of toxoplasmosis is most often made by the presence of multiple subcortical lesions on CT scan. Noncontrast CT is often used as the initial study in the ED because addition of contrast has been shown to be of marginal value in patients with completely normal noncontrast CT scans.[59] In those patients with suspicious lesions, or those with a high suspicion for clinical pathology but equivocal or negative noncontrast scans, a contrast CT may be helpful. In the presence of contrast, toxoplasmosis lesions are ring-enhancing with surrounding areas of edema. MRI is considered even more sensitive in detecting the number and extent of lesions, but is usually not indicated in the ED.[65]

Clinical and radiologic features often cannot reliably distinguish CNS toxoplasmosis from a wide variety of other

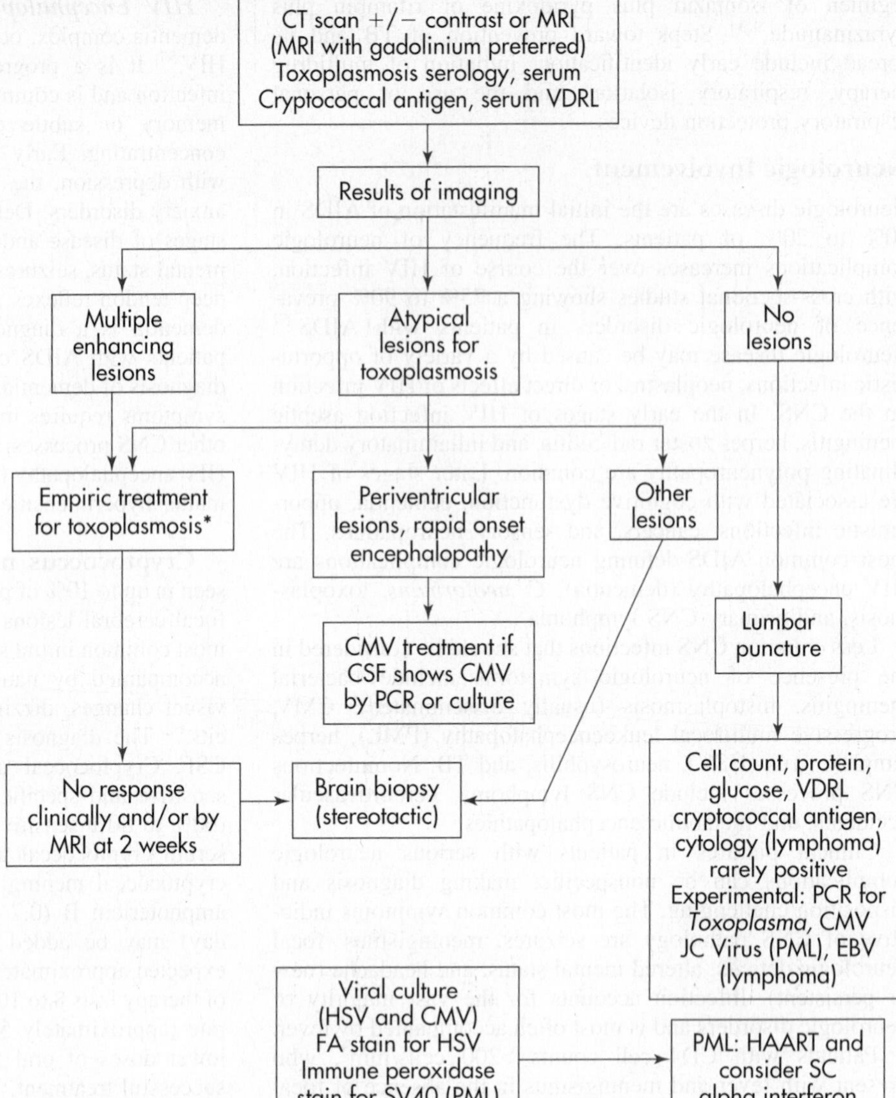

Figure 126-1. **Advanced HIV infection plus altered mental status, new seizures, headache (severe or persistent), or focal neurologic deficits.** *Modified from McArthur J, Bartlett JG. In Bartlett JG, editor:* 1999 Medical management of HIV infection, *Baltimore, 1999, Port City Press.*

* Serology for *Toxoplasma gondii* is positive 85-90% with toxoplasmic encephalitis. Clinical response to empiric treatment is anticipated within one week. Negative serology, atypical presentation, and/or delayed clinical response should prompt early biopsy.

FA, Fluorescent antibody.

causes (lymphoma, cerebral TB, fungi, progressive multifocal leukoencephalopathy, CMV, KS, and hemorrhage).[63,64] General patterns have been described that may be helpful in determining the most likely cause. Toxoplasmosis tends to have a greater number of lesions with a predilection for the basal ganglia and corticomedullary area, versus lymphomas, which are more often singular lesions located in the periventricular matter or corpus callosum. TB is characterized by an inflammatory appearance on CT, with a thick isodense exudate filling the basal cisterns.

Patients with suspected toxoplasmosis should be admitted and treated with pyrimethamine (100 to 200 mg PO loading dose, followed by 50 to 100 mg/day PO), plus sulfadiazine (4 to 8 g/day PO) with folinic acid (10 mg/day PO) to reduce the incidence of pancytopenia. Short courses of high-dose steroids are beneficial in cases in which significant edema or mass effect is noted; seizure prophylaxis with phenytoin may also be used in these cases.[65] Failure to respond to treatment suggests an alternate diagnosis that may require biopsy. As with cryptococcal meningitis, chronic suppressive treatment is usually indicated because of the high likelihood of relapse after successful therapy. Pyrimethamine, sulfadiazine, and folinic acid are recommended. For those patients with positive toxoplasmosis serology and CD4 cell counts <100 cells/mm^3, prophylaxis with TMP-SMX (one DS tablet PO qd) plus folinic acid is indicated; dapsone can be substituted for TMP-SMX in those patients who are intolerant of sulfa drugs.[66]

HIV Neuropathy HIV infection is also associated with a variety of disorders of the peripheral nervous system. These are rarely emergent but require appropriate referral. The most common peripheral disorder to be aware of is HIV neuropathy, which is characterized by painful sensory symptoms in the feet. Treatment in the ED should be directed toward analgesia. Ibuprofen may be used as first-line therapy, although narcotics may be required in more severe cases. Amitriptyline and phenytoin have been shown to be helpful but should be used judiciously because of their potential for causing delirium in patients with concurrent HIV dementia.

Gastrointestinal Involvement

Approximately one half of all patients with AIDS have symptoms produced by infection of the gastrointestinal (GI) tract at some time during the course of their illness. The most common symptoms are abdominal pain, bleeding, and diarrhea. Evaluation of specific causes is often difficult until objective studies are obtained. There is often more than one source of infection present, and this may further complicate establishing the diagnosis. Treatment in the ED focuses on supportive care, fluid and electrolyte repletion, and appropriate studies for further investigation.

Oropharynx Oral involvement is common and may include a variety of causes, including fungal infections (oral candidiasis, histoplasmosis, cryptococcosis, penicilliosis), viral lesions (HSV, herpes zoster virus [HZV], CMV, hairy leukoplakia, papillomavirus), bacterial lesions (periodontal disease, necrotizing stomatitis, TB, MAC, bacillary angiomatosis), neoplasms (KS, lymphoma, Hodgkin's lymphoma), and autoimmune or idiopathic lesions (e.g., salivary gland disease, aphthous ulcers). Oral lesions such as candidiasis and hairy leukoplakia are indicators of disease progression.[67,68]

Oral candidiasis affects more than 80% of patients with AIDS. It typically involves the tongue and buccal mucosa, and may be asymptomatic. Symptoms may include soreness, burning, and dysphagia. Candidiasis can be distinguished from hairy leukoplakia by its characteristic whitish lacy plaques, which are easily scraped away from an erythematous base. Three forms of candidiasis may be seen, including pseudomembranous (thrush), erythematous, and angular cheilitis. Microscopic examination of the material on potassium hydroxide smear can confirm the diagnosis in the ED. Most oral lesions can be managed symptomatically on an outpatient basis. Clotrimazole troches (10 mg PO five times daily for 14 days) are the preferred treatment for oral candidiasis. Other treatment options include nystatin vaginal tablets, which may be dissolved slowly in the mouth four times daily, or nystatin pastilles (2 pastilles dissolved in the mouth five times daily). Systemic therapy may be used for resistant lesions, such as ketoconazole, fluconazole, or itraconazole. Nystatin suspension is not recommended because of inadequate duration of application in the oropharynx.

Hairy leukoplakia is also commonly seen and typically produces white, corrugated or filiform, thickened lesions on the lateral aspects of the tongue. Because it is often asymptomatic, therapy is not necessary, but when indicated treatment may be initiated with acyclovir, ganciclovir, foscarnet, or tretinoin (Retin-A). Lesions commonly reoccur after cessation of therapy.

HSV causes painful oral and perioral ulcerations. It can be tentatively diagnosed in the ED by the identification of multinucleated giant cells in scrapings of the lesions, and can later be diagnosed definitively by culture. Therapy should be initiated with acyclovir.

MAC may also cause painful oral ulcerative lesions. The diagnosis of MAC can be established if an acid-fast stain yields positive findings.

Oral KS may appear as nontender, well-circumscribed, slightly raised, violaceous, or erythematous lesions anywhere in the oropharynx. Definitive diagnosis requires biopsy. Treatment may include surgical excision, localized chemotherapy, sclerosing agents, or radiation therapy.

Periodontal disease may be seen in up to 10% of patients, including gingival erythema or necrotizing periodontal disease. Outpatient treatment may be instituted, including local irrigation and mouth rinses, and oral antibiotics such as amoxicillin-clavulanate, or clindamycin. Dental follow-up is essential.

Aphthous ulcerations, often painful and recurrent, have an unknown etiology, but are thought to be related to immune deficiency. Other causes of ulcerations, such as fungal or mycobacterial infection, HSV, CMV, and lymphoma, should be excluded. Aphthous ulcers usually respond to topical steroids, such as 0.05% fluzinamide ointment mixed 50% with an oral topical anesthetic.

Esophagus Complaints of dysphagia, odynophagia, or chest pain may be indicative of esophageal involvement. *Candida,* HSV, and CMV infection may all cause painful esophagitis. Other causes may include KS, idiopathic entities, MAC, or reflux esophagitis. Although treatment may be initiated empirically based on symptomatology, it may be necessary to perform endoscopy, or to obtain fungal stains, viral cultures, and occasionally biopsies in order to definitively establish the diagnosis. An air-contrast barium swallow can be obtained as part of the ED evaluation. An ulcerative pattern with plaques, often separated by normal mucosa, is characteristic of *Candida* esophagitis. Herpes esophagitis typically produces easily seen "punched-out" ulcerations without associated "heaped-up" plaques.

Esophageal candidiasis, the most common cause of esophageal complaints, may be treated presumptively based on the symptoms and should include either fluconazole (100 to 200 mg PO daily for 2 to 3 weeks) or ketoconazole (200 to 400 mg PO daily for 2 to 3 weeks).[69,70] Alternative therapies may include clotrimazole or itraconazole. Relapses are common after cessation of treatment. Intravenous amphotericin B may be used for refractory cases. Disseminated candidiasis is managed with intravenous amphotericin B and flucytosine. Fluconazole has been shown to be effective in prophylaxis against fungal infections in patients with CD4 counts $<100/mm^3$,[71] although survival is unaffected by prophylactic therapy, and any benefit gained by prophylaxis must be carefully weighed against risks of potentially significant adverse drug reactions.

Intestine Diarrhea is the most common GI complaint in patients with AIDS and is estimated to occur in 50% to 90%. Diarrhea can vary in severity from a few loose stools per day to massive fluid loss with prostration, fever, chills, and weight loss. Potential pathogens include parasites (*Cryptosporidium parvum, Enterocytozoon bieneusi, Isospora belli, Giardia lamblia, Entamoeba histolytica, Microsporidia, Cyclospora,* and others), bacteria (*Salmonella, Shigella, Campylobacter, Helicobacter pylori, M. tuberculosis,* MAC, *Clostridium* *difficile,* and others), viruses (CMV, HSV, HIV, and others), and fungi (*H. capsulatum, C. neoformans, Coccidiodes immitis,* and others). Significant GI bleeding and dehydration have been associated with many pathogens, particularly CMV. *Salmonella* infection can be of particular concern in HIV-infected patients, often producing recurrent bacteremia and other significant clinical disease. Neoplastic GI involvement with KS or lymphoma may produce dysphagia, obstruction, intussusception, or diarrhea.

Cryptosporidium and *Isospora* infections are commonly associated with HIV infection, and both organisms may produce prolonged watery diarrhea.[72,73] Diagnosis may be sought using acid-fast staining of stool samples, by monoclonal antibody, or by enzyme-linked immunoabsorbent assays. Treatment of these disorders is clinically variably successful. Symptoms may be treated with diet modification or loperamide. *Cryptosporidium* infections may be treated with some success with paromomycin (500 to 750 mg PO four times daily for 2 to 4 weeks) or azithromycin (2400 mg/day on day 1, followed by 1200 mg/day for 4 weeks, followed by 600 mg/day maintenance therapy). *Isospora* infections are often successfully treated with TMP-SMX (1 DS tablet PO tid for 10 days, followed by twice weekly therapy for 3 weeks).[74] Pyrimethamine or metronidazole may be used as alternative therapy.

ED management should include repletion of fluid and electrolytes and appropriate diagnostic studies. These may include microscopic examination of stool samples for leukocytes, ova, and parasites; bacterial culture; and acid-fast stain. If indicated, outpatient anoscopy, proctoscopy, or sigmoidoscopy (with or without biopsy) may be arranged for patients who require further evaluation but do not require immediate admission. Management of symptoms of severe diarrhea not requiring specific therapy may include attapulgite (Kaopectate), psyllium (Metamucil), diet modification, or diphenoxylate hydrochloride with atropine (Lomotil).

Liver Hepatomegaly is common and occurs in up to 50% of patients with AIDS. Jaundice is less common. Hepatitis B is common among patients with AIDS, especially in intravenous drug users. Previous hepatitis B infection may become reactivated or acquired with increased prevalence following HIV infection. Several opportunistic organisms, including CMV, MAI, *M. tuberculosis,* and *H. capsulatum,* can produce a hepatitis-like syndrome in patients with HIV infection. Most commonly, these patients have an elevation in the alkaline phosphatase level that is disproportionate to levels of other liver enzymes.

Anorectum Proctocolitis is common in patients with AIDS and may be caused by one or several of a long list of organisms, including *Campylobacter jejuni, Shigella* spp., *Salmonella* spp., *Giardia,* HSV, *E. histolytica, Chlamydia,* and *Neisseria gonorrhoeae.* Diagnostic tests may include standard stool cultures, microscopic examination for leukocytes, ova and parasites, and appropriate cultures or immunoassays for gonorrhea and chlamydial infections. The diagnosis of anal gonorrhea can be confirmed on a Gram's stain of stool by the presence of leukocytes and intracellular organisms. HSV can be diagnosed by viral cultures or by identification of multinucleated giant cells on scrapings of anal lesions.

Cutaneous Involvement

Several common cutaneous manifestations of AIDS are likely to be seen in the ED. Preexisting dermatologic conditions may be exacerbated by HIV infection. Common infections and conditions may occur in an atypical fashion. Generalized cutaneous complaints such as xerosis (dry skin) and pruritus are common and may be manifested before any AIDS-defining illness. Treatment of patients with these conditions is identical to that of noninfected patients. Xerosis may be treated with emollients. Pruritus may be treated with oatmeal baths and, if necessary, antihistamines.

Infections including *S. aureus* (manifested as bullous impetigo, ecthyma, or folliculitis), *P. aeruginosa* (with chronic ulcerations and macerations), HSV, HZV, syphilis, and scabies must always be considered and are generally treated with standard methods.

KS is the second most common manifestation of AIDS and has involved approximately 25% of the known cases to date. It is found commonly among homosexual or bisexual men. The disease is usually widely disseminated with mucous membrane involvement, although it rarely is primarily fatal. Four categories of KS exist: classic, endemic African, iatrogenic, and AIDS-associated. KS typically occurs in HIV-infected patients with any variation of mucocutaneous involvement, lymph node involvement, or involvement of the GI tract or other organs. The typical appearance of cutaneous involvement is pink, red, or purple papules, plaques, nodules, and tumors. Several staging systems have been developed based on cutaneous involvement, lymph node or visceral involvement, systemic signs or symptoms, and CD4 cell count.[75-77] Treatment of KS is based on sites and extent of involvement. Treatments available include cryotherapy, radiotherapy, infrared coagulation, sclerosing agents, intralesional vinblastine, or systemic chemotherapy such as adriamycin, bleomycin, and vincristine.

Varicella zoster eruptions involving several dermatomes are commonly seen in patients with AIDS. Although seropositivity is common in all adults (90%), reactivation causing clinical disease is more common in HIV-infected people, who are 17 times more likely to develop dermatomal zoster reactivation than the general population.[78] Recurrent episodes and multidermatomal involvement are common. In the HIV-infected patient with simple dermatomal zoster infection, outpatient management should be initiated with oral famciclovir (5 mg PO bid or tid for 7 days), acyclovir (800 mg five times daily), or valacyclovir (1000 mg bid for 7 days).[79] Admission is warranted in any patient with systemic involvement, ophthalmic zoster, or severe dermatomal zoster. Intravenous acyclovir is administered at a dosage of 10 mg/kg every 8 hours. Varicella immune globulin may be useful in patients with primary infection and visceral involvement.

HSV infections are very prevalent among HIV-infected patients: 95% of homosexual HIV-infected persons in the United States and Europe are seropositive for HSV-1, HSV-2, or both, and 40% to 60% of injection drug users for HSV-2.[80] Both HSV-1 and HSV-2 may be seen as local infection and systemic involvement. As is the case with many other dermatologic abnormalities, HSV may manifest in an atypical fashion. Frequently the clinical picture includes fever, adenopathy, malaise, and ulcerative lesions of mucosal and cutaneous sites. Common sites of involvement include oral

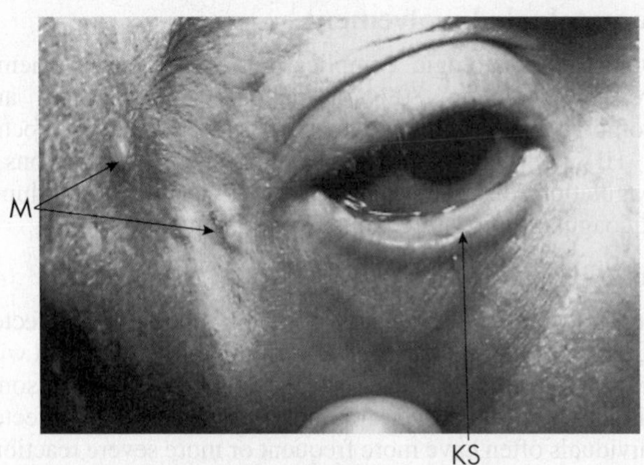

Figure 126-2. **Molluscum contagiosum (*arrows*) and Kaposi's sarcoma (*arrow*) simultaneously in the same patient.** *Courtesy Dr. Antoinette Hood, Johns Hopkins Hospital.*

mucosa, genital areas, and rectum. HSV and HZV may be difficult to distinguish clinically, and cultures may be required to differentiate the two. Reactivation is common. HSV infections respond well to standard therapies, and toxic effects are uncommon. Oral famciclovir (750 mg PO tid) or acyclovir (200 mg five times daily for 10 days) is effective for mucocutaneous infection. For disseminated infection or neurologic involvement, intravenous acyclovir is recommended (5 to 10 mg/kg IV every 8 hours for 7 to 21 days). For acyclovir-resistant lesions, famciclovir, penciclovir, foscarnet, or valacyclovir may be substituted. Suppressive therapy is effective. Patients with these viral infections should be assigned to isolation beds.

Molluscum contagiosum causes small flesh-colored papules with a whitish core and is commonly seen in HIV-infected individuals (Figure 126-2). Treatment may consist of cryotherapy or curettage. Therapy is recommended only for symptomatic lesions because cure is difficult.

Intertriginous infections with either *Candida* or *Trichophyton* are common and may be diagnosed by microscopic examination of scrapings in potassium hydroxide. Treatment may include topical imidazole creams (e.g., clotrimazole, miconazole, or ketoconazole).

Scabies should be considered in all HIV-infected patients, particularly those who have dermatitis with excoriations or pruritus. The yield of microscopically evident mites is high. Preferred treatment is with 5% permethrin in a single application. Sexual and household contacts should also be treated. Norwegian scabies is particularly difficult to treat and should be considered if lesions consistent with scabies fail to respond to traditional therapy. Treatment should be undertaken in consultation with an infectious disease specialist.

Seborrheic dermatitis is a common eruption, particularly among patients with AIDS-associated dementia. Lesions may include erythematous, hyperkeratotic, scaling plaques involving the scalp, face (especially involving the nasolabial folds), ears, chest, and genitalia. Treatment with topical steroids is effective in many patients, although less successfully than in the general population. Alternative therapy includes topical or oral ketoconazole.

Human papillomavirus infections occur with increased frequency in immunocompromised patients. Treatment is cosmetic or symptomatic and may include cryotherapy, topical therapy, or in extreme cases laser therapy.

Other dermatologic disorders occur with increased frequency in patients with AIDS. Psoriasis, atopic dermatitis, and alopecia are common. Any preexisting dermatologic disorder may be exacerbated by HIV infection.

Ophthalmologic Manifestations

Ocular findings are common in the HIV-infected patient. Cotton-wool spots in the retina are the most common eye finding in patients with AIDS and do not require intervention. Other common ophthalmologic manifestations of HIV include CMV retinitis and KS of eyelids or conjunctiva.

CMV retinitis occurs in 10% to 30% of HIV-infected patients and is the most common cause of blindness in patients with AIDS.[81] With advances in HAART, reduced incidences of CMV retinitis have been observed, but discontinuation of HAART may result in intraocular inflammation.[82] CMV retinitis typically produces severe necrotic vasculitis and retinitis. When present, it may be asymptomatic or cause diminished visual acuity, photophobia, scotoma, redness, or pain. It is diagnosed by its characteristic appearance on indirect ophthalmoscopy of fluffy white retinal lesions, often perivascular. Differential diagnosis includes toxoplasmosis, syphilis, HSV infection, HZV infection, and TB. Treatment should be initiated with ganciclovir 5 mg/kg every 12 hours for 2 weeks, followed by 6 mg/kg/day maintenance therapy. Foscarnet may also be used, at a dosage of 90 mg/kg every 12 hours. Similar rates of efficacy are achieved with ganciclovir and foscarnet.[83] Ganciclovir-containing intravitreal implants are another therapeutic option that provides higher intravitreal concentrations.[84,85] Chronic suppressive therapy with ganciclovir or foscarnet may be indicated. Patients with serum antitoxoplasma antibodies should receive prophylaxis for CD4 cell counts $<100/mm^3$, with TMP-SMX.[35]

Cardiovascular Involvement

Clinically significant cardiac disease in the patient with AIDS is relatively uncommon. Autopsy findings suggest cardiac involvement in up to 73% of deceased patients with AIDS.[86,87] The pericardium is the most common site of cardiac involvement, although many patients have clinically insignificant effusions. Pericardial effusions may be secondary to malignancies, uremia, lymphatic obstruction, or infections such as *M. tuberculosis, S. pneumoniae, S. aureus,* or a host of other bacterial, viral, fungal, or protozoal infections. Cardiomyopathies may occur and are commonly associated with advanced HIV infection. Causes of cardiomyopathies may include primary HIV infection; viral, mycobacterial, fungal, or protozoal infection; drugs; immunologic problems; or ischemia. Cardiac neoplasms may also occur, typically either KS or lymphoma. Neoplasms may be clinically silent or may be associated with symptoms such as congestive heart failure, tamponade, or arrhythmias.

Renal Involvement

Renal insufficiency in the patient with AIDS typically follows one of three patterns. Prerenal azotemia is the most common renal abnormality, especially in conjunction with volume loss related to systemic or GI infection. Acute renal failure may also occur and is often secondary to drug nephrotoxicity (e.g., pentamidine, aminoglycosides, sulfa drugs, foscarnet, rifampin, dapsone, and amphotericin B). Chronic renal insufficiency may be caused by HIV-associated nephropathy (HIVAN), vasculitis, or other systemic infection. Postrenal azotemia may result from tubular, ureteral, or pelvic obstruction, from lymphoma, stone, fungus ball, blood clot, or sloughed papilla.

ED evaluation should include urinalysis, assessment of fluid status, and blood urea nitrogen (BUN) and creatinine levels. If indicated, ultrasound or intravenous pyelogram (IVP) may demonstrate the site and degree of obstruction. Renal biopsy may be indicated for patients with proteinuria and undiagnosed renal disease. Treatment depends on the causative agent. Therapies that have demonstrated limited benefit for HIVAN include corticosteroids,[88] angiotensin converting enzyme (ACE) inhibitors, and dialysis. Treatment with these modalities should be initiated in conjunction with a nephrologist.

Psychiatric Considerations

The diagnosis of AIDS involves complex psychological and social issues, in addition to physiologic, neurologic, and psychiatric abnormalities. Interactions with family and friends may be dramatically changed, and issues of confronting chronic illness and death may prove devastating. Depression is common among patients with AIDS and is often responsive to hospitalization and psychosocial intervention. Patients with a history of depression are at increased risk. Depressed patients generally have lower CD4 cell counts and may report more AIDS-related symptoms.[89] Depression may result in suicidal ideation and may bring the patient to the ED after a suicide attempt, such as a drug overdose. Antidepressant therapy may be considered if symptoms of depression continue longer than 2 weeks.

AIDS psychosis is a poorly delineated entity, with the presence of psychiatric symptoms such as hallucinations, delusions, or other abnormal behavioral changes. The cause is unclear at this time, and treatment has been identical to that of other psychoses.

Sexually Transmitted Diseases

Sexually transmitted diseases may be associated with HIV infection. In addition to testing for the more common entities (e.g., gonorrhea, *Chlamydia,* and herpes), serologic testing for syphilis should be performed for all patients who have symptoms suggestive of possible sexually transmitted disease. Because a normal antibody response may be absent in HIV-infected individuals, care must be taken to identify potential cases of syphilis, even among those with negative serologic findings. An alternate means of diagnosis may include dark-field microscopy. Empiric therapy may be instituted, even without laboratory proof of infection. The recommended treatment of primary or secondary syphilis of less than 12 months duration is a single intramuscular dose of benzathine penicillin, 2.4 million units. For latent syphilis or unknown duration of secondary syphilis, three weekly injections are recommended. Patients with neurosyphilis should be treated with 12 to 24 million units of intravenous penicillin G daily for 10 to 14 days. Patients with known or suspected syphilis should be evaluated for the presence of neurosyphilis, which has an increasing incidence among HIV-infected individuals.[90]

Hematologic Involvement

Common hematologic complications may include anemia (present in up to 80% of patients), neutropenia, and thrombocytopenia. Hematopoieses may be adversely affected by HIV or other infections, tumors, or medications.[91] Coagulation disorders may be seen secondary to lupus anticoagulant, viral infections, or idiopathic etiologies.

Drug Reactions

Drug reactions are extremely common among HIV-infected patients for two reasons: first, they are commonly treated with a variety of drugs known to produce adverse effects in some individuals, and second, for unclear reasons, HIV-infected individuals often have more frequent or more severe reactions to commonly used medications. Dermatologic reactions are particularly common.[92,93] Antimicrobial drugs are most frequently implicated. Potential drug interactions should always be considered when prescribing new medications.[94] Drug reactions must *always* be considered as a possible cause of new symptoms. Reactions are numerous and current references should be consulted when drug reactions are suspected. Table 126-2 contains a brief summary of common drug reactions in the HIV-infected patient.

MANAGEMENT

Antiretroviral Therapy and Chemoprophylaxis

Antiretroviral therapy for HIV infection is constantly evolving, now requiring subspecialty training for infectious disease clinicians. The emergency physician should have a basic understanding of the classes of drugs available, the rationale for treatment, and the decision making involved in starting therapy and choosing drugs.

There are three classes of antiretroviral drugs. These include the nucleoside analog reverse transcriptase inhibitors (NRTIs), the nonnucleoside reverse transcriptase inhibitors (NNRTIs), and the protease inhibitors (PIs). Each group of agents independently interrupts the normal life cycle of the HIV. When used with appropriate timing and in combination, these agents have been shown to significantly delay progression of disease and prolong life.

The first drug demonstrated to have antiretroviral activity belonged to the NRTIs, which interfere with the viral enzyme reverse transcriptase. Several controlled trials showed zidovudine (Azidothymidine, AZT, Retrovir) to decrease the number and severity of opportunistic infections.[95-97] Although zidovudine was also found to decrease the rate of AIDS progression in patients with early symptomatic HIV infection, no significant change in survival was found.[98,99] This finding, coupled with the recognition of the emergence of drug resistance and the appearance of significant side effects, led to the development of other NRTIs. Combination therapy, employing zidovudine and another NRTI, resulted not only in prevention of disease progression, but also resulted in decreased mortality.[100] The Food and Drug Administration (FDA) has approved at least seven agents in this class, each with its own unique adverse effect profile. The most common side effects to be aware of include macrocytic anemia with zidovudine; distal sensory peripheral neuropathy with didanosine (Videx), stavudine (Zerit), and zalcitabine (Hivid); and pancreatitis with didanosine.[100] See Table 126-3 for a list of the more common agents and their side effects.

The NNRTIs bind to reverse transcriptase and block RNA-dependent and deoxyribonucleic acid (DNA)–dependent DNA polymerase activity. There are three NNRTIs currently available; the most commonly used are nevirapine (Viramune) and efavirenz (Sustiva). Target organisms have a high propensity for developing resistance to these agents, which are recommended for use only as part of a three-drug (or more) regimen. Rash is the most common side effect associated with the NNRTIs, with a small minority of patients (<5%) developing Stevens-Johnson syndrome.[101]

The enzyme HIV protease activates the HIV proteins, which are required for infectivity, by cleaving the inactive viral polypeptide precursors. PIs block this step, thus preventing HIV particles from becoming infectious. Five PIs are currently approved for clinical use in the United States. Introduction of this class of drugs is believed to be responsible in large part for the marked decline in mortality rates for HIV infection, which was first realized in 1996. PIs have also been associated with a high frequency of side effects. Short-term effects are principally GI (including nausea, diarrhea, and bloating); long-term effects are metabolic, the most common of which are hyperglycemia, hyperlipidemia, and fat redistribution.[33]

In May 1999 the Department of Health and Human Services published guidelines for use of antiretroviral agents in HIV-infected adults and adolescents.[102] In general, multiple goals of antiretroviral therapy include virologic, immunologic, clinical, and therapeutic goals. Since virologic (HIV RNA levels) and immunologic (CD4 cell count) parameters are independent predictors of clinical outcomes, therapeutic recommendations are based on both of these factors. The virologic goal is to reduce viral load as much as possible, halt disease progression, and prevent development of resistant HIV variants. Immunologic goals are to achieve both quantitative (CD4 cell count) and qualitative (pathogen-specific immune response) immune reconstitution. The principal clinical goals of therapy are to prolong and improve quality of life. The therapeutic goal is to achieve the other three goals by choosing a sequence of drugs that maintains therapeutic options, minimizes side effects, and optimizes the likelihood of patient compliance with the chosen regimen.

Expert consensus on the timing of initiation of HAART continues to evolve. For patients who have symptoms of immunosuppression (e.g., thrush, wasting, or any opportunistic infection) treatment is mandatory, regardless of viral load or CD4 cell count. Similarly for those with recognized primary HIV infection antiretroviral therapy is recommended, because early treatment is believed to decrease the number of infected cells, maintain or restore immune response, and perhaps lower the viral "set point," resulting in improved course of the disease.[100] Guidelines for asymptomatic patients are more controversial. Most experts recommend treatment for any patient with either a CD4 count of <500 cells/mm^3 or an HIV viral load of >5000 to 10,000 copies/ml.[103] However, while some practitioners choose to treat all patient who have a detectable viral load, others may choose to withhold therapy based on concerns associated with treatment complexity, adherence, side effects, resistance, and long-term complications.

Selection of an appropriate combination of drugs is also a complex issue for which no definitive recommendations exist. There are currently 14 FDA-approved drugs to choose from. Recommended first-line regimens include two NRTIs and a PI (or two PIs), or two NRTIs and an NNRTI. Again, therapy should be individualized with consideration to tolerability, adverse effect profile, likely drug-to-drug interactions, convenience, and likelihood of adherence. Recent advances in genotypic analysis of HIV strains will soon make selection based on drug resistance patterns a part of therapeutic decision making.

Chemoprophylaxis is directed toward preventing initial and subsequent episodes of certain opportunistic infections (i.e., primary and secondary prophylaxis). Emphasis on measures to prevent opportunistic infections is critical because of the inherent limitations of HAART and the recognition that these infections are a significant cause of morbidity and mortality in the HIV-positive population. CD4 cell count is the best predictor of the risk for opportunistic infections and is used most often in making decisions about initiating or maintaining antimicrobial prophylaxis. The most serious and common infections for which antimicrobial prophylaxis has been shown to be effective include PCP, toxoplasmosis, TB, and MAC. Specific timing and choice of agents are described in the clinical sections above; a more comprehensive review can be found in the recent Public Health Service and Infectious Disease Society Revised Guidelines for the Prevention of Opportunistic Infections.[34] The emergency physician can play a critical role in recognizing those patients who require initiation of chemoprophylaxis, and then working with the patient's primary care doctors or an infectious disease consultant to begin therapy.

Immunizations

In general, HIV-infected patients should not receive live-virus or live-bacteria vaccines. Response to immunizations may be variable among individual patients.[104] Pneumococcal vaccine is recommended for all patients over 2 years of age.[105] Influenza vaccine should be considered, although antibody response may be poor. Hepatitis B vaccination is indicated for patients at risk of exposure, although due to variable immune response follow-up serologic testing is indicated. Hepatitis A vaccination should also be considered because of increased risk of severe liver damage among patients previously infected with hepatitis B or C.[106] Measles-mumps-rubella (MMR) vaccination may be considered, because studies have not documented an increased incidence of adverse effects. If polio vaccine is indicated, enhanced inactivated polio vaccine may be administered. Although recent evidence suggests that the expression of HIV may be transiently increased by administration of tetanus toxoid, the clinical significance of this is unknown.[107] The potential risks and benefits should be considered when making decisions regarding immunization.

Ethical Considerations

Numerous ethical issues arise in the management of HIV-infected patients. General issues relevant to many patients include issues of confidentiality, discrimination, access to health care, justice, informed consent, respect for autonomy, and advance directives. Additionally, concerns specific to HIV infection may arise, such as questions related to prenatal testing, abortion, euthanasia, suicide, access to experimental therapies, and role in clinical trials. In general, commonly accepted principles of medical ethics may be applied, which include principles of beneficence, nonmaleficence, respect for autonomy, and justice.[108] Additionally, codes of ethical conduct developed by the American College of Emergency Physicians (ACEP) and the Society for

Academic Emergency Medicine (SAEM) may be of general guidance.[109,110]

Testing of patients to detect HIV has some controversial aspects. Routine HIV testing initiated in the ED is often not appropriate because of difficulties assuring appropriate pretest and posttest counseling, and confidentiality. However, recommendations and referral for testing are often indicated for patients with risk factors or clinical evidence of HIV infection. Each institution should have appropriate mechanisms arranged for these referrals.

Occupational exposures to blood and body fluids may necessitate testing of patients and health care workers in the ED to expedite initiation of antiretroviral therapy. In such cases, institutions should implement uniform policies and procedures for testing, which assure pretest and posttest counseling and ensure confidentiality of results.

Confidentiality of ED patients' identities and diagnoses is of paramount importance, particularly for HIV-infected patients for whom there may be numerous clinical, social, psychological, career, and insurability effects of breached confidentiality.

Public health responsibilities may at times override the duty of the physician to maintain strict confidentiality. AIDS is a reportable disease in most states, and state guidelines for reporting should be followed as a public health measure, even if this breaches confidentiality (such as in cases of child abuse, gunshot wounds, or other infectious diseases). In addition, the physician who is aware of potentially contagious practices of an infected individual has an obligation to counsel the individual. Additionally, infected patients should be encouraged to share knowledge of their disease state with sexual or needle-sharing partners. In many states the physician has the discretion to inform public health officials of practices, to allow partners potentially at risk to be informed.[111]

The potential value of aggressive interventions in critical care settings must be determined on an individual case basis. Some clinicians believe that in the advanced stages of AIDS, resuscitative measures are not appropriate because of the uniformly poor prognosis. Many patients may agree as they approach the terminal stages of their disease. Appropriate advance directives should be completed prior to entry into the resuscitation setting. However, many patients fail to complete advance directives. Decisions regarding the withholding of extraordinary resuscitation efforts may be difficult to make in the ED because of insufficient information about the wishes, disease state, and prognosis of an individual patient, and the judgment and intentions of the primary care and consulting physicians. Although some ethicists argue against the excessive use of extensive resource allocation for this class of patients,[112] emergency medical decisions should be largely unbiased and based on the appropriate factors relevant to the individual case. As with all patients with clinical indications for invasive monitoring or interventions, decisions should be made based on factors including the patient's wishes (if known) or a surrogate's assessment of the patient's wishes, expected outcome, and potential risks of the intervention. Interventions should not be withheld or discontinued based merely on the diagnosis of AIDS.

If certain diagnostic and therapeutic interventions are withheld, particular attention should be paid to ensure adequate control of pain and other symptoms. Psychosocial, religious, and cultural needs should also be addressed.

The courts have considered increasing numbers and varieties of cases regarding the treatment of AIDS and HIV-related illness. The AIDS Litigation Project (a review of cases) has shown increasing numbers of cases of litigation involving areas of AIDS education, blood supply, epidemiologic surveillance, criminal law, public places, products, fraud, torts, court system, family law, confidentiality, prisons, military, fear of exposure, homelessness, and discrimination.[113]

In general, the same ethical principles of respect for autonomy, beneficence, nonmaleficence, justice, confidentiality, communication, informed consent, and research ethics should be honored when treating HIV-infected patients, as with all ED patients.

Emergency Department Disposition

When there is doubt about diagnostic or management options, consultation with specialists is appropriate. Consultations with an infectious disease specialist, neurologist, psychiatrist, AIDS specialist, and others may be indicated. Although symptomatic patients currently are predominantly cared for by AIDS specialists, the increasing numbers of symptomatic patients will shift the focus of primary care to nonspecialists.

Disposition decisions for HIV-infected patients are based, as for any patient, on clinical condition, availability of outpatient resources, and ability to arrange adequate follow-up observation. Any patient to be discharged must demonstrate the ability for self-care or have sufficient in-home assistance available. In the AIDS population, particular attention should be given to ability to ambulate and tolerate oral intake, as well as availability of timely and appropriate medical follow-up.

Although the AIDS epidemic has raised concerns regarding the economic impact of the disease, financial considerations should not be a factor in determining management or disposition. Guidelines for admission and discharge are given in Box 126-3.

Box 126-3 Considerations for Disposition Decisions for HIV-Infected Patients

Conditions Suggesting Admission

New presentation of fever of unknown origin
Hypoxemia (worse than baseline) (Pao_2 <60 mm Hg)
Suspected *Pneumocystis carinii* pneumonia
Suspected tuberculosis
New central nervous system symptoms
Intractable diarrhea
Suicidal
Suspected cytomegalovirus retinitis
Ophthalmicus zoster
Cachexia or weakness
Unable to care for self or receive adequate care
Unable to assure appropriate follow-up

Suggested Conditions for Considering Discharge

Normal or baseline vital signs
Stable medical condition
Able to take oral medications and is not orthostatic
Follow-up and referral arranged
Patient or caregiver understands instructions
Patient, home caregiver, or hospice able to care for patient

PRECAUTIONS AND POSTEXPOSURE PROPHYLAXIS (PEP) FOR HEALTH CARE WORKERS

Health care workers are often exposed to the blood and body secretions of HIV-infected patients or of other individuals who are at high risk of harboring HIV and other infectious pathogens. The overall risk of having any occupational blood exposure is not insignificant, with more than half of emergency physicians reporting at least one occupational exposure during a 2-year period.[114]

The overall risk of contracting HIV remains small. Worldwide a total of 94 cases of documented occupationally acquired HIV infection and 170 cases of possible occupationally acquired infection have been reported as of September 1997. Fifty-two of the documented cases and 114 of the possible cases occurred in the United States, with the majority of cases occurring in nurses following percutaneous exposure.[115] The efficacy of transmission is estimated at 0.25% to 0.3% via percutaneous exposure and <0.1% for mucocutaneous exposure.

The proportion of patients infected with a pathogen varies by geographic setting and practice locale. One recent survey conducted at a Baltimore inner city hospital found that up to 11% of patients were infected with HIV, and nearly 24% were infected with HIV or hepatitis B or C.[6] It is important to note, however, that numerous studies have demonstrated that a substantial number of patients in the ED have unsuspected HIV infection, and HIV seroreactivity cannot be accurately predicted even with the aid of risk factor assessment.[116,117]

Numerous studies have demonstrated that health care workers can significantly reduce their risk of exposure to blood-borne pathogens by following universal precautions. CDC guidelines for universal precautions include the use of protective equipment (including gloves, gown, mask, and eye protection) for any situation in which the potential for exposure exists. A recent study showed that protective equipment is indicated for most ED procedures, including examination of the bleeding patient, chest tube placement, LP, and other commonly performed procedures in which contact with blood or body fluids is likely.[118] Although significant improvement has been made in emergency physicians' observance of universal precautions, recent studies indicate that continued education and improvements in work environments are required to ensure consistent compliance.[118,119]

HIV transmission by health care workers to patients appears to be extremely rare. There have been only seven cases to date, six of which occurred from a single dentist's practice,[120] and one from a patient who apparently acquired HIV during orthopedic surgery. At this time, routine screening of health care workers is not indicated.[117]

The CDC provides explicit guidelines for PEP for occupational exposure to HIV.[121] These recommendations are based on a retrospective case-control study of needle stick injuries from an HIV-infected source to a health care worker. Results showed a 79% reduction in HIV transmission, after controlling for other risk factors for HIV transmission among subjects who had received zidovudine prophylaxis.[122] Other studies have demonstrated decreased rates of perinatal transmission for women who were given zidovudine during pregnancy, labor, and delivery.[123]

HIV PEP decision-making is a two-step process, requiring categorization of the exposure risk and HIV status of the source. Higher risk exposures associated with an increased likelihood of transmission include deep injuries, visible blood on a device, and injuries sustained when placing a catheter in a vein or artery. High-risk sources are those patients with late stages of HIV infection, which would usually reflect increased viral load and increased infectivity.[124]

Current guidelines advise case-by-case determination of the risk of the exposure in order to determine whether PEP should be recommended, offered, or not recommended. CDC recommends PEP only for percutaneous exposures that involve large volumes of blood or blood containing high HIV titers. PEP is offered for most other percutaneous exposures, and for mucous membrane exposures involving visible blood, tissue, or certain potentially infectious fluids such as semen or vaginal secretions. The CDC does not recommend PEP for other mucus membrane exposures or for the great majority of cutaneous exposures. Current recommendations include administration of combination therapy with zidovudine and lamivudine (3TC); for highest risk exposures, a three-drug regimen including protease inhibitors (e.g., indinavir) is advised, although there is no direct evidence to support this practice. It is recommended that PEP be initiated as soon as possible after the exposure; although no definitive data exist, guidelines suggest starting treatment within 1 to 2 hours and generally restrict therapy to those who seek treatment within 36 hours of exposure. Antiretroviral therapy may be given after 36 hours postexposure in particularly high-risk incidents. Duration of PEP is 4 weeks. Constitutional and GI side effects may be significant and often lead to early termination of treatment.

Because early initiation of PEP is critical for efficacy, the ED is often the site of referral for patients, because services are available at any time. Many EDs are developing protocols and starter treatment packets for PEP, but choice of intervention and regimen is usually best accomplished in consultation with an infectious disease specialist and the patient's primary physician, because this allows arrangement for appropriate medical follow-up and counseling.

Recent interest in the use of PEP for nonoccupational exposure has emerged, because the probability of HIV transmission by certain sexual or injection drug exposures is of the same order of magnitude as percutaneous exposures, for which the CDC recommends PEP.[125] For most cases in which the individual is likely to have continuing risk for exposure, recommendations consist of referral to risk-reduction programs rather than offering PEP. Recommendations regarding the use of PEP for sporadic exposures remain in flux.[126] The CDC is an invaluable resource for information on both occupational and nonoccupational exposures, providing a 24-hour hotline for physicians who need assistance with decision making (1-888-448-4911).

KEY CONCEPTS

- The seroprevalence of HIV and AIDS among ED patients in large metropolitan areas is 2% to 11%. Many of these are undiagnosed cases, so compliance of ED staff with universal precautions is extremely important.
- Acute HIV seroconversion syndrome commonly follows exposure by 2 to 6 weeks and presents with common, nonspecific symptoms such as fever, fatigue, diarrhea, weight loss, adenopathy, and rash. Patients fitting this profile should be screened for HIV risk factors and appropriately referred for HIV testing.
- PCP is the most common opportunistic infection in AIDS patients. It often presents as progressive dyspnea on

exertion associated with a nonproductive cough. The chest x-ray commonly shows a diffuse interstitial infiltrate, but may be normal. Blood gas analysis usually reveals hypoxemia that is often more pronounced after exercise.

- CNS disease is common in HIV-infected patients and is caused by the disease itself, opportunistic infections, and malignancy. An approach to evaluating HIV-infected patients with severe or prolonged headache, altered mentation, new-onset seizures, or focal neurologic deficits is shown in Figure 126-1.
- The evaluation and management of HIV-infected patients with acute symptoms are often complex and best accomplished either in the hospital or in the outpatient setting with close follow-up. Conditions suggesting admission are listed in Box 126-3.

REFERENCES

1. Centers for Disease Control and Prevention: 1993 revised classification system for HIV infection and expanded surveillance case definition for AIDS among adolescents and adults, *MMWR* 41(RR-17):1, 1993.
2. Joint United Nations Programme on HIV/AIDS: *AIDS epidemic update: December, 1999,* Available at www.unaids.org.
3. Palella FJ et al: Declining morbidity and mortality among patients with advanced human immunodeficiency virus, *N Engl J Med* 338:853, 1998.
4. Centers for Disease Control and Prevention: *HIV/AIDS Surveillance Report,* Available at *www.cdc.gov/nchstp/hiv_aids/stats/hasrlink.htm.*
5. Centers for Disease Control and Prevention: HIV/AIDS Surveillance Report, 8:1, 1996.
6. Kelen GD et al: Trends in human immunodeficiency (HIV) virus infection among a patient population in an inner-city emergency department: implications for emergency department screening programs for HIV infection, *Clin Infect Dis* 21:867, 1995.
7. Centers for Disease Control and Prevention: Transmission of HIV possibly associated with exposure of mucous membrane to contaminated blood, *MMWR* 46:620, 1997.
8. Carpenter CC et al: Antiretroviral therapy in adults: updated recommendations of the International AIDS Society—USA Panel, *JAMA* 283:3, 381.
9. Sloand EM et al: HIV testing: State of the art, *JAMA* 266:2861, 1991.
10. Busch MP, Satten GA: Time course of viremia and antibody seroconversion following human immunodeficiency virus exposure, *Am J Med* 102:117, 1997.
11. Roy MJ et al: Absence of true seroreversion of HIV-1 antibody in seroreactive individuals, *JAMA* 269:2876, 1993.
12. Identification of HIV-1 group O infection—Los Angeles County, California, *MMWR* 45:561-565, 1996.
13. Irwin K et al: Performance characteristics of a rapid HIV antibody assay in a hospital with a high prevalence of HIV infection, *Ann Intern Med* 125:471, 1996.
14. Koster, FT: Infection in the HIV-positive patient. In Brillman JC, Quenzer RW, editors: *Infectious diseases in emergency medicine,* Philadelphia, 1998, Lippincott-Raven.
15. Meyer KB, Pauker SG: Screening for HIV: can we afford the false positive rate? *N Engl J Med* 317:238, 1987.
16. Celum CL, Coombs RW: Indeterminate HIV-1 Western blots: implications and considerations for widespread HIV testing, *J Gen Intern Med* 7:640, 1992.
17. Moran GJ: ED management of blood and body fluid exposures, *Ann Emerg Med* 31:47, 1997.
18. Irwin K et al: Performance characteristics of a rapid HIV antibody assay in a hospital with a high prevalence of HIV infection, *Ann Intern Med* 125:471, 1996.
19. Kelen GD, Shahan JB, Quinn TC: ED-based HIV screening and counseling: experience with rapid and standard serologic testing, *Ann Emerg Med* 33:147-155, 1999.
20. Kelen GD et al: Feasibility of an emergency department-based risk-targeted voluntary HIV screening program, *Ann Emerg Med* 27:687-692, 1996.
21. Redfield RR et al: The Walter Reed staging classification for HTLV-III/LAV infection, *N Engl J Med* 314:131, 1986.
22. Stein DS et al: CD4+ lymphocyte cell enumeration for prediction of clinical course of human immunodeficiency virus disease: a review, *J Infect Dis* 165:352, 1992.
23. Phillips AN et al: Serial CD4 lymphocyte counts and development of AIDS, *Lancet* 337:389, 1991.
24. Tindall B et al: Characterization of the acute clinical illness associated with human immunodeficiency virus infection, *Arch Intern Med* 148:945, 1988.
25. Kinloch-de Loes S et al: Symptomatic primary infection due to human immunodeficiency virus type I: review of 31 cases, *Clin Infect Dis* 17:59, 1993.
26. Pantaleo G et al: Studies in subjects with long-term nonprogressive human immunodeficiency virus infection, *N Engl J Med* 332:209, 1995.
27. Saah AJ et al: Predictors of the risk of development of acquired immunodeficiency syndrome within 24 months among gay men seropositive for human immunodeficiency virus type 1: a report from the multicenter AIDS cohort study, *Am J Epidemiol* 135:1147, 1992.
28. Miller V et al: Relations among CD4 lymphocyte count nadir, antiretroviral therapy, and HIV-1 disease progression: results from the EuroAIDS study, *Ann Intern Med* 130:570, 1999.
29. De Wolf F et al: Numbers of CD4+ cells and the levels of core antigens of antibodies to the human immunodeficiency virus as predictors of AIDS among seropositive homosexual men, *J Infect Dis* 158:615, 1988.
30. Fahey JL et al: The prognostic value of cellular and serologic markers in infection with human immunodeficiency virus type 1, *N Engl J Med* 322:166, 1990.
31. MacDonell KB et al: Predicting progression to AIDS: combined usefulness of CD4 lymphocyte counts and p24 antigenemia, *Am J Med* 89:706, 1989.
32. Lin HJ et al: Multicenter evaluation of quantification methods for plasma human immunodeficiency virus type 1 RNA, *J Infect Dis* 170:553, 1994.
33. Hovanessian HC: New developments in the treatment of HIV disease: an overview, *Ann Emerg Med* 33:546, 1999.
34. US Department of Health and Human Services, Panel on Clinical Practices for Treatment of HIV Infection: *Guidelines for the use of antiretroviral agents in HIV-infected adults and adolescents,* Available at: *www.hivatis.org.*
35. Palestine AG et al: Ophthalmic involvement in acquired immunodeficiency syndrome, *Ophthalmology* 91:1092, 1984.
36. Murray JF et al: Pulmonary complications of the acquired immunodeficiency syndrome: report of the Second National Heart, Lung and Blood Institute Workshop, *Am Rev Respir Dis* 135:504, 1987.
37. Masur H et al: Advances in pneumocystis pneumonia: from bench to clinic, *Ann Intern Med* 111:813, 1989.
38. Goodman PC: *Pneumocystis carinii* pneumonia, *J Thorac Imaging* 6:16, 1991.
39. Woolfenden JM et al: Acquired immunodeficiency syndrome: GA-67 citrate imaging, *Radiology* 162:383, 1987.
40. Hartman B et al: *Pneumocystis carinii* pneumonia in the acquired immunodeficiency syndrome (AIDS): diagnosis with bronchial brushings, biopsy, and bronchoalveolar lavage, *Chest* 87:603, 1985.
41. Ng VL et al: Rapid detection of *Pneumocystis carinii* using a direct fluorescent monoclonal antibody stain, *J Clin Microbiol* 128:2228, 1990.
42. Masur H: Drug therapy: prevention and treatment of pneumocystis pneumonia, *N Engl J Med* 327:1853, 1992.
43. NIH-UC Expert Panel for Corticosteroids as Adjunctive Therapy for Pneumocystis Pneumonia: Consensus statement for use of corticosteroids as adjunctive therapy for pneumocystis pneumonia in AIDS, *N Engl J Med* 323:1500, 1990.
44. Gagnon S et al: Corticosteroids as adjunctive therapy for severe *Pneumocystis carinii* pneumonia in the acquired immunodeficiency syndrome: a double-blind placebo-controlled trial, *N Engl J Med* 323:1444, 1990.
45. Gordino FM et al: Adverse reactions to trimethoprim-sulfamethoxazole in patients with acquired immunodeficiency syndrome, *Ann Intern Med* 100:945, 1984.

46. Kovacs JA, Masur H: Prophylaxis against opportunistic infections in patients with human immunodeficiency virus infection, *N Engl J Med* 342:1416, 2000.
47. Decker CF, Masur H: Pneumocystis and other protozoa. In DeVita VT et al, editors: *AIDS: etiology, diagnosis, treatment and prevention,* ed 4, Philadelphia, 1997, Lippincott-Raven.
48. Braun MM et al: Increasing incidence of tuberculosis in a prison inmate population: association with HIV infection, *JAMA* 261:393, 1989.
49. Centers for Disease Control: Summary of notifiable diseases, United States, 1993, *MMWR* 42:1, 1994.
50. Rigsby MO, Friedland G: Tuberculosis and human immunodeficiency virus infection. In DeVita VT et al, editors: *AIDS: etiology, diagnosis, treatment and prevention,* ed 4, Philadelphia, 1997, Lippincott-Raven.
51. Keiper MD et al: CD4 T lymphocyte count and the radiographic presentation of pulmonary tuberculosis, *Chest* 107:74, 1995.
52. Catanzaro A et al: The role of clinical suspicion in evaluating a new diagnostic test for active tuberculosis, *JAMA* 283:639, 2000.
53. Pitchenis AE, Fertel D: Tuberculosis and nontuberculous mycobacterial disease, *Med Clin North Am* 76:121, 1992.
54. Goble M et al: Treatment of 171 patients with pulmonary tuberculosis resistant to isoniazid and rifampin, *N Engl J Med* 328:527, 1993.
55. Frieden TR et al: The emergence of drug-resistant tuberculosis in New York City, *N Engl J Med* 328:521, 1993.
56. Havlir DV, Barnes PN: Tuberculosis in persons with human immunodeficiency virus infection, *N Engl J Med* 340:367, 1999.
57. Lanska DJ: Epidemiology of human immunodeficiency virus infection and associated neurologic illness, *Semin Neurol* 19:105-111, 1999.
58. Rothman RE et al: A decision guideline for emergency department utilization of noncontrast head CT in HIV-infected patients, *Acad Emerg Med* 6:1010, 1999.
59. Barber CJ et al: Clinical utility of cranial CT in HIV positive and AIDS patients with neurological disease, *Clinical Radiology* 42:164, 1990.
60. Post MJD et al: Cranial CT in acquired immunodeficiency syndrome: spectrum of disease and optimal contrast enhancement technique, *AJR* 145:929, 1989.
61. Zuger A et al: Cryptococcal infections in patients with acquired immunodeficiency syndrome, *Am J Med* 81:19, 1986.
62. Davis LE: Fungal infections of the central nervous system, *Neurol Clin* 17:761, 1999.
63. Navia BA et al: Cerebral toxoplasmosis complicating the acquired immune deficiency syndrome: clinical and neuropathological findings in 27 patients, *Ann Neurol* 19:224, 1986.
64. Haverkos HW: Assessment of therapy for toxoplasma encephalitis, *Am J Med* 82:907, 1987.
65. Murri R: A randomized trial of cotrimoxazole and dapsone-pyrimethamine for primary prophylaxis of *P. carinii* pneumonia (PCP) and toxoplasmosis encephalitis (TE), *Int Conf AIDS* 12:298, 1998.
66. Katz MH et al: Progression to AIDS in HIV-infected homosexual and bisexual men with hairy leukoplakia and oral candidiasis, *AIDS* 6:95, 1992.
67. Klein RS et al: Oral candidiasis in high-risk patients as the initial manifestation of the acquired immunodeficiency syndrome, *N Engl J Med* 311:354, 1984.
68. Masouredis CM et al: Prevalence of HIV-associated periodontitis and gingivitis in HIV-infected patients attending an AIDS clinic, *J Acquir Immune Defic Syndr* 5:479, 1992.
69. Bonacini M, Laine LA: Esophageal disease in patients with AIDS, *Gastrointest Endosc Clin N Am* 8:811-821, 1998.
70. Manfredi R et al: Fluconazole as prophylaxis against fungal infection in patients with advanced HIV infection, *Arch Intern Med* 157:64, 1997.
71. Powderly WG et al: A randomized trial comparing fluconazole with clotrimazole troches for the prevention of fungal infections in patients with advanced human immunodeficiency virus infection, *N Engl J Med* 332:700, 1995.
72. White AC et al: Paromomycin for cryptosporidiosis in AIDS: a prospective double-blind trial, *J Infect Dis* 170:419, 1994.
73. Bissuel R et al: Paromomycin: an effective treatment for cryptosporidial diarrhea in patients with AIDS, *Clin Infect Dis* 18:447, 1994.
74. Centers for Disease Control and Prevention Update: Acquired immunodeficiency syndrome—United States, *MMWR* 35:757, 1986.
75. Chachoua A et al: Prognostic factors and staging classification of patients with epidemic Kaposi's sarcoma, *J Clin Oncol* 7:774, 1989.
76. Redfield RR et al: The Walter Reed staging classification for HTLV-III/LAV infection, *N Engl J Med* 314:131, 1986.
77. Safai B: Kaposi's sarcoma and acquired immunodeficiency syndrome. In DeVita VT et al, editors: *AIDS: etiology, diagnosis, treatment and prevention,* ed 4, Philadelphia, 1997, Lippincott-Raven.
78. Tyring S et al: Famciclovir for the treatment of acute herpes zoster: effects on acute disease and postherpetic neuralgia: a randomized, double-blind, placebo-controlled trial. Collaborative Famciclovir Herpes Zoster Study Group, *Ann Intern Med* 123:89, 1995.
79. Berger TG: Dermatologic manifestations of HIV infection. In Cohen PT et al, editors: *The AIDS knowledge base,* Waltham, Mass, 1990, Massachusetts Medical Society.
80. Straus SE et al: Oral acyclovir to suppress recurring herpes simplex virus infections in immunodeficient patients, *Ann Intern Med* 100:522, 1984.
81. Henderly DE, Jampol LM: Diagnosis and treatment of cytomegalovirus retinitis, *J Acquir Immune Defic Syndr* 1:S6, 1991.
82. Whitcup SM: Cytomegalovirus retinitis in the era of highly active antiretroviral therapy, *JAMA* 283:653, 2000.
83. Walmsley S et al: Treatment of cytomegalovirus retinitis with trisodium phosphonoformate hexahydrate (foscarnet), *J Infect Dis* 157:569, 1988.
84. Martin DF et al: Treatment of cytomegalovirus retinitis with an intraocular sustained release ganciclovir implant: a randomized controlled clinical trial, *Arch Ophthalmol* 112:1531, 1994.
85. Dhillon B et al: Intravitreal sustained-release ganciclovir implantation to control cytomegalovirus retinitis in AIDS, *Int J STD AIDS* 9:227-230, 1998.
86. Yunis N, Stone VE: Cardiac manifestations of HIV/AIDS: a review of disease spectrum and clinical management, *J Acquir Immune Defic Syndr* 18:145, 1998.
87. Milei J et al: Cardiac involvement in acquired immunodeficiency syndrome—a review to push action, *Clin Cardiol* 21:465-472, 1998.
88. Smith MC et al: Effect of corticosteroid therapy on human immunodeficiency virus-associated nephropathy, *Am J Med* 97:145, 1994.
89. Lyketsos CG et al: Depressive symptoms as predictors of medical outcomes in HIV infection, *JAMA* 270:2563, 1993.
90. Musher DM et al: Effect of human immunodeficiency virus (HIV) infection on the course of syphilis and on the response to treatment, *Ann Intern Med* 113:872, 1990.
91. Moses A et al: The influence of human immunodeficiency virus-I on hematopoiesis, *Blood* 91:1479, 1998.
92. Harb GE et al: Pharmacoepidemiology of adverse drug reactions in hospitalized patients with human immunodeficiency virus disease, *J Acquir Immune Def Syndr* 6:919, 1993.
93. Hennessy S et al: Predicting cutaneous hypersensitivity reactions to cotrimoxazole in HIV-infected individuals receiving primary *Pneumocystis carinii* pneumonia prophylaxis, *J Gen Intern Med* 10:380, 1995.
94. Tseng AL, Foisy M: Management of drug interactions in patients with HIV, *Ann Pharmacother* 31:1040, 1997.
95. Fischl MA et al: A randomized controlled trial of a reduced dose of zidovudine in patients with the acquired immunodeficiency syndrome, *N Engl J Med* 323:1009, 1990.
96. Kinloch-de Loes S et al: A controlled trial of zidovudine in primary human immunodeficiency virus infection, *N Engl J Med* 333:408, 1995.
97. Volberding PA et al: A comparison of immunity with deferred zidovudine therapy for asymptomatic HIV-infected adults with CD4 counts of 500 or more per cubic millimeter, *N Engl J Med* 333:401, 1995.
98. Hamilton JD et al: A controlled trial of early versus late treatment with zidovudine in symptomatic human immunodeficiency virus infection, *N Engl J Med* 326:437, 1992.
99. The Delta Coordinating Committee: Delta: a randomized control trial comparing combinations of zidovudine plus didanosine or zalcitabine with zidovudine alone in HIV-infected individuals, *Lancet* 348:283, 1996.

100. Carpenter CC et al: Antiretroviral therapy in adults: updated recommendations of the International AIDS Society—USA Panel, *JAMA* 283:381, 2000.
101. Warren KJ et al: Nevirapine-associated Stevens-Johnson syndrome, *Lancet* 351:567, 1998.
102. US Public Health Service (USPHS) and Infectious Disease Society of America (IDSA): 1999 USPHS/IDSA guidelines for the prevention of opportunistic infections in persons infected with human immunodeficiency virus, *MMWR* 48(RR-10):1, 1999.
103. Wolfe PR: Practical approaches to HIV therapy: recommendations for the year 2000, *Post Grad Med* 107:1, 2000.
104. Cohen PT: Immunization of HIV-infected persons. In Cohen PT et al, editors: *The AIDS knowledge base,* Waltham, Mass, 1990, Massachusetts Medical Society.
105. Centers for Disease Control: Prevention of pneumococcal disease: recommendations of the Advisory Committee on Immunization Practices (ACIP), *MMWR* 46(RR-8):1-24, 1997.
106. Vento S et al: Fulminant hepatitis associated with hepatitis A virus superinfection in patients with chronic hepatitis C, *N Engl J Med* 338:286, 1998.
107. Stanley SK et al: Effect of immunization with a common recall antigen on viral expression in patients infected with human immunodeficiency virus type 1, *N Engl J Med* 334:1222, 1996.
108. Beauchamp T, Childress J: *Principles of biomedical ethics,* ed 4, New York, 1994, Oxford University Press.
109. American College of Emergency Physicians: *Code of ethics for emergency physicians,* Dallas, Tex, 1997, American College of Emergency Physicians.
110. Larkin GL: A code of conduct for academic emergency medicine, *Acad Emerg Med* 6:45, 1999.
111. Lo B: Ethical dilemmas in HIV infection: what have we learned? *Law Med Health Care* 20:92, 1992.
112. Casarett DJ, Lantos JD: Have we treated AIDS too well? Rationing and the future of AIDS exceptionalism, *Ann Intern Med* 128:756, 1998.
113. Gostin LO: The AIDS litigation project: a national review of court and Human Rights Commission decisions I. The social impact of AIDS, *JAMA* 263:1961, 1990.
114. Goldberg R et al: Antibody titers to hepatitis B surface antigen among vaccinated emergency physicians: three years' experience with a wellness booth, *Ann Emerg Med* 33:156, 1999.
115. Ippolito G et al: Occupational human immunodeficiency virus infection in health care workers: worldwide cases through September 1997, 28:365-383, 1999.
116. Marcus R et al: Frequency of emergency care provider's contact with blood of patients infected with human immunodeficiency virus, *Ann Emerg Med* 19:454, 1990 (abstract).
117. Phillips KA et al: The cost-effectiveness of HIV testing of physicians and dentists in the United States, *JAMA* 271:851, 1994.
118. Kelen GD et al: Determinants of emergency department procedure- and condition-specific universal (barrier) protection requirements for optimal provider protection, *Ann Emerg Med* 25:743, 1995.
119. Lee CH et al: Occupational exposures to blood among emergency medicine residents, *Acad Emerg Med* 6:1036, 1999.
120. Ciesielski C et al: Transmission of human immunodeficiency virus in a dental practice, *Ann Int Med* 116:798, 1992.
121. Centers for Disease Control and Prevention: Guidelines for the use of antiretroviral agents in HIV-infected adults and adolescents, *MMWR* 46(RR-5):43, 1997.
122. Cardo DM et al: A case-control study of HIV seroconversion in health care workers after percutaneous exposure. Centers for Disease Control and Prevention Needlestick Surveillance Group, *N Engl J Med* 337:1485, 1997.
123. Conner EM et al: Reduction of maternal-infant transmission of human immunodeficiency virus type 1 with zidovudine treatment, *N Engl J Med* 331:1173, 1994.
124. Moran GJ: Emergency department management of blood and body fluid exposures, *Ann Emerg Med* 35:47, 2000.
125. Katz MH, Gerberding JL: Postexposure treatment of people exposed to the human immunodeficiency virus through sexual contract of infection-drug use, *N Engl J Med* 336:1097, 1997.
126. Lurie P et al: Postexposure prophylaxis after nonoccupational HIV exposure: clinical, ethical and policy considerations, *JAMA* 280:1769, 1998.

127 Parasites

Bruce M. Becker
John D. Cahill
W. Brian Gibler

PERSPECTIVE

The Challenge

Parasitology, once a subject of eclectic interest to the emergency physician, has become an increasingly important problem in the United States. During the last few decades there has been a dramatic increase in the immigration of individuals from Southeast Asia, Central and South America, and Africa into urban and rural regions of the United States and Europe. These people have been fleeing from civil unrest, war, economic hardship, and environmental destruction in their own countries. Many of these emigrating populations have come from areas where parasitic infections are endemic. Business and adventure travel, including ecotourism, frequently transports immunologically innocent and vulnerable hosts to sites rich in parasitic disease (Figure 127-1). The prevalence of acquired immunodeficiency syndrome (AIDS) has increased geometrically in the world population. Most parasitic illness is more devastating clinically and more cryptic in symptomatology in patients suffering from AIDS. Patients with AIDS who travel to countries where parasitic illness is endemic are at higher risk of contracting these illnesses. Patients with AIDS who emigrate or travel to the United States or Europe may harbor a host of devastating parasitic illnesses. There also continues to be a significant prevalence of endemic parasitic disease in many rural areas of the southeastern and southwestern United States and in some parts of Europe. Patients with parasitic illness may seek treatment initially in the ED.

The diagnosis and treatment of parasitic disease can be quite satisfying; correct diagnosis and chemotherapy given

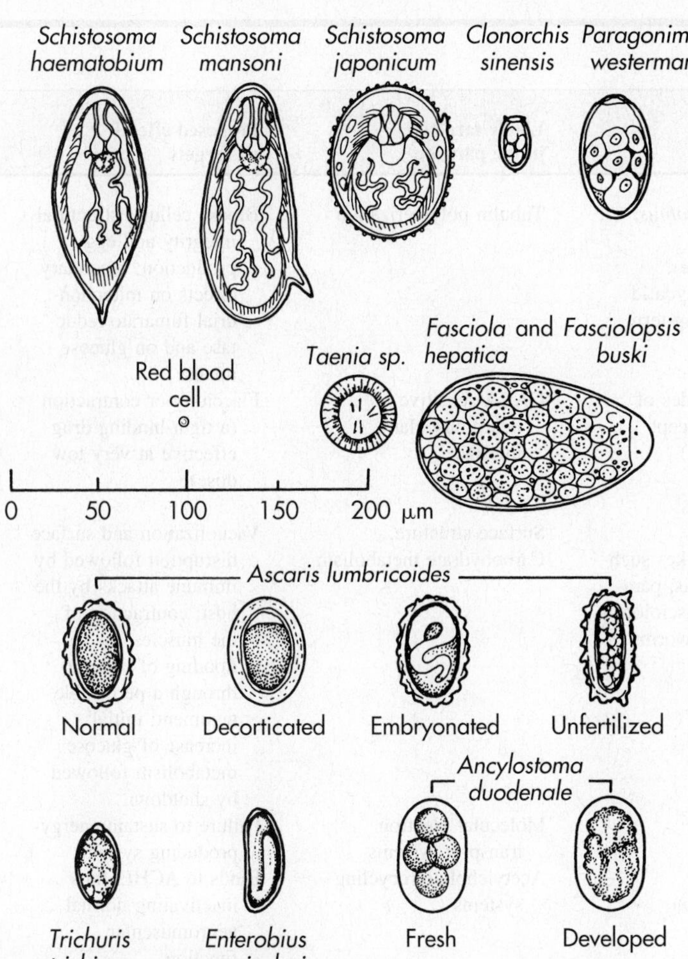

Figure 127-1. **Eggs of major parasitic worms causing disease in humans.**

early in the course of illness often result in rapid recovery. However, mismanagement of parasitic illness can be disastrous. As William Osler often quipped, "Early in the course of disease, diagnosis is difficult and treatment easy; late in the course, diagnosis is easy and treatment difficult." His wisdom applies strongly to parasitic illness, which often begins insidiously and pursues a long, chronic course resulting eventually in end-organ damage and severe morbidity and mortality in the host. The emergency physician must play detective, obtaining a thorough travel history, performing a detailed physical examination, ordering appropriate laboratory studies, and comparing these findings with a strong understanding of the basic life cycles of parasites, their usual and unusual presentations, and the intersecting geography of the organism and host.

The ED is a rogue's gallery of symptoms and signs. To maximize utility for the emergency physician, we have chosen to focus on patient clinical pictures, highlighting affected organ systems and associated symptoms. Some life cycles of important parasites will be briefly discussed. This practical approach will be most useful in the treatment of the sick patient being evaluated in the ED. We suggest identifying and reviewing the appropriate signs and symptoms section for a specific ED patient, and then looking up the pharmacologic interventions in Table 127-1. For readers interested in more detail about individual parasites, we strongly suggest the classic text, Bell's *Tropical Medicine,*[1] or Guerrant, Walker, and Weller's *Tropical Infectious Diseases.*[2]

The Travel History

Parasitic illness should be kept in the differential diagnosis of almost every complaint imaginable, particularly in patients who have recently spent time in areas of the world with endemic parasitic illnesses. As a result, a travel history should be included in the evaluation of most, if not all, ED patients (Table 127-2).

For patients with a recent travel history, the following questions should be asked: What were the exact dates of travel? What countries did the patient visit? How much time was spent in each country? What was the patient doing in the country and where were they living? Were they tourists, adventure travelers, workers? Did they stay in cities, rural villages? Were they sleeping in hotels or tents? Did they engage in protected or unprotected intercourse? What did they eat and drink? Did they receive pretravel immunizations? Did they take prophylactic medications and comply with the regimen? Was mosquito repellent and netting scrupulously employed? Do they have underlying chronic medical problems? What medications do they take? When did symptoms start?

For patients who recently immigrated to the United States, the following questions should be asked: When did the patient arrive and from where? What illnesses, both acute and chronic, had they had previously while living in their country of origin? What treatment did they receive there? If they were refugees, what countries did they pass through and what were the living conditions (especially relevant for patients who

Table 127-1. Drug Classes and Modes of Action

Type of drug	Specific example of drug(s)	Useful in the treatment of	Likely target(s) in the parasite	Proposed effects on targets
Anthelmintics	Thiabendazole Mebendazole Albendazole	*Ascaris, Enterobius,* hookworm, *Strongyloides, Trichuris,* hydatid disease (long-term therapy)	Tubulin polymerization	Blocks cellular structural integrity and egg production; secondary effects on mitochondrial fumarate reductase and on glucose uptake
	Ivermectin* (Stromectol)	Many nematodes of humans (except hookworms) Filariasis Onchocerciasis	GABA-sensitive neuromuscular interface	Flaccidity or contraction (a tight-binding drug effective at very low dose)
Trematodicides	Praziquantel (Biltricide)	Schistosomes Most other flukes such as clonorchis, paragonimus, fasciolopsis (many tapeworms of humans)	Surface structure; Carbohydrate metabolism	Vacuolization and surface disruption followed by immune attacks by the host; contraction of the muscles due to flooding of calcium through a permeable tegument; initial increase of glucose metabolism followed by shutdown
Antiprotozoals	Metronidazole (Flagyl) Tinidazole Niridazole	Amebiasis Balantidiasis Giardiasis *S. haematobium*	Molecular electron transport systems Acetylcholine recycling systems	Failure to sustain energy-producing systems Binds to ACHE, thus inactivating normal neuromuscular function
Antimalarials	Chloroquine phosphate (Aralen)	Many species of susceptible malaria	Parasite digestive vacuole hemoglobinase	Local pH is changed so that enzyme becomes inoperative
	Chloroguanide Pyrimethamine Trimethoprim and combinations of antifolate and sulfa drug (e.g., sulfadoxine/ pyrimethamine [Fansidar])	Many species of susceptible malaria Various malaria species partially or totally refractory to chloroquine	Dihydrofolate reductase step in folate synthesis or incorporation of PABA in folic acid	Blocks normal folate synthesis and eventually one-carbon metabolism

*Presently available from CDC Drug Service, Centers for Disease Control and Prevention, Atlanta, Ga, 30333, telephone: 404-639-3670 (evenings, weekends, and holidays: 404-639-2888).

have lived in a number of refugee camps)? For all patients, note the season that the patient was in the countries (e.g., monsoon versus dry). Ask about animal exposures and bites. Be particularly persistent in uncovering exposure to fresh water, either in work or recreational activities. The incubation period for the development of symptoms for parasitic diseases ranges from days (falciparum malaria) to months (vivax malaria) to years (filariasis). Uncovering parasitic illness depends heavily on Olser's principle—to *make* the diagnosis, one must first *think* of the diagnosis.

PRINCIPLES OF THERAPY

New and more effective antiparasitic agents are continually being developed. The list of drugs used to treat parasitic infestations is large and varied (Table 127-3). The reader should refer to this table as each organism and disease entity is discussed in the chapter. The selections in this table include some of the newest pharmaceutical agents, in addition to many medications that, although still recommended, have now become almost obsolete.

Fortunately, the newer antiparasitic drugs are less toxic to the patient. Parasite biochemical pathways are sufficiently different from those of the human host to allow selective interference with these pathways by chemotherapeutic agents in relatively small doses. In many instances, single-dose treatment can eradicate an entire parasite burden, and this approach has led to mass treatment programs of infected populations in underdeveloped endemic areas. Treatment and disposition in the ED, however, focus on the individual patient and a particular disease entity. Most parasitic

Table 127-2. Parasites According to Geographic Location and Portal of Entry

Parasite	Geographic distribution	Common infective stage and portal of entry
Protozoa		
Entamoeba histolytica	Cosmopolitan, especially prevalent in warm climates	Cyst via mouth
Balantidium coli	Warm climates	Cyst via mouth
Giardia lamblia	Cosmopolitan, especially prevalent in warm climates	Cyst via mouth
Trichomonas vaginalis	Cosmopolitan, United States	Trophozoite via vulva or urethra
Leishmania tropica	Mediterranean area to western India	Leptomonas via skin
Leishmania braziliensis	Mexico to northern Argentina	Leptomonas via skin
Leishmania donovani	China, India, Africa, Mediterranean area, continental Latin America	Leptomonas via skin
Trypanosoma gambiense	West and Central Africa	Trypanosome via skin
Trypanosoma rhodesiense	Central and East Africa	Trypanosome via skin
Trypanosome cruzi	Continental Latin America	Trypanosome via skin
Plasmodium vivax	Warm and cooler climates	Sporozoite via skin
Plasmodium malariae	Warm climates	Sporozoite via skin
Plasmodium falciparum	Warm climates	Sporozoite via skin
Nematodes		
Trichinella spiralis	Cosmopolitan, common in the United States	Encysted larva in pork via mouth
Trichuris trichiura	Warm, moist climates	Embryonated egg via mouth
Strongyloides stercoralis	Warm, moist climates	Filariform larva via skin
Necator americanus	Common in warm climates	Filariform larva via skin
Ancylostoma duodenale	Western South America	Filariform larva via skin
Enterobius vermicularis	Cosmopolitan, common in the United States	Embryonated egg via mouth
Ascaris lumbricoides	Cosmopolitan, common in the United States	Embryonated egg via mouth
Wuchereria bancrofti	Prevalent in warm climates	Filariform larva via skin
Brugia malayi	Asia	Filariform larva via skin
Onchocerca volvulus	Tropical Africa, Mexico, Central America, and northern South America	Filariform larva via skin
Loa loa	Tropical Africa	Filariform larva via skin
Dracunculus medinensis	Tropical Eastern Hemisphere	Larva in arthropod hose via mouth
Cestodes		
Taenia saginata	Cosmopolitan, United States	Cysticercus in beef via mouth
Taenia solium		
1. Adult worm	Cosmopolitan, United States	1. Cysticercus in pork via mouth
2. Cysticercus stage	Cosmopolitan, United States	2. Eggs human infections via mouth
Echinococcus granulosus	Cosmopolitan, United States	Eggs from canines via mouth
Echinococcus multilocularis	Central Europe, Asia, Alaska	Eggs from foxes via mouth
Hymenolepis nana	Warm climates	Eggs human infections via mouth
Hymenolepis diminuta	Warm climates	Larva in arthropod host via mouth
Diphyllobothrium latum	North Temperate Zone, Argentina, Chile, Australia	Sparganum larva fish flesh via mouth
Trematodes		
Fasciola hepatica	Sheep-raising countries	Larva on vegetation via mouth
Fasciolopsis buski	Asia	Larva encysted on water nuts
Clonorchis sinensis	Asia	Larva encysted in freshwater fish
Opisthorchis felineus	Europe, Asia	Larva encysted in freshwater fish
Opisthorchis viverrini	Thailand	Larva encysted in freshwater fish
Paragonimus westermani	Primarily oriental, also South America and Africa	Larva encysted in crabs or crayfishes via mouth
Schistosoma japonicum	Asia	Cercarial larva in water via skin
Schistosoma mansoni	Africa, Latin America	Cercarial larva in water via skin
Schistosoma haematobium	Africa to India, southern Portugal	Cercarial larva in water via skin

Modified from Beaver PC et al: *Clinical parasitology,* ed 9, Philadelphia, 1984, Lea & Febiger.

infections (with certain very important exceptions such as falciparum malaria) pursue a chronic course and are not acutely life-threatening. Remember that the evolutionary goal of the successful parasite is to live with and at the expense of the living host. A parasite that kills its host has no survival advantage. In spite of the subacute or chronic nature of most parasitic infections, once a diagnosis (or a diagnostic plan) has been made and chemotherapy instituted, the emergency physician must arrange careful follow-up and repeat laboratory examinations in order to assure a cure. When the parasites are not promptly eliminated, repeat doses or alternative drugs should be considered, because drug resis-

Text continued on p. 1868

Table 127-3. Drugs for Treatment of Parasitic Infections

Infection	Drug	Adult dosage	Pediatric dosage
Amebiasis (*Entamoeba histolytica*)			
Asymptomatic			
Drug of choice:	Iodoquinol	650 mg tid × 20 days	30-10 mg/kg/day in 3 doses × 20 days
Alternative:	Diloxanide furoate	500 mg tid × 10 days	20 mg/kg/day in 3 doses × 7 days
	Paromomycin	25-30 mg/kg/day in 3 doses × 7 days	25-30 mg/kg/day in 3 doses × 7 days
Mild to moderate intestinal disease			
Drug of choice:	Metronidazole	750 mg tid × 10 days	35-50 mg/kg/day in 3 doses × 10 days
Alternative:	Tinidazole	2 g/day × 3 days	50 mg/kg (maximum 2 g) qd × 3 days
Severe intestinal disease, hepatic abscess			
Drug of choice:	Metronidazole	750 mg tid × 10 days	35-50 mg/kg/day in 3 doses × 10 days
Alternative:	Tinidazole	600 mg bid or 800 mg tid × 5 days	50 mg/kg or 60 mg/kg (maximum 2 g) qd × 3 days
Amebic meningoencephalitis, primary (*Naegleria* spp.)			
Drug of choice:	Amphotericin B	1 mg/kg/day IV, uncertain duration	1 mg/kg/day IV, uncertain duration
Anisakiasis (*Anisakis*)			
Treatment of choice:	Surgical or endoscopic removal		
Ascariasis (*Ascaris lumbricoides*, roundworm)			
Drugs of choice:	Mebendazole	100 mg bid × 3 days	100 mg bid × 3 days
	Or pyrantel pamoate	11 mg/kg once (maximum 1 g)	11 mg/kg once (maximum 1 g)
Balantidiasis (*Balantidium coli*)			
Drug of choice:	Tetracycline	500 mg qid × 10 days	40 mg/kg/day in 4 doses × 10 days (maximum 2 g/day)
Alternatives:	Iodoquinol	650 mg tid × 20 days	40 mg/kg/day in 3 doses × 20 days
	Metronidazole	750 mg tid × 5 days	35-50 mg/kg/day in 3 doses × 5 days
Cutaneous larva migrans (creeping eruption)			
Drug of choice:	Thiabendazole	Topically and/or 50 mg/kg/day in 2 doses (maximum 3 g/day) × 2-5 days	Topically and/or 50 mg/kg/day in 2 doses (maximum 3 g/day) × 2-5 days
***Dracunculus medinensis* (guinea worm)**			
Drug of choice:	Metronidazole	750 mg tid × 5-10 days	25 mg/kg/day (maximum 750 mg/day) in 2 doses × 10 days
Alternative:	Thiabendazole	50-75 mg/day in 2 doses × 3 days	50-75 mg/kg/day in 2 doses × 3 days
***Enterobius vermicularis* (pinworm)**			
Drugs of choice:	Pyrantel pamoate	11 mg/kg once (maximum 1 g); repeat after 2 weeks	11 mg/kg once (maximum 1 g); repeat after 2 weeks
	Mebendazole	A single dose of 100 mg; repeat after 2 weeks	A single dose of 100 mg; repeat after 2 weeks

Modified from Drugs for parasite infections, *Med Lett Drug Ther* 37:99, 1995.

*Some drugs available from CDC Drug Service, Centers for Disease Control and Prevention, Atlanta, Ga, 30333, telephone: 404-639-3670 (nights, weekends, and holidays: 404-639-2888).

Table 127-3. Drugs for Treatment of Parasitic Infections—cont'd

Infection	Drug	Adult dosage	Pediatric dosage
Filariasis			
Wuchereria bancrofti, Brugia malayi			
Drug of choice:	Diethylcarbamazine	Day 1: 50 mg PO Day 2: 50 mg tid Day 3: 100 mg tid Days 4 through 21: 6 mg/kg/day in 3 doses	Day 1: 1 mg/kg PO Day 2: 1 mg/kg tid Day 3: 1-2 mg/kg tid Days 4 through 21: 6 mg/kg/day in 3 doses
Loa loa			
Drug of choice:	Diethylcarbamazine	Day 1: 50 mg PO Day 2: 50 mg tid Day 3: 100 mg tid Days 4 through 21: 9 mg/kg/day in 3 doses	Day 1: 1 mg/kg PO Day 2: 1 mg/kg tid Day 3: 1-2 mg/kg tid Days 4 through 21: 6 mg/kg/day in 3 doses
Onchocerca volvulus			
Drug of choice:	Ivermectin*	150 μg/kg PO once, repeated every 3-12 months	150 μg/kg PO once, repeated every 3-12 months
Fluke, hermaphroditic			
Clonorchis sinensis (Chinese liver fluke)			
Drug of choice:	Praziquantel	75 mg/kg/day in 3 doses × 1 day	75 mg/kg/day in 3 doses × 1 day
Fasciola hepatica (sheep liver fluke)			
Drug of choice:	Bithionol	30-50 mg/kg on alternate days × 10-15 doses	30-50 mg/kg on alternate days × 10-15 doses
Fasciolopsis buski (intestinal fluke)			
Drug of choice:	Praziquantel	75 mg/kg/day in 3 doses × 1 day	75 mg/kg/day in 3 doses × 1 day
Opisthorchis felineus			
Drug of choice:	Praziquantel	75 mg/kg/day in 3 doses × 1 day	75 mg/kg/day in 3 doses × 1 day
Paragonimus westermani (lung fluke)			
Drug of choice:	Praziquantel	75 mg/kg/day in 3 doses × 2 days	75 mg/kg/day in 3 doses × 2 days
Alternative:	Bithionol	30-50 mg/kg on alternate days × 10-15 doses	30-50 mg/kg on alternate days × 10-15 doses
Giardiasis (*Giardia lamblia*)			
Drug of choice:	Metronidazole	250 mg tid × 5 days	15 mg/kg/day in 3 doses × 5 days
Alternatives:	Furazolidone	100 mg qid × 7-10 days	6 mg/kg/day in 4 doses × 7-10 days
	Tinidazole	2 g as a single daily dose for 1-3 days	50 mg/kg as a single daily dose for 1-3 days
Hookworm infection (*Ancylostoma duodenale, Necator americanus*)			
Drugs of choice:	Mebendazole	100 mg bid × 3 days	100 mg bid × 3 days
	Or pyrantel pamoate	11 mg/kg (maximum 1 g) × 3 days	11 mg/kg (maximum 1 g) × 3 days
Leishmaniasis			
Leishmania braziliensis, L. mexicana, L. tropica, L. donovani (kala azar)			
Drug of choice:	Stibogluconate sodium	20 mg/kg/day IV or IM × 20-28 days	20 mg/kg/day IV or IM × 20-28 days
Alternative:	Amphotericin B	0.25-1 mg/kg by slow infusion daily or every 2 days for up to 8 weeks	0.25-1 mg/kg by slow infusion daily or every 2 days for up to 8 weeks

Continued

Table 127-3. Drugs for Treatment of Parasitic Infections—cont'd

Infection	Drug	Adult dosage	Pediatric dosage
Malaria, treatment of (*Plasmodium falciparum, P. ovale, P. vivax,* and *P. malariae*)			
All Plasmodium except chloroquine-resistant P. falciparum			
Oral			
Drug of choice:	Chloroquine phosphate	600 mg base (1 g), then 300 mg base (500 mg) 6 hr later, then 300 mg base (500 mg) at 24 and 48 hr	10 mg base/kg (maximum 600 mg base), then 5 mg base/kg 6 hr later, then 5 mg base/kg at 24 and 48 hr
Parenteral			
Drugs of choice:	Quinine dihydrochloride	20 mg/kg loading dose in 10 mg/kg 5% dextrose over 4 hr followed by 10 mg/kg over 2-4 hr q8hr (maximum 1800 mg/day) until oral therapy can be started	Same as adult dose
	Or quinidine gluconate	10 mg/kg loading dose (maximum 600 mg) in normal saline slowly over 1-2 hr, followed by continuous infusion of 0.02 mg/kg/min for 3 days maximum	Same as adult dose
Alternative:	Chloroquine hydrochloride	200 mg base (250 mg) IM q6hr if oral therapy cannot be started	0.83 mg base/kg/hr × 30 hr continuous infusion or 3.5 mg base/kg q6hr IM or SC
Chloroquine-resistant P. falciparum			
Oral			
Drugs of choice:	Quinine sulfate plus	650 mg tid × 3 days	25 mg/kg/day in 3 doses × 3-7 days
	Pyrimethamine-sulfadoxine	3 tablets at once on last day of quinine	<1 yr: ¼ tablet 1-3 yr: ½ tablet 4-8 yr: 1 tablet 9-14 yr: 2 tablets
	Or plus tetracycline	250 mg qid × 7 days	20 mg/kg/day in 4 doses × 7 days
	Or plus clindamycin	900 mg tid × 3-5 days	20-40 mg/kg/day in 3 doses × 3-5 days
Alternative:	Mefloquine	1250 mg once	25 mg/kg once (<45 kg)
Parenteral			
Drugs of choice:	Quinine dihydrochloride Quinidine gluconate	Same as above Same as above	Same as above Same as above
Prevention of relapses: P. vivax and P. ovale only			
Drug of choice:	Primaquine phosphate	15 mg base (26.3 mg)/day × 14 days or 45 mg base (79 mg)/wk × 8 wk	0.3 mg base/kg/day × 14 days
Malaria, prevention of			
Drug of choice:	Chloroquine phosphate	300 mg base (500 mg salt) PO, once a week beginning 1 wk before and continuing for 4 wks after last exposure	5 mg/kg base (8.3 mg/kg salt) once a week, up to adult dose of 300 mg base, same schedule as adult
Chloroquine-resistant areas			
Drug of choice:	Mefloquine	250 mg tablet PO once a week × 4 wk, then every other week continuing for 4 wk after last exposure	Same schedule as adults using the following dosing guidelines: 15-19 kg: ¼ tablet, 20-30 kg: ½ tablet, 31-45 kg: ¾ tablet, and >45 kg: 1 tablet

Modified from Drugs for parasite infections, *Med Lett Drug Ther* 37:99, 1995.

Continued

Table 127-3. Drugs for Treatment of Parasitic Infections—cont'd

Infection	Drug	Adult dosage	Pediatric dosage
Chloroquine-resistant areas—cont'd			
	or chloroquine phosphate	Same as above	Same as above
	Plus pyrimethamine-sulfadoxine for presumptive treatment	Carry a single dose (3 tablets) for self-treatment of febrile illness when medical care is not immediately available	Same single-dose approach as adults using the following dosing guidelines: <1 yr: ¼ tablet 1-3 yr: ½ tablet 4-8 yr: 1 tablet 9-14 yr: 2 tablets
	Plus proguanil (in Africa south of the Sahara)	200 mg daily starting 1-2 days before exposure and continuing for 7 days after cessation of exposure	Same schedule as adults using the following dosing guidelines: <2 yr: 50 mg daily 2-6 yr: 100 mg daily 7-10 yr: 150 mg daily >10 yr: 200 mg daily
	Or doxycycline	100 mg daily during exposure and for 4 weeks afterward	>8 years of age: 2 mg/kg/day PO, up to 100 mg/day
Schistosomiasis			
Schistosoma haematobium			
Drug of choice:	Praziquantel	40 mg/kg/day in 2 doses × 1 day	40 mg/kg/day in 2 doses × 1 day
S. japonicum			
Drug of choice:	Praziquantel	60 mg/kg/day in 3 doses × 1 day	60 mg/kg/day in 3 doses × 1 day
S. mansoni			
Drug of choice:	Praziquantel	40 mg/kg/day in 2 doses × 1 day	40 mg/kg/day in 2 doses × 1 day
Alternate:	Oxamniquine	15 mg/kg once	20 mg/kg/day in 2 doses × 1 day
S. mekongi			
Drug of choice:	Praziquantel	60 mg/kg/day in 3 doses × 1 day	60 mg/kg/day in 3 doses × 1 day
Strongyloidiasis (*Strongyloides stercoralis*)			
Drugs of choice:	Thiabendazole	50 mg/kg/day in 2 doses (maximum 3 g/day) × 2 days	50 mg/kg/day in 2 doses (maximum 3 g/day) × 2 days
	Or ivermectin	200 µg/kg/day × 1-2 days	200 µg/kg/day × 1-2 days
Tapeworm infection—adult (intestinal stage)			
Diphyllobothrium latum (fish), Taenia saginata (beef), Taenia solium (pork), Dipylidium caninum (dog)			
Drug of choice:	Praziquantel	5-10 mg/kg once	5-10 mg/kg once
Hymenolepis nana (dwarf tapeworm)			
Drug of choice:	Praziquantel	25 mg/kg once	25 mg/kg once
Larval (tissue) stage			
Echinococcus granulosus (hydatid cysts)			
Drug of choice:	Albendazole	400 mg bid × 28 days, repeated as necessary	15 mg/kg/day × 28 days, repeated as necessary
Echinococcus multilocularis			
Treatment of choice:	Surgical excision		
Cysticercus cellulose (cysticercosis)			
Drugs of choice:	Praziquantel	50 mg/kg/day in 3 doses × 15 days	50 mg/kg/day in 3 doses × 15 days
	Or albendazole	15 mg/kg/day in 2-3 doses × 8-28 days, repeated as necessary	15 mg/kg/day in 2-3 doses × 8-28 days, repeated as necessary
Alternative:	Surgery		

Continued

Table 127-3. Drugs for Treatment of Parasitic Infections—cont'd

Infection	Drug	Adult dosage	Pediatric dosage
Trichinosis (*Trichinella spiralis*)			
Drugs of choice:	Steroids for severe symptoms		
	Plus mebendazole	200-400 mg tid × 3 days, then 400-500 mg tid × 10 days	Same as adult
Trichomoniasis (*Trichomonas vaginalis*)			
Drug of choice:	Metronidazole	2 g once or 250 mg tid or 375 mg bid PO × 7 days	15 mg/kg/day PO in 3 doses × 7 days
Trichuriasis (*Trichuris trichiura*, whipworm)			
Drugs of choice:	Mebendazole	100 mg bid × 3 days	100 mg bid × 3 days
	Or albendazole	400 mg once	400 mg once
Trypanosomiasis			
Trypanosoma cruzi (South American trypanosomiasis, Chagas' disease)			
Drug of choice:	Nifurtimox	8-10 mg/kg/day PO in 4 doses × 120 days	1-10 yr: 15-20 mg/kg/day in 4 doses × 90 days 11-16 yr: 12.5-15 mg/kg/day in 4 doses × 90 days
Alternative:	Benznidazole	5-7 mg/kg/day × 30-120 days	Same as adult
T. brucei gambiense, T. b. rhodesiense (African trypanosomiasis, sleeping sickness) hemolymphatic stage			
Drug of choice:	Suramin	100-200 mg (test done) IV, then 1 g IV on days 1, 3, 7, 14, and 21	20 mg/kg on days 1, 3, 7, 14, and 21
Alternative:	Pentamidine isethionate	4 mg/kg/day IM × 10 days	4 mg/kg/day IM × 10 days
Late disease with CNS involvement			
Drug of choice:	Melarsoprol	2-3.6 mg/kg/day IV × 3 days; after 1 wk 3.6 mg/kg/day IV × 3 days; repeat again after 10-21 days	18-25 mg/kg total over 1 month; initial dose of 0.36 mg/kg IV, increasing gradually to maximum 3.6 mg/kg at intervals of 1-5 days for total of 9-10 doses
Alternatives: (*T. b. gambiense* only)	Tryparsamide	One injection of 30 mg/kg (maximum 2 g) IV every 5 days to total of 12 injections; course may be repeated after 1 month	Unknown
	Plus suramin	One injection of 10 mg/kg IV every 5 days to total of 12 injections; course may be repeated after 1 month	Unknown
Visceral larva migrans (toxocariasis)			
Drug of choice:	Diethylcarbamazine	6 mg/kg/day in 3 doses × 7-10 days	6 mg/kg/day in 3 doses × 7-10 days
Alternatives:	Mebendazole	100-200 mg bid × 5 days	Same as adult
	Or albendazole	400 mg bid × 3-5 days	400 mg bid × 3-5 days

Modified from Drugs for parasite infections, *Med Lett Drug Ther* 37:99, 1995.

tance is becoming increasingly common. Referral should be made to a geographic medicine clinic or an infectious disease clinic. Any patient who appears clinically ill or has presumptive falciparum malaria (by symptoms or travel history) should be admitted to the hospital for initial diagnosis, treatment, and observation.

FEVER

Malaria

Principles of Disease The febrile patient with shaking chills and a time-appropriate history of travel to an endemic region should be evaluated for malaria. *Plasmodium falciparum, P. ovale, P. vivax,* and *P. malariae* are responsible for human malaria. Over 41% of the world's population lives in areas where malaria is transmitted (e.g., parts of Africa, Asia, Oceania, Central America, and South America). Approximately 300 to 500 million clinical infections occur annually, resulting in 1.5 to 2.7 million deaths.[3] The female *Anopheles* mosquito is the arthropod vector that can transmit malaria after ingesting gametocytes from infected persons. After sexual reproduction in the gut of the mosquito, sporozoites are released from the salivary glands of the arthropod into the human host during a blood meal. Within the human host, the sporozoites rapidly penetrate the liver parenchymal cells. The protozoans, now termed cryptozoites or exoerythrocytic schizonts, rapidly multiply. Eventual lysis of the hepatic cells results in the release of merozoites that invade erythrocytes once in the bloodstream. In *P. vivax* and *P. ovale* infection, repeated cycles of exoerythrocytic reproduction develop within the hepatocytes, and this cycling is responsible for recrudescent febrile episodes that may occur years after initial infection.

After invading red blood cells (RBCs), the merozoites transform into trophozoites, which feed on the cells' hemoglobin. These trophozoites mature into schizonts that may divide asexually into additional merozoites. The RBCs undergo lysis, releasing many merozoites into the blood. While some merozoites are destroyed by the body's immune apparatus, many enter new erythrocytes. After several repetitions of this erythrocytic cycle, the cyclic process changes and male microgametocytes or female macrogametocytes may develop instead of merozoites. These gametes subsequently complete the reproductive cycle by fusion, sexually, within the gut of a new female *Anopheles* mosquito after she has taken a blood meal from an infected individual. A human contracts malaria from an infected vector mosquito in an endemic region. Other means of transmission have been reported, including blood transfusions, intravenous drug abuse with contaminated syringes, perinatal transmission, organ transplantation, and so-called *airport malaria.* There have been several reports of people acquiring malaria who have never been in an endemic area but live near or work in an international airport. The infected mosquito is transported from the endemic region and released when the plane arrives at its destination.[4-6]

Clinical Features The important difference between *P. falciparum* and the other species is the capacity of *P. falciparum* to cause severe and complicated disease or death. Irregular fevers are the hallmark of malaria. Other symptoms may include anemia, headache, nausea, chills, lethargy, abdominal pain, and upper respiratory complaints.[7] Acute falciparum infection can have the following complications: cerebral malaria, hypoglycemia (especially in children), metabolic acidosis, severe anemia, renal failure, pulmonary edema, disseminated intravascular coagulation (DIC), and death.

In chronic malaria, hepatosplenomegaly occurs secondary to increased cellularity from the immune response. Within the liver, parasites and malarial pigment distend the Kupffer's cells. Parasitized RBCs also adhere to the sinusoidal system of the spleen, reducing its immunologic effectiveness. Anemia results from acute and chronic hemolysis. Blackwater fever, hemoglobinuria caused by severe hemolysis, occurs in patients with chronic falciparum malaria, although it can also occur acutely.[8]

Diagnostic Strategies Thick and thin blood films are the gold standard for the diagnosis of malaria. Viewing several slides may be necessary if the parasite burden is not overwhelming. Giemsa or Wright's stains are both adequate for this purpose when used with ordinary light microscopy. The diagnosis often can be made in a simply equipped laboratory. Even if the parasite is not visualized, the physician should still treat for malaria if clinically suspected.

Management In the past, chloroquine phosphate was the treatment of choice for acute, uncomplicated attacks of malaria. Resistance to chloroquine has been steadily increasing, and now the drug should be used only in regions of known chloroquine sensitivity. Quinine and doxycycline given together are the drugs currently recommended for the treatment of falciparum malaria. Quinine can be given orally or parenterally for more serious and life-threatening infections. When given intravenously, too rapid infusion of quinine can cause profound hypoglycemia. Intravenous quinidine can also be used for life-threatening infections. Pyrimethamine-sulfadoxine is another agent that can be used; however, plasmodia in many regions are now resistant. Mefloquine or halofantrine are other alternative drugs.

Although not used in the United States, the artemisinin agents are excellent antimalarials and are available in enteral and parenteral preparations. They have a rapid onset of action and are tolerated very well. Primaquine is used to expunge the hepatic phases of *P. ovale* and *P. vivax,* preventing recrudescent disease. Before starting primaquine, the patient must be tested for glucose-6-phosphate dehydrogenase (G6PD) enzyme deficiency to avoid precipitating severe hemolysis. Prompt diagnosis and therapeutic intervention are necessary with falciparum malaria to avoid coma and death.[9,10]

Babesiosis

Babesiosis is a malaria-like illness that is becoming increasingly prevalent in the northeastern United States (*Babesia microti*), the northwestern United States (*B. gibsoni*), and Europe (*B. divergens*). The organism is a protozoan similar in structure and life cycle to the plasmodia. It is transmitted by the deer tick, *Ixodes dammini,* the vector of Lyme disease. Several cases have been attributed to transfusion with infected blood.[11] Patients develop fatigue, anorexia, malaise, myalgia, chills, high spiking fevers, sweats, headache, emotional lability, and dark urine. They have hepatosplenomegaly, anemia, thrombocytopenia, leukopenia, elevated liver enzyme levels, and signs of hemolysis with hyperbilirubinemia and decreased haptoglobin. In the healthy host the disease may remit spontaneously.[12] In asplenic patients, the elderly, and those with immunocompromise (especially patients with AIDS and patients taking corticosteroids), up to 85% of RBCs may contain organisms. There is massive hemolysis, jaundice, renal failure, DIC, hypotension, and adult respiratory distress syndrome.[13,14] Diagnosis rests on clinical suspicion, multiple thin and thick blood smears, and serologic testing. The treatment of choice is quinine and clindamycin. Patients infected with *B. divergens* tend to be sicker and require more supportive care. Coinfection with

Borrelia burgdorferi, the agent that causes Lyme disease, results in more severe and prolonged illness.[15] Babesia resemble plasmodia in blood smears. The history will make the diagnosis.

Other Parasites Causing Fever

Other parasitic illnesses that commonly cause significant fever include schistosomiasis, fascioliasis, trypanosomiasis, leishmaniasis, and amebic liver abscess. "Katayama fever" may be the initial phase of schistosomiasis. These patients will report brief exposures to fresh water in endemic areas. They have spiking fevers, diaphoresis, and cough. Eosinophilia is common.[16] Fascioliasis caused by the liver fluke, *Fasciola hepatica,* is endemic throughout Asia, the former Soviet Union, southern Europe, and South America. Infection begins with the ingestion of the metacercariae. Within 6 weeks patients will manifest right upper quadrant abdominal pain, fever, and eosinophilia.[17]

American trypanosomiasis (Chagas' disease) is endemic to Central and South America. The vector, the reduviid bug, sheds the trypomastigotes in its feces proximal to the bite site, leading to local infection and subsequent systemic spread in the host. Acute Chagas' disease begins with the chagoma, the infected and swollen bite site, often periorbital, and quickly progresses to fever, malaise, facial swelling, and pedal edema. Parasitization of cardiac muscle causes the dysrhythmias and ventricular dysfunction that are classically found in late disease (chronic Chagas' cardiopathy).[18] Leishmaniasis, spread to humans by the sandfly as vector, is found in the Middle East, several regions in North and East Africa, and Brazil. Although leishmaniasis can involve the skin (cutaneous) and the mucosa (mucosal), fever is seen only in visceral leishmaniasis, or kala azar. Symptoms also include massive hepatosplenomegaly, neutropenia, and weight loss.[19] Amebic liver abscesses frequently manifest with high fevers, elevated liver function tests, right upper quadrant pain, and an elevated white blood cell count.[20]

NEUROLOGIC SYMPTOMS

Cerebral Malaria

Principles of Disease and Clinical Features Cerebral malaria is a common, life-threatening complication of *P. falciparum* infection. Parasitized RBCs express malarial cell surface glycoproteins called *knobs* that are sticky and cause capillary sludging in the cerebral microvasculature, localized ischemia, capillary leak, and petechial hemorrhages. Patients have fever, altered mentation, and occasionally seizures. A careful history and early diagnosis and therapy are essential to prevent severe morbidity and mortality.

Management Treatment of cerebral malaria includes intravenous quinine and artemisinin; supportive care, including mechanical ventilation for comatose patients and those with noncardiogenic pulmonary edema; antiepileptics; and treatment of acidosis and hypoglycemia (associated with quinine use and cerebral malaria). Mortality is high, especially in children (up to 30%), but if the patient recovers, neurologic sequelae are rare (less than 10%).[21,22] Corticosteroids, including dexamethasone, are not beneficial and are potentially harmful in cerebral malaria.

Cysticercosis

Principles of Disease Cysticercosis is a disease caused by the larval form of *Taenia solium,* a common central nervous system (CNS) pathogen in many tropical areas. *T. solium* (pork tapeworm) is acquired by humans after eating pork containing the larval form *Cysticercus cellulosae* or by ingesting food or water contaminated by eggs from the adult helminth. Eating pork infected with *C. cellulosae* results in the development of adult worms within the human small intestine. Adult worms subsequently produce egg-filled segments that infect pigs or humans when ingested, allowing completion of the life cycle. Accidental consumption of tapeworm eggs or reflux of adult worms into the stomach through reverse peristalsis results in the primary clinical manifestation of this disease. Gastric juice dissolves the egg's outer coat, allowing release of larval oncospheres. The oncospheres penetrate the intestinal wall, subsequently traveling through the bloodstream to multiple body tissues, particularly muscle and occasionally brain.[23-25]

Clinical Features Within the brain, the larvae of *T. solium* form an expanding cyst that induces an immunologic reaction from the host, including inflammation, fibrosis, and ultimately calcification. Neurologic findings develop when the involved neural tissue cannot adequately accommodate the enlarging cyst. Seizure activity is often the first indication of cysticercosis and should be considered in any adult patient with undiagnosed seizures. The diagnosis of *T. solium* is established by finding characteristic eggs, proglottids (gravid segments), or scolices (worm heads) in stool preparations.

Diagnostic Strategies and Management Cranial computed tomography (CT) scan can reveal an enhancing ring lesion with contrast injection. Such lesions can appear similar to a CNS abscess, metastasis, or a primary tumor such as glioblastoma multiforme. Praziquantel is the treatment of choice, and corticosteroids may be necessary during therapy with praziquantel, particularly if CNS cysts are present. Neurosurgical consultation should be sought when treating neurocysticercosis, for acute obstructive hydrocephalus may occur.[1]

Echinococcosis

Principles of Disease and Clinical Features *Echinococcus granulosus* is another tapeworm capable of causing CNS disease. Cerebral hydatid cysts are loculated structures containing *E. granulosus* scolices (heads) and remains of germinal epithelium, termed hydatid sand. Common types of exposure include ingestion of food or water contaminated by the ova from feces of sheep or cattle infected by the adult worm, or close contact with a sheepdog. Infection results in the liberation of the embryo oncosphere into the small intestine. After penetrating the intestinal wall, the larvae travel through the bloodstream to multiple sites for encystment. The liver is the target organ in nearly two thirds of the cases, but the brain is involved in approximately 1 in 14 cases. In the brain, infection with *E. granulosus* is manifested by compressive effects or seizures caused by enlarging cysts.

Diagnostic Strategies and Management The diagnosis of hydatid cyst disease is suggested by localization of the cyst on ultrasound or CT scan. Serologic evaluation, such as serum or cerebrospinal fluid (CSF) complement fixation, confirms the diagnosis. Aspiration of the cyst should not be attempted, because widespread metastatic cysts may develop. Treatment options include using the drug albendazole and surgical resection if warranted. Resection of the cyst may cause an anaphylactoid reaction if there is spillage of hydatid sand.[26]

Trypanosomiasis

Principles of Disease African sleeping sickness is caused by *Trypanosoma brucei gambiense* and *T. b. rhodesiense.* The endemic region for this infection is limited to several areas of East and West Africa. These motile organisms are transmitted by the bite of the *Glossina* (tsetse) fly, which introduces the infective form of the trypanosome into the host blood. A small lesion or boil may develop and persist for several days. The flagellated organism travels throughout the bloodstream, invading the lymph nodes and spleen.

Clinical Features Winterbottom's sign, which is posterior cervical lymphadenopathy, is usually apparent at the time treatment is sought. The patient is often febrile, and trypanosomes are demonstrable in a thick peripheral blood smear. After invasion of nervous tissue intercellular spaces, severe headache may result that may be secondary to CNS inflammation. Some patients may manifest psychiatric symptoms, progressing eventually to extreme sleepiness and lethargy. Coma and death are inevitable in untreated patients, usually as a result of starvation and trypanotoxins.[27-29]

Diagnostic Strategies and Management The diagnosis of African trypanosomiasis requires an appropriate exposure history and characteristic symptoms. Demonstration of trypanosomes in peripheral blood, CSF, or lymph node and bone marrow aspirates establishes the diagnosis. The presence of parasites in the CSF indicates advanced progression of the disease. Suramin sodium is the treatment of choice for early infection with *T. b. rhodesiense.* Pentamidine isethionate is the preferred treatment for early *T. b. gambiense.* Trivalent arsenicals such as melarsoprol, which can penetrate the blood-brain barrier, are used in advanced disease with neurologic sequelae.[2]

Other Parasites Causing Neurologic Symptoms

CNS involvement with *Trichinella spiralis* has been reported in severe cases, following larval migration of this parasite into the brain and meninges. Serious consequences are meningitis, encephalitis, seizures, paresis, coma, and death. The pathophysiology may reflect obstruction of small arterioles by migrating larvae, with subsequent vasculitis or cerebral edema from immunologic reaction to the larvae or larval fragments. Therapy for trichinosis with severe muscle or CNS involvement includes mebendazole or thiabendazole coupled with steroids, which depress the host immune response to infection.[30,31]

Amebic abscess of the brain or meningoencephalitis caused by *Entamoeba histolytica* is a rare complication of infection with this intestinal parasite. Infestation occurs through intake of food or drink contaminated with cysts of this protozoan. Spread of amebae to the brain or meninges from the colonized large bowel wall is rare, but should be considered in any patient with amebiasis and subsequent neurologic impairment. The diagnosis may be made through microscopic identification of trophozoites (motile amebae) in CSF; however, biopsy of affected tissue is more specific. CNS amebiasis is treated with intravenous metronidazole.

Naegleria and *Acanthamoeba* are free-living amebae in freshwater that can be contracted while swimming and diving in ponds and lakes. The amebae are thought to invade the CNS through the olfactory neuroepithelium or cornea (violated by abrasion or associated with contact lens wear), causing an amebic meningoencephalitis. Amphotericin B and miconazole in combination are currently the treatment of choice once motile amebae are identified in CSF.[32]

Strongyloides stercoralis is a very common infection in the tropics. The worm is introduced through the skin and eventually makes its way to the small bowel. Infection with *Strongyloides* is more clinically significant in the immunosuppressed patient who may suffer larval dissemination throughout the body with encephalitis and pyogenic meningitis in the CNS. *Strongyloides* is treated with thiabendazole or albendazole.[33]

Granulomas may occur in the brain from egg deposition by *Schistosoma japonicum.* Generally they do not cause major symptoms; however, several cases of transverse myelitis with paraplegia have been reported.[34]

ANEMIA

Malaria

Malaria infection is often associated with some degree of anemia. Severe anemia is seen more often in children <5 years old. Anemia may develop quickly, linked to an acute infection with massive hemolysis, or it may be more insidious, developing over months. Parasitized RBCs lyse when the merozoite phase is mature. Uninfected RBCs undergo immune destruction from cell surface antibodies produced in response to parasite-associated changes in RBC surface proteins. This process of destruction is abetted by increased reticuloendothelial activity. The reticulocyte response in infected individuals is blunted by inhibition of erythropoietin secretion.[35,36] The antimalarial drug primaquine can precipitate hemolysis in patients who have G6PD deficiency, which is not uncommon in black Africans and some Asians.

Whipworm and Hookworm

Infestation by the whipworm *Trichuris trichiura* and the two human hookworms *Necator americanus* and *Ancylostoma duodenale* may cause iron deficiency anemia. Hookworm infection has been recognized as a major cause of anemia worldwide. Adult worms penetrate into intestinal mucosa and feed, causing significant ongoing luminal blood loss. Eggs defecated in the soil mature through a rhabditiform larval form to the infective filariform larva. These larvae penetrate the human skin, usually through the feet. In trichuriasis, anemia is seen only with massive parasite infestation. Ova from the whipworm are ingested through stool-contaminated food and water. Diagnosis of these infections requires identification of characteristic ova in the stool. As with most helminthic infections, peripheral eosinophilia is common. Mebendazole or albendazole effectively controls trichuriasis and hookworm infections in adults and children. The patient should also be treated with iron if there is an intercurrent anemia.

Tapeworm

Infection with the fish tapeworm *Diphyllobothrium latum* is associated with pernicious anemia. This tapeworm competes with the human host for absorption of vitamin B_{12}. The ingestion of raw freshwater fish that contains the embryo plerocercoid larva in its muscle fibers is followed by the development of a large adult tapeworm within the human small intestine. The diagnosis is made by demonstrating the characteristic ova in the feces. Praziquantel is the drug of choice in adults and children.

PERIPHERAL EDEMA

Elephantiasis

Principles of Disease Elephantiasis, or filariasis, is the development of massive edema with subsequent chronic distention of the overlying skin. It is caused by infestation with the filarial worms *Wuchereria bancrofti* or *Brugia malayi.* The infection is confined to humans and is widely distributed in the warmer parts of the world, including Africa, Asia, South America, and Oceania. More than 90% of all infections are found in Asia, where the disease has reached epidemic proportions in some cities. Infected mosquitoes introduce microfilariae into the bloodstream of the human host during a blood meal. Upon entering the host, the worms migrate into the lymphatic system and mature into coiled, gravid adults. The presence of the adult worm within the lymphatic vessels, particularly of the lower extremities and genitalia, stimulates a profound immunologic reaction. The macrophages, lymphocytes, plasma cells, giant cells, and eosinophils congregate around the constricted lymphatic vessel. This event usually results in an erythematous, edematous, tender lymphatic tract. Its presence in patients at risk should suggest the diagnosis of filariasis.

Clinical Features Chronic manifestations of filariasis include fibrosis of the lymphatic vessel, which sometimes encloses a dead or calcified worm. Subsequent mechanical blockage of the lymphatic system leads inevitably to severe lower extremity and genital edema accompanied by thickening of the skin. Recurrent cellulitis can be a problem in many of these patients; meticulous skin care is essential to prevent this complication.[37]

Diagnostic Strategies and Management The adult female worm produces microfilariae, which periodically are released into the peripheral blood via the lymphatics accompanied by shaking chills and fever. Thick peripheral blood smears may demonstrate infection, particularly at night, when the release of microfilariae is most likely. Diethylcarbamazine (DEC) rapidly clears the microfilariae from the peripheral blood and slowly sterilizes the gravid female nematode. Established elephantiasis of the scrotum can be successfully treated surgically. Lymphatic obstruction of the limbs rarely responds to operative intervention.[38]

DERMATOLOGIC SYMPTOMS

Cutaneous Leishmaniasis

Principles of Disease Cutaneous leishmaniasis is among the most important causes of chronic ulcerating skin lesions in the world. *Leishmania braziliensis* and *L. mexicana* are responsible for "New World" leishmaniasis, whereas *L. tropica* causes "Old World" leishmaniasis. The female *Phlebotomus* sand fly transmits the promastigote form of this parasite during a blood meal. Once in the human host, the leishmanial form of this parasite resides in the macrophages of the skin and subcutaneous tissue.

Clinical Features Skin papules and nodules are seen early in leishmaniasis at the site of the insect bite. A raised macule can also appear, which subsequently develops central ulceration and a raised border. Lymphocyte and macrophage invasion of the epidermis and dermis cause the induration that occurs at the ulcer border. Secondary bacterial infections of these ulcers increase the associated scarring. *L. braziliensis braziliensis* (subspecies of *L. braziliensis*) attacks the mucocutaneous skin borders such as in the nose and mouth. Mutilation of the face occurs after massive tissue destruction, including nasal cartilage. The larynx and trachea also can be involved, compromising the airway. Disseminated cutaneous leishmaniasis (*L. mexicana amazonensis* in South America and *L. tropica aethiopica* in Ethiopia) is characterized by diffuse nodules and papules resembling lepromatous leprosy. Individuals with this manifestation of leishmaniasis are thought to have a defect in their cell-mediated immunity response.[39-41]

Diagnostic Strategies and Management Definitive diagnosis of leishmaniasis is made by direct visualization of the parasite under the microscope. Diagnosis can be made by indirect fluorescent antibody test. An intradermal skin test exists (Montenegro), but it is often negative during the acute stages of the disease. Many forms of cutaneous leishmaniasis, especially *L. tropica* and *L. mexicana,* are self-limited and require no treatment unless the wounds become secondarily infected. Treatment options include sodium stibogluconate, meglumine antimonate, or amphotericin B. These treatments are rarely initiated in the ED.

Dracunculiasis

Principles of Disease and Clinical Features The "fiery serpent," *Dracunculus medinensis,* causes disease as the adult worm migrates through the subcutaneous tissues of the lower extremity. The head of the gravid adult female erodes through the skin of the lower extremity of the human host, and sensing immersion of the affected limb (as the human host wades in a pond or open well) releases larvae into the water. The larvae promptly infect the Cyclops water flea. Humans who drink water containing the infected crustacean complete the cycle of infection.

The patient may complain of rash, intense pruritus, nausea, vomiting, dyspnea, and diarrhea before the female worm ruptures through the lower extremity skin.

Management The typical treatment in developing countries is to wind the worm around a stick and slowly extract the parasite over the course of a day or two. If the worm breaks while being extracted in this fashion, the patient will experience an intense inflammatory reaction with cellulitis along the worm tract. Diagnosis is made when microscopic larvae are found in the fluid of the cutaneous ulcer or when the adult female worm is identified extruding from the skin. The use of metronidazole to shorten the time of extraction is controversial. The World Health Organization has set a goal of eradication of this disease through public health awareness, covered wells, filtered well water (removing the fleas), and keeping the skin lesions out of potable water (keeping the host out of potable water).

Other Parasites Causing Dermatologic Symptoms

Cutaneous larva migrans, the "creeping eruption," occurs in the host's epidermis after penetration by *Ancylostoma braziliense* (dog or cat hookworm) larvae into the skin. Exposure usually occurs after walking barefoot or lying on beaches or other warm soil contaminated by animal feces. The diagnosis is suggested by the presence of a characteristic meandering track on the skin surface caused by larval migration. Visceral larva migrans occurs in young children after ingestion of soil containing ova from the dog ascarid *Toxocara canis.* Thiabendazole, ivermectin, or albendazole is given for cutaneous larva migrans, and antipruritics give symptomatic relief. DEC treats visceral larva migrans. An alternative is thiabendazole.[42]

Swimmer's itch is a dermatitis that occurs after skin penetration by the nonhuman schistosome of avians and mammals, usually from swimming in northern U.S. freshwater lakes. The infection spontaneously resolves, because the nonhuman schistosome is not tolerated by the human host's immune system. Similar dermatitis can also occur after infection with human schistosomes. Treatment is symptomatic.

VISUAL SYMPTOMS

Onchocerciasis

Principles of Disease Onchocerciasis, or "river blindness," is a major cause of blindness in the world. Ninety-five percent of all cases are found in Africa.[43] The parasite is found only in humans and is transmitted by the bite of the Simulium fly. These flies live near rivers, hence the name *river blindness.* Microfilariae of *Onchocerca volvulus* are released by adult nematodes, which coil in subcutaneous nodules in the infected host; the microfilariae then migrate through the dermis and epidermis. The presence of adult worms invokes an allergic response, including the infiltration of lymphocytes, macrophages, plasma cells, and eosinophils.

Clinical Features The skin becomes chronically edematous and pruritic; it atrophies, resulting in loose, thin folds of skin. Patients with nodules in close proximity to the eyes are more likely to develop river blindness. In the eyes an immune sclerosing keratitis, often associated with an iritis, is initiated by the host's immune defenses reacting to foreign tissue that is deposited in the iris musculature when the microfilaria dies during its migration. The death of the microfilaria in the iris muscle is the major cause of ocular destruction and blindness.

Diagnostic Strategies and Management The diagnosis of onchocerciasis requires identification of characteristic microfilariae in skin snipped from the patient. Ivermectin is the drug of choice. In many of the countries where the disease is endemic, the manufacturers of ivermectin have donated the drug in an attempt to eradicate it. Surgical excision of the subcutaneous nodules is recommended when they are located on the head.

Loiasis

Principles of Disease and Clinical Features Another filarial infection that causes ocular problems is loiasis. Loiasis is confined to forest areas in West and Central Africa. Transmission of *Loa loa* occurs through the bite of flies of the genus *Chrysops*. The edema initially associated with the migrating worm is called Calabar swelling. The disease is caused by a migrating adult worm in the subcutaneous tissue. To the patient's distress, the adult worm occasionally migrates through the subconjunctival tissues. This meandering worm can be surgically excised from the conjunctiva. Although upsetting to the patient, the disease often is fairly benign. The adult worm releases sheathed microfilariae into the peripheral bloodstream during the daytime.

Diagnostic Strategies and Management These microfilariae can be detected with a thick blood smear, thus clinching the diagnosis of loiasis. The treatment of choice for *L. loa* is DEC. Corticosteroids or antihistamines often must supplement specific chemotherapy because of the intense allergic reaction that occurs when the killed adult worms and microfilariae disintegrate.[44,45]

Other Parasites Causing Ocular Symptoms

T. canis has a trophism for the host's eyes. Toxocariasis is a roundworm infection often found in urban dogs. Humans ingest the eggs by the fecal-oral route. The larvae migrate and often enter the retina where they become trapped. They stimulate an immune response that culminates in granuloma formation. These granulomata can impair vision and sometimes are mistaken for retinal tumors. There is no means of direct diagnosis short of tissue biopsy. Treatment is with albendazole; larvae visible in the retina can be destroyed with a laser.[1]

Toxoplasma gondii can cause vitreal inflammation with retinal hemorrhages and tears. Immunocompromised patients may develop chorioretinitis and optic neuritis with visual field defects and ocular palsies. Erythrocytes with sticky "knobs" from *P. falciparum* infection can cause retinal vascular congestion and ischemia with hemorrhage, exudate, infarction, and macular destruction. Cerebral malaria can cause cortical blindness. Mucocutaneous leishmaniasis can involve the lids, tear glands, retina, or iris and may result in total ocular destruction. *Acanthamoeba* species can cause a dangerous keratitis in contact lens wearers. The patient will complain of severe pain, tearing, and photophobia. Early infection may be misdiagnosed as herpetic keratitis. The infection may become chronic and require keratoplasty. A number of worms migrate to or through the eye causing inflammation, tissue destruction, and blindness. These include *Ascaris* and hookworm. *Echinococcus* and *Cysticercus* can cause destructive cystic lesions in the eye.

PULMONARY SYMPTOMS

Patients with *P. falciparum* may initially seek treatment for fever and cough. Early in the course of treatment of severe malaria the patient may develop noncardiogenic pulmonary edema or adult respiratory distress syndrome requiring mechanical ventilation with positive end-expiratory pressure (PEEP).[46,47]

E. histolytica can cause sympathetic pleural effusions, direct pulmonary or pleural involvement by extension or rupture of an amebic liver abscess, or direct hematogenous seeding of the lungs leading to considerable additional morbidity and mortality for the patient with underlying amebic infection.[48] *Pneumocystis carinii* pneumonia (PCP) is one of the most common causes of respiratory opportunistic infection (OI) in patients with human immunodeficiency virus (HIV) in the United States and Europe; however, it is responsible for less than 10% of pulmonary OI in Africa and the developing world. The reason for this is unclear. Many patients with AIDS in these countries die with CD4 cell counts that are higher than those associated with PCP disease in the United States.[49]

Löffler's syndrome, characterized by persistent, nonproductive cough, substernal chest pain, wheezing, rales, pulmonary infiltrates on chest x-ray (CXR), and marked eosinophilia,[50] is often seen when larvae from the roundworm *Ascaris lumbricoides,* the hookworms *Necator americanus* and *Ancylostoma duodenale,* and the threadworm *S. stercoralis* transit the lungs as part of their developmental cycles. *Ascaris* larvae penetrate the small intestinal wall to gain entry into the small venules of the gastrointestinal (GI) tract and then migrate to the lungs. *Strongyloides* and the hookworm filariform larvae penetrate through the skin of the feet, entering small cutaneous venules before migration to the lungs. The pulmonary infiltrates and symptoms are transient, resolving within 2 weeks. Diagnosis depends on discovering larvae in sputum or gastric aspirates. Negative stool examinations are nondiagnostic because eggs will not appear in the stool for at least a month following initial infection.[51]

Patients' immune responses to the microfilariae of *Wuchereria bancrofti* and *Brugia malayi* cause tropical eosinophilic pneumonia.[52] These patients present with malaise, weight loss, new-onset nocturnal wheezing and asthma, shortness of breath, and chest discomfort. Chest x-ray films may show nodular or interstitial infiltrates, consolidations, or cavitation. Microfilariae can be seen in lung biopsy material. Untreated infection may result in obstructive or restrictive lung disease. Patients will have marked eosinophilia and elevations of serum immunoglobulin E (IgE).[53]

Paragonimus westermani and echinococcal species are trophic for the lungs in their human hosts. *P. westermani* eggs are shed in stool, hatch in fresh water, and as miracidia infect a snail intermediary. After further development, cercariae are released from the snail, penetrating and encysting in freshwater crab or crayfish. After consumption by the human host, metacercariae from the crab or crayfish excyst within the duodenum, penetrating the duodenal wall into the abdominal cavity. The larvae migrate from the peritoneal cavity through the diaphragm into the pleural cavity, finally migrating to the lungs causing hemorrhage, necrosis, and a granulomatous response. Early in the process patients may have infiltrates and eosinophilia; later disease is marked by bronchiectasis, chronic bronchitis, fever, hemoptysis, and cachexia. Pulmonary nodules and cysts may cavitate.[54] Many of these patients may have positive purified protein derivative (PPD) tests, and their symptoms and radiographs may mimic tuberculosis. Sputum is often blood-streaked and flecked with dark brown particles containing diagnostic ova. Radiography, stool examination, and immune testing of sputum and blood can help make the diagnosis.[55] Praziquantel is the treatment of choice.

E. granulosus causes pulmonary hydatid cyst disease that remains asymptomatic until a cyst grows large enough to cause a mass effect, becomes superinfected, or leaks cyst material, which is highly immunogenic, causing a severe anaphylactoid reaction. Pulmonary hydatid cysts can also be associated with cough, chest pain, and hemoptysis.[56] Primary hydatid disease in the liver can metastasize to the lungs or brain. A thoracic CT scan will show a unilocular lung cyst; the plain radiograph of a ruptured cyst is said to resemble a water lily and is pathognomonic. Cysts can be treated with careful surgical excision and pharmacotherapy.

Early schistosomal disease, "Katayama fever," can cause fever, cough, eosinophilia, and diffuse pulmonary nodules as the schistosomulae pass through the lungs. In long-standing disease, ova shed from worm pairs can lodge in the vasculature of the lungs, causing pseudotubercles, granulomatous lung disease, pulmonary hypertension, and cor pulmonale. In patients who are started on corticosteroids or immunosuppressive therapy who have long-standing, latent, and asymptomatic *Strongyloides stercoralis* infections, the helminth disseminates widely. Fatal, massive pulmonary infections with radiographic whiteouts and insupportable respiratory failure have been reported in patients who have received organ transplants; this clinical disaster occurs more commonly in patients who originally came from developing countries and were never worked up for *Strongyloides* infection prior to transplant.[57,58] Ironically, *Strongyloides* infection can be misdiagnosed as bronchospasm and asthma, prompting the clinician to prescribe steroids that may precipitate dissemination.[59]

CARDIOVASCULAR SYMPTOMS

Chagas' Disease

Principles of Disease *Trypanosoma cruzi* infection causes acute and chronic myocarditis. *T. cruzi* is endemic in South and Central America and causes Chagas' disease. The vector is the reduviid, or "kissing bug," which inhabits the walls and roofs of thatched dwellings built adjacent to forest. Once a disease of rural populations, urban transmigration has expanded the epidemiologic scope of Chagas' disease. The reduviid's bite is no longer the only source of Chagas' disease; transfusion with blood containing live trypanosomes from infected hosts is a growing source of infection.[60,61] The reduviid bites the patient, often in the periorbital region, and excretes feces containing the trypomastigote of *T. cruzi.* The trypanosome enters the inflamed bite wound or other mucosal or conjunctival surfaces, causing local swelling, called a chagoma. Romaña's sign, painless unilateral periorbital edema, is pathognomonic but rarely seen. The trypomastigote migrates to trophic tissues including smooth muscle, cardiac muscle, and autonomic ganglia in the heart, esophagus, and colon, causing local inflammation and tissue destruction.

Clinical Features Acute infection is heralded by fever, facial and dependent extremity edema, hepatosplenomegaly, lymphadenopathy, malaise, lymphocytosis on peripheral blood smear, and elevated liver transaminases. At this stage, fatal left ventricular dysfunction and dysrhythmias are uncommon. Early illness lasts 1 to 2 months and resolves spontaneously to a latency known as the *indeterminate phase,* which can persist throughout the patient's lifetime. Approximately 25% of patients will progress to chronic Chagas' disease, principally cardiopathy and GI disease (GI manifestations of Chagas' will be discussed in the next section). Amastigotes invade cardiac muscle and the cardiac conduction system. There is chronic inflammation, mononuclear cell infiltration, and fibrosis. Patients may develop atrial brady-dysrhythmias, fibrillation, right and left bundle branch blocks, complete heart block, and ventricular dysrhythmias including ventricular fibrillation. There is right and left ventricular dysfunction with dilated cardiomyopathy; cardiac muscle is replaced by fibrosis and scarring. Mural thrombi are not uncommon; thromboembolic disease manifesting as pulmonary embolism, stroke, or peripheral arterial embolism can be the first indication of long-standing asymptomatic infection. Congestive heart failure is rapidly progressive, and fatal within months without aggressive pharmacologic intervention and transplantation.[62]

Diagnostic Strategies Acute Chagas' disease can be diagnosed by the presence of motile trypomastigotes in anticoagulated blood specimens. The organism can also be cultured in special liquid media. Chronic Chagas' disease can be diagnosed using several serologic tests including complement fixation, enzyme-linked immunosorbent assay (ELISA), or indirect immunofluorescence. The assays are nonspecific, cross-reacting with malaria, syphilis, and leishmaniasis, as well as some collagen vascular diseases; consequently, at least two immunologic assays must be positive to confirm the presence of *T. cruzi*. Polymerase chain reaction (PCR) technology is improving and soon will provide the gold standard for diagnosis.[63]

Management Both nifurtimox and benznidazole (Radimil) are used for treating *T. cruzi*. Cure rates rarely exceed 50%. Nifurtimox must be taken for a long time and has many severe side effects. Its production has been discontinued; however, it is the only antitrypanosomal medication available in the United States today (it can be obtained from the Centers for Disease Control and Prevention [CDC]). Benznidazole has fewer side effects. It is now recommended for indeterminate phase treatment. Late complications of chronic diseases are modulated by autoimmune activity and do not respond to antiparasitic pharmacotherapy. Both nifurtimox and benznidazole have been associated with lymphoma in an animal model.[64,65] Chronic Chagas' disease of the heart, esophagus, or colon is treated symptomatically. Patients receiving immunosuppressive therapy to prevent rejection after cardiac transplant have demonstrated recurrent disease in the transplanted myocardium.

GASTROINTESTINAL SYMPTOMS

Diarrhea

Diarrhea is one of the most common symptoms for which travelers seek medical attention. S. L. Gorbach wrote, "Travel expands the mind and loosens the bowels."[66] Diarrhea is also the leading cause of death in children under 5 years old in developing countries and a major source of morbidity for older children and adults. Most diarrheal disease is viral or bacterial; however, there are some noteworthy parasites that cause diarrhea.

Cryptosporidium parvum and *Cyclospora cayetanensis* are food- and water-borne coccidians that cause watery diarrhea. Both are particularly significant causes of morbidity in malnourished children and patients with AIDS. In these populations in the developing world the prevalence may approach 50%[67,68] Cryptosporidial oocysts can be seen in stool, and ELISA and immunofluorescent assays of stool are available. Paromomycin decreases stooling in patients with AIDS, who often have prolonged illness. Treatment is symptomatic for immunocompetent hosts.[69] *Cyclospora* oocysts can be detected in stool samples using a Ziehl-Neelsen stain. Trimethoprim-sulfamethoxazole treats the infection.[70]

E. histolytica causes an invasive or inflammatory diarrhea. Patients will complain of fever, tenesmus, abdominal pain, and watery stool containing blood and mucus. Untreated disease can progress to widespread colitis and perforation of the bowel wall with peritonitis and death.[71] Stool examination will reveal mobile trophozoites containing ingested RBCs. Immune assays of stool can now differentiate between *E. histolytica* and nonpathogenic ameba species. Metronidazole is the drug of choice for amebiasis. *Balantidium coli* is the other protozoan that can cause invasive diarrhea. It has trophism for the terminal ileum, sometimes appearing to be appendicitis. Tetracycline and metronidazole are active against *B. coli*.[72]

Giardia lamblia can cause persistent diarrhea, abdominal bloating, cramps, flatulence, and weight loss. The organism is ingested and reproduces exponentially in the small bowel. In severe infection the entire jejunum becomes covered with organisms, and the patient suffers from malabsorption with steatorrhea. The organisms are rarely seen in fresh stool preparations because they quickly break down and become indiscernible. As a result, direct immunofluorescence and ELISA assays of stool are used to confirm the diagnosis. *Giardia* has many animal reservoirs, including the beaver. Campers who drink unfiltered, pure mountain spring water in the United States commonly contract *Giardia*. Metronidazole and tinidazole treat the disease.

S. stercoralis, Capillaria philippinensis, T. trichiura, and *Schistosoma* have all been associated with diarrhea. Hyperinfection or dissemination of *Strongyloides* can cause persistent diarrhea, weight loss, and abdominal pain. *Trichuris* causes diarrhea when the parasite load in the intestine is very high. Schistosomiasis can cause a chronic granulomatous colitis, which may resemble inflammatory bowel disease or an acute, bloody, febrile colitis associated with "Katayama fever" in the immunologically naive patient.

In chronic schistosomiasis, worm pairs in patients' mesenteric and portal venous systems lay eggs that become ensnared in the liver, causing intense local inflammation and scarring and the classic "pipe stem" cirrhosis with periportal fibrosis. These patients develop portal hypertension, ascites, and esophageal varices. Upper GI bleeding is not as common as in patients with alcoholic cirrhosis; however, the number of patients infected with schistosomiasis in endemic regions is great, and variceal bleeding is an important cause of GI hemorrhage.[73,74]

Abdominal Pain

Parasitic infection was the cause of appendicitis in 3% of cases in an extensive review; pathologic examination revealed enterobiasis, amebiasis, ascariasis, trichuriasis, and taeniasis.[75]

A. lumbricoides can cause significant persistent or recurrent abdominal pain in adults and partial intestinal obstruction in children with significant worm loads. Anthelminthics and conservative, supportive therapy usually obviate the problem without requiring surgical intervention.[76,77] The diagnosis of ascariasis is made by identifying eggs in the stool. Patients with large worm loads may excrete adult worms, especially after therapy is started. Severe intestinal amebiasis can be complicated by colonic perforation and peritonitis.

Angiostrongylus costaricensis, a nematode known as the rat lung worm, is common in Central America. Infected children may clinically appear to have Meckel's diverticula or acute appendicitis. They suffer from nausea, vomiting, fever, abdominal pain localized to the right lower quadrant, and a tender mass. Surgical exploration may uncover abscesses, obstruction, or intestinal infarction.[78]

Anisakiasis is characterized by severe abdominal pain after eating raw fish (sushi and sashimi primarily). *Anisakis marina,* a nematode that burrows into the intestine, is responsible.[79]

The liver fluke, *F. hepatica,* causes a syndrome that mimics viral hepatitis: right upper quadrant pain, fever, nausea and vomiting, jaundice, a tender enlarged liver, and elevated transaminases. Patients also have eosinophilia and urticaria. Imaging studies, including CT scan, will show the tracks of burrowing flukes. Serologic testing makes the diagnosis because the patient's stool may not contain eggs for several months after ingestion.[80] As noted in the discussion of GI bleeding, the eggs of schistosomes become trapped in the portal venules and trigger an inflammatory response, leading to granulomatous liver disease, fibrosis, and cirrhosis. Hepatic granulomas are also seen in disseminated strongyloidiasis and biliary ascariasis.

E. histolytica can cause hepatic abscess. Patients with abscesses typically do not have amebic dysentery and do not shed *Entamoeba* in their stool. Serology is almost always positive in patients with abscesses. Patients have fever, weight loss, anorexia, and right-sided abdominal pain, but no jaundice. Treatment is with metronidazole or tinidazole and a luminal amebicide such as iodoquinol.[81] *Echinococcus granulosus* causes hydatid cysts of the liver that on CT imaging are seen as septations and so-called *daughter cysts.* Pharmacotherapy with albendazole and careful excision remain the treatments of choice. Leaking cyst material will cause a severe anaphylactoid reaction in the host.

Jaundice may result from hemolysis secondary to direct infection of RBCs with *Plasmodium* or *Babesia,* or from biliary obstruction. *Ascaris* can cause biliary colic, pyogenic cholangitis, pancreatitis, or liver abscess. Dead worms can be the nidus for gallstone formation. Biliary imaging and endoscopic retrograde cholangiopancreatography (ERCP) will show worms in the biliary tree. Mechanical removal by endoscopy and anthelminthic therapy is curative.[82] *Clonorchis sinensis* and *F. hepatica* are trophic for the biliary tree. They can be present without symptoms for years before eventually precipitating cholecystitis, cholangitis, or cholangiocarcinoma.[83]

Pruritis Ani

Enterobius vermicularis, or pinworm, causes pruritus ani, a syndrome of intense perianal itch seen primarily in children. Autoinfection is common because children (and adults) will scratch the pruritic anal area and then bite their nails or put their fingers in their mouth. The worm has a worldwide distribution. Diagnosis is clinical and is confirmed by finding the small adult worms wriggling about on the anal verge. Eggs are rarely seen in the stool but can be visualized using the scotch tape test: tape touched to the perianal region will collect eggs that can be seen with light microscopy. Mebendazole is the treatment of choice.

PARASITIC COINFECTIONS IN PATIENTS WITH HIV AND AIDS

Perspective

HIV infection and AIDS are more prevalent in the tropics of developing countries. Heterosexual and perinatal transmission are much more common, thus young children and young adults of both sexes are primarily infected. The clinician may encounter patients who are coinfected with HIV and any other infectious agent, including all of the parasites discussed in this chapter. HIV coinfection may worsen the symptoms and outcome, alter the presentation, increase the virulence, or assist the infective process.

AIDS causes abnormalities in almost every aspect of a host's immune response to infection; cell-mediated immunity (which is quite important in combating parasitic infection) is most affected.[84] The diagnosis and response to therapy of many parasitic infections are monitored serologically. HIV infection interferes with this response, rendering many of these tests unreliable. Therapies that are very effective in the normal host may be ineffective in the patient with HIV infection. Pharmacologic agents may have to be given for long periods of time or for the patient's entire life.

Specific Parasitic Infections

Malaria has not been shown to be an opportunistic infection in patients with AIDS; however, many patients, especially children, with recurrent malaria and anemia from hemolysis have required transfusions from blood supplies not screened for HIV and have become infected.[85] Treating febrile patients for malaria in areas where it is endemic is a common practice. In patients with AIDS, fever alone is not predictive of malaria; diagnosis should precede therapy. (Patients with AIDS have more and more severe allergic reactions to drugs, especially sulfonamides.) Patients with HIV infection are at greater risk for severe clinical manifestations of babesiosis.[86]

Visceral leishmaniasis is more commonly disseminated and fatal in patients with AIDS. Patients can have reactivation of latent leishmanial infections, and a prolonged febrile illness in an HIV-positive patient with a lifetime history of travel in areas of the world where leishmaniasis is endemic should be worked up for this coinfection.[87] Chagas' disease in the indeterminate phase can be reactivated in patients infected with HIV. They frequently have CNS involvement with meningoencephalitis and severe myocarditis.[88] Single-drug therapy may be insufficient; benznidazole penetration into the CSF may not be adequate. *T. gondii* is well recognized throughout the world as a common OI of patients with AIDS, having a particular trophism for the CNS.

The coccidial organisms *Isospora belli, C. parvum,* and *C. cayetanensis* all have been associated with prolonged diarrhea in patients with AIDS. These organisms are difficult to treat and almost impossible to eradicate in these patients. The diarrhea is extremely debilitating and can be as profuse as that seen in cholera. *E. histolytica* has a high prevalence in the male homosexual population who practice unprotected anal intercourse; however, invasive amebiasis is not an OI associated with HIV infection. Schistosomiasis enhances the pathogenesis of HIV and is more difficult to treat and eradicate in patients who are HIV-positive.[89] *S. stercoralis* is more likely to manifest as hyperinfection and disseminated disease in patients who are HIV-positive.[90] In patients who are at risk for HIV (everyone) and parasitic illness, the clinician must always consider coinfection in the differential diagnosis.

KEY CONCEPTS

- Parasitic diseases may present with almost any symptom or constellation of symptoms. As a result, a travel history should be obtained in all patients with clinically significant symptoms of unclear etiology. The combination of presenting symptoms and recent site of travel can lead to early diagnosis of most parasitic infections.
- Parasitic coinfections are particularly common in patients with HIV and AIDS.
- Acute malaria should be suspected in patients with irregular high fevers associated with headache, abdominal pain, or respiratory symptoms. Patients who are clinically ill, or who are suspected of having falciparum malaria, should be hospitalized for evaluation and treatment.
- Cysticercosis should be considered in the differential diagnosis of new-onset seizures.
- *Giardia* should be suspected in patients with diarrhea who have recently been camping or drinking unfiltered mountain spring water.

REFERENCES

1. Bell DR: *Tropical medicine,* ed 4, Oxford, 1995, Blackwell Science.
2. Guerrant RL et al: *Tropical infectious diseases,* ed 1, Philadelphia, 1999, Churchill Livingstone.
3. Danis M, Gentilini M: Malaria, a worldwide scourge, *Rev Prat* 48:254-257, 1998.
4. Isaacson M: Airport malaria: a review, *Bulletin of the World Health Organization* 67:737-743, 1989.
5. Van den Ende et al: A cluster of airport malaria in Belgium in 1995, *Acta Clin Belg* 53:259-263, 1998.
6. Iftikhar SA, Roistacher K: Indigenous *Plasmodium falciparum* in Queens, NY, *Arch Int Med* 155:1099-1101, 1995.
7. Cahill J et al: Malaria in Rhode Island, *Journal of Travel Medicine* 7:112-118, 2000.
8. Molyneux ME, Fox R: Diagnosis and treatment of malaria in Britain, *BMJ* 306:1175-1180, 1993.
9. Gilles HM, Warrell DA: *Bruce-Chwatt's essential malariology,* ed 3, London, 1993, Edward Arnold.
10. Tran TH et al: A controlled trial of artemether or quinine in Vietnamese adults with severe falciparum malaria, *N Engl J Med* 335:76-83, 1996.
11. Mintz ED et al: Transfusion-transmitted babesiosis: a case report from a new endemic area, *Transfusion* 31:365, 1991.
12. Ruebush TK et al: Human babesiosis on Nantucket Island: evidence for self-limited and sub-clinical infections, *N Engl J Med* 297:825, 1977.
13. Golightly LM et al: Fever and headache in a splenectomized woman, *Rev Infect Dis* 11:629, 1989.
14. Benezra D et al: Babesiosis and infection with human immunodeficiency virus (HIV), *Ann Intern Med* 107:944, 1987.
15. Piesman J et al: Concurrent *Borrelia burgdorferi* and *Babesia microti* infection in nymphal *Ixodes dammini, J Clin Microbiol* 24:446, 1986.
16. Doherty JF et al: Katayama fever: an acute manifestation of schistosomiasis, *BMJ* 313:1071, 1996.
17. Arjona R et al: Fascioliasis in developed countries: a review of classic and aberrant forms of the disease, *Medicine (Baltimore)* 74:13, 1995.
18. Kirchof LV: American trypanosomiasis in Central American immigrants, *Am J Med* 82:915-920, 1987.
19. Evans T et al: American visceral leishmaniasis, *West J Med* 142:777-781, 1985.
20. Maltz G, Knauer CM: Amebic liver abscess: a 15 year experience, *Am J Gastroenterol* 86:704, 1991.
21. van Hensbroek MB et al: A trial of artemether or quinine in children with cerebral malaria, *N Engl J Med* 335:69-75, 1996.
22. Nagatake T et al: Pathology of falciparum malaria in Vietnam, *Am J Trop Med Hyg* 47:259-264, 1992.
23. McCormick GF et al: Cysticercosis cerebri, *Arch Neurol* 39:534, 1982.
24. Garcia HH et al: Diagnosis of cysticercosis in endemic regions, *Lancet* 338:549-551, 1991.
25. Vaquez V, Sotelo J: The course of seizures after treatment for cerebral cysticercosis, *N Engl J Med* 327:696-701, 1992.
26. Morris DL, Richards KS: *Hydatid disease, current medical and surgical management,* ed 1, Oxford, 1992, Butterworth-Heinemann.
27. Epidemiology and control of African trypanosomiasis, 1986 Technical Report Series 793, Geneva, 1986, World Health Organization.
28. Ekwanzala M et al: In the heart of darkness: sleeping sickness in Zaire, *Lancet* 348:1427, 1996.
29. Fairlamb AH: Novel approaches to the chemotherapy of trypanosomiasis, *Trans R Soc Trop Med Hyg* 84:613, 1990.
30. Gay T et al: Fatal CNS trichinosis, *JAMA* 247:1024, 1982.
31. Evans RW, Pattern BM: Trichinosis associated with superior sagittal sinus thrombosis, *Ann Neurol* 11:216, 1982.
32. Seidel JS et al: Successful treatment of primary amebic meningoencephalitis, *N Engl J Med* 306:346, 1982.
33. Grove DI: *Strongyloidiasis: a major roundworm infection,* ed 1, London, 1989, Taylor & Francis.
34. Kirchhoff LV, Nash TE: A case of *Schistosomiasis japonica:* resolution of CAT-scan detected cerebral abnormalities without specific therapy, *Am J Trop Med Hyg* 33:1155, 1984.
35. Burgmann H et al: Serum levels of erythropoietin in acute *Plasmodium falciparum* malaria, *Am J Trop Med Hyg* 54:280, 1996.
36. Newton C et al: Severe anemia in children living in a malaria endemic area of Kenya, *Trop Med Int Health* 2:165, 1997.
37. WHO expert committee on filariasis fifth report: Lymphatic filariasis: the disease and its control, Technical Report Series 821, Geneva, 1992, World Health Organization.
38. Ottesen EA et al: A controlled trial of ivermectin and diethylcarbamazine in lymphatic filariasis, *N Engl J Med* 322:1113, 1990.
39. Carvalho EM et al: Immunologic markers of clinical evolution in children recently infected with *Leishmania donovani chagasi, J Infect Dis* 165:535, 1992.
40. Melby PC et al: Cutaneous leishmaniasis: review of 59 cases seen at the National Institutes of Health, *Clin Infect Dis* 15:924, 1992.
41. Gustafson TL et al: Human cutaneous leishmaniasis acquired in Texas, *Am J Trop Med Hyg* 34:58, 1985.
42. Caumes E et al: A randomized trial of ivermectin versus albendazole for the treatment of cutaneous larva migrans, *Am J Trop Med Hyg* 49:641, 1993.
43. Abiose A et al: Reduction in incidence of optic nerve disease with annual ivermectin to control onchocerciasis, *Lancet* 341:130-134, 1993.
44. Natman TB et al: Diethylcarbamazine prophylaxis for human loiasis: results of a double-blind study, *N Engl J Med* 319:752, 1988.
45. Martin PY et al: Tolerance and efficacy of single high dose ivermectin for the treatment of loiasis, *Am J Trop Med Hyg* 48:186-192, 1993.
46. Johnson S et al: Acute tropical infections and the lung, *Thorax* 49:7214, 1994.
47. Charoenpan P et al: Pulmonary edema in severe falciparum malaria: hemodynamic study and clinicophysiologic correlation, *Chest* 97:1190, 1990.
48. Kubitschek KR et al: Amebiasis presenting as pleuropulmonary disease, *West J Med* 142:203, 1985.
49. Malin AS: *Pneumocystis carinii* pneumonia in Africa, *Lancet* 347:127, 1996.
50. Loffler W: Transient lung infiltrations with blood eosinophilia, *Int Arch Allergy Immunol* 8:54, 1956.
51. Allen JN, Davis WB: Eosinophilic lung diseases, *Am J Respir Crit Care Med* 150:1423, 1994.
52. Ottesen EA, Nutman TB: Tropical pulmonary eosinophilia, *Annu Rev Med* 43:417, 1992.
53. Enzenauer RJ et al: Tropical pulmonary eosinophilia, *South Med J* 93:69, 1990.
54. Im JG et al: Pleuropulmonary paragonimiasis: radiologic findings in 71 patients, *AJR* 159:39, 1992.
55. Yee B et al: Pulmonary paragonimiasis in Southeast Asians living in the central San Joaquin Valley, *West J Med* 156:423, 1992.
56. Jerray M et al: Hydatid disease of the lungs: study of 386 cases, *Am Rev Respir Dis* 146:185, 1992.
57. Morgna JS et al: Opportunistic strongyloidiasis in renal transplant recipients, *Transplantation* 42:518-524, 1986.

58. Scoggin CH, Call NB: Acute respiratory failure due to disseminated strongyloidiasis in a renal transplant recipient, *Ann Intern Med* 87:456-458, 1977.
59. Nowokolo C, Imohiosen EAF: Strongyloidiasis of the respiratory tract presenting as asthma, *BMJ* 2:153, 1973.
60. Dunlap NE et al: Strongyloidiasis manifested as asthma, *South Med J* 77:77-78, 1984.
61. Schumis GA: *Trypanosoma cruzi,* the etiologic agent of Chagas' disease: status in the blood supply in endemic and non-endemic countries, *Transfusion* 31:547-557, 1991.
62. Amorim DS: Chagas' disease, *Prog Cardiol* 8:235-279, 1979.
63. Kirchoff LV et al: Comparison of PCR and microscopic methods for detecting *Trypanosoma cruzi, J Clin Microbiol* 34:1171-1175, 1996.
64. Teixera ARI et al: Malignant, non-Hodgkin's lymphoma in *Trypanosoma cruzi* infected rabbits treated with nifurtimox, *J Comp Pathol* 103:37-48, 1990.
65. Teixera ARI et al: Chagas' disease: lymphoma growth in rabbits treated with benznidazole, *Am J Trop Med Hyg* 43:146-158, 1990.
66. Gorbach SL: Traveler's diarrhea, *N Engl J Med* 307:881-883, 1982.
67. Colebunders R et al: Persistent diarrhea strongly associates with HIV infection in Kinshasha, Zaire, *Am J Gastroenterol* 82:859-864, 1987.
68. Molbak K et al: Cryptosporidiosis in infancy and childhood mortality in Guinea-Bissau, West Africa, *BMJ* 307:417-420, 1993.
69. White AC et al: Paromomycin for cryptosporidiosis in AIDS: a prospective, double-blind trial, *J Infect Dis* 170:419-424, 1994.
70. Hoge CW et al: Placebo-controlled trial of clotrimazole for *Cyclospora* infections among travelers and foreign residents in Nepal, *Lancet* 345:691-693, 1995.
71. Wanke C et al: Epidemiologic and clinical features of invasive amebiasis in Bangladesh: a case-control comparison with other diarrheal diseases and post-mortem findings, *Am J Trop Med Hyg* 38:335-341, 1998.
72. Garcia-Laverde A, de Bonilla L: Clinical trials with metronidazole in human balantidiasis, *Am J Trop Med Hyg* 24:781-783, 1975.
73. Strickland GT: Gastrointestinal manifestations of schistosomiasis, *Gut* 35:1334-1337, 1994.
74. Saad AM et al: Oesophageal varices in a region of the Sudan endemic for *Schistosoma mansoni, Br J Surg* 78:1252-1253, 1991.
75. Gupta SC et al: Pathology of tropical appendicitis, *J Clin Pathol* 42:1169-1172, 1989.
76. Hamed AD, Akinola O: Intestinal ascariasis in the differential diagnosis of peptic ulcer disease, *Trop Geogr Med* 42:37-40, 1990.
77. Pinus J: Surgical complications of ascariasis, *Prog Pediatr Surg* 15:79-86, 1982.
78. Hulbert TV et al: Abdominal angiostrongyliasis mimicking acute appendicitis and Meckel's diverticulum: report of a case in the United States and review, *Clin Infect Dis* 14:836, 1992.
79. Kark AE, McAlpine JC: Anisakiasis as a cause of acute abdominal crisis, *Br J Clin Pract* 48:216-217, 1994.
80. Han JK et al: Radiological findings in human fascioliasis, *Abdom Imaging* 18:261, 1993.
81. Barnes PF et al: A comparison of amebic and pyogenic abscess of the liver, *Medicine* 66:472, 1987.
82. Rocha MS et al: CT identification of *Ascaris* in the biliary tract, *Abdom Imaging* 20:317, 1995.
83. Harinasuta T et al: Trematode infections: opisthorchiasis, clonorchiasis, fascioliasis, and paragonimiasis, *Infect Dis Clin North Am* 7:699, 1993.
84. Morrow RH et al: Interactions of HIV infection with endemic tropical diseases, *AIDS* 3:S79, 1989.
85. Greenburg AE et al: The association between malaria, blood transfusions, and HIV seropositivity in a pediatric population in Kinshasa, Zaire, *JAMA* 259:545, 1988.
86. Falagas ME, Klempner MS: Babesiosis in patients with AIDS: a chronic infection presenting as fever of unknown origin, *Clin Infect Dis* 22:809, 1996.
87. Laguna F et al: Gastrointestinal leishmaniasis in human immunodeficiency virus-infected patients: report of five cases and review, *Clin Infect Dis* 19:48, 1994.
88. Rocha A et al: Pathology of patients with Chagas' disease and AIDS, *Am J Trop Med Hyg* 50:261, 1994.
89. Karanja DMS et al: Studies on schistosomiasis in Western Kenya: II. Efficacy of Praziquantel on treatment of schistosomiasis in persons co-infected with human immunodeficiency virus-1, *Am J Trop Med Hyg* 59:307, 1998.
90. Newton RC et al: *Strongyloides stercoralis* hyper-infection in a carrier of HTLV-1 virus with evidence of selective immunosuppression, *Am J Med* 92:202, 1992.

128 Tick-Borne Illnesses

Edward B. Bolgiano
Joseph Sexton

PERSPECTIVE

Ticks are hematophagous parasites of humans and animals, distributed worldwide. They transmit rickettsial, bacterial, spirochetal, viral, and protozoal diseases and cause disease via their own toxins (Table 128-1). As vectors of human disease, ticks rank second in importance only to mosquitoes. Patients may have traveled during the summer months and returned from endemic areas with tick-borne disease. In addition, recent reports of infection acquired within urban areas emphasize the need to consider tick-borne illness even in the absence of a history of travel to high-risk areas.[1]

Reports on ticks, their feeding habits, and their possible relation to disease can be found from early historical time.[2] Pliny (77 AD), in *Historia naturalis,* referred to "an animal living on blood with its head always fixed and swelling, being one of the animals which has no exit [anus] for its food, it bursts with over repletion and dies from actual nourishment." Tick-borne illness was first recognized on the North American continent by Native Americans. According to legend, Shoshone men avoided the "evil spirits" that caused illness by sending only women into certain areas of the Rocky Mountain region known to be especially hazardous. The etiologic association of the tick vector with Rocky Mountain spotted fever was noted by missionaries and by early settlers, who named the affliction "tick fever." Physicians in Idaho and Montana recorded the classic clinical descriptions of the disease in 1899.

Table 128-1. Tick-Borne Illnesses

Type	Disease	Pathogen	Arthropod vector	Geographic distribution
Bacterial (including spirochetal)	Lyme disease	*Borrelia burgdorferi*	*Ixodes scapularis* *I. pacificus* *I. ricinus*	Northeastern United States Upper midwestern United States Pacific coast Europe
	Tularemia	*Francisella tularensis*	*Dermacentor variabilis* *Amblyomma americanum*	Southern United States
	Relapsing fever	*Borrelia hermsii*	*Ornithodoros hemsii*	Western United States
Rickettsial	Rocky Mountain spotted fever	*Rickettsia rickettsii*	*D. andersoni* *D. variabilis*	Predominantly south-eastern United States
	Eastern spotted fever*	*R. conorii* *R. sibirica* *R. australis*		Eastern hemisphere
	Q fever	*Coxiella burnetii*	*D. andersoni*	Worldwide
	Ehrlichiosis	*Ehrlichia canis*	*Rhipicephalus sanguineus*	Southern and eastern United States Worldwide
Parasitic (protozoal)	Babesiosis	*Babesia microti*	*I. scapularis*	Coastal New England
Viral†	Colorado tick fever	Orbivirus	*D. andersoni*	Mountain areas of western United States and Canada
	Tick-borne encephalitis	Flavivirus	*I. marxi* *I. cookei*	Northern United States and Canada
Miscellaneous	Tick paralysis	Neurotoxin	*D. andersoni* *D. variabilis* *A. americanum*	Worldwide
	Pajaroello tick bites	Salivary toxin	*O. coriaceus*	Southern California and Mexico

*Several species of ixodid ticks serve as vectors for Eastern spotted fevers.
†Many other viruses are transmitted to humans by ticks. In the United States only Colorado tick fever occurs with any significant frequency.

PRINCIPLES OF DISEASE

Identification of Ticks

Identification of an arthropod as a tick and subsequent categorization into family and genus are not difficult (Figures 128-1 and 128-2). However, tick identification has limited importance in clinical decision making.

Physiology

Blood-sucking arthropods are divided into two groups according to their method of acquiring blood. The solenophagic feeders insert their mouthparts directly into capillaries and feed on blood alone. Telmophagic feeders insert their mouthparts indiscriminately, lyse tissue, and feed on tissue and extracellular fluids until, eventually, capillary walls are broken down and a pool of blood is produced, from which they feed. Ticks are telmophagic feeders.

In the capitulum of ticks, the sucking structure—the chelicerae—is surrounded by a sheath from which it protrudes during feeding. Sense organs on the capitulum, or podomeres, help locate a host with chemoreceptors. Hair or setae on the legs act as tactile and temperature receptors. A special sensory structure, Haller's organ, is located on the first set of legs and is a humidity and olfactory receptor.[3]

When a suitable location is found, adjacent cheliceral digits incise the skin, and the chelicera and barbed hypostome are inserted. Two mechanisms prevent the tick from being removed from the skin: the barbed hypostome and a cement-like salivary secretion composed of lipoproteins and glycoproteins from the base of the hypostome. This allows the ixodid to attach for as long as 2 weeks. Because argasids are much faster feeders, they have no such cement substance.

Trauma and salivary gland products during a bite can cause local inflammation, hyperemia, edema, hemorrhage, and skin thickening. The saliva injected during feeding contains many different substances. Both hard and soft ticks produce a histolytic secretion that liquefies tissue, which is then sucked into the gut. Eventually, the secretion breaks down the walls of the dermal blood vessels and the released blood is then ingested. To prevent hemostasis, the saliva contains a thrombokinase inhibitor, apyrase, which prevents platelet aggregation by depleting adenosine diphosphate (ADP), prostaglandin (PG)E_2, and prostacyclin to prevent vasoconstriction, and cytolysins. *Ixodes scapularis* has a carboxypeptidase that destroys other inflammatory mediators such as anaphylatoxins and bradykinin, as well as anticomplement C3 factor. These factors would normally cause further inflammation, which would enhance hemostasis. All infectious agents, as well as excretory liquids from some argasids, are transmitted through this saliva. The neurotoxins responsible for tick paralysis are also found in tick saliva.

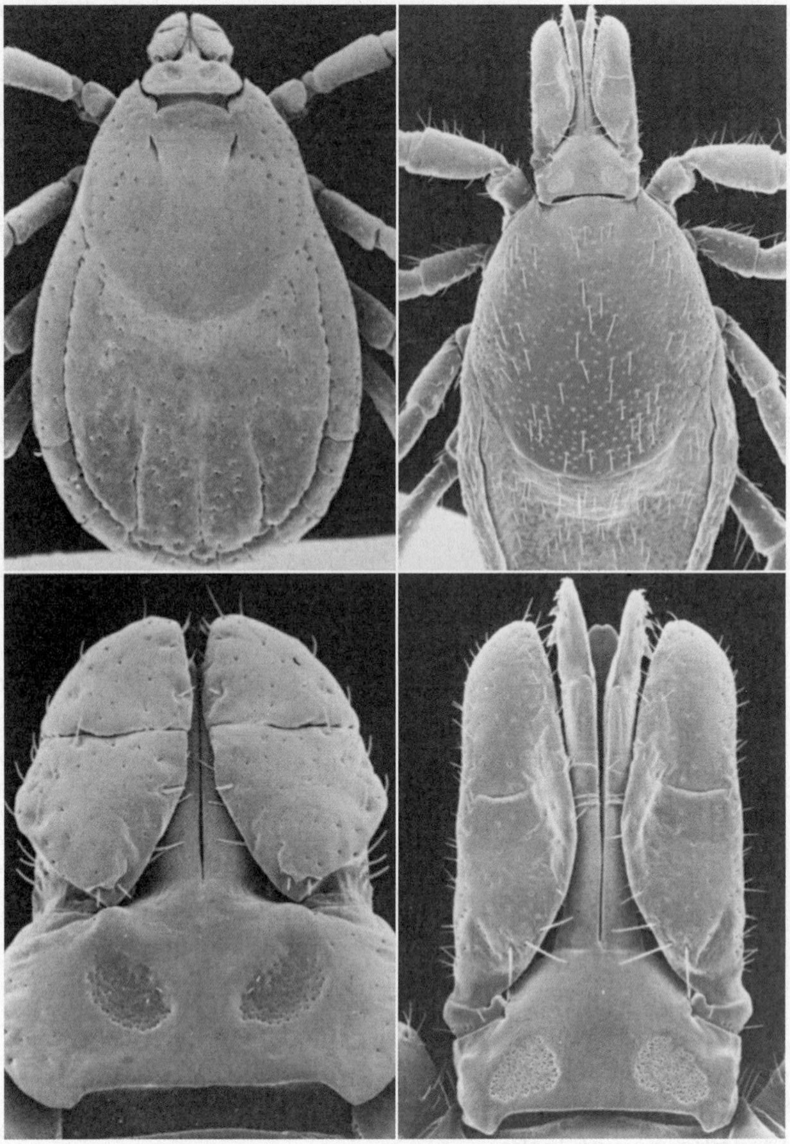

Figure 128-1. **Scanning electron micrographs of two tick species. A, Dorsal view of adult female *Dermacentor variabilis.* B, Dorsal view of adult female *Ixodes scapularis.* C, Dorsal close-up of head. D, Dorsal close-up of head.** ***Courtesy Dr. J.E. Keirans, Georgia Southern University, Statesboro, Georgia.***

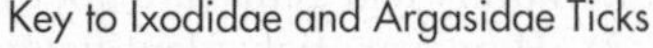

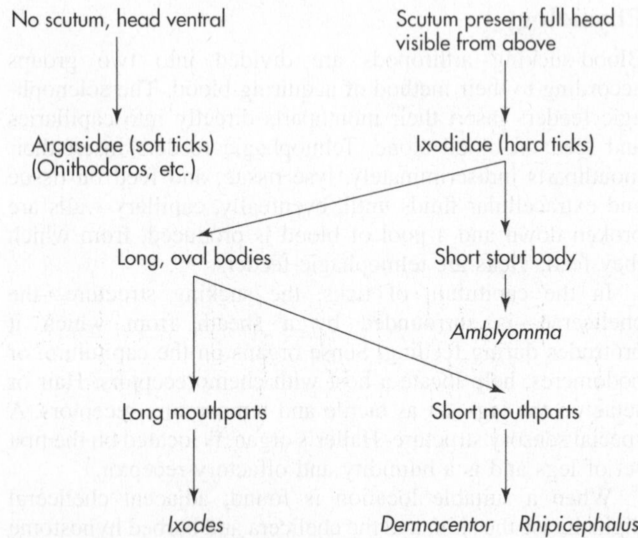

Figure 128-2. **Identification scheme for geni within Ixodidae and Argasidae, the two primary disease-transmitting families of ticks.**

Argasids are short, rapid feeders with preformed distensible endocuticles and therefore need to feed for only minutes to hours for a full meal. As a result, they tend to be found in nests and burrows, where their hosts visit frequently. *Ixodes* ticks need to form a new exocuticle (phase I of feeding), and thus they feed slowly in the first 12 to 24 hours. Once fully formed, the new endocuticle allows for rapid feeding (phase II) and significant engorgement.

LYME DISEASE

Perspective

Lyme disease, the most common vector-borne disease in the United States, is a tick-borne illness caused by the spirochete *Borrelia burgdorferi.* The story of Lyme disease began in 1975, when health officials at the Connecticut State Department of Health and physicians at Yale were alerted by two skeptical mothers to an unusually large number of cases of apparent juvenile rheumatoid arthritis (JRA) occurring in their small coastal community of Old Lyme, Connecticut. Investigation led to the description of a "new" entity, called Lyme arthritis by Steere et al.[4]

Lyme disease occurs worldwide and has been reported on every continent except Antarctica.[5] It now accounts for more than 95% of all reported vector-borne illness in the United States.[6] The number of reported cases of Lyme disease rose from 9896 in 1992 to 16,802 in 1998 (Figure 128-3).[7] The actual overall incidence of Lyme disease is unknown because many cases go unreported. Lyme disease occurs in people of all ages but is more common in children less than 15 years old and in adults 30 to 60 years old.[8]

Persons at greatest risk live or vacation in endemic areas. In the United States, there are three distinct endemic foci: the coastal Northeast (Massachusetts to Maryland), the Midwest (Minnesota and Wisconsin), and the West (California, Oregon, Utah, and Nevada). In 1995, eight states accounted for more than 90% of the total number of cases in the United States.[8]

The principal tick vectors are *I. scapularis* in the Northeast and Midwest and *I. pacificus* in the West. Nymphal *Ixodes* ticks satisfy all known epidemiologic requirements for the zoonosis as it exists in nature. There is no compelling evidence for alternate arthropod vectors of infection.

Tick population density depends on that of their preferred hosts: the white-footed field mouse, *Peromyscus leucopus,* for the larval and nymphal forms and the white-tailed deer, *Odocoileus virginianus,* for the adult form. The white-footed mouse readily becomes infected after being bitten by infected ticks and remains highly infectious for periods of time that approach their life span in nature, thus providing an important reservoir for *B. burgdorferi.*[9] Adult *I. scapularis* ticks feed primarily on deer, which are key hosts in the tick life cycle and in whose fur the adult tick may survive the winter. The relatively recent repopulation of several areas in the United States by white-tailed deer preceded the recent emergence of Lyme disease in those regions.[10]

Although all stages of the tick may feed on humans, the nymph is primarily responsible for the transmission of Lyme disease. It is not surprising that most patients with Lyme disease do not recall a tick bite (less than one third), given the small size (1 to 2 mm) of nymphs (Figure 128-4). The nymph feeds in the spring and summer, which correlates with a peak incidence of early Lyme disease occurring between May and August. In addition, recreational and occupational exposure is greatest during this time. Later manifestations of Lyme disease may appear throughout the year.

Principles of Disease

The spirochete *B. burgdorferi* persists and multiplies in the midgut of its tick vector, *I. scapularis.* Transmission of the spirochete to humans occurs during feeding, generally about 2 days after attachment.[11] Transmission of the spirochete probably occurs via infectious saliva or, alternatively, via periodic regurgitation of gut fluids during the feeding process.[12]

After an incubation period that lasts several days to several weeks, spirochetemia develops and *Borrelia* may migrate outward via blood or lymph to virtually any site in the body. The spirochete appears to be tropic for synovial tissue, skin,

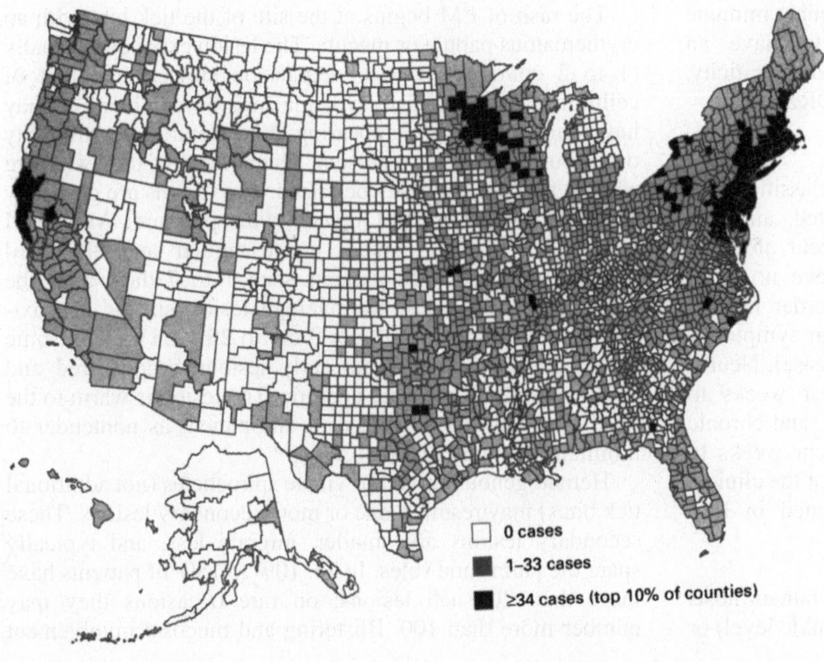

Figure 128-3. **Number of reported cases of Lyme disease by county, United States, 1982-1998.** ***From Surveillance for Lyme Disease—United States, 1992-1998,*** **MMWR 49:1, 2000.**

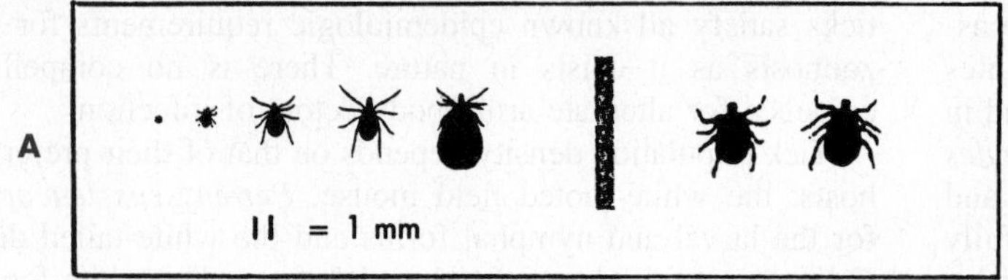

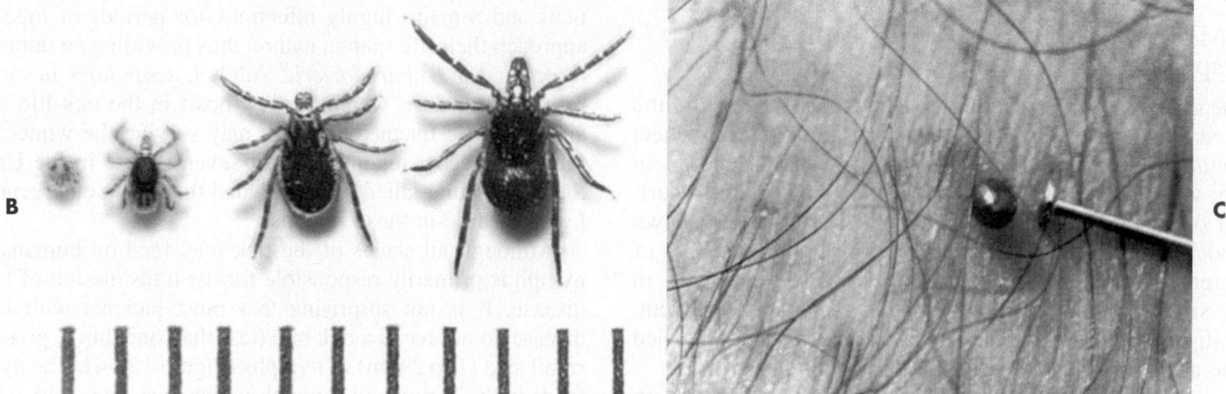

Figure 128-4. **A,** Actual size, *left to right,* of larva, nymph, adult male, adult female, and engorged adult female *Ixodes* sp. ticks, and adult male and female *Dermacentor* sp. ticks. **B,** Larva, nymph, adult male, and adult female of *Ixodes scapularis* on millimeter scale. **C,** Engorged *Ixodes scapularis* nymph, shown in relation to the size of a common pin, in the act of drawing blood. *Drawing courtesy Pfizer Central Research; photographs courtesy M. Fergione.*

and cells of the nervous system, but the mechanism of this tropism is not yet understood. Infection by the spirochete itself accounts for early clinical manifestations. It remains unclear whether late disease manifestations require the continued presence of viable spirochetes or whether an ongoing host immune response to initial infection is sufficient to cause some late disease manifestations. Although the exact roles of infecting spirochetes, spirochetal antigens, and host immune responses are unknown, it is likely that persistent live spirochetes are responsible for most later manifestations of the disease. The variable severity of Lyme disease may in part result from genetic variations in the human immune system. Patients with chronic Lyme arthritis have an increased frequency of human leukocyte antigen specificity, in particular HLA-DR4 and, less often, HLA-DR2.

Clinical Features

Lyme disease, a multisystem disorder, can be classified into three stages: early localized, early disseminated, and late disease. Virtually any clinical feature may occur alone or recur at intervals, and some patients who have no early symptoms may have late symptoms. The disorder usually begins with a rash and associated constitutional symptoms, suggesting a "viral syndrome" (early Lyme disease). Neurologic, joint, or cardiac symptoms may appear weeks to months later (early disseminated Lyme disease), and chronic arthritic and neurologic abnormalities may occur weeks to years later (late Lyme disease). The time course of the clinical features of untreated Lyme disease is illustrated in Figure 128-5.

Early Lyme Disease Ticks may attach to human hosts at the initial point of contact (generally around ankle level) or may move about until they encounter an obstruction. The groin, popliteal fossae, gluteal folds, axillary folds, and ear lobes are common sites of attachment. After transmission of *B. burgdorferi* through a tick bite, the initial site of infection is the skin at the site of the bite. After an incubation period of about 1 week (range, 1 to 36 days), the spirochetes cause a gradually spreading localized infection in skin and a resultant skin lesion, erythema migrans (EM). EM is the most characteristic clinical manifestation of Lyme disease, and it is recognized in 90% or more of patients. EM may go unnoticed if the entire skin surface is not examined.[13]

The rash of EM begins at the site of the tick bite with an erythematous papule or macule. The lesion expands gradually (1 to 2 cm/day, a rate of expansion slower than that of cellulitis). The patch of erythema may be confluent or may have bands of normal-appearing skin. Central clearing may occur but is not always present. The borders of the lesion are usually flat, but they may be raised. The lesions are generally sharply demarcated and blanch with pressure. Most EM lesions are oval or round, but triangular and elongated patches may occur. In patients seen 1 to 7 days after the appearance of lesions, the average lesion size is approximately 8×10 cm (range, 2×3 cm to 25×25 cm). In some cases, the centers of some early lesions become red and indurated or vesicular and necrotic. The lesion is warm to the touch and may be described by the patient as nontender to minimally tender (Figure 128-6).[14]

Hematogenous spread of viable spirochetes (not additional tick bites) may result in one or more secondary lesions. These secondary lesions are smaller, migrate less, and typically spare the palms and soles. In all, 10% to 15% of patients have more than 20 such lesions; on rare occasions they may number more than 100. Blistering and mucosal involvement

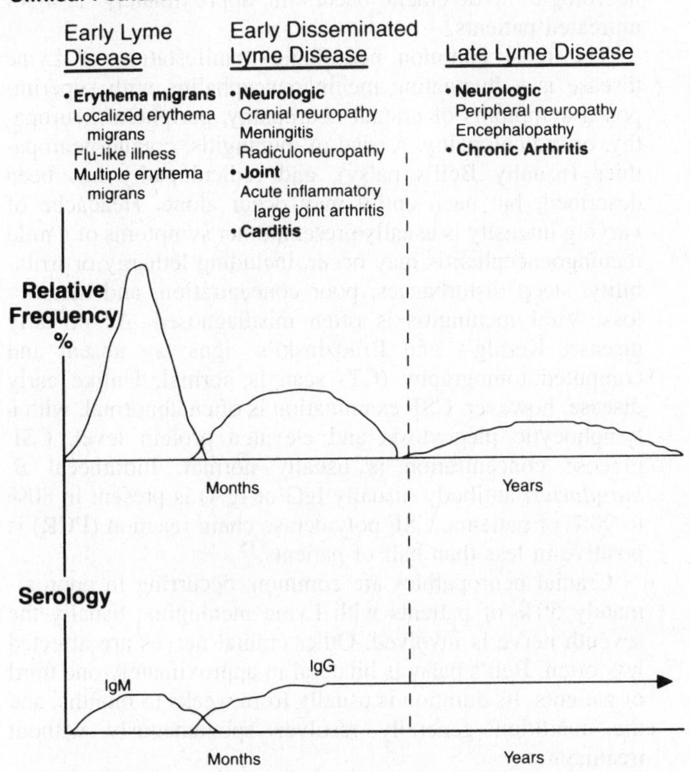

Figure 128-5. **Natural history of serologic response in untreated Lyme disease.** ***From Rahn DW, Evans J: Lyme disease, Philadelphia, 1998, American College of Physicians.***

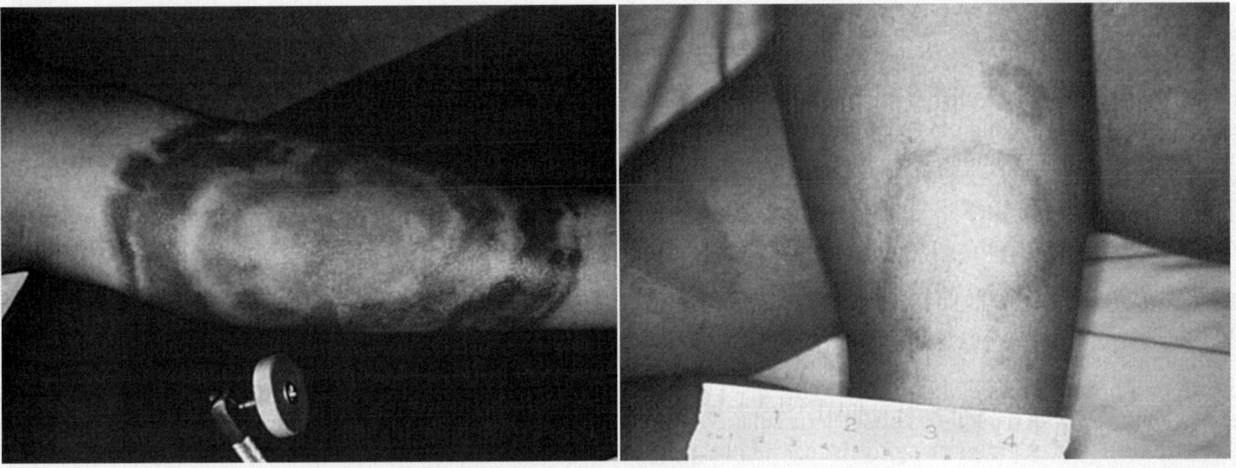

Figure 128-6. **Erythema migrans.**

do not occur. The primary and secondary skin lesions generally fade after about 28 days (range, 1 week to 14 months) without treatment and within several days of antibiotic therapy. Recurrent lesions may develop in patients who do not receive antibiotic therapy, but apparently not in those who receive appropriate antibiotics.[14]

Constitutional symptoms commonly appear in early Lyme disease. Malaise, fatigue, and lethargy are most common (approximately 80% of patients) (Table 128-2) and may be severe. Fever is typically low grade and intermittent. Lymphadenopathy is usually regional in the distribution of EM or may be generalized; splenomegaly may occur. Musculoskeletal complaints such as arthralgias and myalgias are common and are typically short-lived and migratory, sometimes lasting only hours in one location. Frank arthritis may occur at this stage, but it is rare.

Symptoms of meningeal irritation commonly occur. Headache, the most common symptom, is usually intermittent and localized. Nausea, vomiting, and photophobia occasionally accompany the headache. Kernig's and Brudzinski's signs are usually absent, and neck stiffness usually occurs only on extreme forward flexion. At this stage, the neurologic examination and cerebrospinal fluid (CSF) assessment (usually) both yield normal findings.

Signs and symptoms of hepatitis, including anorexia, abdominal pain, right upper quadrant tenderness, nausea, and

Table 128-2. Early Clinical Manifestations of Lyme Disease

	Patients N	(N = 314) (%)
Signs		
ECM*	314	(100)
Multiple annular lesions	150	(48)
Lymphadenopathy		
Regional	128	(41)
Generalized	63	(20)
Pain on neck flexion	52	(17)
Malar rash	41	(13)
Erythematous throat	38	(12)
Conjunctivitis	35	(11)
Symptoms		
Malaise, fatigue, lethargy	251	(80)
Headache	200	(64)
Fever and chills	185	(59)
Stiff neck	151	(48)
Arthralgias	150	(48)
Myalgias	135	(43)
Backache	81	(26)
Anorexia	73	(23)
Sore throat	53	(17)
Nausea	53	(17)
Dysesthesia	35	(11)
Vomiting	32	(10)

From Steere AC et al: *Ann Intern Med* 99:76, 1983.
*Erythema chronicum migrans was required for inclusion in this study.

vomiting, may occur. Mild pharyngitis may be present, but other upper respiratory symptoms such as rhinorrhea do not occur. Although the systemic symptoms of early Lyme disease are often described as flulike, this term can be misleading because clinically significant cough usually does not occur. Conjunctivitis develops in approximately 10% of patients.[14]

The incidence of Lyme disease without EM appears to be approximately 10%.[13] Given the variety of nonspecific signs and symptoms at this stage, in the absence of the characteristic rash or a history of a tick bite, early Lyme disease may be easily confused with a viral or collagen-vascular disease. The intermittent and rapidly changing nature of the early signs and symptoms of Lyme disease may be a helpful distinguishing feature, especially in a patient from an endemic area. If untreated, early symptoms usually last for several weeks but may persist for months.

Acute Disseminated Infection Shortly after disease onset, hematogenous spread can cause a variety of systemic symptoms and secondary sites of infection. Organ systems commonly affected are the nervous system, heart, and joints. Less commonly, eye, liver, skeletal muscle, subcutaneous tissue, and spleen are infected.

Neurologic Manifestations A relatively symptom-free interval usually occurs between early and disseminated infection; however, neurologic signs and symptoms may be the presenting manifestations of Lyme disease or may overlap with early or late manifestations. Beginning an average of 4 weeks (range, 0 to 10 weeks) after the onset of EM, neurologic involvement occurs in approximately 15% of untreated patients.

The most common neurologic manifestation of Lyme disease is a fluctuating meningoencephalitis with superimposed symptoms of cranial neuropathy, peripheral neuropathy, or radiculopathy. A triad of meningitis, cranial neuropathies (usually Bell's palsy), and radiculopathy has been described, but each entity may occur alone. Headache of varying intensity is usually present; other symptoms of a mild meningoencephalitis may occur, including lethargy or irritability, sleep disturbances, poor concentration, and memory loss. Viral meningitis is often misdiagnosed. As in early disease, Kernig's and Brudzinski's signs are absent and computed tomography (CT) scan is normal. Unlike early disease, however, CSF examination is often abnormal, with a lymphocytic pleocytosis and elevated protein level. CSF glucose concentration is usually normal. Intrathecal *B. burgdorferi* antibody (usually IgG or IgA) is present in 80% to 90% of patients. CSF polymerase chain reaction (PCR) is positive in less than half of patients.[15]

Cranial neuropathies are common, occurring in approximately 50% of patients with Lyme meningitis; usually the seventh nerve is involved. Other cranial nerves are affected less often. Bell's palsy is bilateral in approximately one third of patients. Its duration is usually from weeks to months, and the condition generally resolves spontaneously without treatment.

Peripheral nervous system manifestations may also occur in early disseminated Lyme disease. The spinal root and plexus and the peripheral nerves may be involved in the form of thoracic sensory radiculitis, brachial plexitis, mononeuritis, and motor radiculoneuritis in the extremities. Patients may complain of weakness, pain, or dysesthesia. Loss of reflexes may occur. Involvement of the extremities is usually asymmetric, but cervical and thoracic dermatomes may be affected. Other rare neurologic abnormalities described in association with Lyme disease include chorea, transverse myelitis, ataxia, and pseudotumor cerebri.[16] Cerebral vasculitis associated with Lyme disease has also been reported.[17]

Cardiac Manifestations Cardiac involvement in Lyme disease is uncommon. Estimates of the incidence of carditis in untreated patients who have Lyme disease range from 4% to 10%.[18] The average time from initial illness to the development of carditis typically is 3 to 5 weeks (range, 4 days to 7 months). Direct myocardial invasion has been demonstrated with endomyocardial biopsy.[19] Electrophysiologic testing has demonstrated widespread involvement of the conduction system.[20]

The most common cardiac manifestation of Lyme disease is atrioventricular (AV) block, although conduction defects may involve any level of the conducting system. Myopericarditis, tachydysrhythmias, and ventricular impairment occur less often. The distribution of AV block in a review of 105 reported cases of Lyme carditis was as follows: 49% third-degree, 16% second-degree, and 12% first-degree.[20] The degree of AV block may fluctuate rapidly.[18]

A commonly observed feature of AV block in patients with Lyme carditis is its gradual resolution, resembling the resolution after acute inferior wall myocardial infarction and presumably related to the resolution of inflammation. Assessment of the level of the AV block is important to determine the prognosis of a patient with Lyme carditis. In most cases, block appears to be at or above the level of the AV node;

therefore, the prognosis is favorable.[21] However, infranodal AV block does occur and may be characterized by slow escape rhythms of wide QRS pattern, asystole, or fluctuating left and right bundle branch block. Other electrocardiographic (ECG) findings include nonspecific ST- and T-wave abnormalities and intraventricular conduction delay.[21]

Patients with high-degree AV block are usually symptomatic. Symptoms include light-headedness, palpitations, syncope, chest pain, and dyspnea on exertion. Physical examination may reveal flow murmurs and murmurs of mild mitral regurgitation, pericardial friction rub, or evidence of congestive heart failure. Associated left ventricular dysfunction may be present and has been documented by two-dimensional echocardiography and radionuclide studies; in most reported cases, it has been mild and transient.

Arthritis Although classically considered a sign of late disease, acute arthritis may begin during the acute disseminated stage. Weeks to months after initial illness, patients may have monoarticular or oligoarticular arthritis primarily in large joints, especially the knee. In an early study of the natural history of Lyme arthritis, about 50% of untreated patients developed one episode or multiple intermittent attacks of arthritis. Acute arthritis typically is monoarticular with involvement of only one knee. The shoulder, elbow, temporomandibular joint, ankle, wrist, hip, and small joints of the hands and feet are involved less commonly. Episodes of arthritis typically are brief (lasting weeks to months) and separated by variable periods of remission.

Arthrocentesis generally is nondiagnostic, yielding an inflammatory synovial fluid with a mean white blood cell (WBC) count of approximately 25,000 cells/mm^3 (75% polymorphonuclear leukocytes). Higher WBC counts can occur, simulating septic arthritis.[22] The synovial glucose concentration is usually normal and protein levels are variable, ranging from 3 to 8 g/dl. Cultures of the fluid rarely identify the causative spirochete.[23] Complement level is generally greater than one third that of serum. Synovial biopsy reveals hypertrophy, vascular proliferation, and a mononuclear cell infiltrate. Findings, therefore, are similar to those in rheumatoid arthritis, except that rheumatoid factor and antinuclear antibody are negative in Lyme arthritis. Radiography may reveal nonspecific abnormalities such as juxtaarticular osteoporosis, cartilage loss, cortical or marginal bone erosions, and joint effusions.

Ophthalmic Manifestations Ocular involvement may also be seen in early disseminated disease, with manifestations including conjunctivitis, keratitis, choroiditis, retinal detachment, optic neuritis, and blindness.[24] These findings may also be seen in late disease.

Late Lyme Disease The chronic phase of Lyme disease is characterized by arthritic and, less commonly, neurologic symptoms. With time, there is a transition from a pattern of episodic inflammation in early disease to a more indolent persistent inflammation. The term *chronic,* or late, *Lyme disease* is used to describe continuous inflammation in an organ system for more than 1 year.[25]

A pattern of exacerbation and remission of arthritis may occur over several years, with a gradual tendency toward less frequent and less severe occurrences. The spontaneous long-term remission rate approximates 10% to 20% annually in untreated patients. However, patients commonly have episodes of periarticular involvement, arthralgias, or fatigue interspersed between attacks of frank arthritis. During the second or third year of illness, attacks of joint swelling sometimes become longer in duration, lasting months rather than weeks. About 10% of patients develop chronic arthritis.[26]

Late neurologic complications include a wide variety of abnormalities of the central and peripheral nervous systems, as well as fatigue syndromes. Diagnosis may be difficult because of the large number of other neurologic conditions that Lyme disease may imitate and because late neurologic symptoms may be the first symptoms of the disease.[16] The manifestations of chronic neuroborreliosis usually appear months to years after the onset of infection.

The most common late neurologic manifestation of Lyme disease is a chronic encephalopathy that presents as a mild to moderately severe impairment of memory and learning. Hypersomnolence and mild psychiatric disturbances (depression, irritability, or paranoia) may also develop.[15]

Peripheral nervous system disease is often seen in late disease with involvement of cranial nerves, spinal roots, plexuses, and peripheral nerves. A predominantly sensory polyradiculoneuropathy that presents as either radicular pain or distal paresthesia is common. Significant overlap occurs with early symptoms. Less commonly, a demyelinating condition resembling multiple sclerosis may appear in late disease. Symptoms are variable and, like multiple sclerosis, may undergo exacerbations and remissions. CT and magnetic resonance imaging may reveal multiple white matter lesions.[16,27]

Chronic inflammation may also occur in the skin, causing a seldom-recognized late cutaneous manifestation of Lyme disease, acrodermatitis chronica atrophicans (ACA).[28] ACA is usually found on distal extremities at the site of a tick bite. It is characterized in its initial stages by an edematous infiltration that progresses to an atrophic lesion resembling localized scleroderma in its more established form. *B. burgdorferi* has been demonstrated in the skin of patients with ACA, as well as positive serologic studies.

Diagnostic Strategies

The diagnosis of Lyme disease is based primarily on clinical and epidemiologic features and is difficult, especially in the early stage. A history of tick bite is present in only approximately one third of cases. EM is present in most patients and, in an endemic area, is considered diagnostic. However, patients may have isolated late symptoms months after the initial infection and may not recall the rash. The disease should be considered in patients who live in or have visited an endemic area and who present during the summer months with nonspecific symptoms suggesting a viral illness or meningitis. In addition, previously healthy patients who develop monoarticular arthritis, multiple neurologic abnormalities, or heart block should raise the suspicion of Lyme disease.

Routine laboratory studies are nonspecific and generally not helpful in diagnosing Lyme disease.[14] Abnormalities may include an elevated erythrocyte sedimentation rate, mild anemia, total WBC count in the normal range with a decreased absolute lymphocyte count, microhematuria, proteinuria, and increased alanine transferase level.[14,29] Culture of blood, tissue, and body fluids (including CSF and synovial fluid) for *B. burgdorferi* and direct visualization techniques are difficult and have such a low yield that they are not clinically useful.[30,31]

Serologic testing is the most practical and useful means of confirming clinical diagnoses of Lyme disease, but it is not without limitations. Results of serologic tests must be interpreted cautiously within the clinical context and should be regarded as only adjuncts in the diagnosis. Current serologic tests measure host antibody response (both immunoglobulin G [IgG] and immunoglobin M [IgM]) to *B. burgdorferi.* Problems with the performance and interpretation of the tests often result in diagnostic confusion. False-negative and especially false-positive results are common. The antibody response to *B. burgdorferi* develops slowly. The peak of IgM titers appears between 3 and 6 weeks after the onset of illness. Earlier in the course of the illness, IgM titers may be negative. IgM returns to nondiagnostic levels 4 to 6 weeks after peak. IgG antibody may be detectable 2 months after exposure and peaks at approximately 12 months. Early antibiotic therapy may blunt or even abolish the antibody response. During the first month of illness, both IgM and IgG titers should be determined, preferably in acute and convalescent serum samples. Approximately 20% to 30% of patients have a positive response in acute samples, whereas even after antibiotic treatment, about 70% to 80% have a positive response in convalescent samples obtained 2 to 4 weeks later. After that time, most patients have a positive IgG antibody response, and a single test is usually sufficient.

In patients with illness for longer than 1 month, a positive IgM test alone is likely to be a false-positive result. Therefore, a positive IgM response should not be used to support the diagnosis after the first month of infection.

Testing with the enzyme-linked immunosorbent assay (ELISA) is the cornerstone of laboratory diagnosis of Lyme disease. Although ELISA alone has a sensitivity of 89% and a specificity of 72%, a positive test result in patients with a pretest probability of Lyme disease of <0.20 is more likely to be a false-positive than a true-positive result.[32] In patients with a positive or equivocal ELISA, a confirmatory Western blot should be ordered.[33] Criteria for positive Western immunoblotting (requiring the presence of bands at particular locations) have been adopted by the Centers for Disease Control and Prevention.[33]

IgG antibody (and occasionally IgM) may persist for several years after adequate treatment and symptom resolution. Persisting seropositivity is not diagnostic of ongoing infection. IgG antibody developed after natural infection does not confer immunity against future infection by *B. burgdorferi.*

False-positive ELISA results are common. Serologic cross-reactivity can occur between *B. burgdorferi* and other spirochetes, most notably *Treponema pallidum.* False-positive results for Lyme disease can also occur with relapsing fever, gingivitis, leptospirosis, enteroviral and other viral illnesses, rickettsial diseases, autoimmune diseases, malaria, and subacute bacterial endocarditis.[34]

In addition, it is estimated that up to 5% of the normal population will "test positive" for Lyme disease by ELISA. Bayes' theorem states that if the pretest likelihood of the disease is low, then the positive predictive value is low: a positive test result is more likely to be a false-positive result. For this reason, screening serologic tests should not be used in the absence of objective clinical evidence of Lyme disease.[34]

In cases of suspected neurologic involvement, CSF should be examined for evidence of meningitis. CSF specimens may be included in ELISA tests on those patients with neurologic manifestations. CSF serologic testing is generally not necessary, however, because almost all patients with neuroborreliosis have positive results on serum serologic testing.[32]

Other diagnostic tests, including PCR and urine antigen testing, have not been clinically validated and are not recommended for routine clinical use at present.

Differential Considerations

Although Lyme disease presents in many ways, each stage has characteristic clinical findings that are helpful in narrowing a differential diagnosis that at first may seem overwhelmingly broad. Early Lyme disease (EM and associated constitutional symptoms) may be easily confused with a variety of other diseases, especially if the characteristic rash of EM is absent. A common clinical situation involves a patient presenting during the summer months with flulike symptoms, including headache, nausea, fever, chills, myalgias, arthralgias, stiff neck, and anorexia. Even in endemic areas during the summer months, most patients with such symptoms do not have Lyme disease. When headache and stiff neck are the predominant symptoms, the principal diagnostic distinction to be made is between Lyme disease and the enteroviral diseases (and other causes of aseptic meningitis). The enteroviral diseases also have their peak incidence during the summer months; however, diarrhea, commonly associated with enteroviral infection, is not a feature of Lyme disease. Abdominal pain, anorexia, and nausea suggest hepatitis; sore throat, adenopathy, and fatigue suggest mononucleosis; and myalgias and arthralgias suggest connective tissue diseases.[35]

The EM rash is characteristic, but not pathognomonic, of Lyme disease. Some patients are not aware of having had EM, and in others its appearance is atypical. Secondary lesions may be confused with the target lesions of erythema multiforme, which are generally smaller and nonexpanding. Erythema multiforme may also involve the mucous membranes, palms, and soles; EM does not. Malar rash may be present in Lyme disease and suggest systemic lupus erythematosus.[14] Erythema nodosum generally causes more painful induration than EM and has a predilection for the extensor surfaces of the legs. Erythema marginatum of acute rheumatic fever is also in the differential diagnosis of EM; the Lyme disease rash differs in having generally fewer, larger, less evanescent lesions that migrate more slowly.[36] Atypical EM presenting as an urticarial rash may suggest hepatitis B infection or serum sickness. Other cutaneous entities in the differential diagnosis of EM include cellulitis, fungal infection, fixed drug-related eruptions, plant dermatitis, and insect or spider bites. Lyme disease must be considered in a patient with any atypical rash accompanied by a "viral syndrome" or meningitis-like illness, especially during the months of peak incidence.

Acute rheumatic fever, coronary artery disease, or viral myocarditis may be suggested by the cardiac manifestations of Lyme disease. The carditis of Lyme disease, like the carditis of rheumatic fever, may follow pharyngitis and migratory polyarthritis. Erythema marginatum usually occurs with the onset of arthritis, in contrast to EM, which usually precedes the carditis. Although some patients with Lyme disease may satisfy the clinical aspects of the Jones' criteria for acute rheumatic fever, they lack evidence of a preceding streptococcal infection; in addition, valvular involvement is not a prominent feature of Lyme carditis.

The differential diagnosis of the neurologic manifestations caused by Lyme disease is extensive and includes aseptic meningitis, herpes simplex encephalitis, Bell's palsy of other causes, multiple sclerosis, Guillain-Barré syndrome, dementia, primary psychosis, cerebral vasculitis, and brain tumor. Neurologic symptoms often occur in the absence of any epidemiologic clues or preceding clinical symptoms to suggest Lyme disease, thus making the diagnosis particularly challenging.

Lyme arthritis may mimic other immune-mediated disorders. The arthritis of Lyme disease is generally asymmetric, oligoarticular, and episodic. In contrast to patients with rheumatoid arthritis, those with Lyme arthritis rarely have symmetric polyarthritis, morning stiffness, a positive test for rheumatoid factor, or subcutaneous nodules. Lyme arthritis is commonly mistaken for seronegative rheumatoid arthritis; however, Lyme arthritis is most similar to the spondyloarthropathies, particularly reactive arthritis.[41] Lyme disease and Reiter's syndrome both commonly cause huge knee effusions, but in Lyme disease, absence of the extraarticular features of Reiter's syndrome (conjunctivitis, urethritis or cervicitis, balanitis, keratosis blennorrhagica) at the time of the arthritis help distinguish it from Reiter's syndrome. In children, Lyme arthritis may mimic juvenile rheumatoid arthritis (JRA), but usually joint involvement in Lyme disease occurs in short, intermittent attacks and iridocyclitis is usually absent. Rheumatoid factor will be negative in both JRA and Lyme disease. The diseases resemble one another closely enough to have been confused at the time of the initial description of Lyme disease. Other diseases in the differential diagnosis of Lyme arthritis include acute gouty arthritis, septic arthritis, gonococcal arthritis, rheumatic fever, polymyalgia rheumatica, and the temporomandibular joint syndrome.

Management

Prompt treatment of early disease can shorten the duration of symptoms and prevent progression to later stages of disease. Most of the various manifestations of Lyme disease can be treated successfully with oral antibiotic therapy, with the exception of neurologic abnormalities, which usually require intravenous therapy. Treatment of Lyme disease is summarized in Table 128-3.

Vaccination Vaccines against infection with *B. burgdorferi* are available and should be considered for people who live in high-risk areas and are frequently exposed to ticks. Vaccination is not recommended for people who live in regions of low endemicity for the infection.[37,38]

The Lyme disease vaccine (LYMErix) is directed against the outer surface protein A (rOspA) of *B. burgdorferi.* LYMErix is administered by injection into the deltoid muscle, 0.5 ml (30 μg). Optimal protection is provided by three doses on a 0-, 1-, and 12-month schedule. In a randomized controlled clinical trial involving more than 10,000 subjects, the vaccine efficacy was 76%.[39] Yearly or every-other-year booster injections may be necessary to maintain adequate immunity. Vaccination will cause a positive ELISA result but a negative Western blot.

Prophylaxis and Asymptomatic Tick Bites The decision to begin antibiotic therapy in an asymptomatic patient who has been bitten by a tick must be made on an individual basis. The authors of several double-blind, placebo-controlled trials involving 600 subjects have concluded that even in an area in which Lyme disease is endemic, routine antibiotic prophylaxis is not warranted.[40,41] An alternative to prophylactic antibiotics, and probably a more reasonable one given the relatively low risk of acquiring the disease even if bitten by a tick in an endemic area, would be patient education regarding expected early signs and symptoms (rash or fever with or without other systemic symptoms such as headache and myalgia). The alternative approach (treating prophylactically following tick bite) is common among many physicians who practice in highly endemic areas.

Early Disease Prompt antibiotic therapy is essential in early Lyme disease because it generally shortens the duration of the rash and associated symptoms and, more important, prevents later illness in most patients. Some patients with severe early disease, however, develop later stages despite courses of antibiotics.

The drug of choice for men, nonpregnant and nonlactating women, and children older than 8 years of age is doxycycline.[5] An advantage of the use of doxycycline is that it is also effective treatment for human granulocytic ehrlichiosis, which is transmitted by the same tick that transmits Lyme disease. Pregnant or lactating women and children less than 8 years old should receive amoxicillin. For patients who cannot tolerate tetracyclines and are allergic to penicillins, erythromycin is recommended but is probably less effective. Cefuroxime axetil has also been shown to be effective.[42] A Jarisch-Herxheimer–type reaction may occur in the first 24 hours of treatment, consisting of fever, chills, myalgias, headache, tachycardia, increased respiratory rate, and mild leukocytosis.[43] Defervescence usually takes place within 12 to 24 hours, and the patient can be managed by bed rest and aspirin. The pathogenesis of this reaction is controversial, but it is probably caused by the killing of spirochetes with release of pyrogens. The Jarisch-Herxheimer reaction occurs more commonly with penicillin and tetracycline than with erythromycin, probably because of their superior spirocheticidal activity.

Early Disseminated Infection

Neurologic disease For patients with relatively mild symptoms (e.g., solitary facial nerve palsy with a normal CSF examination), doxycycline or amoxicillin can be used in the same dosage as for early disease, but the duration of therapy should be extended to 30 days. The use of prednisone for facial nerve palsy from Lyme disease has been suggested but is not currently recommended.

For patients with other objective neurologic abnormalities (e.g., meningitis or encephalitis, peripheral neuropathies, or cranial neuritis other than facial nerve palsy) or evidence of the spirochete in the CSF, parenteral antibiotic therapy is required. Ceftriaxone may be used. Ceftriaxone may be more effective than penicillin, and many recommend longer courses (e.g., up to 4 weeks).[44] In cases of penicillin or cephalosporin allergy, oral doxycycline for 30 days may be used.

Cardiac disease Patients with mild cardiac conduction system involvement (first-degree AV block with a PR interval less than 0.30 seconds) and no other significant symptoms

Table 128-3. Treatment of Lyme Disease

	Drug	Adult dosage	Pediatric dosage*
Early Lyme disease	Doxycycline†	100 mg PO bid for 10-21 days	
	or		
	Amoxicillin	250-500 mg PO tid for 10-21 days	25-50 mg/kg/day divided tid
Alternative	Cefuroxime axetil	500 mg PO bid for 10-21 days	250 mg bid
	or		
	Erythromycin (less effective than doxycycline or amoxicillin)	250 mg PO qid for 10-21 days	
Neurologic disease			
Facial nerve paralysis	For an isolated finding, oral regimens for early disease, used for at least 30 days, may suffice. For a finding associated with other neurologic manifestations. IV therapy is warranted (see below).		
Lyme meningitis‡	Ceftriaxone	2 gm IV by single dose for 14-21 days	75-100 mg/kg/day IV
	Penicillin G	20 million units daily in divided doses for 10-21 days	300,000 U/kg/day IV
Alternative	Chloramphenicol	1 gm IV every 6 hr for 10-21 days	
Cardiac disease			
Mild§	Doxycycline†	100 mg PO bid	
	or		
	Amoxicillin	250-500 mg PO tid	25-50 mg/kg/day divided tid
More severe	Ceftriaxone	2 gm IV daily by single dose for 14-21 days	75-100 mg/kg/day IV
	or		
	Penicillin G	20 million units daily in divided doses for 14-21 days	300,000 U/kg/day IV
Arthritis			
Oral	Doxycycline†	100 mg PO bid for 30 days	
	or		
	Amoxicillin	500 mg PO tid for 30 days	50 mg/kg/day divided tid
Parenteral	Ceftriaxone	2 gm IV by single dose for 14-21 days	75-100 mg/kg/day IV
	or		
	Penicillin G	20 million units daily in divided doses for 14-21 days	300,000 U/kg/day IV

Modified from Abramowitz M, editor: *Med Lett* 34:95, 1992; and Rahn DW, Malawista SE: *Ann Intern Med* 114:472, 1991.
*Pediatric dosage should not exceed adult dosage.
†Tetracycline, 250 to 500 mg PO qid, may be substituted for doxycycline. Neither oxycycline nor any other tetracycline should be used for children less than 8 years old or for pregnant or lactating women.
‡Regimens for radiculoneuropathy, peripheral neuropathy, and encephalitis are the same as those for meningitis.
§Oral regimens are reserved for mild cardiac involvement (see text).

can usually be treated safely as outpatients with oral doxycycline or amoxicillin for 21 to 30 days.

Patients with higher degrees of AV block, including first-degree block with a PR interval greater than 0.30 seconds or evidence of global ventricular impairment, should be hospitalized for cardiac monitoring and treated with parenteral antibiotics. Either penicillin G or ceftriaxone may be used.

The benefit of adjuvant use of aspirin or prednisone in treating patients with Lyme carditis is uncertain. Temporary cardiac pacing may be necessary in patients who have severe heart block with hemodynamic instability. The block generally resolves completely with antibiotic treatment; thus, the recognition of Lyme carditis in young patients with unexplained heart block is critical to avoid unnecessary permanent pacemaker implantation.

Late Infection

Arthritis In established Lyme arthritis, the response to antibiotic therapy may be delayed for several weeks or months. The use of intravenous penicillin G has been effective in patients with established Lyme arthritis.[45] Ceftriaxone was more effective than penicillin G in one randomized trial and is effective in some patients who do not respond to penicillin.[46,47]

Thirty-day oral regimens with doxycycline or amoxicillin may also be used. Both regimens may be as effective as parenteral penicillin or ceftriaxone and, for reasons of cost and convenience, may be selected as first-line therapy on an outpatient basis before considering parenteral antibiotic therapy. Refractory arthritis may resolve after retreatment with the same or an alternative antibiotic regimen. A small percentage of patients with Lyme arthritis, particularly those with HLA-DR4 specificity or antibody reactivity with OspA, may have persistent joint inflammation despite treatment with either oral or intravenous antibiotics.[26] Patients such as these are often resistant to any antibiotic therapy and may require arthroscopic synovectomy.

Neurologic disease Patients with late neurologic complications, including focal central nervous system (CNS) disease and fatigue syndromes, may be resistant to therapy. Variable success has been reported with high-dose parenteral penicillin G or ceftriaxone.[48] Some patients with peripheral neuropathy and chronic fatigue refractory to penicillin have been treated successfully with ceftriaxone.[47]

Lyme Disease and Pregnancy

A major concern with Lyme disease is its potential effect when contracted during pregnancy. Similar to the spirochetal agents of syphilis and relapsing fever, *B. burgdorferi* can be passed transplacentally. In rare cases, Lyme disease acquired during pregnancy may lead to infection of the fetus and possibly to stillbirth, but adverse effects to the fetus have not been documented conclusively. Counseling termination of a pregnancy because of maternal Lyme disease is unwarranted and unjustified.

Lyme disease contracted during pregnancy can be treated and cured. Most women give birth to normal infants despite documented Lyme borreliosis during their pregnancies.[49] Pregnant women with Lyme disease should be treated aggressively with antibiotics according to the stage of their disease (see Table 128-3). A full course of antibiotics should be used. EM in pregnancy can be treated safely with amoxicillin for 3 to 4 weeks. Concerns about fetal wastage and malformations associated with Lyme disease acquired during pregnancy prompt some physicians to offer a 10-day course of oral amoxicillin to asymptomatic pregnant women bitten by ticks; however, there are no data to support this practice.[13]

RELAPSING FEVER

Perspective

Relapsing fever is caused by bacteria of *Borrelia* species, which belong to the order Spirochaetales. Human *Borrelia* infections occur worldwide and all are associated with arthropod vectors. The epidemic (louse-borne) form of relapsing fever is caused solely by *Borrelia recurrentis.* The endemic (tick-borne) form of relapsing fever is caused by a group of closely related *Borrelia* species, their names derived from the species names of *Ornithodoros* tick vectors that carry them. The more common ones in North America are *B. hermsii, B. turicatae,* and *B. parkeri.*[50] *B. burgdorferi* has been recognized as the etiologic agent of the third and most recently described borrelial disease, Lyme disease.

Principles of Disease

Endemic (tick-borne) relapsing fever is maintained in an animal reservoir consisting primarily of wild rodents, including squirrels, mice, rats, chipmunks, and rabbits. The tick vectors are argasids belonging to several species of the genus *Ornithodoros,* which routinely reside in the nests and burrows of their mammalian hosts. Ticks acquire the infection by feeding on a spirochetemic rodent. The borreliae remain viable in the ticks for several years and can be passed transovarially to the next generation; thus, the tick is a major reservoir and vector. These soft ticks feed for brief periods (15 to 30 minutes), usually at night, and their painless bite generally is unnoticed by the sleeping victim. Transmission occurs by injection of infected saliva through the bite site or intact skin. Less common modes of transmission (e.g., via venipuncture equipment in intravenous drug abusers) have been reported.

In the United States, relapsing fever occurs primarily in the western mountain states. Persons who come in contact with infected ticks from wild rodents are at greatest risk. Outbreaks have been reported among groups sleeping overnight in hunting cabins inhabited by wild rodents.[50,51]

Clinical Features

After a postbite incubation period of 4 to 18 days, during which time the host concentration of spirochetes increases, fever occurs abruptly and is often accompanied by shaking chills, headache, arthralgias, myalgias, nausea, and vomiting. Occasionally a pruritic eschar may be present at the site of the tick bite, but this is usually absent by the onset of clinic symptoms. Consequently, the nonspecific nature of the clinical presentation often leads to the misdiagnosis of a viral illness. The temperature is high (usually 38.5° to 40° C), and generalized muscle weakness and lethargy are common. Hepatomegaly, splenomegaly, and jaundice may be seen. Neurologic involvement is less common but may include delirium, nuchal rigidity, peripheral neuropathy, and pupillary abnormalities. A macular or petechial skin rash, more apparent on the trunk than on the extremities, may be present.

In tick-borne relapsing fever, the initial febrile episode lasts 3 days. This is followed by a variable asymptomatic period of approximately 7 days, during which patients generally feel better and may return to their usual daily activity levels under the assumption that they have recovered from "another viral illness." Relapse then occurs, with symptoms that mimic the original illness. With tick-borne relapsing fever, this cycle repeats itself three to five times. Each successive relapse is usually less severe.

Relapse is caused by the spirochete's ability to undergo antigenic variation within the body of the infected host. Each successive antigenic variation is cleared from the bloodstream by specific host antibodies, and a characteristic relapsing febrile course results.[50,51]

Diagnostic Strategies

The definitive diagnosis of relapsing fever depends on the demonstration of borreliae in the peripheral blood during a febrile episode. In most patients the spirochetes are readily visible on a routine blood smear stained with Wright's or Giemsa stain. Thick or thin blood smears prepared for malaria evaluation are also satisfactory. The organisms lie in the plasma spaces between blood cells or may overlie the blood cells. Several organisms per high-power field are typically visible in febrile patients with relapsing fever.[50] Smears should be obtained as the temperature curve swings up, and repeated samples may be required before obtaining a positive result. Spirochetes may also be visible in wet mounts with the use of phase contrast microscopy. Cultures, although the most sensitive test available, require a special medium and do not yield rapid results, and so are not commonly performed.

Differential Considerations

On initial presentation, the differential diagnosis is extensive; however, it narrows with the occurrence of relapse. A history of possible tick exposure together with recurrent fever should suggest the diagnosis. Other conditions that might be initially considered include malaria, typhus, dengue, yellow fever, Colorado tick fever, and tularemia. Careful examination of blood smears, together with clinical data and other laboratory tests, will aid in making the correct diagnosis.

Management

Relapsing fever is treated effectively with tetracycline or erythromycin. Tetracycline should be avoided in children younger than 8 years old and in pregnant women. Tetracycline or erythromycin should be given in an oral dose of 500 mg for 5 to 10 days; single-dose therapy is also effective.[50] Other treatment regimens, including doxycycline, chloramphenicol, and streptomycin, have been recommended. Treatment with penicillin G has been associated with an increased rate of relapses. Success with ceftriaxone has been reported in a patient with relapsing fever who did not respond to penicillin.

As many as one third of patients may experience a Jarisch-Herxheimer–type reaction after treatment with antibiotics. The reaction may be severe, especially with louse-borne relapsing fever. This phenomenon may be related to administration of cytokine intermediaries or endogenous opioids. Approximately 4 hours after antibiotic treatment and coinciding with the clearance of spirochetes from the blood, the patient usually experiences an increase in temperature, severe rigors, a drop in leukocyte and platelet counts, and hypotension. Anticipation of the reaction is crucial because IV volume expansion with saline solution may be required to maintain the blood pressure; the reaction may be more threatening than the disease itself. Meptazinol, an opioid antagonist with agonist properties, has been proposed for use in treatment of this reaction.

Prognosis is good in treated patients with relapsing fever, with approximately 95% achieving complete recovery. Bad prognostic signs include the presence of jaundice, high spirochete counts in the blood, and hypotension.[50] Transplacental transmission and spontaneous abortion may occur in infected pregnant women. Death is rare and is limited to infants and elderly persons.[52]

TULAREMIA

Perspective

Tularemia was first described in 1837 by Soken, who described a febrile illness with generalized lymphadenopathy in people who had eaten infected rabbit meat.[53] In 1912 McCoy first isolated *Francisella tularensis* from rodents in Tulare County, California, giving rise to the name of the disease. Francis, for whom the genus *Francisella* is named, contributed much to the understanding of the bacteriology and epidemiology.

Tularemia occurs worldwide and is endemic between 30 and 71 degrees north latitude. Ticks, lagomorphs (hares, rabbits), and rodents (mice, rats) are believed to be the most important sources of transmission to humans; however, the organism has been recovered from more than 100 animals, with significant epidemics linked to contact with a variety of them, including domestic cats.[54,55] Insect sources such as flies and spiders may play a marginal role in transmission.

Transmission can also occur by direct contact with or ingestion of infected soil, water, or fomites.[53] Inhalation of dust or water aerosol can also induce infection. Nonimmune laboratory workers who work with *F. tularensis* can acquire the disease. Person-to-person transmission is rare. Tularemia has a bimodal prevalence in the United States, with an increased incidence in May to August associated with tick-borne transmission and a December to January peak associated with hunting and skinning of infected mammals (primarily rabbits).

In the United States, tularemia has been seen in every state but is most common in the southwest central region (Arkansas, Louisiana, Oklahoma, Texas, and Mississippi). It is more common in men than in women. Individuals at increased risk for infection include hunters, trappers, butchers, agricultural workers, campers, sheepherders, mink farmers, and laboratory workers.[54] The incidence of tularemia is low; there are approximately 200 cases annually in the United States.[56] Tularemia was removed from the national list of notifiable diseases in 1995, but as of 1998, 36 states have maintained it on their lists. Fifty percent of reported cases have come collectively from Missouri, Oklahoma, Kansas, and Arkansas.[57]

Principles of Disease

Two types of *F. tularensis* organisms exist and may be distinguished on the basis of geographic distribution, fermentation reactions, and virulence. They are called Jellison type A and B and are serologically identical. Jellison type A (*F. tularensis* biovar *tularensis*), the predominant biovar in North America, is associated with ticks and rabbits and causes severe disease in humans. Strain B (*F. tularensis* biovar *palaeartica*) occurs in Asia, Europe, and, to a minor extent, North America; it is associated with rodents and causes milder disease in humans.

Tularemia presents in different ways, depending on the portal of entry of the organism. The primary route of infection by *F. tularensis* is through the skin. This may occur through hair follicles or through small cuts and abrasions that may be contaminated by exposure to an infected animal; tick exposure may also introduce the bacteria.[54] Because the bacterium has not been isolated from the salivary glands of ticks, it is thought that they may transmit the organism through their feces.[53] Scratching after a tick bite introduces the infected feces into the skin. Inhalation or ingestion of the organism or transmission through the conjunctivae may also cause infection. The incubation period is approximately 2 to 6 days, depending on the size of the inoculum.

After penetration of the skin or epithelial membrane, the organism usually spreads to the regional lymph nodes. An erythematous tender papule develops at the primary infection site, followed by inflammation and skin ulceration. The regional nodes enlarge, necrose, and may rupture. The necrotic, purulent, painful lymph node is termed a bubo. In the ulceroglandular form of the infection, the organism may not spread farther than the regional lymph nodes. If the inoculum is sufficiently large or the host defenses inadequate, bacteremia occurs with dissemination to phagocytic cells of the reticuloendothelial system.

Pulmonary tularemia may result from inhalation of small particle aerosols containing *F. tularensis* or by hematogenous dissemination. Small areas of localized pneumonitis most commonly result; lobar consolidation or abscess formation is rare. Oculoglandular tularemia occurs when the conjunctiva becomes infected from an ulcer or contaminated finger. Typhoidal tularemia follows systemic spread of *F. tularensis* from the oropharynx and probably the gastrointestinal tract when a large inoculum is swallowed.

Clinical Features

Tularemia has six clinical presentations, depending on whether disease is localized to an entry site and its regional lymph nodes (ulceroglandular, glandular, oculoglandular, oropharyngeal) or is more invasive and generalized (typhoidal and pulmonary).

Ulceroglandular tularemia is the most common form of the disease (approximately 80% of cases). Typically, a skin lesion on an extremity at the site of primary inoculation begins as an erythematous papule, which then ulcerates 2 to 3 days later.[54] The ulcer is slow to heal and is often still present when the subsequent regional lymphadenopathy and fever develop. The distribution of the regional adenopathy reflects the primary entry site; patients with tick-borne tularemia usually have inguinal or femoral adenopathy, whereas those who acquire rabbit-associated tularemia have axillary or epitrochlear nodal involvement. Generalized lymphadenopathy may also occur. Occasionally nodes may suppurate and drain.[54]

Glandular tularemia, the second most common form, is characterized by the development of lymphadenopathy (usually cervical) without an associated skin ulcer. *Oculoglandular tularemia* is seen in 1% to 2% of cases and is characterized by unilateral conjunctivitis with regional adenopathy involving preauricular lymph nodes. *Oropharyngeal tularemia* presents as severe exudative pharyngitis with associated cervical lymphadenitis. It has been known to cause acute glaucoma.[58]

Typhoidal tularemia is a systemic form of the disease in which no obvious entry site can be found; it occurs in approximately 10% of tularemia cases. It is this form of the disease that is expected to result from biological warfare tactics through introduction of *Francisella* organisms. Only 10 to 50 organisms are required to induce disease; incubation time is 2 to 10 days.[59] Symptoms may include fever, chills, constipation or diarrhea, abdominal pain, and weight loss.

Pulmonary tularemia is common and has symptoms similar to those of other bacterial pneumonias: fever and chills, cough (usually nonproductive), substernal burning, dyspnea, malaise, and prostration. It may result from either direct inhalation of aerosolized organisms or bacteremic spread from another site. Patchy bilateral infiltrates are usually seen on chest roentgenograms; consolidation and abscesses are less common.

Uncommon complications of tularemia include pericarditis, meningitis, endocarditis, peritonitis, appendicitis, perisplenitis, and osteomyelitis.[54] Guillain-Barré syndrome associated with tularemia has been reported.[60]

Diagnostic Strategies

Diagnosis of tularemia is based on clinical findings and serologic testing. Antibody titers begin to rise approximately 7 to 10 days after exposure and peak in 3 to 4 weeks. In a patient clinically thought to have tularemia, a single specimen with an antibody titer of 1:160 or greater is diagnostic. Confirmatory evidence is provided by a fourfold or greater rise in titer in a second sample obtained 2 weeks later. PCR testing is now available.[61,62]

Aspiration of affected lymph nodes for culture is not routinely recommended because of the associated risk to laboratory personnel. If tularemia is suspected, the laboratory should be alerted so that appropriate precautions are taken in handling and so that enriched medium can be used.

Management

Isolation of patients with tularemia is not required. Streptomycin is the drug of choice for all forms of tularemia; when given intramuscularly in a dose of 30 to 40 mg/kg/day in two divided doses every 12 hours, it usually produces symptomatic improvement and resolution of fever in 1 to 2 days.[54] After the third treatment day, half that dose may then be given for a total course of 7 to 14 days.[53,54] With this regimen, relapses are unusual.

Ulcers and tender lymph nodes usually heal within 7 to 10 days; however, enlarged nodes occasionally develop into fluctuant sterile buboes, requiring incision and drainage after completion of the course of antibiotics. Gentamicin is also effective for treatment (3 to 5 mg/kg/day for 10 to 14 days).[59] Tetracycline and chloramphenicol are effective; however, the risk of relapse is greater than that associated with the aminoglycosides. Imipenem-cilastatin, an antibiotic without nephrotoxicity, has been used successfully to treat pulmonary tularemia in a patient with acute renal failure. Ceftriaxone is not effective against *F. tularensis* infections.[63]

A live vaccine is available for human tularemia, but protection is not complete and the vaccine itself can induce illness.[64]

The mortality rate in untreated cases ranges from approximately 5% to 30%; the higher figure is associated with severe disease or significant pulmonic involvement. With appropriate antibiotic treatment, death is rare (<1%).

ROCKY MOUNTAIN SPOTTED FEVER

Perspective

Rocky Mountain spotted fever (RMSF) is an acute, febrile, systemic tick-borne illness caused by *Rickettsia rickettsii.* The clinical severity of RMSF ranges from mild or even subclinical illness to a fulminant disease with vascular collapse and death within several days of onset. It is the only rickettsiosis still associated with significant mortality, causing approximately 40 deaths in the United States each year.[65]

The recorded history of RMSF dates to Native American inhabitants of wooded Rocky Mountain regions who were afflicted by the disease. Early settlers named the affliction tick fever after missionaries noted the association of the tick vector with the disease. In 1899, RMSF was described as "an acute, endemic, noncontagious but probably infectious, febrile disease, characterized by a continuous moderately high fever, severe arthritic and muscle pains, and a profuse petechial or purpuric eruption in the skin, appearing first on the ankles, wrists, and forehead, but rapidly spreading to all parts of the body." In 1906 the causative organism, *Rickettsia rickettsii,* was identified by Ricketts, who also described the importance of the tick vector in transmission to humans.

Although RMSF was first described in Montana and Idaho, it is now relatively rare in the Rocky Mountain states. Endemic in all 48 contiguous states except Maine, the disease continues to be most prevalent in the southeastern United States. RMSF has been reported in Canada, Central America,

Mexico, and South America but never outside the Western Hemisphere. In 1987, four cases of RMSF were reported among residents of the Bronx in New York City; none of the affected individuals had recently traveled to an area known for endemic disease, thus raising the possibility that other urban foci of RMSF may exist.

RMSF also tends to be focally endemic, with clustering of cases within a larger endemic area that may correspond to "islands" of infected ticks. These areas, ecologically distinct from surrounding areas, may be ideally suited to ticks; they usually consist of fields, deciduous forests with thick ground cover and poor water drainage, and uncultivated areas. In areas with frequent occurrence of RMSF (Oklahoma, North and South Carolina, Tennessee, and Pennsylvania), an infectivity rate of 2% to 15% of the tick population has been reported.[66]

R. rickettsii are obligate intracellular bacteria that often occur in pairs and possess a cell wall similar in structure and chemical composition to that of gram-negative bacteria.[67] *R. rickettsii* contain both ribonucleic acid (RNA) and deoxyribonucleic acid (DNA) and, in contrast to other rickettsial organisms, can invade the nucleus as well as the cytoplasm.

The ticks feed on virtually any available warm-blooded animal, and the occurrence of *R. rickettsii* in the United States does not depend on the presence of any given order of mammal. Infected ticks feed on human beings, dogs, mice, rabbits, weasels, deer, horses, and farm animals. Domestic dogs become infected with *R. rickettsii* and may develop clinical illness similar to that in humans. Although dogs do not play an important role in the amplification cycle of RMSF, they may serve as a conduit for infected ticks, carrying them into close contact with pet owners. Humans serve only as accidental participants in the cycle of infection. A recent retrospective study revealed that none of 10 recipients of blood products found to be from donors with either confirmed or probable RMSF contracted the disease.[68]

Principles of Disease

After introduction of *R. rickettsii* into the host by the tick vector, the organisms invade and multiply in the vascular endothelial cells. They then enter deeper areas of the vessel walls and infect vascular smooth muscle. Rickettsial organisms move from cell to cell by actin-based motility.[69] Damage to endothelial cells not only exposes subendothelium but also releases tissue plasminogen activator and von Willebrand factor, thereby causing microhemorrhage, microthrombus formation, and increased vascular permeability. In addition, antibody forms with antigen activating the complement system (type III immune response) and a cellular response is recruited.

These widespread vascular lesions form the basis for most of the clinical features associated with RMSF. Hypotension, edema, and increased extravascular fluid space result from the increased small vessel permeability. The early rash results from the vasculitis and the associated changes in permeability; later petechial and hemorrhagic lesions are secondary to the vasculitis and thrombocytopenia. Microinfarcts and focal lesions occur in various organs, including the brain, heart, lungs, kidneys, adrenal glands, liver, and spleen. Rickettsial encephalitis and diffuse microinfarcts are usual features of CNS involvement. An interstitial pneumonitis caused by direct lung invasion by the organism may occur, and the adult respiratory distress syndrome (ARDS) may ensue. Acute renal failure and hypovolemic shock, the primary causes of death, can occur as early as the second week of illness.

Clinical Features

A history of tick bite or presence in possible tick-infested areas is elicited in only 60% to 70% of patients with RMSF. The incubation period ranges from 2 to 14 days, with a mean of 7 days.[67] A short incubation period may indicate a more serious infection.

Onset of symptoms is usually abrupt but may be gradual in approximately one third of patients (Table 128-4). Early symptoms are nonspecific and similar to those of many acute infectious diseases, making early diagnosis very difficult. "Typical" patients have a sudden onset of fever, severe headache, myalgias, prostration, nausea, and vomiting. Tenderness may be present in large muscle groups. As many as 80% of patients may have gastrointestinal complaints, secondary to myositis of the abdominal wall. Fever (39° C to 40° C) is nearly always present during the first 2 to 3 days of illness and may precede other signs by a week or more.[67,70] Occasionally, the onset of illness is mild, with lethargy, headache, anorexia, and low-grade fever; these patients may remain ambulatory. The triad of fever, rash, and tick bite occurs in only 3% of cases.[71] An extreme complication of RMSF is gangrene, which is probably induced by small-vessel occlusion.[72]

Cutaneous Manifestations Vasculitis secondary to rickettsial invasion of vascular endothelial cells causes the rash commonly associated with RMSF; however, the rash is

Table 128-4. Symptoms and Signs in 262 Persons with RMSF

Symptom or sign	Present during illness: Any time (%)	First 3 days (%)
Fever (100°-102° F)	99	73
Headache, mild to moderate	91	71
Fever (≥102° F)	90	63
Any rash	88	49
Myalgia, mild to moderate	83	57
Rash, maculopapular	82	46
Rash, palms/soles	74	28
Triad of fever/rash/history of tick exposure	67	3
Nausea/vomiting	60	38
Headache, severe	57	40
Abdominal pain	52	30
Rash, petechial and hemorrhagic	49	13
Myalgia, severe	47	25
Conjunctivitis	30	13
Lymphadenopathy	27	13
Stupor	26	6
Diarrhea	19	9
Edema	18	3
Ataxia	18	7
Meningismus	18	5

From Helmick CG, Bernard KW, D'Angelo LJ: *J Infect Dis* 150:480, 1984.

reportedly absent from 4% to 16% of laboratory-confirmed cases, referred to as Rocky Mountain spotless fever. In addition, the rash may be unnoticed in dark-skinned patients. It usually appears on the fourth febrile day but can emerge as early as the second and as late as the sixth day.[67] The initial lesions are generally restricted to the wrists, ankles, palms, soles, and forearms. They are pink, nonfixed, irregular macules 2 to 6 mm in size. At this initial stage, the lesions fade on pressure and are not palpable. A warm compress applied to the area enhances the rash. After 6 to 12 hours, the rash spreads centripetally to involve the axillae, buttocks, trunk, neck, and face. After 2 to 3 days, the rash becomes maculopapular and changes to a deeper red; at this stage, the rash may be felt by light palpation. By about the fourth day, the rash becomes petechial and fails to fade on pressure. Applying tourniquets for several minutes or taking the blood pressure may cause additional petechiae distal to the site of occlusion (Rumpel-Leede phenomenon). Occasionally the lesions coalesce to form large ecchymotic areas that may slough and form indolent ulcers (Figures 128-7 and 128-8).

Prompt institution of specific therapy may cause the initial nonfixed lesions to disappear rapidly, unlike the later fixed lesions. Patients who have had the typical rash may exhibit brownish discolorations at the site during the convalescent period.[67]

Cardiopulmonary Manifestations Echocardiographic evidence of decreased left ventricular contractility secondary to myocarditis commonly occurs and often is detectable even before clinical signs appear. Clinical manifestations of left ventricular dysfunction are uncommon, however, and hypotension and pulmonary edema, when present, usually have noncardiogenic causes. Chest roentgenograms may demonstrate cardiac enlargement. ECG changes include low-voltage, nonspecific ST-T changes, first-degree AV block, dysrhythmias (sinus and nodal tachycardia, paroxysmal atrial tachycardia, atrial fibrillation), and left ventricular hypertrophy. Most cardiac abnormalities are transient, but persistent echocardiographic changes have been described.

Interstitial pneumonitis and increased pulmonary capillary permeability may result from infection of the pulmonary capillaries with rickettsiae. Nonproductive cough and dyspnea secondary to pneumonitis may be seen on presentation. Chest roentgenogram abnormalities are identified in approximately 25% of patients. These abnormalities include interstitial infiltrates, patchy alveolar infiltrates, pleural effusions, and cardiomegaly with pulmonary edema. Pulmonary consolidation is rare.[67] Severe cases may progress to noncardiogenic pulmonary edema and ARDS.

Neurologic Manifestations Neurologic manifestations of RMSF range from mild headache and lethargy to seizures and coma. Acute disseminated encephalomyelitis has been described.[73] Headache, generally severe in nature, is common, occurring in 50% to 90% of cases. Meningismus is present in 16% to 29% of patients. The CSF may be normal or show slight protein elevation and pleocytosis of both lymphocytes and polymorphonuclear cells (usually 8 to 35 cells/ml). Glucose level and opening pressure are usually normal. Resolution of eosinophilic meningitis during RMSF after appropriate antibiotic treatment has been reported. Fewer than 40% of patients will have a positive CSF result.

Cerebral thrombovasculitis may cause focal neurologic deficits, which are usually transient. Seizures may occur, especially during the acute phase of the illness. Generalized

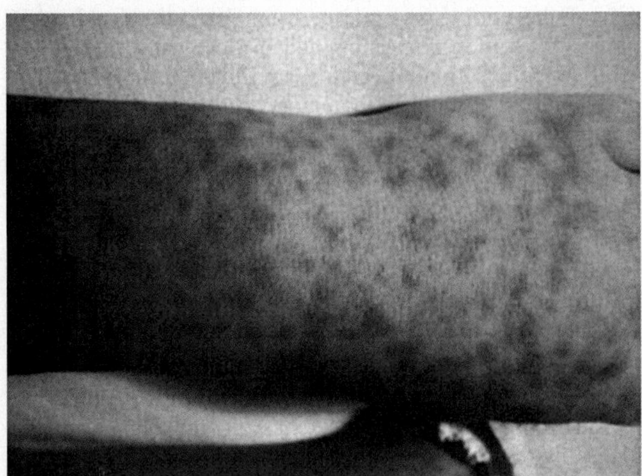

Figure 128-7. **Early appearance of rash: wrist and hand of child with Rocky Mountain spotted fever.** ***Courtesy Centers for Disease Control and Prevention.***

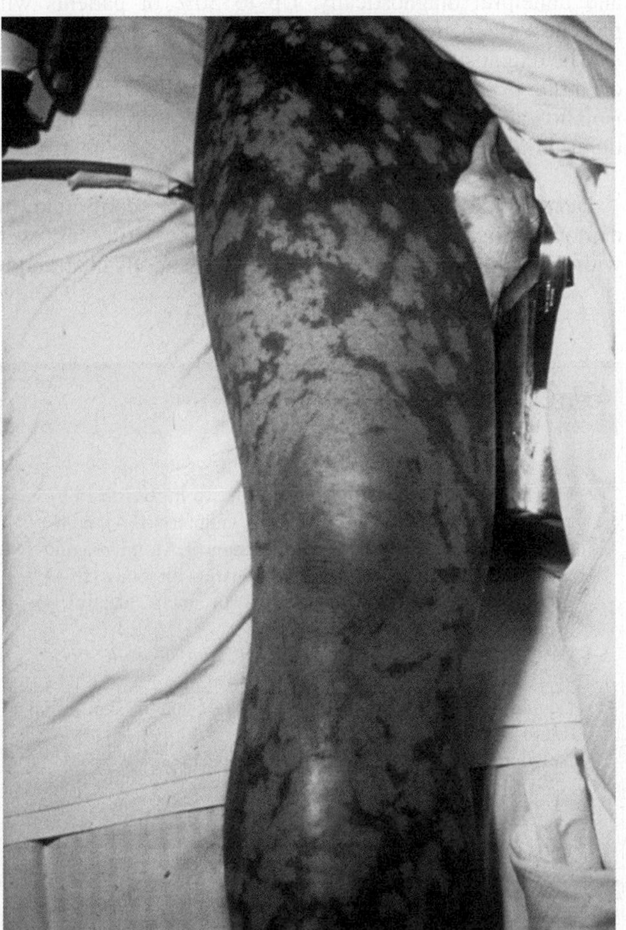

Figure 128-8. **Late appearance of rash: Rocky Mountain spotted fever manifesting on lower extremity.** ***Courtesy Theodore Woodward, MD.***

cerebral dysfunction ranging from lethargy to coma may occur secondary to systemic toxicity (fever, hypotension, hyponatremia) or secondary to vasculitic lesions involving the CNS. Coma is a late finding in severe disease and is seen in fewer than 10% of cases. There have been reports of patients who remain alert but are amnesic about their illness after recovery.

Other reported neurologic manifestations include transient deafness, tremor, rigidity, athetoid movements, paralysis, ataxia, opisthotonos, aphasia, and blindness. Generally, neurologic signs abate without residua; permanent neurologic deficits have been reported rarely.[67] Behavioral disturbances and learning disabilities have been reported in children who develop coma with RMSF.

Diagnostic Strategies

Most immediately available laboratory tests provide little help in diagnosing RMSF. Early in the course of the illness, the diagnosis is based primarily on clinical evidence and depends on the emergency physician's ability to correlate epidemiologic features with clinical signs and symptoms. The initial presentation of RMSF is similar to that of many acute febrile infectious diseases, and almost invariably a therapeutic decision must be made on clinical grounds alone, without the luxury of confirmatory laboratory evidence. Abnormalities such as thrombocytopenia and hyponatremia may be detected by routine laboratory tests, but they are nonspecific and unhelpful diagnostically. Up to 30% of patients will present with anemia.[71]

The diagnosis of RMSF requires positive results using one or more of several tests: serology, skin biopsy, or direct isolation and identification of the organism. Specific diagnostic criteria are summarized in Box 128-1.

Serology Rickettsial infection may be confirmed by demonstrating antibody rise in paired sera. However, even with the most sensitive serologic tests, elevations in antibody titers do not occur until approximately 5 to 7 days after the onset of initial symptoms. As a result, serodiagnosis is retrospective. It is achieved by comparing acute serum that generally yields negative findings with convalescent serum that yields positive results for antibodies. Currently available serologic tests include immunofluorescent antibody (IFA), complement fixation (CF), latex agglutination (LA), microagglutination (MA), and indirect hemagglutination (IHA). A bedside dipstick test is now available, which measures both IgM and IgG antibodies by enzyme immunoassay.[74,75]

Convalescent blood is best obtained 2 to 3 weeks after the onset of clinical illness. Antibiotic therapy does not affect the time of appearance of antibodies or their ultimate titer if such treatment is begun several days after onset of the illness. However, if antibiotic therapy is initiated early in the course of the illness, the rise in titers may be delayed for 4 weeks or more. Under these circumstances, antibody titers should be tested again at 4 to 6 weeks after the onset of illness.

Skin Biopsy Identification by immunofluorescent assay (IFA) and immunoperoxidase staining of *R. rickettsii* in biopsy specimens of the skin rash are the best rapid diagnostic tests currently available for RMSF.[76] In experienced laboratories, the diagnosis of RMSF can be confirmed as soon as 4 hours after the specimen is obtained. The organisms can be detected as early as the third day of clinical illness and as late as the tenth day. Unfortunately, this technique can be used only when a rash is visible for accurate localization of the biopsy site. Biopsy specimens are generally obtained with a 3-mm punch in the center of the skin lesion. Immunofluorescent demonstration of rickettsiae in frozen sections of skin biopsies has a sensitivity of 70%. Immunohistochemical (IHC) staining of tissues at autopsy was positive in all fatal cases in one study, while IFA was negative in the majority of cases.[77] Failure to obtain a biopsy specimen of a rickettsial cutaneous lesion or failure to obtain sections through its center yields false-negative results. Treatment with antirickettsial drugs for 24 hours does not appreciably alter the sensitivity of the test; however, after 48 hours, rickettsiae are substantially reduced in numbers.

Isolation of Organism For most pathogenic infections, the "gold standard" of diagnosis is isolation and identification of the etiologic organism from the patient's blood or tissues. This is seldom attempted in rickettsioses, however, because the isolation procedures are time-consuming, expensive, and hazardous to laboratory personnel. In addition, primary isolation of rickettsiae by inoculation in the yolk sac of the chick embryo usually fails because of the small number of organisms in the patient's blood.

Box 128-1 Diagnostic Criteria

Laboratory criteria for diagnosis of RMSF are:

- Fourfold or greater rise in antibody titer to *Rickettsia rickettsii* antigen by immunofluorescence antibody (IFA), complement fixation (CF), latex agglutination (LA), microagglutination (MA), or indirect hemagglutination antibody (IHA) test in acute- and convalescent-phase specimens, ideally taken ≥3 weeks apart, or
- Positive polymerase chain reaction (PCR) assay to *R. rickettsii,* or
- Demonstration of positive immunofluorescence of skin lesion (biopsy) or organ tissue (autopsy), or
- Isolation of *R. rickettsii* from clinical specimen

Case classification is defined as:

Probable: a clinically compatible case with a single IFA serologic titer of ≥64 or a single CF titer ≥16 or other supportive serology (fourfold rise in titer or a single titer ≥320 by Proteus OX-19 or OX-2 or a single titer ≥128 by an LA, IHA, or MA test)

Confirmed: a clinically compatible case that is laboratory confirmed (CDC Case Definitions 1997)

Differential Considerations

Delayed diagnosis or misdiagnosis is the principal cause of the significant mortality rate associated with RMSF. Clinical diagnosis is difficult, especially early in the course of the illness, because of the nonspecific presentation of the illness. To prevent avoidable mortality, a diagnosis of RMSF must be considered whenever a patient has an unexplained febrile illness (with or without a rash and headache), even if there is neither history of tick bite nor travel to an area known to be endemic for the disease. An atypical presentation or manifestation of RMSF must also be considered during the differential diagnosis including (1) absent rash (Rocky

Mountain "spotless fever") or late appearance of a rash, (2) predominant gastrointestinal features or abdominal pain suggestive of an acute condition in the abdomen, (3) cough and pulmonary congestion suggestive of pneumonitis, and (4) meningismus suggestive of viral meningitis.[65] A presumed diagnosis must be made and specific therapy initiated well before specific confirmatory laboratory values are available.[65]

A wide variety of other infections with similar exanthems can be confused with RMSF. The most common include meningococcal infection, measles (rubeola) and atypical measles, gonococcemia, infectious mononucleosis, toxic shock syndrome, and enteroviral infections. Less common diseases include dengue, leptospirosis, murine typhus, and epidemic typhus.

Management

Treatment of RMSF consists of antibiotic therapy, supportive care, and possibly administration of steroids. An understanding of the underlying pathophysiologic changes and an appreciation of the systemic complications that may occur in the patient afflicted with RMSF are necessary for the formulation of a balanced therapeutic regimen. The course of the disease may be complicated by circulatory collapse, coma, renal failure, and electrolyte imbalances. Although often absent from the mildly ill patient in whom antibiotic therapy alone usually suffices, these complications should be anticipated in the seriously ill patient, especially those first recognized late in the disease.[67]

The most important factor contributing to the persistent case-fatality rate of 5% is delayed administration of specific antibiotic therapy. In one review of fatal cases of RMSF, all patients treated before the fifth day of illness survived, whereas more than 60% of those treated after the sixth day died.[78]

For a select group of early, mildly ill patients, outpatient therapy with oral antibiotics can be successful if the patients are reliable and close follow-up observation is arranged. More severely ill patients in whom the diagnosis is uncertain should receive hospital care with IV antibiotics.[67]

Antibiotics Antibiotic therapy is most effective when initiated during the early stages of disease, coincident with the initial appearance of the rash. If antibiotic therapy is delayed until the rash has become widespread and hemorrhagic, the response is less dramatic.[67] Either tetracycline or chloramphenicol given orally or parenterally is the current drug of choice (Table 128-5). Some authors recommend doxycycline as the drug of choice and chloramphenicol as the alternative.[71,79] Fluoroquinolones have been used successfully in the pediatric population.[80] No study has directly compared the treatment outcome of patients randomized to either agent. Both chloramphenicol and the tetracyclines are rickettsiostatic agents; neither antibiotic kills the organism, but replication is halted, allowing the host's immune response to successfully clear the infection.

The effectiveness of therapy depends on both the duration of therapy and the interval between the onset of illness and initiation of therapy. Treatment should begin as early as possible and continue for 7 to 10 days or until the patient is afebrile for 2 to 5 days. Patients who are clinically ill should be hospitalized for parenteral antibiotic treatment. Response to treatment, as manifested by decreased fever and improved rash, generally occurs 36 to 48 hours after beginning antibiotic therapy. Resistance to either chloramphenicol or the tetracyclines has not been reported.[65] Penicillin, erythromycin, cephalosporins, aminoglycosides, clindamycin, and sulfonamides are ineffective against RMSF. In fact, empiric use of these agents for presumed bacterial infections may permit progression of the illness.

If secondary bacterial infection occurs, administration of sulfonamides should be avoided because these drugs inhibit paraamino benzoic acid (an early and relatively ineffective treatment of RMSF) and may worsen the primary RMSF infection. The role of the new quinolones as potential replacements for tetracycline and chloramphenicol in the treatment of RMSF is as yet unproved.

Supportive Care Major complications of RMSF such as shock, congestive heart failure, disseminated intravascular coagulation (DIC), and ARDS should be anticipated and standard supportive measures instituted when appropriate. Circulatory collapse is common in patients with severe illness and is a major cause of morbidity and mortality in RMSF. Hypotension unresponsive to fluid administration may require the use of vasopressors such as dopamine. In the critically ill patient with widespread vasculitis, however, a delicate balance exists between maintenance of effective circulating volume and excessive leakage of fluids into the tissues, including the lungs and brain. Under these circum-

Table 128-5. Antibiotic Therapy of RMSF

	Antibiotic		
	Tetracycline*†	Chloramphenicol‡	
Patient	Oral	IV	Oral/IV
Adult	2 g/day	(Maximum 1 g/day)	50 mg/kg/day
Child <8 years			50 mg/kg/day
Child >8 years	25-50 mg/kg/day	10-20 mg/kg/day (maximum 1 g/day)	50 mg/kg/day

*Tetracycline should be avoided in children less than 8 years old, pregnant women, and patients with hepatic or renal dysfunction.
†Alternatively, doxycycline 100 mg PO twice daily may be used.
‡Chloramphenicol should be avoided in patients with thrombocytopenia.

stances, the excessive administration of IV fluids can be catastrophic.[65] Isolation of the patient is unnecessary, unless the diagnosis is still uncertain and other highly communicable illnesses such as meningococcemia or measles have not been excluded.

Steroids The use of steroids in RMSF is controversial and is not recommended in the routine care. However, they should be used for severe cases of RMSF complicated by extensive vasculitis, encephalitis, and cerebral edema.[65] In these critically ill patients, short-term, high-dosage steroid therapy is recommended, along with concomitant specific antibiotic therapy.[67]

Q FEVER

Principles of Disease

Q fever was first described in 1937 in Australia as an occupational disease of abattoir workers and dairy farmers. Cattle, sheep, goats, and ticks are the primary reservoirs of *Coxiella burnetii,* but many other species may be infected.[81] The disease is endemic worldwide, although it is rare in Scandinavian countries. The Q fever rickettsiae are extremely resistant to desiccation and to physical and chemical agents and may survive for long periods in the inanimate environment.

C. burnetii is extremely infectious for humans and animals, with a single inhaled organism sufficient to initiate infection in guinea pigs and probably in humans as well. For this reason, it has been considered as an agent of biological warfare. This organism's infectivity and estimated casualty rate have been compared with those of anthrax.[59] Humans are most commonly infected by inhalation of aerosolized particles from contaminated environments. Q fever patients rarely have a history of tick bite.

Clinical Features

The incubation period of Q fever ranges from 14 to 39 days, with an average of 20 days. The clinical manifestations include severe retrobulbar headache, a fever to 40° C (104° F) or higher, shaking chills, general malaise, myalgia, and chest pain. Although it is widely regarded as primarily a respiratory disease, the reported incidence of pulmonary involvement in patients with Q fever varies from 0 to 90%. The reasons for variation in the occurrence of pulmonary involvement are unclear, but explanations include geographic strain variation; plasmids that may regulate virulence; and the source, route, and dose of the agent. Hepatic involvement may be common, but liver dysfunction is usually minimal. Acute renal failure and a lymphocytic meningitis secondary to *C. burnetii* have been described.[82,83]

Q fever may also be a chronic infection, with or without an antecedent acute episode. The chronic forms of the disease include granulomatous hepatitis and culture-negative endocarditis. Endocarditis has been documented in up to 68% of patients with chronic Q fever and the mortality rate among this groups approaches 25%.[84] Most Q fever patients in whom endocarditis develops have a history of valvular heart disease, particularly affecting the aortic valve. These individuals should be especially cognizant of the potential hazards of Q fever infection and should be restricted from certain at-risk occupational settings. Patients with aneurysms and vascular grafts are also at risk. The most common presentations of patients with Q fever endocarditis are fever and congestive heart failure.[85] Human fetal demise and deaths have been attributed to *C. burnetii* infection.[86] Individuals infected with human immunodeficiency virus are at increased risk for contracting Q fever.[87]

Diagnostic Strategies

The diagnosis of Q fever should be suspected in any patient with a severe febrile illness without obvious cause, especially someone who has had recent contact with sheep, cattle, goats, or animal by-products. Because of the laboratory hazards associated with cultivation of Q fever rickettsiae, isolation of *C. burnetii* is not recommended for routine diagnosis. Rather, serologic studies such as IFA and ELISA are the preferred diagnostic tests, but the results are not identifiable until 2 to 3 weeks after the onset of illness.[59,88]

C. burnetii displays an antigenic phase variation (phase I to phase II). In patients with acute Q fever, phase II antibodies dominate the humoral immune response and are detectable by the second week of illness, whereas phase I antibodies are prominent only in patients with chronic Q fever. The finding of "ring granulomas" on bone marrow biopsy can be characteristic of Q fever.[88]

Management

As with other rickettsial diseases, the tetracyclines and chloramphenicol are both effective in treatment of acute Q fever. Most acute Q fever infections resolve without treatment, but the risk of chronic infection makes treatment advisable. The mortality rate is < 1% in untreated patients and lower still in those treated with antibiotics. The prognosis is worse in those patients with protracted illness and hepatic involvement or endocarditis. No current therapy has been shown to completely eradicate *Coxiella* in patients with endocarditis.[87] Inactivated whole cell vaccines for Q fever have proven effective for as long as 5 years.[89] Vaccination can afford considerable protection to slaughterhouse and dairy workers and others at risk.

EHRLICHIOSIS

Perspective

There are presently two major forms of human ehrlichioses in the United States: human monocytic ehrlichiosis (HME) and human granulocytic ehrlichiosis (HGE). Before 1986, *Ehrlichia sennetsu* was the only member of the genus of these organisms thought to infect humans, having been isolated in Japan in 1954 as the causative agent of sennetsu fever, a mononucleosis-like illness. *E. canis* is the causative organism, and the brown dog tick, *Rhipicephalus sanguineus,* is the only known vector. HME was discovered in 1986 and HGE in 1994. Both are identified as emerging diseases by the Centers for Control and Prevention (CDC). A third species, *E. ewingii,* has been shown to cause human disease in the United States.[90]

As of December 1999, only 18 states treat ehrlichiosis as a notifiable disease and five more routinely report it.[91] Both HME and HGE peak around June through August. High-risk populations are similar to those found in Lyme disease, including those living in endemic areas or with frequent contact with wildlife and/or rural, wooded areas. A unique case series of ehrlichiosis in a group of golfers showed that those who spent more time in the rough and wooded areas searching lost balls were at higher risk.[92] HME has predominantly been reported in the south central and southeastern United States; HGE is mostly found in the upper Midwest and northeastern United States.[91,93]

Principles of Disease

The causative agents in the ehrlichioses are gram-negative, obligate intracellular rickettsia-like coccobacilli. Transmitted from the midguts and salivary glands of their tick vectors,[94] these organisms reside in specific circulating leukocytes in human and other mammalian hosts. Reservoirs include the white-tailed deer and the white-footed mouse. One species, *E. equina,* has been isolated in California elk. HME, transmitted by the Lone Star tick, *Amblyomma americanum,* is caused by the organism *Ehrlichia chaffeensis* (named after Fort Chaffee, Arkansas), which invades monocytes. *E. chaffeensis* has recently been isolated from *I. pacificus* ticks in California. *E. phagocytophila* and *E. equi,* both responsible for HGE, invade neutrophils (granulocytes) and are transmitted by the tick *I. scapularis.* Both *I. scapularis* and *I. pacificus* (U.S West Coast counterpart of *I. scapularis*) ticks are also the vectors for Lyme disease.

Clinical Features

HME and HGE appear with similar clinical presentations. The average onset of symptoms (for HME) from time of tick discovery is 9 days but ranges from 0 to 34 days.[95] More than 90% of patients with HME report a history of tick bite.[96] More than 80% appear with fever, headache, and myalgias and 70% with myalgias. Leukopenia, thrombocytopenia, and elevated liver function tests can be seen in anywhere from 50% to 90% of patients. Rashes occur in approximately one third of patients with HME but in only 2% to 11% of those with HGE. Rashes in Lyme disease occur in 85% of patients. Other findings such as ARDS, meningitis, pancarditis, renal failure, and DIC have been reported.[95] The largest data pool available, from the CDC, shows case fatality ratios from 20 states to be 2.7% for HME and 0.7% for HGE.[91] Approximately 45% of HGE patients are hospitalized.

A small series of pediatric patients (average age, 7.4 years) with HME revealed a rash rate of 67%. The majority suffered permanent cognitive or other neurologic damage.[97]

Diagnostic Strategies

The initial diagnoses of HME and HGE are largely based on clinical presentation. Most tests are either retrospective or rarely immediately available. Cytopenia and abnormal liver function usually resolve after the acute phase of illness. Microscopic identification of mulberry-like clusters, called morulae, inside leukocytes on peripheral blood smears is helpful but is usually negative after the first week of illness with HGE, especially if treated with doxycycline. The most common mode of diagnosis is confirmation of IgG antibodies with IFA. Unfortunately, IgM assays are not presently established. Results are therefore often retrospective. EIA and confirmatory tests with Western blot have been developed.[98] PCR testing for DNA fragments, although not readily available in most hospitals, is probably most reliable in the acute phase of illness (1 week).[99] Cultures take up to 2 weeks to grow the organisms.[100] Diagnostic serologic testing is available at the CDC through state health departments.[91]

Confirmation of disease requires a fourfold rise or fall in IFA antibody titer, a positive PCR test, or findings of morulae with a single IFA titer of >63. Probable disease requires a single titer of >63 or the presence of morulae within infected cells. All require compatible clinical suspicion.[91] Most patients with clinical symptoms have IFA titers between 160 and 1280 at presentation.[101]

Management

Tetracycline, which has been shown to be effective in canine ehrlichiosis, is also effective in human ehrlichiosis. Doxycycline and tetracycline regimens for 7 to 14 days are curative. For pediatric patients, the concern for teeth staining is obvious, although it has been argued that most of this effect is seen only with multiple dosing periods. Most patients respond rapidly after treatment is begun, and fever subsides within 24 to 48 hours. Data supporting the use of chloramphenicol are still inconclusive. Rifampin and trovofloxacin have proved effective only in vitro.[102,103] Although more than half of patients with confirmed human ehrlichiosis require hospitalization, almost all recover without residual problems.

BABESIOSIS

Perspective

Babesiosis is a tick-borne, malaria-like, acute febrile illness caused by intraerythrocytic protozoan parasites of the genus *Babesia.* Babesiosis has long been recognized as an important veterinary disease and was probably known in ancient times; in fact, it has been proposed that the fifth plague described in the Book of Exodus was actually babesiosis.

The first human cases of babesiosis were reported in Montana in 1904; investigators seeking the cause of Rocky Mountain spotted fever examined blood smears from local inhabitants and described parasitic forms now known to be characteristic of *Babesia.* Since the late 1950s, several widely scattered cases (mostly in Europe) of human babesiosis have been reported in splenectomized individuals. *B. divergens,* a species primarily infecting cattle, is the most common agent reported; but other species have been implicated as well, including *B. bovis, B. equi,* and a single case of *B. caucasia* infection. Two other strains, WA-1, related to a canine pathogen *B. gibsoni,* and MO1, related to *B. divergens,* have also now been found to cause disease in humans.[94] In all these cases, the course was fulminant and usually fatal.

Since the late 1960s, more than 200 cases have been documented in the United States. Almost all of these cases were caused by *B. microti,* a rodent parasite, and almost all occurred in the coastal regions of southern New England, where *B. microti* is endemic, including Cape Cod and the offshore islands of Massachusetts (Nantucket, Martha's Vineyard) and Rhode Island (Block Island). Babesiosis has also been reported in Maryland, Virginia, Georgia, Wisconsin, Minnesota, California, and Washington. These cases differ from the European cases in that most (approximately 80%) have occurred in individuals with intact spleens. In addition, many of the patients in the United States had little morbidity despite lack of specific therapy.

Principles of Disease

B. microti is associated with deer and mice rather than cattle. The ecology of *B. microti* is similar to that of *Borrelia burgdorferi,* the etiologic agent of Lyme disease, with the same major vector, *Ixodes dammini,* and the same mammalian reservoirs: white-footed mice, which host the larval and nymphal stages of the tick, and white-tailed deer, which host the adult ticks.

Human babesiosis results from accidental human intrusion

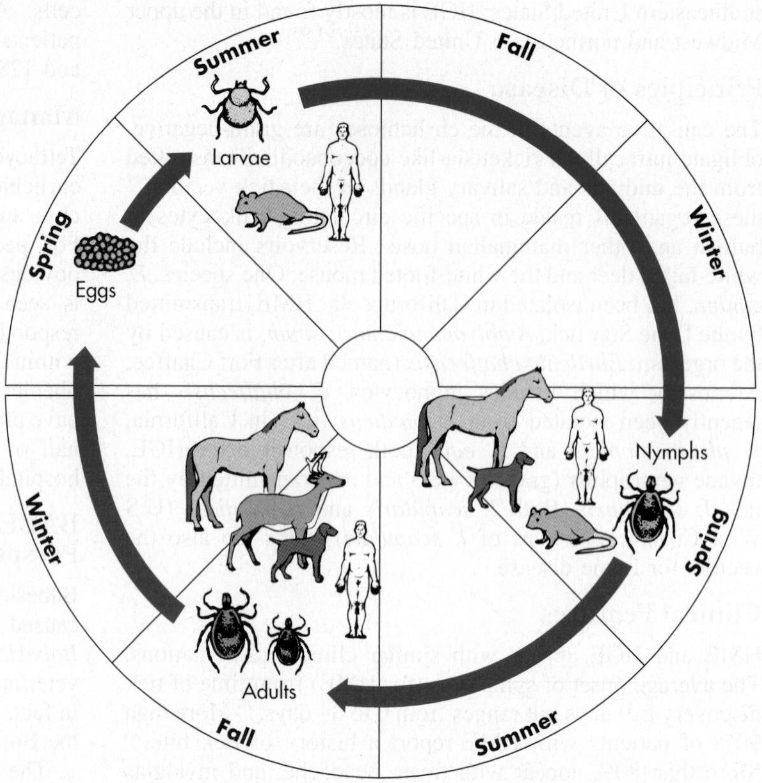

Figure 128-9. **The life cycle of *Ixodes scapularis*. *From Tick Information Sheet: The deer tick. In Hoskins JD, editor:* Tick-transmitted diseases: veterinary clinics of North America*, Philadelphia, 1991, WB Saunders.***

on the natural cycle of infection. The nymphal form of the *Ixodes* tick most commonly transmits the disease to humans, although babesiosis can also be transmitted by the adult stage. Nymphal *I. scapularis* measure only 1 to 2 mm long and thus may be easily overlooked by the patient (Figure 128-9). In more than half of all cases of babesiosis, patients cannot recall tick exposure. As is true for other tick-borne illnesses, the peak incidence of babesiosis is between May and August, coinciding with the nymphal feeding period and also the time of maximal human exposure in endemic areas. Babesiosis acquired by blood transfusion has also been reported.

Clinical Features

Babesiosis has an incubation period of 1 to 4 weeks after tick exposure. Nonspecific flulike symptoms, including fever, chills, headache, fatigue, and anorexia, usually occur. Other less common symptoms are nausea, diaphoresis, depression, photophobia, myalgias, arthralgias, dark urine, emotional lability, and hyperesthesias. Unlike Lyme disease, rash is not a feature of the illness. Physical examination usually reveals normal findings, except for fever, which is usually present, and splenomegaly, which occurs in some patients. Meningeal signs are absent. More severe disease occurs in splenectomized patients[104]; severe hemolytic anemia, hemoglobinuria, jaundice, renal insufficiency, ARDS, and DIC may be seen in these cases. Some patients with babesiosis are only mildly ill, and asymptomatic infection may also occur, as demonstrated by serologic surveys in endemic areas. In a review of 139 patients from New York, mortality approached 6.5%.[105] The diagnosis of babesiosis should be considered in any febrile patient from an endemic area during the tick season and should be part of the differential diagnosis of posttransfusion infections.

Diagnostic Strategies

The diagnosis is established by examination of thick and thin Giemsa-stained blood smears. Characteristic intraerythrocytic forms (pyriform, ring, tetrad) may be present. Malaria may be excluded by the absence of intracellular pigment granules, schizonts, and gametocytes. The presence of parasites in budding tetrad formation, like a Maltese cross, is more suggestive of babesiosis, although this finding is uncommon. Because parasitemia may vary, in suspected cases serial smears over the course of several days may be necessary. The diagnosis can be confirmed by serologic studies. IFA antibody to *B. microti* is available through the CDC, and titers usually rise to 1:1,024 or greater within the first few weeks of illness. IgM-indirect IFA is 91% sensitive and 99% specific in acute babesiosis.[106] Serologic tests for Lyme disease, which shares a common tick vector with babesiosis, should also be obtained on these patients because cases of babesiosis concurrent with Lyme disease have been reported.[19] Some areas have reported that up to 10% of patients with Lyme disease are coinfected with babesial organisms. PCR is also now available and is thought to be highly sensitive and specific.[107] Other laboratory findings include mild to moderate hemolytic anemia, which is present in most patients, and resultant mild elevation in bilirubin and serum lactate dehydrogenase.

Management

Patients who have not had splenectomies generally recover without specific therapy, although prolonged malaise and fatigue are commonly seen. In patients with severe disease or in those who have had splenectomies, the combination of quinine, 650 mg orally, and clindamycin, 600 mg IV, both given every 6 hours, has been shown to be effective and is currently the treatment of choice. Antibiotic therapy is recommended only for patients with severe disease and those who have had splenectomies. Therapy should be continued for a minimum of 7 to 10 days. Other antimalarial drugs such as chloroquine and quinacrine are not effective. Another therapeutic option that may be considered under some circumstances is exchange transfusion; fulminantly ill patients with marked degrees of parasitemia and hemolysis have benefited from this treatment. Effective living vaccines have been developed for bovine babesiosis but not yet for human disease.

COLORADO TICK FEVER

Perspective

Endemic to the Rocky Mountain area, Colorado tick fever (CTF) is an acute tick-borne viral infection characterized by headache, back pain, biphasic febrile course, and leukopenia. The etiologic agent of CTF is a small RNA virus of the genus *Orbivirus,* family Reoviridae. It is one of more than 500 viruses in the heterogeneous group of arthropod-borne viruses (arboviruses).[108] CTF has a sharply defined endemic zone encompassing mountainous and highland areas, from an altitude of about 4,000 to more than 10,000 feet, in the Canadian provinces of British Columbia and Alberta and in at least 11 western states (California, Colorado, Idaho, Montana, Nevada, New Mexico, Oregon, South Dakota, Utah, Washington, and Wyoming).[109] The largest number of cases has generally been reported in Colorado. The distribution of the virus coincides with that of its principal tick vector, *Dermacentor andersoni.* Although RMSF is transmitted by the same vector, that disease is far less common in Colorado: The cases of RMSF are outnumbered at least twenty-fold by cases of CTF.

Principles of Disease

The CTF virus has been isolated from at least eight species of ticks, but *D. andersoni* is the only proven vector for humans. The tick is a significant reservoir for the virus because transstadial transmission (from larva to nymph to adult) of virus occurs, and the tick remains infected and infectious for life (up to 3 years). The primary vertebrate host species for CTF virus maintenance are the chipmunk, *Tamias minimus,* and the golden-mantled ground squirrel, *Spermophilus lateralis;* many other vertebrate hosts have been identified as well, including a species of porcupine in Rocky Mountain National Park. Larval and nymphal stages of *D. andersoni* ticks are responsible for transmission of CTF virus among rodents, and wintering of the virus is accomplished by nymphal and adult *D. andersoni.* Only adult ticks transmit CTF virus to humans.

Several hundred cases per year are reported in the United States.[109] The actual incidence is undoubtedly much higher because many cases are diagnosed as nonspecific "viral illness," and other cases may be very mild or wholly subclinical. Human susceptibility to CTF is universal, but it occurs most commonly in young men, reflecting greater occupational and recreational tick exposure.

Clinical Features

After an incubation period of approximately 3 to 5 days (range, 0 to 14 days), a moderate to severe flulike illness occurs abruptly, with signs and symptoms similar to the early stage of RMSF. Fever, chills, headache, myalgia, lethargy, anorexia, and nausea are common; vomiting and abdominal pain are seen occasionally. Early physical findings are nonspecific. A macular or maculopapular rash has been reported in 5% to 12% of patients, but unlike the rash of RMSF, the rash of CTF is not a prominent feature of the illness.

A distinct feature of the illness is a biphasic course that occurs in approximately 50% of patients, causing a characteristic "saddleback" fever curve. Initial symptoms resolve after 2 to 3 days, and the patient feels relatively well for 1 or 2 days, after which there is a return of fever, headache, and myalgias. The second phase may be more intense than the first phase and generally lasts 2 to 4 days. There may even be a third febrile period. Alternatively, a single prolonged febrile illness may occur. Recovery from CTF usually occurs within 2 weeks, but a convalescence may be prolonged, especially in patients more than 30 years old.

CTF is a self-limited disease, and virtually all patients recover without sequelae. Reports of severe complications such as meningoencephalitis and hemorrhagic diathesis have been limited to children. Only a few fatalities have been recorded.[108]

Diagnostic Strategies

The peripheral leukocyte count is often depressed during the acute illness to as low as 1,000/mm^3 with a relative lymphocytosis. Transient thrombocytopenia may accompany the leukopenia, and less often a mild anemia can occur. These hematologic abnormalities normalize during convalescence, but persistence of the virus in red cells causes a prolonged viremia even when clinical recovery is complete. Transfusion-acquired infection has been reported; it is caused by this persistent viremia in asymptomatic blood donors. No one should donate blood for at least 6 months after recovery from CTF.[108]

The diagnosis of CTF can be confirmed by serologic testing (IFA, neutralizing antibody, CF, enzyme immunoassay) of acute and convalescent samples, but serologic study is of little help acutely because of the slow rise of titers.[110] The most rapid confirmation of CTF, and thus elimination of concern about possible RMSF, is provided by direct immunofluorescent staining of virus in red blood cells in peripheral blood smears.

Management

Treatment for CTF is entirely supportive. Most patients do not require hospitalization, but if RMSF remains a diagnostic possibility, initial treatment with tetracycline or chloramphenicol and a period of observation are necessary until the diagnosis of RMSF can be ruled out.

TICK PARALYSIS

Perspective

Tick paralysis occurs when an adult female tick attaches and releases a neurotoxin that can produce cerebellar dysfunction or an ascending paralysis. Tick paralysis was recognized as early as the beginning of the nineteenth century. Hovell, while traveling through Australia, wrote in 1824 of "the small insect called the tick, which buries itself in the flesh, and would in the end destroy either human or beast if not removed in time."[111]

Tick paralysis has been reported worldwide, but most cases occur in the southeastern and northwestern regions of the United States, western Canada, and Australia. Forty-three species of ticks have been found to cause tick paralysis in humans, other mammals, or birds. Most cases in North America are caused by *Dermacentor* species; in Australia, *Ixodes holocyclus* is primarily associated. Both Ixodidae (hard ticks) and Argasidae (soft ticks) have been implicated. Tick paralysis usually occurs in the spring and summer months, and most cases occur in children, primarily girls, probably because ticks are more easily concealed in longer hair. However, among adults, more men than women acquire the disease.

Principles of Disease

Tick paralysis is thought to be caused by a toxin secreted from the salivary glands of the tick during a blood meal.[112] The mechanism of action of the toxin is poorly understood, but it appears to produce a conduction block in the peripheral branches of motor fibers, resulting in a failure of release of acetylcholine at the neuromuscular junction. Possible central sites of action of the toxin have been postulated to explain cases in which the clinical picture is dominated by cerebellar dysfunction.

Clinical Features

Onset of symptoms usually occurs from 4 to 7 days after the tick attaches. Initially, restlessness and irritability may be seen, followed by ascending flaccid paralysis, acute ataxia, or a combination of the two. Deep tendon reflexes are almost invariably lost. These symptoms can progress rapidly over a few days, with bulbar involvement, respiratory paralysis, and ultimately death, if the tick is not detected and removed.

The ascending nature of tick paralysis has been noted in most descriptions of it; however, ataxia and associated cerebellar findings in the absence of muscle weakness may occur. Thus, tick paralysis may sometimes present as "tick ataxia." Isolated facial paralysis has been reported in patients with ticks embedded behind the ear. Fever, other systemic symptoms, and sensory deficits are unusual.

Differential Strategies

The paralysis should be considered in the differential diagnosis of any patient thought to have Guillain-Barré syndrome, Eaton-Lambert syndrome, myasthenia gravis, poliomyelitis, botulism, diphtheritic polyneuropathy, or any disease with an ascending flaccid paralysis or acute ataxia.

Management

Treatment in the United States consists simply of removing the tick; improvement is generally seen within a few hours and complete recovery within 48 hours. The recommended procedure for the removal is summarized in Box 128-2. Supportive care, including mechanical ventilation, may be necessary. The mortality rate is approximately 10%; nearly all those who die are children.

Tick paralysis in Australia is often more devastating than in the United States. Symptoms of illness caused by the Australian tick, *I. holocyclus,* are not resolved and often worsen after tick removal. Hyperimmune serum is available in Australia and is often needed because symptoms may worsen up to 48 hours after removal.

Prophylaxis with Insect Repellents Insect repellents have long been used to prevent mosquito bites. With recent increased public awareness and concern about tick-borne illness, especially Lyme disease, skin and clothing repellents are now also being marketed for tick protection.

Box 128-2 Recommended Method for Tick Removal

1. Remove an embedded tick by grasping it with blunt forceps or tweezers as close to the point of attachment as possible.
2. Do not use bare fingers to remove ticks from animals or humans; when tweezers are unavailable, fingers should be shielded with a tissue, paper towel, or rubber glove.
3. Apply gentle, steady, upward traction with the forceps; do not twist or jerk the tick. Avoid squeezing or crushing the tick.
4. Do not handle the tick with bare hands. After removing the tick, thoroughly disinfect the bite site and wash hands with soap and water.
5. Dispose of ticks by placing them in a container of alcohol or flushing them down the toilet.

From Needhan GR: *Pediatrics* 75:997, 1985.

The most effective topical insect repellent known is N,N-diethyl-m-toluamide, commonly called DEET. Although effective, DEET is absorbed through the skin into the systemic circulation and may cause allergic and toxic effects in children and adults, especially when used on the skin repeatedly in high concentrations.

Permethrin, actually a pesticide rather than a repellent, can be used as a clothing spray for protection against ticks. Applied to the clothing as an aerosol, it is nonstaining, nearly odorless, and resistant to degradation by light, heat, or immersion in water. Permethrin is toxic to the nervous system of insects, but in mammals it is poorly absorbed and rapidly inactivated. Reported adverse effects have been limited to the skin and are uncommon.

Both topical DEET and clothing impregnated with permethrin have been shown to be effective in field trials when used alone. Wearing protective clothing treated with permethrin, in addition to using DEET on exposed skin, provides the greatest degree of protection against tick bites.[113]

KEY CONCEPTS

- Tick-borne illnesses are frequently misdiagnosed as viral or bacterial infections. Early diagnosis can be facilitated by considering these diagnoses and patients who live in or have recently traveled to endemic areas, and by routinely asking for a history of recent tick or insect bites in patients who present with febrile illnesses.
- Lyme disease should be suspected in patients who present with signs of a viral illness, monoarticular arthritis, meningitis, multiple neurologic abnormalities, or heart block. Diagnosis can be confirmed with serologic testing of acute and convalescent serum samples.
- Relapsing fever should be suspected in patients who present with recurrent viral-like illness associated with high fever. The diagnosis can be confirmed by identifying spirochetes on a blood smear obtained during a period of rising temperature.
- Ulceroglandular tularemia should be suspected in patients

with slow-healing extremity ulcers associated with large regional adenopathy (bubos). The diagnosis can be confirmed with serologic testing.

- Rocky Mountain spotted fever should be suspected in patients who present with a fever associated with typical rash and signs of cardiopulmonary or neurologic dysfunction. In patients who are severely ill, chloramphenicol or tetracycline should be included in broad-spectrum antibiotic coverage pending laboratory confirmation of the diagnosis.

ACKNOWLEDGMENTS

The authors gratefully acknowledge the expert review of the Lyme disease section by Dr. Daniel Rahn.

REFERENCES

1. Magnarelli LA et al: *Borrelia burgdorferi* in an urban environment: white-tailed deer with infected ticks and antibodies, *J Clin Microbiol* 33:541, 1995.
2. Arthur DR: Ticks in Egypt in 1500 BC? *Nature* 206:1060, 1965.
3. Cupp EW: Biology of ticks, *Vet Clin North Am* 21:1, 1991.
4. Steere AC et al: Lyme arthritis: an epidemic of oligaarticular arthritis in children and adults in three Connecticut communities, *Arthritis Rheum* 20:7, 1977.
5. Rahn DW, Egherman WP: Lyme disease: unmasking the great masquerader, *East Med Reports* 10:13, 1989.
6. Dennis DT: Epidemiology, ecology, and prevention of Lyme disease. In Rahn D, Evans J, editors: *Lyme disease,* Philadelphia, 1998, American College of Physicians.
7. Centers for Disease Control: Surveillance for Lyme disease—United States, 1992-1998, *MMWR* 49(SS03):1, 2000.
8. Centers for Disease Control: Lyme disease: United States, 1995, *MMWR* 45:481, 1996.
9. Donahue JG, Piesman J, Spielman A: Reservoir competence of white-footed mice for Lyme disease spirochetes, *Am J Trop Med Hyg* 36:92, 1987.
10. Steere AC et al: Longitudinal assessment of the clinical and epidemiological features of Lyme disease in a defined population, *J Infect Dis* 154:295, 1986.
11. Speilman A et al: Ecology of *Ixodes dammini*–borne human babesiosis and Lyme disease, *Annu Rev Entomol* 30:439, 1985.
12. Burgdorfer W, Hayes SF, Corwin D: Pathophysiology of the Lyme disease spirochete, *Borrelia burgdorferi,* in Ixodid ticks, *Rev Infect Dis* 11:S1442, 1989.
13. Nadelman RB, Wormser GP: Management of tick bites in early Lyme disease. In Rahn D, Evans J, editors: *Lyme disease,* Philadelphia, 1998, American College of Physicians.
14. Steere AC et al: The early clinical manifestations of Lyme disease, *Ann Intern Med* 99:76, 1983.
15. Logigian EL: Neurologic manifestations of Lyme disease. In Rahn D, Evans J, editors: *Lyme disease.* Philadelphia, 1998, American College of Physicians.
16. Pachner AR: *Borrelia burgdorferi* in the nervous system: the new "great imitator," *Ann N Y Acad Sci* 539:56, 1988.
17. Brogan GX, Homan CS, Viccellia P: The enlarging clinical spectrum of Lyme disease: Lyme cerebral vasculitis, a near disease entity, *Ann Emerg Med* 19:572, 1990.
18. Evans J: Lyme carditis. In Rahn D, Evans J, editors: *Lyme disease,* Philadelphia, 1998, American College of Physicians.
19. Marcus LC et al: Fatal pancarditis in a patient with coexistent Lyme disease and babesiosis: demonstration of spirochetes in the myocardium, *Ann Intern Med* 103:374, 1985.
20. van der Linde MR et al: Range of atrioventricular conduction disturbances in Lyme borreliosis: a report of four cases and review of other published reports, *Br Heart J* 63:162, 1990.
21. McAlister HF et al: Lyme carditis: an important cause of reversible heart block, *Ann Intern Med* 110:339, 1989.
22. Jacobs JC, Stevens, M, Duray PH: Lyme disease simulating septic arthritis, *JAMA* 256:1138, 1986.
23. Snydman DR et al: *Borrelia burgdorferi* in joint fluid in chronic Lyme arthritis, *Ann Intern Med* 104:798, 1986.
24. Aaberg TM: The expanding ophthalmologic spectrum of Lyme disease, *Am J Ophthalmol* 107:77, 1989.
25. Rahn D: Natural history of Lyme disease. In Rahn D, Evans J, editors: *Lyme disease,* Philadelphia, 1998, American College of Physicians.
26. Steere AC: Musculoskeletal features of Lyme disease. In Rahn D, Evans J, editors: *Lyme disease,* Philadelphia, 1998, American College of Physicians.
27. Ackerman R et al: Chronic neurologic manifestations of erythema migrans borreliosis, *Ann N Y Acad Sci* 539:16, 1988.
28. Kaufman LD et al: Late cutaneous Lyme disease: acrodermatitis chronica atrophicans, *Am J Med* 86:828, 1989.
29. Duffy J: Lyme disease, *Infect Dis Clin North Am* 1:511, 1987.
30. Steere AC et al: The spirochetal etiology of Lyme disease, *N Engl J Med* 308:733, 1983.
31. Shrestha M, Grodzicki RL, Steere AC: Diagnosing early Lyme disease, *Am J Med* 78:235, 1985.
32. American College of Physicians: Guidelines for laboratory evaluation in the diagnosis of Lyme disease, *Ann Intern Med* 127:1106, 1997.
33. Centers for Disease Control: Recommendations for test performance and interpretation from the Second International Conference of Serologic Diagnosis of Lyme Disease, *MMWR* 44:590, 1995.
34. Sigal LH: Use of the laboratory in the confirmation and management of Lyme disease. In Rahn DW, Evans J, editors: *Lyme disease,* Philadelphia, 1998, American College of Physicians.
35. Malawista SE: Lyme disease. In Wyngaarden JB, Smith LH, editors: *Cecil textbook of medicine,* ed 18, Philadelphia, 1988, WB Saunders.
36. Steere AC et al: Erythema chronicum migrans and Lyme arthritis: the enlarging clinical spectrum, *Ann Intern Med* 86:685, 1977.
37. Centers for Disease Control: Recommendations for the use of Lyme disease vaccine: recommendations of the Advisory Committee on Immunization Practices (ACIP), *MMWR* 48(No. RR07):1, 1999.
38. Thanassi W, Schoen RT: The Lyme disease vaccine: conception, development, and implementation, *Ann Intern Med* 132:661, 2000.
39. Steere AC et al: Vaccination against Lyme disease with recombinant *Borrelia burgdorferi* outer-surface lipoprotein A with adjuvant. Lyme Disease Vaccine Study Group, *N Engl J Med* 339:209, 1998.
40. Shapiro ED et al: A controlled trial of antimicrobial prophylaxis for Lyme disease after deer-tick bites, *N Engl J Med* 327:1769, 1992.
41. Agre F, Schwartz R: The value of early treatment of deer tick bite for the prevention of Lyme disease, *Am J Dis Child* 147:945, 1993.
42. Nadelman RB et al: Comparison of cefuroxime axetil and doxycycline in the treatment of early Lyme disease, *Ann Intern Med* 117:273, 1992.
43. Moore JA: Jarish-Herxheimer reaction in Lyme disease, *Cutis* 39:397, 1987.
44. Luft BJ et al: New chemotherapeutic approaches in the treatment of Lyme borreliosis, *Ann NY Acad Sci* 539:352, 1988.
45. Steere AC et al: Successful parenteral penicillin therapy of established Lyme arthritis, *N Engl J Med* 312:869, 1985.
46. Dattwyler RJ et al: Treatment of late Lyme borreliosis: randomized comparison of ceftriaxone and penicillin, *Lancet* 1:1191, 1988.
47. Dattwyler RJ et al: Ceftriaxone as effective therapy in refractory Lyme disease, *J Infect Dis* 155:1322, 1987.
48. Skoldenberg B et al: Treatment of late Lyme borreliosis with emphasis on neurological disease, *Ann N Y Acad Sci* 539:317, 1988.
49. Maraspin V et al: Treatment of erythema migrans, in pregnancy, *Clin Infect Dis* 22:788, 1996.
50. Butler T: Relapsing fever. In Wyngaarden JB, Smith LH, editors: *Cecil textbook of medicine,* ed 18, Philadelphia, 1988, WB Saunders.
51. Perine PL: Relapsing fever. In Braunwald E et al, editors: *Harrison's principles of internal medicine,* ed 11, New York, 1987, McGraw-Hill.
52. Horton JM, Blaser MJ: The spectrum of relapsing fever in the Rocky Mountains, *Arch Intern Med* 145:871, 1985.
53. Marcus LC: Wilderness-acquired zoonoses. In Auerbach PS, Gehr EC, editors: *Management of wilderness and environmental emergencies,* ed 2, St Louis, 1989, Mosby.
54. Kaye D: Tularemia. In Braunwald E et al, editors: *Harrison's principles of internal medicine,* ed 11, New York, 1987, McGraw-Hill.
55. Liles WC: Tularemia from domestic cats, *West J Med* 158:619, 1993.
56. Gill V, Cunha B: Tularemia pneumonia, *Semin Respir Infect* 12:61, 1997.

57. Centers for Disease Control: Summary of notifiable diseases, United States, 1997, *MMWR* 46:3, 1998.
58. Parssinen O, Rummukainen M: Acute glaucoma and acute corneal oedema in association with tularemia, *Acta Ophthalmol Scand* 75:732, 1997.
59. Franz DR et al: Clinical recognition and management of patients exposed to biological warfare agents, *JAMA* 278:399, 1997.
60. Syrjala H et al: Guillain-Barré syndrome and tularemia pleuritis with high adenosine deaminase activity in pleural fluid (case report), *Infection* 17:152, 1989.
61. Dolan SA, Dommaraju CB, DeGuzman GB: Detection of *Francisella tularensis* in clinical specimens by use of polymerase chain reaction, *Clin Infect Dis* 26:764, 1998.
62. Sjostedt A et al: Detection of *Francisella tularensis* in ulcers of patients with tularemia by PCR, *J Clin Microbiol* 35:1045, 1997.
63. Cross JT, Jacobs RF: Tularemia: treatment failures with outpatient use of ceftriaxone, *Clin Infect Dis* 17:976, 1993.
64. Drabick JJ et al: Passive protection of mice against lethal *Francisella tularensis* (live tularemia vaccine strain) infection by the sera of human recipients of the live tularemia vaccine, *Am J Med Sci* 308:83, 1994.
65. Woodward TE: Rocky Mountain spotted fever: epidemiological and early clinical signs are keys to treatment and reduced mortality, *J Infect Dis* 150:465, 1984.
66. Dalton MJ et al: National surveillance for Rocky Mountain spotted fever, 1981-1992: epidemiologic summary and evaluation of risk factors for fatal outcome, *Am J Trop Med Hyg* 52:405, 1995.
67. Woodward TE: Rickettsial diseases. In Braunwald E et al, editors: *Harrison's principles of internal medicine,* ed 11, New York, 1987, McGraw-Hill.
68. Arguin PM et al: An investigation into the possibility of transmission of tick-borne pathogens via blood transfusion: Transfusion-Associated Tick-Borne Illness Task Force, *Transfusion* 39:828, 1999.
69. Hackstadt T: The biology of rickettsiae, *Infect Agents Dis* 5:127, 1996.
70. Haynes RE, Sanders DY, Cramblett HG: Rocky Mountain spotted fever in children, *J Pediatr* 76:685, 1970.
71. Walker DH: Rocky Mountain spotted fever: a seasonal alert, *Clin Infect Dis* 20:111, 1995.
72. Kirkland KB et al: Rocky Mountain spotted fever complicated by gangrene: report of six cases and review, *Clin Infect Dis* 16:629, 1993.
73. Wei TY, Baumann RJ: Acute disseminated encephalomyelitis after Rocky Mountain spotted fever, *Pediatr Neurol* 21:503, 1999.
74. Hilton E et al: Seroprevalence and seroconversion for tick-borne diseases in a high-risk population in the northeast United States, *Am J Med* 106:404, 1999.
75. PanBioInDx, Inc. Internet address: www.indxdi.com/indx1110.htm, February 2000.
76. Procop GW et al: Immunoperoxidase and immunofluorescent staining of *Rickettsia rickettsii* in skin biopsies, *Arch Pathol Lab Med* 121:894, 1997.
77. Paddock CD et al: Hidden mortality attributable to Rocky Mountain spotted fever: immunohistochemical detection of fatal, serologically unconfirmed disease, *J Infect Dis* 179:1469, 1999.
78. Hattwick MAW et al: Fatal Rocky Mountain spotted fever, *JAMA* 240:1499, 1978.
79. Cale DF, McCarthy MW: Treatment of Rocky Mountain spotted fever in children, *Ann Pharmacother* 31:492, 1997.
80. Tsai TF, Olson JG: Rickettsial spotted fever infections: another pediatric indication for quinolones, *Pediatr Infect Dis* 14:635, 1995.
81. Fournier P-E, Marrie TJ, Raoult D: Minireview: diagnosis of Q fever, *J Clin Microbiol* 36:1823, 1998.
82. Morovic M: Acute renal failure as the main complication of acute infection with *Coxiella burnetti, Nephron* 64:335, 1993.
83. Schattner A: Lymphocytic meningitis as the sole manifestation of Q fever, *Postgrad Med J* 69:36, 1993.
84. Brouqi P: Chronic Q fever, *Arch Intern Med* 153:642, 1993.
85. Fournier P-E et al: *Coxiella burnetii* infection of aneurysms or vascular grafts: report of seven cases and review, *Clin Infect Dis* 26:116, 1998.
86. Raoult D: Q fever during pregnancy: a risk for women, fetuses, and obstetricians, *N Engl J Med* 330:371, 1994.
87. Raoult D: Q fever and HIV infection, *AIDS* 7:81, 1993.
88. Yale SH: Unusual aspects of acute Q fever–associated hepatitis, *Mayo Clin Proc* 69:769, 1994.
89. Ackland JR: Vaccine prophylaxis of Q fever, *Med J Aust* 160:704, 1994.
90. Hmiel SP et al: Human infection with *Ehrlichia ewingii,* the agent of Ozark canine granulocytic ehrlichiosis: proceedings of the First International Conference on Emerging Infectious Diseases; March 8-11; Atlanta, Georgia; Addendum 4 [Abstract], 1998.
91. McQuiston JH et al: Centers for Disease Control and Prevention: the human ehrlichioses in the United States, *Emerg Infect Dis* 5, 1999.
92. Standaert SM et al: Ehrlichiosis in a golf-oriented retirement community, *N Engl J Med* 333:452, 1995.
93. Centers for Disease Control and Prevention: Table 1. Summary: provisional causes of notifiable diseases, United States, cumulative, week ending January 1, 2000, *MMWR* 48:1183, 2000.
94. Walker DH: Tick-transmitted infectious diseases in the United States, *Annu Rev Public Health* 19:237, 1998.
95. Fritz CL et al: Ehrlichiosis, *Infect Dis Clin North Am* 12:1:123, 1998.
96. Eng TR et al: Epidemiologic, clinical, and laboratory findings of human ehrlichiosis in the United States, 1988, *JAMA* 264:2251, 1990.
97. Schutze GE, Jacobs RF: Human monocytic ehrlichiosis in children, *Pediatrics* 100:E10, 1997.
98. Ravyn MD: Immunodiagnosis of human granulocytic ehrlichiosis by using culture-derived human isolates, *J Clin Microbiol* 36:1480, 1998.
99. Comer JA et al: Serologic testing for human granulocytic ehrlichiosis at a national referral center, *J Clin Microbiol* 37:558, 1999.
100. Chu FK: Rapid and sensitive PCR-based detection and differentiation of aetiologic agents of human granulocytotropic and monocytotropic ehrlichiosis, *Mol Cell Probes* 12:93, 1998.
101. IGeneX, Inc. Palo Alto, Ca 94303: Ehrlichiosis: interpretation of laboratory results for ehrlichiosis. Internet address, www.igenex.com/tickopt2.htm. January 3, 2000.
102. Dumler JS, Bakken JS: Human ehrlichiosis: newly recognized infections transmitted by ticks, *Annu Rev Med* 49:201, 1998.
103. Klein MB, Nelson CM, Goodman JL: Antibiotic susceptibility of the newly cultivated agent of human granulocytic ehrlichiosis: promising activity of quinolones and rifamycins, *Antimicrob Agents Chemother* 41:76, 1997.
104. Meldrum SC et al: Human babesiosis in New York State: an epidemiological description of 136 cases, *Clin Infect Dis* 15:1019, 1992.
105. White DJ et al: Human babesiosis in New York State: review of 139 hospitalized cases and analysis of prognostic factors, *Arch Intern Med* 158:2149, 1998.
106. Krause PJ et al: Efficacy of immunoglobulin M serodiagnostic test for rapid diagnosis of acute babesiosis, *J Clin Microbiol* 34:2014, 1996.
107. Krause PJ et al: Concurrent Lyme disease and babesiosis: evidence for increased severity and duration of illness, *JAMA* 275:1657, 1996.
108. Emmons RW: Ecology of Colorado tick fever, *Annu Rev Microbiol* 42:49, 1988.
109. Bowen GS: Colorado tick fever. In Monath TP, editor: *The epidemiology of arthropod-borne viral diseases,* Boca Raton, Fla, 1988, CRC.
110. Calisher CH et al: Diagnosis of Colorado tick fever virus infection by enzyme immunoassays for immunoglobulin M and G antibodies, *J Clin Microbiol* 22:84, 1985.
111. Hovell WH: Journal kept on the journey from Lake George to Port Phillip, 1824-1825, *R Aust Hist Soc* 7:358, 1921.
112. Gothe R, Kunze K, Hoogstraal H: The mechanisms of pathogenicity in the tick paralyses, *J Med Entomol* 16:357, 1979.
113. Abramowicz M, editor: Insect repellents, *Med Lett* 31:45, 1989.

129 Tuberculosis

Dennis Chan

PERSPECTIVE

History and Epidemiology

Tuberculosis (TB) has plagued humankind throughout recorded history. Archaeologic excavations and medical anthropologic studies document the presence of TB in ancient civilizations. Clear evidence of tuberculous lesions of bone have been found in Egyptian mummified human remains that date to 3400 BC.[1] The presence of TB has been microscopically confirmed in the mummies of small children, one from the dynastic period of Egyptian history and one from pre-Columbian southern Peru around 700 AD.[1-3]

Hippocrates (460-370 BC) is credited for providing the first accurate clinical description of TB. He coined the term *phthisis* (to melt and to waste away) to describe the wasting character of the disease, which was also associated with fever and incurable lung ulcerations.[4] Aristotle (384-322 BC) accurately described the contagious nature of the disease, noticing that the phthisis-stricken patient had a "pernicious air" and that "one takes the disease because there is in this air something that is disease-producing to others in the proximity."[5]

TB did not become a major public health problem until the Industrial Revolution. The urbanization of European cities led to overcrowding, widespread poverty, and poor hygienic conditions that were ideal for the epidemic spread of the disease throughout western Europe from the early 1600s through the 1800s.[6] Approximately 25% of all adult deaths in Europe were caused by TB during this period, and in 1861 Oliver Wendell Holmes named it "the white plague."[1] TB gradually became a global epidemic as Europeans colonized North America and explored and colonized other parts of the world.[6] This TB epidemic peaked in western Europe in the early 1800s and by 1900 had peaked in the Americas. Globally, the disease still has not reached a peak in some developing countries in Africa and Asia.[7]

Laennec, who invented the stethoscope in 1816, accurately described the evolution of TB from the small initial tubercle through all of its pathologic manifestations in 1819.[4] Twenty years later, Schöenlein, also recognizing the tubercle as the fundamental anatomic lesion, named the disease tuberculosis.[8] Koch identified the tubercle bacillus in 1882, and Roentgen's subsequent discovery of x-rays in 1895 greatly improved the ability to promptly diagnose TB.[1,4]

The TB epidemic provided fertile ground for quackery. Treatment of TB has progressed from homemade concoctions, the royal touch of a king, bleeding, purging, sweating, and poultices to sanatoriums, artificial pneumothorax, other surgical intervention, and finally modern chemotherapy.[1]

In 1892, Biggs instituted a comprehensive program of TB control in New York City that included public education, systemic surveillance, isolation of patients, nursing follow-up, improved sanitation, and free sputum testing.[8,9] These types of programs and the subsequent introduction of the antituberculous drugs led to an impressive decline in the incidence of TB throughout the twentieth century. Between 1953 and 1985, TB cases decreased by an average of 5.8% per year.[10] As recently as the 1970s, U.S. health officials believed that TB was well under control and could soon be eradicated.[11] Unfortunately, as the incidence and perceived importance of the disease decreased, so did the public health programs to control it.[12] The premature decline in government support for TB control programs made it impossible to appropriately manage the disease. The decline of the infrastructure dedicated to TB control combined with other events during the late 1980s and early 1990s (the human immunodeficiency virus/acquired immunodeficiency syndrome [HIV/AIDS] epidemic, increasing immigration from countries with high TB prevalence, increasing occurrence of TB in institutional living settings, escalating poverty, substance abuse, homelessness, and urban overcrowding) led to a resurgence of TB in the United States from 1986 through 1992 and contributed to the emergence of drug-resistant strains of *Mycobacterium tuberculosis* (MTB).[12]

Worldwide, the disease had become so widespread that in 1993 the World Health Organization (WHO) declared TB a global emergency. TB is still the world's leading single infectious cause of death. One third of the world's population has been infected by TB, and each year more than 8 million people develop active TB and nearly 3 million die.[13]

Elderly people who currently harbor dormant infection that reactivates are the main reservoir of MTB in the United States.[14] Debilitating disease or immunosenescence may predispose to reactivation. Thus, nursing homes are particularly vulnerable to TB outbreaks because reactivation disease in remotely infected individuals may be followed by epidemic spread among the many susceptible hosts living in close quarters.

Immigration from endemic countries is another factor. The largest numbers of people with TB originate from Mexico, the Philippines, and Vietnam.[12] Homelessness has also contributed to the spread of TB in major urban centers. Homelessness is often associated with conditions that decrease resistance to TB, such as malnutrition, alcoholism, or substance abuse. MTB infection in the homeless population may quickly progress to active TB.[15] Last, the HIV epidemic has had the greatest impact on the reemergence of TB in the United States.[16] The pandemic of HIV-related TB has led to an increase in TB cases among non-HIV-infected people owing to the greater numbers of source cases in the community.[13] The rate of TB disease among patients who are HIV-infected and TB-skin-test positive is approximately 200 to 800 times higher than the rate of TB estimated for the US population overall.[17]

The reemergence of TB has also affected children. Between 1962 and the mid-1980s, the rates of childhood TB in the United States decreased an average of 6% a year.[18,19] This trend has reversed along with the young urban adult trend, and the number of cases reported in children 4 years of age or younger increased 36% from 1985 through 1992.[10] This increase reflected an ongoing transmission of TB in the community because TB in young children must result from recent infection.[10]

After a 32-year decline, the number of TB cases in the United States increased 20% between 1986 and 1992. By 1992, roughly 14% more cases (26,673) were reported over the 1985 nadir. This trend, however, reversed in 1993, largely owing to the mobilization of new federal resources provided to the states for TB control and prevention.[12] The number of reported cases during 1996 decreased in each age group as well as all ethnic groups[20]; 1997 marked the fifth consecutive year of decline and the lowest number of TB cases and case rate ever reported in the United States.[12] Investigators from New York City reported a 21% decrease in cases after fortifying the TB control bureau, showing that effective public health programs help control TB even in an area where immunosuppression and nonadherence to therapy are common.[9] Although the rapid resurgence of TB appears to be subsiding in the United States, there is no justification for complacency. Rates of newly diagnosed TB are still significant in different regions of the country and in certain demographic groups.[21]

The populations most likely to develop and transmit TB commonly are seen by emergency physicians who will necessarily play a key role in identification, prevention, and treatment.

Etiology

Tuberculosis in humans is caused by one of the following three pathogenic mycobacteria: *M. bovis, M. africanum,* or *M. tuberculosis. M. bovis* is transmitted by drinking milk from diseased cows, but since pasteurization, it has become a relatively rare cause of TB. *M. africanum* is also a rare cause of human TB and has been documented only in Africa.[22] Worldwide, MTB remains the major causative agent.

Humans are the sole known reservoir for MTB. This pathogen is a primarily intracellular, aerobic, nonmotile, non-spore-forming bacillus with a waxy lipid coat.[22] This coat makes MTB resistant to decolorization with acid alcohol after staining, and thus the term *acid-fast bacillus* (AFB). MTB grows slowly. Its generation time is 15 to 20 hours compared with 20 minutes for some common bacteria; cultures take 4 to 6 weeks to grow on standard media.[22,23]

MTB produces neither endotoxins nor exotoxins. Its cell components are immunoreactive; some are immunosuppressive, and others lead to granuloma formation, macrophage activation, host toxicity, and modification of the immune response.[24]

PRINCIPLES OF DISEASE

Transmission

TB is transmitted primarily via the respiratory route, although other routes, such as direct inoculation, occur primarily among health care workers. Patients with active disease expel MTB in liquid droplets during coughing, sneezing, and vocalizing. The droplets rapidly evaporate and the desiccated bacilli circulate airborne for prolonged periods. These infective particles, or droplet nuclei, measure 1 to 5 μm in diameter, contain one to three tubercle bacilli, and can travel to the distal alveoli.

The susceptible host may become infected when only a few of these droplet nuclei are inhaled. Fomites are not important in the transmission of the disease, so patients' rooms, eating utensils, and bed clothes do not require special decontamination procedures.[22] Because the infectious droplet nuclei are airborne, exchanging contaminated air is the most important environmental control. In addition, MTB is susceptible to ultraviolet radiation, and transmission rarely occurs outdoors because of the dilution of infectious particles and possible exposure to ultraviolet radiation.[25]

The risk for TB transmission increases when source patients have airway and cavitary disease. Infectivity correlates with the number of organisms seen on sputum smear, the extent of pulmonary disease, and the frequency of cough.[22] After institution of proper chemotherapy (three or four drugs) for 2 weeks, patients with initially AFB-negative sputum smears can be considered noncontagious. However, after 2 weeks of treatment, patients who were initially smear-positive may still have viable MTB detectable in their posttreatment sputum cultures, and patients with extensive disease may still have AFB detectable on their posttreatment sputum smears. These latter two groups should still be considered contagious.[26] There is currently no clear epidemiologic evidence to better define the contagiousness of patients after they are started on effective therapy.[26]

Extrapulmonary tuberculosis may also be infectious. Transmission of MTB to health care workers caring for a patient with a draining tuberculous abscess is reported. Irrigation of the abscess may aerosolize the bacilli forming infectious droplet nuclei.[27]

Pathogenesis

Once infectious droplet nuclei are inhaled, the airflow through the bronchial tree tends to deposit them in the midlung zone on the respiratory surface of the alveoli.[22] This launches a complex series of immunologic events. Dannenberg[28] has organized the complex pathogenesis of TB into four stages.

Stage 1 The first stage begins when an alveolar macrophage phagocytoses the recently inhaled bacillus. A macrophage from a resistant host can immediately destroy a less virulent bacillus. In these cases, no tuberculous infection develops and the process ends. If a virulent bacillus can overcome a macrophage's microbicidal capability, the infection may progress to the next stage.

Stage 2 When the alveolar macrophage is unable to destroy the inhaled tubercle bacilli, the bacilli replicate until the macrophage lyses. Circulating monocytes are attracted to this site of infection by the released bacilli, cellular debris, and various chemotactic factors. The monocytes differentiate into macrophages and ingest the free bacilli. Initially, these new macrophages are not activated and cannot destroy or inhibit the mycobacteria. The bacilli grow logarithmically within macrophages and accumulate at the primary focus of infection, now called a tubercle.[29] The infected macrophages may also be transported via lymphatics to regional lymph nodes and from there they can access the bloodstream and spread.

During this lymphohematogenous dissemination, the pathogens tend to distribute preferentially to lymph nodes, kidney, epiphyses of long bones, vertebral bodies, meningeal areas, and the apical posterior areas of the lungs.[22] These sites may be favored because of a high oxygen tension.[30] Others believe that the lung apices are favored because of impaired clearance mechanisms from poor lymph flow.[31]

Stage 3 The third stage of TB begins 2 to 3 weeks after the initial infection, with development of the immune response that terminates the unimpeded growth of MTB.[28] Cell-mediated immunity (CMI) occurs via CD4 helper T cells.[32] When the T cell encounters mycobacterial antigens, it is activated and produces an expanded population of specific T cells. These T cells secrete cytokines (e.g., interferon-γ, tumor necrosis factor) that attract and activate monocyte/macrophages. Once activated, the macrophages, containing previously ingested mycobacteria and their progeny, kill the bacilli. The destruction of the mycobacteria is associated with the formation of epithelioid cell granulomas and clearance of the organisms.[29]

Delayed-type hypersensitivity (DTH) is mediated by cytotoxic CD8 suppressor T cells.[32] The cytotoxic cells kill nonactivated macrophages laden with mycobacteria and thus cause local tissue destruction as well. DTH results in the formation of caseating necrotic granulomas. This stops bacillary growth; mycobacteria, now extracellular, cannot multiply in this acidic, anoxic, extracellular environment.[29] Tubercle bacilli can survive, dormant, in this solid caseous material for years.[29] The host's resistance determines whether the disease remains dormant or immediately progresses to active disease.

In the immunocompetent host with strong CMI, the primary lesion is effectively walled off by epithelioid cells. Eventually, the caseous center inspissates, and the disease is arrested, often for a lifetime.[28] Similarly, at sites of lymphohematogenous spread, the mycobacteria are quickly destroyed with little caseous necrosis by a rapid CMI response.[28] The rapid destruction of the mycobacteria by CMI terminates the infectious process, and the only evidence of the infection will be the conversion to a positive tuberculin (PPD) skin test.[22]

This sequence of events from stage 1 to stage 3 represents the pathogenesis of primary TB in the immunocompetent patient.[32] In most cases, primary TB is subclinical and self-limited. In the immunocompromised host, however, clinically active primary disease may develop rapidly after the initial MTB infection.

The less resistant host with weak CMI relies more on DTH to control the infection. The primary lesion is surrounded by nonactivated macrophages, so it is not effectively walled off, and the caseous center expands, compromising more lung tissue.[30] If these patients eventually contain the infection, it may also go unnoticed and be evident only radiographically as healed parenchymal calcifications of the primary or Ghon focus and of the regional lymph nodes.[22] If host defenses are unable to contain the primary infection, however, as can occur in infants and immunosuppressed adults, the primary focus may become an area of advancing pneumonia.[22] This process is called primary progressive TB. In addition, this host may be unable to control the infection at the sites of lymphohematogenous spread and may form multiple uncontrolled caseous tubercles and develop disseminated TB.[29] HIV-infected patients are particularly susceptible to primary progressive TB because HIV specifically targets CD4+ cells and macrophages.

Stage 4 The final stage usually occurs months to decades after an apparent recovery from the initial infection. TB may progress to stage 4 even when residing in immunocompetent hosts. Usually host factors lead to decreased resistance and reactivation of dormant foci of MTB. The progression is due to liquefaction and cavity formation.

The liquefied tubercle serves as an excellent growth medium for the mycobacteria. The large numbers of extracellular bacilli stimulate DTH that secondarily causes local damage. The tubercle eventually erodes through the bronchial wall and drains its contents, forming a cavity. The liquefied caseous material, teeming with mycobacteria, enters other parts of the lung and the outside environment. The spilling of this liquefied material within the lung may produce a caseous bronchopneumonia.[29]

The cavity formed at the site of the initial focus remains a significant lesion. Cavities provide optimal conditions for mycobacterial growth. The oxygen tension is increased, and the host's defenses are ineffective at interrupting the multiplication of the mycobacteria within a cavity.[29]

CLINICAL FEATURES

The initial infection with MTB is most often asymptomatic in healthy individuals. Mild fever and malaise may develop in association with the immune response at 4 to 6 weeks, but generally the primary infection is clinically insignificant.[33] Conversion to a positive PPD skin test may be the only means of diagnosing the infection. Clinically active TB will develop in 8% to 10% of otherwise healthy PPD converters who do not take prophylactic agents, 3% to 5% in the first 2 years (acute primary TB), and another 5% during the remainder of life (reactivation TB).[16] In contrast, persons also infected with HIV will proceed to acute primary TB at a rate of 37% within 6 months, and then will develop active TB at a rate of 7% to 10% per year.[16]

Reactivation of dormant foci is responsible for the major clinical manifestations of TB.[33] Exogenous reinfection of patients with well-documented prior TB infection causes clinical disease indistinguishable from reactivation TB.[34] Because it may be incorrect to label all late-onset cases as reactivation disease, *postprimary TB* is the preferred term. Postprimary TB is active or chronic disease in a patient previously infected. In the United States and other developed countries, reactivation is thought to be the primary mechanism of postprimary TB. Exogenous reinfection has played a role where contagion levels are high, as in outbreaks of TB and in developing countries.[34]

Patient History

History of Present Illness Clinically significant pulmonary TB is often indolent, and symptoms are absent or minimal until the disease advances. The patient may also have a systemic reaction to the infection. This systemic reaction, thought to be mediated by cytokines, especially tumor necrosis factor-α, causes the constitutional symptoms of anorexia, weight loss, fatigue, irritability, malaise, weakness, headache, chills, and most commonly, fever.[33,35] The fever usually develops in the afternoon, and the patient defervesces while sleeping, which causes the classic night sweats.[33]

Cough is the most common symptom of pulmonary TB. Initially it may be nonproductive, but as caseation necrosis and liquefaction develop, mucopurulent and nonspecific sputum is usually produced.[22,33,35] Hemoptysis, caused by caseous sloughing or endobronchial erosion, is usually minor but often indicates extensive involvement.[22] Many asymptomatic patients present for care because they are alarmed by the hemoptysis.

Patients may also complain of pleuritic chest pain, which is caused by parenchymal inflammation adjacent to the pleural surface. Dyspnea with chest pain may indicate a spontaneous pneumothorax.[36] Shortness of breath from parenchymal lung involvement is unusual, however, and if present, indicates extensive parenchymal disease or tracheobronchial obstruction.[33] Table 129-1 shows the frequency of symptoms found in one study of patients with culture-proven pulmonary TB.[37]

Any vague systemic disorder or fever of unknown etiology may be TB.[16] Atypical presentations are particularly common in infants, the elderly, and immunocompromised persons.

Infants and young children tend to develop large hilar lymph nodes, which may compress a bronchus leading to atelectasis and possibly obstructive pneumonia; they may have a "brassy cough." A node may also erode through the bronchial wall causing symptomatic endobronchial disease and allowing endobronchial spread of tuberculous pneumonia to other areas of the lungs.[22]

In contrast, fewer elderly people tend to present with respiratory symptoms. The diagnosis may be masked by coexistent diseases and nonspecific presenting symptoms.[38] Pulmonary TB should be considered in elderly people with a chronic cough and failure to thrive.[14]

Clinical manifestations of TB in patients coinfected with HIV are even more subtle and nonspecific, especially because these patients are vulnerable to opportunistic infections and neoplasms that can cause the same constitutional symptoms as TB. There is a synergy between the two infections (MTB and HIV) that leads to a greatly increased viral load.[13] Active TB with HIV coinfection has been associated with an increased risk for opportunistic infections and death.[17] Patients with advanced HIV infection also commonly have extrapulmonary involvement (30%) as well as combined pulmonary and extrapulmonary TB (32%).[35]

Risk Factors All patients in the ED who have been coughing should be screened for the presence of TB risk factors (Box 129-1).[39]

Table 129-1. Frequency of Symptoms in Pulmonary TB

Symptom	# with symptom	# Evaluated	Percentage with symptom
Cough	144	185	78
Weight loss	134	181	74
Fatigue	112	165	68
Tactile fever	109	183	60
Night sweats	98	177	55
Chills	92	180	51
Anorexia	76	167	46
Chest pain	71	179	40
Dyspnea	64	173	37
Hemoptysis	51	181	28
No respiratory symptoms	13	186	7
None of above symptoms	9	187	5

From Barnes et al: *Chest* 94:316, 1988.

Risks for acquiring TB may also be stratified by age. Infants and toddlers have poorly developed CMI, so they have a much higher incidence of TB than adults. Children 5 to 10 years of age are relatively resistant to TB. Infants and toddlers commonly have extrapulmonary disease and acute lower and midlung bronchopneumonia that rarely progresses to cavitary disease. Young adults show the adult pattern of apical pulmonary disease, including cavity formation, suggesting reactivation. Because of decreased immunocompetence, the elderly tend to manifest the disease similar to young children.[22] Patients with a history of PPD conversion should be asked about the presence of medical conditions that would put them at risk for developing active postprimary disease via reactivation (Box 129-2).[39]

Patients with a history of active TB should be asked about all antituberculous medications taken or currently being taken and about their compliance. Failure to improve on an appropriate regimen after 2 months may signal nonadherence to therapy or the presence of a resistant strain.[40]

Box 129-1 TB Risk Factors

- Close contacts of known case
- Persons with HIV infection
- Foreign-born from Asia, Africa, Latin America
- Medically underserved, low-income populations
- Elderly persons
- Residents of long-term care facilities (nursing homes, correctional facilities)
- Injection drug users
- Groups identified locally (homeless, migrant farmworkers)
- Persons who have occupational exposure

From CDC: *TB care guide highlights from core curriculum on tuberculosis,* Atlanta, 1994, United States Department of Health and Human Services.

Box 129-2 Risk Factors for Developing Active TB in the Previously Infected

- HIV infection
- Recent TB infection (within past 2 years)
- Chest x-ray study suggestive of prior TB in a person not treated
- Injection drug use
- Diabetes mellitus
- Silicosis
- Prolonged corticosteroid therapy
- Immunosuppressive therapy
- Head or neck cancer
- Hematologic and reticuloendothelial diseases
- End-stage renal disease
- Intestinal bypass or gastrectomy
- Chronic malabsorption syndromes
- Low body weight (10% or more below the ideal)

Modified from CDC: *TB core highlights from core curriculum on tuberculosis,* Atlanta, 1994, United States Department of Health and Human Services.

Physical Findings

Examination of the chest is unlikely to establish the extent of disease. Over areas of infiltration, one may hear rales when the patient breathes in after a short cough (posttussive rales), and bronchial breath sounds may be present over areas of lung consolidation. Distant, hollow breath sounds that can be heard over cavities are called amphoric breath sounds.[22,33]

Erythema nodosum or phlyctenular keratoconjunctivitis (severe unilateral inflammation of an eye) may appear with the onset of tuberculin hypersensitivity. These self-limited, allergic manifestations are not common in the United States.[22] The patient's overall appearance and state of health may be the most useful indicators when evaluating for the potential presence of TB. General signs include pallor secondary to anemia, fever, and cachexia with weight loss.

Complications

Pneumothorax Spontaneous pneumothorax is not common (fewer than 5% of patients with severe cavitary disease) but may occur when a tuberculous cavity ruptures and creates a bronchopleural fistula or when a bleb ruptures into the pleural space (Figure 129-1).[41] Delayed tube thoracostomy and suction result in progressive infection and fibrosis of the pleura that leads to trapping of the lung.[33]

Empyema TB patients with extensive, progressive parenchymal disease and cavitation may develop an empyema. Although rare (1% to 4%), empyema is more common late in the course of the disease in debilitated patients.[33] Rupture of a cavity into the pleural space is usually catastrophic and often associated with bronchopleural fistula formation. An untreated empyema can result in spontaneous pleurocutaneous fistula, a chest wall mass, or rib and vertebra destruction.[41]

Endobronchial Spread Endobronchial spread is the most common complication of cavitary disease. It manifests radiographically as 5- to 10-mm, poorly defined nodules clustered in dependent portions of the lungs. These nodules may rapidly coalesce into parenchymal consolidation, the so-called galloping consumption.[41]

Airway Tuberculosis When a cavity drains its highly infectious material into the bronchial tree, the airways not only spread the infection but also develop endobronchial TB. Bronchiectasis commonly complicates endobronchial TB. Bronchial stenosis may result from extensive damage caused by endobronchial TB or from direct extension of infection from tuberculous adenitis or from lymphatic dissemination to the airway.[22,41] Tuberculous bronchostenosis may appear radiographically as persistent segmental or lobar collapse, lobar hyperinflation, and obstructive pneumonia.[41]

Tracheal and laryngeal TB are less common than endobronchial TB. Laryngeal disease is the most infectious form of TB; it results from the proximal extension of lower airway disease, pooling of infected secretions in the posterior larynx, or hematogenous dissemination to the anterior larynx. Patients with laryngeal TB also usually have active pulmonary disease.[41]

Superinfection Extensive TB infection often heals with open cavities and areas of bronchiectasis.[33] Superinfection may occur with a wide variety of organisms, including *Aspergillus fumigatus*.[42] The characteristic finding on chest radiographs is the aspergilloma or "fungus ball" (Figure 129-2). Aspergillomas are particularly significant because they may cause massive and fatal hemoptysis.[33]

Hemoptysis Mild hemoptysis is a common complication of acute infection. TB is also a major cause of massive hemoptysis. The destroyed lung parenchyma does not support blood vessels that can rupture. Healing also stimulates the growth of fragile neovascularity.[43] A tuberculous lesion or cavity may erode into a pulmonary artery, leading to

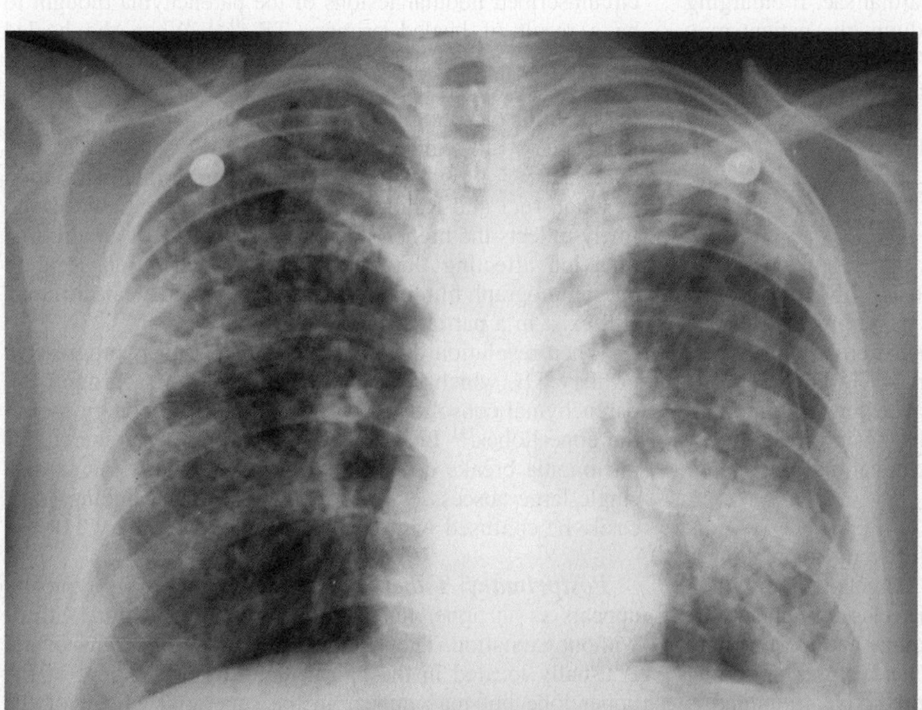

Figure 129-1. **Chest radiograph demonstrating cavitary TB with left-sided pneumothorax, later diagnosed as a bronchopleural fistula.** *Courtesy John Pearce, MD.*

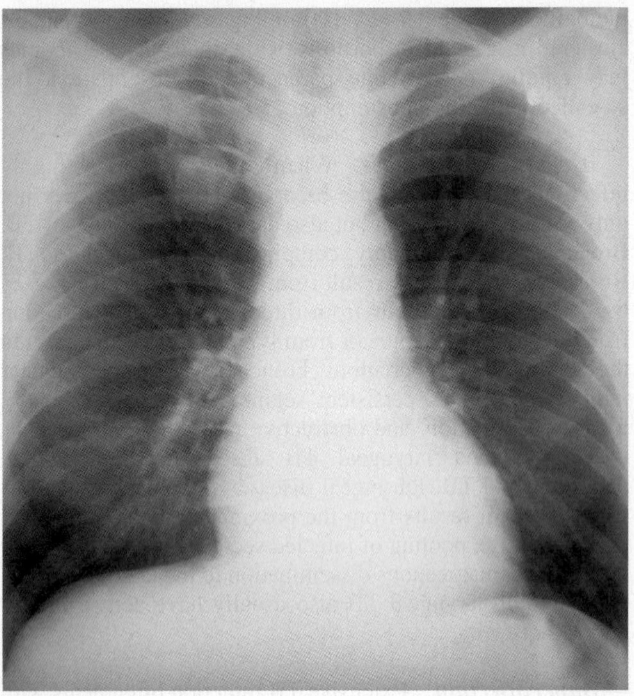

Figure 129-2. **Superinfection of healed tuberculous cavity. An aspergilloma can be seen in the right upper lung.** *Courtesy John Pearce, MD.*

pseudoaneurysm formation (Rasmussen aneurysm) and potentially fatal hemoptysis.[41] Alternatively, superinfection of cavities by invasive organisms or tumor development in scarred lung may erode bronchial or pulmonary vessels and cause major hemorrhage. These patients often require emergency surgical resection or selective embolization.[43]

Primary Tuberculous Pericarditis This complication results from the close anatomic relationship of the mediastinal lymph nodes to the posterior pericardial sac. If enlarging lymph nodes rupture into the pericardium, the patient may have acute pericardial tamponade.[44] Pericardial involvement may also be the result of the hematogenous spread secondary to acute miliary TB.[44] Emergency echocardiography reliably confirms the presence of pericardial fluid.[45]

DIAGNOSTIC STRATEGIES

Laboratory Tests

Routine laboratory studies generally are not useful in suggesting or establishing the diagnosis.[33] Normochromic normocytic anemia, elevated erythrocyte sedimentation rate (ESR) and serum globulin level, hyponatremia, and hypercalcemia can all occur in active pulmonary TB, but these tests are nonspecific.[33,42,46] Tuberculin skin testing is important epidemiologically as a modality for diagnosing MTB infection but is a poor indicator of active clinical disease.[42]

Diagnostic Imaging

The chest radiograph is the most useful study for making a presumptive diagnosis of pulmonary TB. Chest radiograph abnormalities are not limited to the classic upper lobe cavitary infiltrates. Primary TB infection and postprimary disease each have distinctive radiographic features. A normal chest radiograph has a high negative predictive value and is therefore useful in screening ED patients for active pulmonary TB. However, the false-negative rate is approximately 1% in immunocompetent adults and increases to 7% to 15% in HIV-positive patients.[20] Therefore, depending on the clinical circumstances, a normal chest radiograph does not always exclude active TB, especially in patients with endobronchial disease and HIV infection.

Primary Tuberculosis The increasing incidence of primary disease in adults has made the diagnosis of active pulmonary TB difficult. As reported in two separate series, chest radiograph manifestations of primary disease in adults are often not recognized as TB.[47,48]

Primary tuberculous infiltrates can occur in any lobe.[31,41,44,49] For any age group, a pneumonic infiltrate with enlarged hilar or mediastinal nodes should strongly suggest the diagnosis.[44] The infiltrate is usually homogenous and most commonly involves a single lobe. Thus, primary TB may appear radiographically identical to a bacterial pneumonia, with the associated lymphadenopathy, if present, being the only distinguishing feature.

Lymphadenopathy is considered the radiologic hallmark of primary TB in children, but it seen less commonly in adults.[20,31,49] When present, adenopathy is usually unilateral and associated with parenchymal infiltrate (Figure 129-3). It may occur bilaterally or, more rarely, may be an isolated finding on chest radiograph.[33] Massive hilar adenopathy is more common in young children. As a result, atelectasis, resulting from airway compression by adjacent enlarged nodes, is a likely finding in children less than 2 years old but is less common in older children and adults.[41]

Other primary TB chest radiograph findings include a moderate to large pleural effusion, often an isolated finding and prevalence increases with age; miliary TB (innumerable, 1 to 3 mm noncalcified nodules dispersed throughout both lungs with mild basilar predominance), which is mainly a threat to children less than 2 years old, immunocompromised patients, and elderly patients; and tuberculomas, well-circumscribed nodular lesions of the parenchyma thought to be a result of healed primary TB.[20,41] When the healed primary focus is visible on chest radiograph as a calcified scar, it is known as the Ghon focus. Calcified secondary foci of infection are known as Simon foci. A Ghon focus associated with calcified hilar nodes is called a Ranke complex.[22,41] A right-sided predominance in the distribution of Ghon foci and Ranke complexes is well recognized and likely reflects the higher statistical probability of an airborne infection affecting the right lung.[20] Calcification seen on chest radiograph film indicates healing, but viable bacilli may still exist in a partially calcified lesion.[44]

When resolution does not occur, the result is progressive primary TB, which radiographically appears as progressive parenchymal consolidation often including secondary foci in the upper lobes.[41] In some patients the primary tuberculous pneumonia breaks down into multiple cavitary lesions or a single large abscess.[44] These chest radiograph findings may easily be confused with the findings in postprimary TB.

Postprimary Tuberculosis Postprimary TB typically appears as an upper lung infiltrate or consolidation with or without cavitation. The lesion may be small or extensive and is usually located in the apical or posterior segment of the upper lobe but may appear in the superior segment of the

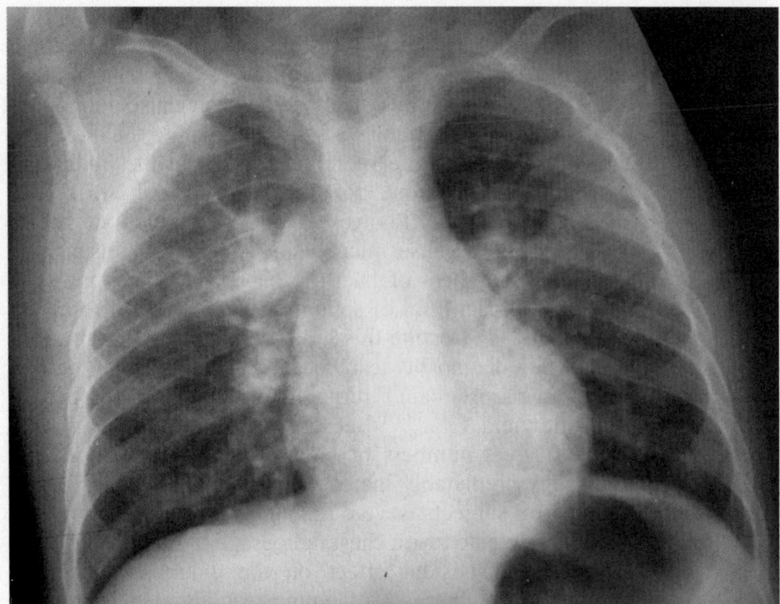

Figure 129-3. **Chest radiographic findings in a child with primary TB. Note active Ghon focus with associated hilar adenopathy, bilateral infiltrates.** ***Courtesy of John Pearce, MD.***

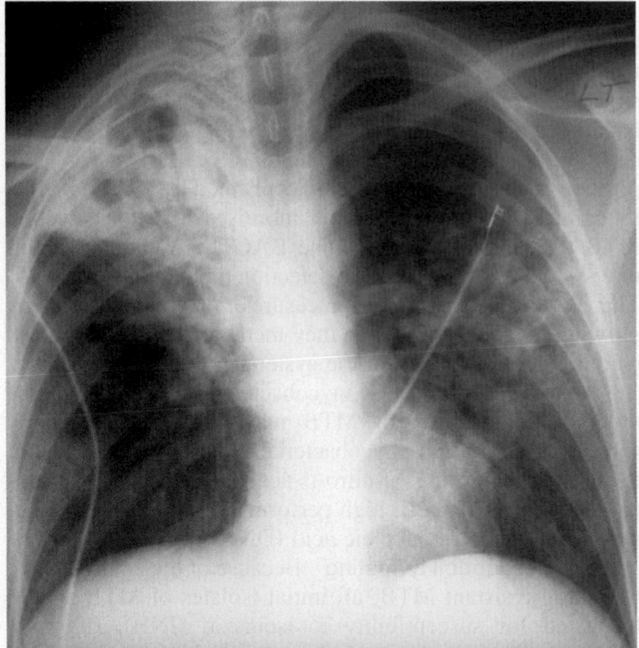

Figure 129-4. **Chest radiograph shows right upper lobe cavitary disease. Also note left-sided infiltrate secondary to endobronchial spread.**

lower lobe.[50] Postprimary disease can and does occur in the lower lung.[31]

In addition, bronchogenic spread can occur, leading to involvement of multiple lobes[50] (Figure 129-4). The patient with bilateral upper lobe disease is extremely likely to have TB.[44] The other important, recognizable characteristics of postprimary disease are fibrosis and cavitation.

The initial lesion of postprimary TB is a poorly defined, heterogenous alveolar opacity called an exudative lesion.[41] These lesions are not purely exudative in that they are associated with a fibrotic pattern of nodules and a few fine, linear densities. Unchecked, the infection may rapidly progress to lobar or complete lung opacification and destruction.[41] Postprimary TB, however, usually runs a chronic course characterized by reactive fibrosis, so in most cases the initial exudative lesions are gradually replaced by more well-defined reticular and nodular opacities or "fibroproductive" lesions.[41,44]

Fibroproductive lesions are often irregular and angular in contour, have strands extending toward the hilum, and have calcification of one or more nodules. This pattern is characteristic of granulomatous disease and is rarely found in other bacterial infections.[31] As fibrosis continues, there may be distortion of normal vascular and mediastinal structures secondary to contraction and shrinkage of the scar. Severe fibrosis with upper lobe volume loss eventually may lead to retraction of the interlobar fissure and upward displacement of the hilum.[44] The chest radiograph appearance at this stage has been variably referred to as "old scarring," "no active disease," or "fibrotic, apparently well-healed TB." Many of these patients have positive sputum, and infectivity cannot be accurately assessed by chest radiograph.[31,41,44] Only serial chest radiographs can reliably differentiate active from inactive disease. Lack of radiographic changes over a 4- to 6-month interval generally indicates "inactive" or more precisely, "radiographically" stable disease.[20]

Cavitation should alert the emergency physician to the high infectivity of the patient and the potential for associated complications such as bronchogenic spread of TB, when an area of caseous necrosis liquifies and communicates with the bronchial tree (see Figure 129-4). Cavities are usually multiple and range in size from a few millimeters to several centimeters in diameter.[41] The walls of the cavities initially are thick and rough, and they become thinner and smoother with healing (Figure 129-5). A hazy, parenchymal reaction around a cavity with an ill-defined wall strongly suggests an active lesion. Most cavities heal by obliteration and may leave a small linear or stellate scar; others remain patent and become thin-walled bullae.[44]

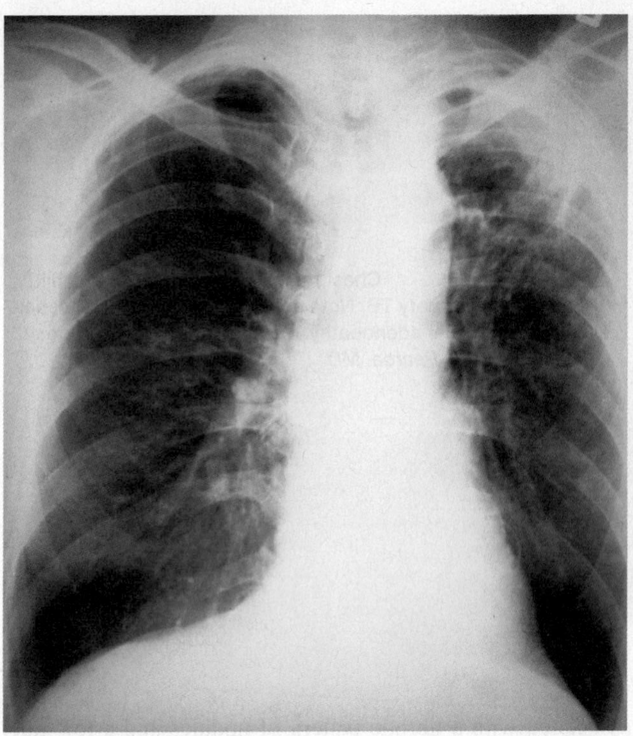

Figure 129-5. **A healed, thin-walled cavity is present in the left upper lobe of this chest film.** *Courtesy of John Pearce, MD.*

Although pulmonary TB usually induces chest radiograph changes, patients with sputum cultures positive for MTB may have normal chest films. In a series of 103 patients, 10 people (9.7%) with confirmed pulmonary TB had normal chest films.[48] Chest films may also be normal in patients with endobronchial TB.[36,51]

Normal chest films appear to be more common in patients with HIV infection.[52] The degree of immunocompromise may influence the incidence of normal films.[53] More commonly, HIV patients tend to demonstrate chest radiograph changes consistent with primary TB.[53] Postprimary changes are uncommon in HIV patients[52] and appear to occur more often in those with early HIV infection, while their cell-mediated immunity is still intact.[52] Severe immunosuppression has been reported to be associated with a miliary pattern of disease on chest radiograph.[20]

Microbiology

Sputum Studies If the clinical or chest radiograph findings suggest the diagnosis of pulmonary TB, the emergency physician should initiate mycobacteriologic studies of the patient's sputum. Spontaneously produced sputum collected under direct supervision is the ideal method of collection.[23] For patients who are not producing sputum, nebulizer induction of sputum and gastric aspiration of swallowed respiratory secretions are the methods of choice.[54] Nebulizer-induced sputums have a higher diagnostic yield than gastric aspirates in adult TB patients, but in some patients, especially children, gastric aspirates may be the only obtainable specimen.

When sputum is not diagnostic in adults, fiberoptic bronchoscopy with bronchial washings, brushings, and bronchoalveolar lavage, or transbronchial biopsy may be necessary to establish the laboratory diagnosis.[54]

Direct Microscopy Direct microscopic examination of a stained sputum specimen is the most rapid laboratory test widely available to support a presumptive diagnosis of TB.[55] Although nontuberculous mycobacteria can cause pulmonary disease, they are rare and vary by geographic location.[42,54] Fluorochrome stains are more sensitive than the traditional Ziehl-Neelson technique for the detection of AFB.[55] A negative AFB smear, however, does not rule out active pulmonary TB because microscopy is relatively insensitive when small numbers of bacilli are present. There must be about 10,000 bacilli/ml of sputum to get a positive result by microscopy.[56,57] Despite this limitation, microscopy remains an essential diagnostic test because of its ease of performance, low cost, rapid turnaround time, and reasonable diagnostic yield.[36,37,58-61] Because cavitary disease is associated with great numbers of bacilli, the diagnostic yield of microscopy predictably increases with cavitation.[37,62]

In control subjects, severe immunocompromise from HIV infection associated with chest radiograph findings of primary TB has no consistent effect on the diagnostic yield of microscopy.[63,64] In cases of pulmonary TB associated with profound immunosuppression from HIV, the unchecked proliferation of bacilli may increase the yield of microscopy more than the presence of cavitation.[54,65,66]

Classically three initial sputum specimens should be obtained to optimize the yield of microscopy.[37,56,59,63,67] The three specimens are obtained on different days.[23,67] A positive smear supports a presumptive diagnosis, and the number of bacilli seen correlates with infectivity.

Culture A presumptive diagnosis of TB based on a positive sputum smear is usually confirmed by isolating MTB by culture. Sputum cultures are more sensitive for detecting MTB than microscopy.[57,59] The BACTEC radiometric culture system has shortened the detection time to 7 to 14 days.[68] The BACTEC instrument measures $^{14}CO_2$ produced by growing mycobacteria when they metabolize the ^{14}C-labeled palmitic acid contained in the system.[69,70]

When the presence of mycobacteria is established, the specific identification of MTB may be accomplished by subjecting the initial mycobacterial isolate to a variety of tests, including the p-nitro-α-acetylamino-β-hydroxypropiophenone (NAP) test, high performance liquid chromatography, and deoxyribonucleic acid (DNA) probes.[68,71]

Drug Susceptibility Testing Because of the emergence of multidrug-resistant MTB, all initial isolates of MTB should be tested for susceptibility to isoniazid (INH), rifampin, streptomycin, ethambutol, and pyrazinamide (PZA).[16] Testing detects selective growth of drug-resistant TB on media containing these primary antituberculous drugs. The BACTEC system can also be used for drug susceptibility testing and is able to complete the tests on the primary drugs in 5 to 7 days, compared with 21 days for conventional testing.[55]

Rapid Diagnostic Tests Recent advances such as the BACTEC system and DNA probes have greatly decreased the time needed to confirm a clinical diagnosis of TB. The identification of MTB, however, still requires 10 to 20 days. All methods for rapid detection of MTB depend on growth of the organism in culture.[69] The development of rapid diagnostic tests may soon use clinical samples to confirm the diagnosis of TB.

Polymerase chain reaction The polymerase chain reaction (PCR) may provide a method for confirming the diagnosis of TB within a few hours. The PCR is a DNA amplification technique that bypasses the delays inherent with mycobacterial cultures. It allows the in vitro synthesis of millions of copies of a specific MTB DNA segment.[70] The PCR amplifies the targeted DNA so that it can be detected by simple laboratory procedures. Diagnostic techniques based on PCR allow direct testing of routine clinical specimens to confirm the diagnosis of TB in hours. Although numerous studies document PCR's ability to detect MTB in clinical samples with a high degree of sensitivity, several technical problems can be encountered with the PCR assay.[72,73] These problems are being resolved but have delayed the approval of PCR for routine clinical use.[72,74-79]

Mycobacterium tuberculosis *direct test* The *Mycobacterium tuberculosis* direct test (MTDT) enzymatically amplifies a 16s ribsomal RNA (rRNA) segment that is specific for MTB complex species. One of its advantages is that there are 2,000 rRNA targets per mycobacterial cell, whereas the PCR assay has only 10 to 16 DNA targets. The amplified product is then identified by hybridization with an acridinium ester-labeled DNA probe. The MTDT has shown excellent sensitivity (75% to 100%) and specificity (95% to 100%) for the rapid identification of MTB in patients who have positive sputum smears for AFB, and results are available in 1 day. Further prospective evaluation is recommended to better define the clinical utility of the MTDT.[80]

Tuberculostearic acid Tuberculostearic acid (TSA) is a fatty acid found only in mycobacteria. It can be detected in clinical specimens containing small numbers of bacilli with gas chromatography/mass spectrometry. Detecting TSA in cerebrospinal fluid (CSF) is the best approach to the rapid diagnosis of tuberculous meningitis, but the equipment and expertise needed to run this test are not widely available outside of specialized research laboratories.[61]

Detection of adenosine deaminase activity Adenosine deaminase (ADA) is released by lymphocytes and macrophages during the cellular immune response. Increased ADA levels can be used as a diagnostic test for tuberculous pleural effusions. The ADA determination is rapid and inexpensive, but because it is relatively nonspecific, it is most useful in populations with a relatively high prevalence of TB.[70,71]

Serology Serodiagnosis of TB could be a minimally invasive approach to rapid diagnosis. Using enzyme-linked immunosorbent assay to diagnose TB from serum may have similar value to direct sputum microscopy.[61] Although this method may be useful in patients who cannot produce sputum, in practice, no serodiagnostic approach to the diagnosis of TB is currently of widespread clinical utility in the United States.[81]

Tuberculin Skin Test While newer diagnostic tests undergo development, the tuberculin skin test remains the only tool available for detecting latent MTB infection.

The tuberculin test is based on the principle that MTB infection induces sensitivity to certain antigens of the bacillus.[82] These antigens are contained in the tuberculin preparation called purified protein derivative (PPD). The individual infected with TB usually turns PPD positive 3 to 8 weeks after the infection, when the immune response is developed.[22]

The standard 0.1-ml dose used in skin testing contains 0.0001 mg of PPD or 5 tuberculin units (TU). This dose is administered intradermally with the needle bevel up, using Mantoux's technique. The properly placed test should leave a blanched, distinct wheal 6 to 10 mm in diameter. An incorrectly administered test may be repeated immediately at a site several centimeters away.[82] Various types of test kits and applicators are available (Heaf and Tine tests), but for diagnostic purposes, the Mantoux test with PPD (5 TU) is superior.[67]

Tests are read 48 to 72 hours after administration. The largest diameter of palpable induration is measured and recorded in millimeters; erythema by itself is not measured. The precise measurement that denotes a positive test depends on the patient's other clinical factors. The current Centers for Disease Control and Prevention (CDC) guidelines use 15 mm of induration as a positive test for people without TB risk factors (Box 129-3).[83]

Some individuals with prior TB infection gradually lose their hypersensitivity reaction to PPD and may react weakly

Box 129-3 Summary of Interpretation of PPD Results

1. An induration of ≥5 mm is classified as positive in:
   - Persons with HIV infection or HIV risk factors but unknown HIV status
   - Close contacts (household, social, unprotected occupational exposure) of persons who have active TB
   - Persons who have fibrotic changes on chest x-ray film (appearance of healed TB)
2. An induration of ≥10 mm is positive in all persons who do not meet any of the above criteria but who have the following risks for TB:

   High-risk groups:
   - Injection drug users known to be seronegative
   - Persons with other medical conditions that may increase the risk for progressing from dormant infection to active TB (e.g., silicosis; gastrectomy or jejunoileal bypass; being ≥10% below ideal body weight; chronic renal failure with dialysis; diabetes mellitus; corticosteroid or immunosuppressive therapy; some hematologic disorders, including malignancies such as leukemias and lymphomas)
   - Children <4 years of age

   High prevalence groups:
   - Persons born in high TB prevalence countries (e.g., Asia, Africa, the Caribbean, and Latin America)
   - Persons from medically underserved, low-income populations
   - Residents of long-term care facilities (e.g., prisons, nursing homes)
   - Persons from high-risk populations in their communities, as determined by local public health authorities
3. An induration of ≥15 mm is classified as positive in persons who do not meet any of the above criteria.
4. Recent converters are defined on the basis of size of induration and age of the person being tested:
   - ≥10 mm increase within a 2-year period is classified as a recent conversion for persons <35 years of age
   - ≥15 mm increase within a 2-year period is classified as a recent conversion for persons ≥35 years of age
5. PPD skin test results in health care workers
   - Generally, the recommendations in sections 1, 2 and 3 of this box should be followed when interpreting skin test results in health care workers. However, the prevalence of TB in the facility should he considered when choosing the appropriate cut-point for defining a positive PPD reaction.

Modified from CDC: *Morb Mortal Wkly Rep* 43 (RR-13):59, 1994.

Box 129-4 Factors Causing Decreased Ability to Respond to Tuberculin

Factors Related to the Person Being Tested

Infections
- Viral (measles, mumps, chickenpox)
- Bacterial (typhoid fever, brucellosis, typhus, leprosy, pertussis, overwhelming tuberculosis, tuberculosis pleurisy)
- Fungal (South American blastomycosis)

Live virus vaccinations (measles, mumps, polio)
Metabolic derangements (chronic renal failure)
Nutritional factors (severe protein depletion)
Diseases affecting lymphoid organs (Hodgkin's disease, lymphoma, chronic lymphocytic leukemia, sarcoidosis)
Drugs (corticosteroids and many other immunosuppressive agents)
Age (newborns, elderly patients with "wanes" sensitivity)
Recent or overwhelming infection with *M. tuberculosis*
Stress (surgery, burns, mental illness, graft versus host reactions)

Factors Related to the Tuberculin Used

Improper storage (exposure to light and heat)
Improper dilutions
Chemical denaturation
Contamination
Adsorption (partially controlled by adding Tween 80)

Factors Related to the Method of Administration

Injection of too little antigen
Delayed administration after drawing into syringe
Injection too close

Factors Related to Reading the Test and Recording Results

Inexperienced reader
Conscious or unconscious bias
Error in recording

Box 129-5 Persons in Whom Tuberculin Testing is Needed

1. Persons with signs (e.g., radiographic abnormality) or symptoms (e.g., cough, hemoptysis, weight loss) suggestive of current tuberculosis disease
2. Recent contacts with known tuberculosis cases or persons suspected of having tuberculosis
3. Persons with abnormal chest roentgenograms compatible with past tuberculosis
4. Persons with medical conditions that increase the risk of tuberculosis (e.g., silicosis, gastrectomy, diabetes, immunosuppressive therapy, lymphomas)
5. Persons with HIV infection
6. Groups at high risk of recent infection with *M. tuberculosis,* such as immigrants from Asia, Africa, Latin America, and Oceania; some inner-city and skid row populations; personnel and long-term residents in some hospitals, nursing homes, mental institutions, and prisons

or not at all. The PPD test, however, can restimulate or enhance their hypersensitivity so that a subsequent test does elicit a positive reaction. This phenomenon is called the booster effect. This boosted reaction may be mistaken for a new infection. To eliminate the booster effect as a confounding factor, a two-step testing method is recommended for persons who undergo serial PPD screening (health care workers). If the result of the first test is negative and the individual does not have a documented negative PPD during the prior 12 months, a second test is done 1 week later using the same dose. If the second test is positive, it is most likely a boosted reaction and the person should be considered previously infected. If the second test result remains negative, the person is considered uninfected and a positive reaction to a subsequent test indicates new infection.[83]

Infection with nontuberculous mycobacteria may cause a false-positive result. False-positive reactions tend to be smaller than the true-positive reaction to MTB infection.[82] Similarly, Bacille Calmette-Guerin (BCG) vaccination may produce a PPD reaction that is generally mild and deteriorates with time. Age at the time of vaccination may be the most important factor determining the subsequent reaction to PPD.[84] Generally, a large reaction to PPD and a long time interval between BCG vaccination and the current skin test make it more likely that the reaction is due to MTB infection.[83]

Many conditions can lead to false-negative reactions to PPD testing (Box 129-4). The incidence of false-negative results in one study was 25% of the 200 patients with active TB.[22] Therefore the clinical significance of a negative PPD is best determined by examining other clinical factors.

Despite some limitations,[85] PPD skin testing remains useful to diagnose individuals, to screen populations, and to evaluate infected persons for prophylactic treatment (Box 129-5).

DIFFERENTIAL CONSIDERATIONS

Pulmonary Tuberculosis

Bacterial Pneumonia A chest radiograph film appearance of segmental or lobar infiltrates in bacterial pneumonia may easily be confused with TB, especially primary disease. Clinically, however, bacterial pneumonias usually present with more profound symptoms of systemic toxicity and symptoms of shorter duration than TB.[42] The white blood cell (WBC) count is often normal in pulmonary TB and there is no prompt response to antibiotics.[77]

Fungal and Nontuberculous
Mycobacterial Infections Histoplasmosis, coccidioidomycosis, and blastomycosis, as well as nontuberculous mycobacterial infections (NMTB) (mainly *M. kansasii* and *M. avium* complex), may be radiologically indistinguishable from TB.[86] The incidence of these infections depends on geographic location.[42,87] NTMB most commonly infects white men in their sixties and seventies who have underlying lung disease; however, during the last decade *M. avium complex* has become an important pathogen in HIV patients.[86,87]

Pneumonias in Patients with HIV Bacterial pneumonias, upper lobe *Pneumocystis carinii* pneumonia (PCP), which can occur in patients taking chronic aerosolized pentamidine, and, rarely, nocardia and rhodococcus infections may mimic TB.[46]

Cavitary Lesions Lung abscess or cavitating pneumonia caused by *Klebsiella pneumoniae, Staphylococcus pyogenes,* or aspiration may appear similar to cavitary TB on chest radiograph.[42] In older patients, especially smokers, bronchogenic carcinoma may mimic TB; this is particularly true of squamous cell carcinoma that tends to cavitate.[42] Because cancer may cause a focus of TB to spread, the two diseases may be present simultaneously.[33]

Other causes of nontuberculous cavitary lesions include pulmonary infarction secondary to pulmonary embolus, Wegener's granulomatosis, and upper lobe bullous disease secondary to emphysema and neurofibromatosis.[42,46]

Upper Lobe Infiltrate with and without Fibrosis This pattern may be seen with atypical mycobacteria, ankylosing spondylitis, silicosis, collagen vascular diseases, lymphomas, and actinomycosis.[46] Upper zone fibrosis and volume loss can occur in the later stages of extrinsic alveolitis, allergic bronchopulmonary aspergillosis, and sarcoidosis. The presence of calcification suggests TB.[42]

Mediastinal Lymphadenopathy The main differential diagnosis of adenopathy is lymphoma and sarcoidosis. In sarcoidosis, lymphadenopathy is usually bilateral, symmetric, and asymptomatic. The nodes in TB tend to be unilateral, or if bilateral, are asymmetric and associated with parenchymal lung disease. Lymphoma tends to have very bulky mediastinal lymphadenopathy.[42]

Extrapulmonary Tuberculosis

Tuberculous infection involving multiple sites is most commonly seen in persons less capable of containing MTB infection such as infants, elderly people, and immunocompromised people.[35] Extrapulmonary TB (EPTB) accounted for roughly 15% of newly diagnosed TB cases in the United States before the HIV epidemic. One study of TB patients with advanced HIV infection reported that 38% had only pulmonary disease, 30% had EPTB alone, and 32% had both pulmonary disease and EPTB.[35]

EPTB may occur in multiple sites; the relative frequencies of the various sites are listed in Table 129-2. The lymph nodes are the most common site of EPTB for both normal and HIV-infected patients. Involvement of the meninges is relatively more common in young children, and the incidence of TB in the remainder of the extrapulmonary sites increases with age.[35] The less commonly involved locations for EPTB include the skin, heart, pericardium, thyroid gland, mastoid cells, sclerae, and adrenal glands.[88,89]

Lymphadenitis Tuberculous lymphadenitis (scrofula) is the most common form of EPTB. Any node can be affected, but the cervical nodes are most commonly involved. Scrofula is common in children but seen most commonly in young adult women, usually Asian/Pacific islanders or African Americans.[22,35]

The patient usually has an enlarging, painless, red, firm mass in the region of one or more lymph nodes, most commonly in the anterior or posterior cervical chain or the supraclavicular fossa.[22,90] Early on, the nodes are described

Table 129-2. Tuberculosis by Predominant Site of Disease

	1979	1989	1992
(% of total cases)			
Pulmonary	85.1	81.5	82
Extrapulmonary	14.9	18.5	17.9
(% of total cases of extrapulmonary TB)			
Lymphatic	35.2	30.7	32.8
Pleural	22.8	24.9	21.1
Bone/joint	9.6	9.8	11.2
Genitourinary	6.1	8.8	8.4
Miliary	9.2	8.6	6.5
Meningeal	4.3	5.1	5.4
Peritoneal	3.5	4.1	4.0
Other sites	9.3	8.0	10.6

From Henderson SO, Mallon WK: *Ann Emerg Med* 26:376, 1995.

as discrete, rubbery masses that are freely mobile, and the overlying skin is normal. Eventually, the nodes may become matted and harder, and the overlying skin inflamed. Fluctuance may be present as well as abscess or sinus tract if a node erodes through the skin. Systemic symptoms are uncommon, except in HIV-positive individuals in whom lymphadenitis is usually generalized.[35] The differential diagnosis includes lymphoma, metastatic cancer, fungal disease, cat-scratch disease, sarcoid, toxoplasmosis, reactive adenitis, or bacterial adenitis.

The diagnosis of scrofula is made by lymph node biopsy or fine needle aspiration.[91] In addition to antituberculous drugs, the definitive treatment recommended for these lesions is complete excision.[22] Incision and drainage should not be done because permanent sinuses and prolonged drainage can result.

Pleural Effusion Pleural EPTB may occur early after primary infection with MTB and present as pleurisy with effusion, or more rarely, it may occur late in postprimary cavitary disease and present as an empyema.[92]

Tuberculous pleurisy often causes no symptoms and resolves spontaneously; however, in the untreated, a 65% relapse rate has been reported with development of active pulmonary or EPTB within 5 years.[22] Dyspnea may occur if the effusion is large, but the effusions are usually small and unilateral. Often the presentation is acute, severe, and indistinguishable from a bacterial pneumonia. In elderly patients, however, the onset is more insidious and likely to be confused with congestive heart failure, cancer, or a pulmonary embolus.[93]

The diagnosis is usually confirmed by examination of pleural fluid or pleural biopsy. WBC counts may range from 100 to 5,000. The fluid is an exudate with a protein usually exceeding 50% of the serum protein, and the glucose may be normal to low. Because there are few bacilli, AFB smears are rarely positive, and cultures grow MTB in only 20% to 40% of patients known to have the disease.[22,35] Pleural biopsy can confirm the diagnosis in approximately 65% to 75% of patients.

Bone and Joint Infection Bone and joint TB remains a disease of older children and young adults in developing countries, while it is increasingly a disease of adults in developed countries.[22] Skeletal TB presumably develops from reactivation of dormant tubercles originally seeded during stage 2 of the primary infection or, in the case of spinal TB, from contiguous spread from paravertebral lymph nodes to the vertebrae. Generally spinal TB (Pott's disease) accounts for 50% to 70% of the reported cases; the hip or knee is involved in 15% to 20% of cases; and the ankle, elbow, wrists, and shoulders and other bones and joints account for 15% to 20% of cases.[35] Approximately 50% of patients have a prior history or concurrent case of pulmonary TB, and the chest radiograph is normal in up to half the cases.

Patients with Pott's disease may simply complain of back pain or stiffness. Examination may show fever, point tenderness, and decreased range of motion. If the initial radiograph is normal, the diagnosis may be delayed, allowing the disease to progress.

The initial lesion usually spreads to the intervertebral disk and then to the adjacent vertebrae, producing the classic radiographic appearance of anterior wedging of two involved vertebral bodies and destruction of the disk. Early changes of spinal TB can be difficult to detect on plain films, so a computed tomography (CT) scan and magnetic resonance imaging (MRI) scan should be used when the disease is suspected.[22,35]

Paraspinal cold abscesses develop in 50% or more of cases, with occasional formation of sinus tracts. The abscess can spread the infection up and down the spine, sometimes sparing vertebral bodies along its course, forming the so-called skip lesions. When imaging the spine for Pott's disease these skip lesions can easily be missed.[94] The main complication of Pott's disease is spinal cord compression.[35]

Surgical treatment is usually reserved for patients with neurologic complications. Most other patients do well when managed conservatively with chemotherapy, modified bed rest, and early ambulation.[22,95]

Renal Disease The kidney is well vascularized, so hematogenous dissemination to that organ is fairly common. After the typical tuberculous lesions develop within the parenchyma, bacilli are secreted into the calyces, renal pelvis, ureters, and bladder. As a result, tuberculous granulomas, scarring, and obstruction can occur anywhere along the urinary tract.[92]

The initial presenting symptoms of urinary involvement are nonspecific. Advanced renal disease and destruction may occur before the diagnosis is made. The urinalysis is often positive for pyuria, hematuria, and albuminuria.

Sterile pyuria is classic for renal TB, but many cases with this finding grow cultures positive for other urinary pathogens. The finding of pyuria in an acid urine with no organisms isolated should increase suspicion of TB.[35]

Complications of renal TB include nephrolithiasis, recurrent bacterial infections, hypertension, and renal insufficiency.[96]

Male Genital Disease Male genital TB is usually associated with coexistent renal TB. Spread of infection from the kidney involves the prostate, seminal vesicles, epididymides, and testes.[22] The patient typically has a painless or slightly painful scrotal mass and possibly symptoms of prostatitis, epididymitis, or orchitis.[35] Epididymal or prostatic calcifications may be clues to the diagnosis.

Female Genital Disease In women, the disease begins in both fallopian tubes.[97] The infection then spreads to the endometrium (50%), ovaries (30%), cervix (5% to 15%), and vagina (1%).[22] Women may have infertility, pelvic pain, menstrual irregularities, and rarely, vaginal discharge. An ulcerating mass may be present on the cervix. There are reports of sexual transmission of TB by individuals with active genital TB.[98] Women with genital TB who become pregnant are at risk for ectopic pregnancy.[22] In the presence of advanced disease, patients are permanently infertile.[99]

Multisystem Disease Acute disseminated tuberculosis refers to active hematogenous spread of MTB to several organs in the body. *Miliary* is a clinical term referring to the massive dissemination that leads to generalized systemic illness.[100] Miliary TB occurs when the host is unable to contain either a recently acquired or a dormant TB infection. In the past, miliary TB occurred mainly in young children after primary infection; today, it is more common in elderly persons and in those infected with HIV.[35]

In young children, the illness is acute and severe. Peritonitis and meningitis may also occur with high frequency in children.[22] In young adults, the acute illness runs a slower course and is usually less severe. Miliary TB is often a subtle disease associated with alcoholism, cirrhosis, neoplasm, pregnancy, collagen vascular disease, and use of corticosteroids or immunosuppressive medications.[22]

The clinical presentations are varied because of the multisystem nature of miliary TB. Systemic symptoms of fever, weight loss, anorexia, and weakness are generally present.[35] The choroidal tubercle is a granuloma in the choroid of the retina, representing the only physical finding specific for disseminated TB.[35]

A presumptive diagnosis can be made rapidly if the chest radiograph shows a miliary infiltrate (Figure 129-6). Unfortunately, the classic miliary pattern is absent in approximately 50% of cases.

Routine laboratory tests are generally not helpful. Hyponatremia from the syndrome of inappropriate secretion of antidiuretic hormone (SIADH) is common and often associated with meningitis. Panculturing usually has a high yield, and HIV patients may have positive blood cultures. Liver biopsy may be the most rapid diagnostic test because caseating granulomas can be seen in 88% of cases. Other potential biopsy sites include lymph nodes, bone marrow, and pulmonary tissue.[100,101]

Mortality for this form of EPTB is higher than for the other forms, with case series reporting rates between 25% and 50%. The high mortality rate is often caused by a delay in treatment, which should always be initiated immediately based on clinical suspicion and not delayed until confirmation of the diagnosis.[101]

A fulminant form of miliary TB may cause the adult respiratory distress syndrome and disseminated intravascular coagulation. In these cases, the addition of corticosteroids (prednisone, 60 to 80 mg/day) is indicated.[22]

Central Nervous System Disease Approximately 4% to 5% of all cases of extrapulmonary TB involve the central nervous system (CNS). It remains one of the more grave

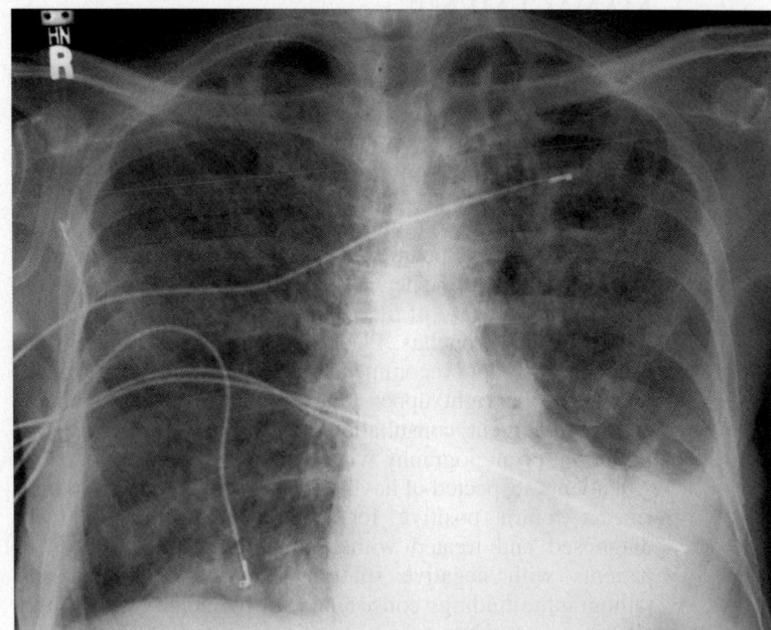

Figure 129-6. **Chest radiograph demonstrates miliary pattern with left pleural effusion.**

consequences of tuberculous infection. The peak incidence of CNS TB is in newborn to 4-year-old children.[35]

Tuberculous Meningitis Tuberculous meningitis usually results from the rupture of a subependymal tubercle into the subarachnoid space rather than direct hematogenous seeding. When developing as a complication of miliary tuberculosis, meningitis usually develops within several weeks.[102] In children, it is an early postprimary event, usually appearing within 6 months. Cerebral involvement is most marked at the base of the brain, and vasculitis of local arteries and veins may lead to aneurysm formation, thrombosis, and focal hemorrhagic infarction. The vessels to the basal ganglia are most commonly involved, leading to lacunar infarcts or movement disorders. Involvement of other vessels, such as the middle cerebral artery, may lead to hemiparesis or hemiplegia.[22]

Clinically, the disease begins with a prodrome of malaise, intermittent headache, and a low-grade fever. Then, 2 to 3 weeks later, the patient develops a protracted headache that may progress to vomiting, confusion, meningismus and focal neurologic signs, and coma.[22] Nuchal rigidity may be absent. Diplopia resulting from the frequent basilar exudate is present in up to 70% of patients. Hyponatremia may be present because SIADH is common. The CSF cell count will range from 0 to 1,500 WBCs, and there is usually a predominance of lymphocytes. Of note, 25% of patients may show a majority of polymorphonuclear cells early in the course. The protein is usually elevated and the CSF glucose has been described as characteristically low, although some case series have observed normal CSF glucose levels. A single lumbar puncture yields a positive AFB culture in only 37% of cases, but pooled samples from multiple lumbar punctures (4) yield a positive culture in 90% of the cases.[22]

CT or MRI may reveal rounded lesions typical of evolving tuberculomas in patients with meningitis, as well as basilar arachnoiditis, cerebral infarction, hydrocephalus, and cerebral edema.[92]

Prognosis is influenced by age, duration of symptoms, and the presence of neurologic deficits. Outcome is also closely linked to the clinical stage at which the disease presents. Complete recovery is the rule in stage I, wherein the alert patient has no focal neurologic signs and no hydrocephalus. Stage II is characterized by confusion and focal neurologic changes, and patients in stage III present stuporous or with dense hemiplegia or paraplegia.[22]

Treatment is with a four-drug regimen because isoniazid (INH) and pyrazinamide (PZA) reach increased concentrations in the CSF in the presence of inflamed meninges. Rifampin also crosses the blood-brain barrier. Corticosteroids should be used in patients who are in clinical stage II or III. Prednisone, 60 to 80 mg, should be given in a daily dose and tapered over 1 to 2 weeks.[22] Ventricular shunting may be needed if hydrocephalus develops.

Spinal Meningitis Tuberculous spinal meningitis is a complication of CNS infection that usually originates via hematogenous dissemination from an outside source, although tuberculous meningitis may extend caudally and involve the spine. Local extension of bony or discal TB has also been described.[103] Presenting symptoms may include focal, motor, or sensory neurologic deficits.

Intracranial Abscess The space-occupying lesions that accompany infection of the CNS by MTB may cause focal or generalized symptoms such as tonic-clonic seizures. Involvement of the CNS parenchyma may be accompanied by meningitis. Imaging reveals either solitary or multiple tuberculomas (Figure 129-7) and areas of TB cerebritis or myelitis that have coalesced into a mature noncaseating tuberculoma.[103]

Treatment includes chemotherapy before surgical removal. Corticosteroids may reduce edema and decrease the symptoms. If MTB is discovered at the time of surgery, postoperative chemotherapy may prevent the further spread of the disease.

Gastrointestinal Disease Gastrointestinal TB occurs secondary to hematogenous or lymphatic spread from distant

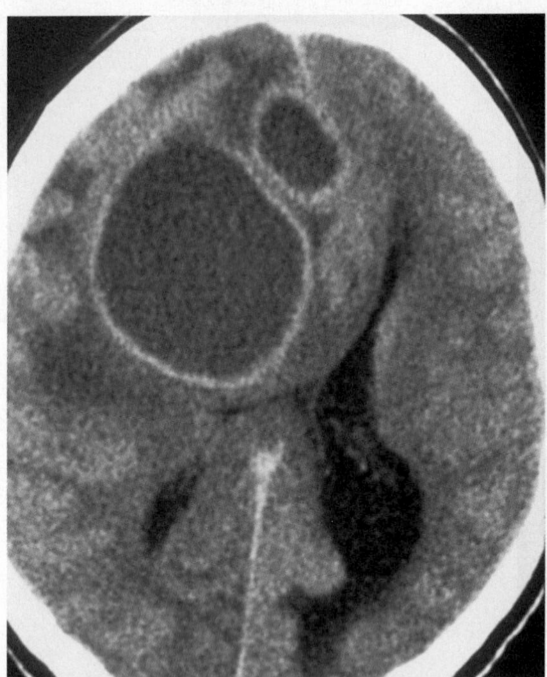

Figure 129-7. **Head CT scan demonstrating tuberculomas in an AIDS patient.**

sites or by direct spread from local sites such as lymph nodes or fallopian tubes. More rarely, it may be due to MTB in swallowed bronchial secretions.[92] TB may occur in any location from the mouth to the anus, but lesions proximal to the terminal ileum are rare. The ileocecal area is the most common site of involvement, producing symptoms of pain, anorexia, diarrhea, obstruction, hemorrhage, and often a palpable mass.

The symptoms and physical findings of this disorder may lead to the misdiagnoses of appendicitis, intestinal obstruction, or cancer. The signs and symptoms are so similar to those of cancer that the diagnosis is often made at surgery. The clinical manifestations of anal TB include fissures, fistulas, and perirectal abscesses.[35]

Peritonitis Tuberculous peritonitis may develop from local spread of MTB from a tuberculous lymph node, intestinal focus, or an infected fallopian tube.[22] In addition, the peritoneum may be seeded in miliary TB, or it may be due to the reactivation of a latent focus.[102,104]

The patient with tuberculous peritonitis commonly has pain and abdominal swelling associated with fever, anorexia, and weight loss. Diagnosis may be confounded by the similarity of this disease to alcoholic hepatitis and by the fact that this disease often coexists with other disorders, especially cirrhosis with ascites.[35] Paracentesis is thus essential. The peritoneal fluid is exudative, with a cell count of 500 to 2,000 cells. Lymphocytes usually predominate with rare exceptions early in the process when polymorphonuclear leukocytes may predominate. Smears of the fluid have a low diagnostic yield, and culture is positive in only 25% of cases. Peritoneal biopsy is often necessary to confirm the diagnosis. Treatment is the same as for pulmonary TB.[22]

MANAGEMENT

ED Management

The most emergent presentation of pulmonary TB is massive hemoptysis, defined as at least 600 ml of blood in 24 hours. Exsanguination rarely occurs, and the major morbidity is due to asphyxiation from aspirated blood.[43] The airway should be secured with a large diameter (8 mm) endotracheal tube (ETT) that can accommodate fiberoptic bronchoscopy. The patient should be positioned with the bleeding lung in a dependent position. The ETT may be positioned above the carina or in the case of bleeding from the right lung into the left mainstem bronchus. Placement into the right mainstem bronchus is not recommended because of the risk of occluding the right upper lobe bronchus.[44] These patients require emergent consultations for bronchoscopy, surgical resection, or angiography with selective embolization.[43]

Patients suspected of having pulmonary TB whose sputum smears return positive for AFB can be presumptively diagnosed and treated with antituberculous therapy.[105] In patients with negative sputum smears but clinical and radiographic findings consistent with pulmonary TB, it may also be appropriate to presumptively initiate treatment for TB.[40,105] Severely ill patients with presumed TB should be treated immediately because a few days on antituberculous agents will not interfere with bacteriologic diagnosis.[106] Local factors, including the prevalence of TB and available resources, help determine the appropriateness of presumptive therapy.[105]

Most TB patients can be managed as outpatients.[107-110] The ideal situation for the patient with newly diagnosed or suspected TB is to be at home, on antituberculosis therapy, with their contacts receiving preventive treatment.[111] The ED discharge instructions should clearly emphasize the importance of adhering to the prescribed treatment regimen and home isolation procedures (avoid meeting new contacts). The patient must be immediately reported to the health department to ensure that the patient has an adequate source of TB care, that support systems and resources are available to complete the care, and that the patient's contacts are investigated and screened.[112] Two weeks of treatment is widely accepted as the minimum time to be rendered noninfectious, but there is no epidemiologic evidence to support this number for all cases of TB (see also under "Transmission").[26,113]

Acutely ill or elderly patients may require hospitalization during the first few days of treatment because adverse reactions are common and may occasionally be life threatening.[113] In addition, severely ill patients may require parenteral drug administration. TB patients have a high rate of HIV coinfection, and the comorbidities associated with HIV, the complex synergy between MTB and HIV, and the potentially harmful drug interactions between the antiretroviral agents and the rifamycins may mandate inpatient treatment for the initial management of these difficult patients.

Hospital admission is also indicated for patients with active MDRTB. These patients commonly require observation during initiation of therapy because of the complexity of the treatment regimens, the toxicity of the drugs, and the need to closely monitor the patient for adherence with treatment and isolation measures.[114] Finally, social issues such as homelessness, households with infants or immunocompromised persons, substance abuse, and inability to care for self

Table 129-3. Antituberculous Medications

	Type	Dose	Side effects
First-line agents			
Isoniazid	Bactericidal	3 to 5 mg/kg (max. 300 mg)	Hepatitis, peripheral neuropathy
Rifampin	Bactericidal	10 mg/kg (max. 600 mg)	Gastrointestinal upset, skin eruptions, hepatitis
Pyrazinamide	Bactericidal	15 to 30 mg/kg (max. 2 g)	Hepatotoxic
Ethambutol	Bacteriostatic	15 to 25 mg/kg	Oculotoxic
Streptomycin	Bactericidal	15 mg/kg (max. 1.5 g)	Ototoxic, nephrotoxic
Second-line agents			
Paraaminosalicylic acid	Bacteriostatic	150 mg/kg (max. 10 to 12 g/day)	Rarely hepatitis
Ethionamide	Bacteriostatic	15 to 20 mg/kg (daily dose 1 g)	Nausea, vomiting, loss of appetite, abdominal pain; occasional hepatitis
Cycloserine	Bacteriostatic	15 to 20 mg/kg (max. 1 g/day)	Behavioral and emotional disturbances
Others:			
Capreomycin			
Kanamycin			
Thiacetazone			

all may necessitate hospitalization. The recalcitrant patient is a potential threat to public health and may require legal measures for involuntary hospitalization.[112]

Surgical Management

The most common indication for surgery is multidrug-resistant TB (MDRTB) with localized disease.[115] When optimal medical therapy based on drug susceptibility testing is given preoperatively and postoperatively, the outcome appears to improve for this difficult group of patients.[115,116] One series reports that more than 90% of 107 patients with MDRTB became sputum-negative after surgery combined with medical therapy.[115] Other indications for surgery include bronchopleural fistula, massive uncontrolled hemoptysis, extensive bronchostenosis, destroyed lung, solitary nodule, trapped lung, complicated cavity, and empyema.[115,116]

Medical Therapy

Antituberculous Medications Controlled clinical trials have yielded three basic therapeutic principles. First, any regimen must contain multiple drugs to which the MTB organism is susceptible. Second, the therapy must be taken regularly. Third, and most problematic, the therapy must continue for a sufficient period.[40]

It is expected that approximately 33% to 50% of patients will fail to follow medical recommendations. Patients at higher risk for noncompliance are those with previous treatment failures; substance abusers; patients with mental, emotional, or physical impairment; and those who have failed preventive treatment.[117] The most effective strategy to ensure compliance is directly observed therapy (DOT). Now the standard of care in the United States, DOT is given two to three times a week, usually after an initial period of daily therapy.[10,40]

Commonly Used Agents The medications most commonly used in the treatment of MTB are summarized in Table 129-3. Although newer agents have been developed, the first-line agents remain the same except in patients coinfected with HIV who are taking protease inhibitors and nonnucleoside reverse transcriptase inhibitors (NNRTIs).[17,118]

The incidence of INH-induced hepatitis, which occurs in 1% to 2% of all patients, increases with patient age.[119] Another adverse effect is peripheral neuropathy. This is uncommon at the 5 mg/kg dose and may be avoided by the administration of pyridoxine, especially to those individuals at risk, namely pregnant women and patients with seizures. Supplemental pyridoxine should also be supplied to those in whom neuropathy is common such as diabetic patients and those with an ethanol use history, uremia, or malnutrition.[40]

Rifampin causes orange discoloration of body fluids, including urine, tears, and sweat. Soft contact lens wearers should be warned of this effect before administration of the medication.

Pyrazinamide works in the acid environment of the macrophage. The chief side effect is hepatotoxicity, but this risk does not increase when 15 to 30 mg/kg of the drug is added to a regimen of INH and rifampin. Visual acuity and red-green color perception should be measured when using ethambutol. Because of the difficulty in visual testing in small children and infants, ethambutol should be avoided in these populations.

Streptomycin must be given parenterally and has a peak of action 1 hour after the intramuscular dose. The chief side effects of this potentially teratogenic agent are ototoxicity and nephrotoxicity.[40]

Fluoroquinolones have played a more recent but limited role in the treatment of TB. They are less effective than the first-line agents and are used mainly in the treatment of drug-resistant disease. If they are used singly, resistance may quickly develop. The agents used are ciprofloxacin, ofloxacin, levofloxacin, and sparfloxacin; the latter two drugs have greater potency. The main side effects are gastrointestinal and CNS symptoms.[118,120]

Fixed Dose Combination Drugs Fixed dose combinations are multiple antituberculous agents packaged into single tablets. They are useful to prevent monotherapy (patient selectively taking only one of prescribed drugs) and the emergence of drug resistance. Rifater contains isoniazid, rifampin, and pyrazinamide. Rifamate contains isoniazid and rifampin. The disadvantages of these combinations are higher cost, the need to take many pills, and the possibility of underdosing.[120]

New Antituberculosis Agents Rifabutin is a rifamycin antibiotic introduced in 1981. It has properties similar to rifamycin and has been used most often for treatment or prophylaxis of infections with *Mycobactrium avium* complex. However, it is also effective against MTB and is active against 30% of rifampicin-resistant MTB strains. Rifabutin may therefore have a role, as of yet not clearly demonstrated, in the treatment of multidrug-resistant TB.[120] The drug's most significant role thus far is in the treatment of TB patients coinfected with HIV who are on protease inhibitors and NNRTIs.[17]

Rifapentine is another rifamycin derivative with excellent activity against MTB and a half-life of 13.2 hours, fivefold greater than rifamycin.[21,118] Its long half-life makes it a good candidate for intermittent therapy regimens (given twice weekly). In initial clinical trials rifapentine was found to be safe and well tolerated, but it had higher relapse rates than those of standard regimens containing rifamycin.[21] The drug has been approved by the Food and Drug Administration for use in intermittent TB treatment regimens in adults without coinfection with HIV, but its exact role is not yet clear.[21,120] An additional rifamycin derivative called KRM-1648 or rifalazil with an extended half-life and increased activity against MTB is also under evaluation in clinical trials.[21]

Other drugs being evaluated for the treatment of MTB include roxithromycin, amoxicillin-clavulanic acid, and interferon-γ.[118]

Initial Therapy

Adults INH has the best combination of effectiveness, low cost, and minor side effects. INH should be included in all treatment regimens as a first-line drug unless there is known resistance or another contraindication. Most therapeutic regimens of less than 6 months duration have an unacceptably high relapse rate. Six months is the shortest standard course of therapy recommended with INH and rifampin. Pyrazinamide improves the efficacy of regimens of less than 9 months, whereas substituting ethambutol or streptomycin for pyrazinamide tends to decrease effectiveness. Intermittent administration of drugs (e.g., four drugs given three times per week) is acceptable and effective treatment after an initial daily regimen has been completed.[40]

The therapy begins with a 2-month period of INH, rifampin, pyrazinamide plus ethambutol or streptomycin unless drug resistance in the community is less than 4%. The INH and rifampin are continued for the remaining 4 months of the therapy, based on drug susceptibility testing. Treatment should be prolonged if the response is suboptimal. In patients who are also HIV-positive, adherence to the regimen plus DOT is recommended.[40] MDRTB therapy must be individualized.[40,119]

Children and Adolescents The treatment of adolescents, children, and infants who are culture positive for MTB is in principle the same as in adults. Some important points in treating children are shown in Box 129-6.

Box 129-6 Treatment of TB in Children

1. Infection with TB in children less than 4 years of age is more likely to disseminate and therefore demands prompt recognition and aggressive management.
2. Sputum smears are a less reliable diagnostic tool. It may be more appropriate to confirm the diagnosis in a child using culture results or results from the adult source. If neither is available, early morning gastric aspirates, bronchoalveolar lavage, or tissue may be used.
3. Because of its ocular toxicity, ethambutol should be avoided in this age group. Pyrazinamide or streptomycin are alternatives.
4. The primary cause of treatment failure in this population is noncompliance. Therefore DOT is preferable, and twice a week regimens are an option.
5. Treat extrapulmonary tuberculosis as described above for pulmonary variety except for infections involving bones or joints, meningitis, and miliary disease when therapy should last 12 months at minimum.

Infant with noncontagious mother The therapy for newborn infants exposed at birth varies depending on the severity of disease in the mother. If the mother is PPD positive without evidence of disease, the infant should be tested with the Mantoux skin test at 4 to 6 weeks old and again at 3 to 4 months old. If the mother has evidence of disease but is no longer infectious, the infant should be tested as mentioned previously and again at 6 months old. Separation of a compliant mother and child is unnecessary. The mother may breastfeed. The infant should begin a course of INH even if the Mantoux and chest radiograph are negative because CMI is not fully developed. If no evidence of disease is evident in the infant after 6 months, the INH may be discontinued.[40]

Infant with contagious mother If the mother has active disease and is contagious, the infant needs to be separated and tested at 4 to 6 weeks old and at 3 to 4 months old. If the mother has any evidence of hematogenous spread of TB, the infant must be separated from the mother and should receive a chest radiograph, skin testing, and 6 months of INH therapy. If any of the skin tests are positive, therapy should continue for a minimum of 9 months.[40]

Extrapulmonary Tuberculosis Clinical experience indicates that 6- to 9-month regimens of therapy are effective treatments except in bone or joint, miliary, and meningeal disease in children. These require a minimum of 12 months of therapy.

Corticosteroids The use of corticosteroids in the treatment of EPTB is more common than in pulmonary disease. Corticosteroids may prevent constriction in tuberculous pericarditis and decrease the neurologic sequelae in all stages of tuberculous meningitis, especially if given early in the disease.[40] In addition, in patients with pulmonary TB, prednisone, 20 to 60 mg/day, may benefit those who continue to spike temperatures and lose weight despite good bacteriologic response to appropriate antituberculous therapy.[121]

Pregnancy Treatment of TB during pregnancy does not jeopardize the fetus. INH, rifampin, and ethambutol all cross the placenta but have no known teratogenic effects. Pyridoxine is recommended for those pregnant women receiving INH. Streptomycin may cause congenital deafness and should therefore be avoided, as should pyrazinamide.

Although these chemotherapeutic agents are present in breast milk, they are not harmful to the infant and are not present in high enough concentrations (approximately 20% of the daily dose) to be therapeutic or preventive.[40]

HIV-Positive Individuals Adequate treatment of active TB in patients coinfected with HIV is critical. It has been observed that immune activation from TB enhances both systemic and local HIV replication and may accelerate the natural progression of HIV infection. Active TB in HIV-infected patients has been associated with increased risk for opportunistic infections and death. TB treatment alone leads to reduction in viral load in these patients.[17] Untreated or inadequately treated TB may result in increased morbidity and mortality, not only from MTB but also from accelerated AIDS. Furthermore, TB can spread rapidly through immunocompromised populations when a source case remains contagious for a prolonged period.[122]

Current CDC and American Thoracic Society guidelines recommend a 6-month treatment regimen for drug-susceptible TB disease in patients coinfected with HIV but suggest prolonged treatment (6 months of treatment after culture conversion) for patients who have a delayed clinical and bacteriologic response to the therapy.[122]

Significant drug interactions between rifamycins used for TB and antiretroviral drugs (protease inhibitors and NNRTIs) used for HIV complicate the treatment of patients with active TB who are coinfected with HIV. These drug interactions are primarily due to changes in the metabolism of the antiretrovirals and the rifamycins secondary to induction or inhibition of the hepatic cytochrome CYP450 enzyme system. The currently available rifamycins are inducers of CYP450, with rifampin being the most potent inducer, rifapentine intermediate, and rifabutin the least potent inducer.[123] Because all the protease inhibitors are metabolized by CYP450, coadministration of rifampin and the protease inhibitors would cause a marked decrease in the blood concentration of the protease inhibitors, likely reducing their antiretroviral activity as well. Conversely, the protease inhibitors are CYP450 inhibitors, so if a potent CYP450 inhibitor such as ritonavir is administered with rifabutin, blood concentrations of rifabutin markedly rise, and rifabutin toxicity could result.[17]

The NNRTIs have similar interactions, but there are major differences in their actions on CYP450 and the degree to which they are substrates of CYP450, so their interactions with rifamycins cannot be summarized as a class.[123] Essentially, serum concentrations of protease inhibitors and NNRTIs need to be at an optimal steady state to prevent resistant mutations of HIV. Because rifampin lowers the levels of these drugs, its use to treat active TB in a patient on a protease inhibitor or an NNRTI is always contraindicated.[17]

To avoid these drug interactions, the CDC recommends, for patients who are taking protease inhibitors or NNRTIs, a 6-month TB regimen that starts with INH, rifabutin, pyrazinamide, and ethambutol for the first 2 months, followed by INH and rifabutin for 4 months. If use of rifamycins is contraindicated, a 9-month regimen is recommended, consisting of INH, streptomycin, pyrazinamide, and ethambutol for 2 months, followed by INH, streptomycin, and pyrazinamide for 7 months.[17]

HIV patients who are not on antiretroviral therapy are advised to take the usual 6-month regimen consisting of INH, rifampin, pyrazinamide, and ethambutol for 2 months, followed by INH and rifampin for 4 months.[17] If INH or rifampin is not tolerated or in cases of drug resistance, therapy should continue for at least 12 months after cultures are negative and for at least 18 months total.[124] DOT has been recommended to ensure adherence and prevent the development of drug resistance. Additionally, pyridoxine, 25 to 50 mg/day or 50 to 100 mg twice a week, should be administered to all HIV-infected patients undergoing TB treatment with INH to decrease the incidence of INH-induced central and peripheral nervous system side effects.[17]

Preventive Therapy Individuals chosen for preventive therapy are those with MTB infection who have a risk of developing TB that outweighs the risks of the therapy itself. These at-risk populations are listed in Boxes 129-1 and 129-2. In addition, preventive therapy may be reasonable for HIV-positive persons who are PPD negative but belong to groups in which the prevalence of TB infection is high.[40]

Preventive therapy consists of INH alone in a single daily dose of 300 mg/day for adults or 3 to 5 mg/kg/day for children, not to exceed the adult dose. Excluding active TB is a critical step before initiating preventive therapy.[124] Effective therapy consists of 9 to 10 months of INH; regimens lasting less than this do not give optimal protection.[125] For HIV-positive patients, at least 9 months of therapy is recommended, and therapy for more than 12 months does not appear to provide additional protection.[17] The most recent CDC guidelines also state that a regimen of rifampin and pyrazinamide administered daily for 2 months is a reasonable treatment option for HIV-infected adults with latent MTB infection.[17]

DOT is recommended in those persons at high risk for developing the disease to decrease possible MDRTB emergence. If daily observation is not an option, INH may be given twice a week at a concentration of 15 mg/kg/day.[124]

Drug-Resistant Tuberculosis Mycobacterial DNA undergoes spontaneous mutations, giving rise to drug-resistant strains, so TB patients who are improperly treated (especially with monotherapy) or nonadherent to their treatment are likely to offer the drug-resistant strains a selective advantage. When these strains predominate, "acquired resistance" has occurred. Patients with acquired resistance can transmit drug-resistant organisms to previously uninfected (never treated) individuals, a process known as primary drug resistance.[126] MDRTB is defined as resistance to two or more first-line antituberculous agents.[127] Multidrug resistance may occur when a single drug is added to a failing regimen, an intervention equivalent to giving monotherapy.[114]

Although all drug-resistant TB can ultimately be traced back to suboptimal treatment, it is the transmission of primary drug resistance from person to person that allows rapid dissemination of drug-resistant strains.[128,129] The spread of primary drug resistance is faster when HIV infection is highly prevalent in a population.[130-132] Because HIV-infected patients progress rapidly from initial TB infection to active disease, those newly infected can quickly become source cases for further transmission of the resistant bacilli.[130,131] In reports from hospital outbreaks of MDRTB, more than 90% of patients had coinfection with HIV, and case fatality rates were as high as 70% to 90%.[133-136]

MDRTB should still be considered a potentially lethal disease with a well-documented ability to spread from patient to patient and from patient to health care worker.[137]

Health care workers should know the prevalence of drug

Box 129-7 Risk Factors for Drug-Resistant MTB[114,126,128,129,138,139]

1. Prior unsuccessful antituberculosis treatment
2. Failure to respond or adhere to a good treatment regimen
3. HIV infection
4. IV drug abuse
5. Close contacts of source cases
6. Recent immigration from area with high prevalence of drug resistance
7. Cavitary lung disease
8. Homelessness
9. Imprisonment
10. Drug malabsorption due to gastrectomy or ileal bypass surgery

resistance in their community and the risk factors (Box 129-7) for drug resistance to identify potential cases.

Rapid identification and prompt isolation of these patients, along with other control measures, can reduce nosocomial transmission of MDRTB to patients and health care workers.[126,133,139] Failure to control drug resistance may lead to wide dissemination of MDRTB and to a public health crisis that physicians will be forced to confront without effective medications.

PREVENTION OF TRANSMISSION IN THE EMERGENCY DEPARTMENT

Patients with TB or TB risk factors commonly receive care in busy, inner-city EDs, where overcrowding and a lack of TB isolation rooms may create an ideal setting for transmission of the disease.[140] Also favoring nosocomial transmission is the fact that ED patients with TB often receive care before the diagnosis is suspected; this risk is particularly high with critically ill patients, who by definition require close, intense contact with multiple emergency care providers. TB is transmitted in both public and community hospital EDs.[140-142]

Early Identification

Triage protocols should be designed to facilitate the immediate identification of active TB patients as they present to the ED, thereby expediting the institution of isolation measures.[83,143] The early suspicion of TB in the ED leads to more rapid isolation and treatment.[143] In addition, the development of policies providing for expedited admission to hospital isolation beds and for improved access to local public health facilities may help decrease TB transmission at virtually no cost.[140] The triage protocol developed by the ED at one institution is shown in Figure 129-8.

Isolation and Environmental Control

In contrast to triage protocols, isolation facilities and environmental control measures are expensive and more difficult to implement. The CDC guidelines specify negative pressure TB isolation rooms with a minimum of 6 but preferably 12 air changes or more per hour, with the air from these rooms venting directly outside. In high prevalence areas recommendations for environmental control in general use and waiting areas include a single-pass, nonrecirculating system that exhausts air to the outside or a recirculation system that passes air through high-efficiency particulate air filters before recirculation. As an adjunct, upper air ultraviolet germicidal irradiation should be added.[83] Although implementation of such measures similar to the CDC guidelines can effectively halt the transmission of MDRTB to health care workers and patients on medical wards, they may not be applicable to a busy ED.[139-144] The cost and space required for these measures render implementation impractical in most overcrowded, public EDs.[139,144] The infection control policies and facilities that are feasible and effective in preventing transmission of TB in the ED remain to be defined.[140,143]

Personal Respiratory Protection Surgical masks prevent TB patients from releasing their infectious secretions into the air. When worn by health care workers, surgical masks may not adequately prevent the inhalation of infectious droplet nuclei.[145] More advanced personal respiratory protection devices range from simple, disposable dust-mist respirators to reusable powered, air-purifying particulate respirators.[83,145] The former are least intrusive and most acceptable to workers, but they offer the least protection because of a higher rate of filter leakage as well as leaks between the face and respirator. Sophisticated respirators offer superior protection but are expensive and bulky, impair verbal communication, and are the least acceptable to health care workers and, presumably, their patients.[25] Their use is warranted, however, during high-risk procedures such as bronchoscopy or sputum induction.[25]

Preventive Therapy After Inadvertent Exposure

Emergency care providers are at high risk for exposure to MTB because they often initiate treatment on patients who have not been screened for active TB.[142]

Based on the evaluation of 33 MTB outbreaks, the recommendations in Box 129-8 can assist physicians in deciding who should be treated after exposure.[146]

Tuberculin Skin Testing Because all ED staff are potentially exposed to MTB, a skin-test program is essential.[83] Skin testing at regular intervals monitors TB transmission among ED staff and targets staff who need prophylactic therapy or treatment.

Bacille Calmette Guerin Vaccine Although the BCG vaccine has been used since 1921, its overall efficacy, duration of protective immunity, and optimal age for administration remain unclear.[147] In the United States, BCG is rarely recommended because of the belief that it would undermine the epidemiologic and diagnostic value of PPD skin testing. Institutional outbreaks of TB and the emergence of MDRTB are sparking reassessment of BCG issue in the United States.[147]

BCG is recommended in the United States only for tuberculin-negative infants and children who cannot take isoniazid and have ongoing exposure to a persistently untreated or inadequately treated patient with active TB, who are continuously exposed to persons with isoniazid- and rifampin-resistant TB, or who belong to groups with rates of new MTB infection exceeding 1% per year.[147]

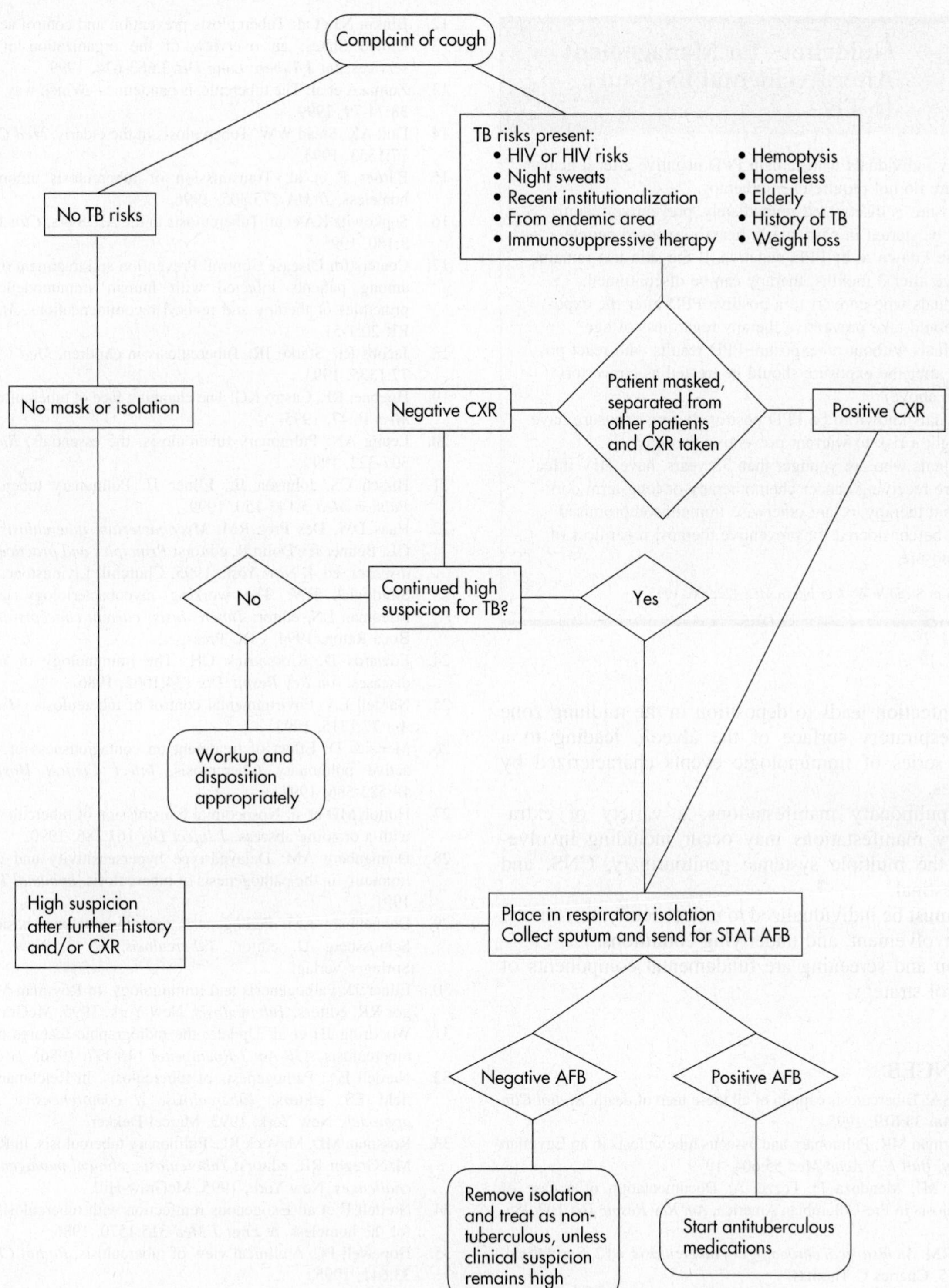

Figure 129-8. **Example of triage protocol for rapid identification of TB patients in the ED.**

A meta-analysis and literature review both support the efficacy of BCG in protecting the health care worker.[147,148] In the United Kingdom, the Joint Tuberculosis Committee of the British Thoracic Society recommends that the health care worker at risk for TB should be protected by BCG vaccination.[149] The vaccine is strongly contraindicated in individuals with HIV infection or other immunosuppressive disease.

KEY CONCEPTS

- The number of tuberculosis cases in the United States as well as worldwide increased between the years 1986 and 1992 after a 32 year decline from 1953 to 1985 (in 1993 the numbers declined again), partially reflecting changing epidemiology. In the United States, immigration and HIV-related TB have been important factors. The reemergence of TB has also affected children.

Box 129-8 Guidelines for Management After Accidental Exposure to TB

1. Healthy individuals who remain PPD negative after a heavy exposure do not require chemotherapy.
2. If exposure is discovered immediately, preventive therapy should be started in particularly heavily exposed people who are known to be PPD negative. If the skin test remains negative after 3 months, therapy can be discontinued.
3. Individuals who convert to a positive PPD after the exposure should take preventive therapy regardless of age.
4. Individuals without preexposure PPD results who react positively after the exposure should be treated as convertors (see #3 above).
5. Individuals known to be PPD positive before exposure have too slight a risk to warrant preventive therapy.
6. Individuals who are younger than 35 years, have HIV infection, are receiving cancer chemotherapy or long-term corticosteroid therapy, or are otherwise immunocompromised should be considered for preventive therapy, regardless of the exposure.

Modified from Stead WW: *Ann Intern Med* 122:906, 1995.

- Droplet infection leads to deposition in the midlung zone on the respiratory surface of the alveoli, leading to a complex series of immunologic events characterized by four stages.
- Beyond pulmonary manifestations, a variety of extrapulmonary manifestations may occur including involvement of the multiple systems: genitourinary, CNS, and gastrointestinal.
- Therapy must be individualized to reflect acuity, sensitivity, system involvement, and underlying conditions.
- Prevention and screening are fundamental components of any control strategy.

REFERENCES

1. Rubin SA: Tuberculosis captain of all these men of death, *Radiol Clin North Am* 33:619, 1995.
2. Zimmerman MR: Pulmonary and osseous tuberculosis in an Egyptian mummy, *Bull N Y Acad Med* 55:604, 1979.
3. Allison MJ, Mendoza D, Pezzia A: Documentation of a case of tuberculosis in Pre-Columbian America, *Am Rev Respir Dis* 107:985, 1973.
4. Burke RM: *An historical chronology of tuberculosis,* ed 2, Springfield, Ill, 1955, Charles C Thomas.
5. Waksman S: *The conquest of tuberculosis,* Berkeley, Calif, 1964, University of California Press.
6. Bates JH, Stead WW: The history of tuberculosis as a global epidemic, *Med Clin North Am* 77:1205, 1993.
7. Stead WW, Dutt AK: Epidemiology and host factors. In Schlossberg D, editor: *Tuberculosis,* ed 3, New York, 1994, Springer-Verlag.
8. Ayvazian FL: History of tuberculosis. In Reichman LB, Hershfield ES, editors: *Tuberculosis: a comprehensive international approach,* New York, 1993, Marcel Dekker.
9. Frieden TR et al: Tuberculosis in New York City—turning the tide, *N Engl J Med* 333:229, 1995.
10. Cantwell MF et al: Epidemiology of tuberculosis in the United States, 1985 through 1992, *JAMA* 272:535, 1994.
11. Bellin E: Failure of tuberculosis control a prescription for change, *JAMA* 271:708, 1994.
12. Binkin NJ et al: Tuberculosis prevention and control activities in the United States: an overview of the organization of tuberculosis services, *Int J Tuberc Lung Dis* 3:663-674, 1999.
13. Zumia A et al: The tuberculosis pandemic—Which way now? *J Infect* 38:74-79, 1999.
14. Dutt AK, Stead WW: Tuberculosis in the elderly, *Med Clin North Am* 77:1353, 1993.
15. Barnes P et al: Transmission of tuberculosis among the urban homeless, *JAMA* 275:305, 1996.
16. Sepkowitz KA et al: Tuberculosis in the AIDS era, *Clin Microbiol Rev* 8:180, 1995.
17. Centers for Disease Control: Prevention and treatment of tuberculosis among patients infected with human immunodeficiency virus: principles of therapy and revised recommendations, *MMWR* 47/No. RR-20:1-51.
18. Jacobs RF, Starke JR: Tuberculosis in children, *Med Clin North Am* 77:1335, 1993.
19. Huebner RE, Castro KG: The changing face of tuberculosis, *Annu Rev Med* 46:47, 1995.
20. Leung AN: Pulmonary tuberculosis: the essentials, *Radiology* 210: 307-322, 1999.
21. Hirsch CS, Johnson JL, Ellner JJ: Pulmonary tuberculosis, *Opin Pulmon Med* 5:143-150, 1999.
22. Haas DW, Des Prez RM: *Mycobacterium tuberculosis.* In Mandell GL, Bennet JE, Dolin R, editors: *Principles and practice of infectious diseases,* ed 4, New York, 1995, Churchill Livingstone.
23. Smithwick RW: The working mycobacteriology laboratory. In Friedman LN, editor: *Tuberculosis: current concepts and treatment,* Boca Raton, 1994, CRC Press.
24. Edwards D, Kirkpatrick CH: The immunology of mycobacterial diseases, *Am Rev Respir Dis* 134:1062, 1986.
25. Nardell EA: Environmental control of tuberculosis, *Med Clin North Am* 77:1315, 1993.
26. Menzies D: Effect of treatment on contagiousness of patients with active pulmonary tuberculosis, *Infect Control Hosp Epidemiol* 18:582-586, 1997.
27. Hutton MD et al: Nosocomial transmission of tuberculosis associated with a draining abscess, *J Infect Dis* 161:286, 1990.
28. Dannenberg AM: Delayed-type hypersensitivity and cell-mediated immunity in the pathogenesis of tuberculosis, *Immunol Today* 12:228, 1991.
29. Dannenberg AM: Pathogenesis and immunology: basic aspects. In Schlossberg D, editor: *Tuberculosis,* ed 3, New York, 1994, Springer-Verlag.
30. Ellner JJ: Pathogenesis and immunology. In Rossman MD, MacGregor RR, editors: *Tuberculosis,* New York, 1995, McGraw-Hill.
31. Woodring JH et al: Update: the radiographic features of pulmonary tuberculosis, *AJR Am J Roentgenol* 146:497, 1986.
32. Nardell EA: Pathogenesis of tuberculosis. In Reichman LB, Hershfield ES, editors: *Tuberculosis: a comprehensive international approach,* New York, 1993, Marcel Dekker.
33. Rossman MD, Mayock RL: Pulmonary tuberculosis. In Rossman MD, MacGregor RR, editors: *Tuberculosis: clinical management and new challenges,* New York, 1995, McGraw-Hill.
34. Nardell E et al: Exogenous reinfection with tuberculosis in a shelter for the homeless, *N Engl J Med* 315:1570, 1986.
35. Hopewell PC: A clinical view of tuberculosis, *Radiol Clin North Am* 33:641, 1995.
36. Hopewell PC, Bloom BR: Tuberculosis and other mycobacterial diseases. In Murray JF, Nadel JA, editors: *Textbook of respiratory medicine,* ed 2, Philadelphia, 1994, WB Saunders.
37. Barnes PF et al: Chest roentgenogram in pulmonary tuberculosis new data on an old test, *Chest* 94:316, 1988.
38. Mathur P et al: Delayed diagnosis of pulmonary tuberculosis in city hospitals, *Arch Intern Med* 154:306, 1994.
39. Centers for Disease Control: *TB care guide highlights from core curriculum on tuberculosis,* Atlanta, 1994, United States Department of Health and Human Services.
40. American Thoracic Society: Treatment of tuberculosis and tuberculosis infection in adults and children, *Am J Respir Crit Care Med* 149:1359, 1994.
41. McAdams HP, Erasmus J, Winter JA: Radiologic manifestations of pulmonary tuberculosis, *Radiol Clin North Am* 33:655, 1995.

42. Omerod LP: Respiratory tuberculosis. In Davies PDO, editor: *Clinical tuberculosis,* New York, 1994, Chapman and Hall Medical.
43. Goldman JM: Hemoptysis: emergency assessment and management, *Emerg Med Clin North Am* 7:325, 1989.
44. Palmer PES: Pulmonary tuberculosis—usual and unusual radiographic presentations, *Semin Roentgenol* 14:204, 1979.
45. Mayron R et al: Echocardiography performed by emergency physicians: impact on diagnosis and therapy, *Ann Emerg Med* 17:156, 1988.
46. Friedman LN, Selwyn PA: Pulmonary tuberculosis: primary, reactivation, HIV related, and non-HIV related. In Friedman LN, editor: *Tuberculosis: current concepts and treatment,* Boca Raton, 1994, CRC Press.
47. Greenbaum M, Beyt BE Jr, Murray PR: The accuracy of diagnosing pulmonary tuberculosis at a teaching hospital, *Am Rev Respir Dis* 121:477, 1980.
48. Counsell SR, Tan JS, Dittus RS: Unsuspected pulmonary tuberculosis in a community teaching hospital, *Arch Intern Med* 149:1274, 1989.
49. Leung AN et al: Primary tuberculosis in childhood: radiographic manifestations, *Radiology* 182:87, 1992.
50. Miller WT: Tuberculosis in the 1990s, *Radiol Clin North Am* 32:649, 1994.
51. Hoheisel G et al: Endobronchial tuberculosis: diagnostic features and therapeutic outcome, *Respir Med* 88:593, 1994.
52. FitzGerald JM, Grzybowski S, Allen EA: The impact of human immunodeficiency virus infection on tuberculosis and its control, *Chest* 100:191, 1991.
53. Greenberg SD et al: Active pulmonary tuberculosis in patients with AIDS: spectrum of radiographic findings (including a normal appearance), *Radiology* 193:115, 1994.
54. Christie JD, Callihan DR: The laboratory diagnosis of mycobacterial diseases: challenges and common sense, *Clin Lab Med* 15:279, 1995.
55. Warren NG, Body BA: Bacteriology and diagnosis. In Rossman MD, MacGregor RR, editors: *Tuberculosis: clinical management and new challenges,* New York, 1995, McGraw-Hill.
56. Yeager HY et al: Quantitative studies of mycobacterial populations in sputum and saliva, *Am Rev Respir Dis* 95:998, 1966.
57. Dutt AK, Stead WW: Smear-negative pulmonary tuberculosis, *Semin Respir Infect* 9:113, 1994.
58. Schluger NW, Rom WN: Current approaches to the diagnosis of active pulmonary tuberculosis, *Am J Respir Crit Care Med* 149:264, 1994.
59. Levy H, Sacho H, Kallenbach J: A reevaluation of sputum microscopy and culture in the diagnosis of pulmonary tuberculosis, *Chest* 95:1193, 1989.
60. Gordin F, Slutkin G: The validity of acid-fast smears in the diagnosis of pulmonary tuberculosis, *Arch Pathol Lab Med* 114:1025, 1990.
61. Daniel TM: The rapid diagnosis of tuberculosis: a selective review, *J Lab Clin Med* 116:277, 1990.
62. Counsell SR, Tan JS, Dittus RS: Unsuspected pulmonary tuberculosis in a community teaching hospital, *Arch Intern Med* 149:1274, 1989.
63. Kramer F et al: Delayed diagnosis of tuberculosis in patients with human immunodeficiency virus infection, *Am J Med* 89:451, 1990.
64. Klein NC et al: Use of mycobacterial smears in the diagnosis of pulmonary tuberculosis in AIDS/ARC patients, *Chest* 95:1190, 1989.
65. Smith RL et al: Factors affecting the yield of acid-fast sputum smears in patients with HIV and tuberculosis, *Chest* 106:684, 1994.
66. Long R et al: The impact of HIV on the usefulness of sputum smears for the diagnosis of tuberculosis, *Am J Public Health* 81:1326, 1991.
67. American Thoracic Society: Diagnostic standards and classification of tuberculosis, *Am Rev Respir Dis* 142:725, 1990.
68. Crawford JT: New technologies in the diagnosis of tuberculosis, *Semin Respir Infect* 9:62, 1994.
69. Chin DP et al: Clinical utility of a commercial test based on the polymerase chain reaction for detecting *Mycobacterium tuberculosis* in respiratory specimens, *Am J Respir Crit Care Med* 151:1872, 1995.
70. Bates JH: New diagnostic methods. In Friedman LN, editor: *Tuberculosis: current concepts and treatment,* Boca Raton, 1994, CRC Press.
71. Pfaller MA: Application of new technology to the detection, identification, and antimicrobial susceptibility testing of mycobacteria, *Am J Clin Pathol* 101:329, 1994.
72. Nolte FS et al: Direct detection of *Mycobacterium tuberculosis* in sputum by polymerase chain reaction and DNA hybridization, *J Clin Microbiol* 31:1777, 1993.
73. Noordhoek GT et al: Sensitivity and specificity of PCR for detection of *Mycobacterium tuberculosis:* a blind comparison study among seven laboratories, *J Clin Microbiol* 32:277, 1994.
74. Macher A, Goosby E: PCR and the misdiagnosis of active tuberculosis, *N Engl J Med* 332:128, 1995.
75. Querol JM et al: The utility of polymerase chain reaction in the diagnosis of pulmonary tuberculosis, *Chest* 107:1631, 1995.
76. Moore DF, Curry JI: Detection and identification of *Mycobacterium tuberculosis* directly from sputum sediments by Amplicor PCR, *J Clin Microbiol* 33:2686, 1995.
77. Vuorinen P et al: Direct detection of *Mycobacterium tuberculosis* complex in respiratory specimens by Gen-Probe amplified *Mycobacterium tuberculosis* direct test and Roche Amplicor *Mycobacterium tuberculosis* test, *J Clin Microbiol* 33:1856, 1995.
78. Beavis KG et al: Evaluation of Amplicor PCR for direct detection of *Mycobacterium tuberculosis* from sputum specimens, *J Clin Microbiol* 33:2582, 1995.
79. Vlaspolder F, Singer P, Roggeveen C: Diagnostic value of an amplification method (Gen-Probe) compared with that of culture for diagnosis of tuberculosis, *J Clin Microbiol* 33:2699, 1995.
80. Galdwin MT, Plorde JJ, Martin TR: Clinical application of the *Mycobacterium tuberculosis* direct test: case report, literature review, and proposed clinical algorithm, *Chest* 114:317-323, 1998.
81. Schluger NW, Rom WN: The polymerase chain reaction in the diagnosis and evaluation of pulmonary infections, *Am J Respir Crit Care Med* 152:11, 1995.
82. Murthy KM, Dutt AK: Tuberculin skin testing: present status, *Semin Respir Infect* 9:78, 1994.
83. CDC: Guidelines for preventing the transmission of *Mycobacterium tuberculosis* in health-care facilities, 1994, *MMWR* 43(RR-13):59, 1994.
84. Menzies R, Vissandjee B: Effect of Bacille Calmette Guerin vaccination on tuberculin reactivity, *Am Rev Respir Dis* 145:621, 1992.
85. Pesanti HL: The negative tuberculin test, tuberculin, HIV, and anergy panels, *Am J Respir Crit Care Med* 149:1699, 1994.
86. Patz EF, Swensen SJ, Erasmus J: Pulmonary manifestations of nontuberculous mycobacterium, *Radiol Clin North Am* 33:719, 1995.
87. Wright PW, Wallace RJ: Nontuberculous mycobacteria. In Davies PDO, editor: *Clinical tuberculosis,* New York, 1994, Chapman and Hall Medical.
88. Singh B, Maharaj TJ: Tuberculosis of the parotid gland: clinically indistinguishable from a neoplasm, *J Laryngol Otolaryngol* 106:929, 1992.
89. Henderson SO, Mallon WK: Tuberculosis as the cause of diffuse parotitis, *Ann Emerg Med* 26:376, 1995.
90. Freixinet J et al: Surgical treatment of childhood mediastinal tuberculosis lymphadenitis, *Ann Thorac Surg* 59:644, 1995.
91. Lau SK et al: Efficacy of fine needle aspiration cytology in the diagnosis of tuberculous cervical lymphadenopathy, *J Laryngol Otolaryngol* 104:24, 1990.
92. Moulding T: Pathophysiology and immunology: clinical aspects. In Schlossberg D, editor: *Tuberculosis,* ed 3, New York, 1994, Springer-Verlag.
93. Epstein DM et al: Tuberculous pleural effusions, *Chest* 91:106, 1987.
94. Sharif HS et al: Role of CT and MR Imaging in the management of tuberculous spondylitis, *Radiol Clin North Am* 33:787, 1995.
95. Miller JD: Pott's paraplegia today (commentary), *Lancet* 346:264, 1995.
96. Narayana AS: Overview of renal tuberculosis, *Urology* XIX:231, 1982.
97. Wehner JH et al: Pulmonary tuberculosis, amenorrhea, and a pelvic mass, *WMJ* 161:515, 1994.
98. Sutherland AM, Glen ES, MacFarlane JR: Transmission of genitourinary tuberculosis, *Health Bull* 40:87, 1982.
99. Schaefer G: Female genital tuberculosis, *Clin Obstet Gynecol* 19:223, 1976.
100. Grieco MH, Chmel H: Acute disseminated tuberculosis as a diagnostic problem, *Am Rev Respir Dis* 109:554, 1974.
101. Proudfoot AT et al: Miliary tuberculosis in adults, *BMJ* 2:273, 1969.

102. Alvarez S, McCabe WR: Extrapulmonary tuberculosis revisited: a review of experience at Boston City and other hospitals, *Medicine* 63:25, 1984.
103. Jinkins RJ et al: MR imaging of central nervous system tuberculosis, *Radiol Clin North Am* 33:771, 1995.
104. Marshall JB: Tuberculosis of the gastrointestinal tract and peritoneum, *J Gastroenterol* 88:989, 1993.
105. Gordin FM et al: Presumptive diagnosis and treatment of pulmonary tuberculosis based on radiographic findings, *Am Rev Respir Dis* 139:1090, 1989.
106. Haas DW, Des Prez RM: Current treatment and management. In Rossman MD, MacGregor RR, editors: *Tuberculosis: clinical management and new challenges,* New York, 1995, McGraw-Hill.
107. Dandoy S: Current status of general hospital use for patients with tuberculosis in the United States, *Am Rev Respir Dis* 126:270, 1982.
108. Brown RE et al: Health-care expenditures for tuberculosis in the United States, *Arch Intern Med* 155:1595, 1995.
109. Gunnels JJ, Bates JH, Swindoll H: Infectivity of sputum-positive tuberculosis patients on chemotherapy, *Am Rev Respir Dis* 109:323, 1974.
110. Bates JH: Ambulatory treatment of tuberculosis—an idea whose time is come, *Am Rev Respir Dis* 109:317, 1974.
111. American Thoracic Society: Control of tuberculosis, *Am Rev Respir Dis* 128:336, 1983.
112. Etkind SC: The role of the public health department in tuberculosis, *Med Clin North Am* 77:1303, 1993.
113. Davies PDO: Problems in the management of tuberculosis. In Davies PDO, editor: *Clinical tuberculosis,* New York, 1994, Chapman and Hall Medical.
114. Goble M: Drug resistance. In Friedman LN, editor: *Tuberculosis: current concepts and treatment,* Boca Raton, 1994, CRC Press.
115. Pomerantz M, Brown J: The surgical management of tuberculosis, *Semin Thorac Cardiovasc Surg* 7:108, 1995.
116. Treasure RL, Seaworth BJ: Current role of surgery in *Mycobacterium tuberculosis, Ann Thorac Surg* 59:1405, 1995.
117. Pozsik CJ: Compliance with tuberculosis therapy, *Med Clin North Am* 77:1289, 1993.
118. Douglas JG, McLeod MJ: Pharmacokinetic factors in the modern drug treatment of tuberculosis, *Clin Pharmacokinet* 37:127-146, 1999.
119. Brausch LM, Bass JB: The treatment of tuberculosis, *Med Clin North Am* 77:1277, 1993.
120. Hershfield E: Tuberculosis: 9. Treatment, *CMAJ* 161:405-411, 1999.
121. Muthuswamy P et al: Prednisone as adjunctive therapy in the management of pulmonary tuberculosis: report of 12 cases and review of the literature, *Chest* 107:1621, 1995.
122. Schluger NW: Issues in the treatment of active tuberculosis in human immunodeficiency virus-infected patients, *Clin Infect Dis* 28:130-135, 1999.
123. Burman WJ, Gallicano K, Peloquin C: Therapeutic implications of drug interactions in the treatment of human immunodeficiency virus-related tuberculosis, *Clin Infect Dis* 28:419-430, 1999.
124. Waxman S, Gang M, Goldfrank L: Tuberculosis in the HIV-infected patient, *Emerg Med Clin North Am* 13:179, 1995.
125. Comstock GW: How much isoniazid is needed for prevention of tuberculosis among immunocompetent adults? *Int J Tuberc Lung Dis* 3:847-850, 1999.
126. O'Brien RJ: Drug-resistant tuberculosis: etiology, management and prevention, *Semin Respir Infect* 9:104, 1994.
127. Kent JH: The epidemiology of multidrug-resistant tuberculosis in the United States, *Med Clin North Am* 77:1391, 1993.
128. Frieden TR et al: The emergence of drug-resistant tuberculosis in New York City, *N Engl J Med* 328:521, 1993.
129. Simone PM, Dooley SW: The phenomenon of multidrug-resistant tuberculosis. In Rossman MD, MacGregor RR, editors: *Tuberculosis: clinical management and new challenges,* New York, 1995, McGraw-Hill.
130. Ellner JJ: Multidrug-resistant tuberculosis, *Adv Intern Med* 40:155, 1995.
131. Daley CL et al: An outbreak of tuberculosis with accelerated progression among persons infected with the human immunodeficiency virus, *N Engl J Med* 326:231, 1992.
132. Small PM et al: Exogenous reinfection with multidrug-resistant *Mycobacterium tuberculosis* in patients with advanced HIV infection, *N Engl J Med* 328:1137, 1993.
133. Bloch AB et al: Nationwide survey of drug-resistant tuberculosis in the United States, *JAMA* 271:665, 1994.
134. Goble M et al: Treatment of 171 patients with pulmonary tuberculosis resistant to isoniazid and rifampin, *N Engl J Med* 328:527, 1993.
135. Fischl MA et al: Clinical presentation and outcome of patients with HIV infection and tuberculosis caused by multiple-drug-resistant bacilli, *Ann Intern Med* 117:184, 1992.
136. Telzak EE et al: Multidrug-resistant tuberculosis in patients without HIV infection, *N Engl J Med* 333:907, 1995.
137. Pearson ML et al: Nosocomial transmission of multidrug-resistant *Mycobacterium tuberculosis* a risk to patients and health care workers, *Ann Intern Med* 17:191, 1992.
138. Ben-Dov I, Mason GR: Drug-resistant tuberculosis in a southern California Hospital: trends from 1969 to 1984, *Am Rev Respir Dis* 135:1307, 1987.
139. Maloney SA et al: Efficacy of control measures in preventing nosocomial transmission of multidrug-resistant tuberculosis to patients and health care workers, *Ann Intern Med* 122:90, 1995.
140. Moran GJ et al: Tuberculosis infection-control practices in United States emergency departments, *Ann Emerg Med* 26:283, 1995.
141. Sokolove PE et al: Exposure of emergency department personnel to tuberculosis: PPD testing during an epidemic in the community, *Ann Emerg Med* 24:418, 1994.
142. Griffith DE et al: Tuberculosis outbreak among healthcare workers in a community hospital, *Am J Respir Crit Care Med* 152:808, 1995.
143. Moran GJ et al: Delayed recognition and infection control for tuberculosis patients in the emergency department, *Ann Emerg Med* 26:290, 1995.
144. Wenger PN et al: Control of nosocomial transmission of multidrug-resistant *Mycobactrium tuberculosis* among healthcare workers and HIV-infected patients, *Lancet* 345:235, 1995.
145. Jarvis WR et al: Respirators, recommendations, and regulations: the controversy surrounding protection of health care workers from tuberculosis, *Ann Intern Med* 122:142, 1995.
146. Stead WW: Management of health care workers after inadvertent exposure to tuberculosis: a guide for the use of preventive therapy, *Ann Intern Med* 122:906, 1995.
147. Colditz GA et al: Efficacy of BCG vaccine in the prevention of tuberculosis. Meta-analysis of the published literature, *JAMA* 271: 698, 1994.
148. Brewer TF, Colditz GA: Bacille Calmette-Guerin vaccination for the prevention of tuberculosis in health care workers, *Clin Infect Dis* 20:136, 1995.
149. Joint Tuberculosis Committee: Control and prevention of tuberculosis in the United Kingdom: code of practice 1994, *Thorax* 49:1193, 1994.

130 Bone and Joint Infections

Brian J. Zink
Jim Edward Weber

PERSPECTIVE

Historically, bone and joint infections have been described in grim terms. *Aids to Surgery,* written in 1919, notes that "acute infective osteomyelitis . . . is a very fatal disease." With septic arthritis "the patient becomes exhausted from toxaemia or pyemia," and "ankylosis is the usual most favourable termination."[1] Advances in diagnostic methods, surgical techniques, and the development of antibiotics have resulted in much better outcomes. In the case of bone infections, the mortality rate has decreased from 15% to 25% in the preantibiotic era to less than 2% today.[2] However, with such advances come new challenges. The type of infections that are encountered today are changing, and management of bone and joint infections is becoming more complex. Emergency physicians must consider many subsets of patients who are at increased risk of infection, including intravenous (IV) drug abusers, patients with acquired immunodeficiency syndrome (AIDS), postsurgical patients, and patients with iatrogenic immunosuppression.[3,4]

The overall occurrence of bone and joint infections appears to have remained constant over the last 3 decades.[5] The incidence of bone infections in hospital patients is approximately 1%. In the United States, the incidence of osteomyelitis in children under the age of 13 is 1 in 5,000, while septic arthritis ranges from 5.5 to 12 per 100,000 individuals.[6] Global epidemiologic data regarding community acquired bone and joint infections in adults vary significantly, with an overall higher incidence in developing countries.

Bone infections show a bimodal age distribution, occurring most commonly in people under 20 or over 50 years old. Joint infections have a similar distribution.[7] No known correlation exists between socioeconomic factors or race and the incidence of bone and joint infections. In children, boys have an increased susceptibility to bone infections, with most series reporting a male/female ratio of 2 to 3:1. Joint infections in the pediatric age group may be slightly more common in boys. In children, bone and joint infections usually occur in previously healthy individuals. The opposite is true in adults in whom risk factors can usually be identified that predispose to both bone and joint infection.

Infectious processes are generally designated as acute, subacute, or chronic. Orthopedic infections are also classified according to the site of involvement and include osseous (osteomyelitis), articular (septic or suppurative arthritis), bursal (septic bursitis), subcutaneous (cellulitis or abscess), muscular (infectious myositis or abscess, and tendinous (infectious tendinitis or tenosynovitis) varieties. The word *osteomyelitis* literally means inflammation of the marrow of the bone, but the term is used to refer to infection in any part of the bone. *Chronic* osteomyelitis may be defined as a bone infection lasting for more than 6 weeks.Septic arthritis is infection of a joint by bacterial or fungal organisms. Bacterial arthritis is sometimes called pyogenic or suppurative arthritis. Several common infectious processes can result in a sterile, secondary inflammation of joints, which is called reactive arthritis. Reactive arthritis is not classified as septic arthritis, but is far more common than septic arthritis. In children, it may occur after infection with human parvovirus, rubella, chickenpox, and probably other viruses. Occasionally, post-infectious arthritis develops after group A streptococcal infection.

Regardless of the anatomic location, the mechanism of contamination with osteomyelitis occurs by one of three routes: (1) hematogenous seeding, (2) seeding from a contiguous source of infection, or (3) direct inoculation of the bone, from surgery or trauma. Recognition of the etiologic mechanism of osteomyelitis may help to guide management and assist in the interpretation of diagnostic imaging examinations.

Septic arthritis usually results from hematogenous migration of bacteria into the joint. In some cases, septic arthritis may result from spread from a contiguous source of infection or by direct inoculation of bacteria. Direct inoculation can result from penetrating trauma or joint aspiration. It is important to consider that septic arthritis may occur concomitantly with osteomyelitis, with infection spreading from bone to joint, and vice versa.

PRINCIPLES OF DISEASE

Bones are comprised of an outer shell, or cortex, of compact bone, and an inner framework of trabeculae, called cancellous, spongy, or medullary bone. On a microscopic level, compact bone is comprised of structural units called haversian systems that are made up of concentric rings of osteocytes. Osteocytes synthesize and maintain the bony matrix. The central haversian canals run parallel to the long axis of the bone and contain the blood supply and reticular connective tissue for the haversian system. Cancellous bone consists of irregular branching trabeculae that enclose marrow cavities. Long bones consist of a diaphysis, or shaft, and two ends, called epiphyses, which communicate with other bones. The metaphysis is the region between the diaphysis and epiphysis (Figure 130-1).

Joints are enclosed within a capsule that consists of two layers. The outer layer is dense fibrous tissue that interweaves with ligaments and the periosteum of articulating bones. The inner layer is the synovial membrane that is made up of secretory cells sitting on a loose fibrous stroma. The synovial membrane extends beyond the epiphysis and attaches to the metaphysis. Because of this special anatomic relationship, infection in the metaphysis femur or humerus may spread more easily into the joint.[8]

In osteomyelitis the suppurative process extends linearly in haversian canals, and local necrosis of bony trabeculae occurs. Infection may proceed laterally through Volkmann's

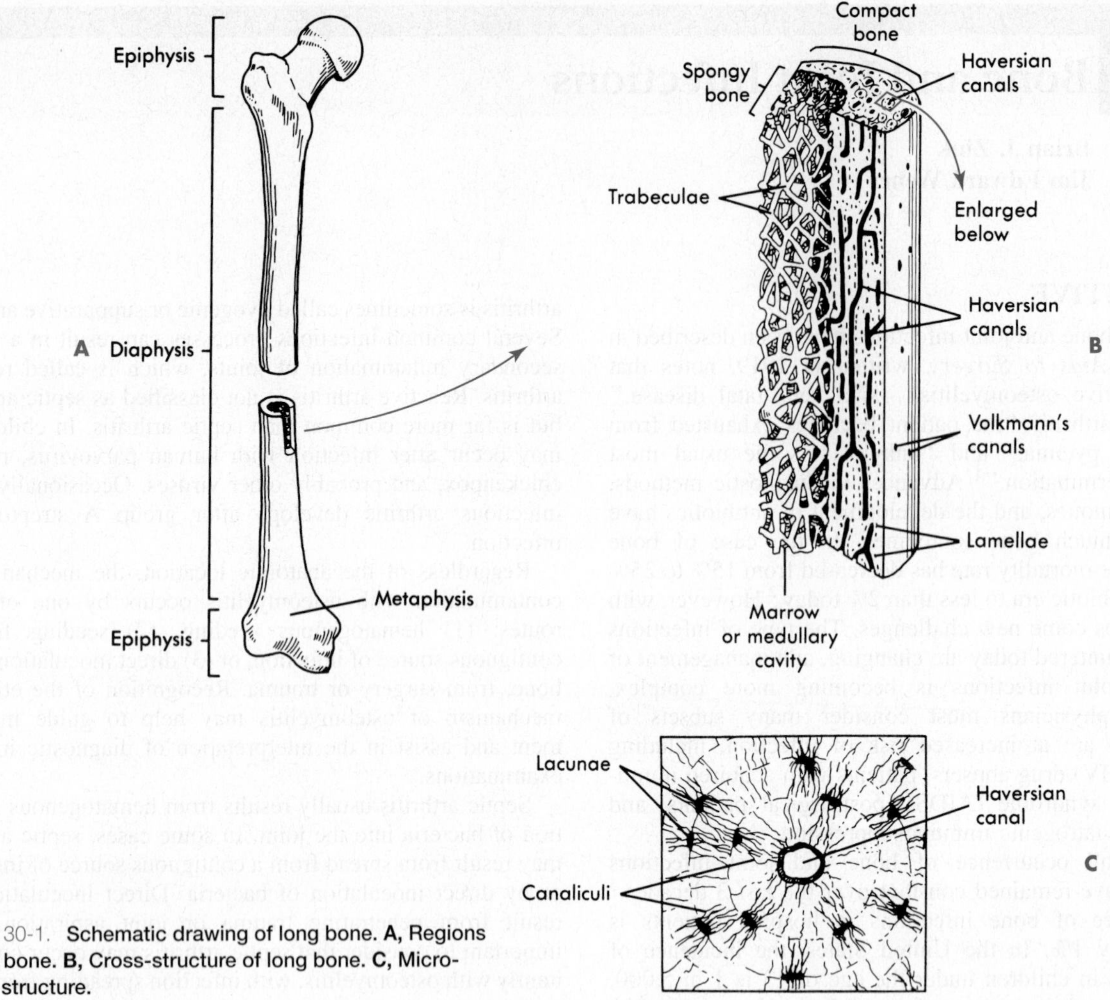

Figure 130-1. **Schematic drawing of long bone. A, Regions of long bone. B, Cross-structure of long bone. C, Microscopic structure.**

canals, which are small channels that run perpendicularly to the haversian canal, and reach the subperiosteal space. As edema and the infectious infiltrate occlude blood supply, larger segments of bone begin to die. In children the lateral spread of infection in the long bone results in a subperiosteal abscess. The periosteum is stimulated, and vigorous formation of new periosteum occurs. This new growth is called an *involucrum.* In adults the periosteum is more firmly adherent to the underlying cortex and has less osteoblastic activity. The formation of subperiosteal abscesses and involucrum is much less common in adult osteomyelitis.[9] If osteomyelitis proceeds unchecked, ischemic segments of bone may disengage from surrounding bone. These separated sections are called *sequestra* and occur only in advanced or chronic osteomyelitis. Pathologic fractures may occur through these areas of devascularized bone. Unchecked chronic osteomyelitis can lead to the development of fistulas that track out to the skin.

Hematogenous osteomyelitis develops when blood-borne bacteria are deposited in bone. This is most common in children and in adults with vertebral osteomyelitis. The pathologic features of hematogenous osteomyelitis differ in the infant, child, and adult. These differences are related, in part, to the particular vascular anatomy of the tubular bones that is evident in each of these three age groups. In the first year of life, arterial vessels from the metaphysis perforate the epiphyseal growth plate and terminate in the epiphysis in venous sinusoids. This communication allows osteomyelitis to advance readily from the metaphysis to the epiphysis and adjacent joint space in infants. After the first year of life there is no longer a vascular connection between the metaphyseal and epiphyseal areas. The metaphyseal arteries end in loops that abut the growth plate. The epiphyseal growth plate is avascular and inhibits the spread of infection to the epiphysis and joint. In the adult, after the closure of the epiphyseal plate, anastomoses form between the metaphyseal and epiphyseal blood vessels, and infection can once again spread from metaphysis to epiphysis and eventually into the synovium and joint space.[2,7,8,10]

A number of local and humoral factors that play a role in determining whether bacteremia progresses to significant skeletal infection are largely unknown. Some sites in the skeletal system are more likely than others to become colonized by bacteria. Bones containing slow-moving venous systems or venous sinusoids, such as the metaphyses of long bones and the vertebral bodies, have increased susceptibility to hematogenous osteomyelitis. In the metaphysis, a relative lack of phagocytic cells in the venous capillaries and sinusoids may further predispose to infection.[2] In the synovial membrane the existence of a deep venous plexus that also has sluggish blood flow may invite deposition of bacteria. The synovium, however, lacks a basement membrane, thus allowing bacteria to penetrate and bind to the exposed surfaces of articular cartilage, bone, and prosthetic devices. A biofilm of polysaccharides is rapidly formed. This film promotes adherence of other bacteria and colony formation.[11,12]

When bacteria begin to destroy bone or the synovium, a dramatic response from local tissues occurs. The surrounding capillaries dilate and become more permeable in response to chemical signals from bacterial toxins or to the release of histamine, bradykinins, and serotonin from damaged cells. Plasma fluids and protein and leukocytes pour into the area.[11-14] Complement proteins play an important role in the response to infection. The activation of complement proteins can occur directly from bacterial accumulation, or via antigen-antibody complexes. Complement proteins enhance the leukocytic response through chemotaxis and opsonization of bacteria. The neutrophil and monocyte (macrophage) are the active cells in phagocytosis of bacteria. Unfortunately, leukocyte migration results in the release of neutrophil elastases, which augment the destruction of the cartilage matrix within the joint.[12] Pressure necrosis from accumulation of purulent synovial fluid may also compromise the synovium and cartilage. Monocytes and T lymphocytes may be less numerous in the cellular response, but have an important role in the production of cytokines, such as tumor necrosis factor and interleukins 1 and 2. Cytokines modulate the sustained inflammatory response to infection.[12-15]

The humoral immune response to bone or joint infection is usually well developed by the time the infection is clinically apparent. B lymphocytes sense bacterial antigens and release antibodies, and an antigen-antibody complex is formed at the site of infection. Via the complement cascade, bacteria are destroyed by neutrophils or macrophages. Bacterial toxins may be destroyed directly by bound antibody.[11-15]

Tissue injury in bone or joint infections can occur by several different mechanisms. Direct tissue destruction by invasive bacteria is the initial insult. After this, microabscesses and edema in infected tissues may lead to vascular occlusion and ischemic necrosis, which is most damaging in the venous capillaries of the metaphysis, where no collateral blood vessels exist to compensate for ischemic injury. If immune complexes become embedded in the bone or cartilage matrix, a prolonged inflammatory response can occur even after the primary infection has been cleared. This is particularly a problem in joints, where articular cartilage can be destroyed. A final type of tissue injury caused by infection is abnormal synthesis of bone or joint matrix and cells. Abnormally synthesized bone or cartilage may be structurally unsound and function poorly.[8,15]

Although hematogenous spread is the most common means of acquiring osteomyelitis in skeletally immature patients, osteomyelitis in the appendicular skeleton of adults occurs more commonly by either spread of the pathogens from a contiguous source of infection or direct implantation. The direction of contamination for contiguous source osteomyelitis is from the soft tissues inward into the bone, and the pathogen is disseminated via haversian and Volkmann's canals to the bone marrow. This is the opposite of hematogenous osteomyelitis, where infection starts in the medullary bone and progresses outward to involve the surrounding structures. The most common sites of this contiguous source osteomyelitis are in the foot and hand. Other common sites affected by this mechanism of infection include the skull, maxilla, and mandible; these osseous infections are usually related to sinus disease and poor dental hygiene.

Most infections caused by direct implantation of bacteria into bones are caused by deep puncture wounds and tend to occur in the hands and feet. Animal bites are another cause of infections that can result in osteomyelitis. Although cats account for only 10% of animal bites, significant infection results from 20% to 50% of cat bites versus only 5% of dog bites. Most human bite injuries are related to fist fights, with the metacarpophalangeal joints representing the most common region of osteomyelitis and secondary joint infection. Osteomyelitis from direct implantation of pathogens can occur with open fractures, and during surgical instrumentation. Artificial joints and other implanted surgical materials can serve as sites for colonization of bacteria.[16,17]

In septic arthritis, infection most likely occurs first in the synovium and then extends into joint fluid, and finally to articular cartilage. The synovial membrane responds to infection by increasing synovial fluid production, resulting in a large joint effusion. Septic arthritis is a closed space infection, and increasing pressure in the joint contributes to a decreased rate of exchange of solutes across the synovial lining. The resultant slow diffusion of nutrients across the synovial membrane may limit the growth of bacteria and may cause bacteria to enter a dormant state. Dormant bacteria may have increased resistance to levels of antibiotics that would normally be bactericidal.[8,13,14]

The most important factor that determines morbidity from septic arthritis is the degree of articular cartilage destruction. Once destroyed, hyaline (articular) cartilage cannot be replaced. Synovial cells and polymorphonuclear leukocytes (PMNs) release lysosomal enzymes into joint fluid. These enzymes contain collagenase and elastase, both of which may degrade cartilage. Other structures that are enclosed within or adjacent to synovium, such as bursae, tendons, and bone, may become damaged in septic arthritis.[8,11-15]

ETIOLOGY AND MICROBIOLOGY OF BONE AND JOINT INFECTIONS

Certain underlying disease states predispose a patient to acquiring bone and joint infections. These conditions include diabetes mellitus, sickle cell disease, AIDS, alcoholism and IV drug abuse (IVDA), chronic corticosteroid use, preexisting joint disease, and other immunosuppressed states. Common to most of the diseases that predispose to bone and joint infections are a decreased ability to mount an inflammatory and immune response, impaired bacterial killing, and poor vasculature. Another subset of patients who are susceptible to bone and joint infections are postsurgical patients—especially those who have had prosthetic devices implanted. In children an association may exist between prior respiratory illness or minor extremity trauma and the development of bone and joint infections.[11,18]

Although most serious bone and joint infections are bacterial, on rare occasions, viruses, fungi, and parasites may be the responsible pathogens.The microbiology of osteomyelitis and septic arthritis is a function of several host and environmental factors. Age is an important variable in determining the bacteria that cause bone and joint infections. A patient's bacterial milieu has some role in determining the incidence of bone and joint infections. For example, people living in crowded conditions where tuberculosis is prevalent are at increased risk for tubercular bone and joint infections.

Elderly patients in hospitals and institutions may be more susceptible to infections with gram-negative bacteria.[7,19] The following points deserve special mention:

1. In all age groups except neonates, *Staphylococcus aureus* is the leading cause of osteomyelitis. It also accounts for more cases of septic arthritis than any other bacterium. In neonates, group B streptococci are common infecting bacteria in bone and joint infections.
2. Before vaccine introduction, *Haemophilus influenzae* type B caused up to 34% of septic arthritis and 13% of osteomyelitis in children under 2 years old.[20] However, since the introduction of the vaccine, *H. influenzae* b has essentially disappeared as a pathogen in hematogenous osteomyelitis and septic arthritis among vaccinated children.[20-22] Another gram-negative coccobacillus within the Neisseriaceae family, *Kingella kingae,* has become more common than *Haemophilus* in causing bone and joint infections in children.[23] *K. kingae* can be part of the normal flora of the nasopharynx, which like *H. influenzae,* can be spread hematogenously to bones and joints. It is a fastidious organism and may be mistaken for *Haemophilus* or *Neisseria* species.[23]
3. Gonococcal arthritis is the most common type of septic arthritis in individuals under 30 years old.
4. In elderly people, gram-negative bacteria account for a higher percentage of cases of bone and joint infections than in younger people.[19]
5. Methicillin-resistant *S. aureus* (MRSA), methicillin-resistant *Staphylococcus epidermidis,* and vancomycin-resistant enterococci (VREC) have emerged as a significant microbiologic problem in the past decade. Multiresistant enterococci pose the greatest potential danger in that no currently available regimen is reliably bactericidal against such organisms.[24]

A typical case of hematogenous osteomyelitis or septic arthritis is caused by a single type of bacterium. In some situations polymicrobial infection is more likely to occur. These include diabetic foot osteomyelitis, posttraumatic osteomyelitis, chronic osteomyelitis, and chronic septic arthritis. Overall, polymicrobial osteomyelitis occurs in 36% to 50% of reported cases.[25] Anaerobic bacteria can complicate polymicrobial infection and may be present in bone and joint infections more often than is commonly recognized. In chronic osteomyelitis, anaerobic bacteria may be present in up to 40% of cases. Culture techniques that are inadequate for isolating anaerobic bacteria may lead to underreporting of infections caused by these agents.[26]

Pseudomonas bacteria are responsible for bone and joint infections in three main settings. The first is in puncture wounds to the foot. *Pseudomonas* does not appear to grow on puncture objects, but rather is intimately associated with shoe gear that may be inoculated into the wound and produce soft-tissue infection and osteomyelitis.[16] Patients in whom prosthetic devices are implanted during orthopedic surgery are at risk for *Pseudomonas* bone and joint infection. IV drug users may develop hematogenous osteomyelitis, often in the spine, from *Pseudomonas* bacteria.[27]

Certain types of trauma may predispose patients to osteomyelitis by particular bacteria. Patients who are wounded or receive open fractures in fresh water are susceptible to infection with the gram-negative bacillus *Aeromonas hydrophila.*[28] People who are bitten by animals, particularly dogs and cats, are at risk for developing osteomyelitis from *Pasteurella multocida.*[17]

Tuberculosis (TB) may occur in bones and joints. The two most common forms of skeletal infection are vertebral osteomyelitis (Pott's disease) and tubercular arthritis. The arthritis of TB is a chronic, low-grade inflammatory process that resembles rheumatoid arthritis more than acute septic arthritis.[29]

Fungal infections have become more common in hospitalized patients because of the use of broad-spectrum antibiotics, immunosuppressive medications, invasive monitoring devices, and total parenteral alimentation. Fungal organisms are responsible for less than 1% of cases of osteomyelitis, but the number of cases reported is increasing. *Candida* osteomyelitis occurs through hematogenous spread or as a postoperative wound infection. Fungal bone infection is indolent and may go through periods of activity and remission.[30] *Aspergillus* has been reported to cause osteomyelitis in vertebrae, hip prostheses, and ribs. In adults the infection is hematogenous. In children *Aspergillus* osteomyelitis is most common in those with prior granulomatous disease and spreads from a primary pulmonary infection. Blastomycosis is usually a pulmonary infection, but the systemic form of the disease has a 14% to 60% incidence of skeletal involvement.[31,32] Similarly, cryptococcal skeletal infection occurs in approximately 10% of patients with the disseminated form of the disease.[33]

Patients with human immunodeficiency virus (HIV) are predisposed to a variety of common and opportunistic pathogens that may cause infections in the bones and joints. One unusual, but particularly characteristic, form of osteomyelitis in HIV-positive patients is bacillary angiomatosis. Bacillary angiomatosis is a gram-negative rickettsia-like organism that frequently leads to osteolytic bone lesions.[34,35]

CLINICAL FEATURES OF OSTEOMYELITIS

Diagnosis

History and Physical Examination The symptoms and signs of osteomyelitis in adults are predictable, although not always present. The predominant symptom is pain over the affected bone. If the leg is involved, the patient will commonly limp; children may refuse to use the limb at all. Localized warmth, swelling, and erythema may be noted by the patient. Fever is inconsistently present, although it is more common in children with osteomyelitis than in adults. Systemic complaints of headache, fatigue, malaise, and anorexia are often reported.

The patient usually does not appear ill. Examination of the involved bone elicits point tenderness over the infected segment. Palpable warmth and soft-tissue swelling with erythema may be present, but these findings are variable. Because osteomyelitis has a propensity to occur in the metaphyses of long bones, it is often difficult to distinguish infection in bone from infection in the neighboring joint. Adding to the confusion, a sympathetic effusion in the adjacent joint may develop in some patients with osteomyelitis who have no joint involvement. In chronic advanced osteomyelitis, the involucrum or sequestrum may be palpated, and sinus tracts that drain through the skin may be noted.

DIAGNOSTIC STRATEGIES

Laboratory Data and Diagnostic Imaging

Laboratory data in patients with osteomyelitis are generally not helpful in establishing a diagnosis. The white blood cell (WBC) count is often, although not always, elevated. Typical values in osteomyelitis range from normal to 15,000/mm^3. The erythrocyte sedimentation rate (ESR) is more helpful than the WBC count. It is a sensitive marker for bone infection; many series report elevated ESRs in more than 90% of patients who have confirmed osteomyelitis.[35] The mean ESR in one large pediatric review was 70 mm/hr. Fewer than 8% of patients with osteomyelitis will have an ESR less than 15 mm/hr. An elevated ESR in the presence of appropriate physical findings should alert the emergency physician to pursue aggressively the diagnosis of osteomyelitis, but a normal or slightly elevated ESR does not eliminate the diagnosis. The ESR is most valuable in following response to treatment. Typically, the ESR falls steadily as osteomyelitis resolves, and increases should it recur.[36] C-reactive protein (CRP), another nonspecific marker of inflammation, may have some use in evaluating patients with bone infections. CRP increases within the first 24 hours of infection, peaks within approximately 48 hours, and is usually normal within 1 week of therapy.[36-38]

Conventional radiography remains the initial imaging test of choice for suspected osteomyelitis. Radiography is readily available, relatively inexpensive, and useful in eliminating other disease entities. In addition, plain radiography is often a helpful adjunct in correctly interpreting secondary imaging studies. Unfortunately, radiography is insensitive to the detection of early osteomyelitis, thereby limiting its utility. Soft tissue edema may be present within 3 to 5 days from the onset of infection. However, fewer than one third of patients have abnormalities on plain radiographs in the first 7 to 10 days after the onset of symptoms. Before lucent areas can be detected radiographically, 30% to 50% of bone mineral must be lost. In more advanced cases, radiographs are helpful. By 28 days from the onset of disease, 90% of the plain radiographs are positive.[39,40] The characteristic early findings on the plain radiograph in osteomyelitis are lucent lytic areas of cortical bone destruction (Figure 130-2). Periosteal reaction is another early sign. It may appear as hypertrophy, or elevation of the periosteum (involucrum) (Figure 130-3). These early periosteal changes are more commonly seen in children than in adults. In advanced disease the lytic lesions are surrounded by dense, sclerotic bone, and sequestra may be noted. Special attention to radiographic appearance of the soft tissues is important in diagnosing osteomyelitis in its early stages. Deep soft-tissue swelling, distorted fascial planes, and altered fat interfaces can be a clue to osteomyelitis in the underlying bone. Because radiographic resolution may lag behind clinical resolution, radiographs are also not helpful in tracking the course of osteomyelitis.[41]

Radionuclide skeletal scintigraphy (bone scanning) is more useful than plain radiographs in the early diagnosis of osteomyelitis. Radionuclide scans can detect osteomyelitis within 48 to 72 hours after the onset of infection. A radioactive tracer is injected into the bloodstream and given time to bind or accumulate in body tissues. A γ-camera or collimator is used to sense released radioactivity, and an image is created that is evaluated for increase or decrease in expected uptake of the radionuclide.

In the ED setting, the most commonly used radionuclide for skeletal scintigraphy is technetium methylene diphosphonate (^{99m}Tc MDP). Technetium-labeled diphosphonates bind to the hydroxyapatite crystals in the bone matrix. The greatest uptake is in immature bone that has increased osteoblastic activity. The standard ^{99m}Tc MDP scan currently is a

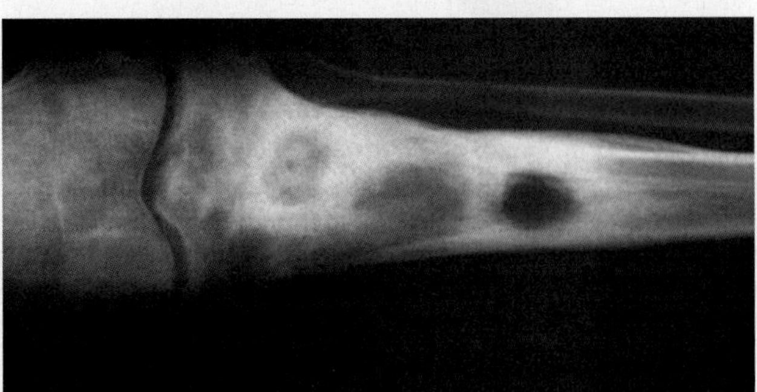

Figure 130-2. **Plain radiograph of tibia. Lucent areas in metaphysis are sites of advanced osteomyelitis. *Courtesy Department of Radiology, University of Cincinnati Medical Center.***

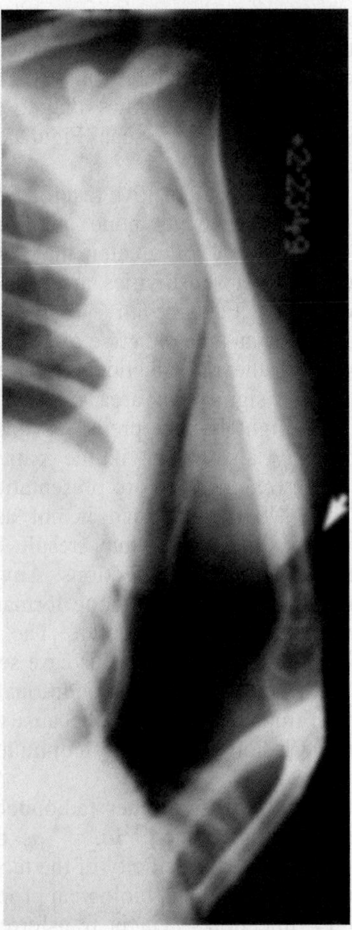

Figure 130-3. **Plain radiograph of humerus. Distal portion of humerus has involucrum formation, representing advanced case of osteomyelitis. *Courtesy Department of Radiology, University of Cincinnati Medical Center.***

Table 130-1. Diagnostic Use of the Three-Phase ^{99m}Tc MDP Bone Scan

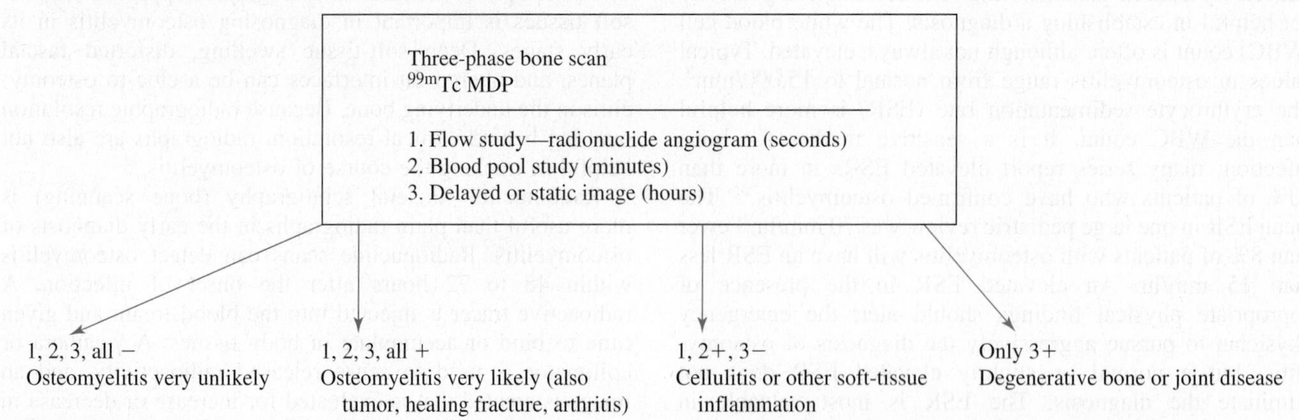

Three-phase bone scan
^{99m}Tc MDP
1. Flow study—radionuclide angiogram (seconds)
2. Blood pool study (minutes)
3. Delayed or static image (hours)
1, 2, 3, all −
Osteomyelitis very unlikely
1, 2, 3, all +
Osteomyelitis very likely (also tumor, healing fracture, arthritis)
1, 2+, 3−
Cellulitis or other soft-tissue inflammation
Only 3+
Degenerative bone or joint disease

Modified from Demopulos GA, Bleck EE, McDougall IR: Role of radionuclide imaging in the diagnosis of acute osteomyelitis, *J Pediatr Orthop* 8(5):558, 1988.

three-phase process. After injection of the ^{99m}Tc MDP, images are obtained within 60 seconds. This is called the radionuclide angiogram and represents the relative blood flow to the area of concern. The second phase involves imaging of the "blood pool" of ^{99m}Tc MDP at 5 to 15 minutes after injection. The third phase is the delayed or static image that is obtained 2 to 4 hours after injection. Areas of osteomyelitis show increased uptake on all three phases of ^{99m}Tc MDP scintigraphy.[42,43] Table 130-1 shows diagnostic categories based on ^{99m}Tc MDP three-phase scan. Figure 130-4 shows a positive ^{99m}Tc MDP scan.

The ^{99m}Tc MDP scan is a sensitive test for osteomyelitis in patients who have no existing bone abnormalities. Most series report a sensitivity of greater than 90% with the three-phase scan. Lower sensitivities are found in cases of neonatal osteomyelitis. False-negative scans are possible if pressure and edema in an area of active osteomyelitis prevent vascular delivery of the radionuclide. The resulting "cold spot" may actually signify an area of aggressive active osteomyelitis but might be interpreted as negative. False-negative scans may also occur if the patient has been receiving antibiotic treatment before presentation. The specificity of a ^{99m}Tc MDP bone scan is not as high as its sensitivity. False-positive scans may result from trauma, surgery, tumors, or soft-tissue infections. Any process that encourages inflammation and new bone formation can be a site of increased uptake of radionuclide. The false-positive rate has been as high as 64% in various case series.[37,38,43] A four-phase ^{99m}Tc MDP study with (an additional) image at 24 hours may further improve specificity, because the amount of activity within the lesion theoretically continues to increase with time.[44]

Additional testing with two other radionuclides, gallium citrate ^{67}Ga and indium oxine ^{111}In,[42,44] is often used to compensate for the limited specificity of the technetium-99m scans. Gallium has chemical and biological properties similar to iron. After IV injection, ^{67}Ga is transferred by plasma proteins (transferrin and lactoferrin) to the membranes of bacteria and neutrophils, and thus accumulates in areas of acute inflammation where WBC concentrations are high. Gallium-67, however, is not very specific for infection. Gallium's fixation to PMNs can give false positive results in

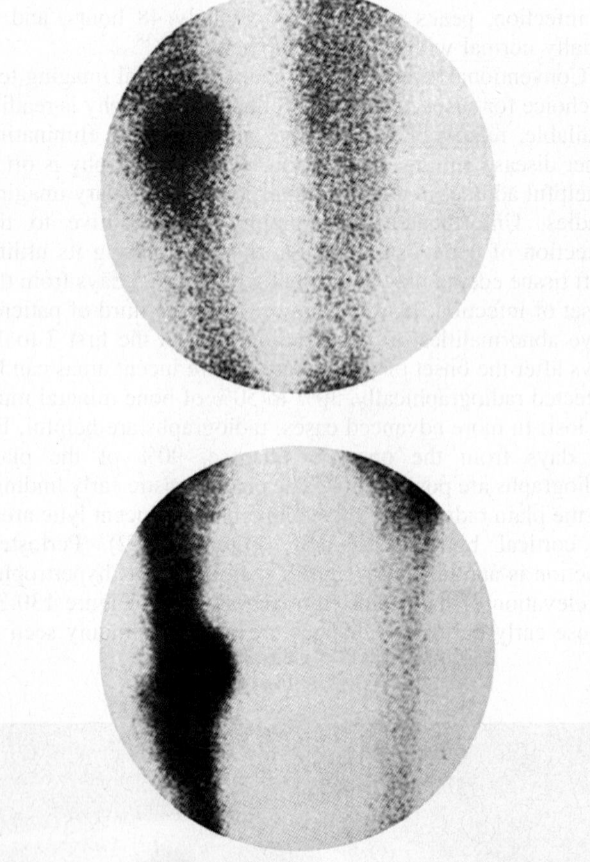

Figure 130-4. **Example of gallium *(top)* and technetium *(bottom)* bone scans in advanced osteomyelitis of tibial metaphysis. Both scans show increased radionuclide uptake. *Courtesy EB Silberstein, Department of Nuclear Medicine, University of Cincinnati.***

inflammatory processes such as rheumatoid arthritis as well as certain neoplasms. This test must be used with caution in patients treated with antibiotics because a false-negative result may occur.[46] When the test is combined with technetium-99, diagnosis of osteomyelitis is considered positive if the gallium-67 uptake is greater than the technetium-99 uptake in the suspected region.[47,48] Overall, the combination of gallium-67 and technetium-99 MDP for establishing a diagnosis of osteomyelitis has a sensitivity of approximately 70% and a specificity of 83% to 93%. The disadvantages of ^{67}Ga for emergency use are the 24- to 48-hour delay in obtaining a final image and the low specificity of the test (see Figure 130-4).[42,47]

^{111}In-labeled WBC scans, when used with technetium-99m, provide added specificity to identify specific sites of infection. These studies are usually reserved for those situations where bone scan findings are equivocal or normal, and osteomyelitis is still a likely consideration. The ^{111}In-labeled WBC scan can distinguish infected bone from bone that has increased turnover from fractures, surgery, prostheses, osteoarthropathy, and tumor. This procedure involves incubating 40 to 60 ml of whole blood with the radionuclide for 2 hours and reinjecting the labeled WBCs. Radiolabeled neutrophils then migrate to areas of infection. Images are obtained at 24 hours. Some investigators also use a 5-hour image that is obtained at the same time as a concurrent ^{99m}Tc MDP delayed image.[49] Labeled leukocytes accumulate only where there is active infection. The disadvantage for emergency use is the delay in final imaging and interpretation. Also, the large amount of blood required for labeling, as well as the high radiation burden, may preclude its use in infants and children.[40,42,47,49]

Recently, the use of technetium-99 hexamethylpropyleneamine oxime (HMPAO)-labeled leukocytes has been popularized in children, because the radiation burden and half-life are significantly shorter than that of indium-111 tagged WBCs. In addition, image acquisition occurs within 4 hours, allowing for earlier diagnosis. Additional studies are necessary to determine the role of HMPAO in imaging of bone infection.[50]

Computed tomography (CT) and magnetic resonance imaging (MRI) are usually considered when there is an indication of localized disease on physical examination or bone scan.[50-52] CT is most commonly used to detect and define areas of possible infection in bones that have a complex anatomy and that are difficult to visualize on plain radiographs and bone scans. The sternum, vertebrae, pelvic bones, and calcaneus are nicely imaged with a CT scan. Osteomyelitis appears as rarefaction, or lucent areas, on the CT scan images. Gas may be seen in bony abscess cavities. The limitation of CT scans for early diagnosis of osteomyelitis is the same as that for plain radiographs. The disease must be present for more than a week for changes to be apparent. An important role of a CT scan in osteomyelitis is to help localize bony lesions that have been found on bone scan. The CT scan can guide the surgeon in debridement and resection of infected bone and in choosing a site for diagnostic bone biopsy.[40]

The anatomic resolution of an MRI scan is far superior to that of bone scans. Soft-tissue contrast is also much greater with the MRI scan than with plain radiographs or the CT scan. An MRI scan is comparable to skeletal scintigraphy in terms of early detection of osteomyelitis. Osteomyelitis produces a diminished intensity of the normal marrow signal on T_1-weighted images and a normal or increased signal on T_2-weighted images. Soft tissue edema, abscesses, and tracts are clearly shown on the MRI scan. Addition of an IV contrast agent such as gadolinium may further distinguish devitalized from normally perfused bone. Metal may sometimes cause distortion of the signal in the area adjacent to a joint prosthesis, but this does not exclude MRI scan in this group of patients (Figures 130-5 and 130-6).

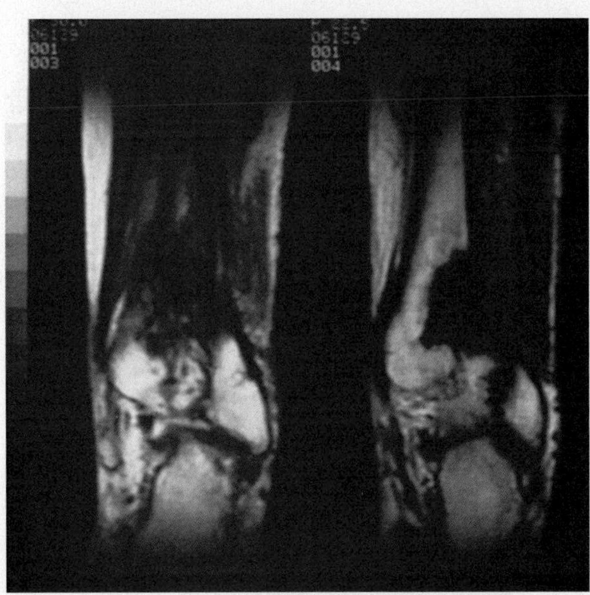

Figure 130-5. **MRI scan of the lower leg in a 32-year-old man, showing altered signal in the distal tibia, consistent with osteomyelitis.** ***Courtesy Department of Radiology, Albany Medical Center.***

Microbiologic Diagnosis

The most direct and often most effective way to diagnose osteomyelitis is to obtain infected bone by needle aspiration or surgical resection. Culture results can then determine specific antimicrobial therapy. Cultures of draining fistulae or sinus tracts are not an acceptable substitute because the organisms cultured from these sites are often different from those in the underlying infected bone.[39] Cultures for fungal and anaerobic organisms should always be obtained.

Particularly in cases of hematogenous osteomyelitis, cultures of blood, urine, cerebrospinal fluid (CSF), and pus from other sites of infection can help uncover the infecting bacteria. Blood cultures in patients with acute untreated osteomyelitis are positive for the offending bacteria approximately 50% of the time.[7] In pediatric patients with osteomyelitis, bacteria are cultured from two or more sources one third of the time.[5]

The likelihood of establishing a bacteriologic diagnosis in acute osteomyelitis is 80% to 90%, but in some cases, even culturing of resected bone yields no organism. Possible reasons for this are poor culture techniques and inadequate preparation of recovered tissue for culture, previous antibiotic treatment, and culturing from necrotic ischemic regions that may be devoid of bacteria.[39]

When the emergency physician is confronted with a patient with possible osteomyelitis, the diagnostic options can seem confusing. The algorithm in Figure 130-7 provides a simplified approach to diagnostic management of the patient with suspected osteomyelitis. A few key points should be considered when using this algorithm:

1. When there is little clinical support for a diagnosis of osteomyelitis and initial skeletal scintigraphy is nega-

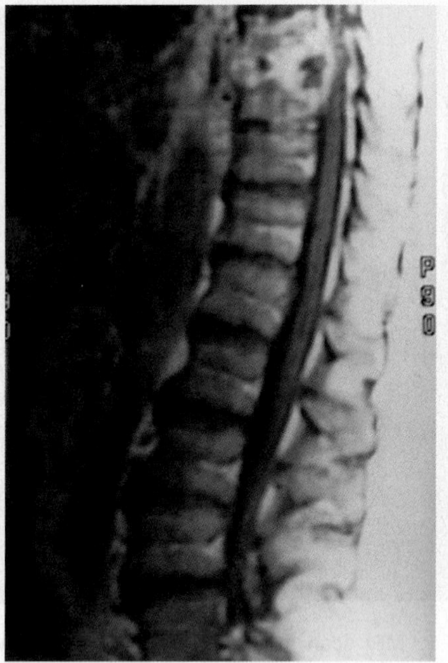

Figure 130-6. **Magnetic resonance image, T_1-weighted with gadolinium contrast, demonstrating increased signal in the eighth and ninth thoracic vertebrae and intervertebral disk, consistent with osteomyelitis and diskitis. The patient was a 71-year-old man with back pain. CT-guided biopsy of the lesion was culture positive for *Staphylococcus aureus*. *Courtesy University of Michigan Health System, Department of Radiology.***

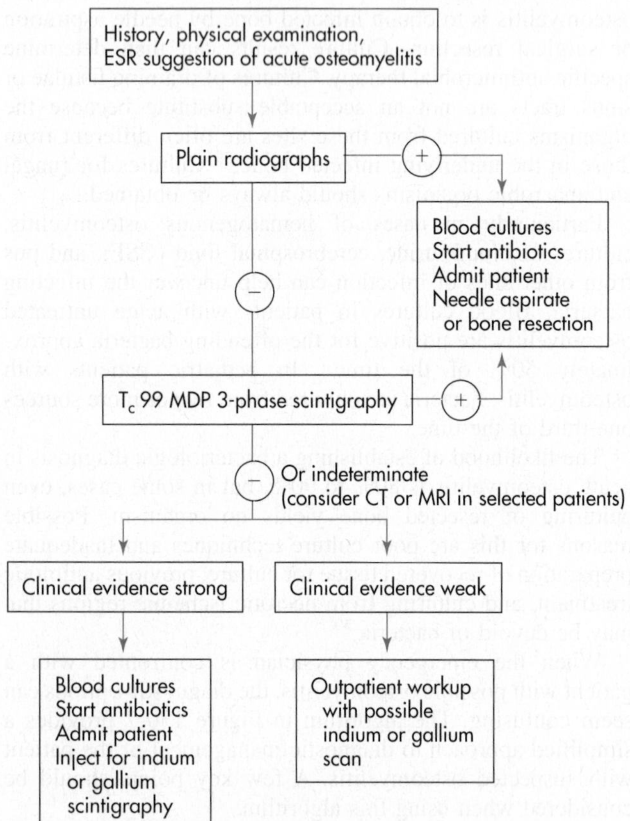

Figure 130-7. **An algorithm for use of imaging studies in ED diagnosis of osteomyelitis.**

tive, it is extremely unlikely that the patient has osteomyelitis.

2. In infants and children the amount of radiation exposure with imaging techniques must be considered.[54]
3. In easily accessible bones, aspiration is a low-risk procedure that will often establish a microbiologic diagnosis.
4. If the clinical presentation strongly suggests osteomyelitis, a lengthy diagnostic workup should not delay treatment. Cultures of blood, urine, and other appropriate sites should be obtained and antibiotic treatment started.[55]
5. The cost of imaging tests for osteomyelitis must be considered in deciding how to pursue the diagnosis. Expense must be weighed against the benefit of early diagnosis of osteomyelitis and the prevention of chronic osteomyelitis.[40]

Clinical Subsets of Osteomyelitis

In some circumstances, osteomyelitis may differ from the classic presentation of acute hematogenous osteomyelitis (AHO). This section reviews some of these special circumstances.

Osteomyelitis in Children Osteomyelitis in children is distinctly different from that in adults, and recommended management varies accordingly. Osteomyelitis in children tends to be acute and hematogenous and can often be treated with antibiotics alone. In contrast, osteomyelitis in adults is often subacute or chronic and is usually secondary to an open wound or as a complication of soft tissue disease. AHO is seen in children as young as 3 months and as old as 16 years. Bacteremia is the presumed cause of bone infection. *S. aureus* is the most common infecting organism in children of all ages except neonates (Table 130-2). Although longitudinal studies performed before or shortly after widespread implementation of the HiB vaccine continue to report *H. influenzae* as a common cause of AHO, the clinical community has witnessed near eradication of the organism.

AHO has a well-established male preponderance (male/female ratio of 2 to 3:1) and involves long bones approximately 80% of the time. The site of infection is usually the distal metaphysis, but up to 30% of AHO occurs in other parts of the bone. The epiphysis may be involved in a "subacute" type of osteomyelitis. Many children (approximately 30%) with AHO have antecedent minor trauma to the involved extremity or a recent upper respiratory illness (URI), although given the high incidence of minor trauma and URIs in this age range, the significance of these findings is unclear. Children with AHO may have fever, chills, vomiting, dehydration, and malaise; but they usually do not appear extremely ill. Most children have characteristic pain, limited use, and point tenderness in the involved limb. The diagnostic evaluation for AHO is listed in Figure 130-7. In 60% of patients with AHO, blood cultures are positive for the bacterial cause of osteomyelitis. A positive blood culture and a physical examination consistent with osteomyelitis may be sufficient to make a diagnosis of AHO. Figures 130-8 and 130-9 show a typical radiograph and bone scan, respectively, of AHO.[2,39,40,55,56]

Neonatal osteomyelitis is increasingly reported and may be difficult to diagnose because of minimal systemic findings. Neonatal osteomyelitis is more commonly seen after abnormal pregnancies or deliveries and often accompanies other

Table 130-2. Microbiology and Initial (Empiric) Antibiotic Treatment of Bone and Joint Infection

	Septic arthritis		Osteomyelitis	
Age group	**Common organisms**	**Antibiotic regimen**	**Common organisms**	**Antibiotic regimen**
Neonate to <3 months	*S. aureus* Group B streptococcus Enterobacteriaceae	PRP + Ceph 3 Alt: PRP + APAG If MRSA is prevalent, use vancomycin in place of PRP	*S. aureus* Group B streptococcus Enterobacteriaceae	PRP + Ceph 3 Alt: PRP + APAG If MRSA is prevalent, use vancomycin in place of PRP
3 months to 14 years	*S. aureus* Group A streptococcus *S. pneumoniae* *H. influenzae*	PRP + Ceph 3 Alt: Vancomycin + Ceph 3	*S. aureus* Group A streptococcus *H. influenzae*	PRP + Ceph 3 Alt: Vancomycin + Ceph 3, Chloramphenicol
14 years to adult	*S. aureus* Streptococcal sp. Enterobacteriaceae	PRP = Ceph 3 Alt: Vancomycin + Ceph 3 or PCN + aminoglycoside or Ceph 3	*S. aureus*	PRP Alt: Vancomycin
Infection subsets				
Sexually active adolescents or adults	*N. gonorrhoeae*	Ceph 3 Alt: Spectinomycin or Penicillin if sensitive		
Sickle cell disease			*Salmonella* sp.	Ceph 3 Alt: FLQ
Intravenous drug abuse	*P. aeruginosa, S. aureus,* Enterobacteriaceae	PRP + FLQ Alt: Vancomycin + FLQ	*S. aureus, P. aeruginosa* Enterobacteriaceae	PRP + FLQ Alt: Vancomycin + FLQ
Plantar puncture wound	*P. aeruginosa*	AP Ceph Alt: FLQ	*P. aeruginosa*	AP Ceph Alt: FLQ
HIV infection	*S. aureus, C. albicans,* Atypical organisms	PRP + Ceph 3, Consider TS and fluconazole or other antifungal	*S. aureus, C. albicans, B. henselae,* acute hematogenous osteomyelitis atypical organisms	PRP + Ceph 3, Consider TS and fluconazole or other antifungal
Human or animal bites	*E. corrodens, P. multocida*	Penicillin +/− AC Alt: Ceph 3, TS	*E. corrodens, P. multocida*	Penicillin +/− AC Alt: Ceph 3, TS

Alt, Alternative antibiotics; *PRP,* penicillinase-resistant penicillin (oxacillin, nafcillin, methicillin, amoxicillin-clavulanate [AC]); *Ceph 3,* third-generation cephalosporin (e.g., ceftriaxone, cefotaxime, cefamandole, ceftizoxime, ceftazidime, moxalactam); *FLQ,* fluoroquinolone; *APAG,* antipseudomonal aminoglycoside; *AP Ceph,* antipseudomonal cephalosporin, (ceftazidime or cefepime); *TS,* trimethoprim sulfamethoxazole; *MRSA,* methicillin-resistant *S. aureus.*
Concurrent treatment for *C. trachomatis* should be given in patients with suspected *N. gonorrhoeae* septic arthritis. Bone and joint infection with *H. influenzae* is now rare in vaccinated children; however, if the Gram stain is suggestive of *H. influenzae,* empiric treatment should be started. Fluoroquinolones are not recommended for use in children.

acute illnesses. Multiple sites of bony involvement are found in approximately half the reported cases. Because of the special vascular anatomy of the neonate, which was previously described, septic arthritis often accompanies osteomyelitis. Osteomyelitis in the neonate is more common in flat bones, such as the facial bones. Group B streptococci are becoming the leading causative bacterium in neonatal osteomyelitis, but staphylococcal species are still common. Skeletal scintigraphy is of limited value in diagnosing neonatal osteomyelitis. The reasons are an inadequate inflammatory response in the neonate, the small size of bones and joints, and active epiphyses that can concentrate the radiolabeled isotope, making it difficult to distinguish infection in the ends of bones. Plain radiographs show abnormalities within days of development of neonatal osteomyelitis and are usually positive by the time the disease is suspected.[41,57]

Two less common forms of osteomyelitis can occur in children: subacute osteomyelitis and chronic recurrent multifocal osteomyelitis (CRMO). Subacute osteomyelitis refers to a form of the disease in which clinical symptoms and signs are slow to appear, and radiographs show small areas of osteomyelitis, usually in the metaphysis of long bones. Cultures of blood and bone are negative more than 50% of the time and, when positive, usually implicate staphylococcal species.[58] Like subacute osteomyelitis, CRMO usually affects older children (6 to 10 years) and adolescents. CRMO is characterized by small foci of infection at various sites in the skeleton. The disease is defined by multiple episodes of indolent infection. Diagnosis is made by radiographs; culture of the bony sites is almost always negative. This disease may be associated with a type of psoriasis.[58,59]

Another subacute form of osteomyelitis that is most common in children and adolescents is *Brodie's abscess.* This

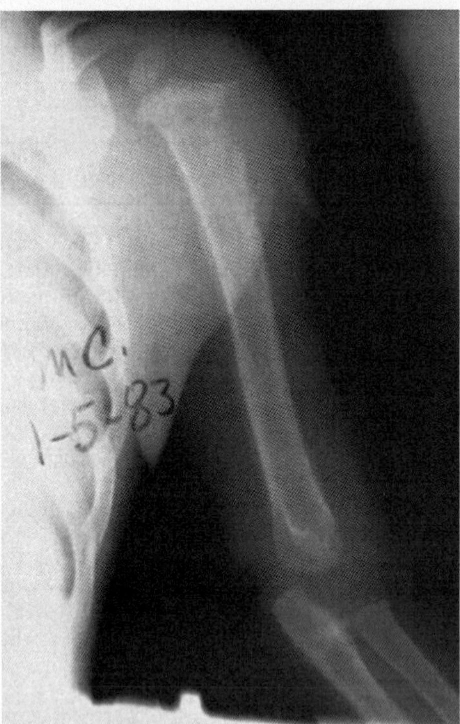

Figure 130-8. **Acute hematogenous osteomyelitis in a child. Proximal humeral metaphysis is affected.** ***Courtesy Department of Radiology, University of Cincinnati Medical Center.***

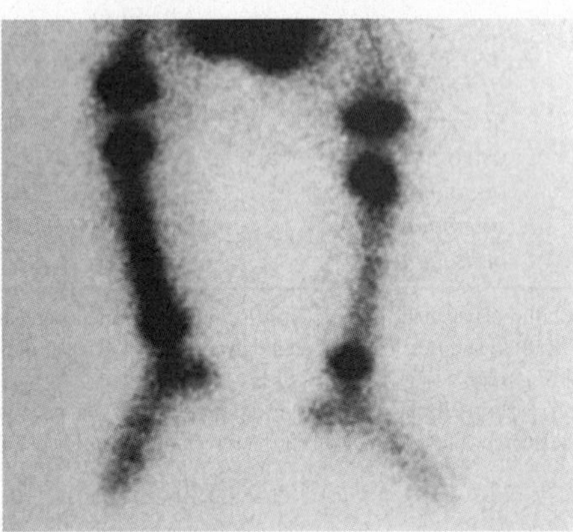

Figure 130-9. **^{99m}Tc-MDP bone scan in a 6-month-old girl demonstrates increased uptake in the left distal tibia, confirming the clinical diagnosis of osteomyelitis.** ***Courtesy Department of Nuclear Medicine, Albany Medical Center.***

is a small round cystic area of osteomyelitis that involves the femoral or tibial metaphysis around the knee. This occurs during the subacute or chronic stage of hematogenous osteomyelitis and may produce minimal symptoms. The causative organism is *S. aureus,* or sometimes *Proteus* or *Pseudomonas* species. On plain radiographs the lesion is lytic, with a well-defined sclerotic margin.[41]

Vertebral Osteomyelitis Vertebral osteomyelitis is a hematogenous disease that usually afflicts older adults in a manner analogous to AHO in children. The venous system surrounding vertebral bodies is valveless (permitting two-way flow of blood) and has transverse and longitudinal anastomoses. Bacteria that reach the spine and enter the venous plexus may be more likely to aggregate and cause infection in this slow-moving system. Infection can readily spread to adjacent vertebral bodies. If pus spreads into the spinal canal and the extradural space, it can cause an epidural abscess. This can lead to cord compression with neurologic deficits and occurs in 10% to 15% of cases of vertebral osteomyelitis. Because intervertebral disks lose their vasculature early in life, hematogenous infection is unlikely. Disks can become infected by direct extension of infection in the vertebral body or by inoculation of bacteria during penetrating procedures or surgery.[60,61]

A clear source of bacterial hematogenous seeding and positive blood cultures occurs in approximately 40% of cases. Genitourinary tract infections that seed the bloodstream are the most common precipitators of vertebral osteomyelitis. Respiratory infections, bacteremia from indwelling venous or arterial catheters, sickle cell disease, and IVDA all predispose to vertebral osteomyelitis. The causative organism is usually staphylococcal, but gram-negative bacteria are commonly isolated. The predominant clinical findings are back pain, stiffness, and point tenderness over vertebral bodies. The lumbar vertebrae are most commonly affected. Only approximately 10% of patients appear septic or toxic; the rest have a subacute presentation.[60,61]

The imaging strategy for diagnosis of vertebral osteomyelitis consists of the sequence of plain radiographs, skeletal scintigraphy, and a CT or MRI scan (Figures 130-6 and 130-10).[60,61] The diagnosis, if strongly suspected, must be confirmed quickly, either through imaging or by direct needle biopsy, to help avert the potentially catastrophic progression to spinal cord compression. Patients who are at increased risk for paralysis include elderly people, those with cervical spine osteomyelitis, and those with serious underlying diseases such as rheumatoid arthritis or diabetes mellitus.[60,61]

A variant of vertebral osteomyelitis that must be distinguished is discitis of childhood. This subacute disease is thought to be a low-grade infection (usually *Staphylococcus* species) within the disk, sometimes extending to the adjacent vertebral plates. The child complains of back pain and sometimes refuses to walk. Bone scintigraphy shows increased uptake in the disk space. Single-photon emission computed tomography (SPECT) imaging and pinhole collimation can accurately identify the site and extent of involvement.[62] Cultures of the disk from needle aspiration are typically negative, and the disease resolves with conservative treatment.[63]

Posttraumatic Osteomyelitis Posttraumatic osteomyelitis is a form of contiguous focus osteomyelitis that results from open fractures, surgery and invasive procedures, burns, bites, and puncture wounds.

At least 10% of open fractures later develop osteomyelitis. The fracture site may be directly contaminated from the environment or iatrogenically during emergency procedures or surgery. The intraoperative implantation of prosthetic devices further increases the chance of infection. Extreme damage to adjacent soft tissues may result in a necrotic nidus of infection that can spread to bone.[64]

Postsurgical osteomyelitis is difficult to diagnose. The sole complaint of the patient may be pain in the region of the previous surgery. Radiologic tests are less helpful because of

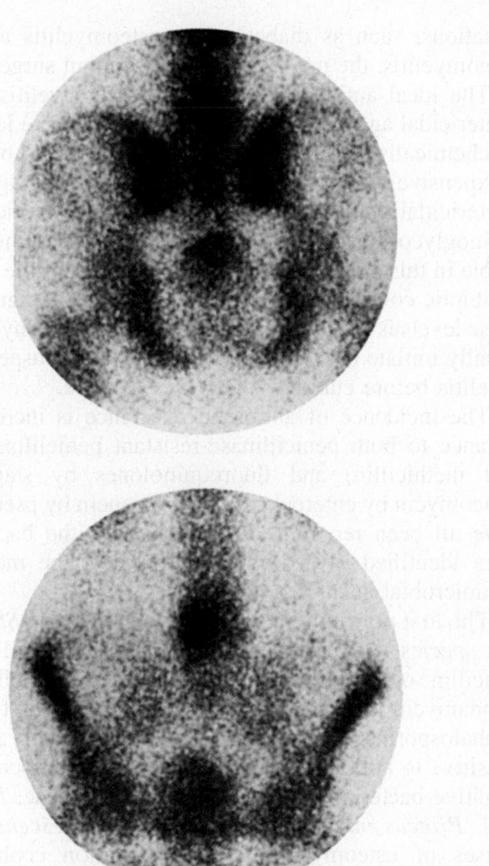

Figure 130-10. Technetium bone scan in vertebral osteomyelitis showing increased uptake in lower lumbar vertebrae. *Courtesy EB Silberstein, Department of Nuclear Medicine, University of Cincinnati.*

the bony changes induced by surgery. The most common form of postsurgical osteomyelitis is infection of a hip prosthesis, which occurs in 1% to 5% of hip replacement surgeries. It has been shown experimentally that bacteria can become immersed in an extremely adherent material called the glycocalyx, which binds to the inert substance of the prosthesis. Systemic antibiotics cannot penetrate this glycocalyx, and the only way to cure the infection is to remove the prosthesis.[65]

Puncture wounds to the feet have approximately a 2% incidence of developing osteomyelitis. The causative organism is usually *Pseudomonas aeruginosa* or *S. aureus.* Other puncture wounds are nosocomial—in the form of subclavian venipuncture, fetal scalp monitors, and other invasive procedures. Osteomyelitis can result from inoculation of bone with bacteria during these punctures.[56]

Diabetic Foot Osteomyelitis The pathologic changes induced by long-standing diabetes mellitus encourage the development of osteomyelitis. The peripheral neuropathy that occurs in 80% of diabetic patients with foot ulcers leads to repetitive trauma and loss of the protective cutaneous barrier of the skin. Once this has occurred, the altered host defense of diabetic patients then allows infection to occur and spread. The small bones and phalanges are most often affected. Infection spreads first to the periosteum and then to the cortex and may finally disrupt medullary bone. The initial phase of the pedal infection in diabetic patients may exacerbate preexisting hyperglycemia, which allows bacteria to replicate at an increased rate and causes defects in leukocyte function. These defects in infection control consist of defective chemotaxis, abnormal phagocytosis, and decreased bactericidal funtion.[66] Defective antibody synthesis and decreased complement levels also exacerbate osteomyelitis. The typical patient with diabetic foot osteomyelitis is more than 50 years old and has advanced insulin-dependent diabetes. More than 60% of such patients have polyneuropathy, more than 50% have retinopathy, and at least 30% have concurrent cardiovascular disease.[2,7,67]

Local findings consist of swelling, erythema, and sometimes pain. Indolent ulcers and frank cellulitis are seen in more than 50% of cases. Because the process is often chronic, radiographic changes have sufficient time to develop. Mottled lytic lesions are typical, and air may be present in the soft tissues. The bone scan is of limited value because of generalized poor perfusion in the area and the frequency of concurrent soft-tissue infection.[2,67] Diabetic foot osteomyelitis is usually polymicrobial. The most common organism is *S. aureus.*[68,69] Other common organisms include streptococci, Enterobacteriaceae, and anaerobes. Surgical treatment is often required, and severe cases often lead to amputation.[2,7,67]

Osteomyelitis in Sickle Cell Disease Patients with sickle cell disease are at increased risk for hematogenous infection, including osteomyelitis. Macrophage function is impaired in sickle cell patients, rendering them susceptible to infections with encapsulated organisms. AHO in children with sickle cell disease differs from that in otherwise normal patients in two major ways. First, infection in sickle cell disease is usually located in the diaphysis of long bones rather than in the metaphysis. Second, in children with sickle cell disease who develop osteomyelitis, *Salmonella* species are the infecting organism in as many as 60% of cases.[70] In some regions of the world such as the Middle East, *Salmonella* is the most commonly reported microbe in sickle cell patients with osteomyelitis.[71] However, domestically, *S. aureus* remains the most common infecting organism. The reason patients with sickle cell disease are predisposed to bone infection with *Salmonella* is not completely understood, although it is postulated that microinfarcts in the bowel allow *Salmonella* bacteremia to seed the bloodstream and become hematogenous osteomyelitis.The differentiation of bone infection from bone infarction in sickle cell patients is a challenge. Fever, a toxic appearance, and an elevated ESR are all more commonly associated with osteomyelitis than with bone infarction. Plain radiographs are not helpful in distinguishing between the two entities. Skeletal scintigraphy may help make the diagnosis. The best method appears to be ^{99m}Tc MDP followed by gallium or indium scanning. Although both infection and infarction may show increased uptake on the technetium scan, the gallium or indium scan should be "hot" with osteomyelitis but "cold" with sickle cell infarction. Another approach is to note the response to conservative therapy: Bone infarctions usually improve within 24 to 48 hours, whereas bone infection worsens.[41]

Chronic Osteomyelitis Historically, chronic osteomyelitis usually resulted from inappropriate or inadequate treatment of acute hematogenous osteomyelitis. However, most chronic bone infections now occur as a complication of internal fixation and joint replacement. Chronic osteomyelitis is more common in posttraumatic and diabetic foot osteomyelitis. A recurrent course, characterized by formation of sequestra and chronic draining tracts or fistulas, indicates that osteomyelitis has become chronic. This infection is almost always polymicrobial and commonly involves anaerobes. Bone scans are of limited use in chronic osteomyelitis; it is difficult to predict improvement or identify active foci of infection on bone scans. Cultures of sinus tracts are useless for predicting which bacteria are active in the underlying bone.[7]

Complications of Osteomyelitis In addition to the development of chronic osteomyelitis, several other complications can arise from acute osteomyelitis. The blood may be seeded with bacteria or bacterial toxins from a focus of osteomyelitis. Sepsis may result, and toxic shock syndrome has been reported with osteomyelitis caused by *S. aureus.*[72] Depending on the location of osteomyelitis, local extension of an invasive, suppurative process can lead to brain abscess, meningitis, spinal cord compression, and pneumonia. In children, osteomyelitis damages the developing skeleton. If infection involves the epiphysis, permanent growth alteration can occur, resulting in a shorter extremity on the affected side. Pathologic fractures may occur through sites of osteomyelitis. Some cases of osteomyelitis may lead to septic arthritis.

DIFFERENTIAL CONSIDERATIONS OF OSTEOMYELITIS

Many different processes involving bone may masquerade as osteomyelitis. Bone tumors may produce local pain, radiographic changes, and even bone scan abnormalities consistent with osteomyelitis. Tumors most likely to mimic osteomyelitis are osteoid osteomas and chondroblastomas. These produce small round radiolucent lesions on radiographs. Ewing's sarcoma is a tumor of bone marrow in children that can be mistaken for osteomyelitis. Metastatic bone tumors and lymphomas should also be considered in the differential diagnosis of osteomyelitis.

Trauma can produce a clinical picture similar to osteomyelitis. In children, when trauma is common and may be occult, the evaluation for osteomyelitis may reveal a buckle fracture.

Other inflammatory and infectious diseases that may be initially confused with osteomyelitis are myositis ossificans, erythema nodosum, cellulitis, and eosinophilic granuloma. This enlarging collection of histiocytes occurs in the marrow cavity and causes lytic destructive lesions.

MANAGEMENT OF OSTEOMYELITIS

The proper management of open fractures in the field is to cut away surrounding clothing, pour sterile saline or water over the exposed bone, and cover the wound with moist sterile gauze bandages or a sterile sheet. Only in the case of severe vascular compromise to the distal limb should an open fracture site be manipulated or realigned because of the danger of further contaminating the wound.

Treatment of osteomyelitis is a combined medical and surgical approach: IV antibiotics and surgical debridement. In some cases, such as acute hematogenous osteomyelitis of children, antibiotics alone can eradicate the infection. In other situations, such as diabetic foot osteomyelitis and chronic osteomyelitis, the use of antibiotics without surgery is futile.

The ideal antibiotic for treating osteomyelitis should be bactericidal against the offending bacteria, have low toxicity, be chemically stable at the site of infection, and be relatively inexpensive. The low pH of infected bone may limit the bactericidal action of some antibiotics, particularly the aminoglycosides. Cephalosporins and penicillins are more stable in this environment. Although it is possible to measure antibiotic concentrations in bone, the clinical significance of these levels is not established. The emergency physician must usually initiate broad-spectrum treatment of suspected osteomyelitis before culture results are available.

The incidence of antibiotic resistance is increasing. Resistance to both penicillinase-resistant penicillins (oxacillin and methicillin) and fluoroquinolones by staphylococci, vancomycin by enterococci, and imipenem by pseudomonads have all been reported. Therefore, once the bacterium has been identified, it is important to select the most specific antimicrobial agent.

The first priority remains adequately treating *Staphylococcus* species with a penicillinase-resistant penicillin such as oxacillin or nafcillin. In patients with penicillin allergy, clindamycin is a good alternative, as are the first-generation cephalosporins. Nonenterococcal streptococci are usually sensitive to antibiotics used to combat staphylococci. Gram-negative bacteria, including Enterobacteriaceae, *Escherichia coli, Proteus mirabilis,* and *Serratia marcescens,* are rarer causes of osteomyelitis. Third-generation cephalosporins, aminoglycosides, imipenem-cilastatin, and ampicillin are the usual choices for broad gram-negative coverage. Beyond this initial broad-spectrum therapy, prospective treatment for anaerobic bacteria, *Pseudomonas, H. influenzae,* and fungal organisms must be based on clinical suspicion.[72,73]

The increase in antimicrobial resistance highlights the need for new antibiotics to expand therapeutic options. Quinupristin/dalfopristin is the first of a unique class of antibiotics called streptogramins. Clinical evidence suggests these agents may be effective against multidrug-resistant organisms including MRSA and VRE.[75] Teicoplanin, a new semisynthetic polypeptide related to vancomycin, has proved effective against various gram-positive infections, with potentially less toxicity.[76] The development of alternative fluoroquinolones that are active against a broad spectrum of gram-positive and gram-negative organisms may improve the future treatment of osteomyelitis.[77] Table 130-2 lists common treatment regimens for the variety of bacteria that cause osteomyelitis. The standard duration of therapy with IV antibiotics for osteomyelitis is 4 to 6 weeks; however, there is no evidence that this regimen is superior to treatment for shorter periods.[73,74,78]

Successful treatment of osteomyelitis correlates best with serum levels of antibiotic, not the route of administration. The standard recommendation is that the antibiotic used should achieve serum levels *eight* times greater than its minimum inhibitory concentration. If the serum concentration of an antibiotic is bactericidal, bactericidal levels in bone will almost always be present.

In many cases of osteomyelitis, antibiotic therapy alone will not cure the infection, and surgical debridement of infected necrotic bone is necessary. This is usually true when osteomyelitis is caused by direct inoculation into bone or spreads from a contiguous focus of infection. If the area of osteomyelitis is small, aspiration or resection of the bone abscess may be both a diagnostic and therapeutic procedure.

Treatment of chronic osteomyelitis is a difficult surgical problem. Instillation of antibiotic-containing beads into infected bone can help eradicate the infection so that bone grafts can be successfully used in chronic osteomyelitis.[79,80] Hyperbaric oxygen therapy (HBO) is reported to be effective in noncontrolled clinical case series, although in animal models it is not as promising. However, differences in bones, organisms, treatment antibiotic(s), routes of antibiotic administration, duration of treatment, adequacy of debridement, and the status of adjacent soft tissues make the results from comparative clinical trials difficult to interpret. In addition, no universal terms for cure, arrest, improvement, and treatment failure currently exist. Mechanistically, HBO appears to be useful for the treatment of osteomyelitis. HBO can elevate the PO_2 in infected bone proportional to vascularity; HBO alleviates hypoxia, which can impair leukocyte bacterial killing and fibroblastic collagen production to support angiogenesis. In addition, HBO enhances antibiotic efficacy in a hypoxic environment.[81,82] Further clinical trials using a standardized staging system are necessary to confirm the favorable results seen in previous clinical trials.

DISPOSITION OF THE PATIENT WITH OSTEOMYELITIS

Several studies demonstrate that osteomyelitis can be treated with oral antibiotics as an outpatient. This is attempted only after a course of IV antibiotics is administered, and it is documented that bactericidal levels in the serum can be achieved with oral antibiotics. IV outpatient antibiotic therapy is another option after the causative bacterium has been isolated and in-hospital bactericidal levels are demonstrated.[78]

CLINICAL FEATURES OF SEPTIC ARTHRITIS

Diagnosis of Septic Arthritis

Septic arthritis usually results from hematogenous migration of bacteria into the joint. In some cases septic arthritis may result from spread from a contiguous focus of infection or by direct inoculation of bacteria. Direct inoculation can result from penetrating trauma or from joint aspiration. Septic arthritis may occur concomitantly with osteomyelitis, with infection spreading from bone to joint, and vice versa. Septic arthritis occurs in all age groups but is most common in children. It is almost always a monoarticular process; polyarticular involvement is present in fewer than 10% of pediatric cases and fewer than 20% of adult cases.[83] In adults polyarticular septic arthritis has a mortality rate of 30%. For reasons yet unknown, septic arthritis is most likely to occur in the joints of the lower extremity. In infants and children, the knee and hip are most often infected; in adults the knee is the site of septic arthritis 40% to 50% of the time. Joints are enclosed within a capsule that consists of two layers. The outer layer is dense fibrous tissue that interweaves with ligaments and the periosteum of articulating bones. The inner layer is the synovial membrane that is made up of secretory cells sitting on a loose fibrous stroma. The synovial membrane lines the entire inner surface of the joint, except for the articular cartilage surfaces, which it does not cover. In most joints the synovium does not extend past the epiphyseal growth plate. In the shoulder and hip joints, however, the synovial membrane extends beyond the epiphysis and attaches to the metaphysis. Because of this special anatomic relationship, infection in the metaphysis of the femur or humerus may spread more easily into the joint.[8]

History and Physical Examination The onset of septic arthritis is usually more acute than is the onset of osteomyelitis. The predominant symptom of septic arthritis is joint pain, which is worse when the joint is moved. Many children who have septic arthritis will not use the limb at all. In patients with underlying joint disease, a careful history may help differentiate chronic joint pain from the acute pain associated with septic arthritis. Immunosuppressed patients, especially those on corticosteroids, may develop septic arthritis with minimal joint pain. Remember that hip pain can be referred to the thigh or knee. Fever is common with septic arthritis. It is present in more than 80% of children and more than 40% of adults. Chills are reported in approximately 25% of cases.[83,85] Constitutional symptoms such as weakness, malaise, anorexia, nausea, and diffuse myalgias are inconsistently present.

It is important to ascertain the presence of underlying joint disease such as osteoarthritis, gout, rheumatoid arthritis, joint surgery, and the presence of other conditions, such as IV drug use, that predispose to septic arthritis. Certain medications, such as antibiotics, antiinflammatory agents, corticosteroids, and analgesics, can alter the course or presentation of septic arthritis.

In a patient with septic arthritis, fever is most commonly present. Tachycardia and hypotension may indicate a generalized septic process. Examination of the skin, nose, ears, and pharynx may reveal a focus of infection. In the neonate or infant, there may be "pseudoparalysis" of the affected limb. In the older child and adult, signs may be more localized. The extremity will usually be held motionless in the position of greatest comfort, which is slight flexion. Swelling, erythema, and warmth are found in almost all cases of septic arthritis. Palpation of the septic joint causes exquisite pain over the synovium, and both flexion and extension of the joint cause severe pain. The affected joint feels warmer than the noninvolved joint, and overlying skin may be reddened. An effusion should be evident by observation and palpation. The hip joint, with its deeper location, may not produce obvious external findings when infected. Periarticular processes such as bursitis, tendonitis, and cellulitis may produce erythema, warmth, and tenderness; but palpation of the joint line and maneuvers that stress the synovium and joint are not usually painful. Periarticular processes do not commonly produce an effusion.[85]

DIAGNOSTIC STRATEGIES OF SEPTIC ARTHRITIS

Joint Aspiration and Joint Fluid Analysis

The diagnosis of septic arthritis requires joint fluid for culture and analysis. It is fortunate that the knee joint is both the most likely to be infected and the easiest to aspirate. Other joints such as the hip may be more difficult to aspirate and may require orthopedic surgical consultation. Ultrasound and fluoroscopy-guided aspiration are adjunct modalities used to obtain fluid from the joint and may be useful in detecting early, less obvious intraarticular fluid collections.[86] (Figure 130-11). However, the absence of sonographic fluid by no means rules out the presence of septic arthritis. Some authors advocate injecting a small amount of contrast material into the joint during aspiration and obtaining an x-ray film to confirm that the needle entered the intraarticular space.[87] The risk of introducing infection into a joint during intraarticular aspiration or injection is very low. Iatrogenic septic arthritis occurs in less than 1 in 10,000 joint injections or aspirations and is most likely to occur in patients with existing joint disease.[86-88]

Because joint fluid analysis is not done as often as other diagnostic tests in the ED, a joint fluid protocol form is useful to ensure that all necessary tests are prepared and ordered properly. Joint fluid cultures must be inoculated as soon as possible after the fluid is obtained. If significant delays occur in the processing of laboratory specimens, the physician may need to inoculate culture media in the ED or take the fluid directly to the microbiology laboratory. Fastidious organisms such as *Neisseria gonorrhoeae* and *H. influenzae* require plating on special media. Anaerobic and fungal media should also be inoculated.

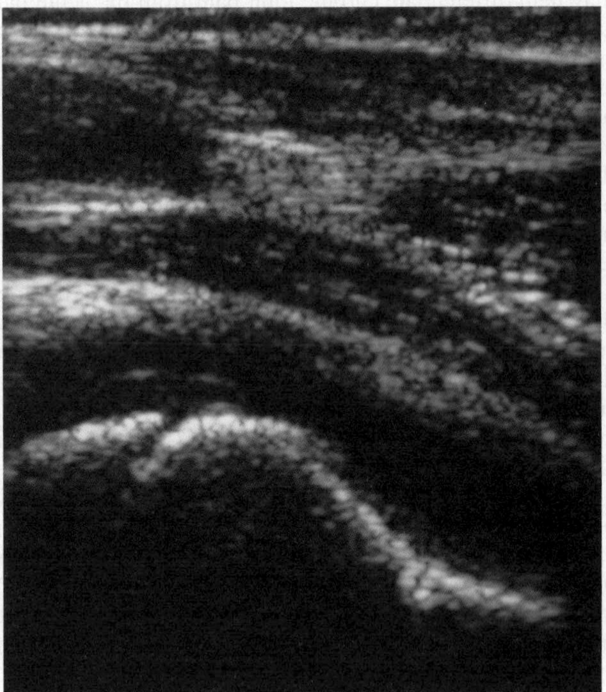

Figure 130-11. **Ultrasound of the right hip in an 8-year-old girl with septic arthritis. A significant joint effusion can be seen just superior to the round contour of the femoral head. Joint aspiration revealed purulent fluid with a white blood cell count of 71,000.**

One method that may increase the yield in isolating bacteria from joint fluid is to inoculate blood culture bottles with joint fluid immediately after joint aspiration. This may allow some bacteria, which would normally die before being inoculated on culture media in the laboratory, to survive and grow in the blood culture bottle (brain-heart infusion broth).[89]

Obtaining synovial tissue by arthroscopy for analysis may be of some benefit in diagnosing septic arthritis. Cultures of this tissue may be positive despite negative joint fluid cultures. Also, the presence of large numbers of neutrophils in the synovial tissue occurs much more commonly in infectious arthritis than in other types of joint inflammation.[8,84,85,90]

Joint fluid culture results in clinically suspected septic arthritis are negative in 20% to 25% of cases. The reasons for this may be an inadequate joint fluid sample, poor culturing techniques, the presence of fastidious organisms, or misdiagnosis of the joint inflammation.[85]

The most helpful joint fluid analysis tests in suspected septic arthritis are the Gram stain, WBC count and differential, and the ratio of the joint fluid glucose to serum glucose. Other tests performed on joint fluid are useful in differentiating inflammatory from noninflammatory joint disease, but they are not helpful in separating infectious inflammatory joint disease from noninfectious inflammatory joint disease. Common joint fluid tests and their results in inflammatory and noninflammatory joints are summarized in Table 130-3. The synovial fluid leukocyte count is usually greater than 50,000 cells/mm^3, with a predominance of PMNs, but other processes can give similar cell counts.[91] The fasting joint fluid glucose level is usually lowered in patients

Table 130-3. Synovial Fluid Findings in Septic Arthritis Compared with Other Joint Diseases

		Inflammatory fluids	
Joint fluid examination	**Noninflammatory fluids**	**Noninfectious**	**Infectious**
Color	Colorless, pale yellow	Yellow	Yellow
Turbidity	Clear, slightly turbid	Turbid	Turbid, purulent
Viscosity	Not reduced	Reduced	Reduced
Mucin clot	Tight clot	Friable	Friable
Cell count (per mm^3)	200 to 1000	3000 to >10,000	10,000 to >100,000
Predominant cell type	Mononuclear	PMN	PMN
Synovial fluid/blood glucose ratio	0.8-1.0	0.5-0.8	<0.5
Lactic acid	Same as plasma	Higher than plasma	Often very high
Gram stain for organism	None	None	Positive*
Culture	Negative	Negative	Positive*

PMN, Polymorphonuclear leukocyte.

*In some cases, especially in gonococcal infection, no organisms may be demonstrated.

From Schmid FR: Principles of diagnosis and treatment of bone and joint infections. In McCarty DJ, editor: *Arthritis and allied conditions, a textbook of rheumatology,* ed 11, Philadelphia, 1989, Lea & Febiger.

with septic arthritis, and the joint fluid/serum glucose ratio is less than 1:2. Other inflammatory joint diseases do not typically cause reduced synovial fluid glucose levels. To reliably interpret the joint fluid/blood glucose ratio, the patient should not have eaten for 6 hours and no glucose-containing IV solutions should be infusing.[9] Another test that is sensitive and specific for joint infection is the joint fluid lactate level. In most cases the lactate level is higher in infected joints than in inflamed joints. This test is not more helpful than the glucose ratio, and in partially treated septic arthritis, joint fluid lactate measurement loses its usefulness. Countercurrent immunoelectrophoresis or latex agglutination provides a method for isolating bacterial antigens from body fluids, which may be helpful in diagnosing septic arthritis. These tests are not widely used in joint fluid analysis.[6,8,25,37,84,85,87,90]

When only a drop or two of synovial fluid can be recovered, the emergency physician must establish priorities for diagnostic tests. The first step is to obtain bacterial cultures. A drop of fluid is then used for a smear and Gram stain. A glucose measurement is the next most helpful test, followed by a cell count. All other tests are nonessential for making a diagnosis of septic arthritis.[8,84,85,90,91]

Blood tests are not consistently helpful in making a diagnosis of septic arthritis. Blood cultures reveal the infecting organism in 25% to 50% of cases, and the ESR is elevated in approximately 90% of cases of septic arthritis.[8,84,85] Typically a WBC count of more than 10,000 cells/mm^3 indicates systemic illness, but is present in only 50% of patients with septic arthritis.[92] Cultures of infectious foci such as the throat and urine may demonstrate the bacteria responsible for septic arthritis.

Plain radiography is not an effective tool for the early evaluation of septic arthritis. Radiographs may reveal a joint effusion that displaces capsular fat planes. This is most helpful in the hip joint, where it is difficult to detect an effusion on physical examination. Medial displacement of the obturator tendon, which lies superior and medial to the hip joint, is a clue to a hip joint effusion. In most joints the small areas of attachment of the synovial membrane to bone are devoid of cartilage. These "bare areas" at the margins of the joint appear as lucencies or erosions early in the course of septic arthritis. Another early radiographic change is periarticular osteopenia, which results from disuse of the extremity and hyperemia of synovium. Bone beneath the articular cartilage may start to erode 1 to 3 weeks into the disease. Radiographs show this erosion and also narrowing of the joint space as articular cartilage is destroyed. These changes may also occur in chronic joint inflammation. Radiographs provide minimal assistance in diagnosing septic arthritis in a patient with existing joint disease. Joint radiographs may detect osteomyelitis in bones adjacent to the joint. Air density in the joint may be a sign of infection with gas-forming organisms or may be the result of a previous joint aspiration.[84,90]

Skeletal scintigraphy has been used in the diagnosis of septic arthritis. Its main advantage is in detecting septic arthritis earlier than other imaging techniques. The specifics of technetium, gallium, and indium scanning have been previously discussed. In septic arthritis, scintigraphy shows symmetric areas of increased uptake on both sides of the joint. In a three-phase ^{99m}Tc scan, all three phases will be "hot" with septic arthritis. It may be difficult to distinguish osteomyelitis in the metaphysis of a long bone from septic arthritis in the adjacent joint. In general, skeletal scintigraphy is used only when there is great enough uncertainty about the diagnosis to warrant further investigation before proceeding with joint aspiration. This is most common in evaluating a hip for septic arthritis. In joints where aspiration is easier, skeletal scintigraphy has little role in diagnosing septic arthritis. There is some risk that the delay associated with obtaining skeletal scintigraphy may lead to further joint destruction before definitive treatment is rendered. MRI provides a detailed image of joint structure and can detect even small effusions.[8,85,90]

Complications of Septic Arthritis

Septic arthritis leads to two types of serious complications: those involving the joint itself and those that are systemic. Children are at great risk for epiphyseal damage if the infection extends through subchondral bone. This can result in impaired growth and length discrepancy in the limbs. Other tissues adjacent to the joint can be invaded. Bursae, tendons, ligaments, and muscles can be destroyed by the suppurative process. Sinus tracts may lead the infection out through the skin. In the hip the pressure and edema of a septic synovial effusion can occlude blood supply, resulting in avascular necrosis of the femoral head. In other joints the end result of uncontrolled septic arthritis is ankylosis. The joint becomes stiff, fused, and devoid of articular cartilage.

In some patients with septic arthritis, the infection causes systemic sepsis. This is most common in elderly and immunocompromised patients.

Clinical Subsets of Septic Arthritis

Septic Arthritis in Infants and Children Septic arthritis is more common in children than in adults, and the incidence of septic arthritis is twice that of osteomyelitis in children.[84] Of pediatric cases, two thirds occur in children less than 2 years old. The bacterial etiologic agent of septic arthritis varies with age. In neonates group B streptococci, *S. aureus,* and gram-negative enteric bacilli are usual pathogens. With treatment, few complications result. *Candida albicans* must also be considered in neonates and premature infants.[93] Since the widespread introduction of the HiB vaccine, *S. aureus* has become the most common cause of septic arthritis in children 3 months to 5 years old. In this age range concomitant respiratory infection or otitis media is often present. If the hip joint is infected, the complication rate is higher, and permanent joint damage is more likely. This is especially true in infants, particularly those who have coexisting septic arthritis and osteomyelitis. Overall, *S. aureus* is the most common infecting organism in all pediatric age groups, followed by group A streptococci and *Streptococcus pneumoniae.*[6] Prior trauma or skin infection may be more common with staphylococcal septic arthritis. Even with full culturing of joint fluid and blood, a causative organism is not discovered in up to 30% of cases of septic arthritis in children. Prior antibiotic treatment in children decreases the yield on synovial fluid cultures from 80% to 38%.[8,83,85,90]

Gonococcal Septic Arthritis *N. gonorrhoeae* is the most common cause of septic arthritis in teenagers and young adults. The incidence of the disease is increasing. A person with gonorrhea of the urethra, cervix, rectum, or pharynx has a 0.5% to 1% chance of developing disseminated gonococcal infection (DGI). Gonococcal septic arthritis is more common in women, especially during pregnancy or after menstruation. The strains of *N. gonorrhoeae* that cause disseminated infection and septic arthritis have different characteristics than those that cause local infection. Those strains that cause disseminated infection contain outer membrane proteins, which make them resistant to serum bactericidal activity. These strains, however, are not more resistant to antibiotics than other types of *N. gonorrhoeae.* The common finding of sterile joint fluid in DGI, even when mucosal cultures are positive, suggests that the host immune response plays a significant role in the development of purulent arthritis.[94,95]

Most, but not all, patients with DGI are symptomatic with their local genital or oral infection. The time for local infection to disseminate can vary from 1 or 2 days to weeks. Symptoms begin soon after gonococcal bacteria enter the bloodstream, *and fever and chills are often present.* The classic triad of DGI is migratory polyarthritis, tenosynovitis, and dermatitis. Asymmetric polyarthralgia, which may be migratory, is the most common presenting complaint, occurring in two thirds of cases; 25% of patients have monoarthralgia.[96] Joint involvement is usually asymmetric and most frequently involves the knee, elbow, wrist, metacarpophalangeal, and ankle joints. Patients with HIV disease may present with involvement of unusual joints, such as the hip and sternoclavicular joint.[97] Tenosynovitis occurs in two thirds of patients with DGI, typically occurring in the hands and fingers. Distribution is usually asymmetric and involves more than one area. Dermatitis is also present in two thirds of patients and may have a number of forms. The most common rash is scattered painless 0.5- to 0.75-cm hemorrhagic macules or papules distributed on the extremities and trunk. A small area of central necrosis may be present in the lesions.[94,95]

Purulent arthritis develops in approximately 40% of patients with disseminated gonococcal infection. In most cases it is monoarticular, but 10% of the time is polyarticular. Some of the strains of *N. gonorrhoeae* that produce disseminated gonococcal infection favor the development of tenosynovitis and dermatitis, whereas others favor the development of purulent arthritis. There is usually not a clear progression of the disease from polyarthralgias to tenosynovitis to purulent monoarticular arthritis. Many patients are afflicted with dermatitis and tenosynovitis without developing true arthritis.[94,95]

Joint fluid analysis in gonococcal arthritis reveals some differences in comparison with other types of bacterial arthritis. The synovial fluid WBC count in gonococcal arthritis is often less than 50,000 cells/mm^3. The joint fluid glucose level is also not usually depressed. Gram stains of aspirated joint fluid are positive for bacteria only 25% of the time in gonococcal arthritis, and cultures of the joint fluid are negative in approximately 50% of cases. This may be due to poor culturing techniques, or it may reflect the fact that a suppurative reactive process can occur in the joint in disseminated gonococcal infections even when bacteria are no longer present. It is important to culture the mucosal surfaces for *N. gonorrhoeae* when clinical suspicion for gonococcal arthritis is high because these may be the only places where bacteria are readily recovered. In 80% of cases, cultures of the genital tract, pharynx, or rectum will be positive. Gonococcal septic arthritis responds rapidly to antibiotic treatment and unlike other types of bacterial arthritis rarely causes permanent damage to the joint.[5,94-96]

Septic Arthritis with Existing Joint Disease Patients with underlying joint disease are more likely to develop septic arthritis. This is especially true for patients with rheumatoid arthritis and crystalline arthritis. Septic arthritis is more likely to be polyarticular and to result in complications in patients with rheumatoid arthritis.[90,98]

The invasion of neutrophils that occurs in septic arthritis probably causes increased precipitation and release of crystals. The clinician who discovers crystals on joint fluid aspiration should not abandon the search for an infectious agent.

Surgical implantation of a joint prosthesis is followed by joint infection in 1% to 5% of cases. The infection is most likely to occur in the first 3 months (50% of cases) after surgery and may be due to bacterial contamination during surgery, spread from a contiguous wound infection, or spread from hematogenous seeding. The prosthesis and cement are foreign bodies and are favorite sites for bacterial colonization. The most common infectious agents are *S. epidermidis* (40% of cases), *S. aureus* (20%), and streptococcal species (20%). The predominant symptom is pain in the joint, and unlike the pain from a loose prosthesis, it is constant and present at rest.[8,90]

The clinical course is variable. With *S. epidermidis* infections, the course is usually indolent. With *S. aureus,* a more aggressive infection results, with more pronounced inflammation, effusion, and systemic symptoms. Radiographic changes that may signify a prosthetic joint infection include widening and lucency of the bone-cement interface to greater than 2 mm, movement of the prosthesis, periosteal reaction, and fractures through the cement. Joint aspiration reveals infection in a prosthetic joint in more than 85% of patients. Aspiration may be more difficult in this situation because of scarring and alteration of the joint space. Patients with prosthetic joints who are undergoing invasive oropharyngeal or genitourinary procedures require antibiotic prophylaxis.[8,90]

Fungal arthritis is uncommon, particularly in children. However, the incidence is rising, principally in hospitalized patients with immune deficiency, underlying malignancy.[84,99] The diagnosis is often delayed for months, and usually made by culture and histologic examination of the synovial tissue.

DIFFERENTIAL CONSIDERATIONS OF SEPTIC ARTHRITIS

Many disease processes can be confused with septic arthritis. Osteomyelitis may mimic septic arthritis because it affects the metaphysis and the neighboring joint may develop an effusion. The two infections can be concurrent. Juvenile rheumatoid arthritis usually produces polyarticular arthritis in children less than 16 years old but may present as a monoarticular process that mimics septic arthritis. Toxic or transient synovitis is another inflammatory process in children that can be confused with septic arthritis. It occurs in the 3-month to 6-year age range, usually affects the hip, and is a self-limiting disease with no long-term morbidity. It may be more common after upper respiratory infections. Children with transient synovitis do not usually appear ill and are not febrile but favor the affected leg. Diagnostic evaluation typically reveals a normal WBC count and sedimentation rate and no radiographic abnormalities. Other diseases of the hip in children that may be mistaken for septic arthritis are Legg-Calvé-Perthes disease (avascular necrosis) and slipped capital femoral epiphysis. Rheumatic fever commonly presents with polyarthritis and may mimic gonococcal arthritis.[8,95] In the adult, osteoarthritis, gout, and pseudogout may produce a joint examination that is similar to septic arthritis. Other arthropathies that must be considered in the differential diagnosis of septic arthritis are Reiter's syndrome, psoriatic arthritis, arthritis associated with inflammatory bowel disease, and ankylosing spondylitis. Collectively, these are known as the seronegative spondyloarthropathies. Trauma to the joint can produce synovitis and hemarthrosis, which may be mistaken for septic arthritis. In a patient with hemophilia hemarthrosis causes joint inflammation and destruction and there may be superimposed infection.[90]

Reactive arthritis has been traditionally considered a sterile inflammatory response to a distant infection. However, recent data support that antigens from the infectious trigger are often present in the joint. Several viral and bacterial microorganisms can produce reactive arthritis. Some of the more common organisms are *Chlamydia, Salmonella, Shigella, Borrelia burgdorferi* (Lyme disease), *Yersinia,* rubella virus, hepatitis B virus, adenoviruses, parvovirus, and Epstein-Barr virus. In reactive arthritis, host factors rather than microbial aggression account for most of the inflammatory process. The pathogenesis of reactive arthritis involves deposition of immune complexes in the joint, persistence of organisms in the joint, and stimulation of the immune system.[100] Strong evidence exists to support a link between the development of reactive arthritis and the HLA-B27 human leukocyte histocompatibility antigen. However, whether the presence of HLA-B27 antigen influences the disease pattern is unknown. Reactive arthritis can usually be distinguished from septic arthritis because reactive arthritis tends to involve multiple joints in a migratory pattern. The severity of the inflammatory process is also less with reactive arthritis. There is less effusion, and the joint is not as hot or tender as it is with septic arthritis. Joint fluid cell counts are usually below 50,000/mm^3, and the joint fluid glucose is not depressed.[8,90,95]

MANAGEMENT OF SEPTIC ARTHRITIS

Septic arthritis is an orthopedic emergency, and it is uniformly accepted that antibiotics should be promptly administered once the diagnosis is made or is strongly suspected. However, considerable disagreement exists regarding medical versus surgical joint decompression. Medical management consists of needle aspiration of the joint. If pus reaccumulates, repeat aspiration is performed. Surgical drainage is accomplished by arthrotomy or arthroscopy. Surgical drainage may involve the placement of tubes in the joint that can be used for irrigation and drainage.[85] The advantages of surgical drainage theoretically are that the joint can be fully cleansed of pus and debris, that loculations can be broken, and that irrigation and drainage tubes can keep the joint free of destructive cells and enzymes. The disadvantages are that arthrotomy usually requires general anesthesia, is a one-time procedure, and can lead to scarring and limitation of joint movement. The advantages of needle aspiration are its simplicity, low morbidity, and the ease with which it can be repeated. Proponents of surgical drainage argue that needle aspiration cannot adequately drain the joint. No randomized controlled studies exist that compare these two approaches to treating the septic joint. However, there is evidence in an animal model that surgical incision and drainage protects the joint from chemical insult better than multiple aspirations.[101]

Although needle aspiration may be adequate treatment for most septic joints, surgical drainage is usually necessary in at least two settings. With septic arthritis of the hip, especially in infants and children, rapid destruction of the joint occurs if drainage is not quickly performed. Needle aspiration is often ineffective in this situation, and it is generally agreed that arthrotomy is the treatment of choice for infected hips.[5,84] Infected joint prostheses also do not respond to conservative therapy and almost always require arthrotomy and drainage.[59]

The only situation in which antibiotics alone can treat a septic joint is in gonococcal septic arthritis. After the diagnostic joint aspiration, almost all cases of gonococcal septic arthritis will quickly resolve with antibiotics alone.[94,95]

The selection of antibiotics for the treatment of septic arthritis is outlined in Table 130-2. In most cases the emergency physician does not know the identity of the causative organism. Because the bacteria that cause septic arthritis vary with the age of the patient, treatment must be tailored to the most likely causative agents. *S. aureus* remains the predominant pathogen for all age groups, and antibiotic selection should always include an antibiotic that has excellent bactericidal activity against *S. aureus,* except when the patient has characteristic gonococcal arthritis. In young adults gonococcal septic arthritis is common. Some strains that cause gonococcal arthritis are resistant to penicillin. In regions where penicillinase-producing *N. gonorrhoeae* is prevalent, gonococcal arthritis is best treated with ceftriaxone. In elderly people, gram-negative septic arthritis is more common, and agents such as the third-generation cephalosporins and aminoglycosides are added to the regimen. Establishing good bactericidal serum levels of antibiotics will ensure that the levels in joint fluid are also bactericidal.[8,90]

DISPOSITION OF THE PATIENT WITH SEPTIC ARTHRITIS

Any patient in whom septic arthritis is suspected requires joint aspiration. In some cases the initial cell counts, glucose level, and Gram stain make the diagnosis of septic arthritis extremely likely. The patient should be given an initial dose of antibiotics in the ED and be admitted. Consultants will then determine the need for further drainage procedures. In many cases joint aspiration in the ED is not diagnostic, and a definitive diagnosis of septic arthritis is impossible. In this situation, if the clinical appearance strongly suggests septic arthritis, the patient should be treated with appropriate antibiotics and admitted to the hospital. If the joint fluid aspirate is not consistent with septic arthritis and clinical findings are equivocal, the patient can be discharged and reevaluated in 24 hours. In some patients, septic arthritis can be difficult to detect. This includes patients on immunosuppressive agents, those with existing joint disease, and those with prosthetic joints. A conservative approach with in-hospital observation and treatment is indicated if there is any possibility of septic arthritis in these patients.

In most cases the prognosis for the patient with septic arthritis is favorable. Two thirds of afflicted patients can expect to cover completely (i.e., full range of motion of the joint and no pain). In approximately one third of cases there is decreased mobility or ankylosis, pain on movement, chronic infection, or overwhelming sepsis and death. The one factor most responsible for poor outcome is any delay in diagnosis and treatment. In infants and children early symptoms can be nonspecific and difficult to assess. Delays in diagnosis and treatment are most serious in infants with septic arthritis of the hip. This group of patients has a disappointingly high rate of complications.[84] In patients with existing joint disease, septic arthritis may be mistaken for another flare-up of the chronic disease.[8,84,90]

KEY CONCEPTS

- Bone and joint infections present a diagnostic challenge to the emergency physician. If any patient has a pain in a bone or joint, the emergency physician must consider skeletal infection in the differential diagnosis. In those cases in which a bone or joint infection exists, early diagnosis and treatment can have a potent impact on the long-term morbidity.
- The vascular anatomy of long bones changes throughout life. In infants and adults, vascular connections exist between the metaphysis and epiphysis, which allow for extension of bone infection into the joint. In children the epiphyseal plate prevents this from happening.
- Joint aspiration is the definitive diagnostic procedure for joint infections. Aspiration or resection of infected bone is the most direct way to diagnose osteomyelitis. Imaging techniques may be helpful in diagnosing osteomyelitis but can be time-consuming and expensive and do not always demonstrate excellent sensitivity.
- Hematologic evaluation is of little value in diagnosing bone and joint infections, with the exception of the ESR, which is elevated in approximately 90% of cases of bone and joint infections.
- When clinical findings suggest the diagnosis of bone or joint infection, the emergency physician should not delay antibiotic treatment. With suspected septic arthritis; joint fluid cultures and blood cultures are obtained as IV antibiotics are ordered. With suspected osteomyelitis, blood cultures are obtained, and IV antibiotics are administered while plans are made for further imaging studies or surgical aspiration or resection of bone.
- The most important aspect of emergency antibiotic treatment of suspected osteomyelitis is to provide potent bactericidal activity against *S. aureus.* In suspected septic arthritis, initial antibiotic treatment must be tailored to the age and clinical characteristics of the patient.

REFERENCES

1. Cunning J, Joll CE: *Aids to surgery,* ed 4, New York, 1919, William Wood.
2. Waldvogel FA, Medoff G, Swatz MN: *Osteomyelitis,* Springfield Ill, 1971, Charles C Thomas.
3. Lee DJ, Sartoris DJ: Musculoskeletal manifestations of human immunodeficiency virus infection: review of imaging characteristics, *Radiol Clin North Am* 32:399-411, 1994.
4. Steinbach LS et al: Human immunodeficiency virus infection: musculoskeletal manifestations, *Radiology* 186:833-838, 1993.
5. Fink CW, Nelson JD: Septic arthritis and osteomyelitis in children, *Clin Rheum Dis* 12:423, 1986.
6. Sonnen GM, Henry NK: Pediatric bone and joint infections, *Pediatr Clin North Am* 43:933-947, 1996.
7. Norman DC, Yoshisawa TT: Infections of the bone, joint, and bursa, *Clin Geriatric Med* 10:703, 1994.
8. Javors JM, Weisman MH: Principles of diagnosis and treatment of joint infections. In Koopman WJ, editor: *Arthritis and allied conditions: a textbook of rheumatology,* ed 13, Baltimore, 1997, Williams & Wilkins.
9. Lew DP, Waldvogel FA: Current concepts: osteomyelitis, *N Engl J Med* 336:999, 1997.
10. Atcheson SG, Ward JR: Acute hematogenous osteomyelitis progressing to septic synovitis and eventual pyoarthrosis: the vascular pathway, *Arthritis Rheum* 21:968, 1978.
11. Gristina AG, Naylor PT, Myrvik QN: Mechanisms of musculoskeletal sepsis, *Orthop Clin North Am* 22:363, 1991.
12. Nair SP, Meghji S, Wilson M: Bacterially induced bone destruction: mechanisms and misconceptions, *Infect Immun* 64:2371, 1996.
13. Gaston H: Synovial lymphocytes and the aetiology of synovitis, *Ann Rheum Dis* 52:S17, 1993.
14. Gillespie WJ, Allardyce RA: Mechanisms of bone degradation in infection: a review of current hypotheses, *Orthopedics* 13:407, 1990.
15. Manolagas SC, Jilka RL: Bone marrow, cytokines, and bone remodeling: emerging insights into the pathophysiology of osteoporosis, *N Engl J Med* 332:305, 1995.
16. Laughlin TJ et al: Soft tissue and bone infections from puncture wounds in children, *West J Med* 166:126-128, 1997.
17. Talan DA et al: Bacteriologic analysis of infected dog and cat bites, *N Engl J Med* 340:85, 1999.
18. Wald ER: Risk factors for osteomyelitis, *Am J Med* 78:206, 1985.
19. Newman ED, Davis DE, Harrington TM: Septic arthritis due to gram-negative bacilli: older patients with good outcome, *J Rheumatol* 15:659, 1988.
20. Howard AW, Viskontas D, Sabbagh C: Reduction in osteomyelitis and septic arthritis related to *Haemophilus influenzae* type b vaccination, *J Pediatr Orthop* 19:705-709, 1999.
21. Adams WG et al: Decline of childhood *Haemophilus influenzae* type b (Hib) disease in the Hib vaccine era, *JAMA* 269:221-226, 1993.
22. Peltola H, Kallio MJ, Unkila-Kallio L: Reduced incidence of septic arthritis in children by *Haemophilus influenzae* type b vaccination. Implications for treatment, *J Bone Joint Surg* 80:471, 1998.
23. Lundy DW, Kehl DK: Increasing prevalence of *Kingella kingae* in osteoarticular infections in young children, *J Pediatr Orthop* 18:262, 1998.
24. Smith TL et al: Emergence of vancomycin resistance in *Staphylococcus aureus, N Engl J Med* 340, 493: 1999.
25. Markus HS: Hematogenous osteomyelitis in the adult: a clinical and epidemiological study, *Q J Med* 71:521, 1989.
26. Hall BB, Rosenblatt JE, Fitzgerald RJ Jr: Anaerobic septic arthritis and osteomyelitis, *Orthop Clin North Am* 15:505, 1984.
27. Broner FA, Carland DE, Zigler JE: Spinal infections in the immunocompromised host, *Orthop Clin North Am* 27:37, 1996.
28. Semel JD, Trenholme G: *Aeromonas hydrophila* water-associated traumatic wound infections: a review, *J Trauma* 30:324, 1990.
29. Berbari EF et al: *Mycobacterium tuberculosis:* a case series and review of the literature, *Am J Orthop* 27:219, 1998.
30. Gathe JC et al: Candida osteomyelitis: report of five cases and a review of the literature, *Am J Med* 82:927, 1987.
31. Moore RM, Green NE: Blastomycosis of bone: a report of six cases, *J Bone Joint Surg* 64A:1097, 1982.
32. Tack KJ et al: Aspergillus osteomyelitis: a report of four cases and a review of the literature, *Am J Med* 73:295, 1982.
33. Behrman RE, Masci JR, Nicholas N: Cryptococcal skeletal infections: case report and review, *Rev Infect Dis* 12:81, 1990.
34. Wyatt SH, Fishman EK: CT/MRI of musculoskeletal complications of AIDS, *Skelet Radiol* 24:481, 1995.
35. Gillespie WJ: Epidemiology in bone and joint infections, *Infect Dis Clin North Am* 4:361, 1990.
36. Unkila-Kallio L et al: Serum C-reactive protein, erythrocyte sedimentation rate, and white blood cell count in acute hematogenous osteomyelitis of children, *Pediatrics* 93:59, 1994.
37. Wall E: Childhood osteomyelitis and septic arthritis, *Curr Opin Pediatr* 10:73, 1998.
38. Roine I, Arguedas A, Faingezicht I: Early detection of sequela-prone osteomyelitis in children with use of simple clinical and laboratory criteria, *Clin Infect Dis* 24:849, 1997.
39. Gentry LO: Osteomyelitis: options for diagnosis and management, *J Antimicrob Chemother* 21:115, 1988.
40. Gold RH, Hawkins RA, Katz RD: Bacterial osteomyelitis: findings on plain radiography, CT, MR, and scintigraphy, *AJR* 157:365, 1991.
41. David R, Barron BJ, Madewell JE: Osteomyelitis, acute and chronic, *Radiol Clin North Am* 25:1171, 1987.
42. Schauwecker DS: The scintigraphic diagnosis of osteomyelitis, *AJR* 158:9, 1992.
43. Holder LE: Clinical radionuclide bone imaging, *Radiology* 176:607, 1990.

44. Boutin RD et al: Update on imaging of orthopedic infections, *Orthop Clin North Am* 29:41, 1998.
45. Mandell GA: Imaging in the diagnosis of musculoskeletal infections in children, *Curr Probl Pediatr* 26:218, 1996.
46. Mettler FA, Guibereau MJ: Tumor and inflammation imaging. In *Essentials of nuclear medicine,* Philadelphia, 1992, WB Saunders.
47. Demopulos GA, Bleck EE, McDougall IR: Role of radionuclide imaging in the diagnosis of acute osteomyelitis, *J Pediatr Orthop* 8:558, 1988.
48. Sorsdahl OA et al: Quantitative bone gallium scintigraphy in osteomyelitis, *Skeletal Radiol* 22:239, 1993.
49. Schauwecker DS: Osteomyelitis: diagnosis with In-111-labeled leukocytes, *Radiology* 171:141, 1989.
50. Lantto EH et al: Tc-99m HMPAO labeled leukocytes superior to bone scan in detection of osteomyelitis in children, *Clin Nucl Med* 17:7, 1992.
51. Munk PL et al: Musculoskeletal infection: findings on magnetic resonance imaging, *Can Assoc Radiol J* 45:355, 1994.
52. Post MJD et al: Magnetic resonance imaging of spinal infection, *Rheum Dis Clin North Am* 17:773, 1991.
53. Mazur JM et al: Usefulness of magnetic resonance imaging for the diagnosis of acute musculoskeletal infections in children, *J Pediatr Orthop* 15:144, 1995.
54. Borman TR, Johnson RA, Sherman FC: Gallium scintigraphy for diagnosis of septic arthritis and osteomyelitis in children, *J Pediatr Orthop* 6:317, 1986.
55. Dagan R: Management of acute hematogenous osteomyelitis and septic arthritis in the pediatric patient, *Pediatr Infect Dis J* 12:88, 1993.
56. Frederiksen B, Chritiansen P, Knudsen FU: Acute osteomyelitis and septic arthritis in the neonate, risk factors and outcome, *Eur J Pediatr* 152: 577, 1993.
57. Asmar BI: Osteomyelitis in the neonate, *Infect Dis Clin North Am* 6:117, 1992.
58. Jones NS, Anderson DJ, Stiles PJ: Osteomyelitis in a general hospital—a five year study showing an increase in subacute osteomyelitis, *J Bone Joint Surg* 69B:779, 1987.
59. Howman-Giles R, Uren R: Multifocal osteomyelitis in childhood review by radionuclide bone scan, *Clin Nuclear Med* 17:274, 1992.
60. Smith AS, Blaser SI: Infectious and inflammatory processes of the spine, *Radiol Clin North Am* 29:809, 1991.
61. Antunes JL: Infections of the spine, *Acta Neurochir (Wien)* 116:179, 1992.
62. Swanson D et al: Diagnosis of discitis by SPECT technetium-99 MDP, *Clin Nucl Med* 12:210-211, 1987.
63. Glazer PA, Hu SS: Pediatric spinal infections, *Orthop Clin North Am* 27:111, 1996.
64. Evans RP, Nelson CL, Harrison BH: The effect of wound environment on the incidence of acute osteomyelitis, *Clin Orthop* 286:289, 1993.
65. Tsukayama DT: Pathophysiology of posttraumatic osteomyelitis, *Clin Orthop* 360:22, 1999.
66. Lipsky BA, Pecorato RE, Ahron JH: Foot ulceration and infections in early diabetics, *Clin Geriatr Med* 6:747, 1990.
67. Caputo GM et al: Assessment and management of foot disease in patients with diabetes, *N Engl J Med* 331:854, 1994.
68. 68. Grayson ML: Diabetic foot infections antimicrobic therapy, *Infect Dis Clin North Am* 9:143, 1995.
69. Hill SL, Holtzman GI, Buse R: The effects of peripheral vascular disease with osteomyelitis in the diabetic foot, *Am J Surg* 177:282, 1999.
70. Burnett MW, Bass JW, Cook BA: Etiology of osteomyelitis complicating sickle cell disease, *Pediatrics* 101:296, 1998.
71. Sadat-Ali M, Sankaran-Kutty, Kutty K: Recent observations on osteomyelitis in sickle cell disease, *Int Orthop* 9:97, 1985.
72. Chen SM, Howes PC: Purulent osteomyelitis associated with empyema and toxic shock syndrome, *J Emerg Med* 6:285, 1988.
73. Dirschl DR, Almekinders LC: Osteomyelitis: common causes and treatment recommendations, *Drugs* 45:29, 1993.
74. Dagan R: Management of acute hematogenous osteomyelitis and septic arthritis in the pediatric patient, *Pediatr Infect Dis J* 12:88, 1993.
75. Low DE: Quinupristin/dalfopristin: spectrum of activity, pharmacokinetics, and initial clinical experience, *Microb Drug Resist* 1:223, 1995.
76. Shea KW, Cunha BA: Teicoplanin, *Med Clin North Am* 79:833, 1995.
77. Galanakis N et al: Chronic osteomyelitis caused by multi-resistant gram negative bacteria: evaluation of treatment with newer quinolones after prolonged follow-up, *Drugs* 51:6, 1996.
78. Tice AD: Outpatient parenteral antimicrobial therapy for osteomyelitis, *Infect Dis Clin North Am* 12:903, 1998.
79. Ostermann PAW, Seligson D, Henry SL: Local antibiotic therapy for severe open fractures: a review of 1085 consecutive cases, *J Bone Joint Surg* 77B:93, 1995.
80. Mader JT, Calhoun J, Cobos J: In vitro evaluation of antibiotic diffusion from antibiotic impregnated biodegradable beads and polymethylmethacrylate beads, *Antimicrob Agents Chemother* 41:415, 1997.
81. 1st European consensus conference on hyperbaric medicine. Wattel F, Mathieu D, editors: *Reports and recommendations,* 1994.
82. Reference deleted in page proofs.
83. Malleson PN: Management of childhood arthritis: part 1: acute arthritis, *Arch Dis Child* 76:460, 1997.
84. Shaw BA, Kasser JR: Acute septic arthritis in infancy and childhood, *Clin Orthop Relat Res* 257:212, 1990.
85. Esterhai JL Jr, Gelb I: Adult septic arthritis, *Orthop Clin North Am* 22:503, 1991.
86. Myers MT, Thompson GH: Imaging a child with a limp, *Pediatr Clin North Am* 44:637-658, 1997.
87. Von Essen R, Savolainen HA: Bacterial infection following intraarticular injection, *Scand J Rheum* 18:7, 1989.
88. Gainor BJ: Septic arthritis: common pitfalls, *Orthop Rev* 28:555, 1989.
89. Von Essen R, Holtta A: Improved method of isolating bacteria from joint fluids by the use of blood culture bottles, *Ann Rheum Dis* 45:454, 1966.
90. Ike RW: Bacterial arthritis. In Koopman WJ, editor: *Arthritis and allied conditions: a textbook of rheumatology,* ed 13, Baltimore, 1997, Williams & Wilkins.
91. Shmerling RH: Synovial fluid analysis: a critical reappraisal, *Rheum Dis Clin North Am* 20:503-512, 1994.
92. Donnatto KC: Orthopedic management of septic arthritis, *Rheum Dis Clin North Am* 24:275, 1998.
93. Barson WJ, Marcon MJ: Successful therapy of *Candida albicans* arthritis with a sequential intravenous amphotericin B and oral fluconazole regimen, *Pediatr Infect Dis J* 15:1119, 1996.
94. Scopelitis E, Martinez-Osuna P: Gonococcal arthritis, *Infect Arthritis* 19:363, 1993.
95. Goldenburg DL: Gonococcal arthritis and other neisserial infections. In Koopman WJ, editor: *Arthritis and allied conditions: a textbook of rheumatology,* ed 13, Baltimore, 1997, Williams & Wilkins.
96. Wise CM et al: Gonococcal arthritis in an era of increasing penicillin resistance, *Arch Intern Med* 154:2690, 1994.
97. Strongin IS et al: An unusual presentation of gonococcal arthritis in an HIV-positive patient, *Ann Rheum Dis* 50:572, 1991.
98. Gardner GC, Weisman MH: Pyarthrosis in patients with rheumatoid arthritis: a report of 13 cases and a review of the literature from the past 40 years, *Am J Med* 88:503, 1990.
99. Cuellar ML, Silveira LH, Espinoza LR: Fungal arthritis, *Ann Rheum Dis* 51:690, 1992.
100. Moreland LW, Koopman WJ: Infection as a cause of arthritis, *Curr Opin Rheum* 3:639, 1991.
101. Goldstein WM, Gleason TF, Barmada R: A comparison between arthrotomy and irrigation and multiple aspirations in the treatment of pyogenic arthritis: a histologic study in a rabbit model, *Orthopedics* 6:1309, 1983.

131 Soft Tissue Infections

Harvey W. Meislin
John A. Guisto

The soft tissue infections seen in the practice of emergency medicine run the gamut from mild superficial infections that require only "tincture of time" to infections that will quickly result in death without immediate diagnosis and resuscitation. Unfortunately, the literature on soft tissue infections is confusing with respect to definition and therapy, in part because the nomenclature has been based on individual names, anatomic areas, or events (e.g., postsurgical gangrene). Also, outcomes and survival in the pre-antibiotic era differ greatly from those of today. Improved culturing techniques for aerobic and anaerobic bacteria, enhanced ability to diagnose and treat soft tissue infections, and modern approaches to analgesia and surgical management all facilitate the diagnosis, treatment, and outcome of soft tissue infections.

This chapter provides emergency physicians with a discussion of soft tissue infections organized on the basis of tissue depth. Thus superficial infections such as cellulitis and impetigo are discussed first. Deeper infections, abscesses, fasciitis, and myositis, follow. As reflected in the soft tissue infection literature, the clinical characteristics often overlap (Table 131-1), allowing such infections to evolve from superficial to deep. In addition, the bacteriologic spectrum may change with time, and thus the clinical manifestations, including systemic symptoms, may be altered. A patient does not strictly have to have an abscess, a cellulitis, or a fasciitis, but can have all of them at any time. A good rule of thumb is this: the deeper the soft tissue infection, the more normal the skin surface appearance.

CELLULITIS

General Cellulitis

Perspective Cellulitis is a soft tissue infection of the skin and subcutaneous tissue usually characterized by erythema, swelling, and tenderness. Cellulitis may be acute, subacute, or, rarely, chronic. Trauma or breaks in the protective cutaneous skin layer may be a predisposing cause, but hematogenous and lymphatic dissemination can account for cellulitis' sudden appearance in previously normal skin.

Principles of Disease and Clinical Features The signs and symptoms of cellulitis are generally pain or tenderness, erythema that blanches on palpation, swelling of the involved area, and local warmth. Cellulitis caused by infection tends to be reproducibly tender in the area of redness. Without therapy it will spread radially both distally and proximally with associated swelling. Cellulitis occurs most often in the lower and then the upper extremities.[1,2] The face is the next most common site. *Staphylococcus aureus* and *Streptococcus pyogenes* are by far the most commonly isolated organisms.[2,3] In children, *Haemophilus influenzae* may cause facial cellulitis, although anaerobic and oral mucosa flora play a role in facial and orbital cellulitis.[1] A portal of entry for the cellulitis is evident in only 50% to 60% of cases.[4]

Ludwig's angina is a cellulitis of the submandibular spaces bilaterally. This deep soft tissue infection caused by oral flora may quickly result in respiratory distress by elevation of the floor of the mouth and the tongue and is often associated with dental abscesses or extractions.[5-7] Cellulitis around the perineum is often the result of anaerobes or fecal flora and may spread rapidly through the soft tissues, producing a necrotizing fasciitis. In general, the bacterial etiology of cellulitis is a reflection of the bacteria found on the skin or mucous membranes of the anatomic site involved.

Differential Considerations Other conditions may simulate the appearance of bacterial cellulitis. They include arthropod and marine envenomation, the inflammatory response to foreign bodies, healing or postsurgical wounds, chemical or thermal burns, septic or inflammatory joints, dermatitis, and the arthritides. Differentiation, especially if the process is early and localized, may be difficult. In nonbacterial cellulitis the inflammation tends to stay localized and is often less tender to palpation.

In bacterial cellulitis, lymphangitis and local lymphadenopathy may be seen. Fluctuance, if present, signifies abscess formation. Fever is uncommon and should prompt the physician to consider secondary bacteremia or systemic involvement. With local involvement, vital signs, other than a slight tachycardia, are usually normal. Unless there is systemic involvement, white blood cell (WBC) counts are usually normal to mildly elevated with little or no shift to the left. One exception is *H. influenzae* B in children. This cellulitis is usually associated with high fever and white blood cell (WBC) counts greater than 15,000/mm^3, with a "left shift."[8,9] Fortunately, the incidence of such infections in children has decreased with the advent of an effective vaccine.

Diagnostic Strategies Bacterial cultures of material obtained by direct needle aspiration of cellulitis, either in the area of greatest erythema intensity or at the leading edge, are uniformly disappointing when no purulence is present. Typically, only 10% to 64% of patients with cellulitis have a positive aspiration culture, even after instillation of sterile saline solution into the involved skin.[1-4] Blood cultures of patients with cellulitis also tend to be disappointing, except in *H. influenzae* B cellulitis, which is associated more than two thirds of the time with bacteremia in children.[1,2]

Soft tissue radiographs and ultrasound may be useful to detect radiopaque foreign bodies, including glass. Computed tomography (CT) or magnetic resonance imaging (MRI) scans are reserved for instances in which deep space infections or abscesses are suspected. For most localized infections, no radiographic procedures are indicated.

Table 131-1. Clinical Characteristics of Soft Tissue Infections

	Cellulitis	Necrotizing fasciitis	Myonecrosis
Depth	Skin, subcutaneous tissue	Skin, subcutaneous tissue, fascia	Fascia, muscle
Predisposing factors	Trauma, superficial infection	Trauma, surgery, diabetes, deep soft tissue infection	Trauma, surgery, contaminated wounds
Skin	Erythema, lymphatic streaking, mildly swollen	Erythema; may have blebs, bullae, or patches of gangrene; severe swelling	Blanched with massive swelling; hemorrhagic bullae to frank necrosis to gangrene
Gas	No	Variable	Often
Pain	Mild	Moderate	Severe
System toxicity	Mild	Moderate to severe	Severe
Bacteriology	Skin flora, one or more agents	Mixed anaerobic and aerobic	Clostridia, anaerobes, aerobes
Therapy	None to local incision	Wide debridement	Radical excision
Mortality	Low	20%-50%	>25%

Management The time-honored treatment for cellulitis includes immobilization, elevation, heat or warm moist packs, analgesics, and antibiotics. Studies do not document any difference in morbidity or resolution with this regimen versus the use of antibiotics alone.

When managing a patient with cellulitis, the emergency physician must attempt to identify the etiologic mechanism. Trauma, puncture wounds, breaks in the skin, lymphatic or venous stasis, immunodeficiency, and foreign bodies are all predisposing factors. Hematogenous or contiguous spread from nearby infected tissue is uncommonly the cause. Most patients respond to appropriate oral antimicrobial agents. Cellulitis in the area of edema from a venous or lymphatic stasis is often difficult to manage and may need aggressive parenteral antibiotic therapy. Secondary bacterial overgrowth is not uncommon.

Disposition Localized cellulitis of an extremity in an immunologically intact, afebrile individual can be treated on an outpatient basis with oral antibiotics. Follow-up is indicated within 24 to 48 hours if the erythematous area is not diminishing in size or if fever develops. In general, antistaphylococcal agents should be selected for outpatient management (Table 131-2) because such agents treat the most common skin organisms that produce cellulitis. Inpatient management with parenteral antibiotics and closer observation are indicated in patients with systemic toxicity and with severe infections involving significant portions of an extremity (particularly the hands and feet), the head and neck, or the perineum. Inpatient management is often likely for significant cellulitis of the lower limb and hand. Patients whose cellulitis continues to worsen after 48 to 72 hours of appropriate outpatient therapy should be treated with parenteral antibiotics. All patients with cellulitis must be monitored closely to ensure that the process is resolving. Patients who are immunocompromised, including those who are diabetic, alcoholic, on chemotherapy or steroid therapy, asplenic, or at either age extreme, need more aggressive monitoring and treatment.

Patients do not have a simple cellulitis if they have a fever, hypotension, confusion, crepitus, or bullae formation of the involved soft tissues. These patients may be septic, with seeding to other sites such as blood, bone, lung, solid organs, or brain. They may have deep soft tissue infections necessitating aggressive surgical debridement. If an infection spreads to deeper tissues either directly or through lymph or blood with distal seeding, the initially localized superficial infection can quickly evolve into a severe systemic illness. Patients with these symptoms should be admitted to the hospital and investigated for deep soft tissue infections and systemic bacteremia.[10]

Special Types of Cellulitis

Periorbital (Preseptal) and Orbital Cellulitis

Perspective Cellulitis of the central face involving the area of the orbits must be treated aggressively. The venous drainage of that area is through communicating vessels into the brain via the cavernous sinus.[11-13] Streptococcal species are currently the most common organisms. The incidence of cellulitis from *H. influenzae* has decreased from previous prominence because of the effective vaccine now available.[14-16]

Principles of Disease and Clinical Features Periorbital (preseptal) cellulitis is an infection lying anterior to the orbital septum. It is usually associated with swelling of the eyelid, discoloration of the orbital skin, redness, and warmth. Conjunctival ecchymosis and injection with occasional discharge, fever, and leukocytosis are seen. Vision, extraocular movements, pupillary findings, and optometric examinations are normal.

Orbital cellulitis tends to have similar but more severe symptoms than preseptal cellulitis. Patients with orbital cellulitis may have proptosis, decreased ocular mobility, ocular pain, and tenderness on eye movement.[17] Retro-orbital gas or abscess formation, seen on CT or MRI scanning, increases the severity of these findings and results in decreased visual acuity.

Both orbital and periorbital cellulitis tends to be associated with youth and to be unilateral. Sinusitis is the leading cause, with up to 81% of cases having coexisting sinus infections.[14] Other etiologies include penetrating or abrading skin trauma, facial fractures, and preexisting vascular or pustular periocular skin infections. Less common causes are chemical agents and dental infections.[11-13]

Table 131-2. Oral Therapy of Superficial Soft Tissue Infections

Drug	Dosage
Streptococcus group A	
Penicillin V (phenoxymethyl penicillin)	250-500 mg qid
First-generation cephalosporin	250-500 mg qid
Erythromycin	250-500 mg qid
Azithromycin	500 mg × 1 dose then 250 mg qd × 4
Clarithromycin	500 mg bid
***Staphylococcus aureus* (not MRSA)**	
Dicloxacillin	125-500 mg qid
Cloxacillin	250-500 mg qid
First-generation cephalosporin	250-500 mg qid
Erythromycin (variable effectiveness)	250-500 mg qid
Azithromycin	500 mg × 1 dose then 250 mg qd × 4
Clarithromycin	500 mg bid
Clindamycin	150-450 mg qid
Amoxicillin/clavulanate	875/125 mg bid or 500/125 mg tid
Ciprofloxacin	500 mg bid
Haemophilus influenzae	
Amoxicillin/clavulanate	250-500 mg tid
Cefaclor	250-500 mg tid
Trimethoprim (TMP)/ sulfamethoxazole (SMX)	160 mg TMP/800 mg SMX bid
Azithromycin	500 mg × 1 dose then 250 mg qd × 4
Clarithromycin	500 mg bid

MRSA, Methicillin-resistant *Staphylococcus aureus.*

Diagnostic Strategies Differentiation of periorbital (preseptal) from orbital cellulitis is an important clinical decision that affects management and prognosis. If orbital cellulitis is suspected based on history and examination, a CT scan of the orbit is the most useful aid to determine retroorbital involvement.[18] Sinus and orbital radiographs tend to be less specific.[19] Causative organisms generally include *Streptococcal* species, *S. aureus,* and, less commonly, *H. influenzae* and anaerobes.[14-16]

Blood cultures and lumbar punctures are indicated in patients with high fevers or those showing signs of meningismus or sepsis.

Management Early periorbital (preseptal) cellulitis may be followed on an outpatient basis for the first 24 to 48 hours of antibiotic therapy, with daily follow-up to determine whether resolution is occurring. A broad-spectrum antistaphylococcal agent provides appropriate coverage. Treatment for orbital cellulitis includes hospitalization, intravenous (IV) antibiotics, and occasionally incision and drainage.[17,19-21] Broad-spectrum antibiotic coverage of *H. influenzae, S. aureus, Streptococcus pyogenes,* and anaerobes is indicated.[6,18]

Streptococcal Cellulitis

Principles of Disease and Clinical Features Streptococcal cellulitis, often termed *ascending cellulitis,* is usually seen after surgery or trauma, but it may occur with no predisposing event. The cause may be as subtle as a break in the skin around the web of the fingers or toes. Ascending cellulitis usually progresses rapidly, with prominent lymphangitic streaking and a swollen extremity. Untreated patients may quickly become toxic (see also discussion of streptococcal toxic shock syndrome).

Management Treatment includes the use of an antistreptococcal agent along with elevation of the involved extremity and warm soaks.

Erysipelas

Principles of Disease and Clinical Features Erysipelas is an acute superficial cellulitis characterized by a sharply demarcated border surrounding skin that is raised, deeply erythematous, indurated, and painful. It usually involves the dermis, lymphatics, and most of the superficial subcutaneous tissue. Erysipelas most often occurs in the very young and those age 50 to 60 years; it is associated with small breaks in the skin, nephrotic syndrome, and postoperative wounds. Patients usually appear toxic with a prodrome of fever, chills, and malaise preceding the eruption of a bright red cellulitis predominantly on the lower extremities or on the face. Group A *Streptococcus,* other streptococcal species, and *S. aureus* are the involved pathogens.[22]

Management The treatment is a first-generation cephalosporin or a macrolide. Diabetic patients may require broader coverage with ampicillin/clavulanic acid or a later-generation cephalosporin.[23]

Staphylococcal Cellulitis

Principles of Disease and Clinical Features *S. aureus* produces various toxins that result in local and systemic effects. Tissue invasion, blister formation, and inflammation are toxin mediated by several substances, such as alpha toxin, hyaluronidase, fibrinolysin, various proteases, and pyrogenic toxin superantigens.[24,25] Staphylococcal cellulitis is usually an indolent infection. The patient often appears less toxic than with streptococcal cellulitis, and the lesions usually appear more localized and result in the formation of an abscess.

Management Antistaphylococcal agents are indicated, along with heat, immobilization, elevation, and incision and drainage if an abscess is present.

Staphylococcal Scalded Skin Syndrome

Principles of Disease and Clinical Features Staphylococcal scalded skin syndrome, also called *staphylococcal epidermal necrolysis,* is caused by an exfoliative toxin produced by phage group II, type 71 staphylococci. This toxin acts on the zona granulosa of the skin to produce a superficial separation that results in widespread painful erythema and blistering of the skin. The syndrome usually occurs in children between ages 6 months and 6 years. Mortality is around 3% in children, but reaches 50% in adults and up to 100% in adults with underlying systemic disease.[26,27] Mucous membranes are usually not involved. Nikolsky's sign, the easy separation of the outer portion of the epidermis from the basal layer when pressure is exerted, is often present. The skin lesion is characterized by the formation of bullae and vesicles leading to the loss of large sheets of superficial epidermis. The resultant appearance is that of scalded skin.[25,28]

Differential Considerations The primary differential diagnosis is toxic epidermal necrolysis (TEN). TEN tends to be a deeper infection, is associated with the use of medication, usually occurs in adults, and does involve mucous membranes.

Diagnostic Strategies The diagnosis is made by clinical features and biopsy or a freshly frozen section of the blister demonstrating subglandular epithelial separation.[26,29] Blister fluid and the skin are usually sterile because this syndrome is toxin generated. *S. aureus* may be cultured from other mucous membrane sites such as the oral and nasal cavities.

Management Treatment of staphylococcal scalded skin syndrome includes adequate hydration, management of fluid and electrolyte balance, and systemic antibiotics with a penicillinase-resistant penicillin.[24,25]

H. Influenzae *Cellulitis*

Principles of Disease and Clinical Features *H. influenzae* cellulitis is usually seen in children under age 5 years and occurs primarily on the face or extremities. The skin often appears red with a violaceous tinge.[30] The patient appears acutely ill, often with high fever; the WBC count is greater than 15,000, and there is a high incidence (75% to 90%) of positive blood cultures. With widespread *H. influenzae* B immunization, there has been a dramatic decrease in *H. influenzae* skin infections.

Management Treatment is parenteral antibiotics with a second- or third-generation cephalosporin followed by ampicillin/clavulanic acid for a total of 10 to 14 days.[31,32]

Gram-Negative and Anaerobic Cellulitis Gram-negative and anaerobic cellulitis usually appears in the immunocompromised patient and occurs around mucous membranes, primarily the perineum, and in chronic wounds that are not kept clean and thus become super-infected. The diagnosis requires culturing. Aggressive debridement and broad-spectrum antimicrobial coverage are indicated.

TOXIC SHOCK SYNDROME

Staphylococcal Toxic Shock Syndrome

Perspective Toxic shock syndrome (TSS) often occurs in menstruating women who use vaginal tampons. Although prevalent in the early 1980s, the incidence of TSS has decreased remarkably since high-absorbency tampons were withdrawn from the market. The incidence of TSS was originally highest in Caucasian menstruating women. Today TSS is also reported in patients of both sexes who have focal soft tissue staphylococcal infections obviously unrelated to menstruation, and nonmenstrual causes are more prevalent.

Principles of Disease and Clinical Features In menstruating women with TSS, *S. aureus* is isolated more than 90% of the time. The clinical manifestations are secondary to a toxin that is produced by a phage group 1 *S. aureus;* other mediators also exist.[25,28,33] Other clinical features include fever, a "sunburn/sandpaper" rash, hypotension, and abnormalities in at least three organ systems. Mucosal inflammation, myalgia, profuse watery diarrhea, and changes in mental status are common (Box 131-1). Differential diagnosis includes Rocky Mountain spotted fever, streptococcal scarlet fever, Kawasaki syndrome, and leptospirosis.[24]

Box 131-1 Toxic Shock Syndrome: Criteria for Diagnosis

Fever of 38.9° C (102° F) or higher
Rash (diffuse macular erythema) that resembles the rash of scarlet fever
Desquamation of skin 1 to 2 weeks after onset of disease
Hypotension (systolic blood pressure less than 90 mm Hg, orthostatic drop of 15 mm Hg or more, or orthostatic dizziness of syncope)
Clinical or laboratory abnormalities in at least three organ systems:
- Gastrointestinal: nausea and vomiting, diarrhea
- Muscular: myalgia or creatine phosphokinase at least two times normal
- Mucous membrane: vaginal, oropharyngeal, or conjunctival hyperemia
- Renal: BUN or creatinine at least twice normal or pyuria greater than five cells per high-power field
- Hepatic: bilirubin, serum transaminases at least twice normal
- Hematologic: thrombocytopenia, <100,000/mm^3
- Neurologic: disorientation or altered consciousness without focal findings

Reasonable evidence for the absence of other causes of illness

Management Treatment includes aggressive fluid resuscitation and the use of α- and β-adrenergic vasoactive agents to maintain blood pressure and urinary output. IV antibiotics that cover for penicillinase-producing *staphylococci,* such as nafcillin or oxacillin, should be used. However, clindamycin and vancomycin are acceptable for patients who are allergic to penicillin.

Tampons and foreign bodies must be removed, focal areas of infection drained, and mucous membranes and other sources cultured for the offending pathogen. Systemic steroids, if administered early, may be beneficial in treating the disease.[25,34,35]

Streptococcal Toxic Shock Syndrome

Perspective Streptococcus has long been known to cause invasive infections. Previously, these infections have been most common and severe in patients with compromised immune systems (e.g., cancer or burns). Since the mid-1980s a streptococcal toxic shock–like syndrome has been described in patients with serious soft tissue infections. Streptococcal toxic shock syndrome (STSS) was first described by Cone in 1987 when he reported two cases of shock caused by isolated *Streptococcal pyogenes* soft tissue infections; he postulated a toxin was responsible for the shock state.[36] Stevens further characterized the syndrome in 1989 as involving otherwise healthy young patients who either presented in shock or progressed to a shock state within 4 hours of admission.[37] These facts seem to indicate an increased virulence of group A β-hemolytic streptococcus. Also, although these cases are predominantly caused by Lancefield group A strains, other groups have also been shown to cause STSS.[38]

Principles of Disease and Clinical Features Route of entry is unknown in up to 50% of cases, with others related to surgery, minor nonpenetrating trauma resulting in hematoma or muscle strain, skin superinfection, or viral infections.[39] In children, STSS most commonly follows chickenpox.[38] There is also an association with the use of nonsteroidal antiinflammatory drugs (NSAIDs), which may mask presenting symptoms, resulting in increased severity of disease.

Patients commonly have pain, which is severe, abrupt in onset, and often present before tenderness or physical findings. Although usually in an extremity, the pain may mimic that associated with pelvic inflammatory disease, pneumonia, acute myocardial infarction, peritonitis, or pericarditis. A minority of patients have influenza-like symptoms of fever, chills, myalgias, and/or diarrhea.

Fever is the most common presenting physical sign. However, if shock is present, the patient may be hypothermic. Tachycardia and hypotension are also frequent. Most patients also have evidence of soft tissue infection: swelling, erythema, bullae, or tenderness. A scarlet fever–like rash is commonly seen[37] (Box 131-2).

These patients often have renal and respiratory failure. The hemodynamic compromise seen in affected patients suggests a cardiotoxic effect of the streptococcal toxins, resulting in normal to low cardiac output, normal systemic vascular resistance, and a reduced left ventricular stroke work index.[40] Mortality approaches 30%.[37,41]

The virulence of these infections is attributed to toxin production, surface proteins, and host factors. *Streptococcal* strains that produce M and T serologic subtypes seem to be associated with overwhelming infection and the production of exotoxins A and B, which allow the process to mimic the staphylococcus toxic shock syndrome.[42-44] The toxins act as superantigens to activate a large population of T cells, bypassing the antigen presentation phase and liberating massive amounts of cytokines TNF-α, IL-1, and IL-6. These cytokines induce the clinical signs of fever, hypotension, shock, rash, and ultimately multiorgan failure.[45] M-1 and M-3 surface proteins have increased in prevalence and provide antiphagocytic properties and increased bacterial adherence to infected tissue, contributing to invasiveness.[39,40]

Box 131-2 Definition of Streptococcal Toxic Shock Syndrome

Must meet criteria from both 1 and 2 below:

1. Isolation of group A streptococcus from:
   a. A normally sterile site such as blood or cerebrospinal fluid is a definite case
   b. A normally nonsterile site such as sputum or skin lesion is a probable case
2. Hypotension and at least two of the following:
   a. Renal impairment
   b. Coagulopathy
   c. Liver involvement
   d. Adult respiratory distress syndrome
   e. Generalized erythematous macular rash that may desquamate
   f. Soft tissue necrosis

Lack of host antibodies to the surface proteins and toxins predispose to infection and increased virulence.

Differential Considerations Differential diagnosis includes staphylococcal TSS and gram-negative sepsis. Staphylococcal infection is unlikely to show cutaneous involvement or extremity pain, may demonstrate a "strawberry tongue," is rarely associated with soft tissue destruction, and has a lower incidence of bacteremia. Endotoxic shock is differentiated by high cardiac output with lowered systemic vascular resistance and a left ventricular stroke work index that is not reduced.

Diagnostic Strategies Creatinine level greater than 2.5 mg/dl indicates renal involvement, which may precede hypotension. Serum creatine kinase correlates well with deep soft tissue involvement, and increasing values may indicate necrotizing fasciitis or myositis (the "flesh-eating bacteria").

Other laboratory abnormalities may include hypoalbuminemia, hypocalcemia, and a sometimes mild leukocytosis with prominent "left shift." Platelets and hematocrit may be initially normal but drop within 48 hours and may be associated with disseminated intravascular coagulation. Blood cultures are positive 60% of the time, and wound cultures 95%.[46]

Management The need for supportive measures mandates admission to the hospital, usually initially into an intensive care setting. Even with appropriate antibiotic therapy and intensive supportive care, the mortality for this disease is 30% to 70%.

It is often difficult to determine initially whether streptococcal or staphylococcal organisms are the offending bacteria, so coverage for both is necessary. Suggested regimens include penicillin plus clindamycin, erythromycin, or ceftriaxone plus clindamycin. Penicillin is only moderately effective against the large inoculum of slow-growing streptococci seen in necrotizing fasciitis or myositis. In vitro studies suggest better results with clindamycin or erythromycin. Clindamycin has several potentially beneficial effects: (1) it is not affected by inoculum size, (2) it can kill cell wall-deficient streptococci (protoplasts), (3) it has a long post-administration efficacy, (4) it suppresses toxin and M-protein production, and (5) it enhances opsonization of streptococcal organisms when they are grown with low concentrations of penicillin.[37,41,47]

Early surgical debridement may be life-saving, and consultation is appropriate as soon as the possible need for surgical intervention is considered.

Use of intravenous gamma globulin remains experimental despite some case reports of success. Gamma globulin preparations contain antibodies to staphylococcal toxins with some cross reactivity to streptococcal toxins. Recommended doses vary; one suggested regimen is 1 g/kg given on the first treatment day and started during surgery if surgery is needed, followed by 0.5 g/kg on the following day.[48] Case reports also indicate there may be some benefit if dexamethasone is given with the globulin, although this benefit is not yet proved.[49]

Currently antibiotic prophylaxis is not recommended for household contacts of patients with this disease, although contact with an infected person increases carrier rates in the young.[38,50] Also, the elderly are at increased risk for invasive disease after contact.[51]

IMPETIGO

Perspective Impetigo is a superficial infection of the skin caused by group A β-hemolytic streptococcus and occasionally coagulase-positive *S. aureus.* There are two distinct subtypes: impetigo contagiosa and bullous impetigo.[52,53] Impetigo is communicable and is the most common cutaneous childhood infection.[54] Most cases occur in late summer and early fall, and the incidence is higher in tropical climates.

Principles of Disease and Clinical Features Insect bites, flies, and infected abrasions may play a role in the nonbullous form of impetigo.[52] The pathogenesis and epidemiology of this infection are a mystery in that inoculation of normal skin does not produce clinical disease. During outbreaks of impetigo, streptococci usually appear on normal skin several days before spreading to the nose or throat. In contrast, staphylococcal colonization of the nose and throat takes place before the development of skin lesions. Streptococci found on the skin are not the same subtype as those that infect the pharynx.[53]

The lesions of impetigo contagiosa begin as tiny papules that rapidly develop into vesicles, which quickly progress to pustules that rupture and crust over within 24 hours. The lesions are usually painless but often pruritic and may coalesce.[52,53] The crusts are usually thick, amber colored, and crumbly. Cultures of early vesicles, pustules, or crusts usually yield β-hemolytic streptococci and occasionally *S. aureus.* After the fifth or sixth day the crusts become thicker and reddish brown. The lesions tend to extend in size, clearing centrally. Lesions are most commonly seen on the legs, with the arms, face, and trunk less commonly affected. Regional lymphadenopathy is common, lymphadenitis is rare, and fever is not usually present.[54]

Bullous impetigo is most commonly seen in neonates. It starts as a small vesicle that quickly enlarges into a bulla, often 1 to 3 cm in diameter. When a bulla ruptures, it leaves a red base with a varnishlike thin crust and scales. Satellite lesions are frequently seen. Nikolsky's sign is not present, and the patient is not toxic.[55] Bullous impetigo occurs most commonly on the face and trunk. Regional lymphadenitis is rare. These lesions generally heal faster than those of impetigo contagiosa.

Differential Considerations Impetigo of Bockhart is a superficial staphylococcal folliculitis consisting of clusters of small pustules surrounding hair follicles.[56]

Ecthyma is closely related to impetigo, except that the infection is usually deeper and heals with scarring. The lesions of ecthyma are usually on the legs and begin as a vesicle that ruptures to form a shallow ulcer. Causative organisms are group A β-hemolytic streptococcus and rarely *S. aureus.* Treatment is 10 to 14 days of penicillin or topical mupirocin.

Diagnostic Strategies Bacteria are usually not seen in Gram's stain of vesicular fluid. *S. aureus* can be found in cultures of denuded skin under the ruptured bullae.[55] Group 2 *S. aureus* usually predominates.[52,55]

Certain strains of streptococci are nephritogenic. Poststreptococcal glomerulonephritis is more likely to follow streptococcal pharyngitis than impetigo. In contrast, acute rheumatic fever is not a consequence of impetigo.[53] Although serologic findings in streptococcal pyoderma may show increases in antibodies to various streptococcal antigens, primarily anti-DNAase B and antihyaluronidase (AH), the serologic response as measured by antistreptolysin O (ASO) is usually poor.[53] The streptozyme test, which measures several streptococcal antibodies, often gives false-negative results.[53]

Management Soaks and wet dressings have not proved useful in treating impetigo. Topical antimicrobial agents such as hexachlorophene or povidone-iodine scrubs or washes are of limited usefulness and may result in the development of satellite lesions.[54] Although various topical antibiotics, including neomycin, bacitracin, polymyxin, erythromycin, and oxytetracycline, have resulted in some improvement of impetigo, topical antibiotics alone or in combination with hexachlorophene have proved ineffective in treating impetigo in military populations. Mupirocin ointment 2% is an effective alternative regimen. Other topical antibiotics may alter antibiotic resistance patterns. The addition of topical steroids to topical antibiotic agents does not improve outcome.

Except for mupirocin, systemic antibiotics are clearly superior to topical antibiotics for treating impetigo contagiosa. Oral erythromycin and phenoxymethyl penicillin are used most commonly. First-generation cephalosporins are also effective, as is clindamycin (see Table 131-2). In some studies, intramuscular benzathine penicillin G is more effective than oral phenoxymethyl penicillin or erythromycin. Although cultures of early lesions often grow only streptococcus, older lesions may yield staphylococcus. Streptococcus seems to be the primary infecting agent, with staphylococcus as a secondary invader. Treatment of impetigo with systemic and topical antibiotics does not prevent poststreptococcal glomerulonephritis, although it clears lesions quickly, reduces local extension and complications such as adenitis, and prevents spread to other individuals.[52]

In cases of bullous impetigo, some topical antibiotic preparations, such as gentamicin and a mixture of polymyxin, neomycin, and bacitracin, are as effective as a combination of oral and intramuscular benzathine penicillin G. Antistaphylococcal agents such as oral cephalosporins and semisynthetic penicillins are usually very effective. In most cases, for a solitary lesion or just a few lesions, a topical antibiotic alone is reasonable therapy.[53]

ABSCESSES

Simple Cutaneous Abscesses

Perspective A cutaneous abscess is a localized collection of pus resulting in a painful fluctuant soft tissue mass surrounded by firm granulation tissue and erythema. Abscesses occur in all areas of the body; approximately 20% are in the head and neck region, 25% in the axillae, 18% in the extremities, 25% in the perirectal area, and 15% in the inguinal area.[57] Most patients complain of pain and the presence of a tender fluctuant mass. Although abscesses may be associated with localized erythema and lymphangitis, the presence of fever or systemic toxicity should alert the emergency physician to the possibility of deeper tissue involvement or systemic bacteremia.[57]

Principles of Disease and Clinical Features The cause of localized abscesses depends on the anatomic region involved.[58] Abscesses on the extremities tend to be associated with interruptions of the integrity of the protective epithelial layer of the skin caused by minor traumas such as cuts, abrasions, or needle punctures. Abscesses of the head, neck, and perineal regions tend to be associated with obstruction of the apocrine sweat glands.[59] The incidence of these abscesses increases in adults because the apocrine and sebaceous glands become active after puberty. Perirectal abscesses arise from bacterial spread from the anal crypts. Vulvovaginal abscesses usually result from obstruction of the Bartholin gland duct. Pilonidal abscesses are caused by plugging of small tears in the skin, usually by hairs around the buttock crease.[60]

Although most abscesses contain bacteria, approximately 5% of abscesses, especially those associated with parenteral drug abuse, may be sterile.[57] Clinically they cannot be differentiated from bacterial abscesses. *Eikenella corrodens* is a microbe often seen with head and neck abscesses associated with IV drug abuse.[61] The bacteria in cutaneous abscesses generally reflect the skin flora of the anatomic area of the body involved (Table 131-3). Anaerobic bacteria, which are known to be part of the normal flora of the skin and mucous membranes, outnumber aerobes 10 to 1 in the oral cavity and 1000 to 1 in the distal colon.[62] Most abscesses that originate from mucous membranes (e.g., perioral, perirectal) tend to be predominantly anaerobic. Bacteria from abscesses in areas more remote from the rectum are primarily constituents of the microflora of the skin. *S. aureus* is the most prevalent aerobe found in abscesses that originate from the skin, yet it is isolated in less than one third of cutaneous abscesses and one half of axillary abscesses.[63] *S. aureus* is not commonly associated with abscesses that originate from mucous membranes (i.e., perirectal, vulvovaginal).[57,63] *Bacteroides fragilis* is one of the few anaerobes resistant to penicillin.[64] Although it is the most common gram-negative anaerobic species in human feces, it is found in fewer than 50% of perineal abscesses.[57] This pathogen, which produces β-lactamase, has been associated with more than 50% of intraabdominal infections. *Escherichia coli* and *Neisseria gonorrhoeae* are rarely found in cutaneous abscesses from any location. Table 131-3 outlines the clinical characteristics of localized aerobic and anaerobic cutaneous abscesses.

Differential Considerations Although abscesses generally tend to be isolated events, recurrent abscesses in the perineal and lower abdominal area may signify the presence of inflammatory bowel disease. Recurring abscesses in the axillae and inguinal areas may represent hidradenitis suppurativa. Finally, recurring abscesses may be associated with immunocompromise such as occurs with neoplasm, corticosteroid therapy, chemotherapy, diabetes mellitus, acquired immunodeficiency syndrome (AIDS), leukemia, vascular insufficiency, trauma, or thermal injury.

Diagnostic Strategies Ultrasound is a useful technique to localize subcutaneous and intramuscular abscesses and foreign bodies that are not radiopaque.[65,66]

The examination material from cutaneous abscesses stained with Gram's stain allows a quick identification of the morphologic type of the offending pathogen. In general, Gram's stain shows one of three patterns: (1) white cells without bacteria, which indicates a sterile abscess; (2) a mixed pattern of gram-positive and gram-negative rods and cocci of varied morphologic types, which indicates mixed aerobic and anaerobic infection; and (3) gram-positive cocci in grapelike clusters, diagnostic of *S. aureus*.[57]

Management The treatment of cutaneous abscesses is simply incision and drainage. Several studies confirm that antibiotics are not indicated in patients with normal host defenses.[2,57,67] Thus a Gram's stain and culture are also unnecessary in these patients. In the immunosuppressed patient, Gram's stain, culture, and antibiotics are indicated. The selection of antibiotics is guided by (1) the flora anticipated at the location of the abscess, (2) the Gram's stain results, (3) the presence of a feculent odor that is indicative of anaerobes, and (4) culture and sensitivity[57,63] (see Table 131-2).

Incision and drainage are generally painful because local anesthetics are less effective in inflamed acidic locations. The use of parenteral or regional analgesia may be indicated in addition to a local anesthetic agent. Nitrous oxide is an option, especially in a self-administered 50% concentration. The incision should be deep enough into the abscess cavity to

Table 131-3. Bacterial Characterization of 135 Outpatient Abscesses

				Types of bacterial growth (% from each area)			Bacterial species per abscess*	
Anatomic areas	**Abscesses (number)**	**Percent of total cultures**	**No growth**	**Aerobes only**	**Anaerobes only**	**Aerobes and anaerobes**	**Aerobes (average no.)**	**Anaerobes (average no.)**
Head and Neck	25	19	4	28	20	48	1	2
Trunk	11	8	0	45	18	36	1	2
Axilla	22	16	0	55	5	41	1	1
Extremity	16	12	19	44	13	25	1	1
Hand	8	6	25	63	0	13	2	0
Inguinal	7	5	0	29	57	14	0	3
Vulvovaginal	13	10	0	15	46	38	1	3
Buttock	12	9	0	33	33	33	1	3
Perirectal	21	16	0	0	33	67	1	5

From Meislin HW et al: *Ann Intern Med* 87:145, 1977.
*Cultures with no growth were excluded.

ensure adequate drainage. Elliptical incisions are preferred by some emergency physicians to prevent premature closure of the cutaneous surface. The cavity should be gently curetted to free all loculated areas of pus, and the cavity should be irrigated. A loose packing should be removed within 48 hours or within 24 hours in cosmetically important areas such as the face. Once the packing is removed, warm soaks are recommended three or four times a day for 10 to 15 minutes for 2 to 3 days.[57,64,68]

Furuncle

A furuncle usually evolves from a superficial folliculitis. It is a deep inflammatory nodule surrounded by an intense local tissue reaction. The abscess tends to be very thin walled, and purulence is present. Skin flora (*S. aureus,* streptococci) are usually isolated.

Carbuncle

A carbuncle is an extensive process of interconnecting deep abscesses that extend into subcutaneous tissues. The microbes are usually aerobic; however, *Pseudomonas aeruginosa* may be present in chronic cases. Predisposing factors include folliculitis, blood dyscrasias, steroids, heavy perspiration, obesity, diabetes, and areas of friction, especially the back of the neck.

Hidradenitis Suppurativa

Perspective Hidradenitis suppurativa is a disease consisting of chronic suppurative abscesses in the apocrine sweat glands. The typical patient is a young adult; the female-to-male ratio is 3:1.[69] An increased incidence may occur in African Americans because of their larger number of apocrine sweat glands.[70] Inflammation begins deep within the acinus or convoluted tubules of the sweat glands as a result of obstruction to apocrine glandular secretions. Additional factors may include obesity, poor hygiene, excessive perspiration, shaving, and irritating deodorants.[71] The axillary location is more common than inguinal and perianal.

Principles of Disease and Clinical Features In most cases the disease manifests as episodic occurrences of a painful subcutaneous nodule, with burning, itching, local cellulitis, swelling, and a malodorous discharge.[68] These nodules drain spontaneously or are surgically incised and followed by drainage of scant pus. Resolution usually occurs within a few days. In some patients, however, the disease tends to be chronic and extensive, with multiple abscesses, sinus tracts, and fistulas. These often heal with hypertrophic scars and may result in a tender, unsightly area.

S. aureus, S. viridans, and common skin anaerobes are usually found. Chronic disease often results in overgrowth with fecal flora in the perineum and *Proteus* with other mixed aerobes and anaerobes in the axilla.[68]

Differential Considerations Hidradenitis suppurativa must be differentiated from a simple cutaneous abscess of the axillary region or perianal and perirectal abscesses. This differentiation is usually accomplished by noting the chronicity of the process, the multiplicity of abscesses, and the lack of involvement with the rectal mucosa.

Management Although clindamycin may provide temporary recession of the disease, the almost inevitable recurrence makes surgery the definitive therapy.[71] Incision and drainage usually suffice in an acute situation. Sinus tracts and fistulas should be unroofed, all loculations excised, and all purulence and necrotic tissue evacuated. Antibiotic coverage is usually unnecessary in patients with normal host defenses and without soft tissue involvement. Chronic or extensive disease often requires extensive surgical removal of all hair-bearing skin in the apocrine gland areas. Coverage requires primary closure, rotated skin flaps, or grafting.[71] Surgical specimens must be examined microscopically because 2% to 3% of hidradenitis cases harbor squamous carcinoma.[72] In cases of extensive perianal disease, some have advised a diverting colostomy before removal of large areas of the skin of the perineal area to prevent fecal contamination.[69]

Hidradenitis suppurativa has been associated with social, personal, and vocational difficulties because of the chronic, uncomfortable, malodorous, and unsightly nature of the disease. Early referral for surgical obliteration of the apocrine glands should be considered in these patients.

Bartholin Cyst Abscess

Principles of Disease and Clinical Features A Bartholin cyst abscess is caused by an obstructed Bartholin duct. The flora is usually a mixture of aerobic and anaerobic flora from the vagina, with *C. trachomatis* and *N. gonorrhoeae* cultured around 10% of the time.[57,62,73-75] The patient usually has a painful cystic mass on the inferior lateral margin of the vaginal introitus. Signs and symptoms are generally localized, but septic shock can occur in rare cases.[76]

Management Abscesses should be drained from the mucosal rather than the cutaneous surface. Doing simple incision and drainage carries a high risk of recurrence, so the cavity should be packed open. The Word catheter is a No. 10 French balloon catheter designed specifically for this purpose, and it is both convenient to use and associated with a high degree of success. After incision and drainage, the catheter is inserted and inflated with 2 to 5 ml of water or saline solution (Figure 131-1). The catheter should be left in place for 4 to 6 weeks so that a sinus will have time to form. Sitz baths help keep the area clean and draining.

Marsupialization is a more complex treatment option, involving incision and drainage of the cavity followed by suturing the walls of the cyst to the skin.

Perirectal Abscess

Principles of Disease and Clinical Features Perirectal abscesses originate in the anal crypts and extend through the ischiorectal space via fistulous tracts into nearby fatty tissue or perimuscular locations.[77,78] Many times, however, the fistulous tracts that connect the abscess site to the anal crypts cannot be traced directly. Patients have pain in the anal region, with a tender mass that may be indurated, fluctuant, or draining. There is usually pain on defecation or with sitting or walking.

Perirectal abscesses occur primarily in adult men, although occasionally they are found in pediatric patients. Inflammatory bowel disease, diabetes, immunodeficiency, malignancies, and pregnancy have been associated with a higher incidence of perirectal abscesses.[79] Fecal flora are causative. The predominant anaerobe is *B. fragilis,* although most

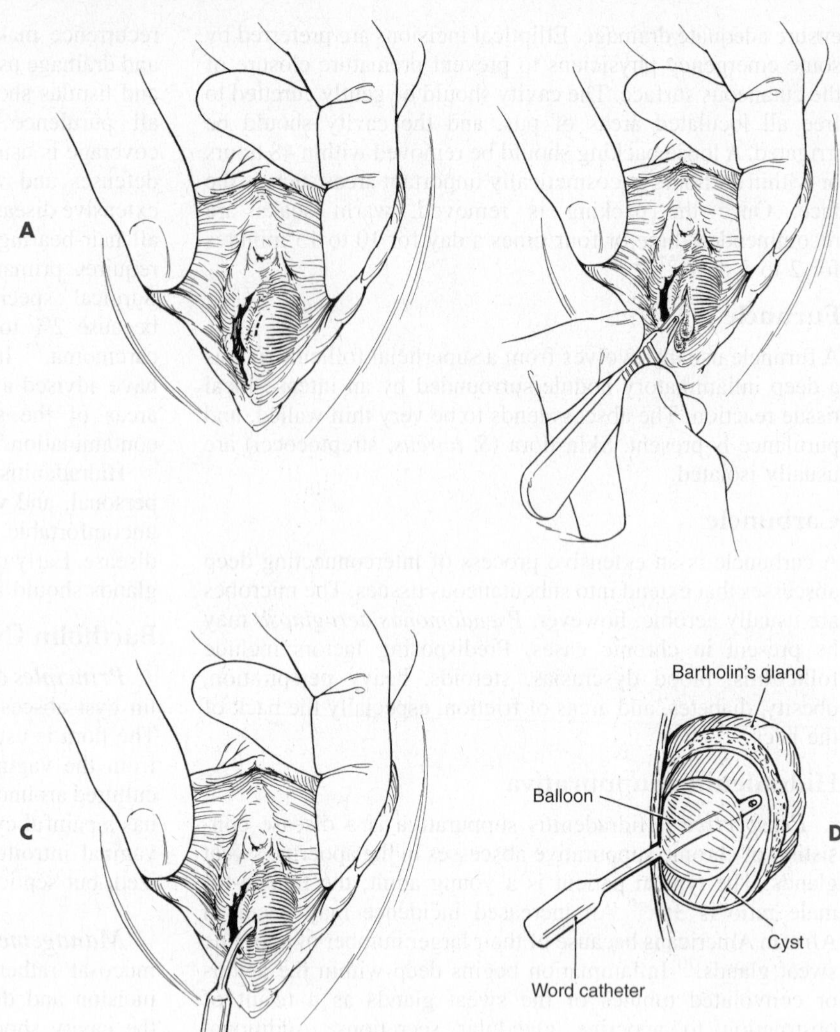

Figure 131-1. **Incision and drainage of Bartholin's abscess. A, Inject local anesthetic into the mucosal surface of the abscess and the mucocutaneous junction of the labia minora. B, Make a 1-cm incision on the mucosal surface. C and D, Insert the Word catheter and inflate the balloon with 5 ml normal saline solution.** *From Campbell CJ: Incision and drainage of Bartholin's cyst. In Rosen P et al, editors:* **Atlas of emergency procedures,** *St. Louis, 2001, Mosby.*

abscesses tend to have mixed anaerobic and aerobic flora.[57,63] Children, unlike adults, demonstrate *E. coli*.

Management The use of antibiotics remains controversial. When there are signs of systemic involvement such as cellulitis, fever, or leukocytosis, antibiotics are indicated.[78] The emergency physician should provide coverage for anaerobes and gram-negative fecal flora before incision and drainage to prevent bacteremia, especially in patients with a history of valvular heart disease or immunocompromise. Postoperative management includes the use of stool softeners, sitz baths, and frequent dressing changes for several days until the incision is healed. Perirectal abscesses are usually classified into four types (Figure 131-2).

Perianal Abscess

A perianal abscess is a tender, swollen, fluctuant mass in the superficial subcutaneous tissue just adjacent to the anus. The patient is usually afebrile, and the process is localized. The treatment is an incision made in a radial direction from the anal opening. If the abscess is extensive or a fistula is identified, the patient should be referred to have the fistulous channel excised and unroofed electively.

Ischiorectal Abscess

An ischiorectal abscess is an infection extending across the external sphincter into the ischiorectal space below the levator ani. Infection may spread superiorly, producing a high abscess that may be difficult to diagnose even when very large because it produces little change in the anorectal skin area. Intrarectal ultrasound appears promising in the diagnosis of complex perirectal abscesses.[80]

Low abscesses tend to burrow down into the fatty tissue between the rectum and ischial tuberosity and produce a perirectal abscess. Perirectal abscesses produce tenderness and bulging, with shiny skin lateral to the anus.

Incision and drainage can be performed on an outpatient basis if the abscess points to the perirectal skin area and the patient is not toxic. If the abscess is large and does not point to the skin or if the patient is toxic, drainage should be performed in the operating theater. These large abscesses must be differentiated from a more extensive fasciitis. High abscesses can be drained only with an incision made deep into the ischiorectal space. Ischiorectal abscesses may burrow into the posterior rectal space, penetrating to the opposite side to form a "horseshoe abscess." These are drained in the operative setting with multiple incisions.

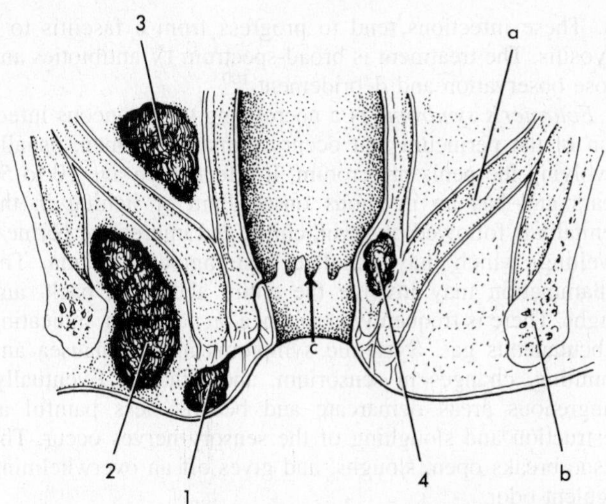

Figure 131-2. Perirectal abscesses. *a,* Levator ani. *b,* Ischial tuberosity. *c,* Anal crypts. *1,* Perianal abscess with anal fistula. *2,* Ischiorectal abscess. *3,* Supralevator ani (pelvirectal) abscess. *4,* Intersphincteric abscess.

Pelvirectal Abscess

Pelvirectal abscesses are also known as *supralevator abscesses.* They form in or spread to the space above the levator ani muscle. These abscesses can result from pelvic inflammatory disease, diverticulitis, or ruptured appendicitis. They are often difficult to diagnose because clinical signs are nonspecific: rectal pain, fever, leukocytosis, and back pain.[81] Endoscopy or barium enema may reveal a bulge in the rectal mucosa. Pelvirectal abscesses are drained in the operating room through an intraanal incision rather than through the ischiorectal space.

Intersphincteric Abscess

Intersphincteric abscesses are often seen as a tender bulge of the rectal mucosa. Incision and drainage are done through a mucosal incision in the distal rectum under general or spinal anesthesia. It may be difficult to differentiate an intersphincteric (submucous) abscess from a high ischiorectal or a supralevator abscess.

Pilonidal Abscess

Principles of Disease and Clinical Features Pilonidal abscesses usually occur in the gluteal fold overlying the coccyx. They result from a minor disruption of the epithelium, with formation of a small pit. Squamous epithelia gradually line this cavity, which then plugs with hair or keratin, preventing drainage and promoting abscess formation.[60,82] These abscesses contain a combination of skin and perineal flora.[57,63] Pilonidal cysts occur more often in men and in dark-skinned or hirsute individuals.[83] These patients complain of tenderness in the gluteal fold. Inspection reveals a tender nodule that is often fluctuant. The process tends to be localized without systemic symptoms.

Management Treatment is incision and drainage, although opinions differ regarding the advisability of a simple incision and drainage versus complete excision of the involved tissue. It is reasonable for the emergency physician to incise and drain any pilonidal abscess that is acutely fluctuant, with referral for more definitive excision if the process tends to be deep or if sinus tracts are present. All hair or keratin plugs must be removed. Recurrence rates after simple drainage range from 10% to 90%. Recurrences take place because of remaining granulation tissue, development of new pits, or the formation of new sinuses. Chronic disease is common and often necessitates inpatient surgical removal of the cysts, sinuses, and granulation tissue. Primary closure or cryosurgery has also been advocated.[83]

FASCIITIS

Principles of Disease and Clinical Features Fasciitis is an infection of the fascia, subcutaneous tissue, and skin. Erythema, marked edema, and, sometimes, areas of gangrene occur (see Table 131-1). Much confusion has surrounded the nomenclature of these necrotizing infections because they have been named for specific bacteria (e.g., hemolytic streptococcal gangrene), after individuals (e.g., Meleney's synergistic gangrene), by anatomic appearance (e.g., necrotizing fasciitis), and for specific circumstances (e.g., postoperative progressive bacterial gangrene). By definition, fasciitis does not involve muscle, but it can spread to invade underlying muscle, causing myonecrosis. Patients with fasciitis manifest moderate to severe systemic toxicity, often out of proportion to the cutaneous findings, with high fever, tachycardia, anxiety, disorientation, and often frank shock. Tissue invasion is rapid, often spreading from a cellulitis to a necrotizing fasciitis within 1 to 2 days. Massive subcutaneous edema and necrosis are common. Early on, the skin may be relatively spared, but as the disease progresses the cutaneous tissues often demonstrate blebs, crepitus, or frank necrosis.[84] Diabetes, peripheral vascular disease, trauma, and recent surgery are predisposing factors. Pain varies because cutaneous nerve endings are quickly destroyed. Thus the absence or cessation of pain may indicate worsening rather than improvement.[85,86]

Management The initial treatment of all of these infections involves fluid resuscitation, parenteral antibiotics, and early surgical incision, drainage, and debridement. Large quantities of crystalloids are often necessary to replace fluid sequestered in the wound. Hemolysis occurs and may require the use of blood replacement products. Disseminated intravascular coagulopathy occurs in severe cases. IV calcium may be necessary to reverse the hypocalcemia that results from necrosis of subcutaneous fat. The usual anaerobic infection has a foul discharge, occurs in locations near mucosal openings (perineum, oral pharynx), may present with gas, and usually has a Gram's stain that shows a polymorphic array of organisms with negative aerobic cultures.[85] The initial choice of antibiotics for necrotizing fasciitis should be guided by the Gram's stain, culture, and anatomic area involved. Use of penicillin, an aminoglycoside, and clindamycin is recommended for a broad spectrum of coverage of aerobes, gram-negative enteric organisms, and anaerobes. If gram-positive organisms are expected or are seen on stain, a penicillinase-resistant penicillin should be added.[87]

Necrotizing Fasciitis

Principles of Disease *Necrotizing fasciitis* is the preferred term for describing these uncommon but potentially lethal infections. This disease usually occurs in men in the lower extremities and may evolve after only minimal local trauma. Although a monobacterial etiology, typically *Clostridium* and *Streptococcus* group A, can be found, the infections are usually produced by mixed flora, both aerobes and anaerobes. During the last two decades, there has been increased recognition of a rapidly spreading necrotizing fasciitis caused by group A β-hemolytic streptococcus (*S. pyogenes*). A substance in the cell wall of streptococci causes a separation of the dermal connective tissue, resulting in continued inflammation and necrosis. Streptococcal necrotizing fasciitis is frequently associated with streptococcal toxic shock syndrome.[88-90]

Early clinical findings are similar to those with most infected wounds, but the involved site quickly becomes erythematous, tender, and edematous; fever is usually present. Numbness or deep pain is often out of proportion to the physical findings. Early on, the skin appears relatively benign, but necrotic patches and bullae may appear between days 2 and 4 as a serosanguinous watery fluid begins to ooze. Deep structures and muscles are not involved. Hypotension, tachycardia, leukocytosis, and hypocalcemia ensue, with systemic toxicity out of proportion to the clinical findings. Radiographs may reveal gas in the tissues. The absence of gas does not exclude the diagnosis of necrotizing fasciitis. Frozen-section biopsy can be useful in diagnosis. MRI helps differentiate acute cellulitis from necrotizing fasciitis.[91-93]

Management Treatment is surgical debridement, fluid and critical care resuscitation, and parenteral antibiotics against *S. aureus, Streptococcus,* gram-negative organisms, and anaerobes as directed by Gram's stains and cultures. Debridement should be aggressive and may have to be repeated. The mortality rate is 20% to 50%.[94-96]

Specific Fasciitis Syndromes

Meleney's synergistic gangrene (progressive bacterial synergistic gangrene) involves superficial and deep fascial planes with thrombosis of the subcutaneous vessels and gangrene of tissues. It is usually seen at the site of a laceration or surgical wound, but sometimes no portal of entry can be found. The skin appears erythematous and may eventually take on a bluish, gangrenous appearance. The patient is toxic, with fever and leukocytosis. Group A streptococcus is found in the skin and blood, although *S. aureus* and gram-negative enteric organisms may be found. Treatment is wide incision and debridement with appropriate antibiotics.[37,93,97-99]

Clostridial cellulitis (anaerobic cellulitis, local gas gangrene) is a gas-forming infection of the skin and subcutaneous tissue that spreads through intrafascial planes. Other bacterial flora may be seen. Healthy muscle is not involved. It results from superinfection of previously traumatized or necrotic tissue. Gas distributes in large bubbles in the fascial plane but not the muscle. Patients show signs of systemic toxicity: fever, tachycardia, edema of the affected part, and pain. Incision and debridement of involved tissue and blebs are necessary. Antibiotic treatment is penicillin or tetracycline. These patients must be hospitalized.

Nonclostridial crepitant cellulitis is similar to clostridial cellulitis except that the flora are usually polymicrobial, with aerobic and anaerobic coliforms such as *E. coli, Klebsiella, Enterobacter, Peptostreptococcus, Peptococcus,* and *B. fragilis.* These infections tend to progress from a fasciitis to a myositis. The treatment is broad-spectrum IV antibiotics and close observation and debridement.[100]

Fournier's syndrome is a necrotizing subcutaneous infection of the perineum that occurs primarily in men, usually involving the penis or scrotum. It affects men age 20 to 50 years and has an insidious onset. Pain or itching in the genitalia is followed by fever, chills, and impressive perineal swelling, which may simulate a strangulated hernia. The inflammation may involve the entire abdomen, back, and thighs. There is frequently crepitance on palpation, indicating subcutaneous gas. Systemic symptoms include nausea and vomiting, changes in sensorium, and lethargy. Eventually, gangrenous areas demarcate and become less painful as destruction and sloughing of the sensory nerves occur. The tissue breaks open, sloughs, and gives off an overwhelming feculent odor.

The most common causal factors are infection or trauma to the perianal area, including anal intercourse, scratches, chemical or thermal injury, and diabetes. Local trauma and perianal disease precede approximately one third of all cases. Cultures demonstrate bacteria of the distal colon, with a complex picture of aerobic and anaerobic bacteria. *B. fragilis* tends to be the predominant anaerobe and *E. coli* the predominant aerobe.

This bacterial invasion of the subcutaneous tissues of the perineum causes obliteration of the small branches of the pudendal arteries that supply the perineal or scrotal skin, resulting in acute dermal gangrene. This combination of erythema, edema, inflammation, and infection in a closed space stimulates anaerobic growth. Management includes Gram's stain and culturing of the wound, antibiotic therapy against anaerobes and gram-negative enterics, and, primarily, wide incision and drainage of the area to remove all the necrotic tissue. Mortality is approximately 5% to 10%.[101-103]

MYOSITIS

Principles of Disease and Clinical Features Myositis, or myonecrosis, is a deep soft tissue infection with death of muscle and a variable degree of inflammation of the overlying tissues (see Table 131-1). The skin may show minimal erythema to frank gangrene, but usually the infection is associated with massive edema. Myositis includes gas gangrene (clostridial myonecrosis), nonclostridial myonecrosis, and synergistic necrotizing cellulitis.

Clostridial myonecrosis, or gas gangrene, is a rapidly progressive muscle-necrosing infection, often with little inflammatory skin reaction but with gas formation. It is usually a result of trauma or recent surgical wounds.[104] Pathogenesis includes the elaboration of exotoxins by Clostridial bacilli. Clostridia are spore-forming, anaerobic, gram-positive bacilli usually found in the soil and in the intestinal tracts of humans and animals. Clostridia produce a toxin that damages and kills muscle, setting up the anaerobic environment that promotes further growth of the bacilli. The incubation period is 1 to 4 days. The patient appears pale and anxious, with a rapid progression to toxemia and shock. The wound becomes painful and markedly swollen, and within hours a brownish, thin exudate develops, with crepitus in the surrounding tissue. A brownish skin discoloration may appear and progress with the development of purplish blebs. An odor described as "sickly sweet" is evident, and the patient becomes anuric.[105] The muscle appears to be cooked or dead and does not bleed when cut or retract when pinched.

Nonclostridial myonecrosis is similar to gas gangrene, except that the flora include anaerobes such as *B. fragilis* and *Peptostreptococcus* along with gram-positive aerobes such as *Staphylococcus.* The prognosis is better than with gas gangrene. Treatment is appropriate debridement and antibiotic coverage. Gas may be present.[87,106]

Synergistic necrotizing cellulitis is a rapidly progressive infection usually of the lower extremities and perineum, commonly seen in patients with diabetes or peripheral vascular disease. Systemic manifestations are variable, from minimal to frank shock. The overlying skin often has a "dishwater" discharge and may show blebs, crepitus, or necrosis. The infection often extends from skin through the muscle. Pain is usually present. The flora that are cultured include aerobes, *Streptococcus, Staphylococcus, Klebsiella, Proteus, E. coli,* and anaerobes, often *Bacteroides* and *Peptostreptococcus.* Hemolysis is common and mortality is high. Treatment includes aggressive fluid and blood product resuscitation, appropriate antibiotics, and rapid surgical debridement.[86,99]

Diagnostic Strategies Gram's stain smears of the area show large gram-positive rods. Radiographs may reveal gas.

Management Treatment is wide debridement and excision of the wound. Parenteral antibiotics should be given to cover anaerobes and enterics; penicillin in large doses, a cephalosporin, or clindamycin is indicated. The mortality rate is high.[106] Hyperbaric oxygen therapy (HBO) may be effective very early in this disease. HBO has been advocated for deep anaerobic infections that result in necrotizing fasciitis and myonecrosis, especially by clostridial species. HBO is also a consideration in cases of nonclostridial involvement and Fournier's syndrome.[107] The definitive benefit of HBO in necrotizing fasciitis remains unproved.[85-87,108] HBO may provide an environment less appropriate for anaerobic growth by reducing the oxygen-reduction potential, decreasing edema via hyperoxic vasoconstriction, enhancing the ability of phagocytes to destroy bacteria, and promoting angiogenesis and subsequent granulation tissue.[107]

KEY CONCEPTS

- The decision to hospitalize patients with soft tissue infections for IV antibiotic treatment should include consideration of the following factors: patient age and immune status, location and extent of local signs of infection, presence of systemic signs, and patient ability for self-care and access to follow-up. In addition, patients who fail to clinically improve after 2 days of outpatient therapy should be admitted for further care and evaluation.
- Orbital cellulitis should be suspected in patients with mid-face infections who exhibit any of the following: proptosis, decreased ocular mobility or ocular pain with eye movement, and diminished visual acuity.
- Antimicrobial prophylaxis should be considered before surgical incision and drainage of perirectal and deep soft tissue abscesses in patients with a history of valvular heart disease or prosthetic heart valves to minimize the chance of endocarditis developing as a result of the bacteremia caused by the procedure.
- Necrotizing fasciitis should be suspected in patients, particularly those who are immunosuppressed, with soft tissue infections accompanied by any of the following factors: rapid spread of infection, systemic toxicity, numbness or deep pain out of proportion to the physical findings, marked local edema, or crepitus and wounds that exhibit necrotic tissue or bullae.

ACKNOWLEDGMENT

Drs. Meislin and Guisto would like to acknowledge and thank Dr. Grace (Tad) McReynolds for her help and assistance with the writing of this chapter.

REFERENCES

1. Fleisher G et al: Cellulitis: bacterial etiology, clinical features and laboratory findings, *J Pediatr* 97:591, 1980.
2. Bobrow BJ et al: Incision and drainage of cutaneous abscesses is not associated with bacteremia in afebrile adults, *Ann Emerg Med* 29:404, 1997.
3. Ginsberg MB: Cellulitis: analysis of 101 cases and review of the literature, *South Med J* 74:530, 1981.
4. Santos J et al: Cellulitis: Treatment with cefoxitin compared with multiple antibiotic therapy, *Pediatrics* 67:887, 1981.
5. Von Ludwig FW: Medizinisches Correspondenz, *Blatt Wurtemberg Arztl Ver* 6:21, 1836.
6. Grodinsky M: Ludwig's angina: an anatomical and clinical study with review of the literature, *Surgery* 5:678, 1939.
7. Moreland LW et al: Ludwig's angina, *Arch Intern Med* 148:461, 1988.
8. Fleisher G et al: Cellulitis: initial management, *Ann Emerg Med* 10:356, 1981.
9. Rapkin RH, Bautista G: *Haemophilus influenzae* cellulitis, *Am J Dis Child* 124:540, 1972.
10. Brook I: Antimicrobial therapy of skin and soft tissue infections in children, *J Am Podiatr Med Assoc* 83:398, 1993.
11. Ogundiya DA et al: Cavernous sinus thrombosis and blindness as a complication of an odontogenic infection, *J Oral Maxillofac Surg* 47:1317, 1989.
12. Price DC et al: Cavernous sinus thrombosis and orbital cellulitis, *South Med J* 64:1243, 1971.
13. Garcia GE et al: The etiologic role of frontal sinusitis in pediatric orbital abscesses, *Am J Otol* 14:449, 1993.
14. Barone ST, Aiuto LT: Periorbital and orbital cellulitis in the *Haemophilus influenzae* vaccine era, *J Pediatr Ophthalmol Strabismus* 34:293, 1997.
15. Donahue SP, Schwartz G: Preseptal and orbital cellulitis in childhood: a changing microbiologic spectrum, *Ophthalmology* 105:1902, 1998.
16. Schwartz GR, Wright SW: Changing bacteriology of periorbital cellulitis, *Ann Emerg Med* 28:617, 1996.
17. Ruben SE et al: Medical management of orbital subperiosteal abscess in children, *J Pediatr Ophthalmol Strabismus* 26:21, 1989.
18. Skedrios DG et al: Subperiosteal orbital abscess in children: diagnosis, microbiology, and management, *Laryngoscope* 103:28, 1993.
19. Siddens JD, Gladstone GJ: Periorbital and orbital infections in children, *J Am Opt A* 92:226, 1992.
20. Powell KR: Orbital and periorbital cellulitis: epidemiology and pathogenesis of periorbital cellulitis, *Pediatr Rev* 16:163, 1995
21. Israele V, Nelson JD: Periorbital and orbital cellulitis, *Pediatr Infect Dis J* 6:404, 1987.
22. Chartier C, Grosshans E: Erysipelas, *Int J Dermatol* 29:459, 1990.
23. Hirschmann JV: Bacterial infections of the skin. In Sams WM, Lynch PJ, editors: *Principles and practice of dermatology,* ed 2, New York, 1996, Churchill Livingstone.
24. Lowy FD: *Staphylococcus aureus* infections. In Review Articles: Medical Progress, *N Engl J Med* 8:520, 1998.
25. Spencer LV, Callen JP: Cutaneous manifestations of bacterial infections, *Dermatol Clin* 7:579, 1989.
26. Ladhani S, Evans RW: Staphylococcal scalded skin syndrome, *Arch Dis Child* 78:85, 1998.

27. Farrell AM: Staphylococcal scalded-skin syndrome, *Lancet* 354:880, 1999.
28. Scott MA: Bacterial skin infections, *Prim Care* 16:591, 1989.
29. Elias PM, Fritsch P, Epstein EH: Staphylococcal scalded skin syndrome, *Arch Dermatol* 113:207, 1977.
30. Dajani AS et al: Systemic *Haemophilus influenzae* disease: an overview, *J Pediatr* 94:355, 1979.
31. Danik SB et al: Cellulitis, *Pediatr Dermatol* 64:157, 1999.
32. Malinow I, Powell KR: Periorbital cellulitis, *Pediatr Ann* 22:241, 1993.
33. Todd J: Staphylococcal toxin syndromes, *Annu Rev Med* 36:337, 1985.
34. Fisher RJ et al: Toxic shock syndrome in menstruating women, *Ann Intern Med* 94:156, 1981.
35. Reingold AL et al: Nonmenstrual toxic shock syndrome: a review of 130 cases, *Ann Intern Med* 96:871, 1982.
36. Cone LA et al: Clinical and bacteriologic observations of a toxic shock–like syndrome due to *Streptococcus pyogenes, N Engl J Med* 317:146, 1987.
37. Stevens DL et al: Severe group A streptococcal infections associated with a toxic shock-like syndrome and scarlet fever toxin A, *N Engl J Med* 321:1, 1989.
38. Schlievert PM et al: Molecular structure of staphylococcus and streptococcus superantigens, *J Clin Immunol* 15:4S, 1995.
39. Stevens DL: The flesh-eating bacterium: What's next? *J Infect Dis* 179(Suppl 2), 1999.
40. Forni AL et al: Clinical and microbiological characteristics of severe group A streptococcus infections and streptococcal toxic shock syndrome, *Clin Infect Dis* 21:333, 1995.
41. Stollerman GH: Changing group A streptococci, the reappearance of streptococcal "toxic shock," *Arch Intern Med* 148:1268, 1988.
42. Nowak R: Flesh-eating bacteria: not new, but still worrisome, *Science* 264:1665, 1994.
43. Erstad BL et al: Toxic shock–like syndrome, *Pharmacotherapy* 12:23, 1992.
44. Torres-Martinez C et al: Streptococcus associated toxic shock, *Arch Dis Child* 67:126, 1992.
45. Manders SM: Toxin-mediated streptococcal and staphylococcal disease, *J Am Acad Dermatol* 39:383.
46. Stevens DL: Invasive group A streptococcus infections, *Clin Infect Dis* 14:2, 1992.
47. Stevens DL et al: The eagle effect revisited: efficacy of clindamycin, erythromycin, and penicillin in the treatment of streptococcal myositis, *J Infect Dis* 158:23, 1988.
48. Perez CM et al: Adjunctive treatment of streptococcal toxic shock syndrome using intravenous immunoglobulin: case report and review, *Am J Med* 102:111, 1997.
49. Chiu CH, Lin TY: Successful treatment of severe streptococcal toxic shock syndrome with a combination of intravenous immunoglobulin, dexamethasone and antibiotics, *Infection* 25:47, 1997.
50. The Working Group on Severe Streptococcal Infections: Defining the group A streptococcal toxic shock syndrome, *JAMA* 269:390, 1993.
51. Davies HD et al: Invasive group A streptococcal infections in Ontario, Canada, *N Engl J Med* 335:547, 1996.
52. Shriner DL et al: Impetigo, *Pediatr Dermatol* 56:30, 1995.
53. Darmstadt GL, Lane AT: Impetigo: an overview, *Pediatr Dermatol* 11:293, 1994.
54. Dagan R: Impetigo in childhood: changing epidemiology and new treatments, *Pediatr Ann* 22:235, 1993.
55. Ginsburg CM: Staphylococcal toxin syndromes, *Pediatr Infect Dis J* 2(Suppl):523, 1983.
56. Becker LE, Tschen E: Common bacterial infections of the skin, *Prim Care* 10:397, 1983.
57. Meislin HW et al: Cutaneous abscesses: anaerobic and aerobic bacteriology and outpatient management, *Ann Intern Med* 87:145, 1977.
58. Brooks I et al: Aerobic and anaerobic bacteriology of wounds and cutaneous abscesses, *Arch Surg* 125:1445, 1990.
59. Anderson DK, Perry AW: Axillary hidradenitis, *Arch Surg* 110:69, 1975.
60. Brealy R: Pilonidal sinus: a new theory of origin, *Br J Surg* 43:62, 1955.
61. Gonzales MH et al: Abscesses of the upper extremity from drug abuse by injection, *J Hand Surg* 18A:868, 1993.
62. Gorbach SL, Bartlett RS: Anaerobic infections: part I, *N Engl J Med* 290:1177, 1974.
63. Meislin HW et al: Management and microbiology of cutaneous abscesses, *J Am Coll Emerg Physicians* 7:186, 1978.
64. Sutter VL, Finegold SM: Susceptibility of anaerobic bacteria to 23 antimicrobial agents, *Antimicrob Agents Chemother* 10:736, 1976.
65. Vincent LM: Ultrasound of soft tissue abnormalities of the extremities, *Radiol Clin North Am* 26:131, 1988.
66. Ginsberg MJ et al: Detection of soft tissue foreign bodies by plain radiography, xerography, computed tomography, and ultrasonography, *Ann Emerg Med* 19:701, 1990.
67. Llera TL, Levy RC: Treatment of cutaneous abscess: a double-blind clinical study, *Ann Emerg Med* 14:15, 1985.
68. Sanders AB et al: Cutaneous infections and abscesses, *Semin Fam Med* 2:75, 1981.
69. Chalfant WP, Nancy TC: Hidradenitis suppurativa of the perineum: treatment by radical excision, *Am Surg* 36:331, 1970.
70. Homma H: On apocrine sweat glands in white and Negro men and women, *Bull Johns Hopkins Hosp* 38:365, 1926.
71. Brown TJ et al: Hidradenitis suppurativa, *South Med J* 91:1107, 1998.
72. Donsky HJ, Mendelson CG: Squamous cell carcinoma as a complication of hidradenitis suppurativa, *Arch Dermatol* 90:488, 1964.
73. Hoosen AA et al: Sexually transmitted diseases including HIV infection in women with Bartholin's gland abscesses, *Genitourinary Med* 71:155, 1995.
74. Bleker OP et al: Bartholin's abscess: the role of *Chlamydia trachomatis, Genitourinary Med* 66:24, 1990.
75. Brook I: Aerobic and anaerobic microbiology of Bartholin's abscess, *Surg Gynecol Obstet* 169:32, 1989.
76. Lopez-Zeno JA et al: Septic shock complicating drainage of a Bartholin's gland abscess, *Obstet Gynecol* 76:915, 1990.
77. Janicke DM, Pundt MR: Anorectal disorders: gastrointestinal emergencies, part II, *Emerg Med Clin North Am* 14:757, 1996.
78. Marcus RH et al: Perirectal abscess, *Ann Emerg Med* 25:597, 1995.
79. Kovalcek PJ et al: Anorectal abscesses, *Surg Gynecol Obstet* 149:884, 1929.
80. Cataldo PA et al: Intrarectal ultrasound in the evaluation of perirectal abscesses, *Dis Colon Rectum* 36:554, 1993.
81. Herr CH, Williams JC: Supralevator anorectal abscess presenting as acute low back pain and sciatica, *Ann Emerg Med* 23:132, 1994.
82. Hanley PH: Acute pilonidal abscesses, *Surg Gynecol Obstet* 150:9, 1980.
83. Allen-Mersh TG: Pilonidal sinus: finding the right track for treatment, *Br J Surg* 77:123, 1990.
84. Goldwag DA, Purcell TB: Necrotizing fasciitis in the pediatric age group: report of a case, *J Emerg Med* 8:299, 1990.
85. Stone DR, Gorbach SL: Necrotizing fasciitis, the changing spectrum, *Infect Dis Dermatol* 15:213, 1977.
86. Urschel JD: Necrotizing soft tissue infections, *Postgrad Med J* 75:645, 1999.
87. Green RJ, Dafoe DC, Raffin TA: Necrotizing fasciitis, *Chest* 110:219, 1996.
88. Feingold DS, Weinberg AN: Group A streptococcal infections, *Arch Dermatol* 132:67, 1996.
89. Guiliano A et al: Bacteriology of necrotizing fasciitis, *Am J Surg* 134:32, 1977.
90. Donaldson PM et al: Rapidly fatal necrotizing fasciitis caused by *Streptococcus pyogenes, J Clin Pathol* 46:617, 1993.
91. Rahmouni A et al: MR imaging in acute infectious cellulitis, *Radiology* 192:493, 1994.
92. Fisher JR et al: Necrotizing fasciitis. Importance of radiographic studies for soft-tissue gas, *JAMA* 241:803, 1979.
93. Zittergruen M, Grose C: Magnetic resonance imaging for early diagnosis of necrotizing fasciitis, *Pediatr Emerg Care* 9:26, 1993.
94. Vorus C et al: Role of early and extensive surgery in the treatment of severe necrotizing soft tissue infection, *Br J Surg* 80:1990, 1993.
95. Brook I, Frazier EH: Clinical and microbiological features of necrotizing fasciitis, *J Clin Microbiol* 33:2382-2387, 1995.

96. Majeski JA, Alexander JW: Early diagnosis, nutritional support, and immediate extensive debridement improve survival in necrotizing fasciitis, *Am J Surg* 145:784, 1983.
97. Aitken DR et al: The changing pattern of hemolytic streptococcal gangrene, *Arch Surg* 117:561, 1982.
98. Wang K, Shih C: Necrotizing fasciitis of the extremities, *J Trauma* 32:179, 1992.
99. Spach DH, Johnson RA: Cellulitis and necrotizing soft tissue infections, *Curr Pract Med* 2:545, 1999.
100. Weinstein L, Barza MA: Gas gangrene, *N Engl J Med* 289:1129, 1973.
101. Mabry RM, Harwood AL: Fournier's disease: necrotizing gangrene of the male genitalia, *J Emerg Med* 1:133, 1983.
102. Nielsen OS, Jensen SK: Fournier gangrene presenting as a gas-forming subcutaneous infection of the scrotum, *Scand J Urol Nephrol* 17:245, 1983.
103. Clayton MD et al: Causes, presentations and survival of fifty-seven patients with necrotizing fasciitis of the male genitalia, *Surg Gynecol Obstet* 170:49, 1990.
104. Parker MT: Postoperative clostridial infections in Britain, *BMJ* 3:671, 1969.
105. Hart GB et al: Gas gangrene. I. A collective review, *J Trauma* 23:991, 1983.
106. Darke SG et al: Gas gangrene and related infections: classification, clinical features and aetiology, management and mortality—a report of 88 cases, *Br J Surg* 64:104, 1977.
107. Riseman JA et al: Hyperbaric oxygen therapy for necrotizing fasciitis reduces mortality and the need for debridements, *Surgery* 108:847, 1990.
108. LeFrock JL, Molavi A: Necrotizing skin and subcutaneous infections, *J Antimicrob Chemother* 9(Suppl A):183, 1982.

132 Sepsis Syndromes

Nathan I. Shapiro
Gary D. Zimmer
Adam Z. Barkin

PERSPECTIVE

Background

Sepsis syndrome represents the systemic inflammatory response triggered by an infection in the host and is mediated by chemical messengers. The causative agent and the host's activated inflammatory cascade cause the body's defenses and regulatory systems to become overwhelmed. Tachycardia, tachypnea, fever, and immune system activation are clinical manifestations. If the body is unable to overcome this insult, cellular injury, tissue damage, shock, multiorgan failure, or death may ensue.

In the past, the term sepsis was broadly used to describe a range of disease states. A unifying effort was made in 1992 at the American College of Chest Physicians/Society of Critical Care Medicine Consensus Conference where clear definitions of sepsis and its sequelae were delineated (Box 132-1).[1] These definitions are essential to today's current understanding of sepsis, and they have served to better focus research efforts.

The spectrum of the sepsis syndromes actually begins with the systemic inflammatory response syndrome (SIRS), "a systemic inflammatory response to a variety of clinical insults."[1] This can occur in the absence of infection, describing the body's response, independent of cause. SIRS is defined by the presence of two or more of the following: tachypnea, hyperthermia or hypothermia, tachycardia, leukocytosis, or bandemia, in response to a variety of clinical insults. These findings should represent a change from the baseline. This syndrome can be due to infectious insults such as bacterial and fungal infections, as well as to noninfectious causes such as pancreatitis, trauma, or ischemia.[1]

Sepsis is SIRS in the setting of an infection. When sepsis progresses to a state of organ dysfunction, hypoperfusion, or hypotension, manifested by acidosis, oliguria, or acute change in mental status, severe sepsis is present. Septic shock is marked by sepsis-induced hypotension (systolic blood pressure <90 mm Hg) despite reasonable fluid resuscitation or sepsis that requires vasopressors or inotropic agents to maintain normotension. In septic shock, tissue oxygen and other nutrient demands exceed their supply, producing lactic acidosis, oliguria, and mental status changes. The ultimate endpoint is multiple organ dysfunction syndrome (MODS). MODS, defined as the "presence of altered organ function in an acutely ill patient such that homeostasis cannot be maintained without intervention,"[1] is the final common pathway for the critically ill.

A landmark study by Rangel-Fausto et al[2] demonstrated this progression of disease in a well-designed prospective study. They demonstrated the clinical progression from SIRS → sepsis → severe sepsis → septic shock by showing both a stepwise progression and increased mortality rates for those developing the more advanced syndromes (Figures 132-1 and 132-2). There was also a direct relationship between the number of SIRS criteria initially fulfilled, the likelihood of progression to more advanced stages of the sepsis syndromes, and increased mortality.

Bacteremia is often seen, but positive cultures are not obligatory in the diagnosis of sepsis. In recent prospective studies, only 17% to 27% of patients with sepsis, 25% to 53% of patients with severe sepsis, and 69% of patients with septic shock actually had positive blood cultures.[2-4] Culture-negative and culture-positive septic populations have similar outcomes in patients given the same degree of sepsis.[2,4,5]

Pneumonia, abdominal abscess with viscus perforation, and urosepsis are common primary causes of sepsis.[2,4,6,7] Gram-positive organisms account for 25% to 50%, gram-negative for 30% to 60%, and fungi for 2% to 10% of sepsis. The most common pathogens are *Escherichia coli, Staphylococcus aureus, Pseudomonas aeruginosa, Enterococcus faecalis, Streptococcus pneumoniae, Klebsiella pneumoniae,*

Box 132-1 Definitions of Sepsis[1]

Bacteremia (fungemia): presence of viable bacteria (fungi) in the blood, as evidenced by positive blood cultures

Systemic inflammatory response syndrome (SIRS): at least two of the following conditions in response to a variety of clinical insults: (1) oral temperature of >38° C or <36° C, (2) respiratory rate of >20 breaths/min or $Paco_2$ of <32 mm Hg, (3) heart rate of >90 beats /min, (4) leukocyte count of >12,000/µl or <4000/µL or >10% immature (band) forms.

Sepsis: The presence of the two or more SIRS criteria in response to an infection

Severe sepsis: sepsis with one or more signs of organ dysfunction, hypoperfusion, or hypotension, such as metabolic acidosis, acute alteration in mental status, oliguria, or adult respiratory distress syndrome.

Septic shock: sepsis with hypotension that is unresponsive to fluid resuscitation plus organ dysfunction or perfusion abnormalities as listed above from severe sepsis

Multiple organ dysfunction syndrome (MODS): dysfunction of more than one organ, requiring intervention to maintain homeostasis

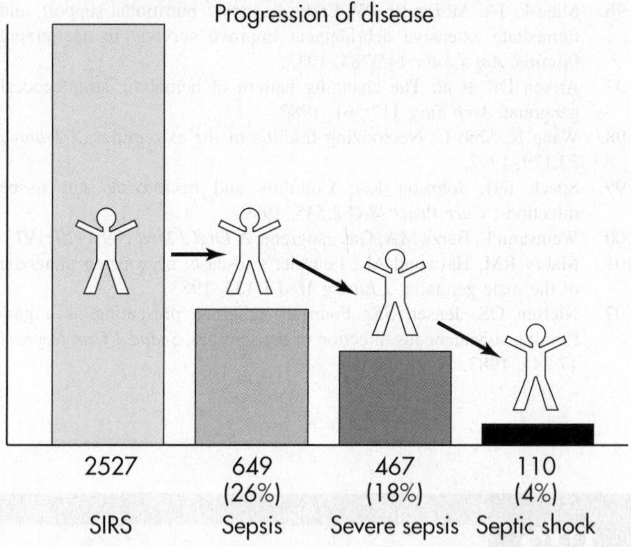

Figure 132-2. **Progression of disease.**

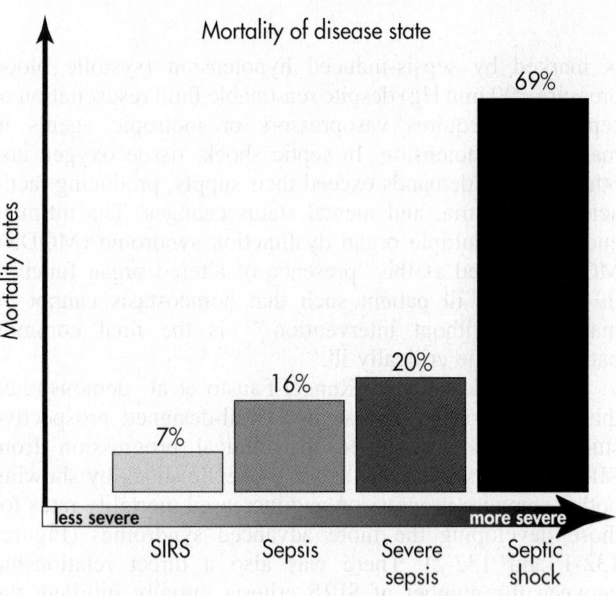

Figure 132-1. **Mortality of disease state.**

Enterobacter species, and coagulase-negative *Staphylococcus* species.[2-4,8,9] The distribution varies with the study, and, more important, host factors such as the host immune system, age, recent hospitalizations, and presence of indwelling vascular catheters.

The health status of the host is a crucial risk factor in the development and progression of sepsis. The elderly and those with multiple comorbidities are more easily overwhelmed by systemic infection. Chemotherapy-induced neutropenia, acquired immunodeficiency syndrome (AIDS), and steroid dependency increase susceptibility to sepsis. Increased use of indwelling devices such as intravascular catheters, prosthetic devices, and endotracheal tubes contributes to the risk of systemic infection and sepsis.

Epidemiology

Sepsis is the most common cause of death in noncardiac intensive care units (ICUs), and the thirteenth most common cause of death overall. There are approximately 500,000 cases per year in the United States, of which about 200,000 progress to septic shock and nearly 100,000 total deaths. Sepsis accounts for two to ten cases per 100 hospital admissions[4,6,8]. The cost of caring for septic patients is estimated at $5 to $10 billion per year in the United States, with a mortality rate estimated between 20% and 50%.[2,6,7,10-13] Deaths from sepsis are on the rise, with the reported rate of death from sepsis increasing from 4.2 to 7.7 per 100,000 population from 1980 to 1992.[11]

PRINCIPLES OF DISEASE

Pathophysiology

Sepsis is the endpoint of a complex process that begins with an infection. The initial host response is to mobilize inflammatory cells, particularly neutrophils and macrophages, to the site of infection. These inflammatory cells then release circulating molecules, most notably cytokines, which trigger a cascade of other inflammatory mediators that result in a coordinated host response. Synthesis of the components of the cascade is increased at many steps along the pathway. If these mediators are not appropriately regulated, sepsis will occur. In the setting of ongoing toxin release, a persistent inflammatory response occurs with ongoing mediator activation, tissue injury, shock, multiorgan failure, and potentially death. This interaction is complex and multifactorial, and our understanding continues to evolve.

A wide variety of organisms can produce sepsis. Gram-negative sepsis is best understood and is clearly initiated by endotoxin, a lipopolysaccharide (LPS) component of the bacterial cell wall. This was demonstrated by Suffredini et al,[14] who injected purified endotoxin into healthy, human volunteers and were able to produce a transient sepsis syndrome: fever, tachycardia, and tachypnea. Kirkland et al[15] showed that pretreatment of mice with antiendotoxin antibodies prevents sepsis when injected with an otherwise lethal dose of endotoxin-containing bacteria. Phagocytosis of endotoxin by macrophages causes the release of cytokines to fight the infection. When sufficient numbers of macrophages are activated by this method, an excess of these inflammatory cytokines is produced and can cause sepsis.

Gram-positive organisms produce an inflammatory response through the direct action of its cell wall components and the indirect action of secreted, soluble substances. Cellular wall components such as peptidoglycan and liptoeichoic acid are thought to initiate the pathway, although the mechanism of action is unproven. Secreted, soluble substances such as exotoxins (e.g., exotoxin A from *P. aeruginosa* and TSS-1 from *S. aureus*) are substances secreted by bacteria and produce a host response through cell membrane receptors. Other extracellular enzymes such as streptokinase are secreted from many gram-positive organisms. As all of these substances circulate freely in the host, they may remain after an active infection has been cleared. Each of these mediators is capable of activating the inflammatory cascade and may lead to the subsequent progression of sepsis.

Mediators of Sepsis In response to toxins, the body reacts by secreting substances such as cytokines, eicosanoids,[16] platelet activation factor,[17,18] oxygen free radicals, complement, and fibrinolysins. Cytokines are cell-signaling peptides with multiple functions. They differ from classic endocrine hormones in that several cell types produce them rather than a dedicated organ; they have little significance in normal homeostasis and are released in response to an exogenous stimulus. Six categories exist: interleukins, tumor necrosis factor (TNF), interferons, colony-stimulating factors, chemotactic factors, and others; the first two have the primary role in sepsis.

Cytokines are primarily pro-inflammatory, antiinflammatory or growth promoting. The molecular mechanisms by which they are regulated are not well understood. The initial cytokine, TNF-α, is found in serum approximately 90 minutes after the administration of endotoxin to healthy volunteers.[19] Interleukin (IL)-6 and IL-8 reach peak levels at approximately 120 minutes. The main pro-inflammatory cytokines are IL-1, TNF, and IL-8. The primary antiinflammatory cytokines are IL-10, IL-6, transforming growth factor β (TGF-β), soluble receptors to TNF, and IL-1 receptor antagonist (IL-1ra).[20-22] If the resultant inflammatory response is adequate, the infection is controlled and cleared. If the response is deficient or excessive, however, a persistent and worsening cascade is produced, ultimately leading to shock, organ failure, and potentially death.

IL-1 and TNF have both been implicated as key mediators in the development of sepsis. Increasing levels of circulating IL-1 and TNF correlate with worsening clinical status.[23] At high doses, both IL-1 and TNF are lethal. They act by stimulating granulocyte-colony stimulatory factors and activating leukocytes.[24] TNF is present first in the bloodstream and it induces the formation of IL-1.[25] Infusing either cytokine into an animal model creates a sepsis syndrome.[26] Selective blockade of either cytokine protects against sepsis in animal models.[27-30]

Antiinflammatory regulators are released in response to rising pro-inflammatory mediators. IL-1 receptor antagonist (IL-1ra) is found in increased levels in healthy volunteers injected with endotoxin and many patients with infection.[31] IL-10 has a purely antiinflammatory role.[32] In experimental models, it has been shown to decrease mortality in the presence of endotoxemia.

Other, noncytokine molecules have been implicated in sepsis. Metabolites of the arachidonic acid pathway are involved in peripheral vasodilation, vasoconstriction, leukocyte, and platelet aggregation.[33] Prostaglandins are responsible for fever.[34] Elevated thromboxane A_2 levels are found in sepsis.[35] Little is known about the actual mechanisms by which eicosanoids participate in sepsis.

Nitric oxide (NO) is a gas that has an important role in septic shock, regulating vascular tone[36] by an indirect effect on smooth muscle cells.[37] NO also contributes to platelet adhesion, insulin secretion, neurotransmission, tissue injury, and inflammation and cytotoxicity.[38-40] Its half-life is quite short (6 to 10 seconds) and it is easily diffused into cells.[37] Although its mechanisms of action are not well understood, it seems to be a key mediator of sepsis. Animal data show that nitric oxide synthase, the enzyme that produces NO, is upregulated in sepsis.[41] The enhanced NO production is thought to contribute to the profound vasodilation found in septic shock.

In the setting of ongoing inflammatory activation, the mediators of sepsis continue to be produced and the cascade perpetuates. Unless appropriately and rapidly controlled, the ultimate effect is a sequence of events starting with cellular dysfunction and ultimately leading to tissue damage, organ dysfunction, and death.

Organ System Dysfunction

Neurologic Patients with sepsis often display neurologic impairment manifested by altered mental status and lethargy, commonly referred to as septic encephalopathy. The incidence has been reported between 10% and 70%.[42,43] The mortality rate in septic patients with encephalopathy is higher than in those without significant neurologic involvement.[44] One prospective case series showed a Glasgow Coma Scale less than 13 correlated with a mortality increase from 20% to 50%.[45] Although the pathophysiology has not been clearly defined, contributing factors include direct bacterial invasion, endotoxemia, altered cerebral perfusion or metabolism, metabolic derangements, multiorgan system failure, and iatrogenesis. Impaired renal or hepatic function in the absence of overt organ failure has been shown to correlate with encephalopathy.[45,46]

Cardiovascular Profound cardiovascular dysfunction is common with sepsis. Gram-negative, gram-positive, and even killed organisms can cause myocardial depression.[47,48] The direct insults of the toxic mediators as well as the mobilization of host-mediators of sepsis produce a distributive shock. Early in sepsis, a hyperdynamic state characterized by increased cardiac output and decreased systemic vascular resistance develops.[49,50] Although the total cardiac output is increased, it is accompanied by ventricular dilation and a decreased ejection fraction. Aggressive fluid resuscitation acts to restore preload in the dilated heart, thus helping to correct for the decreased ejection fraction in the dilated heart, and ultimately improve the cardiac index, even late in shock.[51] Much of the cardiovascular compromise from septic shock is reversible and normal cardiovascular function usually returns within 10 days.[52]

Box 132-2 Definition of ARDS[55]

- Impaired oxygenation, defined as a ratio of partial pressure of arterial oxygen to fractional inspired oxygen ≤200 irrespective of how much positive end-expiratory pressure is used
- Bilateral pulmonary infiltrates of frontal chest x-ray study
- Pulmonary artery occlusion pressure ≤18 mm Hg or no clinical evidence of elevated left atrial pressures

Pulmonary Pulmonary compromise is common and often lethal. The exact mechanism by which sepsis causes respiratory failure is unclear. Sepsis produces a highly catabolic state and places significant demands on the respiratory system. At the same time, airway resistance is increased and muscle function is impaired.[53] Irrespective of whether pneumonia is the etiology of sepsis, the common pulmonary endpoint is the acute respiratory distress syndrome (ARDS).[54] ARDS is defined clinically (Box 132-2) and correlates with the pathologic finding of diffuse alveolar damage. The development of ARDS occurs 4 to 24 hours after radiographic abnormalities develop.[56] Because of alveolar-capillary membrane damage, fluid accumulates in the alveoli. Rather than being a diffuse disease, ARDS is a heterogeneous process that results in interspersed damaged and normal alveoli. Significant right-to-left shunting, arterial hypoxemia, and intractable hypoxemia occur.

Gastrointestinal The hollow viscus is significantly affected by the shock state. A prolonged ileus accompanies hypoperfusion and persists beyond the malperfused state. Splanchnic blood flow is dependent on mean arterial pressure because there is relatively little autoregulation. Therefore, hemodynamic dysfunction may have a profound effect on viscus metabolism.

Solid organ involvement is also common. Even in the previously normal host, elevations in aminotransferases and bilirubin are common early in sepsis, although frank hepatic failure is quite rare. The liver has also been implicated in the pathogenesis of sepsis; some of the mediators of sepsis are produced by the liver.[57]

Endocrine The incidence of adrenocortical dysfunction in sepsis is unclear. Depending on the balance of circulating cytokines, augmentation or suppression of the hypothalamic-pituitary axis is possible. IL-1 and IL-6 both activate the hypothalamic-pituitary-adrenal axis. TNF-α and corticostatin depress pituitary function. Other factors that may contribute to adrenal insufficiency in sepsis include decreased blood flow to the adrenal cortex, decreased pituitary function, and decreased pituitary secretion of adrenocorticotrophic hormone due to severe stress. As a result of these interactions, the hypothalamic thermoregulatory mechanism may be reset, and temperature lability may develop.

Hematologic Sepsis causes abnormalities in many parts of the coagulation system. Endotoxin, TNF-α and IL-1 are the key mediators. Pathologic activation of the extrinsic (tissue-factor dependent) pathway and protein C-protein S and fibrinolysis lead to consumption of essential factors causing disseminated intravascular coagulation (DIC). The activation of the coagulation cascade produces fibrin deposition and microvascular thrombi. If not corrected, these depositions can compromise organ perfusion and contribute to organ failure.

Tissue factor expression on monocytes is increased. This results in fibrin deposition and perhaps contributes to an increased incidence of multiorgan failure due to microvascular thrombi. In one study, the degree of tissue factor expression was found to portend a poorer prognosis.[58]

Protein C and protein S also play a significant role in the genesis of DIC. In an experimental model, the inhibition of the protein C–protein S system increased the potency of endotoxin and increased the likelihood of DIC and fatal septic shock.[59]

In response to the fibrin deposition, the fibrinolytic pathway is activated. Common laboratory findings are low plasma levels of the fibrinolytic proteins and increased fibrin-split products.[60] In late sepsis, the fibrinolytic system is suppressed.[61] This sequence of events leads to consumption of coagulation factors and DIC.

CLINICAL FEATURES

Symptoms and Signs

The approach to a patient with potential or presumed sepsis relies on identifying the presence of a systemically acting infection, as well as localizing the source of the initial infection. This enables appropriately aggressive and directed treatment to the infection source. Often, the source is not readily apparent, but early identification of the septic state allows implementation of broad-spectrum antibiotics that may be potentially lifesaving.

The emergency physician must initially evaluate the stability of the airway, breathing, and circulation (ABCs). Patients with altered consciousness who are unable to protect their airway need to be intubated. Septic patients with severe tachypnea or hypoxia with impending or current respiratory failure also require intubation for positive pressure ventilation. Patients needing hemodynamic blood pressure support must be identified and rapidly and aggressively treated with fluids and vasopressor and inotropic support as needed.

The septic patient manifests signs of systemic infection through tachycardia, tachypnea, hyperthermia or hypothermia, and, if severe, hypotension. A septic patient will often have flushed skin with warm, well-perfused extremities secondary to the early vasodilation and hyperdynamic state. Alternatively, the severely hypoperfused patient with an advanced shock state may appear mottled and cyanotic. In the very early patient presentation, vital sign changes such as tachycardia and tachypnea may be the only early indicators of sepsis.

If the patient is in shock, the etiology should be identified and differentiated from hypovolemic or cardiogenic shock. In approaching septic shock, one should remember the etiology: a pathogenic insult resulting in a dysregulated inflammatory cascade with release of pro-inflammatory and antiinflammatory mediators. These will cause vasodilation and a hyperdynamic cardiovascular system. Thus, a septic patient will classically appear flushed with warm, well-perfused extremities. This should be distinguished from patients with hypovolemic or cardiogenic shock who will appear cool, clammy, and sometimes diaphoretic with poorly perfused extremities. Neck veins will be flat and the pulse rapid and thready. A complete detailed clinical examination should allow the physician to discriminate the etiology of the shock state (see Chapter 4).

The emergency physician should identify risk factors such as immunocompromised states (AIDS infection, malignancy, diabetes, splenectomy, and concurrent chemotherapy), elderly patients, debilitation or institutionalization, and multiple comorbidities. A history of fevers or chills in the setting of intravenous drug abuse (IVDA), an artificial valve, or mitral valve prolapse should increase the suspicion of endocarditis. An examination revealing a murmur, especially if new or in the presence of other stigmata of endocarditis (e.g., splinter hemorrhages, Roth's spots, Janeway lesions) points toward endocarditis.

The respiratory system is the most common focus of infection in the septic patient. History of a productive cough, fevers, chills, upper respiratory symptoms, and throat and ear pain should be elicited. Examination should include detailed evaluation, looking for focal infection such as exudative tonsillitis, sinus tenderness, tympanic membrane injection, and crackles or dullness on lung auscultation. Also, pharyngeal thrush should be noticed as a marker of an immunocompromised state.

The gastrointestinal system is the second-most common source of sepsis. A history of abdominal pain including its description, location, timing, and palliating and aggravating factors should be obtained. Further history, including last bowel movement and the presence of nausea, vomiting, and diarrhea should be noted. A careful physical examination, looking for signs of peritoneal irritation, abdominal tenderness, and hyperactive or hypoactive bowel sounds is critical in identifying the source of abdominal sepsis. Particular attention must be paid to physical examination findings suggestive of common sources of infection or disease: Murphy's sign indicating cholecystitis, pain at McBurney's point indicating appendicitis, left lower quadrant pain suggesting diverticulitis, or rectal examination revealing a rectal abscess or prostatitis.

The neurologic system is examined by looking for signs of meningitis including nuchal rigidity, fevers, and change in consciousness. A detailed neurologic examination is important. Lethargy or altered mentation may indicate primary neurologic process or may be the result of decreased brain perfusion from a shock state.

The genitourinary history includes flank pain, dysuria, polyuria, discharge, Foley catheter placement, and instrumentation. A sexual history should assess sexually transmitted disease (STD) risk. Genitalia should be evaluated for ulcers, discharge, and other penile or vulvar lesions, looking specifically for the woody induration of Fournier's gangrene. A rectal examination should be performed, looking for a tender, boggy prostate consistent with prostatitis. A red and friable cervix, cervical discharge, or cervical motion tenderness is consistent with an STD. Adnexal tenderness in a toxic-appearing female potentially represents a tuboovarian abscess.

Musculoskeletal history includes any localizing symptoms to a particular joint. Redness, swelling, and warmth over a joint, especially with decreased range of motion in that joint, are concerning; septic arthritis may mandate further investigation, including arthrocentesis. A patient should be completely exposed and the skin examined for evidence of cellulitis, abscess, wound infection, or traumatic injury. Deep injuries, foreign bodies, and fasciitis may be difficult to identify clinically. The origin of insult, initial location, and rate of spread should be delineated from a patient with cellulitis. The physician should look for crepitus representing the presence of a more aggressive, gas-forming organism. Local lymphadenopathy, swelling, and streaking should also be noted as signs of an advancing infection. Petechiae and purpura may represent a *Neisseria meningitides* infection or disseminated intravascular coagulopathy. Generalized erythroderma and rash may represent an exotoxin from pathogens such as *S. aureus* or *Streptococcus pyogenes*.

DIAGNOSTIC STRATEGIES

The use of diagnostic testing in patients with sepsis syndromes or suspected syndromes is twofold. First, the clinician should use diagnostic studies to identify the type and location of the infecting organisms. Diagnostic tests are also mandatory to define the extent of infection and state of sepsis to assist in focusing therapy. There is no uniform diagnostic approach; diagnostics must be tailored to the particular patient.

Laboratory

Hematology The white blood cell count (WBC) is a marker of inflammation and activation of the inflammatory cascade. Leukocytosis is associated with infection and incorporated in the consensus definition of sepsis; however, it is often insensitive and nonspecific, limiting its absolute utility in the ED. The febrile neutropenic patient has been shown to be at increased risk for severe infection. Thus a neutrophil count < 500 cells/mm^3 should prompt admission, isolation, and empiric intravenous antibiotics in most chemotherapy patients. A bandemia (>10% bands on a peripheral smear) represents the release of immature cells from the bone marrow and is considered to be a sign of infection and inflammation; it is also part of the consensus sepsis definition. Like the WBC, it is an imperfect indicator of infection. The hemoglobin and hematocrit should be obtained to ensure adequate oxygen delivery in shock. Patients should be maintained with a hematocrit >30% and hemoglobin >10 g/dl. Platelets are an acute-phase reactant and may be elevated in the presence of infections. Conversely, a low platelet count has been found in one study to be a significant predictor of bacteremia in patients with shock.[62] Thrombocytopenia, elevated prothrombin time (PT), an elevated activated partial thromboplastin time, decreased fibrinogen, and increased fibrin split products are associated with DIC and severe sepsis syndrome.

Chemistry Electrolyte abnormalities should be identified and corrected. Low bicarbonate suggests acidosis and inadequate perfusion. An elevated anion gap acidosis in the setting of sepsis syndrome commonly represents lactic acidosis or diabetic ketoacidosis, but other causes need to be ruled out. A high creatinine level is indicative of renal dysfunction or failure, which, if due primarily to sepsis, indicates organ failure and a worse prognosis. Calcium, magnesium, and phosphorous levels should be checked.

The presence of an elevated lactate is associated with inadequate perfusion, shock, and a poorer prognosis.[63] A multicenter prospective study of ICU patients showed an overall 3-day mortality rate of 59% for patients with a lactic acidosis. An arterial blood gas may be helpful in identifying and classifying acid-base disturbances. A metabolic acidosis suggests inadequate tissue perfusion. A low PO_2, specifically a Pao_2 <75 mm Hg, is part of the consensus sepsis syndromes definition. Liver function tests may be used to identify liver failure or dysfunction. An elevated bilirubin may suggest the gallbladder as an etiology for sepsis. An elevated amylase and lipase may represent pancreatitis as the cause of noninfectious SIRS.

Microbiology Obtaining proper blood cultures, sputum cultures, urine cultures, cerebrospinal fluid (CSF) cultures, and other tissue cultures is important in guiding therapy. Although not useful to the ED physician, cultures should be obtained soon after administration of antibiotics in the patient with sepsis syndrome. It is important to stress that the initiation of antibiotic therapy is not delayed while waiting for cultures to be obtained. One well-designed, prospective, inpatient-based study suggests that the following factors are predictive of a positive blood culture: fever >38.3° C, the presence of a rapidly (<1 month) or ultimately (<5 years) fatal disease, shaking chills, IVDA, acute abdomen, or major comorbidity.[3] These factors have not been validated in independent populations. The yield of blood cultures obtained in all patients remains low (5% to 10%) due to a lack of reliable discriminatory guidelines for obtaining blood cultures in the ED.[2,3,6,8,9] Among patients with clinical sepsis, only 30% to 60% of patients will have positive cultures.[4,6,12] Currently, all patients with suspected sepsis syndrome should have at least two sets of blood cultures sent from the ED, along with any clinically indicated sputum, urine, CSF, catheter, or wound cultures.

A Gram stain of sputum, CSF, or abscess drainage may help in the early prediction of a suspected pathogen and guide initial antibiotic therapy. A urinalysis showing a leukocytosis or bacteria is suggestive of a urinary tract infection and potential urosepsis. A lumbar puncture with CSF leukocytosis is indicative of meningitis.

Special Procedures The Swan-Ganz catheter is not a mandatory part of the ED management. The physiologic measurements may be useful in identifying the etiology of shock and guiding fluid and inotropic therapy. Low systemic vascular resistance and high cardiac output are most commonly associated with sepsis, although this may vary with the stage of shock and the individual patient. A central venous pressure (CVP) line may guide fluid resuscitation, with a low CVP indicating the need for continued fluid repletion. An arterial line is useful for close monitoring of hypotensive patients, especially when one or more vasopressors are being titrated to maintain an adequate blood pressure. Although potentially useful monitoring adjuncts, none are mandatory to ED management

Radiology Radiographic studies focus on identifying the source of infection. A chest x-ray study should be obtained in all patients with suspected sepsis syndrome, looking not only for a focal infiltrate representing pneumonia but also for the fluffy, bilateral infiltrates indicative of ARDS. An upright chest x-ray study should be obtained for suspected bowel perforation to detect free air under the diaphragm. The presence of pneumomediastinum is suggestive of esophageal perforation and current or impending mediastinitis.

Soft tissue plain films should be obtained looking for air in the soft tissues associated with necrotizing or gas-forming infection. Periosteal thickening or bone erosion may be seen on plain film of patients with osteomyelitis; a bone scan may be diagnostic. A computed tomography (CT) scan of the abdomen and pelvis may identify abdominal or pelvic pathology, provided there is no clear clinical indication for immediate operative intervention. Suspected diseases such as diverticulitis, appendicitis, necrotizing pancreatitis, microperforation of the stomach or bowel, or formation of an intra-abdominal abscess may be best diagnosed by CT scan. A head CT scan may identify septic emboli from endocarditis or increased intracranial pressure from a mass before performing a lumbar puncture. An abdominal ultrasound may be indicated for suspected cholecystitis, and a pelvic ultrasound for tubo-ovarian abscess or endometritis. A transesophageal echo should be obtained if endocarditis is suspected to detect the presence of any valvular vegetations. Magnetic resonance imaging may be useful to identify soft tissue infections such as necrotizing fasciitis or epidural abscess.

MANAGEMENT

The initial resuscitation phase in the ED is centered on supportive care. Appropriate airway management, intravenous access, oxygen, antibiotics, and fluid resuscitation are the primary modalities available to the emergency physician. After the immediate stabilization, there are three main goals in the therapy of sepsis and septic shock: maintenance of adequate mean arterial pressure, antibiotics and surgical drainage of the infection, and interruption of the cascade leading to septic shock.

Currently, the goal of resuscitation is to normalize tissue oxygenation and perfusion. Clinical endpoints include a mean arterial pressure of 60 to 70 mm Hg, reversal of lactic acidosis, and maintenance of urine output at 0.5 to 1 cc/kg/hr and a normal (or improving) pH. Recent, evidence-based recommendations by the Society of Critical Care Medicine and the American College of Critical Care Medicine are summarized in Table 132-1.

Respiratory Support

Altered mental status is common in septic shock and patients may require rapid airway protection. Patients with a respiratory rate greater than 30 breaths per minute are likely to develop respiratory collapse, irrespective of arterial oxygenation. Wheeler et al[65] reported that 85% of patients with "severe sepsis" will require mechanical ventilation during their hospital course. As patients with impending respiratory failure consume a disproportionately large amount of energy for the muscles of respiration, improved oxygen delivery to other organs is achieved by intubation and mechanical ventilation, sedation and paralysis. Although there are no clear intubation guidelines, hypercapnea, persistent hypoxemia, airway compromise, and profound acidosis are valid indicators.

In addition to airway protection, intubation and mechanical support provide positive pressure ventilation. The pattern of injury is such that normal lung parenchyma is adjacent to affected tissue. Therefore, increased airway pressures are required to maintain normal oxygen delivery. Current recommendations are to maintain transalveolar pressures (measured as plateau pressures) below 35 cm H_2O, as increased pressures are associated with ventilator-induced

Table 132-1. Management Recommendations for Hemodynamic Support

Basic Principles	• ICU admission • Arterial cannulation in patients with shock • Resuscitation to target arterial pressure, heart rate, urine output, mental status, and tissue perfusion • Central venous or pulmonary arterial catheter placement to assess cardiac filling pressures
Fluid Resuscitation	• Fluids are the primary modality to resuscitation[C] • Colloids and crystalloids are equally effective[C] • Invasive monitoring for patients not responding to initial resuscitation with target pulmonary capillary wedge pressure of 12 to 15 mm Hg[D] • Hemoglobin concentrations should be maintained above 8 to 10 g/dl[D]
Vasopressor Therapy	• Dopamine is the first-line agent in shock unresponsive to aggressive fluid resuscitation[E] • Dopamine and norepinephrine are equally effective. Phenylephrine is an alternative[C] • Epinephrine is reserved for refractory hypotension[D] • Routine low-dose (<5 µg/kg/min) dopamine is not recommended, but it is effective in increasing renal blood flow when combined with norepinephrine[E]
Inotropic Therapy	• Dobutamine is the first choice for patients with refractory low cardiac index[E] • Dobutamine may improve cardiac index and organ perfusion, but empiric use is not recommended[D] • Vasopressors and inotropes can be titrated separately to maintain mean arterial pressure and cardiac output[D] • Epinephrine and high-dose dopamine can be used as inotropes, but splanchnic perfusion may be compromised[C]

Modified from Hollenberg S et al: Practice parameters for hemodynamic support of sepsis in adult patients with sepsis, *Crit Care Med* 27:639-660, 1999.
[A]Supported by at least two randomized, controlled trials with clear results.
[B]Supported by one randomized controlled trial with clear results.
[C]Supported by small, randomized trials with uncertain results.
[D] Supported by at least one nonrandomized, contemporaneous trial.
[E]Supported by nonrandomized trials with historical controls and expert opinion or case series.
NOTE: There are no trials that meet criteria A or B.

lung injury.[66,67] Maintaining relatively low transalveolar pressure with increasing end-expiratory pressure (PEEP) is an effective way to increase arterial oxygen delivery.[68]

Cardiovascular Support

Oxygen Delivery Early work by Shoemaker et al[69] showed that supranormal blood oxygen levels in "high-risk" surgical patients decreased mortality. Recent large, prospective, multicenter trials in sepsis have failed to show a mortality benefit of supranormal oxygen delivery.[70,71] Based on existing evidence, routine elevation of oxygen delivery cannot be recommended. Therapy needs to be guided by changes in cardiac output and mixed venous oxygen saturation.

Adequate oxygen carrying capacity is the next key. Organ hypoperfusion is a result of global and distributive changes in both systemic blood flow and the microvasculature. As a result of marrow suppression and dilution with crystalloid fluids, most patients with sepsis have a hemoglobin between 8 and 10 g/dl after initial resuscitation. A hematocrit between 27% and 30% has been reported to be most effective,[72] although other studies challenge this recommendation.[73-76] A recent consensus from the Society of Critical Care Medicine states that patients with hemoglobin less than 8 g/dl "may benefit from blood transfusion, but transfusing to a predefined threshold to increase oxygen delivery cannot be recommended on the basis of existing data."[64] Indicators of clinically significant sepsis include excessive tachycardia, persistent lactic acidosis, cardiac dysfunction, and underlying coronary artery disease.

Fluid Resuscitation Patients with sepsis often require large volumes of intravenous fluid to maintain adequate perfusion.[77] The primary reasons for this intravascular hypovolemia are venodilation and diffuse capillary leak.[78] As much as 6 to 10 L of crystalloid may be required in the first 24 hours.[77] Fluid replacement should be titrated to clinical parameters such as heart rate, blood pressure, change in mental status, capillary refill, cool skin, and adequate urine output (0.5 to 1 cc /kg/hr). Normal (0.9%) saline and lactated Ringer's solutions are equally effective and neither worsens lactic acidosis. Colloids are equally effective as crystalloids, but they are far more expensive and, in the case of pooled human albumin, present an exposure risk.[77] Experience with hypertonic saline is limited and no recommendation on its use can made based on current literature.[64]

In patients who do not respond rapidly to fluid boluses, invasive hemodynamic monitoring in the form of a CVP catheter or pulmonary artery catheter is recommended. The goal is left heart filling pressures between 12 and 15 mm Hg.[79] There has been no conclusive evidence to show that pulmonary edema occurs more frequently with crystalloids unless high cardiac filling pressures are necessary to maintain adequate tissue perfusion.[64] Systemic edema is a common side effect.

There have been recent efforts to identify ways to measure regional perfusion more directly. In particular, direct measurement of splanchnic blood flow has been proposed. Even in the absence of global hypoxia and impaired tissue perfusion, there is evidence that regional hypoperfusion and ischemia exist.[80] Although further study is necessary, there is early evidence that therapy guided toward maintaining splanchnic perfusion can decrease mortality.[81]

Bicarbonate Bicarbonate supplementation was previously the standard of care for those with presumed lactic acidosis. Current consensus is that it should be reserved for severe acidemia (pH <7.0 to 7.2), as there may be a paradoxical decrease in intracellular pH as a result of diffusion of soluble CO_2 across the cell membrane. Alternatively, hyperventilation has been suggested to help increase systemic pH.[82]

Vasopressors

If appropriate fluid resuscitation has failed, vasopressor support may be required. Only in profound hypotension should vasopressors be started before adequate fluid resuscitation. Using mean arterial pressure alone as an indicator of overall efficacy of therapeutic intervention is not helpful.[82] A mean arterial pressure of 60 to 70 mm Hg has been recommended in otherwise healthy, normovolemic adult patients but must be correlated with other indicators of adequate perfusion such as mental status and urine output. Patients with previously uncontrolled hypertension may require mean arterial pressures of 75 mm Hg or even higher. A summary of the commonly used agents and their doses are found in Table 132-2.

Table 132-2. Dosing of Vasoactive Therapy

Drug	Dose
Dobutamine	5-15 μg/kg/min
Dopamine	2-20 μg/kg/min
Epinephrine	5-20 μg/min
Norepinephrine	5-20 μg/min
Phenylephrine	2-20 μg/min

Dopamine Dopamine should be the first agent used for septic shock that is unresponsive to adequate volume expansion. Dopamine is the immediate precursor of norepinephrine and epinephrine. It is primarily a β_1 and dopaminergic agonist. Although not definitively proven, low doses of dopamine may be used in combination with other agents listed below, in an effort to preserve renal and splanchnic blood flow. Doses above 20 μg/kg/min may produce significant vasoconstriction. Persistent tachycardia, decreased PaO_2, and increased pulmonary artery occlusion pressure are common side effects of dopamine use. Dopamine has been shown to increase oxygen delivery better than other catecholamines.[83,84] Based on its mechanism of action, it is most useful in patients who have depressed cardiac output.

Norepinephrine Norepinephrine is a mixed α and β agonist with minimal β_2 activity. Its primary function is to increase cardiac output and systemic vascular resistance. Recommended doses are from 0.01 to 3 μg/kg/min. At least one controlled trial showed norepinephrine to be more effective than dopamine at reversing hypotension for at least 6 hours.[85] There was no difference in adverse effects between norepinephrine and dopamine. When compared with dopamine in septic patients, norepinephrine increases glomerular filtration and urine output equally well.[86-88] Norepinephrine has been studied as a rescue drug to dopamine and has had consistent, replicated improvement in hemodynamics, although mortality benefit has not been shown. It is an important component of the therapy for septic shock, either as a sole vasopressor or in conjunction with dopamine.[64]

Phenylephrine Phenylephrine is a selective α_1-agonist, increasing systemic vascular resistance without significant changes in cardiac output. It can produce a reflexive bradycardia or suppression in cardiac output. A single, small study has shown that phenylephrine is effective in restoring perfusion in patients with septic shock refractory to dopamine or dobutamine.[89] Phenylephrine does not impair cardiac and renal function and may be a good choice when significant tachyarrhythmia limits the use of other agents.[64]

Epinephrine Epinephrine a very potent, mixed α and β agonist. Epinephrine infusion is also associated with increased oxygen consumption, increased systemic lactate concentrations, and decreased splanchnic blood flow. Studies that have shown this rise in lactate were all short-term and there is no evidence about the long-term effects.[90,91] As a result of all of the possible adverse effects of epinephrine, it is currently recommended only for those patients who are unresponsive to other vasopressors.

Dobutamine Dobutamine is a mixed α and β agonist. In dose ranges from 2 to 28 μg/kg/min, cardiac index is increased at the expense of heart rate. In addition, decreased splanchnic blood flow is common.[92] Its use should be reserved for patients with depressed cardiac index and persistent hypoperfusion in spite of adequate volume expansion and other vasopressor agents.

In summary, all of the vasopressor and inotropic agents can produce a decrease in blood flow to the splanchnic and renal vasculature. Administration should begin with a goal of improving mean arterial pressure to the lower limit of normal and then should follow other indices of adequate perfusion. The current recommendation from the Society of Critical Care Medicine is that dopamine is the primary vasopressor for patients with septic shock that is unresponsive to appropriate, aggressive crystalloid therapy.[64] The next most effective agents are norepinephrine and phenylephrine. Epinephrine may be used as a third-line agent for refractory hypotension. Dobutamine may be combined in the setting of persistently depressed cardiac index.

Antibiotics

Early and appropriate antibiotic therapy should target the nidus of infection and reduces mortality, perhaps by as much as 30%.[93-95] If the patient's condition permits, appropriate cultures should be drawn before the administration of broad-spectrum antibiotics (Table 132-3). Surgically correctable conditions, such as intra-abdominal abscess, perforated viscus, retained products of conception, or retained foreign body (such as a tampon) should be treated concurrently.

In the absence of an obvious source of infection, the use of broad-spectrum antibiotics is recommended. The specific agent depends on many variables including institutional preference and local resistance patterns. As results from cultures become available, therapy should be modified. There is no consensus about the need for double or triple antibiotic coverage for particular organisms, although it is common practice to double-cover virulent organisms, such as *P. aeruginosa,* as well as areas that are commonly infected with multiple organisms such as the peritoneum.

Table 132-3. Suggested Initial Antibiotic Management Pending Microbiologic Identification of Organism and Sensitivity

Infection	Modifying factors	Antibiotic
Sepsis unknown source	Immunocompetent	Antipseudomonal cephalosporin, *plus* aminoglycoside or fluoroquinolone; *or* Antipseudomonal penicillin, *plus* aminoglycoside or fluoroquinolone; *or* Carbapenem, *plus* aminoglycoside or fluoroquinolone
	Anaerobic Infection	Add metronidazole or clindamycin to above regimen
	Methicillin resistant *Staphylococcus aureus* (MRSA)	Add vancomycin to above regimen
	Neutropenia	Antipseudomonal penicillin *plus* aminoglycoside or fluoroquinolone; *or* Carbapenem, *plus* aminoglycoside or fluoroquinolone
	Splenectomy	Cefotaxime *or* Ceftriaxone
	HIV infection	Ticarcillin-clavulanate *plus* tobramycin
Pneumonia	Immunocompetent	2nd/3rd generation cephalosporin, *plus* second generation macrolide *or* Fluoroquinolone
	Legionella suspected	Azithromycin or fluoroquinolone or high-dose erythromycin
Abdominal infection	Immunocompetent	Ampicillin, *plus* aminoglycoside, *plus* metronidazole
	Multidrug resistant organism suspected	Ticarcillin/clavulanate carbapenem *or* piperacillin/ tazobactam, *plus* aminoglycoside
Urinary tract source		Fluoroquinolone; *or* third generation cephalosporin; *or* Ampicillin *plus* aminoglycoside
Cellulitis	Not necrotizing fasciitis	Cefazolin *or* nafcillin
	MRSA Possible	Vancomycin
Necrotizing fasciitis (surgical drainage)		Ampicillin/sulbactam; *or* Ticarcillin/clavulanate; *or* Piperacillin, *plus* aminoglycoside, *plus* clindamycin; *or* Carbapenem
IV catheter infection (remove catheter)	Outpatient acquired	Third generation cephalosporin
	MRSA suspected	Add Vancomycin
Fungal infection		Amphotericin B
Cerebrospinal infection	Immunocompetent	Ceftriaxone *plus* vancomycin
	Elderly or immunocompromised	Add ampicillin
Intravenous drug abuse	MRSA not suspected	Nafcillin *plus* aminoglycoside
	MRSA suspected	Vancomycin *plus* aminoglycoside

MRSA, Methicillin-resistant *Staphylococcus aureus.*

Novel Therapies

As our understanding of the pathogenesis of sepsis has improved, efforts to block individual mediators have been undertaken. Numerous glucocorticoid and nonglucocorticoid antiinflammatory trials have been conducted. Other novel therapies are directed at specific endpoints of sepsis such as nitric oxide synthase inhibitors to restore blood pressure, extracorporeal membrane oxygenation (ECMO) to supplement failed lungs, and new catecholamines such as dopexamine. Unfortunately, despite initial in vitro and experimental model success of many of these agents, none have demonstrated improved outcomes in clinical trials at the present time.

Antiinflammatory Agents It has been nearly 30 years since the first attempt to block inflammation in sepsis. Hydrocortisone became the mainstay of therapy[96] but has subsequently fallen out of favor. Multiple, subsequent trials have shown that there is, at best, no benefit to high-dose glucocorticoid therapy for sepsis. In fact, only one subsequent study was able to show a statistically significant decrease in mortality.[97] Unfortunately, subsequent attempts to block individual mediators of sepsis have not yielded significantly better results. At least 20 large-scale, randomized trials have been reported: antiendotoxin strategies,[98-102] monoclonal antibodies against TNF,[103-107] bradykinin antagonists,[108] platelet-activating factor antagonists,[110,111] prostaglandin antagonists,[112,113] and IL-1ra.[94,114,115] None of these studies shows a significant mortality benefit compared to placebo. Based on individual analysis and meta-analyses,[116] there is either no benefit or a small benefit to these agents. In addition, analysis has failed to identify a subpopulation that may benefit from nonglucocorticoid antiinflammatory therapy for sepsis.[117]

Nitric Oxide Synthase Inhibitors Nitric oxide synthase inhibitors have been studied for several years in animal and human models. Numerous, small human trials show an increase in mean arterial pressure.[118,119] Unfortunately, there is no human or animal data to show a decrease in mortality.[119,120] Investigation is ongoing and more recent animal data suggest that further human trials are warranted.

ECMO There are no reports of controlled trials of the efficacy of ECMO circuits in adults. Its clinical use is based on several small animal and human trials. Animal models have shown promising results that, in certain clinical settings, ECMO can increase hemofiltration of endotoxin and decrease serum concentrations of TNFα, lactate, and eicosanoids.[121-123] Retrospective studies of children and neonates have shown decreased mortality in the setting of refractory septic shock, but no prospective trials have been recorded.[124-126] No adult studies have evaluated the effect of ECMO on mortality. Although several small studies have shown improved clearance of the mediators of septic shock, whether that will translate into a mortality benefit is unknown.[64]

Dopexamine Dopexamine is a synthetic catecholamine that has been available in Europe for several years. It is a strong β- and dopaminergic agonist but has little α-adrenergic action. It is theorized to increase hepatosplanchnic perfusion, although this benefit is at the expense of tachycardia. Hypotension has been seen as a result of its β_2 activity. There are small but promising studies that show possible benefit,[127] but based on current pooled data, it is not recommended for routine use.[64]

As our understanding of the pathogenesis of sepsis grows, future agents will likely be developed to combat specific mediators of sepsis. Given the high mortality rate from sepsis, it is clear that much work remains, and there is hope that further study will yield a drug with specific and significant value in combating sepsis-related mortality.

DIFFERENTIAL CONSIDERATIONS

The sepsis syndromes represent a spectrum of disease and clinical presentation. SIRS is defined by hemodynamic and laboratory parameters alone, whereas sepsis must include an infectious etiology. Often, noninfectious etiologies can cause a syndrome that mimics sepsis; thus, one must keep in mind a broad differential when approaching these patients. Box 132-3 provides differential considerations in the patient with sepsis syndromes. A detailed history and physical examination are always the first step in narrowing the differential diagnosis to identify the true etiology. Regardless of the source, SIRS and sepsis must be taken seriously and treated aggressively.

DISPOSITION

Patients with sepsis syndromes should have consultation from the admitting service while in the ED as dictated by their clinical presentation and course. Once the ED management is complete, antibiotics are given, and the need for emergent operative intervention or procedure has been excluded, patients with sepsis should be admitted to the hospital. Patients with severe sepsis and septic shock should be admitted to an ICU, and those with SIRS or impending sepsis may be admitted to a monitored floor with close supervision or an ICU.

Box 132-3 Differential Considerations for Sepsis and Septic Shock

Sepsis
- Dehydration
- ARDS
- Anemia
- Ischemia
- Hypoxia
- Congestive heart failure
- Vasculitis
- Toxicologic
  - Poisonings
  - Overdose
  - Drug-induced
- Pancreatitis
- Hypothalamic injury
- DIC
- Anaphylaxis
- Metabolic
  - Hyperthyroidism
  - DKA
  - Adrenal dysfunction
- Environmental
  - Burn
  - Heat exhaustion/stroke
- Trauma
  - Blood loss
  - Cardiac contusion
- Neuroleptic malignant syndrome

Septic shock
- Hypovolemic shock
  - Acute blood loss
  - Severe dehydration
- Cardiogenic shock
  - Pulmonary embolus
  - Myocardial infarction
  - Pericardial tamponade
  - Tension pneumothorax
- Vasogenic shock
  - Anaphylaxis
  - Paralysis

ARDS, Acute respiratory distress syndrome; *DIC,* disseminated intravascular coagulation; *DKA,* diabetic ketoacidosis.

KEY CONCEPTS

- Sepsis is a progression of disease ranging from SIRS → sepsis → severe sepsis → septic shock → multisystem organ dysfunction syndrome (MODS), all of which are due to a dysregulated inflammatory cascade
- The elderly, immunocompromised, neutropenic, and those with multiple comorbidities are at increased risk for development of sepsis syndromes.
- Early and appropriate antibiotics are essential in the treatment of sepsis syndromes.
- Patients with septic shock should be treated with aggressive fluid resuscitation and vasopressor therapy as needed.

REFERENCES

1. Bone R: American College of Chest Physicians/Society of Critical Care Medicine Consensus Conference: definitions for sepsis and organ failure and guidelines for the use of innovative therapies in sepsis, *Crit Care Med* 20:864-874, 1992.
2. Rangel-Frausto M et al: The natural history of the systemic inflammatory response syndrome (SIRS), *JAMA* 273:117-123, 1995.
3. Bates D et al: Predicting bacteremia in hospitalized patients: a prospectively validated model, *Ann Intern Med* 113:495-500, 1990.
4. Brun-Buisson C et al: Incidence, risk factors, and outcome of severe sepsis and septic shock in adults, *JAMA* 274:968-974, 1995.
5. Perl T et al: Long-term survival and function after suspected gram-negative sepsis, *JAMA* 274:338-345, 1995.
6. Sands K et al: Epidemiology of sepsis syndrome in 8 academic medical centers, *JAMA* 278:234-240, 1997.

7. Friedman G et al: Has the mortality of septic shock changed with time? *Crit Care Med* 26:2078-2086, 1998.
8. Geerdes H et al: Septicemia in 980 patients at a university hospital in Berlin: prospective studies during 4 selected years between 1979 and 1989, *Clin Infect Dis* 15:991-1002, 1992.
9. Leibovici Let al: Septic shock in bacteremia patients: risk factors, features and prognosis, *Scand J Infect Dis* 29:71-75, 1997.
10. Parrillo J: Pathogenetic mechanisms of septic shock, *N Engl J Med* 328:1471-1477, 1993.
11. Pinner R et al: Trends in infectious diseases mortality in the United States, *JAMA* 275:189-193, 1996.
12. Rangel-Frausto M: The epidemiology of bacterial sepsis, *Infect Dis Clin North Am* 13:299-312, 1999.
13. Sharkey R et al: Toxic shock syndrome following influenza A infection, *Intern Care Med* 25:335-336, 1999.
14. Suffredini AF et al: The cardiovascular response of normal humans to the administration of endotoxin, *N Engl J Med* 321:280-287, 1989.
15. Kirkland T et al: An immunoprotective monoclonal antibody to lipopolysaccharide, *J Immunol* 132:2590, 1984.
16. Lefer A: Significance of lipid mediators in shock states, *Circ Shock* 27:3-12, 1989.
17. Chang S et al: Platelet-activating factor mediates hemodynamic changes and lung injury in endotoxin-treated rats, *J Clin Invest* 79:1498-1509, 1987.
18. Terashita Z et al: Is platelet activating factor (PAF) a mediator of endotoxin shock? *Eur J Pharm* 109:257-261, 1985.
19. Deventer SV et al: Experimental endotoxemia in humans: analysis of cytokine release and coagulation, fibrinolytic and complement pathways, *Blood* 76:2520-2526, 1990.
20. Doughty L et al: The IL-10 response in pediatric sepsis and organ failure, *Crit Care Med* 24(suppl):A32, 1996.
21. Platzer C et al: Upregulation of monocytic IL-10 by tumor necrosis factor-a and cAMP elevating drugs, *Int Immunol* 7:517-523, 1995.
22. Dinarello CA et al: The role of interleukin-1 in disease [published erratum appears in *N Engl J Med* 1993 Mar 11;328:744] *N Engl J Med* 328:106-113, 1993.
23. Cannon G et al: Circulating interleukin-1 and tumor necrosis factor in septic shock and experimental endotoxin fever, *J Infect Dis* 161:79-84, 1990.
24. Dinarello C: The proinflammatory cytokines interleukin-1 and tumor necrosis factor and the treatment of septic shock syndrome, *J Infect Dis* 163:1177-1184, 1991.
25. Dinarello C et al: Tumor necrosis factor (Cachectin) is an endogenous pyrogen and induces production of interleukin-1, *J Exp Med* 163:1433, 1986.
26. Okusawa S et al: Interleukin-1 induces a shock-like state in rabbits: synergism with tumor necrosis factor and the effect of cyclooxygenase inhibition, *J Clin Invest* 81:1162, 1988.
27. Ohlsson K et al: Interleukin-1 receptor antagonist reduces mortality from endotoxic shock, *Nature* 348:550, 1990.
28. Tracey K et al: Anti-cachectin/TNF monoclonal antibodies prevent septic shock during lethal bacteremia, *Nature* 330:662, 1987.
29. van der Meer J et al: A low dose of recombinant interleukin-1 protects granulocytopenic mice from lethal gram-negative infection, *Proc Natl Acad Sci* 85:1620-1623, 1988.
30. Alexander H et al: Treatment with recombinant human tumor necrosis factor-alpha protects rats against the lethality, hypotension and hypothermia of gram-negative sepsis, *J Clin Invest* 88:34-39, 1991.
31. Fischer E et al: Interleukin-1 receptor antagonist circulates in experimental inflammation and in human disease, *Blood* 79:2196-2200, 1992.
32. Howard M et al: Interleukin-10 protects mice from endotoxemia, *J Exp Med* 177:1205-1208, 1993.
33. Holtzman M: Arachidonic acid metabolism: implications of biological chemistry for lung function and disease, *Am Rev Respir Dis* 143:188-203, 1991.
34. Arons M et al: Effects of ibuprofen on the physiology and survival of hypothermic sepsis, *Crit Care Med* 27:699-707, 1999.
35. Bernard G et al: Prostacyclin and thromboxane A2 formation is increased in human sepsis syndrome: effects of cyclooxygenase inhibition, *Am Rev Respir Dis* 144:1095-1101, 1991.
36. Palmer R et al: Nitric oxide release accounts for the biologic activity of endothelium-derived relaxing factor, *Nature* 327:524-526, 1987.
37. Lowenstein C et al: Nitric oxide: a physiologic messenger, *Ann Intern Med* 120:227-237, 1994.
38. Murad F: Signal transduction using nitric oxide and cyclic guanosine monophosphate, *JAMA* 276:1189-1192, 1996.
39. Nguyen T et al: DNA damage and mutation in human cells exposed to nitric oxide in vitro, *Biochemistry* 89:3030-3034, 1992.
40. Van Dervort A et al: Nitric oxide regulates endotoxin-induced TNF alpha production in human neutrophils, *J Immunol* 152:4102-4109, 1994.
41. Beasley D et al: Interleukin-1 induces prolonged L-arginine-dependent cyclic guanosine monophoshate and nitrite production in rat vascular smooth muscle cells, *J Clin Invest* 87:602-608, 1991.
42. Young G et al: The encephalopathy associated with septic illness, *Clin Invest Med* 13:297-304, 1990.
43. Sprung C et al: Impact of encephalopathy on mortality in the sepsis syndrome, *Crit Care Med* 18:801-806, 1990.
44. Bleck T et al: Neurologic complications of critical medical illnesses, *Crit Care Med* 21:98-103, 1993.
45. Eidelman L et al: The spectrum of septic encephalopathy: definitions, etiologies, and mortalities, *JAMA* 275:470-473, 1996.
46. Bowton D: Central nervous system effects of sepsis, *Crit Care Clin* 5:785-792, 1989.
47. Hoffman W et al: Role of endotoxemia in cardiovascular dysfunction and lethality: virulent and nonvirulent *Escherichia coli* challenges in a canine model of septic shock, *Infect Immunol* 64:406-412, 1996.
48. Natanson C et al: Role of endotoxemia in cardiovascular dysfunction and mortality: *Escherichia coli* and *Staphylococcus aureus* challenges in a canine model of septic shock, *J Clin Invest* 83:243-251, 1989.
49. Gunnar R et al: Hemodynamic measurements in bacteremia and septic shock in man, *J Infect Dis* 128: 295-298, 1973.
50. Hess M et al: Spectrum of cardiovascular function during gram-negative sepsis, *Prog Cardiovasc Dis* 23:279, 1981.
51. Parker M et al: Serial cardiovascular variables in survivors and nonsurvivors of human septic shock: heart rate as an early predictor of prognosis, *Crit Care Med* 15:923-929, 1987.
52. Ognibene F et al: Depressed left ventricular performance: response to volume infusion in patients with sepsis and septic shock, *Chest* 93:903, 1988.
53. Field S et al: The oxygen cost of breathing in patients with cardiorespiratory disease, *Am Rev Respir Dis* 126:9-13, 1982.
54. Kaplan R et al: Incidence and outcome of the respiratory distress syndrome in gram-negative sepsis, *Arch Intern Med* 139:867-869, 1979.
55. Bernard G et al: The American-European consensus conference on ARDS: definitions, mechanisms, relevant outcomes, and clinical trial coordination, *Am J Respir Crit Care Med* 149:818-824, 1994.
56. Aberle D et al: Radiologic considerations in the adult respiratory distress syndrome, *Clin Chest Med* 11:737-754, 1990.
57. Pastor C et al: Liver injury during sepsis, *J Crit Care* 10:183-197, 1995.
58. Osterud B et al: Increased tissue thromboplastin activity in monocytes of patients with meningococcal infections related to unfavourable prognosis, *Thromb Haemost* 49:5-7, 1983.
59. Taylor F et al: Protein C prevents the coagulopathic and lethal effect of *Escherichia coli* infusion in the baboon, *J Clin Invest* 79:918-925, 1987.
60. Levi M et al: Pathogenesis of disseminated intravascular coagulation in sepsis, *JAMA* 270:975-979, 1993.
61. Voss R et al: Activation and inhibition of fibrinolysis in septic patients in an internal medicine intensive care unit, *Br J Haematol* 75:99-102, 1990.
62. Peduzzi P et al: Predictors of bacteremia and gram-negative bacteremia in patients with sepsis, *Arch Intern Med* 152:529-535, 1992.
63. Stacpoole P et al: Natural history and course of acquired lactic acidosis in adults, *Am J Med* 97:47-54, 1994.
64. Hollenberg S et al: Practice parameters for hemodynamic support of sepsis in adult patients with sepsis, *Crit Care Med* 27:639-660, 1999.
65. Wheeler A et al: Treating patients with severe sepsis, *N Engl J Med* 340:207-214, 1999.

66. Hickling K et al: Low mortality associated with low volume pressure limited ventilation with permissive hypercapnia in severe adult respiratory distress syndrome, *Intern Care Med* 16:372-377, 1990.
67. Roupie E et al: Titration of tidal volume and induced hypercapnea in acute respiratory distress syndrome, *Am J Respir Crit Care Med* 152:121-128, 1995.
68. Dellinger R: Current therapy for sepsis, *Infect Dis Clin North Am* 13:495-509, 1999.
69. Shoemaker W et al: Prospective trial of supranormal values of survivors as therapeutic goals in high-risk surgical patients, *Chest* 94:1176-1186, 1988.
70. Hayes M et al: Elevation of systemic oxygen delivery in the treatment of critically ill patients, *N Engl J Med* 330:1717-1722, 1994.
71. Gattinoni L et al: A trial of goal-oriented hemodynamic therapy in critically ill patients, *N Engl J Med* 333:1025-1032, 1995.
72. Czer L et al: Optimal hematocrit value in critically ill patients, *Surg Gynecol Obstet* 147:363-368, 1978.
73. Steffes C et al: Blood transfusion and oxygen consumption in surgical sepsis, *Crit Care Med* 19:512-517, 1991.
74. Mink R et al: Effect of blood transfusion on oxygen consumption in pediatric septic shock, *Crit Care Med* 18:1087-1091, 1990.
75. Conrad S et al: Effect of red cell transfusion on oxygen consumption following fluid resuscitation in septic shock, *Circ Shock* 31:419-429, 1990.
76. Hebert P: A multicenter, randomized, controlled clinical trial of transfusion requirements in critical care, *N Engl J Med* 340:409-417, 1999.
77. Rackow E et al: Fluid resuscitation in shock: a comparison of cardiorespiratory effects of albumin, hetastarch and saline solutions in patients with hypovolemic shock, *Crit Care Med* 11:839-850, 1983.
78. Rackow Eet al: Mechanisms and management of septic shock, *Crit Care Clin* 9:219-237, 1993.
79. Packman M et al: Optimum left heart filling pressure during fluid resuscitation of patients with hypovolemic and septic shock, *Crit Care Med* 11:165-169, 1983.
80. De Backer D et al: Does hepato-splanchnic VO_2/DO_2 dependency exist in critically ill septic patients? *Am J Respir Crit Care Med* 157:1219-1225, 1998.
81. Gutierrez G et al: Gastric intramucosal pH as a therapeutic index of tissue oxygenation in critically ill patients, *Lancet* 339:195-199, 1992.
82. Shoemaker Wet al: Therapy of shock based on pathophysiology, monitoring, and outcome prediction, *Crit Care Med* 18:S19-S25, 1990.
83. Hannemann L et al: Comparison of dopamine to dobutamine and norepinephrine for oxygen delivery and uptake in septic shock, *Crit Care Med* 23:1962-1970, 1995.
84. Meier-Hellmann A et al: The effects of low-dose dopamine on splanchnic blood flow and oxygen utilization in patients with septic shock, *Intern Care Med* 23:31-37, 1997.
85. Martin C et al: Norepinephrine or dopamine for the treatment of hyperdynamic septic shock, *Chest* 103:1826-1831, 1993.
86. Desjars P et al: Norepinephrine therapy has no deleterious renal effects in human septic shock, *Chest* 17:426-429, 1989.
87. Martin C et al: Renal effects of norepinephrine used to treat septic shock patients, *Crit Care Med* 18:282-285, 1990.
88. Redl-Wenzl E et al: The effects of norepinephrine on hemodynamics and renal function in severe septic shock states, *Intern Care Med* 19:151-154, 1993.
89. Gregory J et al: Experience with phenylephrine as a component of the pharmacologic support of septic shock, *Crit Care Med* 19:1395-1400, 1991.
90. Day N et al: The effects of dopamine and adrenaline infusions on acid-base balance and systemic hemodynamics in severe infection, *Lancet* 348:219-223, 1996.
91. Wilson W et al: Septic shock: does adrenaline have a role as a first-line inotropic agent? *Anaesth Intensive Care* 20:470-474, 1992.
92. Gutierrez G et al: Effect of dobutamine on oxygen consumption and gastric mucosal pH in septic patients, *Am J Respir Crit Care Med* 150:324-329, 1994.
93. Aube H et al: Risk factors for septic shock in the early management of bacteremia, *Am J Med* 93:283-288, 1992.
94. Opal S et al: Confirmatory interleukin-1 receptor antagonist trial in severe sepsis: a phase III, randomized, double-blind, placebo-controlled, multicenter trial, *Crit Care Med* 25:1115-1124, 1997.
95. Pittet D et al: Bedside prediction of mortality from bacteremic sepsis: a dynamic analysis of ICU patients, *Am J Respir Crit Care Med* 153:684-693, 1996.
96. Group CS: The effectiveness of hydrocortisone in the management of severe infection, *JAMA* 183:462-465, 1963.
97. Schumer W: Steroids in the treatment of clinical septic shock, *Ann Surg* 184:333-341, 1976.
98. Hellman J et al: Antiendotoxin strategies, *Infect Dis Clin North Am* 13:371-386, 1999.
99. Greenman RM et al: A controlled clinical trial of E5 murine monoclonal IgM antibody to endotoxin in the treatment of gram-negative sepsis: the XOMA sepsis study group, *JAMA* 266:1097-1102, 1991.
100. McCloskey R et al: Treatment of septic shock with human monoclonal antibody HA-1A: a randomized, double-blind, placebo-controlled trial. CHESS Trial Study Group, *Ann Intern Med* 121:1-5, 1994.
101. Warren H et al: Antiendotoxin monoclonal antibodies, *N Engl J Med* 326:1153-1157, 1992.
102. Ziegler E et al: Treament of gram-negative bacteremia and septic shock with HA-1A human monoclonal antibody against endotoxin, *N Engl J Med* 324:429-436, 1991.
103. Fisher C et al: Influence of anti-tumor necrosis factor monoclonal antibody on cytokine levels in patients with sepsis, *Crit Care Med* 21:318-327, 1993.
104. Reinhart K et al: Assessment of the safety and efficacy of the monoclonal anti-tumor necrosis factor antibody fragment, MAK 195, in patients with sepsis and septic shock: a multicenter, randomized, placebo-controlled, dose-ranging study, *Crit Care Med* 24:733-742, 1996.
105. Dhainaut J et al: CDP571, a humanized antibody to human tumor necrosis factor-alpha: safety, pharmacokinetics, immune response, and influence of the antibody on cytokine concentrations in patients with septic shock, *Crit Care Med* 23:1461-1469, 1995.
106. Abraham E et al: Efficacy and safety of monoclonal antibody to human tumor necrosis factor alpha in patients with sepsis syndrome: a randomized, controlled, multicenter clinical trial. TNF-a MAb Sepsis Study Group, *JAMA* 273:934-941, 1995.
107. Cohen J et al: INTERSEPT: an internation, multicenter, placebo-controlled trial of monoclonal antibody to human tumor necrosis factor-alpha in patients with sepsis. International Sepsis Trial Study Group, *Crit Care Med* 24:1431-1440, 1996.
108. Fein A et al: Treatment of severe systemic inflammatory response syndrome and sepsis with a novel bradykinin antagonist, Deltibant (CB-0127), *JAMA* 277:482-487, 1997.
109. Reference deleted in proofs.
110. Dhainaut J et al: Platelet-activating factor receptor antagonist BN 52021 in the treatment of severe sepsis: a randomized, double-blind, placebo-controlled, multicenter clinical trial, *Crit Care Med* 22:1720-1728, 1994.
111. Dhainaut J et al: Confirming phase III clinical trial to study the efficacy of a PAF antagonist, BN52021, in reducing mortality of patients with severe Gram-negative sepsis, *Am J Respir Crit Care Med* 151:A447, 1995.
112. Abraham E et al: p55 Tumor necrosis factor receptor fusion protein in the treatment of patients with severe sepsis and septic shock: a randomized controlled multicentre trial. Ro 45-2081 Study Group, *JAMA* 277:1531-1538, 1997.
113. Fisher C et al: Treatment of septic shock with the tumor necrosis factor receptor: Fc fusion protein, *N Engl J Med* 334:1697-1702, 1996.
114. Fisher C et al: Initial evaluation of human recombinant interleukin-receptor antagonist in the treatment of sepsis syndrome: a randomized, open-label, placebo-controlled multicenter trial, *Crit Care Med* 22:12-21, 1994.
115. Fisher C et al: Recombinant human interleukin-1 receptor antagonist in the treatment of patients with sepsis syndrome: results from a randomized, double-blind, placebo-controlled trial. Phase III rhIL-1RA Sepsis Syndrome Study Group, *JAMA* 271:1836-1843, 1994.

116. Natanson C: Anti-inflammatory therapies to treat sepsis and septic shock: a reassessment (editorial), *Crit Care Med* 25:1097-1101, 1997.
117. Natanson C et al: Selected treatment strategies for septic shock based on proposed mechanisms of pathogenesis, *Ann Intern Med* 120:771-783, 1994.
118. Lorente J et al: L-arginine pathway in the sepsis syndrome, *Crit Care Med* 21:1287-1295, 1993.
119. Petros A et al: Effects of a nitric oxide synthase inhibitor in humans with septic shock, *Cardiovasc Res* 28:34-39, 1995.
120. Nava E et al: The role of nitric oxide in endotoxic shock: effects of N(G-monomethyl-L-arginine), *J Cardiovasc Pharm* 20:S132-S134, 1992.
121. Griffen M et al: Extracorporeal membrane oxygenation for gram-negative septic shock in the immature pig, *Circ Shock* 33:195-199, 1991.
122. Grootendorst A et al: High volume hemofiltration improves right ventricular function in endotoxin-induced shock in the pig, *Intensive Care Med* 18:235-240, 1992.
123. Stein B et al: Influence of continuous haemofiltration on haemodynamics and central blood volume in experimental endotoxic shock, *Intensive Care Med* 16:494-499, 1990.
124. Goldman A et al: Extracorporeal support for intractable cardiorespiratory failure due to meningococcal disease, *Lancet* 349:466-469, 1997.
125. Beca J et al: Extracorporeal membrane oxygenation for refractory septic shock in children, *Pediatrics* 93:726-729, 1994.
126. McCune S et al: Extracorporeal membrane oxygenation therapy in neonates with septic shock, *J Pediatr Surg* 25:479-482, 1990.
127. Hannemann L et al: Dopexamine hydrochloride in septic shock, *Chest* 109:756-760, 1996.

Index

E

H

T

X

Y

Z